PRINCIPLES of PHARMACOLOGY
THE PATHOPHYSIOLOGIC BASIS OF DRUG THERAPY

Fourth Edition

PRINCIPLES of PHARMACOLOGY
THE PATHOPHYSIOLOGIC BASIS OF DRUG THERAPY

Fourth Edition

David E. Golan, MD, PhD
Editor-in-Chief

Ehrin J. Armstrong, MD, MSc
April W. Armstrong, MD, MPH
Associate Editors

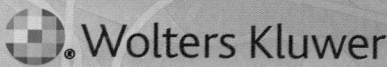

Philadelphia • Baltimore • New York • London
Buenos Aires • Hong Kong • Sydney • Tokyo

Acquisitions Editor: Matthew Hauber
Product Development Editor: John Larkin
Marketing Manager: Mike McMahon
Production Project Manager: Bridgett Dougherty
Design Coordinator: Holly McLaughlin
Manufacturing Coordinator: Margie Orzech
Prepress Vendor: Absolute Service, Inc.

Fourth edition

Library of Congress Cataloging-in-Publication Data

Names: Golan, David E., editor. | Armstrong, Ehrin J., editor. | Armstrong,
  April W., editor.
Title: Principles of pharmacology : the pathophysiologic basis of drug
  therapy / David E. Golan, editor in chief ; Ehrin J. Armstrong, April W.
  Armstrong, associate editors.
Other titles: Principles of pharmacology (Golan)
Description: Fourth edition. | Philadelphia : Wolters Kluwer Health, [2017] |
  Includes bibliographical references and index.
Identifiers: LCCN 2015048962 | ISBN 9781451191004
Subjects: | MESH: Pharmacological Phenomena | Drug Therapy
Classification: LCC RM301 | NLM QV 38 | DDC 615/.1—dc23 LC record available at http://lccn.loc.gov/2015048962

To our students and the patients they will serve

Contents

Preface

The editors are grateful for many helpful suggestions from readers of the first, second, and third editions of *Principles of Pharmacology: The Pathophysiologic Basis of Drug Therapy*. The fourth edition features many changes to reflect the rapidly evolving nature of pharmacology and drug development. We believe that these updates will continue to contribute to the learning and teaching of pharmacology both nationally and internationally:

- Comprehensive updates of *full-color figures* throughout the textbook—about 450 in all. Every figure has been updated and colorized, and over 50 figures are new or substantially modified to highlight advances in our understanding of physiologic, pathophysiologic, and pharmacologic mechanisms. As in the first three editions, our collaboration with a single illustrator creates a uniform "look and feel" among the figures that facilitates understanding and helps the reader make connections across broad areas of pharmacology.
- Comprehensive updates and additions in the *fundamentals of pharmacology*. Along with extensive updates in the chapters on drug–receptor interactions, pharmacodynamics, pharmacokinetics, drug metabolism, drug toxicity, and pharmacogenomics, a new chapter on *drug transporters* has been added. The first section of the textbook now provides a comprehensive framework for the fundamental principles of pharmacology that serve as the foundation for material in all subsequent chapters.
- Comprehensive updates of all 37 *drug summary tables*. These tables, which have been particularly popular with readers, group drugs and drug classes according to mechanism of action and list clinical applications, serious and common adverse effects, contraindications, and therapeutic considerations for each drug discussed in the chapter.
- Comprehensive *updates of all chapters*, including new drugs approved through 2014–2015. We have focused especially on newly discovered and revised mechanisms that sharpen our understanding of the physiology,

pathophysiology, and pharmacology of the relevant system. Sections throughout the book contain substantial amounts of new and updated material, especially the chapters on drug–receptor interactions; drug toxicity; pharmacogenomics; adrenergic pharmacology; local anesthetic pharmacology; the pharmacology of serotonergic and central adrenergic neurotransmission; the pharmacology of analgesia; the pharmacology of cholesterol and lipoprotein metabolism; the pharmacology of volume regulation; the pharmacology of vascular tone; the pharmacology of hemostasis and thrombosis; the pharmacology of the thyroid gland; the pharmacology of the endocrine pancreas and glucose homeostasis; the pharmacology of bone mineral homeostasis; the pharmacology of bacterial DNA replication, transcription, and translation; the pharmacology of bacterial and mycobacterial cell wall synthesis; the pharmacology of viral infections; the pharmacology of cancer; the pharmacology of eicosanoids; the pharmacology of immunosuppression; the fundamentals of drug development and regulation; and protein therapeutics.

As with the third edition, we have recruited a panel of new, expert chapter authors who have added tremendous strength and depth to the existing panel of authors, and the editorial team has reviewed each chapter in detail to achieve uniformity of style, presentation, and currency across the entire text.

Finally, we would like to acknowledge the immeasurable contributions of the late Armen H. Tashjian, Jr., MD, to the conception, design, and implementation of this text. Armen was our friend, mentor, and close colleague, and his indomitable spirit lives on in this fourth edition of *Principles of Pharmacology: The Pathophysiologic Basis of Drug Therapy*.

David E. Golan, MD, PhD
Ehrin J. Armstrong, MD, MSc
April W. Armstrong, MD, MPH

Preface

to the First Edition

This book represents a new approach to the teaching of a first or second year medical school pharmacology course. The book, titled *Principles of Pharmacology: The Pathophysiologic Basis of Drug Therapy*, departs from standard pharmacology textbooks in several ways. *Principles of Pharmacology* provides an understanding of drug action in the framework of human physiology, biochemistry, and pathophysiology. Each section of the book presents the pharmacology of a particular physiologic or biochemical system, such as the cardiovascular system or the inflammation cascade. Chapters within each section present the pharmacology of a particular aspect of that system, such as vascular tone or eicosanoids. Each chapter presents a clinical vignette, illustrating the relevance of the system under consideration; then discusses the biochemistry, physiology, and pathophysiology of the system; and, finally, presents the drugs and drug classes that activate or inhibit the system by interacting with specific molecular and cellular targets. In this scheme, the therapeutic and adverse actions of drugs are understood in the framework of the drug's mechanism of action. The physiology, biochemistry, and pathophysiology are illustrated using clear and concise figures, and the pharmacology is depicted by displaying the targets in the system on which various drugs and drug classes act. Material from the clinical vignette is referenced at appropriate points in the discussion of the system. Contemporary directions in molecular and human pharmacology are introduced in chapters on modern methods of drug discovery and drug delivery and in a chapter on pharmacogenomics.

This approach has several advantages. We anticipate that students will use the text not only to learn pharmacology but also to review essential aspects of physiology, biochemistry, and pathophysiology. Students will learn pharmacology in a conceptual framework that fosters mechanism-based learning rather than rote memorization, and that allows for ready incorporation of new drugs and drug classes into the student's fund of knowledge. Finally, students will learn pharmacology in a format that integrates the actions of drugs from the level of an individual molecular target to the level of the human patient.

The writing and editing of this textbook have employed a close collaboration among Harvard Medical School students and faculty in all aspects of book production, from student–faculty co-authorship of individual chapters to student–faculty editing of the final manuscript. In all, 43 HMS students and 39 HMS faculty have collaborated on the writing of the book's 52 chapters. This development plan has blended the enthusiasm and perspective of student authors with the experience and expertise of faculty authors to provide a comprehensive and consistent presentation of modern, mechanism-based pharmacology.

David E. Golan, MD, PhD
Armen H. Tashjian, Jr., MD
Ehrin J. Armstrong, MD, MSc
Joshua M. Galanter, MD
April W. Armstrong, MD, MPH
Ramy A. Arnaout, MD, DPhil
Harris S. Rose, MD
FOUNDING EDITORS

Acknowledgments

The editors are grateful for the support of students and faculty from around the world who have provided encouragement and helpful suggestions.

Stuart Ferguson continued his exemplary work as an executive assistant by managing all aspects of project coordination, including submission of chapter manuscripts, multiple layers of editorial revisions, coordination of figure generation and revision, and delivery of the final manuscript. We are extraordinarily grateful for his unwavering dedication to this project.

Rob Duckwall did a superb job to update the full-color figures. Rob's standardization and coloration of the figures in this textbook reflect his creativity and expertise as a leading medical illustrator. His artwork is a major asset and highlight of this textbook.

Quentin Baca electronically rendered the striking image on the cover of this textbook. We are most grateful for his creativity and expertise.

The editors would like to thank the publication, editorial, and production staff at Wolters Kluwer for their expert management and production of this handsome volume.

David Golan would like to thank the many faculty, student, and administrative colleagues whose support and understanding were critical for the successful completion of this project. Members of the Golan laboratory and faculty and staff in the Department of Biological Chemistry and Molecular Pharmacology at Harvard Medical School and in the Hematology Division at Brigham and Women's Hospital and the Dana-Farber Cancer Institute were gracious and supportive throughout. Deans Jeffrey Flier and John Czajkowski were especially supportive and encouraging. Laura, Liza, and Sarah provided valuable insights at many critical stages of this project and were constant sources of support and love.

Ehrin Armstrong would like to thank colleagues at the University of Colorado and the Denver Veterans Administration Medical Center for providing academic support and guidance. Greg Schwartz and Jim Beck were especially encouraging. Kiffany, Larry, and Ginger were a constant source of support and love throughout.

April Armstrong would like to thank Drs. David Golan and Laura Green for their constant support over the years. She thanks her dedicated coauthors Eryn Royer, Elizabeth Brezinski, and Chelsea Ma for their hard work. She also thanks Drs. David Norris, David West, and Fu-Tong Liu for fostering her career. She is grateful for the love of her family—Amy, Yanni, and Susan.

Credit lines identifying the original source of a figure or table borrowed or adopted from copyrighted material, and acknowledging the use of noncopyrighted material, are gathered together in a list at the end of the book. We thank all of these sources for permission to use this material.

Contributors

Gail K. Adler, MD, PhD
Associate Professor of Medicine
Harvard Medical School
Associate Physician
Division of Endocrinology, Diabetes
    and Hypertension
Department of Medicine
Brigham and Women's Hospital
Boston, Massachusetts

Francis J. Alenghat, MD, PhD
Assistant Professor
Department of Medicine, Section of
    Cardiology
University of Chicago
Chicago, Illinois

Seth L. Alper, MD, PhD
Professor of Medicine
Harvard Medical School
Renal Division and Molecular and
    Vascular Medicine Division
Department of Medicine
Beth Israel Deaconess Medical Center
Boston, Massachusetts

April W. Armstrong, MD, MPH
Associate Dean for Clinical Research
Director of Clinical Research, Southern
    California Clinical and Translational
    Science Institute (SC CTSI)
Vice Chair, Department of Dermatology
Associate Professor of Dermatology
University of Southern California
Los Angeles, California

Ehrin J. Armstrong, MD, MSc
Associate Professor of Medicine
Division of Cardiology
University of Colorado School
    of Medicine
Denver, Colorado

Sarah R. Armstrong, MS, DABT
Consultant in Toxicology
Amherst, Massachusetts

Ramy A. Arnaout, MD, DPhil
Assistant Professor of Pathology
Harvard Medical School
Associate Director, Clinical
    Microbiology
Department of Pathology
Beth Israel Deaconess Medical Center
Boston, Massachusetts

Alireza Atri, MD, PhD
Ray Dolby Endowed Chair in Brain
    Health Research
Ray Dolby Brain Health Center
California Pacific Medical Center
San Francisco, California
Visiting Scientist in Neurology
Harvard Medical School
Boston, Massachusetts

Jerry Avorn, MD
Professor of Medicine
Harvard Medical School
Chief, Division of
    Pharmacoepidemiology
Brigham and Women's Hospital
Boston, Massachusetts

Quentin J. Baca, MD, PhD
Chief Resident in Anesthesia
Department of Anesthesiology,
    Perioperative and Pain Medicine
Stanford University School of
    Medicine
Palo Alto, California

David A. Barbie, MD
Assistant Professor of Medicine
Harvard Medical School
Associate Physician
Department of Medical Oncology
Dana-Farber Cancer Institute
Boston, Massachusetts

Robert L. Barbieri, MD
Kate Macy Ladd Professor of
    Obstetrics, Gynecology and
    Reproductive Biology
Department of Obstetrics, Gynecology
    and Reproductive Biology
Harvard Medical School
Chairman, Department of Obstetrics
    and Gynecology
Brigham and Women's Hospital
Boston, Massachusetts

Elizabeth A. Brezinski, MD
Resident in Dermatology
Harvard Combined Dermatology
    Residency Training Program
Boston, Massachusetts

Lauren K. Buhl, MD, PhD
Clinical Fellow in Anaesthesia
Harvard Medical School
Resident in Anaesthesia
Beth Israel Deaconess Medical Center
Boston, Massachusetts

Michael S. Chang, MD
Assistant Professor of Orthopedic
    Surgery
University of Arizona College of
    Medicine
Complex Spine Surgeon
Sonoran Spine Center
Phoenix, Arizona

William W. Chin, MD
Bertarelli Professor of Translational
    Medical Science, Emeritus
Harvard Medical School
Boston, Massachusetts
Chief Medical Officer and Executive
    Vice President
Pharmaceutical Research and
    Manufacturers of America
Washington, DC

Janet Chou, MD
Instructor, Department of Pediatrics
Harvard Medical School
Assistant in Medicine
Department of Immunology
Children's Hospital Boston
Boston, Massachusetts

David E. Clapham, MD, PhD
Aldo R. Castañeda Professor of
    Cardiovascular Research
Professor of Neurobiology
Harvard Medical School
Chief, Basic Cardiovascular Research
Department of Cardiology
Children's Hospital Boston
Boston, Massachusetts

Donald M. Coen, PhD
Professor of Biological Chemistry and
    Molecular Pharmacology
Harvard Medical School
Boston, Massachusetts

David E. Cohen, MD, PhD
Robert H. Ebert Professor of Medicine
    and Health Sciences and
    Technology
Director, Harvard-Massachusetts
    Institute of Technology Division of
    Health Sciences and Technology
Harvard Medical School
Director of Hepatology
Division of Gastroenterology,
    Hepatology and Endoscopy
Department of Medicine
Brigham and Women's Hospital
Boston, Massachusetts

Michael W. Conner, DVM
Vice President
Theravance Biopharma, U.S., Inc.
South San Francisco, California

Susannah B. Cornes, MD
Assistant Professor, Department
    of Neurology
University of California, San Francisco
Department of Neurology
UCSF Medical Center
San Francisco, California

Amber Dahlin, PhD, MMSc
Instructor in Medicine
Harvard Medical School
Associate Epidemiologist
Channing Division of Network
    Medicine, Department of Medicine,
    Brigham and Women's Hospital
Boston, Massachusetts

George D. Demetri, MD
Professor of Medicine
Department of Medical Oncology
Co-Director, Ludwig Center
Harvard Medical School
Department of Medical Oncology
Dana-Farber Cancer Institute
Boston, Massachusetts

Catherine Dorian-Conner, PharmD, PhD
Consultant in Toxicology
Half Moon Bay, California

David M. Dudzinski, MD, JD
Clinical Fellow in Medicine
Harvard Medical School
Fellow, Department of Cardiology
Massachusetts General Hospital
Boston, Massachusetts

Baran A. Ersoy, PhD
Instructor in Medicine
Harvard Medical School
Investigator
Brigham and Women's Hospital
Boston, Massachusetts

Hua-Jun Feng, MD, PhD
Instructor in Anaesthesia
Harvard Medical School
Assistant in Pharmacology
Massachusetts General Hospital
Boston, Massachusetts

Stuart A. Forman, MD, PhD
Associate Professor of Anesthesia
Harvard Medical School
Boston, Massachusetts

David A. Frank, MD, PhD
Associate Professor of Medicine
Harvard Medical School
Departments of Medicine and
    Medical Oncology
Dana-Farber Cancer Institute
Boston, Massachusetts

Joshua M. Galanter, MD
Assistant Professor, Department of
    Medicine
University of California, San Francisco
San Francisco, California

Rajesh Garg, MD
Assistant Professor of Medicine
Harvard Medical School
Associate Physician
Division of Endocrinology, Diabetes
    and Hypertension
Department of Medicine
Brigham and Women's Hospital
Boston, Massachusetts

Nidhi Gera, PhD
Research Fellow
Department of Biological Chemistry
    and Molecular Pharmacology
Harvard Medical School
Boston, Massachusetts

David E. Golan, MD, PhD
Professor of Biological Chemistry and
    Molecular Pharmacology
George R. Minot Professor of Medicine
Dean for Basic Science and
    Graduate Education
Special Advisor for Global Programs
Harvard Medical School
Senior Physician, Hematology
    Division, Brigham and
    Women's Hospital and
    Dana-Farber Cancer Institute
Department of Biological Chemistry
    and Molecular Pharmacology,
    Department of Medicine
Harvard Medical School
Boston, Massachusetts

Mark A. Goldberg, MD
Associate Professor of Medicine,
    Part-time
Harvard Medical School
Boston, Massachusetts
Advisor
Medical and Regulatory Strategy
Synageva BioPharma Corp.
Lexington, Massachusetts

Laura C. Green, PhD, DABT
President and Senior Toxicologist
Green Toxicology, LLC
Brookline, Massachusetts

Edmund A. Griffin, Jr., MD, PhD
Assistant Professor of Clinical
    Psychiatry
Department of Psychiatry
Columbia University
Attending Psychiatrist
New York-Presbyterian Hospital
New York, New York

Robert S. Griffin, MD, PhD
Clinical Assistant Professor of
    Anesthesiology
Weill Cornell Medical College
Assistant Attending Anesthesiologist
Hospital for Special Surgery
New York, New York

F. Peter Guengerich, PhD
Professor, Department of Biochemistry
Vanderbilt University School of
    Medicine
Nashville, Tennessee

Stephen J. Haggarty, PhD
Associate Professor of Neurology
Harvard Medical School
Director, Chemical Neurobiology
    Laboratory
Center for Human Genetic Research
Massachusetts General Hospital
Boston, Massachusetts

Sarah P. Hammond, MD
Assistant Professor of Medicine
Harvard Medical School
Associate Physician
Brigham and Women's Hospital
Boston, Massachusetts

Keith A. Hoffmaster, PhD
Director, Global Program
    Management
Translational Clinical Oncology
Novartis Institutes for Biomedical
    Research
Cambridge, Massachusetts

Anthony Hollenberg, MD
Professor of Medicine
Harvard Medical School
Chief, Division of Endocrinology,
    Diabetes and Metabolism
Beth Israel Deaconess Medical Center
Boston, Massachusetts

David L. Hutto, DVM, PhD, DACVP
Corporate Senior Vice President and
    Chief Scientific Officer—Safety
    Assessment
Charles River Laboratories, Inc.
Wilmington, Massachusetts

Louise C. Ivers, MD, MPH, DTM&H
Associate Professor of Medicine
Harvard Medical School
Associate Physician
Department of Medicine
Brigham and Women's Hospital
Boston, Massachusetts

Ursula B. Kaiser, MD
Professor of Medicine
Harvard Medical School
Chief, Division of Endocrinology,
    Diabetes and Hypertension
Brigham and Women's Hospital
Boston, Massachusetts

Lloyd B. Klickstein, MD, PhD
Head of Translational Medicine
New Indications Discovery Unit
Novartis Institutes for
    Biomedical Research
Cambridge, Massachusetts

Vidyasagar Koduri, MD, PhD
Clinical Fellow in Hematology/
    Oncology
Dana Farber Cancer Institute/Harvard
    Cancer Center
Boston, Massachusetts

Tibor I. Krisko, MD
Instructor
Department of Medicine
Harvard Medical School
Boston, Massachusetts
Staff Gastroenterologist
Department of Gastroenterology/
    Medicine
Boston VA Medical Center
Jamaica Plain, Massachusetts

David W. Kubiak, PharmD
Adjunct Clinical Assistant Professor
    of Pharmacy Practice
Massachusetts College of Pharmacy
    and Health Sciences
Adjunct Assistant Professor of
    Pharmacology
Massachusetts General Hospital
    Institute of Health Professions
Adjunct Clinical Assistant Professor
    of Pharmacy Practice
Northeastern University Bouvé
    College of Heath Sciences
Co-Director of Antimicrobial
    Stewardship and Advanced Practice
    Infectious Diseases Pharmacy
    Specialist
Brigham and Women's Hospital
Boston, Massachusetts

Alexander E. Kuta, PhD
Vice President and Head of US
    Regulatory Affairs
EMD Serono, Inc.
Rockland, Massachusetts

Robert Langer, ScD
David H. Koch Institute Professor
Departments of Chemical Engineering
    and Bioengineering
Massachusetts Institute of Technology
Cambridge, Massachusetts
Senior Lecturer on Surgery
Children's Hospital Boston
Boston, Massachusetts

Stephen Lazarus, MD
Professor of Medicine
Division of Pulmonary and Critical
    Care Medicine
Director, Training Program in Pulmonary
    and Critical Care Medicine
University of California, San Francisco
San Francisco, California

Benjamin Leader, MD, PhD
Chief Executive Officer
ReproSource
Woburn, Massachusetts

Jonathan Z. Li, MD, MMSc
Assistant Professor of Medicine
Harvard Medical School
Brigham and Women's Hospital
Boston, Massachusetts

Eng H. Lo, PhD
Professor of Radiology
Harvard Medical School
Director, Neuroprotection
    Research Laboratory
Departments of Radiology
    and Neurology
Massachusetts General Hospital
Boston, Massachusetts

Joseph Loscalzo, MD, PhD
Hersey Professor of the Theory and
    Practice of Medicine
Harvard Medical School
Chairman, Department of Medicine
    and Physician-in-Chief
Brigham and Women's Hospital
Boston, Massachusetts

Daniel H. Lowenstein, MD
Professor, Department of Neurology
University of California, San Francisco
Director, UCSF Epilepsy Center
UCSF Medical Center
San Francisco, California

Chelsea Ma, MD
Resident Physician
Internal Medicine
Beth Israel Deaconess Medical Center
Harvard Medical School
Boston, Massachusetts

Jianren Mao, MD, PhD
Richard J. Kitz Professor of
    Anaesthesia Research
Harvard Medical School
Chief, Division of Pain Medicine
Massachusetts General Hospital
Boston, Massachusetts

Peter R. Martin, MD
Professor, Departments of Psychiatry
    and Pharmacology
Vanderbilt University
Director, Division of Addiction
    Psychiatry and Vanderbilt
    Addiction Center
Vanderbilt University Medical Center
Nashville, Tennessee

Elizabeth Mayne, MD, PhD
Resident in Pediatrics and Child
    Neurology
Department of Pediatrics
Stanford University School of
    Medicine
Palo Alto, California

Alexander J. McAdam, MD, PhD
Associate Professor of Pathology
Harvard Medical School
Medical Director
Infectious Diseases Diagnostic
    Laboratory
Boston Children's Hospital
Boston, Massachusetts

James M. McCabe, MD
Assistant Professor of Medicine
University of Washington
Director, Cardiac Catheterization
    Laboratory
University of Washington Medical
    Center
Seattle, Washington

Keith W. Miller, MA, DPhil
Edward Mallinckrodt Professor
    of Pharmacology
Department of Anaesthesia
Harvard Medical School
Pharmacologist, Department of
    Anesthesia, Critical Care and
    Pain Medicine
Massachusetts General Hospital
Boston, Massachusetts

Joshua D. Moss, MD
Assistant Professor of Medicine
Heart Rhythm Center
University of Chicago Medical Center
Chicago, Illinois

Dalia S. Nagel, MD
Clinical Instructor, Department
    of Ophthalmology
Mount Sinai School of Medicine
Attending Physician
Department of Ophthalmology
Mount Sinai Hospital
New York, New York

William M. Oldham, MD, PhD
Instructor in Medicine
Harvard Medical School
Associate Physician
Pulmonary and Critical Care Medicine
Brigham and Women's Hospital
Boston, Massachusetts

Sachin Patel, MD, PhD
Assistant Professor, Departments
    of Psychiatry and Molecular
    Physiology and Biophysics
Vanderbilt University Medical Center
Nashville, Tennessee

Roy H. Perlis, MD, MSc
Director, Center for Experimental
    Drugs and Diagnostics
Center for Human Genetic Research
    and Department of Psychiatry
Massachusetts General Hospital
Associate Professor of Psychiatry
Harvard Medical School
Boston, Massachusetts

Maarten Postema, PhD
Director of Chemistry
EISAI Inc.
Andover, Massachusetts

Giulio R. Romeo, MD
Instructor in Medicine
Harvard Medical School
Staff Physician, Adult Diabetes
    Section
Joslin Diabetes Center
Staff Physician, Division of
    Endocrinology BIDMC
Boston, Massachusetts

Eryn L. Royer, BA
Medical Student
University of Colorado School of
    Medicine
Aurora, Colorado

Edward T. Ryan, MD
Professor of Medicine
Harvard Medical School
Professor of Immunology and
    Infectious Diseases
Harvard T.H. Chan School of
    Public Health
Director, Tropical Medicine
Massachusetts General Hospital
Boston, Massachusetts

Joshua M. Schulman, MD
Assistant Professor of Dermatology
University of California, Davis
Director of Dermatopathology
Sacramento VA Medical Center
Sacramento, California

Charles N. Serhan, PhD
Simon Gelman Professor of
    Anaesthesia (Biological Chemistry
    and Molecular Pharmacology)
Department of Anesthesiology,
    Perioperative and Pain Medicine
Harvard Medical School
Director, Center for Experimental
    Therapeutics and Reperfusion Injury
Brigham and Women's Hospital
Boston, Massachusetts

Helen M. Shields, MD
Professor of Medicine
Harvard Medical School
Physician, Department of Medicine
Brigham and Women's Hospital
Boston, Massachusetts

Steven E. Shoelson, MD, PhD
Professor of Medicine
Harvard Medical School
Associate Director of Research,
    Section Head, Cellular and
    Molecular Physiology
Joslin Diabetes Center
Boston, Massachusetts

David M. Slovik, MD
Associate Professor of Medicine
Harvard Medical School
Endocrine Unit
Massachusetts General Hospital
Boston, Massachusetts
Chief, Division of Endocrinology
Newton-Wellesley Hospital
Newton, Massachusetts

David G. Standaert, MD, PhD
John N. Whitaker Professor and Chair,
    Department of Neurology
University of Alabama at Birmingham
Director, Division of
    Movement Disorders
University Hospital
Birmingham, Alabama

Gary R. Strichartz, PhD
Professor of Anaesthesia
    (Pharmacology),
Harvard Medical School
Director, Pain Research Center,
    Department of Anesthesiology,
    Perioperative and Pain Medicine
Brigham and Women's Hospital
Boston, Massachusetts

Victor W. Sung, MD
Associate Professor, Department of
  Neurology, Division of Movement
  Disorders
The University of Alabama at
  Birmingham
Birmingham, Alabama

Kelan Tantisira, MD, MPH
Associate Professor of Medicine
Harvard Medical School
Associate Physician
Channing Division of Network
  Medicine and Division of
  Pulmonary and Critical Care
  Medicine
Brigham and Women's Hospital
Boston, Massachusetts

Hakan R. Toka, MD, PhD
Assistant Professor of Medicine
Division of Nephrology and
  Hypertension
Eastern Virginia Medical School
Norfolk, Virginia

John L. Vahle, DVM, PhD, DACVP
Senior Research Pathologist, Department
  of Toxicology and Pathology
Lilly Research Laboratories
Indianapolis, Indiana

Anand Vaidya, MD
Assistant Professor of Medicine
  (Endocrinology)
Harvard Medical School
Division of Endocrinology, Diabetes,
  and Hypertension
Brigham and Women's Hospital
Boston, Massachusetts

Vishal S. Vaidya, PhD
Associate Professor of Medicine
Head, Systems Toxicology
  Program, Laboratory of Systems
  Pharmacology
Harvard Medical School
Brigham and Women's Hospital
Associate Professor of Environmental
  Health
Harvard T.H. Chan School of
  Public Health
Boston, Massachusetts

Andrew J. Wagner, MD, PhD
Assistant Professor, Department of
  Medicine
Harvard Medical School
Medical Director, Ambulatory Oncology
Center for Sarcoma and Bone Oncology
Dana-Farber Cancer Institute
Boston, Massachusetts

Clifford J. Woolf, MB, BCh, PhD
Professor of Neurology
  and Neurobiology
Harvard Medical School
Director, F.M. Kirby
  Neurobiology Center
Children's Hospital Boston
Boston, Massachusetts

Jacob Wouden, MD
Radiologist, Washington Hospital
  Medical Staff
Washington Hospital Healthcare Group
Fremont, California

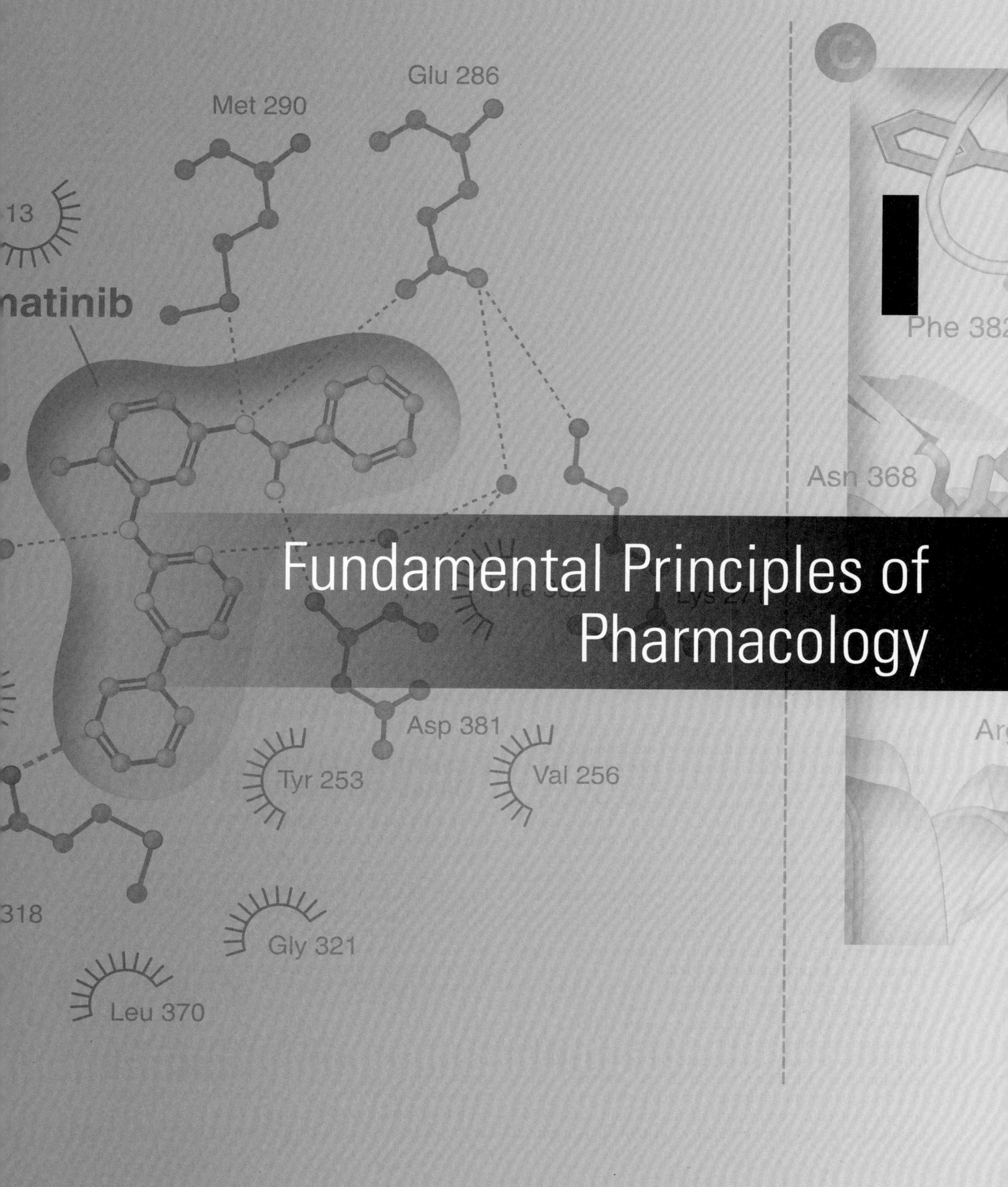

Fundamental Principles of
Pharmacology

1

Drug–Receptor Interactions

Francis J. Alenghat and David E. Golan

INTRODUCTION

Why is it that one drug affects cardiac function and another alters the transport of specific ions in the kidney? Why do antibiotics effectively kill bacteria but rarely harm patients? These questions can be answered by first examining the interaction between a drug and its specific molecular target and then considering the role of that action in a broader physiologic context. This chapter focuses on the molecular details of drug–receptor interactions, emphasizing the variety of receptors and their molecular mechanisms. This discussion provides a conceptual basis for the action of the many drugs and drug classes discussed in this book. It also serves as a background for Chapter 2, Pharmacodynamics, which discusses the quantitative relationships between drug–receptor interactions and pharmacologic effect.

Although drugs can theoretically bind to almost any three-dimensional target, most drugs achieve their desired (**therapeutic**) effects by interacting selectively with target molecules that play important physiologic or pathophysiologic roles. In many cases, selectivity of drug binding to receptors also determines the undesired (**adverse**) effects of a drug. In general, **drugs** are molecules that interact with specific molecular components of an organism to cause biochemical and physiologic changes within that organism.

Drug receptors are macromolecules that, upon binding to a drug, mediate those biochemical and physiologic changes.

CONFORMATION AND CHEMISTRY OF DRUGS AND RECEPTORS

An understanding of why a drug binds to a particular receptor can be found in the structure and chemical properties of the two molecules. This section discusses the basic determinants of receptor structure and the chemistry of drug–receptor binding. The discussion here focuses primarily on the interactions of drugs that are small molecules with target receptors that are mainly macromolecules (especially proteins), but many of these principles also apply to the interactions of antibody- or other protein-based therapeutics with their molecular targets (see Chapter 54, Protein Therapeutics).

Because many human and microbial drug receptors are proteins, it is useful to review the four major levels of protein structure (Fig. 1-1). At the most basic level, proteins consist of long chains of amino acids, the sequences of which are determined by the sequences of the DNA that code for the proteins. A protein's amino acid sequence is referred to as its **primary structure**. Once a long chain of amino acids has been synthesized on a ribosome, many of the amino acids

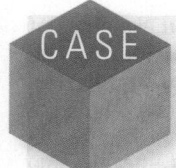

Intent on enjoying his newly found retirement, Mr. B has made a point of playing tennis as often as possible during the past year. For the past 3 months, however, he has noted increasing fatigue. Moreover, he is now unable to finish a meal, despite his typically voracious appetite. Worried and wondering what these symptoms mean, Mr. B schedules an appointment with his doctor. On physical examination, the physician notes that Mr. B has an enlarged spleen, extending approximately 10 cm below the left costal margin; the physical exam is otherwise within normal limits. Blood tests show an increased total white blood cell count (70,000 cells/mm^3) with an absolute increase in neutrophils, band forms, metamyelocytes, and myelocytes, but no blast cells (undifferentiated precursor cells). Cytogenetic analysis of metaphase cells demonstrates that 90% of Mr. B's myeloid cells possess the Philadelphia chromosome (indicating a translocation between chromosomes 9 and 22), confirming the diagnosis of chronic myeloid leukemia. The physician initiates therapy with **imatinib**, a highly selective inhibitor of the BCR-Abl tyrosine kinase fusion protein that is encoded by the Philadelphia chromosome. Over the next month, the cells containing the Philadelphia chromosome disappear completely from Mr. B's blood, and he begins to feel well enough to compete in a seniors tennis tournament. Mr. B continues to take imatinib every day, and he has a completely normal blood count and no fatigue. He is not sure what the future will bring, but he is glad to have been given the chance to enjoy a healthy retirement.

Questions

1. How does imatinib interrupt the activity of the BCR-Abl tyrosine kinase fusion protein?
2. Unlike imatinib, most of the older therapies for chronic myeloid leukemia (such as interferon-α) had significant "flu-like" adverse effects. Why did these therapies cause significant adverse effects in most patients, whereas (as in this case) imatinib causes adverse effects in very few patients?
3. Why is imatinib a selective therapy for chronic myeloid leukemia? Is this selectivity related to the lack of adverse effects associated with imatinib therapy?
4. How does the BCR-Abl protein affect intracellular signaling pathways?

begin to interact with nearby amino acids in the polypeptide chain. These interactions, which are typically mediated by hydrogen bonding, give rise to the **secondary structure** of a protein by forming well-defined conformations such as the α helix, β pleated sheet, and β barrel. As a result of their highly organized shape, these structures often pack tightly with one another, further defining the overall shape of the protein. **Tertiary structure** results from the interaction of amino acids more distant from one another along a single amino acid chain. These interactions include hydrogen bond and ionic bond formation as well as the covalent linkage of sulfur atoms to form intramolecular disulfide bridges. Finally, polypeptides may oligomerize to form more complex structures. The conformation that results from the interaction of separate polypeptides is referred to as the **quaternary structure**.

Different portions of a protein's structure generally have different affinities for water, and this feature has an additional effect on the protein's shape. Because both the extracellular and intracellular environments are composed primarily of water, **hydrophobic** protein segments are often drawn to the inside of the protein or shielded from water by insertion into lipid bilayer membranes. Conversely, **hydrophilic** protein segments are often located on a protein's exterior surface. After all of this twisting and turning is completed, each protein has a unique shape that determines its function, location in the body, relationship to cellular membranes, and binding interactions with drugs and other macromolecules.

The site on the receptor at which the drug binds is called its **binding site**. Each binding site has unique chemical characteristics that are determined by the specific properties of the amino acids that make up the site. The three-dimensional structure, shape, and reactivity of the site, and the inherent structure, shape, and reactivity of the drug, determine the orientation of the drug with respect to the receptor and govern how tightly these molecules bind to one another. Drug–receptor binding is the result of multiple chemical interactions between the two molecules, some of which are fairly weak (such as van der Waals forces) and some of which are extremely strong (such as covalent bonding). The sum total of these interactions provides the specificity of the overall drug–receptor interaction. The favorability of a drug–receptor interaction is referred to as the **affinity** of the drug for its binding site on the receptor. This concept is discussed in more detail in Chapter 2. The chemistry of the local environment in which these interactions occur—such as the hydrophobicity, hydrophilicity, and pK_a of amino acids near the binding site—may also affect the affinity of the drug–receptor interaction. The primary forces that contribute to drug–receptor affinity are described below and in Table 1-1.

van der Waals forces, resulting from the polarity induced in a molecule by the shifting of its electron density in response to the close proximity of another molecule, provide a weak attractive force for drugs and their receptors. This induced polarity is a ubiquitous component of all molecular interactions. **Hydrogen bonds** have substantial strength and are often important for drug–receptor association. This type of bond is mediated by the interaction between positively polarized hydrogen atoms (which are covalently attached to more electronegative atoms such as nitrogen or oxygen) and negatively polarized atoms (such as oxygen, nitrogen, or sulfur that are covalently attached to less electronegative atoms such as carbon or hydrogen). **Ionic interactions**,

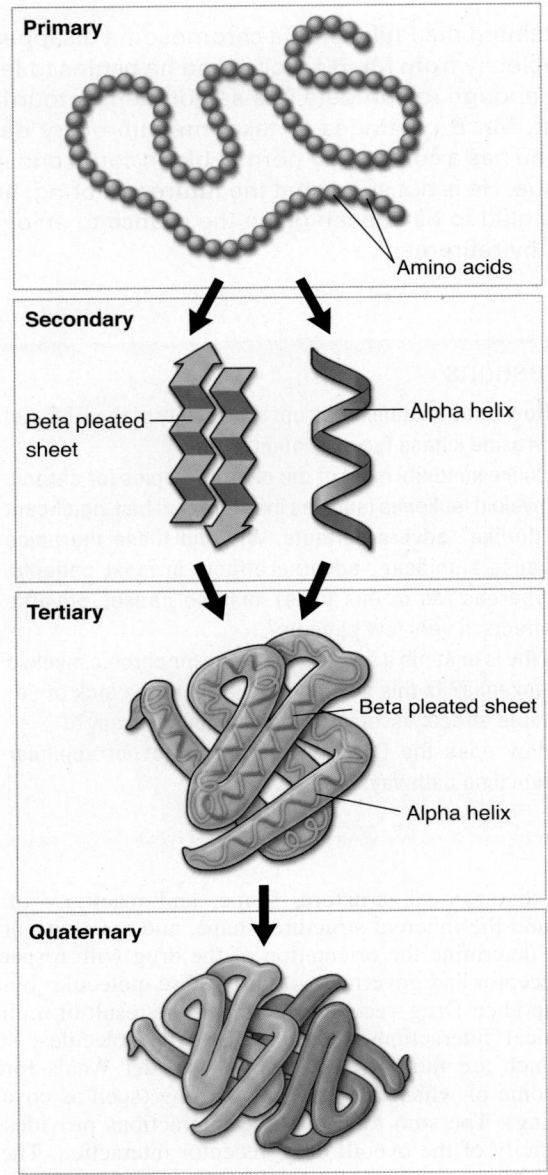

FIGURE 1-1. Levels of protein structure. Protein structure can be divided into four levels of complexity, referred to as *primary, secondary, tertiary,* and *quaternary* structure. Primary structure is determined by the sequence of amino acids that make up the polypeptide chain. Secondary structure is determined by the interaction of positively polarized hydrogen atoms with negatively polarized atoms (such as oxygen) on the same polypeptide chain. These interactions result in a number of characteristic secondary patterns of protein conformation, including the α helix and β pleated sheet. Tertiary structure is determined by the interactions of amino acids that are relatively far apart on the protein backbone. These interactions, which include ionic bonds and covalent disulfide linkages (among others), give proteins their characteristic three-dimensional structure. Quaternary structure is determined by the binding interactions among two or more independent protein subunits.

which occur between atoms with opposite charges, are stronger than hydrogen bonds but less strong than covalent bonds. **Covalent bonding** results from the sharing of a pair of electrons between two atoms on different molecules. Covalent interactions are so strong that, in most cases, they are essentially irreversible. Table 1-1 indicates the mechanism

of interaction and relative strength of each of these types of bonds. As noted above, the environment in which drugs and receptors interact also affects the favorability of binding. The **hydrophobic effect** refers to the mechanism by which the unique properties of the ubiquitous solvent water cause the interaction of a hydrophobic molecule with a hydrophobic binding site to be enhanced.

Rarely is drug–receptor binding caused by a single type of interaction; rather, it is a combination of these binding interactions that provides drugs and receptors with the forces necessary to form a stable drug–receptor complex. In general, multiple weak forces comprise the majority of drug–receptor interactions. For example, imatinib forms many van der Waals interactions and hydrogen bonds with the ATP-binding site of the BCR-Abl tyrosine kinase. The sum total of these relatively weak forces creates a strong (high affinity) interaction between this drug and its receptor (Fig. 1-2). Ionic and hydrophobic interactions exert force at a greater distance than van der Waals interactions and hydrogen bonds; for this reason, the former interactions are often critical to initiate the association of a drug and receptor.

Although relatively rare, covalent interactions between a drug and its receptor are a special case. The formation of a covalent bond is often essentially irreversible, and in such cases, the drug and receptor form an inactive complex. To regain activity, the cell must synthesize a new receptor molecule to replace the inactivated protein; and the drug molecule, which is also part of the inactive complex, is generally not available to inhibit other receptor molecules. Drugs that modify their target receptors (often enzymes) through this mechanism are sometimes called **suicide substrates**. Aspirin is an example of such a drug; it irreversibly acetylates cyclooxygenases to reduce the production of prostaglandins (anti-inflammatory effect) and thromboxanes (antiplatelet effect) (see Chapter 43, Pharmacology of Eicosanoids).

The molecular structure of a drug dictates the physical and chemical properties that contribute to its specific binding to the receptor. Important factors include hydrophobicity, ionization state (pK_a), conformation, and stereochemistry of the drug molecule. All of these factors combine to determine the complementarity of the drug to the binding site. Receptor binding pockets are highly specific, and small changes in the drug can have a large effect on the affinity of the drug–receptor interaction. For example, the **stereochemistry** of the drug has a great impact on the strength of the binding interaction. **Warfarin** is synthesized and administered as a racemic mixture (a mixture containing 50% of the right-handed molecule and 50% of the left-handed molecule); however, the S enantiomer is four times more potent than the R because of a stronger interaction of the S form with its binding site on vitamin K epoxide reductase. Stereochemistry can also affect toxicity in cases where one enantiomer of a drug causes the desired therapeutic effect and the other enantiomer causes an undesired toxic effect, perhaps due to an interaction with a second receptor or to metabolism to a toxic species. Although it is sometimes difficult for pharmaceutical companies to synthesize and purify individual enantiomers on a large scale, a number of currently marketed drugs are produced as individual enantiomers in cases where one enantiomer has higher efficacy and/or lower toxicity than its mirror image.

TABLE 1-1 Relative Strength of Bonds between Receptors and Drugs

BOND TYPE	MECHANISM	BOND STRENGTH
van der Waals	Shifting electron density in areas of a molecule, or in a molecule as a whole, results in the generation of transient positive or negative charges. These areas interact with transient areas of opposite charge on another molecule.	+
Hydrogen	Hydrogen atoms bound to nitrogen or oxygen become more positively polarized, allowing them to bond to more negatively polarized atoms such as oxygen, nitrogen, or sulfur.	++
Ionic	Atoms with an excess of electrons (imparting an overall negative charge on the atom) are attracted to atoms with a deficiency of electrons (imparting an overall positive charge on the atom).	+++
Covalent	Two bonding atoms share electrons.	++++

Impact of Drug Binding on the Receptor

How does drug binding produce a biochemical and/or physiologic change in the organism? In the case of receptors with enzymatic activity, the binding site of the drug is often the **active site** at which an enzymatic transformation is catalyzed, and the catalytic activity of the enzyme is inhibited by drugs that prevent substrate binding to the site or that covalently modify the site. In cases where the binding site is not the active site of the enzyme, drugs can cause a change by preventing the binding of endogenous ligands to their receptor binding pockets. In many drug–receptor interactions, however, the binding of a drug to its receptor results in a change in the **conformation** of the receptor. Altering the shape of the receptor can affect its function, including enhancing the affinity of the drug for the receptor. Such an interaction is often referred to as **induced fit**, because the receptor's conformation changes so as to improve the quality of the binding interaction.

The principle of induced fit suggests that drug–receptor binding can have profound effects on the conformation of the receptor. By inducing conformational changes in the receptor, many drugs not only improve the quality of the binding interaction but also alter the action of the receptor. The change in shape induced by the drug is sometimes identical to that caused by the binding of an endogenous ligand. For example, exogenously administered **insulin analogues** all stimulate the insulin receptor to the same extent, despite their slightly different amino acid sequences. In other cases, drug binding alters the shape of the receptor so as to make it more or less functional than normal. For example, imatinib binding to the BCR-Abl tyrosine kinase causes the protein to assume an enzymatically inactive conformation, thus inhibiting the kinase activity of the receptor.

Another way to describe the induced fit principle is to consider that many receptors exist in multiple conformational states—such as inactive (or closed), active (or open), and desensitized (or inactivated)—and that the binding of a

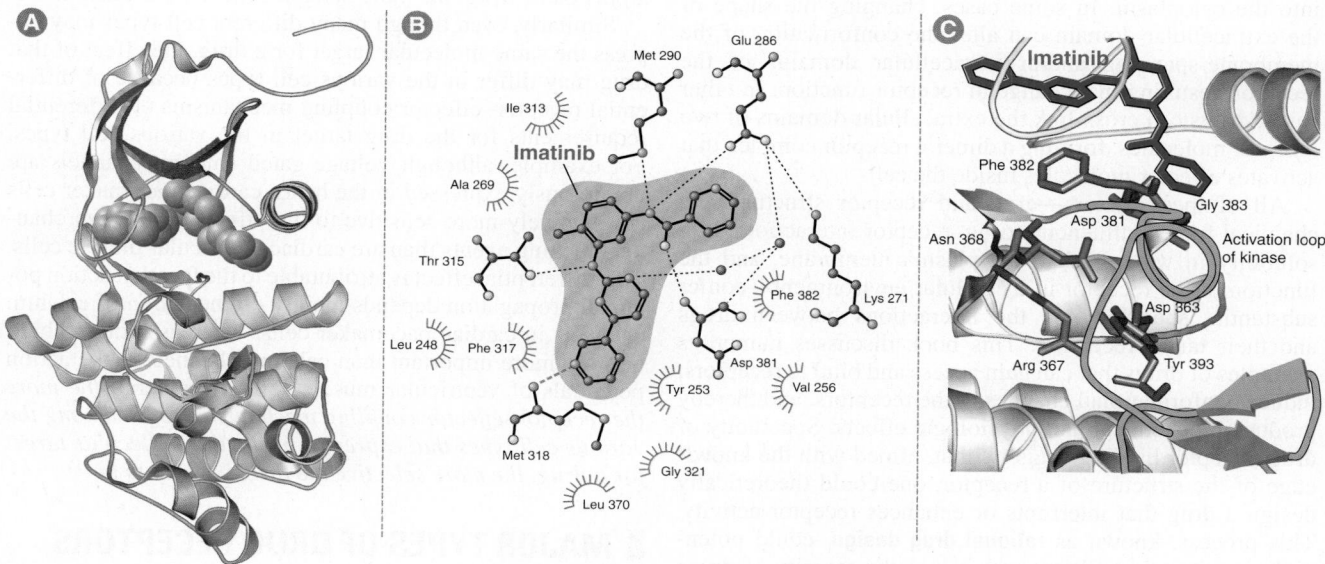

FIGURE 1-2. Structural basis of specific enzyme inhibition: imatinib interaction with the BCR-Abl kinase. A. The kinase portion of the BCR-Abl tyrosine kinase is shown in a ribbon format (*gray*). An analogue of imatinib, a specific inhibitor of the BCR-Abl tyrosine kinase, is shown as a space-filling model (*blue*). **B.** Detailed diagram of the intermolecular interactions between the drug (*shaded in purple*) and amino acid residues in the BCR-Abl protein. Hydrogen bonds are indicated by dashed lines, while van der Waals interactions (indicated by halos around the amino acid name and its position in the protein sequence) are shown for nine amino acids with hydrophobic side chains. **C.** The interaction of the drug (*blue*) with the BCR-Abl protein (*gray*) inhibits phosphorylation of a critical activation loop (*green-highlighted ribbon format*), thus preventing catalytic activity.

drug to the receptor stabilizes one or more of these conformations. Quantitative models that incorporate these concepts of drug–receptor interactions are discussed in Chapter 2.

Membrane Effects on Drug–Receptor Interactions

The structure of the receptor also determines where the protein is located in relationship to cellular boundaries such as the plasma membrane. Proteins that have large hydrophobic domains are able to reside in the plasma membrane because of the membrane's high lipid content. Many receptors that span the plasma membrane have lipophilic domains that are located in the membrane and hydrophilic domains that reside in the intracellular and extracellular spaces. Other drug receptors, including a number of transcription regulators (also called **transcription factors**), have only hydrophilic domains and reside in the cytoplasm, nucleus, or both.

Just as the structure of the receptor determines its location in relationship to the plasma membrane, *the structure of a drug affects its ability to gain access to the receptor.* For example, many drugs that are highly water-soluble are unable to pass through the plasma membrane and bind to target molecules in the cytoplasm. Certain hydrophilic drugs are able to pass through transmembrane channels (or use other transport mechanisms) and gain ready access to cytoplasmic receptors. Drugs that are highly lipophilic, such as many steroid hormones, are often able to pass through the hydrophobic lipid environment of the plasma membrane without special channels or transporters and thereby gain access to intracellular targets.

Drug-induced alterations in receptor shape can allow drugs bound to cell surface receptors to affect functions inside cells. Many cell surface receptors have extracellular domains that are linked to intracellular effector molecules by receptor domains that span the plasma membrane and extend into the cytoplasm. In some cases, changing the shape of the extracellular domain can alter the conformation of the membrane-spanning and/or intracellular domains of the receptor, resulting in a change in receptor function. In other cases, drugs can cross-link the extracellular domains of two receptor molecules, forming a dimeric receptor complex that activates effector molecules inside the cell.

All of these factors—drug and receptor structure, the chemical forces influencing drug–receptor interaction, drug solubility in water and in the plasma membrane, and the function of the receptor in its cellular environment—confer substantial **specificity** on the interactions between drugs and their target receptors. This book discusses numerous examples of drugs that can gain access and bind to receptors, induce conformational changes in the receptors, and thereby produce biochemical and physiologic effects. Specificity of drug–receptor binding suggests that, armed with the knowledge of the structure of a receptor, one could theoretically design a drug that interrupts or enhances receptor activity. This process, known as **rational drug design**, could potentially increase the efficacy and reduce the toxicity of drugs by optimizing their structure so that they bind more selectively to their targets. Rational drug design was first used to develop highly selective agents such as the antiviral protease inhibitor ritonavir and the antineoplastic tyrosine kinase inhibitor imatinib. Indeed, further rounds of rational drug design have led to the development of second-generation

protease inhibitors and antineoplastics with high affinity for the mutated drug targets that can evolve in patients who develop resistance to first-generation drugs. The rational drug design approach is discussed in greater detail in Chapter 51, Drug Discovery and Preclinical Development.

▌ MOLECULAR AND CELLULAR DETERMINANTS OF DRUG SELECTIVITY

The ideal drug would interact only with a molecular target that causes the desired therapeutic effect but not with molecular targets that cause unwanted adverse effects. Although no such drug has yet been discovered (i.e., all drugs currently in clinical use have the potential to cause adverse effects as well as therapeutic effects; see Chapter 6, Drug Toxicity), pharmacologists can take advantage of several determinants of drug **selectivity** in an attempt to reach this goal. Selectivity of drug action can be conferred by at least two classes of mechanisms, including (1) the cell-type specificity of receptor subtypes and (2) the cell-type specificity of receptor–effector coupling.

Although many potential receptors for drugs are widely distributed among diverse cell types, some receptors are more limited in their distribution. Systemic administration of drugs that interact with such localized receptors can result in a highly selective therapeutic effect. For example, drugs that target ubiquitous processes such as DNA synthesis are likely to cause significant toxic side effects; this is the case with many currently available chemotherapeutics for the treatment of cancer. Other drugs that target cell-type restricted processes such as acid generation in the stomach may have fewer adverse effects. Imatinib, for example, is an extremely selective drug because the BCR-Abl protein is not expressed in normal (noncancerous) cells. In general, *the more restricted the cell-type distribution of the receptor targeted by a particular drug, the more selective the drug is likely to be.*

Similarly, even though many different cell types may express the same molecular target for a drug, the effect of that drug may differ in the various cell types because of differential receptor–effector coupling mechanisms or differential requirements for the drug target in the various cell types. For example, although voltage-gated calcium channels are ubiquitously expressed in the heart, cardiac pacemaker cells are relatively more sensitive to the effects of calcium channel blocking agents than are cardiac ventricular muscle cells. This differential effect is attributable to the fact that action potential propagation depends mainly on the action of calcium channels in cardiac pacemaker cells, whereas sodium channels are more important than calcium channels in the action potentials of ventricular muscle cells. In general, *the more the receptor–effector coupling mechanisms differ among the various cell types that express a particular molecular target for a drug, the more selective the drug is likely to be.*

▌ MAJOR TYPES OF DRUG RECEPTORS

Given the great diversity of drug molecules, it might seem likely that the interactions between drugs and their molecular targets would be equally diverse. This is only partly true. In fact, *most of the currently understood drug–receptor interactions can be classified into six major groups.* These groups comprise the interactions between drugs and (1) transmembrane

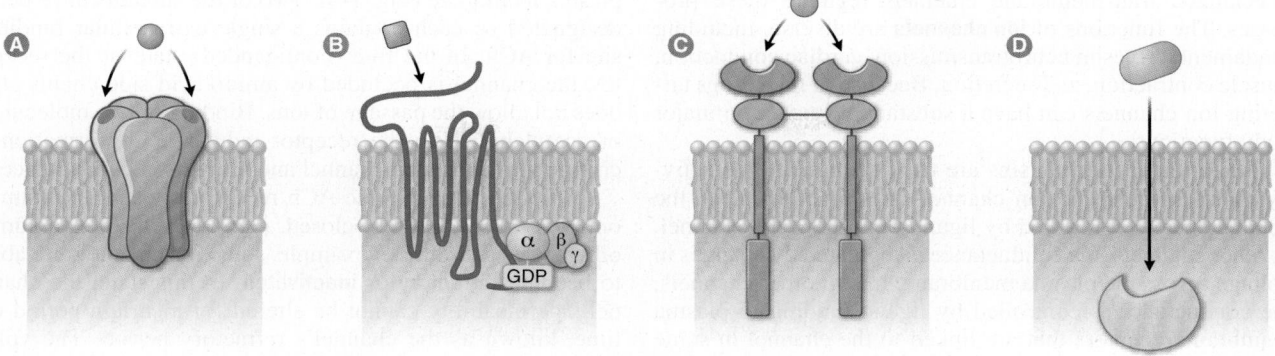

FIGURE 1-3. Major types of interactions between drugs and receptors. Most drug–receptor interactions can be divided into six groups, four of which are shown here. **A.** Drugs can bind to ion channels spanning the plasma membrane, causing an alteration in the channel's conductance. **B.** Heptahelical receptors spanning the plasma membrane are functionally coupled to intracellular G proteins. Drugs can influence the actions of these receptors by binding to the extracellular surface or transmembrane region of the receptor. **C.** Drugs can bind to the extracellular domain of a transmembrane receptor and cause a change in signaling within the cell by activating or inhibiting an enzymatic intracellular domain (*rectangular box*) of the same receptor molecule. **D.** Drugs can diffuse through the plasma membrane and bind to cytoplasmic or nuclear receptors. This is often the pathway used by lipophilic drugs (e.g., drugs that bind to steroid hormone receptors). Additionally, drugs can bind to enzymes and other targets in the extracellular space and to cell surface adhesion receptors without the need to cross the plasma membrane (*not shown*).

ion channels; (2) transmembrane receptors coupled to intracellular G proteins; (3) transmembrane receptors with linked enzymatic domains; (4) intracellular receptors, including enzymes, signal transduction molecules, transcription factors, structural proteins, and nucleic acids; (5) extracellular targets; and (6) cell surface adhesion receptors (Fig. 1-3). Table 1-2 provides a summary of each major interaction type.

Knowing whether and to what extent a drug activates or inhibits its target provides valuable information about the interaction. Although **pharmacodynamics** (the effects of drugs on the human body) is covered in detail in the next chapter, it is useful to state briefly the major pharmacodynamic relationships between drugs and their targets before examining the molecular mechanisms of drug–receptor interactions. *Agonists are molecules that, upon binding to their targets, cause a change in the activity of those targets.* **Full agonists** bind to and activate their targets to the maximal extent possible. For example, acetylcholine binds to the nicotinic acetylcholine receptor and induces a conformational change in the receptor-associated ion

channel from a nonconducting to a fully conducting state. **Partial agonists** produce a submaximal response upon binding to their targets. **Inverse agonists** cause constitutively active targets to become inactive. *Antagonists inhibit the ability of their targets to be activated (or inactivated) by physiologic or pharmacologic agonists.* Drugs that directly block the binding site of a physiologic agonist are called **competitive antagonists**; drugs that bind to other sites on the target molecule, and thereby prevent the conformational change required for receptor activation (or inactivation), may be either **noncompetitive** or **uncompetitive antagonists** (see Chapter 2). As the mechanism of each drug–receptor interaction is outlined in the next several sections, it will be useful to consider at a structural level how these different pharmacodynamic effects could be produced.

Transmembrane Ion Channels

Many cellular functions require the passage of ions and other hydrophilic molecules across the plasma membrane.

TABLE 1-2 Six Major Types of Drug–Receptor Interactions			
RECEPTOR TYPE	**SITE OF DRUG–RECEPTOR INTERACTION**	**SITE OF RESULTANT ACTION**	**EXAMPLES**
Transmembrane ion channel	Extracellular, intrachannel, or intracellular	Cytoplasm	Amlodipine, diazepam, lidocaine, omeprazole
Transmembrane linked to intracellular G protein	Extracellular or intramembrane	Cytoplasm	Albuterol, loratadine, losartan, metoprolol
Transmembrane with linked enzymatic domain	Extracellular or intracellular	Cytoplasm	Erlotinib, insulin, nesiritide, sunitinib
Intracellular	Cytoplasm or nucleus	Cytoplasm or nucleus	Atorvastatin, doxycycline, levothyroxine, paclitaxel
Extracellular target	Extracellular	Extracellular	Dabigatran, donepezil, etanercept, lisinopril
Adhesion	Extracellular	Extracellular	Eptifibatide, natalizumab

Specialized transmembrane channels regulate these processes. The functions of **ion channels** are diverse, including fundamental roles in neurotransmission, cardiac conduction, muscle contraction, and secretion. Because of this, drugs targeting ion channels can have a substantial impact on major body functions.

Three major mechanisms are used to regulate the activity of transmembrane ion channels. In some channels, the conductance is controlled by ligand binding to the channel. In other channels, the conductance is regulated by changes in voltage across the plasma membrane. In still other channels, the conductance is controlled by ligand binding to plasma membrane receptors that are linked to the channel in some way. The first group of channels is referred to as **ligand-gated**, the second as **voltage-gated**, and the third as **second messenger-regulated**. Table 1-3 summarizes the mechanism of activation and function of each channel type.

Channels are generally highly selective for the ions they conduct. For example, action potential propagation in neurons of the central and peripheral nervous systems occurs as a result of the synchronous stimulation of voltage-gated ion channels that permit the selective passage of Na^+ ions into the cell. When the membrane potential in such a neuron becomes sufficiently positive, the voltage-gated Na^+ channels open, allowing a large influx of extracellular sodium ions that further depolarizes the cell. The role of ion-selective channels in action potential generation and propagation is discussed in Chapter 8, Principles of Cellular Excitability and Electrochemical Transmission.

Most ion channels share some structural similarity, regardless of their ion selectivity, the magnitude of their conductance, or their mechanism of activation (gating) or inactivation. Ion channels are pore-forming macromolecules consisting of one or more protein subunits that pass through the plasma membrane. The **ligand-binding domain** can be extracellular, within the channel, or intracellular, whereas the domain that interacts with other receptors or modulators is most often intracellular. The structures of several ion channels have been determined to atomic resolution; the nicotinic acetylcholine (ACh) receptor provides an example of the structure of an important ligand-gated ion channel. This receptor consists of five subunits, each of which crosses the plasma membrane (Fig. 1-4). Two of the subunits have been designated α; each contains a single extracellular binding site for ACh. In the free (nonliganded) state of the receptor, the channel is occluded by amino acid side chains and does not allow the passage of ions. Binding of two molecules of acetylcholine to the receptor induces a conformational change that opens the channel and allows ion conductance.

Although the nicotinic ACh receptor appears to assume only two states, open or closed, many ion channels assume other states as well. For example, some ion channels are able to become **refractory** or **inactivated**. In this state, the channel's permeability cannot be altered for a certain period of time, known as the channel's refractory period. The voltage-gated sodium channel undergoes a cycle of activation, channel opening, channel closing, and channel inactivation. During the inactivation (refractory) period, the channel

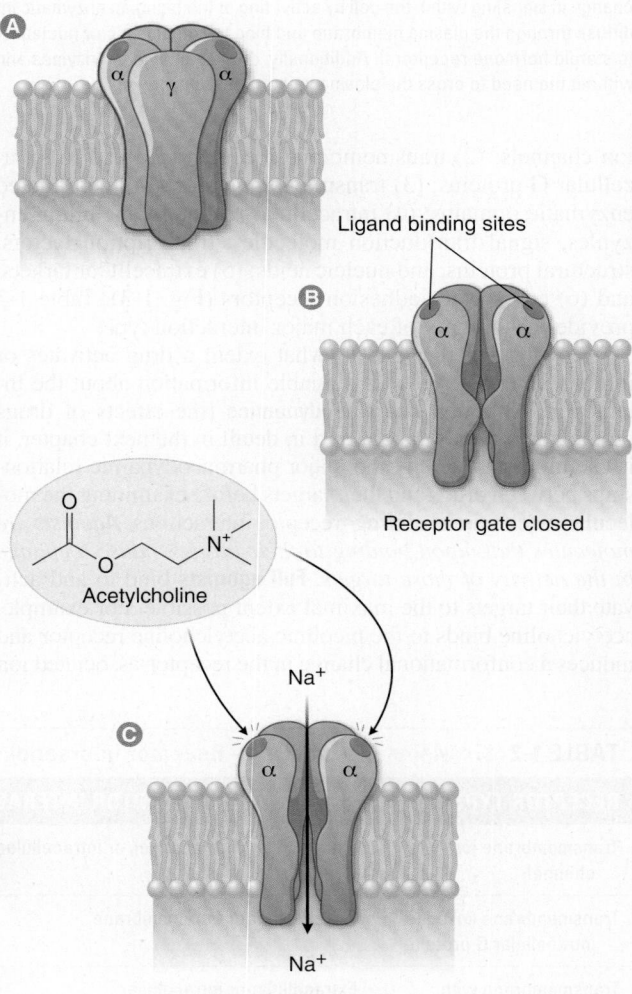

FIGURE 1-4. Ligand-gated nicotinic acetylcholine receptor. A. The plasma membrane acetylcholine (ACh) receptor is composed of five subunits—two α subunits, a β subunit, a γ subunit, and a δ subunit. **B.** The γ subunit has been removed to show an internal schematic view of the receptor, demonstrating that it forms a transmembrane channel. In the absence of ACh, the receptor gate is closed, and cations (most importantly, sodium ions [Na^+]) are unable to traverse the channel. **C.** When ACh is bound to both α subunits, the channel opens, and sodium can pass down its concentration gradient into the cell.

TABLE 1-3 Three Major Types of Transmembrane Ion Channels

CHANNEL TYPE	MECHANISM OF ACTIVATION	FUNCTION
Ligand-gated	Binding of ligand to channel	Altered ion conductance
Voltage-gated	Change in transmembrane voltage gradient	Altered ion conductance
Second messenger-regulated	Binding of ligand to transmembrane receptor with G protein-coupled cytosolic domain, leading to second messenger generation	Second messenger regulates ion conductance of channel

cannot be reactivated for a number of milliseconds, even if the membrane potential returns to a voltage that normally stimulates the channel to open. Some drugs bind with different affinities to different states of the same ion channel. This **state-dependent binding** is important in the mechanism of action of some local anesthetic and antiarrhythmic drugs, as discussed in Chapters 12 (Local Anesthetic Pharmacology) and 24 (Pharmacology of Cardiac Rhythm), respectively.

Two important classes of drugs that act by altering the conductance of ion channels are the local anesthetics and the benzodiazepines. Local anesthetics block the conductance of sodium ions through voltage-gated sodium channels in neurons that transmit pain information from the periphery to the central nervous system, thereby preventing action potential propagation and, hence, pain perception (nociception). Benzodiazepines also act on the nervous system, but by a different mechanism. These drugs inhibit neurotransmission in the central nervous system by potentiating the ability of the neurotransmitter gamma-aminobutyric acid (**GABA**) to increase the conductance of chloride ions across neuronal membranes, thereby driving the membrane potential further away from its threshold for activation.

Transmembrane G Protein-Coupled Receptors

G protein-coupled receptors are the most abundant class of receptors in the human body. These receptors are exposed at the extracellular surface of the plasma membrane, traverse the membrane, and possess intracellular regions that activate a unique class of signaling molecules called **G proteins**. (G proteins are so named because they bind the guanine nucleotides GTP and GDP.) G protein-coupled signaling mechanisms are involved in many important processes, including vision, olfaction, and neurotransmission.

G protein-coupled receptors have seven transmembrane regions within a single polypeptide chain. Each transmembrane region consists of a single α helix, and the α helices are arranged in a characteristic structural motif that is similar in all members of this receptor class. The extracellular domain of this class of proteins usually contains the ligand-binding region, although some G protein-coupled receptors bind ligands within the transmembrane domain of the receptor. G proteins have α and βγ subunits that are noncovalently linked in the resting state. Stimulation of a G protein-coupled receptor causes its cytoplasmic domain to bind and activate a nearby G protein, whereupon the α subunit of the G protein exchanges GDP for GTP. The α-GTP subunit then dissociates from the βγ subunit, and the α or βγ subunit diffuses along the inner leaflet of the plasma membrane to interact with a number of different effectors. These effectors include adenylyl cyclase, phospholipase C, various ion channels, and other classes of proteins. Signals mediated by G proteins are usually terminated by the hydrolysis of GTP to GDP, which is catalyzed by the inherent GTPase activity of the α subunit (Fig. 1-5).

One major role of the G proteins is to activate the production of **second messengers**; that is, signaling molecules that convey the input provided by the first messenger—usually an endogenous ligand or an exogenous drug—to cytoplasmic effectors (Fig. 1-6). The activation of cyclases such as **adenylyl cyclase**, which catalyzes the production of the second messenger cyclic adenosine-3′,5′-monophosphate (**cAMP**), and **guanylyl cyclase**, which catalyzes the production of cyclic guanosine-3′,5′-monophosphate (**cGMP**), constitutes the most common pathway linked to G proteins. In addition, G proteins can activate the enzyme **phospholipase C** (PLC), which, among other functions, plays a key role in regulating the concentration of intracellular

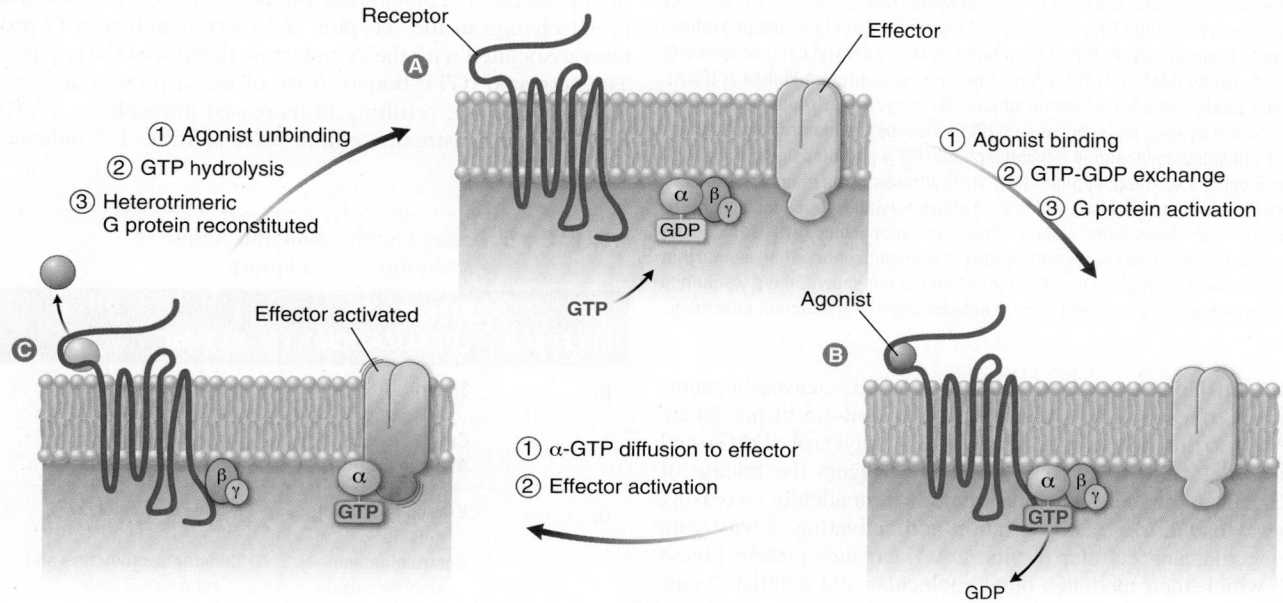

FIGURE 1-5. Receptor-mediated activation of a G protein and the resultant effector interaction. A. In the resting state, the α and βγ subunits of a G protein are associated with one another, and GDP is bound to the α subunit. **B.** Binding of an extracellular ligand (agonist) to a G protein-coupled receptor causes the exchange of GTP for GDP on the α subunit. **C.** The βγ subunit dissociates from the α subunit, which diffuses to interact with effector proteins. Interaction of the GTP-associated α subunit with an effector activates the effector. In some cases (*not shown*), the βγ subunit can also activate effector proteins. Depending on the receptor subtype and the specific Gα isoform, Gα can also inhibit the activity of an effector molecule. The α subunit possesses intrinsic GTPase activity, which leads to hydrolysis of GTP to GDP. This leads to reassociation of the α subunit with the βγ subunit, and the cycle can begin again.

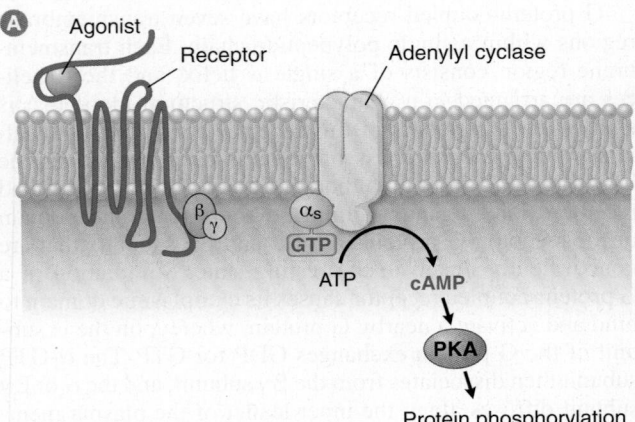

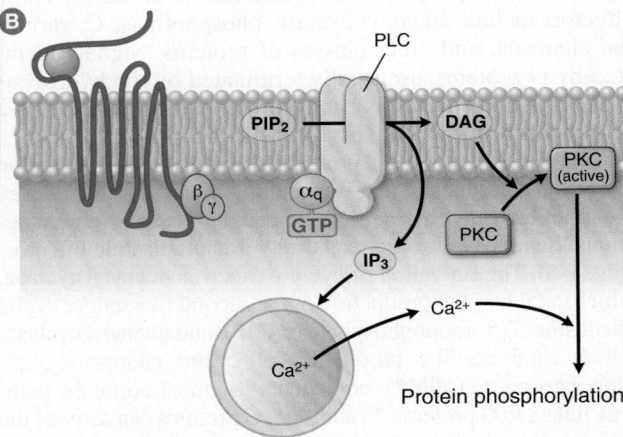

FIGURE 1-6. Activation of adenylyl cyclase (AC) and phospholipase C (PLC) by G proteins. G proteins can interact with several different types of effector molecules. The subtype of Gα protein that is activated often determines which effector the G protein will activate. Two of the most common Gα subunits are Gα$_s$ and Gα$_q$, which stimulate adenylyl cyclase and phospholipase C, respectively. **A.** When stimulated by Gα$_s$, adenylyl cyclase converts ATP to cyclic AMP (cAMP). cAMP then activates protein kinase A (PKA), which phosphorylates a number of specific intracellular proteins. **B.** When stimulated by Gα$_q$, phospholipase C (PLC) cleaves the membrane phospholipid phosphatidylinositol-4,5-bisphosphate (PIP$_2$) into diacylglycerol (DAG) and inositol-1,4,5-trisphosphate (IP$_3$). DAG diffuses in the membrane to activate protein kinase C (PKC), which then phosphorylates specific cellular proteins. IP$_3$ stimulates release of Ca^{2+} from the endoplasmic reticulum into the cytosol. Calcium release also stimulates protein phosphorylation events that lead to changes in protein activation. Although not shown, the βγ subunits of G proteins can also affect certain cellular signal transduction cascades.

calcium. Upon activation by a G protein, PLC cleaves the membrane phospholipid phosphatidylinositol-4,5-bisphosphate (PIP$_2$) to the second messengers diacylglycerol (DAG) and inositol-1,4,5-trisphosphate (IP$_3$). IP$_3$ triggers the release of Ca^{2+} from intracellular stores, thereby dramatically increasing the cytosolic Ca^{2+} concentration and activating downstream molecular and cellular events. DAG activates protein kinase C, which then mediates other molecular and cellular events including smooth muscle contraction and transmembrane ion transport. All of these events are dynamically regulated, so that the different steps in the pathways are activated and inactivated with characteristic kinetics.

A large number of Gα protein isoforms have been identified, each with unique effects on its targets. Based on the primary sequence of the Gα subunit, these isoforms can

TABLE 1-4 The Major G Protein Families and Examples of Their Actions

G PROTEIN	ACTIONS
G-stimulatory (G$_s$)	Activates Ca^{2+} channels, activates adenylyl cyclase
G-inhibitory (G$_i$)	Activates K$^+$ channels, inhibits adenylyl cyclase
G$_o$	Inhibits Ca^{2+} channels
G$_q$	Activates phospholipase C
G$_{12/13}$	Diverse ion transporter interactions

be grouped into five major families—G-stimulatory (G$_s$), G-inhibitory (G$_i$), G$_o$, G$_q$, and G$_{12/13}$. Examples of the effects of these isoforms are shown in Table 1-4. The differential functioning of these G proteins, some of which may couple in different ways to the same receptor in different cell types, is likely to be important for the potential selectivity of future drugs. The βγ subunits of G proteins can also act as second messenger molecules, although their actions are not as completely characterized.

One important class in the G protein-coupled receptor family is the β-adrenergic receptor group. The most thoroughly studied of these receptors have been designated β$_1$, β$_2$, and β$_3$. As discussed in more detail in Chapter 11, Adrenergic Pharmacology, β$_1$ receptors play a role in controlling heart rate; β$_2$ receptors are involved in the relaxation of smooth muscle; and β$_3$ receptors play a role in the mobilization of energy by fat cells. Each of these receptors is stimulated by the binding of endogenous catecholamines, such as **epinephrine** and **norepinephrine**, to the extracellular domain of the receptor. **Epinephrine** binding induces a conformational change in the receptor and thereby activates G proteins associated with the cytoplasmic domain of the receptor. The activated (GTP-bound) form of the G protein activates adenylyl cyclase, resulting in increased intracellular cAMP levels and downstream cellular effects. Table 1-5 indicates

TABLE 1-5 Tissue Localization and Action of β-Adrenergic Receptors

RECEPTOR	TISSUE LOCALIZATION	ACTION
β$_1$	Sinoatrial (SA) node of heart	Increases heart rate
	Cardiac muscle	Increases contractility
	Adipose tissue	Increases lipolysis
β$_2$	Bronchial smooth muscle	Dilates bronchioles
	Gastrointestinal smooth muscle	Constricts sphincters and relaxes gut wall
	Uterus	Relaxes uterine wall
	Bladder	Relaxes bladder
	Liver	Increases gluconeogenesis and glycolysis
	Pancreas	Increases insulin release
β$_3$	Adipose tissue	Increases lipolysis

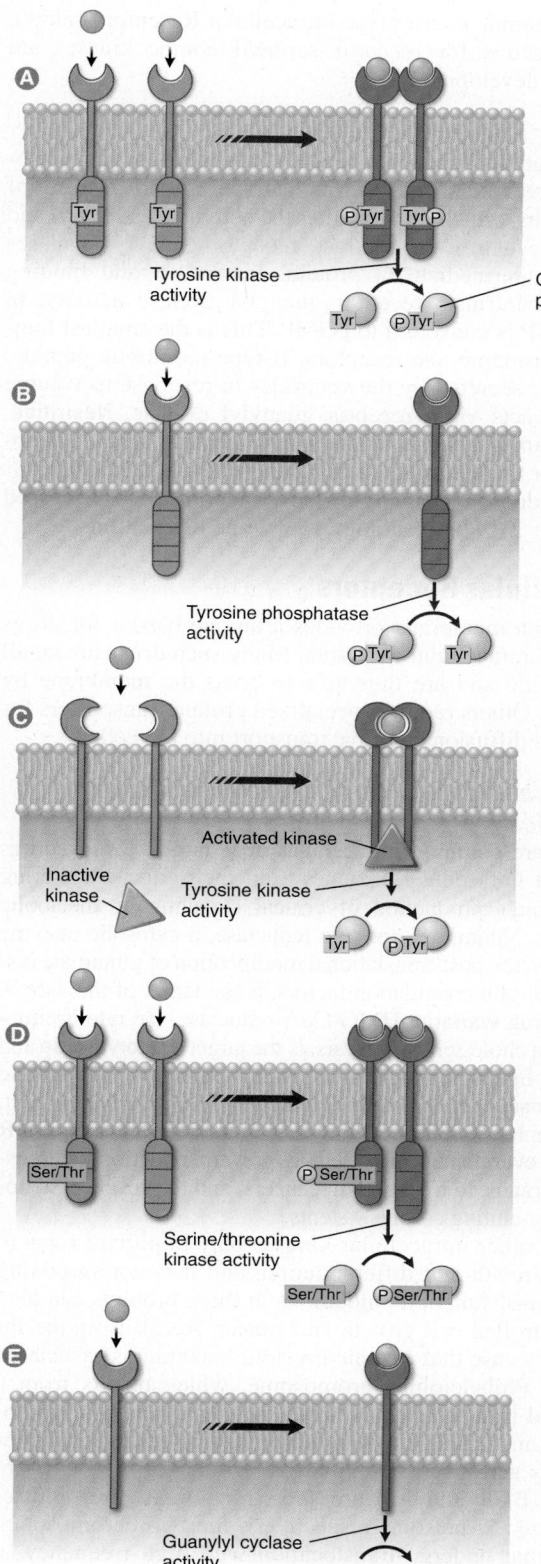

FIGURE 1-7. Major types of transmembrane receptors with linked enzymatic domains. There are five major categories of transmembrane receptors with linked enzymatic domains. **A.** The largest group is composed of **receptor tyrosine kinases**. After ligand-induced activation, these receptors dimerize and transphosphorylate tyrosine residues in the receptor and, often, on target cytosolic proteins. Examples of receptor tyrosine kinases include the insulin receptor and many growth factor receptors. **B.** Some receptors can act as tyrosine phosphatases. These receptors dephosphorylate tyrosine residues either on other transmembrane receptors or on cytosolic proteins. Many cells of the immune system have receptor tyrosine phosphatases. **C.** Some tyrosine kinase-associated receptors lack a definitive enzymatic domain, but binding of ligand to the receptor triggers activation of receptor-associated protein 1 (termed **nonreceptor tyrosine kinases**) that then phosphorylate tyrosine residues on certain cytosolic proteins. **D.** Receptor serine/threonine kinases phosphorylate serine and threonine residues on certain target cytosolic proteins. Members of the TGF-β superfamily of receptors are in this category. **E.** Receptor guanylyl cyclases contain a cytosolic domain that catalyzes the formation of cGMP from GTP. The receptor for B-type natriuretic peptide is one of the receptor guanylyl cyclases that has been well characterized.

some of the diverse tissue localizations and actions of the β-adrenergic receptors.

Transmembrane Receptors with Linked Enzymatic Domains

The third major class of cellular drug targets consists of transmembrane receptors that transduce an extracellular ligand-binding interaction into an intracellular action through the activation of a linked enzymatic domain. The enzymatic domain may be part of the receptor itself or part of a cytosolic protein that is recruited to the receptor in response to receptor activation. Such receptors play roles in a diverse set of physiologic processes, including cell metabolism, growth, and differentiation. Receptors that have a linked enzymatic domain can be grouped into five major classes based on their cytoplasmic mechanism of action (Fig. 1-7). All of these receptors are single–membrane-spanning proteins, in contrast to the seven–membrane-spanning motif present in G protein-coupled receptors. Many receptors with enzymatic cytosolic domains form dimers or multisubunit complexes to transduce their signals.

Many receptors with linked enzymatic domains modify proteins by adding or removing phosphate groups to or from specific amino acid residues. *Phosphorylation is a ubiquitous mechanism of protein signaling.* The large negative charge of phosphate groups can dramatically alter the three-dimensional structure of a protein and thereby change that protein's activity. In addition, phosphorylation is easily reversible, thus allowing this signaling mechanism to act specifically in time and space.

Receptor Tyrosine Kinases

The largest group of transmembrane receptors with enzymatic cytosolic domains is the receptor tyrosine kinase family. These receptors transduce signals from many hormones and growth factors by phosphorylating tyrosine residues on the cytoplasmic tail of the receptor. This leads to recruitment and subsequent tyrosine phosphorylation of cytosolic signaling molecules. When aberrantly expressed or overexpressed, growth factor-responsive receptor tyrosine kinases (such as epidermal growth factor receptor [EGFR], HER2/neu, and vascular endothelial growth factor receptor [VEGFR]) are associated with a wide array of cancers; these receptor tyrosine kinases are the targets of several monoclonal antibody and small-molecule inhibitor drugs (see Chapter 40, Pharmacology of Cancer: Signal Transduction).

The insulin receptor is a well-characterized receptor tyrosine kinase. This receptor consists of two extracellular α subunits that are covalently linked to two membrane-spanning β subunits. Binding of insulin to the α subunits results in a change in conformation of the adjacent β subunits, causing the β subunits to move closer to one another on the intracellular side of the membrane. The proximity of the two β subunits promotes a transphosphorylation reaction, in which one β subunit phosphorylates the other (autophosphorylation). The phosphorylated tyrosine residues then act to recruit other cytosolic proteins, known as insulin receptor substrate (IRS) proteins. Type 2 diabetes mellitus may, in some cases, be associated with defects in post-insulin receptor signaling; thus, understanding the insulin receptor signaling pathways is relevant for the potential design of rational therapeutics. The mechanism of insulin receptor signaling is discussed in more detail in Chapter 31, Pharmacology of the Endocrine Pancreas and Glucose Homeostasis.

Receptor Tyrosine Phosphatases

Just as receptor tyrosine kinases phosphorylate the tyrosine residues of cytoplasmic proteins, receptor tyrosine phosphatases remove phosphate groups from specific tyrosine residues. In some cases, this may be an example of receptor convergence (discussed later), where the differential effects of two receptor types can negate one another. However, receptor tyrosine phosphatases possess novel signaling mechanisms as well. Many receptor tyrosine phosphatases are found in immune cells, where they regulate cell activation. These receptors are discussed further in Chapter 46, Pharmacology of Immunosuppression.

Tyrosine Kinase-Associated Receptors

Tyrosine kinase-associated receptors constitute a diverse family of proteins that, although lacking inherent catalytic activity, recruit active cytosolic signaling proteins in a ligand-dependent manner. These cytosolic proteins are also called (somewhat confusingly) **nonreceptor tyrosine kinases**. Ligand activation of cell surface tyrosine kinase-associated receptors causes the receptors to cluster together. This clustering event recruits cytoplasmic proteins that are then activated to phosphorylate other proteins on tyrosine residues. Thus, the downstream effect is much like that of receptor tyrosine kinases, except that tyrosine kinase-associated receptors rely on a nonreceptor kinase to phosphorylate target proteins. Important examples of tyrosine kinase-associated receptors include cytokine receptors and a number of other receptors in the immune system. These receptors are discussed in detail in Chapter 46.

Receptor Serine/Threonine Kinases

Some transmembrane receptors are capable of catalyzing the phosphorylation of serine or threonine residues on cytoplasmic protein substrates. Ligands for such receptors are typically members of the transforming growth factor β (TGF-β) superfamily. Many receptor serine/threonine kinases are important mediators of cell growth and differentiation that have been implicated in cancer progression and metastasis. While there are many approved drugs that target *cytosolic*

serine/threonine kinases (see Intracellular Receptors below), drugs selective for *receptor* serine/threonine kinases are mainly in development.

Receptor Guanylyl Cyclases

As illustrated in Figure 1-6, the stimulation of G protein-coupled receptors may cause activation and release of Gα subunits, which, in turn, alter the activity of adenylyl and guanylyl cyclases. In contrast, receptor guanylyl cyclases have no intermediate G protein. Instead, ligand binding stimulates intrinsic receptor guanylyl cyclase activity, in which GTP is converted to cGMP. This is the smallest family of transmembrane receptors. B-type natriuretic peptide, a hormone secreted by the ventricles in response to volume overload, acts via a receptor guanylyl cyclase. **Nesiritide**, a recombinant version of the native peptide ligand, is approved for the treatment of decompensated heart failure (although it does not reliably improve outcomes), as discussed in Chapter 21, Pharmacology of Volume Regulation.

Intracellular Receptors

The plasma membrane provides a unique barrier for drugs that have intracellular receptors. Many such drugs are small or lipophilic and are thus able to cross the membrane by diffusion. Others require specialized protein transporters for facilitated diffusion or active transport into the cell.

Intracellular Enzymes and Signal Transduction Molecules

Enzymes are common intracellular drug targets. Many drugs that target intracellular enzymes exert their effect by altering the enzyme's production of critical signaling or metabolic molecules. Vitamin K epoxide reductase, a cytosolic enzyme involved in the post-translational modification of glutamate residues in certain coagulation factors, is the target of the anticoagulant drug **warfarin**. HMG-CoA reductase, the rate-limiting enzyme in cholesterol synthesis, is the target of **atorvastatin** and the other lipid-lowering statins. Many inhibitors of cytosolic **signal transduction molecules** are approved or in development. For example, inhibitors of the serine/threonine kinase mTOR (such as **everolimus**) are used to prevent rejection of transplanted organs, to treat certain cancers, and to prevent restenosis in drug-eluting coronary stents.

Many other intracellular kinases play important roles in cellular growth and differentiation, and it is not surprising that "gain-of-function" mutations in these proteins can lead to uncontrolled cell growth and cancer. Recall from the introductory case that chronic myeloid leukemia is associated with the Philadelphia chromosome, which results from a reciprocal translocation between the long arms of chromosomes 9 and 22. The mutant chromosome codes for a constitutively active tyrosine kinase referred to as the BCR-Abl protein. (BCR and Abl are short for "break-point cluster region" and "Abelson," respectively, the two chromosomal regions that undergo translocation with high frequency in this form of leukemia.) The constitutive activity of this kinase results in phosphorylation of a number of cytosolic proteins, leading to dysregulated myeloid cell growth and chronic myeloid leukemia. **Imatinib** is a selective therapy for chronic myeloid leukemia because it selectively targets the BCR-Abl protein; the drug inhibits BCR-Abl activity by neutralizing its ability to phosphorylate substrates. Imatinib was the first example of a drug targeted selectively to tyrosine kinases, and its success has led to the development of a number of drugs that act by similar mechanisms. Such drugs include second-generation drugs such as **dasatinib** and **nilotinib** that are used to treat CML patients with imatinib-resistant BCR-Abl isoforms, as well as the inhibitors of growth factor-responsive receptor tyrosine kinases discussed above. Indeed, the kinase targets of antineoplastic drugs are diverse. For instance, **sorafenib** targets both receptor tyrosine kinases and intracellular serine/threonine kinases, and **vemurafenib** is a recently approved late-stage melanoma treatment that targets a specific mutant of the serine/threonine kinase B-RAF. As a final example, **idelalisib** is a recently approved phosphatidylinositol-4,5-bisphosphate 3-kinase (PI3K) inhibitor used to treat certain leukemias and lymphomas (see Chapter 40).

Transcription Factors

The transcription regulatory factors are important intracellular receptors that are targeted by lipophilic drugs. All proteins in the body are encoded by DNA. The transcription of DNA into RNA and the translation of RNA into protein are controlled by a diverse set of molecules. Transcription of many genes is regulated, in part, by the interaction between lipid-soluble signaling molecules and transcription regulatory factors. Because of the fundamental role played by control of transcription in many biological processes, **transcription regulators** (also called **transcription factors**) are the targets of some important drugs. **Steroid hormones** are a class of lipophilic drugs that diffuse readily through the plasma membrane and act by binding to transcription factors in the cytoplasm or nucleus (Fig. 1-8).

Just as the shape of a transcription factor governs the drugs to which it binds, the shape also determines where on the genome the transcription factor attaches and which coactivator or corepressor molecules bind to it. By activating or inhibiting transcription, thereby altering the intracellular or extracellular concentrations of specific gene products, drugs that target transcription factors can have profound effects on cellular function. The cellular responses to such drugs, and the effects that result from these cellular responses in tissues and organ systems, provide links between the molecular drug–receptor interaction and the effects of the drug on the organism as a whole. Because gene transcription is a relatively slow and long-lasting process (minutes to hours), drugs that target transcription factors often require a longer period of time for the onset of action to take place, and have longer lasting effects, than do drugs that alter more transient processes such as ion conductance (seconds to minutes).

Structural Proteins

Structural proteins are another important class of intracellular drug targets. For example, the antimitotic vinca alkaloids bind to tubulin monomers and prevent the polymerization of this molecule into microtubules. Inhibition of microtubule formation arrests the affected cells in metaphase, making the vinca alkaloids useful antineoplastic drugs.

Nucleic Acids

Nucleic acids are a fourth subset of intracellular drug targets. Some small-molecule drugs bind directly to RNA or ribosomes; these include important antibiotics (such as **doxycycline** and **azithromycin**) that block translation in target microorganisms. DNA- and RNA-binding chemotherapeutic

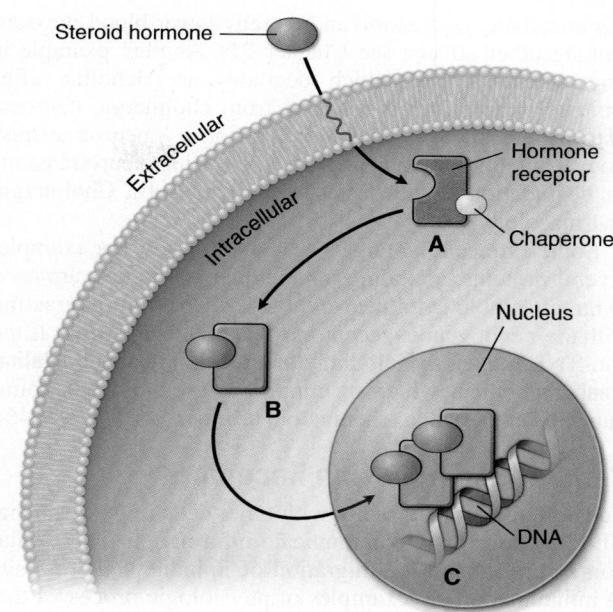

FIGURE 1-8. Lipophilic molecule binding to an intracellular transcription factor. A. Small lipophilic molecules can diffuse through the plasma membrane and bind to intracellular transcription factors. In this example, steroid hormone binding to a cytosolic hormone receptor is shown, although some receptors of this class may be located in the nucleus before ligand binding. **B.** Ligand binding triggers a conformational change in the receptor (and often, as shown here, dissociation of a chaperone repressor protein) that leads to transport of the ligand–receptor complex into the nucleus. In the nucleus, the ligand–receptor complex typically dimerizes. In the example shown, the active form of the receptor is a homodimer (two identical receptors binding to one another), but heterodimers (such as the thyroid hormone receptor and the retinoid X receptor) may also form. **C.** The dimerized ligand–receptor complex binds to DNA and may then recruit coactivators or corepressors (*not shown*). These complexes alter the rate of gene transcription, leading to a change (either up or down) in cellular protein expression.

agents (such as **doxorubicin**) are mainstays of treatment for many cancers. Drugs composed of nucleic acids can also target nucleic acids. **Antisense therapeutics** (such as the recently approved drug **mipomersen**) bind target mRNA to block transcription of specific proteins. With continued development of such antisense approaches and of related RNA interference (RNAi) therapeutics, such targeting could someday enable physicians to routinely modify the expression levels of specific gene transcripts. To date, technical challenges in delivering such therapeutics to their targets have limited their utility to specialized applications.

Extracellular Targets

Many important drug receptors are enzymes with active sites located outside the plasma membrane. The extracellular environment consists of a milieu of proteins and signaling molecules. Many of these proteins serve a structural role, and others are used to communicate information between cells. Enzymes that modify the molecules mediating these important signals can influence physiologic processes such as vasoconstriction and neurotransmission. One example of this class of receptors is the **angiotensin converting enzyme** (ACE), which converts angiotensin I to the potent vasoconstrictor angiotensin II. **ACE inhibitors** are drugs that inhibit this enzymatic conversion and thereby lower blood pressure (among other effects; see Chapter 21). Another example is **acetylcholinesterase**, which degrades acetylcholine after this neurotransmitter is released from cholinergic neurons. **Acetylcholinesterase inhibitors** enhance neurotransmission at cholinergic synapses by preventing neurotransmitter degradation at these sites (see Chapter 10, Cholinergic Pharmacology).

Some extracellular targets are not enzymes. For example, several proteins, including monoclonal antibodies, are used to target soluble cytokines and block them from interacting with their endogenous receptors. One set of such drugs is the anti-TNF-α agents, including **etanercept**, **infliximab**, **adalimumab**, and others, which are commonly used to treat autoimmune diseases such as rheumatoid arthritis (see Chapter 46).

Cell Surface Adhesion Receptors

Cells often interact directly with other cells to perform specific functions or to communicate information. The formation of tissues and the migration of immune cells to a site of inflammation are examples of physiologic processes that require cell–cell adhesive interactions. A region of contact between two cells is termed an **adhesion**, and cell–cell adhesive interactions are mediated by pairs of **adhesion receptors** on the surfaces of the individual cells. In many cases, several such receptor–counter-receptor pairs combine to secure a firm adhesion, and intracellular regulators control the activity of the adhesion receptors by changing their affinity or by controlling their expression and localization on the cell surface. Adhesion receptors also mediate adhesion of cells to the extracellular matrix. Several adhesion receptors involved in the inflammatory response are attractive targets for selective inhibitors. Inhibitors of a specific class of adhesion receptors, known as **integrins**, have entered the clinic in recent years, and these drugs are used in the treatment of a range of conditions including thrombosis (**abciximab**, **eptifibatide**), inflammatory bowel disease (**vedolizumab**), and multiple sclerosis (**natalizumab**) (see Chapter 23, Pharmacology of Hemostasis and Thrombosis, and Chapter 46).

PROCESSING OF SIGNALS RESULTING FROM DRUG–RECEPTOR INTERACTIONS

Many cells in the body are continuously inundated with multiple inputs, some stimulatory and some inhibitory. How do cells integrate these signals to produce a coherent response? G proteins and other second messengers appear to provide important points of integration. As noted above, relatively few second messengers have been identified, and it is unlikely that many more remain to be discovered. Thus, second messengers are an attractive candidate mechanism for providing cells with a set of common points upon which numerous outside stimuli could converge to generate a coordinated cellular effect (Fig. 1-9).

Ion concentrations provide another point of integration for cellular effects because the cellular concentration of a particular ion is the result of the integrated activity of *multiple* ionic currents that both increase and decrease the concentration of the ion within the cell. For example, the contractile state of a smooth muscle cell is a function of the intracellular calcium ion concentration, which is determined by several different Ca^{2+} conductances. These conductances include calcium ion leaks into the cell and calcium currents into and out of the cytoplasm through specialized channels in the plasma membrane and smooth endoplasmic reticulum.

Because the magnitude of cellular response is often considerably greater than the magnitude of the stimulus that caused the response, cells appear to have the ability to amplify the effects of receptor binding. G proteins provide an excellent example of signal amplification. Ligand binding to a G protein-coupled receptor activates a single G protein molecule. This G protein molecule can then bind to and activate many effector molecules, such as adenylyl cyclase, which can then generate an even greater number of second messenger molecules (in this example, cAMP). Another example of signal amplification is "trigger Ca^{2+}" or calcium-induced calcium release, in which a small influx

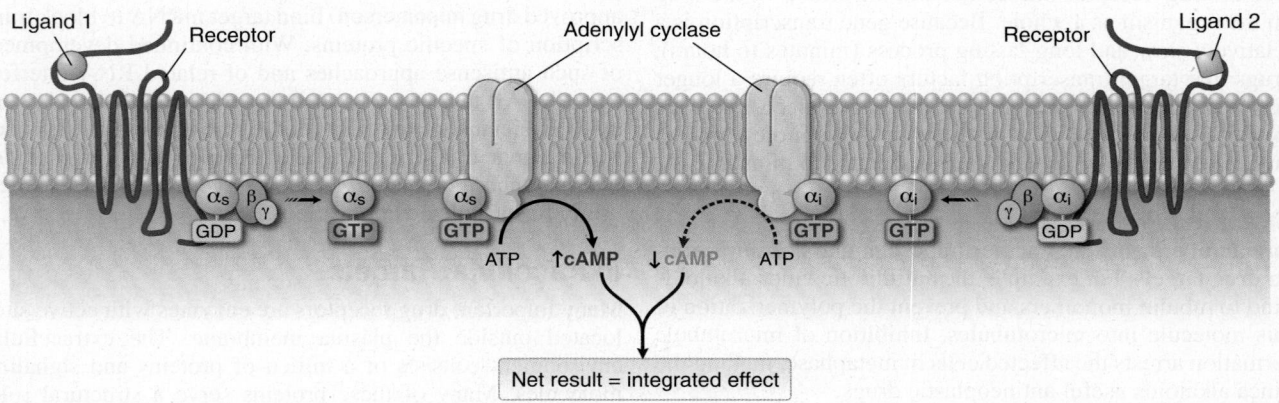

FIGURE 1-9. Signaling convergence of two receptors. A limited number of mechanisms are used to transduce intracellular signal cascades. In some cases, this allows for convergence, where two different receptors have opposite effects that tend to negate one another in the cell. In a simple example, two different G protein-coupled receptors could be stimulated by different ligands. The receptor shown on the left is coupled to $G\alpha_s$, a G protein that stimulates adenylyl cyclase to catalyze the formation of cAMP. The receptor shown on the right is coupled to $G\alpha_i$, a G protein that inhibits adenylyl cyclase. When both of these receptors are activated simultaneously, they can attenuate or even neutralize each other, as shown. Sometimes, signaling through a pathway may alternate as the two receptors are sequentially activated.

of Ca^{2+} through voltage-gated Ca^{2+} channels in the plasma membrane "triggers" the release of larger amounts of Ca^{2+} from intracellular stores into the cytoplasm.

CELLULAR REGULATION OF DRUG–RECEPTOR INTERACTIONS

Drug-induced activation or inhibition of a receptor often has a lasting impact on the receptor's subsequent responsiveness to drug binding. Mechanisms that mediate such effects are important because they prevent overstimulation that could lead to cellular damage or adversely affect the organism as a whole. Many drugs show diminishing effects over time; this phenomenon is called **tachyphylaxis**. In pharmacologic terms, the receptor and the cell become **desensitized** to the action of the drug. Mechanisms of desensitization can be divided into two types: **homologous**, in which the effects of agonists at only one type of receptor are diminished, and **heterologous**, in which the effects of agonists at two or more types of receptors are coordinately diminished. Heterologous desensitization is thought to be caused by drug-induced alteration in a common point of convergence in the signaling pathways activated by the involved receptors, such as a shared effector molecule.

Many receptors exhibit desensitization. For example, the cellular response to repeated stimulation of β-adrenergic receptors by epinephrine diminishes steadily over time (Fig. 1-10). β-Adrenergic receptor desensitization is mediated by epinephrine-induced phosphorylation of the cytoplasmic tail of the receptor. This phosphorylation promotes the binding of β-arrestin to the receptor; in turn, β-arrestin inhibits the receptor's ability to stimulate the G protein G_s. With lower levels of activated G_s present, adenylyl cyclase produces less cAMP. In this manner, repeated cycles of ligand–receptor binding result in smaller and smaller cellular effects. Other molecular mechanisms have even more profound effects, completely turning off the receptor to stimulation by ligand. The latter phenomenon, referred to as **inactivation**, may also result from phosphorylation of the receptor; in this case, the phosphorylation completely blocks the signaling activity of the receptor or causes removal of the receptor from the cell surface.

Another mechanism that can affect the cellular response caused by drug–receptor binding is called *refractoriness*. Receptors that assume a **refractory** state following activation require a period of time to pass before they can be stimulated again. As noted above, voltage-gated sodium channels, which mediate the firing of neuronal action potentials, are subject to refractory periods. After channel opening induced by membrane depolarization, the voltage-gated sodium channel spontaneously closes and cannot be reopened for some period of time (called the **refractory period**). This inherent property of the channel determines the maximum rate at which neurons can be stimulated and transmit information.

The effect of drug–receptor binding can also be influenced by drug-induced changes in the number of receptors on or in a cell. One example of a molecular mechanism by which receptor number can be altered is called **down-regulation**. In this phenomenon, prolonged receptor stimulation by ligand induces the cell to endocytose and sequester receptors

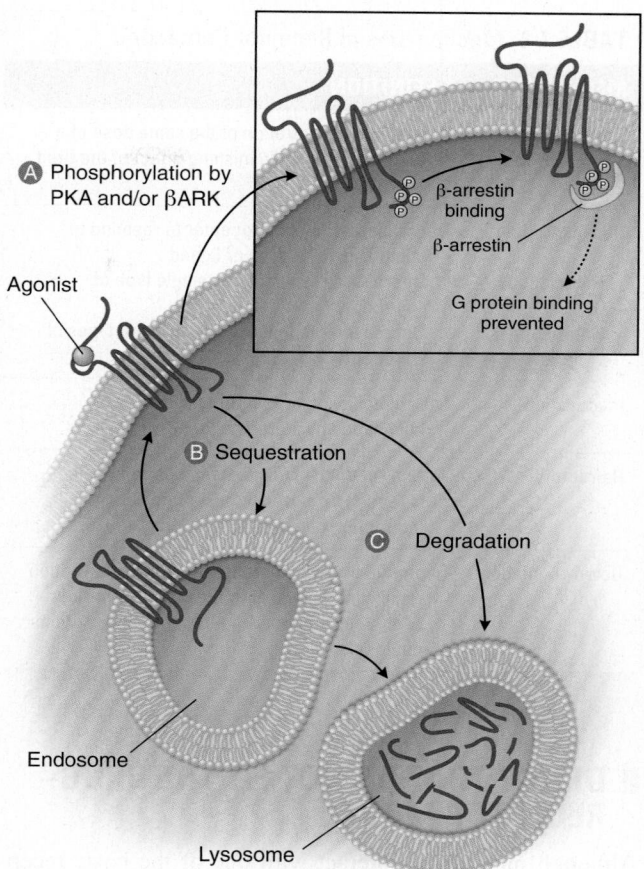

FIGURE 1-10. β-Adrenergic receptor regulation. Agonist-bound β-adrenergic receptors activate G proteins, which then stimulate adenylyl cyclase activity (*not shown*). **A.** Repeated or persistent stimulation of the receptor by agonist results in phosphorylation of amino acids at the C-terminus of the receptor by protein kinase A (PKA) and/or β-adrenergic receptor kinase (βARK). β-Arrestin then binds to the phosphorylated domain of the receptor and blocks G_s binding, thereby decreasing adenylyl cyclase (effector) activity. **B.** Binding of β-arrestin also leads to receptor sequestration into endosomal compartments via clathrin-mediated endocytosis (*not shown*), effectively neutralizing β-adrenergic receptor signaling activity. The receptor can then be recycled and reinserted into the plasma membrane. **C.** Prolonged receptor occupation by an agonist can lead to receptor down-regulation and eventual receptor degradation. Cells can also reduce the number of receptors by inhibiting the transcription or translation of the gene coding for the receptor (*not shown*).

in endocytic vesicles. This sequestration prevents the receptors from coming into contact with ligands, resulting in cellular desensitization. When the stimulus that caused the receptor sequestration subsides, the receptors can be recycled to the cell surface and thereby rendered functional again (Fig. 1-10). Cells also have the ability to alter the rates of synthesis or degradation of receptors and thereby to regulate the number of receptors available for drug binding. Receptor sequestration and alterations in receptor synthesis and degradation occur on a longer time scale than does phosphorylation and have longer lasting effects as well. Table 1-6 provides a summary of the mechanisms by which the effects of drug–receptor interactions can be regulated.

TABLE 1-6 Mechanisms of Receptor Regulation

MECHANISM	DEFINITION
Tachyphylaxis	Repeated administration of the same dose of a drug results in a diminishing effect of the drug over time
Desensitization	Decreased ability of a receptor to respond to stimulation by a drug or ligand
Homologous	Decreased response at a single type of receptor
Heterologous	Decreased response at two or more types of receptor
Inactivation	Loss of ability of a receptor to respond to stimulation by a drug or ligand
Refractory	After a receptor is stimulated, a period of time is required before the next drug–receptor interaction can produce an effect
Down-regulation	Repeated or persistent drug–receptor interaction results in removal of the receptor from sites where subsequent drug–receptor interactions could take place

DRUGS THAT DO NOT FIT THE DRUG–RECEPTOR MODEL

Although most drugs interact with one of the basic receptor types outlined above, others act by nonreceptor-mediated mechanisms. Two examples are the osmotic diuretics and the antacids.

Diuretics control fluid balance in the body by altering the relative rates of water and ion absorption and secretion in the kidney. Many of these drugs act on ion channels. One class of diuretics, however, alters water and ion balance not by binding to ion channels or G protein-coupled receptors but by changing the osmolarity in the nephron directly. The sugar **mannitol**, which is used mainly to treat increased intracranial pressure, is secreted into the lumen of the nephron and increases the osmolarity of the urine to such a degree that water is drawn from the peritubular blood into the lumen. This fluid shift serves to increase the volume of urine while decreasing the blood volume.

Another class of drugs that does not fit the drug–receptor model is the antacids, which are used to treat gastroesophageal reflux disease and peptic ulcer disease. Unlike antiulcer agents that bind to receptors involved in the physiologic generation of gastric acid, antacids act nonspecifically by absorbing or chemically neutralizing stomach acid. Examples of these agents include bases such as $NaHCO_3$ and $Mg(OH)_2$.

CONCLUSION AND FUTURE DIRECTIONS

Although the molecular details of drug–receptor interactions vary widely among drugs of different classes and receptors of different types, the fundamental mechanisms of action described in this chapter serve as paradigms for the principles of pharmacodynamics. The ability to classify drugs based on their receptors and mechanisms of action makes it possible to simplify the study of pharmacology, because the molecular mechanism of action of a drug can usually be linked to its cellular, tissue, organ, and system levels of action. In turn, it becomes easier to understand how a given drug mediates its therapeutic effects and its unwanted or adverse effects in a particular patient. The major aim of modern drug development is to identify drugs that are highly selective by tailoring drug molecules to unique targets responsible for disease. As knowledge of drug development and the genetic and pathophysiologic basis of disease progresses, physicians and scientists will learn to combine the *molecular* specificity of a drug with the *genetic* and *pathophysiologic* specificity of the drug target to provide more and more selective therapies.

Acknowledgment

We thank Josef B. Simon, Christopher W. Cairo, and Zachary S. Morris for their valuable contributions to this chapter in the First, Second, and Third Editions of *Principles of Pharmacology: The Pathophysiologic Basis of Drug Therapy*.

Suggested Reading

Alexander SP, Mathie A, Peters JA. Guide to Receptors and Channels (GRAC), 5th ed. *Br J Pharmacol* 2011;164(suppl 1):S1–S324. (*Brief overviews of molecular targets for drugs, organized by types of receptors.*)

Katritch V, Cherezov V, Stevens RC. Structure-function of the G protein-coupled receptor superfamily. *Annu Rev Pharmacol Toxicol* 2013;53:531–556. (*Reviews recent structural insights into G protein-coupled receptors.*)

Kole R, Krainer AR, Altman S. RNA therapeutics: beyond RNA interference and antisense oligonucleotides. *Nat Rev Drug Discov* 2012;11:125–140. (*Highlights early successes, therapeutic mechanisms, and remaining challenges in the development of RNA-based therapies.*)

Lagerström MC, Schiöth HB. Structural diversity of G protein-coupled receptors and significance for drug discovery. *Nat Rev Drug Discov* 2008;7:339–357. (*Discusses the five families of G protein-coupled receptors, with an eye toward future drug development.*)

Pratt WB, Taylor P, eds. *Principles of drug action: the basis of pharmacology.* 3rd ed. New York: Churchill Livingstone; 1990. (*Contains a detailed discussion of drug–receptor interactions.*)

Venkatakrishnan AJ, Deupi X, Lebon G, Tate CG, Schertler GF, Babu MM. Molecular signatures of G protein-coupled receptors. *Nature* 2013;494:185–194. (*Comparative analysis of structures, ligand binding, and conformational changes of G protein-coupled receptors.*)

Zhang J, Yang PL, Gray NS. Targeting cancer with small molecule kinase inhibitors. *Nat Rev Cancer* 2009;9:28–39. (*Discusses dysregulation of protein kinases in cancer and targeting of these molecules by drugs such as imatinib.*)

Agonist

Competitive
antagonist

2

Pharmacodynamics

Quentin J. Baca and David E. Golan

INTRODUCTION

Pharmacodynamics is the term used to describe the effects of a drug on the body. These effects are typically described in quantitative terms. The previous chapter considered the molecular interactions by which pharmacologic agents exert their effects. The integration of these molecular actions into an effect on the organism as a whole is the subject addressed in this chapter. It is important to describe the effects of a drug quantitatively in order to determine appropriate dose ranges for patients, as well as to compare the potency, efficacy, and safety of one drug to that of another.

DRUG–RECEPTOR BINDING

The study of pharmacodynamics is based on the concept of drug–receptor binding. When either a drug or an endogenous ligand (such as a hormone or neurotransmitter) binds to its receptor, a response may result from that binding interaction. When a sufficient number of receptors are bound (or "occupied") on or in a cell, the cumulative effect of receptor "occupancy" may become apparent in that cell. At some point, all of the receptors may be occupied, and a maximal response may be observed (an exception is the case of spare receptors; see below). When the response occurs in many cells, the effect can be seen at the level of the organ or even the patient. But this all starts with the binding of drug or ligand to a receptor (for the purpose of discussion, "drug" and "ligand" will be used interchangeably for the remainder of this chapter). A model that accurately describes the binding of drug to receptor would therefore be useful in predicting the effect of the drug at the molecular, cellular, tissue (organ), and organism (patient) levels. This section describes one such model.

Consider the simplest case, in which the receptor is either free (unoccupied) or reversibly bound to drug (occupied). We can describe this case as follows:

$$L + R \underset{k_{off}}{\overset{k_{on}}{\rightleftharpoons}} LR \qquad \text{Equation 2-1}$$

where L is ligand (drug), R is free receptor, and LR is bound drug–receptor complex. At equilibrium, the fraction of receptors in each state is dependent on the dissociation constant, K_d, where $K_d = k_{off}/k_{on}$. K_d is an intrinsic property of any given drug–receptor pair. Although K_d varies with temperature, the temperature of the human body is relatively constant, and it can therefore be assumed that K_d is a constant for each drug–receptor combination.

According to the law of mass action, the relationship between free and bound receptor can be described as follows:

$$K_d = \frac{[L][R]}{[LR]} \text{ , rearranged to } [LR] = \frac{[L][R]}{K_d} \qquad \text{Equation 2-2}$$

where $[L]$ is free ligand concentration, $[R]$ is free receptor concentration, and $[LR]$ is ligand–receptor complex concentration. Because K_d is a constant, some important properties of the drug–receptor interaction can be deduced from this equation. First, as ligand concentration is increased, the concentration of bound receptors increases. Second, and not so obvious, is that as free receptor concentration is increased (as may happen, for example, in disease states or upon repeated exposure to a drug), bound receptor concentration also increases. Therefore, *an increase in the effect of a drug can result from an increase in the concentration of either the ligand or the receptor.*

The remainder of the discussion in this chapter, however, assumes that the total concentration of receptors is a

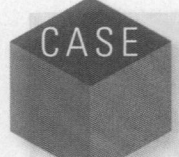

CASE

Admiral X is a 66-year-old retired submarine captain with a 70 pack–year smoking history (two packs a day for 35 years) and a family history of coronary artery disease. He takes daily atorvastatin to reduce his cholesterol level and aspirin to reduce his risk of coronary artery occlusion.

One day, while working in his wood shop, Admiral X begins to feel tightness in his chest. The feeling rapidly becomes painful, and the pain radiates down his left arm. He calls 911, and an ambulance transports him to the local emergency department. After evaluation, it is determined that Admiral X is having an anterior myocardial infarction. Because Admiral X cannot be transferred to a hospital with a cardiac catheterization laboratory within 120 minutes of first medical contact, and he has no relative contraindications to thrombolytic therapy (such as uncontrolled hypertension, history of stroke, or recent surgery), the physician initiates therapy with both a thrombolytic agent, tissue-type plasminogen activator (tPA), and an anticoagulant, heparin. Because of their low therapeutic indices, improper dosing of both of these drugs can have dire consequences (hemorrhage and death). Therefore, Admiral X is closely monitored, and the pharmacologic effect of the heparin is measured periodically by testing the partial thromboplastin time (PTT). Admiral X's symptoms resolve over the next several hours, although he remains in the hospital for monitoring. He is discharged after 4 days in the hospital; his discharge medications include atorvastatin, aspirin, atenolol, lisinopril, and clopidogrel for secondary prevention of myocardial infarction.

Questions

1. How does the molecular interaction of a drug with its receptor determine the potency and efficacy of the drug?
2. Why does the fact that a drug has a low therapeutic index mean that the physician must use greater care in its administration?
3. What properties of certain drugs, such as aspirin, allow them to be taken without monitoring of plasma drug levels, whereas other drugs, such as heparin, require such monitoring?

constant, so that $[LR] + [R] = [R_o]$. This allows Equation 2-2 to be arranged as follows:

$$[R_o] = [R] + [LR] = [R] + \frac{[L][R]}{K_d}$$

$$= [R]\left(1 + \frac{[L]}{K_d}\right) \qquad \textbf{Equation 2-3}$$

Solving for $[R]$ and substituting Equation 2-3 into Equation 2-2 yields:

$$[LR] = \frac{[R_o][L]}{[L] + K_d}, \textbf{rearranged to}$$

$$\frac{[LR]}{[R_o]} = \frac{[L]}{[L] + K_d} \qquad \textbf{Equation 2-4}$$

Note that the left side of this equation, $[LR]/[R_o]$, represents the fraction of all available receptors that are bound to ligand.

Figure 2-1 shows two plots of Equation 2-4 for the binding of two hypothetical drugs to the same receptor. These plots are known as **drug–receptor binding curves**. Figure 2-1A shows a linear plot, and Figure 2-1B shows the same plot on a semilogarithmic scale. Because drug responses occur over a wide range of doses (concentrations), the semilog plot is often used to display drug–receptor binding data. The two drug–receptor interactions are characterized by different values of K_d. In this case, $K_{dA} < K_{dB}$.

Notice from Figure 2-1 that maximal drug–receptor binding occurs when $[LR]$ is equal to $[R_o]$, or $[LR]/[R_o] = 1$. Also notice that, according to Equation 2-4, when $[L] = K_d$, then $[LR]/[R_o] = K_d/2K_d = \frac{1}{2}$. Thus, K_d can be defined as the concentration of ligand at which 50% of the available receptors are occupied.

■ DOSE–RESPONSE RELATIONSHIPS

The pharmacodynamics of a drug can be quantified by the relationship between the dose (concentration) of the drug and the organism's (patient's) response to that drug. One might intuitively expect the dose–response relationship to be related closely to the drug–receptor binding relationship, and this turns out to be the case for many drug–receptor combinations. Thus, a useful assumption at this stage of discussion is that *the response to a drug is proportional to the concentration of receptors that are bound (occupied) by the drug.* This assumption can be quantified by the following relationship:

$$\frac{\text{response}}{\text{max response}} = \frac{[DR]}{[R_o]} = \frac{[D]}{[D] + K_d} \qquad \textbf{Equation 2-5}$$

where $[D]$ is the concentration of free drug, $[DR]$ is the concentration of drug–receptor complexes, $[R_o]$ is the concentration of total receptors, and K_d is the equilibrium dissociation constant for the drug–receptor interaction. (Note that the right side of Equation 2-5 is equivalent to Equation 2-4, with $[D]$ substituted for $[L]$.) The generalizability of this assumption is examined below.

There are two major types of dose–response relationships—graded and quantal. The difference between the two types is that graded dose–response relationships describe the effect of various doses of a drug on an individual, whereas quantal relationships show the effect of various doses of a drug on a population of individuals.

Graded Dose–Response Relationships

Figure 2-2 shows graded dose–response curves for two hypothetical drugs that elicit the same biological response.

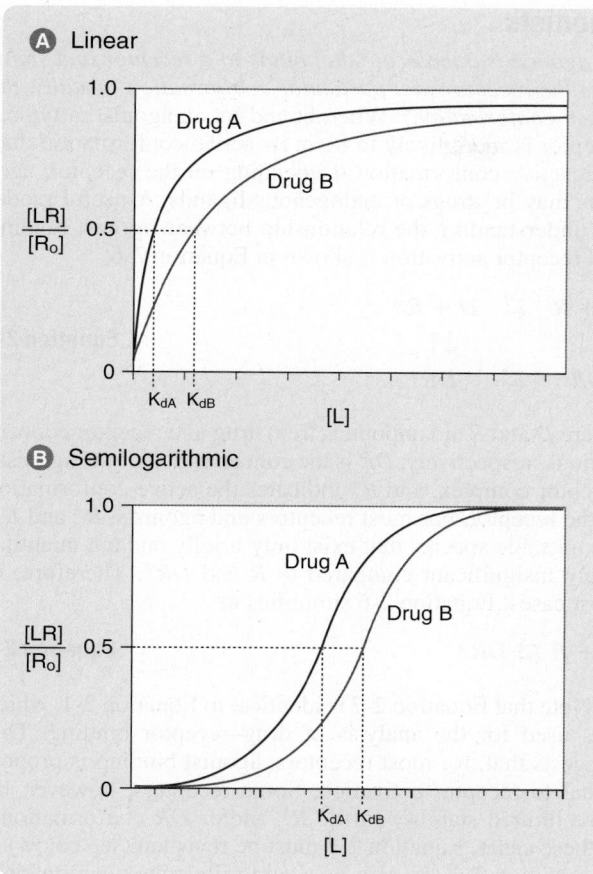

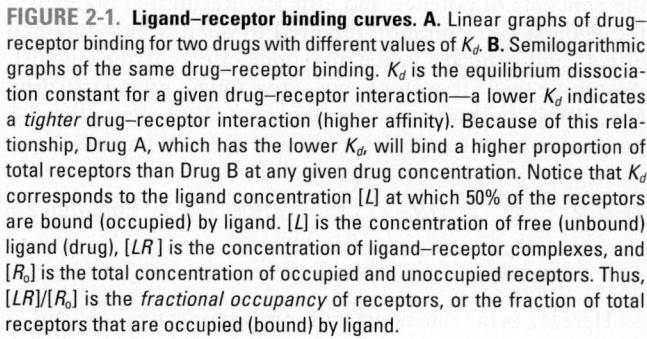

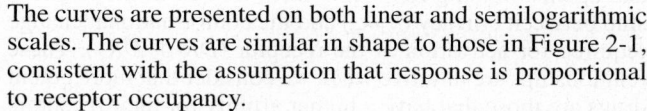

FIGURE 2-1. Ligand–receptor binding curves. A. Linear graphs of drug–receptor binding for two drugs with different values of K_d. **B.** Semilogarithmic graphs of the same drug–receptor binding. K_d is the equilibrium dissociation constant for a given drug–receptor interaction—a lower K_d indicates a *tighter* drug–receptor interaction (higher affinity). Because of this relationship, Drug A, which has the lower K_d, will bind a higher proportion of total receptors than Drug B at any given drug concentration. Notice that K_d corresponds to the ligand concentration [L] at which 50% of the receptors are bound (occupied) by ligand. [L] is the concentration of free (unbound) ligand (drug), [LR] is the concentration of ligand–receptor complexes, and [R_o] is the total concentration of occupied and unoccupied receptors. Thus, [LR]/[R_o] is the *fractional occupancy* of receptors, or the fraction of total receptors that are occupied (bound) by ligand.

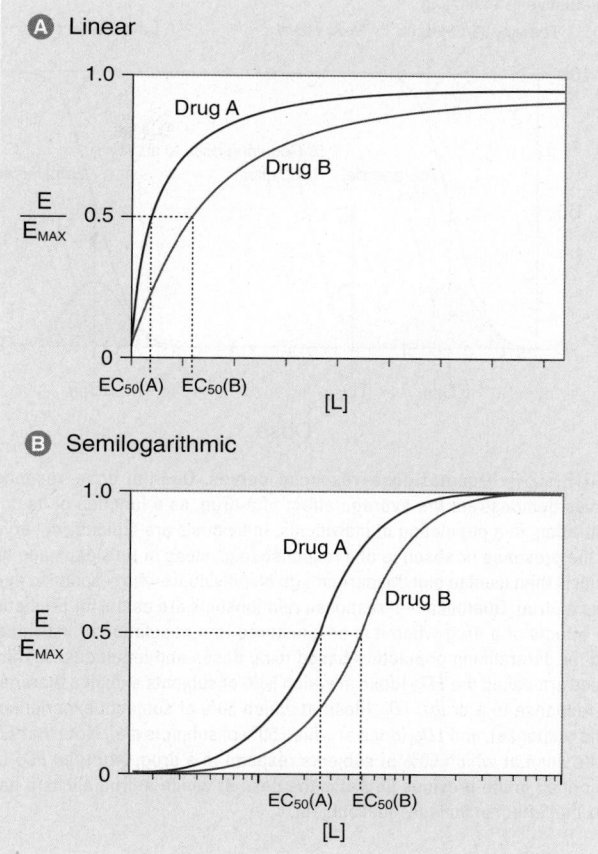

FIGURE 2-2. Graded dose–response curves. Graded dose–response curves demonstrate the effect of a drug as a function of its concentration. **A.** Linear graphs of graded dose–response curves for two drugs. **B.** Semilogarithmic graphs of the same dose–response curves. Note the close resemblance to Figure 2-1: the fraction of occupied receptors [LR]/[R_o] has been replaced by the fractional effect E/E_{max}, where E is a quantifiable response to a drug (e.g., an increase in blood pressure). EC_{50} is the potency of the drug, or the concentration at which the drug elicits 50% of its maximal effect. In the figure, Drug A is more potent than Drug B because it elicits a half-maximal effect at a lower concentration than Drug B. Drugs A and B exhibit the same efficacy (the maximal response to the drug). Note that potency and efficacy are not intrinsically related—a drug can be extremely potent but have little efficacy, and vice versa. [L] is drug concentration, E is effect, E_{max} is efficacy, and EC_{50} is potency.

The curves are presented on both linear and semilogarithmic scales. The curves are similar in shape to those in Figure 2-1, consistent with the assumption that response is proportional to receptor occupancy.

Two important parameters—potency and efficacy—can be deduced from the graded dose–response curve. The **potency (EC_{50})** of a drug is *the concentration at which the drug elicits 50% of its maximal response*. The **efficacy (E_{max})** is *the maximal response produced by the drug*. In accordance with the assumption stated above, efficacy can be thought of as the state at which receptor-mediated signaling is maximal and, therefore, additional drug will produce no additional response. This usually occurs when all the receptors are occupied by the drug. Some drugs, however, are capable of eliciting a maximal response when less than 100% of the drug's receptors are occupied; the remaining receptors can be called **spare receptors**. This concept is discussed further in the text

that follows. Note again that the graded dose–response curve of Figure 2-2 bears a close resemblance to the drug–receptor binding curve of Figure 2-1, with EC_{50} replacing K_d and E_{max} replacing R_o.

Quantal Dose–Response Relationships

The quantal dose–response relationship plots the fraction of the population that responds to a given dose of drug as a function of the drug dose. Quantal dose–response relationships describe the concentrations of a drug that produce a given effect in a population. Figure 2-3 shows an example of quantal dose–response curves. Because of differences in biological response among individuals, the effects of a drug are seen over a range of doses. The responses are defined as either present or not present (i.e., *quantal*, not *graded*). Endpoints such as "sleep/no sleep" or "alive at

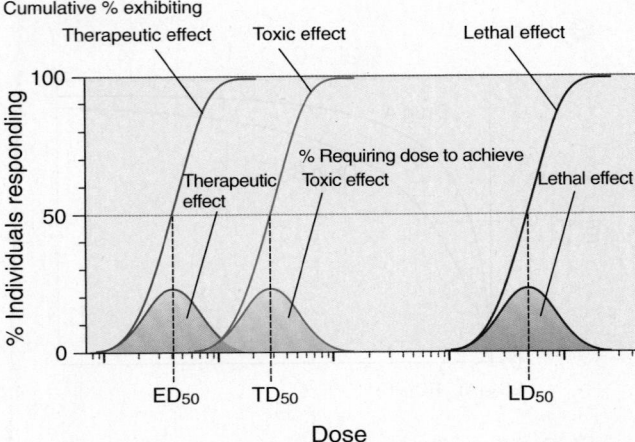

FIGURE 2-3. Quantal dose–response curves. Quantal dose–response curves demonstrate the average effect of a drug, as a function of its concentration, in a population of individuals. Individuals are typically observed for the presence or absence of a response (e.g., sleep or no sleep), and this result is then used to plot the percentage of individuals who respond to each dose of drug. Quantal dose–response relationships are useful for predicting the effects of a drug when it is administered to a population of individuals and for determining population-based toxic doses and lethal doses. These doses are called the ED_{50} (dose at which 50% of subjects exhibit a therapeutic response to a drug), TD_{50} (dose at which 50% of subjects experience a toxic response), and LD_{50} (dose at which 50% of subjects die). Note that ED_{50} is the dose at which 50% of subjects respond to a drug, whereas EC_{50} (as described in the previous figure) is the dose at which a drug elicits a half-maximal effect in an individual subject.

12 months/not alive at 12 months" are examples of quantal responses; in contrast, graded dose–response relationships are generated using scalar responses such as change in blood pressure or heart rate. The goal is to generalize a result to a population rather than to examine the graded effect of different drug doses on a single individual. Types of responses that can be examined using the quantal dose–response relationship include effectiveness (therapeutic effect), toxicity (adverse effect), and lethality (lethal effect). The doses that produce these responses in 50% of a population are known as the **median effective dose (ED_{50})**, **median toxic dose (TD_{50})**, and **median lethal dose (LD_{50})**, respectively.

DRUG–RECEPTOR INTERACTIONS

Many receptors for drugs can be modeled as having two conformational states that are in reversible equilibrium with one another. These two states are called the **active state** and the **inactive state**. Many drugs function as ligands for such receptors and affect the probability that the receptor exists preferentially in one conformation or the other. The pharmacologic properties of drugs are often based on their effects on the state of their cognate receptors. A drug that, upon binding to its receptor, favors the active receptor conformation is called an **agonist**; a drug that prevents agonist-induced activation of the receptor is referred to as an **antagonist**. Some drugs do not fit neatly into this simple definition of agonist and antagonist; these include **partial agonists** and **inverse agonists**. The following sections describe these pharmacologic classifications in more detail.

Agonists

An agonist is a molecule that binds to a receptor and stabilizes the receptor in a particular conformation (usually, the active conformation). When bound by an agonist, a typical receptor is more likely to be in its active conformation than its inactive conformation. Depending on the receptor, agonists may be drugs or endogenous ligands. A useful model for understanding the relationship between agonist binding and receptor activation is shown in Equation 2-6:

$$D + R \rightleftarrows D + R^*$$
$$\updownarrow \qquad\qquad \updownarrow$$
$$DR \rightleftarrows DR^*$$

Equation 2-6

where D and R are unbound (free) drug and receptor concentrations, respectively, DR is the concentration of the agonist–receptor complex, and R^* indicates the active conformation of the receptor. For most receptors and agonists, R^* and DR are unstable species that exist only briefly and are quantitatively insignificant compared to R and DR^*. Therefore, in most cases, Equation 2-6 simplifies to

$$D + R \rightleftarrows DR^*$$

Equation 2-7

Note that Equation 2-7 is identical to Equation 2-1, which was used for the analysis of drug–receptor binding. This suggests that, for most receptors, agonist binding is proportional to receptor activation. Some receptors, however, do have limited stability in the R^* and/or DR conformations; in these cases, Equation 2-6 must be revisited (see below).

Equation 2-6 can also be used to illustrate quantitatively the concepts of potency and efficacy. Recall that potency is the agonist concentration required to elicit a half-maximal effect, and efficacy is the maximal effect of the agonist. Assuming that a receptor is not active unless bound to a drug (i.e., R^* is insignificant compared to DR^*), Equation 2-8 provides a quantitative description of potency and efficacy:

$$D + R \underset{k_{off}}{\overset{k_{on}}{\rightleftarrows}} DR \underset{k_\beta}{\overset{k_\alpha}{\rightleftarrows}} DR^*$$
$$\text{Potency} \qquad\qquad \text{Efficacy}$$

Equation 2-8

Here, k_α is the rate constant for receptor activation, and k_β is the rate constant for receptor deactivation. This equation demonstrates the relationship between potency ($K_d = k_{off}/k_{on}$) and agonist binding ($D + R \rightleftarrows DR$), as well as the relationship between efficacy (k_α/k_β) and the conformational change required for activation of the receptor ($DR \rightleftarrows DR^*$). These relationships are intuitive when we consider that more potent drugs are those that have a higher affinity for their receptors (lower K_d), and more efficacious drugs are those that cause a higher fraction of receptors to be activated.

Antagonists

An antagonist is a molecule that inhibits the action of an agonist but has no effect in the absence of the agonist. Figure 2-4 shows one approach to classifying the various types of antagonists. Antagonists can be divided into receptor and nonreceptor antagonists. A **receptor antagonist** binds to either the active site (agonist binding site) or an allosteric site on a receptor. Binding of an antagonist to the active site prevents the binding of the agonist to the receptor, whereas binding

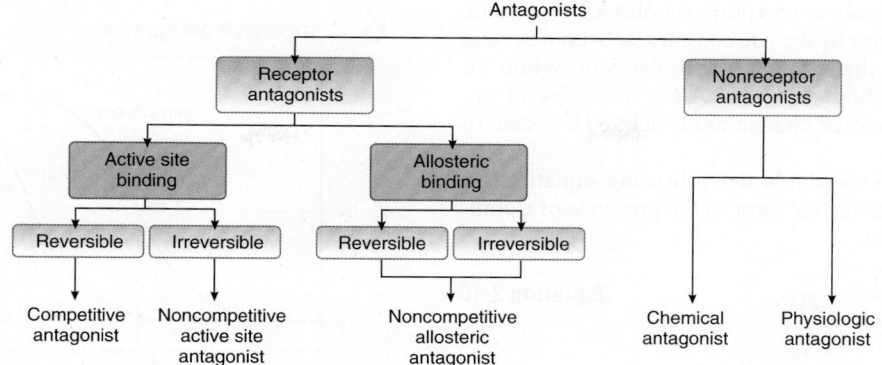

FIGURE 2-4. Antagonist classification. Antagonists can be categorized based on whether they bind to a site on the receptor for agonist (receptor antagonists) or interrupt agonist–receptor signaling by other means (nonreceptor antagonists). Receptor antagonists can bind either to the agonist (active) site or to an allosteric site on the receptor; in either case, they do not affect basal receptor activity (i.e., the activity of the receptor in the absence of agonist). Agonist (active) site receptor antagonists prevent the agonist from binding to the receptor. If the antagonist competes with the ligand for agonist site binding, it is termed a *competitive antagonist*; high concentrations of agonist are able to overcome competitive antagonism. Noncompetitive active site antagonists bind covalently or with very high affinity to the agonist site, so that even high concentrations of agonist are unable to activate the receptor. Allosteric receptor antagonists bind to the receptor at a site other than the agonist site. They do not compete directly with agonist for receptor binding, but rather alter the K_d for agonist binding or inhibit the receptor from responding to agonist binding. High concentrations of agonist are generally unable to reverse the effect of an allosteric antagonist. Nonreceptor antagonists fall into two categories. Chemical antagonists sequester agonist and thus prevent the agonist from interacting with the receptor. Physiologic antagonists induce a physiologic response opposite to that of an agonist, but by a molecular mechanism that does not involve the receptor for agonist.

of an antagonist to an allosteric site either alters the K_d for agonist binding or prevents the conformational change required for receptor activation. Receptor antagonists can also be divided into **reversible** and **irreversible antagonists**; that is, antagonists that bind to their receptors reversibly and those that bind irreversibly. Figure 2-5 illustrates the general effects of these antagonist types on agonist binding; more detail is provided in the following sections.

A **nonreceptor antagonist** does not bind to the same receptor as an agonist, but it nonetheless inhibits the ability of an agonist to initiate a response. At the molecular level, this inhibition can occur by inhibiting the agonist directly (e.g., using antibodies), by inhibiting a downstream molecule in the activation pathway, or by activating a pathway that opposes the action of the agonist. Nonreceptor antagonists can be divided into chemical antagonists and physiologic antagonists. **Chemical antagonists** inactivate an agonist before it has the opportunity to act (e.g., by chemical neutralization);

physiologic antagonists cause a physiologic effect opposite to that induced by the agonist.

Competitive Receptor Antagonists

A **competitive antagonist** *binds reversibly to the active site of a receptor.* Unlike an agonist, which also binds to the active site of the receptor, a competitive antagonist does not stabilize the conformation required for receptor activation. Therefore, the antagonist blocks an agonist from binding to its receptor, while maintaining the receptor in the inactive conformation. Equation 2-9 is a modification of Equation 2-7 that incorporates the effect of a competitive antagonist (*A*).

$$AR \rightleftarrows A + D + R \rightleftarrows DR^* \qquad \textbf{Equation 2-9}$$

In this equation, a fraction of the free receptor molecules (*R*) are unable to form a drug (agonist)–receptor complex (*DR**), because receptor binding to the antagonist results in the

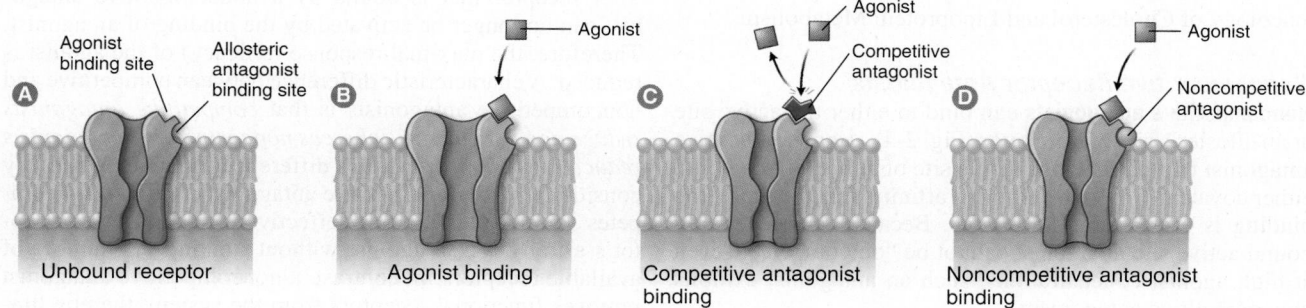

FIGURE 2-5. Types of receptor antagonists. A schematic illustrating the differences between agonist (active) site and allosteric antagonists. **A.** The unbound inactive receptor. **B.** The receptor activated by agonist. Note the conformational change induced in the receptor by agonist binding, for example, the opening of a transmembrane ion channel. **C.** Agonist site antagonists bind to the receptor's agonist site but do not activate the receptor; these agents block agonist binding to the receptor. **D.** Allosteric antagonists bind to an allosteric site (different from the agonist site) and thereby prevent receptor activation, even when the agonist is bound to the receptor.

formation of an antagonist–receptor complex (AR) instead. In effect, the formation of the AR complex sets up a second equilibrium reaction that competes with the equilibrium for agonist–receptor binding. Note that AR is incapable of undergoing a conformational change to the active (R*) state of the receptor.

Quantitative analysis yields the following equation for agonist (D) binding to the receptor in the presence of a competitive antagonist (A):

$$\frac{[DR]}{[R_o]} = \frac{[D]}{[D] + K_d\left(1 + \dfrac{[A]}{K_A}\right)}$$

Equation 2-10

Equation 2-10 is similar to Equation 2-4, except that the effective K_d has been increased by a factor of $(1 + [A]/K_A)$, where K_A is the dissociation constant for binding of the antagonist to the receptor (i.e., $K_A = [A][R]/[AR]$). Because an increase in K_d is equivalent to a decrease in potency, *the presence of a competitive antagonist (A) reduces the potency of an agonist (D) by a factor of $(1 + [A]/K_A)$*. Although the potency of an agonist decreases as the concentration of competitive antagonist increases, the efficacy of the agonist is unaffected. This occurs because the agonist concentration [D] can be increased to counteract ("outcompete") the antagonist, thereby "washing out" or reversing the effect of the antagonist. Figure 2-6A shows the effect of a competitive antagonist on the agonist dose–response relationship. Note that the competitive antagonist has the effect of shifting the agonist dose–response curve to the right, causing a decrease in agonist potency while maintaining agonist efficacy.

Atorvastatin, the drug used in the case at the beginning of this chapter to lower Admiral X's cholesterol, is an example of a competitive antagonist. Atorvastatin is a member of the HMG-CoA reductase inhibitor (statin) class of lipid-lowering drugs. HMG-CoA reductase is an enzyme that catalyzes the reduction of HMG-CoA, which is the rate-limiting step in cholesterol biosynthesis. The similarity between the chemical structures of statins and HMG-CoA allows the statin molecule to bind to the active site of HMG-CoA reductase and thereby to prevent HMG-CoA from binding. This inhibition is reversible because no covalent bonds are formed between the statin and the enzyme. Inhibition of HMG-CoA reductase decreases endogenous cholesterol synthesis and lowers the patient's cholesterol levels. For a more detailed discussion of the mechanism of action of atorvastatin and other HMG-CoA reductase inhibitors, see Chapter 20, Pharmacology of Cholesterol and Lipoprotein Metabolism.

Noncompetitive Receptor Antagonists

Noncompetitive antagonists can bind to either the active site or an allosteric site of a receptor (Fig. 2-4). A noncompetitive antagonist that binds to the active site of a receptor can bind either covalently or with very high affinity; in either case, the binding is effectively irreversible. Because an irreversibly bound active site antagonist cannot be "outcompeted," even at high agonist concentrations, such an antagonist exhibits noncompetitive antagonism.

A noncompetitive allosteric antagonist acts by preventing the receptor from being activated, even when the agonist is bound to the active site. An allosteric antagonist exhibits noncompetitive antagonism regardless of the reversibility of its binding, because such an antagonist acts not by competing

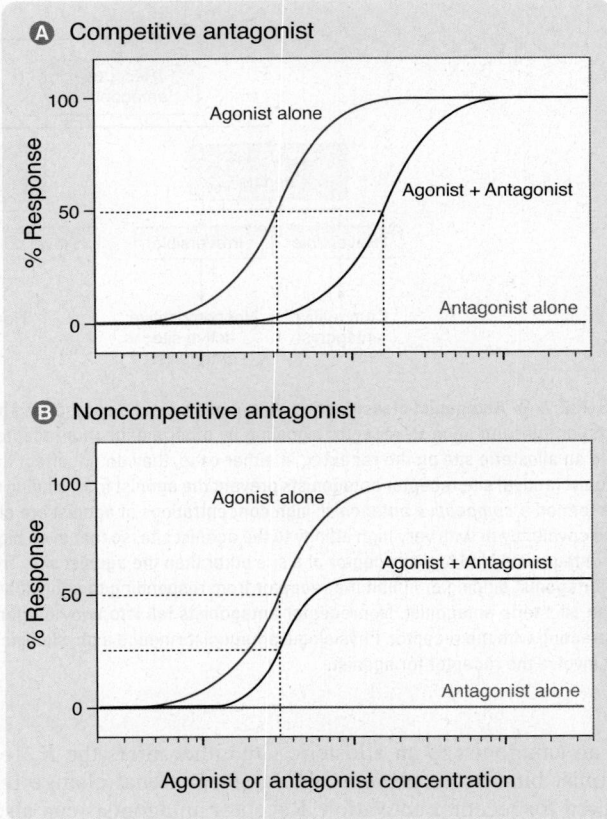

FIGURE 2-6. Antagonist effects on the agonist dose–response relationship. Competitive and noncompetitive antagonists have different effects on potency (the concentration of agonist that elicits a half-maximal response) and efficacy (the maximal response to an agonist). **A.** A competitive antagonist reduces the potency of an agonist, without affecting agonist efficacy. **B.** A noncompetitive antagonist reduces the efficacy of an agonist. As shown here, most allosteric noncompetitive antagonists do not affect agonist potency.

with the agonist for binding to the active site, but rather by preventing receptor activation. The reversibility of antagonist binding is nonetheless important, because the effect of an irreversible antagonist does not diminish when the free (unbound) drug is eliminated from the body, whereas the effect of a reversible antagonist can be "washed out" over time as it dissociates from the receptor (see Equation 2-9).

A receptor that is bound by a noncompetitive antagonist can no longer be activated by the binding of an agonist. Therefore, the maximal response (efficacy) of the agonist is reduced. A characteristic difference between competitive and noncompetitive antagonists is that *competitive antagonists reduce agonist potency, whereas noncompetitive antagonists reduce agonist efficacy*. This difference can be explained by considering that a competitive antagonist continuously competes for receptor binding, effectively reducing the receptor's affinity for an agonist without limiting the number of available receptors. In contrast, a noncompetitive antagonist removes functional receptors from the system, thereby limiting the number of available receptors. Figures 2-6A and 2-6B compare the effects of competitive and noncompetitive antagonists on the agonist dose–response relationship.

Aspirin is one example of a noncompetitive antagonist. This agent irreversibly acetylates cyclooxygenase, the enzyme responsible for generating thromboxane A_2 in platelets. In the absence of thromboxane A_2 generation, platelet aggregation is inhibited. Because the inhibition is irreversible and platelets are not capable of synthesizing new cyclooxygenase molecules, the effects of a single dose of aspirin last for 7 to 10 days (the time required for the bone marrow to generate new platelets), even though the free drug is cleared from the body much more rapidly.

Nonreceptor Antagonists

Nonreceptor antagonists can be divided into chemical antagonists and physiologic antagonists. A **chemical antagonist** inactivates the agonist of interest by modifying or sequestering it, so that the agonist is no longer capable of binding to and activating the receptor. **Protamine** is an example of a chemical antagonist; this basic protein binds stoichiometrically to the acidic **heparin** class of anticoagulants and thereby inactivates these agents (see Chapter 23, Pharmacology of Hemostasis and Thrombosis). Because of this chemical antagonism, protamine can be used to terminate the effects of heparin rapidly.

A **physiologic antagonist** either blocks a receptor that mediates the physiologic response of the receptor for agonist or activates a receptor that mediates a response physiologically opposite to that of the receptor for agonist. For example, in the treatment of hyperthyroidism, **β-adrenergic antagonists** are used as physiologic antagonists to counteract the tachycardic effect of excess thyroid hormone. Excess thyroid hormone produces tachycardia, at least in part, via up-regulation of cardiac β-adrenoceptors, and blocking β-adrenergic stimulation relieves the tachycardia (see Chapter 11, Adrenergic Pharmacology, and Chapter 28, Pharmacology of the Thyroid Gland).

Partial Agonists

A **partial agonist** is a molecule that binds to a receptor at its active site but produces only a partial response, even when all of the receptors are occupied (bound) by the agonist. Figure 2-7A shows a family of dose–response curves for several full and partial agonists. Each agonist acts by binding to the same site on the muscarinic acetylcholine (ACh) receptor. Note that butyl trimethylammonium (TMA) is not only more potent than longer chain derivatives at stimulating muscle contraction but also more efficacious than some of the derivatives (e.g., the heptyl and octyl forms) at producing a greater maximal response. For this reason, butyl TMA is a *full agonist* at the muscarinic ACh receptor, whereas the octyl derivative is a *partial agonist* at this receptor.

Because partial agonists and full agonists bind to the same site on a receptor, a partial agonist can reduce the response produced by a full agonist. In this way, the partial agonist can act as a competitive antagonist. For this reason, partial agonists are sometimes called *partial antagonists* or even *mixed agonist-antagonists*.

It is interesting to consider how an agonist could produce a less-than-maximal response if a receptor can exist in only the active or the inactive state. This is an area of current investigation, for which several hypotheses have been proposed. Recall that Equation 2-6 was simplified to Equation 2-7 based on the assumption that R and DR^* are much more stable than R^* and DR. But what would happen if a drug (call it a partial agonist) could stabilize DR as well

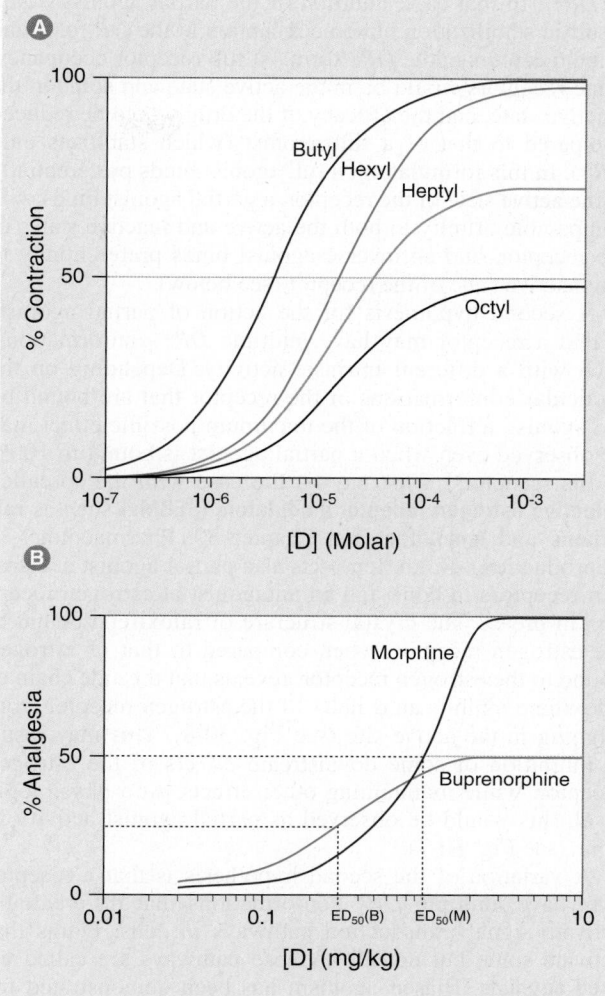

FIGURE 2-7. **Full and partial agonist dose–response curves.** There are many instances in which drugs that all act at the agonist site on the same receptor produce different maximal effects. **A.** Various alkyl derivatives of trimethylammonium all stimulate muscarinic acetylcholine (ACh) receptors to cause muscle contraction in the gut, but they produce different maximal responses, even when all receptors are occupied. In this example, the butyl and hexyl trimethylammonium derivatives are full agonists— although they have different potencies, they are both capable of eliciting a maximal response. Agonists that produce only a partial response, such as the heptyl and octyl derivatives, are called **partial agonists**. Note that the dose–response curves of these partial agonists plateau at values less than those of full agonists. ACh acts as a full agonist in this system (*not shown*). **B.** Partial agonists may be more or less potent than full agonists. In this case, buprenorphine (ED_{50} = 0.3 mg/kg) is more potent than morphine (ED_{50} = 1.0 mg/kg), although it cannot achieve the same maximal response as the full agonist. Buprenorphine is used clinically in the treatment of opioid addiction, where it is desirable to use a partial agonist that is less efficacious than an addicting opioid such as heroin or morphine. Low concentrations of the partial agonist buprenorphine bind tightly to the opioid receptor and competitively inhibit the binding of the more efficacious opioids. Very high doses of buprenorphine show a paradoxically diminished analgesic effect that may be due to lower affinity interactions of the drug with non–mu-opioid receptors (*not shown*).

as DR^*? In that case, addition of the partial agonist would result in stabilization of some receptors in the DR form and some receptors in the DR^* form. At full receptor occupancy, some receptors would be in the active state and some in the inactive state, and the efficacy of the drug would be reduced compared to that of a full agonist (which stabilizes only DR^*). In this formulation, a full agonist binds preferentially to the active state of the receptor, a partial agonist binds with comparable affinity to both the active and inactive states of the receptor, and an inverse agonist binds preferentially to the inactive state of the receptor (see below).

A second hypothesis for the action of partial agonists is that a receptor may have multiple DR^* conformations, each with a different intrinsic activity. Depending on the particular conformations of the receptor that are bound by the agonist, a fraction of the maximum possible effect may be observed even when a partial agonist is bound to 100% of the receptors. This may be the case with the so-called **selective estrogen receptor modulators (SERMs)** such as **raloxifene** and **tamoxifen** (see Chapter 30, Pharmacology of Reproduction). Raloxifene acts as a partial agonist at estrogen receptors in bone and an antagonist at estrogen receptors in breast. The crystal structure of raloxifene bound to the estrogen receptor, when compared to that of estrogen bound to the estrogen receptor, reveals that the side chain of raloxifene inhibits an α helix of the estrogen receptor from aligning in the active site (see Fig. 30-8). This may result in inhibition of some downstream effects of the estrogen receptor, while maintaining other effects. At a physiologic level, this would be observed as partial agonist activity in bone (see Fig. 30-7).

A variation of the second hypothesis is that a receptor may have multiple DR^* conformations that differentially activate signal transduction pathways in cells. Drugs that activate some but not all of these pathways are called **biased agonists**. Biased agonism has been demonstrated for experimental compounds interacting with G protein-coupled receptors and may be relevant for some partial agonists in clinical use.

A study of partial agonists acting on ligand-gated ion channels has suggested yet another model, in which the receptor requires a "priming" conformational change that must occur before activation of the receptor is possible. In this model, although a partial agonist may bind to the receptor with high affinity, it is less efficient than a full agonist at inducing the "primed" conformation of the receptor. Because this "primed" conformation is a prerequisite for activation of the receptor, a partial agonist causes the receptor to spend less time in the open conformation than a full agonist does, and the partial agonist has lower efficacy than the full agonist.

The relative potency of full agonists and partial agonists may be clinically relevant (Fig. 2-7B). A partial agonist with high affinity for its receptor (such as buprenorphine) may be more potent but less efficacious than a full agonist with lower affinity for the same receptor (such as morphine). This characteristic is leveraged clinically when the partial agonist buprenorphine is used to treat opioid addiction. Buprenorphine, with its high affinity for the mu-opioid receptor, can be administered to outcompete other opioids taken by a patient and can therefore help to prevent relapse of opioid addiction. Buprenorphine must be carefully administered to a patient who is currently addicted to full-agonist opioids such as heroin or morphine, because it can outcompete these opioids and cause withdrawal symptoms.

Inverse Agonists

The action of inverse agonists can be understood by considering Equation 2-6 again. As noted above, in some cases, receptors can have inherent stability in the R^* state. In these cases, there is intrinsic activity ("tone") of the receptor system, even in the absence of an endogenous ligand or an exogenously administered agonist. *An **inverse agonist** acts by abrogating this intrinsic (constitutive) activity of the free (unoccupied) receptor.* Inverse agonists may function by binding to and stabilizing the receptor in the DR (inactive) form. This has the effect of deactivating receptors that had existed in the R^* form in the absence of drug. The physiologic importance of receptors that have inherent stability in the R^* state is currently under investigation; receptors with mutations that render them constitutively active may become attractive targets for inverse agonist approaches.

Consider the similarities and differences between the actions of inverse agonists and competitive antagonists. Both types of drug act to reduce the activity of a receptor. In the presence of a full agonist, both competitive antagonists and inverse agonists act to reduce agonist potency. Recall, however, that a competitive antagonist has no effect in the absence of an agonist, whereas an inverse agonist deactivates receptors that are constitutively active in the absence of an agonist. Using Equations 2-6 through 2-9 as models, these concepts can be summarized by stating that *full agonists stabilize DR**, partial agonists stabilize both DR and DR* (or alternate forms of DR* or "primed" forms of DR), inverse agonists stabilize DR, and competitive antagonists "stabilize" R (or AR) by preventing full, partial, and inverse agonists from binding to the receptor.*

Spare Receptors

Recall that the initial discussion of drug–receptor binding assumed that 100% receptor occupancy is required for an agonist to exert its maximal effect. Now, consider the possibility that a maximal response could be achieved with less than 100% receptor occupancy. Figure 2-8 shows an example of a drug–receptor binding curve and a dose–response curve that illustrate this situation. In this example, a maximal effect is achieved at a lower dose of agonist than that required for receptor saturation, that is, the EC_{50} is less than the K_d for this system. This type of discrepancy between the drug–receptor binding curve and the dose–response curve signifies the presence of **spare receptors**. At least two molecular mechanisms are thought to be responsible for the spare receptor phenomenon. First, the receptor could remain activated after the agonist departs, allowing one agonist molecule to activate several receptors. Second, the cell signaling pathways described in Chapter 1, Drug–Receptor Interactions, could allow for significant amplification of a relatively small signal, and activation of only a few receptors could be sufficient to produce a maximal response. The latter is true, for example, with many G protein-coupled receptors; activation of a single $G\alpha_s$ molecule can stimulate adenylyl cyclase to catalyze the formation of dozens of molecules of cAMP.

The presence of spare receptors alters the effect of a noncompetitive antagonist on the system. At low antagonist

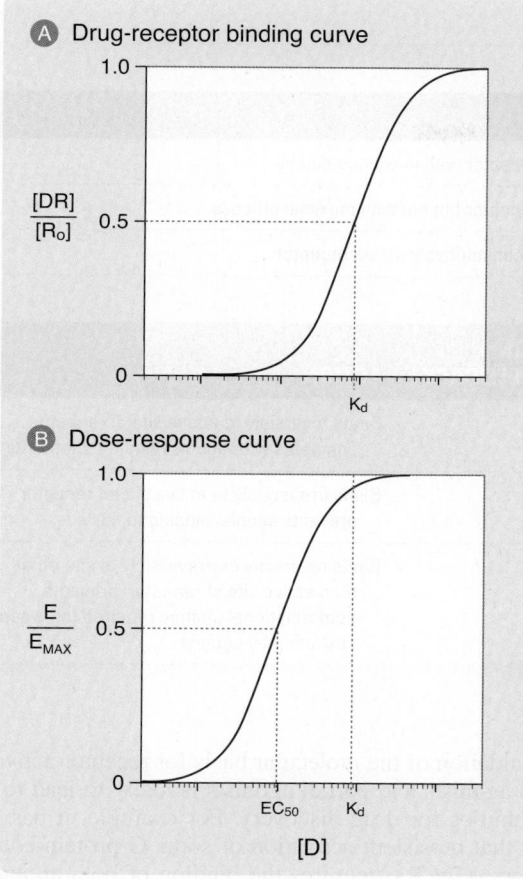

FIGURE 2-8. **Comparison between a drug–receptor binding curve and a dose–response curve in the presence of spare receptors.** In the absence of spare receptors, there often exists a close correlation between a drug–receptor binding curve and a dose–response curve—the binding of additional drug to the receptor causes an incremental increase in response, and EC_{50} is approximately equal to K_d. In situations with spare receptors, however, a half-maximal response is elicited when less than half of all receptors are occupied (the term *spare* implies that occupation of every receptor with drug is not necessary to elicit a full response). **A.** Drug–receptor binding curve. **B.** Dose–response curve for the same drug, in the presence of spare receptors. Note that the maximal response occurs at a lower agonist concentration than does maximal binding, and $EC_{50} < K_d$. These two relationships confirm the presence of spare receptors. D is drug, R is receptor, and $[DR]/[R_o]$ is fractional receptor occupancy. E is response (effect), E_{max} is maximal response (efficacy), and E/E_{max} is fractional response. EC_{50} is potency, and K_d is the equilibrium dissociation constant for drug–receptor binding.

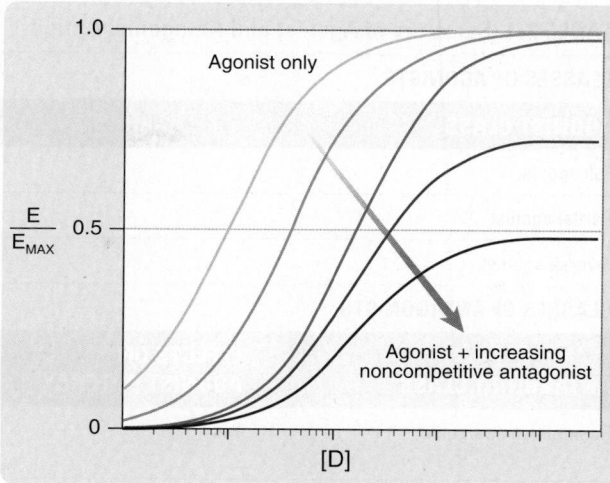

FIGURE 2-9. **Effect of a noncompetitive antagonist on the agonist dose–response curve in the presence of spare receptors.** In a system without spare receptors, a noncompetitive antagonist causes efficacy to decrease at all concentrations of the antagonist (see Fig. 2-6B). In a system with spare receptors, however, potency is decreased but efficacy is unaffected at low concentrations of the antagonist, because a sufficient number of unoccupied receptors is available to generate a maximal response. As increasing concentrations of antagonist bind noncompetitively to more and more receptors, the antagonist eventually occupies all of the "spare" receptors, and efficacy is also reduced.

CONCEPTS IN THERAPEUTICS

Therapeutic Index and Therapeutic Window

The **therapeutic window** is the range of doses (concentrations) of a drug that elicits a therapeutic response, without unacceptable adverse effects (toxicity), in a population of patients. For drugs that have a small therapeutic window, plasma drug levels must be monitored closely to maintain effective dosing without exceeding the level that could produce toxicity. The next chapter discusses some of the techniques used in clinical therapeutics to maintain plasma concentrations of drugs within the therapeutic window.

The therapeutic window can be quantified by the **therapeutic index (TI)** (sometimes called the **therapeutic ratio**), commonly defined as

$$\text{Therapeutic Index (TI)} = \frac{TD_{50}}{ED_{50}} \qquad \textbf{Equation 2-11}$$

where TD_{50} is the dose of drug that causes a toxic response in 50% of the population, and ED_{50} is the dose of drug that is therapeutically effective in 50% of the population. The TI provides a single number that quantifies the relative safety margin of a drug in a population of people. A large TI represents a large (or "wide") therapeutic window (e.g., a thousand-fold difference between the therapeutic and toxic doses), and a small TI represents a small (or "narrow") therapeutic window (e.g., a twofold difference between the therapeutic and toxic doses).

In the case at the beginning of this chapter, the potential for toxicity associated with the use of heparin and tPA is indicated by the low TIs of these drugs. For example, the dose of heparin that can cause major bleeding in a patient is often

concentrations, the noncompetitive antagonist binds receptors that are not required to produce a maximal response; therefore, the efficacy of the agonist is not decreased. The potency of the agonist is affected, however, because potency is proportional to the fraction of available receptors that must be occupied to produce a 50% response. A noncompetitive antagonist reduces the number of available receptors, thereby increasing the fraction of receptors that must be bound at any agonist concentration to produce the same response. At high antagonist concentrations, the noncompetitive antagonist binds not only the "spare" receptors but also receptors that are required to produce a maximal response, and the efficacy and potency of the agonist are both decreased. Figure 2-9 illustrates this concept.

TABLE 2-1 Summary of Agonist and Antagonist Action

CLASSES OF AGONISTS

AGONIST CLASS	ACTION
Full agonist	Activates receptor with maximal efficacy
Partial agonist	Activates receptor but not with maximal efficacy
Inverse agonist	Inactivates constitutively active receptor

CLASSES OF ANTAGONISTS

ANTAGONIST CLASS	EFFECTS ON AGONIST POTENCY	EFFECTS ON AGONIST EFFICACY	ACTION
Competitive antagonist	Yes	No	Binds reversibly to active site of receptor; competes with agonist binding to this site
Noncompetitive active site antagonist	No	Yes	Binds irreversibly to active site of receptor; prevents agonist binding to this site
Noncompetitive allosteric antagonist	No	Yes	Binds reversibly or irreversibly to site other than active site of receptor; prevents conformational change required for receptor activation by agonist

less than twice the dose needed for a therapeutic effect; heparin can therefore be defined as having a therapeutic index of less than two. For this reason, patients treated with heparin must have their PTT, a marker of the coagulation cascade, monitored every few hours. Aspirin's high TI is indicative of its relative safety. Note that the pharmacologic effect of heparin was monitored periodically in the case, whereas aspirin could be administered without the need to monitor its plasma drug level.

CONCLUSION AND FUTURE DIRECTIONS

Pharmacodynamics is the quantitative study of the effects of drugs on the body. Several tools have been developed to compare the efficacy and potency of drugs, including the graded and quantal dose–response relationships. The former is used to examine the effects of various drug doses on an individual, whereas the latter is used to examine the effects of various drug doses on a population. The therapeutic window and therapeutic index are used to compare the concentrations of drugs that produce therapeutic effects and toxic (adverse) effects.

In the study of pharmacodynamics, drugs can be divided into two broad classes—agonists and antagonists. Most agonists cause a receptor to maintain its conformation in the active state, whereas antagonists prevent activation of the receptor by agonists. Antagonists are further divided according to the molecular location of their effect (i.e., receptor or nonreceptor), the site at which they bind to the receptor (i.e., active site or allosteric site), and the mode of their binding to the receptor (i.e., reversible or irreversible). Table 2-1 provides a summary of the various types of agonists and antagonists presented in this chapter.

Elucidation of the molecular basis for receptor activation by full agonists and partial agonists is likely to lead to new opportunities for drug discovery. For example, it has been shown that persistent activation of some G protein-coupled receptors (GPCRs) requires the binding of both an agonist and a G protein to the GPCR. This knowledge may be useful in designing new drugs that modulate the function of specific GPCRs with greater selectivity.

Acknowledgment
We thank Harris S. Rose for his valuable contributions to this chapter in the First and Second Editions of *Principles of Pharmacology: The Pathophysiologic Basis of Drug Therapy.*

Suggested Reading
Cowan A, Doxey JC, Harry EJ. The animal pharmacology of buprenorphine, an oripavine analgesic agent. *Br J Pharmacol* 1977;60:547–554. (*Provides an experimental demonstration of the variation in potency and efficacy of full and partial agonists.*)

Kenakin T, Williams M. Defining and characterizing drug/compound function. *Biochem Pharmacol* 2014;87:40–63. (*Summarizes how the complex drug–receptor interactions of partial agonists, inverse agonists, biased agonists, and allosteric antagonists help to inform drug discovery.*)

Lape R, Colquhoun D, Sivilotti LG. On the nature of partial agonism in the nicotinic receptor superfamily. *Nature* 2008;454:722–727. (*Suggests a mechanistic model for the effect of partial agonists on ligand-gated ion channels.*)

Leff P. The two-state model of receptor activation. *Trends Pharmacol Sci* 1995;16:89–97. (*Provides the theoretical grounding for Equation 2-6; discusses quantitative treatment of drug–receptor interactions.*)

Pratt WB, Taylor P, eds. *Principles of drug action: the basis of pharmacology.* 3rd ed. New York: Churchill Livingstone; 1990. (*Contains an in-depth discussion of pharmacodynamics.*)

Sprang SR. Cell signaling: binding the receptor at both ends. *Nature* 2011;469:172–173. (*Summarizes the finding that persistent activation of some GPCRs requires binding of both agonist and G protein molecules to the receptor.*)

3

Pharmacokinetics

Quentin J. Baca and David E. Golan

INTRODUCTION

Even the most promising of pharmacologic therapies will fail in clinical trials if the drug is unable to reach its target organ at a concentration sufficient to have a therapeutic effect. Many of the characteristics that render the human body resistant to harm by foreign invaders and toxic substances also limit the ability of modern drugs to combat pathologic processes within a patient. An appreciation of the many factors that affect a drug's ability to act within a patient and the dynamic nature of these factors over time is vitally important to the clinical practice of medicine.

All drugs must meet certain minimal requirements to achieve clinical effectiveness. A successful drug must be able to cross the physiologic barriers that limit the access of foreign substances to the body. Drug **absorption** may occur by a number of mechanisms that are designed either to exploit or to breach these barriers. After absorption, the drug uses **distribution** systems within the body, such as the blood and lymphatic vessels, to reach its target organ in an appropriate concentration. The drug's ability to act on its target is also limited by several processes within the patient. These processes fall broadly into two categories: **metabolism**, in which the body typically inactivates the drug through enzymatic degradation (primarily in the liver), and **excretion**, in which the drug is eliminated from the body (primarily by the kidneys and liver, and in the feces). This chapter presents a broad overview of the pharmacokinetic processes of absorption, distribution, metabolism, and excretion (often abbreviated as **ADME**; Fig. 3-1), with a conceptual emphasis on basic principles that, when applied to an unfamiliar situation, should enable the student or physician to understand the pharmacokinetic basis of drug therapy.

PHYSIOLOGIC BARRIERS

A drug must overcome physical, chemical, and biological barriers to reach its molecular and cellular sites of action. The epithelial lining of the gastrointestinal tract and other mucous membranes is one sort of barrier; additional barriers are encountered after the drug enters the blood and lymphatics. Most drugs must distribute from the blood into local tissues, a process that may be impeded by structures such as the blood–brain barrier. Typically, drugs leave the intravascular compartment at the level of the postcapillary venules, where there are gaps between the endothelial cells through which the drug can pass. Drug distribution occurs mainly through passive diffusion, the rate of which is affected by local ionic and cellular conditions. This section describes the major physical, chemical, and biological barriers to drug transport in the body and the properties of drugs that affect their ability to overcome these barriers.

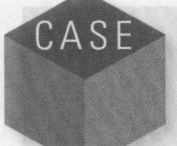

CASE

Mr. W is a 66-year-old technology consultant who makes frequent trips as part of his job in the telecommunications industry. His only medical problem is chronic atrial fibrillation, and his only chronic medication is **warfarin**. On the last night of a consulting trip abroad, he attends a large dinner featuring kebabs and other foods he does not often eat. The next day, he develops profuse, watery, foul-smelling diarrhea. A physician makes a diagnosis of traveler's diarrhea and prescribes a 7-day course of **trimethoprim-sulfamethoxazole**.

Mr. W feels entirely well 2 days into the course of antibiotics, and 4 days later (while still taking his antibiotics), he meets with some clients at another lavish dinner. Mr. W and his guests become intoxicated at the dinner, and Mr. W stumbles and falls on the curb as he is leaving the restaurant. The next day, Mr. W has a markedly swollen right knee that requires evaluation in a local emergency department. Physical examination and imaging studies are consistent with a moderate-sized hemarthrosis of the right knee. Laboratory studies show a markedly elevated international normalized ratio (INR), which is a standardized measure of prothrombin time and, in this clinical setting, a surrogate marker for plasma warfarin level. The emergency physician advises Mr. W that his warfarin level is in the supratherapeutic (toxic) range and that this effect is likely due to adverse drug–drug interactions involving his warfarin, his antibiotics, and his recent alcohol intoxication.

Questions

1. How does a patient with well-established therapeutic levels of a chronic medication suddenly develop clinical manifestations of drug toxicity?

2. Could this situation have been avoided? If so, how?

Biological Membranes

All human cells are limited by a lipid bilayer membrane. The membrane lipids consist mainly of phospholipids, sterols (especially cholesterol), and glycolipids. The amphiphilic nature of the membrane lipids and the aqueous intracellular and extracellular environments cause the membrane to assume a structure with a hydrophobic core and two hydrophilic surfaces. In addition to lipid components, biological membranes contain proteins that may span the membrane (transmembrane proteins) or be exposed only at the extracellular or intracellular membrane surface. The membrane's semipermeable lipid bilayer structure provides a barrier to the transport of molecules and has important implications for drug therapy.

Traversing the Membrane

The hydrophobic core of a biological membrane presents the major barrier to drug transport. Small nonpolar molecules, such as steroid hormones, are able to diffuse easily through membranes. However, passive diffusion is ineffective for the transport of many large polar molecules and drugs. Some transmembrane proteins in the **human solute carrier (SLC)** superfamily—which includes 52 families of proteins such as organic anion transporters, organic cation transporters, peptide transporters, and nucleoside transporters—allow transport of polar drugs and molecules across the membrane. Transmembrane carrier proteins may be specific for a drug and related endogenous molecules; upon binding of the drug to the extracellular surface of the protein, the protein undergoes a conformational change that may be energy-independent (**facilitated diffusion**) or require energy (**active transport**). This conformational change allows the bound drug access to the interior of the cell, where the drug molecule is released from the protein. Alternatively, some drugs bind to specific cell surface receptors and trigger **endocytosis**, a process in which the cell membrane involutes around the molecule to form a vesicle from which the drug is subsequently released into the cell interior.

Membrane Diffusion

In the absence of other factors, a drug will enter a cell until the intracellular and extracellular concentrations of the drug are equal. The rate of diffusion depends on the concentration gradient of the drug across the membrane and on the thickness, area, and permeability of the membrane. Fick's law of diffusion states that the net drug flux across the membrane is:

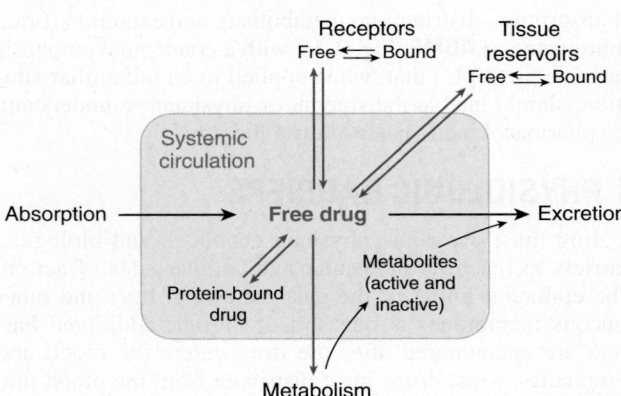

FIGURE 3-1. Drug absorption, distribution, metabolism, and excretion (ADME). The basic principles of pharmacokinetics affect the amount of free drug that ultimately reaches the target site. To elicit an effect on its target, a drug must be absorbed and then distributed to its target before being metabolized and excreted. At all times, free drug in the systemic circulation is in equilibrium with tissue reservoirs, plasma proteins, and the target site (which usually consists of receptors); only the fraction of drug that binds to specific receptors will have a pharmacologic effect. Note that metabolism of drug can result in both inactive and active metabolites; active metabolites may also exert a pharmacologic effect, either on the target receptors or sometimes on other receptors.

$$\text{Flux} = \frac{(C2 - C1) \times (\text{Area} \times \text{Permeability})}{\text{Thickness}_{\text{membrane}}}$$ **Equation 3-1**

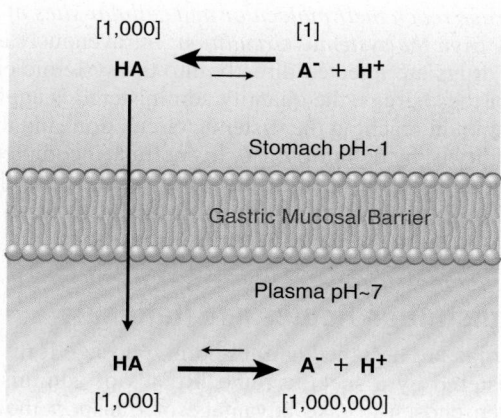

[1,000] HA ⟵ **[1]** A⁻ + H⁺

Stomach pH~1

Gastric Mucosal Barrier

Plasma pH~7

HA ⟶ A⁻ + H⁺
[1,000] **[1,000,000]**

FIGURE 3-2. **pH trapping across lipid bilayers.** In the example shown, consider a hypothetical drug with pK_a = 4. Although this drug is a weak acid, in the highly acidic environment of the stomach, it is largely protonated. If the stomach pH is approximately 1, then for every 1,001 molecules of drug, 1,000 molecules are protonated (and neutral) and only 1 is deprotonated (and negatively charged). The protonated, neutral form of the drug is able to diffuse across the gastric mucosal barrier into the blood. Because the blood plasma has a pH of approximately 7 (it is actually 7.4), and the drug has a pK_a of 4, the vast majority of drug now exists in the deprotonated (negatively charged) form: for every 1,001 molecules of drug, only 1 molecule is protonated (and neutral), while 1,000 molecules are deprotonated (and negatively charged). The negatively charged form of the drug is no longer able to diffuse across the lipid bilayers of the gastric mucosa, and the drug is effectively trapped in the plasma.

where $C1$ and $C2$ are the intracellular and extracellular concentrations of the drug, respectively. This definition applies to an ideal situation where there is an absence of complicating factors such as ionic, pH, and charge gradients across the membrane. In vivo, however, these additional factors affect the ability of a drug to enter cells. For example, a higher concentration of drug outside the cell would ordinarily favor net drug entry into the cell, but if both the cell interior and the drug are negatively charged, then net drug entry into the cell may be impeded. In contrast, a negatively charged cell interior could favor entry of a positively charged drug.

Net diffusion of acidic and basic drugs across lipid bilayer membranes may also be affected by a charge-based phenomenon known as **pH trapping**, which depends on the drug's acid dissociation constant (pK_a) and the pH gradient across the membrane. For weakly acidic drugs, such as phenobarbital and aspirin, the protonated, electrically neutral form of the drug is predominant in the highly acidic environment of the stomach. The uncharged form of the drug can pass through the lipid bilayers of the gastric and duodenal mucosa, speeding the drug's absorption (Fig. 3-2). The weakly acidic drug is then effectively trapped as it is deprotonated to its electrically charged form in the more basic environment of the plasma.

In quantitative terms, the pK_a of a drug represents the pH value at which one-half of the drug is present in its ionic form. The Henderson–Hasselbalch equation describes the relationship between the pK_a of an acidic or basic Drug A and the pH of the biological medium containing the drug:

$$pK_a = \text{pH} + \log \frac{[HA]}{[A^-]}$$ **Equation 3-2**

where HA is the protonated form of Drug A. For example, consider the hypothetical case of a weakly acidic drug with a pK_a of 4. In the stomach, which has a pH of approximately 1, Equation 3-2 becomes:

$$pK_{a_{drug}} = \text{pH}_{stomach} + \log \frac{[HA]}{[A^-]},$$

which simplifies to:

$$3 = \log \frac{[HA]}{[A^-]},$$

and finally:

$$1,000 = \frac{[HA]}{[A^-]}.$$

The protonated form of the drug is present at 1,000 times the concentration of the deprotonated form, and 99.9% of the drug is in the neutral form. Conversely, in the plasma, where the pH is approximately 7.4, more than 99.9% of the drug is in the deprotonated form (see Fig. 3-2).

Central Nervous System

The central nervous system (CNS) presents special challenges to pharmacologic therapy. Unlike most other anatomic regions, the CNS is particularly well insulated from foreign substances. The **blood–brain barrier** uses specialized tight junctions to prevent the passive diffusion of most drugs from the systemic to the cerebral circulation. Therefore, drugs designed to act in the CNS must either be sufficiently small and hydrophobic to traverse biological membranes easily or use existing transport proteins in the blood–brain barrier to penetrate central structures. Hydrophilic drugs that fail to target facilitated or active transport proteins in the blood–brain barrier cannot penetrate the CNS. The blood–brain barrier can be bypassed using intrathecal drug delivery, in which drugs are delivered directly into the cerebrospinal fluid (CSF). Although this approach can be used, for example, to treat infectious meningitis or to provide spinal anesthesia for a cesarean delivery, the intrathecal route is impractical for drugs that must be taken regularly by a patient.

▌ ABSORPTION

The human body presents formidable obstacles to invasion by microorganisms. The integument has a keratinized outer layer and defensins in the epithelium. Mucous membranes are protected by mucociliary clearance in the trachea, lysozyme secretion from lacrimal ducts, acid in the stomach, and base in the duodenum. These nonspecific defense mechanisms present barriers to drug absorption and may limit the drug's **bioavailability** at target organs. Bioavailability, or the fraction of administered drug that reaches the systemic circulation, may depend on the route by which the drug is administered, the chemical form of the drug, and a number of patient-specific factors such as gastrointestinal and hepatic transporters and enzymes.

Bioavailability is defined quantitatively as:

$$\text{Bioavailability} = \frac{\text{Quantity of drug reaching systemic circulation}}{\text{Quantity of drug administered}}$$ **Equation 3-3**

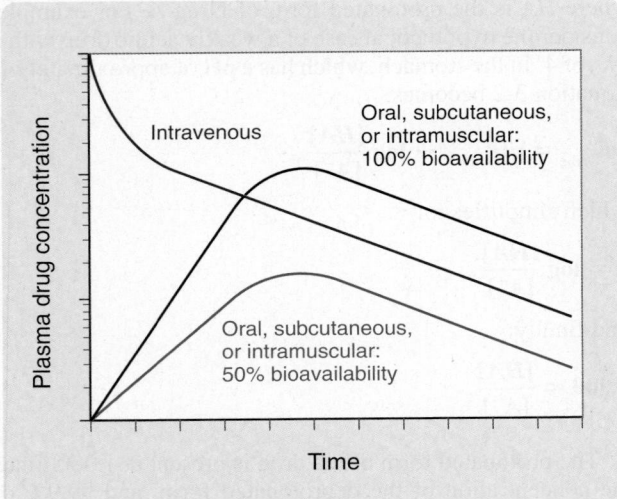

FIGURE 3-3. Bioavailability after administration of a single dose of drug. An intravenously administered drug is immediately available in the circulation. In this example, the drug is then distributed to other body compartments (see Fig. 3-7) and eliminated by first-order kinetics (see Fig. 3-6). In contrast, other routes of administration (e.g., oral, subcutaneous, and intramuscular) demonstrate slower entry of drug into the blood. In addition, nonintravenous routes of administration must take into account bioavailability—for example, many orally administered drugs are incompletely absorbed or undergo first-pass metabolism in the liver. If a drug has 100% bioavailability, the total amount of drug reaching the systemic circulation will be the same for all routes of drug administration, but nonintravenous routes will require a longer period of time to reach a peak concentration of drug in the plasma. If the bioavailability of an oral, subcutaneous, or intramuscular dosage form is less than 100%, then the dose of the drug would have to be increased in order for the total amount of drug reaching the systemic circulation to be the same as that of an intravenous dose. Note that the total amount of drug reaching the systemic circulation can be quantified by integrating the **area under the curve (AUC)** of the plasma drug concentration versus time plot. Thus, although different routes of administration (e.g., oral, subcutaneous, and intramuscular) can have different rates of drug absorption and therefore differ in the kinetics of plasma drug concentration over time (Fig. 3-4), if these routes exhibit the same level of bioavailability, then they will have the same AUC.

This definition of bioavailability is based on the fact that *most drugs reach their molecular and cellular sites of action directly from the systemic circulation.* Intravenously administered drugs are injected directly into the systemic circulation; for these drugs, the quantity administered is equivalent to the amount reaching the systemic circulation, and the bioavailability is, by definition, 1.0. In contrast, incomplete gastrointestinal absorption and "first-pass" hepatic metabolism (see below) typically cause the bioavailability of an orally administered drug to be less than 1.0 (Fig. 3-3).

Administration Routes and Rationale

New drugs are designed and tested in a dosage form that is administered by a specific route. Routes of administration are often chosen to take advantage of transport molecules and other mechanisms that permit the drug to enter body tissues. This section discusses the advantages and disadvantages of drug administration by enteral (oral), parenteral, mucous membrane, and transdermal routes (Table 3-1).

Enteral

Enteral drug administration, or the administration of a drug by mouth, is the simplest of drug routes. The enteral route of administration exploits existing weaknesses in human barrier defenses, but it exposes the drug to harsh acidic (stomach) and basic (duodenum) environments that could limit its absorption. This route provides many advantages for the patient: oral drugs are easily and conveniently self-administered, and these dosage forms are less likely than other methods to introduce systemic infection as a complication of treatment.

An orally administered drug must be stable during its absorption across the gastrointestinal tract epithelium. Gastrointestinal epithelial cell junctions make paracellular transport across an intact epithelium difficult. Instead, ingested substances (such as drugs) must usually traverse the cell membrane at both apical and basal surfaces before entering the blood. The efficiency of this process is determined by drug size and hydrophobicity and sometimes by the presence

TABLE 3-1 Routes of Drug Administration

ROUTE	ADVANTAGES	DISADVANTAGES
Enteral (e.g., aspirin)	Simple, inexpensive, convenient, painless, no infection	Drug exposed to harsh gastrointestinal (GI) environments and first-pass metabolism, requires GI absorption, slow delivery to site of pharmacologic action
Parenteral (e.g., morphine)	Rapid delivery to site of pharmacologic action, high bioavailability, not subject to first-pass metabolism or harsh GI environments	Irreversible, infection, pain, fear, skilled personnel required
Mucous membrane (e.g., nitroglycerin)	Rapid delivery to site of pharmacologic action, not subject to first-pass metabolism or harsh GI environments, often painless, simple, convenient, low infection, direct delivery to affected tissues possible	Few drugs have chemical characteristics or formulations that allow them to be administered via this route
Transdermal (e.g., nicotine)	Simple, convenient, painless, excellent for continuous or prolonged administration, not subject to first-pass metabolism or harsh GI environments	Requires highly lipophilic drug, slow delivery to site of pharmacologic action, may be irritating

of carriers through which the drug may enter and/or exit the cell. *In general, hydrophobic and neutral drugs cross cell membranes more efficiently than hydrophilic or charged drugs, unless the membrane contains a carrier molecule that facilitates the transport of hydrophilic substances.*

Upon traversing the gastrointestinal epithelium, drugs are carried by the portal system to the liver before entering the systemic circulation. While the portal circulation protects the body from the systemic effects of ingested toxins by delivering these substances to the liver for detoxification, this system may complicate drug delivery. All orally administered drugs are subjected to **first-pass metabolism** in the liver. In this process, liver enzymes may inactivate a fraction of the ingested drug. Any drug that exhibits significant first-pass metabolism must be administered in a quantity sufficient to ensure that an effective concentration of active drug exits the liver into the systemic circulation, from which it can reach the target organ. Drugs administered by nonenteral routes are not subjected to first-pass liver metabolism.

Parenteral

Parenteral administration, in which a drug is introduced directly into the systemic circulation, cerebrospinal fluid, vascularized tissue, or some other tissue space, immediately overcomes barriers that can limit the effectiveness of orally administered drugs (Table 3-2). Tissue administration results in a rate of onset of drug action that differs among the various body tissues, depending on the rate of blood flow to the tissue. Subcutaneous (SC) administration of a drug into poorly vascularized adipose tissue results in a slower onset of action than injection into well-vascularized intramuscular (IM) spaces. Drugs that are soluble only in oil-based solutions are often administered intramuscularly. Direct introduction of a drug into the venous (intravenous [IV]) or arterial (intra-arterial [IA]) circulation or into the cerebrospinal fluid (intrathecal [IT]) results in the drug reaching its target organ the fastest. Unlike subcutaneous and intramuscular injections, intravenous injection is not typically limited in the amount of drug that can be delivered. Continuous intravenous infusions can allow tight control over peak and steady-state plasma concentrations during drug delivery.

Parenteral administration may be associated with several potential disadvantages, including an increased risk of infection and the requirement for administration by a health care professional. The onset of action of parenterally administered drugs is often rapid, potentially resulting in increased toxicity when such drugs are administered too rapidly or in incorrect doses. These disadvantages must be weighed against the advantages of parenteral administration (such as speed of onset and control of the delivered dose) and the urgency of the indication for pharmacologic therapy.

Mucous Membrane

Administration of drugs across mucous membranes can potentially provide rapid absorption, low incidence of infection, convenience of administration, and avoidance of harsh gastrointestinal environments and first-pass metabolism. Sublingual, ocular, pulmonary, nasal, rectal, urinary, and reproductive tract epithelia have all been used to deliver drugs in the form of liquid drops, rapidly dissolving tablets, aerosols, and suppositories (among other dosage forms). The mucous membranes are highly vascular, permitting the drug to enter the systemic circulation rapidly and to reach its target organ with minimal delay. Drugs may also be administered directly into the target organ, resulting in virtually instantaneous onset of action. This is advantageous in critical conditions such as acute asthma, where drugs such as β-adrenergic agonists are administered via aerosol directly into the airways.

Transdermal

A limited number of drugs have sufficiently high lipophilicity that passive diffusion across the skin is a viable route of administration. Transcutaneously administered drugs are absorbed from the skin and subcutaneous tissues directly into the blood. This route of administration is ideal for a drug that must be slowly and continuously administered over extended periods. There is no associated risk of infection, and drug administration is simple and convenient. The success of transdermal nicotine, estrogen, and scopolamine patches demonstrates the utility of this route of administration (see Chapter 55, Drug Delivery Modalities, for more details on transdermal drug delivery).

Local, Regional, and Systemic Factors Affecting Absorption

The rate and extent of absorption of a drug are affected by local, regional, and systemic factors. In general, a large or rapidly administered dose creates a high local concentration of a drug. A large concentration gradient between the site of administration and the surrounding tissue drives the distribution of the drug into the nearby tissue and/or vasculature. Any factor that decreases the concentration gradient at the site of administration will diminish the driving force of the gradient and may reduce the amount of drug that is distributed into the local tissues. Regional blood flow has the greatest effect in this regard; in a highly perfused region, drug molecules crossing into that compartment are rapidly removed. This effect maintains the drug concentration at a low level in the compartment, allowing the driving force for entry of new drug molecules into the compartment to remain high (see Equation 3-1). For example, volatile general anesthetics are administered via inhalation. The lungs are highly perfused, and the anesthetic is removed rapidly from the lungs into the systemic circulation. Anesthetic does not accumulate in the local circulation, and a concentration

TABLE 3-2 Routes of Parenteral Drug Administration

PARENTERAL ROUTE	ADVANTAGES	DISADVANTAGES
Subcutaneous (e.g., lidocaine)	Slow onset, may be used to administer oil-based drugs	Slow onset, small volumes
Intramuscular (e.g., haloperidol)	Intermediate onset, may be used to administer oil-based drugs	Can affect lab tests (creatine kinase), intramuscular hemorrhage, painful
Intravenous (e.g., morphine)	Rapid onset, controlled drug delivery	Peak-related drug toxicity
Intrathecal (e.g., methotrexate)	Bypasses blood–brain barrier	Infection, highly skilled personnel required

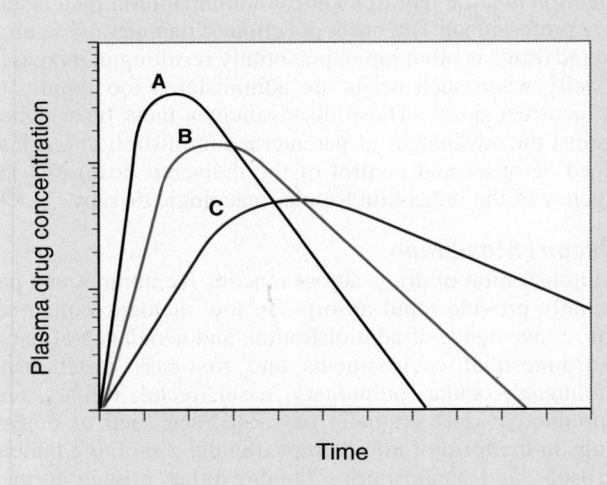

FIGURE 3-4. Effect of rate of absorption on peak plasma concentration of drug and on duration of drug action. The duration of action and peak plasma concentration of a drug can be affected markedly by the drug's absorption rate. In this example, three drugs with identical bioavailability, volume of distribution, and clearance are administered in identical doses. The drugs demonstrate different rates of absorption—Drug A is absorbed quickly, Drug C is absorbed slowly, and Drug B's absorption rate is between those of Drugs A and C. Drug A reaches the highest peak plasma concentration, since all of the drug is absorbed before significant elimination can take place. Drug C is absorbed slowly and never achieves a high plasma concentration, but it persists in the plasma for longer than Drugs A or B because absorption continues during the elimination phase. It should be noted that the hypothetical Drugs A, B, and C could all be the same drug administered by three different routes. For example, curve A could represent intravenous glucocorticoid administration, curve B could be an intramuscular injection, and curve C could be a transdermal formulation of the same drug.

gradient promoting diffusion of anesthetic into the blood is maintained (see Chapter 17, General Anesthetic Pharmacology, for more details). In an individual with greater body mass, both the increased surface area for absorption and the larger tissue volumes available for distribution tend to remove a drug from the site of administration faster and increase the rate and extent of drug absorption. The rate of drug absorption affects both the local concentration of a drug (including its plasma concentration) and its duration of action (Fig. 3-4).

▌DISTRIBUTION

Absorption of a drug is a prerequisite for establishing adequate plasma drug levels, but the drug must also reach its target organ(s) in therapeutic concentrations to have the desired effect on a pathophysiologic process. Drug distribution is achieved primarily through the circulatory system; a minor component is contributed by the lymphatic system. Once a drug has been absorbed into the systemic circulation, it is then capable of reaching any target organ (with the possible exception of sanctuary compartments such as the central nervous system and testes). The concentration of drug in the plasma is typically used to define and monitor therapeutic drug levels, because the concentration of drug in the target organ is often difficult to measure. Even in cases where the plasma concentration of a drug is very different from the

TABLE 3-3 Drug Distribution to Different Body Compartments

COMPARTMENT	EXAMPLES
Total body water	Small water-soluble molecules (e.g., ethanol)
Extracellular water	Larger water-soluble molecules (e.g., mannitol)
Blood plasma	Highly plasma protein-bound molecules, very large molecules, highly charged molecules (e.g., heparin)
Adipose tissue	Highly lipid-soluble molecules (e.g., propofol)
Bone and teeth	Certain ions (e.g., fluoride, strontium)

tissue concentration, the effect of the drug in the target tissue often correlates well with the plasma drug concentration.

Organs and tissues vary widely in their capacity to take up different types of drugs (Table 3-3) and in the proportion of systemic blood flow they receive (Table 3-4). In turn, these factors affect the concentration of the drug in the plasma and determine the amount of drug that must be administered to achieve the desired plasma drug concentration. The ability of nonvascular tissues and plasma proteins to take up and/or bind the drug must be accounted for in designing dosing regimens to achieve and maintain therapeutic drug levels.

Volume of Distribution

The **volume of distribution** (V_d) describes the extent to which a drug partitions between the plasma and tissue compartments. In quantitative terms, V_d represents the fluid volume that would be required to contain the total amount of absorbed drug in the body at a concentration equivalent to that in the plasma at steady state:

$$V_d = \frac{\text{Dose}}{[\text{Drug}]_{\text{plasma}}} \qquad \text{Equation 3-4}$$

The volume of distribution is an extrapolated volume based on the concentration of drug in the plasma, not a physical volume. Thus, V_d is low for drugs that are retained

TABLE 3-4 Total and Weight-Normalized Tissue Blood Flow in an Adult

ORGAN PERFUSED	BLOOD FLOW (mL/min)	ORGAN MASS (kg)	NORMALIZED BLOOD FLOW (mL/min/kg)
Liver	1,700	2.5	680
Kidneys	1,000	0.3	3,333
Brain	800	1.3	615
Heart	250	0.3	833
Adipose	250	10.0	25
Other (muscle, etc.)	1,400	55.6	25
Total	5,400	70.0	—

primarily within the vascular compartment and high for drugs that are highly distributed into adipose and other non-vascular compartments. For very highly distributed drugs, the volume of distribution is often much greater than the volume of total body water, reflecting the low concentration of drug in the vascular compartment at steady state. Some drugs have very large volumes of distribution; examples include amiodarone (4,620 liters [L] for a 70-kg person), azithromycin (2,170 L), chloroquine (9,240 L), and digoxin (645 L), among others.

The capacity of the blood and the various organs and tissues to take up and retain a drug depends on both the volume (mass) of the tissue and the concentrations of specific and nonspecific binding sites for the drug within that tissue. A drug that is taken up in large quantities by tissues such as adipose will preferentially distribute out of the systemic circulation and into these tissues at steady state. In many cases, these tissues must be saturated before plasma levels of such drugs can increase sufficiently to affect the drug's target organ. Thus, for drugs of equal potency, a drug that is more highly distributed among body tissues generally requires a higher initial dose to establish a therapeutic plasma concentration than does a drug that is less highly distributed.

Plasma Protein Binding

The capacity of adipose tissue to absorb a drug increases the tendency of the drug to diffuse from the blood into nonvascular compartments, but this tendency can be counteracted to some extent by plasma protein binding of the drug. Albumin is the most abundant plasma protein (~4 g/dL) and is the protein responsible for most drug binding. Many drugs bind with low affinity to albumin through both hydrophobic and electrostatic forces. Plasma protein binding tends to reduce the availability of a drug for diffusion or transport into the drug's target organ because, in general, only the free or unbound form of the drug is capable of diffusion across membranes (Fig. 3-5). Plasma protein binding may also reduce the transport of drugs into nonvascular compartments such as adipose tissue. Because a highly protein-bound drug tends to remain within the vasculature, such a drug often has a relatively low volume of distribution (typically, 7 to 8 L for a 70-kg person).

Theoretically, plasma protein binding could be important as a mechanism for some drug–drug interactions. Coadministration of two or more drugs that bind to plasma protein could result in a higher-than-expected plasma concentration of the free form of either or both drugs as the coadministered drugs compete for the same binding sites. The increased free drug concentration could potentially cause increased therapeutic and/or toxic effects of the drug. In such cases, the dosing regimen of one or both of the drugs would need to be adjusted to keep the free drug concentration in the therapeutic range. In practice, however, it has been difficult to demonstrate clinically significant drug–drug interactions caused by competitive binding of drugs to plasma proteins, possibly because of the increased clearance of the free drugs as they are displaced from their plasma protein binding sites (see below). An important exception is the contraindication to the use of the antibiotic **ceftriaxone** in neonates with hyperbilirubinemia, since ceftriaxone displaces bilirubin from its binding sites on albumin and thereby exacerbates the hyperbilirubinemia.

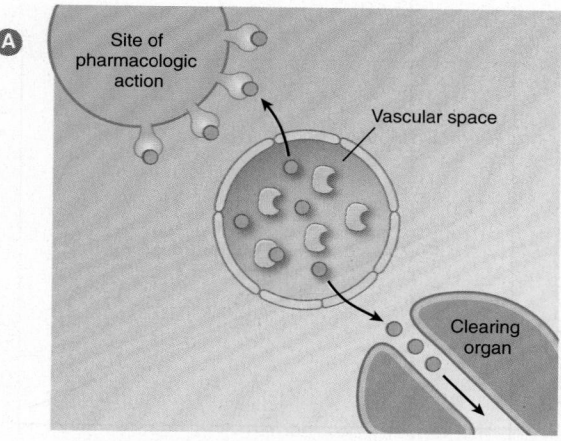

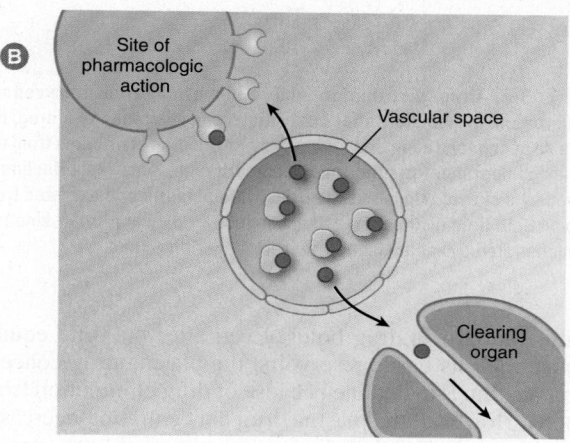

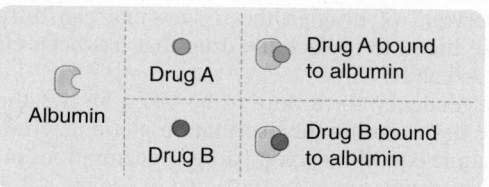

FIGURE 3-5. Protein binding and drug trapping. A drug that is bound to albumin or other plasma proteins cannot diffuse from the vascular space into surrounding tissues. **A.** Drugs that do not bind plasma proteins appreciably (shown here as Drug A) diffuse readily into tissues. This results in both a high level of binding to the site of pharmacologic action (usually receptors) and a high rate of elimination (represented by flux through a clearing organ). Examples of such drugs include acetaminophen, acyclovir, nicotine, and ranitidine. **B.** In contrast, for drugs that exhibit high levels of binding to plasma proteins (shown here as Drug B), a higher total plasma drug concentration is required to ensure an adequate concentration of free (unbound) drug in the circulation, since only a small fraction of the drug can diffuse into the extravascular space. Examples of such drugs include amiodarone, fluoxetine, naproxen, and warfarin. *It should be emphasized that plasma protein binding is only one of many variables that determine drug distribution.* Drug molecule size, lipophilicity, and rate of metabolism are other important parameters that must be taken into account when considering the pharmacokinetics of a particular drug.

Modeling the Kinetics of Drug Distribution

Most drugs are distributed rapidly from the systemic circulation (intravascular compartment) to other compartments in the body. This **distribution phase** results in a sharp decrease in the plasma drug concentration shortly after intravenous

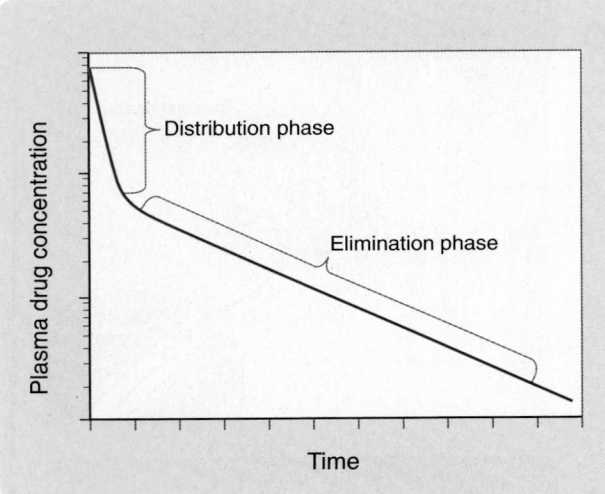

FIGURE 3-6. Drug distribution and elimination after intravenous administration. Immediately after intravenous administration of a drug, the plasma drug concentration declines rapidly as the drug distributes from the vascular compartment to other body compartments. This rapid decline is followed by a slower decline as the drug is metabolized and excreted from the body. Both drug distribution and elimination display first-order kinetics, as demonstrated by linear kinetics on a semilogarithmic plot.

administration of a drug bolus. Even after the drug equilibrates among its tissue reservoirs, the plasma drug concentration continues to decline because of drug elimination from the body. However, the plasma drug concentration decreases more slowly during the elimination phase, in part due to a "reservoir" of drug in the tissues that can diffuse back into the blood to replace the drug that has been eliminated (Figs. 3-6 and 3-7).

The tendency for a drug to be taken up by adipose and muscle tissue during the distribution phase determines a set of dynamic equilibria among drug concentrations in the various body compartments. As shown in Figure 3-8, the rapid decline of plasma drug concentration after administration of an intravenous bolus of drug can be approximated by using a four-compartment model consisting of the blood and vessel-rich, muscle-rich, and adipose-rich tissues. The vessel-rich group is the first extravascular compartment in which the concentration of drug increases, because the high blood flow received by this group *kinetically* favors drug entry into this compartment. However, the muscle-rich group and adipose-rich group often have a higher *capacity* for taking up drug than the vessel-rich group, with the adipose-rich group accumulating the greatest amount of drug at the slowest rate.

The capacity of a compartment for a drug and the rate of blood flow to the compartment also affect the rate at which the drug exits from the compartment. Drugs tend to exit first from the vessel-rich group, followed by the muscle group and then the adipose group. A complex and dynamic pattern of changing blood concentrations may develop, and the pattern is specific for each drug. The pattern may also be patient-specific, depending on factors such as the size, age, and fitness level of the patient. For example, an older patient typically has less skeletal muscle mass than a younger patient, decreasing the contribution of muscle uptake to changes in the plasma concentration of drug. An opposite effect may be seen in an elite athlete, who would be expected

to have both greater muscle mass and greater proportional muscle blood flow. As a third example, an obese person typically exhibits higher capacity for drug uptake into adipose tissue.

More complicated approaches to modeling the kinetics of drug distribution throughout the body can include an exhaustive number of compartments. Some approaches model each organ or vascular bed individually to describe more precisely the drug concentration at specific target sites over time.

METABOLISM

Several organs are capable of metabolizing drugs to some extent, using enzymatic reactions that are discussed in Chapter 4, Drug Metabolism. The kidneys, gastrointestinal tract, lungs, skin, and other organs all contribute to systemic drug metabolism. However, the liver contains the greatest diversity and quantity of metabolic enzymes, and the majority of drug metabolism occurs there. The ability of the liver to modify drugs depends on the amount of drug that enters the hepatocytes. Highly hydrophobic drugs can generally enter cells readily (including liver cells), and the liver preferentially metabolizes hydrophobic drugs. However, the liver contains a multitude of transporters in the human solute carrier (SLC) superfamily that allow entry of some hydrophilic drugs into hepatocytes as well. Hepatic enzymes chemically modify a variety of substituents on drug molecules, thereby either rendering the drugs inactive or facilitating their elimination. These modifications are collectively referred to as **biotransformation**. Biotransformation reactions are classified into two types, termed **oxidation/reduction reactions** and **conjugation/hydrolysis reactions**. (Although biotransformation reactions are often called **phase I** and **phase II** reactions, in this book we typically use the more precise terms *oxidation/reduction* and *conjugation/hydrolysis*; see Chapter 4.)

Oxidation/Reduction Reactions

Oxidation/reduction reactions modify the chemical structure of a drug; typically, a polar group is added or uncovered. The most common pathway, the microsomal **cytochrome P450 enzyme system** in the liver, mediates a large number of oxidative reactions. Some drugs may be administered in inactive (**prodrug**) form and are altered metabolically by oxidation/reduction reactions to the active (drug) form in the liver. This prodrug strategy can facilitate oral bioavailability, decrease gastrointestinal toxicity, and/or prolong the elimination half-life of a drug.

Conjugation/Hydrolysis Reactions

Conjugation/hydrolysis reactions hydrolyze a drug or conjugate a drug to a large, polar molecule in order to inactivate the drug or, more commonly, to enhance the drug's solubility and excretion in the urine or bile. Occasionally, hydrolysis or conjugation can result in the metabolic activation of prodrugs. The most commonly added groups include glucuronate, sulfate, glutathione, and acetate.

As described in more detail in the next chapter, the effects of oxidation/reduction and conjugation/hydrolysis reactions on a particular drug also depend on the presence of other drugs that are being taken concomitantly by the patient. Certain classes of drugs, such as barbiturates, are powerful

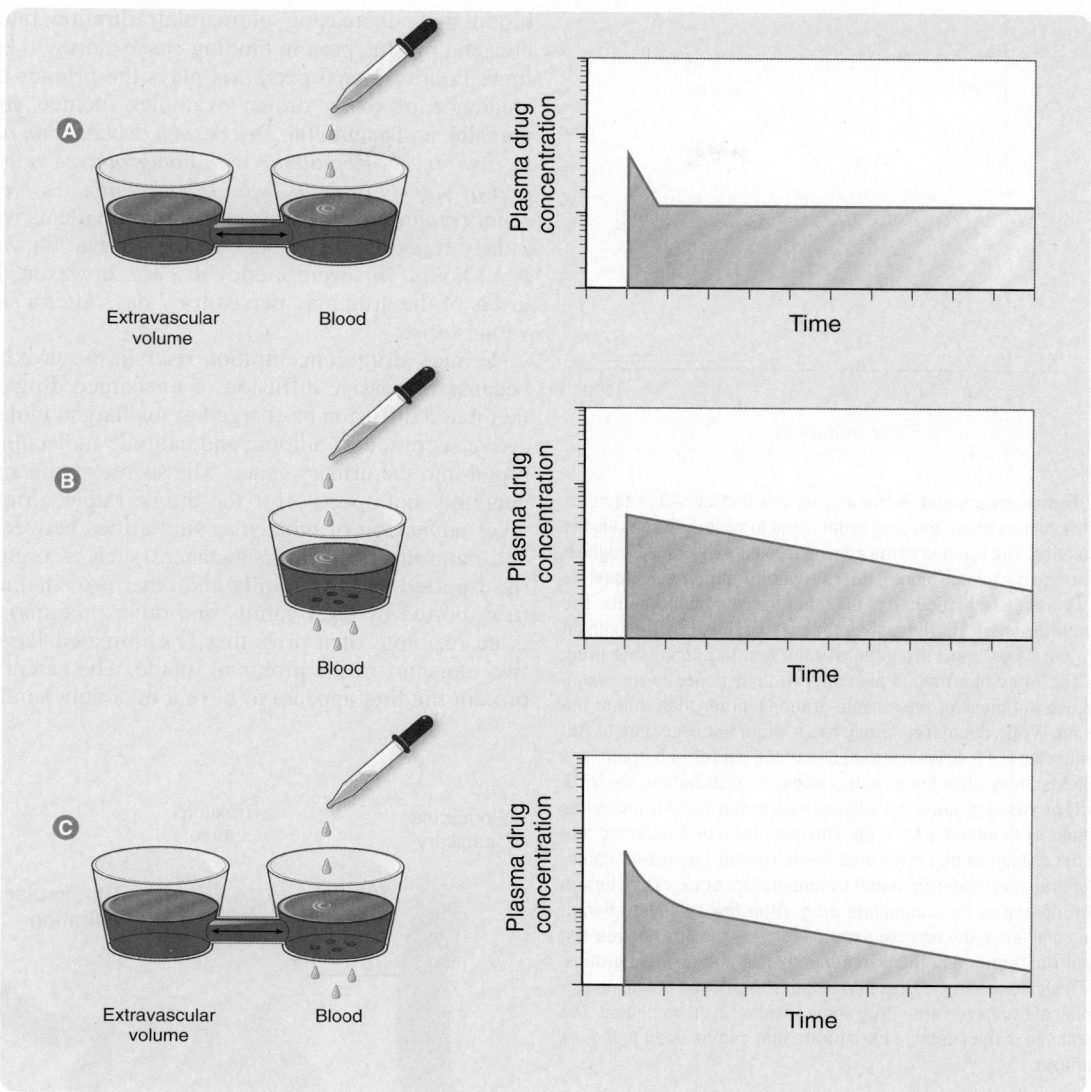

FIGURE 3-7. Schematic model of drug distribution and elimination. A two-compartment pharmacokinetic model can be used to describe drug distribution and elimination after administration of a single intravenous dose. The drug concentration rises rapidly as the drug is added to the first compartment. **A.** In the absence of elimination, the initial rise in drug concentration is followed by a rapid decline to a new plateau as the drug equilibrates (distributes) between the two compartments. **B.** If the distribution of the drug is confined to the blood volume, then the plasma drug concentration declines more slowly as the drug is eliminated from the body. In both cases, as the concentration of drug in the plasma decreases, the forces driving **(A)** drug distribution and **(B)** elimination decrease, and the absolute amount of drug distributed or eliminated per unit time decreases. Therefore, the kinetics of both distribution and elimination appear as straight lines on a semilogarithmic plot; this is the definition of *first-order kinetics*. Note that the half-time for drug elimination is generally longer than the half-time for drug distribution. **C.** When drug distribution and elimination are occurring simultaneously, the decline of plasma drug concentration with time is represented by the sum of the two processes. Note that the curve in **(C)** is the sum of the two first-order processes shown in **(A)** and **(B)**. In the schematics on the left of the figure, the volume in the "Blood" compartment represents plasma drug concentration, the volume in the "Extravascular volume" compartment represents tissue drug concentration, the dropper above the "Blood" compartment represents absorption of drug into the systemic circulation, and the drops below the "Blood" compartment represent elimination of drug by metabolism and excretion.

inducers of enzymes that mediate oxidation/reduction reactions; other drugs are capable of inhibiting these enzymes (see Table 4-3). An understanding of these **drug–drug interactions** is an essential prerequisite to the appropriate dosing of drug combinations.

Physicians and researchers have begun to elucidate the important role of genetic differences among individuals in the various transporters and enzymes responsible for drug absorption, distribution, excretion, and especially metabolism. For example, an individual's complement of cytochrome

P450 enzymes in the liver and their specific genetic polymorphisms determine the rate and extent to which that individual can metabolize numerous therapeutic agents. This topic is discussed in detail in Chapter 7, Pharmacogenomics.

EXCRETION

Oxidation/reduction and conjugation/hydrolysis reactions enhance the hydrophilicity of a hydrophobic drug and its metabolites, enabling such drugs to be excreted along a final

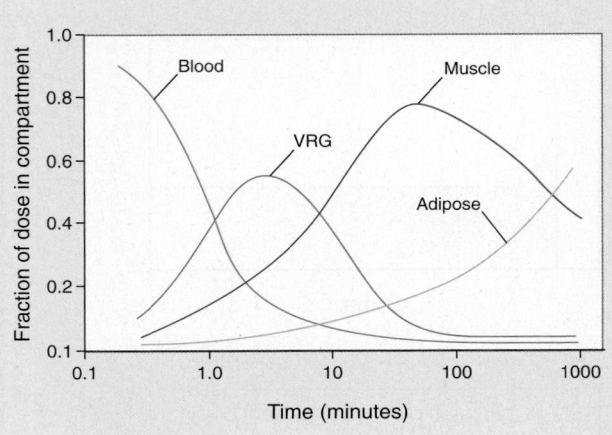

FIGURE 3-8. Four-compartment model of drug distribution. After administration of an intravenous bolus, the drug is delivered to various tissues via the systemic circulation. The fraction of the administered dose is initially highest in the vascular compartment (blood), but the blood fraction subsequently falls rapidly as the drug is distributed to the other tissue compartments. The most vessel-rich tissues (i.e., the tissues that are supplied by the highest fraction of the cardiac output) are generally the first to accumulate drug. However, the tissue compartments also vary in their capacity for taking up drug. Because the mass of the muscle group is larger than that of the vessel-rich group (VRG), the muscle group has a larger uptake capacity. But because the muscles are less well perfused than the vessel-rich group, this effect is manifested only after the drug has begun to distribute to the VRG. The most poorly perfused group is the adipose-rich group, but this group has the highest capacity to accumulate drug. The peak level of drug in the adipose group is not as high as that in the muscle-rich group, because a significant amount of drug has been eliminated by metabolism or excretion before the adipose group begins to accumulate drug. After the administration of drug has been completed, the reverse pattern is seen—the drug leaves first from the vessel-rich group and then from the muscle and adipose groups, respectively. This pattern emphasizes that adipose tissue can provide a significant reservoir of drug even after drug administration is discontinued. The drug in this example is thiopental, a barbiturate that can be used to induce general anesthesia.

common pathway with drugs that are intrinsically hydrophilic. Most drugs and drug metabolites are eliminated from the body through renal and biliary excretion. Renal excretion is the most common mechanism of drug excretion, and it relies on the hydrophilic character of a drug or metabolite. Only a relatively small number of drugs are excreted primarily in the bile or through respiratory and dermal routes. Many orally administered drugs are incompletely absorbed from the upper gastrointestinal tract, and residual drug is eliminated by fecal excretion.

Renal Excretion

Renal blood flow comprises about 25% of total systemic blood flow, ensuring that the kidneys are continuously exposed to any drug found in the blood. The rate of drug elimination through the kidneys depends on the balance of drug filtration, secretion, and reabsorption rates (Fig. 3-9). The afferent arteriole introduces both free (unbound) drug and plasma protein-bound drug into the glomerulus. Typically, however, only the free drug form is filtered into the renal tubule. Therefore, renal blood flow, glomerular filtration rate, and drug binding to plasma protein all affect the amount of drug that enters the tubule at the glomerulus. Enhancing

blood flow, increasing glomerular filtration rate, and decreasing plasma protein binding cause a drug to be excreted more rapidly. Renal excretion plays the primary role in the clearance of many drugs; examples include **vancomycin**, **atenolol**, and **ampicillin**. *Drugs such as these can accumulate to toxic levels in patients with compromised renal function and in elderly patients (who often manifest some degree of renal compromise).* For example, in individuals with normal kidney function, the typical dosing interval for vancomycin is 12 hours. In severe kidney disease, however, therapeutic levels of the drug may persist for 7 days after a single intravenous dose.

Urinary drug concentration rises in the proximal tubule because of passive diffusion of uncharged drug molecules, facilitated diffusion of charged or uncharged molecules, and active secretion of anionic and cationic molecules from the blood into the urinary space. The secretory mechanisms are generally not specific for the drugs; rather, drug secretion takes advantage of molecular similarities between the drug and naturally occurring substances such as organic anions (transported by OAT family and other proteins) and cations (transported by OCT family and other proteins). **Penicillin** is an example of a drug that is eliminated largely by active transport in the proximal tubule. The extent of plasma protein binding appears to have a relatively small effect on

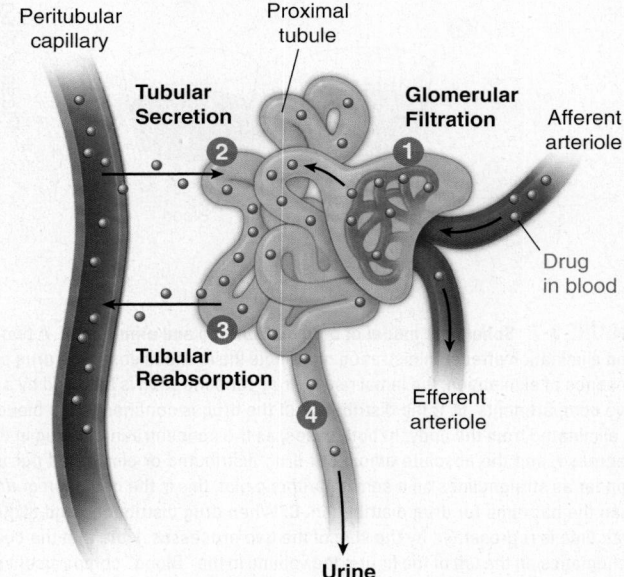

FIGURE 3-9. Drug filtration, secretion, and reabsorption in the kidney. Drugs may be (1) filtered at the renal glomerulus, (2) secreted into the proximal tubule, (3) reabsorbed from the tubular lumen and transported back into the blood, and (4) excreted in the urine. The relative balance of filtration, secretion, and reabsorption rates determines the kinetics of drug elimination by the kidney. Enhancing blood flow, increasing glomerular filtration rate, and decreasing plasma protein binding all cause a drug to be excreted more rapidly, because all these changes result in increased filtration of drug at the glomerulus. Some drugs, such as penicillin, are actively secreted into the proximal tubule. Although reabsorption can decrease the elimination rate of a drug, many drugs exhibit pH trapping in the distal tubule and are therefore efficiently excreted in the urine. For drugs that are dependent on the kidney for elimination, compromised renal function can result in higher plasma drug concentrations, and the dose and frequency of drug administration must be altered accordingly.

drug secretion into the proximal tubule, because the highly efficient transporters that mediate active tubular secretion rapidly remove free (unbound) drug from the peritubular capillaries and thereby alter the equilibrium between free and protein-bound drug at these sites.

The urinary concentration of a drug may fall as the drug is reabsorbed in the proximal and distal tubules. Reabsorption is limited primarily by **pH trapping**, as described above. The renal tubular fluid is typically acidic in and beyond the proximal tubule, which tends to favor trapping of the ionic form of weak bases. Because this region of the tubule contains transporter proteins that are different from those in preceding segments of the nephron, ionic drug forms resist facilitated diffusional reabsorption, and their excretion is thereby enhanced. Drug reabsorption in the tubule can be enhanced or inhibited by chemical adjustment of the urinary pH. Changing the rate of urine flow through the tubules can also modify the rate of drug reabsorption. An increased rate of urine output tends to dilute the drug concentration in the tubule and to decrease the amount of time during which facilitated diffusion can occur; both of these effects tend to decrease drug reabsorption. For example, aspirin is a weak acid that is excreted by the kidney. Aspirin overdose is treated by administering sodium bicarbonate to alkalinize the urine (and thus trap aspirin in the tubule) and by increasing the urine flow rate (and thus dilute the tubular concentration of the drug). Both of these clinical maneuvers result in faster elimination of the drug.

Biliary Excretion

Drug reabsorption also plays an important role in biliary excretion. Some drugs are secreted from the liver into the bile by members of the **ATP binding cassette (ABC)** superfamily of transporters, which includes seven families of proteins such as the **multidrug resistance (MDR)** family. Because the bile duct enters the gastrointestinal tract in the duodenum, such drugs must pass through the length of the small and large intestine before being eliminated. In many cases, these drugs undergo **enterohepatic circulation**, in which they are reabsorbed in the small intestine and subsequently retained in the portal and then the systemic circulation. Drugs such as steroid hormones, digoxin, and some cancer chemotherapeutic agents are largely excreted in the bile.

■ CLINICAL APPLICATIONS OF PHARMACOKINETICS

The dynamic interactions among drug absorption, distribution, metabolism, and excretion determine the plasma concentration of a drug and dictate the ability of the drug to reach its target organ in an effective concentration. Often, the desired duration of drug therapy exceeds that achievable by a single dose, and multiple doses are needed to provide a relatively constant plasma concentration of drug within the limits of efficacy and toxicity. The results of clinical trials of drugs under development, as well as clinical experience using US Food and Drug Administration (FDA)-approved drugs, suggest standard doses of a drug in the average patient. However, pharmacokinetic and other differences among patients (such as disease status and pharmacogenomic profile) must also be considered in designing a dosing regimen for a drug or drug combination in the individual patient.

Clearance

The clearance of a drug is the pharmacokinetic parameter that most significantly limits the time course of action of the drug at its molecular, cellular, and organ targets. Clearance can be conceptualized in two complementary ways. First, it is defined as the rate of elimination of the drug from the body relative to the concentration of the drug in plasma. Alternatively, clearance is the rate at which plasma would have to be cleared of the drug to account for the observed kinetics of change of the total amount of drug in the body, assuming that all the drug in the body is present at the same concentration as that in the plasma. Therefore, clearance is expressed in units of volume/time, as follows:

$$\text{Clearance} = \frac{\text{Metabolism} + \text{Excretion}}{[\text{Drug}]_{\text{plasma}}} \qquad \textbf{Equation 3-5}$$

where metabolism and excretion are expressed as rates (amount/time).

Although metabolism and excretion are distinct physiologic processes, the pharmacologic endpoint is equivalent—a reduction in circulating levels of active drug. As such, metabolism and excretion are often referred to collectively as clearance mechanisms, and the principles of clearance can be applied to both:

$$\text{Clearance}_{\text{total}} = \text{Clearance}_{\text{renal}} + \text{Clearance}_{\text{hepatic}}$$
$$+ \text{Clearance}_{\text{Other}} \qquad \textbf{Equation 3-6}$$

Metabolism and Excretion Kinetics

The rate of drug metabolism and excretion by an organ is limited by the rate of blood flow to that organ. The majority of drugs demonstrate **first-order kinetics** when used in standard therapeutic doses; that is, the amount of drug that is metabolized or excreted in a given unit of time is directly proportional to the concentration of drug in the systemic circulation at that time. Because the clearance mechanisms for most drugs are not saturated under ordinary circumstances, increases in plasma drug concentration are matched by increases in the rate of drug metabolism and excretion (see Equation 3-5). The first-order elimination rate (where elimination includes both metabolism and excretion) follows Michaelis-Menten kinetics:

$$E = \frac{V_{\max} \times C}{K_m + C} \qquad \textbf{Equation 3-7}$$

where $V_{\max}$ is the maximum rate of drug elimination, K_m is the drug concentration at which the rate of elimination is $\frac{1}{2} V_{\max}$, C is the concentration of drug in the plasma, and E is the elimination rate (Fig. 3-10). Because elimination is usually a first-order process, a semilogarithmic plot of plasma drug concentration versus time typically shows a straight line during the elimination phase (see Fig. 3-6).

A small number of drugs (e.g., phenytoin and ethanol) demonstrate **saturation kinetics**, in which the clearance mechanisms become saturated at or near the therapeutic concentration of the drug. Once saturation occurs, the clearance rate fails to increase with increasing plasma drug concentrations (**zero-order kinetics**). This can result in dangerously elevated plasma concentrations of the drug, which can cause toxic (or even lethal) effects.

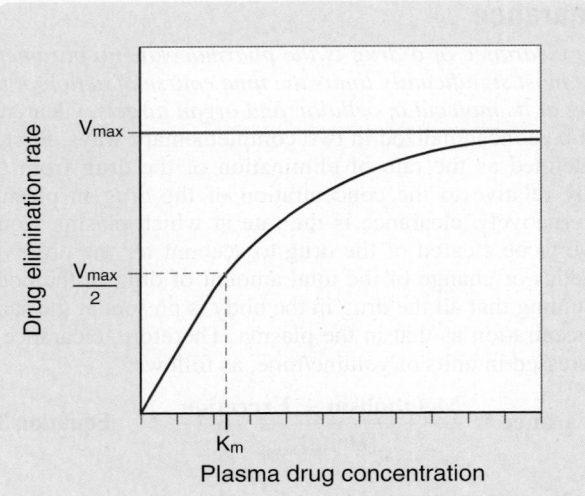

FIGURE 3-10. Michaelis-Menten kinetics. Drug elimination typically follows Michaelis-Menten (first-order) kinetics. The rate of drug elimination increases as the plasma drug concentration increases, until the elimination mechanisms become saturated and reach a maximal elimination rate (V_{max}) at high plasma concentrations. The Michaelis-Menten constant, K_m, is the drug concentration at which the drug elimination rate is ½ V_{max}.

The extent to which an organ contributes to drug clearance is quantified by its **extraction ratio**, which compares the drug levels in plasma immediately before entering and just after exiting the organ:

$$\text{Extraction} = \frac{C_{in} - C_{out}}{C_{in}} \qquad \textbf{Equation 3-8}$$

where C is the concentration. An organ that contributes substantially to drug clearance is expected to have a higher extraction ratio (closer to 1) than an organ that does not participate substantially in drug clearance (closer to zero). For example, the liver extraction ratio is high for drugs that have substantial first-pass metabolism.

Half-Life

By decreasing the concentration of active drug in the blood, drug metabolism and excretion shorten the time during which a drug is capable of acting on a target organ. The **elimination half-life** of a drug is defined as *the amount of time over which the drug concentration in the plasma decreases to one-half of its original value.* Knowledge of a drug's elimination half-life allows the clinician to estimate the frequency of dosing required to maintain the plasma concentration of the drug in the therapeutic range (see below). There are many potentially confounding factors in any clinical situation, and it is useful to consider here the simplest of cases. Because most drugs are eliminated by first-order kinetics, the body can often be modeled as a single compartment with a volume that is equivalent to the volume of distribution. In this model, the elimination half-life ($t_{1/2}$) depends only on the volume of distribution and clearance of the drug:

$$t_{1/2} = \frac{0.693 \times V_d}{\text{Clearance}} \qquad \textbf{Equation 3-9}$$

where V_d is the volume of distribution and 0.693 is an approximation of ln 2.

Thus, all of the factors outlined above that affect the volume of distribution and clearance of a drug also affect the half-life of the drug. A decrease in drug clearance or increase in volume of distribution tends to prolong the elimination half-life and thereby enhance the effect of the drug on the target organ. The half-life must be carefully considered in designing any dosing regimen, as the effects from a drug with a long half-life may last for a number of days. For example, the half-life of chloroquine is more than 1 week and that of amiodarone is more than 1 month.

Factors Altering Half-Life

Physiologic and pathologic changes in the volume of distribution must be considered when determining the appropriate drug dose and dosing interval (Table 3-5). As patients age, their skeletal muscle mass decreases, which could decrease the volume of distribution. In contrast, an obese person has an increase in the capacity for drug uptake by adipose tissue, and a drug that distributes into fat may need to be given in a higher dose in order to reach therapeutic plasma drug levels. As a third example, if drug dosing is based on total body weight but the adipose group does not take up the drug, then potentially toxic drug levels could be reached in an obese individual. Finally, some drugs may partition preferentially into pathologic fluid spaces such as ascites or a pleural effusion, causing long-term toxicity if the drug dosage is not adjusted accordingly.

Physiologic and pathologic processes may also affect drug clearance. For example, the cytochrome P450 enzymes responsible for drug metabolism in the liver can be induced, increasing the rate of drug inactivation, or inhibited, decreasing the rate of drug inactivation. Specific P450 enzymes are induced by some drugs (such as **carbamazepine**, **phenytoin**, **prednisone**, and **rifampin**) and inhibited by others (such as

TABLE 3-5 Factors Affecting Drug Half-Life

FACTORS AFFECTING HALF-LIFE	MOST COMMON EFFECT ON HALF-LIFE
Effects on Volume of Distribution	
Aging (decreased muscle mass → decreased distribution)	Decreased
Obesity (increased adipose mass → increased distribution)	Increased
Pathologic fluid (increased distribution)	Increased
Effects on Clearance	
Cytochrome P450 induction (increased metabolism)	Decreased
Cytochrome P450 inhibition (decreased metabolism)	Increased
Cardiac failure (decreased clearance)	Increased
Hepatic failure (decreased clearance)	Increased
Renal failure (decreased clearance)	Increased

cimetidine, ciprofloxacin, diltiazem, and fluoxetine); see Table 4-3 for a list of notable inducers and inhibitors of specific enzymes. Organ failure is another critical factor in determining appropriate dosing regimens. Hepatic failure may both alter liver enzyme function and decrease biliary excretion. Decreased cardiac output reduces the amount of blood that reaches clearance organs. Renal failure decreases drug excretion because of decreased drug filtration and secretion into the renal tubules. In summary, *hepatic, cardiac, and renal failure can each lead to a decreased ability to inactivate or eliminate a drug and thereby increase the elimination half-life of the drug.*

Therapeutic Dosing and Frequency

The basic principles of pharmacokinetics—absorption, distribution, metabolism, and excretion—influence the design of an optimal dosing regimen for a drug. Absorption determines the potential route(s) of administration and helps to determine optimal drug dose. For two drugs with the same potency, the more highly absorbed drug—as evidenced by a higher bioavailability—generally requires a lower dose than the more poorly absorbed drug. In contrast, a more highly distributed drug—as evidenced by a higher volume of distribution—generally necessitates higher drug dosing. The elimination rate of a drug influences its half-life and thereby determines the frequency of dosing required to maintain therapeutic plasma drug levels.

In general, *therapeutic dosing of a drug seeks to maintain the peak (highest) plasma drug concentration below the toxic concentration and the trough (lowest) drug concentration above the minimally effective level* (Fig. 3-11). This can be accomplished most efficiently using continuous drug delivery by intravenous (continuous infusion), subcutaneous (continuous pump or implant), transcutaneous (dermal patch), oral (sustained-release tablet), and other routes of administration, as described in more detail in Chapter 55. In many cases, however, the dosing regimen must also consider

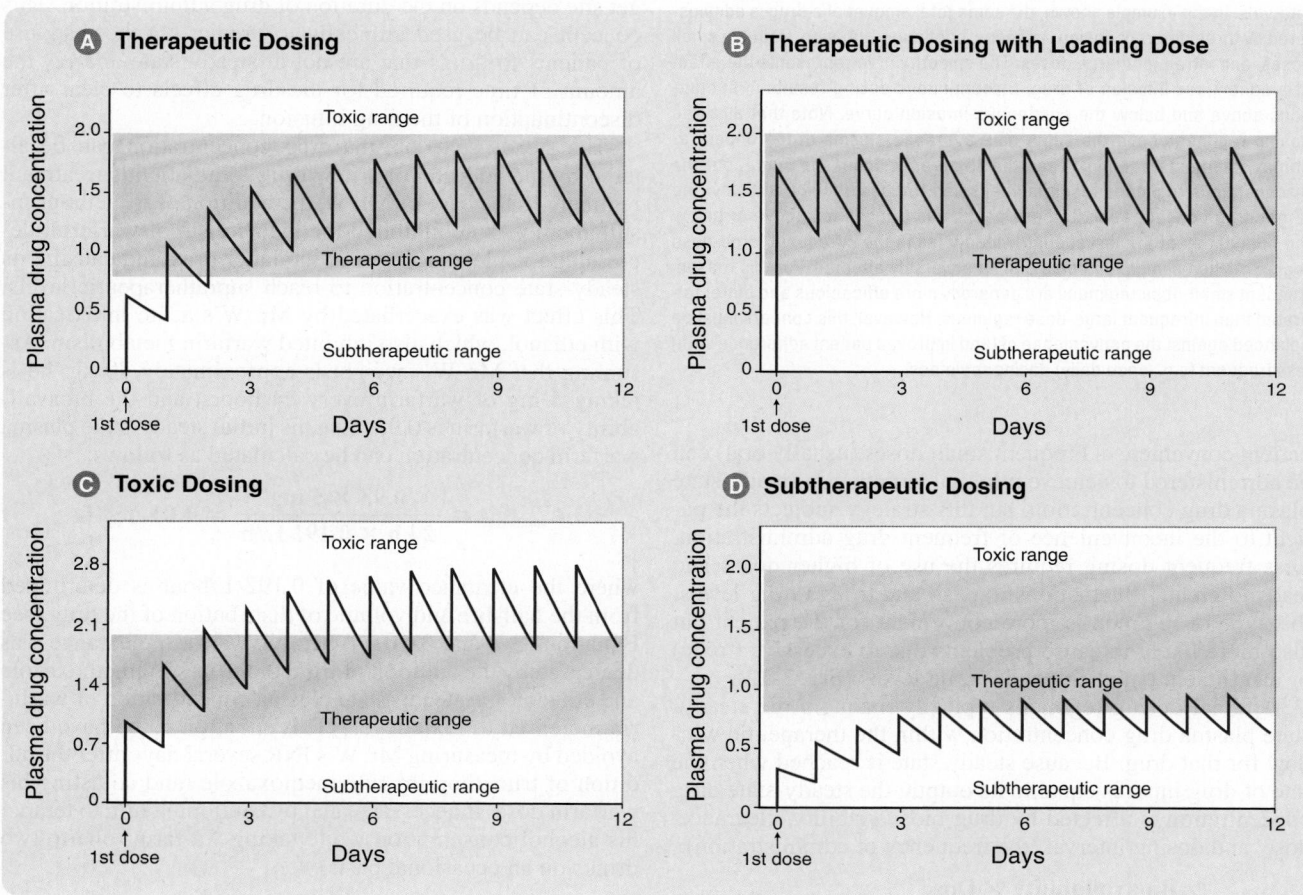

FIGURE 3-11. Therapeutic, subtherapeutic, and toxic drug dosing. From a clinical perspective, drug concentrations in plasma can be divided into subtherapeutic, therapeutic, and supratherapeutic or toxic ranges. The goal of most drug-dosing regimens is to maintain the drug at concentrations within the therapeutic range (referred to as the *therapeutic window*). **A.** The first several doses of a drug are typically subtherapeutic as the drug equilibrates to its steady-state concentration (approximately four elimination half-lives are required to achieve steady state). Appropriate drug dosing and dosing frequency result in steady-state drug levels that are therapeutic, and the maximal and minimal concentrations of the drug remain within the therapeutic window. **B.** If the initial (loading) dose is larger than the maintenance dose, the drug reaches therapeutic concentrations more rapidly. The magnitude of the loading dose is determined by the volume of distribution of the drug. **C.** Excessive maintenance doses or dosing frequency result in drug accumulation and toxicity. **D.** Insufficient maintenance doses or dosing frequency result in subtherapeutic steady-state drug concentrations. In all four panels, the drug is administered once daily, distributed very rapidly to the various body compartments, and eliminated with first-order kinetics.

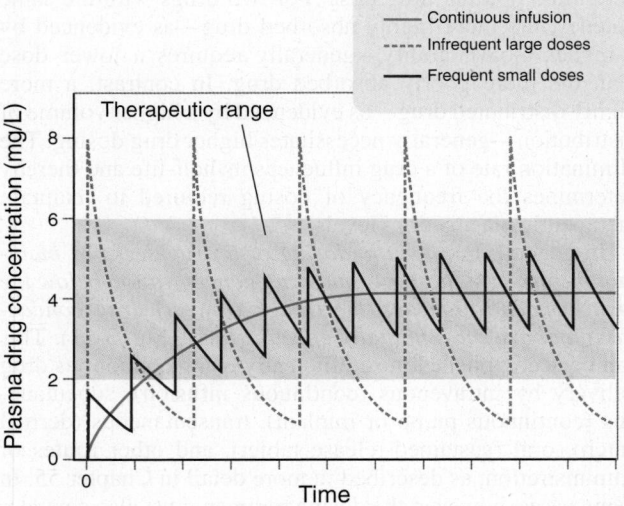

FIGURE 3-12. Fluctuations in steady-state drug concentration depend on dosing frequency. The same average steady-state plasma drug concentration can be achieved using a variety of different drug doses and dosing intervals. In the example shown, the same total amount of a drug is administered by three different dosing regimens: continuous infusion, frequent small doses, and infrequent large doses. The smooth curve represents the effect of a continuous infusion of drug. Discontinuous dosing results in fluctuations above and below the continuous-infusion curve. Note that all three dosing regimens have the same time-averaged plasma drug concentration at steady state (4 mg/L) and the same area under the curve, but the discontinuous regimens result in peaks and troughs above and below the target drug concentration. If these peaks and troughs fall above or below the boundaries of the therapeutic window (as in the infrequent large-dose regimen), then clinical outcome can be adversely affected. For this reason, frequent small-dose regimens are generally more efficacious and better tolerated than infrequent large-dose regimens. However, this concern must be balanced against the convenience of (and improved patient adherence with) less frequent (e.g., once daily) dosing regimens.

patient convenience. Frequent small doses (usually oral) can be administered to achieve minimal variation in steady-state plasma drug concentration, but this strategy subjects the patient to the inconvenience of frequent drug administration. Less frequent dosing requires the use of higher doses and leads to greater fluctuations in peak and trough drug levels; this type of regimen is more convenient for the patient but also more likely to cause problems due to excessive (toxic) or insufficient (subtherapeutic) drug levels (Fig. 3-12).

Optimal dosing regimens typically maintain the steady-state plasma drug concentration within the therapeutic window for that drug. Because steady state is reached when the rate of drug input is equal to its output, the steady-state drug concentration is affected by drug bioavailability, clearance, dose, and dosing interval (the frequency of administration):

$$C_{\text{steady state}} = \frac{\text{Bioavailability} \times \text{Dose}}{\text{Interval}_{\text{dosing}} \times \text{Clearance}} \qquad \textbf{Equation 3-10}$$

where C is the plasma concentration of the drug.

Immediately after the initiation of drug therapy, the rate of drug entry into the body (k_{in}) is much greater than the elimination rate (k_{out}); therefore, the drug concentration in the blood increases. Assuming that elimination follows first-order kinetics, the rate of elimination also increases as the plasma drug concentration increases, because the elimination rate is proportional to the plasma drug concentration. Steady state is reached when the two rates (k_{in} and k_{out}) are equal. Because k_{in} is a constant, *the approach to steady state is governed by k_{out}, the composite rate for all drug clearance mechanisms.* (k_{out} can also be called k_e, the composite rate for drug elimination.) In most dosing regimens, drug levels accumulate after each successive dose, and the steady state is reached only when the amount of drug entering the system is equal to the amount being removed from the system (see Fig. 3-11). Clinically, this principle must be remembered when the dosing regimen is altered, because approximately four elimination half-lives must pass before the new steady state is reached.

The concept of **context-sensitive half-life** describes the dynamic half-life of elimination of drug from its target site from the beginning of dosing to the time at which steady state is reached. This concept is important clinically, particularly for continuous infusions of drugs such as opioid analgesics or intravenous anesthetics such as propofol. Often, these drugs are administered as continuous infusions for periods of time that are insufficiently long to reach steady state. In these cases, the half-life of elimination of drug from a target site depends on the duration of drug administration. This concept can be used clinically to predict (1) the response of patients to drugs that are not at steady state and (2) the amount of time required for the drug effects to clear after discontinuation of the drug infusion.

The steady-state plasma drug concentration can be altered by the addition of a new drug to a patient's treatment regimen. In the case of Mr. W, the addition of trimethoprim-sulfamethoxazole inhibited the metabolism of warfarin, decreasing the clearance rate of the latter drug and causing its steady-state concentration to reach supratherapeutic levels. This effect was exacerbated by Mr. W's acute intoxication with ethanol, which also inhibited warfarin metabolism. Assuming that Mr. W's weight is approximately 70 kg, he is taking 5 mg of warfarin every 24 hours, and the bioavailability of warfarin is 0.93, then his initial steady-state plasma warfarin concentration can be calculated as follows:

$$C_{\text{steady state}} = \frac{0.93 \times 5 \text{ mg}}{24 \text{ h} \times 0.192 \text{ L/h}} = 1.01 \text{ mg/L}$$

where the clearance value of 0.192 L/hour is determined from the half-life and volume of distribution of the drug (see Equations 3-9 and 3-10). When his warfarin clearance was decreased by the addition of trimethoprim-sulfamethoxazole and ethanol, the steady-state plasma concentration of warfarin increased to toxic levels. This situation could have been avoided by measuring Mr. W's INR several days after the addition of trimethoprim-sulfamethoxazole (and adjusting his warfarin dose, if necessary) and by cautioning him to temper his alcohol consumption while taking warfarin (one to two drinks on an occasional basis).

Loading Dose

After administration of a drug by any route, the plasma concentration of the drug initially increases. Distribution of drug from the vascular (blood) compartment to body tissues then causes the plasma drug concentration to decrease. The rate and extent of this decrease are significant for drugs with high volumes of distribution. If the administered dose of drug fails to take account of the volume of distribution, instead accounting only for the blood volume, then therapeutic drug levels will not be reached promptly. Initial (loading) doses of drug are often administered to compensate for drug distribution into the tissues. Such doses may be much higher than would be required if the drug were retained in the vascular compartment. Loading doses may be used to achieve therapeutic levels of drug (i.e., levels at the desired steady-state concentration) with only one or two doses of drug:

$$\text{Dose}_{\text{loading}} = V_d \times C_{\text{steady state}} \qquad \textbf{Equation 3-11}$$

where V_d is the volume of distribution and C is the desired steady-state plasma concentration of the drug.

In the absence of a loading dose, approximately four elimination half-lives are required for the tissue distribution and plasma concentration of a drug to reach steady state. Use of a loading dose circumvents this process by providing a sufficient amount of drug to attain an appropriate (therapeutic) drug concentration in the blood and tissues after only one or two doses of drug. For example, **lidocaine** has a volume of distribution of 77 L in a 70-kg person. Assuming that a steady-state plasma concentration of 3.5 mg/L is needed to control ventricular arrhythmias, the appropriate loading dose of lidocaine in this person can be calculated as:

$$\text{Dose}_{\text{loading}} = 77 \text{ L} \times 3.5 \text{ mg/L} = 269.5 \text{ mg}$$

Maintenance Dose

Once steady-state drug concentrations are achieved in the plasma and the tissues, subsequent doses need to replace only the amount of drug that is lost through metabolism and excretion. The maintenance dose rate of a drug is dependent on the drug clearance, according to the principle that *rate in = rate out at steady state*:

$$\text{Dose}_{\text{maintenance}} = \text{Clearance} \times C_{\text{steady state}} \qquad \textbf{Equation 3-12}$$

Administration of a dose rate greater than the calculated maintenance dose rate would provide a drug input greater than the drug clearance, and the drug could accumulate to toxic levels within the tissues. In Mr. W, the calculated maintenance dose for warfarin is:

$$\text{Dose}_{\text{maintenance}} = 0.192 \text{ L/h} \times 1.01 \text{ mg/L}$$
$$= 0.194 \text{ mg/h} = 4.65 \text{ mg/day}$$

The appropriate maintenance dose for Mr. W is therefore 4.65 mg/day. Because warfarin is only 93% bioavailable, Mr. W should take 5 mg/day to maintain an adequate steady-state plasma concentration. (Note also that, because warfarin has a low therapeutic index and toxic levels of the drug can lead to potentially fatal hemorrhage, the biological activity of warfarin should be monitored carefully by periodic measurement of the INR.)

For a small number of drugs, the body's capacity to eliminate the drug (e.g., through hepatic metabolism) may become saturated at therapeutic or only slightly supratherapeutic plasma drug concentrations. In these cases, the kinetics of drug elimination may change from first-order to zero-order (also called **saturation kinetics**; see above). Continued administration of drug results in rapid drug accumulation in the plasma, and drug concentrations may reach toxic levels (Fig. 3-13).

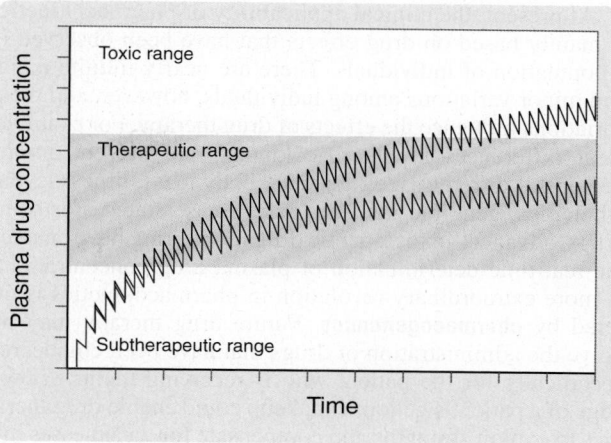

FIGURE 3-13. Saturation kinetics and drug toxicity. Drug elimination typically follows first-order Michaelis-Menten kinetics, increasing as the plasma drug concentration increases. At optimal dosing, the steady-state plasma drug concentration remains within the therapeutic range (*bottom curve*). However, excessive drug dosing may saturate the body's capacity to eliminate the drug, for example, by overwhelming the hepatic cytochrome P450 enzyme system (*top curve*). In this case, the elimination rate of the drug does not increase with increasing plasma drug concentration (i.e., elimination follows zero-order rather than first-order kinetics). Continued administration of the drug results in drug accumulation, and the plasma drug concentration may reach toxic levels.

CONCLUSION AND FUTURE DIRECTIONS

This chapter has provided an overview of the pharmacokinetic processes of absorption, distribution, metabolism, and excretion (ADME). An understanding of the factors that determine a drug's ability to act in an individual patient and the changing nature of these factors over time is vitally important to the safe and efficacious use of drug therapy. The key equations governing the relationships among dosing, clearance, and plasma drug concentration (Table 3-6) are important to consider when making therapeutic decisions about drug regimens.

TABLE 3-6 Summary of Key Pharmacokinetic Relationships

Initial concentration	$= \dfrac{\text{Loading dose}}{\text{Volume of distribution}}$
Steady-state concentration	$= \dfrac{\text{Fraction absorbed} \times \text{Maintenance dose}}{\text{Dosing interval} \times \text{Clearance}}$
Elimination half-life	$= \dfrac{0.693 \times \text{Volume of distribution}}{\text{Clearance}}$

At present, the clinical applicability of pharmacokinetics is mainly based on drug effects that have been observed in a population of individuals. There are nearly infinite major and minor variations among individuals, however, and these variations influence the effects of drug therapy. For example, clear differences in pharmacokinetics are present among persons of different ages, genders, body mass, fitness levels, ethnicities, genomic makeup, and disease states. For some drugs, advances in therapeutic drug monitoring have enabled the real-time determination of plasma drug concentrations. A more extraordinary revolution in pharmacokinetics is offered by **pharmacogenomics**. Future drug therapy may involve the administration of drugs that have been engineered specifically for the patient who is receiving them. Knowledge of a patient's genomic makeup could enable drug therapies to exploit strengths and compensate for weaknesses in a host of patient-specific variables. For example, genetic tests for variants of the P450 enzymes that metabolize warfarin are now available, and clinical trials are underway to study whether pharmacogenetic testing can better predict dosing requirements to maintain therapeutic levels of this drug. This topic is discussed in Chapter 7.

Finally, it should be noted that the use of proteins and other macromolecules as drugs presents unique pharmacokinetic opportunities and challenges compared to the use of small molecules as drugs. Some of the challenges include protein absorption and stability, protein distribution to sites of therapeutic action, and protein clearance by enzymatic degradation and other mechanisms. The study of the mechanisms involved in determining the pharmacokinetics of protein therapeutics is in its infancy compared to the considerable knowledge that exists regarding the pharmacokinetics of small molecules and provides opportunities for discovery and optimization of macromolecular therapies. This topic is discussed in more detail in Chapter 54, Protein Therapeutics.

Acknowledgment

We thank John C. LaMattina for his valuable contributions to this chapter in the First and Second Editions of *Principles of Pharmacology: The Pathophysiologic Basis of Drug Therapy*.

Suggested Reading

Ezan E. Pharmacokinetic studies of protein drugs: past, present and future. *Adv Drug Deliv Rev* 2013;65:1065–1073. (*Overview of the opportunities and challenges presented by the pharmacokinetics of protein therapeutics.*)

Godin DV. Pharmacokinetics: disposition and metabolism of drugs. In: Munson PL, ed. *Principles of pharmacology.* New York: Chapman & Hall; 1995. (*A solid introductory text, this chapter illustrates the various aspects of pharmacokinetics with many examples of specific drugs.*)

Hediger MA, Clémençon B, Burrier RE, Bruford EA. The ABCs of membrane transporters in health and disease (SLC series): introduction. *Mol Aspects Med* 2013;34:95–107. (*Reviews and introduces a special issue on the 52 families of proteins in the human solute carrier superfamily.*)

Klaasen CD, Aleksunes LM. Xenobiotic, bile acid, and cholesterol transporters: function and regulation. *Pharmacol Rev* 2010;62:1–96. (*Reviews the function, regulation, and substrates of ABC-superfamily, SLC-superfamily, and other transporters that mediate the cellular uptake and efflux of drugs and other molecules.*)

Pratt WB, Taylor P, eds. *Principles of drug action: the basis of pharmacology.* 3rd ed. New York: Churchill Livingstone; 1990, Chapters 3 and 4. (*This text provides a comprehensive treatment of pharmacokinetics and pharmacokinetic principles.*)

Rees DC, Johnson E, Lewinson O. ABC transporters: the power to change. *Nat Rev Mol Cell Biol* 2009;10:218–227. (*Reviews the molecular mechanisms of ABC-superfamily transporters.*)

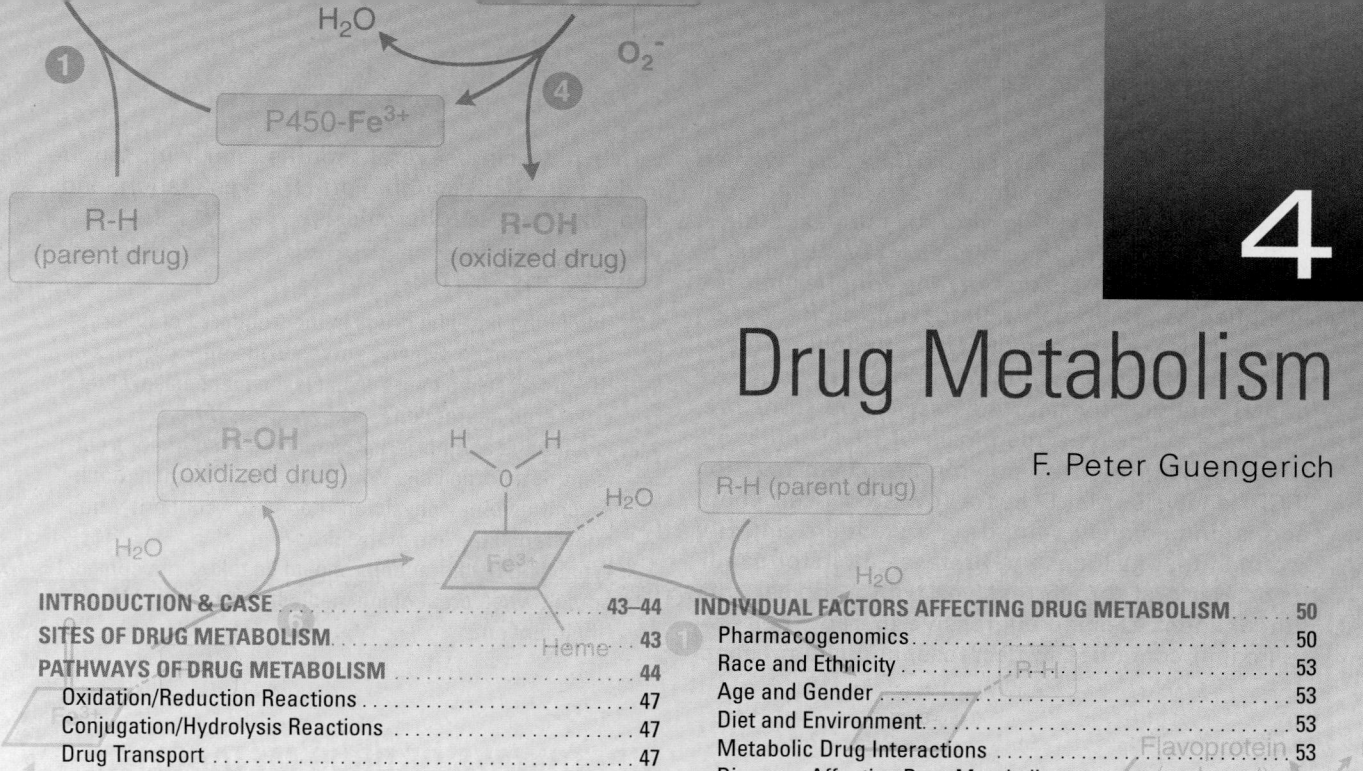

4

Drug Metabolism

F. Peter Guengerich

INTRODUCTION

Our tissues are exposed on a daily basis to **xenobiotics**—foreign substances that are not naturally found in the body. Most drugs are xenobiotics that are used to modulate bodily functions for therapeutic ends. Drugs and other environmental chemicals that enter the body are modified by a vast array of enzymes. The biochemical transformations performed by these enzymes can alter the compound to render it beneficial, harmful, or simply ineffective. The processes by which biochemical reactions alter drugs within the body are collectively called **drug metabolism** or **drug biotransformation**.

The previous chapter introduced the importance of renal clearance in the pharmacokinetics of drugs. Although the biochemical reactions that alter drugs to renally excretable forms are an essential part of drug metabolism, drug metabolism encompasses more than this one function. Drug biotransformation can alter drugs in four important ways:

- An *active drug* may be converted to an *inactive drug*.
- An *active drug* may be converted to an *active* or *toxic metabolite*.
- An *inactive prodrug* may be converted to an *active drug*.
- An *unexcretable drug* may be converted to an *excretable metabolite* (e.g., to enhance renal or biliary clearance).

This chapter presents the major processes of drug metabolism. Following the case is an overview of the sites of drug metabolism, focusing principally on the liver. The two major types of biotransformation are then discussed; these are often termed **phase I** and **phase II reactions**, although the terminology is imprecise and it incorrectly implies a temporal order of the reactions. (In addition, **phase III** is sometimes used to describe the process of drug transport.) In this chapter,

we use *oxidation/reduction* and *conjugation/hydrolysis* to describe these processes more accurately. The chapter concludes with a discussion of the factors that can lead to differences in drug metabolism among individuals.

SITES OF DRUG METABOLISM

The liver is the main organ of drug metabolism. This fact figures prominently in the phenomenon known as the **first-pass effect**. Orally administered drugs are often absorbed in the gastrointestinal (GI) tract and transported directly to the liver via the portal circulation (Fig. 4-1). In this manner, the liver has the opportunity to metabolize drugs before they reach the systemic circulation and, therefore, before they reach their target organs. The first-pass effect must be taken into account when designing dosing regimens because, if hepatic metabolism is extensive, the amount of drug that reaches the target tissue is much less than the amount (dose) that is administered orally (see Chapter 3, Pharmacokinetics). Certain drugs are inactivated so efficiently upon their first pass through the liver that they cannot be administered orally and must be given parenterally. One such drug is the antiarrhythmic lidocaine, which has a bioavailability of only 3% when taken orally (see Chapter 12, Local Anesthetic Pharmacology).

Although the liver is quantitatively the most important organ in metabolizing drugs, every tissue in the body is capable of drug metabolism to some degree. Particularly active sites include the skin, the lungs, the gastrointestinal tract, and the kidneys. The gastrointestinal tract deserves special mention because this organ, like the liver, can contribute to the first-pass effect by metabolizing orally administered drugs before they reach the systemic circulation.

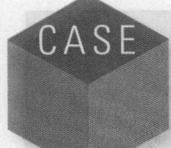

CASE Ms. B is a 32-year-old Caucasian woman who complains of sore throat and difficulty swallowing for the past 5 days. Physical examination reveals creamy white lesions on the tongue that are identified as oral thrush, a fungal infection. Her history includes sexual activity with multiple partners, inconsistent use of condoms, and continuous use of oral contraceptives for the past 14 years. The presentation suggests a diagnosis of HIV-1 infection, which is confirmed by polymerase chain reaction (PCR) analysis. Ms. B has a low CD4 T-cell count and is immediately started on a standard anti-HIV regimen that includes the protease inhibitor saquinavir. Her oral thrush resolves with a topical antifungal agent. Despite aggressive therapy, her CD4 cell count continues to decrease, and she presents to her physician several months later with fatigue and a persistent cough. Further investigation leads to a diagnosis of tuberculosis.

Questions

1. One of the first-line drugs in the treatment of tuberculosis is rifampin, which decreases the effectiveness of HIV protease inhibitors. What is the mechanism of this drug–drug interaction?
2. Isoniazid is another drug commonly used in the treatment of tuberculosis. Why does Ms. B's ethnic background give her physician reason for concern when considering the use of this drug?
3. What dietary interactions should be taken into consideration when prescribing medications to treat Ms. B's HIV infection?

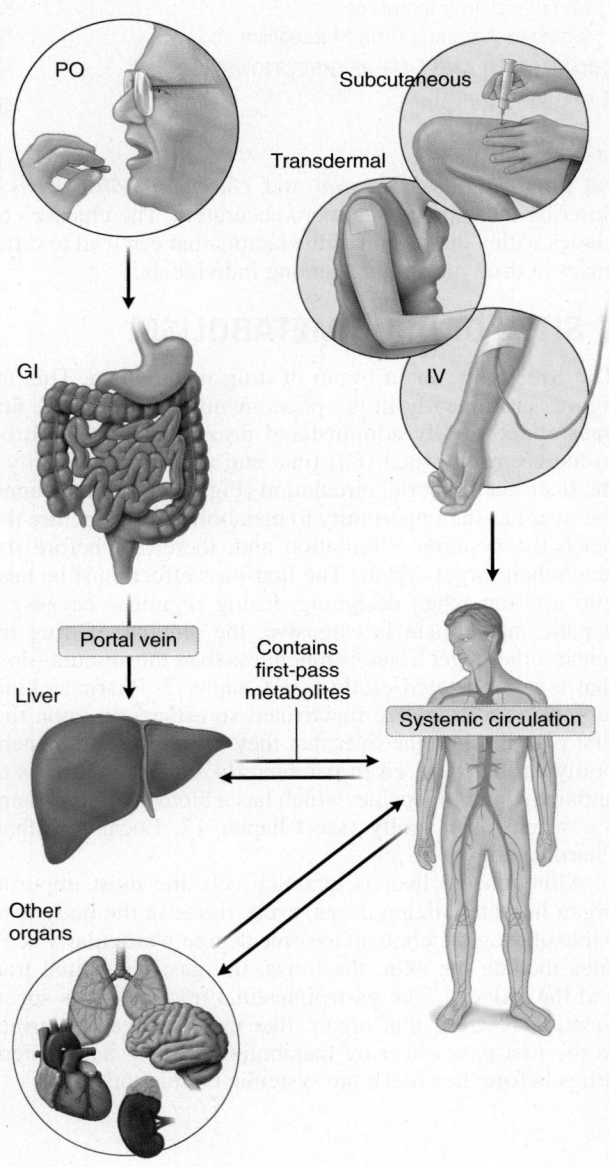

FIGURE 4-1. Portal circulation and the first-pass effect. Drugs administered by mouth (*per os*, or PO) are absorbed in the GI tract and then delivered, via the portal vein, to the liver. This pathway allows the liver to metabolize drugs before they reach the systemic circulation, a process responsible for the **first-pass effect**. In contrast, drugs that are administered intravenously (IV), transdermally, or subcutaneously enter the systemic circulation directly and can reach their target organs before hepatic modification. The first-pass effect has important implications for bioavailability; the oral formulation of a drug that undergoes extensive first-pass metabolism must be administered in a much larger dose than the equivalent IV formulation of the same drug.

PATHWAYS OF DRUG METABOLISM

Drugs and other xenobiotics undergo biotransformation before excretion from the body. Many pharmaceuticals are lipophilic, enabling the drug to diffuse across cell membranes, such as those of the intestinal mucosa or of the target tissue. Unfortunately, the same chemical property that enhances bioavailability of drugs may also make renal excretion difficult, because clearance by the kidney requires that these drugs be made more hydrophilic so that they can dissolve in the aqueous urine. Thus, biotransformation reactions often enhance the hydrophilicity of compounds to render them more susceptible to renal excretion.

Biotransformation reactions have been classically divided into two main types: oxidation/reduction (phase I) and conjugation/hydrolysis (phase II). Oxidation reactions typically transform the drug into more hydrophilic metabolites by adding or exposing polar functional groups such as hydroxyl (-OH) or amine ($-NH_2$) groups (Table 4-1). Such metabolites are often pharmacologically inactive and, without further modification, may be excreted. Some products of oxidation and reduction reactions, however, require further modifications prior to excretion. Conjugation (phase II) reactions modify compounds through attachment of hydrophilic groups, such as glucuronic acid, to create more polar conjugates (Table 4-2). It is important to note that these conjugation reactions occur independently of oxidation/reduction reactions, and the enzymes involved in oxidation/reduction and conjugation/hydrolysis reactions often compete for substrates.

TABLE 4-1 Oxidation and Reduction Reactions

REACTION CLASS	STRUCTURAL FORMULA	REPRESENTATIVE DRUGS
I. Cytochrome P450-Dependent Oxidations		
1. Aliphatic Hydroxylation	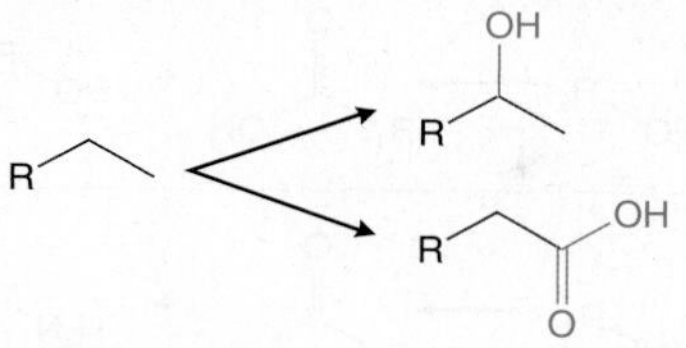	Barbiturates Digitoxin Cyclosporine
2. Aromatic Hydroxylation	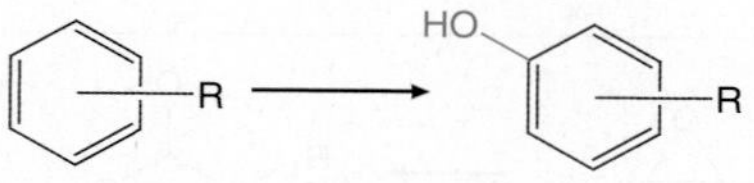	Propranolol Phenytoin
3. N-Dealkylation	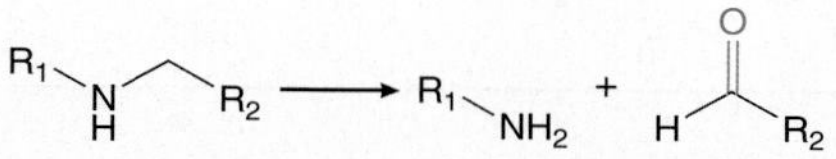	Methamphetamine Lidocaine
4. O-Dealkylation	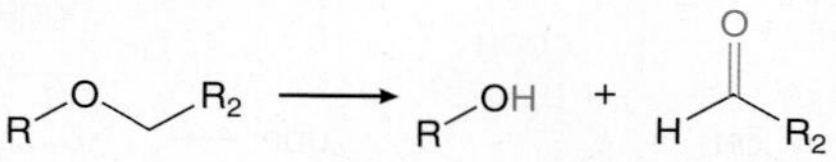	Codeine
5. S-Oxidation	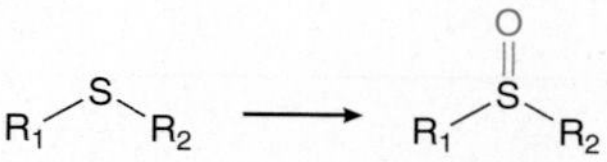	Phenothiazine Cimetidine
6. N-Oxidation	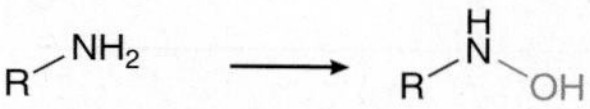	Quinidine
7. Desulfuration	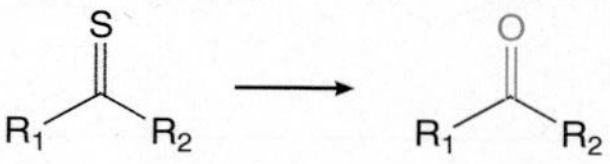	Thiopental
8. Epoxide Formation	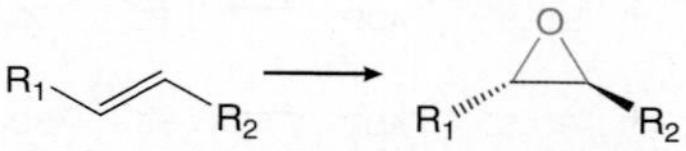	Carbamazepine
II. Cytochrome P450-Independent Oxidations		
1. Alcohol Dehydrogenation/ Aldehyde Dehydrogenation	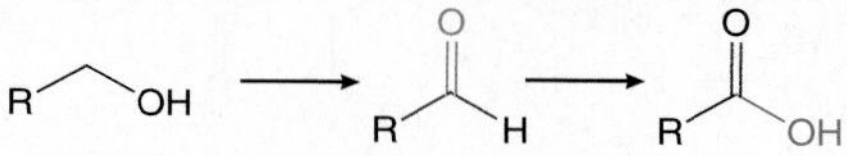	Ethanol Pyridoxine
2. Oxidative Deamination	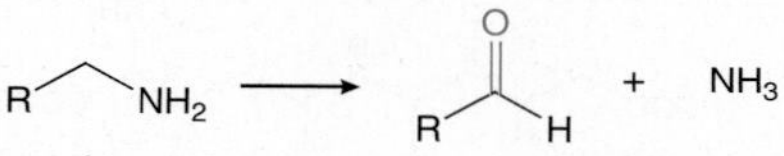	Histamine Norepinephrine
3. Decarboxylation	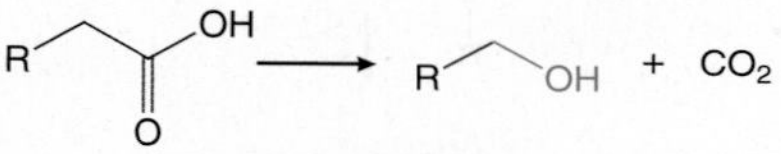	Levodopa
III. Reductions		
1. Nitro Reduction	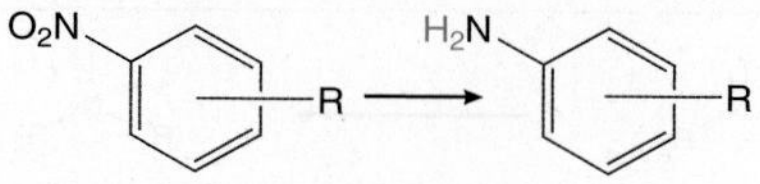	Nitrofurantoin Chloramphenicol
2. Dehalogenation	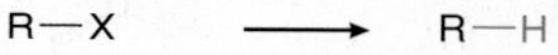	Halothane Chloramphenicol
3. Carbonyl Reduction	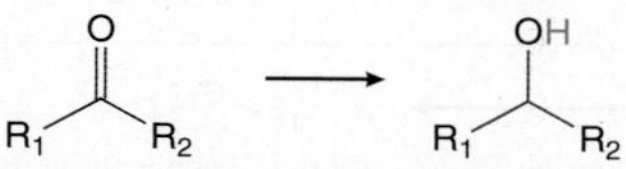	Methadone Naloxone

TABLE 4-2 Hydrolysis and Conjugation Reactions

REACTION CLASS	STRUCTURAL FORMULA	REPRESENTATIVE DRUGS
I. Hydrolysis		
1. Ester Hydrolysis		Procaine Aspirin Succinylcholine
2. Amide Hydrolysis		Procainamide Lidocaine Indomethacin
3. Epoxide Hydrolysis		Carbamazepine (epoxide metabolite)
II. Conjugation		
1. Glucuronidation		Diazepam Digoxin Ezetimibe
2. Acetylation		Isoniazid Sulfonamides
3. Glycine Conjugation		Salicylic acid
4. Sulfate Conjugation		Estrone Methyldopa
5. Glutathione Conjugation (and processing to mercapturic acids)		Ethacrynic acid Dichloroacetic acid Acetaminophen (metabolite) Chlorambucil
6. N-Methylation		Methadone Norepinephrine
7. O-Methylation		Catecholamines
8. S-Methylation		Thiopurines

Oxidation/Reduction Reactions

Oxidation reactions involve membrane-associated enzymes expressed in the endoplasmic reticulum (ER) of hepatocytes and, to a lesser extent, of cells in other tissues. The enzymes that catalyze these phase I reactions are typically oxidases; the majority of these enzymes are **heme protein monooxygenases** of the **cytochrome P450** class. Cytochrome P450 enzymes (sometimes abbreviated CYP) are also known as *microsomal mixed-function oxidases* and are involved in the metabolism of approximately 75% of all drugs used today. (The term P450 refers to the 450-nm absorption peak characteristic of these heme proteins when they bind carbon monoxide.)

The net result of a cytochrome P450-dependent oxidation reaction is:

$$\text{Drug} + O_2 + \text{NADPH} + H^+ \rightarrow$$

$$\text{Drug-OH} + H_2O + \text{NADP}^+ \quad \textbf{Equation 4-1}$$

The reaction proceeds when the drug binds to the oxidized (Fe^{3+}) cytochrome P450 to form a complex, which is then reduced in two sequential oxidation/reduction steps as outlined in Figure 4-2A. Nicotinamide adenine dinucleotide phosphate (NADPH) donates the electrons in both of these steps via a flavoprotein reductase. In the first step, the donated electron reduces the cytochrome P450–drug complex. In the second step, the electron reduces molecular oxygen to form an activated oxygen–cytochrome P450–drug complex. Finally, as the complex becomes more active through rearrangement, the reactive oxygen atom is transferred to the drug, resulting in the formation of the oxidized drug product and recycling oxidized cytochrome P450 in the process. The mechanism of these reactions is illustrated in Figure 4-2B.

Most liver cytochrome P450 oxidases exhibit broad substrate specificity (Table 4-1). This is due in part to the activated oxygen of the complex, which is a powerful oxidizing agent that can react with a variety of substrates. The names of the cytochrome P450 enzymes are sometimes designated by "P450" followed by the number of the P450 enzyme family, capital letter of the subfamily, and an additional number to identify the specific enzyme (e.g., P450 3A4). Many of the P450 enzymes have partially overlapping specificities that together allow the liver to recognize and metabolize a wide array of xenobiotics.

Together, P450-mediated reactions account for more than 95% of oxidative biotransformations. Other pathways may also oxidize lipophilic molecules. A pertinent example of a non-P450 oxidative pathway is the **alcohol dehydrogenase** pathway that oxidizes alcohols to their aldehyde derivatives as part of the overall process of excretion. These enzymes are also the basis for the toxicity of methanol. Methanol is oxidized by alcohol dehydrogenase to formaldehyde, which can do considerable damage to some tissues. The optic nerve is particularly sensitive to formaldehyde, and methanol toxicity can cause blindness.

Another important non-P450 enzyme is **monoamine oxidase (MAO)**. This enzyme is responsible for the oxidation of amine-containing endogenous compounds such as catecholamines and tyramine (see Chapter 11, Adrenergic Pharmacology) and some xenobiotics, including drugs.

Conjugation/Hydrolysis Reactions

Conjugation and hydrolysis reactions provide a second set of mechanisms for modifying compounds for excretion (Fig. 4-3). Although hydrolysis of ester- and amide-containing drugs is sometimes included among the phase I reactions (in the older terminology), the biochemistry of hydrolysis is more closely related to conjugation than to oxidation/reduction. Substrates for these reactions include both metabolites of oxidation reactions (e.g., epoxides) and compounds that already contain chemical groups appropriate for conjugation, such as hydroxyl (-OH), amine ($-NH_2$), or carboxyl (-COOH) moieties. These substrates are coupled by transfer enzymes to endogenous metabolites (e.g., glucuronic acid and its derivatives, sulfuric acid, acetic acid, amino acids, and the tripeptide glutathione) in reactions that often involve high-energy intermediates (Table 4-2). The conjugation and hydrolysis enzymes are located in both the cytosol and the endoplasmic reticulum of hepatocytes (and other tissues). In most cases, the conjugation process makes the drug more polar. Virtually all of the conjugated products are pharmacologically inactive, with some important exceptions (e.g., morphine glucuronide).

Some conjugation reactions are important clinically in the case of neonates, who have not yet fully developed the capacity to carry out this set of reactions. UDP-glucuronyl transferase (UDPGT) is responsible for conjugating bilirubin in the liver and facilitating its excretion. A relative deficiency of this enzyme at the time of birth puts infants at risk for neonatal jaundice, which results from increased serum levels of unconjugated bilirubin. Neonatal jaundice is a problem because neonates have not only underdeveloped activity of this enzyme but also an undeveloped blood–brain barrier. Unconjugated bilirubin is water-insoluble and very lipophilic; it binds readily to the unprotected neonatal brain and is capable of causing significant damage to the central nervous system. This pathologic condition is known as *bilirubin encephalopathy* or **kernicterus**. Neonatal hyperbilirubinemia (unconjugated) can be treated with phototherapy with 450-nm light, which converts circulating bilirubin to an isomer that is more rapidly excreted. Another effective treatment is the administration of small doses of the barbiturate **phenobarbital**, which powerfully up-regulates the expression of the enzyme UDPGT and thereby reduces serum levels of unconjugated bilirubin. This example illustrates a recurring theme: understanding drug metabolism can help predict both adverse and potentially advantageous drug–drug interactions.

It is important to note that conjugation and hydrolysis reactions do not necessarily constitute the last step of biotransformation. Since the conjugation of these highly polar moieties occurs intracellularly, they often require active transport across cellular membranes to be excreted (active transport of the parent drug can also occur). Moreover, some conjugation products may be subjected to further metabolism.

Drug Transport

Although many drugs are sufficiently lipophilic to cross cell membranes passively, it is now appreciated that many drugs need to be transported actively into cells. This fact has significant consequences for oral bioavailability (transport into enterocytes or active excretion into the intestinal lumen), hepatic metabolism (transport into hepatocytes for enzymatic metabolism and for excretion into bile), and renal

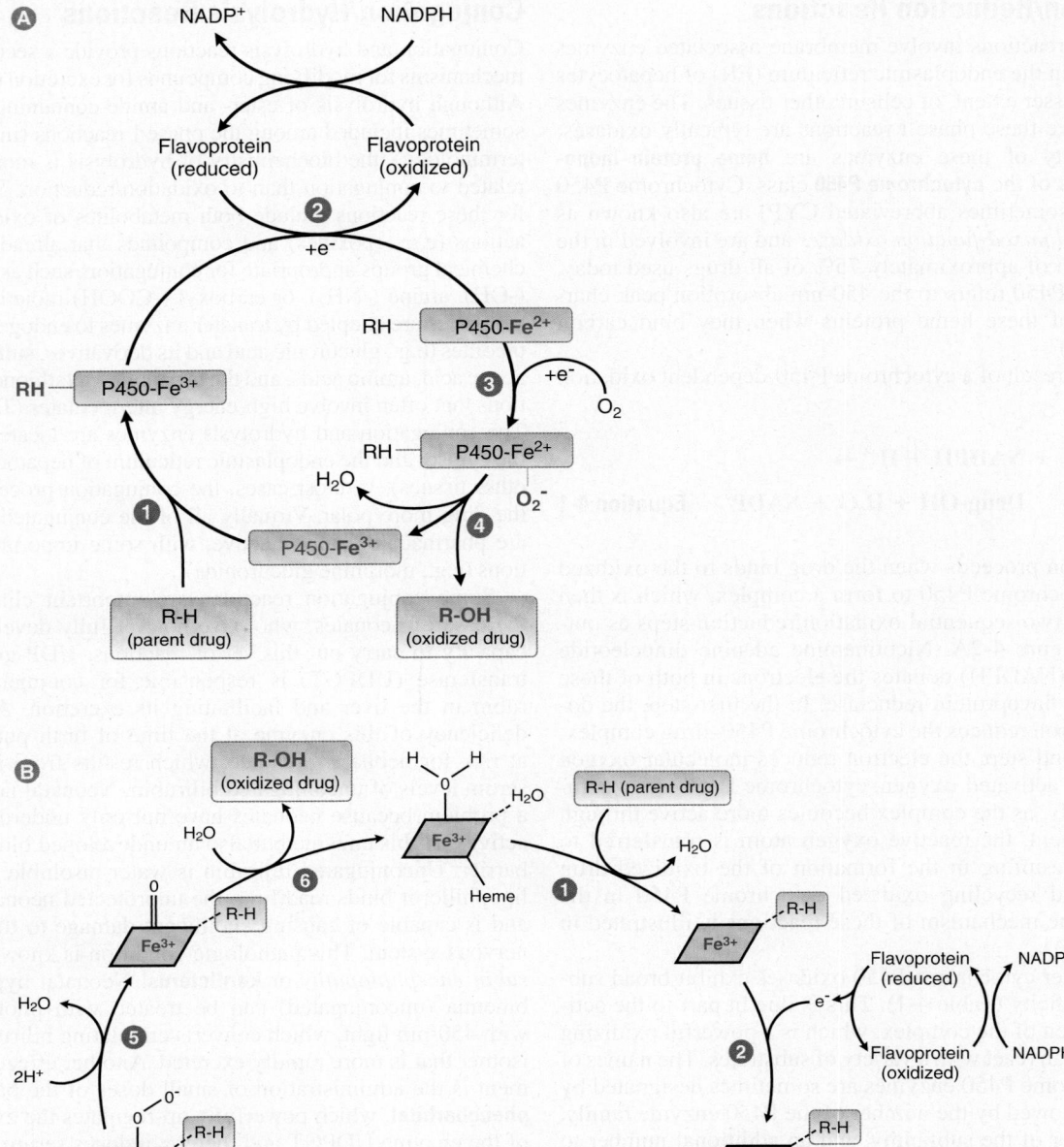

FIGURE 4-2. Cytochrome P450-mediated drug oxidation. Many drug metabolism reactions involve a system of hepatic P450 microsomal enzymes that catalyze the oxidation of drugs. **A.** An overview of the reaction involves a set of oxidation/reduction steps in which an iron moiety in the P450 enzyme acts as an electron carrier to transfer electrons from NADPH to molecular oxygen. The reduced oxygen is then transferred to the drug, resulting in an additional -OH group on the now-oxidized drug (for this reason, P450 enzymes are sometimes referred to colloquially as "oxygen guns" or even "nature's blowtorch"). The addition of the -OH group results in increased drug hydrophilicity and an increased rate of drug excretion. **B.** The detailed mechanism of the P450 reaction can be divided into six steps: (1) drug complexes with oxidized cytochrome P450; (2) NADPH donates an electron to the flavoprotein reductase, which reduces the P450-drug complex; (3 and 4) oxygen joins the complex, and NADPH donates another electron, creating the activated oxygen–P450 substrate complex; (5) iron is oxidized, with the loss of water; and (6) the oxidized drug product is formed. There are multiple P450 enzymes; each has a somewhat different specificity for substrates (such as drugs). Five of the human P450s (1A2, 2C9, 2C19, 2D6, and 3A4) account for approximately 90% of the oxidative metabolism of drugs.

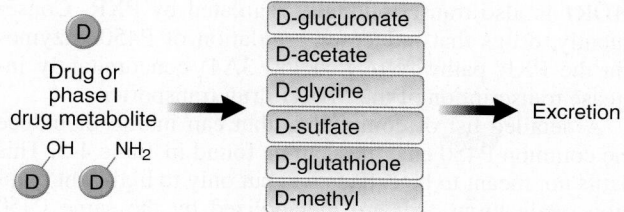

FIGURE 4-3. Conjugation reactions. In these reactions, a drug (represented by D) or drug metabolite (represented by D-OH and D-NH$_2$) is conjugated to an endogenous moiety. Glucuronic acid, a sugar, is the most common group that is conjugated to drugs, but conjugations of acetate, glycine, sulfate, glutathione, and methyl groups are also common. The addition of one of these moieties makes the resulting drug metabolite more hydrophilic and often enhances drug excretion. (Methylation, an important exception, does not increase drug hydrophilicity.) Transport mechanisms also play a major role in the elimination of drugs and their metabolites.

clearance (transport into proximal tubular cells and excretion into the tubular lumen). Several important molecules mediate these processes. The **multidrug resistance protein 1 (MDR1)**, or **P-glycoprotein**, which is a member of the ABC family of efflux transporters, actively transports compounds back into the intestinal lumen. This process limits the oral bioavailability of several important drugs, including digoxin and HIV-1 protease inhibitors. The metabolism of drugs from the portal circulation (i.e., the first-pass effect) often requires the transport of compounds into hepatocytes via the **organic anion transporting polypeptide (OATP)** and the **organic cation transporter (OCT)** family of proteins. These transporters are particularly relevant for the metabolism of several 3-hydroxy-3-methylglutaryl-coenzyme A (HMG-CoA) reductase inhibitors (statins), which are used in the treatment of hypercholesterolemia. For example, metabolism of the

HMG-CoA reductase inhibitor pravastatin is dependent on the transporter OATP1B1, which transports the drug into hepatocytes. Drug uptake into hepatocytes via OATP1B1 is thought to be the rate-limiting step in the clearance of pravastatin from the bloodstream. The uptake of pravastatin on its first pass through the liver also provides a potential advantage by keeping the drug out of the systemic circulation, from which it could be taken up by muscle cells and thereby cause toxic effects such as rhabdomyolysis. The **organic anion transporter (OAT)** family of transporters is responsible for renal secretion of many clinically important anionic drugs, such as β-lactam antibiotics, nonsteroidal anti-inflammatory drugs (NSAIDs), and antiviral nucleoside analogs.

Induction and Inhibition

The use of phenobarbital to prevent neonatal jaundice demonstrates that drug metabolism can be influenced by the expression levels of drug-metabolizing enzymes. Although some P450 enzymes are constitutively active, others can be induced or inhibited by various compounds. Induction or inhibition can be incidental (a side effect of a drug) or deliberate (the desired effect of therapy).

The primary mechanism of P450 enzyme induction is an increase in the expression of the enzyme chiefly through increased transcription, although augmented translation and decreased degradation can also have minor roles. The induction of P450 enzymes by a wide array of drugs reflects the biology of xenobiotic receptors that act as the body's surveillance system to metabolize potentially toxic compounds. Drugs, environmental pollutants, industrial chemicals, and even foodstuffs can enter hepatocytes and bind to several different xenobiotic receptors, such as the pregnane X receptor (PXR), constitutively active/androstane receptor (CAR), and aryl hydrocarbon receptor (AhR) (Fig. 4-4).

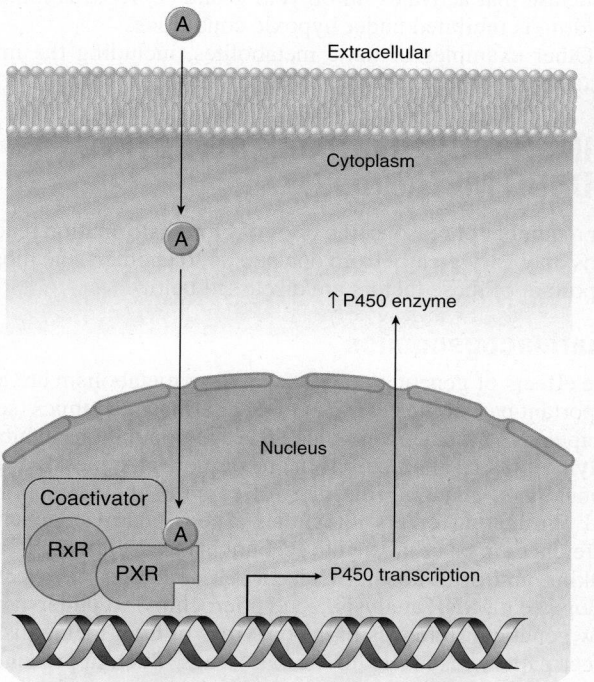

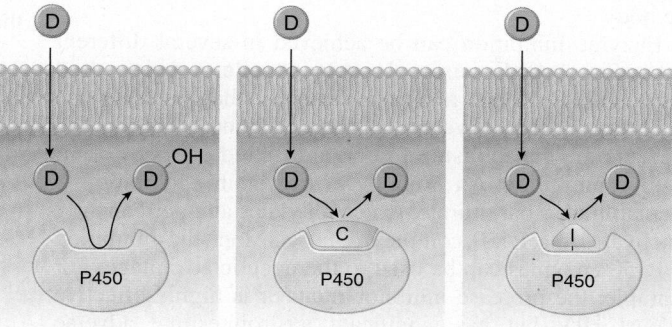

FIGURE 4-4. Conceptualization of P450 induction and inhibition. Drugs can both induce the expression and inhibit the activity of P450 enzymes. Some drugs can induce the synthesis of P450 enzymes (*left panel*). In this example, Drug A activates the pregnane X receptor (PXR), which heterodimerizes with the retinoid X receptor (RXR) to form a complex with coactivators and initiate transcription of the P450 enzyme. Induction can also occur via the constitutively active/androstane receptor (CAR) or the aryl hydrocarbon receptor (AhR) (*not shown*). Drug D enters the cell and is hydroxylated by a P450 enzyme (*right panel*). The P450 enzyme can be inhibited by a second drug acting as a competitive inhibitor (Drug C) or an irreversible inhibitor (Drug I). The mechanism by which a drug inhibits P450 enzymes is not necessarily predictable from the drug's chemical structure; the mechanism can only be determined experimentally. In addition, metabolites of Drugs A, C, and I can play a role in enzyme induction and inhibition (*not shown*).

These molecules are nuclear hormone receptors; when a xenobiotic compound binds to and activates the receptor, the complex is translocated to the nucleus, where it binds to the enhancer regions of various biotransformation enzymes, promoting increased expression of P450 enzymes via transcription. By a similar mechanism, nuclear hormone receptor activation can also increase the expression of drug transporters that aid in clearing the compounds from the body, such as MDR1 and OATP1.

There are multiple consequences of P450 enzyme induction. *First*, a drug can increase its own metabolism. For example, **carbamazepine**, an antiepileptic drug, not only induces P450 3A4 but also is metabolized by P450 3A4. Hence, carbamazepine increases its own metabolism by inducing P450 3A4. *Second*, a drug can increase the metabolism of a co-administered drug. For example, P450 3A4 is responsible for metabolizing almost 50% of all clinically prescribed drugs. Should such a drug be co-administered with carbamazepine, its metabolism would also be increased. This situation can be problematic, because the increased P450 3A4 activity can reduce drug concentrations below their therapeutic levels if standard doses of the drugs are administered. In Ms. B's case, the administration of **rifampin** in conjunction with her HIV therapy could be detrimental, because rifampin induces P450 3A4 and thereby increases the metabolism of protease inhibitors such as saquinavir, thus reducing the therapeutic effectiveness of the protease inhibitor. *Third*, induction of P450s or some of the other biotransformation enzymes can result in the production of toxic levels of reactive drug metabolites, resulting in tissue damage or other adverse effects.

Just as certain compounds can induce P450 enzymes, other compounds can inhibit these enzymes. *An important consequence of enzyme inhibition is the decreased metabolism of drugs that are metabolized by the inhibited enzyme.* Such inhibition can both allow drug levels to reach toxic concentrations and prolong the presence of active drug in the body.

Enzyme inhibition can be achieved in several different ways (Fig. 4-4). For example, **ketoconazole**, a widely used antifungal drug, has a nitrogen moiety that binds to the heme iron in the active site of P450 enzymes; this binding prevents the metabolism of co-administered drugs by competitive inhibition. An example of irreversible inhibition is **secobarbital**, a barbiturate, which alkylates and permanently inactivates the P450 complex. On occasion, the inhibition of P450 enzymes can be used to therapeutic advantage. For example, the protease inhibitor **ritonavir** is highly effective against HIV but has significant gastrointestinal adverse effects that limit its use as a chronic treatment. However, because ritonavir is a potent inhibitor of P450 3A4, it can be used clinically in doses that are below the threshold for gastrointestinal adverse effects but high enough to inhibit P450 3A4. Inhibition of P450 3A4 "boosts" the effective concentrations of other HIV protease inhibitors that are metabolized by this P450 enzyme. For example, lopinavir cannot achieve therapeutic levels as a single agent because of extensive first-pass metabolism, but co-administration with ritonavir allows lopinavir to reach therapeutic concentrations.

Drug transporters can also be induced or inhibited by other drugs. For example, macrolide antibiotics can inhibit MDR1, and this inhibition can lead to increased serum levels of drugs, such as digoxin, that are excreted by MDR1.

MDR1 is also transcriptionally regulated by PXR. Consequently, drugs that induce up-regulation of P450 enzymes via the PXR pathway (e.g., P450 3A4) concomitantly increase transcription of the MDR1 drug transporter.

A detailed list of compounds that can inhibit or induce the common P450 enzymes can be found in Table 4-3. This list is not meant to be exhaustive, but only to highlight common medications that are metabolized by the same P450 enzymes. New drugs are extensively tested for drug interactions, both in the laboratory (in vitro) and in clinical trials, as required by the US Food and Drug Administration.

Active and Toxic Metabolites

Knowing the routes by which therapeutic agents are metabolized can affect the choice of drug to prescribe in a particular clinical situation. This is true both when the metabolite is active, in which case the administered agent may be acting as a **prodrug**, and when the agent has **toxic metabolites** (see Chapter 6, Drug Toxicity).

Prodrugs are inactive compounds that are metabolized by the body into their active, therapeutic forms. One example of a prodrug is the selective estrogen receptor modulator **tamoxifen**; this drug has little activity until it is hydroxylated to become 4-hydroxytamoxifen, a metabolite that is 30- to 100-fold more active than the parent compound. Another example is the angiotensin II receptor antagonist **losartan**; the potency of this drug is increased tenfold upon oxidation of its alcohol group to a carboxylic acid by P450 2C9.

The strategy of selective prodrug activation can be used for therapeutic benefit in cancer chemotherapy. One example of this strategy is the use of **mitomycin C**, a naturally occurring compound that is activated to a powerful DNA alkylating agent after it is *reduced* by several enzymes including a cytochrome P450 *reductase*. Mitomycin C selectively kills hypoxic cancer cells in the core of solid tumors because (1) these cells have increased levels of the cytochrome P450 reductase that activates mitomycin C and (2) reoxidation of the drug is inhibited under hypoxic conditions.

Other examples of toxic metabolites, including the important case of **acetaminophen**, are discussed in Chapter 6.

▌ INDIVIDUAL FACTORS AFFECTING DRUG METABOLISM

For a number of reasons, the rates of biotransformation reactions may vary greatly from one person to another. The most important of these factors are discussed below.

Pharmacogenomics

The effects of genetic variability on drug metabolism are an important part of the new science of pharmacogenomics (see Chapter 7, Pharmacogenomics). Certain populations exhibit polymorphisms or mutations in one or more enzymes of drug metabolism, changing the rates of some of these reactions and eliminating others altogether. These pharmacogenetic differences must be taken into account in therapeutic decision making and drug dosing. Current research uses new technology (e.g., SNP analysis, gene microchips) to understand how genetic differences in the enzymes of drug metabolism affect patient responses to various drugs. Such approaches are already employed extensively in pharmaceutical development and are beginning to be applied in clinical practice.

TABLE 4-3 Some Pharmacologic Substrates, Inhibitors, and Inducers of Cytochrome P450 Enzymes

P450 ENZYME	SUBSTRATES	INHIBITORS	INDUCERS
P450 3A4	**Anti-HIV agents** Indinavir Nelfinavir Ritonavir Saquinavir **Benzodiazepines** Alprazolam Midazolam Triazolam **Calcium channel blockers** Diltiazem Felodipine Nifedipine Verapamil **Immunosuppressants** Cyclosporine Tacrolimus **Macrolide antibiotics** Clarithromycin Erythromycin **Statins** Atorvastatin Lovastatin **Others** Finasteride Loratadine Losartan Quinidine Sildenafil Tadalafil	**Antifungal agents (azoles)** Itraconazole Ketoconazole **Anti-HIV agents** Delavirdine Indinavir Ritonavir Saquinavir **Calcium channel blockers** Diltiazem Verapamil **Macrolide antibiotics** Clarithromycin Erythromycin Troleandomycin (not azithromycin) **Others** Cimetidine Grapefruit juice Mifepristone Nefazodone Norfloxacin	**Antiepileptics** Carbamazepine Oxcarbazepine Phenobarbital Phenytoin **Anti-HIV agents** Efavirenz Nevirapine **Rifamycins** Rifabutin Rifampin Rifapentine **Others** St. John's wort
P450 2D6	**5-HT reuptake inhibitors** Fluoxetine Paroxetine **Antiarrhythmic agents** Flecainide Mexiletine Propafenone **Antidepressants** Amitriptyline Clomipramine Desipramine Imipramine Nortriptyline **Antipsychotics** Haloperidol Perphenazine Risperidone Venlafaxine **Beta-adrenergic antagonists** Alprenolol Bufuralol Carvedilol Metoprolol Penbutolol Propranolol Timolol **Opioids** Codeine Dextromethorphan	**5-HT reuptake inhibitors** Fluoxetine Paroxetine **Antiarrhythmic agents** Amiodarone Quinidine **Antidepressants** Clomipramine **Antipsychotics** Haloperidol	**None identified**

continues

TABLE 4-3 Some Pharmacologic Substrates, Inhibitors, and Inducers of Cytochrome P450 Enzymes *(continued)*

P450 ENZYME	SUBSTRATES	INHIBITORS	INDUCERS
P450 2C19	**Antidepressants** Clomipramine Imipramine **Proton pump inhibitors** Lansoprazole Omeprazole Pantoprazole **Others** Clopidogrel Propranolol R-Warfarin	**Proton pump inhibitors** Omeprazole **Others** Fluoxetine Ritonavir Sertraline	Norethindrone Prednisone Rifampin
P450 2C9	**Angiotensin II receptor antagonists** Irbesartan Losartan **Nonsteroidal anti-inflammatory drugs (NSAIDs)** Ibuprofen Suprofen **Others** S-Warfarin Tamoxifen	**Antifungal agents (azoles)** Fluconazole Miconazole **Others** Amiodarone Phenylbutazone	Rifampin Secobarbital
P450 2E1	**General anesthetics** Enflurane Halothane Isoflurane Methoxyflurane Sevoflurane **Others** Acetaminophen Ethanol	Disulfiram	Ethanol Isoniazid
P450 1A2	**Antidepressants** Amitriptyline Clomipramine Clozapine Imipramine **Others** R-Warfarin Tacrine	**Quinolones** Ciprofloxacin Enoxacin Norfloxacin Ofloxacin **Others** Fluvoxamine	Char-grilled meat Cruciferous vegetables Insulin Omeprazole Tobacco smoke

For example, most pharmaceutical companies avoid development of a drug that is metabolized primarily by a highly polymorphic enzyme, because such polymorphisms may lead to wide interindividual variability in drug response.

One clinically important example of pharmacogenetic variability involves the plasma enzyme cholinesterase. One in every 2,000 Caucasians carries a genetic alteration in cholinesterase, which metabolizes the muscle relaxant **succinylcholine** (among other functions). This altered form of the enzyme has an approximately 1,000-fold reduced affinity for succinylcholine, resulting in slowed elimination and prolonged circulation of the active drug. Should a sufficiently high plasma concentration of succinylcholine be reached, respiratory paralysis and death can occur unless the patient is supported with artificial respiration until the drug is cleared.

A similar situation can occur with **isoniazid**, one of the drugs considered for treatment of Ms. B's tuberculosis. Genetic variability, in the form of a widespread autosomal recessive trait that results in decreased synthesis of an enzyme, causes the metabolism of this drug to be slowed in certain subsets of the US population. The enzyme at issue is *N*-acetyltransferase, which inactivates isoniazid by an acetylation (conjugation) reaction. The "slow acetylator" phenotype is expressed by 45% of whites and blacks in the United States and by some Europeans living in high northern latitudes. The "fast acetylator" phenotype is found in more than 90% of Asians and in Inuits in the United States. Blood levels of isoniazid are elevated fourfold to sixfold in slow acetylators relative to fast acetylators. Moreover, because the free drug acts as an inhibitor of P450 enzymes, slow acetylators are more susceptible to adverse drug interactions. If Ms. B expresses the slow acetylator phenotype and her dose of isoniazid is not decreased accordingly, then the addition of isoniazid to her drug regimen could potentially have a toxic effect.

A third example involves **clopidogrel**, an antiplatelet drug that promotes blood vessel patency after strokes or coronary angioplasty. The loss of efficacy of this medication may lead to re-stenosis or thrombosis of a vessel or stent, often with severe consequences. Clopidogrel is a prodrug that is metabolized to its active form via P450 enzymes, including P450 2C19. Polymorphisms of P450 2C19 have recently been associated with both decreased antiplatelet effect and increased cardiovascular morbidity. In addition, because many proton pump inhibitors are also metabolized by P450 2C19, co-administration of clopidogrel with one of these commonly prescribed medications may lead to a decrease in the plasma levels of active clopidogrel.

Race and Ethnicity

Some genetic aspects of race and/or ethnicity affect drug metabolism. In particular, differences in drug action among races/ethnicities have been attributed to polymorphisms in specific genes. For example, P450 2D6 is functionally inactive in 8% of Caucasian individuals but in only 1% of Asians. Moreover, African Americans have a high frequency of a P450 2D6 allele that encodes an enzyme of reduced activity. These observations are clinically relevant, in that P450 2D6 is responsible for the oxidative metabolism of about 20% of drugs—including many beta-antagonists and tricyclic antidepressants—and for the conversion of codeine to morphine.

In some cases, a polymorphism in the target gene is the basis for racial differences in drug action. The activity of the enzyme vitamin K epoxide reductase (VKORC1), which is the target of the anticoagulant **warfarin**, is affected by single nucleotide polymorphisms (SNPs) that render an individual either more or less sensitive to warfarin and that dictate administration of lower or higher doses of the drug, respectively. In one study, Asian American populations were found to be enriched in haplotypes (inherited combinations of individual base/SNP differences) associated with increased sensitivity to warfarin, while African American populations exhibited haplotypes associated with increased resistance to warfarin. Perhaps the most prominent example of a race-based therapeutic is the combination of fixed-dose **isosorbide dinitrate** and **hydralazine** (also known as *BiDil*). This combination of vasodilators was reported to cause a 43% decrease in mortality in African Americans with heart failure. Although the biochemical basis of this effect is not known, these clinical data demonstrate that race may be a key consideration in choosing drug treatments and doses.

Age and Gender

Drug metabolism can also differ among individuals as a result of age and gender differences. Many reactions of biotransformation are slowed in both young children and the elderly. At birth, neonates are capable of carrying out many but not all oxidative reactions; however, most of these drug-metabolizing enzyme systems mature gradually over the first 2 weeks of life and throughout childhood. Recall that neonatal jaundice results from a deficiency of the bilirubin-conjugating enzyme UDPGT. Another example of a conjugating enzyme deficiency that puts infants at risk for toxicity is the so-called **gray baby syndrome**. *Haemophilus influenzae* infections in infants were once treated with the antibiotic **chloramphenicol**; excretion of this drug requires an oxidative transformation followed by a conjugation reaction. The oxidation metabolite of chloramphenicol is toxic; if this metabolite fails to undergo conjugation, it can build up in the plasma and may reach toxic concentrations. Toxic levels of the metabolite can cause neonates to experience shock and circulatory collapse, leading to the pallor and cyanosis that give the syndrome its name.

In the elderly, a general decrease in metabolic capacity is observed. As a result, particular care must be taken in prescribing drugs for this segment of the population. The elderly's decline in metabolic capacity has been attributed to age-related decreases in liver mass, hepatic blood flow, and possibly hepatic enzyme activity. Another therapeutic consideration is that the elderly are frequently taking multiple medications, with a consequent increase in the risk of drug–drug interactions.

There is some evidence for gender differences in drug metabolism, although the mechanisms are not well understood and data from experimental animals have not been particularly illuminating. Decreased oxidation of ethanol, estrogens, benzodiazepines, and salicylates has been reported anecdotally in women relative to men and may be related to androgenic hormone levels.

Diet and Environment

Both diet and environment can alter drug metabolism by inducing or inhibiting enzymes of the P450 system. An interesting example is grapefruit juice. The psoralen derivatives and flavonoids in grapefruit juice inhibit both P450 3A4 and MDR1 in the small intestine. Inhibition of P450 3A4 significantly decreases the first-pass metabolism of co-administered drugs that are also metabolized by this enzyme, and inhibition of MDR1 significantly increases the absorption of co-administered drugs that are substrates for export (efflux) by this enzyme. The **grapefruit juice effect** is important when grapefruit juice is ingested together with drugs that are acted upon by these enzymes. Such drugs include some protease inhibitors, macrolide antibiotics, HMG-CoA reductase inhibitors (statins), and calcium channel blockers. **Saquinavir** is one of the protease inhibitors that is both metabolized by P450 3A4 and exported by MDR1. In the case that opens this chapter, Ms. B should be alerted to the fact that the simultaneous ingestion of grapefruit juice and saquinavir could inadvertently lead to toxic serum levels of the protease inhibitor.

Herbal medications can also have significant effects on the P450 system. One such example is **St. John's wort**, a popular herbal preparation used for mood stabilization. Many observational studies have noted that St. John's wort can induce P450 expression and thereby decrease the efficacy of other drugs. Compounds from herbs and spices may also inhibit P450s. One example is piperine (the essential chemical in black pepper), which has been shown to inhibit P450 3A4 and the MDR protein in animal models; the clinical importance of this effect remains uncertain.

Because many endogenous substances used in the conjugation reactions are ultimately derived from the diet (and also require energy for the production of the appropriate cofactors), nutrition can affect drug metabolism by altering the pool of such substances available to the conjugating enzymes. Pollutant exposures can produce similarly dramatic effects on drug metabolism; one common example is the AhR-mediated P450 enzyme induction by polycyclic aromatic hydrocarbons in cigarette smoke.

Metabolic Drug Interactions

Drugs can potentially affect oral bioavailability, plasma protein binding, hepatic metabolism, and renal excretion of co-administered drugs. Among the categories of drug–drug interactions, the effects on biotransformation have special clinical importance. The concept of P450 enzyme induction and inhibition has already been introduced. A common clinical situation that must take this type of drug–drug interaction into consideration is the prescription of certain antibiotics to women who are already using hormonal contraception. For example, enzyme induction by the antibiotic **rifampin** can cause estrogen-based hormonal contraception to be ineffective at standard doses because P450 3A4 is induced by rifampin and this is the main enzyme involved in the metabolism of the common estrogenic component 17α-ethynylestradiol. In this situation, other means of birth control should be recommended during the course of rifampin therapy. Ms. B should be made aware of this interaction if rifampin is added to her therapeutic regimen. Another phenomenon associated with enzyme induction is **tolerance**, which can occur when a drug induces its own metabolism and thus reduces its efficacy over time (see the discussion of carbamazepine above and the discussion of tolerance in Chapter 19, Pharmacology of Drugs of Abuse).

Because drugs are often prescribed in combination with other pharmaceuticals, careful attention should be paid to drugs that are metabolized by the same hepatic enzymes. The concomitant administration of two or more drugs that are metabolized by the same enzyme will generally result in higher serum levels of the drugs. The mechanisms of drug–drug interaction can involve competitive substrate inhibition, allosteric inhibition, or irreversible enzyme inactivation; in any case, drug levels can increase acutely, possibly leading to deleterious results. For example, **erythromycin** is metabolized by P450 3A4, but the resulting nitrosoalkane metabolite can form a complex with P450 3A4 and inhibit the enzyme. This inhibition can lead to potentially fatal drug–drug interactions. A notable example is the interaction between erythromycin and **cisapride**, a drug that stimulates GI tract motility. Toxic concentrations of cisapride can inhibit hERG potassium channels in the heart and thereby induce potentially fatal cardiac arrhythmias; for this reason, cisapride was withdrawn from the market in 2000. Before its withdrawal, cisapride was often well tolerated as a single agent. However, because cisapride is metabolized by P450 3A4, when the activity of P450 3A4 was compromised due to the concomitant administration of erythromycin or another inhibitor of P450 3A4, serum cisapride concentrations could increase to levels associated with arrhythmia induction.

In other cases, drug interactions may be beneficial. For example, as noted above, the ingestion of **methanol** (a component of wood alcohol) can result in blindness or death because its metabolites (formaldehyde, an embalming agent, and formic acid, a component of ant venom) are highly toxic. One treatment for methanol poisoning is the administration of **ethanol**, which competes with methanol for oxidation by alcohol dehydrogenase (and, to a lesser extent, by P450 2E1). The resulting delay in oxidation allows the methanol to be cleared renally before its toxic byproducts can form in the liver.

Diseases Affecting Drug Metabolism

Many disease states can affect the rate and extent of drug metabolism in the body. Because the liver is the main site of biotransformation, many liver diseases significantly compromise drug metabolism. Hepatitis, cirrhosis, cancer, hemochromatosis, and fatty infiltration of the liver each impair

cytochrome P450s and other hepatic enzymes that are crucial to drug metabolism. As a result of this slowed metabolism, the levels of the active forms of many drugs may be significantly higher than intended and thereby cause toxic effects. Thus, the doses of many drugs may need to be lowered for individuals with hepatic disease.

Concomitant cardiac disease can also affect drug metabolism. The rate of metabolism of many drugs, such as the antiarrhythmic lidocaine and the opioid morphine, is dependent on drug delivery to the liver via the bloodstream. Because blood flow is commonly compromised in cardiac disease, there must be heightened awareness of the potential for supratherapeutic levels of drugs in patients with heart failure. In addition, some antihypertensive agents selectively reduce blood flow to the liver and can thereby increase the half-life of a drug such as lidocaine, leading to potentially toxic levels.

Thyroid hormone regulates the basal metabolic rate of the body, which, in turn, affects drug metabolism. Hyperthyroidism can increase the rate of metabolism of some drugs, whereas hypothyroidism can do the opposite. Other conditions, such as pulmonary disease, endocrine dysfunction, and diabetes, are also thought to affect drug metabolism, but the mechanisms for these effects are not yet completely understood.

▌ CONCLUSION AND FUTURE DIRECTIONS

This chapter has reviewed a number of issues relating to drug metabolism, including the sites of biotransformation, the transport and enzymatic metabolism of drugs at those sites, and individual factors that can affect those reactions. The case of Ms. B illustrates the clinical implications of drug metabolism, including the possible influences of ethnicity and drug–drug interactions on pharmacologic therapy. Understanding drug metabolism, and particularly the interactions of drugs within the body, allows the principles of biotransformation to be applied in the design and use of therapeutics. As pharmacogenomics and rational drug design lead pharmacology research into the future, increased understanding of biotransformation will also render the pharmacologic treatment of disease more individualized, efficacious, and safe. This topic is discussed in Chapter 7.

Acknowledgment

We thank Cullen Taniguchi for his valuable contributions to this chapter in the Second and Third Editions of *Principles of Pharmacology: The Pathophysiologic Basis of Drug Therapy*.

Suggested Reading

Burchard EG, Ziv E, Coyle N, et al. The importance of race and ethnic background in biomedical research and practice. *N Engl J Med* 2003;348:1170–1175. (*Current understanding regarding ethnic variability in response to drug administration.*)

Gong IY, Kim RB. Impact of genetic variation in OATP transporters to drug disposition and response. *Drug Metab Pharmacokinet* 2013;28:4–18. (*Review of the crucial role played by drug transporters in drug metabolism.*)

Johansson I, Ingelman-Sundberg M. Genetic polymorphism and toxicology—with emphasis on cytochrome P450. *Toxicol Sci* 2011;120:1–13. (*Review of toxicity issues with some drugs and the role of P450 variations.*)

Katsanis SH, Javitt G, Hudson K. Public health. A case study of personalized medicine. *Science* 2008;320:53–54. (*A discussion of aspects of the use of personalized medicine, including roles of P450 genes.*)

Kirchheiner J, Seeringer A. Clinical implications of pharmacogenetics of cytochrome P450 drug metabolizing enzymes. *Biochim Biophys Acta* 2007;1770:489–494. (*Discussion of clinical issues with several drugs and P450s.*)

Mega JL, Close SL, Wiviott SD, et al. Cytochrome P450 polymorphisms and response to clopidogrel. *N Engl J Med* 2009;360:354–362. (*Example of P450 genetic polymorphisms and clinical efficacy of clopidogrel.*)

Rendic S, Guengerich FP. Survey of human oxidoreductases and cytochrome P450 enzymes involved in the metabolism of xenobiotic and natural chemicals. *Chem Res Toxicol* 2015;28:38–42. (*Analysis of fractions of drugs metabolized by different cytochrome P450 enzymes.*)

Seden K, Dickinson L, Khoo S, Back D. Grapefruit-drug interactions. *Drugs* 2010;70:2373–2407. (*Review of P450 interactions with grapefruit.*)

Shi S, Klotz U. Drug interactions with herbal medicines. *Clin Pharmacokinet* 2012;51:77–104. (*Review of P450 interactions with herbal medicines.*)

Wienkers L, Pearson P, eds. *Handbook of drug metabolism.* 2nd ed. New York: Marcel Dekker; 2009. (*Collection of articles on aspects of drug metabolism.*)

Wilke RA, Lin DW, Roden DM, et al. Identifying genetic risk factors for serious adverse reactions: current progress and challenges. *Nat Rev Drug Discov* 2007;6:904–916. (*Review of current status of use of genetics for predicting adverse reactions.*)

Wilkinson GR. Drug metabolism and variability among patients in drug response. *N Engl J Med* 2005;352:2211–2221. (*An excellent basic review of the P450 system and drug–drug interactions.*)

Zhang D, Zhu M, Humphreys WG, eds. *Drug metabolism in drug design and development: basic concepts and practice.* Hoboken, NJ: John Wiley & Sons; 2007. (*Drug metabolism as it pertains to development of new pharmaceuticals.*)

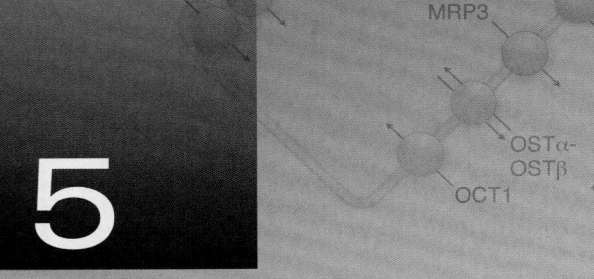

5

Drug Transporters

Baran A. Ersoy and Keith A. Hoffmaster

INTRODUCTION

Membrane transporters are proteins that facilitate the transport of soluble small molecules across lipid bilayers. These transporters regulate the tissue and plasma distribution as well as the excretion of drugs and endogenous compounds and therefore affect their pharmacokinetic profile (i.e., absorption, distribution, metabolism, and excretion). Transporters are generally classified as **uptake** or **efflux** proteins depending on the direction in which they move substrates across the membranes of cells. They include several protein families that exhibit broad substrate specificity and tissue distribution. The function of transporters depends on the tissue in which they are expressed as well as their subcellular localization to the apical or basolateral membrane (Fig. 5-1). Whereas transporters expressed in organs of elimination (e.g., liver or kidney) can facilitate the clearance of drugs and/or metabolites from the systemic circulation, efflux transporters in non-eliminating organs such as the central nervous system and placenta primarily function to minimize the exposure of the brain and the developing fetus, respectively, to potentially harmful exogenous substrates. In some cases, intestinal efflux transporters expressed at the apical membrane of the enterocyte can limit the oral bioavailability of drugs; in other cases, uptake transporters expressed at this membrane can aid in the systemic absorption of compounds, thereby enhancing their oral bioavailability. Transporter function in the liver often facilitates drug clearance, but efficient active uptake into the liver after an oral dose can also affect drug bioavailability by contributing to first-pass hepatic metabolism and elimination. Because drugs can both inhibit and induce transporters, concurrent administration of multiple drugs may alter the pharmacokinetics and pharmacodynamics of the other compounds depending on transporter affinity, specificity, and alternate mechanisms of drug disposition. Therefore, identifying the specific transporter(s) for which a novel drug is a substrate (or inhibitor) may not only help to devise optimization and formulation strategies that improve drug bioavailability and efficacy, but may also prevent adverse effects by anticipating and limiting drug–drug interactions. There are over 400 transporters in the human genome. This chapter provides an overview of this effective but complex system by focusing on a select number of well-characterized transporters involved in drug disposition and in the flux of endogenous substrates and on those that may become the sites of drug–drug interactions.

The Human Genome Organisation (HUGO) Gene Nomenclature Committee (HGNC) has approved standard acronyms for both solute carrier (SLC) and ATP-binding cassette (ABC) families of transporters. However, many drug transporters, especially those discussed in greater detail in this chapter, were initially cloned and named based on their pharmacologic attributes such as substrate specificity and association with drug resistance. For instance, the ABCB1 gene was originally named and is more commonly referred to as P-glycoprotein (P-gp) because it was initially identified as a glycoprotein that controls cell membrane permeability (P). Ensuing studies have also led to its characterization as a multidrug resistance (MDR) protein encoded by the MDR1 gene. Therefore, P-gp, MDR1, and ABCB1 are all synonyms for the same transporter. In this chapter, the transporters are referred to using popular names, with HGNC nomenclature

CASE

Mr. H is a 47-year-old mildly overweight man who comes to the walk-in clinic complaining of muscle pain and weakness in his arms and legs. He has been taking a statin medication for the past 4 years and has been able to manage his cholesterol levels effectively with this medication and diet modifications. When asked about any recent changes to his medications or diet, he indicates that his primary care physician started him 3 weeks ago on medical therapy to help control his triglyceride levels. In addition to the recent muscle pain, Mr. H has noticed a mild rash on his torso over the past 3 weeks since starting the new medication prescribed to help control his triglycerides.

Questions

1. Without knowing the specific medications that Mr. H is taking, which drug–drug interactions do you suspect might be contributing to his new symptoms?
2. Consultation with Mr. H's primary care physician reveals that Mr. H is also taking a fixed-dose combination of lopinavir/ritonavir to manage his HIV infection. How might this complicate the drug–drug interaction suspected in question 1?

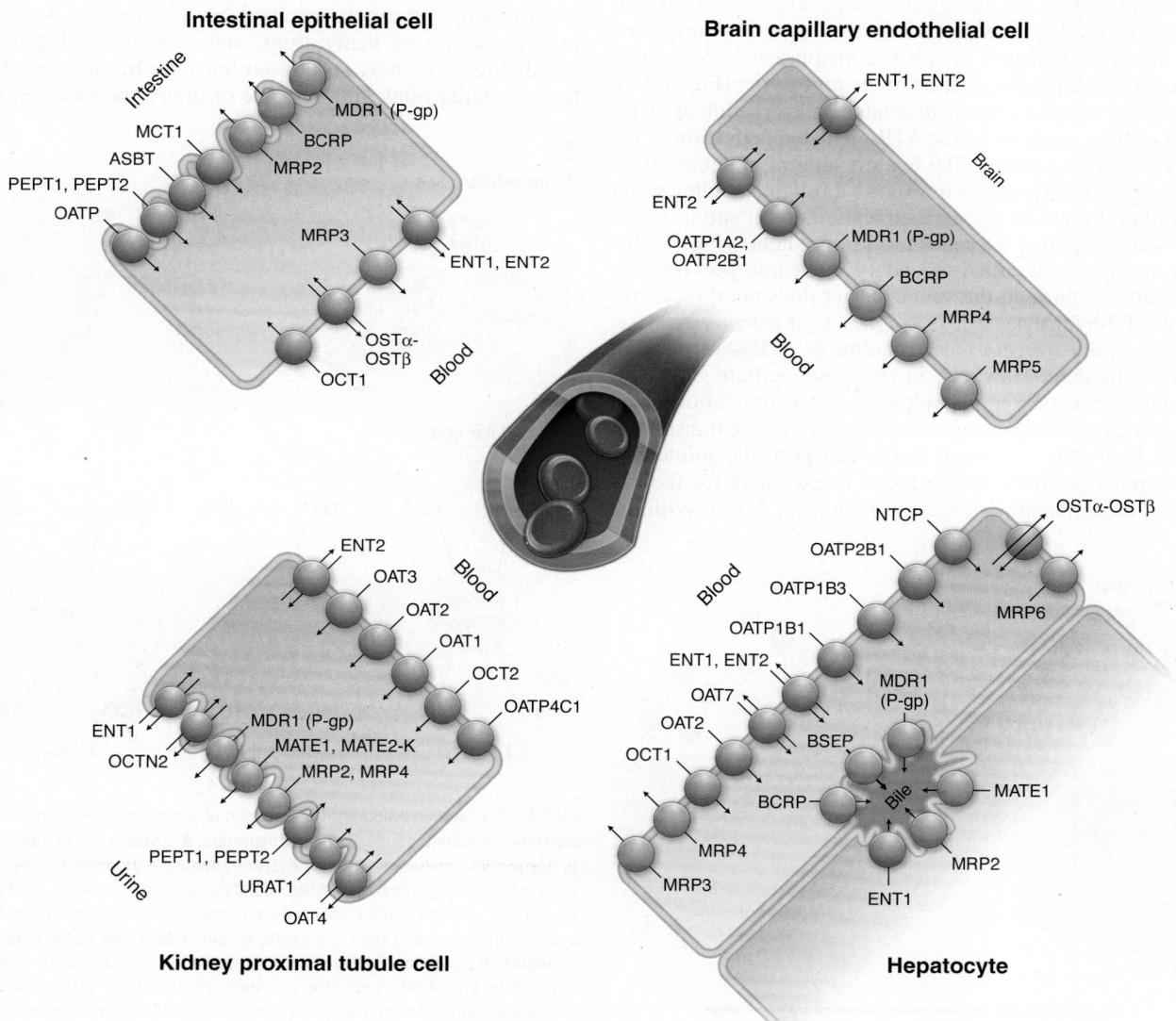

FIGURE 5-1. Major transporters of drugs and endogenous compounds in the intestine, kidney, liver, and blood–brain barrier. Uptake transporters are shown in blue and efflux transporters are shown in red. Bidirectional transport is denoted by double arrows. See text for abbreviations.

and other acronyms stated in parentheses. Additional details on nomenclature and synonyms/previous names can be found at http://www.genenames.org/genefamilies/ABC and http://www.genenames.org/genefamilies/SLC.

UPTAKE AND EFFLUX TRANSPORTERS

Drugs and endogenous compounds cross cellular membrane barriers by simple diffusion, passive transport, or active transport. Simple diffusion (also called *passive diffusion*) can occur when small, partially water-soluble solutes such as certain polar lipids pass freely through a membrane bilayer, driven by their concentration gradient across the membrane (Fig. 5-2). However, many molecules require the assistance of membrane transporters to move across membranes. Solute carriers facilitate the passive transport of substrates down their concentration gradient (Fig. 5-3). In contrast, the transport of substrates against their concentration gradient requires active transporters (Fig. 5-4). *Primary active transport* utilizes the energy of hydrolysis of adenosine triphosphate (ATP); the substrate first binds to the transporter, and substrate transport across the membrane is completed upon ATP-mediated activation of the transporter (Fig. 5-4A). *Secondary active transport* depends on the creation of an inward sodium gradient by the ATP-mediated activation of the Na^+/K^+-ATPase pump. The inward sodium gradient drives the coupled transport (co-transport) through a solute carrier of sodium (down its electrochemical gradient) and of a second solute (against its concentration gradient) (Fig. 5-4B). This mechanism is called secondary active transport because the transport through the solute carrier does not directly require ATP hydrolysis but is coupled to a primary ATPase. *Tertiary active transport* also requires an ATPase-dependent sodium gradient. However, in this case, sodium influx facilitates the diffusion and intracellular accumulation of an anion such as bicarbonate via a secondary active transporter. In the final step of tertiary active transport, the solute carrier exports the intracellular anion in exchange for the uptake of an extracellular organic anion (Fig. 5-4B). With the

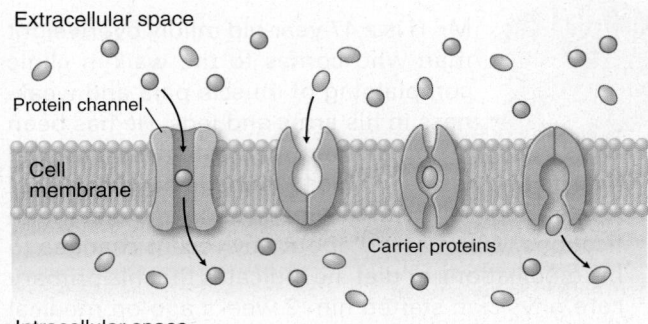

FIGURE 5-3. Passive transport. In this process, protein channels or carrier proteins facilitate the transport of substrates down their concentration gradient.

exception of OSTα-OSTβ (which transports bile acids; see below), all known uptake transporters lack ATPase activity and belong to the solute carrier (SLC) family. Secondary or tertiary active transport mechanisms are required for cellular absorption of many drugs, nutrients, and endogenous metabolites. The next section outlines the transporters that have essential roles in the uptake of drugs and endogenous

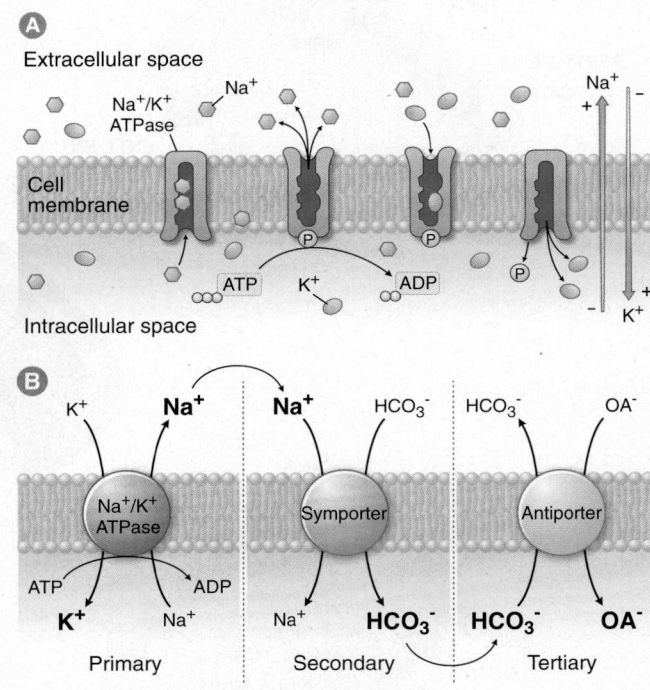

FIGURE 5-4. Active transport. The transport of substrates against their concentration gradient requires active transporters. **A. Primary active transport.** In this process, the energy of hydrolysis of adenosine triphosphate (ATP) is used to transport solutes against their concentration gradients; for example, the Na^+/K^+-ATPase pump drives sodium (outward) and potassium (inward) against their concentration gradients. **B. Secondary and tertiary active transport.** In secondary active transport, the creation of an inward sodium gradient by the ATPase-mediated activation of the Na^+/K^+-ATPase drives the coupled transport (co-transport) through a solute carrier (symporter) of sodium (down its concentration gradient) and a second solute (against its concentration gradient). Here, the second solute is bicarbonate (HCO_3^-). In tertiary active transport, a second solute carrier (antiporter) facilitates the export of the second solute (here, HCO_3^-) in exchange for the uptake of an extracellular organic anion (OA^-). Font size reflects the relative concentration of the solute in the extracellular space and the intracellular space.

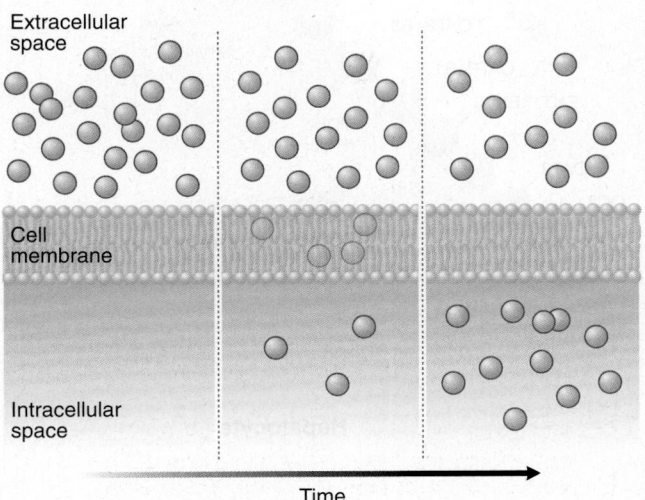

FIGURE 5-2. Simple diffusion. In this process, small, partially water-soluble solutes pass freely through a membrane bilayer, driven by their concentration gradient across the membrane. This process is also called *passive diffusion.*

compounds in key tissues that are involved in the absorption, distribution, and elimination of drugs. These tissues include the intestine, liver, kidney, and endothelial cells of the blood–brain barrier.

Uptake Transporters

Organic Anion-Transporting Polypeptide (OATP) Family

OATPs (SLCO, former SLC21) are expressed in all epithelial cells. These transporters facilitate the uptake of large hydrophobic and amphiphilic organic compounds, such as bile acids, thyroid hormones, conjugated steroids, and eicosanoids (Table 5-1). Although OATPs are primarily responsible for the transport of anionic compounds, some members of the OATP family transport bulky type II organic cations such as rocuronium. The accumulation of substrates such as bile acids within the liver is a concentrating process, and OATPs move substrates into cells by a tertiary active transport mechanism. Of the 11 family members, 5 have been implicated in the transport of xenobiotics. OATP1B1, OATP1B3, and OATP2B1 mediate the uptake of drugs (e.g., **statins**) across the sinusoidal membrane of hepatocytes, whereupon the drugs can be metabolized by enzymes such as cytochrome P450s (CYPs) and/or secreted into the bile or back into the systemic circulation (Fig. 5-1). Inhibition of hepatic OATPs has been implicated as a potential mechanism of drug–drug interactions. The potential for these interactions has resulted in revised dosing guidelines for some statins when they are administered with drugs that inhibit OATPs (e.g., **cyclosporine**, **gemfibrozil**, **lopinavir/ritonavir**). OATP1A2 is ubiquitously expressed and contributes primarily to drug absorption from the intestinal lumen into intestinal epithelial cells. OATP4C1 facilitates the uptake of drugs such as **digoxin** from the circulation into kidney proximal tubule cells, from which the drugs are eliminated via the urine (Fig. 5-1).

In the introductory case, Mr. H was most likely started on a drug that inhibited the hepatic uptake of his statin, and thereby increased the systemic bioavailability of the statin, via a transporter-related drug–drug interaction. Fibrates such as **gemfibrozil** are commonly used to reduce triglyceride levels when statins and diet modification prove insufficient. Concurrent administration of statins with gemfibrozil can cause myopathy, however, in part due to inhibition of OATP1B1-mediated hepatic uptake of statins by gemfibrozil. This drug–drug interaction results in increased blood levels of the statin and consequent systemic toxicity. Mr. H was also taking a fixed dose of lopinavir/ritonavir, which is an inhibitor of OATP1B1- and OATP1B3-mediated drug uptake into the liver; this combination of HIV protease inhibitors may have further contributed to drug–drug interactions and exacerbated systemic adverse effects of Mr. H's statin after initiation of treatment for hypertriglyceridemia.

Organic Anion Transporter (OAT) Family

OATs, which belong to the SLC22A family, mediate the cellular uptake of small organic anions such as conjugated steroids, biogenic amines, and cGMP as well as a broad range of xenobiotics such as antivirals, antibiotics, ACE inhibitors, and anticancer drugs (Table 5-1). Despite their classification as uptake transporters, OAT isoforms 1–4 and 7 have essential roles in drug clearance by facilitating the uptake of drugs from the systemic circulation into the liver and kidneys, where they can be metabolized and excreted (Fig. 5-1). Uptake of anions into cells against their electrochemical gradient requires OATs to function as tertiary active transporters. OAT1, OAT3, and OAT4 exchange intracellular 2-oxoglutarate, and OAT7 exports intracellular short-chain fatty acids such as butyrate in exchange for their extracellular substrates. OAT1, OAT2, and OAT3 clear many organic anions from the systemic circulation into the kidney proximal tubule, from which the anions are eliminated in the urine. OAT2 and OAT7 are expressed mainly on the sinusoidal membrane of hepatocytes. Unlike OAT1, OAT2, and OAT3, OAT4 and the urate anion exchanger 1 (URAT1) are expressed on the apical (brush border) membrane of the kidney proximal tubule, where they mediate the reabsorption of uric acid from urine. Therefore, drugs that inhibit OAT4 and URAT1 may decrease blood uric acid levels and thereby provide therapeutic benefit (e.g., in the treatment of gout by the URAT1 inhibitor **probenecid**; see Chapter 49, Integrative Inflammation Pharmacology: Gout) and may potentially cause enhanced elimination of OAT4 substrates.

Organic Cation Transporter (OCT) Family

Like OATs, OCTs belong to the SLC22A family and contribute to the renal clearance of xenobiotics such as antiviral drugs. OCTs also mediate the transport of a diverse group of small organic cations such as catecholamines, hormones, and neurotransmitters (Table 5-1). Transport of cations by OCTs occurs down the electrochemical gradient of the solute and does not depend on ATP hydrolysis or ion exchange; instead, the transport is thought to be driven by differences in membrane potential. OCT isoforms can have overlapping substrates, and the transport of solutes can be bidirectional depending on the electrochemical gradient. There is strong evidence for the roles of OCT1, OCT2, and OCT3 in drug disposition (Table 5-1; Fig. 5-1). OCT1 is highly expressed in the sinusoidal (basolateral) membrane of hepatocytes. OCT2 is expressed mostly in the kidney proximal tubule and it contributes to the uptake of metabolites from the blood into the tubule. In contrast, OCT3 exhibits broad tissue distribution; its highest expression is in the intestine, liver, and kidney, where it facilitates intestinal absorption and hepatic and renal secretion of drugs, respectively. All three transporters mediate the uptake of a wide array of therapeutic agents, including sedatives, antidepressants, β-blockers, and antidiabetic drugs such as **metformin**. OCTs are also an important site of drug–drug interactions. In certain cases, OCT-mediated renal uptake can contribute to the adverse effects of nephrotoxic drugs, which can be prevented by the concomitant administration of an OCT inhibitor.

Bile Acid Transporters

A significant fraction of bile acids are recycled via three main transporter mechanisms in the liver and gastrointestinal (GI) tract. Na^+/taurocholate co-transporting polypeptide (NTCP, SLC10A1) is exclusively expressed at the sinusoidal membrane of hepatocytes and is a key mechanism in the transport of conjugated and unconjugated bile acids from the circulation into the liver (Fig. 5-1). Whereas OATPs are responsible for the sodium-independent uptake of bile acids, NTCP is responsible for sodium-dependent secondary active bile acid transport that is coupled to the activation of Na^+/K^+-ATPase. In addition to bile acids, NTCP mediates

TABLE 5-1 Uptake Transporters

TRANSPORTER	ORGAN/LOCATION (SEE FIG. 5-1)	ENDOGENOUS SUBSTRATES	DRUG SUBSTRATES	INHIBITORS
OATP1B1 (SLCO1B1)	Hepatocytes (sinusoidal)	Steroid hormones, thyroid hormones, bilirubin glucuronide, bilirubin, bile acids, prostaglandin E2	Repaglinide, valsartan, olmesartan, cerivastatin, pitavastatin, rosuvastatin, temocaprilat, enalapril	Saquinavir, ritonavir, lopinavir, rifampicin, cyclosporine, gemfibrozil, clarithromycin
OATP1B3 (SLCO1B3)	Hepatocytes (sinusoidal)	Steroid hormones, bile acids	Pitavastatin, rosuvastatin, fexofenadine, valsartan, telmisartan, olmesartan, enalapril, erythromycin, valsartan	Rifampicin, cyclosporine, ritonavir, lopinavir, erythromycin
OATP1A2 (SLCO1A2)	Brain, kidney, liver, intestine, endothelium	Bile salts, cholic acid, DHEAS, prostaglandin E2, taurocholate, bilirubin, conjugated steroids, peptides	Aliskiren, erythromycin, fexofenadine, imatinib, levofloxacin, lopinavir, methotrexate, rosuvastatin, pitavastatin, ouabain, saquinavir, sulfobromophthalein, unoprostone, acebutolol, atenolol, atrasentan, celiprolol, sotalol, talinolol, tebipenem, digoxin	Naringin, hesperidin, quercetin, ritonavir, lopinavir, saquinavir, rifampicin, rifamycin, verapamil, apigenin
OATP2B1 (SLCO2B1)	Hepatocytes (sinusoidal), placenta, heart, brain, kidney, lung, small intestine, endothelium	Bile acids, steroid hormones, taurocholate	Glyburide, rosuvastatin, fexofenadine, bosentan, rifampicin	Rifampin, cyclosporine, naringin, hesperidin, quercetin
OAT1 (SLC22A6)	Kidney proximal tubule, placenta	Uric acid, folate, cyclic nucleotides, prostaglandins E2 and F2α	Adefovir, cidofovir, zidovudine, lamivudine, zalcitabine, acyclovir, tenofovir, ciprofloxacin, cephaloridine, methotrexate, pravastatin	Probenecid, novobiocin
OAT3 (SLC22A8)	Kidney proximal tubule, choroid plexus, blood–brain barrier	Uric acid, bile acids, prostaglandins	Nonsteroidal anti-inflammatory drugs (NSAIDs), fexofenadine, methotrexate, ceftizoxime, cefaclor	Probenecid, novobiocin
OCT1 (SLC22A1)	Hepatocytes (sinusoidal), intestine (apical), neurons	Choline, acetylcholine, monoamine neurotransmitters	Metformin, oxaliplatin, acyclovir, ganciclovir	Quinine, quinidine, disopyramide, cimetidine, atropine, prazosin
OCT2 (SLC22A2)	Kidney proximal tubule, neurons	Choline, acetylcholine, monoamine neurotransmitters, creatinine, bile acids	Metformin, pindolol, procainamide, ranitidine, amantadine, amiloride, oxaliplatin, varenicline, cisplatin, debrisoquine, propranolol, guanidine, D-tubocurarine, pancuronium	Cimetidine, pilsicainide, cetirizine, testosterone, quinidine, rifampicin, naringin, ritonavir
OCT3 (SLC22A3)	Liver, kidney, placenta, small intestine	Creatinine, guanidine, neurotransmitters, hormones	Atropine, prazosin, diphenhydramine, ranitidine, amantadine, ketamine, memantine, phencyclidine, nicotine, clonidine, dizocilpine, metformin, cimetidine, verapamil, procainamide, D-amphetamine	Cimetidine, quinidine, rifampicin, prazosin, phenoxybenzamine, corticosterone, progesterone, β-estradiol
PEPT1 (SLC15A1)	Kidney proximal tubule, intestinal enterocytes	Dipeptides and tripeptides	Cephalexin, cefadroxil, bestatin, enalapril, captopril, valacyclovir, β-lactam antibiotics, ACE inhibitors	Glycylproline, 4-aminomethylbenzoic acid
PEPT2 (SLC15A2)	Kidney proximal tubule, choroid plexus, lung	Dipeptides, tripeptides	Cephalexin, cefadroxil, ubenimex, valacyclovir, enalapril, captopril, β-lactam antibiotics, ACE inhibitors	Zofenopril, fosinopril, cefadroxil, captopril, losartan

TRANSPORTER	ORGAN/LOCATION (SEE FIG. 5-1)	ENDOGENOUS SUBSTRATES	DRUG SUBSTRATES	INHIBITORS
NTCP (SLC10A1)	Hepatocytes (sinusoidal)	Taurocholate, bile salts, steroids, thyroid hormones	Rosuvastatin	Cyclosporine, gemfibrozil, propranolol, furosemide, ketoconazole, rifamycin, glibenclamide, ritonavir, bosentan, efavirenz, saquinavir
ASBT (SLC10A2)	Intestine	Taurocholate, bile acids	Dimeric bile acid analogues	Dihydropyridine, calcium channel blockers, statins
OSTα-OSTβ	Intestine (apical), hepatocytes (sinusoidal)	Bile acids	Digoxin, rosuvastatin	Rifamycin SV

Data compiled from: Giacomini KM, Huang SM, Tweedie DJ, et al.; International Transporter Consortium. Membrane transporters in drug development. *Nat Rev Drug Discov* 2010;9:215–236. Knowledge Center, Solvo Biotechnology; http://www.solvobiotech.com/knowledge-center. König J, Müller F, Fromm MF. Transporter and drug–drug interactions: important determinants of drug disposition and effects. *Pharmacol Rev* 2013;65:944–966. US Food and Drug Administration. Drug development and drug interactions: table of substrates, inhibitors, and inducers. http://www.fda.gov/drugs/developmentapprovalprocess/developmentresources/druginteractionslabeling/ucm093664.htm.

partial uptake of some statins (e.g., **rosuvastatin**; Table 5-1). The apical sodium-dependent bile acid transporter (ASBT, SLC10A2) is expressed at the apical membrane of the epithelial cells of the distal small intestine and mediates the uptake of bile acids from the intestinal lumen (Fig. 5-1, Table 5-1). OSTα-OSTβ is the only uptake transporter that does not belong to the SLC family. It comprises a heterodimer of two different subunits and can function as either an efflux transporter or an uptake transporter depending on the electrochemical gradient of its substrates. However, the major function of the transporter is to contribute to the enterohepatic recirculation of bile acids: OSTα-OSTβ mediates the efflux of bile acids and conjugated steroids from intestinal epithelia into the circulation, from which the bile acids are taken up by hepatocytes (Fig. 5-1, Table 5-1).

Peptide Transporter (PEPT) Family

PEPT family transporters (SLC15A) are proton-driven symporters that are highly expressed in the intestine and kidney. PEPT1 has a key role in the absorption of dietary nitrogen, in the form of dipeptides and tripeptides, from the lumen of the small intestine into enterocytes. Peptide-like metabolites or drugs such as β-lactam antibiotics and ACE inhibitors exhibit high bioavailability due largely to PEPT1-mediated absorption (Table 5-1). Both PEPT1 and PEPT2 are expressed in the kidney, where they mediate reuptake of small peptides at the apical membrane of the kidney proximal tubule and regulate systemic nitrogen balance (Fig. 5-1).

Concentrative and Equilibrative Nucleoside Transporter (CNT and ENT) Families

CNT (SLC28) family members CNT1, CNT2, and CNT3 mediate sodium-dependent uptake of nucleosides by epithelial cells. CNT1 and CNT2 specifically transport pyrimidine and purine nucleosides, respectively, whereas CNT3 is capable of transporting both classes of nucleosides. In contrast, ENT (SLC29) family members provide bidirectional transport of purine and pyrimidine nucleosides. The direction of ENT-mediated transport depends on the concentration gradient of the nucleosides and functions to equilibrate extracellular and intracellular nucleoside levels. Whereas intracellular nucleoside accumulation contributes to nucleotide synthesis, CNT- and ENT-mediated nucleoside uptake may also limit the activation of extracellular nucleoside signaling events, such as the activation of adenosine receptors. In addition to endogenous nucleosides, CNTs and ENTs transport nucleoside analogues such as cytotoxic anticancer (e.g., **gemcitabine**) and antiviral (e.g., **zidovudine**) drugs. Therefore, factors or compounds that reduce the expression or activity of these transporters on target tissues may reduce the efficacy of nucleoside anticancer and antiviral drugs.

Glucose Transporters

The glucose transporter family (GLUT, SLC2) regulates the distribution of glucose between the plasma and tissues. Among the several family members, GLUT1–4 isoforms are the most studied and most relevant to glucose metabolism. GLUT1 has broad tissue expression and is responsible for sustaining basal cellular glucose levels with a slow uptake rate. GLUT2 is expressed in the organs that participate in the regulation of plasma glucose levels, such as kidney, liver, intestine, and pancreas. GLUT2 mediates the uptake of dietary glucose in the intestine. Because it has relatively low affinity for glucose, GLUT2 acts as a sensor for glucose levels within the pancreatic beta cells that secrete insulin in response to increases in plasma glucose. GLUT2 exhibits bidirectional transport capability, allowing for the influx or efflux of glucose across the cell membrane. The efflux transporter activity of GLUT2 at the sinusoidal membrane of hepatocytes is essential for the transport of glucose produced in the liver into the plasma in order to maintain plasma glucose homeostasis during starvation or fasting. GLUT3 is enriched in neurons; it exhibits high relative affinity for glucose in order to provide a constant influx of glucose from the circulation into neuronal cells, even at low plasma glucose concentrations. GLUT4 mediates insulin-sensitive glucose uptake and storage in the adipose tissue and striated muscle. Under conditions of low plasma insulin concentrations, such as fasting, GLUT4 is sequestered in intracellular vesicles and does not transport glucose. Insulin stimulation causes GLUT4 to translocate to the plasma membrane, where it initiates glucose uptake (see Fig. 31-4).

Sodium glucose transport protein (SGLT, SLC5) family members 1 and 2 are symporters that transport glucose against its concentration gradient via a secondary active mechanism. SGLT1 at the intestinal brush border and SGLT1 and SGLT2 at the kidney proximal tubule brush border mediate glucose absorption from the intestinal lumen and the renal filtrate, respectively. In turn, GLUT2 efflux activity at the apical membrane of these tissues facilitates glucose transport from the cells into the circulation. SGLT2 is responsible for more than 90% of glucose reuptake from the renal filtrate, and inhibition of SGLT2 reduces plasma glucose levels. SGLT2 has been targeted for pharmacologic intervention in the management of diabetes. **Dapagliflozin** selectively inhibits SGLT2 over SGLT1; this selective inhibition facilitates reduction of plasma glucose levels without impairing SGLT1-mediated intestinal glucose absorption, potentially limiting adverse effects such as diarrhea that may be associated with elevated intestinal glucose levels.

Efflux Transporters

Oral drug administration generally provides the most convenient and affordable route for the systemic delivery of therapeutic agents; high, reproducible oral bioavailability minimizes variability in drug exposure across patient populations. After oral administration, drugs typically are absorbed from the intestinal lumen, delivered into the mesenteric blood supply, and then circulated through the hepatic portal system via the portal vein before entering the systemic circulation (see Chapter 3, Pharmacokinetics). Efflux transporters can affect oral bioavailability (1) by limiting the amount of drug that is absorbed across the enterocyte and/or (2) by transporting drug from the liver into the bile and thereby contributing to a first-pass effect. Whereas efflux transporters expressed on the canalicular membrane of the hepatocyte facilitate the excretion of xenobiotics into the bile, efflux transporters expressed on the sinusoidal (basolateral) membrane can promote the flux of drug and metabolites back into the systemic circulation (Fig. 5-1). Compounds eliminated into the bile across the canalicular membrane of the hepatocyte are concentrated in the gall bladder and released into the small intestine, where both parent drug and possibly metabolites can be absorbed across the intestine (a process known as **enterohepatic recirculation**) or eliminated into the feces. However, the same first-pass mechanisms (i.e., absorption, efflux, metabolism, and biliary excretion) that limited the compound's ability to reach the systemic circulation and the peripheral tissues still exist. The oral bioavailability of compounds that undergo extensive enterohepatic recirculation may appear extremely low; however, in cases where the target tissue is either the liver (e.g., statins) or intestine, these compounds may have desired pharmacologic effects despite limited systemic exposure. For drugs that are high-affinity substrates for intestinal and hepatic transporters, alternative routes of administration (such as intravenous and subcutaneous) can circumvent the first-pass effect and possibly increase the systemic exposure. However, even when drug delivery is used to avoid a first-pass effect, the drugs that reach the systemic circulation must nevertheless transit through the hepatobiliary system and may still be cleared rapidly due to efficient drug efflux processes. Compounds in the systemic circulation can also be eliminated in the kidney via active efflux into the urine. Because the transport of compounds from within the intracellular space is often against a concentration gradient, the process requires active transport; the majority of efflux pumps belong to the ATP-binding cassette (ABC) family of active transporters. This section outlines the efflux transporters that have major roles in drug disposition as well as those that facilitate the transport of endogenous compounds.

ATP-Binding Cassette (ABC) Transporter Family

ABC transporters constitute the largest transporter superfamily. They are active transporters that mediate efflux of various substrates—such as phospholipids, steroids, and drugs—out of cells against their concentration gradient. The superfamily is divided into seven families, of which only members of the ABCB, ABCC, and ABCG families have essential roles in drug disposition. ABCA and ABCD proteins transport only endogenous substrates and regulate cellular cholesterol and fatty acid metabolism, and ABCE and ABCF family members lack transmembrane domains and are not involved in the transport of drugs or endogenous compounds across the membranes of cells.

P-Glycoprotein and Bile Salt Export Pump (ABCB Family)

The ABCB family, also known as *multidrug resistance/transporters associated with antigen processing (MDR/TAP)*, consists of 11 members and includes perhaps the most studied drug transporter, P-glycoprotein (P-gp, also known as *MDR1 or ABCB1*). P-gp was initially discovered and characterized as a protein that mediates anticancer drug resistance. Its expression is elevated in many cancer cells, and P-gp contributes to multidrug resistance against antineoplastic therapeutics. P-gp is also expressed in the apical membrane of the small intestine, liver, kidney, endothelial cells of the blood–brain barrier, and placenta (Fig. 5-1), and it both limits exposure of substrates to certain organs and serves as a mechanism to eliminate xenobiotics from the body. P-gp has broad substrate specificity and it exhibits high affinity for cationic and amphiphilic compounds such as phospholipids (Table 5-2).

Although P-gp may have evolved as a defense mechanism to protect organisms against exogenous toxins, other ABCB family members such as MDR3 are important for phospholipid homeostasis in cell membranes. The bile salt export pump (BSEP, ABCB11) is an ABCB efflux transporter that is expressed at high levels on the hepatocyte canalicular membrane (Fig. 5-1). BSEP facilitates transport of bile salts and bile salt conjugates such as taurocholate from hepatocytes into the bile, and bile flow rate is largely regulated by the activity of BSEP. BSEP has also been shown to export statins such as **pravastatin** into the bile; by this mechanism, such drugs may be cleared from the liver (Table 5-2). Although its interaction with pravastatin suggests that BSEP may play a role in drug disposition, a more immediate concern is that a xenobiotic can inhibit BSEP and potentially contribute to cholestasis and intracellular accumulation of bile acids in hepatocytes. Clinical studies suggest that the endothelin receptor antagonist **bosentan** inhibits BSEP and may thereby induce cholestasis due to intracellular accumulation of cytotoxic bile salts.

TABLE 5-2 Efflux Transporters

TRANSPORTER	ORGAN/LOCATION (SEE FIG. 5-1)	ENDOGENOUS SUBSTRATES	DRUG SUBSTRATES	INHIBITORS
P-gp (MDR1, ABCB1)	Intestine (apical), kidney proximal tubule, hepatocytes (canalicular), blood–brain barrier	Steroids, phospholipids, bilirubin, bile acids	Digoxin, loperamide, quinidine, vinblastine, talinolol, berberine, irinotecan, doxorubicin, paclitaxel, fexofenadine, seliciclib, telithromycin, clarithromycin	Cyclosporine, quinidine, tariquidar, verapamil, ketoconazole, nelfinavir, ritonavir, tacrolimus, valspodar, saquinavir, elacridar, reserpine
MDR3 (ABCB4)	Liver (canalicular)	Phosphatidylcholine	Digoxin, paclitaxel, vinblastine	Verapamil, cyclosporine
BSEP (ABCB11)	Liver (canalicular)	Bile acids, taurocholate	Pravastatin, vinblastine	Bosentan, cyclosporine, rifampin, glibenclamide, glyburide
BCRP (ABCG2)	Intestine, liver (canalicular), breast, placenta, blood–brain barrier, stem cells	Uric acid, vitamins, dietary flavonoids, porphyrins, estrone 3-sulfate	Daunorubicin, doxorubicin, topotecan, irinotecan, methotrexate, imatinib, rosuvastatin, sulfasalazine, nucleoside analogues	Elacridar, imatinib, novobiocin, estrone, 17β-estradiol, ritonavir, omeprazole
MRP2 (ABCC2)	Intestine, liver, kidney, brain	Bilirubin, cholecystokinin, estrone 3-sulfate, glutathione and glucuronide conjugates	Glutathione and glucuronide conjugates, indinavir, cisplatin, methotrexate, etoposide, mitoxantrone, valsartan, olmesartan	Cyclosporine, delavirdine, efavirenz, emtricitabine, benzbromarone
MRP3 (ABCC3)	Intestine (brush border), liver (sinusoidal), kidney, placenta, adrenal gland	Bile salts, estradiol-17β-glucuronide, leukotriene C4	Etoposide, methotrexate, teniposide, fexofenadine, glucuronide conjugates, acetaminophen, vincristine	Delavirdine, efavirenz, emtricitabine, lamivudine, tenofovir, indomethacin, furosemide, probenecid, nevirapine
MRP4 (ABCC4)	Prostate, kidney, placenta, liver, blood–brain barrier	Taurocholate, cAMP, cGMP, urate, DHEAS, prostaglandins E1 and E2	Acyclovir, ritonavir, tenofovir, topotecan, PMEA, methotrexate, furosemide, ceftizoxime, cefazolin, 6-mercaptopurine	Indomethacin, MK571, diclofenac, celecoxib, sulfinpyrazone, quercetin
MATE1 (SLC47A1)	Kidney proximal tubule, liver (canalicular), skeletal muscle	Creatinine, guanidine, nucleosides	Metformin, cephalexin, acyclovir, ganciclovir, fexofenadine, oxaliplatin	Quinidine, cimetidine, verapamil, procainamide
MATE2-K (SLC47A2)	Kidney proximal tubule	Estrone sulfate, creatinine	Metformin, cimetidine, procainamide	Cimetidine, quinidine, pramipexole

Data compiled from same sources as in Table 5-1.

Multidrug Resistance-Associated Proteins (ABCC Family)

The ABCC family, also known as the *multidrug resistance-associated protein (MRP/CFTR) family*, consists of 9 members that exhibit high specificity for organic anions such as glutathione- and glucuronide-conjugated drugs. ABCC family members are localized to the apical and basolateral membranes of hepatocytes, enterocytes, kidney proximal tubule, endothelial cells of the blood–brain barrier, and placenta (Fig. 5-1). Similar to P-gp, MRPs are abundantly expressed in tumors and cause resistance to anticancer drugs. MRP2 mediates hepatobiliary clearance of drugs including **methotrexate** and statins. In addition to its expression on the canalicular membrane of hepatocytes, MRP2 is expressed on the apical membrane of the intestine and the kidney proximal tubule. In contrast, MRP3 and MRP4 are expressed on the basolateral membrane of the liver and are responsible for the transport of compounds from the liver back into the blood.

Several pathophysiologic consequences of hereditary MRP deficiency have been reported, the most notable of which is **Dubin-Johnson syndrome**. In this syndrome, MRP2 deficiency results in the clinical manifestation of conjugated hyperbilirubinemia. MRPs transport not only exogenous molecules but also a wide array of endogenous compounds such as leukotrienes, bilirubin glucuronides, prostaglandins, cAMP, cGMP, and steroids (Table 5-2). Moreover, MRPs likely have a role in the disposition and elimination of drug metabolites, especially charged anionic glucuronide and sulfate conjugates.

The cystic fibrosis transmembrane conductance regulator (CFTR) is also a member of the ABCC family. CFTR transports chloride ions across the membrane of mucus-secreting epithelial cells in the lung, digestive system, pancreas, reproductive system, and other organs and tissues. Mutations in CFTR disrupt chloride transport, which leads to impaired mucus formation and flow, and are the cause of cystic fibrosis in humans.

Breast Cancer Resistance Protein (ABCG Family)

Among the five ABCG family members, breast cancer resistance protein (BCRP, ABCG2) is the only one implicated in the disposition of drugs and xenobiotics (Table 5-2). BCRP is expressed in several tissues, including the intestinal tract, blood–brain barrier, liver canalicular membrane, kidney proximal tubule, testis, and placenta (Fig. 5-1). The substrate specificity of BCRP overlaps with that of P-gp; as such, BCRP can enhance the xenobiotic barrier function where these transporters are co-expressed. Despite its name, BCRP has relatively low levels of expression in breast cancers, but it has been shown to confer drug resistance in several other tumor types (e.g., leukemia, lung cancer, and melanoma). In addition to its role in drug disposition, BCRP exports urea into the urinary tract and mediates secretion of vitamins into breast milk.

Other ABCG family members are involved in endogenous functions (see Chapter 20, Pharmacology of Cholesterol and Lipoprotein Metabolism). ABCG5 and ABCG8 form a heterodimer that controls biliary sterol and lipid secretion in the canalicular membrane of the liver as well as clearance of sterols in the small intestine. ABCG1 promotes efflux of cholesterol from macrophages to high-density lipoprotein (HDL) particles.

ABCA and ABCD Families

ABCA and ABCD family members mediate the transport of endogenous substrates. For example, ABCA1 of the ABCA family mediates cellular lipid efflux by transporting cholesterol and phospholipids out of hepatocytes and macrophages, contributing to the biogenesis of HDL. ABCD transporters are expressed on the membrane of peroxisomes and regulate fatty acid uptake by these organelles. This suggests that some transporters may have evolved to regulate trafficking of endogenous compounds between plasma and tissues and to eliminate toxic byproducts of cellular metabolism, whereas a subset of transporters may have adapted to also promote the elimination of nutrients, xenobiotics, and their metabolites.

Solute Carrier (SLC) Family
Multi-Antimicrobial Extrusion Protein (MATE) Family

Multi-antimicrobial extrusion proteins, also known as *multidrug and toxic compound extrusion proteins* (*MATEs*), are a family of multidrug efflux transporters that exhibit affinity for organic cations. They function as proton/drug antiporters that import a proton into the intracellular medium as a counterion for the export of a drug molecule out of the cell. MATE1 (SLC47A1) is expressed on the canalicular membrane of hepatocytes and on kidney proximal tubule cells, where it exports exogenous compounds into bile and urine, respectively (Fig. 5-1). MATE2-K (SLC47A2) is expressed only in the kidney proximal tubule, where it mediates clearance of exogenous substrates alongside MATE1 (Fig. 5-1). Both transporters exhibit selectivity for compounds that are substrates for OCTs, such as **metformin** and tetraethylammonium. Their endogenous substrates include organic cations such as guanidine and creatinine (Table 5-2).

■ CLINICAL PERSPECTIVES ON DRUG TRANSPORTERS

The pharmacokinetic, pharmacodynamic, and toxicologic properties of drugs are characterized and optimized initially through a comprehensive series of *in silico* predictions, in vitro cell culture, and membrane preparation studies and then through in vivo animal models and clinical trials. Membrane uptake and efflux transporters can influence the absorption, distribution, and excretion of xenobiotics and may therefore have substantial impact on the efficacy and safety of drugs. Drugs can act as substrates for transporters and may also alter the activity of transporters through inhibition or induction of transport processes, which could result in the impaired or enhanced transport of endogenous substrates. Moreover, much as in the case of drug-metabolizing enzymes, the concomitant administration of several drugs can lead to drug–drug interactions if one agent alters the transport of the other. This could potentially reduce the clearance of the co-administered drug, affect the drug's oral bioavailability, and lead to adverse effects or lack of efficacy due to unexpected changes in drug exposure. Understanding the specific transporters that govern the absorption, distribution, and clearance of new therapeutic agents will help anticipate and minimize the unexpected impact of these mechanisms on drug disposition and potential drug–drug interactions.

There are apparent species differences in drug transporters as well as lack of direct orthologs for some human transporters (e.g., OATP1B1 and OATP1B3), and several human transporters have therefore been cloned and expressed in cell lines. Transgenic mouse models expressing human transporter genes have also been created to enable preclinical studies designed to help predict clinical outcomes. These models, together with known substrates and inhibitors of drug transporters (Tables 5-1 and 5-2), can aid in understanding the clinical relevance of these mechanisms for drug disposition.

Drug–Drug Interactions

Since the discovery of P-gp as a multidrug resistance gene against anticancer drugs, many other hydrophobic and cationic drugs have been identified as its substrates (Table 5-2). The cardiac glycoside **digoxin** is considered to be a prototypical P-gp substrate, and the potential drug–drug interactions due to inhibition of P-gp by novel drug entities can be determined by measuring the plasma levels of digoxin upon co-administration of the novel drugs. Drugs that inhibit P-gp, such as the antiarrhythmic agent **quinidine** and the antiviral drug **ritonavir**, elevate intestinal uptake and reduce biliary and renal clearance of digoxin in vivo and thereby increase plasma levels of digoxin (Table 5-3). Because P-gp is the primary transporter preventing the entry of exogenous compounds into the central nervous system, substrates for P-gp are often unable to cross the blood–brain barrier. Inhibition of P-gp at the blood–brain barrier has been reported in some preclinical studies, but the ability to inhibit P-gp at the human blood–brain barrier does not yet have proven clinical relevance, likely because the compounds are unable to achieve high enough unbound concentrations in the systemic circulation to inhibit blood–brain barrier P-gp in vivo.

Like P-gp, BCRP was initially characterized as a multidrug resistance gene expressed in neoplastic cell lines. In animal studies, BCRP not only limits the efficacy of anticancer drugs such as **topotecan** but also substantially reduces the intestinal uptake of non-cancer drugs such as **atorvastatin**. **Elacridar** is a potent BCRP inhibitor that can be used to test whether new drugs are cleared by BCRP or to increase the bioavailability of known BCRP substrates. For example,

TABLE 5-3 Clinically Observed Drug–Drug Interactions Due to Transporters

TRANSPORTER	INHIBITOR OR *INDUCER	AFFECTED DRUG	PHARMACOKINETIC CHANGES DUE TO AFFECTED DRUG
OATP1B1 (SLCO1B1)	Lopinavir/ritonavir	Bosentan	AUC↑5-48-fold
	Cyclosporine	Pravastatin	AUC↑9.9-fold, C_{max}↑7.78-fold
	Rifampin (single dose)	Glyburide	AUC↑2.3-fold
OATP1B3 (SLCO1B3)	Cyclosporine	Pitavastatin	AUC↑4.6-fold, C_{max}↑6.6-fold
	Cyclosporine	Rosuvastatin	AUC↑7.1-fold
	Lopinavir/ritonavir	Rosuvastatin	AUC↑2.1-fold, C_{max}↑4.65-fold
OATP1A2 (SLCO1A2)	Grapefruit juice	Fexofenadine	AUC↓2.7-fold, C_{max}↓2.63-fold
	Orange juice	Fexofenadine	AUC↓3.3-fold, C_{max}↓3-fold
	Apple juice	Fexofenadine	AUC↓3.7-fold, C_{max}↓3.57-fold
	Naringin	Aliskiren	AUC↓1.6-fold, C_{max}↓2.44-fold
OATP2B1 (SLCO2B1)	Orange juice	Aliskiren	AUC↓2.6-fold
	Apple juice	Aliskiren	AUC↓2.6-fold
OAT1 (SLC22A6)	Probenecid	Cephradine	AUC↑3.6-fold
	Probenecid	Cidofovir	AUC↑1.5-fold, CL_r↓1.47-fold
	Probenecid	Acyclovir	AUC↑1.4-fold, CL_r↓1.47-fold
OAT3 (SLC22A8)	Probenecid	Furosemide	AUC↑2.9-fold
OCT2 (SLC22A2)	Cimetidine	Dofetilide	AUC↑1.5-fold, CL_r↓1.5-fold
	Cimetidine	Pindolol	AUC↑1.5-fold, CL_r↓1.5-fold
	Cimetidine	Metformin	AUC↑1.4-fold, CL_r↓1.37-fold
	Cimetidine	Varenicline	AUC↑1.3-fold
	Cimetidine	Pilsicainide	AUC↑1.3-fold, CL_r↓1.39-fold
P-gp (MDR1, ABCB1)	Dronedarone	Digoxin	AUC↑2.6-fold, C_{max}↑1.75-fold
	Quinidine	Digoxin	AUC↑1.7-fold, CL_r↓1.5-2-fold
	Ritonavir	Digoxin	AUC↑1.86-fold, CL_r↓1.54-fold
	Ranolazine	Digoxin	AUC↑1.6-fold, C_{max}↑1.46-fold
	Clarithromycin	Digoxin	AUC↑1.7-fold, C_{max}↑1.75-fold
	*Rifampin	Digoxin	AUC↓1.4-fold, C_{max}↓1.6-fold
	*St. John's wort	Digoxin	AUC↓1.4-fold, C_{max}↓1.56-fold
	*Rifampin	Talinolol	AUC↓1.5-fold, C_{max}↓1.6-fold
	*St. John's wort	Talinolol	AUC↓1.3-fold
	*Tipranavir/ritonavir	Loperamide	AUC↓2-fold
	*Tipranavir/ritonavir	Saquinavir/ritonavir	AUC↓5-fold
BCRP (ABCG2)	Elacridar	Topotecan	AUC↑2.4-fold, C_{max}↑3.8-fold

the oral administration of elacridar with topotecan substantially increases plasma concentrations of topotecan (Table 5-3). Similar to the limited significance of P-gp inhibition at the human blood–brain barrier, BCRP inhibition at the blood–brain barrier is thought to have limited effect on drug distribution to the brain.

Among the uptake transporters, OAT1 and OAT3 are implicated in the transport and clearance via the kidney proximal tubule of a broad range of drugs such as antivirals, antibiotics, statins, and anticancer drugs. **Probenecid** is a well-established inhibitor of both transporters and, when co-administered with furosemide or methotrexate, increases the bioavailability of these OAT substrates. Probenecid is also used to prevent renal injury by blocking OAT1-mediated renal uptake of the nephrotoxic antiviral drug **cidofovir** (Table 5-3).

OCTs and MATEs often work in concert to facilitate drug transport across the liver and kidney (Fig. 5-1, and see the following discussion). These two transporter families also share the common inhibitors **cimetidine** (histamine receptor

antagonist), **pyrimethamine** (antiprotozoal and antimalarial dihydrofolate reductase inhibitor), and the chemotherapeutic tyrosine kinase inhibitors **imatinib** and **erlotinib** (Tables 5-1 and 5-2). Although cimetidine has been largely supplanted by proton pump inhibitors in the treatment of acid reflux, it may prove useful for the study of drug–drug interactions in vivo. Both cimetidine and pyrimethamine exhibit higher selectivity and increased potency for MATE compared to OCT family members; therefore, any drug–drug interaction involving these drugs could depend on the dose of the co-administered inhibitors. OCTs facilitate drug uptake from the blood into the liver and kidney, and MATEs contribute to drug secretion from these tissues into the bile and urine, respectively. Therefore, for example, low-dose cimetidine co-administration, which would inhibit only MATE-mediated excretion, may result in increased **metformin** localization to the liver and kidneys. As a second example, high-dose cimetidine co-administration inhibits not only MATE-mediated drug excretion but also OCT2-mediated renal uptake of the anticancer drug **cisplatin** from the blood, thereby increasing cisplatin plasma levels and protecting the kidneys against the nephrotoxic adverse effects of this drug.

Inhibition of drug uptake into the liver and kidney can result in increased plasma levels and improved efficacy of the drug. This generalization does not hold, however, if the site of action of the drug *is* the liver or kidney. For example, the liver is the target tissue for statins such as **atorvastatin**, **pravastatin**, and **rosuvastatin**, where these agents inhibit HMG-CoA reductase to reduce cholesterol synthesis. The uptake of statins into hepatocytes is mediated by OATP1B1 and OATP1B3 (Fig. 5-1). Co-administered drugs that inhibit these uptake transporters impair statin uptake by the liver and increase statin plasma concentration (Table 5-3). This may not only lead to reduced efficacy of the statin in the liver but also increase the risk of adverse effects such as rhabdomyolysis; the combination of these effects could decrease the therapeutic index of the drug.

Foods as well as drugs can interfere with transporter activity. Grapefruit juice was initially identified as an inhibitor of the drug-metabolizing enzyme CYP3A4. However, recent studies show that grapefruit juice and other fruit juices such as orange juice and apple juice may also impair OATP-mediated uptake transport. **Naringin**, the active component of grapefruit juice, inhibits OATP1A2 and OATP1B1 and leads to reduced drug bioavailability in clinical studies. In addition, the **hesperidin** and **quercetin** constituents of orange juice and apple juice, respectively, may be responsible for inhibiting OATP1A2 and OATP2B1. Although co-administration of certain fruit juices with drugs that are OATP substrates may reduce drug bioavailability, clinical effects have been observed only when the drugs are taken together with large volumes of these juices (Table 5-3). In vitro studies have started to explore the potential for foods to alter the function of other transporters, but these observations have yet to translate into clinical outcomes. For example, grapefruit juice has been shown to inhibit P-gp activity in vitro, but clinical studies do not demonstrate inhibition of P-gp when grapefruit juice is co-administered with digoxin.

Drugs are also capable of inducing the expression of transporters. Similar to the induction of P450 enzyme expression, drug transporter expression can be regulated by the nuclear pregnane X receptor (PXR), constitutive androstane receptor (CAR), farnesoid X receptor (FXR), and vitamin D receptor. Relative to the effect of transporter inhibition, the overall impact of transporter induction on clinically relevant drug interactions is minimal, and most drug interactions involving induction have been attributed to the induction of P-gp in the intestine. **St. John's wort** and **rifampin** are strong PXR agonists, and the co-administration of **digoxin** with St. John's wort or rifampin results in reduced digoxin plasma levels (Table 5-3). Similarly, rifampin preadministration reduces plasma concentrations of **talinolol** and **carvedilol**, likely due to P-gp induction. In all of these cases, enhanced expression of P-gp would be expected to reduce the systemic exposure of the drug and thereby reduce the efficacy of the drug.

Drug Interference with Endogenous Metabolite Trafficking

Several drugs have been implicated in the disruption of endogenous metabolite trafficking and homeostasis, most likely

TABLE 5-4 Adverse Drug Reactions Due to Transporter–Drug Interactions

TRANSPORTER	DRUG	ADVERSE REACTION
P-gp (MDR1, ABCB1)	Cyclosporine	Nephrotoxicity
	Tacrolimus	Nephrotoxicity
	Loperamide	Respiratory depression
BSEP (ABCB11)	Bosentan	Cholestatic liver injury
	Cyclosporine	Cholestatic liver injury
	Glibenclamide	Cholestatic liver injury
	Rifampin	Cholestatic liver injury
	Troglitazone	Cholestatic liver injury
MRP2 (ABCC2)	Irinotecan	Diarrhea
	Methotrexate	Nephrotoxicity
BCRP (ABCG2)	Irinotecan	Myelosuppression
OAT1 (SLC22A6)	Adefovir	Nephrotoxicity
	Cidofovir	Nephrotoxicity
	Tenofovir	Nephrotoxicity
OCTs	Metformin	Hyperlactacidemia, lactic acidosis
OCT2 (SLC22A2)	Cisplatin	Nephrotoxicity
OATP1B1 (SLCO1B1)	Mycophenolate mofetil	Leukopenia, anemia, thrombocytopenia, diarrhea, nausea, vomiting, infection
	Simvastatin	Myopathy

Adapted from Table 4 of König J, Müller F, Fromm MF. Transporter and drug–drug interactions: important determinants of drug disposition and effects. *Pharmacol Rev* 2013;65:944–966.

stemming from the inhibitory effect of these drugs on transporters. For example, inhibition of the bile salt transporter BSEP could impair bile formation and flow, resulting in elevated hepatic bile acids and leading to cholestatic liver injury (Table 5-4). URAT1 and OAT4 are essential for establishing systemic uric acid balance, and inhibition of URAT1 has been exploited as a treatment for gout. However, compounds such as **losartan** can inhibit both URAT1 and OAT4 and may therefore cause undesirable adverse effects such as the formation of kidney stones. The HIV protease inhibitor **ritonavir** blocks GLUT4, and this could result in hyperglycemia in prediabetic patients treated with ritonavir. Pharmacologic inhibition of SGLT2 results in osmotic diuresis due to the increased glucose load in the urine and has been linked to increased urination and thirst in clinical studies. One such SGLT2 inhibitor, **dapagliflozin**, may cause hypotension and light-headedness due to excessive dehydration. Additional adverse effects related to transporter–drug interactions are listed in Table 5-4.

Pharmacogenomics

Genotype-dependent alterations in drug-metabolizing enzymes (such as CYPs) are well documented. Similar to CYPs, uptake and efflux transporters are subject to single nucleotide polymorphisms (SNPs), which can result in altered pharmacokinetics for certain drugs such as **statins** and antidiabetics. The OATP1B1 polymorphism N130D has been shown to result in elevated serum bilirubin levels and reduced hepatic uptake of OATP1B1 drug substrates, such as statins. Patients who carry one or two copies of the V174A variant of OATP1B1 exhibit 2- and 12-fold increased risk of developing myopathy, respectively, in the setting of daily simvastatin treatment. The Q141K variant of BCRP is also associated with altered statin pharmacokinetics; increased plasma levels of the drug are due to reduced efflux activity at the intestinal lumen. The A270S variant of OCT2 has been implicated in reduced renal uptake and clearance of the antidiabetic drug **metformin**. Because such SNPs represent common variants that occur in more than 1% of the population, a large number of patients could potentially be affected by altered pharmacokinetics. Therefore, genetic analysis of specific drug transporters could provide a valuable advance toward personalized medicine.

INTEGRATION OF DRUG TRANSPORTER SCIENCE INTO DRUG DISCOVERY AND DEVELOPMENT

Progress in our understanding of mechanisms of drug transport aids in designing drugs with optimal transport properties, predicting drug–drug and drug–disease interactions, and determining optimal routes of administration (Box 5-1). A new drug entity may be optimized for maximum potency against its biological target by structural modification of moieties on the molecule and pharmacologic testing of the derivative compounds in cell culture or *in silico* systems. However, the efficacy of a potential drug candidate with exquisite in vitro potency may be severely impeded in clinical trials if it does not also have an optimal pharmacokinetic profile. For drug candidates that are substrates for one or more of the major drug transporters, the transporter(s) can influence the pharmacokinetic profile of the drug by limiting or enhancing the ability of the drug to reach its biological target in vivo. Therefore, in drug discovery, an understanding of whether a compound (or compound class) is a substrate or inhibitor of a drug transporter can aid in early optimization of the compound's chemical structure. For oral administration, it is important to take into account the contribution of intestinal drug efflux transporters (e.g., P-gp, BCRP, and MRP2) relative to the contribution of passive intestinal permeability, since these transporters can reduce overall intestinal permeability and contribute to low oral bioavailability.

Drug disposition can be improved not only by avoiding efflux channels but also by optimizing for transport by uptake channels. Because the target organ of statins is the liver, optimal uptake from the plasma into hepatocytes would be expected to improve the pharmacodynamics of these HMG-CoA reductase inhibitors. The substrate preference of CNTs/ENTs and PEPTs for nucleosides and peptides, respectively, has been exploited to enhance the absorption of drugs that otherwise exhibit high clearance rates. The oral bioavailability of ganciclovir is tenfold less than its optimized peptide conjugate (prodrug) **valganciclovir**, which is a substrate for PEPT1. As a final example, the chemotherapeutic efficacy of a cytotoxic nucleoside analogue such as **gemcitabine** may depend on its cellular uptake into tumors by ENT1. Patients whose tumors exhibit low levels of ENT1 expression respond poorly to treatment with gemcitabine.

The identification of transporters that may have primary roles in the uptake and elimination of new drug entities is key to understanding the disposition as well as the potential for drug–drug interactions of a novel therapeutic agent. Advances in drug transporter research have also contributed to awareness by regulatory agencies that transport is an important consideration in the evaluation of new drugs. The US Food and Drug Administration (FDA), European Medicines Agency (EMA), and the Japanese Pharmaceuticals and Medical Devices Agency (PMDA) have offered updated clinical and nonclinical guidelines on drug transporters to consider in drug development. Increased awareness and recognition of transporter-dependent drug–drug interactions has led to the inclusion of these interactions in drug labels, along with the precautions that must be taken in the setting of multidrug therapies. The International Transporter Consortium (ITC) has proposed decision trees that could guide and help interpret preclinical studies assessing the potential role of specific transporters in the disposition of new drug entities and extrapolate whether additional clinical studies for drug–drug interactions are warranted. There is now general consensus around the importance of testing the transport of new drugs—especially by the well-established transporters P-gp, BCRP, OCT2, OAT1, OAT3, OATP1B1, and OATP1B3—in order to better predict clinical outcomes and drug–drug interactions.

CONCLUSION AND FUTURE DIRECTIONS

Significant advances have been made in our understanding of drug–transporter interactions in recent years, and the majority of key transporters essential in drug disposition and drug–drug interactions have been identified. The impact (or lack thereof) of many of these transporters has been tested and demonstrated clinically, and both drug development strategies and regulatory guidelines continue to be established and refined based on our evolving scientific understanding of drug transporters. As listed in Tables 5-1 and 5-2, transporter inhibitors that are currently available for use in vitro and in vivo exhibit overlapping specificities. This limits the use of nonspecific inhibitors to screen for interactions in cell culture and animal models. Discovery of more selective inhibitors would help to establish and standardize in vitro and in vivo techniques and should lead to consistent characterization of drug disposition and drug–drug interactions for novel therapeutics. These efforts should be assisted by computational approaches that predict transporter–substrate interactions based on the chemical structures of the molecules using molecular docking simulations as well as established crystal structures of transporters. With the continued and expanding use of polypharmacy to treat complex diseases, there is an urgent need to understand the potential for transporter-mediated drug interactions together with metabolic drug interactions. Emerging in vitro and in vivo tools to study drug disposition, such as 3-D tissue-engineered organ models, coupled with our growing insights into the basic science of drug transporters, should enable better predictions of the clinical impact of transporter-related mechanisms on the patient.

BOX 5-1 Drug Development Case

A pharmaceutical lab is developing a new drug for the treatment of hypercholesterolemia. The approach is to inhibit a key enzyme involved in the cholesterol biosynthesis pathway. This enzyme, HMG-CoA reductase, is localized to the liver and it serves as the rate-controlling enzyme of the mevalonate pathway, the metabolic pathway that produces cholesterol and other isoprenoids. The main strategy for the program is to utilize the liver's capacity for active uptake of xenobiotics in order to target the liver selectively. Data from recent studies with the company's lead compounds have recently been presented. Figure A shows the uptake of four compounds into suspended rat hepatocytes. Each of the compounds was incubated with the cells at 37°C for up to 30 seconds.

The project team decides to conduct follow-up studies in rats. These in vivo studies show significant differences among the compounds in bioavailability after oral administration (%F), acute hyperbilirubinemia with Compound A, and a transient increase in serum bile acids with Compound D (Figure B). Given the high in vitro potency of the four compounds (Figure B), the pharmacologist on the project team is also keen to determine their in vivo efficacy in rats. Results show that, when administered at 5 mg/kg orally, the efficacy of the compounds is rank-ordered as follows: A (most efficacious) > D >> B >> C (least efficacious).

Questions and Discussion

1. Based on the data shown in Figure A, by which mechanism is each compound likely entering the hepatocytes?

    Compound A and Compound B could be taken up by multiple uptake transporters (e.g., OATPs, OATs, or OCTs) that are expressed on the sinusoidal membrane of hepatocytes. Transporter-mediated uptake could be tested by measuring the uptake of each compound into suspended hepatocytes in the presence of selective transporter inhibitors or by measuring the uptake of the compounds in cell lines that express a specific transporter compared to the uptake in a control cell line. Compound C and Compound D likely enter

Compound	In vitro potency (nM)	Oral bioavailability (%F)	In vivo observations
A	35	3.1	Elevated conjugated bilirubin
B	41	28	No adverse events
C	0.2	2.2	No adverse events
D	121	97	Increased serum bile acids

FIGURE B. In vitro and in vivo data for Compounds A, B, C, and D after oral administration of 30 mg/kg in rats.

the cell through passive diffusion or could be transported by a low-affinity, high-capacity transporter at a very slow uptake rate.

2. Why is the bioavailability of Compounds A and C low, whereas the bioavailability of Compound D is high?

    Compound A most likely undergoes enterohepatic recirculation, and only a limited amount of the drug makes it into the systemic circulation. Compound C exhibits both low hepatic uptake and low bioavailability, so the majority of the compound might simply not be absorbed in the intestine and instead be eliminated in the feces. Compound D has minimal uptake into hepatocytes and nearly complete oral bioavailability. Complete absorption of Compound D across the intestine, with a minimal first-pass hepatic transport or metabolism effect, would explain the high oral bioavailability in rats.

3. Assuming that Compound A is acidic and is charged at physiologic pH, which specific active-transport mechanisms (uptake and/or efflux) are likely responsible for the transport of Compound A from the plasma into the bile?

    If Compound A is acidic and charged at physiologic pH (anionic), then it is more likely to be transported into hepatocytes by uptake transporters that exhibit relatively high affinity for anionic substrates, such as OATP1B1. MRP2 may mediate its excretion into bile, since this efflux transporter also has relatively high affinity for anionic substrates.

4. What are potential mechanisms by which Compounds A and D cause hyperbilirubinemia and cholestasis, respectively?

    Impaired clearance of bilirubin via the hepatobiliary route can result in hyperbilirubinemia. Compound A increases conjugated bilirubin, suggesting that the compound has minimal impact on the transport of bilirubin into the hepatocyte and limited impact on the metabolism of bilirubin to bilirubin glucuronide. Compound A likely inhibits a mechanism involved in the excretion of conjugated bilirubin into the bile, likely via MRP2. MRP2 inhibition studies in

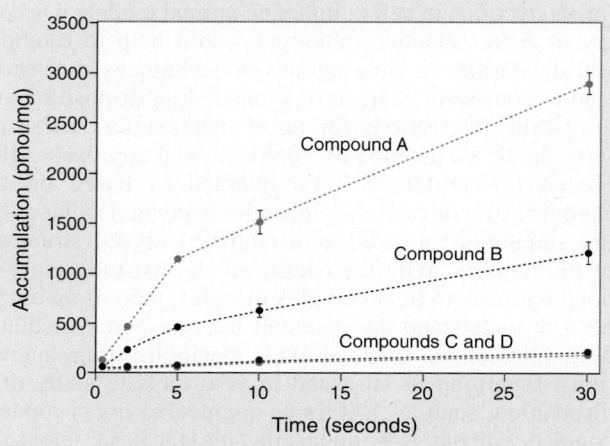

FIGURE A. Accumulation of four lead HMG-CoA reductase inhibitors in suspended rat hepatocytes over 30 seconds.

BOX 5-1 Drug Development Case (continued)

transfected cell lines, combined with in vivo studies in rats with cannulated bile ducts, would help to support this hypothesis. Compound D does not appear to be a substrate for hepatic transport based on the suspended hepatocyte data; nonetheless, the compound could inhibit transporters involved in bile acid disposition. Inhibition of either NTCP at the sinusoidal membrane or BSEP at the canalicular membrane of hepatocytes would explain the in vivo results. Further studies of uptake inhibition of bile acids (e.g., taurocholate) into suspended hepatocytes, or inhibition of BSEP (measured by taurocholate transport) in BSEP-expressing vesicles or in sandwich-cultured hepatocytes, would help to determine the mechanism that is more likely to be involved.

5. The team is allowed to advance only one of the four lead compounds into clinical trials. Which compound would be the preferred agent for clinical-trial testing?

Compound A should be advanced into clinical studies. This compound exhibits the highest efficacy in vivo, likely due to its effective uptake into the liver—which is the target site of action for the inhibition of HMG-CoA reductase. Compound A is likely to be associated with a relatively low level of systemic adverse effects due to its enterohepatic recirculation, and the observed hyperbilirubinemia in rats could potentially be avoided by dose adjustment. Given the likely involvement of hepatic transporters in Compound A disposition, Compound A may need to be studied further in patients with hepatic impairment in order to understand any potential impact on safety and efficacy. Compound D exhibits low hepatic uptake and high bioavailability, suggesting that higher levels of systemic exposure would be required to achieve a pharmacologic effect comparable to that of Compound A. The need for higher systemic exposure would warrant a careful assessment of off-target effects that could contribute to dose-limiting toxicities in the clinic. Moreover, the observation of altered bile acid disposition in rats suggests that further investigation of the mechanism of cholestasis would be warranted, as well as evaluation of the potential for translation to humans if the compound were to move further into development. Compound B exhibits good hepatic uptake and in vitro potency. Although the lack of adverse effects makes it a potential candidate for advancement to clinical trials, its efficacy in vivo is significantly lower than that of Compounds A and D. Higher doses of Compound B may be permissible due to the apparent lack of toxicity, but the physicochemical properties of the compound will at some point limit the dose that can be absorbed/administered. Compound C is the least promising candidate due to its low hepatic uptake and low in vivo efficacy. For all of the compounds, the potential for species differences in transporter activity should be considered (both as substrates and inhibitors), and analogous studies with human transporters should be conducted to better predict the likelihood that the results of the rodent studies will translate faithfully to the clinic. ■

Suggested Reading

Brouwer KL, Keppler D, Hoffmaster KA, et al.; International Transporter Consortium. In vitro methods to support transporter evaluation in drug discovery and development. *Clin Pharmacol Ther* 2013;94:95–112. (*In vitro methods for the identification of drug transporters involved in the disposition of new drug entities.*)

Giacomini KM, Huang SM, Tweedie DJ, et al.; International Transporter Consortium. Membrane transporters in drug development. *Nat Rev Drug Discov* 2010;9:215–236. (*The initial white paper from the International Transporter Consortium.*)

Giacomini KM, Huang SM. Transporters in drug development and clinical pharmacology. *Clin Pharmacol Ther* 2013;94:3–9. (*Reviews roles of drug transporters in drug absorption, distribution, and elimination.*)

König J, Müller F, Fromm MF. Transporter and drug–drug interactions: important determinants of drug disposition and effects. *Pharmacol Rev* 2013;65: 944–966. (*Reviews the role of transporters in drug–drug interactions.*)

Morrissey KM, Wen CC, Johns SJ, Zhang L, Huang SM, Giacomini KM. The UCSF-FDA TransPortal: a public drug transporter database. *Clin Pharmacol Ther* 2012;92:545–546. (*http://dbts.ucsf.edu/fda transportal*)

Nigam SK. What do drug transporters really do? *Nat Rev Drug Discov* 2015;14:29–44. (*Reviews endogenous functions of drug transporters.*)

Palmeira A, Sousa E, Vasconcelos MH, Pinto MM. Three decades of P-gp inhibitors: skimming through several generations and scaffolds. *Curr Med Chem* 2012;19:1946–2025. (*Overview of P-gp activity modulators for the reversal of multidrug resistance in cancer.*)

Roth M, Obaidat A, Hagenbuch B. OATPs, OATs and OCTs: the organic anion and cation transporters of the *SLCO* and *SLC22A* gene superfamilies. *Br J Pharmacol* 2012;165:1260–1287. (*Extensive review of the biology and pharmacology of organic anion and cation transporters.*)

6

Drug Toxicity

Michael W. Conner, Catherine Dorian-Conner,
Vishal S. Vaidya, Laura C. Green, and David E. Golan

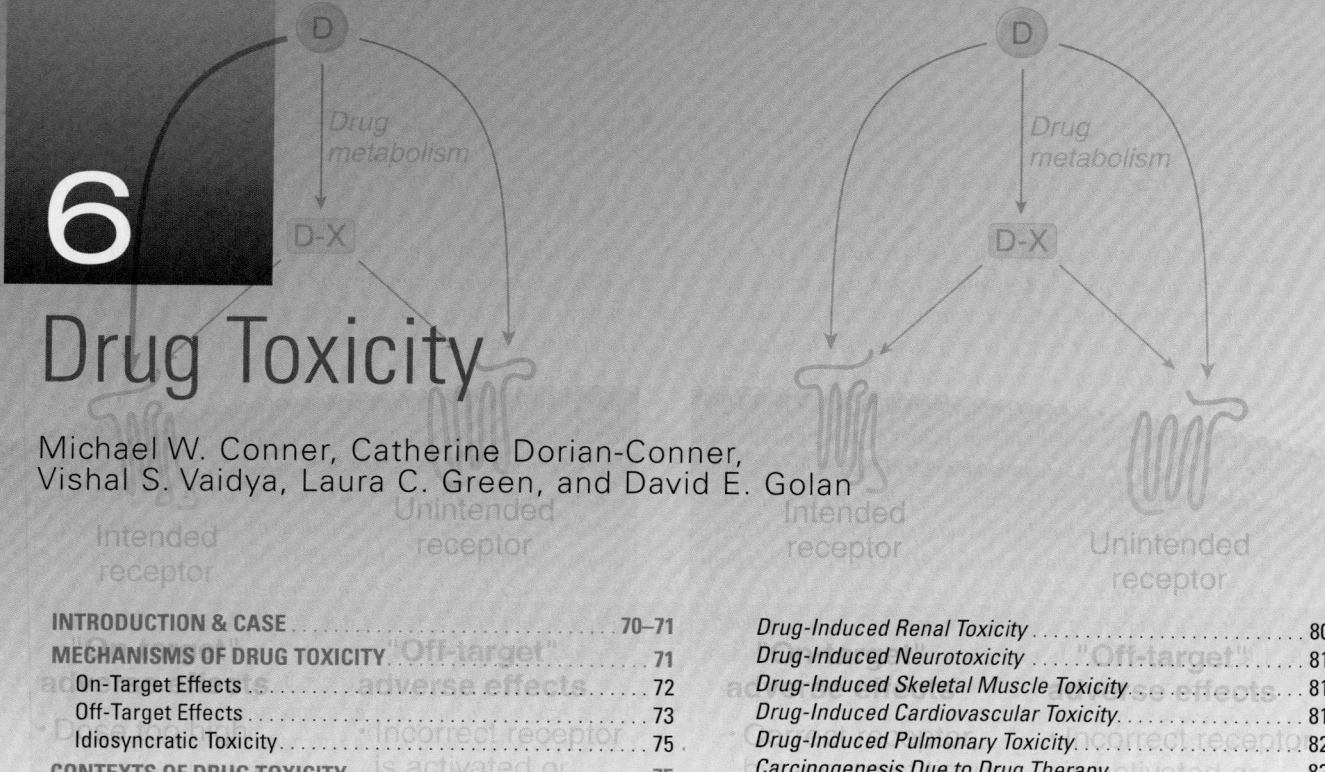

INTRODUCTION

Like many medical interventions, the use of drugs for therapeutic benefit is subject to the law of unintended consequences. These consequences—termed **side effects**, **adverse effects**, or **toxic effects**—are a function of the mechanisms of drug action, the size of the drug dose, and the characteristics and health status of the patient. As such, the principles of pharmacology, presented in the preceding chapters, apply to drug toxicology as well. Many subsequent chapters contain Drug Summary Tables that list, among other properties, the specific adverse effects that can be caused by each drug. This chapter focuses on the mechanisms underlying these adverse effects.

As a general matter, adverse effects range from those that are common and relatively benign to those that pose serious risk of organ damage or death. Even the former group of adverse effects, however, can cause considerable discomfort and lead patients to avoid or reduce their use of medication. Also, in general, the type and risk of adverse effects depend on the **margin of safety** between the dose required for efficacy and the dose that causes adverse effects. When the margin of safety is large, toxicity results primarily from overdoses; when this margin is small or nonexistent, adverse effects may be manifest at otherwise therapeutic doses. These principles apply both to prescription medications and to over-the-counter drugs such as acetaminophen and aspirin. Note

that safety margins are a function not only of the drug but also of the patient, in that genetic or other characteristics—such as polymorphisms in enzymes that detoxify harmful metabolites, comorbidities, or reduced functional reserve in key organs—render patients more or less capable of defending against toxicity. This is one reason why, all other things being equal, new medications should be initiated at the lowest doses likely to be therapeutic.

Drug toxicity is critically important in drug development (see Chapter 51, Drug Discovery and Preclinical Development, and Chapter 52, Clinical Drug Evaluation and Regulatory Approval). Early in drug development, preclinical and clinical studies are used to evaluate compound potency, selectivity, pharmacokinetic and metabolic profiles, and toxicity. Prior to marketing, the regulatory agencies responsible for drug approval review the test data and decide whether the benefits of the drug outweigh its risks. Once a drug is marketed and many more patients are exposed, the appearance of unexpected types or frequencies of adverse effects may cause a reevaluation of the drug, such that its use may be restricted to specific patient populations or withdrawn entirely (as in the cases, for example, of the nonsteroidal anti-inflammatory drug **rofecoxib** and the antidiabetic drug **troglitazone**).

In this chapter, categories of drug toxicities that derive from inappropriate activation or inhibition of the intended drug target (**on-target adverse effects**) or unintended targets

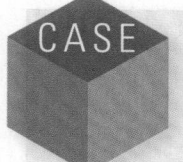
CASE

Ms. G is an 80-year-old piano teacher with progressively severe right leg pain over a period of 5 to 10 years. She has continued to teach in her studio but at the cost of increasing pain and fatigue. Imaging studies reveal severe osteoarthritis of the right hip. She is scheduled for elective replacement of the right hip with a prosthetic joint.

The total hip replacement is performed without immediate complications. During the first few days after the operation, Ms. G is given low-molecular-weight heparin and warfarin as prophylaxis against deep vein thrombosis. Six days after the operation, she develops excruciating pain in the area of the operation. Right lateral hip and buttock swelling is noted on physical examination. A complete blood count reveals significant blood loss (drop in hematocrit from 35% to 25%), and she is taken back to the operating room for evacuation of a large hematoma around the prosthetic joint. Although the hematoma does not appear to be grossly infected, cultures of the hematoma are positive for *Staphylococcus aureus*.

Because prosthetic joint infections are difficult to treat successfully without removal of the prosthesis, Ms. G is started on an aggressive 12-week course of combination antibiotics in which intravenous vancomycin and oral rifampin are administered for 2 weeks followed by oral ciprofloxacin and rifampin for 10 weeks. She tolerates the first 2 weeks of antibiotics without complications. However, 36 hours after switching her antibiotic from vancomycin to ciprofloxacin, she develops a high fever to 103°F

and extreme weakness. Aspiration of the hip reveals only a scant amount of straw-colored (i.e., nonpurulent) fluid. Ms. G is therefore admitted to the hospital for close observation.

Twelve hours after her admission, Ms. G develops an extensive maculopapular rash over her chest, back, and extremities. Her ciprofloxacin and rifampin are discontinued, and vancomycin is restarted. Gradually, over the next 72 hours, her temperature returns to normal and her rash begins to fade. There is no growth in the culture of the right hip aspirate. Ms. G is continued on vancomycin as a single agent for the next 4 weeks without incident; rifampin is restarted, again without incident; and the 12-week antibiotic course is eventually completed using a combination of trimethoprim-sulfamethoxazole and rifampin.

Four months after her hip surgery, Ms. G is back to teaching her piano students and making slow but steady progress in her rehabilitation program.

Questions

1. How likely was it that Ms. G's high fever, weakness, and skin rash represented a drug reaction to ciprofloxacin?
2. What was the rationale for co-administration of low-molecular-weight heparin and warfarin in the immediate postoperative period?
3. Was there a cause-and-effect relationship between administration of the prophylactic anticoagulants and Ms. G's life-threatening bleeding complication?

(**off-target adverse effects**) are discussed first. The phenotypic effects of these drug toxicities are then discussed at the physiologic, cellular, and molecular levels. General principles and specific examples are also illustrated in this chapter and throughout the book. The development of rational therapeutic strategies often requires an understanding of the mechanisms of both drug action and drug toxicity.

MECHANISMS OF DRUG TOXICITY

Whether a drug will do more harm than good in an individual patient depends on many factors, including the patient's age, genetic makeup, and preexisting conditions; the dose of the drug administered; and other drugs that the patient may be taking. For example, the very old or very young may be more susceptible to the toxic effects of a drug because of age-dependent differences in pharmacokinetic profiles or drug-metabolizing enzymes. As discussed in Chapter 4, Drug Metabolism, genetic factors may determine individual characteristics of drug metabolism, receptor activity, or repair mechanisms. Adverse drug reactions may be more likely in patients with preexisting conditions, such as liver or kidney dysfunction, and, of course, in patients allergic to specific

drugs. Concomitant medications can confound both efficacy and toxicity of drugs, particularly when these medications share or modulate the same metabolic pathways or transporters. Drug interactions with health supplements are also an important but often under-recognized cause of drug toxicity. Drug–drug and drug–herb interactions are discussed later in this chapter. The clinical determination of a drug's toxicity may not always be straightforward: as in the case of Ms. G, for example, a patient being treated with an antibiotic to combat an infection can develop a high fever, skin rash, and significant morbidity due either to recurrence of the infection or, instead, to an adverse reaction to the antibiotic.

Although a spectrum of adverse effects may be associated with the use of any drug or drug class, it is helpful to conceptualize the mechanisms of drug toxicity based on several general paradigms:

- "On-target" adverse effects, which are the result of the drug binding to its intended receptor, but at an inappropriate concentration, with suboptimal kinetics, or in the incorrect tissue (Fig. 6-1)
- "Off-target" adverse effects, which are caused by the drug binding to a target or receptor for which it was not intended (Fig. 6-1)

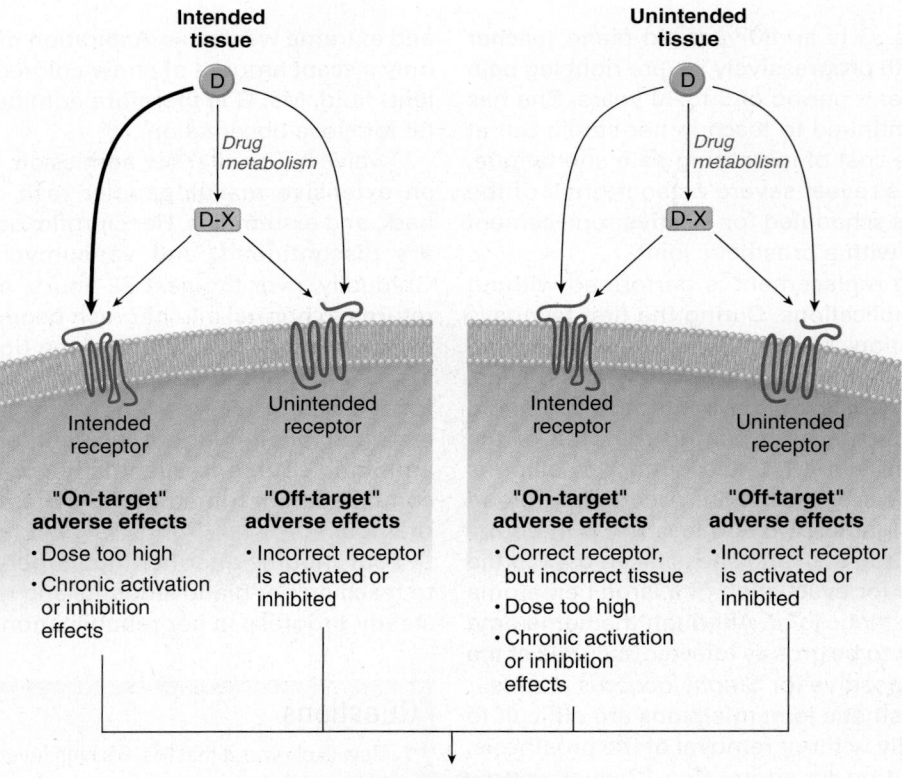

FIGURE 6-1. On-target and off-target adverse drug effects. Drug D is intended to modulate the function of a specific receptor (*intended receptor*) in a particular tissue (*intended tissue*). On-target adverse effects in the intended tissue could be caused by a supratherapeutic dose of the drug or by chronic activation or inhibition of the intended receptor by Drug D or its metabolite D–X. The same on-target effects could occur in a second tissue (*unintended tissue*); in addition, the intended receptor could mediate an adverse effect because the drug is acting in a tissue for which it was not designed. Off-target effects occur when the drug and/or its metabolites modulate the function of a target (*unintended receptor*) for which it was not intended.

- Adverse effects mediated by the immune system (Fig. 6-2)
- Idiosyncratic responses for which the mechanism is not known

These four mechanisms are discussed below. Note that many drugs can have both on-target and off-target effects, and adverse effects observed in patients can be due to multiple mechanisms.

On-Target Effects

An important concept in drug toxicity is that an adverse effect may be an exaggeration of the desired pharmacologic action as a result of changes in exposure or sensitivity to the drug (see Fig. 6-1). This can occur due to deliberate or accidental overdoses, alterations in the pharmacokinetics of the drug (e.g., due to liver or kidney disease or to interactions with other drugs), or changes in the pharmacodynamics of the drug–receptor interaction that alter the pharmacologic response (e.g., an increase in receptor number). All such changes can lead to an increase in the effective concentration of the drug and thus to an increased biological response. Because on-target effects are mediated via the desired mechanism of action of the drug, these effects are often shared by every member of the therapeutic class and are thus also known as **class effects**.

An important set of on-target adverse effects may occur because the drug, or one of its metabolites, interacts with the

appropriate receptor but in tissues other than those affected by the disease condition being treated (Fig. 6-1). Many drug targets are expressed in more than one cell type or tissue. For example, the antihistamine **diphenhydramine** is an H_1 receptor antagonist used to ameliorate the effects of histamine release in allergic conditions. This drug also crosses the blood–brain barrier to antagonize H_1 receptors in the central nervous system, leading to somnolence. This adverse effect led to the design of second-generation H_1 receptor antagonists that do not cross the blood–brain barrier and thus do not induce drowsiness. Notably, the first of these second-generation H_1 antagonists, **terfenadine**, produced an off-target effect (interaction with cardiac potassium channels) that led to a different and serious adverse effect—an increased risk of cardiac death. This example is discussed later in this chapter.

Local anesthetics such as **lidocaine** and **bupivacaine** provide a second example of an on-target adverse effect. These drugs are intended to prevent axonal impulse transmission by blocking sodium channels in neuronal membranes near the site of injection. Blockade of sodium channels in the central nervous system (CNS) following overdose or inappropriate administration (e.g., intravascular administration) can lead to tremors, seizures, and death. These on-target effects are discussed in greater detail in Chapter 12, Local Anesthetic Pharmacology.

The antipsychotic agent **haloperidol** is thought to produce its beneficial effect through blockade of mesolimbic and mesocortical D_2 receptors. One consequence of blocking D_2

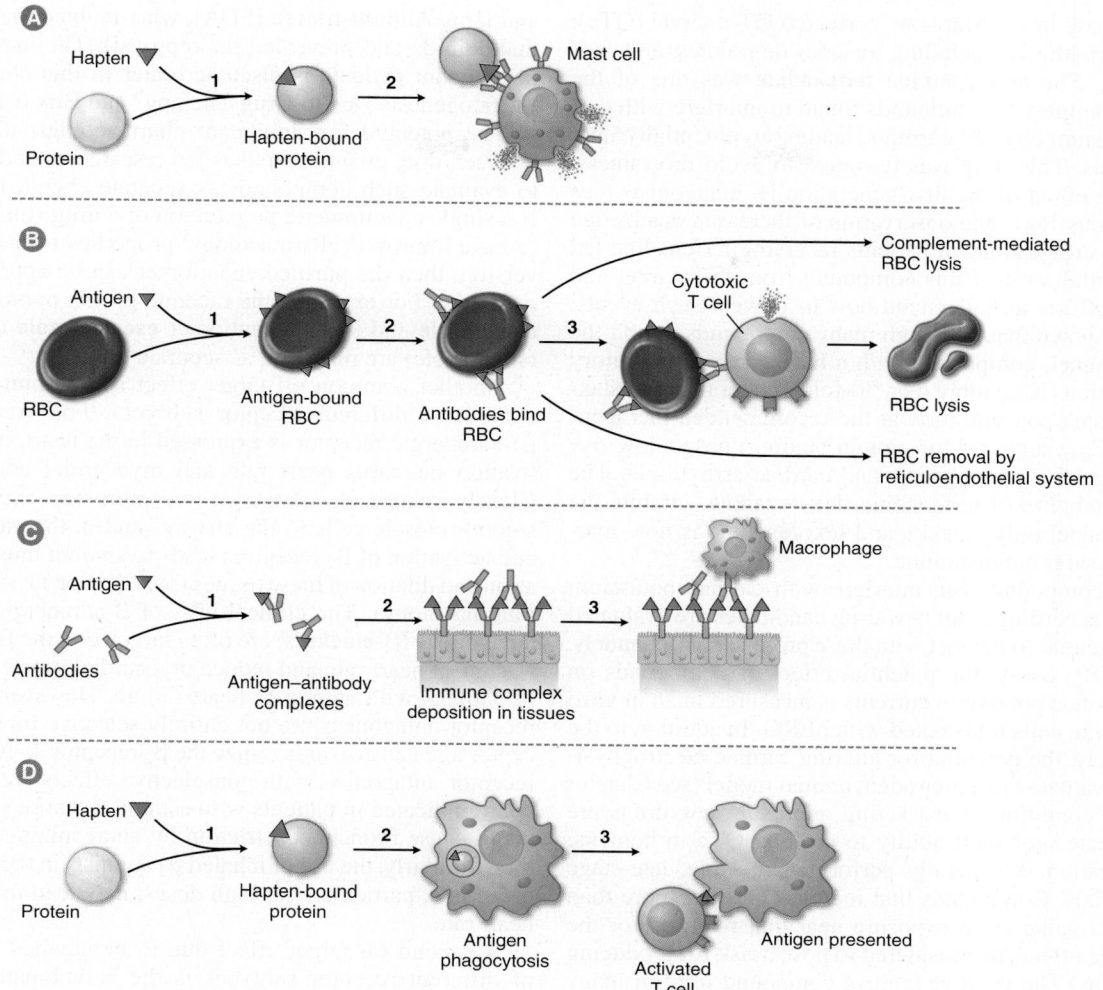

FIGURE 6-2. Mechanisms of hypersensitivity reactions. A. Type I hypersensitivity reactions occur when a hapten binds to a protein (1). The antigen cross-links IgE antibodies on the surface of a mast cell, leading to mast cell degranulation (2). Mast cells release histamine and other inflammatory mediators. **B.** Type II hypersensitivity reactions occur when an antigen binds to the surface of a circulating blood cell, usually a red blood cell (RBC) (1). Antibodies to the antigen then bind the surface of the RBC (2), attracting cytotoxic T cells (3), which release mediators that lyse the RBC. Binding of antibody to RBCs can also directly activate complement-mediated RBC lysis and RBC removal by the reticuloendothelial system. **C.** Type III hypersensitivity reactions occur when antibodies bind to a soluble toxin, acting as an antigen (1). The antigen–antibody complexes are then deposited in the tissues (2), attracting macrophages (3) and activating a complement-mediated reaction sequence (*not shown*). **D.** Type IV hypersensitivity reactions occur when a hapten binds to a protein (1) and the hapten-bound protein is phagocytosed by a Langerhans cell (2). The Langerhans cell migrates to a regional lymph node, where it presents the antigen to a T cell, thereby activating the T cell (3).

receptors in the pituitary gland is an increase in prolactin secretion, leading in some cases to amenorrhea, galactorrhea, sexual dysfunction, and osteoporosis. These on-target effects are discussed in Chapter 14, Pharmacology of Dopaminergic Neurotransmission.

Sometimes, on-target adverse effects unmask important functions of the biological target. A prominent example of this phenomenon occurs with administration of hydroxymethylglutaryl-coenzyme A (HMG-CoA) reductase inhibitors (so-called **statins**), which are used to decrease cholesterol levels. The intended target tissue of these drugs is the liver, where they inhibit HMG-CoA reductase, the rate-limiting enzyme of isoprenoid synthesis. A rare adverse effect of statin therapy is muscle toxicity, including rhabdomyolysis and myositis; the fact that this effect occurs highlights the physiologic role of HMG-CoA reductase in regulating the post-translational modification of several muscle proteins through a lipidation process called *geranylgeranylation*. Statins, as examples of drugs causing skeletal muscle injury, are also referenced later in this chapter.

Off-Target Effects

Very few drugs are so selective that they interact with only one molecular target. Off-target adverse effects occur when a drug interacts with unintended targets (Fig. 6-1). A prominent example of an off-target effect is the interaction of numerous compounds with cardiac I_{Kr} potassium channels. (Because the human ether-à-go-go-related gene [hERG] codes for one subunit of the human I_{Kr} channel, these channels are also called *hERG channels*.) Inhibition of potassium currents carried by I_{Kr} channels can lead to delayed repolarization of cardiac myocytes (see Chapter 24, Pharmacology of Cardiac Rhythm). In turn, delayed repolarization can lead to an increase in the heart-rate corrected QT interval (QTc), cardiac arrhythmias including torsades de pointes, and sudden death. The antihistamine **terfenadine** was one of the earliest examples of compounds found to interfere with cardiac potassium channel currents, leading to potentially fatal arrhythmias. This drug was designed to avoid drowsiness, an adverse effect of the first-generation H_1 antagonists (see earlier discussion). The observation of increased deaths due to cardiac arrhythmias in patients receiving terfenadine led to both withdrawal of this compound from the market and vigorous efforts to understand how to prevent such events. It is now known that, although many compounds inhibit the hERG channel, compounds with a half-maximal inhibitory concentration (IC_{50}) more than 30-fold greater than the maximum plasma concentration at the recommended therapeutic dose (C_{max}, adjusted for protein binding) pose a low risk of causing QTc prolongation and cardiac arrhythmia. The active metabolite of terfenadine, **fexofenadine**, inhibits the hERG channel only weakly, and fexofenadine is now marketed as a safer antihistamine.

Many compounds can interfere with cardiac potassium channels; accordingly, all new drug candidates are evaluated for the potential to interact with these promiscuous channels. In the hERG assay, the potential effect of compounds on human cardiac potassium currents is measured in an in vitro system using cells transfected with hERG. In addition to the hERG assay, the potential for altering cardiac electrophysiology is evaluated in a nonrodent animal model (see Chapter 51). As a condition of marketing approval, new drugs are also evaluated for their ability to prolong QTc in humans; this evaluation is generally performed in large, late-stage clinical trials. Compounds that increase QTc by more than a specified value at an exposure near that required for the therapeutic effect are considered to pose a risk for producing arrhythmias. The positive control compound used in many of these "thorough QTc studies" is **moxifloxacin**, an antibiotic that increases QTc at clinical doses (but confers a low risk of arrhythmogenesis). While the approach of relying most heavily on hERG inhibition in vitro and on thorough QTc clinical trials has prevented the recent introduction of "torsadogenic" drugs, this approach has been criticized for its low sensitivity, cost, and lack of assessment of the impact of other ion channel effects that mitigate or enhance the effects of compounds on QTc. Based on these concerns, alternative approaches are being considered, including preclinical evaluations that study a broader range of ion channel effects and clinical studies at an earlier stage of drug development.

Enantiomers (mirror-image isomers) of a drug can also cause off-target effects. As described in Chapter 1, Drug–Receptor Interactions, drug receptors are exquisitely sensitive to the three-dimensional structure of the drug molecule; therefore, receptors can often distinguish between enantiomers of a drug. A tragic and well-known example of this phenomenon occurred with the administration of racemic **thalidomide** (mixture of [R]- and [S]-enantiomers) in the 1960s as a treatment for morning sickness in pregnant women. While the [R]-enantiomer of thalidomide was an effective sedative, the [S]-enantiomer was a potent teratogen that caused severe birth defects such as amelia (absence of limbs) and various degrees of phocomelia in an estimated 10,000 newborns in 46 countries (but not in the United States, thanks to Frances Kelsey at the Food

and Drug Administration [FDA], who doubted the safety of thalidomide and prevented its approval). The use of drugs in pregnant patients is discussed later in this chapter (see "Teratogenesis Due to Drug Therapy" and Box 6-1).

The potential for significant pharmacologic differences between drug enantiomers has led researchers and the FDA to evaluate such compounds as separate chemical entities. If a single enantiomeric preparation of a drug can be shown to have improved pharmacologic properties over a racemic version, then the purified enantiomer can be approved as a new drug. For example, the racemic proton pump inhibitor **omeprazole** and its [S]-enantiomer **esomeprazole** (as in [S]-omeprazole) are marketed as separate drugs.

Another common off-target effect is the unintended activation of different receptor subtypes. For example, the β_1-adrenergic receptor is expressed in the heart, and its activation increases heart rate and myocardial contractility. Closely related β_2-adrenergic receptors are expressed in smooth muscle cells in the airways and in the vasculature, and activation of β_2 receptors leads to smooth muscle relaxation and dilation of these tissues (see Chapter 11, Adrenergic Pharmacology). The clinical uses of β-adrenergic receptor antagonists (**β-blockers**) are often targeted to the β_1 receptor to control heart rate and reduce myocardial oxygen demand in patients with angina or heart failure. However, some β_1 receptor antagonists are not entirely selective for the β_1 receptor and can also antagonize the β_2 receptor. β-Adrenergic receptor antagonists with nonselective effects are therefore contraindicated in patients with asthma, because such drugs could cause bronchoconstriction by antagonizing β_2 receptors. Similarly, the use of inhaled β_2 agonists in the treatment of asthma, particularly at high doses, may lead to increased heart rate.

A second off-target effect due to unintended activation of different receptor subtypes is the valvulopathy caused by the anorectic agent **fenfluramine**. This drug's primary mechanism of action appears to involve release of serotonin (5-hydroxytryptamine [5-HT]) and inhibition of 5-HT reuptake in brain areas that regulate feeding behavior. However, the compound also activates 5-HT_{2B} receptors, leading to proliferation of myofibroblasts in the atrioventricular valves. Pulmonary hypertension can develop and, in some cases, lead to death. Because of this adverse effect, fenfluramine has been withdrawn from the market (see "Drug-Induced Cardiovascular Toxicity").

The potential off-target effects of some drugs can be explored by using genetically modified laboratory mice or rats in which the intended target receptor has been deleted (sometimes only in specific tissues). If the drug nonetheless affects the physiology of these rodents, then targets other than the intended target must be involved.

Off-target effects of some drugs and drug metabolites can be determined only empirically, underscoring the importance of extensive drug testing both in preclinical experiments and in clinical trials. Despite such testing, some rare drug toxicities are discovered only when exposure occurs in a much larger population than that required for clinical trials. For example, **fluoroquinolones**, a class of broad-spectrum antibiotics derived from nalidixic acid, displayed minimal toxicities in preclinical studies and clinical trials. Wider clinical use of these drugs, however, led to reports of anaphylaxis, QTc prolongation, and potential cardiotoxicity, resulting in the removal of two drugs of this class, **temafloxacin** and

grepafloxacin, from the market. Use of another fluoroquinolone, **trovafloxacin**, is significantly restricted due to hepatic toxicity. In comparison, **ciprofloxacin** and **levofloxacin** are generally well tolerated and are frequently used in the treatment of bacterial infections. As seen in the introductory case, however, even these agents can occasionally cause a severe drug hypersensitivity reaction.

Idiosyncratic Toxicity

Idiosyncratic drug reactions are adverse effects that appear unpredictably, in a small fraction of patients, for unknown reasons. These effects are not typically manifest in premarketing testing in either laboratory animals or patients. The appearance of idiosyncratic injury leading to permanent organ dysfunction and/or death, even if rare, often prompts withdrawal of the drug from the market, precisely because susceptible patient populations cannot be identified. The systematic study of patient variations in response to different drugs may help to elucidate the genetic or other mechanisms that underlie idiosyncratic drug reactions.

▌ CONTEXTS OF DRUG TOXICITY

Drug Overdose

The Swiss physician and alchemist Paracelsus noted nearly 500 years ago that "all substances are poison; there is none which is not a poison. The right dose differentiates a poison and a remedy." In some cases, such as a suicide or homicide, the overdose of a drug is intentional. Most cases of overdose, however, are accidents. Adverse drug events due to medication errors are estimated to affect some 7 million people each year, with associated costs of $21 billion annually. This significant cost to both the patient and the health care system has led to systematic efforts intended to minimize errors in prescribing and dosing practices.

Drug–Drug Interactions

As the population has aged and increasing numbers of patients have been prescribed multiple medications, the potential for drug–drug interactions has grown. Numerous adverse interactions have been identified, and the mechanisms often involve pharmacokinetic or pharmacodynamic effects. Drug–herb interactions are also an important subset of drug–drug interactions.

Pharmacokinetic Drug–Drug Interactions

Pharmacokinetic interactions arise when one drug changes the absorption, distribution, metabolism, or excretion of another drug, thereby altering the concentration of active drug in the body. As discussed in Chapter 4, some drugs can inhibit or induce hepatic P450 enzymes. If two drugs are metabolized by the same P450 enzyme, competitive or irreversible inhibition of that P450 enzyme by one drug can result in an increase in the plasma concentration of the second drug. On the other hand, induction of a specific P450 enzyme by one drug can lead to a decrease in the plasma concentrations of other drugs that are metabolized by the same enzyme. The antifungal drug **ketoconazole** is a potent inhibitor of cytochrome P450 3A4 (CYP3A4). Co-administration of drugs that are also metabolized by CYP3A4 may result in reduced metabolism of these drugs and higher plasma drug levels. If the co-administered drug has a low therapeutic index, toxicity may occur. Because of its potent inhibition of CYP3A4, ketoconazole is often used in clinical studies designed to assess the importance of pharmacokinetic drug–drug interactions.

In addition to altering the activity of P450 enzymes, drugs can affect the transport of other drugs into and out of tissues (see Chapter 4 and Chapter 5, Drug Transporters). For example, **P-glycoprotein (P-gp)**, encoded by the multidrug resistance 1 (MDR1) gene, is an efflux pump that transports drugs into the intestinal lumen. Administration of a drug that inhibits or is a substrate for P-gp can lead to an increase in the plasma concentration of other drugs that are normally pumped out of the body by this mechanism. Since P-gp also plays a role in transport of drugs across the blood–brain barrier, compounds that inhibit P-gp can affect drug transport into the CNS. Other transporters, such as the **organic anion transporting polypeptide 1** (**OATP1**), mediate uptake of drugs into hepatocytes for metabolism and transport of drugs across the tubular epithelium of the kidney for excretion; both of these mechanisms promote clearance of drugs from the body. Interactions of a drug or one of its metabolites with these classes of transporters can lead to inappropriately high plasma concentrations of other drugs that are handled by the same transporter.

A pharmacokinetic interaction can sometimes be desirable. For example, because **penicillin** is cleared via tubular secretion in the kidney, the elimination half-life of this drug can be increased if the drug is given concomitantly with **probenecid**, an inhibitor of renal tubular transport. A second example is the combination of **imipenem**, a broad-spectrum antibiotic, with **cilastatin**, a selective inhibitor of a renal brush border dipeptidase (dehydropeptidase I). Because imipenem is rapidly inactivated by dehydropeptidase I, co-administration of imipenem with cilastatin is used to achieve therapeutic plasma concentrations of the antibiotic.

A drug that binds to plasma proteins (such as albumin) may displace a second drug from the same proteins to increase its free plasma concentration and thereby increase its bioavailability to target and nontarget tissues. This effect can be enhanced in a situation in which circulating albumin levels are low, such as liver failure or malnutrition (decreased albumin synthesis) or nephrotic syndrome (increased albumin excretion).

Pharmacodynamic Drug–Drug Interactions

Pharmacodynamic interactions arise when one drug changes the response of target or nontarget tissues to another drug. Toxic pharmacodynamic interactions can occur when two drugs activate complementary pathways, leading to an exaggerated biological effect. Such a drug interaction occurs upon co-administration of **sildenafil** (for erectile dysfunction) and **nitroglycerin** (for angina pectoris). Sildenafil inhibits phosphodiesterase type 5 (PDE5) and thus prolongs the action of cyclic GMP (cGMP), and nitroglycerin stimulates guanylyl cyclase to increase cGMP levels in vascular smooth muscle. Co-exposure to the two drugs increases cGMP to an even greater degree, increasing the risk of severe hypotension (see Chapter 22, Pharmacology of Vascular Tone).

A second example is the co-administration of antithrombotic drugs. After hip replacement surgery, patients are often treated with prophylactic warfarin for a number of weeks to prevent the development of postoperative deep vein thrombosis. Because plasma warfarin concentrations may not reach a therapeutic level for several days, patients are sometimes co-administered low-molecular-weight heparin and warfarin during this time. As seen in the case of Ms. G, however, significant bleeding may result if the effects of the heparin and warfarin synergize to produce supratherapeutic levels of anticoagulation. Newer antithrombotic drugs used for prophylaxis after orthopedic surgery (e.g., apixaban, rivaroxaban) may avoid this increased risk of bleeding because they reach therapeutic concentrations rapidly and do not require co-administration with another antithrombotic drug such as heparin.

Drug–Herb Interactions

The safety and efficacy of a drug may also be altered by co-exposure with various nonpharmaceuticals, such as foods, beverages, and herbal and other dietary supplements. Many herbal products are complex mixtures of biologically active compounds, and their safety and effectiveness have rarely been tested in controlled studies. The wide use of unregulated herbal products among the public should lead clinicians to inquire about patient use of such products.

The literature contains some reports of therapeutic failure of drugs taken in conjunction with herbal products and some reports of toxicity. For example, the herbal preparation **ginkgo biloba** (from the tree of the same name) inhibits platelet aggregation. Concomitant use of ginkgo and **nonsteroidal anti-inflammatory drugs (NSAIDs)**, which also inhibit platelet aggregation, may increase the risk of bleeding. In combination with **selective serotonin reuptake inhibitors**, **St. John's wort** may cause serotonin syndrome.

Cellular Mechanisms of Toxicity: Apoptosis and Necrosis

Cells are equipped with various mechanisms to avoid or repair damage: toxicity occurs if and when these defenses are overwhelmed. In some cases, toxicity can be minimized in the short term, but repeated insults (e.g., those leading to fibrosis) can eventually compromise organ function.

The primary cellular responses to a potentially toxic drug are illustrated in Figure 6-3A and 6-3B, using the hepatocyte as an example. Depending on the severity of the toxic insult, a cell may undergo **apoptosis** (programmed cell death) or **necrosis** (uncontrolled cell death). Apoptosis allows the cell to undergo ordered self-destruction by the coordinated activation of a number of dedicated proteins. Apoptosis can be beneficial when it eliminates damaged cells without damage to surrounding tissue. Inhibition of apoptosis is common in many cancer cells.

If the toxic insult is so severe that ordered cell death cannot be accomplished, the cell may undergo **necrosis**. Necrosis is characterized by enzymatic digestion of cellular contents, denaturation of cellular proteins, and disruption of cellular membranes. While apoptotic cells undergo cell death with minimal inflammation and disruption of adjacent tissue, necrotic cells attract inflammatory cells that can damage nearby healthy cells.

Organ and Tissue Toxicity

Most chapters in this book contain tables that list the serious and common adverse effects of the drugs discussed in that chapter. Here, we consider common mechanisms of injury and repair pertaining to the toxic effects of drugs on the major organ systems. This chapter cannot catalogue every known or suspected injury to each organ or organ system, since the range of drug-associated organ and tissue toxicity is quite large. Instead, a few specific examples of injury are provided to demonstrate the general features of drug toxicity.

Harmful Immune Responses and Immunotoxicity

Stimulation of the immune system plays a role in the toxicity of several drugs and drug classes. Drugs can be responsible for immune reactions (the classic type I through type IV reactions), syndromes that mimic some features of immune responses (red man syndrome), and skin rashes (eruptions)—including severe and life-threatening conditions such as Stevens-Johnson syndrome and toxic epidermal necrolysis. Drugs can also compromise the normal function of the immune system (immunotoxicity), leading to secondary effects such as increased risk of infection.

Some drugs may be recognized by the immune system as foreign substances. Small-molecule drugs with a mass of less than 600 daltons are not direct immunogens but can act as **haptens**, such that the drug binds (often covalently) to a protein in the body and is then capable of triggering an immune response. If a drug is sufficiently large (e.g., a therapeutic peptide or protein), it may directly activate the immune system. The two principal immune mechanisms by which drugs can produce damage are **hypersensitivity responses** (allergic responses) and **autoimmune reactions**.

The hypersensitivity responses are classically divided into four types (Fig. 6-2). Table 6-1 provides information about the mediators and clinical manifestations of the four types of hypersensitivity reactions. Prior exposure to a substance is required for each of the four types of reactions.

Type I hypersensitivity responses (**immediate hypersensitivity** or **anaphylaxis**) result from the production of IgE antibody after exposure to an antigen. The antigen may be a foreign protein, such as the bacterially derived thrombolytic drug **streptokinase**, or it may be an endogenous protein modified by a **hapten** to become immunogenic. **Penicillin** fragments—either in the administered drug formulation or formed in vivo—can act as haptens and activate the immune system. Subsequent exposure to the antigen causes mast cells to degranulate, releasing inflammatory mediators such as histamine, serotonin, and leukotrienes that promote bronchoconstriction, vasodilatation, and inflammation. Type I hypersensitivity responses manifest as a **wheal-and-flare reaction** in the skin. Symptoms of "hay fever" such as conjunctivitis and rhinitis may develop in the upper respiratory tract, while asthmatic bronchoconstriction may occur in the lower respiratory tract (see Chapter 48, Integrative Inflammation Pharmacology: Asthma).

Type II hypersensitivity responses (**antibody-dependent cytotoxic hypersensitivity**) occur when a drug binds to cells, usually red blood cells, and is recognized by an antibody, usually IgG or IgM. The antibody triggers cell lysis by complement fixation, phagocytosis by macrophages, or cytolysis by cytotoxic T cells. Type II responses are rare adverse responses to several drugs, including penicillin and **quinidine**.

Type III hypersensitivity responses (**immune complex-mediated hypersensitivity**) occur when antibodies, usually IgG or IgM, are formed against soluble antigens. The antigen–antibody complexes are deposited in tissues such as kidneys, joints, and lung vascular endothelium. These complexes

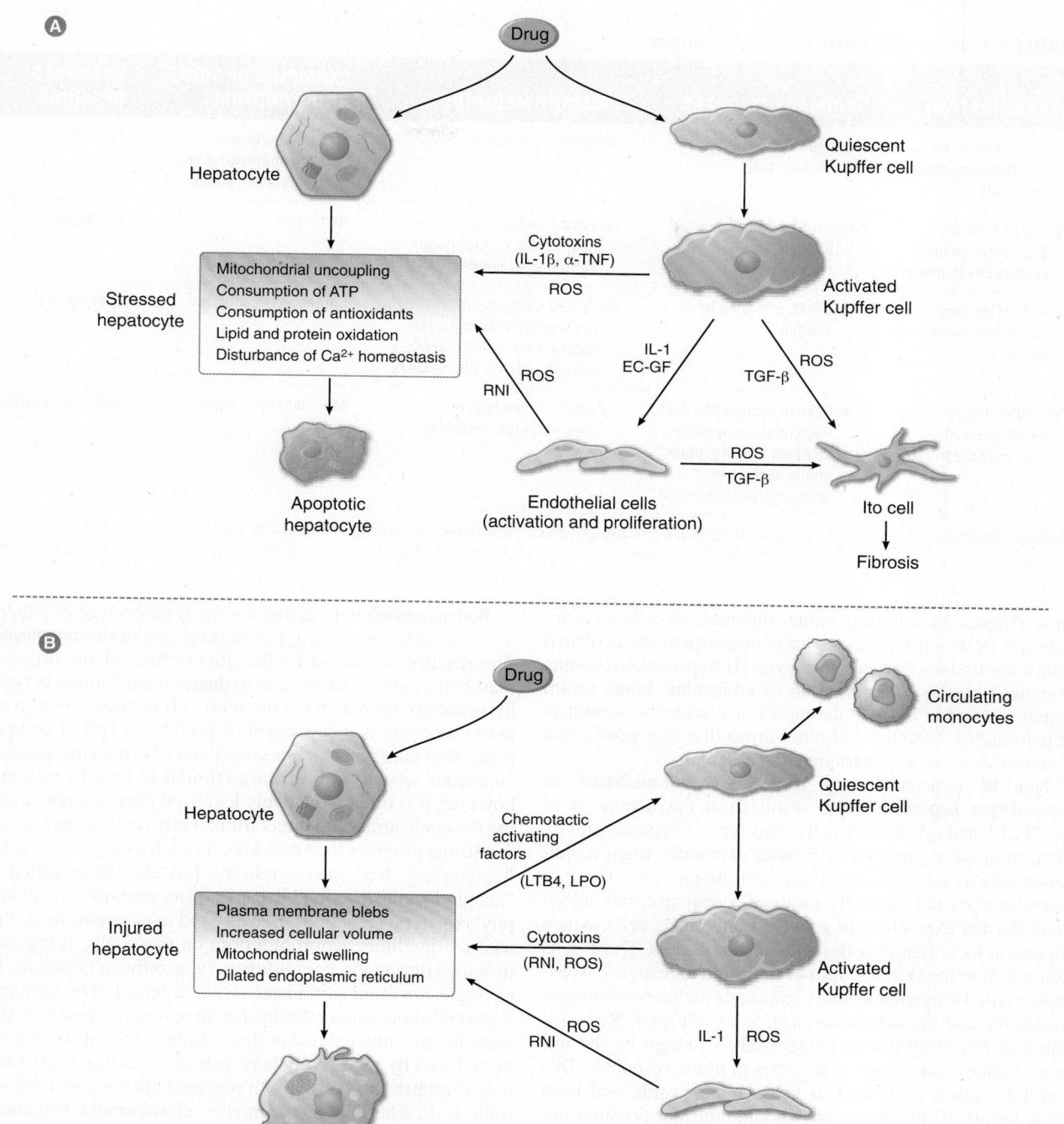

FIGURE 6-3. Subtoxic and toxic damage to hepatocytes in response to moderate and high doses of drug. A. Subtoxic damage. Moderate doses of a potentially toxic drug activate Kupffer cells and are metabolized by hepatocytes. The resulting hepatocyte stress may be exacerbated by the effects of reactive oxygen species (ROS) and reactive nitrogen intermediates (RNI) elaborated by activated endothelial cells. Hepatocyte apoptosis and Ito cell activation may result, leading to fibrosis. **B. Toxic damage.** High doses of a toxic drug are metabolized by hepatocytes to reactive metabolites that can induce cell injury. Chemotactic activating factors released by the injured hepatocytes activate Kupffer cells and endothelial cells, which elaborate toxic ROS and RNI. The end result of this toxic cascade is hepatocyte necrosis. EC-GF, endothelial cell growth factor; IL-1, interleukin-1; IL-1β, interleukin-1β; LPO, lipid peroxidation; LTB4, leukotriene B4; TGF-β, transforming growth factor β; α-TNF, tumor necrosis factor α.

TABLE 6-1 Types of Hypersensitivity Reactions

CLASSIFICATION	PRIMARY TRIGGERS	PRIMARY MEDIATORS	EXAMPLES OF SIGNS AND SYMPTOMS	EXAMPLES OF DRUGS
Type I or immediate-type hypersensitivity (humoral)	Antigen-binding IgE on mast cells	Histamine, serotonin	Hives and urticaria, bronchoconstriction, hypotension, shock	Penicillin
Type II or antibody-dependent cellular cytotoxicity (humoral)	IgG, IgM, and cell-bound antigen	Activated complement; neutrophils, macrophages, natural killer cells	Hemolysis	Cefotetan
Type III or immune-complex disease (humoral)	IgG, IgM, and soluble antigen	Activated complement; neutrophils, macrophages, natural killer cells; reactive oxygen species, chemokines	Cutaneous vasculitis	Mitomycin C
Type IV or delayed-type hypersensitivity (cell-mediated)	Antigen in association with major histocompatibility complex (MHC) protein on the surface of antigen-presenting cells	Cytotoxic T lymphocytes, macrophages, cytokines	Macular rash, organ failure	Sulfamethoxazole

Adapted from Table 2 in Bugelski PJ. Genetic aspects of immune-mediated adverse drug effects. *Nat Rev Drug Discov* 2005;4:59–69.

cause damage by initiating **serum sickness**, an inflammatory response in which leukocytes and complement are activated within the tissues. For example, type III hypersensitivity can be caused by the administration of **antivenins**, horse serum proteins obtained by inoculating a horse with the venom to be neutralized. Examples of other drugs that may pose a risk of serum sickness are **bupropion** and **cefaclor**.

Type IV hypersensitivity responses (**cell-mediated** or **delayed-type hypersensitivity**) result from the activation of T_H1, T_H17, and cytotoxic T cells. This type of hypersensitivity most commonly presents as **contact dermatitis** when a substance acts as a hapten and binds to host proteins. The first exposure does not normally produce a response, but subsequent dermal exposure can activate Langerhans cells, which migrate to local lymph nodes and activate T cells. The T cells then return to the skin and initiate an immune response. Well-known type IV hypersensitivity responses include reactions to poison ivy and the development of latex allergies. Repeated exposure to a drug that is recognized as foreign by the immune system can trigger a massive immune response. This "cytokine storm" can lead to fever, hypotension, and even organ failure. Thus, physicians should consider possible immune reactions to all administered drugs, even those that have appeared to be safe in large populations. In the case presented at the beginning of the chapter, Ms. G's fever and rash were likely caused by a T-cell-mediated hypersensitivity reaction to ciprofloxacin. Once this was recognized and the ciprofloxacin was stopped, her fever and rash resolved as well.

Autoimmunity results when a person's immune system attacks her or his own cells (see Chapter 46, Pharmacology of Immunosuppression). Several drugs and other chemicals can initiate autoimmune reactions. **Methyldopa** can cause hemolytic anemia by eliciting an autoimmune reaction against the Rhesus antigens (Rh factors) on red blood cells. Several other drugs, such as **hydralazine**, **isoniazid**, and **procainamide**, can cause a lupus-like syndrome by inducing antibodies to myeloperoxidase (hydralazine and isoniazid) or DNA (procainamide).

Red man syndrome occurs in a small percentage of patients receiving intravenous drugs such as the antibiotic **vancomycin**. The reaction is caused by the direct effect of the drugs on mast cells, causing these cells to degranulate. Unlike in type I hypersensitivity reactions, the mast cell degranulation in red man syndrome is independent of preformed IgE or complement. Red man syndrome is associated with the emergence of cutaneous wheals and urticaria (similar to type I reactions); however, it is often a relatively localized phenomenon affecting the neck, arms, and upper trunk. Only rarely does red man syndrome progress to severe toxicity such as angioedema and hypotension. Red man syndrome has also been called an "anaphylactoid reaction" because of its resemblance to anaphylaxis (type I reaction). Because red man syndrome is initiated by the direct action of a drug on mast cells, it typically develops during the drug infusion (vancomycin infusions, for example, are often administered over a period of 60 minutes). The syndrome usually diminishes in severity or resolves after reducing the infusion rate or discontinuing the infusion; it can be reduced by the prophylactic use of antihistamines; and it may diminish in severity with repeated intravenous administrations. In addition to vancomycin, **ciprofloxacin**, **amphotericin B**, and **rifampin** can cause this reaction. Red man syndrome is also associated with certain excipients used in intravenous formulations; one such excipient is **Cremophor** (also known as **Kolliphor®**), an excipient for **paclitaxel**, **cyclosporine**, and several other drugs.

Many drugs can elicit the development of **skin rashes**, which are usually diagnosed as erythema multiforme. The more severe (sometimes life-threatening) conditions known as **Stevens-Johnson syndrome** and **toxic epidermal necrolysis** have been reported with barbiturates, sulfonamides, antiepileptics (**phenytoin**, **carbamazepine**), nonsteroidal anti-inflammatory drugs (**ibuprofen**, **celecoxib**, **valdecoxib**), **allopurinol**, and other drugs. The pathogenesis of Stevens-Johnson syndrome is not completely understood, but the morphologic appearance of mucous membrane and skin inflammation, with the development of blisters and separation of the epidermis from the dermis, is consistent with an immune etiology. A temporal relationship may exist between the administration of a drug and the development of skin lesions, but some cases of Stevens-Johnson syndrome are idiopathic or related to infection. Thus, not every case of Stevens-Johnson syndrome can be attributed to drug exposure.

Immunotoxicity, or injury to the immune system, can occur either as an adverse effect of therapy or as the specific intent of therapy. Cytotoxic agents used in cancer chemotherapy are designed to kill proliferating neoplastic cells but also routinely damage proliferating normal cells in the bone marrow, lymphoid tissues, gastrointestinal tract, and hair follicles at concentrations of drug that are required for efficacy. For these agents, there is generally little safety margin for damage to normal tissues, and successful therapy depends on a greater sensitivity of the cancer cells compared to normal tissues (see Chapter 33, Principles of Antimicrobial and Antineoplastic Pharmacology). An increased risk of infection often accompanies therapy with agents that are cytotoxic to white blood cells. The margin between adverse effects and therapeutic effects may be increased by the use of agents that stimulate leukocyte production (e.g., **filgrastim**).

Targeting of the immune system may be appropriate when the disease is caused or exacerbated by a deleterious immune response (see Chapter 46). For example, inhaled corticosteroids may be used to control symptoms in patients with frequent, severe exacerbations of chronic obstructive pulmonary disease (see Chapter 48). By inhibiting immune responses to pathogenic microorganisms, however, such treatment is also associated with an increased risk of pneumonia.

Some immunotherapies target specific cell types in the immune system and are associated with an increased risk of serious infection. **Rituximab** is a monoclonal antibody (mAb) that targets CD20-positive B cells, which are involved in the pathogenesis of non-Hodgkin's lymphoma (malignant CD20-positive B cells) and rheumatoid arthritis (antibody-producing CD20-positive B cells). Two potentially serious adverse effects that have been observed with the use of rituximab are progressive multifocal leukoencephalopathy (PML), an infection caused by a polyomavirus, the JC virus (JCV), and hepatitis B reactivation with the potential for fulminant hepatitis. These infectious agents are generally present in latent form in patients prior to treatment with rituximab, but the loss of immunocompetence as a result of treatment allows expression of these serious infections. Similarly, **efalizumab** is a monoclonal antibody that targets CD11a, the α subunit of leukocyte function-associated antigen-1 (LFA-1), which is expressed on all leukocytes. By decreasing the cell surface expression of CD11a and inhibiting the binding of LFA-1 to intercellular adhesion molecule-1 (ICAM-1), efalizumab inhibits leukocyte adhesion and is an effective immunotherapy for psoriasis. However, because CD11a is also expressed on the surface of B cells, monocytes, neutrophils, natural killer cells, and other leukocytes, efalizumab can affect the activation, adhesion, migration, and destruction of these cells as well. Like rituximab, efalizumab has been associated with PML; this serious adverse effect led to its withdrawal from the market in 2009. A similar increase in the frequency of PML has been found in patients receiving **natalizumab** for multiple sclerosis. Natalizumab binds to the α4 subunit of α4β1 and α4β7 integrins expressed on the surface of all leukocytes except neutrophils; by inhibiting the α4-mediated adhesion of leukocytes to their target cells, leukocyte recruitment and activation are prevented.

Cytotoxic antineoplastic agents often decrease the proliferation not only of the target cancer cells but also of proliferating cells of normal tissues (see earlier discussion). Targeted antineoplastic therapies may reduce the impact on normal proliferating cell populations (see Chapter 33), but immunosuppression and infection remain risks. In recent years, numerous **tyrosine kinase inhibitors** have been developed for the treatment of malignant tumors. The mechanism of action of these compounds is competitive inhibition with ATP at the ATP-binding site of the kinases. The role of tyrosine kinases in cancer is presented in detail in Chapter 40, Pharmacology of Cancer: Signal Transduction. **Sunitinib** is an example of an anticancer tyrosine kinase inhibitor. This agent is approved for use in gastrointestinal stromal tumors, advanced renal cell carcinoma, and well-differentiated pancreatic neuroendocrine tumors. Although sunitinib is selective for VEGF and other receptor tyrosine kinases expressed in these cancers, its adverse effects include serious infections of the perineum, respiratory tract, urinary tract, and skin as well as sepsis and septic shock. These infections may occur with or without neutropenia, and necrotizing fasciitis of the perineum may lead to death. Increased risk of infections has also been observed with the tyrosine kinase inhibitors **afatinib**, **bosutinib**, **ibrutinib**, and **ponatinib**.

Drug-Induced Hepatotoxicity

Many drugs are metabolized in and/or excreted by the liver, and some of these metabolites can cause liver damage. A clinically significant example is **acetaminophen**, a widely used analgesic and antipyretic. In its therapeutic dose range, acetaminophen is metabolized predominantly by glucuronidation and sulfation, resulting in readily excreted metabolites; a small fraction of the dose is also excreted unchanged. As shown in Figure 6-4, however, acetaminophen can also be oxidized to a reactive and potentially toxic species, **N-acetyl-p-benzoquinoneimine (NAPQI)**. Glutathione can conjugate with and thereby detoxify NAPQI, but overdosing with acetaminophen depletes glutathione reserves (as can other conditions), leaving NAPQI free to attack cellular and mitochondrial proteins, resulting ultimately in the necrosis of hepatocytes. Timely (within about 10 hours of acetaminophen overdosing) administration of the antidote **N-acetylcysteine (NAC)** replenishes glutathione stores and can avert liver failure and death. This example underscores the importance of **dose**: although acetaminophen is used safely by millions of individuals every day, the same drug, when taken in excess, is responsible for some 50% of the cases of acute liver failure in the United States.

The liver metabolizes and excretes many endogenous compounds as well as drugs. Of particular interest with regard to drug-induced hepatotoxicity are the hepatocyte transporters and enzymes responsible for bile acid absorption from the blood, bile acid processing within the hepatocyte, and bile acid secretion into the bile canaliculi (see Chapter 5). Some drugs share these pathways with the endogenous bile acids. Inhibition of bile acid transporters by a drug or its metabolites can lead to decreased bile acid secretion, with subsequent increases in intracellular and plasma concentrations of bile acids and accompanying hepatocellular injury. Inhibition of the bile salt export pump (BSEP) was a contributing factor in the hepatotoxicity that caused

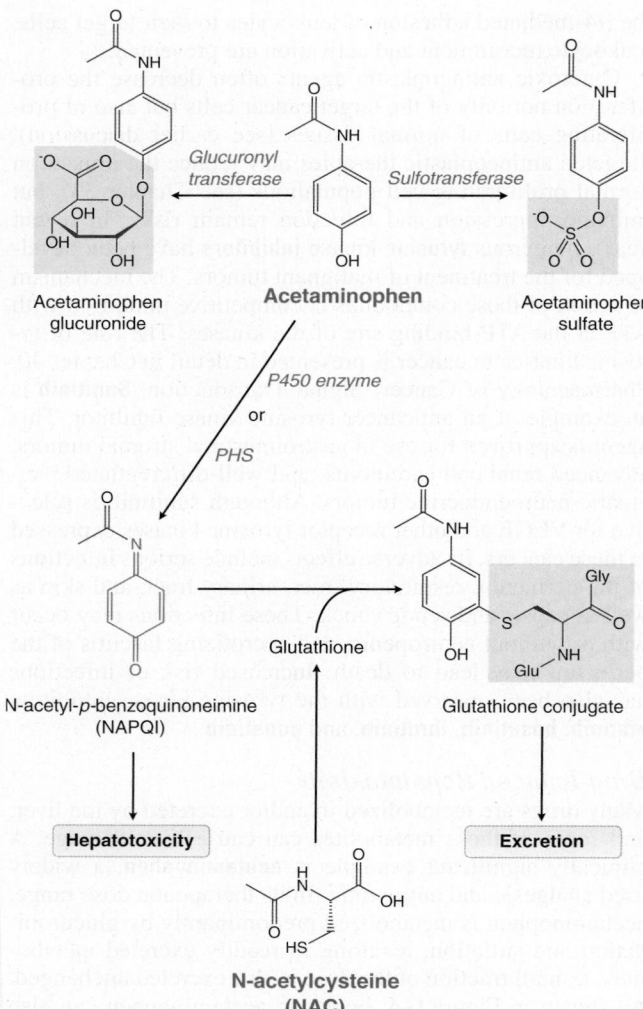

FIGURE 6-4. Mechanism of acetaminophen poisoning and treatment. Therapeutic doses of acetaminophen are nontoxic, but one metabolite formed at supratherapeutic doses can cause potentially lethal hepatotoxicity. Under ordinary circumstances, acetaminophen is metabolized primarily by glucuronidation (~55–60%) and sulfation (~30–35%); another 5% or less is excreted unchanged. The remaining 5–10% is oxidized to a reactive intermediate, *N*-acetyl-*p*-benzoquinoneimine (NAPQI). This oxidation is catalyzed by cytochrome P450 enzymes (CYP), primarily CYP2E1, as well as CYP3A4 and CYP1A2, and by prostaglandin H synthase (PHS). At therapeutic doses, NAPQI reacts rapidly with glutathione to form a nontoxic metabolite that is readily excreted. Under conditions of overdosing, however, NAPQI formation exceeds glutathione production, allowing free NAPQI to attack mitochondrial and cellular proteins. If this process is unchecked, hepatocyte necrosis and acute liver failure can result. Timely administration of the antidote *N*-acetylcysteine (NAC) can be lifesaving (within ~10 hours of acetaminophen overdosing), in that NAC both reacts directly with NAPQI (*not shown*) and serves as a precursor to glutathione.

troglitazone, an insulin-sensitizing agent developed to treat diabetes, to be withdrawn from the market.

Unexpected hepatotoxicity is the most frequent reason for drug withdrawals in the United States. Many cases of fulminant hepatitis after drug therapy are idiosyncratic—that is, the mechanism by which the patient develops hepatic injury is not known—making it difficult to identify at-risk patients. In some cases, failure to determine the mechanism(s) responsible for hepatic injury is due to the inability to reproduce the injury in laboratory animals. A further challenge is that hepatotoxicity may not be anticipated based on preclinical studies, because compounds exhibiting significant hepatotoxicity in animal studies at doses near the anticipated therapeutic exposures in humans are generally withdrawn from development. Further confounding the prevention of hepatotoxicity is that clinical trials of a drug typically include a few thousand patients, even though a risk of drug-induced hepatotoxicity in the range of 1 in 10,000 to 1 in 100,000 patients would be of sufficient concern to result in withdrawal from the market. In other words, many clinical trials are too small, or have been designed with exclusion criteria that are not maintained once the drug is marketed, to detect unacceptable risks of hepatotoxicity. Withdrawal of troglitazone, for example, occurred only after it was noted that approximately 1 in 10,000 patients taking the drug died from acute liver failure.

The serum levels of certain enzymes (alanine aminotransferase [ALT], aspartate aminotransferase [AST], and alkaline phosphatase [ALP]) and bilirubin are often used to monitor for potential hepatotoxicity in patients. The combination of hepatocellular injury (indicated by increased serum levels of ALT, AST, and ALP) and decreased hepatic function (indicated by elevated bilirubin) is the best predictor of outcome for drug-induced hepatotoxicity. Elevation of serum ALT to >3 times the upper limit of normal, combined with elevation of serum bilirubin to >2 times the upper limit of normal, is associated with a mortality rate of at least 10%. This predictor has become known as Hy's rule, named for the hepatologist Hyman Zimmerman.

Drug-Induced Renal Toxicity

The kidney is the major route of excretion of many drugs and their metabolites. Nephrotoxicity may manifest as alterations in renal hemodynamics, tubular damage and obstruction, glomerular nephropathy, and interstitial nephritis. Progressive renal failure, characterized by progressive increases in serum creatinine, may result from loss of function of a sufficient number of nephrons. Examples of drug classes that can cause renal failure include certain antibiotics, NSAIDs, antineoplastic agents, immunomodulators, and angiotensin converting enzyme (ACE) inhibitors. Here, we describe the mechanisms of nephrotoxicity caused by the aminoglycoside antibiotic **gentamicin** and the antifungal agent **amphotericin B**. Renal injury is a common adverse effect of treatment with both of these agents.

Gentamicin causes renal injury in part through its inhibition of lysosomal hydrolases (sphingomyelinase, phospholipases) in proximal tubules of the kidney, leading to the lysosomal accumulation of electron-dense lamellar structures containing undegraded phospholipids. This process is called *renal phospholipidosis*. Lysosomal rupture leads to cell death in the form of *acute tubular necrosis*. Renal tubular injury by gentamicin and other aminoglycoside antibiotics is reversible upon cessation of treatment, provided that the initial injury is not too severe.

The polyene **amphotericin B** damages fungal cell membranes by interacting with ergosterol and forming membrane pores through which potassium leaks, leading to cell death. Amphotericin-induced renal injury appears to occur via a similar mechanism, with initial binding of drug to sterols in the membranes of renal tubular epithelial cells. Because the mechanism responsible for efficacy is shared by the mechanism responsible for toxicity, the margin between the exposures required for antifungal activity and those required for renal injury is small, leading to a high frequency of renal injury in patients receiving amphotericin B. Liposomal formulations of amphotericin B have been developed in an attempt to reduce this toxicity and to increase the plasma half-life of the drug. If the initial injury is not too severe, cessation of treatment with amphotericin often results in recovery of renal function.

Contrast media is administered intra-arterially or intravenously to provide radiographic delineation of the vasculature in organs such as the heart and the brain. These agents appear to cause renal injury both by direct toxicity to renal tubular epithelial cells and by constriction of the vasa recta, leading to reduced renal medullary blood flow. The nephrotoxicity of contrast media is dose-related, and patients with preexisting reductions in medullary blood flow—due, for example, to renal insufficiency, intravascular volume depletion, heart failure, diabetes, or diuretic or NSAID use—are at higher risk.

Drug-Induced Neurotoxicity

Drug-induced neurotoxicity is most often associated with the use of cytotoxic cancer chemotherapeutic agents. In most cases, neurotoxicity manifests in the peripheral nerves, but the central nervous system may be affected as well. Peripheral neuropathy has been associated with vinca alkaloids (e.g., **vincristine**, **vinblastine**), taxanes (e.g., **paclitaxel**), and platinum compounds (e.g., **cisplatin**). The neuropathy caused by vinca alkaloids and taxanes is directly related to their primary mechanism of action, microtubule disruption (see Chapter 39, Pharmacology of Cancer: Genome Synthesis, Stability, and Maintenance). In peripheral nerves, microtubule disruption is thought to result in altered axonal trafficking and both sensory and motor neuropathy. Platinum-containing compounds may have direct toxic effects on peripheral nerves. **Methotrexate** use has been associated with serious toxicity in the CNS (e.g., leukoencephalopathy, seizures).

Drug-Induced Skeletal Muscle Toxicity

Drugs and drug classes associated with skeletal muscle injury include HMG-CoA reductase inhibitors (**statins**), corticosteroids (**dexamethasone**, **betamethasone**, **prednisolone**, **hydrocortisone**), **zidovudine**, and **daptomycin**. Statin-induced myopathy appears to relate to the inhibition of geranyl-geranylation of several muscle proteins. Corticosteroid-induced muscle injury is complex, involving altered carbohydrate metabolism, decreased protein synthesis, and alterations in mitochondrial function that reduce oxidative capacity. Patients treated with corticosteroids can manifest weakness, atrophy, myalgia, and microscopic decreases in muscle fiber size. Corticosteroid-associated muscle injury is reversible, albeit slowly. Understanding the pathogenesis of zidovudine-induced myopathy is complicated by the ability of HIV, the retroviral infection for which zidovudine is administered, to induce myopathy in the absence of drug therapy. Nonetheless, the improvement in muscle function upon withdrawal of zidovudine and the independent demonstration of zidovudine-induced myopathy in rodents suggest that the drug itself causes myopathy, at least in some patients. The mechanism of zidovudine-associated myopathy is not well understood, but accumulation of the drug in skeletal muscle, disruption of mitochondrial cristae, and decreased oxidative phosphorylation are thought to play a role.

Daptomycin is a cyclic lipopeptide antibiotic active against Gram-positive bacteria. Its mechanism of action is a subject of active investigation. Daptomycin binds to the cell membrane of bacteria. It appears to induce the formation of curved patches of membrane, leading to aberrant recruitment of proteins involved in cell division, membrane ion leaks, membrane depolarization, and bacterial cell death. Its spectrum of action is thought to result from the higher content of negatively charged anionic phospholipids in the membranes of Gram-positive bacteria compared to Gram-negative bacteria. In preclinical studies of daptomycin, skeletal muscle was the main target organ of toxicity. The degree of skeletal myopathy was related to both the frequency of dosing (i.e., the incidence and severity of toxicity increased if the once-daily dose was divided into several smaller doses) and the total exposure to drug (expressed as the area under the curve [AUC]). The mechanism of skeletal muscle injury by daptomycin is not fully understood. It is hypothesized that daptomycin disrupts muscle cell membranes, consistent with its lipophilic nature and its mechanism of action in bacteria. The membrane injury causes leakage of creatine kinase (CK), and increased CK activity in the serum is a clinical indicator of myotoxicity. Myopathy associated with an increase in CK has been observed in patients as well as in animals and is reversible upon discontinuation of daptomycin. Myopathy seldom occurs in patients administered once-daily doses.

Drug-Induced Cardiovascular Toxicity

Three major mechanisms of drug-induced cardiovascular toxicity have been recognized. First, as discussed earlier, many drugs interact with cardiac potassium channels to cause QTc prolongation, delayed repolarization, and cardiac arrhythmias. Second, some drugs are directly toxic to cardiac myocytes. The anthracycline antineoplastic agent **doxorubicin** avidly binds to iron; in the presence of oxygen, the iron can cycle between the iron(II) and iron(III) states, leading to the production of reactive oxygen species (ROS). These ROS promote cytotoxicity and death of cardiac myocytes; the mechanism of cell death may relate to the low activity of antioxidant enzyme systems in these cells. Cardiotoxicity, leading to heart failure and arrhythmia, is often the dose-limiting toxicity in patients receiving this drug. Third, as noted earlier, some drugs are toxic to heart valves. The amphetamine analog **fenfluramine** exerts its desired anorectic effect by increasing the release and decreasing the uptake of serotonin. Fenfluramine and its metabolite norfenfluramine also bind with high affinity to 5-HT$_{2B}$ receptors. Drug binding to 5-HT$_{2B}$ receptors in heart valves activates mitogenic pathways, resulting in proliferation of valvular myofibroblasts that form myxoid plaques on the atrioventricular valves, leading to valvular insufficiency and death in some patients. The increased serotonergic activity of fenfluramine can also increase vascular resistance and remodel the pulmonary arterial system, leading to pulmonary hypertension. As noted earlier, the severe adverse effects of fenfluramine have caused the drug to be withdrawn from the market. Because of the potential severity of all these cardiovascular toxicities, there is a concerted effort to avoid selection of compounds for drug development that exhibit significant prolongation of the QTc interval or binding affinity for 5-HT$_{2B}$ receptors.

Drug-Induced Pulmonary Toxicity

Adverse effects in the lungs range from acute, reversible exacerbations of asthmatic symptoms to chronic injury characterized by remodeling and/or fibrosis. Reversible airway obstruction can be associated with β-adrenoceptor antagonist therapy, whereas chronic injury is observed in some patients receiving the chemotherapeutic agent **bleomycin** or the antiarrhythmic drug **amiodarone**. The response to injury after cellular damage is largely determined by the regenerative capacity of the target organ. Repeated insults to the lung, particularly to the epithelial cells lining conducting airways and alveoli, may be followed by regeneration. However, repeated cycles of epithelial injury can also lead to excessive deposition of collagen and extracellular matrix proteins in alveolar septa and the alveolar spaces, causing **fibrosis**. Pulmonary fibrosis is manifested as loss of lung function. Bleomycin and amiodarone are contraindicated in patients with existing disease of the lung parenchyma because both of these agents can cause pulmonary fibrosis.

Carcinogenesis Due to Drug Therapy

Drugs (and other agents) that can cause cancer are termed *carcinogens*. More broadly, a **carcinogen** is a chemical, physical, or biological insult that acts by causing specific types of DNA damage (these agents are termed *initiators*) or by facilitating proliferation of cells carrying precancerous mutations (these agents are **promoters**). *Initiators* act by damaging DNA, interfering with DNA replication, or interfering with DNA repair mechanisms. Most initiators are reactive species that covalently modify the structure of DNA, preventing accurate replication and, if unrepaired or misrepaired, leading to one or more mutations. If the mutation affects a gene that controls cell cycle regulation, neoplastic transformation may be initiated. Carcinogenesis is a complex process, involving multiple genetic and epigenetic changes, that usually takes place over years or decades.

For most therapeutic areas, compounds that cause direct DNA damage are avoided. Yet DNA damage and/or interference with DNA repair is the desired therapeutic effect of many agents used to treat neoplasia. Damage to normal blood cell progenitors is an important on-target adverse effect of cytotoxic alkylating agents used in cancer chemotherapy (**chlorambucil**, **cyclophosphamide**, **melphalan**, **nitrogen mustards**, and **nitrosoureas**). These agents can cause myelodysplasia and/or acute myeloid leukemia (AML). Indeed, 10% to 20% of cases of AML in the United States arise secondary to treatment of other cancers with such anticancer drugs.

Tamoxifen, a nongenotoxic estrogen receptor modulator, is an effective treatment in patients with estrogen-sensitive breast cancer. However, this agent also increases the risk of some tumors. Although tamoxifen is an antagonist of estrogen receptors in the breast, it is a *partial agonist* in other tissues that express the estrogen receptor, most notably the uterus. Therefore, an adverse effect of breast cancer treatment with tamoxifen can be the development of endometrial cancer. Newer estrogen receptor modulators, such as **raloxifene**, do not stimulate uterine estrogen receptors and may be used to treat or prevent breast cancer with a lower risk of endometrial cancer (see Chapter 30, Pharmacology of Reproduction).

Product labels describe the preclinical assessment of each drug in the section of the label entitled "Carcinogenesis, Mutagenesis, Impairment of Fertility." In this section, it is not unusual to find descriptions of rodent studies that suggest carcinogenic potential for drugs. Since mutagens are not typically developed as drugs (with the exceptions noted above), the treatment-related tumors observed in these lifetime studies in rodents administered high doses of drug are generally attributed to nongenotoxic (epigenetic) mechanisms. To assess whether the rodent findings represent a risk to the intended patient population, it is important to understand the mechanism by which these tumors occur. The proton pump inhibitor **omeprazole**, for example, causes tumors of the gastric enterochromaffin-like (ECL) cells in rodents. The development of these tumors results from a dose-related and sustained increase in gastrin, which is secondary to the desired effect of the compound (decreased acid secretion). However, the exposures required for sustained gastrin elevation and tumor formation in rodents far exceed the exposures required for efficacy in patients. Further, the gastrin elevations noted in patients are of low magnitude and are not sustained. Thus, the carcinogenic finding in the rodent studies is not considered to signal a risk for tumor development in patients treated with omeprazole.

Teratogenesis Due to Drug Therapy

Drugs given to pregnant patients may adversely affect the fetus. **Teratogenesis** is the induction of structural defects in the fetus, and a **teratogen** is a substance that can induce such defects. The fetus's exposure to a drug is determined by maternal absorption, distribution, metabolism, and excretion of the drug and by the ability of the active teratogen to cross the placenta. These issues are further discussed in Box 6-1.

Drugs that might have few adverse effects on the mother may cause substantial damage to the fetus. Because development of the fetus is precisely timed, the teratogenic effect of any substance is dependent on the developmental timing of the exposure. In humans, **organogenesis** generally occurs between the third and eighth weeks of gestation, and it is during this period that teratogens have the most profound effects. Before the third week, most toxic compounds result in death to the embryo and spontaneous abortion, whereas after organogenesis, teratogenic compounds may affect growth and functional maturation of organs but do not affect the basic developmental plan. For example, **retinoic acid** (vitamin A) possesses significant on-target teratogenic toxicity. Retinoic acid activates nuclear retinoid receptors (RARs) and retinoid X receptors (RXRs) that regulate a number of key transcriptional events during development. Given the severity of birth defects that can occur, women who take RAR/RXR agonists such as **isotretinoin** for acne must sign FDA-mandated informed consent forms to demonstrate that they are aware of the risk of serious drug-related birth defects.

Another example of an on-target teratogenic effect is in utero exposure of the fetus to **ACE inhibitors**. Although ACE inhibitors were previously not contraindicated in the first trimester of pregnancy, recent data indicate that fetal exposure during this period significantly increases the risks of cardiovascular and central nervous system malformations. ACE inhibitors can cause a group of conditions including oligohydramnios, intrauterine growth retardation, renal dysplasia, anuria, and renal failure, reflecting the importance of the angiotensin pathway on renal development and function.

BOX 6-1 Application to Therapeutic Decision Making: Drugs in Pregnancy

Prescribing drugs to women who are, or might become, pregnant requires a risk–benefit evaluation for both the mother and the fetus. However, many drugs have not been systematically studied in pregnant populations, so such risk–benefit evaluations may be uncertain. The FDA places drugs into five "pregnancy categories" based on data from studies in laboratory animals, observations from well-controlled epidemiologic studies (or lack thereof), and/or case reports. These categories appear on drug labels and are listed below. Note that the categories are not strictly scaled according to risk; although Category A drugs are typically the safest for use in pregnancy, and Category X drugs are, as the name suggests, contraindicated, drugs in Category B—for which, by definition, human data are limited or inadequate—are not necessarily "almost as safe" as those in Category A.

Category A
Adequate and well-controlled studies have failed to demonstrate a risk to the fetus in the first trimester of pregnancy (and there is no evidence of risk in later trimesters).

Category B
Animal reproduction studies have failed to demonstrate a risk to the fetus, and there are no adequate and well-controlled studies in pregnant women.

Category C
Animal reproduction studies have shown an adverse effect on the fetus, and there are no adequate and well-controlled studies in humans, but potential benefits may warrant use of the drug in pregnant women despite potential risks.

Category D
There is positive evidence of human fetal risk based on adverse reaction data from investigational or marketing experience or studies in humans, but potential benefits may warrant use of the drug in pregnant women despite potential risks.

Category X
Studies in animals or humans have demonstrated fetal abnormalities and/or there is positive evidence of human fetal risk based on adverse reaction data from investigational or marketing experience, and the risks involved in use of the drug in pregnant women clearly outweigh potential benefits.

Category X drugs include not only teratogens but also drugs that have no proper use in pregnant patients. Statins are in this category, for example, because the normal physiologic increase in serum cholesterol that occurs during pregnancy should not be suppressed.

Despite their long history of use, the label categories remain a source of confusion, even occasionally within the FDA itself. For example, the antibiotic **tigecycline** is classified in Category D, but the absence of controlled data from humans indicates that it should instead be placed in Category C. More generally, the FDA pregnancy categorization of drugs, like any such scheme, is not perfect and may fail to capture the nuances of some drug-specific and patient-specific circumstances. Thus, the physician should also rely on his or her own judgment, keeping in mind the following issues:

- What are the risks to both fetus and mother of *not* treating the illness for which the drug is being considered?
- Is the drug known to cross the placenta? Based on its molecular weight, charge, hydrophobicity, and/or potential for carrier-mediated transport, is it likely to cross the placenta?
- Is there a pharmacologic rationale for how the drug could affect the fetus (e.g., through effects on organogenesis, organ development, organ function, or a delivery complication) should the fetus be exposed?

When appropriate, drugs that have proven effective for treating a patient's condition should be continued. To minimize fetal risk, drugs should be prescribed at the lowest therapeutic dose, taking into account the metabolic and physiologic changes that occur during pregnancy. ∎

PRINCIPLES FOR TREATING PATIENTS WITH DRUG-INDUCED TOXICITY

Treatment of drug-induced toxicity may include (1) reducing or eliminating exposure to the drug, (2) administering specific treatments based on antagonizing the mechanism of action of the drug or altering its metabolism, and/or (3) providing supportive measures.

Reduction of exposure to a therapeutic agent in a patient who experiences adverse effects may seem intuitive, but it is not always the correct choice. The appearance of an adverse effect during therapy does not necessarily indicate that the effect is due to the drug, despite the temporal relationship between the initiation of therapy and the appearance of the adverse effect. Even if the adverse effect most likely occurred because of the drug, the risks of cessation must be weighed against the benefits of continuing the drug. Cessation of therapy is more obviously a correct choice when the adverse effects have been previously associated with the

drug and are life-threatening, such as anaphylaxis due to a beta-lactam antibiotic. Needless to say, for such patients, future therapy with this class of antibiotics would also be contraindicated. Adverse effects that are irreversible and/or likely to increase in severity with continued treatment may also lead to the appropriate decision to terminate therapy. Many adverse effects, however, are considered tolerable and reversible. Depending on the severity of the disease condition being treated, it may be that the overall benefit to the patient is greater with drug treatment than without. An example of such circumstances is the leukopenia that often occurs in patients receiving chemotherapy with cytotoxic drugs. Thus, the decision to withdraw or reduce therapy can be complex and often requires evaluation of many factors affecting the patient's immediate and long-term health.

Therapies designed to counteract the adverse effects produced by a drug are often based on antagonizing the pharmacologic (on-target) activity of the drug or interfering with effects related to metabolism of the drug. Antagonizing the pharmacologic activity of a drug is a useful approach in overdoses of opioids, benzodiazepines, and acetylcholinesterase (AChE) inhibitors. Interference with the toxic effects of drug metabolites is a useful approach in the treatment of acetaminophen toxicity. These examples are briefly discussed below.

Conceptually, the simplest treatment for drug overdose is the administration of an antagonist that blocks the action of the drug (see Fig. 2-4). For example, an opioid overdose can be treated with **naloxone**, a competitive antagonist at the μ-opioid receptor. By competitively binding to opioid receptors, naloxone prevents or reverses the toxic effects of natural or synthetic opioids, including respiratory depression, sedation, and hypotension. Naloxone has a rapid onset of action and is highly potent; indeed, if no clinical improvement is observed within 10 minutes after naloxone doses of up to 10 mg, a different diagnosis or multiple toxic entities should be considered. Naloxone has a relatively short half-life, so it must be given every 1 to 4 hours to provide adequate receptor antagonism while the opioid is being cleared.

Flumazenil, a competitive antagonist at the $GABA_A$ (benzodiazepine) receptor, is used to treat benzodiazepine overdose. Flumazenil acts by competitive antagonism at benzodiazepine receptors in the central nervous system to completely or partially reverse the sedative effects of benzodiazepines. Like naloxone, it has a rapid onset of action and is highly potent; its effects should be seen within 5 minutes at a dose of not more than 3 mg. Flumazenil also has a short half-life (approximately 1 hour) and must be given frequently to provide adequate receptor antagonism while the benzodiazepine is being cleared.

Pharmacologic antagonism can also be used when the toxic agent is not a direct agonist but instead indirectly increases the concentration of the natural ligand for a receptor. AChE inhibitors produce a supraphysiologic concentration of acetylcholine at cholinergic synapses and a characteristic toxidrome of cholinergic excess—bradycardia, miosis, hypersalivation, sweating, diarrhea, vomiting, bronchoconstriction, weakness, respiratory paralysis, and convulsions. Although it is sometimes possible to restore AChE activity, the treatment of AChE inhibition generally depends on administering an anticholinergic agent such as **atropine**. By antagonizing the muscarinic acetylcholine receptor, atropine restores cholinergic balance and prevents bronchoconstriction, the most common cause of death in patients exposed to AChE inhibitors.

As noted earlier, a consequence of acetaminophen overdose is depletion of intracellular glutathione by the drug's metabolite *N*-acetyl-*p*-benzoquinoneimine (NAPQI). Glutathione stores can be replenished by administering **N-acetylcysteine** (NAC), a metabolic precursor of glutathione (see Fig. 6-4 for details). In addition to supportive therapy (gastric lavage and/or charcoal), NAC is given orally or intravenously within about 10 hours after ingestion of a potentially hepatotoxic dose of acetaminophen to prevent or lessen hepatic injury.

Finally, supportive therapy can be provided in the face of drug-induced toxicity. One example is the administration of intravenous fluids to patients with renal injury in order to maintain adequate renal blood flow. In cases of severe renal injury, dialysis may be required until renal function is regained. Another example is the treatment of bone marrow suppression resulting from the administration of cytotoxic agents in cancer chemotherapy. **Filgrastim**, a recombinant human granulocyte colony-stimulating factor (G-CSF), can be used to stimulate leukocyte production and provide supportive therapy until endogenous production of leukocytes resumes in the bone marrow.

▌ TOWARD EARLY DETECTION AND PREDICTION OF DRUG TOXICITY

A key element of the US FDA's strategic plan of August 2011 states: "Modernizing toxicology and continually improving the ability of nonclinical tests, models, and measurements to predict product safety issues will increase the likelihood that toxicity risks will be identified earlier in product development, assuring patient safety, and mitigating the need to withdraw previously approved products." One effective approach toward early detection and prediction of drug toxicity is the use of sensitive, specific, and qualified translational biomarkers.

Many current approaches to detect and predict drug toxicity in animal studies use a combination of microscopic tissue examination and measurement of "traditional" biomarkers to assess organ injury. As described above, examples of traditional biomarkers include serum concentrations of urea nitrogen and creatinine to evaluate potential adverse renal effects and serum activities of alanine aminotransferase (ALT), aspartate aminotransferase (AST), and gamma-glutamyltransferase (GGT) and serum concentrations of bilirubin and bile acids to evaluate potential adverse hepatic effects. However, these traditional markers are now viewed as relatively insensitive, particularly those for monitoring renal injury. Because of renal reserve, for instance, creatinine may not increase until there has been considerable (greater than 70%) loss of renal function. Of additional concern is drug-induced renal injury in patients with preexisting renal dysfunction, since these patients have diminished reserve capacity. It is also important to note that the degree of loss of renal function in drug studies cannot be equated with the potential for reversibility of the morphologic changes that may accompany the loss of function. As noted above, nonclinical studies and clinical experience have demonstrated that drug-induced renal injury is often reversible, depending on the extent of injury.

With these considerations in mind, the goal of recent efforts is to identify safety biomarkers that may improve the detection and prediction of drug toxicity by (1) identifying toxicity early in drug development, thereby reducing the rate of attrition of drug candidates during later stage clinical trials, and (2) providing markers to monitor toxicity in patients, with the goal of reducing the entry of drugs into the market that have unacceptable toxicity and facilitating the management of patients who suffer organ damage or injury.

Over the last decade, consortia such as the European Innovative Medicines Initiative (IMI), Predictive Safety Testing Consortium (PSTC), and Health and Environmental Sciences Institute (HESI) have dedicated resources to identifying translational biomarkers for early detection of toxicity. In 2008, the US FDA, European Medicines Agency (EMA), and Japanese Pharmaceuticals and Medical Devices Agency (PMDA) jointly announced the qualification of seven urinary biomarkers to monitor kidney toxicity in preclinical studies. This international effort showed that, in many instances, kidney injury molecule-1 (KIM-1), clusterin (CLU), albumin, total protein, β2-microglobulin, cystatin C, and trefoil

TABLE 6-2 Online Resources for Information on Drug Toxicity

TYPE OF INFORMATION	SOURCE	WEBSITE
Product labels	Physician's Desk Reference Drug manufacturer	http://csi.micromedex.com/Login.asp Various websites by manufacturer
Regulatory agencies	US Food and Drug Administration European Medicines Agency (EMA)	http://www.fda.gov/ http://www.ema.europa.eu/

Government databases	National Library of Medicine
	National Toxicology Program
	TOXNET
	International Conference on Harmonization
	   of Technical Requirements for
	   Registration of Pharmaceuticals for
	   Human Use (ICH)
		http://www.ncbi.nlm.nih.gov/pubmed/
		http://ntp.niehs.nih.gov/
		http://toxnet.nlm.nih.gov/
		http://www.ich.org/products/guidelines.html

Commercial databases	Pharmapendium Medscape DiscoveryGate INCHEM	https://www.pharmapendium.com/ http://www.medscape.com/ https://www.discoverygate.com http://www.inchem.org

factor 3 (TFF3) provide an earlier signal than traditional biomarkers and also add significant information with regard to potential localization of the adverse renal effects. Notably, these newer biomarkers correlated with the "gold standard" of kidney toxicity, quantitative histopathology. Thus, although the newer biomarkers generally do not offer higher sensitivity in nonclinical models, they do provide important perspective on which biomarkers would be useful to monitor in both clinical studies (before drug approval) and in patients (after drug approval) in order to better understand potential risks to humans.

As with traditional biomarkers, decisions on whether to withdraw therapy for individual patients or to continue clinical development of a drug in which increases in these biomarkers have been observed still require a risk–benefit analysis (see "Principles for Treating Patients with Drug-Induced Toxicity" earlier in this chapter). The kidney biomarker qualification process has led some pharmaceutical companies to include an assessment of newer biomarkers in nonclinical and clinical data submitted for review to regulatory agencies in the United States, Europe, and Japan. Similar efforts are underway to identify safety biomarkers for liver, heart, skeletal muscle, testicular, and vascular toxicity, including an evaluation of the performance of these biomarkers in diagnosis and prognosis of toxicity in clinical studies.

CONCLUSION AND FUTURE DIRECTIONS

This chapter has presented a mechanism-based approach to understanding drug toxicity and provided examples to illustrate these principles in major organ systems. Drug development aims to discover compounds that are both effective and highly selective and thus less likely to cause serious or otherwise undesirable off-target effects. The challenges of the future lie particularly with understanding the basis for variability of therapeutic and toxic responses to drugs. In an attempt to predict which patient populations will be most susceptible to an adverse drug reaction, one approach under evaluation is to find correlations between individual single nucleotide polymorphisms (SNPs) and possible adverse reactions by comparing the SNPs of patients who have adverse reactions with those who do not. The identification of patients with genetic variants of the molecular target (and closely related targets) of a drug could provide useful information about patients who might be more likely to experience adverse effects.

Predicting efficacy and safety in individual patients remains a challenge to the treating physician. The decision to use drug therapy requires knowledge of the potential benefits and risks of the therapy. Moreover, physicians have the responsibility to communicate these risks and benefits to the patient so that the full range of therapeutic options can be considered. One challenge to the physician is where to find this information. Sources include the scientific literature, the product label, direct communications to prescribing physicians, and reviews of the preclinical and clinical data prepared by the FDA during its review of a New Drug Application (NDA; see Chapter 52).

The key toxicity information, both preclinical and clinical, is contained in the product label. Revisions of the label may occur as serious adverse events are attributed to drugs during postmarketing surveillance, and it is incumbent on the physician to consult the most recent version of the product label. Alerts of serious consequences may also be transmitted in the form of direct communications to prescribing physicians, and the FDA website can be consulted for current regulatory actions related to a drug's safety. The European Medicines Agency (EMA) website contains information regarding regulatory actions for medicines marketed in Europe. Table 6-2 lists some of the online sources that can be consulted for in-depth information about drug toxicity. Good sources of detailed information on preclinical toxicity and clinical adverse events are the documents prepared by the FDA pharmacologist (preclinical) and medical reviewer (clinical) as part of their review of the NDA.

Acknowledgment

We thank Cullen Taniguchi, Sarah R. Armstrong, Vivian Gonzalez Lefebre, and Robert H. Rubin for their valuable contributions to this chapter in the First, Second, and Third Editions of *Principles of Pharmacology: The Pathophysiologic Basis of Drug Therapy*.

Suggested Reading

Agranat I, Caner H, Caldwell J. Putting chirality to work: the strategy of chiral switches. *Nat Rev Drug Discov* 2002;1:753–768. (*An overview of enantiomeric-specific properties of drugs and the strategies of switching drugs from achiral to chiral preparations.*)

Bonventre JV, Vaidya VS, Schmouder R, Feig P, Dieterle F. Next-generation biomarkers for detecting kidney toxicity. *Nat Biotechnol* 2010;28:436–440. (*Reviews potential new biomarkers for assessing renal function in both nonclinical and clinical studies.*)

Bugelski PJ. Genetic aspects of immune-mediated adverse drug effects. *Nat Rev Drug Discov* 2005;4:59–69. (*Overview of immune-mediated adverse effects, including detailed mechanistic information.*)

Campion S, Aubrecht J, Boekelheide K, et al. The current status of biomarkers for predicting toxicity. *Expert Opin Drug Metab Toxicol* 2013;9:1391–1408. (*Reviews sensitivity and utility of currently used biomarkers for assessment of toxicity during drug development.*)

Elangbam CS. Current strategies in the development of anti-obesity drugs and their safety concerns. *Vet Pathol* 2009;46:10–24. (*Provides examples of drug development guided by knowledge of mechanisms of toxicity.*)

Fujimoto K, Kumagai K, Ito K, et al. Sensitivity of liver injury in heterozygous Sod2 knockout mice treated with troglitazone or acetaminophen. *Toxicol Pathol* 2009;37:193–200. (*Demonstrates use of genetically engineered animals to study mechanisms of toxicity.*)

Hondeghem LM. QTc prolongation as a surrogate for drug-induced arrhythmias: fact or fallacy? *Acta Cardiol* 2011;66:685–689. (*Commentary on relative utility of drug-induced changes in QTc as a predictor of arrhythmogenic potential of drugs.*)

International Conference on Harmonisation of Technical Requirements for Registration of Pharmaceuticals for Human Use. ICH harmonised tripartite guideline: immunotoxicity studies for human pharmaceuticals S8, 2005. http://www.ich.org/fileadmin/Public_Web_Site/ICH_Products/Guidelines/Safety/S8/Step4/S8_Guideline.pdf. (*Summary of principles and guidelines for evaluating potential immunotoxicity of drug candidates.*)

Liebler DC, Guengerich FP. Elucidating mechanisms of drug-induced toxicity. *Nat Rev Drug Discov* 2005;4:410–420. (*Introduces the concept of a mechanism-based approach to drug toxicity.*)

Morgan RE, Trauner M, van Staden CJ, et al. Interference with bile salt export pump function is a susceptibility factor for human liver injury in drug development. *Toxicol Sci* 2010;118:485–500. (*Correlation between drug-induced inhibition of bile salt export protein (BSEP) and hepatotoxicity in patients.*)

Morgan RE, van Staden CJ, Chen Y, et al. A multifactorial approach to hepatobiliary transporter assessment enables improved therapeutic compound development. *Toxicol Sci* 2013;136:216–241. (*Describes in vitro approaches for reducing risk of hepatotoxicity during selection of candidates for drug development.*)

Navarro VJ, Senior JR. Drug-related hepatotoxicity. *N Engl J Med* 2006;354:731–739. (*Overview of pharmacogenomic approaches to understanding and predicting drug hepatotoxicity.*)

Owczarek J, Jasińska M, Orszulak-Michalak D. Drug-induced myopathies: an overview of the possible mechanisms. *Pharmacol Rep* 2005;57:23–34. (*Overview of mechanisms leading to skeletal muscle toxicity.*)

Sager PT, Gintant G, Turner JR, Petit S, Stockbridge N. Rechanneling the cardiac proarrhythmia safety paradigm: a meeting report from the Cardiac Safety Research Consortium. *Am Heart J* 2014;167:292–300. (*A summary of new initiatives to better evaluate risk of arrhythmogenic potential of drugs and reduce the need for thorough QTc studies.*)

U.S. Food and Drug Administration. *Pregnancy, lactation, and reproductive potential: labeling for human prescription drug and biological products—content and format.* June 2015. Washington, DC: U.S. Department of Health. (*Reviews proposals to revise product labels to better describe reproductive and developmental risks.*)

7

Pharmacogenomics

Amber Dahlin and Kelan Tantisira

INTRODUCTION

Modern pharmacologic agents are used to treat or control diseases that range from hypertension to human immunodeficiency virus (HIV) infection. In many cases, the same drug regimens are used for populations of people. Large variations among individuals are often found in response to drug therapy, however. These variations range from potentially life-threatening adverse drug reactions to equally serious lack of therapeutic efficacy. Many factors influence the drug response phenotype, including age, gender, and underlying disease, and genetic variation plays an important role. Interindividual differences in the genes that encode drug targets, drug transporters, and enzymes that catalyze drug metabolism can profoundly affect the success or failure of pharmacotherapy.

Pharmacogenetics is the study of the role of inheritance in variation in drug response. The convergence of recent advances in genomic science and equally striking advances in molecular pharmacology has resulted in the evolution of pharmacogenetics into pharmacogenomics. The promise of pharmacogenetics-pharmacogenomics is the possibility that knowledge of a patient's DNA sequence could be used to enhance pharmacotherapy, maximize drug efficacy, and reduce the incidence of adverse drug reactions. Therefore, pharmacogenetics and pharmacogenomics represent an important aspect of the aspiration to "personalize" or "individualize" medicine—in this case, drug therapy. This chapter describes the principles of pharmacogenetics and pharmacogenomics as well as recent developments in this discipline. Several key examples are cited in which knowledge of pharmacogenetics-pharmacogenomics may help to individualize drug therapy.

PHYSIOLOGY

Genomic Variation and Pharmacogenomics

The human genome contains approximately 3 billion nucleotides. According to current estimates, the genome contains approximately 19,000–20,000 protein-coding genes that, through alternative splicing and post-translational modification, may encode 100,000 or more proteins. On average, any two people differ at about one nucleotide in every 1,000 in their genome, totaling an average interindividual difference of 3 million base pairs throughout the genome. The majority of these differences are so-called **single nucleotide polymorphisms** or **SNPs** (pronounced "snips"), in which one nucleotide is exchanged for another at a given position. SNPs and other differences in DNA sequence can occur anywhere in the genome, in both coding regions and noncoding regions. If a SNP changes the encoded amino acid, it is called a *nonsynonymous coding SNP* (cSNP). The remaining differences in DNA sequence involve insertions, deletions, duplications, and reshufflings, sometimes of just one or a few nucleotides but occasionally of whole genes or larger DNA segments that include many genes. Functionally significant DNA sequence differences that we currently understand tend to fall within genes, either within their coding sequences or in the promoters, enhancers, splice sites, or other sequences that control gene transcription or mRNA stability. Heritable genetic regulation that does not occur through DNA sequence changes, termed *epigenetics*, also contributes to functionally significant variation in genes and gene expression. Taken together, these differences constitute each person's genetic individuality. Some of that individuality affects the way in which each person will respond to drug treatment.

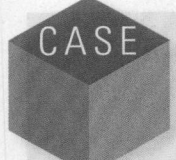

CASE

Robert H, a 66-year-old man, is shoveling snow one wintry morning in Minnesota when he slips and falls on a patch of ice. He immediately feels pain in his left hip and is unable to stand. He is brought to the hospital, where x-rays reveal that he has fractured his hip. He undergoes surgery the next day and is discharged to a rehabilitation hospital 3 days later. After less than 24 hours at the rehabilitation hospital, Mr. H develops the sudden onset of pleuritic chest pain. He is brought to the emergency department, where a computed tomography (CT) scan with intravenous contrast reveals a pulmonary embolus. He is treated with heparin and is anticoagulated with warfarin at a starting dose of 5 mg each day, with a target international normalized ratio (INR) of 2.0–3.0. Mr. H is discharged back to his rehabilitation hospital and referred to his local physician. When the INR is subsequently measured, it is 6.2, a value associated with an increased risk of hemorrhage. He is taking no other medication that might interfere with plasma levels of warfarin. The physician advises Mr. H to stop taking warfarin for 2 days. After multiple attempts at adjusting his dose of warfarin, Mr. H eventually reaches a stable INR of 2.5 when taking 1 mg of warfarin each day.

Questions

1. What molecular mechanisms could be responsible for the apparent sensitivity of Mr. H to warfarin?
2. What additional laboratory information could assist in anticoagulating this patient?
3. Would that information have helped in the selection of Mr. H's initial warfarin dose?

▌ PHARMACOLOGY

The concept that inheritance might be an important determinant of individual variation in drug response emerged half a century ago. It originally grew out of clinical observations of striking differences among patients in their response to "standard" doses of a drug. Those observations, coupled with twin and family studies that showed inherited variations in plasma drug concentrations and other pharmacokinetic parameters, led to the birth of pharmacogenetics. Many of those original examples of pharmacogenetic variation, and many of the most striking examples even today, involve *pharmacokinetics*—factors that influence the concentration of drug reaching its target(s). However, examples of pharmacogenetic variation in the drug target, so-called pharmacodynamic factors, are also being reported with increasing frequency. Pharmacogenetic variation related to unpredicted (idiosyncratic) adverse effects from drugs has also been described. While not detailed further in this chapter, an example of an idiosyncratic pharmacogenetic effect is provided by the serious hypersensitivity reaction associated with the HLA-B*5701 allele in patients taking abacavir, a reverse transcriptase inhibitor and anti-HIV agent (see Chapter 38, Pharmacology of Viral Infections). Predrug testing for HLA-B*5701 has been shown to nearly eliminate such hypersensitivity reactions.

Variation in Enzymes of Drug Metabolism: Pharmacokinetics

Inherited variation in enzymes that catalyze drug metabolism is the most common factor responsible for pharmacogenetic variation in response to medications. The enzymes involved in drug metabolism are discussed in Chapter 4, Drug Metabolism. There are two broad categories of drug-metabolizing enzymes: those that catalyze phase I reactions (functionalization reactions that typically involve oxidation or reduction) and those that catalyze phase II reactions (typically, conjugation reactions that add groups, such as glucuronic acid, that enhance drug solubility and thus drug excretion).

Phase I and phase II reactions do not necessarily occur in that order, and metabolic intermediates resulting from both types of reactions may be pharmacologically active. In fact, some medications are administered as inactive prodrugs that must undergo phase I and/or phase II metabolism before they can exert their pharmacologic effect.

Genetic polymorphisms are common in enzymes that catalyze drug metabolism, and clinically significant polymorphisms have been found in nearly all of the major enzymes involved in both phase I and phase II reactions (Table 7-1). Two "classic" examples are provided by the inherited variations in the enzymatic hydrolysis of the short-acting muscle relaxant **succinylcholine** by the enzyme butyrylcholinesterase (BChE; also known as *serum cholinesterase*) and the enzymatic acetylation of drugs such as the antituberculosis drug **isoniazid** (see Chapter 35, Pharmacology of Bacterial and Mycobacterial Infections: Cell Wall Synthesis). Patients with variations in BChE have a decreased rate of metabolism of succinylcholine, resulting in prolonged paralysis after drug exposure. A genetically polymorphic phase II enzyme, N-acetyltransferase 2 (NAT2), catalyzes the acetylation of isoniazid. Patients treated with isoniazid can be classified as either "slow acetylators," who metabolize isoniazid slowly and have high blood drug levels, or "fast acetylators," who metabolize isoniazid rapidly and have low blood drug levels. Family studies have shown that the rate of isoniazid biotransformation is inherited.

The slow-acetylator phenotype is associated with drug toxicities that result from excessive drug accumulation; examples include hydralazine- and procainamide-induced lupus and isoniazid-induced neurotoxicity and liver injury. Although the antihypertensive agent **hydralazine** is rarely used today in the treatment of hypertension, this drug has recently reemerged as one of the two active components in BiDil, a combination drug approved for the treatment of patients with symptomatic heart failure. It is of interest that the US Food and Drug Administration (FDA) has approved BiDil for use only in patients of African ancestry, presumably because of an ethnically dependent genetic difference in response to this drug.

TABLE 7-1 Examples of Genetic Polymorphisms and Drug Metabolism

ENZYME	AFFECTED DRUG, CLASS, OR COMPOUND
Phase I (Oxidation/Reduction) Enzyme	
CYP1A2	Acetaminophen, caffeine, propranolol
CYP1B1	Estrogens
CYP2A6	Halothane, nicotine
CYP2B6	Cyclophosphamide
CYP2C8	Paclitaxel, retinoic acid
CYP2C9	Nonsteroidal anti-inflammatory drugs, phenytoin, warfarin
CYP2C19	Omeprazole, phenytoin, propranolol
CYP2D6	Antidepressants, β-adrenergic antagonists, codeine, debrisoquine, dextromethorphan
CYP2E1	Acetaminophen, ethanol
CYP3A5	Calcium channel blockers, cyclosporine, dapsone, etoposide, lidocaine, lovastatin, macrolides, midazolam, quinidine, steroids, tacrolimus, tamoxifen
Phase II (Conjugation) Enzyme	
N-Acetyltransferase 1	Sulfamethoxazole
N-Acetyltransferase 2	Dapsone, hydralazine, isoniazid, procainamide, sulfonamides
Sulfotransferases (SULTs)	Acetaminophen, dopamine, epinephrine, estrogens
Catechol-O-methyltransferase	Catecholamines, levodopa, methyldopa
Histamine N-methyltransferase	Histamine
Thiopurine S-methyltransferase	Azathioprine, mercaptopurine, thioguanine
UDP-glucuronosyltransferases	Androgens, ibuprofen, irinotecan, morphine, naproxen

Early examples of the importance of pharmacogenetic variation, such as those represented by BChE and NAT2, served as a stimulus to search for additional examples. Most of the second-generation examples continued to be associated with pharmacokinetics and continued to be recognized from clinical observations—often from adverse drug responses. They were most often studied either by administering a "probe drug" to a group of subjects and measuring plasma or urinary drug and/or metabolite concentrations or by directly assaying a drug-metabolizing enzyme in an easily accessible tissue such as the red blood cell (e.g., a series of methyltransferase enzymes). Two prototypic examples that have become pharmacogenetic "icons" are the **cytochrome P450 2D6 (CYP2D6)** and **thiopurine S-methyltransferase (TPMT)** genetic polymorphisms. Because of the clinical implications of these polymorphisms, the FDA in its 2003 "Guidance on Pharmacogenomic Data" cited CYP2D6 and TPMT as examples of valid pharmacogenomic biomarkers.

CYP2D6 is a member of the cytochrome P450 (CYP) family of microsomal, phase I drug-metabolizing enzymes. CYP2D6 contributes to the metabolism of a large number of medications, including antidepressants, antipsychotics, antiarrhythmics, and analgesics. The CYP2D6 polymorphism was originally described by two different laboratories studying two different probe drugs: the antihypertensive **debrisoquine** and the oxytocic agent **sparteine**. The frequency distribution of the debrisoquine urinary metabolic ratio, the ratio of the parent drug to its oxidized metabolite, is shown in Figure 7-1A for a Northern European population. Shown at the far right of the figure is a group of "poor metabolizers" of debrisoquine, subjects homozygous for recessive alleles (genes) coding for enzymes with decreased activity or for deletion of the *CYP2D6* gene; shown in the middle is the large group of "extensive metabolizers," subjects heterozygous or homozygous for the "wild-type" allele; and shown at the far left is a small subset of "ultrarapid metabolizers," some of whom have multiple copies of the *CYP2D6* gene.

Several molecular genetic mechanisms are responsible for variation in CYP2D6 enzyme activity, including nonsynonymous cSNPs, gene deletion, and gene duplication; some ultrarapid metabolizers can have up to 13 copies of the gene. It has been estimated that 6% to 10% of Caucasians are CYP2D6 poor metabolizers. Among East Asians, in contrast, the poor-metabolizer phenotype is present at a frequency of just 1% to 2%. The ultrarapid-metabolizer phenotype, rare in most Caucasian populations, has a frequency of 3% in Spaniards and up to 13% in Ethiopians. These ethnic differences have potentially important medical implications because CYP2D6 metabolizes many commonly prescribed medications, including the β-adrenergic blocker **metoprolol**,

A CYP2D6 pharmacogenetics

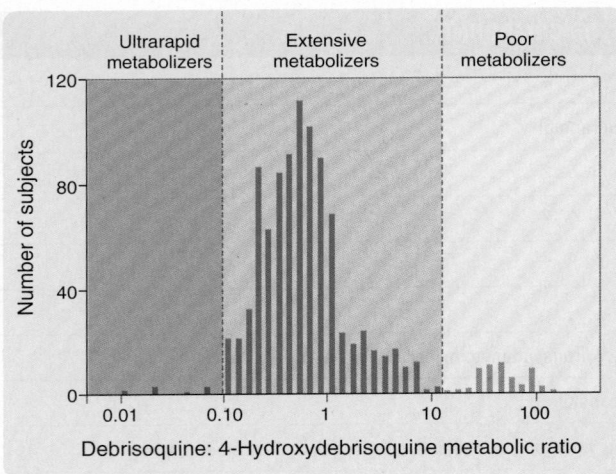

B AmpliChip CYP450 array

FIGURE 7-1. CYP2D6 pharmacogenetics. A. Frequency distribution of the metabolic ratio for the cytochrome P450 2D6 (CYP2D6)-catalyzed metabolism of debrisoquine to form its 4-hydroxy metabolite. Data for 1,011 Swedish subjects are plotted as the ratio of metabolites in the urine. Most subjects metabolize debrisoquine extensively, while some subjects metabolize the compound ultrarapidly and others metabolize the compound poorly. **B.** The AmpliChip CYP450 array can be used to determine variant genotypes for cytochrome P450 genes that influence drug metabolism.

the neuroleptic **haloperidol**, the opioids **codeine** and **dextromethorphan**, and the antidepressants **fluoxetine**, **imipramine**, and **desipramine**, among many others (Table 7-1). Therefore, poor metabolizers for CYP2D6 can potentially experience an adverse drug effect when treated with standard doses of agents such as metoprolol that are inactivated by CYP2D6, whereas codeine is relatively ineffective in poor metabolizers because it requires CYP2D6-catalyzed metabolism to form the more potent opioid morphine. Conversely, ultrarapid metabolizers may require unusually high doses of drugs that are inactivated by CYP2D6, but those same subjects can be "overdosed" with codeine, suffering respiratory depression or even respiratory arrest in response to "standard" doses. In one tragic case, a nursing infant whose mother was an ultrarapid CYP2D6 metabolizer died when the mother was prescribed a standard dose of codeine and the baby was overdosed on morphine present in the breast milk. For ultrarapid

and poor metabolizers, alternative analgesics are now recommended as substitutes for codeine.

CYP2D6 genetic polymorphisms are also important for the efficacy of the breast cancer drug **tamoxifen**. Tamoxifen is used to block the estrogen receptor (ER) in approximately 60% of breast cancer patients with ER-positive tumors. However, tamoxifen is a prodrug that requires metabolic activation to form 4-hydroxytamoxifen and 4-hydroxy-N-desmethyltamoxifen (endoxifen) (Fig. 7-2A). These metabolites are approximately 100 times more potent as antagonists of the ER than the parent drug. As a result, patients who are CYP2D6 poor metabolizers (Fig. 7-1) are relatively unable to form the active 4-hydroxy metabolites of tamoxifen. Poor-metabolizer patients have worse outcomes with respect to breast cancer recurrence than do CYP2D6 extensive metabolizers (EMs) (Fig. 7-2B). Furthermore, if EM patients are co-administered other drugs such as antidepressants that are good CYP2D6 substrates, they may receive less benefit from tamoxifen therapy than do CYP2D6 EMs who are not co-administered drugs that compete with tamoxifen for CYP2D6-catalyzed metabolism.

In the past, an individual's genotype for *CYP2D6* and many other genes encoding drug-metabolizing enzymes was inferred from phenotype (e.g., the urinary metabolic ratio that can be measured by assaying the urinary excretion of a specific metabolite after the administration of a probe drug) (Fig. 7-1A). As discussed below, genotype assignment is now increasingly dependent on DNA-based tests performed with commercially available, direct-to-consumer testing devices such as the genotyping "chip" shown in Figure 7-1B.

TPMT represents another example of an important and clinically relevant genetic polymorphism for drug metabolism. TPMT catalyzes the S-methylation of thiopurine drugs such as **6-mercaptopurine** and **azathioprine** (see Chapter 39, Pharmacology of Cancer: Genome Synthesis, Stability, and Maintenance). Among other indications, these cytotoxic and immunosuppressive agents are used to treat acute lymphoblastic leukemia and inflammatory bowel disease. Although thiopurines are useful drugs, they have a narrow therapeutic index (i.e., the ratio between the toxic dose and the therapeutic dose is small), with occasional patients suffering from life-threatening thiopurine-induced myelosuppression.

In Caucasians, the most common variant allele for TPMT is *TPMT*3A*; the frequency of this allele is approximately 5%, so 1 in 300 subjects carries two copies of the *TPMT*3A* allele. *TPMT*3A* is predominantly responsible for the trimodal frequency distribution of the level of red blood cell TPMT activity shown in Figure 7-3. *TPMT*3A* has two nonsynonymous cSNPs, one in exon 7 and another in exon 10 (Fig. 7-3). The presence of *TPMT*3A* results in a striking decrease in tissue levels of TPMT protein. Mechanisms responsible for the observed decrease in TPMT*3A protein level include both accelerated TPMT*3A degradation and intracellular TPMT*3A aggregation, probably as a result of protein misfolding. As a result, drugs such as 6-mercaptopurine are poorly metabolized and may reach toxic levels. *Subjects homozygous for TPMT*3A are at greatly increased risk for life-threatening myelosuppression when treated with standard doses of thiopurine drugs.* These patients should be treated with approximately one-tenth to one-fifteenth the standard dose.

There are striking ethnic differences in the frequency of variant alleles for TPMT. For example, *TPMT*3A* is rarely observed in East Asian populations, whereas *TPMT*3C*, which has only the exon 10 SNP, is the most common variant

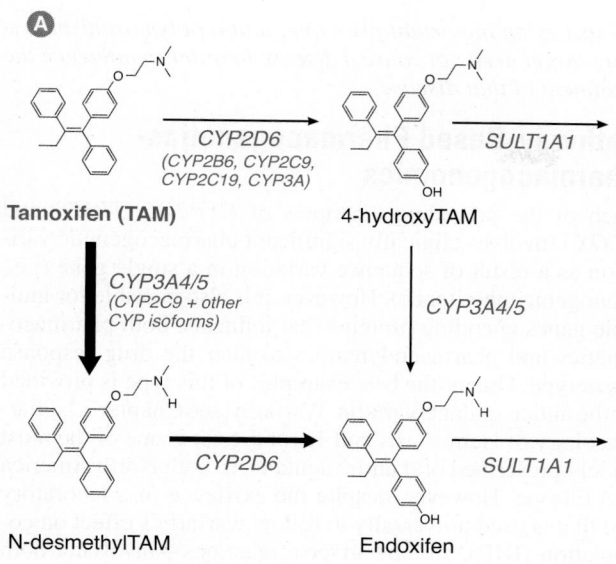

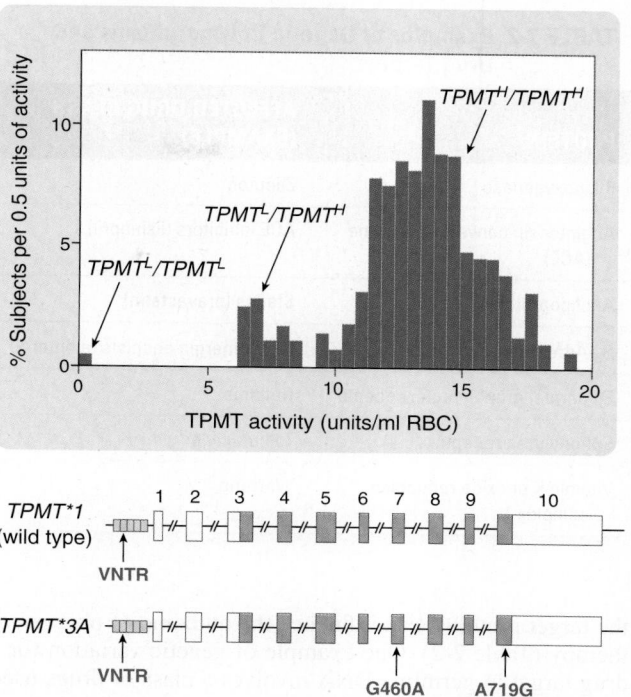

FIGURE 7-3. TPMT pharmacogenetics. Frequency distribution of red blood cell (RBC) thiopurine S-methyltransferase (TPMT) activity for 298 unrelated Caucasian subjects. *TPMT^L* indicates an allele or alleles for the trait of low activity, while *TPMT^H* refers to the "wild type" (*TMPT*1*) allele for the trait of high activity. The observed trimodal frequency distribution for RBC TPMT activity is due mainly to the effect of *TPMT*3A*, the most common variant allele for low activity in a Caucasian population. *TMPT*1* and *TPMT*3A* differ by two nonsynonymous single nucleotide polymorphisms (SNPs), one in exon 7 and one in exon 10. VNTR, variable number tandem repeat.

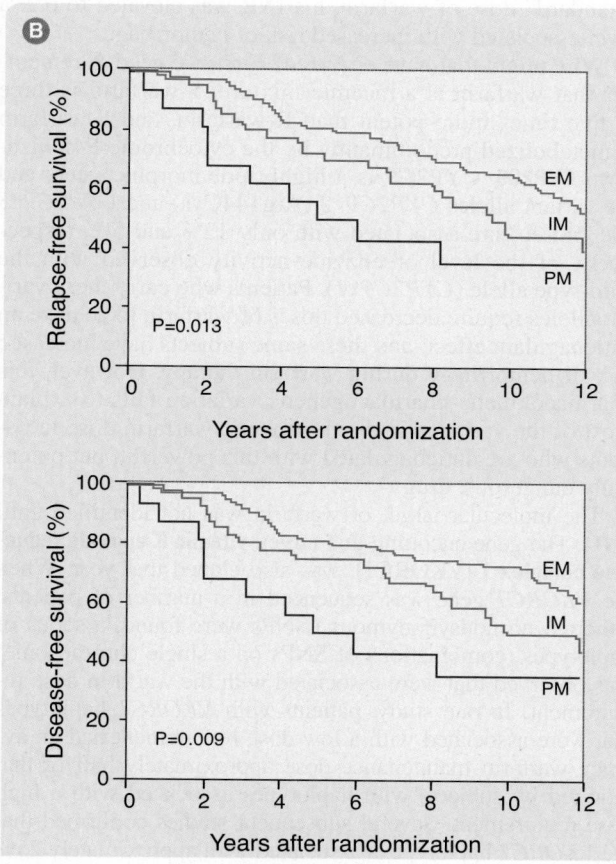

FIGURE 7-2. Tamoxifen pharmacogenetics. A. Tamoxifen is metabolized by two cytochrome P450 pathways to form the active metabolites 4-hydroxy-tamoxifen (4-hydroxyTAM) and endoxifen, which are further metabolized by sulfotransferase (SULT) 1A1 (*not shown*). Genetic variations in CYP2D6 can influence the extent of tamoxifen metabolism. **B.** Kaplan-Meier curves showing the influence of CYP2D6 "metabolizer" status on the survival of women with estrogen receptor-positive (ER[+]) breast cancer who were treated with tamoxifen. Patients who were extensive metabolizers (EM) of tamoxifen had improved relapse-free survival and disease-free survival relative to intermediate metabolizers (IM) and poor metabolizers (PM).

allele in those populations. For these populations, alternative agents or dose reductions are recommended for thiopurine drugs. Because of its clinical significance, TPMT was the first example selected by the FDA for public hearings on the inclusion of pharmacogenetic information in drug labeling. For the same reason, clinical testing for TPMT genetic polymorphisms is widely available. The phenomenon of marked changes in the level of a protein as a result of the alteration of only one or two amino acids in the protein has been observed repeatedly for multiple other genes of pharmacogenetic significance and is a common explanation for the functional effects of nonsynonymous cSNPs within these genes.

The BChE, NAT2, CYP2D6, and TPMT genetic polymorphisms all behave as monogenic (single-gene) Mendelian traits, as do many other early examples from pharmacogenetics. However, pharmacogenetics-pharmacogenomics has now moved beyond monogenic traits with pharmacokinetic phenotypes, and the focus increasingly involves functionally and clinically significant variation in drug targets as well as drug-metabolizing enzymes. Variation can also involve multiple genes and pathways that influence both pharmacokinetics and pharmacodynamics.

Variation in Drug Targets: Pharmacodynamics

Drugs generally exert their effects by interacting with specific target proteins. Therefore, genetic variations in these target proteins, or in signaling pathways downstream from

TABLE 7-2 Examples of Genetic Polymorphisms and Drug Targets

PROTEIN	AFFECTED DRUG CLASS (EXAMPLE)
5-Lipoxygenase	Zileuton
Angiotensin converting enzyme (ACE)	ACE inhibitors (lisinopril)
Apolipoprotein E	Statins (pravastatin)
β_2-Adrenergic receptor	β-Adrenergic agonists (albuterol)
Epidermal growth factor receptor	Gefitinib
Sulfonylurea receptor	Tolbutamide
Vitamin K epoxide reductase complex 1	Warfarin

the target proteins, can influence the outcome of pharmacotherapy (Table 7-2). One example of genetic variation for a drug target in germline DNA involves a class of drugs used to treat asthma. As noted in Chapter 48, Integrative Inflammation Pharmacology: Asthma, the anti-asthma medication **zileuton** decreases airway inflammation by inhibiting the enzyme **5-lipoxygenase**, an enzyme encoded by the gene *ALOX5*. Variations in 5-lipoxygenase illustrate the point that variation in many areas of a gene can affect protein function. Polymorphisms in gene regulatory regions, such as the gene promoter, can influence transcription and thereby alter protein expression. The promoter of the *ALOX5* gene displays variation in the number of tandem repeats of the sequence GGGCGG. These repeat sequences bind the transcription factor complex Sp1, which up-regulates *ALOX5* transcription.

The most common *ALOX5* allele contains five repeats and is present in about 77% of *ALOX5* transcripts. As a result, approximately 94% of the population has at least one copy of the five-repeat allele. The most common variant alleles contain four and three repeats and are present at frequencies of about 17% and 4%, respectively. Because of increased Sp1 binding, people who carry the five-repeat allele are thought to express more 5-lipoxygenase than those who lack it. Interestingly, there seems to be no relationship between the presence or absence of the five-repeat allele and the severity of asthma in the population; that is, this *ALOX5* promoter polymorphism does not seem to affect the disease process itself. However, in trials of zileuton and closely related 5-lipoxygenase inhibitors, only subjects who had at least one copy of the five-repeat allele responded to the drug. This result suggests that zileuton-like compounds are unlikely to help the 6% of the population who lack the five-repeat allele and that identifying this subgroup would allow the use of alternative, more effective medications. The *ALOX5* example demonstrates that pharmacodynamic-pharmacogenetic variation (i.e., variation in genes encoding drug targets) can be just as important, if not more important, than the pharmacokinetic-pharmacogenetic variation represented by *CYP2D6* and *TPMT*. Table 7-2 lists several drug target proteins with genetic polymorphisms that have been associated with variation in drug response. *This example also*

illustrates an important principle, that a polymorphism in a drug target need not cause a disease in order to influence the treatment of that disease.

Pathway-Based Pharmacogenetics-Pharmacogenomics

Each of the preceding examples of *CYP2D6*, *TPMT*, and *ALOX5* involves clinically significant pharmacogenetic variation as a result of sequence variation in a single gene (i.e., monogenic inheritance). However, it is also possible for multiple genes encoding proteins that influence both pharmacokinetics and pharmacodynamics to alter the drug response phenotype. One of the best examples of this type is provided by the anticoagulant **warfarin**. Warfarin (see Chapter 23, Pharmacology of Hemostasis and Thrombosis) is one of the most widely prescribed oral anticoagulants in both North America and Europe. However, despite the existence of a laboratory test that is used universally to follow warfarin's effect on coagulation (INR), serious adverse reactions—involving both hemorrhage and undesired thrombosis—continue to complicate warfarin therapy. These complications are illustrated by the case of Mr. H at the beginning of this chapter: after a "standard" dose of warfarin, his INR was elevated to 6.2, a level associated with increased risk of hemorrhage.

Why might that have occurred? First, we need to remember that warfarin is a racemic mixture. S-warfarin is three to five times more potent than R-warfarin, and S-warfarin is metabolized predominantly by the cytochrome P450 isoform **CYP2C9**. CYP2C9 is a highly polymorphic gene, and the variant alleles *CYP2C9*2* (Arg144Cys) and *CYP2C9*3* (Ile358Leu) are associated with only 12% and 5%, respectively, of the level of enzyme activity observed with the wild-type allele (*CYP2C9*1*). Patients who carry these variant alleles require decreased doses of warfarin to achieve an anticoagulant effect, and these same subjects have increased risk of hemorrhage during warfarin therapy. However, this pharmacokinetic-pharmacogenetic variation fails to explain most of the variance in the therapeutic warfarin dose in patients who are anticoagulated with this powerful, but potentially dangerous, drug.

The molecular target of warfarin was not identified until 2004. The gene encoding that target, **vitamin K epoxide reductase complex 1** (VKORC1), was also cloned that year. When the *VKORC1* gene was sequenced in a number of patients, although no nonsynonymous cSNPs were found, a series of haplotypes (combinations of SNPs on a single chromosome) was observed that were associated with the warfarin dose requirement. In one study, patients with *VKORC1* haplotypes that were associated with a low dose requirement had an average warfarin maintenance dose approximately half of that required by subjects with haplotypes associated with a high dose requirement. Several subsequent studies confirmed that the *VKORC1* haplotype is associated with approximately 25% to 30% of the variance in the warfarin maintenance dose, while 5% to 15% can be explained by the *CYP2C9* genotype. The roles of CYP2C9 and VKORC1 in warfarin pharmacokinetics and pharmacodynamics are shown schematically in Figure 7-4. Because the genes encoding both of these proteins contribute to variation in drug response, genotyping for *CYP2C9* and haplotyping for *VKORC1* represent potentially useful strategies for the determination of an initial warfarin dose for Mr. H.

An initial analysis of combined data for over 5,000 patients worldwide who were anticoagulated with warfarin

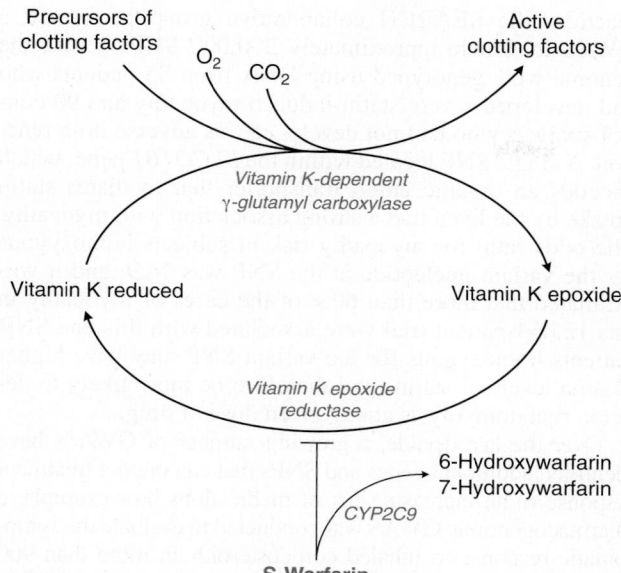

as clinical variables are important for anticoagulant therapy, in 2010, the FDA guidelines for warfarin recommended that patient genotypes (if known) should be considered in warfarin dose selection and monitoring. However, the question of whether genotype-guided dosing regimens are superior to dosing regimens that utilize clinical variables alone is not yet answered. In particular, two of three recent multicenter randomized controlled clinical studies to evaluate the efficacy of including patient genotype information in clinical dosing regimens demonstrated little improvement over clinical dosing protocols or algorithms in terms of time spent within the therapeutic range. It remains uncertain whether genotype-guided warfarin dosing improves clinical outcomes and prevents the bleeding complications associated with supra-therapeutic warfarin dosing. To date, such efficacy measures have been associated with genotype guidance, but only in a study comparing a large cohort of subjects with historical controls.

Warfarin provides an important example of a situation in which pharmacokinetic-pharmacogenetic data may prove inadequate for clinical translation because those data explain too little of the variation in therapeutic drug dose. Thus, warfarin may represent, probably in a simplified form, the type of polygenic, pathway-based pharmacogenetic-pharmacogenomic model (i.e., one that combines pharmacokinetic and pharmacodynamic variants) that may become increasingly common in the future.

Role of Epigenetics in Pharmacogenetics-Pharmacogenomics

Epigenetics is an emerging area of pharmacogenomics (Fig. 7-5). Epigenetics refers to heritable changes in gene function and expression that are not a result of DNA sequence changes. Several recent studies show that, in addition to DNA sequence changes, epigenetic changes including DNA

FIGURE 7-4. Warfarin pharmacokinetics and pharmacodynamics. Vitamin K is a required cofactor for the post-translational γ-carboxylation of glutamate residues in certain clotting factor precursors (see Chapter 23). Vitamin K is oxidized to the inactive epoxide as a consequence of the carboxylation reaction. The enzyme vitamin K epoxide reductase (VKORC1) converts the inactive epoxide into the active, reduced form of vitamin K. Warfarin acts as an anticoagulant by inhibiting VKORC1 and thereby preventing the regeneration of reduced vitamin K. S-warfarin is metabolized to 6-hydroxywarfarin and 7-hydroxywarfarin by cytochrome P450 2C9 (CYP2C9).

and were genotyped for both *CYP2C9* and *VKORC1* showed that adding genotype data to clinical variables provided a superior prediction of the warfarin dose requirement than an algorithm that used only clinical data such as age, diet, and weight. Due to the increasing evidence that genetic as well

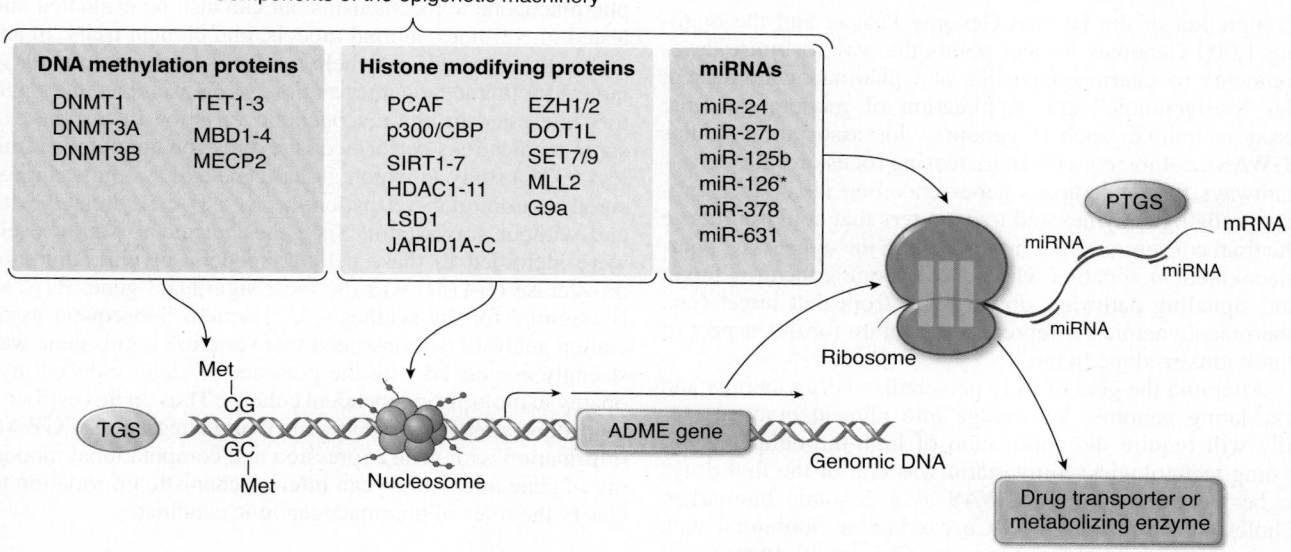

FIGURE 7-5. Epigenetic control of absorption, distribution, metabolism, and excretion (ADME) genes. The molecules that regulate epigenetic effects include a host of proteins for DNA methylation (DNMT1, DNMT3A, DNMT3B, TET1-3, MBD1-4, MECP2), histone modification (HDAC1-11, p300/CBP, PCAF, SIRT1-7, EZH1/2, DOT1L, MLL2, and others), and miRNAs (miR-24, miR-27b, miR-125b, miR-126*, miR-378, and miR-631). Collectively, these proteins and miRNAs contribute to transcriptional gene silencing (TGS) and post-transcriptional gene silencing (PTGS) of drug transporters and metabolizing enzymes. Down-regulation of expression of ADME genes can lead to variations in the pharmacokinetic and pharmacodynamic profiles of the drugs that interact with their gene products.

methylation, histone modification, and post-transcriptional regulation via noncoding RNAs (including micro RNAs [miRNAs]) can regulate the expression of genes involved in pharmacokinetic and pharmacodynamic responses. Furthermore, since DNA variation alone cannot entirely explain interindividual differences in drug response and adverse drug event phenotypes, investigation of epigenetic mechanisms is likely to have clinical benefit.

The most common form of epigenetic change is DNA methylation. DNA methyltransferases (DNMTs) add a methyl group from S-adenosylmethionine to cytosine in specific promoter sites called *CpG sites*. In the human genome, up to 80% of the CpG sites are methylated. Large regions of unmethylated CpG sites, called *CpG islands*, are present near promoters and are associated with increased transcription, whereas methylation of CpG sites within promoters is associated with gene silencing. Examples of *pharmacoepigenetic* mechanisms related to variation in drug responses may include altered methylation of specific CpG sites in promoters of genes involved in drug absorption, distribution, metabolism, and excretion (ADME). For instance, differential methylation of the CYP3A4 promoter correlates with its hepatic gene expression. Drug- and toxin-related changes in CYP1A1 and CYP1B1 expression are also directly related to altered methylation patterns of these genes. In one investigation, treatment of HepG2 liver cells with the anticancer agent decitabine (a DNA methyltransferase inhibitor) led to partial demethylation of the CYP1B1 promoter and restored CYP1B1 inducibility.

Evidence also exists for the role of tissue-specific miRNAs in regulating the expression of multiple pharmacokinetic enzymes and transporters, including CYP3A4, CYP1B1, ABCB1, ABCG2, and ABCC1. Clarifying the role of miRNAs in the control of ADME gene expression will improve mechanistic understanding of variation in drug levels and pharmacodynamic effects and help in identifying new potential therapeutic targets.

Modern Pharmacogenomics

Completion of the Human Genome Project and the ongoing 1,000 Genomes Project points the way to future developments in pharmacogenetics and pharmacogenomics in the "postgenomic" era. Application of modern genomic assay techniques such as genome-wide association studies (GWAS), combined with an increasing focus on pathways—pathways that encompass genes encoding all of the drug-metabolizing enzymes and transporters that could influence the final concentration of drug reaching the target (i.e., pharmacokinetics), together with genes encoding the drug target and signaling pathways downstream from that target (i.e., pharmacodynamics)—represent the future for this aspect of "individualized medicine."

Attaining the goal of truly personalized drug therapy and translating genomic knowledge into clinical practice rapidly will require the application of high-throughput genotyping technologies. Simvastatin was one of the first drugs to be identified through GWAS as a genomic biomarker. Cholesterol-lowering HMG-CoA reductase inhibitors, such as **simvastatin** and **atorvastatin** (see Chapter 20, Pharmacology of Cholesterol and Lipoprotein Metabolism), are among the most widely prescribed drugs worldwide. Although these drugs are generally very safe, statins can rarely cause serious myopathy with rhabdomyolysis and renal failure. In an attempt to predict and prevent this serious adverse drug reaction, the SEARCH collaborative group performed a GWAS in which approximately 300,000 SNPs across the genome were genotyped using DNA from 85 patients who had developed severe statin-induced myopathy and 90 control subjects who had not developed this adverse drug reaction. A single SNP located within the *SLCO1B1* gene, which encodes an organic anion transporter that mediates statin uptake by the liver, had a strong association with myopathy. The odds ratio for myopathy risk in subjects homozygous for the variant nucleotide at the SNP was 16.9, and it was estimated that more than 60% of the cases of myopathy in this 12,064-patient trial were associated with this one SNP. Patients homozygous for the variant SNP may have higher plasma levels of statins and therefore be more likely to develop rhabdomyolysis at any given dose of drug.

Over the last decade, a growing number of GWASs have identified additional genes and SNPs that can predict treatment response to an increasing list of medications. For example, a pharmacogenomic GWAS was conducted to evaluate the symptomatic response to inhaled corticosteroids in more than 900 patients with asthma. That study identified a functional SNP in the promoter region of *GLCCI1*, a suspected mediator of glucocorticoid-induced apoptosis. Patients who carried the SNP had worse therapeutic responses to inhaled glucocorticoids after 4–8 weeks of therapy and were therefore at higher risk of developing treatment-resistant asthma and asthma exacerbations.

While GWAS has successfully identified multiple genes that may explain a portion of the variability observed in therapeutic responses to various drugs, these genes alone fail to account for the majority of the heritability in therapeutic response. The variability observed in drug responses is likely due to the coordinated effects of functional SNP genotypes, gene pathways, epigenetic effects, and environmental factors. In recent years, *integrative pharmacogenomics* and *systems biology* approaches have been utilized to integrate diverse data types and to perform predictive modeling of the most important interactions that contribute to clinical response phenotypes. These models not only provide insight into the pharmacogenetic mechanisms but can also be evaluated and tested in cell lines, animal models, and clinical trials. In addition, these models may help to identify new potential drug targets for therapeutic intervention. As an example, investigators interested in pharmacogenetic variation in response to statin medications performed an expression quantitative trait loci (QTL) study in which global gene expression was measured in immortalized patient-derived B cells treated with and without simvastatin. Six genes related to statin levels were identified in these cellular models; glycine amidinotransferase (*GATM*) was the most significant gene. (GATM is essential for the synthesis of creatine.) Subsequent association analyses demonstrated that variation in this gene was strongly associated with the presence of statin-induced myopathy in multiple independent cohorts. Thus, in this evolving field, downstream approaches involving integration of GWAS information with gene expression and computational modeling of gene interactions can infer mechanistic information to clarify the roles of pharmacogenomic candidates.

Pharmacogenomics and Regulatory Science

To achieve individualized drug therapy, we need not only to understand the science underlying pharmacogenetics and pharmacogenomics and to develop state-of-the-art technologies to detect and assay DNA sequence data but also to translate that knowledge into the clinic. That translation process will require the active involvement of the FDA and the pharmaceutical industry, which develops virtually all new drugs. Early efforts by the FDA began with thiopurine drugs and TPMT and were followed by hearings on a genetic polymorphism in *UGT1A1*, a gene encoding a phase II enzyme involved in biotransformation of the antineoplastic agent irinotecan. Public hearings have also been held on *CYP2C9*, *VKORC1*, and warfarin—resulting in relabeling—and on tamoxifen and *CYP2D6*.

Incorporating information from pharmacogenetics could also contribute to postmarketing surveillance, not only to help avoid adverse reactions but also to "rescue" drugs that might be of benefit to groups of patients selected on the basis of genetic variation in drug response. The latter situation was highlighted by reports that a polymorphism in the β_1-adrenoceptor influences response to the β_1-adrenergic antagonist **bucindolol**—both in vitro and in patients with heart failure. This β-antagonist had initially failed in a clinical trial that did not include genotyping, perhaps because only patients with the wild-type β_1-adrenoceptor genotype displayed the desired clinical response.

CONCLUSION AND FUTURE DIRECTIONS

Pharmacogenetics and pharmacogenomics involve the study of ways in which DNA sequence variation affects the response of individual patients to medications. The goal of pharmacogenetics and pharmacogenomics is to maximize efficacy and minimize toxicity based on knowledge of an individual's genetic composition. Although many factors other than inheritance influence differences among patients in their response to drugs, the past half-century has demonstrated that genetics is an important factor responsible for variation in the occurrence of adverse drug reactions or the failure of individual patients to achieve the desired therapeutic response. Pharmacogenetics has evolved during that half-century from classical examples, such as CYP2D6 and TPMT, to include more complex situations such as that represented by the pharmacogenetics of warfarin, a drug that displays both pharmacokinetic and pharmacodynamic pharmacogenetic variation, and that represented by new loci and SNPs related to pharmacogenomic phenotypes identified through GWAS. The areas of genomic medical science, epigenetics, and systems biology also present unique challenges

in translation into the clinic. However, there can no longer be any doubt that pharmacogenetics and pharmacogenomics will be applied to clinical medicine with increasing breadth and depth and that, ultimately, they will enhance our ability to individualize drug therapy.

Acknowledgment

The authors would like to acknowledge Liewei Wang and Richard M. Weinshilboum, the authors of this chapter in the Second and Third Editions of *Principles of Pharmacology: The Pathophysiologic Basis of Drug Therapy*, who provided the template for and insight into the construction of this chapter.

Suggested Reading

Caudle KE, Klein TE, Hoffman JM, et al. Incorporation of pharmagenomics into routine clinical practice: the Clinical Pharmacogenetics Implementation Consortium (CPIC) guideline development process. *Curr Drug Metab* 2014;15:209–217. (*Overview of metrics used to determine which pharmacogenetic variants are suitable for clinical implementation.*)

Drazen JM, Yandava CN, Dube L, et al. Pharmacogenetic association between *ALOX5* promoter genotype and the response to anti-asthma treatment. *Nat Med* 1999;22:168–171. (*Original study that showed different pharmacologic responses in people with different polymorphisms of the ALOX5 gene.*)

Ingelman-Sundberg M, Zhong XB, Hankinson O, et al. Potential role of epigenetic mechanisms in the regulation of drug metabolism and transport. *Drug Metab Dispos* 2013;41:1725–1731. (*Review of emerging evidence for the role of epigenetics in drug transport and metabolism.*)

Mallal S, Phillips E, Carosi G, et al. HLA-B*5701 screening for hypersensitivity to abacavir. *N Engl J Med* 2008;358:568–579. (*A double-blind randomized study of a genetic biomarker for an idiosyncratic adverse drug response.*)

Mangravite LM, Engelhardt BE, Medina MW, et al. A statin-dependent QTL for GATM expression is associated with statin-induced myopathy. *Nature* 2013;502:377–380. (*Investigation of pharmacogenetic variation in response to statin medications.*)

SEARCH Collaborative Group. SLCO1B1 variants and statin-induced myopathy—a genomewide study. *N Engl J Med* 2008;359:789–799. (*The first genome-wide association study of a drug response.*)

Tantisira KG, Lasky-Su J, Harada M, et al. Genomewide association between GLCCI1 and response to glucocorticoid therapy in asthma. *N Engl J Med* 2011;365:1173–1183. (*The first genome-wide association study to evaluate lung function changes in response to corticosteroid treatment in asthma.*)

Zineh I, Pacanowski M, Woodcock J. Pharmacogenetics and coumarin dosing—recalibrating expectations. *N Engl J Med* 2013;369:2273–2275. (*Perspective on caveats for adopting genotype-guided dosing regimens for anticoagulants.*)

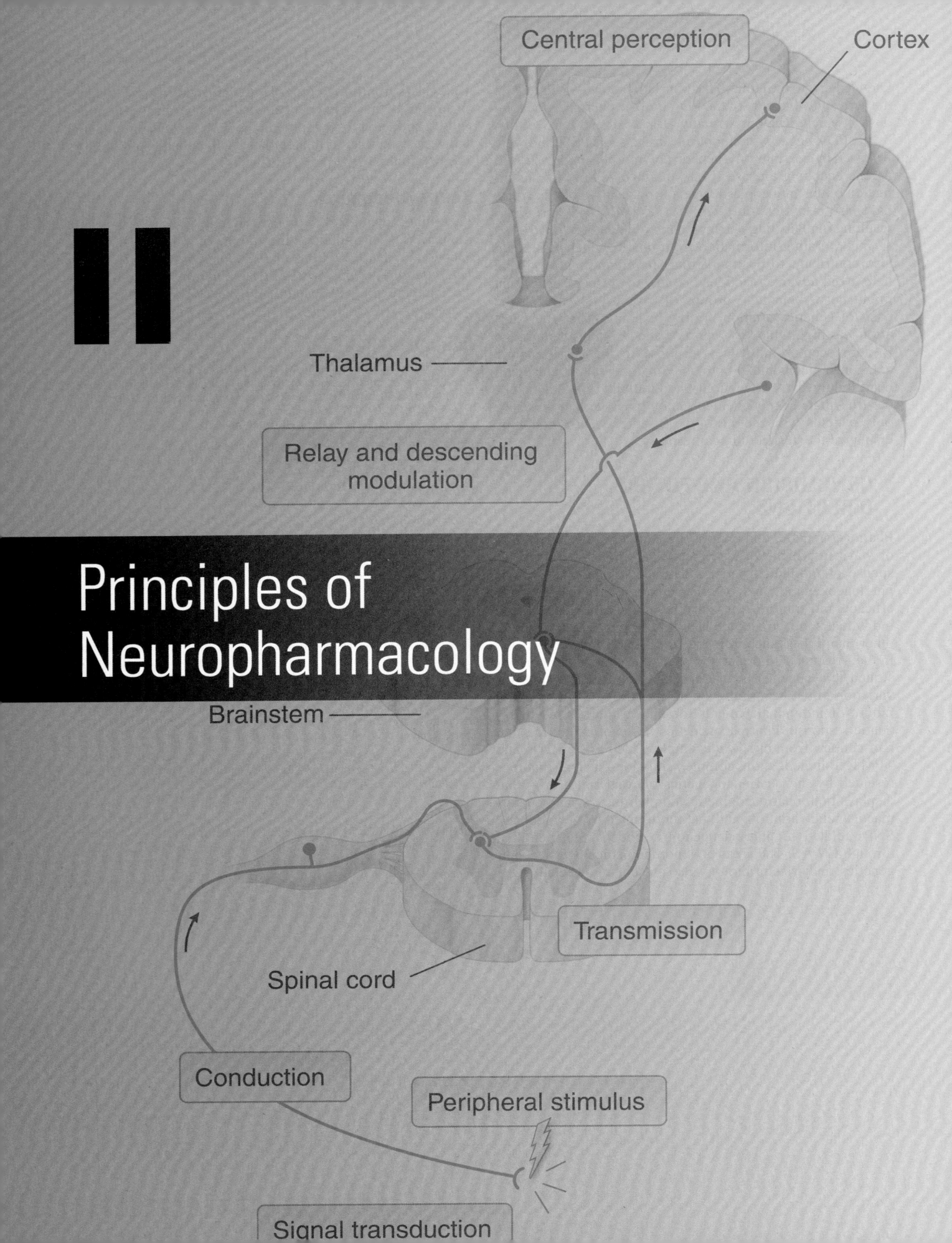

II

Principles of
Neuropharmacology

Acetylcholine

Nicotinic
receptors

Fundamental Principles of Neuropharmacology

Acetylcholine

Muscarinic

Nicotinic

8

Principles of Cellular Excitability and Electrochemical Transmission

Elizabeth Mayne, Lauren K. Buhl, and Gary R. Strichartz

INTRODUCTION

Cellular communication is essential for the effective functioning of any complex multicellular organism. The major mode of *intercellular* communication is the transmission of chemical signals, such as neurotransmitters, neuropeptides, and hormones. In excitable tissues, such as nerves and muscles, rapid *intracellular* communication relies on the propagation of electrical signals—action potentials—along the plasma membrane of the cell. Both chemical and electrical transmission commonly involve the movement of ions across the plasma membrane or across the membranes of internal organelles such as the endoplasmic reticulum. Ionic movements can directly change the cytoplasmic concentration of ions, such as Ca^{2+}, that are key regulators of biochemical and physiologic processes like phosphorylation, secretion, and contraction. Ionic movements also change the electrical potential across the membrane through which the ions flow, thus regulating various **voltage-dependent** functions including the opening of other ion channels. Some of these events are brief, with durations and actions of several milliseconds (0.001 sec). Others can take many seconds, with biochemical consequences—for example, phosphorylation of proteins—that can persist for minutes or hours. Even gene expression can be regulated by changes in ion concentrations, resulting in long-term changes in cellular physiology, growth, differentiation, and death.

Many drugs modify chemical or electrical signaling to increase or decrease cellular excitability and electrochemical transmission. To appreciate how such drugs act, the present chapter explains the electrochemical foundations that underlie signaling within and between electrically active cells. These general principles are applicable to many areas of pharmacology, including those discussed in Chapters 10 to 12 (Section IIB, Principles of Autonomic and Peripheral Nervous System Pharmacology), Chapters 13 to 19 (Section IIC, Principles of Central Nervous System Pharmacology), and Chapter 24, Pharmacology of Cardiac Rhythm.

CELLULAR EXCITABILITY

Excitability refers to the ability of a cell to generate and propagate electrical **action potentials**. Neuronal, cardiac, smooth muscle, skeletal muscle, and many endocrine cells have an excitable character. Action potentials may propagate over large distances, as in peripheral nerve axons that conduct over several meters, or they may stimulate activity in cells of much smaller size such as the 30- to 50-μm-diameter interneurons that are contained within a single autonomic ganglion. The function of action potentials differs depending on the cell in which they occur. Propagating waves of action potentials rapidly conduct encoded information with fidelity over long distances along axons. Within a small cell, action potentials excite the whole cell at once, causing an increase

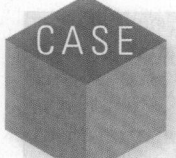

CASE

During a business trip to Japan, Karl G attends a dinner in his honor at a restaurant that specializes in fugu fish. Karl is impressed because he has heard that this special dish is not available in the United States and is an expensive delicacy in Japan.

Before the meal is over, Karl notes an unusual and delightful sensation of tingling and numbness in his mouth and around his lips. His hosts are pleased that he is experiencing the desired effect of fugu fish ingestion.

Karl is fascinated and somewhat fearful of the potential toxic effects of the fugu neurotoxin (tetrodotoxin) as they are described to him by his knowledgeable hosts. However, his hosts assure him that the sushi chef at the restaurant is fully licensed to prepare fugu fish and is certified by the government.

Karl is relieved when he awakens the next morning without any signs of weakness or paralysis. However, he decides that he will politely forgo seafood for the rest of the trip and ask for Kobe beef instead.

Questions

1. What is the molecular mechanism of action of tetrodotoxin?
2. What is the effect of tetrodotoxin on the action potential?

in intracellular ions (e.g., Ca^{2+}) followed by a rapid release of chemical transmitter molecules or hormones. These chemicals then travel to specific receptors, near or far from the releasing cell, to effect **chemical transmission**, which is discussed in the second part of this chapter.

Cellular excitability is fundamentally an electrical event. Therefore, an understanding of basic electricity is necessary to explain the biological processes of excitability and synaptic transmission. The following sections present basic principles of electricity as applied to two important cellular components—the plasma membrane and ion-selective channels.

Ohm's Law

The magnitude of a current (**I**, measured in amperes) flowing between two points is determined by the potential difference (**V**, measured in volts) between those two points and the resistance to current flow (**R**, measured in Ohms):

$$I = V/R \qquad \text{Equation 8-1a}$$

For example, current may flow from the extracellular to the intracellular compartment in response to an electrical potential difference (also known as a *voltage difference*) across the plasma membrane. Voltage can be thought of as a potential energy or as the propensity for charged particles to flow from one area to another. Resistance is the obstacle to this flow. Decreased resistance allows greater ion flow and therefore increased current (current has units of charge/time). When this relationship, known as *Ohm's law*, is applied to biological membranes such as the plasma membrane, the electrical resistance is often replaced by its reciprocal, the conductance (**g**, measured in reciprocal ohms, or siemens [**S**]):

$$I = gV \qquad \text{Equation 8-1b}$$

For simplicity, assume that all resistive elements in the cell membrane behave in an "ohmic way"; that is, their current–voltage (I-V) relationship is described by Equations 8-1a, b. In this case, the I-V relationship is linear, with a slope given by the conductance, **g**. Figure 8-1 represents the transmembrane current (**I**) measured at different transmembrane potentials (**V**) in a hypothetical cell. The slope of the **I-V** curve equals the conductance. From a conceptual perspective, current increases as voltage increases because a higher voltage results in a greater potential energy difference between the

inside and outside of the cell, which in turn favors an increased rate of charge movement across the membrane.

The convention used in most texts and in this chapter is that the voltage across a membrane, the "membrane potential," is expressed as the difference between the intracellular and extracellular potentials ($V_m = V_{in} - V_{out}$). For most normal cells, V_m is negative when the cell is at rest ($V_{in} < V_{out}$). The membrane is termed **hyperpolarized** when V_m is more negative than at rest, and it is described as **depolarized** when V_m is more positive than at rest. Current is conventionally defined with respect to the direction in which positive charge flows. Positive charge moving from inside to outside is called *outward current* and is represented graphically by positive values. Positive charge moving from outside to inside is called *inward current* and is represented graphically by negative values. Movement of negative charge is defined in the exact opposite way. Note that an efflux of K^+ cations is electrically equivalent to an influx of Cl^- anions; both are outward currents.

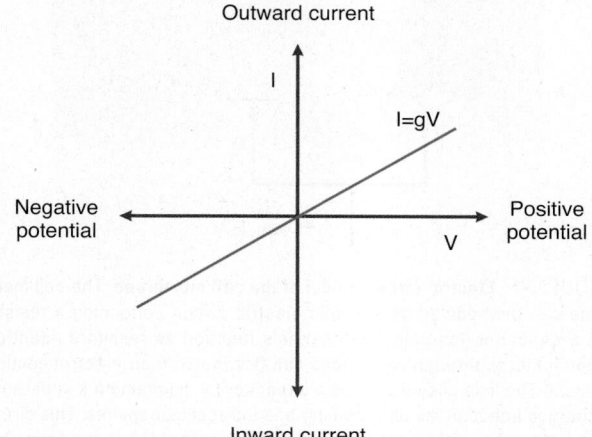

FIGURE 8-1. Ohm's law. Ohm's law states that there is a linear relationship between current (*I*) and voltage (*V*) and that the slope of the *I* versus *V* plot yields the conductance (*g*). By convention, outward current is the flow of positive charge from inside the cell to outside the cell. Transmembrane potential is defined by the difference in electric potential (voltage) between the inside and outside of the cell. For most cells, the resting potential inside the cell is negative relative to that outside the cell. Conductance, *g*, is the reciprocal of resistance.

Ion Channels

How does current actually flow across a cell membrane? Biological membranes are composed of a lipid bilayer within which some proteins are embedded and to which other proteins are attached (schematically represented in Fig. 8-2). Pure lipid membranes are virtually impermeable to most polar or charged substances, thus having a very high intrinsic resistance. From an electrical perspective, the lipid bilayer also acts as a capacitor by separating the extracellular and intracellular ions. To enable the passage of ions that carry electrical current, ion channels span the membrane. Most ion channels are gated—that is, they remain closed until specific signals dictate their opening. Once open, they exhibit ion selectivity, allowing only certain ions or types of ions to pass. From an electrical perspective, a set of gated ion channels is a variable conductor: it provides many individual conductances for different ions to flow between the extracellular and intracellular environments. The magnitude of the overall conductance depends on the fraction of channels in the open state and the conductance of the individual open channels.

Channel Selectivity, the Nernst Equation, and the Resting Potential

By itself, the hypothetical I-V relation in Figure 8-1 does not explain the electrical behavior of most real cells. If a cell behaved according to Equation 8-1, then the potential difference across the membrane would be zero in the absence of an externally applied current. Instead, most cells maintain a negative potential difference across their plasma membrane.

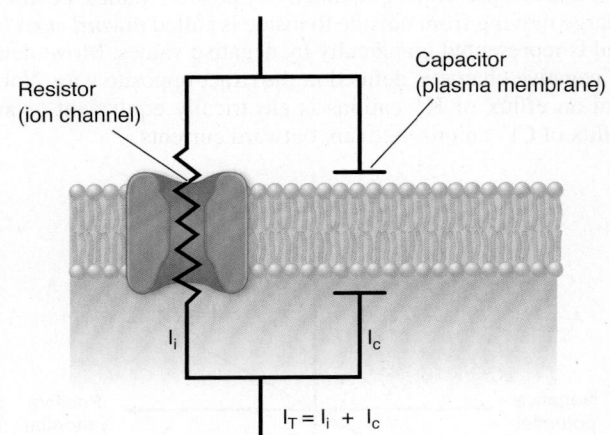

FIGURE 8-2. Electric circuit model of the cell membrane. The cell membrane can be modeled as a simple electric circuit containing a resistor and a capacitor. Ion-selective channels function as resistors (identical to conductors), through which ions can flow down their electrochemical gradient. The lipid bilayer acts as a capacitor by maintaining a separation of charges between the extracellular and intracellular spaces. This circuit (referred to as an *RC*, or *resistor-capacitor*, circuit) changes the timing between the flow of charges across the membrane (current) and changes in transmembrane potential (voltage), because the lipid bilayer, acting as a capacitor, stores some of the charge that passes across the membrane. Time is required to store this charge; therefore, the initial change in voltage associated with a step of current is slow. As the capacitor (lipid bilayer) fills with charges and the voltage change grows, more of the charge passes through the resistor, until a new steady state is reached and the current–voltage relationship becomes more linear. (I_c, capacitor current; I_i, ionic current; I_T, total current.)

This voltage difference is most pronounced in neuronal and cardiac ventricular cells, where a resting potential (the voltage difference across the membrane in the absence of external stimuli) of -60 to -90 mV can be recorded. The resting potential results from three factors: (1) an unequal distribution of positive and negative charges on each side of the plasma membrane, (2) a difference in selective permeabilities of the membrane to the various cations and anions, and (3) the current-generating action of active (energy-requiring) and passive pumps that help to maintain the ion gradients. The effects of these interrelated factors can be explained best with an example.

Consider the case when there are only potassium ions (K^+) and protein-bound anions (A^-) inside the cell and no other ions outside the cell (Fig. 8-3). If this cell's membrane is permeable to potassium alone, due to the presence of channels that are open at rest and pass only K^+ ions, then K^+ will flow outward, while A^- will remain inside. The K^+ ions flow outward because of a **chemical gradient**; that is, K^+ efflux is energetically favorable because the K^+ concentration inside the cell is greater than that outside the cell. A potential efflux of the anion, A^-, is also favored by its chemical gradient, but the absence of transmembrane channels permeable to A^- prevents this anion from flowing across the membrane. Because of this selective permeability for K^+, every K^+ ion that exits the cell leaves one net negative charge (an A^- ion) on the inside of the cell and adds one net positive charge (a K^+ ion) on the outside of the cell. This separation of charges across the membrane creates a negative membrane potential.

If a negative membrane potential were not established as K^+ leaves the cell, then K^+ ions would continue to exit until the extracellular concentration of K^+ was equal to the intracellular concentration of K^+. However, the establishment of a voltage difference creates an **electrostatic force** that eventually prevents net K^+ efflux (Fig. 8-3B). Thus, the electrical gradient (V_m) and the chemical gradient "pull" the K^+ ions in opposite directions: the electrical gradient favors an inward flow of K^+ ions, while the chemical gradient favors an outward flow of K^+ ions. These forces combine to create an **electrochemical gradient**, which is equal to the sum of the electrical gradient and the chemical gradient. *The transmembrane electrochemical gradient is the net driving force for passive ion movement across biological membranes.*

As a result of the electrochemical gradient, the extracellular concentration of K^+ does not equalize with the intracellular concentration. Instead, an equilibrium is established in which the electrostatic force "pulling" K^+ back into the cell is balanced exactly by the chemical gradient driving K^+ efflux. The electrical potential at which this equilibrium occurs, for any permeant ion X, is a function of the charge of the ion (z), the temperature (T), and the intracellular and extracellular concentrations of the ion. This relationship is expressed as the **Nernst equation**:

$$V_x = V_{in} - V_{out} = \frac{RT}{zF} \ln \frac{[X]_{out}}{[X]_{in}} \qquad \textbf{Equation 8-2}$$

where V_x is the transmembrane potential that a membrane selectively permeable to ion X would reach at equilibrium (i.e., the **Nernst potential** for that ion), $V_{in} - V_{out}$ is the transmembrane voltage difference, RT/zF is a constant for a given temperature and charge (this number simplifies to 26.7 mV for a charge of $+1$ at a temperature of $37°C$), and $[X]_{out}$ and $[X]_{in}$ are the extracellular and intracellular

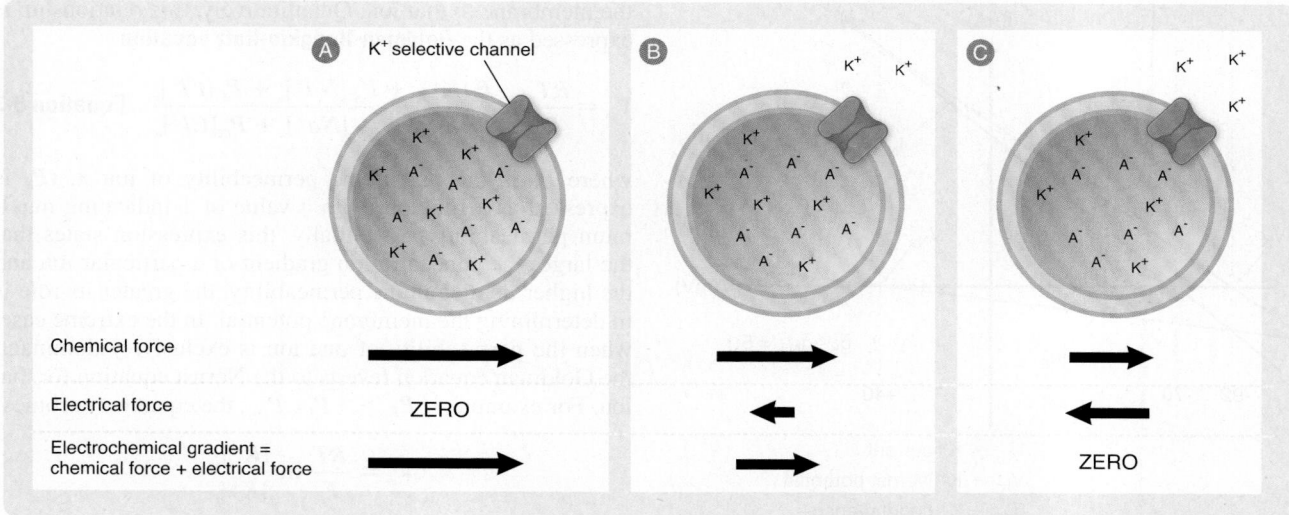

FIGURE 8-3. Electrochemical basis of the resting membrane potential. A. Consider a prototypical cell that initially contains equal concentrations of intracellular potassium ions (K$^+$) and impermeant anions (A$^-$). Assume further that ions can exit the cell only via a single K$^+$-selective channel. In this case, there is a strong chemical gradient for K$^+$ to exit the cell, but there is no electrical force favoring ion flow because the electrical sum of the intracellular charges is zero. **B.** K$^+$ begins to exit the cell through the K$^+$-selective channel, but A$^-$ remains inside the cell because it has no exit route. Therefore, the K$^+$ chemical gradient across the membrane becomes smaller. As K$^+$ exits the cell, the net negative charge from the A$^-$ remaining inside the cell produces a negative membrane potential that exerts an electrical force opposing K$^+$ efflux. This force is opposite in direction to that of the chemical gradient; as a result, the total electrochemical gradient (the sum of the chemical force and the electrical force) is less than the chemical gradient alone. **C.** When the electrical gradient is equal and opposite to the chemical gradient, the system is in equilibrium and no net ion flow occurs. The voltage resulting from the separation of charges at equilibrium is referred to as the **Nernst potential**.

concentrations, respectively, of ion X. The electrochemical driving force on ion X is equal to the difference between the actual membrane potential and the Nernst potential for that ion, $V_m - V_x$.

The third determinant of the resting membrane potential is the active and passive ion pumps that move ions across the membrane. These pumps govern the concentration of ions inside and outside the cell and act as generators of net current by moving net charge across the membrane, termed **electrogenic transport**. Numerous pumps play an important physiologic role in maintaining ion gradients; these include the ATP-dependent Na$^+$/K$^+$ pump (which uses the energy of ATP hydrolysis to extrude three Na$^+$ ions for every two K$^+$ ions that enter the cell) and the Na$^+$/Ca^{2+} exchanger (which extrudes one Ca^{2+} for every three Na$^+$ ions that enter the cell). The coordinated action of these pumps closely regulates the intracellular and extracellular concentrations of all biologically important cations and anions. By knowing the values of these ion concentrations, it is possible to calculate

the Nernst potentials for these cations and anions at physiologic temperature and, hence, the value of the transmembrane potential at which the net driving force for each ion is equal to zero (Table 8-1).

Variations in the magnitude and direction of transport for each ion (mediated by pumps and exchangers in the plasma membrane) and differences in the membrane permeability for each ion (mediated by channels selective for each ionic species) generate the distinct intracellular and extracellular concentrations for each of the four key ions. The relative ionic permeabilities of the neuronal membrane at rest are K$^+$ >> Cl$^-$ > Na$^+$ >> Ca^{2+}. Because the plasma membrane contains K$^+$-selective channels that are open under resting conditions while most other channels are closed, the resting membrane potential most closely approximates the Nernst potential for K$^+$ (about -90 mV). In reality, the additional, weak permeabilities of other ionic species raise the resting membrane potential above that for K$^+$. Thus, although K$^+$ is the most permeant ion, the permeability of the other ions and

TABLE 8-1 Nernst Equilibrium Potentials for Major Ions

ION	EXTRACELLULAR CONCENTRATION	INTRACELLULAR CONCENTRATION	NERNST EQUATION FOR ION	NERNST POTENTIAL FOR ION
Na$^+$	145 mM	15 mM	26.7 ln (145/15)	$V_{Na^+} = +61$ mV
K$^+$	4 mM	140 mM	26.7 ln (4/140)	$V_{K^+} = -95$ mV
Cl$^-$	122 mM	4.2 mM	-26.7 ln (122/4.2)	$V_{Cl^-} = -90$ mV
Ca^{2+}	1.5 mM	$\approx 1 \times 10^{-5}$ mM	26.7/2 ln (1.5/1 $\times 10^{-5}$)	$V_{Ca^{2+}} = +159$ mV

The calculated values of the Nernst potential are typical of mammalian skeletal muscle. Many human cells have similar transmembrane ion gradients.

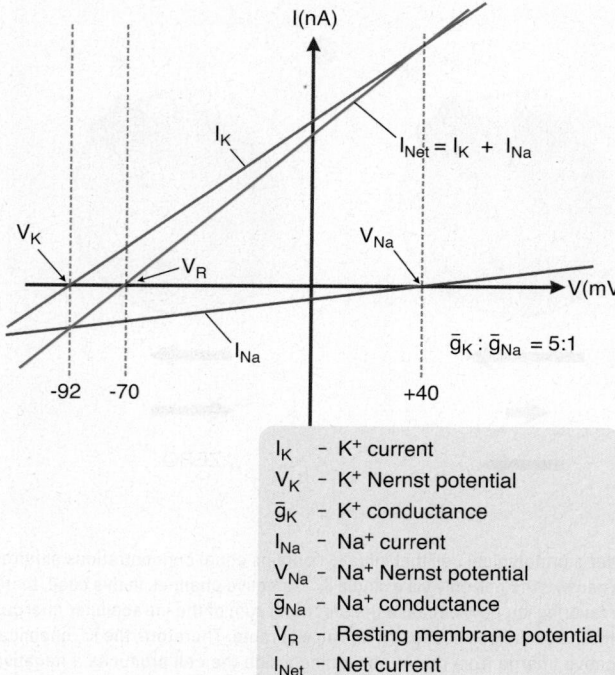

I_K	- K⁺ current
V_K	- K⁺ Nernst potential
$\bar{g}_K$	- K⁺ conductance
I_{Na}	- Na⁺ current
V_{Na}	- Na⁺ Nernst potential
$\bar{g}_{Na}$	- Na⁺ conductance
V_R	- Resting membrane potential
I_{Net}	- Net current

FIGURE 8-4. Relative contribution of K⁺ and Na⁺ to the resting membrane potential. The relative membrane permeabilities of K⁺, Na⁺, and other ions, and the Nernst (electrochemical equilibrium) potentials of these ions, together determine the resting membrane potential. In the example shown, the conductance of K⁺ is five times greater than the conductance of Na⁺ (shown by the slopes of the *I* versus *V* lines for I_K and I_{Na}, respectively). That is, the membrane is five times more permeable to K⁺ than to Na⁺. The K⁺ current is described by I_K [$I_K = \bar{g}_K(V - V_K)$], while the Na⁺ current is described by I_{Na} [$I_{Na} = \bar{g}_{Na}(V - V_{Na})$]. (In this example, $\bar{g}_K$ and $\bar{g}_{Na}$ are constant conductances over all voltages.) I_{Net}, the net membrane current, is the sum of these two currents ($I_{Net} = I_K + I_{Na}$). The "resting" membrane potential (V_R) is the value of V at which I_{Net} equals zero. In this example, note that V_R is close to, but greater than, V_K. This is because, although K⁺ is the primary determinant of the resting potential, the minor Na⁺ current depolarizes V_R to a value more positive than V_K.

the action of the "electrogenic" pumps also contribute to the overall resting potential. At the *steady state* that describes the true resting membrane potential (Fig. 8-4), V_m does not equal the Nernst potential for any of the individual ions, and each ionic species experiences a net electrochemical force. In other words, ($V_m - V_{ion}$) is nonzero, and small ion fluxes occur. The algebraic sum of these inward and outward currents is small and is balanced by currents from active, electrogenic pumps, so there is no *net* current across the resting membrane. It has been estimated that up to 25% of all cellular energy in excitable tissues is expended in maintaining ion gradients across cellular membranes.

The Goldman Equation

The example shown in Figure 8-3 addresses a situation where only one ionic species flows across the plasma membrane. In reality, many cells possess a number of different channels that are selective for different ions, all of which contribute to the overall resting membrane potential. When the resting potential is determined by two or more species of ions, the influence of each species is governed by its concentrations inside and outside the cell and by the relative permeability of

the membrane to that ion. Quantitatively, this relationship is expressed as the **Goldman-Hodgkin-Katz equation**:

$$V_m = \frac{RT}{F} \ln \frac{P_K[K^+]_o + P_{Na}[Na^+]_o + P_{Cl}[Cl^-]_i}{P_K[K^+]_i + P_{Na}[Na^+]_i + P_{Cl}[Cl^-]_o} \quad \text{Equation 8-3}$$

where P_x is the membrane permeability of ion x. (P_x is expressed as a fraction, with a value of 1 indicating maximum permeability.) Essentially, this expression states that the larger the concentration gradient of a particular ion and the higher its membrane permeability, the greater its role is in determining the membrane potential. In the extreme case, when the permeability of one ion is exclusively dominant, the Goldman equation reverts to the Nernst equation for that ion. For example, if $P_K >> P_{Cl}, P_{Na}$, the equation becomes

$$V_m = \frac{RT}{F} \ln \frac{[K^+]_o}{[K^+]_i}$$

Alternatively, if P_{Na} greatly exceeds P_K, P_{Cl}, then $V_m \sim V_{Na}$, and the membrane is strongly depolarized. This important concept links changes in ion channel permeability to changes in membrane potential. *Whenever an ion-selective channel opens, the membrane potential shifts toward the Nernst potential for that ion.* The relative contribution of a given channel to the overall membrane potential depends on the extent of ion flow through that channel. Time-dependent changes in the membrane permeabilities of Na⁺ and K⁺ (and, in cardiac cells, Ca²⁺) account for the major distinguishing feature of electrically excitable tissues—the action potential.

The Action Potential

According to Ohm's law, passage of current across a cell membrane causes the voltage across the membrane to change, reaching a new steady-state value that is determined by the membrane's resistance (see above). The time course of this voltage change is exponential, determined by the product of the resistance r_m and the capacitance c_m of the membrane, with a rate constant equal to $[r_m \times c_m]^{-1}$. (The membrane's capacitance results from having an insulator, the hydrocarbon core of the phospholipids in the membrane, between two conductors, the ionic solutions on either side of the membrane [see Fig. 8-2]. Capacitors store charge at both surfaces and require time to change the magnitude of this charge.) If the stimulated potential change is less than the **threshold** value for triggering an action potential (see below), then the membrane voltage changes smoothly and returns to its resting value when the stimulating current is turned off (Fig. 8-5A). On the other hand, if the membrane voltage changes positively by more than the threshold value, then a dramatic event occurs: the membrane voltage rises much more rapidly, to a value of approximately +50 mV, and then drops to its resting value of approximately −80 mV (Fig. 8-5B). This "suprathreshold" event is known as the **action potential (AP)**. Importantly, hyperpolarizing stimuli cannot trigger an AP (Fig. 8-5C).

In most neurons, the balance between voltage-gated Na⁺ and K⁺ channels regulates the AP. (In cardiac cells and many secretory cells, voltage-gated Ca²⁺ channels are also involved in AP regulation; see Chapter 24.) Voltage-gated Na⁺ channels conduct an inward current that depolarizes the cell at the beginning of the AP. Voltage-gated K⁺ channels conduct an outward current that repolarizes the cell at the end of the AP, in preparation for the next excitatory event.

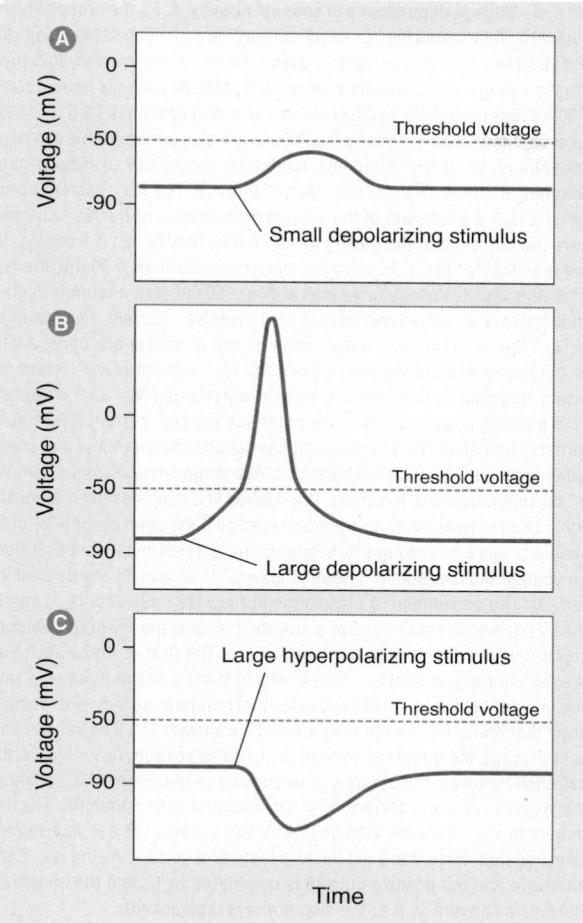

FIGURE 8-5. The action potential. A. In the example shown, a resting cell has a membrane potential of approximately −80 mV. If a small depolarizing stimulus is applied to the cell (e.g., a stimulus that opens a few voltage-gated Ca^{2+} channels), the membrane slowly depolarizes in response to the influx of Ca^{2+} ions. Once the stimulus ends and the Ca^{2+} channels close, the membrane returns to its resting potential. The time course of the voltage change is determined by the membrane capacitance (see Fig. 8-2). **B.** If a larger depolarizing stimulus is applied to the cell, such that the membrane potential exceeds its "threshold" voltage, the membrane rapidly depolarizes to about +50 mV and then returns to its resting potential. This event is known as an **action potential**; its magnitude, time course, and shape are determined by voltage-gated Na^+ and K^+ channels that open in response to membrane depolarization. **C.** In comparison, application of a hyperpolarizing stimulus to a cell does not generate an action potential, regardless of the magnitude of hyperpolarization.

Figure 8-6 shows the current–voltage (I-V) relationships for the voltage-gated Na^+ channel and the "resting" K^+ channel. The total Na^+ conductance of the membrane is the product of the constant conductance of a single open Na^+ channel, the total number of Na^+ channels, and the probability that an individual Na^+ channel is open, P_o. P_o depends on the membrane potential and increases with depolarization (shown in Fig. 8-6A), and it is this voltage dependence that enables a cell to overcome the resting K^+ conductance to generate and propagate action potentials in response to depolarizing inputs. The open channel probability represents the fraction of all Na^+ channels that open (albeit transiently, see below) in response to a single voltage step. For example, at very negative potentials (e.g., −85 mV), essentially no Na^+ channels

are open; as the membrane is rapidly depolarized through 0 mV, most or all Na^+ channels open; and fast depolarizations to −25 mV open about half of the Na^+ channels. These are the relations that occur when a constant depolarization is imposed on the membrane (in a process called **voltage-clamping**); when the brief depolarization of an AP stimulates the membrane, fewer Na^+ channels have time to reach the open state, and a large reserve of unopened channels provides a "margin of safety" for impulse transmission.

Recall that ionic current is the product of the ionic conductance (g) and a potential difference. For ions, the potential difference is the same as the electrochemical driving force, $V_m - V_x$, where V_x is the Nernst potential for the specified ion. For example, for Na^+ current:

$$I_{Na} = g_{Na}(V_m - V_{Na})$$

or

$$I_{Na} = \bar{g}_{Na}P_o(V_m - V_{Na})$$

Equation 8-4

Here, $\bar{g}_{Na}$ is the Na^+ conductance of the membrane when all Na^+ channels are open, and P_o is, as above, the probability that any individual Na^+ channel is open. The graphic illustration of this equation is shown in Figure 8-6B, where the Na^+ current for a "fully activated" membrane is described by the straight line that passes with positive slope through V_{Na}. If there were no voltage dependence to the Na^+ conductance (i.e., if g_{Na} were always equal to $\bar{g}_{Na}$), this line would extend throughout the negative voltage range, as shown by its dashed-line extrapolation. However, the voltage dependence of P_o (Fig. 8-6A) causes the actual Na^+ conductance g_{Na} to be voltage-dependent, resulting in deviation of the actual I_{Na} from this theoretical "fully activated" condition. Thus, increasing depolarizations from rest (caused, for example, by an applied stimulus) result in inward Na^+ currents that first become larger as more channels open and then become smaller as V_m approaches V_{Na}, reducing the driving force through open channels (Fig. 8-6B).

Potassium channels conduct outward currents that oppose the depolarizing actions of inward Na^+ currents. Although there are many types of K^+ channels with diverse "gating" properties, only two types need to be considered in order to appreciate the role of K^+ channels in excitability. These two K^+ channel types include the voltage-independent "leak" channels and the voltage-gated "delayed rectifier" channels. **Leak channels** are the K^+ channels that contribute to the resting membrane potential by remaining open throughout the negative range of membrane potentials. The K^+ current that flows through these channels is shown by the dashed line labeled I_K in Figure 8-6B; for these channels, K^+ current will flow for all V_m not equal to V_K.

The summation of I_{Na} and $I_{K(leak)}$ is represented by the dashed blue line in Figure 8-6C. Three important points on this line define three critical aspects of the AP. The net ionic current (I_{Net}) is zero at all three of these points. First, at rest, $V_m \approx V_K$. Under this condition, small, transient membrane *depolarizations* caused by "external" stimuli increase the driving force for K^+ ions, resulting in net *outward* currents from ion conductances through leak channels that repolarize the membrane back to rest when the external stimulus ends. Second, at $V_m = V_T$, the outward potassium currents are matched by inward sodium currents, and the net current is also zero. Under this condition, however, even a *small further depolarization* results in a *net inward current* that

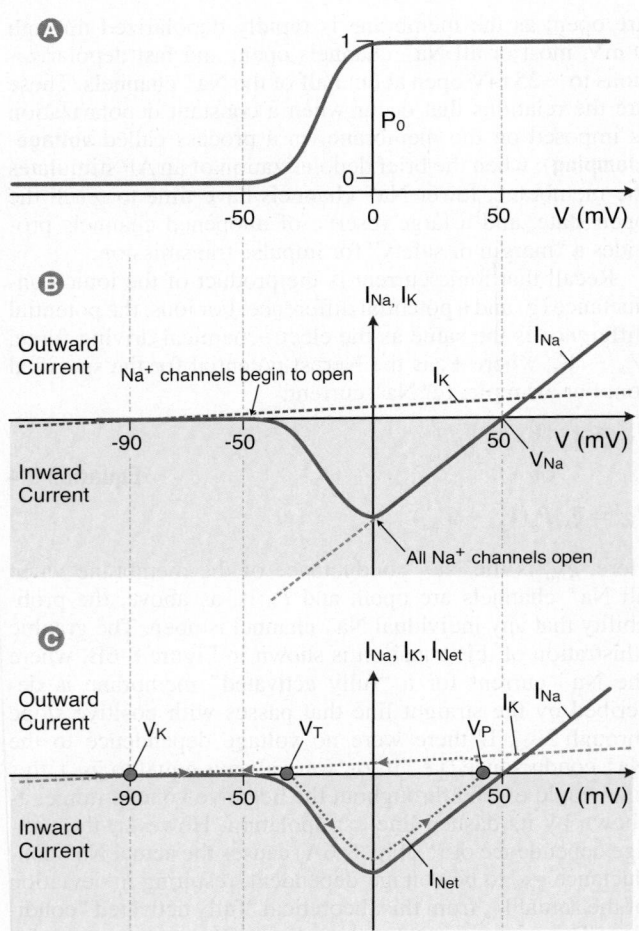

FIGURE 8-6. Voltage dependence of channel activity. A. P_o, the probability that an individual voltage-gated Na^+ channel will open, is a function of the membrane voltage (V). At voltages more negative than -50 mV, there is a very low probability that a voltage-gated sodium channel will open. At voltages more positive than -50 mV, this probability begins to increase and approaches 1.0 (i.e., a 100% chance of opening) at 0 mV. These probabilities are also generalizable to a population of voltage-gated Na^+ channels, so that virtually 100% of voltage-gated Na^+ channels in the membrane will open at 0 mV. **B.** The Na^+ current across a membrane (I_{Na}) is a function of the voltage dependence of the Na^+ channels that carry the current and the driving force (that is, how far V_m is from V_{Na}, the reversal potential for Na^+). At voltages more negative than -50 mV, the Na^+ current is zero. As the voltage increases above -50 mV, Na^+ channels begin to open, and there is an increasing inward (negative) Na^+ current. The maximum inward Na^+ flux is reached at 0 mV, when all the channels are open. As the voltage continues to increase above 0 mV, the Na^+ current is still inward, but decreasing, because inward flow of the positively charged Na^+ ions is opposed by the increasingly positive intracellular potential. The Na^+ current is zero at V_{Na} (the Nernst potential for Na^+) because, at this voltage, the electrical and chemical gradients for Na^+ ion flow are balanced. At voltages more positive than V_{Na}, the Na^+ current is outward (positive). The dashed line indicates the relationship that would exist between Na^+ current and voltage if the open probability of the Na^+ channels were not voltage-dependent. The potassium current that flows through voltage-independent K^+ "leak channels" is shown by the dashed line labeled I_K. **C.** The summation of plasma membrane Na^+ currents (I_{Na}) and K^+ currents (I_K) demonstrates three key transition points in the I-V graph (*denoted by blue circles*) at which the net current is zero. The first of these points occurs at a membrane potential of -90 mV, where $V = V_K$. At this voltage, a small increase in potential (i.e., a small depolarization) results in an outward (positive) K^+ current that brings the membrane potential back toward V_K. The second point occurs at $V_{Threshold}$, the threshold voltage (V_T). At this voltage, $I_{Na} = -I_K$; further depolarization results in the opening of more voltage-dependent Na^+ channels and a net negative (inward) current, which initiates the action potential. The third point occurs at V_{Peak}, the peak voltage (V_P). At this voltage, the transition occurs from a net negative current to a net positive (outward) current. As the Na^+ channels inactivate, the net positive current is dominated by I_K, and the membrane potential returns toward V_K (i.e., the membrane is repolarized).

further depolarizes the membrane, which leads to a larger inward current and further membrane depolarization. *This positive feedback loop constitutes the rising phase of the AP.* Thus, the AP occurs in response to any rapid depolarization beyond V_T, which is defined as the **threshold potential**. Third, V_p is the potential at the peak of the AP. As the membrane approaches V_p, it moves further from V_K and closer to V_{Na}, so the driving force for sodium influx decreases while that for potassium efflux grows. Once V_m reaches this maximum depolarization, the net current switches sign from inward to outward, and consequently, the membrane begins to be repolarized.

Voltage-gated (**delayed rectifier**) K^+ channels contribute to the rapid repolarization phase of the AP. Although membrane depolarization opens these channels, they open and close more slowly than do Na^+ channels in response to depolarization. Therefore, inward Na^+ current dominates the early (depolarization) phase of the AP, and outward K^+ current dominates the later (repolarization) phase (Fig. 8-7). This is why the AP is characterized by an initial rapid depolarization (caused by fast inward Na^+ current) followed by a prolonged repolarization (caused by slower and more sustained outward K^+ current).

The final feature determining membrane excitability is the limited duration of Na^+ channel opening in response to membrane depolarization. After opening in response to rapid membrane depolarization, most Na^+ channels enter a closed state in which they are **inactivated** (i.e., prevented from subsequent opening). Recovery from inactivation

occurs only when the membrane is repolarized, whereupon the Na^+ channels return relatively slowly to the closed, resting state from which they can then open in response to a stimulus. This inactivation of Na^+ conductance, combined with the slowly decaying voltage-gated K^+ conductance, produces dynamic changes in membrane excitability. Following just one AP, fewer Na^+ channels are available to open (i.e., $\overline{g}_{Na}$ is temporarily smaller), more K^+ channels are open (i.e., g_K is larger), the corresponding ionic currents are changed, and V_T *is therefore more positive than it was before the AP.* An excitable membrane is in its so-called **refractory state** during this period, which lasts from just after the AP until the conditions of fast g_{Na} inactivation and slow g_K activation have returned to their resting values. Very slow depolarizing stimuli will fail to induce an AP, even when the membrane reaches the threshold potential defined by a rapid depolarizing stimulus, because of the accumulation of inactivated Na^+ channels during the slow depolarizing stimulus.

The inactivation property of Na^+ channels is important in the concept of **use-dependent block**, as discussed in Chapter 12, Local Anesthetic Pharmacology, and Chapter 24. Also, under pathologic conditions, cells may express Na^+ channels that inactivate incompletely and therefore continue to carry an inward current after termination of the AP. Such currents may be adequate to raise the membrane potential above V_T and thus induce repetitive firing. Diseases such as myotonia and certain types of neuropathic pain appear to arise from expression of this type of altered Na^+ channel.

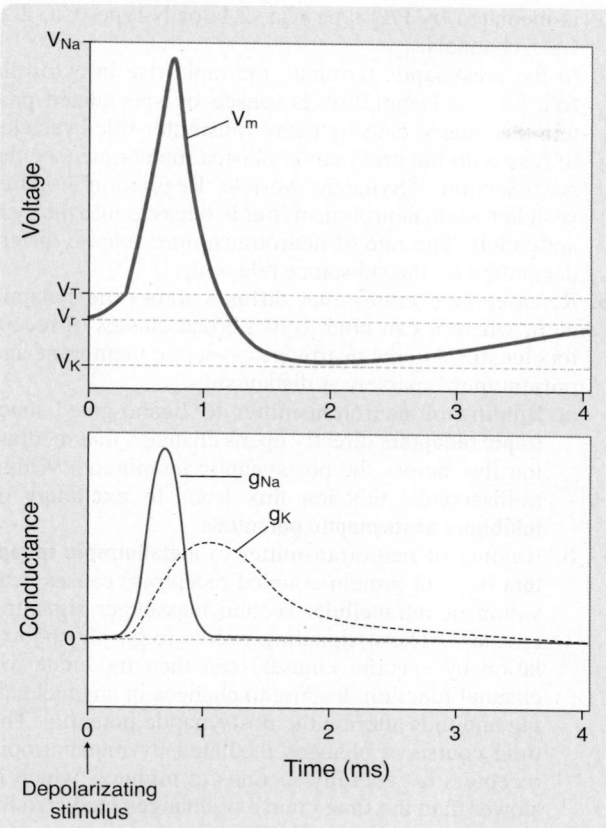

FIGURE 8-7. Time course of voltage-dependent Na⁺ and K⁺ conductances. During the course of an action potential, the transmembrane voltage (V_m) first increases rapidly from V_T toward V_{Na}, then decreases below V_T, and more slowly approaches V_K. The shape and duration of the action potential can be explained by the differential time courses of the voltage-dependent Na⁺ and K⁺ currents. In response to a depolarizing stimulus, the Na⁺ conductance (g_{Na}) increases rapidly because of the rapid opening of voltage-gated Na⁺ channels, then decreases because of Na⁺ channel inactivation. The K⁺ conductance (g_K) increases concurrently with g_{Na} but takes a longer time to reach its maximum conductance because there is a slower rate constant for opening of voltage-dependent K⁺ channels. Eventually, g_K is greater than g_{Na}, and the membrane repolarizes. (V_{Na}, V_K, Nernst potentials for Na⁺ and K⁺, respectively; V_r, resting membrane potential; V_T, threshold potential for action potential firing.)

PHARMACOLOGY OF ION CHANNELS

Many drugs act directly on ion channels to produce changes in membrane excitability. For example, local anesthetics are injected locally at high concentrations to block Na⁺ channels in peripheral and spinal neurons; this Na⁺ channel block inhibits AP propagation and prevents sensory transmission (e.g., pain) and motor nerve impulses by these nerves (see Chapter 12). At much lower concentrations, these and structurally similar antiarrhythmic drugs act systemically to suppress abnormal APs in the heart and to treat neuropathic pain and some forms of myotonia (see Chapter 24). Drugs that block K⁺ channels are used to treat certain types of cardiac arrhythmias and may be used in the future to overcome nerve conduction deficits secondary to demyelinating conditions such as multiple sclerosis and spinal cord injury. Calcium channels are blocked directly by some drugs used in the treatment of hypertension; such drugs act by relaxing vascular smooth muscle and

lowering systemic vascular resistance. Some cardiovascular diseases are also treated by selective blockers of cardiac Ca²⁺ channels (see Chapter 22, Pharmacology of Vascular Tone). Highly potent and selective blockers of a certain class of neuronal Ca²⁺ channel have been purified from the venom of a marine snail (*Conus* sp.) and administered into the spinal fluid to treat severe cases of neuropathic pain. **Tetrodotoxin**, the fugu neurotoxin from the introductory case, blocks most neuronal voltage-gated Na⁺ channels with high affinity. As a result, tetrodotoxin can inhibit AP propagation in the nervous system, leading to fatal paralysis if ingested in sufficient amounts. Ion channel function can also be modified through pharmacologic modulation of the receptors that regulate the channels, as described below.

ELECTROCHEMICAL TRANSMISSION

Neurons communicate with one another and with other cell types through the regulated release of small molecules or peptides known as **neurotransmitters**. Neurotransmitters may be released into the circulation, from which they can act on distant organs, or they may diffuse only a short distance to act on juxtaposed target cells at specialized connections called **synapses**. Synaptic transmission thus integrates electrical signals (voltage changes in the plasma membrane of the presynaptic cell) with chemical signals (release of neurotransmitter by the presynaptic cell and subsequent binding of the transmitter to receptors in the membrane of the postsynaptic cell). For this reason, synaptic transmission is often referred to as **electrochemical transmission**.

The general sequence of processes essential for electrochemical transmission is as follows (Fig. 8-8):

1. Neurotransmitters are synthesized by cytoplasmic enzymes and stored in the neuron. Common neurotransmitters include acetylcholine, norepinephrine, γ-aminobutyric acid (GABA), glutamate, dopamine, and serotonin. Most neurons are specialized to release only one type of neurotransmitter, and this specialization is determined largely by the synthetic enzymes expressed in that neuron. After synthesis, neurotransmitters are actively transported from the cytoplasm into intracellular vesicles (often called **synaptic vesicles**) in which they reach high concentrations. Loading of these vesicles is accomplished by the coordinated activity of a number of vesicular membrane proteins. In most cases, an ATP-dependent transporter pumps protons from the cytoplasm into the vesicle, thereby creating a proton gradient across the vesicle membrane. The electrochemical energy in this proton gradient is used to provide specialized neurotransmitter transporters with the fuel for active transport of neurotransmitter molecules from the cytoplasm into the vesicle. Neurotransmitter-filled vesicles undergo a docking process and are primed at the "active zone" inside the plasma membrane of the presynaptic terminal, a cellular structure that is specialized for neurotransmitter release.

2. When the threshold condition is reached in the neuron, an AP is initiated and propagated along the axonal membrane to the presynaptic nerve terminal.

3. Depolarization of the nerve terminal membrane causes opening of voltage-dependent Ca²⁺ channels and influx of Ca²⁺ through these open channels into the presynaptic nerve terminal. In many neurons, this Ca²⁺ influx

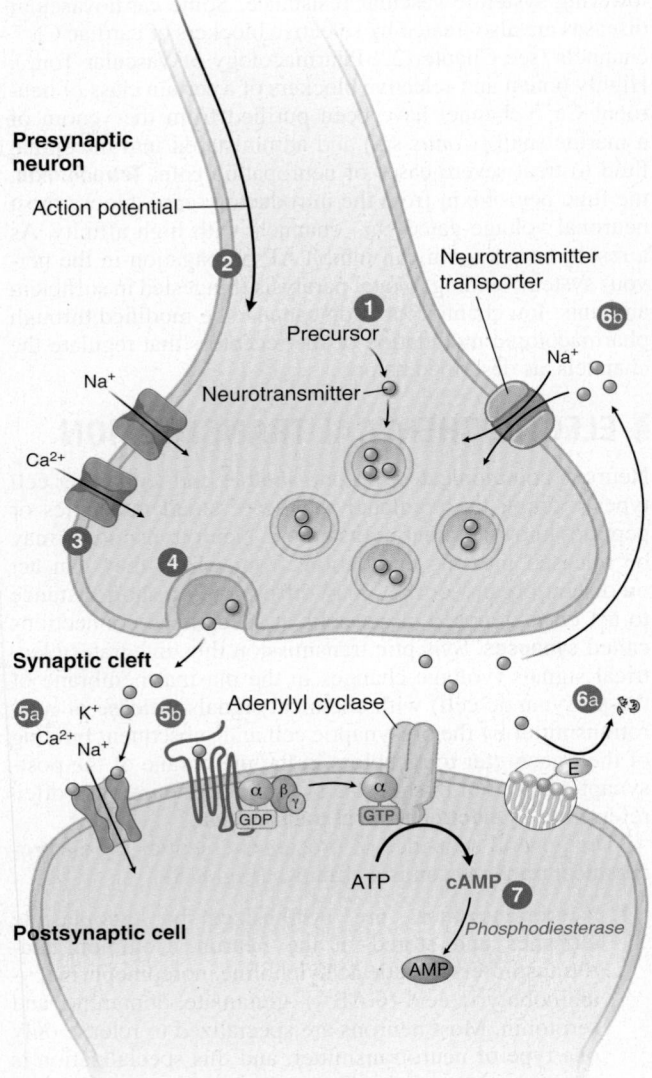

FIGURE 8-8. Steps in synaptic transmission. Synaptic transmission can be divided into a series of steps that couple electrical depolarization of the presynaptic neuron to chemical signaling between the presynaptic and postsynaptic cells. **1.** Neuron synthesizes neurotransmitter from precursors and stores the transmitter in vesicles. **2.** An action potential traveling down the neuron depolarizes the presynaptic nerve terminal. **3.** Membrane depolarization activates voltage-dependent Ca^{2+} channels, allowing Ca^{2+} entry into the presynaptic nerve terminal. **4.** The increased cytosolic Ca^{2+} stimulates vesicle fusion with the plasma membrane of the presynaptic neuron, with subsequent release of neurotransmitter into the synaptic cleft. **5.** Neurotransmitter diffuses across the synaptic cleft and binds to one of two types of postsynaptic receptors. **5a.** Neurotransmitter binding to ionotropic receptors causes channel opening and changes the permeability of the postsynaptic membrane to ions. This may also result in a change in the postsynaptic membrane potential. **5b.** Neurotransmitter binding to metabotropic receptors on the postsynaptic cell activates intracellular signaling cascades; the example shows G protein activation leading to the formation of cAMP by adenylyl cyclase. In turn, such a signaling cascade can activate other ion-selective channels (*not shown*). **6.** Signal termination is accomplished by removal of transmitter from the synaptic cleft. **6a.** Transmitter can be degraded by enzymes (E) in the synaptic cleft. **6b.** Alternatively, transmitter can be recycled into the presynaptic cell by reuptake transporters. **7.** Signal termination can also be accomplished by enzymes (such as phosphodiesterase) that degrade postsynaptic intracellular signaling molecules (such as cAMP).

is mediated by P/Q-type (Ca_v 2.1) or N-type (Ca_v 2.2) Ca^{2+} channels.

4. In the presynaptic terminal, the rapid rise in cytosolic free Ca^{2+} concentration is sensed by specialized protein machinery, causing neurotransmitter-filled vesicles to fuse with the presynaptic plasma membrane (see the next section, "Synaptic Vesicle Regulation"). After vesicle fusion, neurotransmitter is released into the synaptic cleft. The rate of neurotransmitter release differs depending on the substance released.

5. Released neurotransmitter diffuses across the synaptic cleft, where it can bind to two broad classes of receptors localized in the nearby postsynaptic membrane and present more sparsely at distant sites:

   a. Binding of neurotransmitter to ligand-gated **ionotropic receptors** directly opens channels that mediate ion flux across the postsynaptic membrane. Within milliseconds, this ion flux leads to **excitatory** or **inhibitory postsynaptic potentials**.

   b. Binding of neurotransmitter to **metabotropic receptors** (e.g., G protein-coupled receptors) causes activation of intracellular second messenger signaling cascades. These signaling events (e.g., phosphorylation by specific kinases) can then modulate ion channel function, leading to changes in channel gating and thus altering the postsynaptic potential. The time course of changes mediated by metabotropic receptors is generally seconds to minutes, which is slower than the time course of changes mediated by ionotropic receptors. Both ionotropic and metabotropic receptors are commonly present on the same cell, accounting for fast and slow changes, respectively, in the postsynaptic membrane potential.

   Some neurotransmitters may also bind to a third class of receptors on the *presynaptic* membrane. These receptors are called **autoreceptors** because they regulate neurotransmitter release.

6. Excitatory postsynaptic potentials (EPSPs) and inhibitory postsynaptic potentials (IPSPs) propagate passively (i.e., without generating an AP) along the membrane of the postsynaptic cell. A large number of EPSPs can summate to raise the postsynaptic membrane potential beyond threshold voltage (V_T). If this occurs, a single or multiple APs can be generated in the postsynaptic cell. (This process is not shown in Fig. 8-8.)

7. Stimulation of the postsynaptic cell is terminated by removal of the neurotransmitter from the synaptic cleft, desensitization of the postsynaptic receptor, or a combination of both. Neurotransmitter removal occurs by two mechanisms:

   a. Degradation of the neurotransmitter by enzymes in the synaptic cleft; and

   b. Uptake of the neurotransmitter by specific transporters into the presynaptic terminal (or the closely surrounding glial cells), which terminates synaptic action and allows the neurotransmitter to be recycled into synaptic vesicles in preparation for a new release event.

8. For G protein-coupled metabotropic receptors in the postsynaptic cell, termination of the response to a transmitter stimulus is also dependent on intracellular enzymes that inactivate second messengers (e.g., phosphodiesterases that convert cAMP to its inactive metabolite AMP) or that reverse phosphorylation of target proteins.

The prototypic chemical synapse is that of the neuromuscular junction (see Fig. 10-4 for more detail). At this junction, terminal branches of the motor axon lie in synaptic troughs on the surface of the muscle cells. When the neuron fires, acetylcholine (ACh) is released from the motor neuron terminals. The released ACh diffuses across the **synaptic cleft** to bind to ligand-gated ionotropic receptors located on the postsynaptic muscle membrane. This binding of ACh to its receptors causes a transient increase in the probability of opening of receptor-associated ion channels. The channel pore is equally permeable to Na^+ and K^+, so these channels have a **reversal potential** (i.e., a potential at which there is no net current flowing through the channel) of approximately -10 mV (the average of the individual Na^+ and K^+ Nernst potentials; see Eq. 8-3). The *net inward current* passing through these open channels depolarizes the muscle cell membrane. Although this particular **end-plate potential**, resulting from one presynaptic AP, is sufficiently large to stimulate an AP in the muscle, such a magnitude is exceptional. Because most neuronal excitatory postsynaptic potentials are too small to stimulate an AP, several neuronal excitatory postsynaptic potentials must occur together, within a short time ($\sim$10 ms) and at closely spaced synapses (allowing temporal and spatial integration), in order for the postsynaptic depolarization to reach the threshold value for firing of an AP.

Many neurons synthesize and release **neuropeptides** in addition to neurotransmitters. Neuropeptides, which are short chains of amino acids, exert effects on other neurons and play key roles in processes as diverse as energy homeostasis and cellular excitability. In contrast to the fast neurotransmission mediated by synaptic vesicle fusion and neurotransmitter release, neuropeptides signal more slowly and are typically released via the regulated secretory pathway. Indeed, the synthesis, storage, and release of neuropeptides are similar to hormone production and secretion, and many neuropeptides were initially identified as hormones acting outside the central nervous system. Like hormones, neuropeptides are synthesized as precursor polypeptides (preproneuropeptides) on ribosomes at the endoplasmic reticulum and subsequently processed enzymatically into the propeptide, sorted, and packaged along with specialized proteases into **dense-core secretory vesicles** in the Golgi apparatus (see below).

As with hormones, the proneuropeptide may include multiple distinct neuropeptides, and a neuron can therefore release more than one neuropeptide. Proteases within the vesicle cleave the proneuropeptide into the individual neuropeptides during fast axonal transport of the vesicle toward the synapse. Unlike classical neurotransmitter vesicles, neuropeptide vesicles do not undergo docking at the synapse, and release may occur at sites other than the synaptic terminal. Exocytosis of neuropeptide vesicles thus tends to occur only in response to sustained Ca^{2+} elevation, which typically requires repeated or prolonged stimuli. Once released, neuropeptides act almost exclusively at metabotropic receptors. Because they are often released extrasynaptically, neuropeptides typically diffuse over longer distances than neurotransmitters to bind to receptors on numerous cells surrounding the release site, a process known as **volume transmission**.

The following discussion highlights steps in the basic processes of neurotransmission that can be modified by pharmacologic agents.

Synaptic Vesicle Regulation

Nerve terminals contain two types of secretory vesicles: small, **clear-core synaptic vesicles** and large, **dense-core synaptic vesicles**. The clear-core vesicles store and secrete small organic neurotransmitters such as acetylcholine, GABA, glycine, and glutamate. Dense-core vesicles are more likely to contain neuropeptide or amine neurotransmitters. As described above, the larger dense-core vesicles are similar to the secretory granules of endocrine cells because their release is not limited to "active zones" on the presynaptic cell. Dense-core vesicle release is also more likely to follow a train of impulses (continuous or rhythmic stimulation) than a single AP. Hence, the smaller clear-core vesicles are involved in rapid chemical transmission, while the larger dense-core vesicles are implicated in slow, modulatory, or distant signaling.

Recently, many of the proteins that control synaptic vesicle trafficking have been identified. Synaptic vesicles interact with a family of proteins called **synapsins** that bind to the actin cytoskeleton in a phosphorylation-dependent manner. Activity at the synapse drives phosphorylation and dephosphorylation of synapsins via a variety of protein kinases and phosphatases, and synapsins are thus thought to regulate the availability of vesicles for Ca^{2+}-dependent exocytosis. Vesicle docking and priming at the active zone are mediated by interactions between proteins in the synaptic vesicle membrane and the plasma membrane. Once docked and primed, Ca^{2+}-sensing proteins called **synaptotagmins** play a key role in exocytosis. For both Ca^{2+}-regulated and Ca^{2+}-independent vesicle exocytosis, fusion between the synaptic vesicle and plasma membranes is mediated by the **SNARE/SM** protein complex present in both the vesicle membrane (synaptobrevin/VAMP) and the plasma membrane (syntaxin-1, SNAP-25) (Fig. 8-9). Certain neurotoxins, such as tetanus toxin and botulinum toxin (see Chapter 10, Cholinergic Pharmacology), appear to act by selectively cleaving SNAREs and thereby inhibiting synaptic vesicle exocytosis. Conversely, a toxin in the venom of the black widow spider binds to specific receptors in presynaptic nerve terminals and oligomerizes to form pores in the presynaptic plasma membrane, thereby bypassing the physiologic regulation of synaptic vesicle fusion to stimulate spontaneous release of neurotransmitters. SNAREs and associated proteins may provide future targets for pharmacologic control of synaptic transmission.

Postsynaptic Receptors

A large number of neuropharmacologic drugs act on neurotransmitter or neuropeptide receptors. These integral membrane proteins fall into two classes: **ionotropic** and **metabotropic**.

Ionotropic receptors, such as nicotinic acetylcholine receptors, AMPA and NMDA glutamatergic receptors, and "A" type GABA receptors, are almost always composed of four to five subunits that oligomerize in the membrane to form a ligand-gated channel. Relatively rapid binding of one or sometimes two ligand molecules to the receptor leads to a slower allosteric conformational change that opens the channel pore. The subunits composing the same functional receptor often differ among different tissues and, as a consequence, the detailed molecular pharmacology of the receptors is tissue-dependent. For example, although acetylcholine is the endogenous transmitter for all nicotinic cholinergic receptors, different synthetic agonists (or antagonists) selectively activate (or inhibit) these receptors in skeletal muscle, autonomic ganglia, or the central nervous system (see Chapter 10). Ionotropic receptors are also found presynaptically, where they modulate neurotransmitter release from the presynaptic terminal.

Metabotropic receptors, which exert their effects through activation of intracellular signaling cascades, are similarly diverse in ligands, location, and effect. They are found both pre- and postsynaptically and commonly coexist with ionotropic receptors. Most metabotropic receptors are G protein-coupled receptors (GPCRs). Classical fast neurotransmitters (glutamate, ACh, and GABA), monoamines (dopamine, serotonin, and norepinephrine), and neuropeptides can all act via metabotropic receptors. A neurotransmitter or peptide may have multiple distinct metabotropic receptors, each with different or even opposing intracellular signaling pathways. For example, dopamine increases cAMP levels via the D1 family of dopamine receptors but decreases cAMP levels via the D2 family of dopamine receptors (see Chapter 14, Pharmacology of Dopaminergic Neurotransmission). The intracellular effects of metabotropic receptor activation are numerous and diverse. Postsynaptically, metabotropic receptor signaling can open ion channels to create slow excitatory or inhibitory postsynaptic currents or modulate channel properties to change cellular excitability. Second messenger cascades regulate the activity of a host of intracellular targets and processes (see Chapter 1, Drug–Receptor Interactions, as well as chapters in Sections IIB and IIC). Activation of presynaptic receptors can regulate the probability of neurotransmitter release at the synapse. The diversity of structure and function of metabotropic receptors makes them prime candidates for development of selective agonists or antagonists that activate or inhibit specific subtypes of metabotropic receptors.

Transmitter Metabolism and Reuptake

Altering the metabolism of the neurotransmitter provides an important mechanism for pharmacologic intervention at the synapse. The two major types of intervention involve inhibition of neurotransmitter degradation and antagonism of neurotransmitter reuptake. Acetylcholinesterase, the enzyme responsible for degrading acetylcholine, is an example of the first type of drug target. **Acetylcholinesterase inhibitors** are the mainstays of treatment for myasthenia gravis (see Chapter 10).

The transporters that facilitate neurotransmitter reuptake from the synaptic cleft into the presynaptic cell are of even greater importance. Because these reuptake transporters are crucial for the termination of synaptic transmission, their inhibition has profound effects. For example, the psychotropic effects of **cocaine** derive from this drug's ability to inhibit dopamine and norepinephrine reuptake in the brain, and the therapeutic benefit of antidepressants such as **fluoxetine** likely results from inhibition of serotonin-selective reuptake

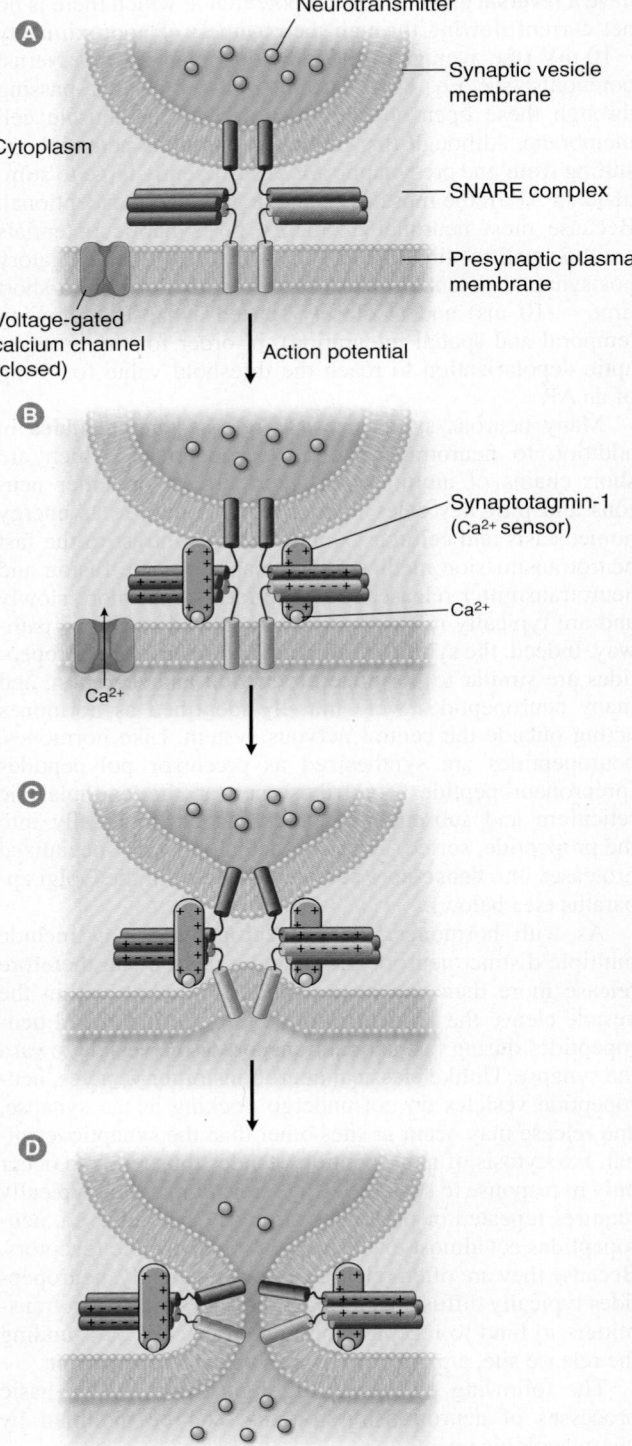

FIGURE 8-9. Current model of neurotransmitter release. A. Synaptic vesicles are tethered close to the plasma membrane of the presynaptic neuron by several protein–protein interactions. The most important of these interactions involve SNAREs (soluble N-ethylmaleimide-sensitive factor attachment protein receptors) and SM (Sec1/Munc18-like) proteins present in both the vesicle membrane and the plasma membrane. The SNARE proteins include synaptobrevin (*red*), syntaxin-1 (*yellow*), and SNAP-25 (*green*). The SM proteins include Munc18-1 and others (*not shown*). Voltage-gated Ca^{2+} channels are located in the plasma membrane in close proximity to these SNARE/SM complexes; this facilitates the sensing of Ca^{2+} entry by Ca^{2+}-binding proteins (synaptotagmin-1, *in blue*) localized to the presynaptic plasma membrane and/or the synaptic vesicle membrane. **B–D.** Voltage-gated calcium channels open in response to an action potential, allowing entry of extracellular Ca^{2+} into the cell. The increase in intracellular Ca^{2+} triggers binding of synaptotagmin-1 to the SNARE/SM complex and fusion of the vesicle membrane with the plasma membrane, releasing neurotransmitter molecules into the synaptic cleft. Several additional proteins (Munc13-1, complexin-1, and others) are also involved in the regulation of synaptic vesicle fusion (*not shown*).

(see Chapter 15, Pharmacology of Serotonergic and Central Adrenergic Neurotransmission). Because reuptake transporters tend to be substrate-specific, it is anticipated that new drugs can be designed to selectively target other specific transporter subtypes as well.

■ CONCLUSION AND FUTURE DIRECTIONS

Cellular excitability is a crucial component of intercellular communication. The fundamental basis for cellular excitability lies in the electrochemical gradients that are established by ion pumps across the lipid bilayer of the plasma membrane and in the ion-selective channels that regulate the permeability of the membrane selectively for different ionic species, allowing a change in membrane voltage to be coupled to a chemical stimulus or response. The action potential, a special type of stereotyped response found in excitable cells, is made possible by the voltage-dependent properties of Na^+ and K^+ channels.

The basic processes of electrochemical transmission provide the substrate for pharmacologic modulation of cellular excitation and communication, topics that are addressed in more detail throughout this book.

Acknowledgment

We thank Michael Ty for his valuable contributions to this chapter in the First and Second Editions of *Principles of Pharmacology: The Pathophysiologic Basis of Drug Therapy.*

Suggested Reading

Catterall WA, Raman IM, Robinson HP, Sejnowski TJ, Paulsen O. The Hodgkin-Huxley heritage: from channels to circuits. *J Neurosci* 2012;32:14064–14073. (*Historical overview of our understanding of the action potential.*)

Choquet D, Triller A. The dynamic synapse. *Neuron* 2013;80:691–703. (*Conceptual overview of synaptic physiology, with an emphasis on recent research advances.*)

Kullmann DM, Waxman SG. Neurological channelopathies: new insights into disease mechanisms and ion channel function. *J Physiol (London)* 2010;588:1823–1827. (*Review of neurologic diseases resulting from alterations in ion channel physiology.*)

Nestler EJ, Hyman SE, Holtzman DM, Malenka RC. *Molecular neuropharmacology: a foundation for clinical neuroscience.* 3rd ed. New York: McGraw-Hill Professional; 2015. (*An overview of neuropharmacology.*)

Südhof TC. Neurotransmitter release: the last millisecond in the life of a synaptic vesicle. *Neuron* 2013;80:675–690. (*Review of events and mechanisms of synaptic vesicle fusion.*)

van den Pol AN. Neuropeptide transmission in brain circuits. *Neuron* 2012;76:98–115. (*Review of neuropeptide functions.*)

Brain capillary

Pericyte

Astroglial process

Basement membrane

Mitochondria

Tight junction

9

Principles of Nervous System Physiology and Pharmacology

Joshua M. Galanter, Susannah B. Cornes, and Daniel H. Lowenstein

◼ INTRODUCTION

The nervous system contains more than 10 billion neurons. Most neurons form thousands of synaptic connections, giving the nervous system complexity unlike that seen in any other organ system. Interactions among neuronal circuits mediate functions ranging from primitive reflexes to language, mood, and memory. To perform these functions, the individual neurons that comprise the nervous system must be organized into functional networks, which, in turn, are organized into larger anatomical units.

The previous chapter reviewed the physiology of individual neurons by describing electrical transmission within a neuron and chemical transmission from one neuron to another. This chapter discusses neuronal systems by examining two levels of organization. First, the gross anatomical organization of the nervous system is presented to place in context the sites of action of pharmacologic agents that act on this system. Second, the major patterns of neuronal connectivity (so-called neuronal tracts) are presented, because knowledge of the ways in which neuronal cells are organized to transmit, process, and modulate signals facilitates a deeper understanding of the actions of drugs on these tracts. This chapter also discusses the major types of neurotransmitters and the blood–brain barrier; these functional and metabolic concepts have important pharmacologic consequences for drugs that act on the nervous system.

◼ NEUROANATOMY

The nervous system can be divided structurally and functionally into peripheral and central components. The **peripheral nervous system** includes all nerves traveling between the central nervous system and somatic and visceral sites. It is divided functionally into the **autonomic** (involuntary) **nervous system** and the **sensory and somatic** (voluntary) **nervous system**.

The **central nervous system (CNS)** includes the cerebrum, diencephalon, cerebellum, brainstem, and spinal cord. The CNS relays and processes signals received from the peripheral nervous system; the processing results in responses that are formulated and relayed back to the periphery. The CNS is responsible for important functions such as perception—including sensory, auditory, and visual processing—wakefulness, language, and consciousness.

Anatomy of the Peripheral Nervous System

The autonomic nervous system regulates involuntary responses of smooth muscle and glandular tissue. For example, it controls vascular tone, heart rate and contractility, pupillary constriction, sweating, salivation, piloerection ("goose bumps"), uterine contraction, gastrointestinal (GI) motility, and bladder function. The autonomic nervous system is

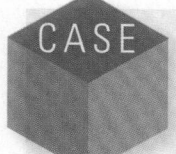

CASE

Martha P is a 66-year-old woman with a 4-year history of worsening Parkinson's disease, a neurological disorder resulting from the progressive degeneration of nigrostriatal neurons that use dopamine as a neurotransmitter. The disease causes a resting tremor, rigidity, difficulty initiating movement, and postural instability. While visiting her physician, Ms. P registers an unusual complaint: "It seems that my Sinemet doesn't work as well when I take it with meals." Ms. P explains that she has recently started on a new "low-carb" diet that has increased her protein intake at the expense of high-carbohydrate foods. Concerned, Ms. P asks, "Could my diet have anything to do with this?" Her physician explains that levodopa, a component of her Sinemet, helps replace a chemical in her brain that is produced in insufficient quantities because of the loss of certain neurons in her brain. Although many factors could lead to the decreased effectiveness of her medication, Ms. P's doctor confirms her suspicion that her high-protein diet could indeed be interfering with the medication's ability to reach her brain. He recommends that she moderate her protein intake, and, if necessary, take a higher dose of Sinemet after a high-protein meal. At her follow-up visit, Ms. P is happy to report that her medication is more effective now that she is eating less protein.

Questions

1. Where is the nigrostriatal tract located? How does the degeneration of a specific group of neurons result in specific symptoms such as those seen in Parkinson's disease?
2. Why is levodopa used in the treatment of Parkinson's disease, and what is the relationship of this compound to dopamine?
3. Why does protein consumption interfere with the action of levodopa?
4. Why does Sinemet contain both levodopa and carbidopa?

divided into the **sympathetic** nervous system, responsible for "fight or flight" responses, and the **parasympathetic** nervous system, responsible for "rest and digest" responses. The sensory and somatic peripheral nervous system carries sensory signals from the periphery to the CNS and motor signals from the CNS to striated muscle; these signals regulate voluntary movement (Fig. 9-1).

Autonomic Nervous System

Autonomic nerve fibers interact with their target organs by a two-neuron pathway. The first neuron originates in the brainstem or spinal cord and is termed a **preganglionic neuron**. The preganglionic neuron synapses outside the spinal cord with a **postganglionic neuron** that innervates the target organ. As discussed below, the anatomical location of these connections differs for neurons of the sympathetic and parasympathetic divisions of the autonomic nervous system.

Anatomy of the Sympathetic Nervous System

The sympathetic nervous system is also known as the **thoracolumbar system**, because its preganglionic fibers arise from the first thoracic segment to the second or third lumbar segment of the spinal cord (Fig. 9-2). Specifically, the preganglionic nerve cell bodies arise from the **intermediolateral** columns in the spinal cord. Preganglionic nerves exit the spinal cord at the ventral roots of each vertebral level and make synaptic connections with postganglionic neurons in sympathetic ganglia. Most sympathetic ganglia are located in the sympathetic chain, which consists of 25 pairs of interconnected ganglia that lie on either side of the vertebral column. The first three ganglia, termed the **superior cervical ganglion**, **middle cervical ganglion**, and **inferior cervical ganglion**, send their postganglionic fibers via the cranial and cervical spinal nerves. The superior cervical ganglion innervates the pupil, salivary glands, and lacrimal glands, as well as blood vessels and sweat glands in the head and face (Fig. 9-2). Postganglionic neurons arising in the middle and inferior cervical ganglia, as well as the thoracic ganglia, innervate the heart and lungs. Fibers arising from the remaining paravertebral ganglia innervate sweat glands, pilomotor muscles, and blood vessels of skeletal muscle and skin throughout the body.

Postganglionic neurons that innervate the GI tract down to the sigmoid colon, including the liver and pancreas, arise from ganglia that are located anterior to the aorta, at the origins of the celiac, superior mesenteric, and inferior mesenteric blood vessels (Fig. 9-2). Hence, these ganglia, collectively known as **prevertebral ganglia**, are named the **celiac ganglion**, **superior mesenteric ganglion**, and **inferior mesenteric ganglion**, respectively. In contrast to the paravertebral ganglia, the prevertebral ganglia have long preganglionic fibers and short postganglionic fibers.

The **adrenal medulla** is contained within the adrenal glands that lie on the superior surface of the kidneys. The adrenal medulla contains postsynaptic neuroendocrine cells (Fig. 9-2). Unlike sympathetic postganglionic neurons, which synthesize and release norepinephrine, neuroendocrine cells of the adrenal medulla synthesize primarily epinephrine (85%) and release this neurotransmitter into the bloodstream rather than at synapses on a specific target organ (see Chapter 11, Adrenergic Pharmacology).

Many pharmacologic agents modulate sympathetic nervous system activity. As discussed in Chapter 11, the sympathetic nervous system has an organ-specific distribution of adrenergic receptor types. This organ-specific receptor expression allows drugs to modulate sympathetic activity selectively. For example, certain sympathetic agonists, such as **albuterol**, can dilate bronchioles selectively, while certain sympathetic antagonists, such as **metoprolol**, can selectively decrease heart rate and contractility.

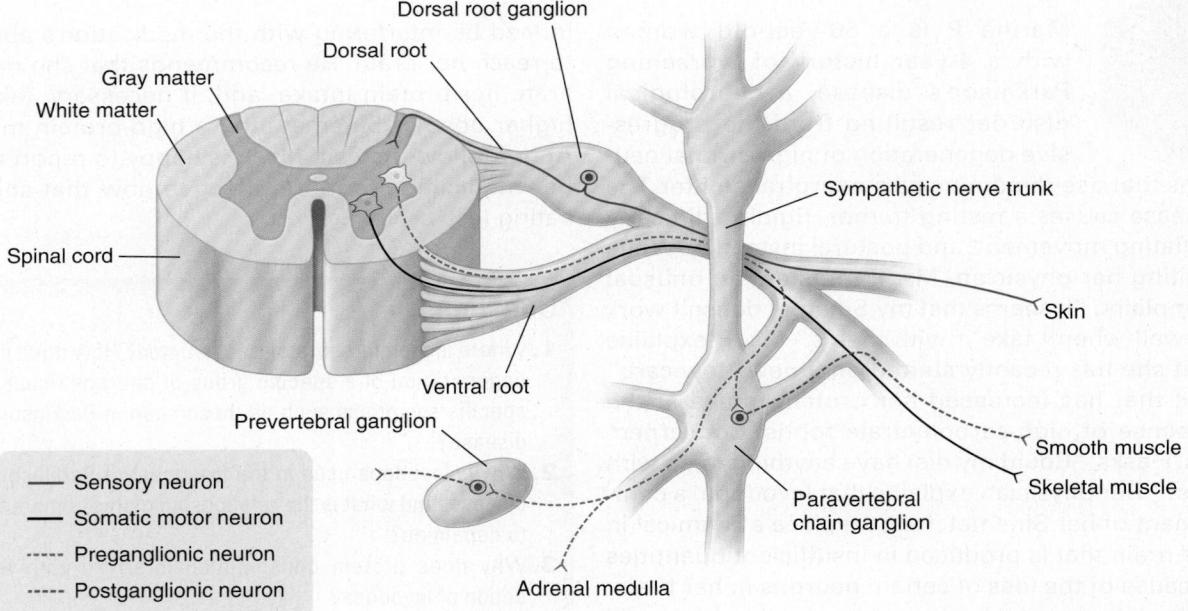

FIGURE 9-1. Organization of the peripheral nervous system. The peripheral nervous system contains sensory, somatic motor, and autonomic components. Sensory neurons (*solid blue line*) arise principally in the skin or joints, have cell bodies and nuclei in the dorsal root ganglia, and project onto neurons located in the dorsal horn of the spinal cord. Somatic motor neurons (*solid black line*) arise in the ventral horn of the spinal cord, exit through the ventral roots, and join fibers of sensory neurons to form spinal nerves, which then innervate skeletal muscle. The autonomic component of the peripheral nervous system consists of a two-nerve system; the two nerves are called *preganglionic* and *postganglionic* neurons, respectively. Sympathetic preganglionic neurons (*dashed gray line*) arise in the ventral horn of the thoracic and lumbar segments of the spinal cord and project onto postganglionic neurons in the paravertebral and prevertebral ganglia. Sympathetic postganglionic neurons (*dashed blue line*) innervate many organs, including smooth muscle. The adrenal medulla is also innervated by preganglionic neurons of the sympathetic nervous system (see Fig. 9-2). Parasympathetic preganglionic neurons (*not shown*) arise in nuclei in the brainstem and the sacral segments of the spinal cord and project onto postganglionic neurons in ganglia located near the innervated organs.

Anatomy of the Parasympathetic Nervous System

Nearly all of the parasympathetic ganglia lie in or near the organs they innervate. The preganglionic fibers of the parasympathetic nervous system arise in the brainstem or in sacral segments of the spinal cord; thus, the parasympathetic system is also called the **craniosacral system** (Fig. 9-2). In some cases, parasympathetic preganglionic neurons can travel almost 1 meter before synapsing with their postganglionic targets. Preganglionic nerve fibers of cranial nerve (CN) III, the **oculomotor nerve**, arise from a region of the midbrain termed the **Edinger-Westphal nucleus** and innervate the pupil, stimulating it to constrict. The medulla of the brain contains nuclei for parasympathetic nerve fibers in CNs VII, IX, and X. Parasympathetic fibers in the facial nerve (CN VII) stimulate salivary secretion by the submaxillary and sublingual glands as well as tear production by the lacrimal gland. Parasympathetic fibers in the ninth cranial nerve, the **glossopharyngeal nerve**, stimulate the parotid gland. The 10th cranial nerve, termed the **vagus nerve**, provides parasympathetic innervation to the major organs in the chest and abdomen, including the heart, tracheobronchial tree, kidneys, and GI system down to the proximal colon. Parasympathetic nerves originating in the sacral region of the spinal cord innervate the remainder of the colon, urinary bladder, and genitalia.

Many pharmacologic agents modulate parasympathetic nervous system activity. For example, **bethanechol** is a parasympathomimetic that promotes GI and urinary tract motility.

Antagonists of parasympathetic activity include **atropine**, a drug used locally to dilate the pupils or systematically to increase heart rate, and **ipratropium**, a drug used to dilate bronchioles. These agents and others are discussed in Chapter 10, Cholinergic Pharmacology.

Peripheral Motor and Sensory Systems

Fibers of the somatic nervous system innervate their target striated muscles directly (Fig. 9-1). The first-order neurons from the motor cortex send projections that cross in the lower medulla and descend through the spinal cord in the lateral corticospinal tract before synapsing on the second-order neurons in the **ventral horns** of the spinal cord. Projections from the second-order neurons exit through the **ventral roots** and join the **dorsal roots**, carrying sensory nerve fibers, to form the **spinal nerves**. Spinal nerves exit the vertebral column through the intervertebral foramina, after which they separate into peripheral nerves. Somatic components of the peripheral nerves innervate muscles directly. Muscles are innervated in a **myotomal distribution**. That is, neurons originating from a particular ventral root level of the spinal cord (e.g., C6) innervate specific muscles (e.g., flexor muscles of the forearm).

Sensory neurons have cell bodies in the **dorsal root ganglia**. The endings of sensory nerves lie in the skin and joints and enter the spinal cord through the **dorsal roots**. Neurons for vibration and position sense (proprioception) ascend through the ipsilateral **dorsal columns** in the spinal cord and synapse with secondary neurons in the contralateral

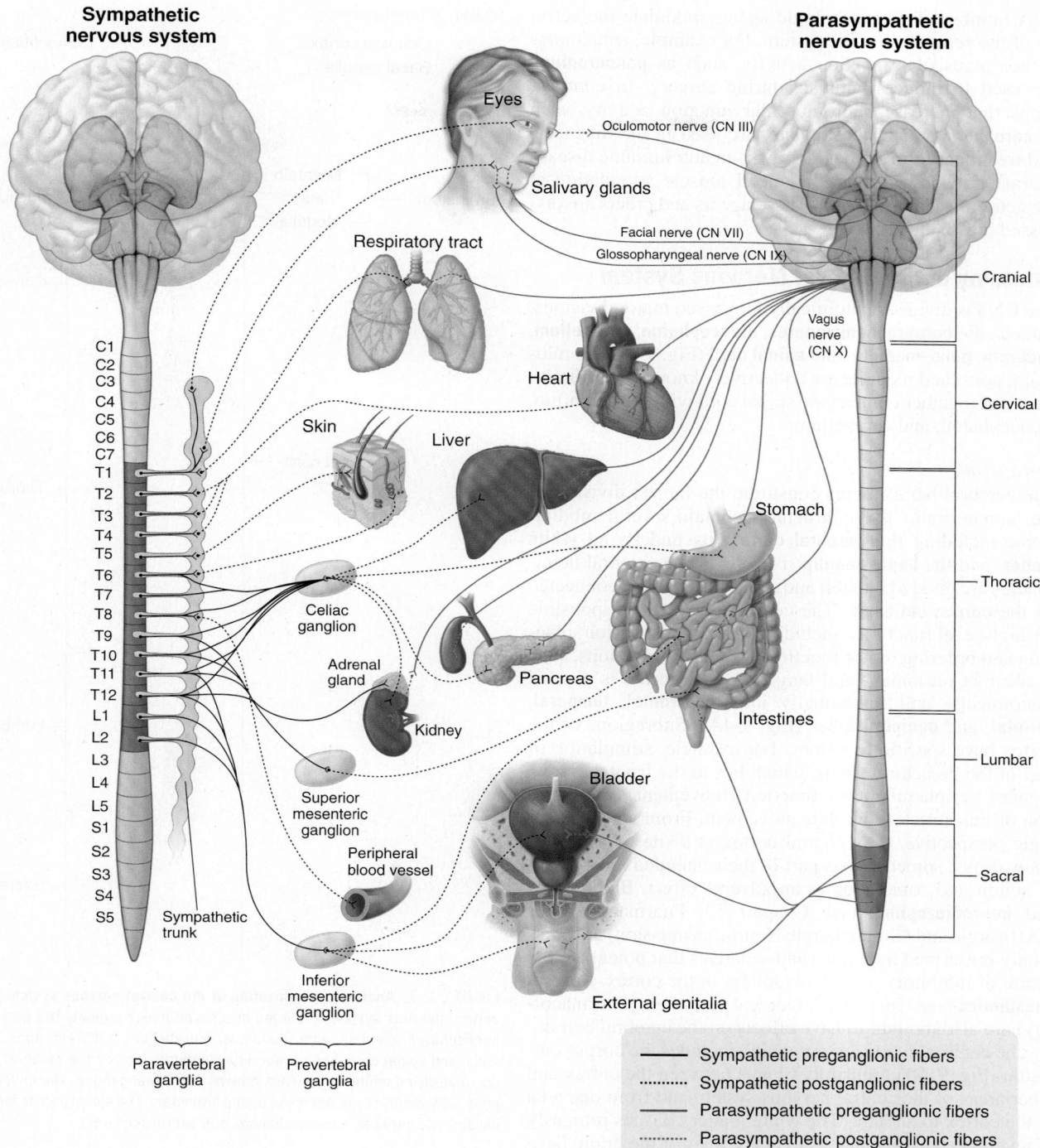

Sympathetic nervous system

Parasympathetic nervous system

Eyes
Oculomotor nerve (CN III)
Salivary glands
Facial nerve (CN VII)
Respiratory tract
Glossopharyngeal nerve (CN IX)

Vagus nerve (CN X)

Heart
Skin
Liver
Stomach

Celiac ganglion
Adrenal gland
Pancreas
Kidney
Intestines

Superior mesenteric ganglion
Peripheral blood vessel
Bladder

Sympathetic trunk
Inferior mesenteric ganglion
External genitalia

C1 C2 C3 C4 C5 C6 C7 T1 T2 T3 T4 T5 T6 T7 T8 T9 T10 T11 T12 L1 L2 L3 L4 L5 S1 S2 S3 S4 S5

Cranial
Cervical
Thoracic
Lumbar
Sacral

Paravertebral ganglia
Prevertebral ganglia

Sympathetic preganglionic fibers
Sympathetic postganglionic fibers
Parasympathetic preganglionic fibers
Parasympathetic postganglionic fibers

FIGURE 9-2. Patterns of sympathetic and parasympathetic innervation. Sympathetic preganglionic neurons arise in the thoracic and lumbar segments of the spinal cord. Sympathetic preganglionic neurons project onto postganglionic neurons in ganglia that lie close to the spinal cord, most notably the paravertebral ganglia, and in the prevertebral ganglia located near the aorta. Parasympathetic ganglia generally lie close to the organs they innervate. Thus, parasympathetic preganglionic neurons, which arise in nuclei in the brainstem and the sacral segments of the spinal cord, are generally long and project onto short postganglionic neurons.

lower medulla. Sensory neurons that carry sensations of pain and temperature synapse with secondary neurons in the **posterior horn** of the spinal cord and then cross within the spinal cord to ascend in the contralateral spinothalamic tract. Both the spinothalamic tract and the dorsal column tracts connect with third-order neurons in the thalamus, part of the

diencephalon (see below), before ultimately reaching the somatosensory cortex. Sensory information is encoded in a **dermatomal distribution**. That is, neurons originating from a particular dorsal root level of the spinal cord (e.g., C6) carry sensory information corresponding to a particular area of the skin (e.g., the lateral aspects of the forearm and hand).

A number of pharmacologic agents modulate the activity of the somatic nervous system. For example, antagonists of neuromuscular junction activity, such as **pancuronium**, are used to induce paralysis during surgery. In contrast, drugs that increase neuromuscular junction activity, such as **edrophonium** and **neostigmine**, are used in the diagnosis and treatment of myasthenia gravis, an autoimmune disease characterized by decreased skeletal muscle stimulation at the neuromuscular junction. These agents and others are discussed in Chapter 10.

Anatomy of the Central Nervous System

The CNS is divided anatomically into seven major divisions, namely, the **cerebral hemispheres**, **diencephalon**, **cerebellum**, **midbrain**, **pons**, **medulla**, and **spinal cord** (Fig. 9-3). The midbrain, pons, and medulla are collectively known as the **brainstem** and together connect the spinal cord with the cerebrum, diencephalon, and cerebellum.

Cerebrum

The cerebral hemispheres constitute the largest division of the human brain. These structures contain several subdivisions, including the **cerebral cortex**, its underlying **white matter**, and the **basal ganglia** (Fig. 9-4). The cerebral hemispheres are divided into left and right sides that are connected by the **corpus callosum**. The cerebral cortex is responsible for high-level functions, including sensory perception, planning and ordering motor functions, cognitive functions, such as abstract reasoning, and language. The cortex is divided anatomically and functionally into the **frontal**, **temporal**, **parietal**, and **occipital** lobes (Fig. 9-4A). Subregions of the cortex have specific functions. For example, stimulation of part of the precentral gyrus, which lies in the frontal cortex, induces peripheral motor function (movement), and ablation of this structure inhibits movement. From a pharmacologic perspective, the cerebral cortex is a site of action of many drugs, sometimes as part of their intended mechanism of action and sometimes as an adverse effect. **Barbiturates** and **benzodiazepines** (see Chapter 13, Pharmacology of GABAergic and Glutamatergic Neurotransmission) are commonly prescribed hypnotics and sedatives that potentiate the action of inhibitory neurotransmitters in the cortex. **General anesthetics** (see Chapter 17, General Anesthetic Pharmacology) are also thought to have effects on the cerebral cortex.

The cerebral white matter, which includes the corpus callosum (Fig. 9-4B), transmits signals between the cortex and other areas of the central nervous system and from one area of the cortex to another. The white matter consists primarily of myelinated axons that, as in other areas of the brain, have an associated vascular network of small arteries, veins, and capillaries. It is around these small vessels that inflammatory cells collect in diseases such as multiple sclerosis, and it is the small arterioles that are especially affected by systemic hypertension.

The basal ganglia consist of three deep nuclei of gray matter (Fig. 9-4C), including the **caudate** and **putamen**—together known as the **striatum**—and the **globus pallidus**. In a general sense, these nuclei help initiate and control cortical actions. These actions include not only intended movement but also behavior and certain rudimentary aspects of cognition. Regions of the basal ganglia responsible for movement ensure that intended actions are carried out and irrelevant movements are inhibited. As seen in the

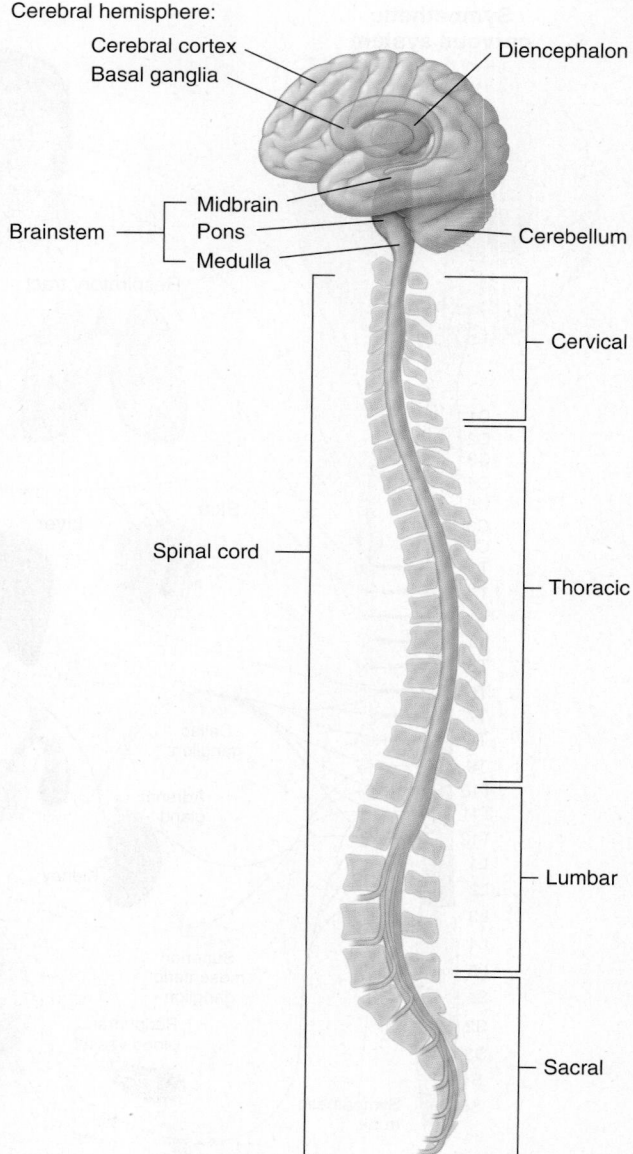

FIGURE 9-3. Anatomic organization of the central nervous system. The central nervous system is divided into seven major regions: the cerebral hemispheres, diencephalon (thalamus), cerebellum, midbrain, pons, medulla, and spinal cord. The cerebral hemispheres include the cerebral cortex, underlying white matter (*not shown*), and basal ganglia. The midbrain, pons, and medulla together make up the brainstem. The spinal cord is further divided into cervical, thoracic, lumbar, and sacral segments.

case of Ms. P, Parkinson's disease is caused by degeneration of a dopaminergic pathway that arises in the **substantia nigra** in the midbrain (see below) and terminates in the striatum (hence its name, the **nigrostriatal tract** or pathway). This degeneration prevents the basal ganglia from properly initiating motor activity—resulting in decreased intended movement and an unintended tremor—and causes the decreased ("flat") affect characteristic of Parkinson's disease. **Levodopa**, a component of Ms. P's Sinemet medication, acts on the striatum to ameliorate these clinical manifestations of the disease (see Chapter 14, Pharmacology of Dopaminergic Neurotransmission).

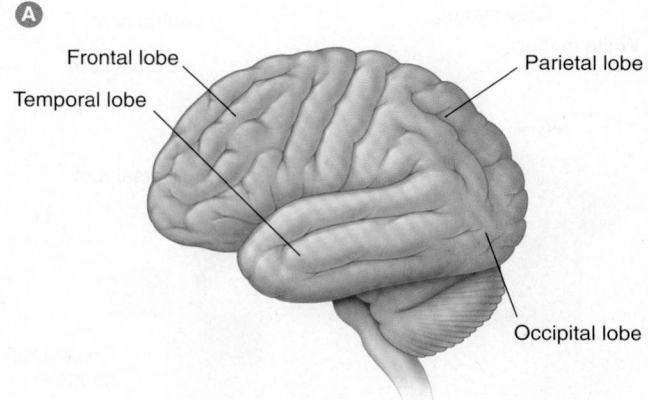

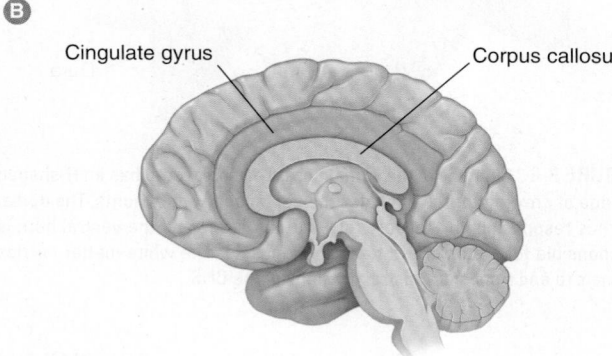

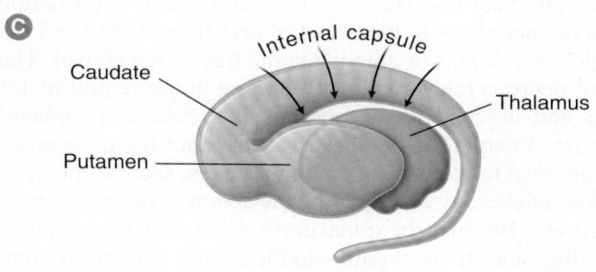

FIGURE 9-4. Anatomy of the cerebral hemispheres. A. In this lateral view, the cerebral hemispheres are divided into four lobes—frontal, parietal, occipital, and temporal—which are structurally and functionally distinct from each other. **B.** A sagittal view of the cerebral hemispheres shows the corpus callosum and cingulate gyrus. The corpus callosum connects the left and right hemispheres and coordinates their actions. The cingulate gyrus is part of the limbic system; it lies immediately superior to the corpus callosum. **C.** The basal ganglia include the caudate and putamen, which are together known as the *striatum*, and the globus pallidus (medial to the putamen, *not shown*). The thalamus lies medial to the basal ganglia. Arrows indicate the trajectory of neurons in the internal capsule, a bundle of white matter that carries motor commands from the cortex to the spinal cord.

A rim or "limbus" around the cortex has "older," more basic functions and is loosely termed the **limbic system**. This system consists of the **cingulate gyrus** (Fig. 9-4B), the **hippocampal formation** (including the **hippocampus** and surrounding structures), and the **amygdala**. These structures are responsible for emotion, social behavior, autonomic control, the perception of pain, and memory. For example, the memory loss associated with Alzheimer's disease is caused by degeneration of the hippocampal formation. Only a few drugs that specifically affect the limbic system are currently

available, although many agents affecting this region of the brain are in development. It should be noted that many drugs of abuse (see Chapter 19, Pharmacology of Drugs of Abuse) stimulate the brain reward pathway, which includes the **nucleus accumbens** and its projections to the limbic system.

Diencephalon

The diencephalon is divided into the **thalamus** and **hypothalamus**. The thalamus, which has several distinct nuclei, is located medially in the brain and inferior to the cerebral cortex. Some thalamic nuclei link sensory pathways from the periphery to the cerebral cortex. Other nuclei act as connections between the basal ganglia and the cortex. The thalamus is not a simple signal relay; rather, it filters and modulates sensory information, in part dictating which signals reach conscious awareness.

The hypothalamus lies ventral to the thalamus. It controls the autonomic nervous system, the pituitary gland, and essential behaviors such as hunger and thermoregulation. Descending pathways from the medial hypothalamus regulate autonomic preganglionic neurons in the medulla and spinal cord. It is generally believed that the antihypertensive effect of **clonidine** is mediated by its action at receptors on brainstem neurons controlled by the hypothalamus (see Chapter 11). Other neurons originating in the medial hypothalamus secrete hormones either directly into the systemic circulation (e.g., **vasopressin** from axon terminals in the posterior pituitary gland) or into a portal system that, in turn, controls hormone secretion by the anterior pituitary gland (see Chapter 27, Pharmacology of the Hypothalamus and Pituitary Gland). The hypothalamus also initiates complex behaviors in response to hunger, extremes in temperature, thirst, and time of day.

Cerebellum

The cerebellum lies inferior to the posterior end of the cerebrum and dorsal to the brainstem. It has three functionally distinct regions: the central **cerebellar vermis**, the lateral **cerebellar hemispheres**, and the small **flocculonodular lobe** (Fig. 9-5). The cerebellum has a relatively well-defined pattern of neural connections, receiving inputs from a wide

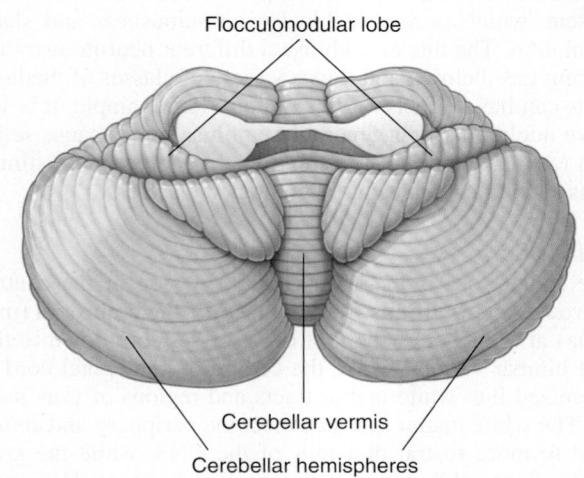

FIGURE 9-5. Anatomy of the cerebellum. The cerebellum is divided into the cerebellar hemispheres (laterally), the vermis (medially), and the small flocculonodular node. The area immediately above the flocculonodular lobe in this drawing is a cross section of the cerebellar peduncles.

variety of sources and sending output primarily to the motor areas of the cerebral cortex via the thalamus. The cerebellum coordinates voluntary movement in space and time, maintains balance, controls eye movement, and has roles in motor learning (for example, hand–eye coordination) and certain cognitive functions such as the timing of repetitive events and language. Few drugs are designed primarily to affect the cerebellum. However, several agents, notably alcohol and certain antiepileptic drugs, are toxic to the cerebellum. These agents especially affect the vermis, which controls balance.

Brainstem

The midbrain, pons, and medulla are collectively known as the **brainstem**. The brainstem connects the spinal cord to the thalamus and cerebral cortex. It is arranged with the midbrain superior, the medulla inferior, and the pons bridging the midbrain and medulla (Fig. 9-3). White matter pathways interconnecting the spinal cord, cerebellum, thalamus, basal ganglia, and cerebral cortex course through this small region of the brain. In addition, the brainstem gives rise to most of the **cranial nerves**. Some of these nerves are conduits for sensation from the head and face, including hearing, balance, and taste. The cranial nerves also control the motor output to the skeletal muscles of mastication, facial expression, swallowing, and eye movement. The brainstem also regulates parasympathetic output to the salivary glands and the iris.

The medulla contains several control centers that are essential for life, including centers that direct the output of the autonomic nuclei, pacemakers that regulate heart rate and breathing, and centers that control reflex actions such as coughing and vomiting. Several relay structures in the pons also play a role (in conjunction with the midbrain) in regulating vital functions such as respiration. The base of the pons contains white matter tracts connecting the cerebral cortex and the cerebellum. Neurons in the **periaqueductal gray**, especially in the midbrain, send descending projections to the spinal cord that modulate pain perception (see Chapter 18, Pharmacology of Analgesia).

Clusters of diffusely projecting neurons lie throughout the brainstem, hypothalamus, and the surrounding base of the brain. These nuclei, which include the **locus ceruleus**, **raphe nucleus**, and several others, comprise the **reticular activating system**, which is responsible for consciousness and sleep regulation. The nuclei each use a different neurotransmitter system (see below), and thus a variety of classes of medications can have effects on this system. For example, it is via these nuclei that first-generation antihistamines cause sedation (see Chapter 44, Histamine Pharmacology) and stimulants such as cocaine cause heightened alertness.

Spinal Cord

The spinal cord is the most caudal division of the central nervous system. It runs from the base of the brainstem (medulla) at the level of the first cervical vertebra down to the first lumbar vertebra. Like the cerebrum, the spinal cord is organized into white matter tracts and regions of gray matter. The white matter tracts connect the periphery and spinal cord to more rostral divisions of the CNS, while the gray matter forms the nuclear columns that lie in an H-shaped pattern in the center of the spinal cord (Fig. 9-6).

Neurons in the spinal cord can be defined by their spatial location relative to the gray matter "H." These neurons include sensory neurons located in the dorsal horns of the "H,"

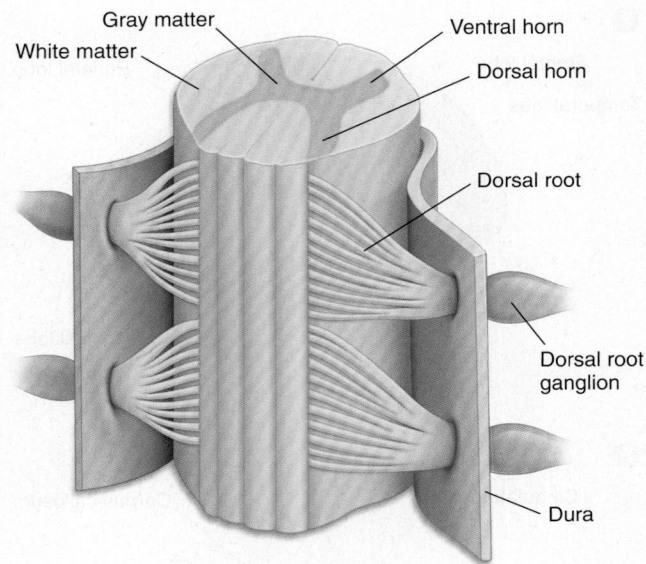

FIGURE 9-6. Anatomy of the spinal cord. The spinal cord has an H-shaped wedge of gray matter that includes the dorsal and ventral horns. The dorsal horn is responsible for sensory relays to the brain, and the ventral horn is responsible for motor relays to skeletal muscle. The white matter carries signals to and from more rostral divisions of the CNS.

motor neurons located in the ventral horns of the "H," and spinal interneurons. The sensory neurons relay information from the periphery to more rostral divisions of the CNS via the dorsal columns or spinothalamic tracts (see above). The motor neurons relay commands arising in the central motor areas and descend in the corticospinal tract to peripheral muscles. Interneurons connect sensory and motor neurons and are responsible for mediating reflexes, such as the deep tendon reflexes, by coordinating the action of opposing muscle groups. Because the spinal cord carries sensory signals—including sensations of pain—to the central nervous system, it is an important target for analgesic drugs such as opioids (see Chapter 18).

Cellular Organization of the Nervous System

Cellular organization in the autonomic and peripheral nervous system involves a limited number of neurons that make few connections. For example, somatic and sensory information is carried directly between the spinal cord and the periphery. Autonomic nerves are slightly more complex, in that the signal must undergo synaptic transmission between a preganglionic and a postganglionic neuron. In both cases, however, few ancillary neuronal connections are made, and little or no modification of information occurs.

In contrast, cellular organization in the central nervous system is far more complex. Information is not simply relayed from one area to another; instead, central neurons receive signals from numerous sources and distribute their own axons widely. Some neurons synapse with hundreds of thousands of other neurons. Moreover, not every synaptic connection is excitatory (i.e., designed to depolarize the postsynaptic neuron). Some connections are inhibitory (i.e., designed to hyperpolarize the postsynaptic neuron). Other neurons projecting onto a target neuron can modulate the relative excitability of the cell, affecting the response of

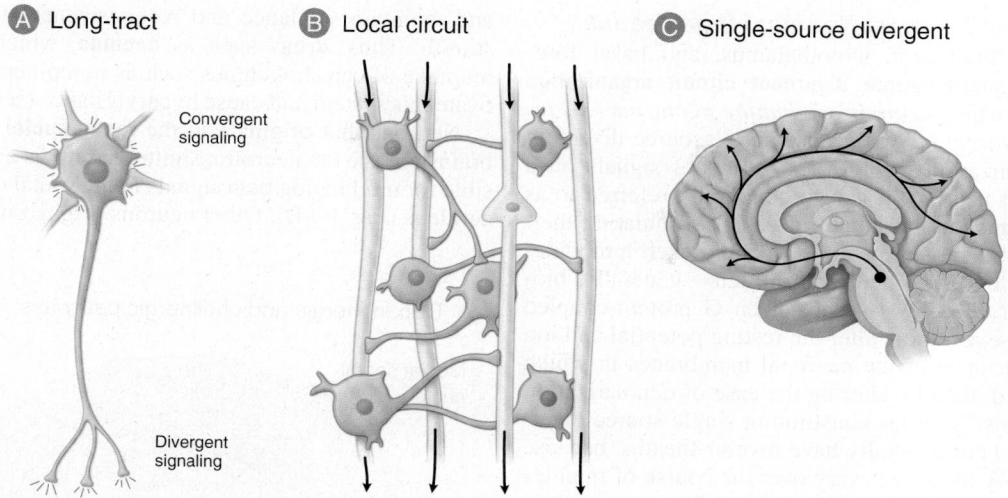

FIGURE 9-7. Cellular organization of the central nervous system. The CNS has three main organizational motifs. **A.** Long-tract neurons act as relays between the periphery and higher sites in the CNS. Long-tract neurons receive signals from many different neurons (convergent signaling) and synapse with many downstream neurons (divergent signaling). **B.** Local circuit neurons show a complicated structural motif, arranged in layers, which includes both excitatory and inhibitory neurons. These circuits are used to process information. **C.** Single-source divergent neurons typically originate in a nucleus in the brainstem and have axonal terminals that innervate thousands of neurons, usually in the cerebral cortex.

the postsynaptic neuron to other signals. The complexity generated by this variability is needed to carry out the many intricate processes performed by the brain.

Although the CNS possesses immense complexity at the level of neuronal connectivity, three major motifs are used to organize neurons into functional units in the nervous system: the **long-tract neuronal systems**, **local circuits**, and **single-source divergent systems** (Fig. 9-7). The peripheral nervous system is organized exclusively as a long-tract system, while the central nervous system uses all three motifs.

Long-Tract Neuronal Organization

Long-tract neuronal organization involves neural pathways that connect distant areas of the nervous system to one another (Fig. 9-7A). It is the organization used by the peripheral nervous system, and it is important for the transmission of signals from one region to another within the central nervous system.

In the peripheral nervous system, signals are transmitted with little modification. Sensory neurons respond to stimuli such as touch, temperature, pressure, vibration, and noxious chemicals and, if the initial membrane depolarization is strong enough, transmit an action potential directly to the spinal cord. There, sensory neurons synapse directly with somatic motor neurons, forming reflex arcs, and with ascending spinal neurons that transmit the information to higher levels. Motor neurons carry information directly from the spinal cord out through the ventral roots and project directly on the motor end plates of the muscles they innervate. The long axon tracts of the peripheral sensory and motor neurons are bundled together and travel as peripheral nerves.

As described above, preganglionic neurons of the autonomic nervous system form synaptic connections with postganglionic neurons at ganglia that are located prevertebrally, paravertebrally, or near the innervated visceral organs. One preganglionic neuron typically makes synaptic connections with up to several thousand postganglionic neurons,

an organization that is termed **divergent signaling**. Although divergent signaling does result in some processing and modification of information, the autonomic nervous system does not generally modify neural signals appreciably.

In contrast to neurons in the peripheral pathways, neurons in long-tract systems of the central nervous system not only relay but also integrate and modify signals. CNS long-tract neurons display divergent signaling like autonomic neurons but also receive synaptic connections from many upstream neurons (**convergent signaling**). The CNS uses both excitatory and inhibitory neurotransmitters to localize a signal, a strategy that is known as **center-surround signaling**. For example, sensory perception in the CNS can precisely localize a signal by activating cortical neurons that map to one area of the body and inhibiting neurons that map to surrounding areas of the body.

Local Circuit Neuronal Organization

Local circuit neurons *maintain connectivity primarily within the immediate area.* These neurons are generally responsible for *modulating* signal transmission (Fig. 9-7B). For example, neurons in the cerebral cortex are organized in layers, usually six in number. While information flows into one layer and out of a different layer through long-tract connections, links between the layers process the signals and interpret the inputs. Local synaptic connections can be both excitatory and inhibitory, ensuring that only certain patterns of inputs are passed along. For example, information originating in the lateral geniculate neurons enters the primary visual cortex through a long-tract connection called the **optic tract**. In an area of the cortex designed to perceive lines, the outgoing neurons will be excited only if the incoming neurons fire in a particular pattern, in this case designating a line in a particular orientation. The outgoing signal might then serve as the input to another area of the brain that recognizes shapes. If this area receives an appropriate pattern of lines from the appropriate sources, it might recognize a particular object, such as the grid on a tic-tac-toe board.

Single-Source Divergent Neuronal Organization

Nuclei in the brainstem, hypothalamus, and basal forebrain follow **single-source divergent circuit organization** (Fig. 9-7C), in which *neurons originating in one nucleus innervate many target cells*. Because single-source divergent neuronal organization involves the action of signals on a wide variety of neurons, it is also commonly referred to as a **diffuse system of organization**. Instead of stimulating their targets directly, divergent neurons typically exert a modulatory influence by using neurotransmitters—generally, biogenic amines (see below)—that act on G protein-coupled receptors. These receptors alter the resting potential and ion channel conductance of the neuronal membranes in which they are located, thereby altering the ease of depolarization of these neurons. Neurons constituting single-source divergent circuits do not generally have myelin sheaths, because their modulatory influences vary over the course of minutes or hours rather than fractions of a second. In addition, their axons are highly branched, enabling synaptic connections with a large number of target neurons.

The principal single-source divergent neuronal systems are summarized in Table 9-1. They include pigmented dopaminergic neurons that originate in the **substantia nigra**, widely innervate the striatum, and are responsible for regulating the activity of neurons that control intended actions (Fig. 9-8A). Specifically, neurons in the nigrostriatal tract excite downstream pathways that initiate movement and inhibit pathways that suppress movement. The nigrostriatal tract degenerates in Parkinson's disease, which is why Ms. P displayed a paucity of movement. Other dopaminergic neurons medial to the substantia nigra project to the prefrontal cortex and influence thought processes.

Another example of a single-source divergent circuit involves the noradrenergic nucleus in the pons termed the **locus ceruleus** (Fig. 9-8B). Neurons originating in this nucleus widely innervate the cerebral cortex and cerebellum and maintain vigilance and responsiveness to unexpected stimuli. Thus, drugs such as **cocaine**, which inhibits the reuptake of catecholamines such as norepinephrine, can activate this system and cause hypervigilance (see Chapter 19).

Neurons that originate in the **raphe nuclei** in the caudal brainstem use the neurotransmitter **serotonin** and are responsible for modulating pain signals in the spinal cord and locus ceruleus (Fig. 9-8B). Other neurons originating in the raphe

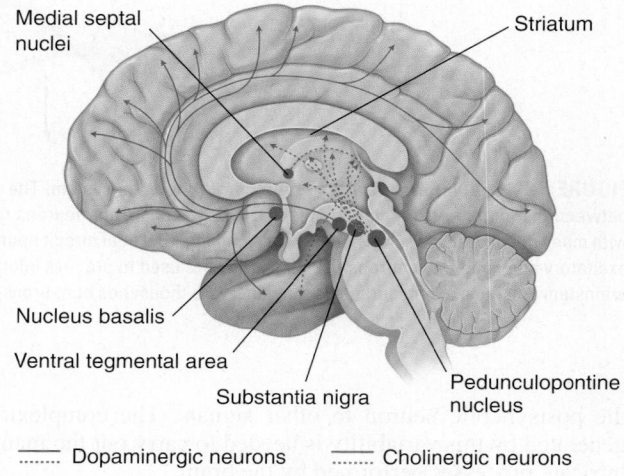

Ⓐ Dopaminergic and cholinergic pathways

Medial septal nuclei — Striatum

Nucleus basalis

Ventral tegmental area

Substantia nigra — Pedunculopontine nucleus

······ Dopaminergic neurons ······ Cholinergic neurons

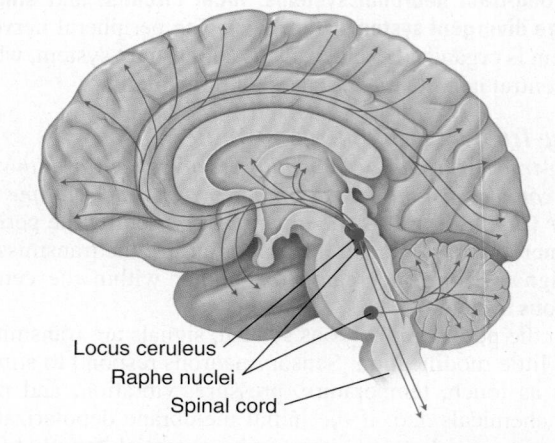

Ⓑ Noradrenergic and serotonergic pathways

Locus ceruleus
Raphe nuclei
Spinal cord

—— Noradrenergic neurons —— Serotonergic neurons

FIGURE 9-8. Diffuse neuronal systems. A. Dopaminergic neurons (*blue*) arise in the substantia nigra and the ventral tegmental area and project to the striatum and the cerebral cortex, respectively. These neurons are associated with the initiation of movement and the brain reward pathways. Cholinergic neurons (*red*) arise in the nucleus basalis, pedunculopontine nucleus, and medial septal nuclei. These neurons, which project widely throughout the brain, are responsible for maintaining sleep–wake cycles and regulating sensory transmission. **B.** Noradrenergic neurons (*blue*) arise in the locus ceruleus and innervate the entire brain. These neurons are responsible for maintaining alertness. Serotonergic neurons (*red*) arise in the raphe nuclei and project to the diencephalon, to the basal ganglia, and, via the basal forebrain, to the cerebral hemispheres as well as the cerebellum and spinal cord. Serotonergic neurons are believed to have a role in modulating affect and pain.

TABLE 9-1 Single-Source Divergent Neuronal Systems

ORIGIN	NEUROTRANSMITTER	FUNCTIONS
Substantia nigra (midbrain)	Dopamine	Enable intended movement; executive function; emotional regulation; memory
Locus ceruleus (pons)	Norepinephrine	Vigilance; responsiveness to unexpected stimuli
Raphe nuclei (medulla, pons, and midbrain)	Serotonin	Perception of pain; responsiveness of cortical neurons; mood (?)
Basal nucleus of Meynert	Acetylcholine	Alertness
Pedunculopontine nucleus	Acetylcholine	Sleep–wake cycles
Tuberomamillary nucleus (hypothalamus)	Histamine	Forebrain arousal

nuclei widely innervate the forebrain, modulating the responsiveness of neurons in the cortex. Serotonergic neurons regulate wakefulness and sleep, and dysfunction of the serotonergic system is hypothesized to be a cause of depression. Because antidepressants block the reuptake of serotonin, this class of drugs may activate the serotonergic raphe pathway (see Chapter 15, Pharmacology of Serotonergic and Central Adrenergic Neurotransmission).

Three other important nuclei that widely innervate the cortex are the **basal nucleus of Meynert**, the **pedunculopontine nucleus**, and the **tuberomamillary nucleus**. The basal nucleus and the pedunculopontine nucleus use **acetylcholine** as a neurotransmitter (Fig. 9-8A). The former nucleus projects to the cortex and regulates alertness, while the latter nucleus controls sleep–wake cycles and arousal. Cells in the basal forebrain that receive inputs from the pedunculopontine nucleus degenerate in several diseases, including Alzheimer's disease. The tuberomamillary nucleus uses the neurotransmitter **histamine** (see below) and may help maintain arousal through its actions on the forebrain. The somnolence induced by first-generation antihistamines—histamine H_1 receptor

antagonists used to treat allergies (see Chapter 44)—may be caused by inhibition of transmission involving tuberomamillary nucleus neurons.

NEUROPHYSIOLOGY

Neurotransmitters

The peripheral nervous system uses only two neurotransmitters: acetylcholine and norepinephrine (Fig. 9-9). In contrast, the CNS uses not only a wide variety of small molecule neurotransmitters, including acetylcholine and norepinephrine (Table 9-2), but also many **neuroactive peptides**. These peptides may be transmitted concurrently with the small molecule neurotransmitters, and they generally have a neuromodulatory role.

The small molecule neurotransmitters can be organized into several broad categories based on both their structure and function (Fig. 9-10). The first category, the **amino acid** neurotransmitters, includes **glutamate**, **aspartate**, **GABA**, and **glycine**. The **biogenic amine** neurotransmitters, which are

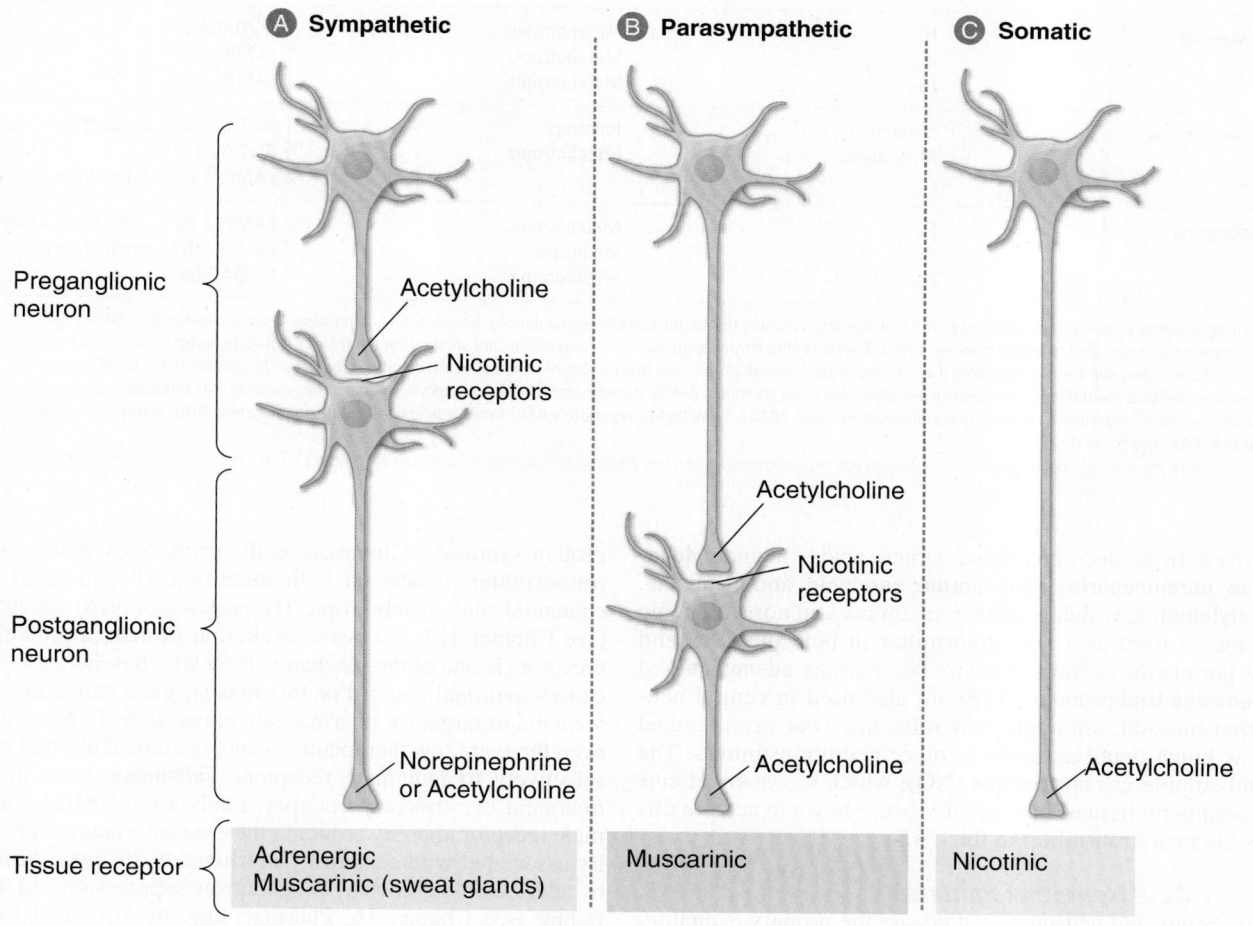

FIGURE 9-9. Neurotransmitters in the peripheral nervous system (A-C). Only two neurotransmitters are required to mediate neurotransmission in the peripheral nervous system. Acetylcholine is released by sympathetic and parasympathetic preganglionic neurons, parasympathetic postganglionic neurons, somatic motor neurons, and sympathetic postganglionic neurons that innervate sweat glands. All other sympathetic postganglionic neurons release norepinephrine. Acetylcholine stimulates nicotinic acetylcholine receptors on sympathetic and parasympathetic postganglionic neurons and at the neuromuscular junction. Acetylcholine stimulates muscarinic acetylcholine receptors on sweat glands and on tissues innervated by parasympathetic postganglionic neurons. Norepinephrine stimulates α- and β-adrenergic receptors on tissues (except for sweat glands) innervated by sympathetic postganglionic neurons.

TABLE 9-2 Small Molecule Neurotransmitters in the Central Nervous System

NEUROTRANSMITTER	RECEPTOR SUBTYPE	RECEPTOR MOTIF	MECHANISM
GABA	$GABA_A$	Ionotropic	$\downarrow$ cAMP
	$GABA_B$	Metabotropic	$\uparrow$ Cl^- conductance
			$\uparrow$ K^+, Cl^- conductance
Glycine	α, β Subunits	Ionotropic	$\uparrow$ Cl^- conductance
Glutamate, Aspartate	AMPA	Ionotropic	$\uparrow$ Na^+, K^+ conductance
	Kainate	Ionotropic	$\uparrow$ Na^+, K^+ conductance
	NMDA	Ionotropic	$\uparrow$ Na^+, K^+, Ca^{2+} conductance
	mGlu (1–7)	Metabotropic	$\downarrow$ cAMP
			$\uparrow$ IP_3/DAG/Ca^{2+}
Dopamine	D1, D5	Metabotropic	$\uparrow$ cAMP
	D2, D3, D4	Metabotropic	$\downarrow$ cAMP; $\uparrow$ K^+, $\downarrow$ Ca^{2+} conductance
Norepinephrine	α_1	Metabotropic	$\uparrow$ IP_3/DAG/Ca^{2+}
	α_2	Metabotropic	$\downarrow$ cAMP; $\uparrow$ K^+, $\downarrow$ Ca^{2+} conductance
	β_1, β_2, β_3	Metabotropic	$\uparrow$ cAMP
Serotonin	$5-HT_1$	Metabotropic	$\downarrow$ cAMP; $\uparrow$ K^+ conductance
	$5-HT_2$	Metabotropic	$\uparrow$ IP_3/DAG/Ca^{2+}
	$5-HT_3$	Ionotropic	$\uparrow$ Na^+, K^+ conductance
	$5-HT_{4-7}$	Metabotropic	$\uparrow$ cAMP
Histamine	H_1	Metabotropic	$\uparrow$ IP_3/DAG/Ca^{2+}
	H_2	Metabotropic	$\uparrow$ cAMP
	H_3	Metabotropic	$\downarrow$ cAMP
Acetylcholine	Nicotinic	Ionotropic	$\uparrow$ Na^+, K^+, Ca^{2+} conductance
	Muscarinic	Metabotropic	$\uparrow$ IP_3/DAG/Ca^{2+}
			$\downarrow$ cAMP; $\uparrow$ K^+ conductance
Adenosine	P_1	Metabotropic	$\downarrow$ cAMP; $\downarrow$ Ca^{2+}, $\uparrow$ K^+ conductance
	P_{2X}	Ionotropic	$\uparrow$ Ca^{2+}, K^+, Na^+ conductance
	P_{2Y}	Metabotropic	$\uparrow$ IP_3/DAG/Ca^{2+}

Neurotransmitters can be organized into several categories, including the amino acids, biogenic amines, acetylcholine, adenosine, and nitric oxide (NO). Each neurotransmitter can bind to one or more receptors. Except for the NO receptor, which is intracellular (*not shown*), the other small molecule receptors are all at the cell surface. These cell surface receptors may be ionotropic or metabotropic. The mechanism of action of each receptor is indicated. In addition to the small molecule neurotransmitters, more than 50 neuroactive peptides have been identified. AMPA, kainate, and NMDA receptors are named after agonists that selectively activate them. AMPA, α-amino-3-hydroxy-5-methyl-4-isoxazolepropionic acid; NMDA, N-methyl-D-aspartate; cAMP, cyclic adenosine-3′,5′-monophosphate; DAG, diacylglycerol; IP_3, inositol-1,4,5-trisphosphate.

derived from decarboxylated amino acids, include **dopamine, norepinephrine, epinephrine, serotonin,** and **histamine.** **Acetylcholine,** which is neither an amino acid nor a biogenic amine, is used as a neurotransmitter in both the CNS and the peripheral nervous system. The purines **adenosine** and **adenosine triphosphate** (ATP) are also used in central neurotransmission, although their roles have not been studied in as much detail as those of other neurotransmitters. The lipid-soluble gas **nitric oxide** (NO), which has many effects in peripheral tissues, has recently been shown to act as a diffusible neurotransmitter in the CNS.

Amino Acid Neurotransmitters

The amino acid neurotransmitters are the primary excitatory and inhibitory neurotransmitters in the CNS. Two types of amino acid neurotransmitters are used: the acidic amino acids glutamate and aspartate, which are primarily excitatory, and the neutral amino acids GABA and glycine, which are primarily inhibitory. Glutamate, aspartate, and glycine are all alpha-amino acids that are also building blocks for

protein synthesis. Glutamate is the primary excitatory neurotransmitter; it acts on both ionotropic (ligand-gated ion channels) and metabotropic (G protein-coupled) receptors (see Chapter 13). Excessive excitation of certain glutamate receptors is one of the mechanisms by which ischemic injury causes neuronal death. For this reason, glutamate receptors are a major target for pharmaceutical research. To date, however, there are few therapeutic agents in clinical use that bind selectively to glutamate receptors. **Felbamate,** used in the treatment of refractory epilepsy, inhibits the NMDA glutamate receptor, thereby reducing the excessive neuronal activity associated with seizures. Unfortunately, its use is limited by adverse effects such as bone marrow suppression and liver failure (see Chapter 16, Pharmacology of Abnormal Electrical Neurotransmission in the Central Nervous System). GABA, which is also discussed in Chapter 13, is the primary inhibitory neurotransmitter in the CNS. Several classes of therapeutic agents, most notably the barbiturates and benzodiazepines, bind to GABA receptors and, by allosteric mechanisms, potentiate the effect of endogenous GABA.

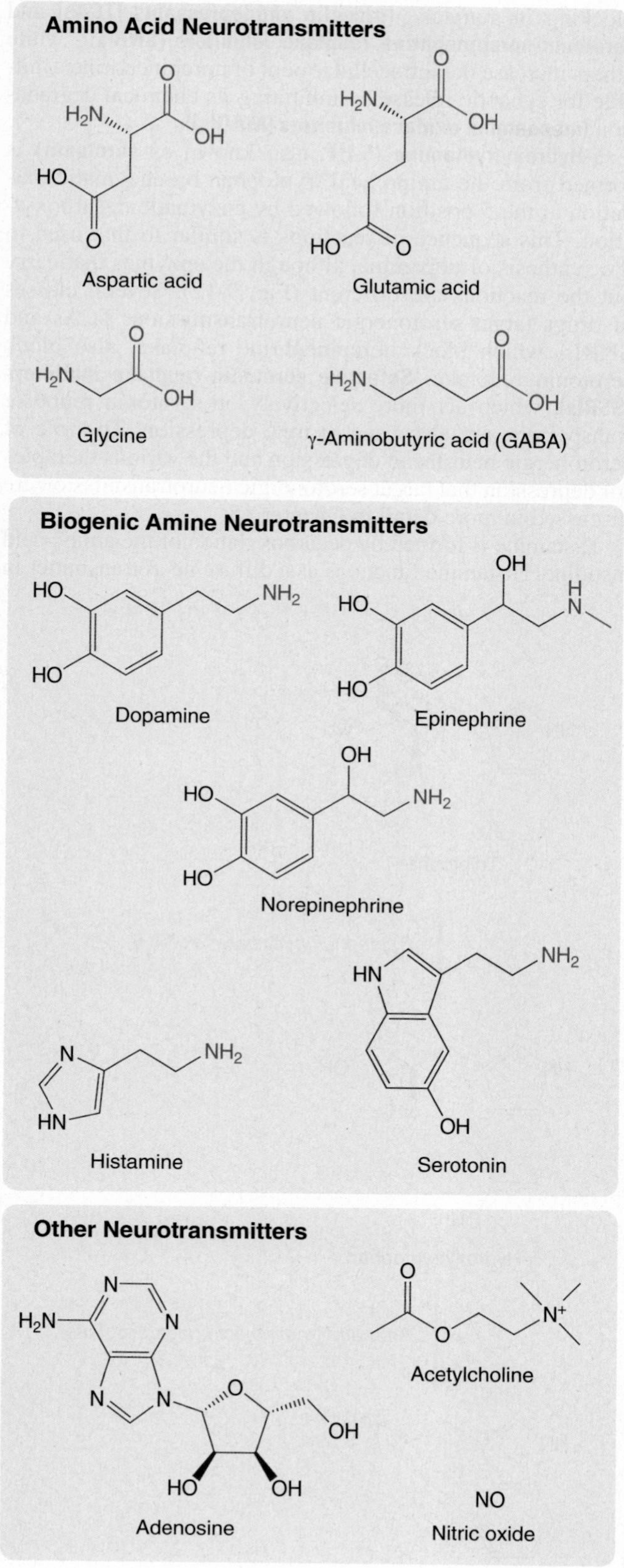

Amino Acid Neurotransmitters

Aspartic acid

Glutamic acid

Glycine

γ-Aminobutyric acid (GABA)

Biogenic Amine Neurotransmitters

Dopamine

Epinephrine

Norepinephrine

Histamine

Serotonin

Other Neurotransmitters

Adenosine

Acetylcholine

NO
Nitric oxide

FIGURE 9-10. Structures of the small molecule neurotransmitters. The principal small molecule neurotransmitters can be divided into two broad categories. Amino acids are the primary excitatory (glutamate and aspartate) and inhibitory (glycine and γ-aminobutyric acid) neurotransmitters in the CNS. Their amino and carboxylic acid groups are shown in blue. Biogenic amines are the primary modulatory neurotransmitters in the CNS. The amine moiety is shown in blue. Dopamine, norepinephrine, and epinephrine share a common catechol group; histamine has an imidazole group; and serotonin has an indole group. Acetylcholine (a neurotransmitter in diffuse modulatory systems in the CNS), adenosine, and nitric oxide (NO) do not fall into either structural category. The bond order is 2.5 for the nitrogen–oxygen bond in NO, intermediate in strength between a double bond and a triple bond.

Biogenic Amines

The biogenic amines (along with acetylcholine) are used by the diffuse neuronal systems to modulate complex central nervous system functions such as alertness and consciousness. In the peripheral nervous system, norepinephrine is released by sympathetic postganglionic neurons to effect the sympathetic response. The adrenal medulla is a neuroendocrine tissue that releases the biogenic amine epinephrine into the circulation in response to stress.

The biogenic amines are all synthesized from amino acid precursors. Based on these precursors, the biogenic amines can be divided into three categories. The catecholamines (dopamine, norepinephrine, and epinephrine) are derivatives of tyrosine. The indoleamine serotonin is synthesized from tryptophan. **Histamine** is formed from histidine. These three categories are described briefly below.

The catecholamines are all derived from tyrosine in a series of biochemical reactions (Fig. 9-11). First, tyrosine is oxidized to **L-dihydroxyphenylalanine (L-DOPA)**. L-DOPA is then decarboxylated to dopamine. In the case of Ms. P, L-DOPA (levodopa) is one of the components of the medication used to compensate for the loss of dopaminergic neurons in the substantia nigra. (Dopamine is not an effective therapeutic for Parkinson's disease because it does not cross the blood–brain barrier; see below.) Central dopaminergic receptors have been the target of a wide variety of therapeutics. For example, both dopamine precursors and direct dopamine receptor agonists are used in the treatment of Parkinson's disease, as discussed in Chapter 14. Dopamine receptor antagonists have been used with success in treating the psychotic symptoms of schizophrenia; this topic is also discussed in Chapter 14. Certain drugs of abuse, such as cocaine and the amphetamines, can activate brain reward pathways that depend on dopaminergic neurotransmission, as discussed in Chapter 19.

Dopamine is synthesized from tyrosine and L-DOPA in the cytoplasm but is then transported into synaptic vesicles. In dopaminergic neurons, the dopamine contained in synaptic vesicles is released as the neurotransmitter. In adrenergic and noradrenergic neurons, dopamine is converted to norepinephrine within the synaptic vesicles by the enzyme **dopamine-β-hydroxylase**. In a small number of neurons and in the adrenal medulla, norepinephrine is then transported back into the cytoplasm, where it is methylated to form epinephrine. Chapter 11 discusses the pharmacology of drugs that target peripheral adrenergic receptors, including both agonists, such as bronchodilators and vasopressors, and antagonists, such as antihypertensives. Several classes of therapeutic agents act on central adrenergic receptors. **Clonidine** is a partial agonist that acts on presynaptic α_2-receptors. Some **antidepressants** increase the synaptic concentration of norepinephrine by

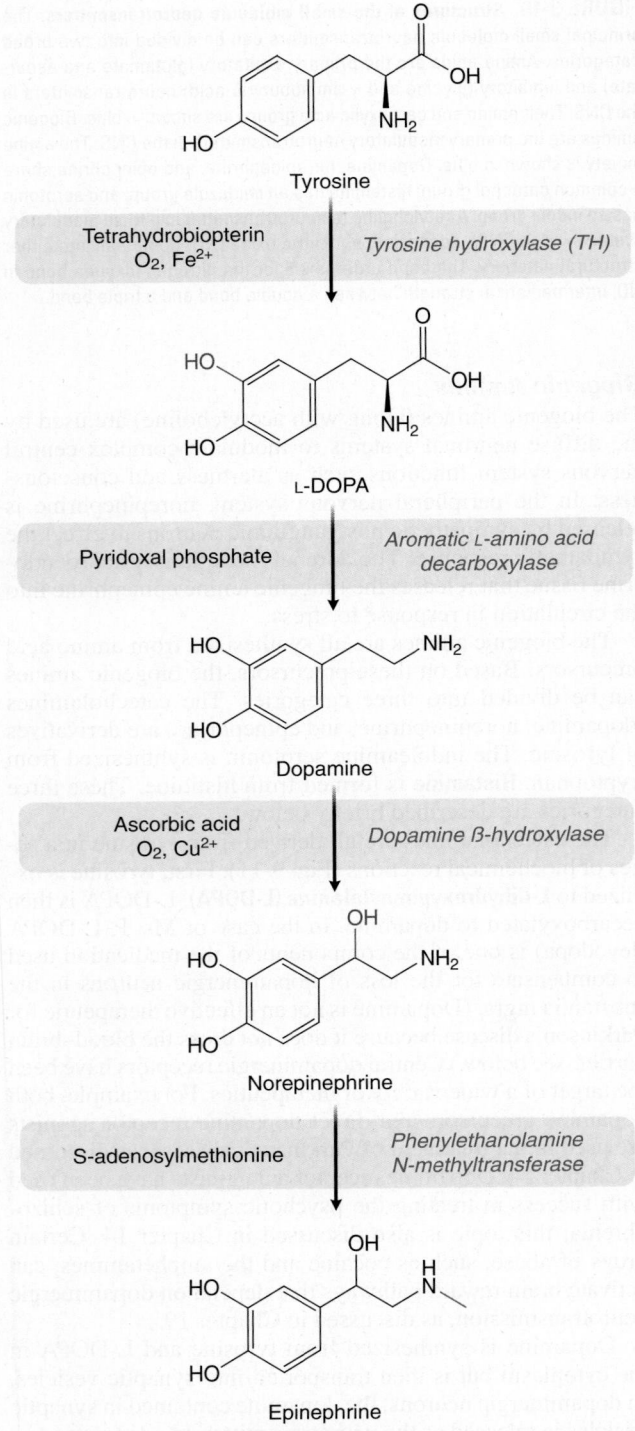

FIGURE 9-11. Synthesis of catecholamines. Catecholamines are all synthesized from tyrosine. Sequential enzymatic reactions result in hydroxylation of tyrosine to form L-DOPA, decarboxylation of L-DOPA to form dopamine, hydroxylation of dopamine to form norepinephrine, and methylation of norepinephrine to form epinephrine. Depending on the enzymes (*shown in blue lettering*) expressed in a particular type of presynaptic neuron, the reaction sequence may stop at any of the last three steps, so that dopamine, norepinephrine, or epinephrine can be the final product that is synthesized and used as a neurotransmitter.

blocking its reuptake (**tricyclic antidepressants [TCAs]** and **serotonin-norepinephrine reuptake inhibitors [SNRIs]**), while others increase the intracellular pool of norepinephrine available for synaptic release by inhibiting its chemical degradation (**monoamine oxidase inhibitors [MAOIs]**).

5-Hydroxytryptamine (**5-HT**, also known as **serotonin**) is formed from the amino acid tryptophan by enzymatic oxidation at the 5 position followed by enzymatic decarboxylation. This sequence of reactions is similar to that used in the synthesis of dopamine, although the enzymes that carry out the reactions are different (Fig. 9-12). Several classes of drugs target serotonergic neurotransmission. TCAs and SNRIs, which block norepinephrine reuptake, also block serotonin reuptake. **Selective serotonin reuptake inhibitors (SSRIs)**, which act more selectively on serotonin reuptake transporters, are also used to treat depression. The role of serotonergic neurons in depression and the various therapies for depression that target serotonergic neurotransmission are discussed in more detail in Chapter 15.

Histamine is formed by decarboxylation of the amino acid histidine. Histamine functions as a diffuse neurotransmitter in

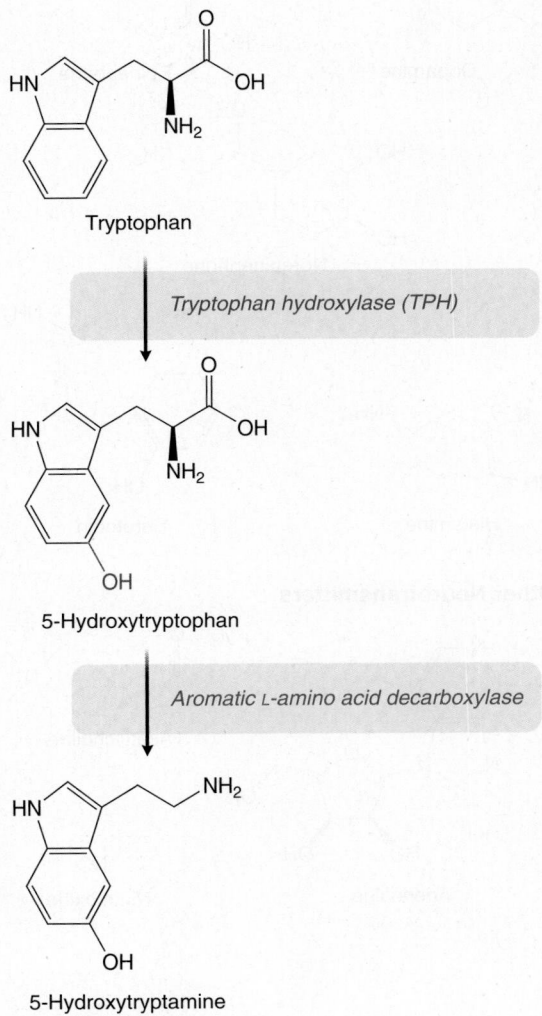

FIGURE 9-12. Synthesis of 5-hydroxytryptamine (serotonin). Tryptophan is first oxidized by tryptophan hydroxylase (TPH) and then decarboxylated by aromatic L-amino acid decarboxylase to yield serotonin.

the CNS; it also has a particular role in the maintenance of arousal via the tuberomamillary nucleus of the hypothalamus and in the sensation of nausea via the area postrema in the floor of the fourth ventricle. Few therapeutics intentionally target central histaminergic neurotransmission. Instead, most drugs in this class act on peripheral histamine H_1 receptors, at which histamine mediates the inflammatory response to allergic stimuli, or on H_2 receptors in the treatment of peptic ulcer disease (see Chapters 44 and 47, Integrative Inflammation Pharmacology: Peptic Ulcer Disease). Peripherally acting antihistamines are sometimes used to effect sedation or as antiemetics, acting via the central neuroanatomic substrates noted above.

Other Small Molecule Neurotransmitters

Acetylcholine plays a major role in peripheral neurotransmission. At the neuromuscular junction, this molecule is used by somatic motor neurons to depolarize striated muscle. In the autonomic nervous system, acetylcholine is the neurotransmitter used by all preganglionic neurons and by parasympathetic postganglionic neurons. The multiple functions of acetylcholine in the peripheral nervous system have spurred the development of a wide range of drugs that target peripheral cholinergic neurotransmission. These include muscle paralytics, which interfere with neurotransmission at the motor end plate, acetylcholinesterase inhibitors, which increase local acetylcholine concentration by interfering with the metabolic breakdown of the neurotransmitter, and receptor-specific agonists and antagonists.

In the CNS, acetylcholine acts as a diffuse-system neurotransmitter. Like the biogenic amines, it is thought to regulate sleep and wakefulness. **Donepezil**, a reversible acetylcholinesterase inhibitor that acts at central cholinergic synapses, helps to "brighten" patients with dementia (see Chapter 10). Peripheral anticholinergic agents may cause central cholinergic blockade and thereby result in major adverse effects. For example, the antimuscarinic drug **scopolamine** can cause drowsiness, amnesia, fatigue, and dreamless sleep. In contrast, cholinergic agonists such as **pilocarpine** can induce adverse effects of cortical arousal and alertness.

The **purinergic** neurotransmitters adenosine and adenosine triphosphate have a role in central neurotransmission. This role is most evident in the effects of **caffeine**, which is a competitive antagonist at adenosine receptors and causes a mild stimulant effect. In this case, the adenosine receptors, which are located on *presynaptic* noradrenergic neurons, act to inhibit the release of norepinephrine. Antagonism of these adenosine receptors by caffeine causes the release of norepinephrine to be disinhibited, which results in the characteristic stimulatory effects of the drug.

Nitric oxide (NO), which has generated significant interest as a peripheral vasodilator, acts in the brain as a neurotransmitter. Unlike the other small molecule neurotransmitters, NO diffuses through the neuronal membrane and binds to its receptors within the target cell. Receptors for NO are thought to reside in presynaptic neurons, allowing NO to act as a retrograde messenger. While many therapeutics target the peripheral vasodilatory effects of NO, none as of yet target its actions as a central neurotransmitter.

Neuropeptides

The neuroactive peptides are the last major class of neurotransmitters. Many neuropeptides also have endocrine, autocrine, and paracrine actions. Major examples of neuroactive peptide families are the **opioids**, **tachykinins**, **secretins**, **insulins**, and **gastrins**. Neuropeptides also include the pituitary hormone release and inhibiting factors, including **corticotropin-releasing hormone (CRH)**, **gonadotropin-releasing hormone (GnRH)**, **thyrotropin-releasing hormone (TRH)**, **growth hormone-releasing hormone (GRH)**, and **somatostatin**. The opioid peptide family includes the **enkephalins**, **dynorphins**, and **endorphins**. Opioid receptors, which are distributed widely in areas of the spinal cord and brain that are involved in pain sensation, are the principal pharmacologic targets of opioid analgesics such as morphine (see Chapter 18) and of some drugs of abuse such as heroin (see Chapter 19).

The Blood–Brain Barrier

In the case of Ms. P, L-DOPA, the immediate precursor of dopamine, is administered rather than the neurotransmitter itself. Unlike L-DOPA, which is able to cross from the blood to the brain tissue where it acts to treat Ms. P's Parkinson's disease, dopamine is unable to cross that boundary. The reason for this exclusion is the existence of a selective filter, termed the **blood–brain barrier,** which regulates the transport of many molecules from the blood into the brain (Fig. 9-13). The blood–brain barrier protects the brain tissue both from toxic substances that circulate in the blood and from neurotransmitters such as epinephrine, norepinephrine, glutamate, and dopamine that have systemic effects in body tissues but that would bind receptors in the CNS and cause undesirable effects if access were permitted.

The structural basis for the blood–brain barrier resides in the unique design of the cerebral microcirculation. In most tissues, there are small gaps, called **fenestrae**, between the endothelial cells that line the microvasculature. These gaps allow water and small molecules to diffuse across the lining without resistance but filter out large proteins and cells. In the CNS, the endothelial cells form tight junctions that prevent diffusion of small molecules across the vessel wall. Also, unlike peripheral endothelial cells, CNS endothelial cells do not generally have pinocytotic vesicles that transport fluid from the blood vessel lumen to the extracellular space. In addition, blood vessels in the CNS are covered by cellular processes derived from **astroglia**. These processes play an important role in selectively transporting certain nutrients from the blood to central neurons.

In the absence of a selective transport mechanism, the blood–brain barrier generally excludes water-soluble substances. In contrast, lipophilic substances, including important lipid-soluble gases such as oxygen and carbon dioxide, can usually diffuse across the endothelial membranes. The oil/water partition coefficient is a good indicator of the ease with which a small molecule can enter the CNS. Lipophilic substances with high oil/water partition coefficients can generally diffuse across the blood–brain barrier, whereas hydrophilic substances with low oil/water partition coefficients are typically excluded (Fig. 9-14).

Many important hydrophilic nutrients, such as glucose and a number of amino acids, would not be able to cross the blood–brain barrier without the existence of specific transporters. Glucose, for example, is transported across the barrier by a **hexose transporter** that allows this nutrient to move down its concentration gradient in a process called **facilitated diffusion**. Amino acids are transported by three different transporters: one for large neutral amino acids such as valine and phenylalanine; one for smaller neutral amino acids and polar amino acids, such as glycine and

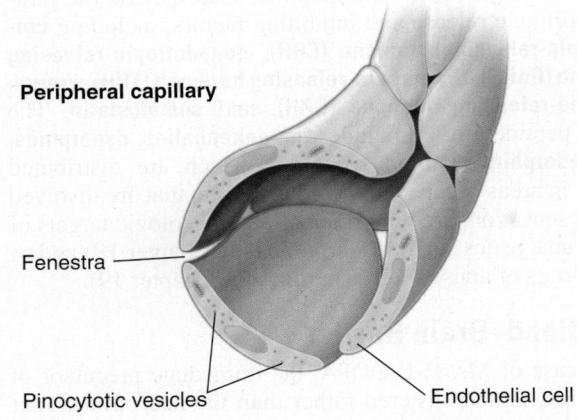

Peripheral capillary

Fenestra

Pinocytotic vesicles

Endothelial cell

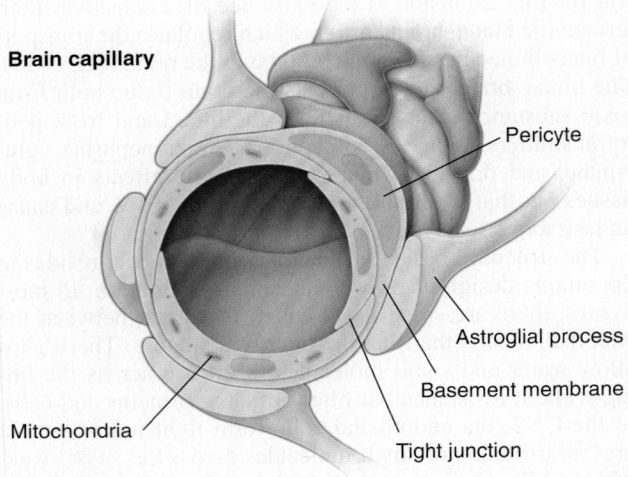

Brain capillary

Pericyte

Astroglial process

Basement membrane

Mitochondria

Tight junction

FIGURE 9-13. Features of capillaries in the central nervous system compared to the peripheral vasculature. In the periphery, capillary endothelial cells have gaps (termed *fenestrae*) between them and use intracellular pinocytotic vesicles to facilitate the transcapillary transport of fluid and soluble molecules. In contrast, CNS vessels are sealed by tight junctions between the endothelial cells. The cells have fewer pinocytotic vesicles and are surrounded by pericytes and astroglial processes. In addition, capillary endothelial cells in the CNS have more mitochondria than those in systemic vessels; these mitochondria may reflect the energy requirements necessary for CNS endothelial cells to transport certain molecules into the CNS and transport other molecules out of the CNS.

glutamate, respectively; and one for alanine, serine, and cysteine. L-DOPA is transported by the large neutral amino acid transporter, but dopamine itself is excluded by the blood–brain barrier. For this reason, L-DOPA is administered in lieu of dopamine to patients with Parkinson's disease. After meals with a high protein content, however, the transporter can become overwhelmed, and its transport of L-DOPA can become ineffective. This explains Ms. P's complaint that her medication was less effective after she began a diet high in protein. The blood–brain barrier also contains a number of ion channels, which ensure that ion concentrations in the brain are maintained at homeostatic levels.

Just as certain vital hydrophilic nutrients are allowed access to the brain tissue via particular transporters, many potentially toxic lipophilic compounds can be excluded from the

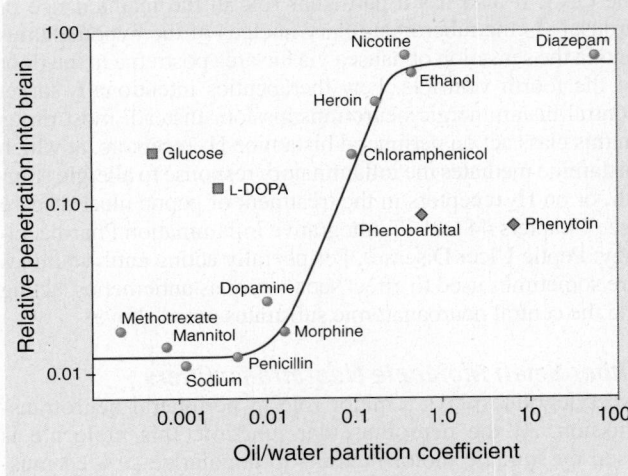

FIGURE 9-14. Relative ability of compounds to enter the brain from the blood. In general, there is a correlation between the oil/water partition coefficient of a compound and its ability to enter the brain from the systemic circulation. Specific transporters facilitate the entry into the brain of certain compounds (*squares*), such as glucose (glucose transporter) and L-DOPA (large neutral L-amino acid transporter). Transporters also pump certain compounds out of the CNS (*diamonds*), such as phenobarbital and phenytoin. The metabolic blood–brain barrier, consisting of a number of drug-metabolizing enzymes, also limits the CNS concentration of certain drugs.

brain by a class of proteins known as **multiple drug resistance (MDR) transporters**. These transporters pump hydrophobic compounds out of the brain and back into the blood vessel lumen. (Note that MDR transporters are present in many cell types, playing an important role in processes such as the resistance of tumor cells to chemotherapeutic agents; see Chapter 5, Drug Transporters.) A **metabolic blood–brain barrier** adds a layer of protection against toxic compounds; this barrier is maintained by enzymes that metabolize compounds transported into CNS endothelial cells. One such enzyme, **aromatic L-amino acid decarboxylase** (sometimes called **DOPA decarboxylase**), metabolizes peripheral L-DOPA to dopamine, which is unable to cross the blood–brain barrier. For this reason, Ms. P's medication includes a second component, **carbidopa**, which is an inhibitor of DOPA decarboxylase. Carbidopa ensures that L-DOPA is not metabolized to dopamine peripherally before crossing the blood–brain barrier. Importantly, carbidopa itself is unable to cross the blood–brain barrier and, therefore, does not interfere with the conversion of L-DOPA to dopamine in the CNS.

■ CONCLUSION AND FUTURE DIRECTIONS

This chapter discusses the anatomical organization of the peripheral and central nervous systems, the transmission and processing of electrical and chemical signals by neurons, the principal neurotransmitters used by CNS neurons, and the structure and function of the blood–brain barrier. Although this chapter introduces some specific drugs as examples, the focus is on the general principles of anatomy and neurotransmission that are important for understanding the action of all pharmacologic agents affecting the nervous system. The remaining chapters in this section discuss specific neurotransmitter systems and specific agents that act on the peripheral and central nervous systems. Thus, Chapters 10 and 11 describe peripheral cholinergic and adrenergic systems, and Chapter 12, Local Anesthetic Pharmacology, discusses the production of local anesthesia by inhibition of electrical transmission through peripheral and spinal neurons. Chapter 13 describes central excitatory and inhibitory neurotransmission. Although few therapeutics currently take advantage of glutamatergic neurotransmission, two major classes of drugs, the benzodiazepines and the barbiturates, affect GABAergic neurotransmission by potentiating the effect of GABA at the GABA$_A$ receptor. Chapter 14 discusses dopaminergic systems, describing in more detail the concept, introduced in the present chapter, that some of the symptoms of Parkinson's disease can be alleviated by drugs that increase dopaminergic transmission. Chapter 14 also explains how inhibiting dopaminergic transmission can alleviate some of the symptoms of schizophrenia, implying that dopamine may play a role in this disease. Chapter 15 discusses drugs that modify affect, the outward manifestations of mood. These agents include antidepressants, which block reuptake or inhibit metabolism of the biogenic amines norepinephrine and serotonin, as well as the "mood stabilizer" lithium, which is thought to affect a signal transduction pathway. Chapter 16 explores the pharmacology of abnormal electrical neurotransmission, including the action of channel blockers, such as **phenytoin**, which block the propagation of action potentials and thereby inhibit many types of seizures. Chapter 17 describes the pharmacology of general anesthetics, agents whose mechanism of action remains an area of active investigation. Chapter 18 discusses the pharmacology of analgesia, including opioid receptor agonists and nonopioid analgesics. To conclude, Chapter 19 focuses on the pharmacology of drugs of abuse.

Suggested Reading

Blumenfeld H. *Neuroanatomy through clinical cases*. 2nd ed. Sunderland, MA: Sinauer Associates, Inc.; 2010. (*Thorough review of human neuroanatomy with an emphasis on clinical correlation; includes many exemplary clinical cases.*)

Squire LR, Berg D, Bloom F, du Lac S, Ghosh A, Spitzer NC, eds. *Fundamental neuroscience*. 4th ed. Waltham, MA: Academic Press; 2013. (*Comprehensive textbook containing detailed information on human neuroanatomy and neurophysiology.*)

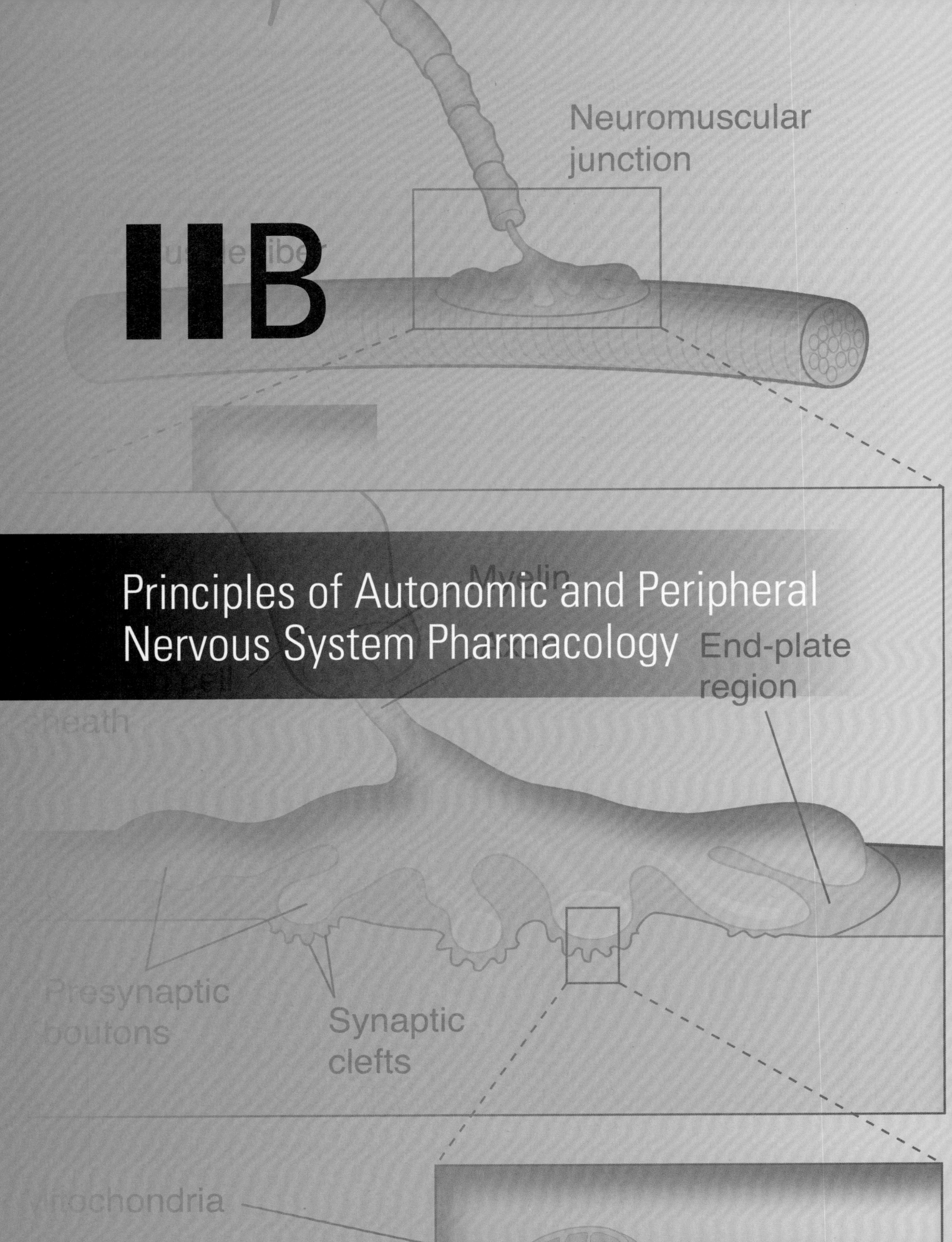

IIB

Principles of Autonomic and Peripheral Nervous System Pharmacology

Neuromuscular junction

End-plate region

Presynaptic boutons

Synaptic clefts

Myelin

Mitochondria

Cholinergic neuron

Na$^+$

Choline

AcCoA + Choline

Hemicholinium

Choline
acetyltransferase

Vesamicol

ACh

Calcium
channel

Calcium
channel

Ca^{2+}

Ca^{2+}

LEMS
(autoantibody)

Botulinum

ACh

10
Cholinergic Pharmacology

Alireza Atri, Michael S. Chang, and Gary R. Strichartz

INTRODUCTION

Cholinergic pharmacology is centered on the properties of the first identified neurotransmitter, **acetylcholine (ACh)**. The functions of cholinergic pathways are diverse; generally, they involve the neuromuscular junction (NMJ), the autonomic nervous system, the central nervous system (CNS), and the non-neuronal cholinergic system (NNCS). In the neuronal cholinergic systems, ACh acts as a neurotransmitter at the NMJ, at autonomic ganglia, at terminal synapses of parasympathetic postganglionic fibers and a few sympathetic postganglionic fibers, and in the CNS. Many non-neuronal cells also express ACh receptors and can thereby serve as effector cells for both neuronally and non-neuronally released ACh.

Despite the many physiologic actions of ACh, the current therapeutic uses for cholinergic and anticholinergic drugs are limited by the ubiquitous nature of cholinergic pathways, and thus, by the inherent difficulty of effecting a specific pharmacologic intervention without inducing adverse effects. Nonetheless, medications with somewhat targeted cholinomimetic and anticholinergic actions are in widespread clinical use for their effects on the brain (especially cognition and behavior), neuromuscular junction, heart, eyes, lungs, and genitourinary and gastrointestinal tracts.

Other chapters that discuss applications of cholinergic pharmacology are Chapter 18, Pharmacology of Analgesia; Chapter 47, Integrative Inflammation Pharmacology: Peptic Ulcer Disease; and Chapter 48, Integrative Inflammation Pharmacology: Asthma.

BIOCHEMISTRY AND PHYSIOLOGY OF CHOLINERGIC NEUROTRANSMISSION

Acetylcholine synthesis, storage, and release follow a similar set of steps in all cholinergic neurons. The specific effects of ACh at a particular cholinergic synapse are largely determined by the ACh receptor type at that synapse. Cholinergic receptors are divided into two broad classes. **Muscarinic acetylcholine receptors (mAChR)** are G protein-coupled receptors that are expressed at the terminal synapses of all parasympathetic postganglionic fibers and a few sympathetic postganglionic fibers, at autonomic ganglia, and in the CNS. **Nicotinic acetylcholine receptors (nAChR)** are ligand-gated ion channels that are concentrated postsynaptically at many excitatory autonomic synapses and presynaptically in the CNS. **Acetylcholinesterase (AChE)**, the enzyme responsible for acetylcholine degradation, is also an important pharmacologic target. In this section, the biochemistry of each of these pharmacologic targets is described and the physiologic effects of acetylcholine at the neuromuscular junction, in the autonomic nervous system, in the CNS, and in the non-neuronal cholinergic system are discussed.

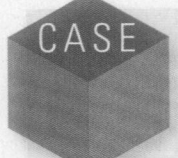

CASE

The year is 1744. Virginian settlers capture Chief Opechancanough, warrior chief of the Powhatans and uncle to Pocahontas. Opechancanough is considered a master tactician and has a reputation as a brutal warrior. One colonial correspondent portrays a different picture of the captured chief, however: "The excessive fatigues he encountered wrecked his constitution; his flesh became macerated; his sinews lost their tone and elasticity and his eyelids were so heavy that he could not see unless they were lifted up by his attendants . . . he was unable to walk; but his spirit, rising above the ruins of his body, directed [his followers] from the litter on which he was carried by his Indians." During the confinement of Opechancanough to a prison in Jamestown, it is discovered that, after a period of inactivity, he is able to raise himself from the ground to a standing position.

It is thought that the story of Opechancanough provides the earliest recorded description of myasthenia gravis, a neuromuscular disease resulting from the autoimmune production of antibodies directed against cholinergic receptors at the neuromuscular junction. In 1934, almost 2 centuries later, the English physician Mary Broadfoot Walker encounters several patients with similar symptoms of muscle weakness, which remind her of the symptoms of patients with tubocurare poisoning. Given her findings, Dr. Walker administers an antidote, physostigmine, to her immobile patients. The results are startling—within minutes, her patients are able to rise and walk across the room. Dr. Walker has discovered the first truly effective medication for myasthenia gravis. Despite the significance of her accomplishment, it is largely ridiculed by the scientific community because the treatment improves the symptoms of myasthenia gravis too rapidly and effectively to be believable. It is not until many years later that the scientific community comes to accept her findings.

Questions

1. Why do tubocurare poisoning and myasthenia gravis produce similar symptoms?
2. How does physostigmine improve the symptoms of myasthenia gravis? Why is it dangerous to administer physostigmine to every patient presenting with muscle weakness?
3. What are the therapeutic uses of anticholinergic drugs in other diseases such as Alzheimer's dementia?
4. What are the advantages and disadvantages of using medications with anticholinergic effects in older individuals and individuals with cognitive impairments?

Synthesis of Acetylcholine

Acetylcholine is synthesized in a single step from choline and acetyl coenzyme A (acetyl CoA) by the enzyme **choline acetyltransferase (ChAT)**:

$$\text{Acetyl Coenzyme A + Choline} \xrightarrow{\text{ChAT}}$$

$$\text{Acetylcholine + Coenzyme A + H}_2\text{O} \qquad \textbf{Equation 10-1}$$

In the CNS, choline used for the synthesis of acetylcholine arises from one of three sources. Approximately 35% to 50% of the choline generated by acetylcholinesterase in the synaptic cleft (see Fig. 10-1 and below) is transported back into the axon terminal, where it comprises about half of the choline used in ACh synthesis. Plasma-based stores of choline may also be transported to the brain as part of phosphatidylcholine (a phospholipid), which is then metabolized to free choline. (The incorporation of choline into phosphatidylcholine is essential, because choline itself cannot cross the blood–brain barrier.) Choline is also stored in phospholipids as phosphorylcholine, where it can be used when needed.

Acetyl CoA for the synthesis reaction is derived mainly from glycolysis and is ultimately produced by the enzyme pyruvate dehydrogenase. Although the synthesis of acetyl CoA occurs at the inner membrane of mitochondria, choline acetyltransferase is located in the cytoplasm. It is hypothesized that citrate serves as the carrier for acetyl CoA from the mitochondrion to the cytoplasm, where the citrate is freed by citrate lyase.

The choline acetyltransferase reaction is not the rate-limiting step in ACh synthesis. Rather, ACh synthesis is limited by the availability of the choline substrate, which depends on uptake of choline into the neuron. Two processes are responsible for choline transport. The first is low-affinity ($K_m = 10–100\ \mu M$) facilitated diffusion. This transport system is not saturable and is found in cells that synthesize choline-containing phospholipids, such as the corneal epithelium. Far more important is a sodium-dependent, high-affinity transport system ($K_m = 1–5\ \mu M$) found specifically in cholinergic nerve terminals. Because the high-affinity transporter is saturated at concentrations of choline $>10\ \mu M$, it sets an upper limit on the supply of choline for ACh synthesis. As the rate-limiting component in ACh synthesis, this transporter is a target for several anticholinergic drugs (e.g., **hemicholinium-3**, see Fig. 10-1).

Storage and Release of Acetylcholine

After its synthesis in the cytoplasm, ACh is transported into synaptic vesicles for storage. An ATPase that pumps protons into the vesicle provides the energy necessary for this process. Transport of protons out of the vesicle (i.e., down the H^+ concentration gradient) is coupled to uptake of ACh into the vesicle (i.e., against the ACh concentration gradient) via an ACh-H^+ antiport channel. This antiporter is a target for some anticholinergic drugs, such as **vesamicol**, and its inhibition results in a deficit of ACh storage and subsequent release (Fig. 10-1). Cholinergic synaptic vesicles contain not only ACh but also ATP and heparan sulfate proteoglycans,

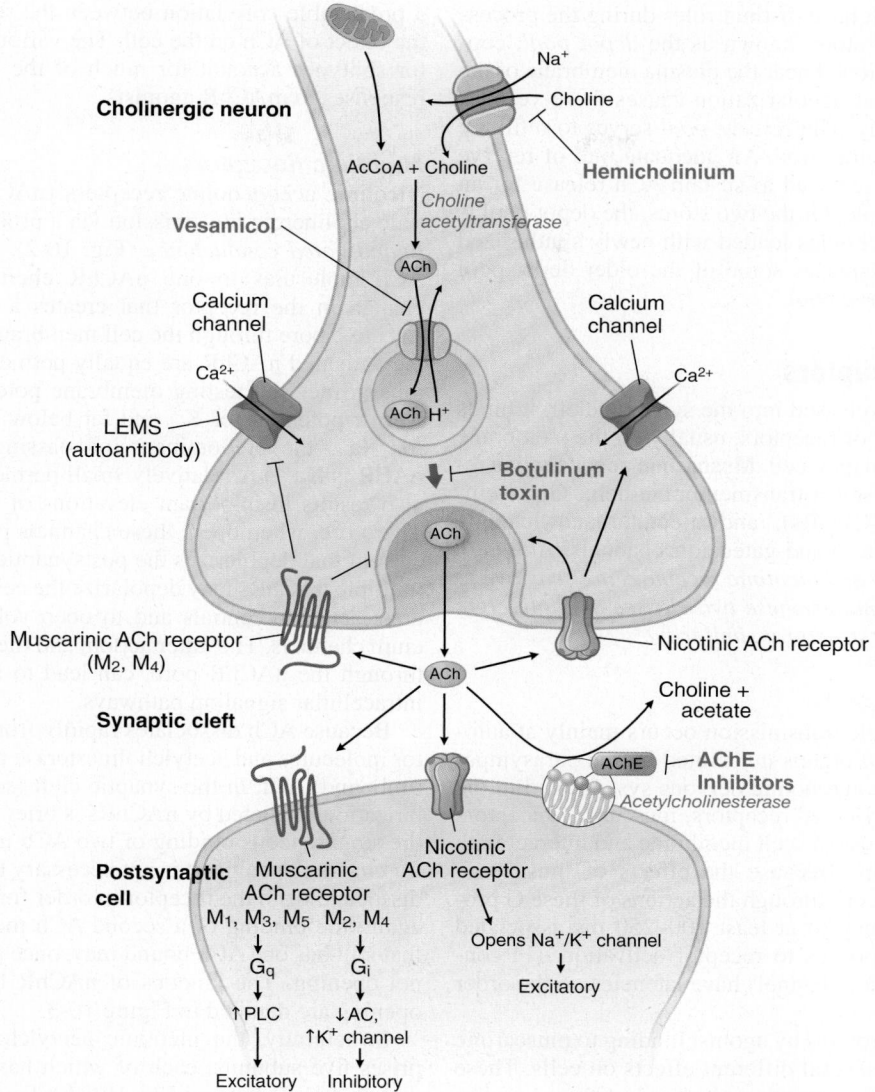

FIGURE 10-1. **Acetylcholine synthesis, storage, release, and degradation pathways and pharmacologic agents that act on these pathways.** Choline is transported into the presynaptic cholinergic nerve terminal by a high-affinity Na^+-choline co-transporter. This transporter is inhibited by hemicholinium. The cytosolic enzyme choline acetyltransferase catalyzes the formation of acetylcholine (ACh) from acetyl coenzyme A (AcCoA) and choline. Newly synthesized ACh is packaged (together with ATP and proteoglycans) into vesicles for storage. Transport of ACh into the vesicle is mediated by a H^+-ACh antiporter, which is inhibited by vesamicol. The ACh-containing vesicles fuse with the plasma membrane when intracellular calcium levels increase in response to a presynaptic action potential, releasing the neurotransmitter into the synaptic cleft. Lambert-Eaton myasthenic syndrome (LEMS) results from an autoantibody that blocks the presynaptic Ca^{2+} channel. Botulinum toxin prevents the exocytosis of presynaptic vesicles, thereby blocking ACh release. Acetylcholine diffuses in the synaptic cleft and binds to postsynaptic and presynaptic receptors. Acetylcholine receptors are divided into nicotinic and muscarinic receptors. Nicotinic receptors are ligand-gated ion channels that are permeable to cations, while muscarinic receptors are G protein-coupled receptors that alter cell signaling pathways, including activation of phospholipase C (PLC), inhibition of adenylyl cyclase (AC), and opening of K^+ channels. Postsynaptic nicotinic receptors and M_1, M_3, and M_5 muscarinic receptors are excitatory; postsynaptic M_2 and M_4 muscarinic receptors are inhibitory. Presynaptic nicotinic receptors enhance Ca^{2+} entry into the presynaptic neuron, thereby increasing vesicle fusion and release of ACh; presynaptic M_2 and M_4 muscarinic receptors inhibit Ca^{2+} entry into the presynaptic neuron, thereby decreasing vesicle fusion and release of ACh. Acetylcholine in the synaptic cleft is degraded by membrane-bound acetylcholinesterase (AChE) into choline and acetate. Numerous inhibitors of AChE exist; most clinically relevant anticholinesterases are competitive inhibitors of the enzyme.

both of which serve as counter-ions for ACh. By neutralizing the positive charge of ACh, these molecules disperse electrostatic forces that would otherwise prevent dense packing of ACh within the vesicle. (Released ATP also acts as a neurotransmitter, through purinergic receptors, to inhibit the release of ACh and norepinephrine from autonomic nerve endings.)

Release of ACh into the synaptic cleft occurs via fusion of the synaptic vesicle with the plasma membrane. This process

depends on axon terminal depolarization and the opening of voltage-dependent calcium channels. The increase in intracellular Ca^{2+} facilitates the binding of synaptotagmin to the SNARE-complex proteins, which together mediate vesicle–membrane attachment and fusion. The result is that the contents of the vesicle are released as discrete "quanta" into the synaptic cleft. (See Chapter 8, Principles of Cellular Excitability and Electrochemical Transmission, for additional details on electrochemical transmission.)

Two stores of ACh have distinct roles during the process of ACh release. One store, known as the *depot pool*, consists of vesicles positioned near the plasma membrane of the axon terminal. Axonal depolarization causes these vesicles to release ACh rapidly. The *reserve pool* serves to refill the depot pool as it is being used. An adequate rate of reserve pool mobilization is required to sustain ACh release for an extended period of time. Of the two stores, the depot pool is replenished first by vesicles loaded with newly synthesized ACh; this process displaces some of the older depot pool vesicles into the reserve pool.

Cholinergic Receptors

After ACh has been released into the synaptic cleft, it binds to one of two classes of receptors, usually on the membrane surface of the postsynaptic cell. **Muscarinic acetylcholine receptors (mAChR)** are seven-transmembrane-helix G protein-coupled receptors (GPCRs), and **nicotinic acetylcholine receptors (nAChR)** are ligand-gated ion channels. *Although muscarinic receptors and nicotinic receptors are sensitive to the same neurotransmitter, these two classes of cholinergic receptors share little structural similarity.*

Muscarinic Receptors

Muscarinic cholinergic transmission occurs mainly at autonomic ganglia, at end organs innervated by the parasympathetic division of the autonomic nervous system, and in the CNS. As G protein-coupled receptors, muscarinic receptors transduce signals across the cell membrane and interact with GTP-binding proteins. Because the effects of muscarinic receptor activation occur through the actions of these G proteins, there is a latency of at least 100–250 ms associated with muscarinic responses to receptor activation. (In contrast, nicotinic receptor channels have latencies on the order of 5 ms.)

Activation of G proteins by agonist binding to muscarinic receptors may have several different effects on cells. These include inhibition of adenylyl cyclase (via G_i) and stimulation of phospholipase C (via $G_{q/11}$), both mediated by an α subunit of the G protein. (See Chapter 1, Drug–Receptor Interactions, for a discussion of these signaling mechanisms.) Muscarinic activation also modulates ion channels via the $\beta\gamma$ subunit of a G protein. The predominant effect of such mAChR stimulation is to increase the opening of specific potassium channels (G protein-modulated inwardly rectifying K^+ channels, or GIRKs), thereby hyperpolarizing the cell. The $\beta\gamma$ subunit of the G_i protein binds to the channel and enhances its probability of being open.

Five distinct cDNAs for muscarinic receptors, denoted M_1–M_5, have been isolated and detected in human cells. These receptor types form two functionally distinct groups. M_1, M_3, and M_5 are coupled to G proteins responsible for the stimulation of phospholipase C. M_2 and M_4, on the other hand, are coupled to G proteins responsible for adenylyl cyclase inhibition and K^+ channel activation. The receptors of each functional group can be distinguished based on their responses to pharmacologic antagonists (Table 10-1). Generally, M_1 is expressed in cortical neurons and autonomic ganglia, M_2 in cardiac muscle, and M_3 in smooth muscle and glandular tissue. Because stimulation of M_1, M_3, and M_5 receptors facilitates excitation of the cell, while stimulation of M_2 and M_4 receptors suppresses cellular excitability, there is a predictable correlation between the receptor subtype and the effect of ACh on the cell. The various muscarinic receptor subtypes account for much of the diversity in cellular responses to mAChR agonists.

Nicotinic Receptors

Nicotinic acetylcholine receptors (nAChRs) mediate nicotinic cholinergic transmission via a process known as *direct ligand-gated conductance* (Fig. 10-2). The binding of two ACh molecules to one nAChR elicits a conformational change in the receptor that creates a monovalent cation-selective pore through the cell membrane. Open channels of the activated nAChR are equally permeable to K^+ and Na^+ ions. (Since the resting membrane potential is close to the Nernst potential for K^+ and far below the Nernst potential for Na^+, the predominant ion passing through the open nACR is Na^+.) A relatively small permeability to Ca^{2+} ions also results in important elevations of intracellular $[Ca^{2+}]$. Therefore, when open, these channels produce a net inward current that depolarizes the postsynaptic cell. Stimulation of multiple nAChRs may depolarize the cell sufficiently to generate action potentials and to open voltage-dependent calcium channels. The latter action, and the direct entry of Ca^{2+} through the nAChR pore, can lead to activation of several intracellular signaling pathways.

Because ACh dissociates rapidly from active-state receptor molecules and acetylcholinesterase rapidly degrades free (unbound) ACh in the synaptic cleft (see below), the depolarization mediated by nAChRs is brief (<10 ms). Although the simultaneous binding of two ACh molecules is required for channel opening, it is not necessary for both molecules to dissociate from the receptor in order for the channel to open again; the binding of a second ACh molecule to a receptor that still has one ACh bound may, once again, result in channel opening. The kinetics of nAChR binding and channel opening are detailed in Figure 10-3.

Structurally, the nicotinic acetylcholine receptor comprises five subunits, each of which has a mass of approximately 40 kilodaltons (Fig. 10-2A). Several types of nAChR subunits have been identified; these are designated α, β, γ, δ, and ε. All of these subunits share 35–50% homology with one another. Each receptor at the NMJ is composed of two α subunits, one β and one δ subunit, and either one γ or one ε subunit. (The $\alpha_2\beta\varepsilon\delta$ form dominates at the neuromuscular junction in mature skeletal muscle, while the $\alpha_2\beta\gamma\delta$ form is expressed in embryonic muscle.) Agonist molecules bind at a hydrophobic pocket that is formed between each α subunit and the adjacent, complementary subunit—this is the structural basis for the binding of two ACh molecules to each receptor. The conformational change in the α subunits induced by the binding of ACh initiates the overall changes in the pore that permit ion flow through the receptor (i.e., that open the channel).

Besides simply opening and closing in response to ACh binding, nicotinic receptors also modulate their responses to various concentration profiles of ACh. The receptors react differently to discrete, brief pulses of ACh than to neurotransmitter that is present continuously. As noted above, under normal conditions, a closed, resting-state channel responds to dual ACh binding by opening transiently, and the low affinity of the receptor for ACh causes rapid dissociation of ACh from the receptor and return of the receptor to its resting conformation. In contrast, continuous exposure

TABLE 10-1 Characteristics of Cholinergic Receptor Subtypes

RECEPTOR	TYPICAL LOCATIONS	RESPONSES	MECHANISM	PROTOTYPE AGONIST	PROTOTYPE ANTAGONIST
Muscarinic M_1	Autonomic ganglia	Late excitatory postsynaptic potential (EPSP)	$G_{q/11} \rightarrow PLC \rightarrow \uparrow IP_3 +$ $\uparrow DAG \rightarrow \uparrow Ca^{2+} +$ $\uparrow PKC$	Oxotremorine	Pirenzepine
	CNS	Complex: at least arousal, attention, analgesia			
Muscarinic M_2	Heart: SA node	Slowed spontaneous depolarization; hyperpolarization	α subunit of $G_i \rightarrow$ inhibits AC; $\beta\gamma$ subunit of $G_i \rightarrow \uparrow$ K^+ channel (GIRK) opening		AF-DX 117
	Heart: AV node	$\downarrow$ Conduction velocity			
	Heart: atrium	$\downarrow$ Refractory period; $\downarrow$ contractile force			
	Heart: ventricle	Slight $\downarrow$ in contractility			
Muscarinic M_3	Smooth muscle	Contraction	As M_1		Hexahydrosiladifenidol
Muscarinic M_4	CNS		As M_2; presynaptic autoreceptors, negative feedback to suppress ACh release		Himbacine
Muscarinic M_5	CNS		As M_1		
Nicotinic N_M	Skeletal muscle at neuromuscular junction (NMJ)	End-plate depolarization; skeletal muscle contraction	Opening of nAChR Na^+/K^+ channels	Phenyltrimethylammonium	Tubocurare
Nicotinic N_N	Autonomic ganglia	Depolarization and firing of postganglionic neuron	Opening of nAChR Na^+/K^+ channels; postsynaptic depolarization and presynaptic interactions with other receptors, calcium channels	Dimethylphenylpiperazinium	Trimethaphan
	Adrenal medulla	Secretion of catecholamines			
	CNS	Complex: at least arousal, attention, analgesia			

Cholinergic receptors are divided into nicotinic and muscarinic receptors. All nicotinic receptors are ligand-gated cation-selective channels, while muscarinic receptors are G protein-coupled receptors. Specific pharmacologic agonists and antagonists exist for most subclasses, although the majority of these agents are currently used only for experimental purposes.

of the receptor to ACh causes it to undergo a change to a "desensitized" conformation in which the channel is locked closed. The desensitized state is also characterized by a greatly increased affinity of the receptor for ACh, so that ACh remains bound to the receptor for a relatively long period of time. This prolonged binding of ACh to the desensitized conformation delays the conversion of the receptor to its resting state and hence prolongs the time during which the receptor is incapable of being activated by agonist.

Nicotinic cholinergic receptors at autonomic ganglia and in the central nervous system (termed N_2 or N_N) are similar to receptors at the NMJ (N_1 or N_M), with the exception that the subunits in N_N receptors are composed solely of α and β subunits. To complicate matters, however, nine different α subunit types (α_2–α_{10}) and three β subunit types (β_2–β_4) have been detected in neuronal tissues. (α_1 and β_1 refer to the distinct subunit types found at the NMJ.) This diversity of α and β subunit combinations is responsible for the variable responses of CNS and autonomic nAChRs to pharmacologic agents. Presynaptic nAChRs in the CNS modulate the release both of ACh itself and of other excitatory and inhibitory neurotransmitters. This effect may involve prolonged elevations

of $[Ca^{2+}]$ in the presynaptic nerve terminals, which lead to inactivation of neuronal calcium channels.

Degradation of Acetylcholine

In order for acetylcholine to be useful for rapid, repeated neurotransmission, there must be a mechanism to limit its duration of action. Degradation of ACh is essential not only to prevent unwanted activation of neighboring neurons or muscle cells but also to ensure proper timing of signaling at the postsynaptic cell. A single receptor molecule is typically capable of distinguishing between two sequential presynaptic release events because degradation of ACh in the synaptic cleft occurs faster than the time course of nAChR activation.

Enzymes collectively known as **cholinesterases** are responsible for degrading acetylcholine. The two types of cholinesterase, **AChE** and **butyrylcholinesterase** (**BuChE**, also known as *pseudocholinesterase* or *nonspecific cholinesterase*), are distributed widely throughout the body. AChE is indispensable for the degradation of ACh and is capable of hydrolyzing about 4×10^5 molecules of ACh per enzyme molecule per minute; its turnover time of 150 μs makes it one

A Overall Structure

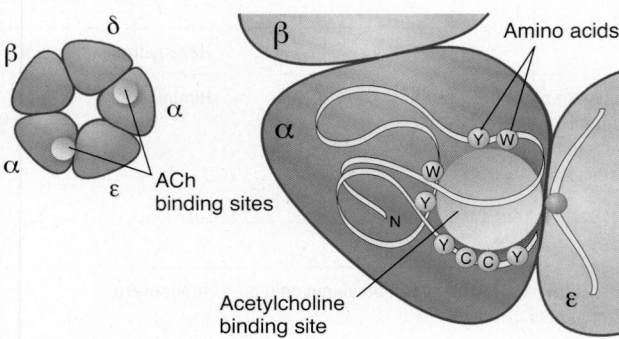

B Acetylcholine Binding Site

C Ion Channel

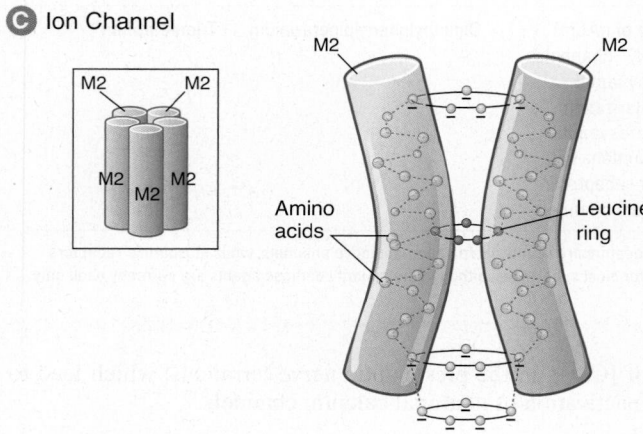

FIGURE 10-2. Structural biology of the nicotinic acetylcholine receptor. A. Overall structure of the nicotinic acetylcholine receptor (N_M type) and its five subunits ($\alpha_2\beta\epsilon\delta$). Each subunit is composed of a transmembrane protein that has four membrane-spanning (hydrophobic) alpha-helical regions (M_1, M_2, M_3, M_4). The large hydrophilic N-terminal domains of the two α subunits contain the binding sites for acetylcholine. **B.** Acetylcholine binding site viewed from above (*inset*: lower magnification). The labeled amino acids of the α subunit hydrophilic domain are particularly important in binding acetylcholine. The conformational change that results from the binding of two acetylcholine molecules opens the channel. **C.** The M_2 domains of the five subunits all face the interior of the protein and together form the transmembrane channel (*inset*). Three negatively charged rings of five amino acids (one from each M_2 subunit) draw positively charged ions through the channel. At the center, an uncharged leucine ring (*purple*) participates in closing the ion channel when the receptor becomes desensitized to acetylcholine.

of the most efficient hydrolytic enzymes known. AChE is concentrated on the postsynaptic membrane, and the choline that it frees there is efficiently transported back into the presynaptic terminal. BuChE has a secondary role in ACh degradation; the enzyme can hydrolyze ACh but at rates much slower than that of AChE. Evidence suggests that BuChE may be involved in early neural development as a co-regulator of ACh and may also be involved in the pathogenesis of Alzheimer's disease. Because of its central importance to cholinergic transmission, a class of drugs known as *acetylcholinesterase inhibitors* has been designed to target AChE.

Physiologic Effects of Cholinergic Transmission

Neuromuscular Junction

Acetylcholine is the principal neurotransmitter at the neuromuscular junction (Fig. 10-4). ACh is released by α motor neurons and it binds to nicotinic receptors in the muscle cell membrane, resulting in motor end-plate depolarization. The extent of depolarization depends on the quantity of ACh released into the synaptic cleft. Release of ACh is quantal in nature; that is, ACh is released in discrete quantities by the presynaptic motor neuron. Each quantum of ACh corresponds to the contents of a single synaptic vesicle and elicits a small depolarization in the motor end-plate termed a **miniature end-plate potential (MEPP)**. Under resting conditions, sporadic MEPPs are detected at the motor end-plate, corresponding to a low baseline level of unstimulated ACh release that arises from spontaneous synaptic vesicle fusion with the motor axon's presynaptic membrane. In contrast, the arrival of an action potential at the motor axon terminal causes many more vesicles (up to thousands) to fuse with the neuronal membrane and release their ACh. At the motor end-plate, the result is a relatively large depolarization termed the **end-plate potential (EPP)** (Fig. 10-5). The magnitude of an EPP is more than sufficient to trigger an action potential that propagates from the end-plate throughout the muscle fiber and, hence, produces a single contraction or "twitch."

Acetylcholine not only triggers muscle contraction as its primary effect at the NMJ, but also modulates its own action at this site. Presynaptic cholinergic receptors, located on the axon terminal of the motor neuron, respond to ACh binding by *facilitating* the mobilization of synaptic vesicles from the reserve pool to the depot pool. This positive feedback loop, in which the release of ACh stimulates additional ACh release, is necessary to ensure sufficient ACh release when the nerve is stimulated with high frequency ($\sim$100 Hz). Despite this mechanism, the ACh output per nerve impulse wanes rapidly during prolonged high-frequency stimulation. Fortunately, because an excess of ACh is released and an excess of ACh receptors is present, there is a large safety margin. Only when 50% or more of the postsynaptic receptors are desensitized is a decline in muscle tension observed during tetanic stimulation (a phenomenon known as **tetanic fade**). Importantly, selective blockade of the modulatory presynaptic cholinergic receptors by antagonists such as **hexamethonium** prevents facilitation and causes rapid tetanic fade to occur under otherwise normal conditions (Fig. 10-6).

Autonomic Effects

Autonomic activity can be classified as either *tonic* activity, which accounts for end organ stimulation at rest, or *phasic* activity, which triggers an elevated response to changing

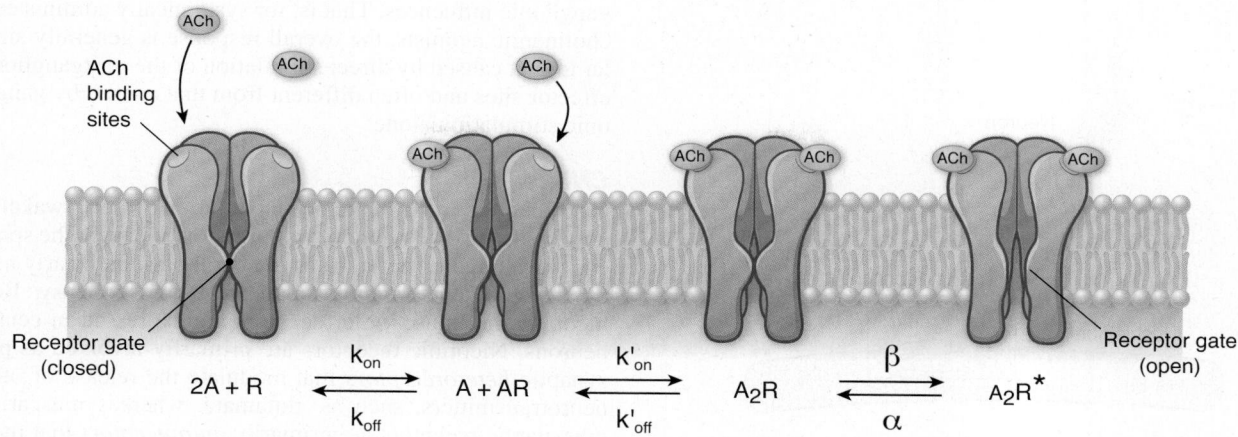

FIGURE 10-3. Kinetics of nicotinic acetylcholine receptor binding and channel opening. Each transition between states of receptor binding and channel opening is completely reversible, and it is not necessary to go through all of the possible conformations before returning to a given state. For example, a receptor with two associated ligands may lose one and then gain another to return to its initial state, without the need for both ligands to dissociate. A, agonist ligand (ACh); R, nicotinic ACh receptor (closed); R*, nicotinic ACh receptor (open); k_{on}, rate constant for association (binding) of the first ACh molecule to the receptor; k'_{on}, rate constant for association of the second ACh molecule to the receptor; k_{off}, rate constant for dissociation of the first ACh molecule from the receptor; k'_{off}, rate constant for dissociation of the second ACh molecule from the receptor; β, rate constant of channel opening after both ACh molecules have bound; α, rate constant of channel closure. Note that channel opening and closing are much faster events than binding and dissociation of ACh to the receptor, so that a receptor with two bound ACh molecules can open and close multiple times before one of the agonists dissociates.

conditions. Neurotransmission through autonomic ganglia is complicated because several distinct receptor types contribute to the complex changes observed in postganglionic neurons. The generalized postsynaptic response to presynaptic impulses can be separated into four distinct components (Fig. 10-7). *The primary event in the postsynaptic ganglionic response is a rapid depolarization mediated by nicotinic ACh receptors in the cell membrane of postganglionic neurons.* The mechanism is similar to that in the NMJ, in that an inward current elicits a near-immediate excitatory postsynaptic potential (EPSP) of 10–50 ms in duration. Typically, the amplitude of such an EPSP is only a few millivolts, and many such events must sum for the postsynaptic cell membrane to reach the threshold for firing an action potential (Fig. 10-7A). The three remaining events of ganglionic transmission modulate this primary signal and are known as *the slow EPSP, the IPSP (inhibitory postsynaptic potential), and the late, slow EPSP.* The **slow EPSP** occurs after a latency of 1 second and is mediated by M_1 muscarinic ACh receptors. The duration of this effect is 10–30 seconds (Fig. 10-7C). The **IPSP** is largely a product of catecholamine (i.e., dopamine and norepinephrine) stimulation of dopaminergic and α-adrenergic receptors (see Chapter 11, Adrenergic Pharmacology), although some IPSPs in a few ganglia are mediated by M_2 muscarinic receptors. The latency and duration of the IPSPs generally vary between those of the fast and slow EPSPs. The **late, slow EPSP** is mediated by a decrease in potassium conductance induced by stimulation of receptors for peptide transmitters (i.e., angiotensin, substance P, and luteinizing hormone-releasing hormone). Lasting for several minutes, the late, slow EPSP is thought to have a role in the long-term regulation of postsynaptic neuron sensitivity to repetitive depolarization.

One pharmacologic consequence of such a complex pattern of depolarization in autonomic ganglia is that drugs selective for the IPSP, slow EPSP, and late, slow EPSP are generally not capable of eliminating ganglionic transmission.

Instead, such agents alter only the efficiency of transmission. For example, **methacholine**, a muscarinic receptor agonist, has modulatory effects on autonomic ganglia that resemble the stimulation of slow EPSPs (see below). Blockade of excitatory transmission through autonomic ganglia relies on inhibition of the nAChRs that mediate fast EPSPs.

The overall effect of ganglionic blockade is complex and depends on the relative predominance of sympathetic and parasympathetic tone at the various end organs (Table 10-2). For example, the heart is influenced at rest primarily by the parasympathetic system, whose *tonic* effect is a slowing of the heart rate. Thus, blockade of autonomic ganglia that innervate the heart by moderate to high doses of the antimuscarinic agent **atropine** results in blockade of vagal slowing of the sinoatrial node and hence in relative *tachycardia*. (It should be noted that in low doses, the central parasympathetic stimulating effects of atropine predominate, initially resulting in *bradycardia* prior to its peripheral vagolytic action.) Blood vessels, in contrast, are innervated only by the sympathetic system. Because the normal effect of sympathetic stimulation is to cause vasoconstriction, ganglionic blockade results in vasodilation. It is important to realize, however, that the responses described above ignore the presence of muscarinic ACh receptors at many of the end organs. When stimulated directly by cholinergic agents, such receptors often mediate a response that overrides the response produced by ganglionic blockade. In general, the expected net cardiovascular effects of muscarinic blockade produced by clinical doses of atropine in a healthy adult with a normal hemodynamic state are mild tachycardia, with or without flushing of the skin, and no profound effect on blood pressure.

The muscarinic receptor subtypes expressed in visceral smooth muscle, cardiac muscle, secretory glands, and endothelial cells mediate highly diverse responses to cholinergic stimulation. These effects are detailed in Table 10-3. In general, these end-organ effects tend to predominate over

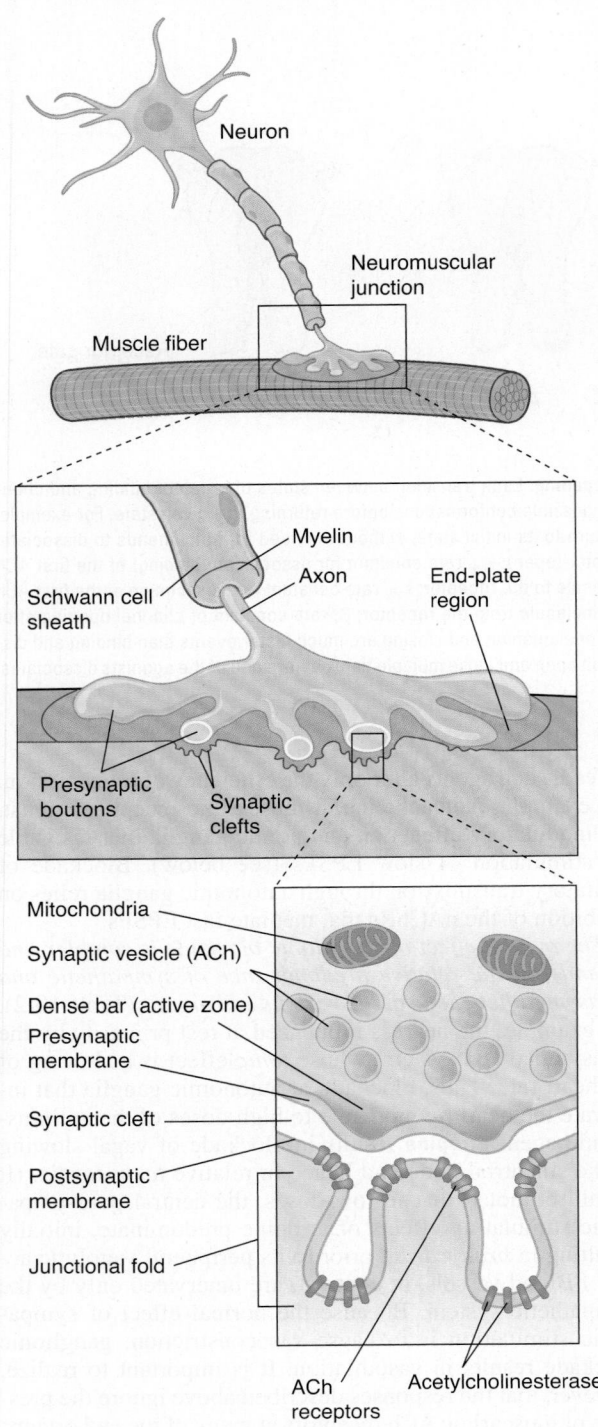

FIGURE 10-4. The neuromuscular junction (NMJ). At the neuromuscular junction, motor neurons innervate a group of muscle fibers. The area of muscle fibers innervated by an individual motor neuron is referred to as the **end-plate** region. Multiple presynaptic terminals extend from the axon of the motor neuron. When the motor neuron is depolarized, its synaptic vesicles fuse with the presynaptic membrane, releasing ACh into the synaptic cleft. ACh receptors of the neuromuscular junction are exclusively nicotinic, and stimulation of these receptors results in depolarization of the muscle cell membrane and generation of an end-plate potential.

ganglionic influences. That is, for systemically administered cholinergic agonists, the overall response is generally similar to that caused by direct stimulation of the postganglionic effector sites and often different from that caused by ganglionic stimulation alone.

CNS Effects

CNS functions of ACh include modulation of sleep, wakefulness, learning, and memory; suppression of pain at the spinal cord level; and essential roles in neural plasticity, early neural development, immunosuppression, and epilepsy. Both nicotinic and muscarinic receptors are expressed in central neurons. Nicotinic receptors are primarily involved as presynaptic *heteroreceptors* that modulate the release of other neurotransmitters, such as glutamate, whereas muscarinic presynaptic receptors are primarily *autoreceptors* that modulate the release of ACh. While the past two decades have improved understanding of the diversity of subunits and molecular properties of neuronal nicotinic receptors, important questions remain about the anatomical distributions and functional roles of different neuronal receptor subtypes in the CNS and of their changes in disease states and during nicotine abuse (as occurs with smoking).

As part of the ascending **reticular activating system**, cholinergic neurons play an important role in arousal and attention (see Fig. 9-8). Levels of ACh throughout the brain increase during wakefulness and REM sleep and decrease during inattentive states and non-REM/slow-wave sleep (SWS). During an awake or aroused state, cholinergic projections from the pedunculopontine nucleus, the lateral tegmental nucleus, and the nucleus basalis of Meynert (NBM) are all active. Because the NBM projects diffusely throughout the cortex and hippocampus (see Fig. 9-8), activation of the NBM causes a global increase in ACh levels. Acetylcholine markedly potentiates the excitatory effects of other inputs to its cortical target cells without affecting the baseline activity of these neurons, an effect that likely derives from its modulation of excitatory neurotransmitter release. This primed state is thought to improve the ability of such neurons to process incoming inputs. For the brain as a whole, the result is a heightened state of responsiveness.

The cholinergic link to memory processes is supported by evidence from diverse experimental models. Whereas elevated ACh levels during wakefulness appear to benefit memory encoding processes, consolidation of hippocampus-mediated, episodic, explicit memories benefit from SWS, when ACh levels are at their minimum. By artificially keeping ACh levels elevated during SWS (e.g., by administration of an AChE inhibitor), consolidation of newly acquired explicit learning and episodic memories can be disrupted. Current understanding of the interplay among ACh, sleep, and memory is as follows. During awake states, ACh prevents interference with initial learning in the hippocampus by suppressing retrieval of previously stored memories (to prevent them from interfering with new encoding), but release of this suppression is necessary to allow consolidation of new memories. During sleep (in particular, during SWS), lower ACh levels are required for proper consolidation of newly acquired memories because stronger excitatory feedback transmission is needed to reactivate memories for consolidation within neocortical brain areas. Therefore, it may be useful to remember to sleep, as sleep is needed to remember, or at least to remember better.

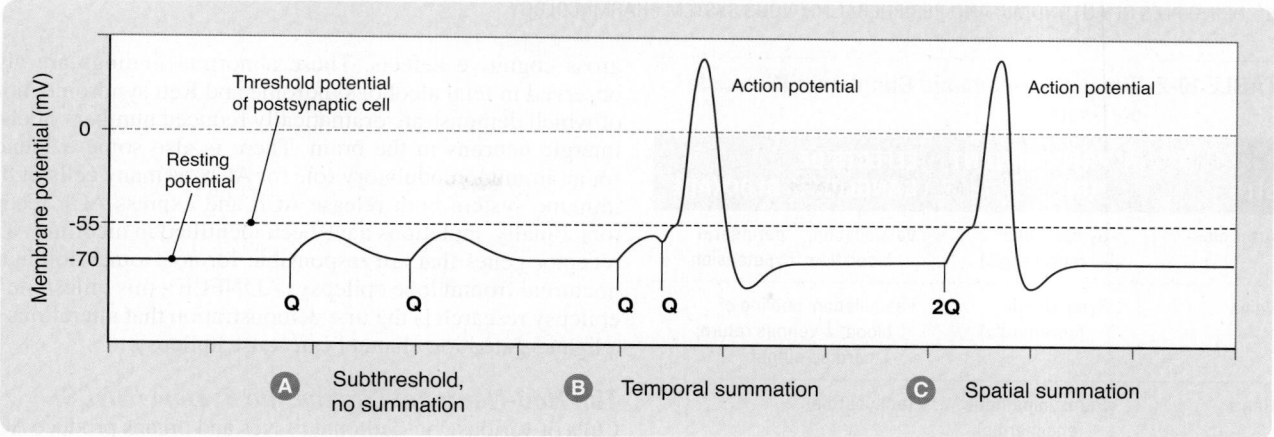

FIGURE 10-5. Quantal release of acetylcholine and muscle contraction. Muscle contraction relies on the accumulation of a sufficient concentration of acetylcholine at the motor end-plate to depolarize the muscle beyond the threshold potential (typically, about -55 mV). After local depolarization occurs, a self-propagating action potential is generated that can spread along the muscle fiber and result in muscle contraction. **A.** As a single cholinergic vesicle releases its contents into the NMJ, a small depolarization (Q), otherwise known as a *miniature end-plate potential* (MEPP), occurs in the local region of the muscle. This MEPP is insufficient to generate an action potential. When a sufficient number of individual cholinergic vesicles empty their contents into the NMJ, either in quick succession (**B**) or simultaneously (**C**), sufficient depolarization occurs (termed the *end-plate potential*, or EPP) that the motor end-plate threshold for action potential generation is exceeded, and muscle contraction occurs. An isolated action potential produces a twitch, while a train of action potentials may produce sustained contraction of the muscle. Note that although this example uses two MEPPs for simplicity, many more than two MEPPs are actually required to achieve threshold-level depolarization. In this figure, the x-axis is time.

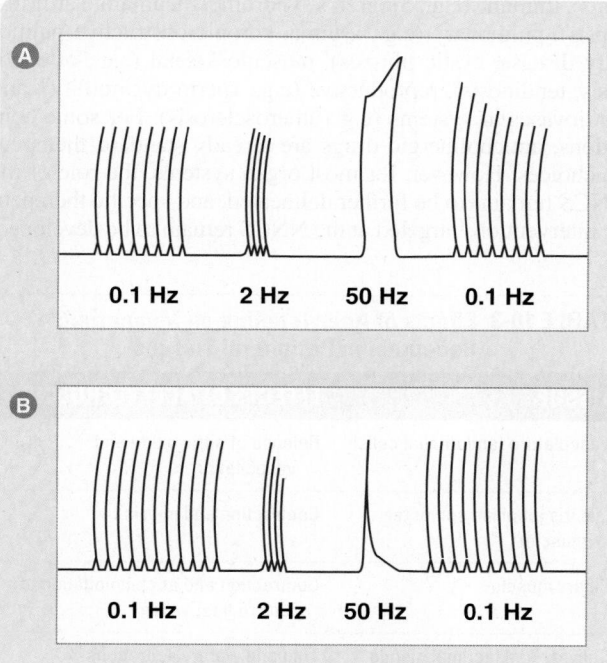

FIGURE 10-6. Tetanic fade and the effects of hexamethonium. A. Control stimulation. Rapid stimulation of muscle contraction relies on presynaptic acetylcholine autoreceptors that provide positive feedback and thereby increase the amount of acetylcholine released with each depolarization. The diagram shows control muscle responses to single-shock stimulation (0.1 Hz), a train of four stimulations (2 Hz), or tetanic stimulation (50 Hz). Positive feedback increases the amount of ACh released with each depolarization during tetanic stimulation, providing enhanced muscle contraction that gradually fades back to baseline during subsequent single-shock stimulation. **B.** Stimulation after the administration of hexamethonium. Note that although the response to isolated (0.1 Hz) stimuli is unchanged in the presence of hexamethonium, the drug prevents the increased effect that normally occurs with higher frequency (50 Hz) stimulation. This is a result of hexamethonium's antagonism of the acetylcholine autoreceptor on the presynaptic terminal that is normally responsible for positive feedback of ACh release.

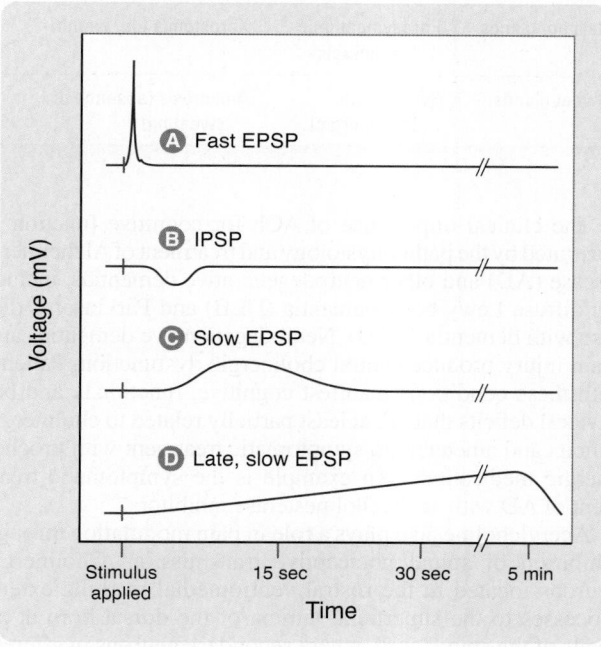

FIGURE 10-7. Four types of synaptic signals in an autonomic ganglion. The response of autonomic ganglia to neurotransmission is a complex event mediated by a number of different neurotransmitters and receptor types and occurring on several distinct time scales. **A.** The primary mode of neurotransmission is the action potential, which is produced by a sufficiently strong (suprathreshold) excitatory postsynaptic potential (EPSP). The fast EPSP is mediated by acetylcholine acting on postsynaptic nicotinic ACh receptors. **B.** The inhibitory postsynaptic potential (IPSP) is a membrane hyperpolarization response. This response is thought to be mediated by several different postsynaptic receptor types, including modulatory dopamine receptors and α-adrenergic receptors as well as M_2 muscarinic ACh receptors. **C.** The slow EPSP is mediated by M_1 muscarinic receptors, has a latency of about 1 second after an initial depolarization, and lasts for 10–30 seconds. **D.** The late, slow EPSP occurs on the order of minutes after a depolarization event. This excitatory response may be mediated by peptides that are co-released with acetylcholine.

TABLE 10-2 Effects of Autonomic Ganglionic Blockade on Tissues

SITE	PREDOMINANT TONE	EFFECTS OF GANGLIONIC BLOCKADE
Arterioles	Sympathetic (adrenergic)	Vasodilation; ↑ peripheral blood flow; hypotension
Veins	Sympathetic (adrenergic)	Vasodilation; pooling of blood; ↓ venous return; ↓ cardiac output
Heart	Parasympathetic (cholinergic)	Tachycardia
Iris	Parasympathetic (cholinergic)	Mydriasis (pupil dilation)
Ciliary muscle	Parasympathetic (cholinergic)	Cycloplegia (focused to far vision)
Gastrointestinal tract	Parasympathetic (cholinergic)	↓ Tone and motility; constipation; ↓ secretions
Urinary bladder	Parasympathetic (cholinergic)	Urinary retention
Salivary glands	Parasympathetic (cholinergic)	Xerostomia (dry mouth)
Sweat glands	Sympathetic (cholinergic)	Anhidrosis (absence of sweating)

The clinical importance of ACh for cognitive function is illustrated by the pathophysiology and treatment of Alzheimer's disease (AD) and other neurodegenerative dementias, including diffuse Lewy body dementia (DLB) and Parkinson's disease with dementia (PDD). Neurodegenerative dementias and brain injury produce central cholinergic dysfunction. Patients with these conditions manifest cognitive, functional, and behavioral deficits that are at least partially related to cholinergic deficits and amenable to symptomatic treatment with procholinergic medications. An example is the symptomatic treatment of AD with acetylcholinesterase inhibitors.

Acetylcholine also plays a role in pain modulation through inhibition of spinal nociceptive transmission. Cholinergic neurons located in the rostral ventromedial medulla extend processes to the superficial lamina of the dorsal horn at all levels of the spinal cord, where secondary neurons in afferent sensory pathways are located. ACh released by the cholinergic neurons is believed to bind to muscarinic ACh receptors located on secondary sensory neurons specific for pain transmission, resulting in suppression of action potential firing in these cells and consequently in analgesia (see Chapter 18). Clinically, the analgesic properties of ACh can be demonstrated by injecting AChE inhibitors into the spinal fluid.

Acetylcholine has CNS effects unrelated to its role as a neurotransmitter. ACh has been observed to inhibit neurite growth. During the early phases of neural development, when such growth is essential, AChE levels are increased. The presence of ACh in chick limb buds and myotomes suggests other, morphogenetic roles for this compound. Lesioning of rat cholinergic neurons during development results in cortical abnormalities, including aberrant growth and positioning of pyramidal cell dendrites, altered cortical connectivity, and

gross cognitive defects. These abnormal findings are also observed in fetal alcohol syndrome and Rett syndrome, both of which demonstrate dramatically reduced numbers of cholinergic neurons in the brain. There is also some evidence for an immunomodulatory role for ACh, as many cells of the immune system both release ACh and express ACh receptors. Finally, mutations have been identified in nicotinic ACh receptor genes that are responsible for autosomal dominant nocturnal frontal lobe epilepsy (ADNFLE); this milestone in epilepsy research is the first demonstration that alterations in a ligand-gated ion channel can cause epilepsy.

The Non-Neuronal Cholinergic System (NNCS)

Cells of various non-neuronal tissues and organs produce ACh (non-neuronal ACh [NN-ACh]). NN-ACh acts in an autocrine and paracrine fashion on nicotinic and muscarinic ACh receptors that are expressed on neighboring ACh-producing or effector cells. The NNCS regulates physiologic processes including cell growth, adhesion, migration, and differentiation. Dysfunction of the NNCS may contribute to the pathogenesis of disease in several organ systems, including the skin (e.g., atopic dermatitis, pemphigus, psoriasis, vitiligo) and the urinary (e.g., overactive bladder syndrome), gastrointestinal (e.g., gastroesophageal reflux disease, peptic ulcer disease, pancreatitis), immune (e.g., Sjogren's syndrome, rheumatoid arthritis, sepsis), pulmonary (e.g., asthma, chronic obstructive pulmonary disease, cystic fibrosis), musculoskeletal (e.g., osteoporosis, tendinosis), reproductive (e.g., sperm dysmotility), and cardiovascular systems (e.g., atherosclerosis). For some conditions, anticholinergic drugs are already standard therapeutic choices. However, for most organ systems, the role of the NNCS remains to be further delineated, and specific therapeutic interventions targeted at the NNCS remain to be developed.

TABLE 10-3 Effects of Acetylcholine on Muscarinic Receptors in Peripheral Tissues

TISSUE	EFFECTS OF ACETYLCHOLINE
Vasculature (endothelial cells)	Release of nitric oxide and vasodilation
Eye iris (pupillae sphincter muscle)	Contraction and miosis
Ciliary muscle	Contraction and accommodation of lens to near vision
Salivary and lacrimal glands	Thin and watery secretions
Bronchi	Constriction; ↑ secretions
Heart	Bradycardia, ↓ conduction velocity, AV block at high doses, slight ↓ in contractility
Gastrointestinal tract	↑ Tone, secretions; relaxation of sphincters
Urinary bladder	Contraction of detrusor muscle; relaxation of sphincter
Sweat glands	Diaphoresis
Reproductive tract, male	Erection
Uterus	Variable

PHARMACOLOGIC CLASSES AND AGENTS

Pharmacologic manipulation of cholinergic transmission has met with only limited success because the complex actions of ACh make it difficult to obtain selective effects. For example, many cholinergic agents are capable of both stimulating and blocking cholinergic receptors through a mechanism known as *depolarizing blockade* (see below). Therefore, only a relatively small fraction of the many cholinergic and anticholinergic agents discovered over the past century are used in clinical practice. These drugs are used primarily for (1) modulation of gastrointestinal motility, (2) xerostomia (dry mouth), (3) glaucoma, (4) motion sickness and antiemesis, (5) neuromuscular diseases such as myasthenia gravis and Eaton-Lambert syndrome, (6) acute neuromuscular blockade and reversal during surgery, (7) ganglionic blockade during aortic dissection, (8) dystonias (e.g., torticollis), headache, and pain syndromes, (9) reversal of vagal-mediated bradycardia, (10) mydriasis, (11) bronchodilation in chronic obstructive pulmonary disease, (12) bladder spasms and urinary incontinence, (13) cosmetic effects on skin lines and wrinkles, and (14) treatment of Alzheimer's disease and other neurodegenerative dementias.

Slight variations in the pharmacologic properties of individual cholinergic and anticholinergic agents are responsible for their large differences in therapeutic utility. The relative selectivity of action of the most useful agents depends on both pharmacodynamic and pharmacokinetic factors, including inherent differences in receptor binding affinity, bioavailability, tissue localization, and resistance to degradation. These variations, in turn, derive from the molecular structure and charge of the drug. The structure of **pirenzepine**, for example, allows the drug to bind M_1 muscarinic receptors (located in autonomic ganglia) with higher affinity than M_2 and M_3 receptors (located at parasympathetic end organs). As a result, the drug's predominant effect at clinically used doses is ganglionic blockade (see Table 10-1). Similarly, the addition of a methyl group to acetylcholine yields **methacholine**, which is more resistant to degradation by AChE and, hence, possesses a longer duration of action. Charged agents such as muscarine generally do not cross membrane barriers. The absorption of such drugs through both the gastrointestinal (GI) mucosa and the blood–brain barrier is significantly impaired, unless specific carriers are available to transport the drug; therefore, such drugs typically have little or no effect on the CNS. In contrast, lipophilic agents have excellent CNS penetration. As one example, the high CNS penetration of **physostigmine** makes this drug the agent of choice for treating the CNS effects of anticholinergic overdose.

The following discussion is ordered mechanistically. For each class of drugs, the selectivity of individual agents within the class is used as a basis to explain the therapeutic uses of each agent.

Inhibitors of Acetylcholine Synthesis, Storage, and Release

Drugs that inhibit the synthesis, storage, or release of ACh have only recently begun to have clinical use (Fig. 10-1). **Hemicholinium-3** blocks the high-affinity transporter for choline and thus prevents the uptake of choline required for ACh synthesis. **Vesamicol** blocks the ACh-H^+ antiporter that transports ACh into vesicles, thereby preventing the storage of ACh. Both of these compounds are utilized only in research settings, however. **Botulinum toxin A**, produced by *Clostridium botulinum*, degrades SNAP-25 and thus prevents synaptic vesicle fusion with the axon terminal (presynaptic) membrane. This paralysis-inducing property is currently used in the treatment of several diseases associated with increased muscle tone, such as torticollis, achalasia, strabismus, blepharospasm, and other focal dystonias. Botulinum toxin is also approved for cosmetic treatment of facial lines or wrinkles and is used to treat various headache and pain syndromes (e.g., by intrathecal delivery into the spinal fluid). Because it degrades a protein common to the synaptic vesicle fusion machinery in multiple types of nerve terminals, botulinum toxin has a general effect on the release of many different neurotransmitters, not just ACh.

Acetylcholinesterase Inhibitors

Agents in this class bind to and inhibit AChE, thereby increasing the concentration of endogenously released ACh in the synaptic cleft. The accumulated ACh subsequently activates nearby cholinergic receptors. Agents in this class are also referred to as *indirectly acting* ACh receptor agonists because they generally do not activate receptors directly. It is important to note that a few AChE inhibitors have a direct action as well. For example, **neostigmine**, a quaternary carbamate, not only blocks AChE but also binds to and activates nAChRs at the neuromuscular junction.

Structural Classes

All indirectly acting cholinergic agonists interfere with the function of AChE by binding to the active site of the enzyme. There are three chemical classes of such agents, including (1) simple alcohols with a quaternary ammonium group, (2) carbamic acid esters of alcohols bearing either quaternary or tertiary ammonium groups, and (3) organic derivatives of phosphoric acid (Fig. 10-8). The most important functional difference among these classes is pharmacokinetic.

Edrophonium is a simple alcohol that inhibits AChE by reversibly associating with the active site of the enzyme. Because of the noncovalent nature of the interaction between the alcohol and AChE, the enzyme–inhibitor complex lasts for only 2–10 minutes, resulting in a relatively rapid but completely reversible block.

The carbamic acid esters **neostigmine** and **physostigmine** are hydrolyzed by AChE, so a labile covalent bond is formed between the drug and the enzyme. However, *the rate at which this reaction occurs is many orders of magnitude lower than for ACh*. The resulting enzyme–inhibitor complex has a half-life of approximately 15–30 minutes, corresponding to an effective inhibition lasting 3–8 hours.

Organophosphates such as **diisopropyl fluorophosphate** have a molecular structure that resembles the transition state formed in carboxyl ester hydrolysis. These compounds are hydrolyzed by AChE, but the resulting phosphorylated enzyme complex is extremely stable and dissociates with a half-life of hundreds of hours. Furthermore, the enzyme–organophosphate complex is subject to a process known as **aging**, in which oxygen–phosphorus bonds within the inhibitor are broken spontaneously in favor of stronger bonds between the enzyme and the inhibitor. Once aging occurs, the duration of AChE inhibition is increased even further. Thus, organophosphate inhibition is essentially irreversible,

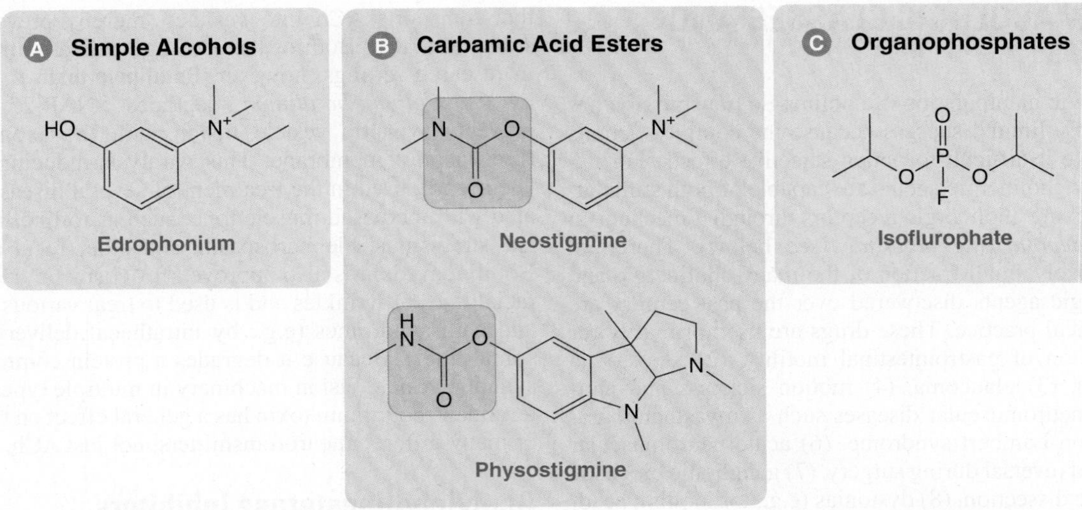

FIGURE 10-8. Structural classes of acetylcholinesterase inhibitors. Acetylcholinesterase (AChE) inhibitors are divided into three structural classes. **A.** Simple alcohols such as edrophonium have a short half-time of AChE inhibition. Edrophonium is used in the diagnosis of myasthenia gravis and other diseases of the neuromuscular junction. **B.** Carbamic acid esters are hydrolyzed by AChE. This results in the formation of a covalent bond between the carbamic acid ester (*boxed*) and AChE and a consequently long half-time of AChE inhibition. Neostigmine is used to treat myasthenia gravis and, during or after surgery, to reverse paralysis induced by nicotinic acetylcholine receptor antagonists. Physostigmine, because it has good CNS penetration, is the agent of choice for treating anticholinergic poisoning. **C.** Organophosphates form an extremely stable phosphorus–carbon bond with AChE. This results in irreversible inactivation of AChE. As a result, many organophosphates are extremely toxic.

and the body must synthesize new AChE molecules to restore AChE activity. However, if strong nucleophiles (such as **pralidoxime**) are administered before aging has occurred, it is possible to displace the organophosphate from the inhibited AChE and recover enzymatic function.

Clinical Applications

Acetylcholinesterase inhibitors have a number of clinical applications, including (1) increasing transmission at the neuromuscular junction, (2) increasing parasympathetic tone, and (3) increasing central cholinergic activity (e.g., to treat symptoms of AD).

Because of their ability to increase the activity of endogenous ACh, AChE inhibitors are especially useful in diseases of the neuromuscular junction, where the primary defect is an insufficient quantity of either ACh or AChR. In myasthenia gravis, autoantibodies are generated against N_M receptors. These antibodies both induce N_M receptor internalization and block the ability of ACh to activate the receptors. As a result, patients with myasthenia gravis present with significant weakness (recall the description of Chief Opechancanough in the introductory case). Eaton-Lambert syndrome is also characterized by muscle weakness, but this disorder is caused by autoantibodies generated against Ca^{2+} channels; both presynaptic Ca^{2+} entry and the subsequent release of ACh in response to axon terminal depolarization are attenuated. Certain anticholinergic drugs, such as tubocurare, also cause weakness or paralysis by acting as competitive antagonists at the nAChR, preventing ACh from binding to the receptor and causing nondepolarizing blockade of cholinergic transmission. Acetylcholinesterase inhibitors (such as the physostigmine used in the introductory case) improve all three of these conditions by increasing the concentration of endogenously released ACh at the neuromuscular junction and thereby increasing ACh signaling.

Because ACh binding to N_M receptors results in muscle cell depolarization, *AChE inhibitors are ineffective at reversing the action of agents that cause paralysis by inducing sustained depolarization, such as succinylcholine* (see below). In fact, AChE inhibitors in sufficiently high doses can exacerbate existing weakness and paralysis caused by depolarizing blockade. Thus, it is of fundamental importance that the cause of the muscle weakness should be determined before treatment is initiated. Short-acting AChE inhibitors such as edrophonium are ideal for such diagnostic purposes. **Edrophonium** mitigates weakness if the blockade is attributable to competitive AChR antagonists or to diseases such as myasthenia gravis or Eaton-Lambert syndrome. In contrast, if muscle strength decreases further with edrophonium administration, then depolarizing blockade may be suspected. The short half-life of edrophonium ensures that exacerbation of the latter condition will last for a minimal amount of time. For chronic treatment of myasthenia gravis, longer acting AChE inhibitors such as **pyridostigmine**, **neostigmine**, and **ambenonium** are the preferred agents.

AChE inhibitors exert other therapeutic effects by potentiating parasympathetic actions in target tissues. Topical application of AChE inhibitors to the cornea of the eye decreases intraocular pressure by facilitating the outflow of aqueous humor. The main effect of AChE inhibitors on the gastrointestinal system is an increase in smooth muscle motility because of enhancement of ganglionic transmission at Auerbach's plexus, although these agents also cause increased secretion of gastric acid and saliva. Neostigmine, the most popular drug for this application, is typically used for relief of abdominal distention. The use of anticholinesterases in reversing anticholinergic drug poisoning is also well established. The agent of choice for this indication is typically **physostigmine**; its tertiary amine structure allows it ready access to the brain and spinal cord, where it can counteract the CNS effects of anticholinergic toxicity.

Acetylcholinesterase inhibitors are also used to treat the symptoms of AD dementia and other conditions causing

TABLE 10-4 Pharmacokinetic and Mechanistic Characteristics of Donepezil, Rivastigmine, Rivastigmine Transdermal Patch, Galantamine, and Galantamine ER

DRUG	BIOAVAILABILITY (%)	T_{MAX} (H)	ELIMINATION HALF-LIFE (H)	HEPATIC METABOLISM	REVERSIBLE INHIBITION OF AChE	OTHER CHOLINOMIMETIC EFFECTS
Donepezil	100	3–5	60–90	Yes	Yes	—
Rivastigmine	40	0.8–1.8	2	No	No*	BuChEI
Rivastigmine Patch	55–65	3.4	8–12	No	No*	BuChEI
Galantamine	85–100	0.5–1.5	5–8	Yes	Yes	nAChR agonist
Galantamine ER	85–100	4.5–5	25–35	Yes	Yes	nAChR agonist

*Rivastigmine is a "pseudo-irreversible" inhibitor of AChE and BuChE.

T_{max}, time to peak plasma concentration; AChE, acetylcholinesterase; BuChEI, butyrylcholinesterase inhibitor; nAChR agonist, allosteric (potentiating) ligand at some nicotinic acetylcholine receptors in the CNS.

dementia (e.g., Parkinson's disease with dementia, diffuse Lewy body dementia, vascular-ischemic dementia), brain injury (e.g., traumatic brain injury), and cognitive impairment (e.g., cognitive impairment associated with multiple sclerosis and schizophrenia). **Donepezil** and **rivastigmine** are second-generation AChE inhibitors indicated for the treatment of AD dementia in the mild, moderate, and severe stages; **galantamine** is a second-generation AChE inhibitor indicated for the treatment of AD dementia in the mild and moderate stages. **Rivastigmine** is also approved by the US Food and Drug Administration (FDA) for the treatment of Parkinson's disease with dementia. **Tacrine** is a first-generation AChE inhibitor that is no longer in clinical use—it had the disadvantage of four-times-daily dosing and it had the potential to cause hepatic toxicity.

In both short-term (24–52 weeks) efficacy trials and long-term clinical effectiveness studies, these AChE inhibitors have demonstrated beneficial effects in producing improvement or stabilization of symptoms and in slowing the progression of cognitive, functional, and behavioral decline in AD dementia. Although there are mechanistic and pharmacokinetic differences among these drugs (Table 10-4), there are no significant differences in their efficacy in the treatment of AD. For example, rivastigmine is a "pseudo-irreversible" cholinesterase inhibitor because it forms a labile carbamoylate complex with AChE (and BuChE), inactivating the enzyme until the covalent bond is broken. While rivastigmine is available as a twice-daily oral preparation, it is now used mostly as a once-daily transdermal patch formulation. Galantamine is both a reversible AChE inhibitor and an allosteric (potentiating) nicotinic receptor ligand. All of these drugs exhibit linear pharmacokinetics, and their time to peak plasma concentration (T_{max}) values and elimination half-lives are prolonged in elderly patients.

With appropriately slow titration, these medications are generally well tolerated and have a favorable adverse effect profile (with the exception of tacrine, which is no longer used clinically; see above). While these medications are relatively selective for AChE in the CNS, the most common adverse effects—including nausea, vomiting, anorexia, flatulence, loose stools, diarrhea, and abdominal cramping—are related to peripheral cholinomimetic effects

on the GI tract. The rivastigmine transdermal patch can also cause skin irritation, redness, and rash at the site of application. The adverse effects of AChE inhibitors may occur in 5–20% of patients, are usually mild and transient, and are related to the dose and rate of dose escalation. For the oral preparations, the adverse GI effects of AChE inhibitors can be minimized by administering the drug after a meal or in combination with memantine, an NMDA channel blocker that is indicated for the treatment of moderate to severe AD. For transdermal rivastigmine, adverse effects can be minimized by applying the patch to a different site each day. These medications may also increase the risk of syncope, particularly in susceptible individuals and with overdose. Use of these agents is contraindicated in patients with unstable or severe cardiac disease (particularly cardiac arrhythmias), uncontrolled epilepsy, unexplained or recurrent syncope, or active peptic ulcer disease.

Receptor Agonists

All cholinergic receptor agonists bind to the ACh binding site of cholinergic receptors. Receptor agonists can be divided into muscarinic and nicotinic receptor-selective agents, although some cross-reactivity exists with virtually all of these agents. Muscarinic receptor agonists are used clinically in the diagnosis of asthma and as miotics (agents that cause pupil constriction). Nicotinic receptor agonists are used clinically for induction of muscle paralysis.

Muscarinic Receptor Agonists

Agents in this class are divided structurally into choline esters and alkaloids (Fig. 10-9). The choline esters are charged, highly hydrophilic molecules that are poorly absorbed by the oral route and inefficiently distributed to the CNS. Choline esters include acetylcholine, methacholine, carbachol, and bethanechol (Table 10-5). Acetylcholine is not administered in clinical settings because of its broad actions and its extremely rapid hydrolysis by AChE and pseudocholinesterase.

Methacholine is at least three times more resistant to hydrolysis by AChE than is ACh. This agent is relatively selective for cardiovascular muscarinic cholinergic receptors, and it has relatively little affinity for nicotinic

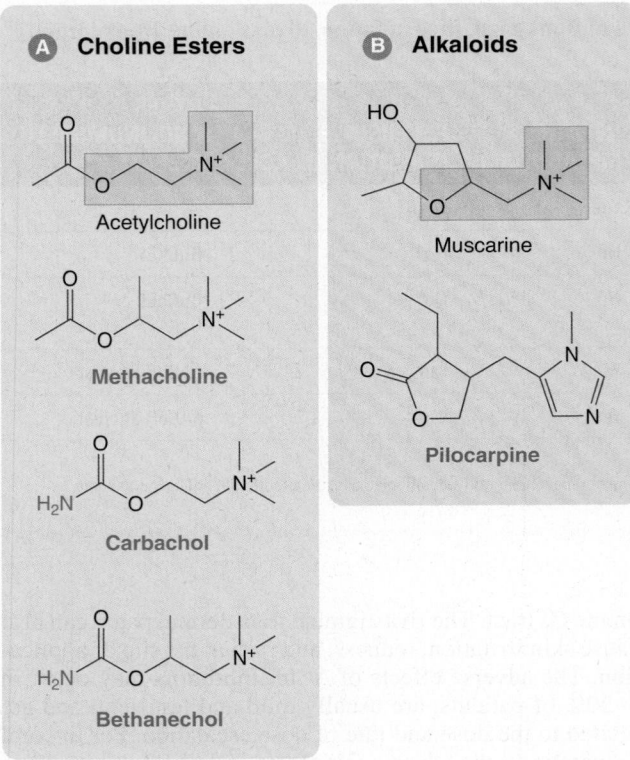

FIGURE 10-9. Structural classes of muscarinic receptor agonists. Muscarinic receptor agonists are divided into choline esters and alkaloids. **A.** Choline esters are charged molecules and therefore have little CNS penetration. Methacholine is highly resistant to AChE and is used in the diagnosis of asthma. Carbachol has both nicotinic and muscarinic receptor activity; it is only used topically for treatment of glaucoma. Bethanechol is highly selective for muscarinic receptors; it is used to promote GI and bladder motility. Shown in blue are groups in the drug molecules that differ from acetylcholine. **B.** Alkaloids have highly variable structures; some have excellent CNS penetration. Muscarine, the prototypical muscarinic receptor agonist, is an alkaloid that is structurally similar to acetylcholine (*boxed areas*). Until recently, pilocarpine was the only alkaloid muscarinic receptor agonist used clinically. It is used to treat xerostomia (dry mouth) in patients with Sjögren's syndrome and postradiation syndromes. Cevimeline, an M_1 and M_3 agonist, is also effective in xerostomia related to Sjögren's syndrome (*not shown*).

cholinergic receptors. Although methacholine can stimulate receptors expressed on cardiovascular tissues, the magnitude of its response is unpredictable. This fact has limited its use as a vasodilator or cardiac **vagomimetic** (i.e., a drug that mimics the cardiac response to vagus nerve [parasympathetic] stimulation, which typically includes bradycardia, decreased contractility, and compensatory sympathetic reflexes). Currently, methacholine is used only in the diagnosis of asthma; in this application, the bronchial hyperreactivity that is characteristic of asthma causes an exaggerated bronchoconstriction response to parasympathomimetics (see Chapter 48).

Both carbachol and bethanechol are resistant to cholinesterases because, in these drugs, a carbamoyl group is substituted for the acetyl ester group of ACh (Fig. 10-9). This resistance to AChE extends their duration of action and allows time for distribution of the intact drug to areas of lower blood flow. **Carbachol** has enhanced nicotinic activity relative to other choline esters. This agent cannot be used systemically because its nicotinic action at autonomic ganglia leads to unpredictable responses. Instead, the agent is used principally as a topical miotic agent, typically in the treatment of glaucoma. Local application of the drug to the cornea of the eye results in both pupillary constriction (miosis) and decreased intraocular pressure.

Bethanechol is almost completely selective for muscarinic receptors. It is an agent of choice for promoting GI and urinary tract motility, particularly for postoperative, postpartum, and drug-related urinary retention and for hypotonic neurogenic bladder.

In contrast to the choline esters, the alkaloids vary greatly in structure. Some are amphipathic, while others are highly charged. Most of these agents are tertiary amines, although a few are quaternary amines with protonated or permanently charged nitrogens substituting for the choline-centered N of ACh. The amphipathic nature of the tertiary amine alkaloids permits absorption through the GI mucosa and penetration into the CNS. **Muscarine** is an example of a quaternary amine alkaloid that has low bioavailability because of its permanently charged nature.

Most alkaloids are primarily of value in pharmacologic research. The most clinically used alkaloid is **pilocarpine**, a miotic agent and a sialagogue (saliva-inducing agent) used to treat xerostomia (dryness of the mouth secondary to reduced salivary secretion). **Cevimeline**, an M_1 and M_3 agonist, is used to treat xerostomia in Sjögren's syndrome.

Nicotinic Receptor Agonists

Succinylcholine is a choline ester that has high affinity for nicotinic receptors and is resistant to AChE. It is used to induce paralysis during surgery by means of **depolarizing blockade**. This effect can be caused by any direct nAChR *agonist* because such drugs activate receptor-associated channels and produce depolarization of the cell membrane.

TABLE 10-5 Relative Pharmacologic Properties of Choline Esters

ESTER	SUSCEPTIBILITY TO AChE	CARDIAC ACTIVITY	GI ACTIVITY	URINARY ACTIVITY	EYE ACTIVITY (TOPICAL)	ATROPINE ANTAGONISM	NICOTINIC ACTIVITY
Acetylcholine	+++	++	++	++	+	+++	++
Methacholine	+	+++	++	++	+	+++	+
Carbachol	−	+	+++	+++	++	+	+++
Bethanechol	−	±	+++	+++	++	+++	−

Note that all actions are mediated by muscarinic receptors, with the exception of nicotinic activity. "−" indicates negligible activity. "±" indicates unpredictable.

TABLE 10-6 Comparison of Nondepolarizing and Depolarizing NMJ-Blocking Agents

EFFECT	NONDEPOLARIZING	DEPOLARIZING
Effect on motor end-plate	Increased activation threshold to ACh; no depolarization	Partial; persisting depolarization
Initial excitatory effect on muscle	None	Transient fasciculations
Muscle response to tetanic stimulation during partial block	Poorly sustained contraction	Well-sustained contraction
Effect of previous administration of a competitive NMJ-blocking agent	Additive effect	Antagonistic effect
Effect of previous administration of a depolarizing NMJ-blocking agent	No effect or antagonistic effect	No effect or additive effect

In order to produce depolarizing blockade, the agent must persist at the neuromuscular junction and activate the nicotinic receptor channels continuously. Note that this effect is unlike the depolarization pattern seen in the generation of a standard action potential or end-plate potential, in which ACh is present at the neuromuscular junction for only a brief period of time.

The overall pattern is a brief period of excitation, manifested by widespread fasciculations in muscle cells, followed by flaccid paralysis. The paralysis occurs for two reasons. First, the open cholinergic channels maintain the cell membrane in a depolarized state, effecting inactivation of voltage-gated sodium channels so that they cannot open to support further action potentials. Second, the agonist-bound nAChRs spontaneously desensitize, preventing their opening and response to any subsequently delivered, additional agonist. Because of this mechanism, *any nAChR agonist, including ACh, is capable of producing depolarizing blockade at sufficiently high concentrations.* Generally, depolarizing blockade with succinylcholine is used for only short durations because prolonged depolarization can lead to life-threatening electrolyte imbalances (caused by prolonged Na^+ influx and K^+ efflux). Table 10-6 compares the effects of depolarizing and nondepolarizing NMJ-blocking agents.

The concept of depolarizing blockade pertains to *all* cholinergic receptors and is *not strictly limited to the NMJ.* For example, this mechanism accounts for the paradoxical suppression of parasympathomimetic activity at autonomic ganglia by high levels of agonists, such as nicotine, that are selective for nicotinic receptors. The potential for inducing depolarizing blockade is partially responsible for the unpredictable effects of nAChR agonists. Although muscarinic receptor agonists can also cause depolarizing blockade at autonomic ganglia, this effect is obscured by the overwhelmingly parasympathomimetic responses seen at other neuroeffector sites.

The toxic effects of cholinergic agents and poisons are described in Box 10-1.

Receptor Antagonists

Antagonists of AChRs act by binding directly to the agonist site and competitively blocking stimulation of the receptor by endogenous ACh or exogenously administered receptor agonists.

Muscarinic Receptor Antagonists

Anticholinergic compounds that act on muscarinic receptors are used to produce a parasympatholytic effect in target organs. By blocking normal cholinergic tone, these compounds allow sympathetic responses to predominate (Table 10-2). The most commonly used anticholinergics are either naturally occurring alkaloids or synthetic quaternary ammonium compounds. The alkaloids are relatively selective for antagonist activity at muscarinic receptors, whereas the synthetic compounds also demonstrate substantial antagonism at nicotinic receptors.

The prototypical muscarinic receptor antagonist is **atropine**, a naturally occurring alkaloid found in the plant *Atropa belladonna*, or deadly nightshade. Belladonna derived its name from Italian for "beautiful woman"—during the Renaissance, women in Italy ingested or applied to their eyes extracts and juices of berries from the plant to cause dilation of the pupils, which was considered a mark of beauty. Atropine is used clinically to induce mydriasis (pupil dilation) for ophthalmologic examinations, to reverse symptomatic sinus bradycardia, to inhibit excessive salivation and mucus secretion during surgery, to prevent vagal reflexes induced by surgical trauma of visceral organs, and to counteract the effects of muscarine poisoning from certain mushrooms (see Box 10-1). Because of its marginal activity at nicotinic receptors, extremely high doses of atropine are required for any effects to be seen at the NMJ. Similarly, because nicotinic receptors are primarily responsible for excitatory transmission at autonomic ganglia, atropine produces only partial block at these sites and only at relatively high doses.

Scopolamine (hyoscine hydrobromide), a tertiary amine, differs from atropine by virtue of its substantial CNS effects. Scopolamine is frequently used for the prevention and treatment of motion sickness, as an antiemetic, and, in the hospice setting, as an adjunct to end-of-life comfort care medications to effect mild sedation and management of oral secretions. A transdermal patch system has been developed to effect slow absorption and long duration of the anti-motion sickness effect while avoiding a rapid rise in plasma levels and adverse CNS effects (e.g., anterograde disruption of novel learning and memory encoding, inattention, and slowing of psychomotor speed). Scopolamine can also be used to ameliorate nausea, particularly that associated with chemotherapy, and can be administered intravenously during procedures in which minimizing oral secretions is desirable.

Methscopolamine and **glycopyrrolate** are quaternary amine antimuscarinics with low CNS penetration that are used for their peripheral effects to decrease oral secretions, decrease GI spasms, and, in the case of glycopyrrolate, prevent bradycardia during surgical procedures. Both drugs have delayed but measurable CNS and cognitive anticholinergic effects. **Pirenzepine**, which is selective for M_1 and M_4 receptors, was a potential alternative to H_2 receptor antagonists in the treatment of peptic ulcer disease, but its use has been supplanted by the advent of the proton pump inhibitors (see Chapter 47).

Ipratropium, a synthetic quaternary ammonium compound, is more effective than β-adrenergic agonists in the treatment of chronic obstructive pulmonary disease (COPD) but less effective in treating asthma. **Tiotropium** has

BOX 10-1 Cholinergic Toxicity

The toxic effects of cholinergic agents are a function of their mechanism of action (e.g., muscarinic versus nicotinic stimulation), dose and duration of exposure, route of absorption, CNS penetration, and metabolism.

Muscarinic Cholinergic Toxicity

Acute toxicity with direct muscarinic agents is often due to ingestion of toxic mushrooms (e.g., mushrooms in the genus *Inocybe*) and drugs such as pilocarpine. Adverse effects of muscarinic overstimulation typically manifest within 15–30 minutes and include nausea, vomiting, diarrhea, sweating, hypersalivation, cutaneous flushing, reflex tachycardia (sometimes bradycardia), and bronchoconstriction. Intoxication with these agents can be treated by competitive blockade using atropine.

Nicotinic Cholinergic Toxicity

Acute toxicity with nicotine, often due to ingestion of cigarettes and insecticides, produces adverse effects on the CNS, skeletal muscle end-plate, and cardiovascular system. Acute nicotinic toxicity can cause CNS hyperexcitation (seizures progressing to coma and respiratory arrest), skeletal muscle depolarization blockade (respiratory arrest), and cardiovascular abnormalities (hypertension and arrhythmias). As little as 40 mg of nicotine (equivalent to 1 mg of pure liquid nicotine, or the amount of nicotine found in two regular cigarettes) can be fatal, especially in infants. Treatment, including antiepileptic drugs and mechanical ventilation, is dictated by symptoms. Atropine may be used to counteract parasympathetic stimulation.

Cholinesterase Inhibitor Poisoning

Acute cholinesterase inhibitor toxicity is often due to exposure to organophosphate pesticides. Such exposures remain an important threat to children and those in the developing world. Initially, signs of muscarinic toxicity predominate, including vomiting, diarrhea, profuse sweating, hypersalivation, miosis, and bronchoconstriction. Signs of nicotinic toxicity often follow rapidly, including confusion and seizures due to CNS hyperexcitation and respiratory compromise due to depolarizing neuromuscular blockade. Treatment includes emergency management of vital signs (particularly maintaining respiratory integrity), decontamination, symptomatic treatment with atropine, and pralidoxime (PAM) administration to regenerate active enzyme from the organophosphorus–cholinesterase complex (mostly at skeletal muscle neuromuscular junctions; PAM does not readily penetrate the CNS). Time is of the essence to maximize the potential for recovery. Large doses of atropine may be necessary in some cases (e.g., when toxicity is due to potent agents such as parathion and chemical nerve agents); 1–2 mg of intravenous atropine is administered every 5–15 minutes until signs of effect (such as reversal of miosis and dry mouth) are noted and maintained. Repeated administration of atropine may be required for hours or days, depending on the elimination half-life of the organophosphate.

Examples of misuse of cholinergic chemical agents include the use of Sarin nerve gas in the 1980s by Iraq against Kurdish civilians and Iranian troops and in 1995 by a Japanese terrorist in an attack on Tokyo subway passengers. **Sarin**, one of a class of nerve agents known as "G" agents that also includes tabun and soman, is a colorless and odorless gas with high toxic potency; as little as 0.5 mg of Sarin is lethal for adults. Time is of the utmost importance in recognizing an exposure, providing rapid decontamination in accordance with hazmat protocols, and administering atropine and pralidoxime. When exposure to nerve agents can be expected, prophylaxis may be achieved with pyridostigmine or physostigmine (e.g., as prophylactically administered to some US troops in the Gulf War). ■

---

similar, and possibly superior, efficacy to ipratropium as a bronchodilator in the treatment of COPD. The superior efficacy of ipratropium and tiotropium in COPD is likely due to the fact that the major reversible bronchoconstrictive component in COPD is mediated by cholinergic neural tone (see Chapter 48). In poorly controlled asthma, the addition of tiotropium to inhaled glucocorticoids and long-acting beta-agonists may significantly increase the time to first severe exacerbation and provide modest sustained bronchodilation.

Some antimuscarinic drugs are used in the treatment of urinary incontinence and overactive bladder syndrome. Muscarinic stimulation promotes voiding by causing (1) detrusor muscle contraction and (2) bladder trigone and sphincter muscle relaxation. Antimuscarinics produce the opposite effects by promoting detrusor relaxation and tightening the bladder sphincter. Antimuscarinics currently approved for the treatment of overactive bladder include **oxybutynin**, **propantheline**, **terodiline**, **tolterodine**, **fesoterodine**, **trospium**, **darifenacin**, and **solifenacin**. Among these agents, oxybutynin, propantheline, tolterodine, fesoterodine, and trospium are nonspecific muscarinic receptor antagonists, whereas darifenacin and solifenacin are selective M_3 receptor antagonists. These agents appear to have similar clinical efficacy. Clinical trials suggest that tolterodine may cause less dry mouth than oxybutynin and that the newer M_3-selective agents darifenacin and solifenacin may cause less dry mouth and constipation than the nonselective agents.

Atropine, from belladonna extract, was one of the drugs first used to treat symptoms of Parkinson's disease (PD). Antimuscarinics are still used at times to ameliorate tremor and rigidity in patients with PD. These medications include **amantadine**, **biperiden**, **benztropine**, **procyclidine**, and **trihexyphenidyl**. Although antimuscarinics may be helpful in the treatment of PD-related tremor and rigidity, the *use of antimuscarinics in elderly and cognitively susceptible patients should be avoided* because of the high risk of potential adverse effects (see Box 10-2). **Benztropine** and **trihexyphenidyl** are commonly used to treat extrapyramidal symptoms, dystonias, and akathisia associated with neuroleptics; these adverse effects are thought to be due to an imbalance between dopaminergic and cholinergic pathways secondary to excessive neuroleptic-induced dopamine antagonism. **Trihexyphenidyl** is also used to treat neuroleptic-induced hypersalivation syndrome.

BOX 10-2 Potential Adverse Effects of Drugs with Anticholinergic Properties in Geriatric and Cognitively Impaired Patients

Drug-related anticholinergic adverse effects are potentially hazardous to elderly patients, especially those with cognitive impairment, and cause significant morbidity in this population. Additive anticholinergic effects from medications can compromise the safety of geriatric patients because (1) many common drugs possess at least a small measure of anticholinergic activity, (2) the elderly, and especially the cognitively impaired elderly, are exquisitely sensitive to cholinergic blockade (due to central cholinergic hypofunction and dysfunction in aging and dementia, respectively), and (3) polypharmacy is a common practice in the geriatric population. Adverse effects from anticholinergic drugs in the elderly may include acute encephalopathy (delirium, confusional state), falls, urinary retention, constipation, and exacerbation and decompensation of underlying cognitive, functional, and behavioral deficits (particularly in patients with dementia) and may necessitate increased care and hospitalization. It should be noted that many over-the-counter medications have anticholinergic effects. For example, a common offender in causing confusion and cognitive dysfunction in the elderly and cognitively impaired individuals is **diphenhydramine**, an antihistamine with anticholinergic properties that is often used as a hypnotic either alone or in combination with acetaminophen. Clinicians and pharmacists should be vigilant to minimize polypharmacy in the geriatric population and to monitor and prevent medication-related anticholinergic adverse events. The updated Beers Criteria of potentially inappropriate drugs for elderly patients identifies medications (many with anticholinergic properties) and classes of medications, and specific medications in patients with certain conditions, that may pose greater potential risks than benefits in persons older than 65 years of age. Particular caution must be used with medications with strong anticholinergic effects; these include diphenhydramine, scopolamine, antimuscarinic agents used for urinary incontinence, antispasmodics, skeletal muscle relaxants, tricyclic antidepressants, and some antipsychotics (Table 10-7). ■

TABLE 10-7 Medications with Anticholinergic Properties That Can Be Inappropriate for Use by Cognitively Impaired Older Adults (2012 AGS Beers Criteria)

Antihistamines	Antiparkinson Agents	Antidepressants
Brompheniramine	Benztropine	Amitriptyline
Carbinoxamine	Trihexyphenidyl	Amoxapine
Chlorpheniramine		Clomipramine
Clemastine	**Skeletal Muscle Relaxants**	Desipramine
Cyproheptadine		Doxepin
Dimenhydrinate	Carisoprodol	Imipramine
Diphenhydramine	Cyclobenzaprine	Nortriptyline
Hydroxyzine	Orphenadrine	Paroxetine
Loratadine	Tizanidine	Protriptyline
Meclizine		Trimipramine

Antispasmodics	Antipsychotics	Antimuscarinics *(urinary incontinence)*
Atropine products	Chlorpromazine	
Belladonna alkaloids	Clozapine	Darifenacin
Dicyclomine	Fluphenazine	Fesoterodine
Homatropine	Loxapine	Flavoxate
Hyoscyamine products	Olanzapine	Oxybutynin
Loperamide	Perphenazine	Solifenacin
Propantheline	Pimozide	Tolterodine
Scopolamine	Prochlorperazine	Trospium
	Promethazine	
	Thioridazine	
	Thiothixene	
	Trifluoperazine	

Adapted with permission from The American Geriatrics Society. American Geriatrics Society updated Beers Criteria for potentially inappropriate medication use in older adults. *J Am Geriatr Soc* 2012;60:616–631. doi:10.1111/j.1532-5415.2012.03923.x.

Antimuscarinic toxicity causes substantial morbidity and functional impairment in the geriatric population (see Box 10-2). Depending on the dose, antimuscarinic agents such as atropine and scopolamine may cause bradycardia and sedation at low to medium levels of muscarinic blockade, and tachycardia and CNS hyperexcitation (with delirium, hallucinations, and seizures) at higher levels. Other adverse effects may include blurred vision (cycloplegia and mydriasis), dry mouth, ileus, urinary retention, flushing and fever, agitation, and tachycardia. Antimuscarinic medications are contraindicated in patients with glaucoma. Patients with angle-closure glaucoma, which may be precipitated in individuals with shallow anterior chambers, are especially at risk. Antimuscarinics should also be used with caution in patients with prostatic hypertrophy and in patients with dementia or cognitive impairment. Antimuscarinic toxicity is considered dangerous in infants and children, who are exquisitely sensitive to the hyperthermic adverse effects caused by an overdose. Symptomatic treatment may include controlled cooling and

antiepileptic drugs, but slow administration of low doses of intravenous physostigmine may also be required.

High doses of quaternary antimuscarinics and short-acting ganglionic blockers (such as trimethaphan) can cause parasympathetic ganglionic toxicity, manifested as autonomic blockade and severe orthostatic hypotension. The antimuscarinic effects may be treated with neostigmine, and the hypotension may require treatment with sympathomimetics such as phenylephrine.

Nicotinic Receptor Antagonists

Selective nicotinic receptor antagonists are used primarily to produce **nondepolarizing (competitive) neuromuscular blockade** during surgical procedures. Nondepolarizing neuromuscular junction (NMJ) blockers, such as **tubocurare**, act by antagonizing nicotinic ACh receptors directly, thus preventing binding of endogenously released ACh and subsequent muscle cell depolarization. This leads to flaccid paralysis that is similar in presentation to the paralysis in myasthenia gravis. In selecting a specific agent, the primary consideration is its duration of action—ranging from very long-lasting agents (**d-tubocurarine, pancuronium**) to intermediate-duration agents (**vecuronium, rocuronium**) to rapidly degraded compounds (**mivacurium**). Because nicotinic receptors are expressed in autonomic ganglia as well as the NMJ, nondepolarizing blocking agents often have variable adverse effects associated with ganglionic blockade. Both the muscular paralysis and the autonomic blockade can be reversed by administration of AChE inhibitors. A new class of agents, epitomized by **sugammadex**, can also be used to accelerate the recovery of blockade by **vecuronium** and **rocuronium**. These agents act by chelating vecuronium or rocuronium in an inactive complex, which is then slowly cleared from the circulation. Sugammadex is investigational in the United States.

In special cases, compounds with relatively selective antagonist activity at nAChRs can be used to induce autonomic blockade. The effects of autonomic ganglionic blockade are discussed above and are listed in detail in Table 10-2. Most commonly, **mecamylamine** and **trimethaphan** are administered when ganglionic blockade is desired. The only current use for these agents is to treat hypertension in patients with acute aortic dissection, because the drugs lower blood pressure while simultaneously blunting the sympathetic reflexes that would normally cause a deleterious rise in pressure at the site of the tear.

◼ CONCLUSION AND FUTURE DIRECTIONS

There are two major classes of cholinergic receptors: nicotinic and muscarinic. Nicotinic receptors are ligand-gated channels that require the direct binding of two acetylcholine molecules to open. These receptors comprise all of the cholinergic receptors at the neuromuscular junction (N_M), and they predominate at autonomic ganglia (N_N). Thus, the primary cholinergic functions mediated by nAChRs include skeletal muscle contraction and autonomic activity. The predominant applications of pharmacologic agents directed at nAChRs are (1) neuromuscular blockade, through competitive antagonists and depolarizing blockers, and (2) ganglionic blockade, which results in effector organ responses that are opposite to those produced by physiologic autonomic tone.

Muscarinic receptors are G protein-coupled receptors that bind acetylcholine and initiate signaling through several intracellular pathways. These receptors are expressed in the autonomic ganglia and effector organs, where they mediate a parasympathetic response. The primary use of muscarinic receptor agonists and antagonists is to modulate autonomic responses of effector organs. Both nicotinic and muscarinic receptors are ubiquitous in the CNS, where the effects of acetylcholine include analgesia, arousal, and attention. The relative roles of mAChRs and nAChRs in the brain and spinal cord are not fully understood, and the most effective currently available CNS drugs increase endogenous cholinergic transmission by inhibiting the action of acetylcholinesterase, the enzyme that hydrolyzes ACh.

Although cholinergic pharmacology is a relatively mature field with several receptor-selective agents, the specificity of action of the various agents continues to be refined. The discovery of muscarinic receptor subtype diversity may lead to the development of agents selective for subtypes that are expressed in a tissue-specific pattern. Similarly, elucidation of the role of nicotinic receptor subunit diversity in the CNS has spurred development of more selective agents that modulate the activity of these receptor subtypes. For example, a selective partial agonist at the α_7 nicotinic ACh receptor is in late-stage clinical trial testing in AD dementia. Another avenue for future investigation involves positive allosteric modulators of nicotinic receptors; these agents may augment endogenous cholinergic tone in a manner that is more spatially and temporally specific, thus potentially providing differential efficacy and improved safety.

Acetylcholinesterase inhibitors are widely used in clinical practice and are standard of care in the treatment of AD and other dementias. They may provide short-term (6–12 month) symptomatic benefits in AD and, when used chronically, slow clinical decline. Several nicotinic and muscarinic agonists and receptor modulators are in clinical development for the treatment of cognitive impairment, AD dementia, neuropathic pain syndromes, and neuroprotection. Nicotinic receptors may also provide targets for future treatment approaches in epilepsy.

Finally, the physiologic and pathophysiologic roles of the non-neuronal cholinergic system remain to be fully delineated, and specific therapies targeted at this system remain to be developed.

Suggested Reading

Abirishami A, Ho J, Wong J, Yin L, Chung F. Sugammadex, a selective reversal medication for preventing postoperative residual neuromuscular blockade. *Cochrane Database Syst Rev* 2009;4:CD007362. (*Reviews clinical trials on the effectiveness of sugammadex in postoperative recovery.*)

Albuquerque EX, Pereira EFR, Alkondon M, Rogers SW. Mammalian nicotinic acetylcholine receptors: from structure to function. *Physiol Rev* 2009;89:73–120. (*Excellent review of nAChR structure, gating, and physiologic roles.*)

Atri A, Shaughnessy LW, Locascio JJ, Growdon JH. Long-term course and effectiveness of combination therapy in Alzheimer disease. *Alzheimer Dis Assoc Disord* 2008;22:209–221. (*Assesses long-term clinical effectiveness of cholinergic and glutamatergic anti-AD medications in slowing the course of AD dementia.*)

Beckmann J, Lips KS. The non-neuronal cholinergic system in health and disease. *Pharmacology* 2013;92:286–302. (*Reviews the non-neuronal cholinergic system and its role in normal and pathologic processes and conditions.*)

Dani JA, Bertrand D. Nicotinic acetylcholine receptors and nicotinic cholinergic mechanisms of the central nervous system. *Ann Rev Pharmacol Toxicol* 2007;47:699–729. (*A thorough review of the nicotinic cholinergic system, with many citations.*)

Kerstjens HA, Engel M, Dahl R, et al. Tiotropium in asthma poorly controlled with standard combination therapy. *N Engl J Med* 2012;367: 1198–1207. (*Replicate clinical trials demonstrating that the addition of tiotropium to inhaled glucocorticoids and long-acting beta-agonists significantly increases time to first severe exacerbation and provides sustained bronchodilation in poorly controlled asthma.*)

Marchi M, Grilli M. Presynaptic nicotinic receptors modulating neurotransmitter release in the central nervous system: functional interactions with other coexisting receptors. *Prog Neurobiol* 2010;92:105–111. (*A brief and readable review.*)

Rountree SD, Atri A, Lopez OL, Doody RS. Effectiveness of antidementia drugs in delaying Alzheimer's disease progression. *Alzheimers Dement* 2013;9:338–345. (*Reviews the evidence base for cholinergic and other medications in AD dementia.*)

Sher E, Chen Y, Sharples TJW, Broad LM. Physiological roles of neuronal nicotinic receptor subtypes: new insights on the nicotinic modulation of neurotransmitter release, synaptic transmission and plasticity. *Curr Topics Med Chem* 2004;4:283–297. (*A thorough treatise on this important topic.*)

Uteshev VV. The therapeutic promise of positive allosteric modulation of nicotinic receptors. *Eur J Pharmacol* 2014;727:181–185. (*Reviews theoretical and practical considerations for the role of positive allosteric modulators of nicotinic ACh receptors.*)

DRUG SUMMARY TABLE: CHAPTER 10 Cholinergic Pharmacology

INHIBITORS OF ACETYLCHOLINE SYNTHESIS, STORAGE, AND RELEASE
Mechanism—Inhibit the synthesis, storage, or release of acetylcholine

DRUG	CLINICAL APPLICATIONS	*SERIOUS* AND COMMON ADVERSE EFFECTS	CONTRAINDICATIONS	THERAPEUTIC CONSIDERATIONS
Hemicholinium-3 **Vesamicol**	None (used experimentally only)	Not applicable	Not applicable	Hemicholinium-3 blocks the high-affinity transporter for choline and thereby prevents the uptake of choline required for ACh synthesis. Vesamicol blocks the ACh-H$^+$ antiporter that transports ACh into synaptic vesicles. Both of these compounds are utilized only in research settings.
Botulinum toxin	Focal dystonias Torticollis Achalasia Strabismus Blepharospasm Headache and pain syndromes Wrinkles Hyperhidrosis	*Cardiac arrhythmia, syncope, hepatotoxicity, anaphylaxis* Injection-site pain, dyspepsia, dysphagia, muscle weakness, neck pain, eyelid ptosis, fever	Hypersensitivity to botulinum toxin Infection at the proposed injection site	Botulinum toxin, produced by *Clostridium botulinum*, degrades synaptobrevin and thus prevents synaptic vesicle fusion with the axon terminal (presynaptic) membrane.

INHIBITORS OF ACETYLCHOLINE DEGRADATION
Mechanism—Inhibit acetylcholinesterase (AChE) by binding to the enzyme's active site

DRUG	CLINICAL APPLICATIONS	*SERIOUS* AND COMMON ADVERSE EFFECTS	CONTRAINDICATIONS	THERAPEUTIC CONSIDERATIONS
Edrophonium **Neostigmine** **Pyridostigmine** **Ambenonium** **Physostigmine**	Diagnosis of myasthenia gravis, reversal of neuromuscular blockade (edrophonium only) Urinary or gastrointestinal motility agent, neuromuscular junction diseases such as myasthenia gravis (pyridostigmine, neostigmine, and ambenonium only) Glaucoma (neostigmine, pyridostigmine, ambenonium, and physostigmine only) Antidote to anticholinergic overdose (physostigmine only)	*Seizure, bronchospasm, cardiac arrhythmia, bradycardia, cardiac arrest* Hypotension or hypertension, salivation, lacrimation, diaphoresis, vomiting, diarrhea, miosis, frequent urination	Hypersensitivity to drug (shared contraindication) Mechanical intestinal or urinary obstruction (edrophonium, neostigmine, pyridostigmine, and physostigmine only) Concomitant choline ester or depolarizing neuromuscular blocker use (ambenonium and physostigmine only) Cardiovascular disease, asthma, diabetes, gangrene (physostigmine only)	Edrophonium is short-acting (2–10 minutes); rapid onset of action makes edrophonium useful for diagnosis of muscle weakness. For chronic treatment of myasthenia gravis, longer acting cholinesterase inhibitors such as pyridostigmine, neostigmine, and ambenonium are preferred. Neostigmine also has direct cholinergic agonist effect at N$_M$ receptors. Topical application of cholinesterase inhibitors to the cornea of the eye decreases intraocular pressure by facilitating the outflow of aqueous humor. Nonpolar structure makes physostigmine useful for treating anticholinergic CNS toxicity.
Diisopropyl fluorophosphates	Not applicable (sometimes encountered as a toxin)	*Respiratory paralysis* Bradycardia, bronchospasm, fasciculations, muscle cramps, weakness, CNS depression, agitation, confusion, delirium, coma, bronchorrhea, salivation, lacrimation, diaphoresis, vomiting, diarrhea, miosis	Not applicable	An organophosphate compound used as an insecticide, as a substrate for the production of organophosphate chemical weapons (nerve gases), and formerly as a topical miotic medication in ophthalmology.

continues

DRUG SUMMARY TABLE: CHAPTER 10 Cholinergic Pharmacology *continued*

DRUG	CLINICAL APPLICATIONS	SERIOUS AND COMMON ADVERSE EFFECTS	CONTRAINDICATIONS	THERAPEUTIC CONSIDERATIONS
Donepezil **Rivastigmine** **Galantamine**	Alzheimer's dementia (shared indication) Dementia associated with Parkinson's disease (rivastigmine only)	*Cardiac arrhythmia (shared adverse effect); gastrointestinal hemorrhage (donepezil and galantamine only); pancreatitis, stroke, seizure, delirium, bronchospasm (rivastigmine only)* Diarrhea, nausea, vomiting, cramps, anorexia, vivid dreams, insomnia	Hypersensitivity to drug	Second-generation AChE inhibitors that provide symptomatic benefits and/or slowing clinical decline in Alzheimer's dementia. Rivastigmine inhibits both acetylcholinesterase and butyrylcholinesterase by forming a carbamoylate complex with the enzymes. Galantamine also acts as an allosteric (potentiating) ligand at nicotinic receptors. Tacrine is a first-generation cholinesterase inhibitor that is no longer used.

MUSCARINIC RECEPTOR AGONISTS
Mechanism—Stimulate muscarinic receptor activity

DRUG	CLINICAL APPLICATIONS	SERIOUS AND COMMON ADVERSE EFFECTS	CONTRAINDICATIONS	THERAPEUTIC CONSIDERATIONS
Methacholine	Diagnosis of asthma	*Dyspnea* Light-headedness, headache, pruritus, throat irritation	Hypersensitivity to methacholine Recent myocardial infarction or stroke Aortic aneurysm Uncontrolled hypertension Low baseline pulmonary function tests	Methacholine is highly resistant to acetylcholinesterase; it is relatively selective for cardiovascular muscarinic cholinergic receptors.
Carbachol **Bethanechol** **Cevimeline** **Pilocarpine**	Glaucoma (carbachol and pilocarpine only) Raised intraocular pressure (carbachol and pilocarpine only) Miosis induction for surgical procedure (carbachol only) Urinary tract motility agent (bethanechol only) Xerostomia in Sjögren's syndrome (cevimeline and pilocarpine only) Radiation-induced xerostomia (pilocarpine only)	*Retinal detachment (carbachol and pilocarpine only); seizure, asthma exacerbation (bethanechol only); pulmonary edema (pilocarpine only)* Clouding of corneal stroma (carbachol only); sweating, shivering, nausea, dizziness, increased frequency of urination, rhinitis (bethanechol, cevimeline, and pilocarpine only)	Hypersensitivity to drug (shared contraindication) Acute iritis (carbachol, pilocarpine, and cevimeline only) Narrow-angle glaucoma (cevimeline and pilocarpine only) Asthma (bethanechol, pilocarpine, and cevimeline only) Bradycardia, hypotension, coronary artery disease, epilepsy, compromised integrity of gastrointestinal or bladder wall, hyperthyroidism, parkinsonism, peptic ulcer (bethanechol only)	Carbachol has enhanced nicotinic action relative to other choline esters; carbachol cannot be used systemically because of its unpredictable nicotinic action at autonomic ganglia; topical application of carbachol to the cornea of the eye results in both pupillary constriction (miosis) and decreased intraocular pressure. Bethanechol is almost completely selective for muscarinic receptors. Pilocarpine and cevimeline (an M_1 and M_3 agonist) are used to treat xerostomia in Sjögren's syndrome.

NICOTINIC RECEPTOR AGONISTS

Mechanism—Stimulate opening of nicotinic ACh receptor channel and produce depolarization of the cell membrane; succinylcholine persists at the neuromuscular junction and activates the nicotinic receptor channels continuously, which results in inactivation of voltage-gated sodium channels so that they cannot open to support further action potentials (sometimes called *depolarizing blockade*)

Drug	Indications	Adverse Effects	Contraindications	Notes
Succinylcholine	Induction of neuromuscular blockade in surgery Intubation	*Cardiac arrhythmia, cardiac arrest, hyperkalemia, malignant hyperthermia, rhabdomyolysis, anaphylaxis, renal failure, respiratory depression* Raised intraocular pressure	Hypersensitivity to succinylcholine Personal or family history of malignant hyperthermia Skeletal muscle myopathies Upper motor neuron injury Extensive denervation of skeletal muscle	Short duration of action makes succinylcholine drug of choice for paralysis during intubation. Causes transient fasciculations.

MUSCARINIC RECEPTOR ANTAGONISTS

Mechanism—Selectively antagonize muscarinic receptors

Drug	Indications	Adverse Effects	Contraindications	Notes
Atropine	Biliary colic Acute symptomatic bradyarrhythmia Gastrointestinal spasm Atrioventricular heart block Mydriasis induction Ureteric colic Organophosphate poisoning Poisoning by other parasympathomimetic drugs or substances (e.g., toxic mushrooms)	*Cardiac arrhythmia, myocardial infarction, anaphylaxis, delirium, hallucinations, seizure, glaucoma, pulmonary edema* Tachycardia, dry mucous membranes, flushing, gastrointestinal upset, xerostomia, dizziness, headache, blurred vision, urinary retention, impotence	Hypersensitivity to atropine Narrow-angle glaucoma Reflux esophagitis, ulcerative colitis, paralytic ileus, or obstructive gastrointestinal disease Unstable cardiovascular status Myasthenia gravis	A naturally occurring alkaloid found in the plant *Atropa belladonna*. Mainly muscarinic activity; marginal nicotinic effect. More effective at reversal of exogenous rather than endogenous cholinergic activity.
Scopolamine	Motion sickness Nausea and vomiting	*Glaucoma, drug-induced psychosis* Somnolence, xerostomia, blurred vision	Hypersensitivity to scopolamine Chronic lung disease Hepatic or renal impairment Narrow-angle glaucoma Prostatic hypertrophy Pyloric obstruction	Significant CNS effects. Delivered via transdermal patch.
Pirenzepine Methscopolamine Glycopyrrolate	Peptic ulcer disease (shared indication) Surgically induced or vagally induced bradycardia (glycopyrrolate only) Chronic drooling associated with neurologic condition (glycopyrrolate only)	*Cardiac arrhythmia, cardiac arrest, malignant hyperthermia, anaphylaxis, seizure, respiratory arrest* Flushing, gastrointestinal upset, xerostomia, urinary retention, decreased sweating, headache	Shared contraindication: Hypersensitivity to drug Methscopolamine and glycopyrrolate only: Gastrointestinal obstruction Obstructive uropathy Narrow-angle glaucoma Myasthenia gravis Unstable cardiovascular status in acute hemorrhage Glycopyrrolate only: Concomitant use of oral potassium chloride Newborns less than 1 month of age	Alternative or additive agents to standard peptic ulcer disease therapies (rarely used for this indication). Methscopolamine and glycopyrrolate have delayed but measurable CNS and cognitive anticholinergic effects.

continues

DRUG SUMMARY TABLE: CHAPTER 10 Cholinergic Pharmacology *continued*

DRUG	CLINICAL APPLICATIONS	*SERIOUS* AND COMMON ADVERSE EFFECTS	CONTRAINDICATIONS	THERAPEUTIC CONSIDERATIONS
Ipratropium **Tiotropium**	Chronic obstructive pulmonary disease (COPD) (shared indication) Nasal discharge (ipratropium only)	*Hypersensitivity reaction, stroke (shared adverse effects); myocardial infarction, bronchospasm (ipratropium only); bowel obstruction (tiotropium only)* Abnormal taste in mouth, xerostomia, bronchitis, sinusitis	Hypersensitivity to ipratropium or tiotropium	Ipratropium is more effective than β-adrenergic agonists in the treatment of COPD but less effective in treating asthma. Relative to ipratropium, tiotropium has similar, and possibly superior, efficacy as a bronchodilator in the treatment of COPD. In poorly controlled asthma, the addition of tiotropium to inhaled glucocorticoids and long-acting beta-agonists may significantly increase the time to first severe exacerbation and provide modest sustained bronchodilation.
Oxybutynin **Propantheline** **Terodiline** **Tolterodine** **Fesoterodine** **Trospium** **Darifenacin** **Solifenacin**	Shared indications: Hyperreflexic and overactive bladder Urge incontinence Propantheline only: Peptic ulcer disease	*Angioedema, immune hypersensitivity reaction (shared adverse effects); hypertensive crisis, Stevens-Johnson syndrome, rhabdomyolysis (trospium only); delirium, hallucinations (trospium and solifenacin only); prolonged QT interval, bowel obstruction (solifenacin only)* Gastrointestinal upset, dry mouth, application-site erythema, pruritus, urinary retention	Shared contraindication: Hypersensitivity to drug Shared contraindication except for terodiline: Narrow-angle glaucoma Gastric retention Urinary retention Propantheline only: Myasthenia gravis Unstable cardiovascular adjustment in acute hemorrhage	Oxybutynin, propantheline, tolterodine, fesoterodine, and trospium are nonspecific muscarinic receptor antagonists, whereas darifenacin and solifenacin are selective M_3 receptor antagonists. Tolterodine may cause less dry mouth than oxybutynin, and the newer M_3-selective agents darifenacin and solifenacin may cause less dry mouth and constipation than nonselective agents.

NICOTINIC RECEPTOR ANTAGONISTS
Mechanism—Selectively antagonize nicotinic receptors, thus preventing endogenous ACh binding and subsequent muscle cell depolarization (sometimes called *nondepolarizing blockade*) (all except sugammadex); chelate vecuronium and rocuronium (sugammadex)

Pancuronium **Tubocurarine** **Vecuronium** **Rocuronium** **Mivacurium**	Induction of neuromuscular blockade in surgery Intubation	*Anaphylaxis, hypertension, respiratory failure (shared adverse effects); prolonged muscle weakness (vecuronium and pancuronium only)* Salivation, flushing (mivacurium only)	Hypersensitivity to drug (shared contraindication) Neonates (pancuronium and mivacurium only)	Pancuronium and tubocurarine are long-acting agents; vecuronium and rocuronium are intermediate-acting agents; mivacurium is a short-acting agent. Nondepolarizing blocking agents have variable adverse effects associated with ganglionic blockade, which can be reversed by administration of AChE inhibitors.

Sugammadex	Reversal of neuromuscular blockade by vecuronium, rocuronium (investigational in US)	Investigational			Sugammadex chelates vecuronium and rocuronium in the circulation, thus accelerating the reversal of blockade and speeding postoperative recovery (investigational in United States).
Trimethaphan Mecamylamine	Hypertension in patients with acute aortic dissection	Investigational	*Paralytic ileus, urinary retention, respiratory arrest, syncope* Orthostatic hypotension, dyspepsia, diplopia, sedation	Shared contraindication: Hypersensitivity to drug Trimethaphan only: Asphyxia Uncorrected respiratory insufficiency Neonates at risk for paralytic or meconium ileus Hypovolemia and shock Mecamylamine only: Coronary insufficiency or recent myocardial infarction Glaucoma Pyloric stenosis Renal insufficiency Patients treated with sulfonamides	Mecamylamine and trimethaphan are administered when ganglionic blockade is desired; these drugs lower blood pressure while simultaneously blunting the sympathetic reflexes that would normally cause a deleterious rise in pressure at the site of the tear in cases of aortic dissection.

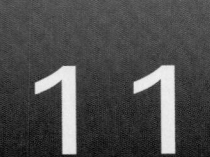

11

Adrenergic Pharmacology

Nidhi Gera, Ehrin J. Armstrong, and David E. Golan

INTRODUCTION

Adrenergic pharmacology involves the study of agents that act on pathways mediated by the endogenous catecholamines norepinephrine, epinephrine, and dopamine. The sympathetic nervous system is the major source of endogenous catecholamine production and release. Signaling through catecholamine receptors mediates diverse physiologic effects, including increasing the rate and force of cardiac contraction, modifying the peripheral resistance of the arterial system, inhibiting the release of insulin, stimulating hepatic release of glucose, and increasing adipocyte release of free fatty acids. Drugs that target the synthesis, storage, reuptake, and metabolism of norepinephrine and epinephrine or that directly target the postsynaptic receptors for these transmitters are frequent therapies for many major diseases, including hypertension, shock, asthma, and angina. This chapter examines the biochemical and physiologic basis for adrenergic action and then discusses the action of the different classes of adrenergic drugs.

BIOCHEMISTRY AND PHYSIOLOGY OF ADRENERGIC FUNCTION

The autonomic nervous system contributes to homeostasis through the concerted action of its sympathetic and parasympathetic branches. Catecholamines are the major effectors of sympathetic signaling. The following discussion presents the biochemistry of catecholamine action, from synthesis to metabolism to receptor activation. The physiologic roles of the endogenous catecholamines epinephrine (adrenaline), norepinephrine (noradrenaline), and dopamine are then discussed, with emphasis on the specificity of receptor expression in different organ systems.

Catecholamine Synthesis, Storage, and Release

Catecholamines are synthesized by sequential chemical modifications of the amino acid tyrosine. This synthesis occurs primarily at sympathetic nerve endings and in chromaffin cells. Epinephrine is predominantly synthesized in chromaffin cells of the adrenal medulla; sympathetic neurons produce norepinephrine as their primary neurotransmitter (Fig. 11-1). Tyrosine, the precursor for catecholamine synthesis, is transported into neurons via an aromatic amino acid transporter that uses the Na^+ gradient across the neuronal membrane to concentrate tyrosine (as well as phenylalanine, tryptophan, and histidine). The first step in catecholamine synthesis, the oxidation of tyrosine to **dihydroxyphenylalanine (DOPA)**, is mediated by the enzyme **tyrosine hydroxylase (TH)**. TH is the rate-limiting enzyme in catecholamine synthesis, and it is regulated by feedback (end-product) inhibition and by kinase-mediated phosphorylation of the enzyme. DOPA is converted to dopamine by a relatively nonspecific aromatic amino acid decarboxylase. Dopamine is then hydroxylated by **dopamine-β-hydroxylase** to yield

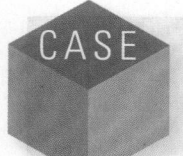

CASE

The year is 1960. Ms. S has felt depressed for a number of years. She has tried several different medications to alleviate her feelings of hopelessness and lack of motivation, but nothing seems to help. Recently, however, her doctor has prescribed iproniazid, a new medication reported to be of benefit in many cases of depression. He tells her that scientists believe that the drug has beneficial effects in depression by inhibiting an enzyme in the brain called *monoamine oxidase* (MAO). MAO is one of the enzymes responsible for catecholamine degradation, and its inhibition significantly increases the available concentrations of catecholamines. Because iproniazid is a new drug, its potential adverse effects are not well defined, so her doctor advises Ms. S to report any unusual effects of the medication.

Hopeful, but not expecting significant changes, Ms. S takes the medication. Within a few weeks, she begins to feel motivated and energetic for the first time in 20 years. Exuberant at her new sense of energy, Ms. S reclaims her past life as a socialite by hosting a gala wine and cheese reception. The best and brightest of the city turn up, expecting a fine evening. As she stands up to give thanks to her attendees, Ms. S celebrates with a large swig of her favorite 1954 Chianti. By the end of the party, Ms. S has a severe headache and nausea. Recalling her doctor's warning, Ms. S has a friend rush her to the nearest hospital. In the emergency department, the attending physician records a blood pressure of 230/160 mm Hg. Recognizing that Ms. S is experiencing a hypertensive emergency, the doctor administers phentolamine (an α-adrenoceptor antagonist). Ms. S's blood pressure quickly normalizes, and the doctor's subsequent clinical investigation identifies a new, and now famous, drug–food interaction involving MAO inhibitors. This potential adverse interaction is shared by some other MAO inhibitors; more recent work on subtype-selective and reversible MAO inhibitors has minimized the incidence of this interaction.

Questions

1. Which enzymes metabolize catecholamines? What are the specificities of isoforms of these enzymes for the various catecholamines?
2. What is the mechanistic explanation for the interaction of MAO inhibitors with red wine and aged cheese?
3. How did phentolamine lower Ms. S's blood pressure?

---

norepinephrine. In tissues that produce epinephrine, norepinephrine is then methylated on its amino group by **phenylethanolamine N-methyltransferase (PNMT)**. Expression of PNMT in the adrenal medulla is largely dependent on the high concentrations of cortisol that flow into the medulla via veins draining the adrenal cortex.

The conversions of tyrosine to DOPA and of DOPA to dopamine occur within the cytoplasm. Dopamine is transported into synaptic vesicles by a 12-helix membrane-spanning proton antiporter called the **vesicular monoamine transporter (VMAT)**. Unlike all the other enzymes in the catecholamine biosynthesis pathways, dopamine-β-hydroxylase is associated with the inner surface of secretory vesicles, and it catalyzes the conversion of dopamine to norepinephrine inside these vesicles.

There are three distinct vesicular transporters that differ in substrate specificity and localization. VMAT1 and VMAT2 (also known as *Uptake 2* [Fig. 11-2]) both transport serotonin (5-HT), histamine, and all catecholamines. The tissue-specific expression of VMAT1 and VMAT2 is mutually exclusive: VMAT1 expression is restricted mainly to nonneuronal cells (adrenal gland, gastric mucosa, intestine, and sympathetic ganglia) and VMAT2 is expressed primarily in the central nervous system (CNS). In addition to these expression differences, the affinity of VMAT2 for histamine (K_m, 3 μM) is significantly higher than that of VMAT1 for histamine (K_m, 436 μM). The vesicular acetylcholine transporter (VAChT) is expressed in cholinergic neurons, including motor nerves (see Chapter 10, Cholinergic Pharmacology). These antiporters use the proton gradient generated by a H+-ATPase in the vesicular membrane to concentrate dopamine (or, in the case of VAChT, acetylcholine) inside the vesicle. Norepinephrine concentrations within the vesicle can reach 100 mM. To stabilize the osmotic pressure resulting from the high concentration gradient for norepinephrine across the vesicle membrane, norepinephrine is thought to condense with ATP. Consequently, ATP and norepinephrine are co-released upon vesicle exocytosis.

In adrenal medullary cells, norepinephrine is transported or diffuses from vesicles back into the cytoplasm, where PNMT converts it to epinephrine. Epinephrine is then transported back into vesicles for storage until its eventual release by exocytosis. The nonselective nature of VMAT1 and VMAT2 has important pharmacologic consequences, as discussed below.

Activation of the sympathetic nervous system and subsequent catecholamine release are initiated by signals originating in an array of processing areas in the CNS, especially the limbic system. These CNS neurons project axons that synapse on sympathetic preganglionic neurons in the intermediolateral columns of the spinal cord. The preganglionic axons project to the sympathetic ganglia. The preganglionic neurons use acetylcholine as the neurotransmitter to activate nicotinic acetylcholine (ACh) receptors, which are cation-selective channels that depolarize the neuronal membrane and thereby generate postsynaptic potentials in postganglionic neurons. Ganglionic blockers such as **hexamethonium** and **mecamylamine** block the ganglionic nicotinic ACh receptor, without significant effects on skeletal muscle ACh receptors (see Chapter 10). The sympathetic postganglionic axons

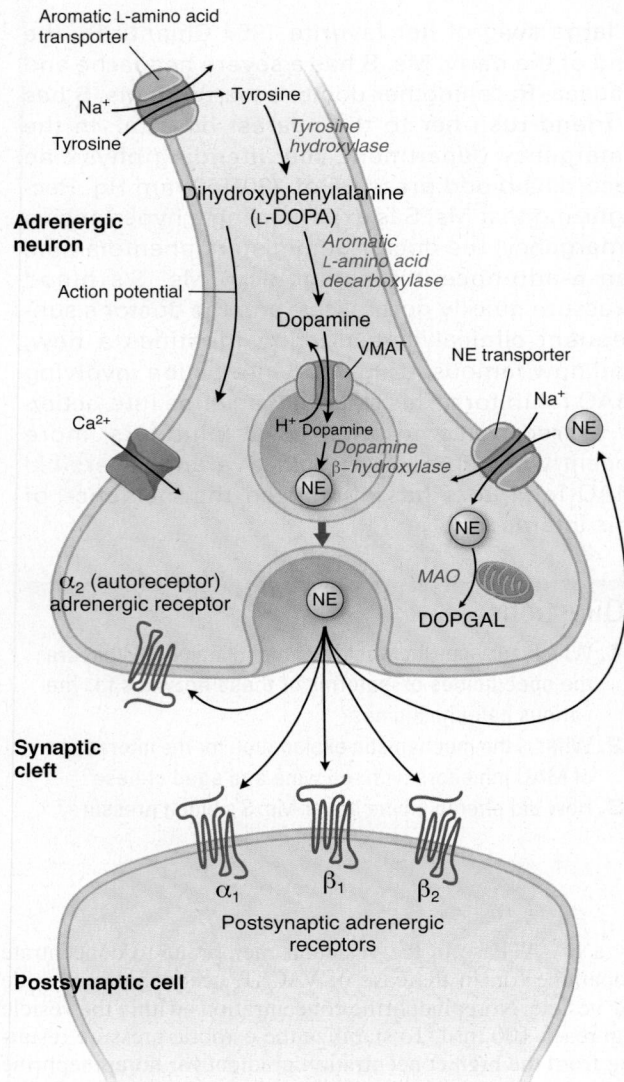

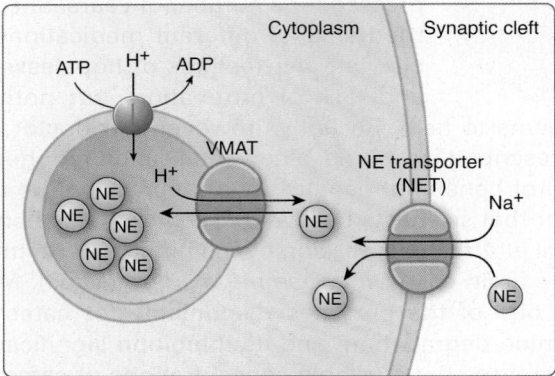

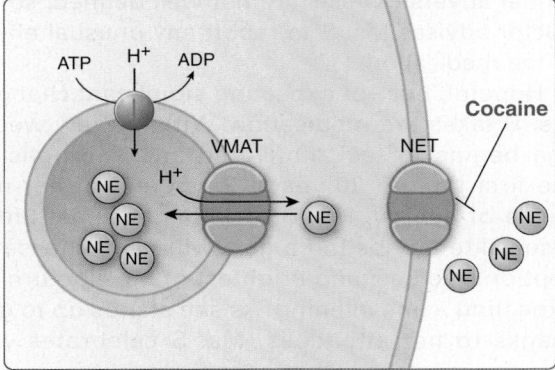

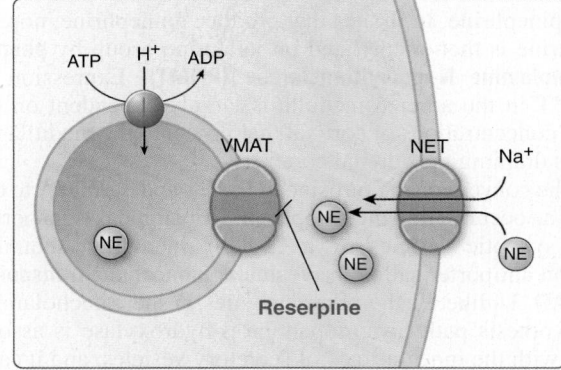

FIGURE 11-1. Catecholamine synthesis, storage, release, and reuptake pathways. The endogenous catecholamines dopamine, norepinephrine, and epinephrine are all synthesized from tyrosine. The rate-limiting step in catecholamine synthesis, the oxidation of cytoplasmic tyrosine to dihydroxyphenylalanine (L-DOPA), is catalyzed by the enzyme tyrosine hydroxylase. Aromatic L-amino acid decarboxylase then converts L-DOPA to dopamine. Vesicular monoamine transporter (VMAT) translocates dopamine (and other monoamines) into synaptic vesicles. In adrenergic neurons, intravesicular dopamine-β-hydroxylase converts dopamine to norepinephrine (NE). Norepinephrine is then stored in the vesicle until release. In adrenal medullary cells, norepinephrine returns to the cytosol, where phenylethanolamine N-methyltransferase (PNMT) converts norepinephrine to epinephrine. The epinephrine is then transported back into the vesicle for storage (*not shown*). α-Methyltyrosine inhibits tyrosine hydroxylase, the rate-limiting enzyme in catecholamine synthesis (*not shown*). Released norepinephrine can stimulate postsynaptic α₁-, β₁-, or β₂-adrenergic receptors or presynaptic α₂-adrenergic autoreceptors. Released norepinephrine can also be taken up into presynaptic terminals by the selective NE transporter. NE in the cytoplasm of the presynaptic neuron can be further taken up into synaptic vesicles by VMAT (*not shown*) or degraded to 3,4-dihydroxyphenylglycoaldehyde (DOPGAL; see Fig. 11-3) by mitochondrion-associated monoamine oxidase (MAO).

FIGURE 11-2. Mechanisms of action of cocaine and reserpine. A. Norepinephrine (NE) that has been released into the synaptic cleft can be taken up into the cytoplasm of the presynaptic neuron by the selective NE transporter (NET), an Na⁺-NE co-transporter. Cytoplasmic NE is concentrated in synaptic vesicles by the nonselective vesicular monoamine transporter (VMAT), an H⁺-monoamine antiporter. An H⁺-ATPase uses the energy of ATP hydrolysis to concentrate protons in synaptic vesicles and thereby generates a transmembrane H⁺ gradient. This H⁺ gradient is used by VMAT to drive monoamine transport into the synaptic vesicle. **B.** Cocaine inhibits the NE transporter, allowing released NE to remain in the synaptic cleft for a longer period of time. By this mechanism, cocaine potentiates neurotransmission at adrenergic synapses. **C.** Reserpine inhibits the vesicular monoamine transporter, preventing the refilling of synaptic vesicles with NE and eventually depleting the adrenergic terminal of neurotransmitter. By this mechanism, reserpine inhibits neurotransmission at adrenergic synapses.

form varicosities or *en passant* connections with target organs. The arrival of an action potential at these endings opens voltage-gated neuronal Ca^{2+} channels, and the ensuing Ca^{2+} influx triggers exocytosis of the catecholamine-containing synaptic vesicles. Various novel substances—including peptides from sea snails—block these Ca^{2+} channels; **ziconotide** is an example of a drug in this class that has efficacy in the treatment of severe pain (see Chapter 18, Pharmacology of Analgesia). Norepinephrine rapidly diffuses away from the sympathetic nerve endings and locally regulates target tissue responses (e.g., smooth muscle tone) by activating adrenergic receptors expressed on target tissues. (An exception is that ACh is the transmitter used at sympathetic nerve endings in sweat glands.) Importantly, adrenergic receptors are also expressed at sympathetic nerve endings; these receptors may serve as an autoregulatory mechanism for modulating the extent of neurotransmitter release.

Reuptake and Metabolism of Catecholamines

The action of a catecholamine molecule at its postsynaptic receptor is terminated by one of three mechanisms: (1) reuptake of catecholamine into the presynaptic neuron, (2) metabolism of catecholamine to an inactive metabolite, and (3) diffusion of the catecholamine away from the synaptic cleft. The first two of these mechanisms require specific transport proteins or enzymes and, therefore, are targets for pharmacologic intervention.

Reuptake of catecholamine into the neuronal cytoplasm is mediated by a selective catecholamine transporter (e.g., **norepinephrine transporter**, or **NET**) that is also known as *Uptake 1* (Fig. 11-2). Approximately 90% of the released norepinephrine is taken up by this process (recycled); the remainder is either metabolized locally or diffuses into the blood. Uptake 1 is a symporter that uses the inward Na^+ gradient to concentrate catecholamines in the cytoplasm of sympathetic nerve endings, thus limiting the postsynaptic response and allowing neurons to recycle the transmitter for subsequent release. Inside the nerve terminal, catecholamines can be further concentrated in synaptic vesicles via VMAT, the same transporter used to transport dopamine into the vesicle for catecholamine synthesis. Thus, *the pool of catecholamines available for release comes from two sources*: molecules that are synthesized *de novo* and molecules that are recycled via neuronal reuptake.

Catecholamine metabolism involves the two enzymes **MAO** and **catechol-O-methyltransferase (COMT)** (Fig. 11-3). MAO is a mitochondrial outer-membrane enzyme that is expressed in most neurons. It exists in two isoforms: MAO-A and MAO-B. The two isoforms have some degree of ligand specificity: MAO-A preferentially degrades serotonin, norepinephrine, and dopamine, while MAO-B degrades dopamine more rapidly than serotonin and norepinephrine. As indicated in the clinical case, MAO inhibitors are efficacious in the treatment of depression. The MAO-A isoform is responsible for detoxifying substances in cheese and wine before they reach the general circulation. COMT is a cytosolic enzyme that is relatively nonspecific and is expressed primarily in the liver.

Catecholamine Receptors

Adrenergic receptors (also called **adrenoceptors**) are selective for norepinephrine and epinephrine. Supraphysiologic concentrations of dopamine can also activate some adrenoceptors. These receptors are divided into three main classes,

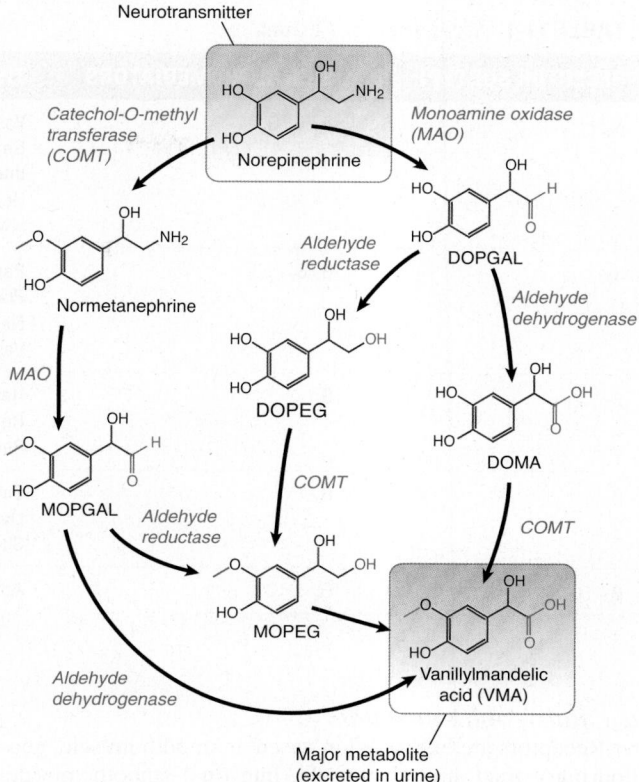

FIGURE 11-3. Norepinephrine metabolism. Norepinephrine is degraded to metabolites by two main enzymes. Catechol-O-methyltransferase (COMT) is a widely distributed cytosolic enzyme; COMT in the liver is particularly important in the metabolism of circulating catecholamines. Monoamine oxidase (MAO), which is localized to the outer surface of mitochondria, is found in many monoaminergic (including adrenergic) neurons. COMT, MAO, aldehyde reductase, and aldehyde dehydrogenase metabolize catecholamines to multiple intermediates (abbreviated as DOPGAL, MOPGAL, DOPEG, DOMA, and MOPEG) that are eventually excreted. Vanillylmandelic acid (VMA) is the major metabolite excreted in urine.

termed α_1, α_2, and β (Table 11-1). Each of these major classes has three subtypes: α_{1A}, α_{1B}, and α_{1D}; α_{2A}, α_{2B}, and α_{2C}; and β_1, β_2, and β_3. Each of the adrenergic receptor subtypes is a member of the G protein-coupled receptor (GPCR) superfamily (also known as *seven-transmembrane helix receptors*). GPCRs regulate complex intracellular signaling networks through intermediate transducing molecules, which are called *G proteins* because of their GTP binding and hydrolysis activity. G proteins are heterotrimeric, with α, β, and γ subunits. In the resting (inactive) state, G_α binds guanosine 5'-diphosphate (GDP) and is associated with $G_{\beta\gamma}$. Binding of agonist to the GPCR triggers the dissociation of GDP and the binding of guanosine 5'-triphosphate (GTP) to the G_α subunit. GTP binding initiates a conformational change that leads to the dissociation of $G_{\beta\gamma}$ and to the activation of G_α. Both G_α and $G_{\beta\gamma}$ can activate downstream effectors. In mammals, at least 27 G_α, 5 G_β, and 13 G_γ subtypes are present, and downstream GPCR signaling depends on the specific $G_{\alpha\beta\gamma}$ combination. On the basis of the primary sequence of the G_α subunit, G proteins can be divided into four major families—G_s, G_i, $G_{q/11}$, and G_{12}—and each family of G_α subunit activates specific downstream signaling pathways (see Chapter 1, Drug–Receptor Interactions).

TABLE 11-1 Adrenoceptor Actions

RECEPTOR SUBTYPE	SIGNALING MEDIATORS	TISSUE	EFFECTS
α_1	$G_q/G_i/G_o$	Vascular smooth muscle	Contraction
		Genitourinary smooth muscle	Contraction
		Intestinal smooth muscle	Relaxation
		Heart	↑ Inotropy and excitability
		Liver	Glycogenolysis and gluconeogenesis
α_2	G_i/G_o	Pancreatic β-cells	↓ Insulin secretion
		Platelets	Aggregation
		Nerve	↓ Norepinephrine release
		Vascular smooth muscle	Contraction
β_1	G_s	Heart	↑ Chronotropy and inotropy
		Heart	↑ AV node conduction velocity
		Renal juxtaglomerular cells	↑ Renin secretion
β_2	G_s	Smooth muscle	Relaxation
		Liver	Glycogenolysis and gluconeogenesis
		Skeletal muscle	Glycogenolysis and K^+ uptake
β_3	G_s	Adipose	Lipolysis

α_1- and α_2-Adrenoceptors

α_1-Receptors are expressed in vascular smooth muscle, genitourinary tract smooth muscle, intestinal smooth muscle, prostate, brain, heart, liver, and other cell types. The prototypical signaling mechanism of α_1-receptors involves $G_{q/11}$, which is generally a stimulatory protein that activates various effectors including phospholipase C, phospholipase D, phospholipase A_2, Ca^{2+} channels, K^+ channels, Na^+/H^+ exchangers, several members of the mitogen-activated protein (MAP) kinase pathways, and a variety of other kinases including phosphatidylinositol 3-kinase. Phospholipase C cleaves phosphatidylinositol-4,5-bisphosphate, generating the two second messengers inositol trisphosphate (IP_3) and diacylglycerol (DAG). IP_3 acts to increase intracellular $[Ca^{2+}]$ via both release of endogenous Ca^{2+} stores and influx of Ca^{2+} from extracellular fluid. Increased intracellular $[Ca^{2+}]$ activates various regulatory proteins that mediate physiologic responses in various tissues. DAG activates protein kinase C, which further activates a variety of protein substrates including ion channels such as Na^+/H^+ exchangers, Ca^{2+} channels, and K^+ channels. Phospholipase D catalyses the hydrolysis of phosphatidylcholine to phosphatidic acid and choline. Phosphatidic acid may act directly as a signaling molecule or be further metabolized to DAG by phosphatidic acid hydrolase. $G_{q/11}$-stimulated activation of phospholipase A_2 is mediated by increased intracellular $[Ca^{2+}]$ or by activation of protein kinase C and MAP kinase pathways. The various α_1-receptor subtypes likely differ in their tissue-specific localization and their capacity to activate downstream signaling pathways.

The downstream signaling pathways activated by α_1-receptors can be complex. Stimulation of α_1-receptors in vascular smooth muscle cells increases intracellular $[Ca^{2+}]$, leading to activation of calmodulin, phosphorylation of myosin light chain, increased actin–myosin interaction, and muscle contraction (see Chapter 22, Pharmacology of Vascular Tone). Therefore, α_1-receptors are important in mediating increases in peripheral vascular resistance, which can increase blood pressure and redistribute blood flow. While α_1-receptor antagonists would seem to be attractive in the therapy of hypertension, their clinical efficacy in preventing the complications of hypertension is uncertain. α_1-Receptor activation also causes contraction of genitourinary smooth muscle, and α_1-receptor antagonists are clinically efficacious in the symptomatic treatment of benign prostatic hyperplasia (BPH) (see below).

α_2-Adrenoceptors activate G_i, an inhibitory G protein. G_i has multiple signaling actions, including inhibition of adenylyl cyclase (thus decreasing cAMP levels), activation of G protein-coupled inward rectifier K^+ channels (causing membrane hyperpolarization), and inhibition of neuronal Ca^{2+} channels. These effects tend to decrease neurotransmitter release from the target neuron. α_2-Receptors are found on both presynaptic neurons and postsynaptic cells. *Presynaptic α_2-receptors function as autoreceptors to mediate feedback inhibition of sympathetic transmission.* α_2-Receptors are also expressed on platelets and pancreatic β-cells, where they mediate platelet aggregation and inhibit insulin release, respectively. The latter observations have led to the development of agents that are selective inhibitors of α_2-receptors. The main pharmacologic approach to α_2-receptors, however, has been in the treatment of hypertension. α_2-Receptor *agonists* act at CNS sites to decrease sympathetic outflow to the periphery, resulting in decreased norepinephrine release at sympathetic nerve terminals and, therefore, decreased vascular smooth muscle contraction.

β-Adrenoceptors

β-Adrenoceptors are divided into three subclasses, termed β_1, β_2, and β_3 (Table 11-1). All three subclasses activate a stimulatory G protein, G_s. G_s activates adenylyl cyclase, which catalyzes the formation of intracellular cAMP from adenosine triphosphate (ATP). Increased intracellular cAMP activates protein kinases, especially protein kinase A (PKA), by binding to the regulatory subunit of the enzyme. This results in the release and activation of the catalytic subunit of PKA, which phosphorylates and activates a variety of intracellular proteins including ion channels and transcription factors. The nature of the signaling differences among the β-adrenoceptor subtypes is unclear since they all appear to couple efficiently to G_s, and stimulation of $β_1$- and $β_2$-adrenoceptors causes increased intracellular cAMP. It has been suggested that specificity may be conferred by differences in the composition of the G protein subunits associated with the two receptors. $β_1$-Adrenoceptors couple exclusively to G_s, but $β_2$-adrenoceptors can also activate effectors via coupling to G_i. Thus, $β_2$-adrenoceptors can limit and spatially restrict cAMP production by switching between G_s- and G_i-mediated signaling, which, in turn, affects PKA-dependent regulation of target proteins.

Pharmacologic selectivity among the β-adrenoceptors appears to reside in the tissue-selective distribution of each β-adrenoceptor subtype. $β_1$-Adrenoceptors are localized primarily in the kidney and heart. In the kidney, they are present mainly on renal juxtaglomerular cells, where receptor activation causes renin release (see Chapter 21, Pharmacology of Volume Regulation). Stimulation of cardiac $β_1$-receptors (which represent 70–80% of all cardiac β-adrenergic receptors) causes an increase in both inotropy (force of contraction) and chronotropy (heart rate). The inotropic effect is mediated by increased phosphorylation of Ca^{2+} channels by protein kinase A, including calcium channels in the sarcolemma and phospholamban in the sarcoplasmic reticulum, and by phosphorylation of troponin I and troponin C, which reduces myofilament sensitivity to Ca^{2+} (see Chapter 25, Pharmacology of Cardiac Contractility). The increased chronotropy results from a $β_1$-mediated increase in the rate of phase 4 depolarization of sinoatrial node pacemaker cells. Both effects contribute to increased cardiac output (recall that cardiac output = heart rate × stroke volume). Activation of $β_1$-receptors also increases conduction velocity in the atrioventricular (AV) node because the $β_1$-stimulated increase in Ca^{2+} entry increases the rate of depolarization of AV node cells.

$β_2$-Adrenoceptors are expressed in smooth muscle (including bronchial smooth muscle), liver, skeletal muscle, and heart. In smooth muscle, receptor activation stimulates G_s, adenylyl cyclase, cAMP, and protein kinase A. Protein kinase A phosphorylates several contractile proteins, especially myosin light chain kinase. Phosphorylation of myosin light chain kinase reduces its affinity for calcium-calmodulin, leading to relaxation of the contractile apparatus. $β_2$-Adrenoceptor activation may also relax bronchial smooth muscle by G_s-independent activation of K^+ channels. Increased K^+ efflux leads to bronchial smooth muscle cell hyperpolarization and, therefore, opposes the depolarization necessary to elicit contraction. In hepatocytes, activation of the G_s signaling cascade initiates a series of intracellular phosphorylation events that result in glycogen phosphorylase activation and glycogen catabolism. The result of $β_2$-adrenoceptor stimulation of hepatocytes is, therefore, an increase in plasma glucose. In skeletal muscle, activation of these same signaling pathways stimulates glycogenolysis and promotes K^+ uptake. Recent studies in cardiac myocytes suggest that $β_2$-adrenoceptor-mediated activation of the $G_{βγ}$ subunit of G_i leads to activation of phosphatidylinositide-3 kinase γ, which, in turn, activates the protein kinase B (also known as *Akt*) pathway that confers anti-apoptotic activity.

$β_3$-Adrenoceptors are expressed in adipose tissue and in the gastrointestinal tract. Stimulation of $β_3$-receptors leads to an increase in lipolysis and thermogenesis in adipocytes and to a decrease in gastrointestinal tract motility. These physiologic actions have led to speculation that $β_3$-agonists may be useful in the treatment of obesity, noninsulin-dependent diabetes mellitus, and other potential indications, but such selective pharmacologic agents remain to be developed for clinical use.

Regulation of Receptor Response

The ability of receptor agonists to initiate downstream signaling is related to the number of receptors activated, and changes in the density of receptors on the cell surface often alter the apparent efficacy of an agonist. Thus, both short-term (desensitization) and long-term (down-regulation) changes in the number of functional adrenoceptors are important in regulating tissue response (see Fig. 1-10).

When an agonist activates an adrenoceptor, the dissociation of its associated heterotrimeric G protein subunits leads not only to downstream signaling, as discussed above, but also to a negative feedback mechanism that limits tissue responses. Activation of β-adrenoceptors recruits GPCR-specific protein kinases (GRKs), which phosphorylate serine and threonine residues in the carboxyl-terminal tail of the receptor. Protein kinase A and protein kinase C can also phosphorylate G protein-coupled receptors. The phosphorylated state of the receptor promotes the translocation to the membrane of a cytosolic protein called **β-arrestin**, which binds to the intracellular domain of the receptor and sterically inhibits interaction between the receptor and the G protein. This effectively silences receptor signaling. β-Arrestins also recruit clathrin and the clathrin adaptor protein AP2 to the phosphorylated receptor, and this complex targets the adrenoceptors to clathrin-coated pits. These pits are pinched off from the membrane with the help of the large GTPase dynamin, and the internalized receptors are then either rapidly recycled, targeted to endosomes and recycled more slowly, or degraded in lysosomes. Each of these processes is important in regulating tissue responsiveness on a short- or long-term basis. Over the last decade, evidence has suggested that β-arrestins can turn on (rather than off) novel signaling pathways by serving as scaffold proteins for signaling complexes that promote G protein-independent pathways involving the activation of Erk1/2, Src, and small GTP-binding proteins. A newly discovered aspect of GPCR signaling is that some antagonists that block G protein signaling pathways may also function as agonists in alternative signaling pathways such as β-arrestin signaling. In this way, both the desensitization/down-regulation and the signaling roles for β-arrestins may be involved in physiologic and pathologic situations.

Physiologic and Pharmacologic Effects of Endogenous Catecholamines

The endogenous catecholamines epinephrine and norepinephrine act as agonists at both α- and β-adrenoceptors. At supraphysiologic concentrations, dopamine can also act as an agonist at α- and β-receptors. The overall effect of each catecholamine is complex and depends on the concentration of the agent and on tissue-specific receptor expression.

Epinephrine

Epinephrine is an agonist at both α- and β-adrenoceptors. *At low concentrations, epinephrine has predominantly $β_1$ and $β_2$*

effects, while at higher concentrations, its α_1 effects become more pronounced. Acting at β_1-receptors, epinephrine increases cardiac contractile force and cardiac output, with consequent increases in cardiac oxygen consumption and systolic blood pressure. Vasodilation mediated by β_2-receptors causes a decrease in peripheral resistance and a decrease in diastolic blood pressure. Stimulation of β_2-receptors also increases blood flow to skeletal muscle, relaxes bronchial smooth muscle, promotes glycogenolysis, and increases the concentrations of glucose and free fatty acids in the blood. Recent studies suggest that β_1-receptors are responsible for vasodilation in large arteries such as the femoral and pulmonary arteries, while β_2-receptors have a predominant role in vasodilation of the arterioles that contribute to peripheral vascular resistance. These β_1 and β_2 effects are all components of the "fight-or-flight" response.

Epinephrine was used to treat acute asthmatic attacks shortly after its discovery more than 100 years ago; other drugs with higher selectivity for β_2-receptors, and which are delivered directly to pulmonary β_2-receptors by inhalation, are now more often used in the treatment of asthma, chronic obstructive pulmonary disease, and other pulmonary conditions. Epinephrine remains a drug of choice for the treatment of anaphylaxis. Locally injected epinephrine causes vasoconstriction and prolongs the action of local anesthetics; for example, it is often used in combination with a local anesthetic in dentistry. It is ineffective orally due to extensive first-pass metabolism. Epinephrine has a rapid onset and a brief duration of action when injected intravenously. Adverse consequences of rapid intravenous infusions include increased cardiac excitability that may lead to cardiac arrhythmias and excessive increases in blood pressure.

Norepinephrine

Norepinephrine is an agonist at α_1- and β_1-receptors but has relatively little effect at β_2-receptors. Because of the lack of action at β_2-receptors, systemic administration of norepinephrine increases not only systolic blood pressure (β_1 effect) but also diastolic blood pressure and total peripheral resistance. Norepinephrine is used in the pharmacologic treatment of hypotension in patients with distributive shock, most frequently due to sepsis.

Dopamine

Although dopamine is a prominent CNS neurotransmitter, systemic administration has few CNS effects because it does not readily cross the blood–brain barrier. Dopamine activates one or more subtypes of catecholamine receptor in peripheral tissues, and the predominant effect is dependent on the local concentration of the compound. At low doses (<2 μg/kg per min), a continuous intravenous infusion of dopamine acts predominantly on D1 dopaminergic receptors in renal, mesenteric, and coronary vascular beds. D1 dopaminergic receptors activate adenylyl cyclase in vascular smooth muscle cells, leading to increased cAMP levels and vasodilation. At higher rates of infusion (2–10 μg/kg per min), dopamine is a positive inotrope via its activation of β_1-adrenergic receptors. At still higher rates of infusion (>10 μg/kg per min), dopamine acts on vascular α_1-adrenergic receptors to cause vasoconstriction.

Dopamine is used in the treatment of shock, particularly in states of shock caused by low cardiac output and accompanied by compromised renal function leading to oliguria. However, efficacy in protecting the kidneys has not been clearly demonstrated.

PHARMACOLOGIC CLASSES AND AGENTS

Pharmacologic intervention is possible at each of the major steps in catecholamine synthesis, storage, reuptake, metabolism, and receptor activation. The following discussion presents the various classes of agents in the order of their action on adrenergic pathways, from neurotransmitter synthesis to receptor activation.

Inhibitors of Catecholamine Synthesis

Inhibitors of catecholamine synthesis have limited clinical utility because such agents nonspecifically inhibit the formation of all catecholamines (see Fig. 11-1). **α-Methyltyrosine** is a structural analogue of tyrosine that is transported into nerve terminals, where it inhibits tyrosine hydroxylase, the first enzyme in the catecholamine biosynthesis pathway. This agent is used occasionally in the treatment of hypertension associated with pheochromocytoma (a tumor of the enterochromaffin cells of the adrenal medulla that produces norepinephrine and epinephrine). Its clinical use is limited, however, because it causes significant orthostatic hypotension and sedation, and many other antihypertensive drugs with fewer adverse effects are available for this indication.

Inhibitors of Catecholamine Storage

Catecholamines originate from two pools—de novo synthesis and recycled transmitter. An agent that inhibits catecholamine storage in vesicles generally has two sequential effects. In the short term, the agent increases the net release of catecholamine from the synaptic terminal, and thus mimics sympathetic stimulation **(sympathomimetic)**. Over a longer time period, however, the agent depletes the pool of available catecholamine and thus acts as a **sympatholytic** (inhibitor of sympathetic activity) (Fig. 11-4).

Reserpine binds tightly to the vesicular antiporter VMAT at or very near the substrate-binding site on the cytoplasmic surface of the transporter. Although the time course of binding is relatively slow, the tight binding results in irreversible inhibition of the antiporter (see Figs. 11-1 and 11-2). VMAT inhibition causes the secretory vesicles to lose their ability to concentrate and store norepinephrine and dopamine. At low doses, reserpine causes neurotransmitter to leak into the cytoplasm, where the catecholamine is destroyed by MAO. At high doses, the rate of transmitter leak can be sufficiently high to overwhelm the MAO in the presynaptic neuron. Under these conditions, there is a high concentration of transmitter in the neuronal cytoplasm, and transmitter can exit from the cytoplasm to the synaptic space through NET acting in reverse. The efflux of catecholamine has a transient sympathomimetic effect. Because reserpine's inhibition of VMAT is irreversible, new storage vesicles must be synthesized and transported to the nerve terminal to restore proper vesicular function. The recovery phase may require days to weeks after an individual stops taking reserpine. Reserpine can also be used experimentally to assess whether drugs need to be concentrated in presynaptic terminals to exert their action. In the past, reserpine was used to treat hypertension. However, the irreversible nature of its action and its association with severe depression make it an unattractive agent now that more efficacious and less toxic drugs are available for the treatment of hypertension. Nonetheless, there has

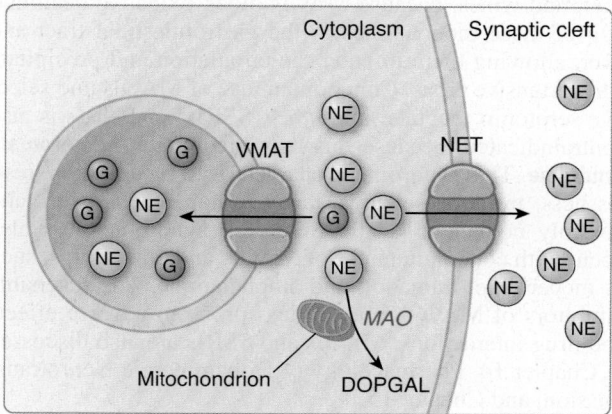

A Acute effect of indirect sympathomimetic

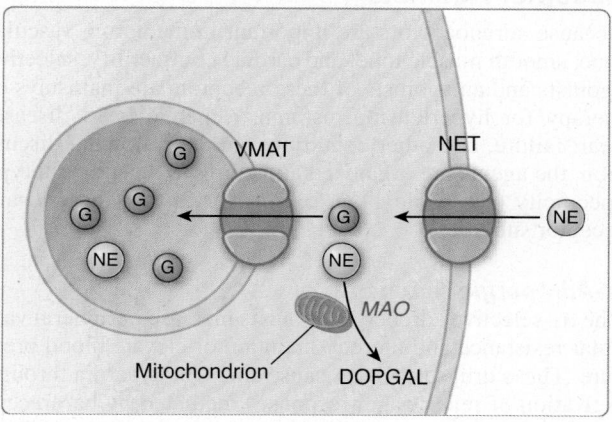

B Chronic effect of indirect sympathomimetic

FIGURE 11-4. Acute and chronic effects of indirect sympathomimetics. Indirect sympathomimetics have different effects on sympathetic outflow depending on whether they are administered acutely or chronically. **A.** Administered acutely, an indirect sympathomimetic such as guanethidine (G) displaces norepinephrine (NE) that is stored in the synaptic vesicles of adrenergic neurons. This results in a massive efflux of norepinephrine through the NE transporter acting in reverse; the resultant flooding of the synapse with norepinephrine causes marked sympathetic stimulation. **B.** Administered chronically, an indirect sympathomimetic such as guanethidine (G) is concentrated in synaptic vesicles and replaces norepinephrine. In addition, monoamine oxidase (MAO) degrades the small pool of norepinephrine that remains in the cytoplasm. Both of these effects contribute to decreased sympathetic stimulation.

been some interest in the possibility that reserpine may be a useful drug for the treatment of hypertension when used at doses lower than those associated with severe depression.

Tyramine is a dietary amine that is ordinarily metabolized by MAO in the gastrointestinal tract and liver. In patients taking MAO inhibitors (MAOIs; see below), tyramine is absorbed in the gut, transported through the blood, and taken up by sympathetic neurons, where it is transported into synaptic vesicles by VMAT. Uptake of tyramine by the synaptic vesicles causes displacement of vesicular norepinephrine and nonvesicular release of norepinephrine from the nerve terminal via reversal of NET. By this mechanism, an acute challenge with large amounts of dietary tyramine, or with modest dietary tyramine in patients taking MAOIs, can cause acute and massive release of norepinephrine from nerve terminals. In turn, the massive norepinephrine release

causes a pressor response with markedly elevated systolic blood pressure. Fermented foods such as red wine and aged cheese possess high concentrations of tyramine; this is why, in the introductory case, Ms. S developed a hypertensive crisis shortly after her wine and cheese party.

Although tyramine itself is poorly retained in synaptic vesicles, its hydroxylated metabolite **octopamine** (the synthesis of which is catalyzed by vesicular dopamine β-hydroxylase) can be stored at high concentrations in the vesicles. Under conditions of chronic MAOI treatment and modest dietary tyramine intake, norepinephrine may gradually be replaced by octopamine in storage vesicles. Because octopamine has little agonist activity at most mammalian adrenoceptors, postsynaptic responses to sympathetic stimulation may gradually be diminished, leading ultimately to postural hypotension. Migraine and cluster headaches have been associated with elevated levels of circulating neurotransmitters and neuromodulators, including tyramine and octopamine.

Like tyramine, **guanethidine** is actively transported by NET into neurons, where it concentrates in transmitter vesicles and displaces norepinephrine, leading to gradual depletion of norepinephrine (Fig. 11-4). Like octopamine, guanethidine is not an agonist at postsynaptic adrenoceptors, so its vesicular release upon sympathetic stimulation does not elicit a postsynaptic response. In the past, guanethidine was used to treat uncontrolled hypertension. Guanethidine inhibits cardiac sympathetic nerves, leading to reduced cardiac output, and it blocks sympathetically mediated vasoconstriction, leading to reduced cardiac preload. Inhibition of these sympathetic responses by guanethidine can lead to symptomatic hypotension following exercise or standing up (postural hypotension).

Guanadrel also acts as a false neurotransmitter. As with guanethidine, this agent can be used in the treatment of hypertension, but it is no longer a first-line agent. The adverse effect profile of guanadrel is similar to that of guanethidine.

Amphetamine has several adrenergic actions: (1) it displaces endogenous catecholamines from storage vesicles (similar to tyramine); (2) it is a weak inhibitor of MAO-A; (3) it competitively inhibits catecholamine reuptake mediated by NET and DAT; and (4) it is an agonist at the trace amine-associated receptor 1 (TAAR1), a G_s/G_q coupled receptor on presynaptic neurons. Stimulation of TAAR1 by amphetamine activates protein kinases A and C, causing DAT phosphorylation and thereby noncompetitively inhibiting dopamine reuptake. Although amphetamine binds to postsynaptic adrenergic receptors, the drug has little agonist action at α- or β-adrenoceptors. Amphetamine has marked behavioral effects including increased alertness, decreased fatigue, depressed appetite, and insomnia. Thus, it has been used to treat depression, attention-deficit hyperactivity disorder (ADHD), and narcolepsy (recurrent attacks of drowsiness and sleep during the daytime) and to suppress appetite. Its adverse effects can be substantial, including fatigue and depression following the period of central stimulation.

Ephedrine, **pseudoephedrine**, and **phenylpropanolamine** are structurally related agents that have some capacity to activate various adrenergic responses. Ephedrine has been used medically for the treatment of persistent hypotension. An herbal source of ephedrine (and various isomers) called *ma huang* was used to treat asthma in China for at least 2,000 years. Pseudoephedrine is used as an over-the-counter decongestant and is found in some cold remedies. Phenyl-propanolamine was removed from the over-the-counter market in the United States due to concerns about an association with cerebral hemorrhage.

Methylphenidate, a structural analogue of amphetamine, is widely used in psychiatry to treat ADHD in children; its major effect is thought to be related to enhanced attention.

Amphetamine can cause psychological and physiologic dependence as well as tolerance. Amphetamine may cause paranoia and hallucinations. **Methamphetamine** ("crank" or "crystal meth") is a major drug of abuse. See Chapter 15, Pharmacology of Serotonergic and Central Adrenergic Neurotransmission, for more detailed discussion of the pharmacology of amphetamine and related drugs.

Inhibitors of Catecholamine Reuptake

Inhibitors of catecholamine reuptake can exert an acute and powerful sympathomimetic effect by prolonging the time that released neurotransmitter remains in the synaptic cleft. **Cocaine** is a potent inhibitor of NET; unlike other uptake inhibitors (such as imipramine and fluoxetine), cocaine essentially eliminates catecholamine transport (see Fig. 11-2). It is used occasionally as a local anesthetic because of its independent activity as an inhibitor of neuronal action potentials (see Chapter 12, Local Anesthetic Pharmacology); in addition, in this setting, cocaine promotes vasoconstriction due to its capacity to inhibit norepinephrine uptake. Cocaine is a controlled substance with high abuse potential. It is a major public health concern because of its role as an agent of abuse (see Chapter 19, Pharmacology of Drugs of Abuse).

Tricyclic antidepressants (TCAs) and **serotonin-norepinephrine reuptake inhibitors (SNRIs)** inhibit NET-mediated reuptake of norepinephrine into presynaptic terminals and thus promote accumulation of norepinephrine in the synaptic cleft. Because of their important role in the treatment of depression, TCAs, SNRIs, and other inhibitors of norepinephrine reuptake are discussed in more detail in Chapter 15.

Inhibitors of Catecholamine Metabolism

Monoamine oxidase inhibitors (MAOIs) prevent secondary deamination of catecholamines that are transported into presynaptic terminals or taken up into tissues such as the liver. In the absence of metabolism, more catecholamine accumulates in presynaptic vesicles for release during each action potential. Most MAOIs are oxidized by MAO to reactive intermediates, which then act as irreversible inhibitors of MAO. Nonselective agents in this class (i.e., agents that inhibit both MAO-A and MAO-B) include **tranylcypromine**, **phenelzine**, and **iproniazid** (the drug used in the introductory case; this drug was later withdrawn from the market in the United States and some other countries). Selective inhibitors include **clorgyline**, which is selective for MAO-A, and **selegiline** and **rasagiline**, which are selective for MAO-B. **Moclobemide** is a reversible inhibitor of MAO-A.

As with the tricyclic antidepressants, MAOIs are used to treat depression. Selegiline and rasagiline are also approved for the treatment of Parkinson's disease; their mechanism of action may include both potentiation of dopamine in the remaining nigrostriatal neurons and decreased formation of neurotoxic intermediates. As noted above, patients taking MAOIs should avoid eating certain fermented or aged foods containing large amounts of tyramine and other monoamines, such as most cheeses and some fishes, poultry, beef, and wines, because MAOIs block oxidative deamination of these monoamines in the gastrointestinal tract and liver, allowing them to enter the circulation and precipitate a hypertensive crisis. Concomitant use of MAOIs and selective serotonin reuptake inhibitors (SSRIs) or SNRIs is also contraindicated, because this may precipitate the **serotonin syndrome**. This syndrome is characterized by agitation, restlessness, tremors, seizures, tachycardia, hypertension, and possibly coma and death. Serotonin syndrome may also occur with concomitant use of MAOIs and other drugs, such as meperidine, tramadol, and amphetamine. The reversible inhibitors of MAO-A may be less prone to adverse effects and drug interactions. MAOIs and SSRIs are also discussed in Chapter 14, Pharmacology of Dopaminergic Neurotransmission, and Chapter 15.

Receptor Agonists

Because adrenoceptors are important in mediating vascular tone, smooth muscle tone, and cardiac contractility, selective agonists and antagonists of these receptors are mainstays of therapy for hypertension, asthma, ischemic heart disease, heart failure, and other conditions. In the following discussion, the agents are organized according to receptor subtype specificity (see Table 11-1 for an overview of the relevant receptor subtypes).

α-Adrenergic Agonists

The α_1-selective adrenergic agonists increase peripheral vascular resistance and thereby maintain or elevate blood pressure. These drugs may also cause sinus bradycardia through activation of reflex vagal responses mediated by baroreceptors. Systemically administered α_1-agonists, such as **methoxamine**, have limited clinical use but are sometimes employed to increase blood pressure in the treatment of shock. A number of topically administered α_1-agonists, such as **phenylephrine**, **oxymetazoline**, and **tetrahydrozoline**, are used in the nonprescription remedies Afrin® and Visine® (and others) to constrict vascular smooth muscle in the symptomatic relief of nasal congestion and ophthalmic hyperemia. Oxymetazoline is also a partial agonist at α_2-receptors. Damage to the nasal mucosa and possible rebound hypersensitivity and return of symptoms often accompany extended use of these medications. Phenylephrine is also used intravenously in the treatment of distributive shock.

Clonidine is an α_2-receptor agonist that lowers blood pressure and decreases heart rate by acting in brainstem vasomotor centers to suppress sympathetic outflow to the periphery. Evidence supporting its capacity to decrease adverse cardiovascular outcomes in patients with hypertension is limited. Clonidine has limited utility in ameliorating symptoms of withdrawal from ethanol and opioid drugs. Adverse effects include bradycardia caused by decreased sympathetic activity and increased vagal activity, as well as dry mouth and sedation. Because sympathetic nervous system activation is an important mechanism in maintaining blood pressure on standing, postural hypotension may also complicate therapy with this drug. Other centrally acting α_2-agonists include the seldom-used agents **guanabenz** and **guanfacine**. These agents have adverse effect profiles similar to that of clonidine.

Dexmedetomidine is an α_2-receptor agonist whose capacity to cause sedation has been exploited as a beneficial effect in surgical patients, because sedation is induced by this drug without additional respiratory depression. Suppression of sympathetic nervous system activity by dexmedetomidine helps to avoid swings in blood pressure in surgical patients, who are carefully monitored by anesthetists during surgical procedures. Dexmedetomidine may also possess analgesic properties. Note that the α_2-mediated effects of sedation and decreased sympathetic activity are adverse effects of clonidine in the setting of outpatient treatment for hypertension but beneficial effects of dexmedetomidine in the controlled setting of the surgical patient.

α-Methyldopa is a precursor (prodrug) to the α_2-agonist α-methylnorepinephrine. Dopamine β-hydroxylase catalyzes the metabolism of methyldopa to methylnorepinephrine, and the α-methylnorepinephrine is then released by the adrenergic nerve terminal, where it can act presynaptically as an α_2-agonist. This action results in decreased sympathetic outflow from the CNS and consequent lowering of blood pressure in hypertensive patients. Methyldopa is also a competitive inhibitor of DOPA decarboxylase, which converts DOPA to dopamine, and thereby reduces adrenergic neurotransmission in the peripheral nervous system. Because α-methyldopa use can be associated with rare hepatotoxicity, autoimmune hemolytic anemia, and adverse CNS effects, this drug is very rarely used in the treatment of hypertension in the United States, with one exception—there is considerable experience with methyldopa as an antihypertensive drug in pregnancy, and it is still used as a preferred drug in that context.

β-Adrenergic Agonists

Stimulation of β_1-adrenergic receptors causes increases in the heart rate and the force of cardiac muscle contraction, resulting in increased cardiac output, while stimulation of β_2-adrenergic receptors causes relaxation of vascular, bronchial, and gastrointestinal smooth muscle. **Isoproterenol** is a nonselective β-agonist. This drug lowers peripheral vascular resistance and diastolic blood pressure (a β_2 effect), while systolic blood pressure remains unchanged or slightly increased (a β_1 effect). Because isoproterenol is a positive inotrope (increases cardiac contractility) and chronotrope (increases heart rate), cardiac output is increased. Isoproterenol can be used to relieve bronchoconstriction in asthma (β_2 effect). However, because isoproterenol is a nonselective activator of β_1- and β_2-adrenoceptors, its use for relief of bronchoconstriction is often accompanied by adverse cardiac effects. Use of this drug in asthma has therefore been supplanted by newer β_2-selective agonists (see below). Isoproterenol may occasionally be used to increase the heart rate in emergency situations of profound bradycardia, typically in anticipation of the placement of an electrical cardiac pacemaker.

The overall effect of **dobutamine** depends on the differential effects of the two stereoisomers contained in the racemic mixture (see Chapter 1 for a discussion of stereoisomers). The (−) isomer acts as both an α_1-agonist and a weak β_1-agonist, whereas the (+) isomer acts as both an α_1-antagonist and a potent β_1-agonist. The α_1-agonist and antagonist properties effectively cancel each other out when the racemic mixture is administered, and the observed clinical result is that of a selective β_1-agonist. This agent has more prominent inotropic than chronotropic effects, resulting in increased contractility and cardiac output. Dobutamine can

be used intravenously in the urgent treatment of severe heart failure. It is also used as a diagnostic agent, in conjunction with imaging of the heart, in the investigation of ischemic heart disease.

β_2-Selective agonists are valuable in the treatment of asthma. These drugs represent pharmacologic improvements over epinephrine (an agonist at all adrenergic receptors) and isoproterenol (an agonist at β_1- as well as β_2-receptors) in that their effects are more limited at nontarget tissues. It is particularly important that these selective drugs have limited capacity to stimulate β_1-adrenoceptors in the heart and, therefore, limited capacity to produce adverse cardiac effects. Specificity for the lung rather than the heart or other peripheral tissues has been further enhanced by generally delivering these drugs via aerosols inhaled into the lungs. Administration of the drugs directly into the lungs lowers the amount of drug that reaches the systemic circulation, again limiting the activation of cardiac β_1-receptors and skeletal muscle β_2-receptors. The most important effects of these agents are relaxation of bronchial smooth muscle and decrease in airway resistance. β_2-Selective agonists are not completely specific for airway β_2-receptors, however, and adverse effects can include skeletal muscle tremor (through β_2-stimulation) and tachycardia (through β_1-stimulation).

Metaproterenol is the prototype β_2-selective agonist. This drug is used to treat obstructive airway disease and acute bronchospasm. **Terbutaline** and **albuterol** are two other agents in this class that have similar efficacy and duration of action. **Salmeterol** is a long-acting β_2-agonist; its effects last for about 12 hours. The clinical utility of β_2-selective agonists is discussed more fully in Chapter 48, Integrative Inflammation Pharmacology: Asthma.

Receptor Antagonists

A broad spectrum of disease states respond to modulation of adrenoceptor activity, and antagonists at α- and β-adrenoceptors are among the most widely used drugs in clinical practice.

α-Adrenergic Antagonists

α-Adrenergic antagonists block the binding of endogenous catecholamines to α_1- and α_2-adrenoceptors. These agents cause vasodilation, decreased blood pressure, and decreased peripheral resistance. The baroreceptor reflex usually attempts to compensate for the fall in blood pressure, resulting in reflex increases in heart rate and cardiac output.

An important laboratory tool since the 1950s, **phenoxybenzamine** is an alkylating agent that blocks both α_1- and α_2-receptors irreversibly. In addition, phenoxybenzamine inhibits catecholamine uptake into both adrenergic nerve terminals and extraneuronal tissues. Because of its many direct and indirect effects on the sympathetic nervous system and target tissues, phenoxybenzamine, once used in the treatment of hypertension and benign prostatic hyperplasia (BPH), is now rarely used clinically. Some physicians use preoperative phenoxybenzamine to prepare patients with pheochromocytoma for surgery with the intent to decrease operative complications. Phenoxybenzamine has been found to cause tumors in laboratory animals, although the implications of these findings for humans are unclear.

Phentolamine is a reversible, nonselective α-adrenoceptor antagonist. This drug can also be used in the preoperative management of pheochromocytoma. Phentolamine was the pharmacologically ideal agent for use in the introductory case, because it blocked the α-adrenergic–mediated vasoconstriction that caused Ms. S's hypertension. However, most physicians have very little clinical experience with phentolamine, and other drugs are more frequently used in the treatment of severe hypertension.

Prazosin has a 1,000-fold higher affinity for α_1-receptors than for α_2-receptors. Its selective blockade of α_1-receptors in arterioles and veins results in decreased peripheral vascular resistance and dilation of the venous (capacitance) vessels. The latter effect decreases venous return to the heart; because of this reduction in cardiac preload, prazosin has little tendency to increase cardiac output and heart rate. Prazosin is an antihypertensive drug. Because patients may experience marked postural hypotension and syncope with the first dose, the drug is generally prescribed initially at a very low dose and is titrated to higher doses depending on the clinical response. Used in this manner, postural hypotension is uncommon, presumably due to the development of tolerance (by an unclear mechanism). Other agents in this class include **terazosin** and **doxazosin**; these agents have a longer half-life than prazosin, allowing less frequent dosing. α_1-Receptor antagonists are not often used clinically in the treatment of hypertension, because comparative studies have suggested that other antihypertensive medications, such as diuretics, may be more effective.

Because α_1-adrenoceptors mediate contraction of genitourinary as well as vascular smooth muscle, some α_1-antagonists have found clinical application in the symptomatic treatment of benign prostatic hyperplasia (BPH). α_1-Adrenoceptor antagonists may be more efficacious than finasteride (a 5α-reductase inhibitor; see Chapter 30, Pharmacology of Reproduction) in the medical treatment of BPH. Also, their onset of action is relatively rapid, whereas that of 5α-reductase inhibitors is generally delayed by months or more. As noted above, there are three subtypes of the α_1-receptor, namely α_{1A}, α_{1B}, and α_{1D}. Evidence points to preferential expression of the α_{1A}-receptor in genitourinary smooth muscle. **Tamsulosin** is a relatively selective antagonist at α_{1A}-receptors; however, the selectivity is modest: the drug binds with approximately sixfold higher affinity to α_{1A}- than to α_{1B}-receptors. The increased selectivity of tamsulosin for α_{1A}-receptors may decrease the incidence of orthostatic hypotension relative to that associated with prazosin and other nonsubtype-selective α_1-adrenoceptor antagonists. However, this modest advantage has been demonstrated only at low doses of tamsulosin.

Selective blockade of α_2-autoreceptors by drugs such as **yohimbine** leads to increased release of norepinephrine, with subsequent stimulation of cardiac β_1-receptors and peripheral vasculature α_1-receptors. α_2-Selective antagonists also cause increased insulin release through blockade of α_2-receptors in the pancreatic islets, which suppress insulin secretion. Yohimbine has been used to treat erectile dysfunction on the basis of very limited data suggesting possible clinical efficacy.

β-Adrenergic Antagonists

β-Adrenergic antagonists block the positive chronotropic and inotropic actions of endogenous catecholamines at β_1-receptors, resulting in decreased heart rate and myocardial contractility. These drugs decrease blood pressure in hypertensive patients but generally do not lower blood pressure in normotensive individuals. Long-term use of β-adrenoceptor blockers decreases peripheral vascular resistance, although

the mechanism of this effect remains unclear. The decreases in peripheral vascular resistance and cardiac output both contribute to the antihypertensive effect of these drugs. Nonselective β-adrenoceptor antagonists also block β_2-receptors in bronchial smooth muscle, which can cause life-threatening bronchoconstriction in patients with asthma. In addition, nonselective β-receptor blockade may mask symptoms of hypoglycemia in diabetic patients. For these reasons, selective inhibitors of β_1-adrenoceptors have been developed.

Pharmacologic antagonists at β-adrenergic receptors can be divided into nonselective β-antagonists, nonselective β-antagonists with concomitant action as α_1-antagonists, β-adrenergic partial agonists, and β_1-selective antagonists (Table 11-2). Selective blockers of β_2-adrenergic receptors have not been developed clinically as there is no obvious indication for selective β_2-receptor antagonism.

Propranolol, **nadolol**, and **timolol** do not distinguish between β_1- and β_2-receptors in their binding affinities. This is the origin of the term "nonselective β-blockers." At clinical doses, these drugs do not block α-receptors. Nonselective β-blockers have been used for many years in the treatment of hypertension and angina. Although nonselective β-blockers are relatively contraindicated in patients with asthma, these drugs are often well tolerated in patients with chronic obstructive pulmonary disease (COPD) and may be initiated cautiously in many such patients if they have a compelling indication (e.g., coronary artery disease). Nadolol is also efficacious in the prevention of bleeding from esophageal varices in patients with cirrhosis. It is pharmacologically attractive for this indication because it has a long half-life,

TABLE 11-2 Selectivity of Some β-Adrenoceptor Antagonists

DRUG	NOTES
Nonselective β-Adrenergic Antagonists	
Propranolol	Short half-life
Nadolol	Long half-life
Timolol	Lipophilic, high CNS penetration
Nonselective β- and α_1-Antagonists	
Labetalol	Also partial agonist at β_2-receptors
Carvedilol	Intermediate half-life
β-Adrenergic Partial Agonists	
Pindolol	β-Nonselective
Acebutolol	β_1-Selective
β_1-Selective Adrenergic Antagonists	
Esmolol	Short half-life (3–4 minutes)
Metoprolol	Intermediate half-life
Atenolol	Intermediate half-life
Celiprolol	Also agonist at β_2-receptors

CNS, central nervous system.

allowing once-daily administration, and, because the drug is excreted primarily by renal elimination without hepatic metabolism, no dosing adjustments are needed on account of hepatic insufficiency. **Penbutolol** is an additional drug in this class. An ocular formulation of timolol is used in the treatment of glaucoma; even when administered to the eye, systemic absorption of the drug may be sufficiently high to cause adverse effects in susceptible patients. **Levobunolol** and **carteolol** are additional nonselective β-blockers that are indicated for administration via eye drops in the treatment of glaucoma.

Labetalol and **carvedilol** block α_1-, β_1-, and β_2-receptors. Labetalol has two chiral centers; the clinically used drug is a combination of four stereoisomers that have differing pharmacologic properties. Two of these isomers are inactive— (S,S) and (R,S). The (S,R) isomer is a powerful α_1-blocker, and the (R,R) isomer is a nonselective blocker at α_1-, β_1-, and β_2-receptors. Because the effect and metabolism of these isomers may vary among individual patients, the relative proportion of α_1- versus β-blockade is variable. The α_1-receptor blockade tends to lower peripheral resistance; β-blockade also contributes to a decrease in blood pressure, as indicated above. An intravenous formulation of labetalol is available for the lowering of blood pressure in patients with hypertensive emergencies. Drug-induced hepatitis is an unpredictable and idiosyncratic adverse effect of labetalol.

In addition to its action as an α_1-, β_1-, and β_2-receptor blocker, carvedilol acts as a G protein-independent, β-arrestin biased ligand at both β_1- and β_2-adrenergic receptors. Moreover, while carvedilol is efficacious in the outpatient management of hypertension, much interest in this drug has been due to its efficacy in the management of heart failure with decreased systolic function. Carvedilol's cardioprotective effect may be related to its action as a β-arrestin biased ligand at β_1-adrenoceptors, leading to transactivation of the epidermal growth factor receptor.

Pindolol is a partial agonist at β_1- and β_2-receptors. The drug blocks the action of endogenous norepinephrine at β_1-receptors and is useful in treating hypertension. As a partial agonist, pindolol also causes partial stimulation of β_1-receptors, leading to overall smaller decreases in resting heart rate and blood pressure than those caused by pure β-antagonists. **Acebutolol** is a partial agonist at β_1-adrenoceptors but has no effect at β_2-receptors. This agent is also used to treat hypertension and ischemic heart disease. While it has been suggested that partial agonists may be less likely to cause adverse effects in patients with bradycardia, the clinical advantages of drugs in this category remain unclear.

Esmolol, **metoprolol**, **atenolol**, and **betaxolol** are β_1-selective adrenergic antagonists. The elimination half-life is the main feature that distinguishes among these agents. Esmolol has an extremely short half-life (3–4 minutes); metoprolol and atenolol have intermediate half-lives (4–9 hours). Because of its short half-life, esmolol may be safer in unstable patients requiring β-blockade. Esmolol is rapidly metabolized by esterases. Clinical trials have shown that some β-blockers, including metoprolol, prolong life expectancy in patients with mild to moderate heart failure and in patients who have survived a first myocardial infarction (see Chapter 26, Integrative Cardiovascular Pharmacology: Hypertension, Ischemic Heart Disease, and Heart Failure). **Nebivolol** is a novel β_1-selective adrenergic antagonist that

has the ancillary property of promoting vasodilation via nitric oxide release from endothelial cells.

Many of the major adverse effects of β-adrenergic antagonists are a predictable extension of their pharmacologic effects. Such effects include worsening of bronchoconstriction in patients with asthma, decreased cardiac output in patients with decompensated heart failure, and potentially impaired recovery from hypoglycemia in diabetic patients receiving insulin. While β_1-selective adrenergic antagonists may have a lower propensity to block β_2-receptors in bronchial smooth muscle, the selectivity of these drugs is modest and may not be a clinically reliable safeguard against adverse effects. With chronic administration of β-receptor antagonists, pharmacologic adaptations may occur that render cells hypersensitive to catecholamines when the drug is stopped suddenly.

■ CONCLUSION AND FUTURE DIRECTIONS

Adrenergic pharmacology encompasses drugs that act at essentially every step of adrenergic neurotransmission, from synthesis of catecholamines to stimulation of α- and β-receptors. Other classes of drugs, such as L-channel Ca^{2+} blockers, interfere with effector responses activated by these receptors. Novel drugs are being developed that selectively inhibit the downstream effector pathways activated by adrenergic receptors. The drugs discussed in this chapter are mainstays of therapy for hypertension, angina, heart failure, shock, asthma, pheochromocytoma, and other conditions. The beneficial pharmacologic actions of these drugs, as well as many of their important adverse effects, can be anticipated from knowledge of their molecular and cellular mechanisms of action and how these actions affect the processes of adrenergic neurotransmission. While nine subtypes of adrenergic receptor have been identified, three in each of the major classes, the clinical relevance of these subtypes has not yet been fully determined and the pharmacologic implications of these discoveries have not been fully exploited. The development of novel, subtype-selective agonists and antagonists may lead to more effective and less toxic therapies. Biased ligands represent an opportunity for the discovery of new drugs that may expand and diversify the therapeutic options available to clinicians.

Acknowledgment

We thank Freddie M. Williams, Timothy J. Turner, and Brian B. Hoffman for their valuable contributions to this chapter in the First, Second, and Third Editions of *Principles of Pharmacology: The Pathophysiologic Basis of Drug Therapy*.

Suggested Reading

DeWire SM, Ahn S, Lefkowitz RJ, Shenoy SK. Beta-arrestins and cell signaling. *Annu Rev Physiol* 2007;69:483–510. (*Review of novel mechanisms of signaling via seven transmembrane receptors.*)

Reiter E, Ahn S, Shukla AK, Lefkowitz RJ. Molecular mechanism of β-arrestin-biased agonism at seven transmembrane receptors. *Annu Rev Pharmacol Toxicol* 2012;52:179–197. (*Review of biased ligands that have the ability to alter the balance between G protein-dependent and β-arrestin-dependent signal transduction.*)

Rosenbaum DM, Rasmussen SG, Kobilka BK. The structure and function of G-protein-coupled receptors. *Nature* 2009;459:356–363. (*Detailed review of the structure of adrenergic receptors.*)

DRUG SUMMARY TABLE: CHAPTER 11 Adrenergic Pharmacology

DRUG	CLINICAL APPLICATIONS	SERIOUS AND COMMON ADVERSE EFFECTS	CONTRAINDICATIONS	THERAPEUTIC CONSIDERATIONS
INHIBITORS OF CATECHOLAMINE SYNTHESIS Mechanism—Inhibit tyrosine hydroxylase, the rate-limiting enzyme in the catecholamine biosynthesis pathway				
α-Methyltyrosine	Pheochromocytoma-associated hypertension	Orthostatic hypotension, sedation	Hypersensitivity to α-methyltyrosine	Used rarely
INHIBITORS OF CATECHOLAMINE STORAGE Mechanism—Inhibit catecholamine storage in synaptic vesicles, resulting in short-term increase in release of catecholamines from the synaptic terminal but long-term depletion of available pool of catecholamines				
Reserpine	Hypertension Agitated psychotic states	*Cardiac arrhythmia, gastrointestinal hemorrhage* Gastrointestinal upset, xerostomia, dizziness, headache, lethargy, depression, nasal congestion	Hypersensitivity to reserpine alkaloids Active gastrointestinal disease Depression, electroshock therapy Renal failure	Irreversibly inhibits VMAT, resulting in vesicles that lose the ability to concentrate and store norepinephrine and dopamine. Used experimentally to assess whether effect of drug requires its concentration in presynaptic terminals. Rarely used as a therapeutic agent due to its irreversible action and its association with depression.
Guanethidine Guanadrel	Hypertension	*Hypertension (guanethidine only)* Orthostatic hypotension, fluid retention, dizziness, impotence (shared adverse effects); nasal congestion, blurred vision (guanethidine only); gastrointestinal upset (guanadrel only)	Hypersensitivity to drug MAOI therapy Heart failure Pheochromocytoma	Guanethidine and guanadrel concentrate in transmitter vesicles and displace norepinephrine, leading to gradual depletion of norepinephrine. Inhibition of cardiac sympathetic nerves leads to reduced cardiac output; inhibition of sympathetic response leads to symptomatic hypotension after exercise.
Amphetamine Methylphenidate	Attention-deficit hyperactivity disorder (ADHD) (shared indication) Narcolepsy (amphetamine only)	*Peripheral vascular disease, decreased body growth, priapism, drug dependence, hypertension, tachyarrhythmia, Gilles de la Tourette's syndrome, seizure, psychotic disorder with prolonged use* Dysphoric mood, rebound fatigue, addiction potential, loss of appetite, erectile dysfunction, nausea, insomnia	Hypersensitivity to drug Advanced cardiovascular disease Glaucoma Hyperthyroidism MAOI therapy Severe hypertension History of drug dependence	Amphetamine and methylphenidate displace endogenous catecholamines from storage vesicles, weakly inhibit MAO, and block catecholamine reuptake mediated by NET and DAT. Amphetamine is also an agonist at TAAR1, which activates PKA- and PKC-mediated DAT phosphorylation and thereby noncompetitively inhibits dopamine reuptake. Dependence and tolerance can occur.
Pseudoephedrine	Allergic rhinitis Nasal congestion	*Atrial fibrillation, ventricular premature beats, myocardial ischemia* Hypertension, tachyarrhythmia, insomnia, anxiety, restlessness	Hypersensitivity to pseudoephedrine Advanced cardiovascular disease MAOI therapy Severe or uncontrolled hypertension	Used as an over-the-counter decongestant; often found in cold remedies and appetite suppressants. Ephedrine and phenylpropanolamine have been restricted in the United States.

INHIBITORS OF CATECHOLAMINE REUPTAKE **Mechanism—Inhibit norepinephrine transporter (NET)-mediated reuptake of catecholamines, potentiating catecholamine action**				
Cocaine **Imipramine** **Amitriptyline**	See Drug Summary Table: Chapter 12 Local Anesthetic Pharmacology See Drug Summary Table: Chapter 15 Pharmacology of Serotonergic and Central Adrenergic Neurotransmission			
MONOAMINE OXIDASE (MAO) INHIBITORS **Mechanism—Inhibit MAO, increasing catecholamine levels by blocking catecholamine degradation**				
Phenelzine **Iproniazid** **Tranylcypromine** **Clorgyline** **Brofaromine** **Befloxatone** **Moclobemide** **Selegiline** **Rasagiline**	See Drug Summary Table: Chapter 15 Pharmacology of Serotonergic and Central Adrenergic Neurotransmission			
α_1-ADRENERGIC AGONISTS **Mechanism—Selectively activate α_1-adrenergic receptors to increase peripheral vascular resistance**				
Methoxamine	Hypotension, shock	*Bradycardia (vagal reflex), ventricular ectopic beat* Hypertension, vasoconstriction, nausea, headache, anxiety	Hypersensitivity to methoxamine Severe hypertension	Very limited clinical use in the treatment of shock.
Phenylephrine **Oxymetazoline** **Tetrahydrozoline**	Ophthalmic hyperemia (shared indication) Nasal congestion (shared indication) Hypotension (phenylephrine only)	*Cardiac arrhythmia, hypertension* Headache, insomnia, nervousness, rebound nasal congestion, mucosal irritation	Hypersensitivity to drug (shared contraindication) Narrow-angle glaucoma (shared contraindication) Severe hypertension or tachycardia (contraindication for IV form of phenylephrine)	Used in the nonprescription remedies Afrin® and Visine® (and others) for relief of nasal congestion and ophthalmic hyperemia; rebound of symptoms often accompanies use of these drugs. Phenylephrine is also used intravenously in the treatment of distributive shock.
α_2-ADRENERGIC AGONISTS **Mechanism—Selectively activate central α_2-adrenergic autoreceptors and thereby inhibit sympathetic outflow from CNS**				
Clonidine **Dexmedetomidine** **Guanabenz** **Guanfacine** **Methyldopa**	Hypertension (clonidine, guanabenz, guanfacine, and methyldopa only) Sedation of surgical and ICU patients without respiratory depression (dexmedetomidine only) Attention-deficit hyperactivity disorder (guanfacine only)	*Cardiac arrhythmias (shared adverse effect); seizure (guanfacine only); heart failure, colitis, pancreatitis, hepatotoxicity, autoimmune hemolytic anemia, systemic lupus erythematosus, parkinsonism (methyldopa only); bronchospasm, pleural effusion, respiratory depression (dexmedetomidine only)* Rash, hypotension, hypertension, xerostomia, sedation, dizziness, headache (shared adverse effects); impotence (methyldopa only)	Hypersensitivity to drug (shared contraindication) MAO inhibitor therapy and active liver disease (methyldopa only)	Clonidine is used for treatment of hypertension and symptoms associated with opioid withdrawal. Methyldopa is drug of choice for treatment of hypertension during pregnancy.

continues

DRUG SUMMARY TABLE: CHAPTER 11 Adrenergic Pharmacology *continued*

DRUG	CLINICAL APPLICATIONS	SERIOUS AND COMMON ADVERSE EFFECTS	CONTRAINDICATIONS	THERAPEUTIC CONSIDERATIONS
β-ADRENERGIC AGONISTS **Mechanism—Activate β-adrenergic receptors**				
Isoproterenol **Dobutamine** **Metaproterenol** **Terbutaline** **Albuterol** **Salmeterol**	See Drug Summary Table: Chapter 25 Pharmacology of Cardiac Contractility See Drug Summary Table: Chapter 48 Integrative Inflammation Pharmacology: Asthma			
α-ADRENERGIC ANTAGONISTS **Mechanism—Block the binding of endogenous catecholamines to α₁- and α₂-adrenoceptors, causing vasodilation, decreased blood pressure, and decreased peripheral resistance**				
Phenoxybenzamine **Phentolamine**	Pheochromocytoma-associated hypertension and sweating (shared indication) Reversal of anesthesia during dental procedure (phentolamine only) Treatment of norepinephrine extravasation reaction (phentolamine only)	*Cardiac arrhythmia, stroke (phentolamine only); seizure (phenoxybenzamine only)* Postural hypotension, tachycardia, gastrointestinal upset, xerostomia, sedation, miosis, absence of ejaculation	Hypersensitivity to drug (shared contraindication) Severe hypotension (shared contraindication) Coronary artery disease (phentolamine only)	Phenoxybenzamine irreversibly blocks both α₁- and α₂-receptors by covalent binding. Phentolamine is a reversible, nonselective α-adrenoceptor antagonist. Used in preoperative management of pheochromocytoma.
Prazosin **Terazosin** **Doxazosin**	Hypertension (shared indication) Benign prostatic hyperplasia (terazosin and doxazosin only)	*Pancreatitis (prazosin only); intraoperative floppy iris syndrome, priapism (terazosin and doxazosin only); hepatitis, angioedema (doxazosin only)* Marked first-dose postural hypotension, palpitations, dizziness, sedation, headache, nasal congestion	Hypersensitivity to prazosin, terazosin, or doxazosin	Prazosin, terazosin, and doxazosin are nonsubtype-selective antagonists of α₁-receptors in arterioles and veins. Reflex tachycardia does not usually occur. Due to potential severe postural hypotension, first dose is generally prescribed in small quantities at bedtime (to ensure that the patient remains supine). Terazosin and doxazosin have a longer half-life than prazosin. Tricyclic antidepressants may increase the risk of postural hypotension.
Tamsulosin	Benign prostatic hyperplasia	*Retinal detachment, priapism* Dizziness, headache, abnormal ejaculation, rhinitis	Hypersensitivity to tamsulosin	Tamsulosin is a subtype-selective α₁A-receptor antagonist that has more specificity toward smooth muscle in genitourinary tract; thus, tamsulosin has lower incidence of orthostatic hypotension.

Drug	Indications	Adverse Effects	Contraindications	Notes
Yohimbine	Organic and psychogenic impotence	*Bronchospasm, nervousness, tremor, anxiety, agitation, increased blood pressure, antidiuresis*	Chronic inflammation of sexual organs or prostate gland; Concurrent use with mood-altering drugs; Gastric and duodenal ulcers; Pregnancy; Psychiatric patients; Renal and liver disease	Yohimbine is an α_2-selective antagonist that leads to increased release of norepinephrine, which stimulates cardiac β_1-receptors and peripheral vascular α_1-receptors. Also leads to increased insulin release due to blockade of α_2-receptors in pancreatic islets.

β-ADRENERGIC ANTAGONISTS

Mechanism—Block β-adrenergic receptors; this class of drugs can be divided into nonselective β-antagonists, nonselective β- and α_1-antagonists, partial agonists, and β_1-selective antagonists

Drug	Indications	Adverse Effects	Contraindications	Notes
Propranolol Nadolol Timolol Penbutolol Levobunolol Carteolol	Shared indication except for levobunolol: Hypertension. Propranolol and nadolol only: Angina. Propranolol and timolol only: Migraine, Postmyocardial infarction syndrome. Propranolol only: Heart failure, Pheochromocytoma, Capillary hemangioma, Essential tremor, Cardiac arrhythmia, Idiopathic hypertrophic subaortic stenosis. Timolol, levobunolol, and carteolol ocular formulations only: Glaucoma	*Cardiac arrhythmias, heart failure (shared adverse effects); bronchospasm (propranolol, levobunolol, carteolol, and timolol only); Stevens-Johnson syndrome (propranolol and levobunolol only); toxic epidermal necrolysis, stroke (propranolol only). Gastrointestinal upset (propranolol and timolol only); sleep disorder (propranolol only); angina, hypotension, rash, blurred vision (timolol and carteolol only); burning sensation in eye (levobunolol and carteolol only); dizziness, headache, conjunctival edema, epiphora (carteolol only)*	Shared contraindications: Hypersensitivity to drug; Severe sinus bradycardia; Bronchial asthma or chronic obstructive pulmonary disease; Cardiogenic shock; Second- and third-degree AV block. Propranolol, nadolol, timolol, levobunolol, and carteolol only: Heart failure. Propranolol only: Hypotension; Pheochromocytoma; Premature infants	Propranolol, nadolol, and timolol block β_1- and β_2-receptors nonselectively. Propranolol is extremely lipophilic; its CNS concentration is sufficiently high that sedation and decreased libido may result. An ocular formulation of timolol is used in the treatment of glaucoma.
Labetalol Carvedilol	Hypertension (shared indication) Heart failure (carvedilol only)	*Heart failure, hyperkalemia, hepatotoxicity, bronchospasm (labetalol only); atrioventricular block, Stevens-Johnson syndrome, toxic epidermal necrolysis, aplastic anemia, intraoperative floppy iris syndrome (carvedilol only); Orthostatic hypotension, dizziness (labetalol only); fatigue (carvedilol only)*	Hypersensitivity to drug; Asthma; Cardiogenic shock; Heart failure; Second- or third-degree atrioventricular block; Severe bradycardia; Severe hepatic impairment	Labetalol and carvedilol block α_1-, β_1-, and β_2-receptors. Labetalol may cause liver damage; liver function tests must be monitored.

continues

DRUG SUMMARY TABLE: CHAPTER 11 Adrenergic Pharmacology *continued*

DRUG	CLINICAL APPLICATIONS	*SERIOUS* AND COMMON ADVERSE EFFECTS	CONTRAINDICATIONS	THERAPEUTIC CONSIDERATIONS
Pindolol **Acebutolol**	Hypertension (shared indication) Ventricular arrhythmias (acebutolol only)	*Heart failure* Edema	Shared contraindications: Hypersensitivity to drug Bradycardia Heart failure Cardiogenic shock Second- or third-degree heart block Pindolol only: Asthma or chronic obstructive pulmonary disease	Pindolol is a partial agonist at β_1- and β_2-receptors; it is preferred in hypertensive patients who have bradycardia or decreased cardiac reserve. Acebutolol is a partial agonist at β_1-adrenoceptors but has no effect at β_2-receptors.
Esmolol **Metoprolol** **Atenolol** **Betaxolol** **Nebivolol**	Hypertension (shared indication) Supraventricular tachycardia (esmolol only) Angina (metoprolol and atenolol only) Acute myocardial infarction (metoprolol and atenolol only) Heart failure (metoprolol only) Primary open-angle glaucoma (betaxolol only)	*Ventricular arrhythmia (betaxolol and nebivolol only); heart failure (atenolol and metoprolol only); thyrotoxicosis, systemic lupus erythematosus (atenolol only); atrioventricular block (betaxolol only).* Hypotension (shared adverse effect); bradyarrhythmia (metoprolol and atenolol only); fatigue (atenolol only); burning sensation in eye (betaxolol only)	Shared contraindications: Hypersensitivity to drug Second- and third-degree AV block Sinus bradycardia Heart failure Cardiogenic shock Metoprolol only: Sick sinus syndrome Peripheral arterial circulatory disorders Hypotension Nebivolol only: Hepatic impairment	Esmolol, metoprolol, and atenolol are β_1-selective adrenergic antagonists. Esmolol has an extremely short half-life (3–4 minutes) and thus is used for emergency β-blockade, as in thyroid storm. Nebivolol has the ancillary property of promoting vasodilation via nitric oxide release from endothelial cells.

12

Epineurium
Perineurium
Endoneurium
Schwann cell

Local Anesthetic Pharmacology

Quentin J. Baca, Joshua M. Schulman, and Gary R. Strichartz

INTRODUCTION

Local anesthetics (LAs) are a class of locally applied chemicals, with similar molecular structures, that can disrupt nerve transmission, inhibit the perception of sensations (importantly, pain), blunt autonomic activity, and prevent movement. They are used for a variety of clinical applications and delivered via many different approaches, ranging from topical application for burns and small cuts, to injections during dental care, to epidural and intrathecal ("spinal") blocks during obstetric procedures and major surgery.

Cocaine, the first local anesthetic, comes from the leaves of the coca shrub (*Erythroxylon coca*). It was first isolated in 1860 by Albert Niemann, who noted its numbing powers. In 1886, Carl Koller introduced cocaine into clinical practice as a topical ophthalmic anesthetic. However, its addictive properties and toxicity prompted the search for substitutes. **Procaine**, the first of these substitutes to prove clinically useful, was synthesized in 1905. Known as Novocain®, it is still used today, although less frequently than some more recently developed LAs.

Local anesthetics exert their effect by blocking voltage-gated sodium channels, thus inhibiting the propagation of action potentials along neurons (see Chapter 8, Principles of Cellular Excitability and Electrochemical Transmission). By inhibiting action potential propagation, LAs prevent transmission of information to and from the central nervous system (CNS). LA actions are not selective for pain fibers; they can also block conduction in other sensory fibers as well as motor and autonomic fibers and action potentials in skeletal and cardiac muscle. This nonselective blockade can serve other useful functions (see Chapter 24, Pharmacology of Cardiac Rhythm) or can be a source of toxicity.

PHYSIOLOGY OF NOCICEPTION

Nociception occurs following the activation of particular primary sensory nerve fibers (nociceptors) by a noxious stimulus representing potential or actual tissue damage. Noxious stimuli include extreme temperatures, intense mechanical perturbations, harsh chemical environments, and certain molecules released by damaged cells (Fig. 12-1). Nociceptors are activated by noxious stimuli at free nerve endings, which are located in the skin, deeper tissues such as joints and tendons, and viscera. When activated, nociceptors transmit impulses from the periphery to the dorsal horn of the spinal cord, where the information is subsequently processed through synaptic circuitry and transmitted to various parts of the brain. Thus, nociceptors are the first, or primary, cells in a chain of neurons ultimately responsible for pain perception. Because nociceptors, among other sensory fibers, transmit information toward the brain, they are termed **afferent neurons**.

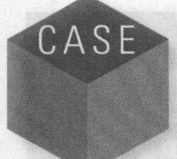

CASE

EM is a 24-year-old graduate student in organic chemistry. While he is working in the lab one evening, a bottle of concentrated hydrochloric acid falls from a shelf above him and smashes his left hand against the lab bench before it shatters and cuts his index finger. Although he reflexively jerks his hand away, some of the acid falls on the fingertips of his hand. He immediately feels a localized sharp pain where the bottle cut his hand followed by a diffuse stinging pain where the acid touched his skin. Although he begins to rinse his hand under running water, he still feels a slowly developing, burning, throbbing ache throughout his hand. EM anxiously telephones 911 and is transported to the emergency department.

On exam in the emergency department, he is noted to have a 1.5-cm laceration of his left index finger and isolated areas of red, tender skin with partial-thickness burn on the fingers exposed to acid. He is in severe pain and his laceration will need to be sutured. After continued irrigation of the acid-exposed areas of his hand, topical EMLA cream (eutectic mixture of local anesthetic—a combination of lidocaine and prilocaine) is applied to the burned areas and a *digital nerve block* of his index finger is performed. After the area is made sterile, 1 cc of 2% lidocaine without epinephrine is injected into the medial and lateral aspects of his finger near the web space to block the digital nerves. The lidocaine injection is directed toward both the palm and the back of his hand in order to block both the dorsal and ventral contributions to the digital nerves that run down the lateral and medial aspects of the finger. He notices that the sharp stinging pain from his cut abates first, followed by the dull throbbing ache in his finger. EM then loses sensation to light touch on his finger and later notes that he cannot feel the needle piercing his skin as the sutures are applied. EM's wounds heal over the next 2 weeks, and the pain, now primarily a result of post-traumatic inflammation, is well controlled with oral ibuprofen. He is able to return to work.

Questions

1. Why did EM initially experience a stinging pain before the dull aching pain, and why did the stinging pain resolve more quickly than the dull pain after lidocaine administration?

2. Why is epinephrine sometimes administered with lidocaine, and why was it not co-administered in this case?

3. What is lidocaine's mechanism of action? To which broader class of drugs does it belong?

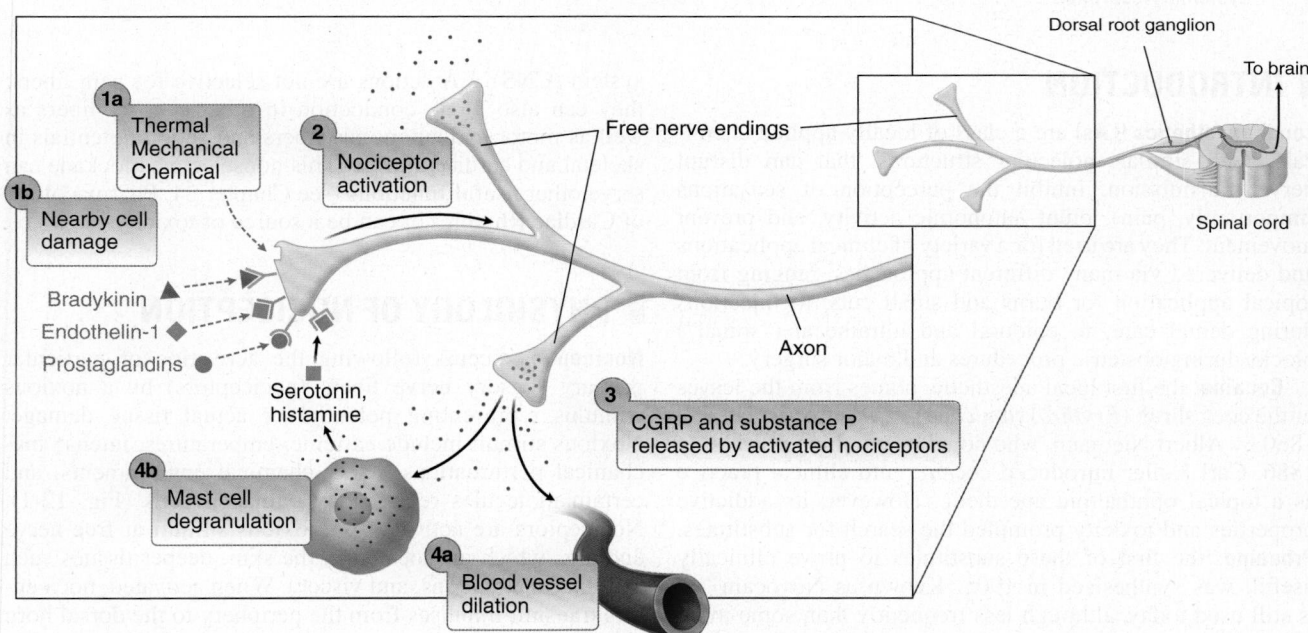

FIGURE 12-1. Nociceptor activation. Nociceptors transduce pain information using a variety of mechanisms. Some receptors on the neuron transduce noxious stimuli (thermal, mechanical, or chemical) into electrical potentials. Other receptors are stimulated by substances that are released when nearby cells are injured (bradykinin, endothelin-1, ATP, prostaglandins). The release of K^+ from nearby damaged cells directly depolarizes nociceptor membranes. All of these stimuli cause nociceptor "sensitization," which decreases the threshold for electrical activation. **1a.** A noxious stimulus leads to nociceptor activation and action potential generation (**2**). **1b.** Concurrent nearby cell damage causes nociceptor sensitization. **3.** Activated nociceptors release substances, including substance P and calcitonin gene-related peptide (CGRP), that contribute to further sensitization and that initiate inflammatory responses to promote healing. For example: **4a.** Blood vessel dilation promotes white blood cell recruitment to the area. **4b.** Mast cell degranulation releases histamine and serotonin, thus increasing sensitization.

Nociceptors are normally not activated by nonnoxious stimuli such as a breeze against one's skin or a handshake (the nerves that are activated in these circumstances are termed **tactile** or **low-** or **medium-threshold mechanoreceptors**). When a noxious stimulus is present at a free nerve ending of a nociceptor, it activates specific transducing receptors that generate inward currents and depolarize the primary neuron (Fig. 12-1; also see Chapter 8). If a noxious stimulus has an intensity above the nociceptor's threshold (e.g., above a certain temperature), an action potential (AP) will be generated. Sensory information is almost always encoded by trains of APs, and the frequency of APs in a train increases as the stimulus intensity increases (e.g., at higher temperatures). If impulses from a nociceptive afferent nerve are sufficiently frequent, or if multiple nociceptors are activated, then the generating stimulus is perceived as "painful." Although lower stimulus intensities may not be perceived, these "subliminal" sensory inputs are still transmitted to the CNS and can influence future sensory coding. Explicitly painful stimuli are able to induce long-lasting increases in responsiveness of the CNS and thus to effect a "memory" of pain. Such *central sensitization* is one component of chronic pain (see Chapter 18, Pharmacology of Analgesia).

Transmission of Pain Sensation

In their simplest form, neurons are composed of dendrites, a cell body, and an axon. Axons transmit information along the neuron to dendrites, which synapse with other neurons. Nerve axons are classified as **A-fibers**, **B-fibers**, or **C-fibers**, ranked in the order of decreasing diameter and having respectively decreasing conduction velocities. A-fibers and B-fibers are myelinated; while C-fibers are nonmyelinated, they are still encased in a peripheral glial Schwann cell that collects up to 10 axons in a Remak bundle (Table 12-1). Myelin is composed of the cell membranes of supportive cells in the nervous system (Schwann cells peripherally and oligodendrocytes in the CNS) that wrap tightly many times around neuronal axons to create an electrically insulating sheath that increases the velocity of impulse transmission. Regular, narrow spacings between the myelinated segments, called *nodes of Ranvier*, contain the voltage-gated

Na^+ channels and are the locations where inward ionic current drives the APs of myelinated fibers.

Distinct types of nociceptors are activated by specific noxious stimuli and transmit information along characteristic classes of axons. Nociceptor axons are generally either **Aδ-fibers** or **C-fibers**. *Thermal* nociceptors are activated at temperatures above 45°C (noxious heat, C-fibers) or below 5°C (noxious cold, Aδ-fibers). *High-threshold mechanical* nociceptors exclusively transmit information indicating injurious force on the skin (Aδ- and some Aβ-fibers). *Polymodal* nociceptors are activated by thermal, mechanical, and chemical stimuli (C-fibers).

First Pain and Second Pain

Myelinated Aδ-fibers transmit impulses faster than nonmyelinated C-fibers do (Fig. 12-2). An Aδ-fiber transmits impulses along its axon at a rate of 5–25 meters per second (m/s), while C-fibers transmit impulses at roughly 1 m/s. Impulse transmission is slower in C-fibers primarily because these fibers are nonmyelinated.

The Aδ-fibers transmit what is called **first pain**, which is perceived within seconds after an injury, is sharp in quality, and is highly localized on the body. The density of nociceptor Aδ-fibers is high on the fingertips, face, and lips but relatively low on the back. Aδ-fibers require a weaker stimulus for excitation than C-fibers do.

The C-fibers transmit what is called **second pain**. Second pain is slower to develop, appearing many seconds after an insult, but lasts much longer than first pain; it often feels dull, throbbing, or burning, is poorly localized, and endures long after the stimulus ends. C-fiber nociceptors are often polymodal, which means that a single fiber can be activated by noxious thermal, mechanical, and chemical stimuli. In the case above, EM experienced an initial stinging first pain transmitted by myelinated Aδ-fibers and a later burning and throbbing second pain transmitted by unmyelinated C-fibers. Afferent activity conducted by C-nociceptors has a pronounced potential to create central sensitization, and it also activates regions of the brain, such as the amygdala and prefrontal cortex, that are involved in the affective, subjective aspect of pain perception.

TABLE 12-1 Types of Peripheral Nerve Fibers

FIBER TYPE	MYELINATED	DIAMETER (μm)	CONDUCTION VELOCITY (m/s)	FUNCTION	SENSITIVITY TO LIDOCAINE
Aα, Aβ	Yes	6–22	10–85	Motor and proprioception (pressure, touch, position)	+, ++
Aγ	Yes	3–6	15–35	Muscle tone	++++
Aδ	Yes	1–4	5–25	First pain and temperature	++++
B	Yes	<3	3–15	Vasomotor, visceromotor, sudomotor, pilomotor	+++
C (sympathetic)	No	0.3–1.3	0.7–1.3	Vasomotor, visceromotor, sudomotor, pilomotor	++
C (dorsal root)	No	0.4–1.2	0.1–2.0	Second pain and temperature	++

Each peripheral nerve fiber type is responsible for transmitting one or more specific modalities. For example, the nociceptors (Aδ and C dorsal root fibers) are responsible for transmitting pain and temperature sensations. These fibers are not activated by pressure, light touch, or position changes. Myelin is an insulator that allows impulses to be conducted at faster speeds along axons. The nonmyelinated C-fibers have a slower conduction velocity than the myelinated fibers do. The different fiber types are affected by local anesthetics with differing degrees of sensitivity.

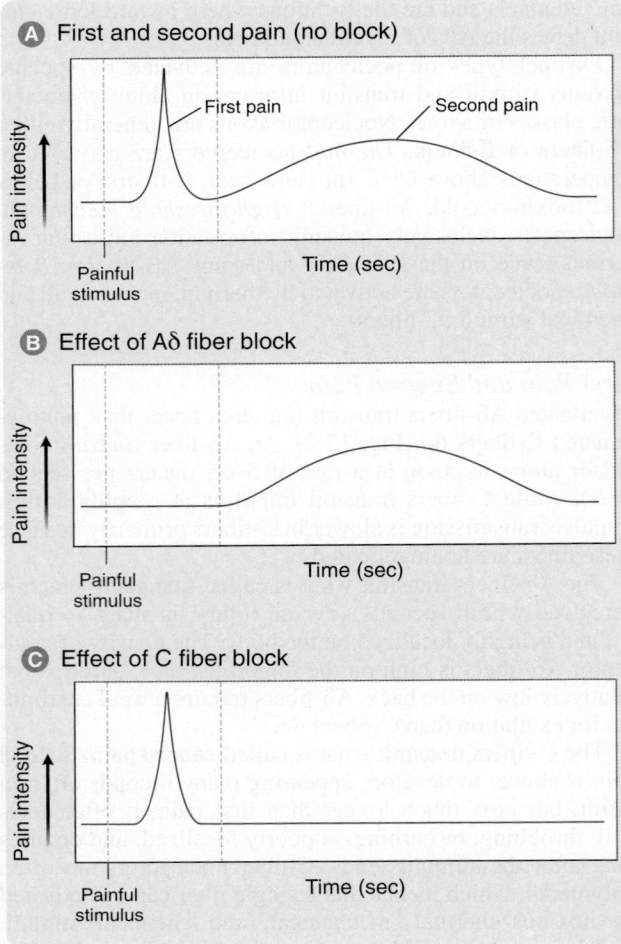

FIGURE 12-2. First and second pain. First pain, which is transmitted by Aδ-fibers, is sharp and highly localizable. Second pain, which is transmitted by C-fibers, is slower in arriving, duller, and longer lasting **(A)**. First pain can be prevented by selective blockade of Aδ-fibers **(B)**, and second pain can be prevented by selective blockade of C-fibers **(C)**. Because Aδ-fibers are more susceptible than C-fibers to blockade by local anesthetics, first pain often disappears at concentrations of anesthetic lower than those required to eliminate second pain.

Pain Perception

Pain is the physical or emotional distress due to perceived actual or potential tissue injury. Pain perception is a complex process that involves activation of nociceptive neurons by a noxious stimulus and central regulation and interpretation of the nociceptive signals in the CNS. Impulses generated in the skin by nociceptor activation are conducted to the dorsal horn of the spinal cord. In the dorsal horn, the nociceptors form synapses with interneurons and second-order neurons. The second-order neurons travel in the lateral areas of the spinal cord and project mainly to the thalamus, a gray matter structure just superior to the brainstem. The thalamus has cells that project to the somatosensory cortex of the parietal lobe and to other areas of the cortex (Fig. 12-3). Nociceptive signals as well as information from non-nociceptive afferent nerves are integrated centrally and interpreted as pain. The subjective sensation of pain is also altered by less tangible central factors including emotional state and higher

executive function. The CNS uses efferent projections within the brain and spinal cord to modulate the incoming nociceptive signals and thus to modify pain perception (see Chapter 18). For example, an athlete focused on an important game might not feel the pain of an injury intensely until after the game is over. Her brain modulates the effect of the input so that the same stimulus is perceived as less painful at certain times than at others.

Analgesia and Anesthesia

Analgesics are specific inhibitors of *pain* pathways, whereas **local anesthetics** are *nonspecific* inhibitors of peripheral sensory (including pain), motor, and autonomic nerve transmission. Analgesics have actions at specific receptors on

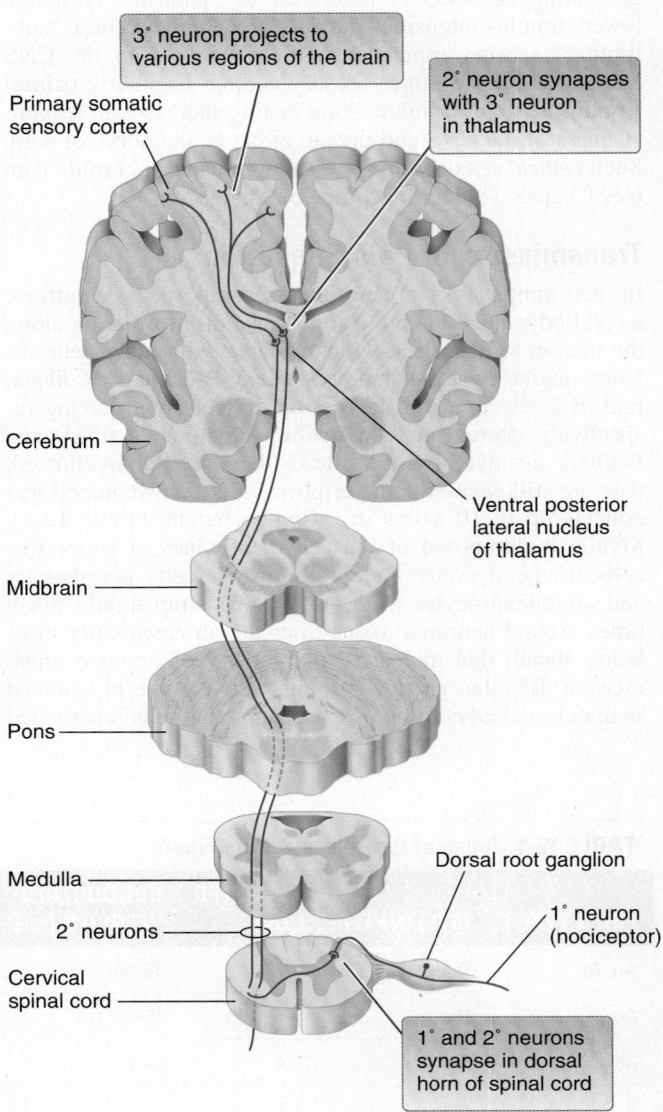

FIGURE 12-3. Pain pathways. Primary (1°) nociceptors have cell bodies in the dorsal root ganglion and synapse with secondary (2°) afferent neurons in the dorsal horn of the spinal cord. Primary afferents use the neurotransmitter glutamate. The 2° afferents travel in the lateral areas of the spinal cord and eventually reach the thalamus, where they synapse with tertiary (3°) afferent neurons. The processing of pain is complex, and 3° afferents have many destinations including the somatosensory cortex (localization of pain) and the limbic system (emotional aspects of pain).

primary nociceptors and in the CNS (see Chapter 18). For example, opioid analgesics activate opioid receptors, which signal cells to increase potassium conductance in postsynaptic neurons and to decrease calcium entry into presynaptic neurons. By these mechanisms, postsynaptic excitability and presynaptic transmitter release are reduced, and pain sensations are not transmitted as effectively to the brain (or within it). Importantly, the transmission of other sensations and motor information is not affected.

Local anesthetics act by a different mechanism. *These agents inhibit conduction of action potentials in all afferent and efferent nerve fibers, usually in the peripheral nervous system.* Thus, pain and other sensory modalities are not transmitted effectively to the brain, and motor and autonomic impulses are not transmitted effectively to muscles and peripheral organs.

PHARMACOLOGIC CLASSES AND AGENTS

Local anesthetics prevent signal transmission by blocking the function of sodium channels in excitable tissues. All LAs share this common mechanism of action and have similar chemical structures. The next section highlights the general principles of LA pharmacology and how the molecular properties of LAs affect their function. Specific LA agents are discussed at the end of the chapter.

Molecular Determinants of Local Anesthetic Action

All local anesthetics have three structural domains: an aromatic group, an amine group, and an ester or amide linkage connecting these two groups (Fig. 12-4). Local anesthetics are structurally classified as **ester-linked LAs** or **amide-linked LAs**. As discussed below, the structure of the aromatic group influences the hydrophobicity of the drug, and the nature of the amine group influences the charge of the drug. Both features define the rate of onset, potency, duration of action, and adverse effects of an individual local anesthetic.

Aromatic Group

To be effective, a local anesthetic must partition into, diffuse across, and finally dissociate from the membrane into the cytoplasm; the compounds most likely to do so have moderate hydrophobicity. All local anesthetics contain an aromatic group that gives the molecule much of its hydrophobic character. Adding alkyl substituents on the aromatic ring, or on the amino nitrogen, also increases the hydrophobicity of these drugs.

Biological membranes have a hydrophobic interior because of their lipid bilayer structure. The hydrophobicity of an LA molecule affects the ease with which the drug passes through nerve cell membranes to reach its target site, which is the *cytoplasmic side of the voltage-gated sodium channel* (Fig. 12-5). Molecules with low hydrophobicity partition very poorly into the membrane because their solubility in the lipid bilayer is so low; such molecules are largely restricted to the polar aqueous environment. As the hydrophobicity of a series of drugs increases, the concentration in the membrane and the correlated permeability of the drugs through the cell membrane also increase. However, at a certain hydrophobicity, this relationship reverses, and a further increase in

hydrophobicity results in a decrease in permeability. This somewhat paradoxical behavior occurs because molecules that are extremely hydrophobic partition so strongly into the cell membrane that they remain there. The same strong hydrophobic forces that concentrate such molecules in the cell membrane cause them to dissociate very slowly from that compartment.

The LA binding site on the sodium channel contains both hydrophilic and hydrophobic residues that are located on transmembrane helices in three of the four domains that form the channel's pore. The fit is not very tight, however, resulting

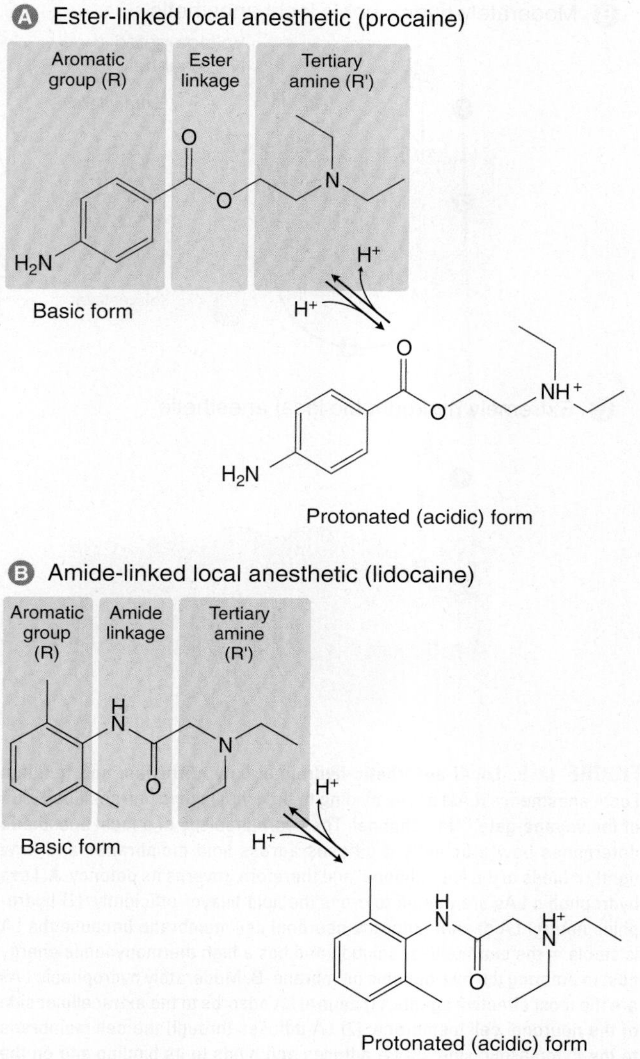

A Ester-linked local anesthetic (procaine)

Aromatic group (R)   Ester linkage   Tertiary amine (R')

Basic form

Protonated (acidic) form

B Amide-linked local anesthetic (lidocaine)

Aromatic group (R)   Amide linkage   Tertiary amine (R')

Basic form

Protonated (acidic) form

FIGURE 12-4. Prototypical local anesthetics. Procaine **(A)** and lidocaine **(B)** are prototypical ester-linked and amide-linked local anesthetics, respectively. Local anesthetics have an aromatic group on one end and an amine on the other end of the molecule; these two groups are connected by an ester (-RCOOR') or amide (-RHNCOR') linkage. In solution at high pH, the equilibrium between the basic (neutral) and acidic (charged) forms of a local anesthetic favors the basic form. At low pH, the equilibrium favors the acidic form. At intermediate (physiologic) pH, nearly equal concentrations of the basic and acidic forms are present. Generally, ester-linked local anesthetics are easily hydrolyzed to a carboxylic acid (RCOOH) and an alcohol (HOR') in the presence of water and esterases. In comparison, amides are far more stable in solution. Consequently, amide-linked local anesthetics generally have a longer duration of action than do ester-linked anesthetics.

A Poorly hydrophobic local anesthetic

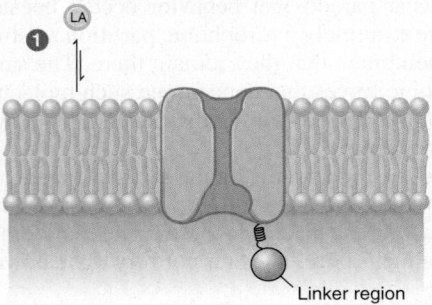

B Moderately hydrophobic local anesthetic

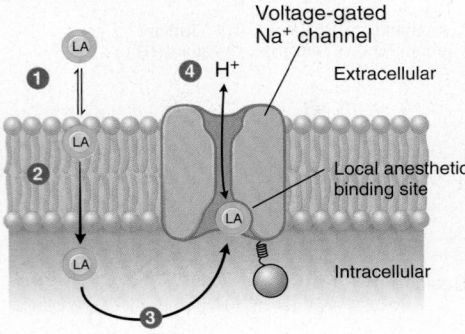

C Extremely hydrophobic local anesthetic

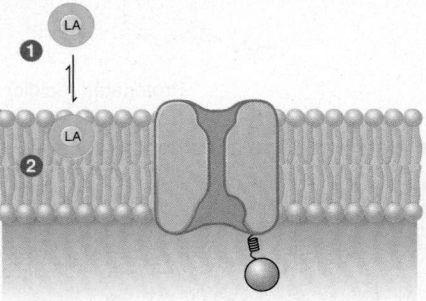

FIGURE 12-5. Local anesthetic hydrophobicity, diffusion, and binding. Local anesthetics (LAs) act by binding to the cytoplasmic (intracellular) side of the voltage-gated Na^+ channel. The hydrophobicity of a local anesthetic determines how efficiently it diffuses across lipid membranes and how tightly it binds to the Na^+ channel and therefore governs its potency. **A.** Less hydrophobic LAs are unable to cross the lipid bilayer efficiently: (1) hydrophilic neutral LA cannot enter the neuronal cell membrane because the LA is stable in the extracellular solution and has a high thermodynamic energy cost to entering the hydrophobic membrane. **B.** Moderately hydrophobic LAs are the most effective agents: (1) neutral LA adsorbs to the extracellular side of the neuronal cell membrane; (2) LA diffuses through the cell membrane to the cytoplasmic side; (3) LA diffuses and binds to its binding site on the voltage-gated sodium channel; and (4) once bound, LA can switch between its neutral and protonated forms by binding and releasing protons. **C.** Extremely hydrophobic LAs become trapped in the lipid bilayer: (1) neutral LA adsorbs to the neuronal cell membrane (2), where it is unlikely to dissociate from or diffuse out of the membrane.

in relatively low LA potency (IC_{50} of 10^{-3} to 10^{-5} M) and only weak stereoselectivity. In general, more hydrophobic drugs bind more tightly to the target site, increasing the potency of the drug. However, because of the practical need for the drug to diffuse across several membranes in order to reach the target site (see below), LAs with moderate

hydrophobicity are the clinically effective molecules. In addition, excessively hydrophobic drugs have limited solubility in the aqueous solutions of their pharmaceutical formulation, and even the molecules that do dissolve remain in the first membrane that is encountered, never reaching the target site in the axon membrane (despite their high affinity for that site). Indeed, access of LAs from the injection site to the axon is so poor, due to permeability barriers and removal by the local circulation, that LA concentrations 20- to 50-fold higher than those effective on an isolated nerve must be injected locally for a successful block.

Amine Group

The amine group of a local anesthetic can exist in either the protonated (positively charged; acid) form or the deprotonated (neutral; base) form.

The pK_a is the pH at which the concentrations of a base and its conjugate acid are equal. LAs are weak bases; their pK_a values range from about 8 to 10. Thus, at the physiologic pH of 7.4, substantial amounts of both the protonated form and the neutral form coexist in solution. As the pK_a of a drug increases, a larger fraction of molecules exists in solution in the protonated form at physiologic pH (see Chapter 1, Drug–Receptor Interactions). Protonation and deprotonation reactions are very rapid in solution (10^3 sec^{-1}), but drugs in membranes or bound to proteins are protonated and deprotonated more slowly.

The neutral forms of LAs diffuse across membranes much more easily than the positively charged forms do. However, the positively charged forms bind with much higher affinity to the drugs' target binding site. This site is located in the pore of the voltage-gated sodium channel and is accessible from the intracellular, cytoplasmic entrance of the channel (Fig. 12-5B). Thus, moderately hydrophobic weak bases are effective as local anesthetics because, at physiologic pH, a significant fraction of the weak base molecules are in the neutral form, which, because of its moderate hydrophobicity, can rapidly diffuse across membranes to enter nerve cells. Once the drug is inside the cell, it can then readily gain a proton, become positively charged, and bind to the sodium channel. The neutral species of LAs can also bind to the channel, but the dissociation of this species from the channel is much faster and its affinity is correspondingly lower. Some nonionizable LA drugs, such as benzocaine, are permanently neutral but are still able to block sodium channels. For these drugs, however, the block is weak and rapidly reversible.

Mechanism of Action of Local Anesthetics

Anatomic Factors in Impulse Blockade

The peripheral nerve is composed of a collection of different types of nerve fibers (A-, B-, and C-fibers) surrounded by three protective membranes, or sheaths: the epineurium, perineurium, and endoneurium. Local anesthetic molecules must pass through these sheaths, which present the same permeation-limiting barriers as the nerve cell membranes, considered above, before they can reach the neuronal membranes to block conduction (Fig. 12-6). The sheaths are made up of connective tissue and cell membranes. LAs are injected outside the most external sheath, the epineurium, to avoid mechanical damage to the nerve, but the major barrier to LA penetration into the nerve is the perineurium, an epithelium-like tissue that bundles axons into separate fascicles. Recall that LAs affect not only nociceptors but also

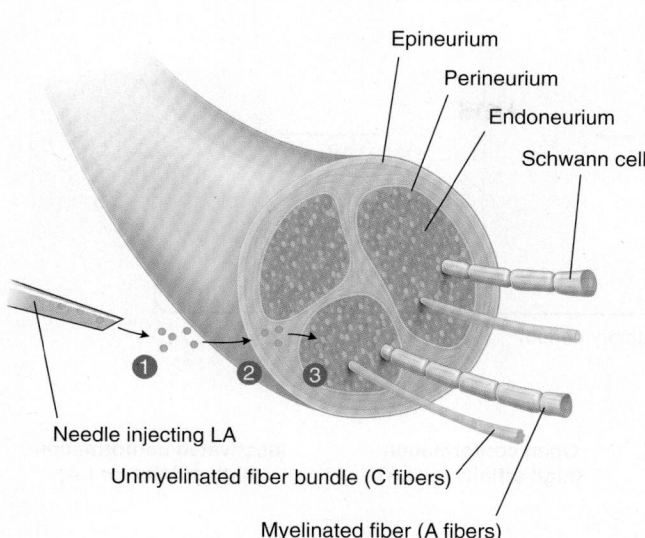

Epineurium
Perineurium
Endoneurium
Schwann cell

Needle injecting LA

Unmyelinated fiber bundle (C fibers)

Myelinated fiber (A fibers)

FIGURE 12-6. Peripheral nerve anatomy. 1. Local anesthetics (LAs) are injected or otherwise applied outside the peripheral nerve epineurium (the outermost sheath of connective tissue containing blood vessels, adipose tissue, fibroblasts, and mast cells). **2.** LA molecules must cross the epineurium to reach the perineurium, another epithelial membrane, which organizes nerve fibers into fascicles. The perineurium is the most difficult layer for local anesthetics to penetrate because of the tight junctions between its cells. **3.** LAs then pass through the endoneurium, which envelops the myelinated and unmyelinated fibers, Schwann cells, and capillaries. Only LAs that have passed through these three sheaths can reach the neuronal membranes where the voltage-gated sodium channels are located. Clinically, a high concentration of local anesthetic must be applied because only a fraction of the molecules reach the target site.

other afferent and efferent, somatic, and autonomic nerve fibers. All of these fibers may be contained within a peripheral nerve, and conduction in all fibers can be blocked by local anesthetics. This is why, in the introductory case, EM experienced not only loss of pain sensation but also a more complete block of all sensation in his left index finger.

In general, more proximal regions of the body (shoulder, thigh) are innervated by axons traveling relatively superficially in a peripheral nerve, while more distal regions (hands, feet) are innervated by axons traveling closer to the core of the nerve. Because local anesthetics are applied to the outside of a peripheral nerve, external to the epineurium, the axons innervating more proximal areas are usually reached first by the local anesthetic that is diffusing radially into the nerve. Consequently, *in the anatomic progression of functional block, proximal areas are numbed before distal areas.* For example, if a nerve block is applied in the brachial plexus, the shoulder and upper arm are numbed before the forearm, hand, and fingers.

During the onset of local anesthesia, different fiber types within a peripheral nerve are also blocked at different rates due to their intrinsic susceptibility to blockade. The general order in which functional deficits occur is as follows: first pain, second pain, temperature, touch, proprioception (pressure, position, or stretch), and finally skeletal muscle tone and voluntary tension. This phenomenon is referred to as **differential functional blockade**. In the introductory case, recall that EM's first pain was blocked before his second pain,

and that block of both sensations preceded the loss of his other sensory modalities. Clinically, if a patient is still able to feel the sharp pain of a pinprick, then the degree of anesthesia is unlikely to be sufficient to block the transmission of long-lasting second pain.

Because locomotor function is resistant to effects of relatively low concentrations of epidural local anesthetics, it is possible to block nociception with relatively little effect on ambulation. The concentration of local anesthetic required to block sensory impulses without inducing a large motor blockade varies for different agents. With lidocaine, for example, it is impossible to block Aδ-fibers without also blocking Aγ-motor fibers (Table 12-1); in contrast, epidural bupivacaine can achieve analgesia at low concentrations without debilitating motor block. For this reason, dilute epidural bupivacaine is frequently used during labor, as it relieves pain while still allowing the parturient to push with contractions.

Voltage-Gated Sodium Channel

Local anesthetics prevent impulse transmission by blocking sodium channels in neuronal membranes. The sodium channel exists in three main conformational states: open, inactivated, and resting. In going from the resting to the open state, the channel also moves through several transient "closed" conformations. The resting neuronal membrane potential is -60 to -70 mV. At this potential, the channels are in equilibrium between the resting state (majority) and the inactivated state (minority). During an action potential, the resting channels move through the closed conformations and finally open briefly to allow sodium ions to enter the cell. This sodium influx results in depolarization of the membrane. After a few milliseconds, the open channel spontaneously undergoes a conformational change to the inactivated state. This halts the influx of sodium, and the membrane repolarizes.

The inactivated state of the channel returns slowly to the resting state in the repolarized membrane. The time needed to make this transition largely determines the length of the refractory period. During the absolute refractory period, there are so few Na^+ channels in the resting state that, even if all the resting-state channels were simultaneously activated to the open state, the activation threshold would not be reached. Thus, no new action potentials can be generated during this period of time (Fig. 12-7A).

Modulated Receptor Hypothesis

The different conformational states of the sodium channel (resting, various closed, open, and inactivated) bind local anesthetics with different affinities. This concept is known as the **modulated receptor hypothesis** (Fig. 12-7B and Table 12-2).

Local anesthetics have a higher affinity for the open and inactivated states of the sodium channel than for the resting state. Although the LA binds at a site in the channel's pore, the molecular mechanism of channel inhibition involves not only the physical occlusion of the pore but also the restriction of the conformational changes that underlie activation of the channel. The binding of drug to the closed states that occur during the sequential activation process seems to restrict the conformational changes of the sodium channel, so that a drug-bound channel cannot undergo the full range of motions necessary to open.

For a drug-bound channel to reopen, the LA must dissociate from the channel and thereby allow the channel to return to its resting state. This dissociation of drug (the rate

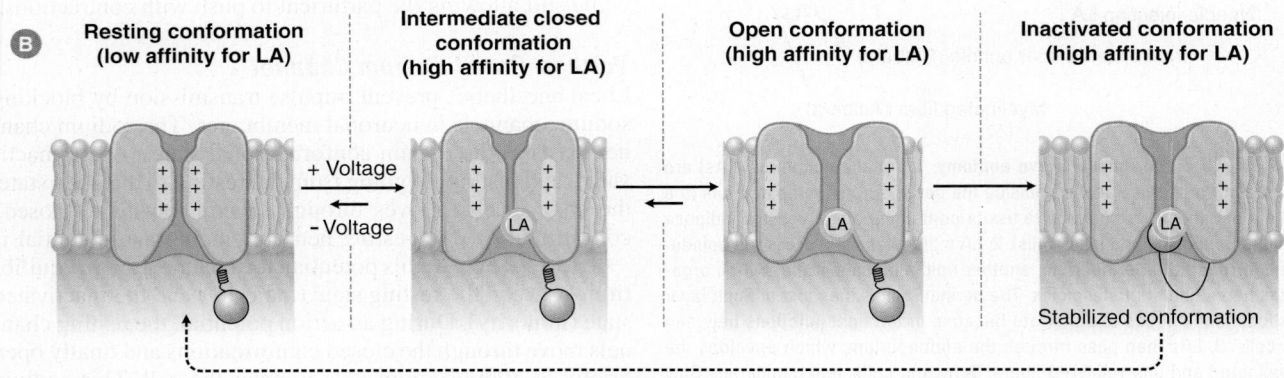

FIGURE 12-7. Local anesthetic binding to different conformations (states) of the sodium channel. A. The sodium channel is composed of one polypeptide chain that has four repeating units. One region, known as the *S4 region*, has many positively charged amino acids (lysine and arginine). These residues give the channel its voltage dependence. At rest, the pore is closed. When the membrane is depolarized, the charged residues move in response to the change in the electric field. This results in several conformational changes (intermediate closed states) that culminate in channel opening. After about 1 ms (the channel open time), the 3–4 amino acid "linker region" plugs the open channel, yielding the inactivated conformation. The inactivated conformation returns to the resting state only when the membrane is repolarized; this conformational change involves the return of the S4 region to its original position and the expulsion of the linker region. The time required for the channel to return from the inactivated state to the resting state is known as the *refractory period*; during this period, the sodium channel is incapable of being activated. **B.** The binding of local anesthetic (LA) alters the properties of the intermediate forms assumed by the sodium channel. Sodium channels in any of the conformations (resting, closed, open, or inactivated) can bind local anesthetic molecules, although the resting state has a low affinity for LA, while the other three states have a high affinity for LA. LA can dissociate from the channel–LA complex in any conformational state, or the channel can undergo conformational changes while associated with the LA molecule. Ultimately, the channel–LA complex must dissociate and the sodium channel must return to the resting state in order to become activated. LA binding extends the refractory period, including both the time required for dissociation of the LA molecule from the sodium channel and the time required for the channel to return to the resting state.

of which varies among the different LAs) is slower than the normal recovery from the inactivated to the resting channel conformation in the absence of LA. Thus, by delaying the inactivated channel's return to the resting state, LAs extend the refractory period of the neuron by about 50- to 100-fold. At high concentrations of LAs, the number of resting channels that are drug-bound (blocked) is sufficient to prevent impulse conduction altogether.

Tonic and Phasic Inhibition

The differential affinity of local anesthetics for different states of the voltage-gated sodium channel has an important pharmacologic consequence: the degree of inhibition of sodium current by the LA depends on the frequency of impulses in the nerve, such that the number of APs in a train is diminished under conditions where single impulses are unaffected. When there is a long interval between action potentials, any additional LA binding that occurred during the preceding impulse has time to fully reverse, and the level of inhibition of each impulse is the same; the inhibition is said to be *tonic*. When the interval between action potentials is short, drug dissociation from additionally bound channels is incomplete, and the number of bound channels increases with each successive impulse; the inhibition is said to be *phasic* or use-dependent (Fig. 12-8).

Tonic inhibition occurs when the time between action potentials is long compared to the time for dissociation of the LA from the sodium channel. Assume, for example, that before an action potential arrives, an equilibrium has been established in which 5% of the sodium channels are bound by local anesthetic molecules. When an action potential arrives, the other 95% of the channels are available to open and subsequently to inactivate. During the brief impulse, some of these channels become bound by local anesthetic molecules.

TABLE 12-2 Modulated Receptor Hypothesis

CHANNEL STATE	AFFINITY FOR LOCAL ANESTHETIC	RELATIVE EFFECT ON CHANNEL
Resting	Low	Prevents channel opening (only at high LA concentrations)
Closed (several)	High	Prevents channel opening (major effect)
Open	High	Blocks channel pore (minor effect)
Inactivated	High	Extends refractory period (major effect)

The voltage-gated sodium channel can assume several different conformations. Local anesthetics (LAs) have different affinities for different conformations of the channel; this differential affinity alters the kinetics of sodium channel activation (see Fig. 12-7).

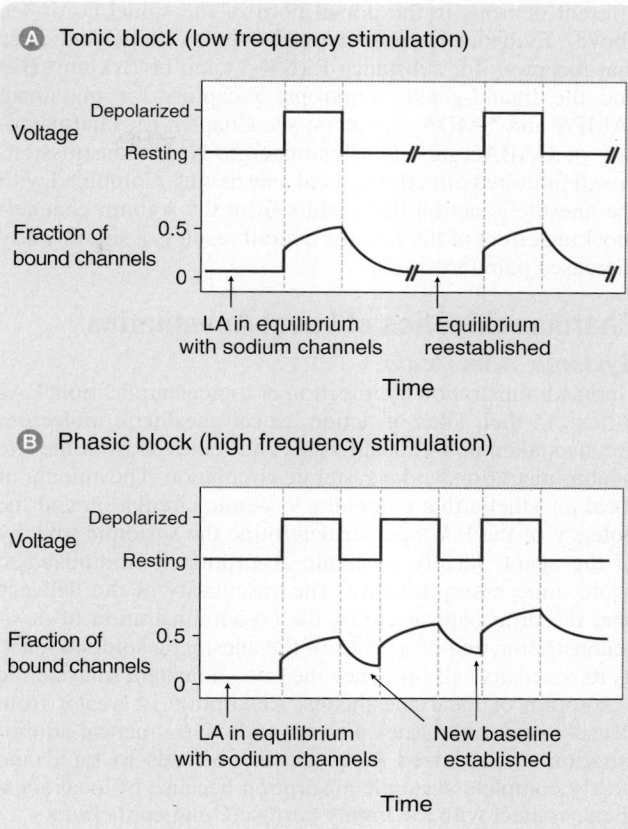

FIGURE 12-8. Tonic and phasic (use-dependent) inhibition. A. In tonic block, depolarizations occur with low frequency, and there is sufficient time between depolarizations for equilibrium binding of local anesthetic (LA) molecules to the various states of the sodium channel to be reestablished. When a depolarization occurs, resting channels (which have low affinity for LA) are converted into open channels and inactivated channels (both of which have high affinity for LA). Thus, there is an increase in the number of LA-bound channels. Once the depolarization ends, there is sufficient time before the next depolarization for equilibrium between LA molecules and sodium channels to be reestablished, and virtually all of the channels return to the resting and unbound state. **B.** In phasic block, depolarizations occur with high frequency, and there is not sufficient time between depolarizations for equilibrium to be reestablished. After each depolarization, a new baseline is established that has more LA-bound channels than the previous baseline, leading eventually to conduction failure. Because high-frequency stimulation of nociceptors occurs in areas of tissue damage, phasic (use-dependent) block causes actively firing nociceptors to be inhibited more effectively than nerve fibers that are only occasionally firing. The frequency dependence of phasic block depends on the rate at which LA dissociates from its binding site on the channel.

However, in the relatively long time before the next impulse arrives at the LA-exposed region, the bound LA can dissociate from the sodium channel, allowing those channels to return to the resting state. Thus, before the next action potential arrives, the 5% binding equilibrium is reestablished. The next action potential will therefore be blocked to the same extent as the previous one.

Phasic inhibition occurs when there is not sufficient time between action potentials for this equilibrium to be reestablished. Rapidly arriving action potentials cause resting sodium channels to open and then inactivate, and some of these channels become bound by LAs. However, because there is not sufficient time between impulses for all the newly formed LA–sodium channel complexes to dissociate, only some of the channels are able to return to the resting state. With each arriving action potential, more and more channels are blocked, until a new steady state of LA–sodium channel binding is reached. This is the phenomenon of phasic, or use-dependent, inhibition. As more of the channels are bound by LA, fewer and fewer channels are available to open when the next action potential arrives. Consequently, *action potential conduction is increasingly inhibited at higher frequencies of impulses.*

The clinical importance of this phenomenon is that tissue injury or trauma causes nociceptors in the area of injury to fire at high frequency. In these situations, application of a local anesthetic tends to block local nociceptors in a phasic manner, inhibiting pain transmission to a greater extent than the transmission of other local sensory or motor impulses that are blocked only tonically.

Other Receptors for Local Anesthetics

In addition to blocking sodium channels, LAs have a wide range of other biochemical and physiologic effects. Local anesthetics can interact with potassium channels, calcium channels, pacemaker channels, ligand-gated channels (such as the ionotropic glutamate receptors), transient receptor potential (TRP) channels, and several G protein-coupled receptors (including muscarinic cholinergic receptors, β-adrenergic receptors, and receptors for substance P). Local anesthetics can also uncouple some G proteins from their cell surface receptors and thus inhibit signal transduction. In most cases, these effects are not significant because LAs have lower affinity for these other receptors than for the sodium channel. But for some types of local anesthetics in some clinical situations, these alternate targets may have important therapeutic and toxic consequences.

For example, in spinal anesthesia, a high concentration of local anesthetic is injected into the cerebrospinal fluid, from which the LA then diffuses into the spinal cord. Neuropeptides (such as **substance P**) and small organic neurotransmitters (such as **glutamate**) mediate the transmission of nociceptive impulses between the primary and secondary afferent neurons in the dorsal horn of the spinal cord (see above). Evidence from in vivo and in vitro studies indicates that receptors for substance P (NK-1) and bradykinin (B2) and the ligand-gated, ionotropic receptors for glutamate (AMPA and NMDA receptors; see Chapter 13, Pharmacology of GABAergic and Glutamatergic Neurotransmission) are all inhibited directly by local anesthetics. Combined with the anesthetic action that results from the sodium channel-blocking effect of the LA, the overall result is a significantly increased pain threshold.

Pharmacokinetics of Local Anesthetics

Systemic Absorption

Upon administration by injection or topical application, LAs diffuse to their sites of action. Local anesthetic molecules are also taken up by local tissues and removed from the site of administration by the systemic circulation. The amount of local anesthetic that enters the systemic circulation and the potency of the LA together determine the systemic toxicity of the agent. Ideally, systemic absorption is minimized to avoid unnecessary toxicity. The vascularity of the delivery site, the drug concentration, the co-administration of a vasoconstrictor, and properties of the anesthetic solution (such as its viscosity) all influence the rate and extent of systemic absorption of local anesthetics. Absorption is greater from densely perfused tissues. For example, intratracheal administration of vaporized local anesthetic leads to rapid and nearly complete systemic absorption because of local anesthetic contact with the highly perfused lung epithelium.

Distribution

After absorption, local anesthetics are distributed throughout the body. Similar to the effect of vascularity on the rate of absorption, the rate of distribution and the peak plasma concentration of anesthetic depend on the vascularity of the nearby tissue. This effect is particularly important for injected local anesthetics, where distribution away from the site of injection is a determinant of LA concentration at the intended site of action (and therefore duration of effect) and of peak LA plasma concentration (and therefore risk of toxicity). For example, a larger total quantity of local anesthetic can be safely given in a peripheral nerve block than in an intercostal block because the high vascularity of the intercostal space results in more rapid distribution of the anesthetic, a higher peak plasma concentration of the anesthetic, and an increased risk of systemic toxicity. Common sites of local anesthetic administration, ranked in order of most vascular to least vascular, include intercostal, caudal epidural space, lumbar epidural space, brachial plexus, femoral nerve, and subcutaneous tissue.

Vasoconstrictors (such as epinephrine) are often administered together with many short-acting or medium-acting local anesthetics. These adjunctive agents reduce blood flow to the area of injection by causing the smooth muscles of the vessels to contract and thereby slow the rate of removal of the LA. In doing so, vasoconstrictors both increase the concentration of anesthetic around the nerve and decrease the peak plasma concentration that is reached in the systemic circulation. The former effect enhances the duration of action of the LA, and the latter effect decreases the LA's systemic toxicity. However, vasoconstriction can also lead to tissue hypoxia and damage if the oxygen supply to the area is reduced too severely. Thus, *vasoconstrictors are not used*

when LAs are administered in the extremities, because there is limited circulation to these areas. In the introductory case, EM was given lidocaine without epinephrine to avoid tissue hypoxia in his digit.

In the circulation, LAs bind reversibly to two major plasma proteins: α-1 acid glycoprotein (an acute-phase protein) and albumin. Local anesthetics also bind to the membranes of all cells in the blood. Binding to plasma proteins decreases as the pH decreases, suggesting that the neutral form binds these proteins with higher affinity. Tissue binding, largely due to membrane uptake and partitioning, occurs at the site of injection as well as other sites. The more hydrophobic the agent is, the greater the extent of tissue binding.

The volume of distribution (V_d) indicates the extent to which a drug distributes to the tissues from the systemic circulation. For the same amount of administered drug, a less hydrophobic LA (e.g., procaine) has a higher plasma concentration (i.e., less is stored in tissues) and therefore a smaller V_d. A more hydrophobic LA (e.g., bupivacaine) has a lower plasma concentration (i.e., more is stored in tissues) and therefore a larger V_d. Local anesthetics with a larger V_d are eliminated more slowly. (See Chapter 3, Pharmacokinetics, for a detailed discussion of the inverse relationship between V_d and the elimination half-life of a drug.)

Metabolism and Excretion

Ester-linked LAs are metabolized by tissue and plasma esterases (pseudocholinesterases). This process is fast (on the order of minutes), and the resulting products are excreted via the kidney.

Amide-linked LAs are primarily metabolized in the liver by cytochrome P450 enzymes. The three major routes of hepatic metabolism are aromatic hydroxylation, N-dealkylation, and amide hydrolysis. Metabolites of amide-linked LAs are returned to the circulation and excreted by the kidney. Alterations in liver perfusion can change the rate at which these agents are metabolized, as can induction or inhibition of the P450 enzymes. Metabolism is slowed in patients with cirrhosis or other liver diseases, and a standard dose of an amide-linked LA can lead to toxicity in such a patient. Some metabolism of amide-linked LAs can also occur extrahepatically, for example, in the lung and kidney.

Administration of Local Anesthetics

The method of administration of local anesthetics can determine both the therapeutic effect and the extent of systemic toxicity. The following is an overview of the most common methods for administering local anesthetics.

Topical Anesthesia

Topical anesthetics provide short-term pain relief when applied to mucous membranes or skin. The drug must cross the epidermal barrier, with the stratum corneum (outermost layer of the epidermis) presenting the major obstacle, to reach the Aδ-fibers and C-fibers in the epidermis. Once across the epidermis, local anesthetics are absorbed rapidly into the circulation, increasing the risk of systemic toxicity. A mixture of tetracaine, adrenaline (epinephrine), and cocaine, known as **TAC**, is a historically common anesthetic that was often used before suturing small cuts. Because of concern about cocaine toxicity and/or addiction from this formulation, alternatives such as **EMLA** are now used (see below). Recent formulations of local anesthetics for transdermal administration include lidocaine patches that deliver the medication over 12–24 hours.

Infiltration Anesthesia

Infiltration anesthesia is used to numb an area of skin or a mucosal surface via injection. The local anesthetic is injected intradermally or subcutaneously, often at several neighboring sites near the area to be anesthetized. This technique produces numbness more rapidly than topical anesthesia, because the agent does not have to cross the epidermis. However, the injection can be painful due to the acidic pH of the local anesthetic solution that is needed to maintain the drug in an ionized, soluble, and chemically stable form. Neutralization of the solution by addition of sodium bicarbonate can reduce the injection pain. The local anesthetics most commonly used for infiltration anesthesia include **lidocaine**, **procaine**, and **bupivacaine**. Infiltration of local anesthetics for dental procedures is discussed in Box 12-1.

Peripheral Nerve Blockade

Peripheral nerve blocks are increasingly used for pain control associated with trauma and surgery. Generally, local anesthetics are injected percutaneously using anatomic landmarks, ultrasound guidance, or fluoroscopic techniques to safely deliver the anesthetic near a particular nerve. Anesthetics can be delivered as bolus injections (single shot or, occasionally, repeated nerve block) or as continuous infusions via catheters that are inserted near the target nerve. As in the case of the digital nerve block for EM, single shot injections may be used to provide short-term anesthesia for a procedure. Alternatively, femoral nerve blocks often use continuous infusions of local anesthetics to control pain from a hip fracture both prior to and for days after surgery.

This technique is particularly helpful in elderly patients who may be sensitive to adverse effects of opioid medications, such as delirium and respiratory depression, that might otherwise be used to control pain. The choice of anesthetic typically depends on the desired duration of action.

Peripheral nerve blocks are also used in the management of trauma. Intercostal nerve blocks can reduce pain after rib fracture, which can improve lung mechanics and reduce rates of pulmonary complications such as pneumonia. Examples of other useful peripheral blocks include transversus abdominis plane (TAP) block for the anterior abdominal wall; interscalene, cervical plexus, and brachial plexus blocks for shoulder and arm surgery; and femoral and popliteal blocks for the distal lower limb.

Central Nerve Blockade

This type of blockade, also called *neuraxial blockade*, involves delivery of drug near the spinal cord. Central nerve blockade includes both epidural and intrathecal (spinal) anesthesia. The early effects of these procedures result primarily from impulse blockade in spinal roots, but in later phases, anesthetic drug penetrates and may act within the spinal cord. **Bupivacaine** is particularly useful as an epidural anesthetic during labor because, at low concentrations, it provides adequate pain relief without significant motor block. Reports of bupivacaine cardiotoxicity have led to decreased use of this agent in high concentrations (>0.5% weight/volume [w:v]), although the dilute solutions used in obstetrics are rarely toxic.

Intravenous Regional and Systemic Anesthesia

Local anesthetic can be injected intravenously into a distal extremity to provide regional anesthesia to that limb. Generally, venous blood is encouraged to drain from the limb by

---

BOX 12-1 Local Anesthetics in Dentistry

Modern dentistry is predicated on the action of local anesthetics: without adequate pain control, patients could not comfortably undergo the majority of dental procedures. Not surprisingly, then, local anesthetics are the most commonly used drugs in dentistry.

Often, both an injected and a topical anesthetic agent are used in dental procedures; the injected agent blocks the sensation of pain during (and sometimes after) the procedure, while the topical agent allows for painless needle penetration when the injected agent is administered.

Topical anesthetics are applied to mucous membranes and penetrate to a depth of 2 to 3 millimeters. Because topical anesthetics must diffuse across this distance, relatively high concentrations are used, and care must be taken to avoid local and systemic toxicity. Benzocaine and lidocaine—two commonly used topical anesthetics—are insoluble in water and poorly absorbed into the circulation, decreasing the likelihood of systemic toxicity.

Injected anesthetics are administered either as local infiltrations or as field or nerve blocks. In a local infiltration, the anesthetic solution is deposited at the site where the dental procedure will be performed. The solution bathes free nerve endings at that site, blocking pain perception. In field and nerve blocks, the

anesthetic solution is deposited more proximally along the nerve, away from the site of incision. These techniques are used when larger regions of the mouth must be anesthetized.

Numerous injected anesthetics are used in dental practice, and the choice of which agent to use for a given procedure reflects factors such as the rate of onset, the duration of action, and the vasodilatory properties of the agent. Lidocaine is the most widely used injected anesthetic; it is notable for a rapid rate of onset, long duration of action, and extremely low incidence of allergic reaction. Mepivacaine is less vasodilating than most other local anesthetics, allowing it to be administered without a vasoconstrictor. This property makes mepivacaine ideally suited for pediatric dentistry, because it is "washed out" of the area of administration more rapidly than agents administered with vasoconstrictors. As a result, mepivacaine provides a relatively short period of soft-tissue anesthesia, minimizing the risk of inadvertent, self-inflicted trauma from biting or chewing on anesthetized tissue. Bupivacaine is a more potent and longer acting anesthetic than lidocaine or mepivacaine. It is used for lengthy dental procedures and for the management of postoperative pain. ■

elevating it above the level of the heart before a proximal tourniquet is applied and the anesthetic is injected into the vein. This allows high local concentrations of anesthetic to reach the nerves in the limb, while limiting the redistribution of the anesthetic and thus preventing systemic toxicity. This type of local anesthesia, also called *Bier block*, is occasionally used for arm and hand surgery. Systemic intravenous lidocaine is used perioperatively to reduce postoperative pain and is also administered for relief of chronic pain from injury or disease (e.g., diabetic neuropathy). Relief of chronic pain often lasts for weeks following a single, brief lidocaine infusion, even though the drug is cleared from the circulation within a few hours. The mechanism underlying this long duration of effect remains uncertain.

Major Toxicities

Local anesthetics can have both systemic and organ-specific toxicities. These include hypersensitivity reactions as well as effects on local tissues, the CNS, peripheral vasculature, and the heart. Toxicity associated with LAs range from mild local tissue irritation to life-threatening complications including CNS excitation and depression and cardiovascular collapse.

Local anesthetics can cause local irritation. For example, skeletal muscle is sensitive to intramuscular LA injection. After intramuscular injection of LAs, plasma levels of creatine kinase are elevated, indicating damage to muscle cells. This effect is usually reversible, and muscle regeneration is complete within a few weeks of the injection. Peripheral nerve blocks and, particularly, spinal blocks with high concentrations of LAs (e.g., 5% lidocaine) frequently cause local neurotoxicity. Some of this toxicity may result from local inflammation of surrounding tissues, but there is also evidence for neuronal apoptosis, perhaps triggered by elevation of intracellular Ca^{+2}.

Local anesthetics can have serious effects on the CNS. LAs are small amphipathic molecules that, as the uncharged species, can rapidly cross the blood–brain barrier. Initially, LAs produce signs of CNS excitement, including perioral numbness or a metallic taste at lower plasma concentrations, followed by shivering, twitching, and seizures at higher concentrations. Cellular studies show that some LAs release Ca^{+2} from intracellular stores and thus stimulate the release of glutamate in the brain, resulting in the excitatory phase of CNS toxicity. CNS excitation is followed by depression. As the concentration of LA increases in the CNS, all neuronal pathways are blocked—excitatory as well as inhibitory—leading to CNS depression. Death can ultimately result from respiratory failure. CNS toxicity is most commonly associated with inadvertent intravascular injection of local anesthetic or with large doses of intrathecal anesthetic.

Local anesthetics have complex effects on the peripheral vasculature. Lidocaine, for example, initially causes vasoconstriction but can subsequently also cause vasodilation. Such biphasic actions may be attributable to separate effects, respectively, on the vascular smooth muscle and on sympathetic nerves that innervate resistance arterioles. Bronchial smooth muscle is also affected in a biphasic manner, with initial bronchoconstriction followed by bronchodilation. The early effect may reflect LA-induced release of calcium ions into the cytoplasm from intracellular stores, while the latter effect may be caused by LA inhibition of plasma membrane sodium and calcium channels (see the following discussion).

The cardiac effects of LAs are complex due to their actions on multiple molecular targets, including Na^+, K^+, Ca^{2+}, and pacemaker channels. An early effect is to reduce the conduction velocity of the cardiac action potential through both conducting and nodal tissues. At very low concentrations, LAs can act as antiarrhythmic drugs because of their ability to prevent ventricular tachycardia and ventricular fibrillation (this is an example of use-dependent block; see above). Lidocaine, for example, is used as both a local anesthetic and a class IB antiarrhythmic (see Chapter 24). Local anesthetics also cause a dose-dependent decrease in cardiac contractility (a negative inotropic effect). The mechanism of this effect is not entirely understood but may be caused by LA-mediated slow release of calcium from the sarcoplasmic reticulum with a consequent reduction in the stores of calcium available to drive subsequent contractions. LAs can also directly block calcium channels in the plasma membrane. The combination of reduced intracellular calcium storage and decreased calcium entry may lead to decreased myocardial contractility.

It has recently been shown that lipid emulsions injected into the circulation may help reverse CNS and cardiac toxicity from LAs. This finding has been demonstrated in animal models of local anesthetic toxicity and in many clinical case reports of successful resuscitation after seizure or cardiac arrest related to local anesthetic overdose. While the mechanism of this effect is unclear, it is thought that the lipid serves as a "sink" for the hydrophobic local anesthetic and allows the local anesthetic to redistribute away from CNS and cardiac tissue and into the lipid. It has become common to have lipid emulsions immediately available for resuscitation in surgical centers where nerve blocks are performed.

Hypersensitivity to local anesthetics is rare. This adverse effect is usually manifested as allergic dermatitis or asthma. LA-induced hypersensitivity occurs almost exclusively with ester-linked LAs. For example, a metabolite of procaine, para-aminobenzoic acid (PABA), is a known allergen (as well as the active agent in many sunscreens).

Individual Agents

Having discussed the general properties of local anesthetics, this section presents examples of individual anesthetics in current clinical use, with an emphasis on the agents' differences in potency and elimination half-life.

Ester-Linked Local Anesthetics

Procaine

Procaine (Novocain®) is a short-acting, ester-linked LA (Fig. 12-4A). Its low hydrophobicity allows for rapid removal of drug from the site of administration via the circulation and results in little sequestration of drug in the local tissue surrounding the nerve. In the bloodstream, procaine is degraded rapidly by plasma pseudocholinesterases, and the metabolites are subsequently excreted in the urine. Procaine's low hydrophobicity also causes it to dissociate rapidly from its binding site on the sodium channel, accounting for the low potency of this agent.

Procaine's primary uses are in infiltration anesthesia and in dental procedures. Occasionally, it is used in diagnostic nerve blocks. Procaine is rarely used for peripheral nerve block because of its low potency, slow onset, and short duration of action. The rapidly hydrolyzed, short-acting homologue of procaine, **2-chloroprocaine** (Nesacaine®), is popular as an obstetric anesthetic that is sometimes administered epidurally to control pain during delivery.

One of the metabolites of procaine is PABA, a compound required by some bacteria for purine and nucleic acid synthesis. The antibacterial sulfonamides are structural analogues of PABA that competitively inhibit the synthesis of an essential metabolite in folate biosynthesis (see Chapter 33, Principles of Antimicrobial and Antineoplastic Pharmacology). Excess PABA can reduce the effectiveness of sulfonamides and therefore exacerbate bacterial infections. As mentioned above, PABA is also an allergen.

Tetracaine

Tetracaine is a long-acting, highly potent, ester-linked LA. Its long duration of action is caused by its high hydrophobicity—it has a butyl group attached to its aromatic group—which allows tetracaine to remain in the tissue surrounding a nerve for an extended period of time. Tetracaine's hydrophobicity also promotes prolonged interaction with its binding site on the sodium channel, accounting for its higher potency than lidocaine and procaine. It is mainly used in spinal and topical anesthesia. Its effective metabolism is slow, despite the potential for rapid hydrolysis by esterases, because it is released only gradually from tissues into the bloodstream.

Cocaine

Cocaine, the prototypical and only naturally occurring LA, is ester-linked. It has an intermediate potency for nerve block (one-half that of lidocaine) and a medium duration of action. Cocaine's structure is slightly unusual for local anesthetics; its tertiary amine is part of a complex cyclic structure to which a secondary ester group is attached.

Cocaine's primary therapeutic uses are in ophthalmic anesthesia and as part of the topical anesthetic TAC (tetracaine, adrenaline, cocaine; see above). Like prilocaine (see below), cocaine has a marked vasoconstrictive action that results from its inhibition of catecholamine uptake in synaptic terminals of both the peripheral and central nervous systems (see Chapter 11, Adrenergic Pharmacology). Inhibition of this uptake system is also the mechanism for cocaine's profound cardiotoxic potential and for the psychotropic "high" associated with cocaine use. Cardiotoxicity and euphoria limit the value of cocaine as a local anesthetic.

Amide-Linked Local Anesthetics
Lidocaine and Prilocaine

Lidocaine, the most commonly used LA and the one used in EM's case, is an amide-linked drug of moderate hydrophobicity (Fig. 12-4B). It has a rapid onset of action and a medium duration of action (about 1–2 hours) and is moderately potent. Lidocaine has two methyl groups on its aromatic ring, bordering the amide bond, which enhance its hydrophobicity relative to procaine and slow its rate of hydrolysis.

Lidocaine has a relatively low pK_a, and a large fraction of the drug is present in neutral form at physiologic pH. This property allows rapid diffusion of the drug through membranes and a rapid block. Lidocaine's duration of action is based on two factors: its moderate hydrophobicity and its amide linkage. The amide linkage prevents degradation of the drug by esterases, and its hydrophobicity allows the drug to remain near the area of administration (i.e., in local tissue) for a long time. Its hydrophobicity also allows lidocaine to bind more tightly than procaine to the LA binding site

on the sodium channel, enhancing its potency. The vasoconstrictive effects of co-administered epinephrine can extend lidocaine's duration of action substantially.

Lidocaine is used in infiltration, peripheral nerve block, epidural, spinal, and topical anesthesia. The mechanism of antiarrhythmic action is its blocking of sodium channels in cardiac myocytes. Lidocaine's slow metabolism in the circulation makes it a useful Class IB antiarrhythmic (see Chapter 24). More potent amide-linked LAs, such as bupivacaine, bind too tightly to cardiac sodium channels to serve as useful antiarrhythmics; such drugs cause either conduction blocks or tachyarrhythmias (see below).

Lidocaine undergoes metabolism in the liver, where it is first N-dealkylated by P450 enzymes (see Chapter 4, Drug Metabolism). Subsequently, it undergoes hydrolysis and hydroxylation. Lidocaine's metabolites have only weak anesthetic activity.

The systemic toxic effects of lidocaine are manifested mainly in the CNS and heart. Adverse effects can include drowsiness, tinnitus, twitching, and even seizures. CNS depression and cardiotoxicity occur at high plasma levels of the drug. Still, lidocaine has a higher therapeutic index than bupivacaine.

Prilocaine is similar to lidocaine, except that it causes less vasodilation and, at high doses, can cause methemoglobinemia. Since it causes less vasodilation, it is often an anesthetic of choice when vasoconstrictive additives such as epinephrine must be avoided.

Bupivacaine

Bupivacaine is an amide-linked LA with a long duration of action. It is highly hydrophobic (and therefore highly potent) as a result of a butyl group attached to the tertiary nitrogen. Dilute bupivacaine (0.125% w:v or lower) administered epidurally has more effect on nociception than on locomotor activity. This property, combined with the drug's long duration of action and high potency, has made bupivacaine useful in spinal, epidural, and peripheral nerve blocks and in infiltration anesthesia. Bupivacaine is metabolized in the liver, where it undergoes N-dealkylation by P450 enzymes. It has been used widely in low concentrations for labor and postoperative anesthesia because it provides 2–3 hours of pain relief with minimal motor blockade. However, because of its cardiotoxicity at higher concentrations, total acceptable doses must be carefully determined and not exceeded when used for these indications. (The drug blocks cardiac myocyte sodium channels during systole but is very slow to dissociate during diastole. Thus, it can trigger arrhythmias through the promotion of reentry pathways.)

Bupivacaine contains a chiral center, and it exists as a racemic mixture of mirror-image R- and S-enantiomers. The R- and S-enantiomers have different affinities for the sodium channel and, therefore, different cardiovascular effects. The S-enantiomer has been separated and marketed as the safer and less cardiotoxic **levobupivacaine**, as has its structurally homologous relative **ropivacaine**.

Articaine

Articaine is a relatively new amide-linked LA that has several interesting structural features. First, along with **prilocaine**, articaine is unique among local anesthetics because of its secondary amine group. (Virtually all other LAs have a tertiary amine group.) Second, articaine is structurally unique because it contains an ester group bound to a thiophene ring;

the presence of the ester group means that articaine can be partially metabolized in the plasma by cholinesterases, as well as in the liver. Its rapid metabolism in the plasma may minimize its potential toxicity. Articaine is currently used in dentistry, where it is becoming an increasingly popular agent, and it may find additional uses as more studies of its clinical applications are performed.

EMLA

EMLA (eutectic mixture of local anesthetic) is a combination of lidocaine and prilocaine that is delivered topically as a cream or patch. EMLA is useful clinically because it has a higher concentration of local anesthetic per drop contacting the skin than standard topical preparations. It is effective in a number of situations including venipuncture, arterial cannulation, lumbar puncture, and dental procedures, and is most commonly used in pediatric settings.

■ CONCLUSION AND FUTURE DIRECTIONS

Local anesthetics are vital to the practice of medicine, surgery, and dentistry because they can block pain sensations regionally. Their clinical actions involve blocking pain neurons called *nociceptors*. Nociceptors are afferent neurons whose axons are classified as either Aδ- or C-fibers. Local anesthetics block all types of nerve fibers in peripheral nerves, including those of nociceptors, by blocking voltage-gated sodium channels in neuronal membranes. LAs act on sodium channels from the cytoplasmic side of the membrane.

In general, local anesthetics have an aromatic group that is connected to an ionizable amine via an ester or amide linkage. This structure is common to almost all local anesthetics and contributes to their function. Both the hydrophobicity, attributable in large part to the aromatic ring and its substituents, and the ionizability (pK_a) of the amine determine the potency of the LA and the kinetics of local anesthetic action. Molecules with pK_a values of 8–10 (weak bases) are the most effective as local anesthetics. The neutral form can cross membranes to reach the LA binding site on the sodium channel, and the protonated form is available to bind with high affinity to that target site.

The sodium channel exists in three main conformational states: open, inactivated, and resting. There are also several transient "closed" states between the resting and open states. Local anesthetics bind with higher affinity to the open and inactivated conformations than to the resting conformation of the sodium channel. This tight binding slows the return of the channel to the resting state after an action potential and thereby extends the refractory period, increasingly inhibiting the transmission of trains of action potentials occurring at high frequency.

Local anesthetics have actions beyond their inhibition of sodium channels. Some of these ancillary effects show therapeutic promise and could potentially lead to other indications for LAs. For example, LAs have been reported to affect wound healing, inflammation, thrombosis, hypoxia/ischemia-induced brain injury, and bronchial hyperactivity. This is particularly important clinically since regional blocks using local anesthetics are becoming more common in surgery. LAs are also being investigated for use in chronic and neuropathic pain management, such as that seen in patients with diabetic neuropathy, postherpetic neuralgia, burns, cancer, and strokes. The development of ultralong-acting LAs (whose effects could last for days) is continuing to be investigated: these studies involve altering LA structure at the molecular level, using a variety of drug delivery systems, and discovering new classes of neuronal impulse blockers.

Lastly, a promising area of current discovery involves nociceptor-specific LAs. Some of these experimental agents bind to particular sodium channel subtypes that are expressed preferentially on Aδ- or C-fibers. Others are charged anesthetics that typically cannot diffuse through neuronal cell membranes; co-administration of these anesthetics with agents that activate other ion channels found preferentially on nociceptors (such as TRPV1) allows the anesthetic molecules to cross the nociceptor membrane through these open channels in a modality-specific fashion. Nociceptor-specific LAs have the potential to block pain perception without affecting motor, autonomic, or other neuronal signaling and may therefore be useful in a variety of clinical settings.

Suggested Reading

Berde CB, Strichartz GR. Local anesthetics. In: Miller RD, Cohen NH, Eriksson LI, Fleisher LA, Wiener-Kronish JP, Young WL, eds. *Miller's anesthesia.* 8th ed. Philadelphia: Elsevier Churchill Livingstone; 2015. (*A more complete mechanistic and, primarily, clinical summary.*)

Crystal CS, McArthur TJ, Harrison B. Anesthetic and procedural sedation techniques for wound management. *Emerg Med Clin North Am* 2007;25: 41–71. (*A clinically oriented review that discusses how to administer LAs at various anatomic sites.*)

McLure HA, Rubin AP. Review of local anaesthetic agents. *Minerva Anestesiol* 2005;71:59–74. (*A clear discussion of both general concepts and individual agents.*)

Mercado P, Weinberg GL. Local anesthetic systemic toxicity: prevention and treatment. *Anesthesiol Clin* 2011;29:233–242. (*Review of LA toxicity and discussion of clinical use of lipid rescue therapy for LA toxicity.*)

Suzuki S, Gerner P, Colvin AC, Binshtok AM. C-fiber-selective peripheral nerve blockade. *Open Pain J* 2009;2:24–29. (*Reviews research on agents that may have selectivity for C-fibers.*)

DRUG SUMMARY TABLE: CHAPTER 12 Local Anesthetic Pharmacology

DRUG	CLINICAL APPLICATIONS	*SERIOUS* AND COMMON ADVERSE EFFECTS	CONTRAINDICATIONS	THERAPEUTIC CONSIDERATIONS
ESTER-LINKED LOCAL ANESTHETICS Mechanism—Inhibit voltage-gated sodium channels in excitable cell membranes				
Procaine 2-Chloroprocaine	Infiltration anesthesia Obstetrical anesthesia, given epidurally before delivery (2-chloroprocaine)	*Cardiac arrest and hypotension from excessive systemic absorption, CNS depression or excitation, respiratory arrest* Contact dermatitis	Hypersensitivity to procaine Use epidural anesthesia with extreme caution in patients with neurologic disease, spinal deformities, septicemia, or severe hypertension	Procaine's low hydrophobicity and rapid peripheral metabolism allow for rapid drug clearance and a short elimination half-life, but its low hydrophobicity also accounts for its low potency. Excess PABA (metabolite of procaine) can reduce the effectiveness of sulfonamides.
Tetracaine	Topical anesthesia (as TAC: tetracaine/epinephrine/cocaine) Spinal anesthesia	*Same as procaine* Additionally, drug-induced keratoconjunctivitis	Hypersensitivity to tetracaine Localized infection at proposed site of topical application	High hydrophobicity confers longer duration of action and higher potency; tetracaine is more potent than lidocaine and procaine. Do not inject large doses in patients with heart block.
Cocaine	Mucosal and ophthalmic local anesthetic Diagnosis of Horner syndrome pupil	*Accelerates coronary atherosclerosis, tachycardia, seizure* CNS depression or excitation, anxiety	Hypersensitivity to cocaine-containing products	Medium potency (one-half that of lidocaine), medium duration of action, marked vasoconstrictive action, cardiotoxic. Cardiotoxicity and euphoria limit the value of cocaine as a local anesthetic.
AMIDE-LINKED LOCAL ANESTHETICS Mechanism—Inhibit voltage-gated sodium channels in excitable cell membranes				
Lidocaine	Infiltration anesthesia Peripheral nerve block Epidural, spinal, and topical anesthesia Postherpetic neuralgia	*Cardiac arrest, arrhythmias, methemoglobinemia* Hypotension, nausea	Hypersensitivity to amide-linked local anesthetics Congenital or idiopathic methemoglobinemia	Lidocaine has a rapid onset of action, a medium duration of action (about 1–2 hours), and is moderately potent, due to its moderate hydrophobicity. Concurrent administration of co-formulated epinephrine prolongs its duration of action.
Prilocaine	Dental infiltration anesthesia and nerve block	*Cardiac arrest, methemoglobinemia, anaphylaxis, seizure, respiratory arrest* Bradyarrhythmia, hypotension, tremor, confusion, dizziness, somnolence, diplopia, tinnitus, nervousness, euphoria	Same as lidocaine	Prilocaine does not require epinephrine to prolong its duration of action, which makes it a good choice for patients in whom epinephrine is contraindicated.

continues

DRUG SUMMARY TABLE: CHAPTER 12 Local Anesthetic Pharmacology *continued*

DRUG	CLINICAL APPLICATIONS	*SERIOUS* AND COMMON ADVERSE EFFECTS	CONTRAINDICATIONS	THERAPEUTIC CONSIDERATIONS
Bupivacaine	Infiltration, regional, epidural, and spinal anesthesia Sympathetic nerve block	*Cardiotoxicity at higher concentrations, bacterial meningitis, sepsis, chondrolysis of articular cartilage, CNS depression or excitation, paraplegia, seizure, respiratory arrest*	Hypersensitivity to bupivacaine Obstetrical paracervical block anesthesia Local infection at the proposed site of spinal anesthesia Contraindicated for use in spinal anesthesia in the presence of septicemia, severe hemorrhage, shock, or arrhythmias such as complete heart block	Highly hydrophobic, high potency, long duration of action. Cardiotoxicity at higher concentrations limits its use. The R-enantiomer and S-enantiomer have different affinities for the sodium channel and, therefore, different cardiovascular effects; the S-enantiomer, which is less toxic and less potent, is levobupivacaine; its structural homologue is ropivacaine.
Articaine	Dental anesthesia Epidural, spinal, and regional anesthesia	*Same as lidocaine*	Infection at site of injection (especially lumbar puncture sites) Shock	Articaine's current clinical application is largely in dentistry.
EMLA (eutectic mixture of lidocaine and prilocaine)	Topical local anesthetic for normal intact skin, mucosal membranes, and dental procedures	*Same as lidocaine*	Hypersensitivity to amide-linked local anesthetics	Delivered topically as a cream, swab, or patch. Useful clinically due to higher concentration of local anesthetic per drop contacting the tissue than standard topical preparations.

IIC

Activated circuit

Inhibitory surround

A

C

Principles of
Central Nervous System Pharmacology

13

Pharmacology of GABAergic and Glutamatergic Neurotransmission

Stuart A. Forman, Hua-Jun Feng, Janet Chou, Jianren Mao, and Eng H. Lo

INTRODUCTION

Inhibitory and excitatory neurotransmitters regulate almost every behavioral process, including consciousness, sleep, learning, memory, and all sensations. Inhibitory and excitatory neurotransmitters are also implicated in pathologic processes such as epilepsy and the neurotoxicity associated with stroke. The interactions among ion channels, the receptors that regulate these channels, and amino acid neurotransmitters in the central nervous system (CNS) constitute the molecular basis for these processes. This chapter discusses the physiology, pathophysiology, and pharmacology of **γ-aminobutyric acid (GABA)** and **glutamate** neurotransmission. Together, these molecules are the two most important amino acid neurotransmitters in the CNS.

OVERVIEW OF GABAERGIC AND GLUTAMATERGIC NEUROTRANSMISSION

The CNS has high concentrations of certain amino acids that bind to postsynaptic receptors and thereby act as inhibitory or excitatory neurotransmitters. Of the two main classes of neuroactive amino acids, γ-aminobutyric acid (GABA) is the major inhibitory amino acid, and glutamate is the primary excitatory amino acid.

Amino acid neurotransmitters elicit inhibitory or excitatory responses by altering the conductance of one or more ion-selective channels. Inhibitory neurotransmitters induce a net outward current, generally hyperpolarizing the membrane. For example, inhibitory neurotransmitters may open K^+ channels or Cl^- channels to induce K^+ efflux or Cl^- influx, respectively.

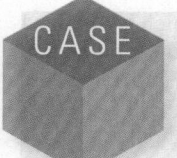

CASE

SB, a 70-year-old man, is having trouble sleeping. He recalls that his sister has been prescribed phenobarbital, a barbiturate, to control her epileptic seizures, and that barbiturates are sometimes also prescribed as sleeping pills. He decides to take "just a few" with some alcohol to help him sleep. Shortly afterward, SB is rushed to the emergency department after his sister finds him minimally responsive. On examination, he is difficult to arouse and dysarthric, with an unsteady gait and impaired attention and memory. His respiratory rate is approximately six shallow breaths per minute. The patient is subsequently intubated to protect him from aspirating gastric contents. Activated charcoal is administered through a nasogastric tube to limit further absorption of phenobarbital. He also receives intravenous sodium bicarbonate to alkalinize his urine to a pH of 7.5 to facilitate renal drug excretion. Three days later, he has recovered sufficiently to return home.

Questions

1. What are the signs of barbiturate poisoning, and how are these signs explained by the drugs' mechanism of action?

2. How do barbiturates act to control epileptic seizures and to induce sleep?

3. How does the patient's age affect the extent of CNS depression caused by barbiturates?

4. What is the interaction of barbiturates and ethanol that results in profound CNS and respiratory depression?

Either type of ion movement—the loss of intracellular cations or the gain of intracellular anions—results in membrane hyperpolarization and decreased membrane resistance (Fig. 13-1), respectively moving the membrane potential further below its threshold value and reducing the ability of inward currents to depolarize the membrane.

Excitatory amino acid neurotransmitters induce a net inward current, generally depolarizing the membrane. For example, excitatory neurotransmitters may open cation-specific channels, such as a sodium channel, and thereby cause a net influx of sodium ions that depolarizes the membrane. An excitatory (depolarizing) response could also result if a neurotransmitter closes potassium "leak channels" to reduce the outward flow of potassium ions and thereby depolarize the membrane (see Chapter 8, Principles of Cellular Excitability and Electrochemical Transmission).

Pharmacologic agents that modulate GABAergic neurotransmission, including **benzodiazepines** and **barbiturates**, are drug classes of major clinical importance. In comparison, pharmacologic agents targeting glutamatergic neurotransmission remain largely experimental. The balance of the discussion is, therefore, addressed at GABAergic physiology and pharmacology; the pathophysiology and pharmacology of glutamatergic neurotransmission is discussed at the end of the chapter.

PHYSIOLOGY OF GABAERGIC NEUROTRANSMISSION

GABA functions as the primary inhibitory neurotransmitter in the mature mammalian CNS. The cell membranes of most vertebrate CNS neurons and astrocytes express GABA receptors, which decrease neuronal excitability through several mechanisms. Because of their widespread distribution, GABA receptors influence many neural circuits and functions. Drugs that modulate GABA receptors affect arousal and attention, memory formation, anxiety, sleep, and muscle tone. Modulation of GABA signaling is also an important mechanism for treatment of focal or widespread neuronal hyperactivity in epilepsy.

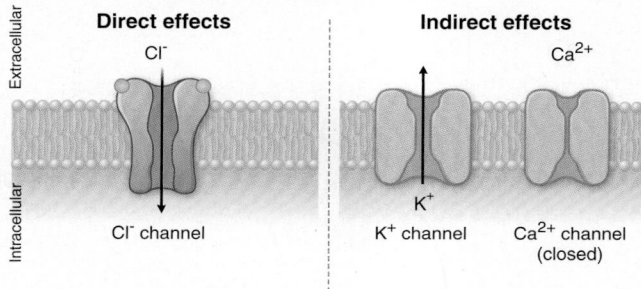

A Effects of inhibitory neurotransmitters

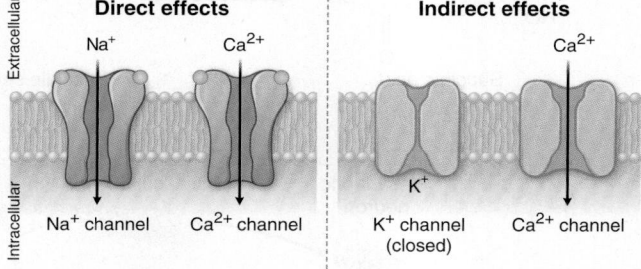

B Effects of excitatory neurotransmitters

FIGURE 13-1. Effects of inhibitory and excitatory neurotransmitters on ion conductances. A. Inhibitory neurotransmitters *hyperpolarize* membranes by inducing a net outward current, by promoting either an influx of anions (e.g., opening a Cl^- channel) or an efflux of cations (e.g., opening a K^+ channel). Opening of chloride or potassium channels also decreases the membrane resistance and thereby lowers the ΔV_m response to excitatory currents, a process called *shunting*. The decreased membrane resistance results in decreased responsiveness (i.e., a smaller change in V_m per change in current) because $\Delta V_m = \Delta i_m \times r_m$, where V_m is the membrane potential, i_m is the excitatory current, and r_m is the membrane resistance. **B.** Excitatory neurotransmitters *depolarize* membranes by inducing a net inward current, either by enhancing inward current (e.g., opening a Na^+ or Ca^{2+} channel) or by reducing outward current (e.g., closing a K^+ channel). Potassium channel closure, independent of changes in the resting membrane potential, also increases the resting membrane resistance and renders the cell more responsive to excitatory postsynaptic currents.

GABA Metabolism and Transport

The synthesis of GABA is mediated by **glutamic acid decarboxylase (GAD)**, which catalyzes the decarboxylation of glutamate to GABA in GABAergic nerve terminals (Fig. 13-2A). Thus, the amount of GABA in brain tissue correlates with the amount of functional GAD. GAD requires pyridoxal phosphate (vitamin B_6) as a cofactor. GABA is packaged into presynaptic vesicles by a vesicular transporter (**VGAT**). (The same transporter, VGAT, is also expressed in nerve terminals that release glycine, another inhibitory neurotransmitter.) In response to an action potential and the presynaptic elevation of intracellular Ca^{2+}, GABA is released into the synaptic cleft by fusion of GABA-containing vesicles with the presynaptic membrane.

Termination of GABA action at the synapse depends on the removal of GABA from the extracellular space. Neurons and glia take up GABA via specific **GABA transporters (GATs)** in the cell membrane. Four GATs have been identified, GAT-1 through GAT-4, each with a characteristic distribution in the CNS. Within cells, the widely distributed mitochondrial enzyme **GABA transaminase (GABA-T)** catalyzes the conversion

of GABA to succinic semialdehyde (SSA), which is oxidized to succinic acid by SSA dehydrogenase. Succinic acid enters the Krebs cycle to become α-ketoglutarate, and GABA-T regenerates glutamate from α-ketoglutarate (Fig. 13-2A).

GABA Receptors

GABA mediates its neurophysiologic effects by binding to GABA receptors. There are two types of GABA receptors. **Ionotropic GABA receptors** (**GABA_A** and **GABA_C**) are multisubunit membrane proteins that bind GABA and open an intrinsic chloride ion channel. **Metabotropic GABA receptors** (**GABA_B**) are heterodimeric G protein-coupled receptors that activate neuronal potassium channels through second messengers.

Ionotropic GABA Receptors: GABA_A and GABA_C

The most abundant GABA receptors in the CNS are ionotropic **GABA_A** receptors, which are members of the superfamily of fast neurotransmitter-gated ion channels. This superfamily includes peripheral and neuronal nicotinic acetylcholine receptors (nAChRs), serotonin type 3A/B (5-HT$_{3A/B}$) receptors,

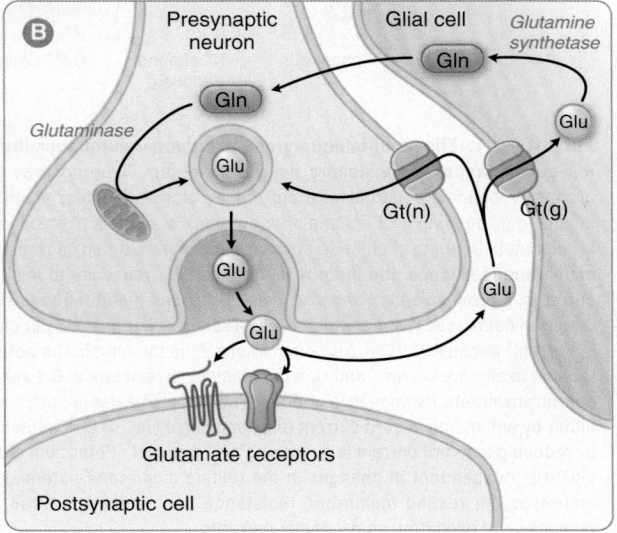

FIGURE 13-2. Glutamate and GABA synthesis and metabolism. A. Glutamate synthesis and metabolism are intertwined with GABA synthesis and metabolism. In one pathway for glutamate synthesis, α-ketoglutarate produced by the Krebs cycle serves as a substrate for the enzyme GABA transaminase (GABA-T), which reductively transaminates intraneuronal α-ketoglutarate to glutamate. The same enzyme also converts GABA to succinic semialdehyde. Alternatively, glutamate is converted to GABA by the enzyme glutamic acid decarboxylase (GAD), changing the major excitatory neurotransmitter to the major inhibitory transmitter. GABA-T is irreversibly inhibited by vigabatrin; by blocking the conversion of GABA to succinic semialdehyde, this drug increases the amount of GABA available for release at inhibitory synapses. GABA-T, GABA transaminase; SSADH, succinic semialdehyde dehydrogenase; GAD, glutamic acid decarboxylase. **B.** Glutamate transporters in neuronal [Gt(n)] and glial [Gt(g)] cell membranes sequester glutamate (Glu) from the synaptic cleft into their respective cells. In the glial cell, the enzyme glutamine synthetase transforms glutamate into glutamine (Gln). Glutamine is then transferred to the neuron, which converts it back to glutamate via mitochondria-associated glutaminase.

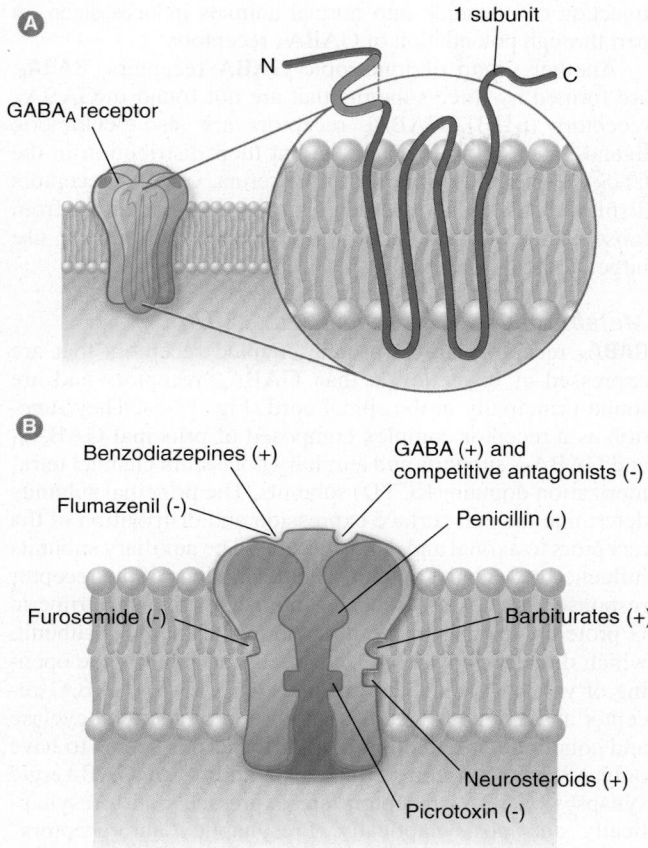

FIGURE 13-3. **Schematic representation of the GABA_A receptor. A.** The pentameric structure of the GABA_A receptor. Each of the five subunits is typically one of three predominant subtypes: α, β, or γ. Activation requires the simultaneous binding of two GABA molecules to the receptor, one to each of the two binding sites at the interface of the α and β subunits. Each subunit of the GABA_A receptor has four membrane-spanning regions and a cysteine loop in the extracellular N-terminal domain (*depicted as a blue segment and a dashed line*). **B.** Drug binding sites on the GABA_A receptor. For most of the exact locations schematically indicated in this diagram, the current evidence is largely indirect. (+) indicates agonist or allosteric modulator action at the GABA_A receptor; (−) indicates competitive or noncompetitive antagonist action.

and glycine receptors. Like other members of this superfamily, GABA_A receptors are pentameric transmembrane glycoproteins that are assembled to form a central ion pore surrounded by five subunits, each of which has four membrane-spanning domains (Fig. 13-3A). Sixteen different GABA_A receptor subunits are currently known (α1–6, β1–3, γ1–3, δ, ε, π, and θ). The number of pentameric ion channels that could be formed by potential combinations of 16 subunits is very large, but only about 20 different subunit combinations have been identified in native GABA_A receptors. Importantly, receptors containing different subunit combinations display distinct distributions at the cellular and tissue levels, and evidence is accumulating that different GABA_A receptor subtypes play distinct roles in specific neural circuits. Most synaptic GABA_A receptors consist of two α subunits, two β subunits, and one γ subunit. "Extrasynaptic" GABA_A receptors have also been identified on dendrites, axons, and neuronal cell bodies. These often contain α5 subunits together with a γ subunit or a δ subunit.

The five subunits of GABA_A receptors surround a central chloride-selective ion pore that opens in the presence of GABA. GABA and other agonists bind to two sites, which are located in extracellular portions of the receptor-channel complex at the interface between the α and β subunits. GABA_A receptors also contain a number of modulatory sites where other endogenous ligands and/or drugs bind (Fig. 13-3B). In many cases, the presence of these sites and the impact of ligand binding depend on the receptor subunit composition.

GABA_A receptor-channel activation follows the binding of two molecules of GABA, one to each of the receptor's agonist sites (Fig. 13-3). Fast **inhibitory postsynaptic currents (IPSCs)** are responses activated by very brief (high-frequency) bursts of GABA release at synapses. Uptake by GAT removes GABA from the synapse in less than 1 ms; IPSCs deactivate over about 12–20 ms, a rate that is determined by both closure of the GABA_A receptor ion channel and dissociation of GABA from the receptor. Prolonged occupation of the agonist sites by GABA also leads to GABA_A receptor **desensitization**, a transition to an inactive agonist-bound state (Fig. 13-4). During burst (or "phasic") firing, the presynaptic nerve membrane releases "quanta" (~1 mM) of GABA by exocytosis of synaptic vesicles, resulting in transient, large-amplitude **inhibitory postsynaptic potentials (IPSPs)**. The diffusion of GABA away from synaptic clefts also results in low concentrations of GABA (up to a few μM) in cerebrospinal fluid and interstitial spaces. Thus, GABA also activates extrasynaptic GABA_A receptors and thereby induces a baseline "tonic" inhibitory current in many neurons.

Because the internal chloride concentration $[Cl^-]_{in}$ of mature neurons is lower than the extracellular Cl^- concentration $[Cl^-]_{out}$, activation of chloride-selective channels (increasing conductance) shifts the neuronal transmembrane voltage toward the Cl^- equilibrium potential ($E_{Cl} \sim -70$ mV). This Cl^- flux *hyperpolarizes* or stabilizes the postsynaptic cell near its normal resting membrane potential ($V_m \sim -65$ mV), reducing the likelihood that excitatory stimuli will initiate action potentials. Open Cl^- channels attenuate the change in membrane potential caused by excitatory synaptic currents, an effect called **shunting**. This is the molecular explanation for the inhibitory effects of GABA signaling via GABA_A receptors.

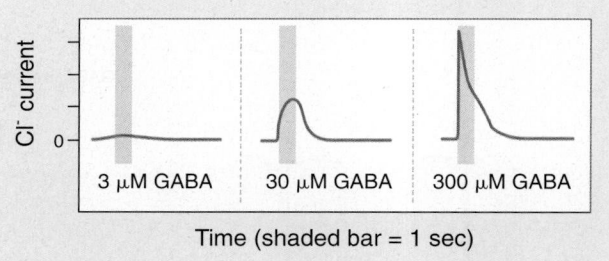

FIGURE 13-4. **Effects of GABA on GABA_A-mediated chloride conductance.** Increasing concentrations of GABA induce both larger Cl^- currents and more rapid receptor desensitization. The latter phenomenon can be observed as the rapid decline from the peak current during continuous exposure to 300 μM GABA (*right panel*). In each panel, the shaded bar indicates the 1-second period during which GABA was applied. Although individual presynaptic endings release GABA for much shorter times, the cumulative GABA released from many presynaptic neurons, stimulated by trains of invading action potentials, can persist for seconds.

In mature neurons, the chloride gradients are maintained by a potassium-chloride (K^+-Cl^-) co-transporter (KCC2). In immature neurons of fetal and neonatal brain, the Cl^- gradient may be reversed due to a difference in the Cl^- transporting pumps (sodium-potassium-chloride [Na^+-K^+-Cl^-] co-transporter, NKCC1). In neurons expressing NKCC1, $GABA_A$ receptors may mediate the outward flow of Cl^- ions, constituting an *inward current* and thus *depolarizing* the neuron. Thus, drugs that activate or potentiate $GABA_A$ receptors may have an excitatory action during brain development rather than the inhibitory effect they have in mature neurons.

The molecular role of $GABA_A$ receptors in neurons is consistent with their known physiologic roles in CNS disease and with their pharmacology. Drugs that inhibit $GABA_A$ receptors produce seizures in animals, and mutations in $GABA_A$ receptor subunits that impair activation at the molecular level are associated with inherited human epilepsy syndromes. Conversely, endogenous or exogenous substances that enhance the activation of $GABA_A$ receptors reduce neuronal excitability and may impair numerous CNS functions. Recent evidence indicates that $GABA_A$ receptors are also expressed in peripheral tissues such as airway epithelium. Activation of these receptors may enhance smooth muscle relaxation (bronchodilation) and could represent a future therapy for asthma.

Certain endogenous substances such as taurine and steroids (also known as **neurosteroids)** allosterically modulate $GABA_A$ receptor activity. The steroid hormones deoxycorticosterone and progesterone are metabolized in the brain to produce pregnenolone, dehydroepiandrosterone (DHEA), 5α-dihydrodeoxycorticosterone (DHDOC), 5α-tetrahydrodeoxycorticosterone (THDOC), and allopregnanolone. Neurosteroids do not act through nuclear receptors like most steroid hormones; instead, they alter $GABA_A$ receptor function by binding to allosteric sites on the receptor protein, causing increased $GABA_A$ receptor activation. DHDOC and THDOC are thought to modulate brain activity during stress. Menstrual variations in allopregnanolone, a metabolite of progesterone, contribute to perimenstrual (catamenial) epilepsy. Sulfation of pregnenolone and DHEA results in neurosteroids that *inhibit* $GABA_A$ receptors. Another endogenous substance that enhances $GABA_A$ receptor activity is **oleamide,** a fatty acid amide found in the cerebrospinal fluid of sleep-deprived animals.

Injection of oleamide into normal animals induces sleep, in part through potentiation of $GABA_A$ receptors.

Another group of ionotropic GABA receptors, **$GABA_C$,** are formed by three subunits that are not found in $GABA_A$ receptors (ρ1–3). $GABA_C$ receptors are also pentameric ligand-gated chloride channels, but their distribution in the CNS is restricted primarily to the retina. $GABA_C$ receptors display distinct pharmacologic properties that differ from those of most $GABA_A$ receptors. No drugs currently in use target $GABA_C$ receptors.

Metabotropic GABA Receptors: $GABA_B$

$GABA_B$ receptors are G protein-coupled receptors that are expressed at lower levels than $GABA_A$ receptors and are found principally in the spinal cord (Fig. 13-5). They function as a receptor complex composed of principal $GABA_{B1}$ and $GABA_{B2}$ subunits and auxiliary potassium channel tetramerization domain (KCTD) subunits. The principal subunits determine the cell surface expression and distribution of the receptors to axonal and dendritic sites. The auxiliary subunits influence the agonist potency and the kinetics of the receptor response. The $GABA_B$ receptor interacts with heterotrimeric G proteins, leading to the dissociation of their βγ subunit, which directly activates K^+ channels and inhibits the opening of voltage-gated Ca^{2+} channels (Fig. 13-5). $GABA_B$ receptor activation also leads to inhibition of adenylyl cyclase and concomitant reduction in cAMP, but this seems to have only minor effects on cellular excitability. At GABAergic synapses, $GABA_B$ receptors are expressed both presynaptically and postsynaptically. Presynaptic "autoreceptors" modulate neurotransmitter release by reducing Ca^{2+} influx, while postsynaptic $GABA_B$ receptors produce slow IPSPs through activation of G protein-activated "inward rectifier" K^+ channels (GIRKs). The slower rates of activation and deactivation of $GABA_B$ currents in comparison to $GABA_A$ currents are due to the relatively slow second messenger signal transduction mechanisms.

Because K^+ has an equilibrium potential near −90 mV, activation of K^+ channels by $GABA_B$-coupled G proteins inhibits neuronal firing. Thus, like increased Cl^- conductance, increased K^+ conductance drives the neuronal transmembrane voltage toward "resting" potentials, reduces the frequency of action potential initiation, and shunts excitatory currents.

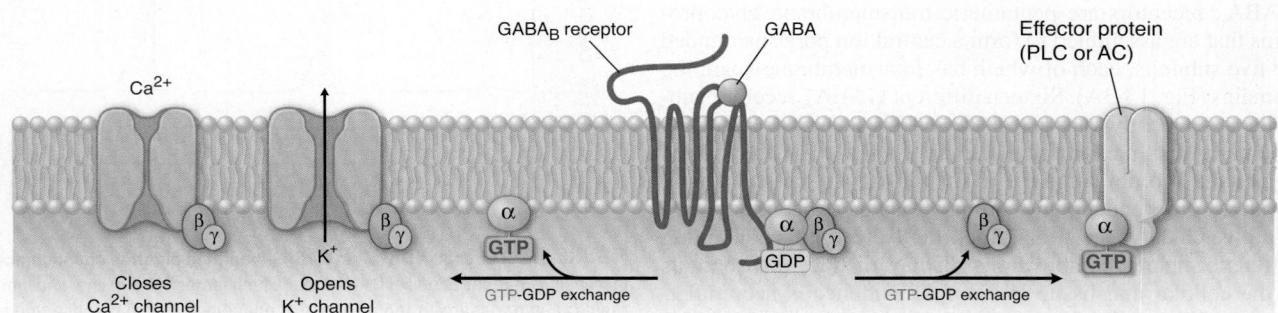

FIGURE 13-5. Downstream signaling of the GABA_B receptor. GABA_B receptor activation alters cytoplasmic G proteins that then dissociate into α and βγ subunits, the latter of which bind directly to K^+ or Ca^{2+} channels (*leftward arrow*). The released α subunits are linked to second messenger systems such as adenylyl cyclase (AC) or phospholipase C (PLC) (*rightward arrow*). The increased K^+ efflux leads to slow, long-lasting inhibitory postsynaptic potentials. The reduced Ca^{2+} influx may account for the ability of GABA_B autoreceptors to inhibit presynaptic neurotransmitter release. The GABA_B receptor functions as an obligate heterodimer of GABA_B1 and GABA_B2 subunits, each of which is a seven-transmembrane-spanning G protein-coupled receptor (*not shown*).

PHARMACOLOGIC CLASSES AND AGENTS AFFECTING GABAERGIC NEUROTRANSMISSION

Pharmacologic agents acting on GABAergic neurotransmission affect GABA metabolism, transport, or receptor activity. The majority of pharmacologic agents affecting GABAergic neurotransmission act on the ionotropic $GABA_A$ receptor. Several drug classes can regulate $GABA_A$ receptors by interacting with the GABA binding sites or with allosteric sites (Fig. 13-3). Therapeutic agents that activate $GABA_A$ receptors are used for sedation, anxiolysis, hypnosis (general anesthesia), neuroprotection following stroke or head trauma, and control of epilepsy. Other agents that modulate GABAergic transmission are used only for experimental purposes (Table 13-1).

Inhibitors of GABA Metabolism and Transport

Tiagabine is a competitive inhibitor of the GABA transporters in neurons and glia, where it may act selectively on GAT-1. Epilepsy is the major clinical indication for tiagabine. By inhibiting GABA reuptake, tiagabine increases both synaptic and extrasynaptic GABA concentrations. The result is nonspecific agonism of both ionotropic and metabotropic GABA receptors, with the major effects at $GABA_A$ receptors.

Tiagabine is an oral medication that is rapidly absorbed with 90% bioavailability and is highly protein bound. Metabolism is hepatic, primarily by CYP3A4. Tiagabine does not induce cytochrome P450 enzymes, but its metabolism is influenced by concomitant use of either inducers or inhibitors of CYP3A4. Adverse effects of tiagabine are those of high GABA activity, including confusion, sedation, amnesia, and ataxia. Tiagabine potentiates the action of $GABA_A$ receptor modulators such as ethanol, benzodiazepines, and barbiturates.

γ-Vinyl GABA (vigabatrin) is a "suicide inhibitor" of GABA transaminase (GABA-T, see Fig. 13-2). Administration of this drug blocks the conversion of GABA to succinic semialdehyde, resulting in high intracellular GABA concentrations and increased synaptic GABA release. Like the effect of tiagabine, enhancement of GABA receptor function by γ-vinyl GABA is not selective because GABA concentrations are increased wherever GABA is released, including the retina.

Vigabatrin is used in the treatment of epilepsy, and it is being investigated for treatment of drug addiction, panic disorder, and obsessive-compulsive disorder. Adverse effects

TABLE 13-1 Partial List of Agents That Modulate GABAergic Transmission

DRUG CLASS	PRESUMED MECHANISM	EFFECTS
GABA Synthesis		
Allylglycine	Inhibits glutamic acid decarboxylase	Convulsant
Isoniazid	Inhibits pyridoxal kinase (antivitamin B_6 effect)	Convulsant at high doses
GABA Release		
Tetanus toxin	Inhibits GABA and glycine release	Convulsant
GABA Metabolism and Transport		
Tiagabine	Inhibits GAT-1	Anticonvulsant
Vigabatrin	Inhibits GABA transaminase	Anticonvulsant
$GABA_A$ Receptor Agonists		
Muscimol	$GABA_A$ receptor agonist	Anticonvulsant, mimics psychosis
Gaboxadol	$GABA_A$ receptor agonist	Anticonvulsant
$GABA_A$ Receptor Antagonists		
Bicuculline	Competitive antagonist	Convulsant
Gabazine	Competitive antagonist	Convulsant
Picrotoxin	Noncompetitive antagonist, pore blocker, occludes the chloride channel	Convulsant
$GABA_A$ Receptor Modulators		
Benzodiazepines	Potentiate GABA binding	Anticonvulsant, anxiolytic
Barbiturates	Increase GABA efficacy, weak agonist	Anticonvulsant, anesthetic
$GABA_B$ Receptor Agonists		
Baclofen	$GABA_B$ receptor agonist	Muscle relaxant

of γ-vinyl GABA include drowsiness, confusion, and headache. The drug has been reported to cause bilateral visual field defects associated with irreversible diffuse atrophy of the peripheral retinal nerve fiber layer. This appears to result from accumulation of the drug in retinal nerves.

GABA$_A$ Receptor Agonists and Antagonists

Agonists such as **muscimol** and **gaboxadol** activate the GABA$_A$ receptor by binding directly to the GABA binding site. Muscimol, first derived from hallucinogenic *Amanita muscaria* mushrooms, is a full agonist at many GABA$_A$ receptor subtypes and is used primarily as a research tool. Purified muscimol (as well as other GABA$_A$ receptor agonists) does not induce hallucinations, which are probably caused by other factors from *Amanita muscaria*. Gaboxadol at high concentrations is a partial agonist at synaptic GABA$_A$ receptors; at low concentrations, gaboxadol selectively activates extrasynaptic receptors containing α4, β3, and δ subunits. Gaboxadol was initially approved for treatment of epilepsy and anxiety, but therapeutic doses were associated with ataxia and sedation. Lower gaboxadol doses, which activate extrasynaptic receptors, induce slow-wave sleep in laboratory animals. Human trials of gaboxadol for treatment of insomnia were halted in 2007 due to concerns about adverse effects such as hallucinations, disorientation, sleepwalking, and sleep-driving.

Bicuculline and **gabazine** are competitive antagonists that bind at the GABA sites on GABA$_A$ receptors. **Picrotoxin** is a noncompetitive inhibitor of GABA$_A$ receptors that blocks the ion pore. All of these GABA$_A$ antagonists induce seizures and are used exclusively for research; they also illustrate the importance of the tonic activity of GABA$_A$ receptors in maintaining a state of relatively normal excitability in the CNS.

GABA$_A$ Receptor Modulators

Benzodiazepines and barbiturates are modulators of GABA$_A$ receptors that act at allosteric binding sites to enhance GABAergic neurotransmission (Fig. 13-3B). **Benzodiazepines** have sedative, hypnotic, muscle relaxant, amnestic, and anxiolytic effects. At high doses, benzodiazepines can cause hypnosis and stupor. However, when used alone, these drugs rarely cause fatal CNS depression. **Barbiturates** constitute a large group of drugs that were first introduced in the mid-twentieth century and continue to be used, albeit with diminishing frequency, for control of epilepsy, as general anesthetic induction agents, and for control of intracranial hypertension.

Benzodiazepines

Benzodiazepines are high-affinity, highly selective drugs that bind at a single site on GABA$_A$ receptors containing α1, α2, α3, or α5 subunits and a γ subunit. In molecular studies, benzodiazepine potency correlates with hydrophobicity. However, benzodiazepines are highly bound to plasma proteins such as albumin, and hydrophobicity enhances protein binding and thereby reduces the drugs' free concentration and transport across the blood–brain barrier. Therefore, highly protein-bound benzodiazepines may appear less potent in vivo even though they display higher potency in molecular studies. Furthermore, in clinical states associated with low albumin, such as acute hemodilution or liver dysfunction, the clinical potency of benzodiazepines may be dramatically increased.

Benzodiazepines act as positive allosteric modulators by enhancing GABA$_A$ receptor channel gating in the presence of GABA (Fig. 13-6). Benzodiazepines *increase the frequency of channel opening* in the presence of low GABA concentrations, and, at GABA concentrations similar to those in synapses,

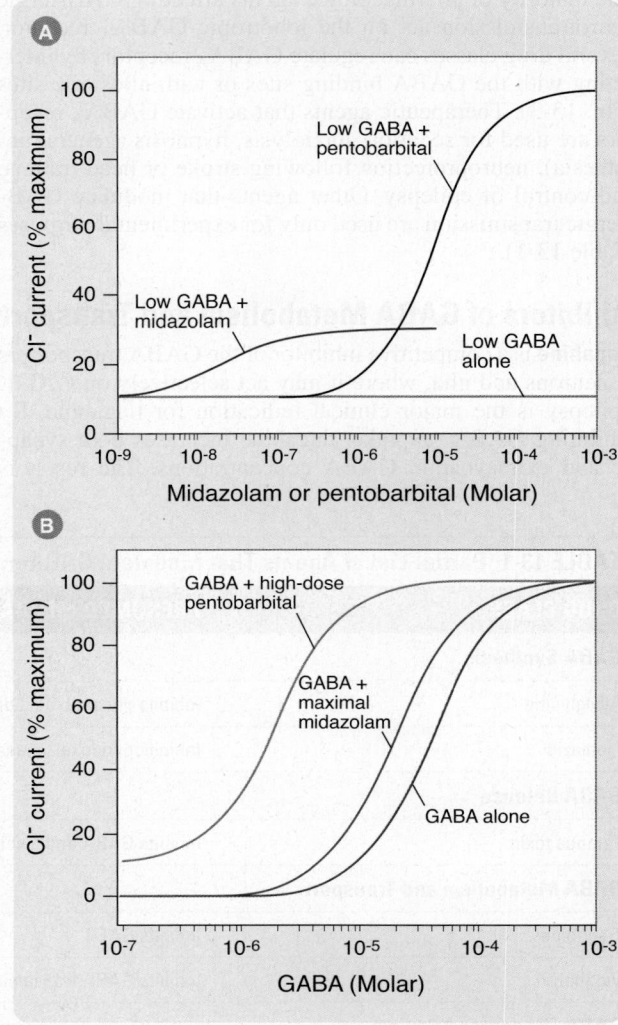

FIGURE 13-6. Effects of benzodiazepines and barbiturates on GABA$_A$ receptor activity. A. Both benzodiazepines and barbiturates enhance GABA$_A$ receptor activation (measured experimentally by Cl$^-$ current), but with different potencies and efficacies. Midazolam (a benzodiazepine) maximally enhances by about threefold the current evoked by 10 μM GABA (low GABA). In contrast, the anesthetic barbiturate pentobarbital increases the current evoked by 10 μM GABA to a much greater extent (near that of a maximal GABA response), but its maximal effect requires concentrations greater than 100 μM. Thus, benzodiazepines such as midazolam are high-potency, low-efficacy modulators of GABA$_A$ receptor activity, while barbiturates such as pentobarbital are low-potency, high-efficacy modulators. **B.** Another way to compare the efficacy of benzodiazepines and barbiturates is to measure the degree to which they enhance the sensitivity of GABA$_A$ receptors to GABA. Maximally effective concentrations of midazolam shift the GABA concentration–response curve modestly to the left, reducing the EC$_{50}$ (increasing the potency) of GABA by about twofold. In contrast, high-dose pentobarbital causes a much greater shift to the left, reducing the EC$_{50}$ of GABA by approximately 20-fold. Pentobarbital at high concentrations also directly activates GABA$_A$ receptors, even in the absence of GABA (note the nonzero Cl$^-$ current at 10^{-7} M GABA). In contrast, the benzodiazepines do not have direct agonist activity.

receptor deactivation is slowed. Both actions result in a net increase in Cl⁻ influx. In addition, GABA$_A$ receptors in the open state have a higher affinity for GABA than in the closed state, so the ability of benzodiazepines to favor channel openness results, secondarily, in an apparently higher agonist affinity.

Benzodiazepines do not activate native GABA$_A$ receptors in the absence of GABA, but they do activate certain mutant receptors and enhance maximal activation by partial agonists, indicating that they are **weak positive allosteric agonists** (Fig. 13-7). This mechanism is consistent with the known location of the benzodiazepine binding site at the interface between the external domains of the α and γ subunits. This site is a structural homologue of the two GABA agonist sites at the interfaces between the β and α subunits.

In GABA concentration–response studies, benzodiazepines shift the response curve to the left, increasing the apparent potency of GABA by up to threefold (Fig. 13-6B). This is a smaller allosteric effect than that caused by other modulators, such as barbiturates or other general anesthetics (see etomidate, below). The limited efficacy of benzodiazepines is accompanied by a reduced potential for fatal overdose. However, the margin of safety decreases when benzodiazepines are co-administered with alcohol or other sedative/hypnotics.

Clinical Applications

Benzodiazepines are used as sleep enhancers, anxiolytics, sedatives, antiepileptics, and muscle relaxants, and for treatment of ethanol withdrawal symptoms (Table 13-2). Benzodiazepines achieve an anxiolytic effect by inhibiting synapses in the limbic system, a CNS region that controls emotional behavior and is characterized by a high density of GABA$_A$ receptors. Benzodiazepines such as **diazepam** and **alprazolam** are used to mitigate chronic, severe anxiety and the anxiety associated with some forms of depression and schizophrenia. Because of the potential for the development of tolerance, dependence, and addiction, benzodiazepine use should be intermittent. In acute-care settings, such as in preparation for invasive procedures, **midazolam** is frequently used as a rapid-onset and short-acting anxiolytic/sedative/amnestic. Benzodiazepines are often adequate as sedatives for brief,

uncomfortable procedures associated with minimal sharp pain, such as endoscopy. When combined with opioids, however, a synergistic potentiation of both sedation and respiratory depression can occur. Given prior to general anesthesia, benzodiazepines reduce the requirement for hypnotic agents.

Many benzodiazepines, including **estazolam**, **flurazepam**, **quazepam**, **temazepam**, and **triazolam**, and other benzodiazepine site agonists, including the so-called **z-drugs** (**zolpidem**, **zaleplon**, **zopiclone**, and **eszopiclone**), are prescribed for treatment of insomnia. Benzodiazepines both facilitate sleep onset and increase the overall duration of sleep. They also alter the distribution of the various sleep stages: they increase the length of stage 2 non-rapid eye movement (NREM) sleep (the light sleep that normally comprises approximately half of sleeping time) and decrease the length of REM sleep (the period characterized by frequent dreams) and slow-wave sleep (the deepest level of sleep). After extended use, these effects may diminish because of tolerance. In a healthy individual, hypnotic doses of benzodiazepines induce respiratory changes comparable to those present during natural sleep and do not cause significant cardiovascular changes. Patients with either pulmonary or cardiovascular disease may experience significant respiratory or cardiovascular depression because of medullary depression from otherwise therapeutic doses of these drugs. Patients who have suffered brain damage from stroke or head trauma may also become profoundly sedated with these drugs.

The sedative benzodiazepines differ in their rates of onset, durations of effect, and tendencies to cause rebound insomnia when withdrawn. For example, **flurazepam** is a long-acting benzodiazepine that facilitates sleep onset and maintenance and increases sleep duration. Although it does not cause significant rebound insomnia, its long elimination half-life (about 74 hours) and the accumulation of active metabolites may cause daytime sedation. **Triazolam** is a fast-onset benzodiazepine that also decreases the time needed to fall asleep. Intermittent rather than chronic administration of this drug is recommended to lessen the rebound insomnia associated with its discontinuation. The so-called **z-drugs** such as **zolpidem** are unique among sedatives used for insomnia in selectively interacting with GABA$_A$ receptors containing

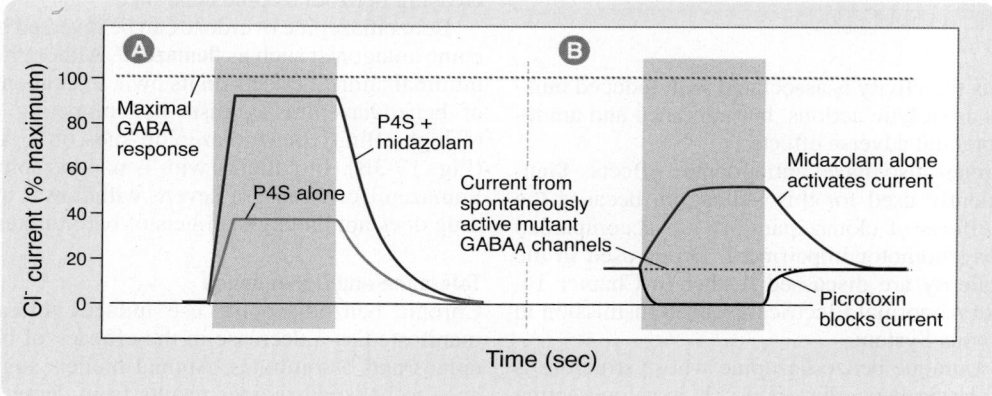

FIGURE 13-7. Evidence that benzodiazepines enhance the GABA$_A$ receptor channel opening probability. A. When GABA$_A$ receptors are activated using saturating concentrations of the partial agonist P4S, midazolam increases the peak current. This indicates that the P4S efficacy (the maximal channel opening probability) is increased by the addition of midazolam. **B.** GABA$_A$ receptors containing a certain point mutation are spontaneously active, which can be demonstrated by the loss of current caused by picrotoxin (a noncompetitive GABA$_A$ receptor antagonist). When these mutant receptors are exposed to midazolam, the amount of current increases, indicating that midazolam directly influences the opening of GABA$_A$ receptors. This effect is not observed in wild-type channels, which exhibit only rare spontaneous openings.

TABLE 13-2 Clinical Uses and Relative Duration of Action of Several Benzodiazepines

BENZODIAZEPINE	CLINICAL USES	DURATION OF ACTION
Clorazepate	Anxiety disorders, seizures	Short-acting (3–8 hours)
Midazolam	Preanesthetic, IV general anesthetic	Short-acting (3–8 hours)
Alprazolam	Anxiety disorders, phobias	Intermediate-acting (11–20 hours)
Lorazepam	Anxiety disorders, status epilepticus, IV general anesthetic	Intermediate-acting (11–20 hours)
Chlordiazepoxide	Anxiety disorders, alcohol withdrawal	Long-acting (1–3 days)
Clobazam	Anxiety disorders, seizures	Long-acting (1–3 days)
Clonazepam	Seizures	Long-acting (1–3 days)
Diazepam	Anxiety disorders, status epilepticus, muscle relaxant, IV general anesthetic, alcohol withdrawal	Long-acting (1–3 days)
Triazolam	Insomnia	Short-acting (3–8 hours)
Estazolam	Insomnia	Intermediate-acting (11–20 hours)
Temazepam	Insomnia	Intermediate-acting (11–20 hours)
Flurazepam	Insomnia	Long-acting (1–3 days)
Quazepam	Insomnia	Long-acting (1–3 days)

α1 subunits. This selectivity is associated with reduced muscle relaxant and anxiolytic actions, but tolerance and amnesia remain as potential adverse effects.

Benzodiazepines also have antiepileptic effects. **Clonazepam** is frequently used for this indication, because the anticonvulsant effects of clonazepam are not accompanied by significant psychomotor impairment. Drugs used in the treatment of epilepsy are discussed further in Chapter 16, Pharmacology of Abnormal Electrical Neurotransmission in the Central Nervous System.

Clobazam is a unique benzodiazepine whose structure is different from classic benzodiazepines. It is a long-acting benzodiazepine used for selective anxiolysis and seizure control. Compared with other benzodiazepines, this agent is less sedating and has fewer negative effects on cognition.

Benzodiazepines reduce skeletal muscle spasticity by enhancing the activity of inhibitory interneurons in the spinal cord. **Diazepam** is used to alleviate muscle spasms caused by physical trauma as well as muscle spasticity associated with neuromuscular degenerative disorders such as multiple sclerosis. The high doses required for these effects also frequently cause sedation.

Pharmacokinetics and Metabolism

Benzodiazepines can be administered via oral, transmucosal, intravenous, and intramuscular routes. The lipophilic nature of benzodiazepines explains their rapid and complete absorption. Although these drugs and their active metabolites are bound to plasma proteins, they do not compete with other protein-bound drugs. Benzodiazepines are metabolized by hepatic microsomal cytochrome P450 enzymes, specifically CYP3A4, and subsequently excreted in the urine as glucuronides or oxidized metabolites. Prolonged benzodiazepine administration does not significantly induce hepatic drug-metabolizing enzyme activity. However, other drugs that inhibit CYP3A4 activity (e.g., ketoconazole and macrolide antibiotics) may enhance the effects of benzodiazepines, while drugs that induce CYP3A4 (e.g., rifampicin, omeprazole, nifedipine) may reduce their effectiveness. Patients with impaired hepatic function, including the elderly and the very young, may experience prolonged effects from benzodiazepine administration. Some benzodiazepine metabolites (e.g., **desmethyldiazepam**) remain pharmacologically active and are cleared more slowly than the parent drug.

Adverse Effects

The adverse effects of benzodiazepines are primarily related to their therapeutic effects in undesirable settings: amnesia, oversedation, and ataxia. In patients with insomnia, rare but sometimes dangerous adverse effects of benzodiazepines and z-drugs include sleepwalking, sleep-driving, and sleep-eating. The relative safety of benzodiazepines derives from their limited efficacy in modulating GABA$_A$ receptors. High doses of benzodiazepines rarely cause death unless administered with other drugs, such as ethanol, CNS depressants, opioid analgesics, or tricyclic antidepressants. The enhanced CNS depression seen with concomitant ethanol and benzodiazepine use is due to both synergistic effects on GABA$_A$ receptors and ethanol-mediated inhibition of CYP3A4. The latter effect occurs when ethanol is consumed rapidly, decreasing benzodiazepine clearance.

Benzodiazepine overdose can be reversed by a benzodiazepine antagonist such as **flumazenil**. Although flumazenil has minimal clinical effects on its own, it antagonizes the effects of benzodiazepine agonists by competing for occupancy of high-affinity benzodiazepine sites on GABA$_A$ receptors (Fig. 13-3B). In patients with benzodiazepine dependence, flumazenil can cause a severe withdrawal syndrome. This drug does not block the effects of barbiturates or ethanol.

Tolerance and Dependence

Chronic benzodiazepine use induces tolerance, which is manifested as a decrease in the efficacy of both benzodiazepines and barbiturates. Animal models suggest that tolerance to benzodiazepines results from decreased expression of benzodiazepine (GABA$_A$) receptors at synapses. Another proposed mechanism for tolerance involves uncoupling of the benzodiazepine binding site from the GABA site. Sudden cessation after chronic benzodiazepine administration can result in a withdrawal syndrome characterized by confusion, anxiety, agitation, and insomnia.

Barbiturates

The CNS sites affected by **barbiturates** are widespread, including the spinal cord, brainstem (cuneate nucleus, substantia nigra, reticular activating system), and brain (cortex, thalamus, cerebellum). Barbiturates reduce neuronal excitability primarily by increasing GABA-mediated inhibition via $GABA_A$ receptors. Barbiturate-enhanced GABAergic transmission in the brainstem suppresses the reticular activating system (discussed in Chapter 9, Principles of Nervous System Physiology and Pharmacology), causing sedation, amnesia, and loss of consciousness. Heightened GABAergic transmission at motor neurons in the spinal cord relaxes muscles and suppresses reflexes. Selectivity for $GABA_A$ receptor subtypes containing specific subunit combinations has not been demonstrated for barbiturates. The stoichiometry of barbiturate binding sites on $GABA_A$ receptors is variable.

The anesthetic barbiturates **thiopental**, **pentobarbital**, and **methohexital** act as both agonists at $GABA_A$ receptors and as enhancers of receptor responses to GABA. Anticonvulsant barbiturates such as **phenobarbital** produce far less direct agonism on native $GABA_A$ receptors. The direct $GABA_A$ receptor activation is not mediated by GABA binding sites but depends on barbiturate-specific sites in the β subunits of the receptor.

At clinically relevant concentrations of barbiturates, the degree of membrane hyperpolarization due to direct activation of $GABA_A$ receptors is far less than that from enhancement of GABA agonism. *The major action of the barbiturates is to enhance the efficacy of GABA by increasing the time that the Cl^- channel stays open, permitting a much greater influx of Cl^- ions for each activated channel* (Fig. 13-6A). This leads to a greater degree of hyperpolarization and to decreased excitability of the target cell. The GABA-enhancing action of barbiturates is greater than that of the benzodiazepines (Fig. 13-6B). The direct-activating and GABA-enhancing actions of barbiturates may be associated with different binding sites or, as shown for etomidate (see below), may reflect actions at a single class of sites. In keeping with their relative efficacy for GABA potentiation, overdoses of the low-efficacy benzodiazepines are deeply sedating but rarely dangerous, whereas barbiturate overdose may produce profound hypnosis, coma, respiratory depression, and death if supportive therapy is not provided.

Barbiturates affect not only $GABA_A$ receptors but also receptors involved in excitatory neurotransmission. Barbiturates decrease activation of glutamate-sensitive AMPA receptors (see Fig. 13-8B), thereby reducing both membrane depolarization and neuronal excitability. At anesthetic concentrations, pentobarbital also decreases the activity of voltage-dependent Na^+ channels, inhibiting high-frequency neuronal firing.

Clinical Applications

Before the discovery of benzodiazepines, the sedative/hypnotic effects of barbiturates were commonly used to treat insomnia or anxiety. Benzodiazepines have largely replaced barbiturates in most clinical applications because benzodiazepines are safer, cause less tolerance, have fewer withdrawal symptoms, and induce less profound effects on drug-metabolizing enzymes. Barbiturates are still used for induction of general anesthesia, as antiepileptic agents, and for neuroprotection (Table 13-3).

The lipid-soluble barbiturates, such as **thiopental**, **methohexital**, and **pentobarbital**, are used to induce general anesthesia. These drugs enter the brain rapidly after intravenous

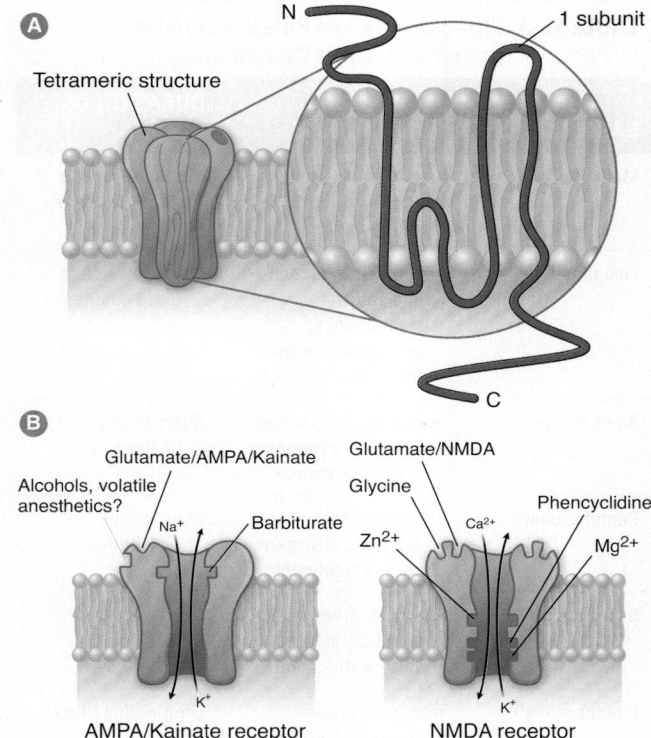

FIGURE 13-8. Schematic representation of the ionotropic glutamate receptors. A. All three ionotropic glutamate receptors are tetrameric complexes composed of the same (termed **homomeric**) or different (termed **heteromeric**) subunits. The structure on the right shows one ionotropic glutamate receptor subunit, which spans the membrane three times and has a partially spanning hairpin turn that, when juxtaposed with homologous turns from the other three subunits, forms the lining of the ion channel's pore. **B.** Major binding sites on the AMPA/kainate and NMDA classes of ionotropic glutamate receptors are shown. Although there is indirect evidence for the location of many of the drug binding sites that are schematically indicated in this diagram, the definitive localization of these sites remains to be determined.

administration and then redistribute to less highly perfused tissues. This redistribution away from the CNS results in a short duration of action after a single bolus administration. The anesthetic barbiturates are also discussed in Chapter 17, General Anesthetic Pharmacology.

Barbiturates such as **phenobarbital** serve as effective antiepileptics. As discussed in Chapter 16, seizures are characterized by rapidly depolarizing CNS neurons that repeatedly fire action potentials. Barbiturates reduce epileptic activity both by enhancing GABA-mediated synaptic inhibition and by inhibiting AMPA receptor-mediated excitatory transmission. Phenobarbital is used to treat focal and tonic–clonic seizures at concentrations that produce minimal sedation.

The profound suppression of neuronal activity by high-dose barbiturates can produce electroencephalographic silence, known as *barbiturate coma*. This state is associated with significantly reduced brain oxygen consumption and reduced cerebral blood flow. These effects can protect the brain from ischemic damage in pathologic conditions associated with reduced oxygen delivery (e.g., hypoxia, profound anemia, shock, brain edema) or increased oxygen demand (e.g., status epilepticus). To produce barbiturate coma, bolus

TABLE 13-3 Clinical Uses and Relative Duration of Action of Several Barbiturates

BARBITURATE	CLINICAL USES	DURATION OF ACTION
Methohexital	Anesthesia induction and short-term maintenance	Ultrashort-acting (5–15 minutes)
Thiopental	Anesthesia induction and short-term maintenance, emergency seizure treatment	Ultrashort-acting (5–15 minutes)
Amobarbital	Insomnia, preoperative sedation, emergency seizure treatment	Short-acting (3–8 hours)
Pentobarbital	Insomnia, preoperative sedation, emergency seizure treatment	Short-acting (3–8 hours)
Secobarbital	Insomnia, preoperative sedation, emergency seizure treatment	Short-acting (3–8 hours)
Phenobarbital	Treatment of seizures, status epilepticus	Long-acting (days)

The duration of action of a barbiturate is determined by the rapidity with which it is redistributed from the brain to other, less vascular compartments, particularly to muscle and fat.

administration is followed by infusion (or multiple additional boluses) to maintain the CNS concentration of drug at therapeutic levels.

Pharmacokinetics and Metabolism

Barbiturates, like benzodiazepines, can be administered orally or intravenously. Oral administration may be associated with significant first-pass metabolism and reduced bioavailability. **Methohexital** can also be absorbed transmucosally. The ability of a barbiturate to cross the blood–brain barrier and enter the CNS is largely determined by its lipid solubility. Consequently, termination of the drug's acute CNS effects depends primarily on its redistribution from the brain, first to such highly perfused areas as the splanchnic circulation, then to skeletal muscle, and, finally, to poorly perfused adipose tissue. As a result, bolus administration of a barbiturate that redistributes rapidly causes only a short-lived effect on the CNS. Chronic administration of the lipophilic barbiturates may have a prolonged effect because of the high uptake capacity of adipose tissue, which leads to a high volume of distribution and a long elimination half-life.

Barbiturates undergo extensive hepatic metabolism before renal excretion. The cytochrome P450 enzymes that metabolize barbiturates are CYP3A4, CYP3A5, and CYP3A7. Chronic barbiturate use greatly up-regulates the expression of these enzymes, thereby accelerating the metabolism of barbiturates (contributing to tolerance) and other substrates for these enzymes. Barbiturate use can thus enhance the metabolism of other sedative/hypnotics, as well as benzodiazepines, phenytoin, digoxin, oral contraceptives, steroid

hormones, bile salts, cholesterol, and vitamins D and K, although the concomitant administration of barbiturates with these agents slows their biotransformation because of substrate competition for the metabolizing enzymes. Elderly patients (who often have impaired liver function) and patients with severe liver disease have reduced barbiturate clearance; even normal doses of sedative/hypnotics may have significantly greater CNS effects in these patients, as experienced by SB in the introductory case. Because acidic compounds such as phenobarbital are excreted faster in alkaline urine, administration of intravenous sodium bicarbonate increases clearance.

Adverse Effects

The multiplicity of sites at which barbiturates act, coupled with their low selectivity and high efficacy for enhancing GABA$_A$ receptor activation, contributes to the relatively low therapeutic index of these drugs. Unlike benzodiazepines, high doses of barbiturates can cause fatal CNS and respiratory depression. The anesthetic barbiturates such as pentobarbital are more likely to induce profound CNS depression than the antiepileptic barbiturates such as phenobarbital (Table 13-4). In addition, as exemplified by the case of SB, the concomitant administration of barbiturates and other CNS depressants, often ethanol, results in CNS depression more severe than that caused by barbiturates alone.

Tolerance and Dependence

Repeated and extended misuse of barbiturates induces tolerance and physiologic dependence. Prolonged barbiturate use increases the activity of cytochrome P450 enzymes and accelerates barbiturate metabolism, thereby contributing to the development of tolerance to barbiturates and cross-tolerance to benzodiazepines, other sedative/hypnotics, and ethanol.

TABLE 13-4 Comparison of Pentobarbital and Phenobarbital

	PENTOBARBITAL	PHENOBARBITAL
Routes of administration	Oral, IM, IV, rectal	Oral, IM, IV
Duration of action	Short-acting (1–4 hours)	Long-acting (days)
Suppression of spontaneous neuronal activity	Yes	Minimal
Activity at GABA$_A$ receptor	Major: Increases efficacy of GABA by increasing open time of Cl⁻ channel Minor: Direct GABA$_A$ receptor activation	Increases efficacy of GABA by increasing open time of Cl⁻ channel
Activity at glutamate receptor	Noncompetitive antagonist at AMPA receptor (2–3 times more potent than phenobarbital)	Noncompetitive antagonist at AMPA receptor
Therapeutic uses	Preoperative sedation Emergency treatment for seizures	Antiepileptic

Development of physiologic dependence results in a drug withdrawal syndrome characterized by tremors, anxiety, insomnia, and CNS excitability. If left untreated, these withdrawal effects may progress to seizures and cardiac arrest.

Etomidate, Propofol, and Alphaxalone

Etomidate, **propofol**, and **alphaxalone** are drugs used for induction of general anesthesia. Etomidate and propofol are also discussed in Chapter 17. Like barbiturates, these intravenous anesthetics act primarily on GABA$_A$ receptors. Etomidate is particularly useful during induction of anesthesia in hemodynamically unstable patients. Propofol is the most widely used anesthetic induction agent in the United States. It is used both for single-bolus induction of anesthesia and for maintenance via continuous intravenous infusion. Alphaxalone is a **neurosteroid** that is rarely used clinically.

Mechanisms of Action

Like barbiturates, etomidate, propofol, and alphaxalone enhance activation of GABA$_A$ receptors by GABA and, at high concentrations, can act as agonists. For etomidate, both of these actions display similar stereoselectivity. Quantitative analysis indicates that both actions are caused by etomidate binding at a single set of two identical allosteric sites per receptor. Similar mechanisms are hypothesized to account for the actions of propofol and alphaxalone.

Etomidate and propofol act selectively at GABA$_A$ receptors that contain β2 and β3 subunits. Based on knock-in animal experiments, in which β3 subunits are expressed as transgenes, β3-containing receptors are the most important for the hypnosis and muscle relaxation associated with general anesthesia. Alphaxalone shows little selectivity among synaptic GABA$_A$ receptors but is more potent at extrasynaptic receptors that contain δ subunits.

Pharmacokinetics and Metabolism

Both etomidate and propofol induce anesthesia rapidly after bolus intravenous injection. Like barbiturates, these hydrophobic drugs cross the blood–brain barrier rapidly. The CNS effect of a bolus dose lasts for only several minutes, because redistribution to muscle and other tissues rapidly reduces the CNS drug concentrations. Propofol has an extremely large volume of distribution, and prolonged continuous infusions may be used without significant changes in the apparent clearance of the drug. Metabolism of etomidate and propofol is primarily hepatic.

Adverse Effects

Etomidate inhibits the synthesis of cortisol and aldosterone. Suppression of cortisol production is thought to contribute to mortality among critically ill patients who receive prolonged etomidate infusions. Etomidate is generally used only for single-dose induction of anesthesia, not for anesthesia maintenance. It is also used rarely at subhypnotic doses for treatment of metastatic cortisol-producing tumors.

The major toxicity of propofol as a general anesthetic is depression of cardiac output and vascular tone. Hypotension is observed in patients who are hypovolemic or, as with many elderly patients, dependent on vascular tone to maintain blood pressure. Propofol is formulated in a lipid emulsion, and hyperlipidemia has been reported in patients receiving prolonged infusions for sedation.

There is growing evidence in fetal and newborn animal models that positive GABA$_A$ receptor modulators lead to neurotoxicity and later neurodevelopmental problems. The mechanism suggested for this toxicity is the depolarizing effect of GABA$_A$ receptors in some fetal and neonatal neurons (see earlier discussion), resulting in excitotoxicity in the presence of GABA$_A$ receptor enhancers. These data have raised concerns about potential damage to the brains of human fetuses and neonates who are exposed to general anesthetics. Long-term clinical studies are underway to assess the functional impact of these effects.

GABA$_B$ Receptor Agonists and Antagonists

Baclofen is the only compound currently in clinical use that targets GABA$_B$ receptors. It was first synthesized as a GABA analogue and screened for antispastic action before GABA$_B$ receptors were discovered. Subsequently, it was found that baclofen is a selective GABA$_B$ receptor agonist. It is used primarily for treatment of spasticity associated with motor neuron diseases (e.g., multiple sclerosis) or spinal cord injury. Oral baclofen is effective for mild spasticity. Severe spasticity may be treated with intrathecal baclofen therapy using doses that are far lower than those required systemically. By activating metabotropic GABA receptors in the spinal cord, baclofen stimulates downstream second messengers to act on Ca^{2+} and K$^+$ channels. Although baclofen is prescribed primarily for treatment of spasticity, clinical observations suggest that it also modulates pain and cognition, and it is being investigated as a therapy for drug addiction.

Baclofen is absorbed slowly after oral administration; peak plasma concentrations are reached after 90 minutes. It has a modest volume of distribution and does not readily cross the blood–brain barrier. Baclofen is primarily cleared from the circulation in unmodified form in the urine; about 15% of the drug is metabolized by the liver and then excreted in bile. The elimination half-time is about 5 hours in patients with normal renal function, and dosing is typically three times daily. After intrathecal injection and infusion, spasmolytic effects are observed at 1 hour and peak effects are observed at 4 hours.

Adverse effects of baclofen include sedation, somnolence, and ataxia. These are worsened when baclofen is taken with other sedative drugs. Reductions in renal function may precipitate toxicity as drug levels rise. Baclofen overdose can produce blurry vision, hypotension, cardiac and respiratory depression, and coma.

Tolerance apparently does not develop to oral baclofen. In contrast, dosing requirements after initiation of intrathecal baclofen often increase over the first 1 to 2 years. Withdrawal from baclofen therapy, especially from intrathecal infusion, can precipitate acute hyperspasticity, rhabdomyolysis, pruritus, delirium, and fever. Withdrawal has also led to multiorgan failure, coagulation abnormalities, shock, and death. If withdrawal symptoms persist, effective treatments reportedly include benzodiazepines, propofol, intrathecal opioid administration, and restarting baclofen.

Nonprescription Uses of Drugs That Alter GABA Physiology

Ethanol

Ethanol acts as an anxiolytic and sedative by causing CNS depression, but it is not without significant potential toxicity. Ethanol appears to exert its effects by acting on multiple targets, including $GABA_A$ and glutamate receptors. Ethanol increases $GABA_A$-mediated Cl^- influx and inhibits the excitatory effects of glutamate at NMDA receptors. Ethanol interacts synergistically with other sedatives, hypnotics, antidepressants, anxiolytics, anticonvulsants, and opioids.

Ethanol tolerance and dependence are associated with changes in $GABA_A$ receptor function. In animal models, chronic ethanol administration blunts the ethanol-mediated potentiation of GABA-induced Cl^- influx in the cerebral cortex and cerebellum. Acute tolerance to ethanol occurs without a change in the number of $GABA_A$ receptors, but chronic ethanol exposure alters $GABA_A$ receptor subunit expression in the cortex and cerebellum. Changes in the subunit composition of $GABA_A$ receptors may be responsible for the changes in receptor function associated with chronic ethanol use.

Other mechanisms proposed for the development of tolerance to ethanol include post-translational modifications of $GABA_A$ receptors and changes in second messenger systems, for example, alterations in the expression patterns of different isoforms of protein kinase C (PKC). The upregulation of NMDA receptor expression that occurs with prolonged ethanol use may account for the hyperexcitability associated with ethanol withdrawal.

Benzodiazepines, such as **diazepam** and **chlordiazepoxide**, reduce the tremors, agitation, and other effects of acute alcohol withdrawal. Use of these medications in a patient experiencing withdrawal from chronic alcohol abuse can also prevent the development of withdrawal seizures (delirium tremens).

Chloral Hydrate, γ-Hydroxybutyric Acid, and Flunitrazepam

Chloral hydrate is an older sedative–hypnotic rarely used today to alleviate insomnia. It has occasionally been employed to incapacitate individuals against their will, for example, to facilitate the commission of a crime. **Gamma (γ)-hydroxybutyric acid** (GHB) is a GABA isomer that has clinical utility as a sedative and treatment for narcolepsy but finds much wider illicit use as a recreational drug and "date rape" drug. There is recent evidence that GHB acts in part by activating $GABA_B$ receptors, but it is also an endogenous molecule that may act as a neurotransmitter at other receptors that have not been identified. Like barbiturates, high doses of GHB can produce deep sedation and coma, and its effects are exacerbated by ethanol. **Flunitrazepam** (Rohypnol®) is a fast-acting benzodiazepine that can cause amnesia and thereby prevent an individual's recall of events that occurred under the drug's influence. This drug has also been reported to facilitate "date rape."

▌PHYSIOLOGY OF GLUTAMATERGIC NEUROTRANSMISSION

Glutamatergic synapses exist throughout the CNS. The binding of glutamate to its receptors initiates excitatory neuronal responses associated with motor neuron activation, acute sensory responses including the development of elevated pain sensation (hyperalgesia), synaptic changes involved in certain types of memory formation, and cerebral neurotoxicity from brain ischemia as well as functional deficits from spinal cord injury. Although the clinical applications of glutamate pharmacology are currently limited, it is anticipated that glutamate pharmacology will become an increasingly important area of neuropharmacology.

Glutamate Metabolism

Glutamate synthesis occurs via two distinct pathways. In one pathway, α-ketoglutarate formed in the Krebs cycle is transaminated to glutamate in CNS nerve terminals, a step that is directly linked to GABA conversion (Fig. 13-2A). Alternatively, glutamine produced and secreted by glial cells is transported into nerve terminals and converted to glutamate by **glutaminase** (Fig. 13-2B).

Glutamate is released via calcium-dependent exocytosis of transmitter-containing vesicles. Glutamate is removed from the synaptic cleft by glutamate reuptake transporters located on presynaptic nerve terminals and on the plasma membrane of glial cells. These transporters are Na^+-dependent and have a high affinity for glutamate. In glial cells, the enzyme **glutamine synthetase** converts glutamate to glutamine, which is recycled into adjacent nerve terminals for conversion back to glutamate. Glutamine generated in glial cells can also enter the Krebs cycle and undergo oxidation; the resulting α-ketoglutarate enters neurons to replenish the α-ketoglutarate consumed during glutamate synthesis (Fig. 13-2B).

Glutamate Receptors and Transporters

As with GABA receptors, glutamate receptors are divided into **ionotropic** and **metabotropic** subgroups.

Ionotropic Glutamate Receptors

Ionotropic glutamate receptors mediate fast excitatory synaptic responses. These receptors are multisubunit, cation-selective channels that, on activation, permit the flow of Na^+, K^+, and, in some channels, Ca^{2+} ions across plasma membranes. Ionotropic glutamate receptors are thought to be tetramers composed of different subunits, with each subunit containing helical domains that span the membrane three times, in addition to a short sequence that forms the channel's pore when the entire tetramer is assembled (Fig. 13-8A).

There are three main subtypes of glutamate-gated ion channels, classified according to their activation by the selective agonists **AMPA**, **kainate**, and **NMDA**. The diversity of ionotropic receptors arises from differences in amino acid sequence because of alternative mRNA splicing and post-transcriptional mRNA editing and from the use of different combinations of subunits to form the receptors (Table 13-5).

AMPA (α-amino-3-hydroxy-5-methyl-4-isoxazole propionic acid) **receptors** are located throughout the CNS, particularly in the hippocampus and cerebral cortex. Four AMPA receptor subunits (GluR1–GluR4) have been identified (Table 13-5). AMPA receptor activation results primarily in Na^+ influx (as well as some K^+ efflux), allowing these receptors to regulate fast, excitatory postsynaptic depolarization at glutamatergic synapses (Fig. 13-8B). Although most AMPA receptors in the CNS have low Ca^{2+} permeability, the absence of certain subunits (such as GluR2) in the receptor complex increases the Ca^{2+} permeability of the channel. Calcium entry through AMPA receptors may play a role in long-term changes in neuronal phenotype and in neuronal damage associated with stroke.

Kainate receptors are expressed throughout the CNS, particularly in the hippocampus and cerebellum. Five kainate receptor subunits have been identified (Table 13-5). Like AMPA receptors, kainate receptors allow Na^+ influx and K^+ efflux through channels that possess rapid activation and deactivation kinetics. The combination of subunits in the

TABLE 13-5 Classification of Ionotropic Glutamate Receptor Subtypes

IONOTROPIC GLUTAMATE RECEPTOR SUBTYPE	SUBUNITS	AGONISTS	ACTIONS
AMPA	GluR1 GluR2 GluR3 GluR4	Glutamate or AMPA	Increase Na^+ and Ca^{2+} influx, increase K^+ efflux; note that receptors with GluR2 have ion channels with low Ca^{2+} permeability
Kainate	GluR5 GluR6 GluR7 KA1 KA2	Glutamate or kainate	Increase Na^+ influx, increase K^+ efflux
NMDA	NR1 NR2A NR2B NR2C NR2D	Glutamate or NMDA and glycine and membrane depolarization	Increase Ca^{2+} influx, increase K^+ efflux

kainate receptor complex determines whether the channel is also permeable to Ca^{2+}. Experiments using receptor-selective agents have allowed the assignment of specific functions to kainate receptors in different regions of the CNS.

NMDA (N-methyl-D-aspartate) **receptors** are expressed primarily in the hippocampus, cerebral cortex, and spinal cord. These receptors consist of multisubunit oligomeric transmembrane complexes. NMDA receptor activation, which requires simultaneous binding of glutamate and glycine, opens a channel that allows K^+ efflux as well as Na^+ and Ca^{2+} influx (Fig. 13-8B). In NMDA receptors that are occupied by glutamate and glycine, Mg^{2+} ions block the channel pore in the resting membrane (Fig. 13-8B). Depolarization of the membrane concurrent with agonist binding is required to relieve this voltage-dependent Mg^{2+} block. Either trains of postsynaptic action potentials or activation of AMPA/kainate receptors in adjacent regions of the membrane can cause postsynaptic membrane depolarization that unblocks the Mg^{2+}-bound NMDA receptor. Therefore, NMDA receptors differ from the other ionotropic glutamate receptors in two important respects—they require the binding of multiple

ligands for channel activation, and their gating depends on more intense presynaptic activity than that required to open AMPA or kainate receptors.

Metabotropic Glutamate Receptors
Metabotropic glutamate receptors (mGluR) consist of a seven-transmembrane-spanning domain protein that is coupled via G proteins to various effector mechanisms (Fig. 13-9). At least eight subtypes of metabotropic glutamate receptors exist; each belongs to one of three groups (groups I, II, and III) according to its sequence homology, signal transduction mechanism, and pharmacology (Table 13-6).

Group I receptors cause neuronal excitation either through phospholipase C (PLC) activation and IP$_3$-mediated release of intracellular Ca^{2+} or through activation of adenylyl cyclase and cAMP generation. (The difference arises from the coupling of different G proteins to the receptors.) Groups II and III receptors inhibit adenylyl cyclase and decrease cAMP production (Table 13-6). These second messenger pathways subsequently regulate ion fluxes of other channels. For example, metabotropic glutamate receptor activation in the

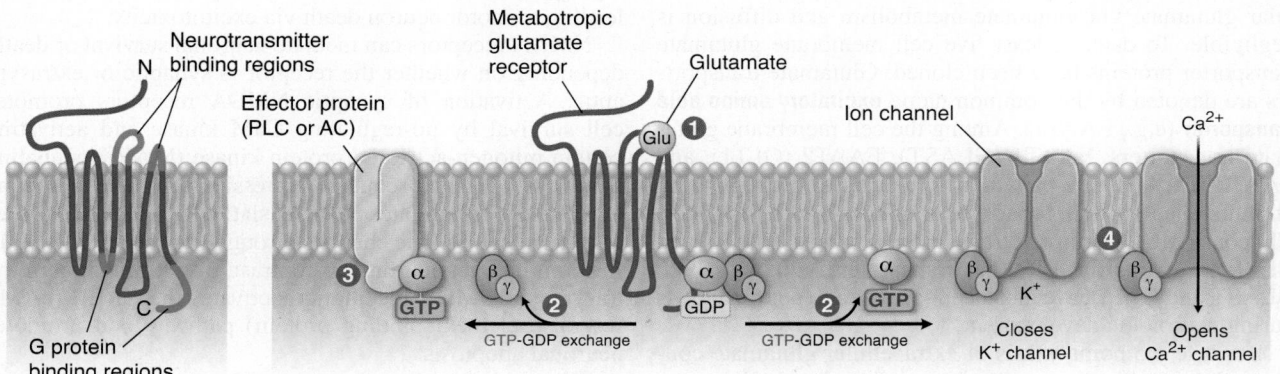

FIGURE 13-9. Schematic representation and downstream signaling of metabotropic glutamate receptors. Left panel: Metabotropic glutamate receptors are seven-transmembrane-spanning proteins with an extracellular ligand binding site and an intracellular G protein binding site. **Right panel: 1-2.** Ligand binding to the metabotropic glutamate receptor results in GTP association with the α subunit of the G protein. The GTP-associated α subunit then dissociates from the β-γ dimer. **3.** G$_α$ and G$_{βγ}$ can then activate effector proteins such as adenylyl cyclase (AC) and phospholipase C (PLC). **4.** G$_{βγ}$ subunits can also open or close ion channels directly.

TABLE 13-6 Metabotropic Glutamate Receptor (mGluR) Subtypes and Their Actions

GROUP	SUBTYPE	ACTIONS
I	mGluR1 mGluR5	Activates adenylyl cyclase → increases cAMP (mGluR1 only) Increases PLC activity → PIP_2 hydrolysis → increases IP_3 and DAG → increases Ca^{2+} levels, stimulates PKC Inhibits K^+ channels
II	mGluR2 mGluR3	Inhibits adenylyl cyclase → decreases cAMP Inhibits voltage-sensitive Ca^{2+} channels Activates K^+ channels
III	mGluR4 mGluR6 mGluR7 mGluR8	Inhibits adenylyl cyclase → decreases cAMP Inhibits voltage-sensitive Ca^{2+} channels

Group I mGluRs activate adenylyl cyclase and phospholipase C (PLC), while group II and group III mGluRs inhibit adenylyl cyclase. The downstream effects of mGluRs on ion channels are complex and varied. Some of the main actions on ion channels are listed. Note that the actions of group I receptors are generally excitatory, while those of groups II and III receptors are generally inhibitory.

hippocampus, neocortex, and cerebellum increases neuronal firing rates by inhibiting a hyperpolarizing K^+ current. Presynaptic mGluRs, such as group II and III receptors in the hippocampus, can function as inhibitory autoreceptors that inhibit presynaptic Ca^{2+} channels and thereby limit presynaptic release of glutamate. (There are also presynaptic ionotropic *cholinergic* receptors in the CNS that act to modulate the release of glutamate.)

Glutamate Transporters

Maintenance of a physiologic range of extracellular glutamate concentration is necessary to prevent glutamate overexcitation and neurotoxicity. Regulation of extracellular glutamate is primarily carried out by an efficient, high-capacity glutamate transporter system, because clearance of extracellular glutamate via glutamate metabolism and diffusion is negligible. To date, at least five cell membrane glutamate transporter proteins have been cloned. Glutamate transporters are denoted by the common name **excitatory amino acid transporter** (e.g., EAAT1). Among the cell membrane glutamate transporters, EAAT1 (GLAST), EAAT2 (GLT1), and EAAC3 (EAAC1) are particularly relevant to the regulation of glutamate uptake in broad CNS regions. EAAC1 is generally considered a neuronal transporter, whereas GLAST and GLT1 are primarily astroglial transporters, although both GLAST and GLT1 have also been localized to neuronal cells during neurologic development.

Because the homeostasis of extracellular glutamate concentration is critically regulated by neuronal and glial transporters, reduced glutamate transporter expression and/or function would be expected to increase extracellular glutamate concentration, with excessive subsequent activation of glutamate receptors and excitotoxicity. To date, numerous studies have shown a detrimental effect of reduced glutamate transporter expression and function on the pathogenesis of neurologic disorders including cerebral ischemia, epilepsy, spinal cord injury, amyotrophic lateral sclerosis, AIDS neuropathy, and Alzheimer's disease.

PATHOPHYSIOLOGY AND PHARMACOLOGY OF GLUTAMATERGIC NEUROTRANSMISSION

Under physiologic conditions, termination of glutamate receptor activation occurs via transmitter reuptake by presynaptic and glial transporters, transmitter diffusion out of the synaptic cleft, or receptor desensitization. As described below, increased release or decreased reuptake of glutamate in pathologic states can lead to a positive feedback cycle involving increased intracellular Ca^{2+} levels, cellular damage, and further glutamate release. Together, these processes can lead to **excitotoxicity**, defined as neuronal death caused by excessive cellular excitation.

Excitotoxicity has been implicated as a pathophysiologic mechanism in many diseases, including neurodegenerative syndromes, stroke and trauma, hyperalgesia, and epilepsy. Although the clinical applications of interrupting excitotoxicity remain limited, it is hoped that better understanding of glutamate-induced excitotoxicity will lead to the development of new approaches for treatment of these diseases.

Neurodegenerative Diseases

Elevated levels of dysregulated glutamate (i.e., excitotoxicity) have been implicated in Huntington's disease, Alzheimer's disease, and amyotrophic lateral sclerosis (ALS). In ALS, motor neurons degenerate in the ventral horn of the spinal cord, brainstem, and motor cortex, resulting in weakness and atrophy of skeletal muscles. The pathogenesis of this disease and the reasons for the selective pattern of neurodegeneration remain uncertain; mechanisms currently proposed for cell death in ALS include excitotoxicity and oxidative stress. The CNS areas affected in ALS express diverse populations of AMPA and NMDA receptors as well as glutamate reuptake transporters. Patients with ALS have impaired glutamate transporters in the spinal cord and motor cortex. These abnormal glutamate transporters permit the accumulation of high glutamate concentrations in the synaptic cleft, possibly leading to motor neuron death via excitotoxicity.

NMDA receptors can mediate neuronal survival or death, depending on whether the receptor is synaptic or extrasynaptic. Activation of synaptic NMDA receptors promotes cell survival by up-regulating CaM kinase and activating certain mitogen-activated protein kinase (MAPK) signaling pathways. The subsequent expression of growth factors (e.g., BDNF) modulates post-translational targets and causes long-term phenotypic changes through transcriptional modification in target neurons. In contrast, overstimulation of extrasynaptic NMDA receptors inactivates the CREB (cAMP response element binding protein) pathway and promotes neuronal apoptosis.

Riluzole is a voltage-gated sodium channel blocker that prolongs survival and decreases disease progression in ALS. Although the exact mechanism of action is uncertain, it appears that riluzole acts in part by reducing Na^+ conductance and thereby decreasing glutamate release. The drug may also directly antagonize NMDA receptors.

Excitotoxicity from excessive glutamate release has also been implicated in progression of dementia in Alzheimer's disease. **Memantine** is a noncompetitive NMDA receptor antagonist (channel blocker) used in the treatment of this disease. In clinical studies, memantine slows the rate of clinical deterioration in patients with moderate to severe Alzheimer's disease.

In Parkinson's disease, reduced dopaminergic transmission to the striatum results in the overactivation of glutamatergic synapses in the CNS. Excessive glutamatergic neurotransmission contributes to the clinical signs of Parkinson's disease, as discussed in Chapter 14, Pharmacology of Dopaminergic Neurotransmission. **Amantadine** is a noncompetitive blocker of NMDA receptor channels, similar in action to memantine. Although amantadine is not an effective treatment as a single agent, the combination of amantadine and **levodopa** reduces the severity of dyskinesia in Parkinson's disease by 60%. It is not clear, however, whether the effect of amantadine derives solely from NMDA receptor blockade.

Stroke and Trauma

In ischemic stroke, interruption of blood flow to the brain leads to deficits in oxygen supply and glucose metabolism that trigger excitotoxicity (Fig. 13-10). In hemorrhagic stroke, high concentrations of glutamate are found in blood leaking into the brain. In traumatic brain injury, the direct rupture of brain cells can release high intracellular stores of glutamate and K^+ into the restricted extracellular space.

Dysregulation of excitatory transmitters such as glutamate leads to widespread membrane depolarization, elevation of intracellular Na^+ and Ca^{2+} concentrations, and triggering of glutamate release from adjacent neurons. Increasing glutamate levels activate Ca^{2+}-permeable NMDA and AMPA receptor-coupled channels. Ultimately, the resultant accumulation of intracellular Ca^{2+} activates many Ca^{2+}-dependent degradation enzymes (e.g., DNAses, proteases, phosphatases, and phospholipases) that lead to neuronal cell death.

Although the highly Ca^{2+}-permeable NMDA receptor was originally viewed as the major contributor to neuronal cell death caused by Ca^{2+} overload, AMPA receptors have also been implicated. Clinical trials of NMDA and AMPA receptor antagonists in patients with stroke have not been successful to date and, in some cases, have led to schizophrenia-like effects, memory impairment, and neurotoxic reactions. Future pharmacologic research will be directed at the development and use of drugs with fewer adverse effects, such as the noncompetitive NMDA receptor antagonist **memantine** or drugs targeted to specific subunits of the NMDA or AMPA receptor complex.

Glutamate released during ischemic or traumatic brain damage can also activate metabotropic glutamate receptors. In animal models of stroke, pharmacologic antagonism of the mGluR1 receptor subtype facilitates recovery and survival of hippocampal neurons and prevents memory and motor loss caused by trauma. These findings suggest that the mGluR1 subunit may represent a potential target for pharmacologic intervention (Figs. 13-10 and 13-11).

Epilepsy

Seizures can result from overstimulation of glutamatergic pathways, beginning with overactivation of AMPA receptors and progressing to overactivation of NMDA receptors. In animal models, inhibition of AMPA receptor activation prevents seizure onset, whereas NMDA receptor antagonists decrease seizure intensity and duration. **Lamotrigine**, a drug used in the treatment of refractory focal seizures (see Chapter 16), stabilizes the inactivated state of the voltage-gated Na^+ channel and thereby reduces membrane excitability, the number of action potentials in a burst, glutamate release, and glutamate receptor activation. **Felbamate** is another antiepileptic that has a variety of actions, including the inhibition of NMDA receptors. Because of associated aplastic anemia and hepatotoxicity, its use is restricted to patients with refractory seizures.

Hyperalgesia

Hyperalgesia is the increased perception of pain, often in response to stimuli that, under normal conditions, cause little or no pain. Hyperalgesia can occur in the presence of peripheral nerve injury, inflammation, surgery, and diseases such as diabetes. Although hyperalgesia is reversed in most cases when the underlying pathophysiology has resolved, it may persist even in the absence of an identified organic source, leading to chronic pain that is physically crippling and psychologically debilitating.

Evidence is accumulating that glutamatergic transmission contributes to the development and/or maintenance of hyperalgesia. NMDA receptors enhance synaptic transmission

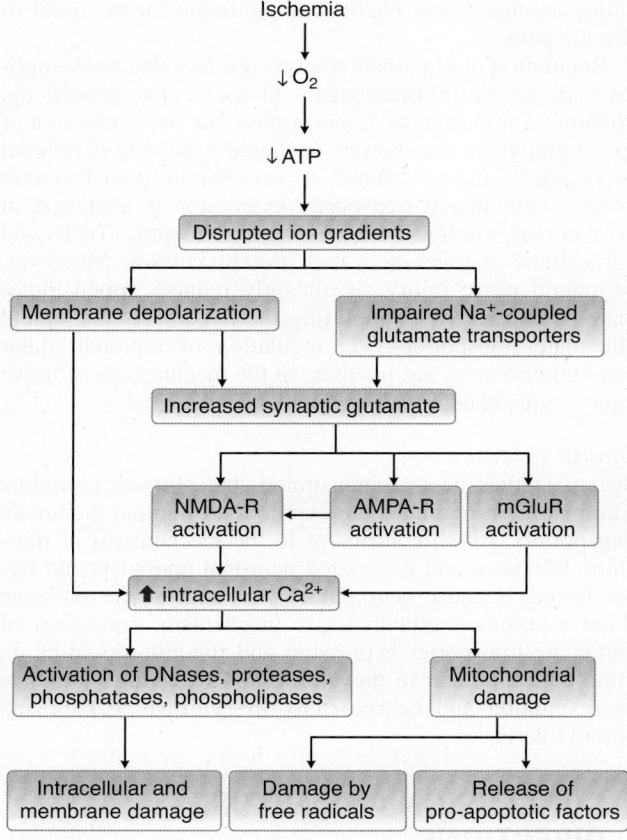

FIGURE 13-10. Role of glutamate receptors in excitotoxicity. A multiplicity of damaging cellular processes occur as a consequence of the decreased ATP levels that result from impaired oxidative metabolism or from the oxidative damage caused by activated neutrophils that invade an ischemic region; only glutamate-mediated processes are depicted here.

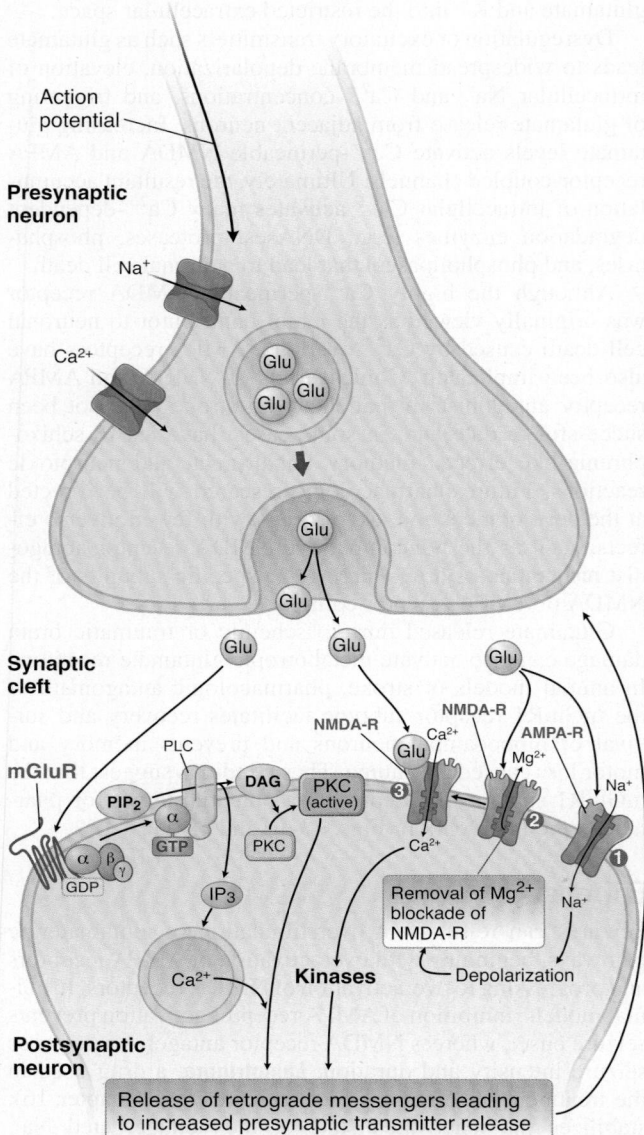

FIGURE 13-11. Interactions among metabotropic, AMPA, and NMDA classes of glutamate receptors. Action potentials depolarize the plasma membrane of presynaptic neurons, leading to opening of voltage-gated Ca^{2+} channels and ultimately to glutamate release into the synaptic cleft. Studies have proposed a "tonic" physiologic role for activation of the metabotropic glutamate receptor (mGluR) during low-frequency stimulation of postsynaptic neurons by glutamate. In contrast, high-frequency presynaptic stimulation "phasically" activates AMPA receptors (*1*) and thereby induces the prolonged membrane depolarization required to relieve the Mg^{2+} blockade of NMDA receptors (*2*). Calcium entering the cell via activated, Mg^{2+}-free NMDA receptors (*3*) is then able to activate downstream kinases independently of the mGluR. Kinases associated with the postsynaptic densities, which act to scaffold the ionotropic receptors to the membrane, phosphorylate AMPA receptor subunits and thereby cause a change in that receptor's composition (*not shown*). AMPA-R, AMPA receptor; DAG, diacylglycerol; IP_3, inositol-1,4,5-trisphosphate; mGluR, metabotropic glutamate receptor; PIP_2, phosphatidylinositol-4,5-bisphosphate; PKC, protein kinase C; PLC, phospholipase C.

between nociceptive afferent fibers and neurons in the dorsal horn of the spinal cord. As discussed in Chapter 18, Pharmacology of Analgesia, experimental hyperalgesia often involves a phenomenon called **central sensitization**, in which repeated nociceptive stimuli in the periphery lead to progressively increasing excitatory postsynaptic responses in postsynaptic pain neurons in the superficial dorsal horn. One mechanism by which this synaptic potentiation occurs involves postsynaptic NMDA receptors that, when stimulated chronically, increase the strength of excitatory connections between presynaptic and postsynaptic neurons in spinal pain circuits. In turn, the Ca^{2+} influx through activated NMDA receptors acts on special localized kinases to effect a phosphorylation-induced switch of the subunits of the AMPA receptor, allowing more Ca^{2+} to enter through AMPA receptors. Increased intracellular Ca^{2+} also activates Ca^{2+}-sensitive transcription factors, such as CREB, and induces changes in protein synthesis via ribosomes located right at the synaptic terminals.

Experimental NMDA receptor antagonists can both prevent and reverse central sensitization in patients. Many of these antagonists, however, also inhibit a wide range of fast excitatory synaptic pathways in the CNS. For this reason, current NMDA receptor drug development focuses on intraspinal or extradural administration of NMDA receptor antagonists to limit the effects of the drug to the dorsal horn of the spinal cord. The high density of kainate receptors in sensory neurons may also modulate transmitter release, providing another future pharmacologic target for the relief of chronic pain.

Regulation of glutamate transporters has also been implicated in the central mechanisms of nociceptive processing. Preclinical studies have demonstrated that the expression of spinal glutamate transporters is altered following peripheral nerve injury and contributes to neuropathic pain behavior in rats. This altered transporter expression is mediated, at least in part, through a tyrosine kinase receptor (TrkB) and intracellular mitogen-activated protein kinases. Moreover, peripheral nerve injury significantly reduces spinal glutamate uptake activity, supporting the hypothesis that spinal glutamate transporters, via regulation of regional glutamate homeostasis, are involved in the mechanisms of nerve injury-induced neuropathic pain behaviors.

Opioid Tolerance

Recent studies have demonstrated that chronic morphine administration regulates the expression of spinal glutamate transporters, which contributes to the mechanisms of morphine tolerance and associated neuronal apoptosis and hyperalgesia. Because neuropathic pain and opioid tolerance share a common glutamatergic mechanism, regulation of glutamate transporter expression and function could be an important approach to preventing and reversing glutamate overexcitation and neurotoxicity in neuropathic pain and opioid tolerance.

■ CONCLUSION AND FUTURE DIRECTIONS

GABA and glutamate represent the major inhibitory and excitatory neurotransmitters in the CNS, respectively. Most drugs that act on GABAergic neurotransmission enhance GABAergic activity and thereby depress CNS functions.

Modulation of GABAergic transmission can occur either presynaptically or postsynaptically. Drugs acting at presynaptic sites primarily target GABA synthesis, degradation, and reuptake. Drugs acting postsynaptically affect GABA receptors directly, either by occupying the GABA binding site or by an allosteric mechanism. Each of the three main GABA receptor types has a distinct pharmacology. The GABA$_A$ receptor is targeted by the largest number of drugs, including GABA binding-site agonists, benzodiazepines, barbiturates, general anesthetics, and neuroactive steroids. GABA$_B$ receptors are currently targeted by only a few therapeutic agents, which are used to treat spasticity. GABA$_B$ receptors have recently been found to influence pain, cognition, and addictive behavior, and interest is growing in drugs that modulate these receptors. GABA$_C$ receptors have not yet been developed as a target of pharmacologic agents.

To improve safety and reduce adverse effects, including ataxia, tolerance, and physical dependence, development of new anxiolytics and sedatives has aimed for low-efficacy compounds (e.g., benzodiazepines) as well as compounds with selective activity at GABA$_A$ receptor subtypes. Animal models with selectively mutated GABA$_A$ receptor subunits have revealed that sedation/hypnosis is produced by enhancing the activity of receptors containing $\alpha1$ subunits. In contrast, anxiolysis is produced by modulation of $\alpha2$- or $\alpha3$-containing receptors, and amnesia is associated with $\alpha5$-containing receptors. There is also evidence for distinct pharmacology and physiology of synaptic GABA$_A$ receptors containing different β subunits.

Because of the potential role of excitatory neurotransmission in a number of pathologic processes, such as neurodegenerative diseases, stroke, trauma, hyperalgesia, and epilepsy, glutamate receptors have become important targets for drug development. The diversity of glutamate receptors and receptor subunits constitutes a potential advantage for the development of glutamate receptor antagonists that are selective for a particular receptor subtype. In the future, highly selective antagonists for glutamate receptor subtypes could potentially protect the CNS in stroke, prevent hyperalgesia after tissue trauma, and treat epileptic seizures.

Although neurotransmitter receptors comprise the traditional targets for drug development, recent experimental studies suggest that targeting scaffolding proteins may also be a promising area for treatment of stroke and other diseases. Postsynaptic cytoskeletal proteins such as postsynaptic density protein-95 (PSD-95) comprise an important part of the dendrite scaffolding structure, and PSD-95 mediates the intracellular signaling that occurs after glutamate receptor activation. In the context of excitotoxicity, PSD-95 can amplify the initial NMDA signal into deleterious cascades of nitric oxide generation. Blockade of PSD-95 reduces ischemic brain injury after experimental stroke in rats.

A clinical trial testing this approach as a therapy for ischemic stroke is now ongoing.

Emerging opportunities also exist for regulation of glutamate transporter expression and activity. This approach may minimize the pathologic impact of glutamate overload while retaining the physiologic role of glutamate. Current research is exploring the cellular and molecular mechanisms of transporter expression and function in relation to the pathogenesis of neuropathic pain, opioid-related problems, and other neurologic disorders. In addition, studies on the role of glutamate transporter regulation in opioid tolerance and dependence may provide new insights into the cellular mechanisms of substance abuse.

Acknowledgment

We thank Gary R. Strichartz for his valuable contributions to this chapter in the First, Second, and Third Editions of *Principles of Pharmacology: The Pathophysiologic Basis of Drug Therapy.*

Suggested Reading

Aarts M, Liu Y, Liu L, et al. Treatment of ischemic brain damage by perturbing NMDA receptor-PSD-95 protein interactions. *Science* 2002; 298:846–850. (*Scaffolding proteins as therapeutic targets for glutamate excitotoxicity and neuropathic pain.*)

Besancon E, Guo S, Lok J, Tymianski M, Lo EH. Beyond NMDA and AMPA glutamate receptors: emerging mechanisms for ionic imbalance and cell death in stroke. *Trends Pharmacol Sci* 2008;29:268–275. (*This review expands on traditional concepts of excitotoxicity to include newly discovered mechanisms of cell death.*)

Foster AC, Kemp JA. Glutamate- and GABA-based CNS therapeutics. *Curr Opin Pharmacol* 2006;6:7–17. (*General overview of pharmacologic strategies in GABAergic and glutamatergic neurotransmission.*)

Herd MD, Belelli D, Lambert JJ. Neurosteroid modulation of synaptic and extrasynaptic GABA$_A$ receptors. *Pharmacol Ther* 2007;116:20–34. (*Reviews physiology of neurosteroids and their interactions with GABA$_A$ receptors.*)

Lo EH, Dalkara T, Moskowitz MA. Mechanisms, challenges and opportunities in stroke. *Nat Rev Neurosci* 2003;4:399–415. (*Advances in pathophysiology of excitotoxicity in stroke.*)

Mizuta K, Xu D, Pan Y, et al. GABA$_A$ receptors are expressed and facilitate relaxation in airway smooth muscle. *Am J Physiol Lung Cell Mol Physiol* 2008;294:L1206–L1216. (*Points to a role for GABA$_A$ receptors in airway tone.*)

Olsen RW, Sieghart W. GABA$_A$ receptors: subtypes provide diversity of function and pharmacology. *Neuropharmacology* 2008;56:141–148. (*Reviews different GABA$_A$ receptor subtypes and their physiologic and pharmacologic roles.*)

Rudolph U, Knoflach F. Beyond classical benzodiazepines: novel therapeutic potential of GABA$_A$ receptor subtypes. *Nat Rev Drug Discov* 2011;10:685–697. (*Reviews evidence that different GABA$_A$ receptor subtypes mediate different benzodiazepine effects.*)

Werner FM, Coveñas R. Classical neurotransmitters and neuropeptides involved in generalized epilepsy: a focus on antiepileptic drugs. *Curr Med Chem* 2011;18:4933–4948. (*Discusses the linked roles of GABA and glutamate and their receptors in epilepsy.*)

DRUG SUMMARY TABLE: CHAPTER 13 Pharmacology of GABAergic and Glutamatergic Neurotransmission

DRUG	CLINICAL APPLICATIONS	SERIOUS AND COMMON ADVERSE EFFECTS	CONTRAINDICATIONS	THERAPEUTIC CONSIDERATIONS
INHIBITORS OF GABA METABOLISM AND TRANSPORT Mechanism—Inhibit GAT-1 (tiagabine) or GABA transaminase (vigabatrin)				
Tiagabine	Focal and tonic–clonic seizures (adjunctive therapy)	*Unexplained sudden death, Stevens-Johnson syndrome, seizure, suicidal thoughts* Confusion, sedation, dizziness, depression, psychosis, tremor, gastrointestinal irritation	None known	Enhances GABA activity by blocking GABA reuptake into presynaptic neurons. Tiagabine potentiates the action of GABA$_A$ receptor modulators such as ethanol, benzodiazepines, and barbiturates.
Vigabatrin	Focal and tonic–clonic seizures (adjunctive therapy) Infantile spasms	*Liver failure, visual field defect, psychotic disorder, suicidal thoughts* Somnolence, tremor	None known	Blocks conversion of GABA to succinic semialdehyde, resulting in high intracellular GABA concentrations and increased synaptic GABA release. Transfer across the blood–brain barrier is slow, and the drug is cleared mainly by renal excretion with a half-life of 5–6 hours.
GABA$_A$ RECEPTOR AGONISTS AND ANTAGONISTS Mechanism—Directly activate GABA$_A$ receptor (muscimol), competitive antagonist at GABA$_A$ receptor (bicuculline, gabazine), noncompetitive antagonist at GABA$_A$ receptor (picrotoxin)				
Muscimol	None (used experimentally only)	Not applicable	Not applicable	Derived from hallucinogenic *Amanita muscaria* mushrooms.
Bicuculline Gabazine Picrotoxin	None (used experimentally only)	Not applicable	Not applicable	Induce seizures.
GABA$_A$ RECEPTOR MODULATORS: BENZODIAZEPINES Mechanism—Allosteric modulators of the GABA$_A$ receptor that act to increase the frequency of receptor opening and potentiate effects of GABA (all except flumazenil); benzodiazepine antagonist (flumazenil)				
Short Acting: Clorazepate Midazolam Triazolam Zolpidem ***Intermediate Acting:*** Alprazolam Estazolam Lorazepam Temazepam	Alcohol withdrawal syndrome (clorazepate, chlordiazepoxide, and diazepam only) Anxiety (clorazepate, midazolam, alprazolam, lorazepam, chlordiazepoxide, clobazam, and diazepam only) Insomnia (triazolam, zolpidem, estazolam, lorazepam, temazepam, flurazepam, and quazepam only)	*Cardiac arrest, agitation, respiratory arrest (midazolam only); hepatotoxicity (triazolam, alprazolam, and zolpidem only); Stevens-Johnson syndrome (alprazolam and clobazam only); toxic epidermal necrolysis (clobazam only); delirium, depression (lorazepam only); drug dependence (temazepam, alprazolam, and flurazepam only); neutropenia (diazepam only); respiratory depression (diazepam and flurazepam only)*	Shared contraindication: Hypersensitivity to drug Clorazepate, midazolam, lorazepam, clonazepam, diazepam, and alprazolam only: Glaucoma Midazolam and triazolam only: Concomitant use with HIV protease inhibitors Triazolam and alprazolam only: Concomitant use with itraconazole, ketoconazole, nefazodone	Metabolized by CYP3A4 and excreted in the urine as glucuronides or oxidized metabolites. Benzodiazepine levels are decreased by carbamazepine or phenobarbital. Patients with impaired hepatic function, including the elderly and the very young, may experience prolonged effects from benzodiazepine administration.

Drug	Therapeutic Indications	Adverse Effects	Contraindications	Therapeutic Considerations

Long Acting:
Chlordiazepoxide
Clobazam
Clonazepam
Diazepam
Flurazepam
Quazepam
	Sedation (midazolam and diazepam only)
	Seizure disorders (clorazepate, lorazepam, clonazepam, and diazepam only)
	Lennox-Gastaut syndrome (clobazam only)
	Premedication for anesthetic procedure (lorazepam)
	Panic disorder (alprazolam and clonazepam only)
	Muscle spasm (diazepam only)
		Excessive somnolence (shared adverse reaction); dizziness (zolpidem, alprazolam, and estazolam only); cognitive dysfunction (alprazolam and chlordiazepoxide only); headache (zolpidem only); dysarthria (alprazolam only); hypotension (temazepam and diazepam only); edema, ataxia, irregular periods (chlordiazepoxide only); muscle weakness (diazepam only); taste disorder, blurred vision (flurazepam only); gastrointestinal upset (chlordiazepoxide, alprazolam, and quazepam only)	Triazolam, estazolam, temazepam, and flurazepam only:
			  Pregnancy
			Lorazepam only:
			  Intra-arterial administration
			  Respiratory insufficiency
			Lorazepam, quazepam, and diazepam only:
			  Sleep apnea syndrome
			Clonazepam and diazepam only:
			  Significant liver disease
			Diazepam only:
			  Myasthenia gravis
			  Pediatric patients less than 6 months of age
				Zolpidem is not technically a benzodiazepine but binds to the same site on GABA$_A$ receptors as benzodiazepines do. Clobazam is less sedating than other benzodiazepines and has fewer effects on cognition.

Flumazenil	Reversal of benzodiazepine activity	*Seizures, death* Diaphoresis, injection site pain, dizziness, headache, blurred vision, agitation	Hypersensitivity to flumazenil Patient being given a benzodiazepine for intracranial hypertension or status epilepticus Patient with serious tricyclic antidepressant overdose	In patients with benzodiazepine dependence, flumazenil can induce a severe withdrawal syndrome.

GABA$_A$ RECEPTOR MODULATORS: BARBITURATES
Mechanism—Potentiate GABA activity at GABA$_A$ receptors. At high concentrations, act as direct agonists at GABA$_A$ receptors; may also antagonize AMPA receptor

Drug	Therapeutic Indications	Adverse Effects	Contraindications	Therapeutic Considerations

Methohexital
Pentobarbital
Thiopental
Secobarbital
Amobarbital
	Induction and maintenance of anesthesia (shared indication)
	Insomnia (pentobarbital, secobarbital, and amobarbital only)
	Seizure (pentobarbital, thiopental, and amobarbital only)
	Increased intracranial pressure (thiopental only)
		Cardiac arrest (methohexital and thiopental only); respiratory depression (methohexital, amobarbital, and thiopental only); shock, thrombophlebitis, seizure (methohexital only); increased intracranial pressure (thiopental only); drug dependence (secobarbital only)
		Injection site reaction (methohexital and thiopental only); hypotension, spasmodic movement (methohexital only); confusion, dizziness, headache, somnolence (amobarbital only)
			Shared contraindications:
			  Hypersensitivity to drug
			  Porphyria
			Secobarbital and amobarbital only:
			  Impaired liver function
			  Respiratory disease
				Lipid-soluble barbiturates that enter the brain rapidly after intravenous administration and then redistribute to less highly perfused tissues.
				Chronic use of CYP3A4 inducers such as phenytoin and rifampin enhances barbiturate metabolism; conversely, CYP3A4 inhibitors such as ketoconazole, erythromycin, cimetidine, and certain SSRIs may reduce barbiturate metabolism and thereby increase sedative effects.

continues

DRUG SUMMARY TABLE: CHAPTER 13 Pharmacology of GABAergic and Glutamatergic Neurotransmission *continued*

DRUG	CLINICAL APPLICATIONS	*SERIOUS* AND COMMON ADVERSE EFFECTS	CONTRAINDICATIONS	THERAPEUTIC CONSIDERATIONS
Phenobarbital	Refractory epilepsy, especially focal and tonic–clonic seizures Sedation	*Erythroderma, barbiturate withdrawal*	Hypersensitivity to barbiturates Porphyria Concomitant use with rilpivirine Impaired liver function Respiratory disease	Phenobarbital is one of the few barbiturates that undergoes both renal and hepatic clearance. Approximately 25% of a phenobarbital dose is cleared as the unchanged drug in the urine, while the liver metabolizes the remaining 75%.
OTHER GABA_A RECEPTOR MODULATORS Mechanism—Modulation of ligand-gated ion channels (most likely)				
Etomidate	Induction and maintenance of anesthesia	*Hypotension* Injection site pain, nausea, vomiting	Hypersensitivity to etomidate	Causes minimal cardiopulmonary depression, possibly due to lack of effect on the sympathetic nervous system
Propofol	Induction and maintenance of anesthesia Sedation of mechanically ventilated patients	*Cardiovascular and respiratory depression, hypertension, pancreatitis, seizure, acute renal failure, priapism, bacterial septicemia* Injection site reaction	Hypersensitivity to propofol	Useful especially in short day-surgery procedures because of its rapid elimination Tolerance to propofol has been reported in pediatric patients receiving frequent (daily) anesthetics for radiation therapy, possibly due to increased clearance rather than reduced sensitivity at the GABA_A receptor.
Alphaxalone	None (used experimentally only)	Not applicable	Porphyria	Alphaxalone is a neuroactive steroid but is rarely used clinically.
GABA_B RECEPTOR AGONIST Mechanism—Activates metabotropic GABA_B receptor				
Baclofen	Spasticity	*Gastrointestinal hemorrhage, aseptic meningitis, coma, seizure, pneumonia, drug withdrawal* Poor muscle tone, asthenia, dizziness, somnolence	Hypersensitivity to baclofen	Clearance is primarily renal in an unmodified form; about 15% of the drug is metabolized by the liver and excreted in bile. Withdrawal from baclofen, especially intrathecal infusion, can precipitate acute hyperspasticity, rhabdomyolysis, pruritus, delirium, and fever.

NMDA RECEPTOR ANTAGONISTS AND OTHER AGENTS AFFECTING GLUTAMATERGIC NEUROTRANSMISSION

Mechanism—Antagonize NMDA receptor (riluzole, memantine, amantadine, felbamate); block voltage-gated sodium channels (riluzole, lamotrigine, felbamate)

Drug	Clinical Applications	Serious and Common Adverse Effects	Contraindications	Therapeutic Considerations
Riluzole	Amyotrophic lateral sclerosis (ALS)	*Cardiac arrest, respiratory depression* Hypertension, tachycardia, circumoral paresthesia, gastrointestinal upset, arthralgia, asthenia, dizziness, somnolence	Hypersensitivity to riluzole	Riluzole is thought both to block voltage-gated sodium channels (thereby reducing sodium conductance and decreasing glutamate release), and to directly antagonize NMDA receptors. Prolongs survival and decreases disease progression in ALS.
Memantine	Alzheimer's disease	*Stroke, seizure, acute renal failure* Constipation, dizziness, headache	Hypersensitivity to memantine	Noncompetitive NMDA receptor antagonist. Slows the rate of clinical progression of moderate to severe Alzheimer's disease.
Amantadine	Parkinson's disease Influenza A prophylaxis and infection Extrapyramidal disease	*Congestive heart failure, malignant melanoma, neuroleptic malignant syndrome, immune hypersensitivity reaction, suicidal ideation* Orthostatic hypotension, edema, insomnia, hallucinations	Hypersensitivity to amantadine	Noncompetitive NMDA receptor antagonist.
Lamotrigine	See Drug Summary Table: Chapter 16 Pharmacology of Abnormal Electrical Neurotransmission in the Central Nervous System			
Felbamate	See Drug Summary Table: Chapter 16 Pharmacology of Abnormal Electrical Neurotransmission in the Central Nervous System			

14

Pharmacology of Dopaminergic Neurotransmission

David G. Standaert and Victor W. Sung

INTRODUCTION

Dopamine (DA) is a catecholamine neurotransmitter that is the therapeutic target for a number of important central nervous system (CNS) disorders, including Parkinson's disease and schizophrenia. DA is also a precursor for the other catecholamine neurotransmitters norepinephrine and epinephrine. The machinery of catecholamine neurotransmission has a number of components that are shared among members of the class, including biosynthetic and metabolic enzymes. There are also components that are specialized for the individual members of the class, including reuptake pumps and presynaptic and postsynaptic receptors. This chapter presents the principles that underlie current therapies for diseases that directly or indirectly involve changes in dopaminergic neurotransmission. The chapter begins with a discussion of the biochemistry and cell biology of dopaminergic neurotransmission and the localization of the major DA systems in the brain. Following this background, the chapter explores the physiology, pathophysiology, and pharmacology of **Parkinson's disease**, which results from the specific loss of neurons in one of these DA systems, and **schizophrenia**, which is currently treated, in part, with drugs that inhibit dopaminergic neurotransmission.

BIOCHEMISTRY AND CELL BIOLOGY OF DOPAMINERGIC NEUROTRANSMISSION

Dopamine belongs to the **catecholamine** family of neurotransmitters. In addition to dopamine, this family includes **norepinephrine (NE)** and **epinephrine (EPI)**. As the name suggests, the basic structure of the catecholamines consists of a catechol (3,4-dihydroxybenzene) moiety connected to an amine group by an ethyl bridge (Fig. 14-1A). Recall from Chapter 9, Principles of Nervous System Physiology and Pharmacology, that catecholaminergic pathways in the brain have "single source-divergent" organization, in that they arise from small clusters of catecholamine neurons that give rise to widely divergent projections. CNS catecholamines modulate the function of point-to-point neurotransmission and affect complex processes such as mood, attentiveness, and emotion.

The neutral amino acid **tyrosine** is the precursor for all catecholamines (Fig. 14-1B). The majority of tyrosine is obtained from the diet; a small proportion may also be synthesized in the liver from **phenylalanine**. The first step in the synthesis of DA is the conversion of tyrosine to **L-DOPA** (**L-3,4-dihydroxyphenylalanine**, or **levodopa**) by oxidation of the 3 position on the benzene ring. This reaction is catalyzed by the enzyme **tyrosine hydroxylase (TH)**, a ferro

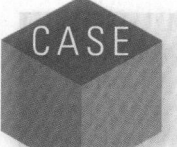

Mark S is a 55-year-old man who goes to see his physician because he notices a tremor in his right hand that has developed gradually over a number of months. He finds he can keep the hand quiet if he concentrates on it, but the shaking quickly reappears if he is distracted. His handwriting has become small and difficult to read, and he has trouble using a computer mouse. His wife complains that he never smiles anymore and that his face is becoming expressionless. She also says that he walks more slowly and he has trouble keeping up with her. As Mr. S enters the examination room, his doctor notices that he is walking hunched over and has a short, shuffling gait. The doctor finds on physical examination that Mr. S has increased tone and cogwheel rigidity in his upper extremities, particularly on the right side, and that he is significantly slower than normal at performing rapid alternating movements. The physician determines that Mr. S's symptoms and signs most likely represent the early stages of Parkinson's disease, and she prescribes a trial of levodopa.

Questions

1. How does the selective loss of dopaminergic neurons result in symptoms such as those Mr. S is experiencing?

2. What will be the effect of levodopa on the course of Mr. S's disease?

3. How will Mr. S's response to levodopa change over time?

4. Is levodopa the best choice for Mr. S at this stage of his disease?

(iron containing)-enzyme that consists of four identical subunits of approximately 60 kDa each. In addition to Fe^{2+}, TH also requires the cofactor tetrahydrobiopterin, which is oxidized to dihydrobiopterin in the course of the reaction. Importantly, oxidation of tyrosine to L-DOPA is the rate-limiting step in the production not only of DA but of all catecholamine neurotransmitters.

The next and final step in the synthesis of DA is the conversion of L-DOPA to DA by the enzyme **aromatic L-amino acid decarboxylase (AADC)**. AADC cleaves the carboxyl group from the α-carbon of the ethylamine side chain, liberating carbon dioxide. AADC requires the cofactor pyridoxal phosphate. Although AADC is sometimes referred to as "DOPA decarboxylase," it is promiscuous in its ability to cleave carboxyl groups from the α-carbons of all aromatic amino acids and is involved in the synthesis of noncatechol transmitters, such as serotonin. AADC is abundant in the brain. It is expressed by dopaminergic neurons, but it is also present in nondopaminergic cells and glia. Furthermore, AADC is expressed throughout the body in almost all cell types.

In dopaminergic neurons, the end product of the catecholamine synthetic pathway is dopamine. In cells that secrete the catecholamine NE, DA is converted to NE by the enzyme **dopamine β-hydroxylase**. In other cells, NE may subsequently be converted to epinephrine by **phenylethanolamine N-methyltransferase**. Dopaminergic neurons lack both of these enzymes, but it is important to keep in mind the entire pathway of catecholamine biosynthesis because pharmacologic manipulation of DA biosynthesis can also alter the production of NE and EPI. For a more complete discussion of the last two steps in NE and EPI synthesis, see Chapter 11, Adrenergic Pharmacology.

Dopamine Storage, Release, Reuptake, and Inactivation

DA is synthesized from tyrosine in the cytoplasm of the neuron and then transported into secretory vesicles for storage and release (Fig. 14-2). Two separate molecular pumps are required for the transport of DA into synaptic vesicles.

A proton ATPase concentrates protons in the vesicle, creating an electrochemical gradient characterized by a low intravesicular pH (i.e., a high proton concentration) and an electropositive vesicle interior. This gradient is exploited by a proton antiporter, the **vesicular monoamine transporter (VMAT)**, which allows protons to move down the gradient (out of the vesicle) while simultaneously transporting DA into the vesicle against its concentration gradient. Upon nerve cell stimulation, the DA storage vesicles fuse with the plasma membrane in a Ca^{2+}-dependent manner, releasing DA into the synaptic cleft. In the cleft, DA can bind to both postsynaptic DA receptors and presynaptic DA autoreceptors (see below).

Several mechanisms exist to remove synaptic DA and terminate the signaling produced by the neurotransmitter. Most of the DA released into the synaptic cleft is transported back into the presynaptic cell by a 12-transmembrane domain protein, the **dopamine transporter (DAT)**. DAT belongs to the family of catecholamine reuptake pumps. DA reuptake involves transport of the neurotransmitter against its concentration gradient and therefore requires an energy source. For this reason, the DAT couples dopamine reuptake to the cotransport of Na^+ down its concentration gradient into the cell. In fact, both Na^+ and Cl^- are co-transported with DA into the cell. Because the Na^+ gradient is maintained by the Na^+/K^+-ATPase pump, DA reuptake depends indirectly on the presence of a functioning Na^+/K^+ pump. DA taken up into the presynaptic cell can either be recycled into vesicles for further use in neurotransmission (by VMAT) or degraded by the action of the enzymes **monoamine oxidase (MAO)** or **catechol-O-methyltransferase (COMT)** (Fig. 14-3).

MAO is a key enzyme that functions to terminate the action of catecholamines in both the brain and the periphery. MAOs exist in two isoforms: MAO-A, which is expressed in the brain as well as the periphery, and MAO-B, which is concentrated in the CNS. Both isoforms of MAO can degrade dopamine as well as a wide range of monoamine compounds. Under normal conditions, MAO-B is responsible for catabolizing most CNS dopamine. The different roles played by the isoforms of MAO are therapeutically important. Selective inhibition of MAO-B is used to augment the function of

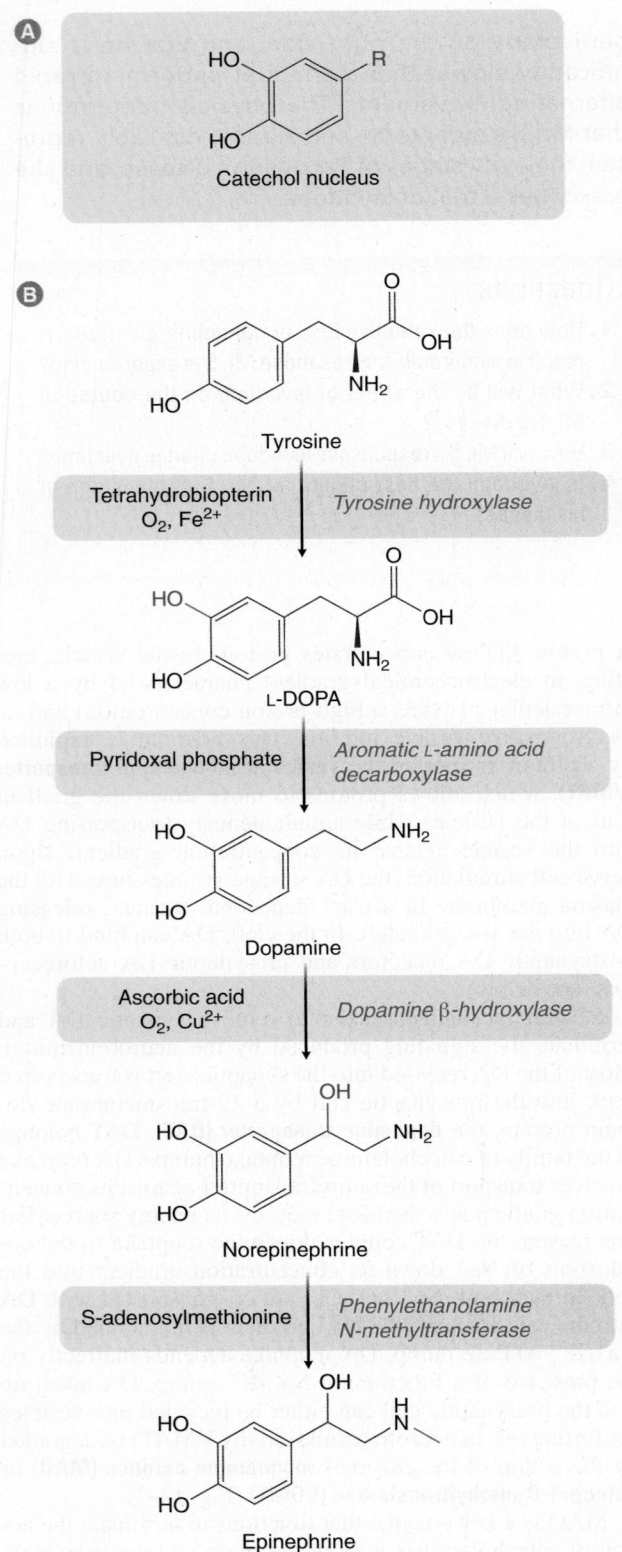

FIGURE 14-1. Catecholamine synthesis. A. Catecholamines consist of a catechol nucleus with an ethylamine side chain (R group). The R group is ethylamine in dopamine, hydroxyethylamine in norepinephrine, and N-methyl hydroxyethylamine in epinephrine. **B.** Dopamine is synthesized from the amino acid tyrosine in a series of step-wise reactions. In cells that contain dopamine β-hydroxylase, dopamine can be further converted to norepinephrine; in cells that also contain phenylethanolamine N-methyltransferase, norepinephrine can be converted to epinephrine.

CNS dopamine and generally is well tolerated. Inhibition of MAO-A, on the other hand, retards the breakdown of all central and peripheral catecholamines; as noted in Chapter 11, MAO-A inhibition may lead to life-threatening toxicity when combined with catecholamine releasers such as the indirect-acting sympathomimetic **tyramine** found in certain wines and cheeses.

Synaptic DA that is not taken up into the presynaptic cell can either diffuse out of the synaptic cleft or be degraded by the action of COMT. COMT is expressed in the brain, liver,

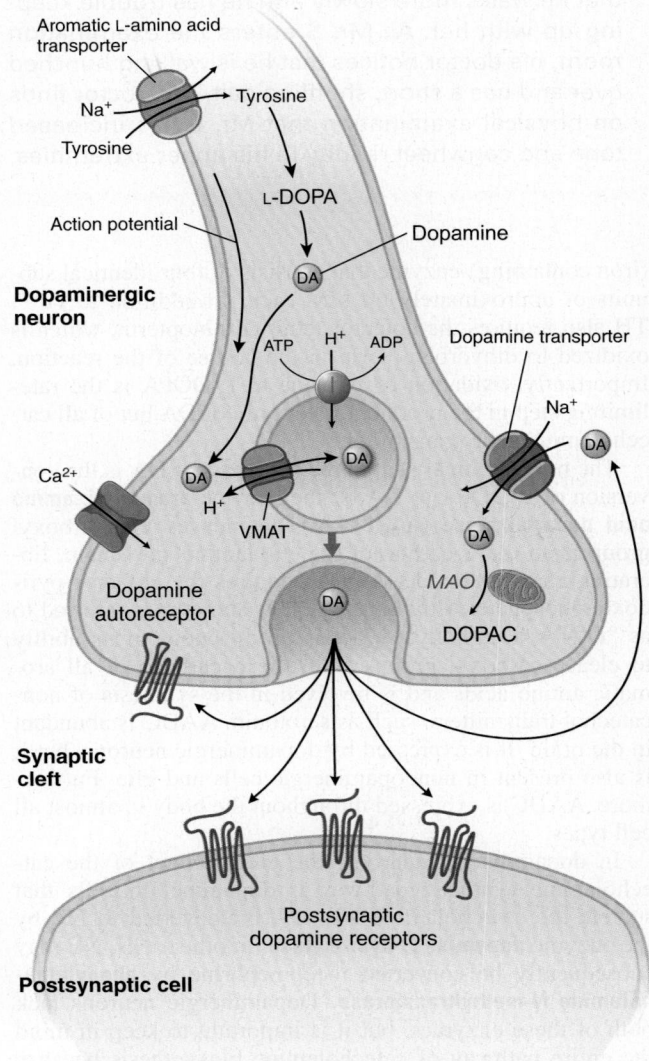

FIGURE 14-2. Dopaminergic neurotransmission. Dopamine (DA) is synthesized in the cytoplasm and transported into secretory vesicles by the action of a nonselective monoamine-proton antiporter (VMAT) that is powered by the electrochemical gradient created by a proton ATPase. Upon nerve cell stimulation, DA is released into the synaptic cleft, where the neurotransmitter can stimulate postsynaptic dopamine receptors and presynaptic dopamine autoreceptors. DA is transported out of the synaptic cleft by the selective, Na$^+$-coupled dopamine transporter (DAT). Cytoplasmic DA is retransported into secretory vesicles by VMAT or degraded by the enzyme monoamine oxidase (MAO).

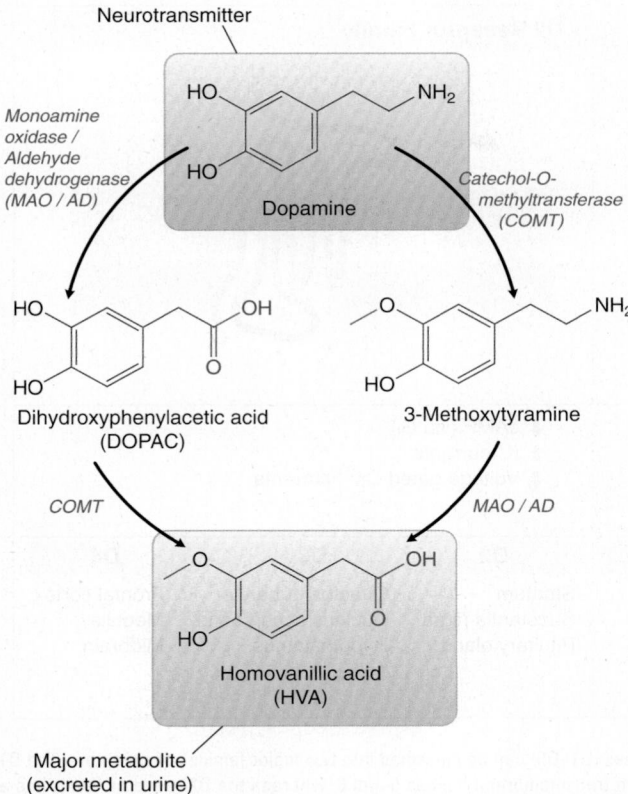

FIGURE 14-3. Catecholamine metabolism. Dopamine is metabolized to homovanillic acid (HVA) in a series of reactions. Dopamine is oxidized to dihydroxyphenylacetic acid (DOPAC) by sequential action of the enzymes monoamine oxidase (MAO) and aldehyde dehydrogenase (AD). Catechol-O-methyltransferase (COMT) then oxidizes DOPAC to HVA. Alternatively, dopamine is methylated to 3-methoxytyramine by COMT and then oxidized to HVA by MAO and AD. HVA, the most stable dopamine metabolite, is excreted in the urine.

kidney, and heart; it inactivates catecholamines by adding a methyl group to the hydroxyl group at the 3 position of the benzene ring. In the CNS, COMT is expressed primarily by neurons. The sequential action of COMT and MAO degrades DA to the stable metabolite **homovanillic acid (HVA)**, which is excreted in the urine (Fig. 14-3).

Dopamine Receptors

Dopamine receptors are members of the G protein-coupled family of receptor proteins. The properties of dopamine receptors were originally classified by their effect on the formation of cyclic AMP (cAMP): activation of D1 class receptors leads to increased cAMP, while activation of D2 class receptors inhibits cAMP generation (Fig. 14-4). Subsequent studies led to cloning of the receptor proteins, revealing five distinct receptors, each encoded by a separate gene. All known DA receptors have the typical structure of G protein-coupled receptors, with seven-transmembrane domains. The **D1** class contains two dopamine receptors (D1 and D5), while the **D2** class contains three receptors (D2, D3, and D4). There are two alternative forms of the D2 protein, D2$_S$ (i.e., short) and D2$_L$ (i.e., long), which represent alternate splice variants of the same gene; their difference lies in the third cytoplasmic loop, which affects G protein interaction but not dopamine binding.

The five different dopamine receptor proteins have distinct distributions in the brain (Fig. 14-5). Both D1 and D2 receptors are expressed at high levels in the **striatum** (caudate and putamen), where they play a role in motor control by the **basal ganglia**, as well as in the **nucleus accumbens** (see Chapter 19, Pharmacology of Drugs of Abuse) and **olfactory tubercle**. D2 receptors are also expressed at high levels on anterior pituitary gland **lactotrophs**, where they regulate prolactin secretion (see Chapter 27, Pharmacology of the Hypothalamus and Pituitary Gland). D2 receptors are thought to play a role in **schizophrenia** because many antipsychotic medications have high affinity for these receptors (see below), although the localization of the D2 receptors involved remains to be elucidated. D3 and D4 receptors are structurally and functionally related to D2 receptors and may also be involved in the pathogenesis of schizophrenia. High levels of D3 receptors are expressed in the **limbic system**, including the nucleus accumbens and olfactory tubercle, while D4 receptors have been localized to the **frontal cortex**, **diencephalon**, and brainstem. D5 receptors are distributed sparsely and expressed at low levels, mainly in the **hippocampus**, **olfactory tubercle**, and **hypothalamus**.

Regulation of cAMP formation is the defining characteristic of the dopamine receptor classes, but dopamine receptors can also affect other aspects of cellular function depending on their localization and linkage to second messenger systems. Most dopamine receptors are expressed on the surface of postsynaptic neurons at dopaminergic synapses. The density of these receptors is tightly controlled through regulated insertion and removal of dopamine receptor proteins from the postsynaptic membrane. DA receptors are also expressed presynaptically on the terminals of dopaminergic neurons. Presynaptic dopamine receptors, most of which are of the D2 class, serve as **autoreceptors**. These autoreceptors sense dopamine overflow from the synapse and reduce dopaminergic tone, both by decreasing DA synthesis in the presynaptic neuron and by reducing the rate of neuronal firing and dopamine release. Inhibition of DA synthesis occurs through cAMP-dependent downregulation of TH activity, while the inhibitory effect on DA release and neuronal firing is due, in part, to a separate mechanism involving the modulation of K^+ and Ca^{2+} channels. Increased K^+ channel opening results in a larger current that hyperpolarizes the neuron, so that a larger depolarization is needed to reach the firing threshold. Decreased Ca^{2+} channel opening results in decreased levels of intracellular Ca^{2+}. Because Ca^{2+} is required for synaptic vesicle trafficking to and fusion with the presynaptic membrane, decreases in intracellular Ca^{2+} levels result in decreased dopamine release.

Central Dopamine Pathways

Most central dopaminergic neurons originate in discrete areas of the brain, as shown in Figure 14-6 (see also Fig. 9-8), and have divergent projections. Three major pathways can be distinguished. The largest DA tract in the brain is the **nigrostriatal** system, which contains about 80% of the brain's DA. This tract projects rostrally from cell bodies in the **pars compacta** of the **substantia nigra** to terminals that richly innervate the caudate and putamen, two nuclei that are collectively called the **striatum**. The striatum is named for the striped appearance of the white fiber tracts that run through it; the substantia nigra is named for the dark

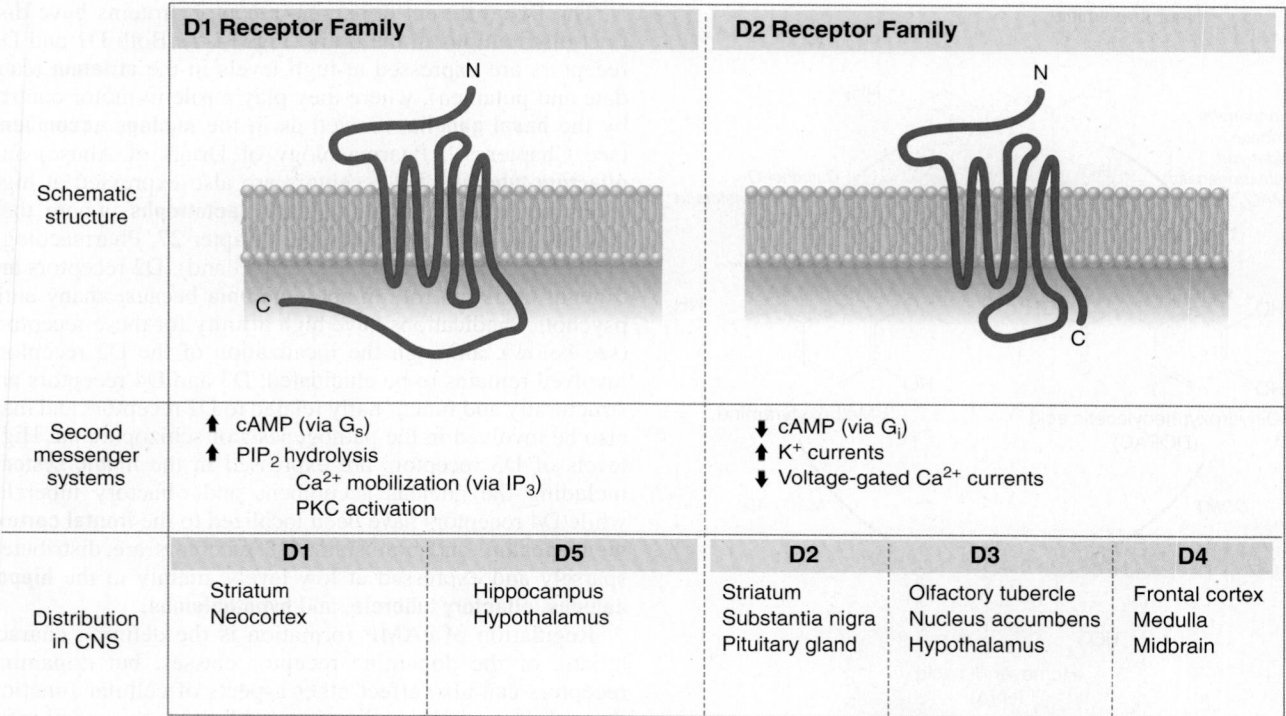

FIGURE 14-4. Dopamine receptor families. The five dopamine receptor subtypes (D1–D5) can be classified into two major families of receptors. The D1 receptor family has a long C-terminal tail and a short cytoplasmic loop between transmembrane helices 5 and 6, whereas the D2 receptor family has a short C-terminal tail and a long cytoplasmic loop between helices 5 and 6. Stimulation of the D1 family is excitatory, increasing cAMP and intracellular Ca^{2+} levels and activating protein kinase C (PKC). Stimulation of the D2 family is inhibitory, decreasing cAMP and intracellular Ca^{2+} levels and hyperpolarizing the cell. The five receptor subtypes exhibit distinctive patterns of distribution in the central nervous system; the major areas of distribution are listed for each subtype. Within the D2 receptor subtype, there are $D2_S$ and $D2_L$ isoforms (*not shown*). IP_3, inositol trisphosphate; PIP_2, phosphatidylinositol-4,5-bisphosphate.

pigmentation that results from the decomposition of DA to melanin. Dopaminergic neurons of the nigrostriatal system are involved in the stimulation of purposeful movement. Their degeneration results in the abnormalities of movement that are characteristic of Parkinson's disease.

Medial to the substantia nigra is an area of dopaminergic cell bodies in the midbrain called the **ventral tegmental area (VTA)**. The VTA has widely divergent projections that innervate many forebrain areas, most notably the cerebral cortex, the nucleus accumbens, and other limbic structures.

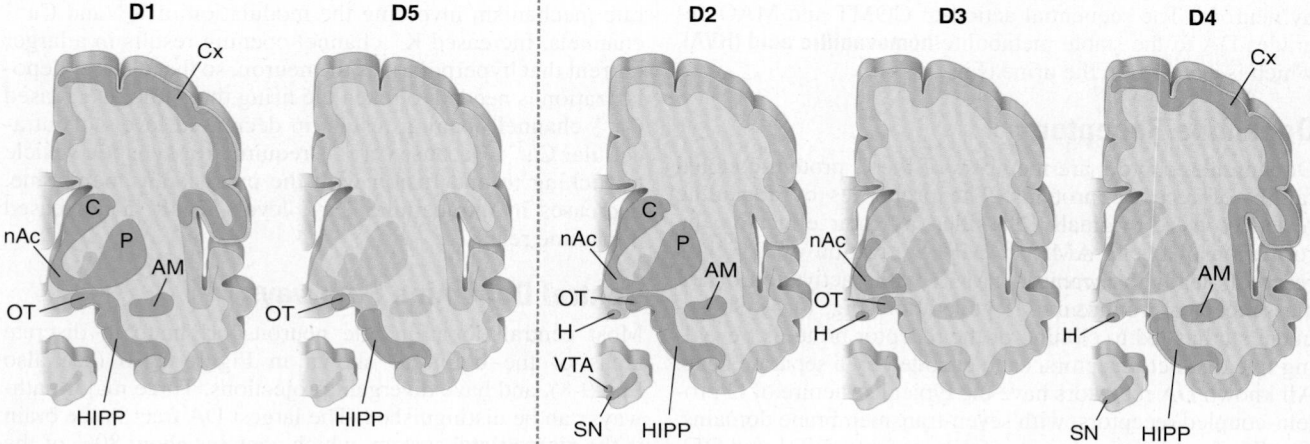

FIGURE 14-5. Location of dopamine receptors in the brain. The location of the five dopamine receptor subtypes in the human brain, as determined by localization of receptor mRNAs in corresponding regions of the rat brain, is shown in *orange* in coronal section. Both D1 and D2 receptors are localized in the caudate and putamen (the striatum), nucleus accumbens, amygdala, olfactory tubercle, and hippocampus. In addition, D1 receptors are present in the cerebral cortex, whereas D2 receptors are present in the substantia nigra, ventral tegmental area, and hypothalamus. AM, amygdala; C, caudate; Cx, cerebral cortex; H, hypothalamus; HIPP, hippocampus; nAc, nucleus accumbens; OT, olfactory tubercle; P, putamen; SN, substantia nigra; VTA, ventral tegmental area.

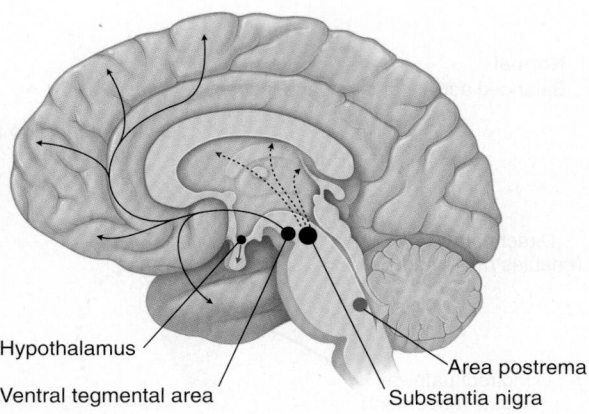

FIGURE 14-6. Central dopamine pathways. Dopaminergic neurons originate in a number of specific nuclei in the brain. Neurons that originate in the hypothalamus and project to the median eminence (*blue arrow*) are tonically active and inhibit prolactin secretion. Neurons that project from the substantia nigra to the striatum (*dashed arrows*) regulate movement. Dopaminergic neurons that project from the ventral tegmental area to the limbic system and prefrontal cortex (*solid black arrows*) are thought to have roles in the regulation of mood and behavior. The area postrema contains a high density of dopamine receptors, and stimulation of these receptors activates the vomiting centers of the brain.

These systems play an important and complex (as yet poorly understood) role in motivation, goal-directed thinking, regulation of affect, and positive reinforcement (reward). Derangement of these pathways may be involved in the development of **schizophrenia**; as discussed below, the blocking of dopaminergic neurotransmission can lead to a remission in psychotic symptoms. (See Chapter 19 for a more complete discussion of the reward pathway.)

DA-containing cell bodies in the **arcuate** and **paraventricular nuclei** of the hypothalamus project axons to the median eminence of the hypothalamus. This system is known as the **tubero-infundibular** pathway. Dopamine is released by these neurons into the portal circulation connecting the median eminence with the anterior pituitary gland and tonically inhibits the release of prolactin by pituitary lactotrophs.

A fourth anatomic structure, the **area postrema** located in the floor of the fourth ventricle, is also a target of dopaminergic therapies. The area postrema contains only a modest number of intrinsic dopamine neurons but a high density of dopamine receptors (mostly of the D2 class). The area postrema is one of the **circumventricular organs** that function as blood chemoreceptors. Unlike the rest of the brain, the blood vessels in the circumventricular organs are fenestrated, allowing communication between the blood and CNS (i.e., the circumventricular organs are "outside" the blood–brain barrier [BBB]). Stimulation of DA receptors in the area postrema activates the vomiting centers of the brain and is one of the causes of **emesis**. Drugs that block dopamine D2 receptors are used to treat nausea and vomiting.

A derangement in any of these dopaminergic systems can result in disease. Parkinson's disease, which arises from dysregulated dopamine neurotransmission, and schizophrenia, which may also result from abnormal dopamine neurotransmission, are two such examples. These two diseases, and the pharmacologic interventions used to treat them, are highlighted below. Because the pharmacologic manipulation

of dopaminergic systems is not always specific to one system, many of the adverse effects of drugs that act on these systems can be predicted based on their effects on the other dopaminergic systems.

DOPAMINE AND CONTROL OF MOVEMENT: PARKINSON'S DISEASE

Physiology of Nigrostriatal Pathways

The basal ganglia have a crucial role in the regulation of purposeful movement and are a site of the pathology in Parkinson's disease. The basal ganglia do not connect directly to spinal motor neurons and thus do not directly control the individual movements of muscles. They appear to function instead by assisting in learning coordinated patterns of movement and by facilitating the execution of learned motor patterns. Dopamine has a central role in the operation of this system, including signaling when desired movements are executed successfully and driving the learning process.

Anatomically, the basal ganglia form a reentrant loop by receiving input from the cerebral cortex, processing this information in the context of dopaminergic input from the substantia nigra, and sending information back to the cortex by way of the thalamus. The internal circuitry of the basal ganglia consists of several components. The striatum (caudate and putamen) is the primary input nucleus of the system, while the globus pallidus pars interna and substantia nigra pars reticulata are the output nuclei. These are interconnected through two internuclei, the subthalamic nucleus and the globus pallidus pars externa.

Much of the information processing performed by the basal ganglia occurs in the striatum. The cortical inputs to this structure are excitatory and use glutamate as a transmitter. The striatum is also the target of the dopaminergic nigrostriatal pathway. The neurons in the striatum are of several types. The majority of neurons are "medium spiny" neurons. These cells are studded with spines that receive input from corticostriatal axons. These medium spiny neurons release the inhibitory transmitter GABA and send their projections to two downstream targets, forming the **direct pathway** and the **indirect pathway** (Fig. 14-7). The striatum also contains several small but important populations of interneurons, including neurons that release acetylcholine. These interneurons participate in the intercommunication between the direct and indirect pathways.

The balance of activity between the direct and indirect pathways regulates movement. The direct pathway, formed by striatal neurons expressing primarily dopamine D1 receptors, projects directly to the output of the basal ganglia, the internal segment of the **globus pallidus**. The latter neurons tonically inhibit the thalamus, which in turn, sends excitatory projections to the cortex that initiate movement. In this manner, activation of the direct pathway disinhibits the thalamus; that is, *the activation of the direct pathway stimulates movement*. The indirect pathway, formed by striatal neurons expressing predominantly D2 receptors, projects to the external segment of the globus pallidus, which in turn, inhibits neurons in the **subthalamic nucleus**. The neurons in the subthalamic nucleus are excitatory glutamatergic neurons that project to the internal segment of the globus pallidus. As a result of this multistep pathway, activation of the indirect pathway disinhibits neurons of the subthalamic nucleus, which, in turn, stimulate neurons in the internal segment of

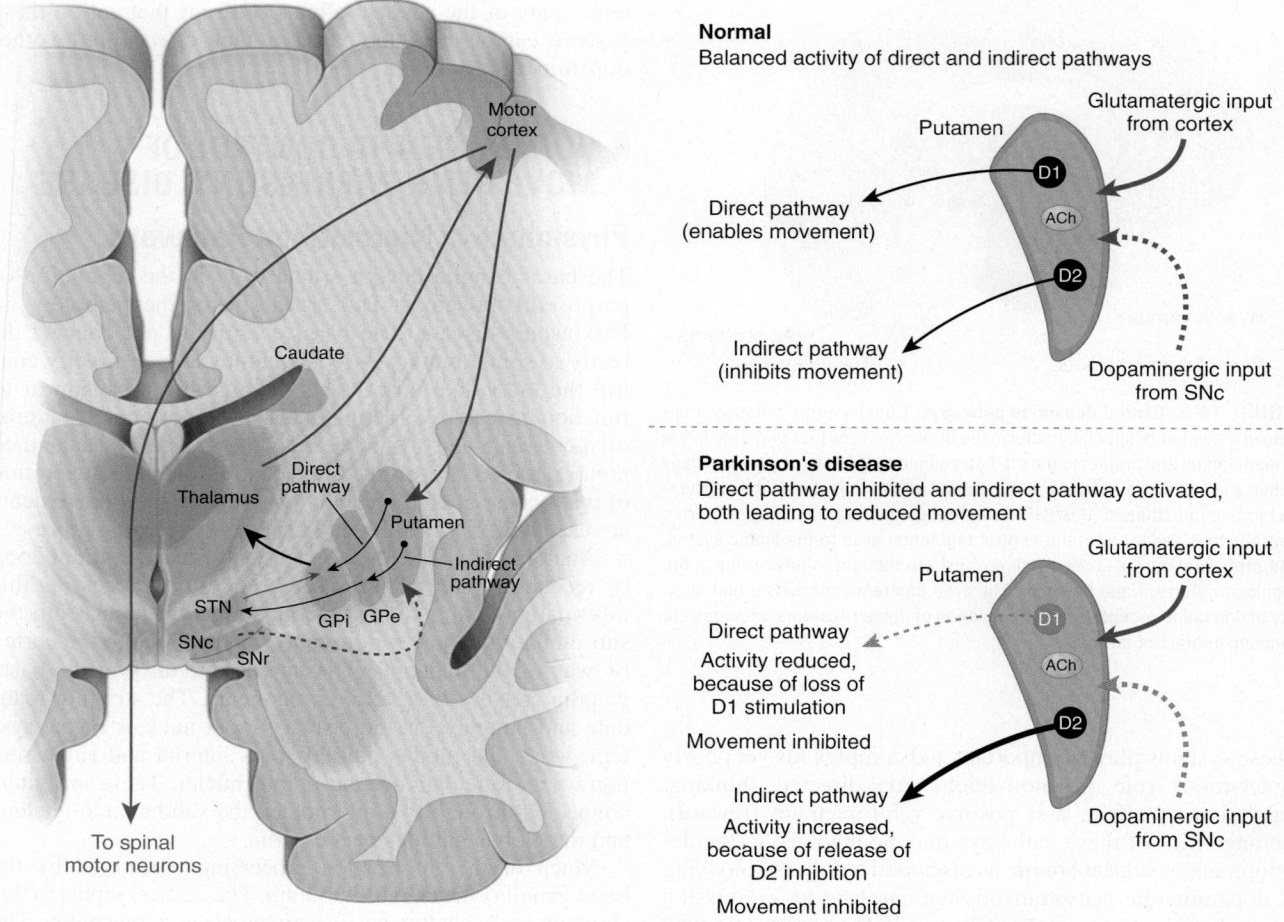

FIGURE 14-7. Effect of Parkinson's disease on dopaminergic pathways that regulate movement. Two principal pathways in the basal ganglia regulate movement: the direct pathway, which enables movement, and the indirect pathway, which inhibits movement. Dopamine stimulates the direct pathway and inhibits the indirect pathway, yielding a net bias that allows purposeful movement. Excitatory pathways are shown in *blue*, and inhibitory pathways are shown in *black*. The direct pathway signals from putamen to GPi to thalamus to cortex, while the indirect pathway signals from putamen to GPe to STN to GPi to thalamus to cortex. GPi, internal segment of the globus pallidus; GPe, external segment of the globus pallidus; SNc, substantia nigra pars compacta; SNr, substantia nigra pars reticulata; STN, subthalamic nucleus. **Inset:** Both direct and indirect pathway neurons in the putamen receive inputs from the nigrostriatal dopaminergic system (*dotted blue arrow*) and from cortical glutamatergic systems (*solid blue arrow*), process these inputs in the context of local cholinergic influences (ACh), and transmit a GABAergic output (*not shown*). Degeneration of dopaminergic neurons in the substantia nigra results in understimulation of the direct (movement-enabling) pathway and underinhibition of the indirect (movement-inhibiting) pathway. The net result is a paucity of movement. *Dotted gray arrow* indicates decreased activity caused by understimulation, and *thick black arrow* indicates increased activity caused by underinhibition.

the globus pallidus to inhibit the thalamus; that is, *the activation of the indirect pathway inhibits movement.*

The differential expression of D1 and D2 receptors within the two pathways leads to differing effects of dopaminergic stimulation. Increased levels of dopamine in the striatum tend to activate the D1-expressing neurons of the direct pathway while inhibiting the D2-expressing neurons of the indirect pathway. Notice that both of these effects promote movement. The opposite effect occurs in Parkinson's disease, a state of dopamine deficiency: the direct pathway shows reduced activity, while the indirect pathway is overactive, leading to reduced movement.

This model of basal ganglia function is greatly simplified, of course, but it has been useful in developing a deeper understanding of how the basal ganglia work. An important prediction of the model is that, in Parkinson's disease, the indirect pathway (and, in particular, the subthalamic nucleus) should be overactive. This prediction has been proven

directly by in vivo electrical recordings in patients with Parkinson's disease. Furthermore, surgical therapies that target the subthalamic nucleus, such as deep brain stimulation in this location, are now often used to treat Parkinson's disease when pharmacologic treatments are inadequate.

Pathophysiology

In Parkinson's disease, there is a selective loss of dopaminergic neurons in the **substantia nigra pars compacta** (Fig. 14-7). The extent of loss is profound, with at least 70% of the neurons destroyed at the time symptoms first appear; often, 95% of the neurons are missing at autopsy. The destruction of these neurons results in the core motor features of the disease: bradykinesia, or slowness of movement; rigidity, a resistance to passive movement of the limbs; impaired postural balance, which predisposes to falling; and a characteristic tremor when the limbs are at rest.

The mechanisms underlying the destruction of DA neurons in the substantia nigra in Parkinson's disease are not fully understood. Both environmental factors and genetic influences have been implicated. In 1983, the unexpected development of Parkinson's disease in abusers of the synthetic opioid meperidine (see Chapter 18, Pharmacology of Analgesia) yielded the first agent known to produce Parkinson's disease directly and the strongest evidence that environmental factors can cause Parkinson's disease. These individuals, who tended to be young and otherwise healthy, suddenly developed severe, levodopa-responsive parkinsonian symptoms. The cases were all linked to a single contaminated batch of meperidine that had been synthesized in a makeshift lab. The contaminant was found to be **1-methyl-4-phenyl-1,2,3,6-tetrahydropyridine (MPTP)**, which forms as an impurity in the synthesis of meperidine when its manufacture is carried out for too long and at too high a temperature. Studies in nonhuman primates have shown that MPTP is oxidized in the brain to MPP^+ (1-methyl-4-phenyl-pyridinium), which is selectively toxic to neurons in the substantia nigra. Despite extensive searches, it does not appear that there is any significant amount of MPTP present in the everyday environment, and MPTP itself is not the cause of most cases of Parkinson's disease. There may, however, be other environmental factors that have a more subtle effect on development of the disease, such as exposure to certain pesticides.

Recent research has established that genetic factors contribute to Parkinson's disease. The best-studied examples are families with mutations in or overexpression of the protein α-synuclein, which lead to autosomal dominant forms of Parkinson's disease. While the function of this protein is not clear, it appears to be involved in the formation of neurotransmitter vesicles and the release of dopamine in the brain. At least four other genes have been identified as causing Parkinson's disease in one or more families. These genetic discoveries have provided important clues into the biology of Parkinson's disease and have allowed the development of transgenic mouse and fruit fly models that serve as a platform for developing new treatments. Although these genetic discoveries have provided insight into the biology of Parkinson's disease, it is important to note that all of the different genetic causes identified so far account for less than 10% of cases, and most cases are still of unknown cause. The etiology of Parkinson's disease in most patients is likely multifactorial, with contributions from both genetic and environmental factors.

Pharmacologic Classes and Agents

Parkinson's disease is a progressive neurodegenerative disorder. Loss of dopaminergic neurons likely begins a decade or more before the symptoms become apparent, and this loss continues relentlessly. Currently available treatments are mostly *symptomatic*, meaning that they treat the symptoms but do not alter the underlying degenerative process. Symptomatic treatments are very useful and can restore function and quality of life for many years, but ultimately, the progression of the disease leads to increasing difficulty in managing the symptoms. In addition, some features of Parkinson's disease do not respond well to current medications, particularly the nonmotor symptoms (such as cognitive impairment and dementia) that characterize the late stages of the disease and that result from an extension of the disease process from the dopaminergic system to other areas of the brain. The goal of

much current research is the development of **neuroprotective** and **neurorestorative** therapies, which might delay or eliminate the need for symptomatic treatment and avoid the late complications of the disorder.

Most of the pharmacologic interventions currently used in Parkinson's disease are aimed at restoring DA levels in the brain. In general, medications used in the management of Parkinson's disease can be divided into DA precursors, DA receptor agonists, and inhibitors of DA degradation. There is a smaller but still useful role for the existing nondopaminergic therapies, such as anticholinergic agents that modify the function of striatal interneurons.

Dopamine Precursors

Levodopa was first used to treat Parkinson's disease over 40 years ago and is still the most effective treatment for the disease. DA itself is not suitable because it cannot cross the BBB. However, DA's immediate precursor, L-DOPA (levodopa), is readily transported across the BBB by the neutral amino acid transporter (see Chapter 9); once in the CNS, L-DOPA is converted to dopamine by the enzyme AADC. Thus, L-DOPA must compete with other neutral amino acids for transport across the BBB, and its availability in the CNS may be compromised by recent high-protein meals (see the introductory case in Chapter 9).

Orally administered levodopa is readily converted into dopamine by AADC in the gastrointestinal tract. This metabolic process both diminishes the amount of levodopa that can reach the blood–brain barrier for transport into the CNS and increases the peripheral adverse effects that result from the generation of dopamine in the peripheral circulation (predominantly nausea, due to binding of this dopamine to receptors in the area postrema). When levodopa is administered alone, only 1–3% of the administered dose reaches the CNS unchanged. In order to boost the levels of levodopa available to the brain and reduce the adverse effects of peripheral levodopa metabolism, levodopa is almost always administered in combination with **carbidopa**, an inhibitor of AADC (Fig. 14-8). *Carbidopa effectively prevents the conversion of levodopa to DA in the periphery.* Importantly, because carbidopa is not able to cross the BBB, it does not interfere with the conversion of levodopa to DA in the CNS. Carbidopa increases the fraction of orally administered levodopa available in the CNS from 1–3% (without carbidopa) to 10% (with carbidopa), allowing a significant reduction in the dose of levodopa and reducing the incidence of peripheral adverse effects.

Many patients with Parkinson's disease show remarkable symptomatic improvement when prescribed the combination of levodopa and carbidopa, especially during the early phase of the disease. In fact, an improvement in symptoms following the initiation of levodopa therapy is considered diagnostic of Parkinson's disease. Over time, however, the effectiveness of levodopa declines. Continued use results in both tolerance and sensitization to the medication, manifested as a drastic narrowing of the therapeutic window. As patients continue on levodopa therapy, they require higher doses to produce a clinically significant improvement in symptoms. They develop fluctuations in motor function that include periods of freezing and increased rigidity, known as "off" periods, alternating with periods of normal or even dyskinetic (excess involuntary) movement, known as "on" periods. These "on" periods generally occur shortly after the

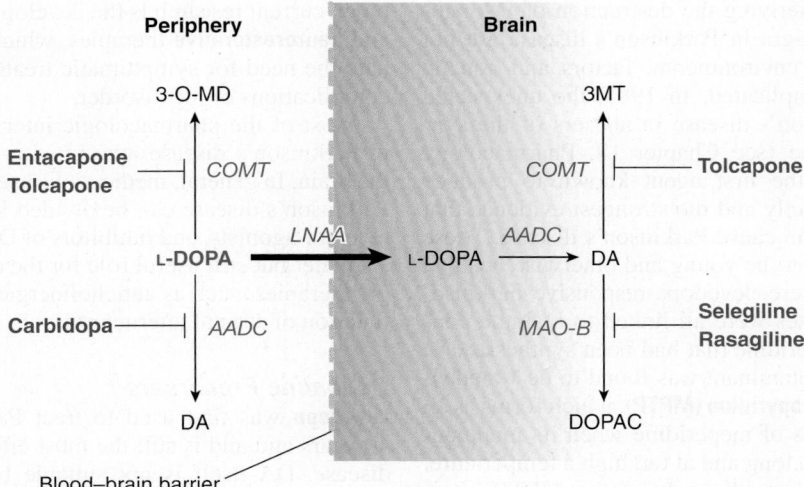

FIGURE 14-8. Effects of carbidopa, COMT inhibitors, and MAO-B inhibitors on the peripheral and central metabolism of levodopa. Orally administered levodopa (L-DOPA) is metabolized in the peripheral tissues and in the gastrointestinal (GI) tract by aromatic L-amino acid decarboxylase (AADC), catechol-O-methyltransferase (COMT), and monoamine oxidase A (MAO-A; *not shown*). This metabolism substantially reduces the effective dose of levodopa available to the brain and substantially increases the adverse peripheral effects of the drug. Carbidopa is an AADC inhibitor that cannot cross the blood–brain barrier. When levodopa is administered in combination with carbidopa, a greater fraction of the levodopa is available to the brain. Therefore, a smaller dose of levodopa is required for clinical efficacy, and the drug has less severe adverse effects in the periphery. By inhibiting COMT in the periphery, entacapone and tolcapone similarly increase the fraction of peripheral levodopa available to the brain. L-DOPA is transported across the blood–brain barrier by the L-neutral amino acid transporter (LNAA) and metabolized to dopamine (DA) by AADC. Within the brain, DA is metabolized by COMT and MAO-B. Tolcapone (COMT inhibitor) and selegiline and rasagiline (selective MAO-B inhibitors) augment the effectiveness of levodopa therapy by inhibiting the metabolism of DA in the brain. 3-O-MD, 3-O-methylDOPA; DOPAC, dihydroxyphenylacetic acid; 3MT, 3-methoxytyramine.

administration of levodopa/carbidopa, when a large bolus of dopamine is delivered to the striatum. The dyskinetic adverse effect of "on" periods can be overcome initially by taking smaller doses of medication, although this increases the likelihood of "off" periods. "Off" periods tend to occur as plasma levels of levodopa decline and can be compensated for by increasing either the dose or frequency of levodopa or by using agents that slow the degradation of dopamine (described below). As the disease progresses, these symptoms become increasingly difficult to manage.

The most profound adverse effect of levodopa is its propensity to cause **dyskinesias**, or uncontrollable rhythmic movements of the head, trunk, and limbs. These appear in at least half of all patients within 5 years of starting the drug, and they generally worsen as the disease progresses. Similar to the "on/off" phenomenon, dyskinesias are usually linked to levodopa dosing, mostly occurring at times of maximal levodopa plasma concentrations. Accordingly, dyskinesias can also be managed initially by using smaller doses of levodopa more frequently. Unfortunately, as the disease progresses, continued therapy leads to worsening of both the dyskinesias and the "on/off" phenomenon, to the point where one or the other is almost always present.

Although levodopa-induced dyskinesias and fluctuations in motor function are complex and poorly understood, at least two factors are thought to contribute to these adverse effects. First, the continued destruction of dopaminergic neurons as Parkinson's disease progresses results in the striatum's increasing inability to store dopamine effectively and reduces the ability of dopamine terminals to buffer the synaptic concentrations of dopamine. Second, chronic therapy with levodopa appears to cause adaptations in postsynaptic neurons in the striatum. Dopamine concentrations in striatal synapses

are normally tightly regulated. The large fluctuations in dopamine concentration produced by intermittent oral levodopa administration induce changes in the cell surface expression of dopamine receptors and in postreceptor signaling events. These postsynaptic adaptations alter the cell's sensitivity to synaptic dopamine levels, further accentuating responses associated with high ("on" period, dyskinesia) and low ("off" period, akinesia) transmitter concentrations.

The predictable decline in efficacy and increase in adverse effects that result from prolonged levodopa therapy have led to discussions about the appropriate time to begin treatment of Parkinson's disease with levodopa and the relative merits of delaying the use of this drug in the early stages of the disease. Recent studies have suggested that there may be advantages to initial treatment with therapies other than levodopa, particularly the dopamine receptor agonists (see below), but these alternatives can lead to more severe adverse effects than levodopa, at least in some patients. In addition, most patients who are initially treated with other therapies generally require levodopa treatment at some point. Levodopa remains the most effective therapy for Parkinson's disease and should be initiated as soon as other therapies are unable to control parkinsonian symptoms effectively. Further delays in levodopa therapy are associated with reduced rates of symptom control and increased mortality.

Dopamine Receptor Agonists

Another strategy for enhancing dopaminergic neurotransmission is to target the postsynaptic DA receptor directly through the use of DA receptor agonists. The earliest therapies in this class were ergot derivatives such as **bromocriptine** (D2 agonist) and **pergolide** (D1 and D2), but these have been found to induce adverse effects, including fibrosis of cardiac valves, and have largely been abandoned in favor of nonergot agonists such as **pramipexole**, **ropinirole**, and **rotigotine** (all D3>D2).

As a class, DA receptor agonists have several advantages. Because they are nonpeptide molecules, they do not compete with levodopa or other neutral amino acids for transport across the BBB. Furthermore, because they do not require enzymatic conversion by AADC, they remain effective late in the course of Parkinson's disease. All of the dopamine receptor agonists in current use have half-lives longer than that of levodopa, which allows for less frequent dosing and a more uniform response to the medications.

The major limitation to the use of the dopamine receptor agonists is their tendency to induce unwanted adverse effects, which may include nausea, peripheral edema, and hypotension. All of the dopamine agonists may also produce a variety of adverse cognitive effects, including excessive sedation, vivid dreams, and hallucinations, particularly in elderly patients. Dopamine receptor agonists may also trigger symptoms of the dopamine dysregulation syndrome, in which patients exhibit impaired impulse control. Common manifestations include pathological gambling, overspending, compulsive eating, and hypersexuality. These behaviors may be socially destructive and require discontinuation of the medications.

Recent studies have examined the use of pramipexole and ropinirole as initial monotherapy for Parkinson's disease. It was thought that, because the dopamine agonists have longer half-lives than levodopa, they might be less likely to induce "off" periods. These studies show that use of the dopamine receptor agonists as initial treatment for Parkinson's disease does delay the onset of "off" periods and dyskinesias, but there is also an increased rate of adverse effects compared to initial treatment with levodopa. At present, many practitioners use dopamine agonists as the initial treatment for Parkinson's disease, especially in younger individuals.

Inhibitors of Dopamine Metabolism

A third strategy that has been employed to treat Parkinson's disease involves the inhibition of DA breakdown. Inhibitors of both MAO-B (the isoform of MAO that predominates in the striatum) and COMT have been used as adjuvants to levodopa in clinical practice (Fig. 14-8). **Selegiline** is an MAO inhibitor that, in low concentrations, is selective for MAO-B. It does not interfere with the peripheral metabolism of monoamines by MAO-A, and it avoids the toxic effects of dietary tyramine and other sympathomimetic amines that are associated with nonselective MAO blockade (see Chapter 15, Pharmacology of Serotonergic and Central Adrenergic Neurotransmission). A drawback of selegiline is that this drug forms a potentially toxic metabolite, amphetamine, which can cause sleeplessness and confusion, especially in the elderly. **Rasagiline**, a newer MAO-B inhibitor that does not form toxic metabolites, is also approved in the United States. Both rasagiline and selegiline improve motor function in Parkinson's disease when used alone, and both can augment the effectiveness of levodopa therapy. There has also been interest in the question of whether MAO inhibitors can limit the formation of reactive free radicals associated with dopamine catabolism and thereby alter the rate of disease progression, but clinical trials of both drugs searching for a "neuroprotective" effect have been inconclusive so far.

Tolcapone and **entacapone** inhibit COMT and thereby inhibit the degradation of levodopa as well as DA. Tolcapone is a highly lipid-soluble agent that can cross the BBB, while entacapone distributes only to the periphery. Both drugs decrease the peripheral metabolism of levodopa and thereby make more levodopa available to the CNS. Tolcapone has the additional property of crossing the blood–brain barrier effectively and inhibiting central as well as peripheral COMT. In clinical trials, both tolcapone and entacapone have been shown to reduce the "off" periods that are associated with decreasing plasma levodopa levels. Although the central effect of tolcapone is an advantage (Fig. 14-8), there have been several reports of fatal hepatic toxicity associated with tolcapone, and it must be used with great care. In practice, therefore, entacapone is the most widely used COMT inhibitor.

Nondopaminergic Pharmacology in Parkinson's Disease

Amantadine, trihexyphenidyl, and benztropine are all drugs that do not clearly affect dopaminergic pathways but are nonetheless effective in the treatment of Parkinson's disease. **Amantadine** was developed and is marketed primarily as an antiviral that reduces the length and severity of influenza A infections (see Chapter 38, Pharmacology of Viral Infections). In patients with Parkinson's disease, however, amantadine is used to treat levodopa-induced dyskinesias that develop late in the course of the disease. The mechanism by which amantadine reduces dyskinesia is thought to involve blockade of excitatory NMDA receptors. **Trihexyphenidyl** and **benztropine** are muscarinic receptor antagonists that reduce cholinergic tone in the CNS. They reduce tremor more than bradykinesia and are therefore more effective in treating patients for whom tremor is the major clinical manifestation of Parkinson's disease. These anticholinergic drugs are thought to act by modifying the actions of striatal cholinergic interneurons, which regulate the interactions of direct and indirect pathway neurons. They also cause a range of anticholinergic adverse effects, which may include dry mouth, urinary retention, and most importantly, impairment of memory and cognition.

Treatment of Patients with Parkinson's Disease

The treatment of patients with Parkinson's disease is an individualized process that must take into account not only the extent of symptoms but also the patient's age, occupation, activities, and perceived disabilities. There is at present no laboratory test that can specifically confirm the diagnosis; instead, diagnosis is based on history and physical examination, along with laboratory studies to exclude other possible diagnoses. In patients with early disease, it may be appropriate to recommend a nonpharmacologic approach to treatment that emphasizes exercise and lifestyle modification. Almost all patients eventually require treatment with medication. In patients with mild symptoms, MAO-B inhibitors, amantadine, or anticholinergic medications may be considered. When symptoms are more advanced, a dopaminergic therapy is indicated. Levodopa is the most effective therapy, but many younger patients are treated first with a dopamine agonist in the hope of delaying the onset of motor fluctuations. Advanced disease with fluctuations requires polypharmacy, often including levodopa, dopamine agonists, entacapone, MAO-B inhibitors, and amantadine.

It is important to be vigilant for the development of cognitive symptoms and adverse effects, which may require modification of the therapeutic approach.

■ DOPAMINE AND DISORDERS OF THOUGHT: SCHIZOPHRENIA

Pathophysiology

Schizophrenia is a thought disorder characterized by one or more episodes of psychosis (impairment in reality testing). Patients may manifest disorders of perception, thinking, speech, emotion, and/or physical activity. Schizophrenic symptoms are divided into two broad categories. **Positive symptoms** involve the development of abnormal functions; these symptoms include **delusions** (distorted or false beliefs and misinterpretation of perceptions), **hallucinations** (abnormal perceptions, especially auditory), **disorganized speech**, and **catatonic behavior**. **Negative symptoms** involve the reduction or loss of normal functions; these symptoms include **affective flattening** (decrease in the range or intensity of emotional expression), **alogia** (decrease in the fluency of speech), and **avolition** (decrease in the initiation of goal-directed behavior). The American Psychiatric Association criteria for schizophrenia are listed in Box 14-1.

Schizophrenia typically begins to affect individuals in their late teens and early 20s. The disorder affects males and females equally. Approximately 4.75 million individuals suffer from schizophrenia in the United States, and 100,000 to 150,000 new cases are diagnosed annually. A genetic component of the disease has been demonstrated, but concordance among identical twins is only 50%. Schizophrenia, therefore, appears to have a multifactorial etiology, with both genetic and environmental components.

The model that is most commonly cited to explain the pathogenesis of schizophrenia is the **dopamine hypothesis**, which states that the illness is caused by increased and dysregulated levels of DA neurotransmission in the brain. This hypothesis arises from the empiric observation that treatment with DA receptor antagonists, specifically D2 antagonists, relieves a number of the symptoms of schizophrenia in many, but not all, patients with the disease. The DA hypothesis is supported by several additional clinical observations. First, some patients taking drugs that increase DA levels or that activate dopamine receptors in the CNS, including **amphetamines**, **cocaine**, and **apomorphine**, develop a schizophrenia-like state that subsides when the dose of the drug is lowered. Second, hallucinations are a known adverse effect of levodopa therapy for Parkinson's disease. Finally, researchers have been able to correlate decreased

---

BOX 14-1 Criteria for Schizophrenia, from the Diagnostic and Statistical Manual of Mental Disorders, Fifth Edition (DSM-5)

A. Characteristic symptoms: Two (or more) of the following, each present for a significant portion of time during a 1-month period (or less if successfully treated). At least one of these should include 1–3:

1. Delusions
2. Hallucinations
3. Disorganized speech
4. Grossly disorganized or catatonic behavior
5. Negative symptoms (i.e., diminished emotional expression or avolition)

B. Social/occupational dysfunction: For a significant portion of the time since the onset of the disturbance, one or more major areas of functioning, such as work, interpersonal relations, or self-care, are markedly below the level achieved before the onset (or when the onset is in childhood or adolescence, failure to achieve expected level of interpersonal, academic, or occupational achievement).

C. Duration of 6 months: Continuous signs of the disturbance persist for at least 6 months. This 6-month period must include at least 1 month of symptoms (or less if successfully treated) that meet Criterion A (i.e., active-phase symptoms) and may include periods of prodromal or residual symptoms. During these prodromal or residual periods, the signs of the disturbance may be manifested by only negative symptoms or two or more symptoms listed in Criterion A present in an attenuated form (e.g., odd beliefs, unusual perceptual experiences).

D. Schizoaffective and mood disorder exclusion: Schizoaffective disorder and mood disorder with psychotic features have been ruled out because either (1) no major depressive, manic, or mixed episodes have occurred concurrently with the active-phase symptoms, or (2) if mood episodes have occurred during active-phase symptoms, their total duration has been brief relative to the duration of the active and residual periods.

E. Substance/general medical condition exclusion: The disturbance is not attributable to the direct physiologic effects of a substance (e.g., a drug of abuse, a medication) or a general medical condition.

F. Relationship to a global developmental delay or autism spectrum disorder: If there is a history of autism spectrum disorder or other communication disorder of childhood onset, the additional diagnosis of schizophrenia is made only if prominent delusions or hallucinations are also present for at least 1 month (or less if successfully treated).

Classification of longitudinal course (the minimum observation period is 1 year; see DSM-5 for full description):

1. First episode, currently in acute episode
2. First episode, currently in partial remission
3. First episode, currently in full remission
4. Multiple episodes, currently in acute episode
5. Multiple episodes, currently in partial remission
6. Multiple episodes, currently in full remission
7. Continuous
8. Unspecified ■

Reprinted with permission from the American Psychiatric Association. *Diagnostic and statistical manual of mental disorders.* 5th ed. Arlington, VA: American Psychiatric Association; 2013.

DA metabolite levels, and by extension decreased DA levels, with clinical improvement in some schizophrenic symptoms.

The dysregulation of dopaminergic neurotransmission in schizophrenia is thought to occur at specific anatomic locations in the brain. The **mesolimbic system** is a dopaminergic tract that originates in the ventral tegmental area and projects to the nucleus accumbens in the ventral striatum, parts of the amygdala and hippocampus, and other components of the limbic system. This system is involved in the development of emotions and memory, and some hypothesize that mesolimbic hyperactivity is responsible for the positive symptoms of schizophrenia. This hypothesis is supported by positron emission tomography (PET) scans of the brains of patients displaying the earliest signs of schizophrenia; these PET images show changes in blood flow to the mesolimbic system that reflect changes in the level of functioning of this system. Dopaminergic neurons of the **mesocortical system** originate in the ventral tegmental area and project to regions of the cerebral cortex, particularly the prefrontal cortex. Because the prefrontal cortex is responsible for attention, planning, and motivated behavior, the hypothesis has been advanced that the mesocortical system plays a role in the negative symptoms of schizophrenia.

All of the evidence implicating DA in the pathogenesis of schizophrenia is circumstantial, however, and much of it is conflicting. Changes in DA levels, particularly in the mesolimbic and mesocortical systems, could simply reflect downstream consequences of a pathologic process in a heretofore undiscovered pathway. One hypothesis involving such an upstream process suggests that an imbalance in glutamatergic neurotransmission plays an important role in schizophrenia. This model is supported by the observation that phencyclidine (PCP) (see Chapter 19), an antagonist at NMDA receptors, causes symptoms similar to those of schizophrenia. In fact, the syndrome seen in patients taking PCP chronically—consisting of psychotic symptoms, visual and auditory hallucinations, disorganized thought, blunted affect, withdrawal, psychomotor retardation, and an amotivational state—has components of both the positive and negative symptoms of schizophrenia. Dopaminergic neurons and excitatory glutamatergic neurons often form reciprocal synaptic connections, which could account for the efficacy of DA receptor antagonists in schizophrenia. Even if this hypothesis is correct, at present, there are no useful therapies for schizophrenia that act at glutamate receptors. Glutamate is the primary excitatory transmitter in the brain, and further research will be required to identify drugs that are sufficiently selective for use in schizophrenia and that have an acceptable adverse effect profile.

Pharmacologic Classes and Agents

Although the biological basis of schizophrenia remains controversial, a number of drugs are effective in treating the illness. When successful, these medications can lead to a remission of psychosis and allow the patient to integrate into society. Patients only rarely return completely to their premorbid state, however. Drugs used in the management of psychosis are often called **neuroleptics** or **antipsychotics**. Although these terms are frequently used interchangeably, they have slight yet important differences in connotation. The term *neuroleptic* emphasizes the drugs' neurological actions that are commonly manifested as adverse effects of treatment. These adverse effects, often called **extrapyramidal effects**,

result from DA receptor blockade in the basal ganglia and include the parkinsonian symptoms of slowness, stiffness, and tremor. The term *antipsychotic* denotes the ability of these drugs to abrogate psychosis and alleviate disordered thinking in schizophrenic patients. The antipsychotics may be further divided into **typical antipsychotics**, older drugs with prominent actions at the D2 receptor, and **atypical antipsychotics**, a newer generation of drugs with less prominent D2 antagonism and consequently fewer extrapyramidal effects.

Typical Antipsychotic Agents

The history of the typical antipsychotic drugs dates back to the approval of **chlorpromazine** in 1954. Approval was based on observations of the drug's effectiveness in schizophrenia, but there was little understanding of its mechanism of action. In the 1960s, as the role of DA in the brain became better understood, the ability of the typical antipsychotic drugs to block dopaminergic neurotransmission in the CNS was first elucidated. Affinity binding studies performed in the 1980s demonstrated that both therapeutic efficacy and extrapyramidal adverse effects of the typical antipsychotics correlate directly with the affinity of these drugs for D2 receptors. As shown in Figure 14-9, drugs with higher affinity for D2 receptors, as represented by lower dissociation constants, tend to require smaller doses to control psychotic symptoms and alleviate schizophrenia.

Mechanism of Action

Although the typical antipsychotics block D2 receptors in all of the CNS dopaminergic pathways, their mechanism of action as antipsychotics appears to involve antagonism of mesolimbic, and possibly mesocortical, D2 receptors. As described above, one hypothesis holds that the positive symptoms of schizophrenia correlate with hyperactivity of the mesolimbic system, and antagonism of mesolimbic dopamine receptors could alleviate these symptoms. The typical antipsychotics are relatively less effective at controlling the negative symptoms of schizophrenia. This relative lack of efficacy at treating the negative symptoms could relate to the hypothesis that the negative symptoms correlate with hypoactivity of mesocortical neurons, because the antagonist action of the antipsychotics would not be expected to correct dopaminergic hypoactivity. Many of the adverse effects of the typical antipsychotics are likely mediated by binding of these drugs to D2 receptors in the basal ganglia (nigrostriatal pathway) and pituitary gland (see below).

The typical antipsychotics fall into several structural classes, of which the most prominent are the **phenothiazines** and the **butyrophenones** (Fig. 14-10). **Chlorpromazine** is the prototypical phenothiazine, and **haloperidol** is the most widely used butyrophenone. Despite differences in structure and D2 receptor affinity, all typical antipsychotics have similar clinical efficacy at their standard doses. In general, aliphatic phenothiazines (such as chlorpromazine) are less potent antagonists at D2 receptors than are butyrophenones, **thioxanthenes** (phenothiazines in which a nitrogen in the phenothiazine nucleus is substituted by a carbon), or phenothiazines functionalized with a piperazine derivative (such as **fluphenazine**). For all of these drugs, the clinical dose can be adjusted to account for the in vitro D2 receptor binding affinity, so that efficacy is unaffected by potency at clinically useful doses. However, the potency of the typical antipsychotics is critical in determining the drugs' adverse effects profiles.

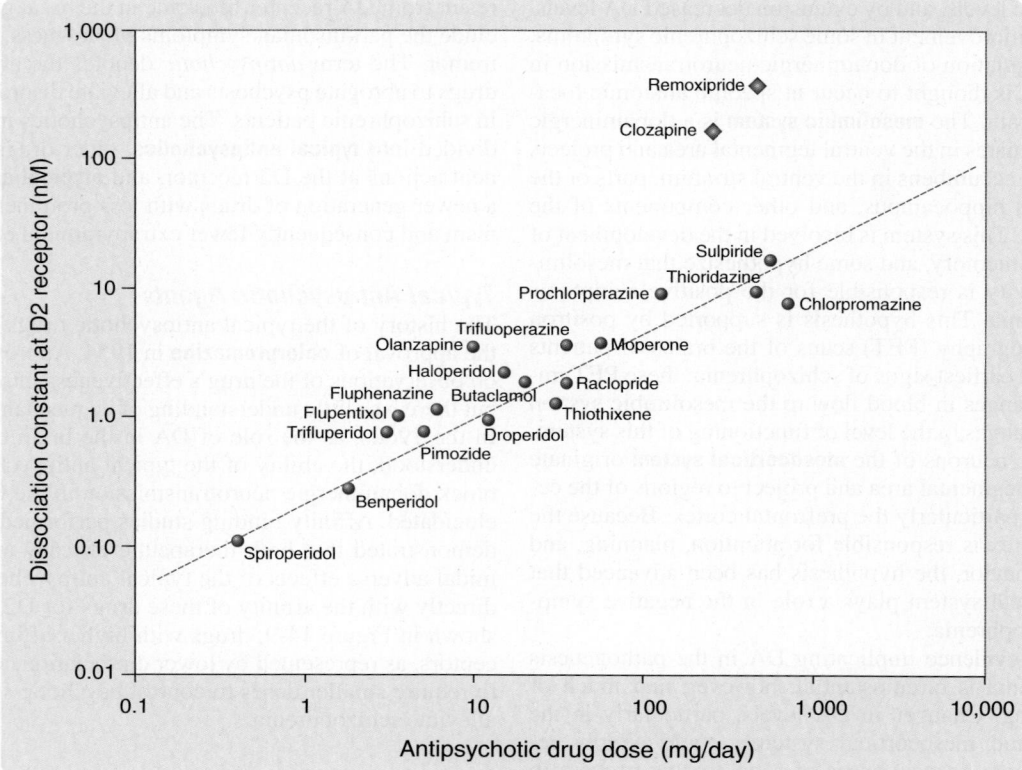

FIGURE 14-9. Antipsychotic potency of dopamine receptor antagonists. Over at least three orders of magnitude, the clinically effective dose of the typical antipsychotics is proportional to the dissociation constant of the drugs at D2 receptors. (Note that a higher dissociation constant represents a lower binding affinity.) Atypical antipsychotics such as clozapine and remoxipride (*blue diamonds*) are exceptions to this rule; these agents have clinical effects at a dose lower than that predicted by their dissociation constants. Data points represent the mean dissociation constant (averaged over multiple studies) at the most common clinically effective dose. The *dotted line* represents the best fit to the data for all of the typical antipsychotics (*blue circles*).

Adverse Effects

The adverse effects of typical antipsychotic drugs can be divided into two broad categories: those caused by antagonist action at dopamine D2 receptors outside the mesolimbic and mesocortical systems (on-target effects) and those caused by nonspecific antagonist action at other receptor types (off-target effects). Given the broad distribution of dopamine receptor expression, it is not surprising that dopamine receptor antagonists have a wide range of on-target adverse effects. As noted above, the most prominent of these effects are often referred to as **extrapyramidal effects**. Because endogenous stimulation of dopamine D2 receptors inhibits the indirect pathway within the basal ganglia, antagonism of D2 receptors by typical antipsychotic drugs can disinhibit the indirect pathway and thereby induce parkinsonian symptoms. Such symptoms can sometimes be treated with the nondopaminergic therapies for Parkinson's disease, such as amantadine and anticholinergic drugs. Dopaminergic drugs are often ineffective because of the high affinity of the antagonists for the D2 receptor and because, when used in this setting, dopaminergic drugs could cause a relapse of schizophrenic symptoms.

The most severe adverse effect of the typical antipsychotics is the so-called **neuroleptic malignant syndrome (NMS)**, a rare but life-threatening syndrome characterized by catatonia, stupor, fever, and autonomic instability; myoglobinemia and death occur in about 10% of these cases. NMS is most commonly associated with the typical antipsychotic drugs that have a high affinity for D2 receptors, such as haloperidol. It can also be seen in patients with Parkinson's disease who abruptly discontinue dopaminergic medications, emphasizing the importance of dopamine in the causation of NMS. The symptoms are thought to arise at least in part from the actions of the antipsychotics on the dopaminergic systems in the hypothalamus, which are essential for the body's ability to control temperature.

Treatment with antipsychotics and other dopamine antagonists can also cause abnormal movements, a condition known as **tardive dyskinesia**. This condition is observed most frequently after prolonged treatment with drugs that have a high affinity for the D2 receptor, such as haloperidol. It is occasionally seen in patients after only short-term treatment and has been reported to occur after a single dose of a D2 receptor antagonist. The syndrome is characterized by repetitive, involuntary, stereotyped movements of the facial musculature, arms, and trunk. The exact mechanism is unknown, but it is believed to involve adaptive hypersensitivity of D2 receptors in the striatum, which, in turn, results in excessive dopaminergic activity. Antiparkinsonian drugs can exacerbate tardive dyskinesia, and discontinuation of antiparkinsonian drugs can ameliorate the symptoms. Administration of high doses of high-potency typical antipsychotics can temporarily suppress the disorder, presumably by overcoming the adaptive response in striatal neurons, but may in the long run lead to worsening of symptoms. In many cases, cessation of all typical antipsychotic medications will

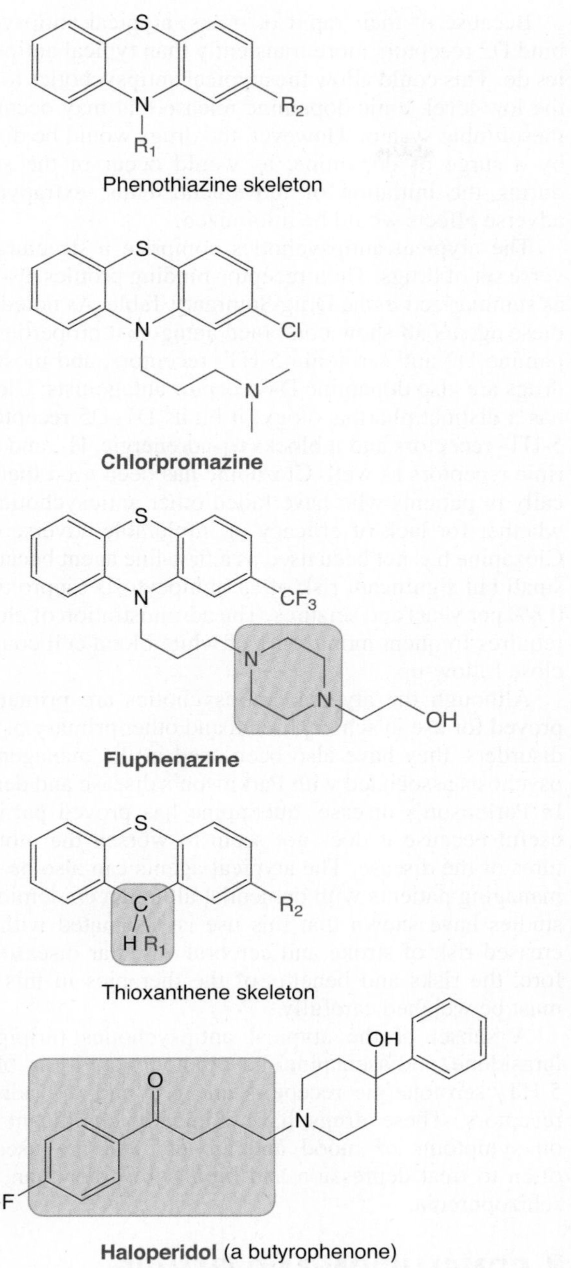

FIGURE 14-10. Chemical structures of the typical antipsychotics. The structure of the phenothiazines is based on a common skeleton, with two variable functional groups. Chlorpromazine, the first approved antipsychotic, has substituted aminopropyl (R_1) and chloride (R_2) side groups. Piperazine (*in blue box*)-substituted phenothiazines, such as fluphenazine, are significantly more potent than aliphatic-substituted phenothiazines, such as chlorpromazine. The fourth structure represents the skeleton of a thioxanthene, which substitutes a carbon (*in blue box*) for the phenothiazine nitrogen. As illustrated by the structure of haloperidol, butyrophenones (*in blue box*) are structurally distinct from phenothiazines and thioxanthenes.

lead to slow reversal of the striatal adaptations, with eventual improvement in the symptoms of tardive dyskinesia. Some patients, however, are left with a permanent and irreversible movement disorder.

Some adverse effects of typical antipsychotics are thought to be caused by antagonist action at dopamine receptors in the pituitary gland, where dopamine tonically inhibits **prolactin** secretion. Antagonism of D2 receptors increases prolactin secretion, leading to amenorrhea, galactorrhea, and false-positive pregnancy tests in women and to gynecomastia and decreased libido in men.

Other adverse effects of the typical antipsychotics result from nonspecific antagonism of muscarinic and α-adrenergic receptors. Antagonism of peripheral muscarinic pathways causes anticholinergic effects, including dry mouth, constipation, difficulty urinating, and loss of accommodation (see Chapter 10, Cholinergic Pharmacology). α-Adrenergic antagonism can cause orthostatic hypotension and, in men, failure to ejaculate. Sedation can also occur because of inhibition of central α-adrenergic pathways in the reticular activating system. When sedation interferes with normal functioning during chronic antipsychotic use, it is considered an adverse effect. In the acutely psychotic patient, however, sedation may be part of the drug's intended spectrum of action.

The adverse effect profiles of the typical antipsychotics depend on their potency. High-potency drugs (whose clinical doses are only a few milligrams) tend to have fewer sedative effects and cause less postural hypotension than drugs with lower potency (i.e., drugs that require high doses to achieve a therapeutic effect). On the other hand, lower potency typical antipsychotics tend to cause fewer extrapyramidal adverse effects. These observations can be rationalized by the fact that high-potency drugs have high affinity for D2 receptors and are therefore more selective in their action. Thus, these drugs are more likely to cause on-target adverse effects mediated by D2 receptors (i.e., extrapyramidal effects) and less likely to cause off-target adverse effects mediated by muscarinic and α-adrenergic receptors (i.e., anticholinergic effects, sedation, and postural hypotension). Conversely, low-potency typical antipsychotics do not bind D2 receptors as tightly and cause fewer extrapyramidal effects, while their lower selectivity results in more prominent anticholinergic and antiadrenergic effects.

Pharmacokinetics, Metabolism, and Drug Interactions

As with many drugs active in the CNS, the typical antipsychotics are highly lipophilic. In part because of this lipophilicity, typical antipsychotics tend to be metabolized in the liver and to exhibit both high binding to plasma proteins and high first-pass metabolism. The drugs are generally formulated as oral or intramuscular dosage forms. The latter are useful in treating acutely psychotic patients who may be a danger to themselves or others, while the oral formulations are generally used for chronic therapy. Elimination half-lives of the typical antipsychotics are erratic because their kinetics of elimination typically follow a multiphasic pattern and are not strictly first-order. In general, however, the half-lives of most typical antipsychotics are on the order of 1 day, and it is common practice to follow a once-daily dosing regimen.

Two drugs, **haloperidol** and **fluphenazine**, are available as decanoate esters. These highly lipophilic drugs are injected intramuscularly, where they are slowly hydrolyzed and released. The decanoate ester dosage forms provide a long-acting formulation that can be administered every 3 to 4 weeks. These formulations are particularly useful for treating poorly adherent patients.

Because typical antipsychotics are antagonists at dopamine receptors, it is logical that these drugs should interact prominently with antiparkinsonian drugs that act either by increasing synaptic dopamine concentrations (levodopa) or through direct stimulation of dopamine receptors (dopamine agonists). Antipsychotics inhibit the action of both of these drug classes, and the administration of typical antipsychotics to patients with Parkinson's disease often leads to a marked worsening of parkinsonian symptoms. In addition, typical antipsychotics potentiate the sedative effects of benzodiazepines and centrally active antihistamines. Because the latter are pharmacodynamic effects that result from the nonspecific binding of typical antipsychotics to cholinergic and adrenergic receptors, the low-potency typical antipsychotics tend to manifest more pronounced sedative effects than their high-potency counterparts.

Atypical Antipsychotic Agents

The so-called atypical antipsychotics have efficacy and adverse effect profiles that differ from those of the typical antipsychotics. The nine principal atypical antipsychotics available in the United States are **risperidone**, **clozapine**, **olanzapine**, **quetiapine**, **ziprasidone**, **aripiprazole**, **iloperidone**, **lurasidone**, and **asenapine**. All of these drugs are more effective than the typical antipsychotics at treating the negative symptoms of schizophrenia. Long-term treatment trials comparing typical antipsychotics to atypical antipsychotics show similar treatment efficacy between the classes and similar rates of discontinuation due to adverse events, although the types of adverse events differ. Atypical antipsychotics cause significantly milder extrapyramidal symptoms than typical antipsychotics but have a much higher incidence of other adverse effects such as metabolic dysfunction, weight gain, and sedation.

The atypical antipsychotics have a relatively low affinity for D2 receptors; unlike the typical antipsychotics, their affinity for D2 receptors does not correlate with their clinically effective dose (Fig. 14-9). Three main hypotheses have emerged to explain this discrepancy. The 5-HT$_2$ hypothesis states that antagonist action at the serotonin 5-HT$_2$ receptor (see Chapter 15), or antagonist action at both 5-HT$_2$ and D2 receptors, is critical for the antipsychotic effect of the atypical antipsychotics. This hypothesis is based on the finding that the US Food and Drug Administration (FDA)-approved atypical antipsychotics are all high-affinity 5-HT$_2$ receptor antagonists. It is not clear, however, how 5-HT$_2$ antagonism contributes to the antipsychotic effect. The second model, the D4 hypothesis, is based on the finding that many of the atypical antipsychotics are also dopamine D4 receptor antagonists. This model suggests that selective D4 antagonism, or a combination of D2 and D4 antagonism, is critical to the mechanism of action of the atypical antipsychotics. Quetiapine does not act as a D4 receptor antagonist, however, so the D4 hypothesis cannot account for the mechanism of action of all atypical antipsychotics. The final hypothesis states that the atypical antipsychotics exhibit a milder extrapyramidal adverse effect profile because of their relatively rapid dissociation from the D2 receptor. As described in Chapter 2, Pharmacodynamics, the binding affinity (K_d) of a drug is equal to the ratio of its rate of dissociation from the receptor (k_{off}) to its rate of association to the receptor (k_{on}):

$$D + R \xrightarrow{\ k_{on}\ } DR \xrightarrow{\ k_{off}\ } D + R$$

$$K_d = \frac{k_{off}}{k_{on}} \qquad\qquad \textbf{Equation 14-1}$$

Because of their rapid off-rates, atypical antipsychotics bind D2 receptors more transiently than typical antipsychotics do. This could allow the atypical antipsychotics to inhibit the low-level, tonic dopamine release that may occur in the mesolimbic system. However, the drugs would be displaced by a surge of dopamine, as would occur in the striatum during the initiation of movement. Thus, extrapyramidal adverse effects would be minimized.

The atypical antipsychotics comprise a structurally diverse set of drugs. Their receptor-binding profiles also differ, as summarized in the Drug Summary Table. As noted above, these agents all show combined antagonist properties at dopamine D2 and serotonin 5-HT$_2$ receptors, and most of the drugs are also dopamine D4 receptor antagonists. Clozapine has a distinct pharmacology; it binds D1–D5 receptors and 5-HT$_2$ receptors and it blocks α_1-adrenergic, H$_1$, and muscarinic receptors as well. Clozapine has been used therapeutically in patients who have failed other antipsychotic drugs, whether for lack of efficacy or intolerable adverse effects. Clozapine has not been used as a first-line agent because of a small but significant risk of agranulocytosis (approximately 0.8% per year) and seizures. The administration of clozapine requires frequent monitoring of white blood cell counts and close follow-up.

Although the atypical antipsychotics are primarily approved for use in schizophrenia and other primary psychotic disorders, they have also been used in the management of psychosis associated with Parkinson's disease and dementia. In Parkinson's disease, quetiapine has proved particularly useful because it does not seem to worsen the motor features of the disease. The atypical agents can also be used in managing patients with dementia, although epidemiological studies have shown that this use is associated with an increased risk of stroke and cerebral vascular disease; therefore, the risks and benefits of the therapies in this setting must be weighed carefully.

A subset of the atypical antipsychotics (aripiprazole, lurasidone, and asenapine) have potent activity in blocking 5-HT$_7$ serotonergic receptors and α_{2A} and α_{2C} adrenergic receptors. These drugs have clinically significant effects on symptoms of mood and anxiety and are used more often to treat depression and bipolar disorder than to treat schizophrenia.

■ CONCLUSION AND FUTURE DIRECTIONS

Treatments for both Parkinson's disease and schizophrenia modulate dopaminergic neurotransmission in the CNS. In Parkinson's disease, the degeneration of dopaminergic neurons that project to the striatum is responsible for motor symptoms, including resting tremor, rigidity, and bradykinesia. In this disease, the direct pathway—which enables movement—is understimulated, whereas the indirect pathway—which inhibits movement—is disinhibited. Pharmacologic treatment of Parkinson's disease depends on agents that increase dopamine release or activate dopamine receptors in the caudate and putamen and thereby help restore the balance between the direct and indirect pathways.

Schizophrenia is treated by inhibiting dopamine receptors at various sites in the limbic system. The pathophysiology of schizophrenia is not fully understood, and this lack of knowledge about etiology limits rational drug development. The clinical effectiveness of the various antipsychotic agents has provided useful clues, however. In particular, the pharmacology of the typical antipsychotic agents has formed the basis of the dopamine model of schizophrenia, which posits that dysregulated levels of dopamine in the brain play a role in the pathophysiology of the disease. The effectiveness of the atypical antipsychotic agents, which affect the function of several different receptor types, has highlighted the fact that the dopamine hypothesis is a simplification. The atypical agents represent an attractive new modality for treating schizophrenia because they have fewer extrapyramidal effects and are more effective for some disease symptoms than the typical antipsychotics.

Future developments in the treatment of Parkinson's disease and schizophrenia are focused on creating more selective agents within the current drug classes and on better elucidating the underlying pathophysiology of the disorders. New dopamine receptor agonists with higher selectivity, particularly those that bind D1 receptors, may one day provide more effective treatment for Parkinson's disease with less severe adverse effects. The development of newer antipsychotics with increased receptor selectivity may similarly expand the therapeutic options for treating schizophrenia. Because Parkinson's disease involves the death of dopaminergic neurons, much effort is currently directed at neuroprotective drugs that may slow the progression of the disease. Further research into a potential role for a glutamate deficit in the pathophysiology of schizophrenia may yield new therapeutics for this disorder. For example, the development of selective glutamate receptor agonists may one day complement or even replace the use of dopamine receptor antagonists. Another important advance in the treatment of schizophrenia will likely result from the elucidation of models for the mechanism of the atypical antipsychotics, which will allow rational development of more effective drugs.

Acknowledgment

We thank Joshua M. Galanter for his valuable contributions to this chapter in the First and Second Editions of *Principles of Pharmacology: The Pathophysiologic Basis of Drug Therapy*.

Suggested Reading

Albin RL, Young AB, Penney JB. The functional anatomy of basal ganglia disorders. *Trends Neurosci* 1989;12:366–375. (*A classic article that describes the concept of "direct" and "indirect" pathways.*)

Connolly BS, Lang AE. Pharmacological treatment of Parkinson disease: a review. *JAMA* 2014;16:1670–1683. (*A comprehensive, evidence-based evaluation of current therapies.*)

George M, Amrutheshwar R, Rajkumar RP, Kattimani S, Dkhar SA. Newer antipsychotics and upcoming molecules for schizophrenia. *Eur J Clin Pharmacol* 2013;69:1497–1509. (*A review of recently approved antipsychotic agents.*)

Goldman JG, Weintraub D. Advances in the treatment of cognitive impairment in Parkinson's disease. *Mov Disord* 2015;30:1471–1489. (*A review of current treatments and future therapeutic opportunities and challenges.*)

Howes OD, Kambeitz J, Kim E, et al. The nature of dopamine dysfunction in schizophrenia and what this means for treatment. *Arch Gen Psychiatry* 2012;69:776–786. (*A review of the evidence for dopamine dysfunction in schizophrenia, emphasizing the presence of presynaptic defects.*)

Kalia LV, Kalia SK, Lang AE. Disease-modifying strategies for Parkinson's disease. *Mov Disord* 2015;30:1442–1450. (*A review of current clinical trials of disease-modifying therapies for Parkinson's disease.*)

Naber D, Lambert M. The CATIE and CUtLASS studies in schizophrenia: implications for clinicians. *CNS Drugs* 2009;23:649–659. (*Discusses the major trials comparing typical and atypical antipsychotics on the basis of efficacy, adverse effect profiles, and cost.*)

Suchowersky O, Reich S, Perlmutter J, et al. Practice parameter: diagnosis and prognosis of new onset Parkinson disease (an evidence-based review). Report of the Quality Standards Subcommittee of the American Academy of Neurology. *Neurology* 2006;66:968–975. (*This "parameter," as well as several others published in the same issue, represents the product of a careful review of the evidence for the effectiveness of various treatments for Parkinson's disease.*)

Thenganatt MA, Jankovic J. Parkinson disease subtypes. *JAMA Neurol* 2014;4:499–504. (*A comprehensive literature review of the spectrum of features seen in Parkinson disease.*)

Trinh J, Farrer M. Advances in the genetics of Parkinson disease. *Nat Rev Neurol* 2013;8:445–454. (*A review of the rapidly evolving genetics of Parkinson's disease.*)

DRUG SUMMARY TABLE: CHAPTER 14 Pharmacology of Dopaminergic Neurotransmission

DRUG	CLINICAL APPLICATIONS	*SERIOUS* AND COMMON ADVERSE EFFECTS	CONTRAINDICATIONS	THERAPEUTIC CONSIDERATIONS
DOPAMINE PRECURSORS **Mechanism—Provide substrate for increased dopamine synthesis; levodopa is transported across the blood–brain barrier by the neutral amino acid transporter and then decarboxylated to dopamine by the enzyme aromatic L-amino acid decarboxylase (AADC)**				
Levodopa	Parkinson's disease	*Dyskinesia, heart disease, orthostatic hypotension, psychotic disorder* Loss of appetite, nausea, vomiting	Hypersensitivity to levodopa Concomitant use of MAO inhibitor	Levodopa, when administered alone, has low availability in CNS due to peripheral metabolism to dopamine; therefore, it is almost always administered in combination with carbidopa, an inhibitor of DOPA decarboxylase. Continued use results in both tolerance and sensitization; patients develop periods of increased rigidity alternating with periods of normal or dyskinetic movement. Dyskinesias are nearly ubiquitous in patients within 5 years of starting levodopa; as the disease progresses, continued levodopa therapy leads to worsening of both the dyskinesias and the "on/off" phenomenon.
DOPAMINE RECEPTOR AGONISTS **Mechanism—These agonists bind to and activate postsynaptic dopamine receptors directly; they are relatively selective for D3>D2 dopamine receptors**				
Pramipexole **Ropinirole** **Rotigotine**	Parkinson's disease Restless leg syndrome	*Heart failure, malignant melanoma, sleep attack* Orthostatic hypotension, constipation, amnesia, asthenia, extrapyramidal movements, somnolence, dizziness, hallucinations, dream disorder	Hypersensitivity to pramipexole, ropinirole, or rotigotine	Dopamine agonists have half-lives longer than that of levodopa, which allows for less frequent dosing. Cognitive effects can include excessive sedation, vivid dreams, and hallucinations. Some studies suggest that use of dopamine agonists rather than levodopa as initial treatment for Parkinson's disease delays the onset of "off" periods and dyskinesias, especially in younger individuals.
INHIBITORS OF LEVODOPA OR DOPAMINE METABOLISM **Mechanism—Inhibit breakdown of dopamine in the CNS by inhibiting MAO-B (rasagiline and selegiline) or COMT (tolcapone); inhibit breakdown of levodopa by COMT in the periphery (entacapone and tolcapone)**				
Rasagiline **Selegiline**	Parkinson's disease	*Hypertension, serotonin syndrome (rasagiline only); atrial fibrillation, hypertensive crisis, suicidal thoughts (selegiline only)* Orthostatic hypotension, dyskinesia, rash, dyspepsia, arthralgia, headache, weight loss (shared adverse effects); somnolence, hallucinations, increased risk of melanoma (rasagiline only); insomnia, application site reaction (selegiline only)	Shared contraindications: Hypersensitivity to rasagiline or selegiline Concomitant use of cyclobenzaprine, mirtazapine, St. John's wort Concomitant use of dextromethorphan due to risk of psychosis Concomitant use of other monoamine oxidase inhibitors (MAOIs) or sympathomimetic amines due to risk of severe hypertensive reactions	Selegiline in low doses is selective for MAO-B, which predominates in the striatum; higher doses inhibit MAO-A as well as MAO-B, with associated risks of toxicity. Selegiline forms the potentially toxic metabolite amphetamine, which may lead to insomnia and confusion (especially in the elderly).

Drug	Indication	Adverse Effects	Contraindications	Therapeutic Considerations
			Concomitant use of meperidine, methadone, propoxyphene, tramadol due to risk of severe hypertension or hypotension, malignant hyperpyrexia, or coma Elective surgery requiring general anesthesia Tyramine-rich foods Selegiline only: Concomitant use of selective serotonin reuptake inhibitors, serotonin-norepinephrine reuptake inhibitors, and tricyclic antidepressants Concomitant use of carbamazepine and oxcarbazepine Concomitant use of cocaine or local anesthesia containing sympathomimetic vasoconstrictors Concomitant use of sympathomimetic amines that contain vasoconstrictors such as pseudoephedrine, phenylephrine, phenylpropanolamine, ephedrine, amphetamine Pheochromocytoma	Rasagiline does not form toxic metabolites. Both rasagiline and selegiline improve motor function when used alone and can augment the effectiveness of levodopa.
Tolcapone **Entacapone**	Parkinson's disease	*Rhabdomyolysis, neuroleptic malignant syndrome, hallucinations [shared adverse effects]; dystonia, fulminant hepatic failure, neoplasm of the skin, sleep attack, pleural effusion, pulmonary fibrosis (tolcapone only)* Gastrointestinal upset, dyskinesia (shared adverse effects); orthostatic hypotension, diaphoresis, muscle cramping, confusion, dizziness, headache, dream disorder, upper respiratory infection (tolcapone only); hyperactive behavior (entacapone only)	Hypersensitivity to tolcapone or entacapone Tolcapone only: History of rhabdomyolysis or hyperpyrexia related to tolcapone Liver disease	Tolcapone is a highly lipid-soluble agent that can cross the blood–brain barrier, while entacapone distributes only to the periphery. COMT inhibitors can be used in combination with carbidopa to further enhance the plasma half-life of levodopa; COMT inhibitors have been shown in some trials to reduce the "off" periods that are associated with decreasing plasma levodopa levels. Rare but fatal hepatic toxicity has been reported with tolcapone use. Entacapone is the more widely used COMT inhibitor.

continues

DRUG SUMMARY TABLE: CHAPTER 14 Pharmacology of Dopaminergic Neurotransmission *continued*

DRUG	CLINICAL APPLICATIONS	SERIOUS AND COMMON ADVERSE EFFECTS	CONTRAINDICATIONS	THERAPEUTIC CONSIDERATIONS
MISCELLANEOUS ANTIPARKINSONIAN DRUGS Mechanism—Amantadine's therapeutic mechanism in the treatment of Parkinson's disease is thought to be related to antagonism of excitatory NMDA receptors; trihexyphenidyl and benztropine are muscarinic receptor antagonists that reduce cholinergic tone in the CNS by modifying the actions of striatal cholinergic interneurons				
Amantadine	Parkinson's disease Influenza A Extrapyramidal disease	*Heart failure, malignant melanoma, leukopenia, neutropenia, immune hypersensitivity reaction, neuroleptic malignant syndrome, exacerbation of mental disorder* Insomnia, dizziness, hallucinations, agitation, orthostatic hypotension, peripheral edema, gastrointestinal upset	Hypersensitivity to amantadine	Amantadine was developed as an antiviral that reduces the length and severity of influenza A infections; in patients with Parkinson's disease, amantadine is used to treat levodopa-induced dyskinesias that develop late in the course of the disease. May exacerbate mental illness in patients with psychiatric illness or substance abuse problems.
Trihexyphenidyl **Benztropine**	Parkinson's disease (shared indication) Extrapyramidal disease (benztropine only)	*Paralytic ileus, confusion (shared adverse effects); glaucoma (trihexyphenidyl only); anhidrosis, heatstroke, psychosis (benztropine only)* Dizziness, blurred vision, nausea, xerostomia (shared adverse effects); nervousness (trihexyphenidyl only); urinary retention (benztropine only)	Hypersensitivity to trihexyphenidyl or benztropine Narrow-angle glaucoma	Trihexyphenidyl and benztropine reduce tremor more than bradykinesia and are therefore effective in treating patients for whom tremor is the major clinical manifestation of Parkinson's disease. May worsen dementia and cognitive impairment in the elderly.
ANTIPSYCHOTIC AGENTS Mechanism—Antagonize mesolimbic, and possibly mesocortical, D2 receptors; adverse effects are likely mediated by binding to D2 receptors in basal ganglia (nigrostriatal pathway) and pituitary gland				
Phenothiazines and derivatives: **Chlorpromazine** **Thioridazine** **Mesoridazine** **Perphenazine** **Fluphenazine** **Thiothixene** **Trifluoperazine** **Chlorprothixene**	Psychotic disorder (shared indication) Nausea and vomiting (chlorpromazine and perphenazine only) Chlorpromazine only: Intractable hiccoughs Acute intermittent porphyria Tetanus	*Systemic lupus erythematosus (shared adverse effect); prolonged QT interval (chlorpromazine, mesoridazine, perphenazine, thiothixene, and trifluoperazine only); ineffective thermoregulation (chlorpromazine, mesoridazine, perphenazine, thiothixene, and trifluoperazine only); paralytic ileus, anemia, leukopenia, jaundice, dystonia, neuroleptic malignant syndrome, seizure, priapism (chlorpromazine only)* Hypotension, gastrointestinal upset, xerostomia, dizziness, parkinsonism, somnolence (shared adverse effects); blurred vision, urinary retention, nasal congestion (thioridazine, mesoridazine, perphenazine, thiothixene, and trifluoperazine only)	Hypersensitivity to phenothiazines Severe toxic central nervous system depression or comatose states (shared contraindications) Concomitant administration of drugs that prolong QT interval or patients with prolonged QT interval (thioridazine and mesoridazine only) Blood dyscrasias (perphenazine, thiothixene, and trifluoperazine only) Bone marrow depression (trifluoperazine and perphenazine only) Circulatory collapse (thiothixene and chlorprothixene only) Subcortical brain damage (perphenazine only) Thioridazine only: History of cardiac arrhythmias Concomitant use with drugs that inhibit CYP2D6 Hypertensive or hypotensive heart disease	In general, aliphatic phenothiazines are less potent antagonists at D2 receptors than butyrophenones, thioxanthenes, or phenothiazines functionalized with a piperazine derivative. The potency of the typical antipsychotics is critical in determining the drugs' adverse effect profile; high-potency drugs tend to have fewer sedative effects and cause less postural hypotension than drugs with lower potency; on the other hand, lower potency typical antipsychotics tend to cause fewer extrapyramidal effects. Fluphenazine is available as decanoate ester, delivered intramuscularly every 3–4 weeks. Administration of typical antipsychotics to patients with Parkinson's disease often leads to marked worsening of parkinsonian symptoms. Typical antipsychotics potentiate the sedative effects of benzodiazepines and centrally active antihistamines.

continues

Butyrophenones: **Haloperidol** **Droperidol**	Psychoses Tourette's syndrome (haloperidol only) Nausea and vomiting; anesthesia adjunct (droperidol only)	*Prolonged QT interval, neuroleptic malignant syndrome, extrapyramidal disease (shared adverse effects); paralytic ileus, seizure, priapism (haloperidol only)* Hypotension, somnolence (shared adverse effects); constipation, xerostomia, blurred vision (haloperidol only); tachycardia, anxiety (droperidol only)	Hypersensitivity to haloperidol or droperidol Parkinson's disease Severe toxic central nervous system depression or comatose states (haloperidol only) QT interval prolongation (droperidol only)	Haloperidol is the most widely used butyrophenone. Haloperidol is available as decanoate ester, delivered intramuscularly every 3–4 weeks; this formulation is useful for treating poorly adherent patients.
Other typical antipsychotics: **Loxapine** **Molindone** **Pimozide**	Psychotic disorders (shared indication) Tourette's syndrome (pimozide only)	*Stroke, parkinsonism (loxapine only); neuroleptic malignant syndrome, tardive dyskinesia (molindone only); parkinsonism, prolonged QT interval, ineffective thermoregulation (pimozide only)* Anticholinergic symptoms, sedation (shared adverse effects); vision alteration (pimozide only)	Hypersensitivity to loxapine, molindone, or pimozide Comatose or severe drug-induced depressed states (shared contraindications) Lung disease associated with bronchospasm (loxapine only) Pimozide only: Concomitant pemoline, methylphenidate, or amphetamines that may cause motor and phonic tics Concomitant dofetilide, sotalol, quinidine, other Class IA and III antiarrhythmics, mesoridazine, thioridazine, chlorpromazine, or droperidol Concomitant sparfloxacin, gatifloxacin, moxifloxacin, halofantrine, mefloquine, pentamidine, arsenic trioxide, levomethadyl acetate, dolasetron mesylate, probucol, tacrolimus, ziprasidone, sertraline, or macrolide antibiotics Concurrent administration with drugs that have demonstrated QT prolongation and inhibitors of CYP3A4 (zileuton, fluvoxamine) Concomitant use of citalopram, escitalopram, sertraline, or nefazodone History of cardiac arrhythmias	Molindone exerts its antipsychotic effects on the ascending reticular activating system in the absence of muscle relaxation and incoordination effects. Pimozide has more specific dopamine receptor antagonism and less α-adrenergic receptor blocking activity than other neuroleptic agents, which results in less potential for inducing sedation and hypotension.

DRUG SUMMARY TABLE: CHAPTER 14 Pharmacology of Dopaminergic Neurotransmission *continued*

DRUG	CLINICAL APPLICATIONS	*SERIOUS* AND COMMON ADVERSE EFFECTS	CONTRAINDICATIONS	THERAPEUTIC CONSIDERATIONS
ATYPICAL ANTIPSYCHOTIC AGENTS **Mechanism—Combined antagonist properties at dopamine D2 and serotonin 5-HT2 receptors; clozapine and olanzapine are also dopamine D4 receptor antagonists.**				
Risperidone **Olanzapine** **Ziprasidone** **Paliperidone** **Quetiapine** **Aripiprazole** **Iloperidone** **Lurasidone** **Asenapine**	Psychotic disorders Bipolar disorder Depression (adjunct) Autism (risperidone and aripiprazole only)	*Hyperglycemia, diabetic ketoacidosis, coma, QT prolongation (shared adverse effects); hyperthermia (risperidone and aripiprazole only); agranulocytosis (risperidone, paliperidone, quetiapine, aripiprazole, and lurasidone only); priapism (risperidone, paliperidone, and quetiapine only); pulmonary embolism (risperidone and olanzapine only); stroke (olanzapine, aripiprazole, and iloperidone only); neuroleptic malignant syndrome (aripiprazole, lurasidone, and asenapine only); suicidal ideation (aripiprazole and iloperidone only); thrombocytopenia (risperidone only); status epilepticus (olanzapine only); rhabdomyolysis (aripiprazole only)* Anticholinergic symptoms, sedation, weight gain, mild extrapyramidal symptoms (shared adverse effects); increased prolactin level (olanzapine, paliperidone, and iloperidone only); gastrointestinal upset (quetiapine, aripiprazole, and lurasidone only); anxiety (quetiapine and aripiprazole only); increased blood pressure (quetiapine only)	Hypersensitivity to the drug Concomitant use with strong CYP3A4 inducers or inhibitors	Atypical antipsychotics are more effective than typical antipsychotics at treating the negative symptoms of schizophrenia. Atypical antipsychotics cause significantly milder extrapyramidal symptoms than typical antipsychotics. Risperidone binds to D2, 5-HT$_2$, α_1, α_2, H$_1$ receptors. Olanzapine binds to D1–D4, 5-HT$_2$, α_1, H$_1$, M1–M5 receptors. Ziprasidone binds to D2, 5-HT$_1$, 5-HT$_2$, α_1, H$_1$ receptors. Paliperidone is the active metabolite of risperidone. Quetiapine binds to D1, D2, 5-HT$_1$, 5-HT$_2$, α_1, α_2, H$_1$ receptors. Aripiprazole is a D2 and 5-HT$_{1A}$ partial agonist and a 5-HT$_{2A}$ antagonist. Iloperidone is a D2 and 5-HT$_{2A}$ antagonist, with higher affinity for 5-HT$_{2A}$ than D2. Quetiapine and clozapine (below) have the lowest incidence of causing extrapyramidal symptoms. Aripiprazole, lurasidone, and asenapine have potent activity in blocking 5-HT$_7$, α_{2A}, and α_{2C} receptors and are most commonly used to augment treatment of depression or bipolar disorder. Asenapine is available only in a sublingual dosage form.
Clozapine	Schizophrenia refractory to other antipsychotics	*Cardiomyopathy, myocarditis, prolonged QT interval, Stevens-Johnson syndrome, diabetes mellitus, diabetic ketoacidosis, agranulocytosis, thrombocytopenia, neuroleptic malignant syndrome, seizure, glaucoma, pneumonia, pulmonary embolism* Anticholinergic symptoms, tachycardia, gastrointestinal upset, sedation, weight gain, fever	History of clozapine-induced agranulocytosis or severe granulocytopenia Myeloproliferative disorders	Clozapine has not been used as a first-line agent because of a small but significant risk of agranulocytosis. Clozapine binds to D1–D5, 5-HT$_2$, α_1, H$_1$, muscarinic receptors.

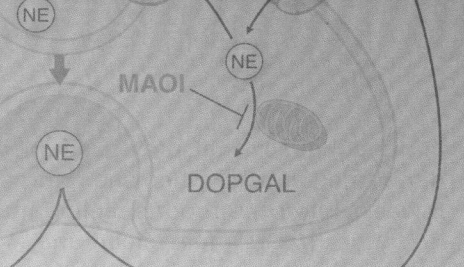

15

Pharmacology of Serotonergic and Central Adrenergic Neurotransmission

Stephen J. Haggarty and Roy H. Perlis

▮ INTRODUCTION

This chapter introduces the neurotransmitter **serotonin** (5-hydroxytryptamine; 5-HT), which is a target for many drugs used to treat psychiatric disorders related to depression and anxiety. Some of these medications also affect **norepinephrine (NE)** neurotransmission, and both neurotransmitter pathways are believed to be central to the modulation of mood. The various mechanisms by which drugs can alter serotonin and norepinephrine signaling are discussed. Although many such drugs function as antidepressants or anti-anxiety medications, interventions in this pharmacologic group are also effective treatments for migraine headache, irritable bowel syndrome, and other conditions. **Lithium** and some other drugs used to treat bipolar disorder are also discussed.

The major mood disorders are defined by the presence of depressive and/or manic or hypomanic episodes. Patients with recurrent depressive episodes and no history of mania or hypomania are said to have **major depressive disorder (MDD)**; patients who have experienced at least one manic or hypomanic episode, with or without an additional history of depressive episodes, are said to have **bipolar disorder (BD)**. The lifetime prevalence of MDD is approximately 17%, whereas that of BD is 1% to 2%. MDD can occur as an isolated illness or can be comorbid with other diseases such as stroke, dementia, diabetes, cancer, and coronary artery disease. Although twin studies suggest that up to 1/3 of the risk for MDD is heritable, environmental stress such as early traumatic experiences are also associated with risk. Aging and cerebral atherosclerosis are also associated with late-onset depression in the elderly. In addition to genetic and environmental triggers, many classes of drugs can precipitate or exacerbate depressive episodes (e.g., interferon, glucocorticoids, and chemotherapeutic agents). BD has a particularly strong heritable risk, even though environmental factors are often triggers for the mood episodes themselves. Although mania is a characteristic of BD, patients spend significant periods of their lives depressed, and depressive symptoms are strongly associated with the elevated risk for suicide among mood disorders. (Of note, in the majority of suicides, a physician [not necessarily a psychiatrist] will have seen the patient less than 1 month before the suicide.)

Both MDD and BD are major causes of morbidity worldwide, resulting in lost productivity and substantial use of medical resources. The World Health Organization (WHO) projects that a major depression will be the leading cause of disease burden by the year 2030, ahead of ischemic heart disease, road traffic incidents, and cerebrovascular disease.

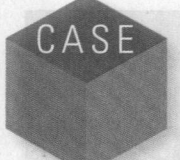

CASE

Mary R is a 27-year-old office worker who presents to her primary care physician, Dr. Lee, with an 8-lb. weight loss over the previous 2 months. Ms. R tearfully explains that she is plagued by near-constant feelings of sadness and by a sense of helplessness and inadequacy at work. She feels so terrible that she has not had a good night of sleep in more than a month. She no longer enjoys living and has recently become scared when new thoughts of suicide enter her mind. Ms. R tells Dr. Lee that she had felt like this once before, but it had passed after several months. Dr. Lee asks her about her sleep patterns, appetite levels, ability to concentrate, energy level, mood, interest level, and feelings of guilt. He asks her specific questions about thoughts of suicide, particularly whether she has formed a specific plan and whether she has ever attempted suicide. Dr. Lee explains to Ms. R that she has major depressive disorder, likely caused by specific abnormalities in the function of her brain circuitry, and he prescribes the antidepressant fluoxetine.

Two weeks later, Ms. R calls to indicate that the medicine is not working. Dr. Lee encourages her to continue taking the medicine, and after 2 more weeks, Ms. R begins to feel better. She no longer feels sad and demoralized; the feelings of helplessness and inadequacy that previously plagued her have diminished. In fact, when she returns to see Dr. Lee 6 weeks later, she reports feeling much better. She no longer needs much sleep and is always full of energy. She is now convinced that she is the most intelligent person in her company. She proudly tells Dr. Lee that she has recently purchased a new sports car and gone on a large shopping spree. After taking a more detailed history, Dr. Lee tells Ms. R that she may be having a manic episode and, in consultation with a psychiatrist, prescribes lithium and gradually tapers the fluoxetine. Ms. R is hesitant to take the new medication, arguing that she feels fine and that she is concerned about the adverse effects of lithium.

Questions

1. How is a depressive episode different from occasionally "feeling blue"?

2. What caused Ms. R's mania? Why is it necessary to treat bipolar disorder if the patient "feels good"?

3. Why is there a delay in the onset of fluoxetine's therapeutic effect?

4. What specific concerns might Ms. R have about the adverse effects of lithium?

■ BIOCHEMISTRY AND PHYSIOLOGY OF SEROTONERGIC AND CENTRAL ADRENERGIC NEUROTRANSMISSION

Serotonin (5-hydroxytryptamine; 5-HT) and norepinephrine (NE) have critical roles in modulating mood, the sleep–wake cycle, motivation and reward, cognitive processing, pain perception, neuroendocrine function, and other physiologic processes. Serotonergic projections to the spinal cord modulate pain perception, visceral regulation, and motor control, while projections to the forebrain are important in modulating mood, cognition, and neuroendocrine function. The noradrenergic system modulates vigilance, stress responses, neuroendocrine function, pain control, and sympathetic nervous system activity. The wide variety of behavioral and psychological processes regulated by these two neurotransmitters explains the similarly wide variety of disorders that can be treated by medications that alter the levels or postsynaptic signaling of 5-HT and/or NE.

5-HT and NE are primarily released from nonsynaptic neuronal varicosities. Unlike synapses, which form tight contacts with specific target neurons, varicosities release large amounts of neurotransmitter from vesicles into the extracellular space, establishing concentration gradients of neurotransmitter in the projection areas of the varicosities. 5-HT-containing cells within the **raphe nuclei** and NE-containing cells within the **locus ceruleus** project broadly throughout the cerebral cortex, while dopamine has a more focused pattern of projections. Each of these systems has prominent presynaptic autoreceptors that control local transmitter concentrations. This autoregulation results in coordinated firing, which causes spontaneous and synchronous waves of activity that can be measured as firing frequencies; for example, the cells within the raphe nuclei usually fire at rates between 0.3 and 7 spikes per second. Because the frequency of basal (tonic) firing does not change rapidly and the quanta of neurotransmitter released with each discharge are fairly well conserved, the neurotransmitter concentration in the vicinity of the varicosities is maintained within a narrow range.

The mean concentration establishes the baseline **tone** of activity in the target neurons that receive 5-HT and NE projections. In addition, specific stimuli can elicit rapid bursts of firing that are superimposed on the baseline tonic activity. Diffusely projecting systems can thus provide two types of information: a rapid and discrete neuronal firing akin to more traditional neurotransmission and a slower tonic firing that presumably allows for integration of information over a longer period of time.

Serotonin Synthesis and Regulation

Serotonin is synthesized from the amino acid tryptophan by the enzyme **tryptophan hydroxylase (TPH)**, which converts tryptophan to **5-hydroxytryptophan**. **Aromatic L-amino acid decarboxylase** then converts 5-hydroxytryptophan to serotonin (Fig. 15-1A). These enzymes are present throughout the cytoplasm of serotonergic neurons, both in the cell body and in cell processes. Serotonin is concentrated and stored within vesicles located in axons, cell bodies, and dendrites.

The biochemistry of norepinephrine synthesis and regulation is discussed in Chapter 11, Adrenergic Pharmacology. For review, the synthesis of norepinephrine is summarized in Figure 15-1B.

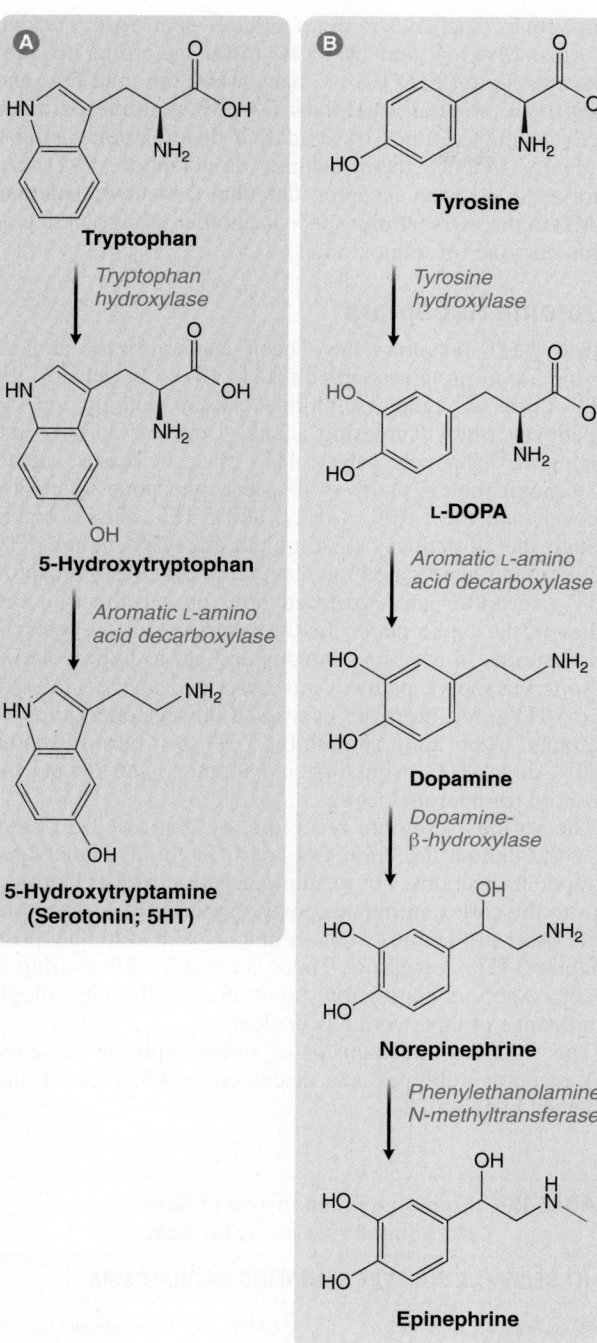

The serotonin metabolic cycle (Fig. 15-2) involves synthesis, uptake into synaptic vesicles, exocytosis, reuptake into the cytoplasm, and then either uptake into vesicles or degradation. The metabolic cycle of norepinephrine is summarized in Figure 15-3. Importantly, regulation of the levels of 5-HT and NE neurotransmission can occur at any of these steps.

For all monoamines, the first synthetic step is rate-limiting. Thus, 5-HT synthesis is rate-limited by **tryptophan hydroxylase (TPH)**, and DA and NE synthesis is rate-limited by **tyrosine hydroxylase (TH)**. Both enzymes are tightly regulated by inhibitory feedback via autoreceptor-mediated signaling. 5-HT presynaptic autoreceptors respond to locally increased 5-HT concentrations by G_i protein signaling, which decreases TPH activity and serotonergic neuron firing. Although other explanations exist, this autoregulatory loop could be one explanation for the observed time course of clinical action of antidepressants, which is discussed below (see "The Monoamine Theory of Depression").

5-HT is transported into vesicles by the vesicular monoamine transporter (VMAT). The transporter is a nonspecific monoamine transporter that is important for the vesicular packaging of dopamine (DA) and epinephrine (EPI) as well

FIGURE 15-1. Synthesis of serotonin and norepinephrine. A. 5-Hydroxytryptamine (serotonin) is synthesized from the amino acid tryptophan in two steps: the hydroxylation of tryptophan to form 5-hydroxytryptophan by tryptophan hydroxylase and the subsequent decarboxylation of this intermediate to produce 5-hydroxytryptamine (5-HT) by aromatic L-amino acid decarboxylase. Tryptophan hydroxylase is the rate-limiting enzyme in this pathway. **B.** Norepinephrine is synthesized from the amino acid tyrosine in a three-step process similar to the synthetic pathway for serotonin. Tyrosine is first oxidized to L-DOPA by the enzyme tyrosine hydroxylase and then decarboxylated to dopamine. After dopamine is transported into the synaptic vesicle, it is hydroxylated by the enzyme dopamine β-hydroxylase to form norepinephrine. The same enzyme decarboxylates 5-hydroxytryptophan and L-DOPA; it is known generically as aromatic L-amino acid decarboxylase. Tyrosine hydroxylase is the rate-limiting enzyme in this pathway.

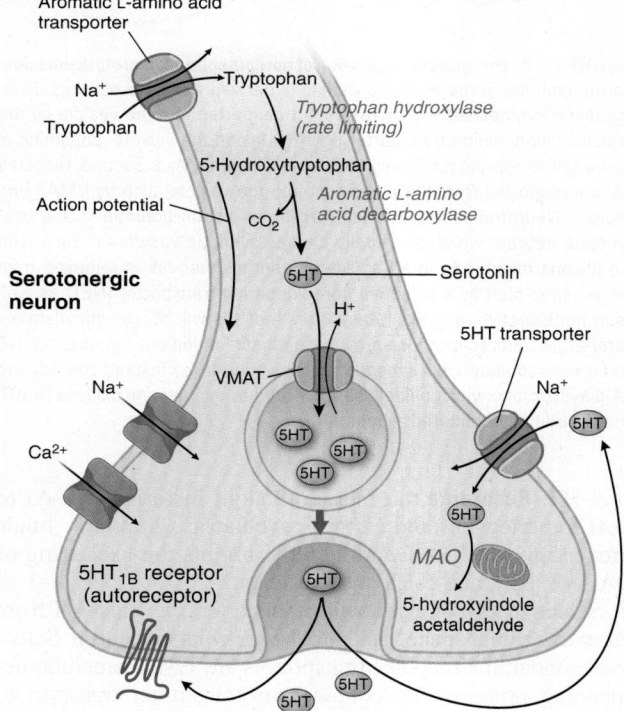

FIGURE 15-2. Presynaptic regulation of serotonin neurotransmission. Serotonin (5-HT) is synthesized from tryptophan in a two-reaction pathway: the rate-limiting enzyme is tryptophan hydroxylase. Both newly synthesized 5-HT and recycled 5-HT are transported from the cytoplasm into synaptic vesicles by the vesicular monoamine transporter (VMAT). Neurotransmission is initiated by an action potential in the presynaptic neuron, which eventually causes synaptic vesicles to fuse with the plasma membrane in a Ca^{2+}-dependent manner. 5-HT is removed from the synaptic cleft by a selective 5-HT transporter (SERT) as well as by nonselective reuptake transporters (not shown). 5-HT can stimulate 5-HT$_{1B}$ autoreceptors on the presynaptic membrane to provide feedback inhibition. Cytoplasmic 5-HT is either sequestered in synaptic vesicles by VMAT or degraded by mitochondrial monoamine oxidase (MAO).

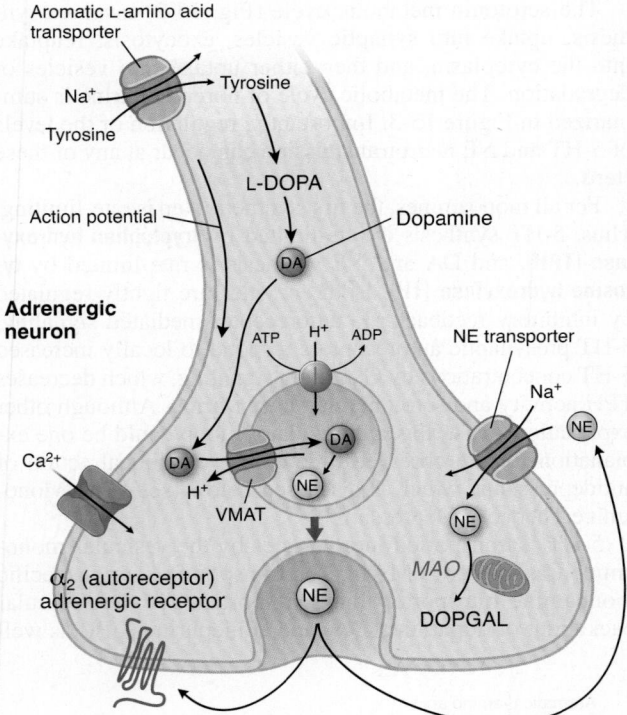

FIGURE 15-3. Presynaptic regulation of norepinephrine neurotransmission. Norepinephrine in the synaptic vesicle is derived from two sources. First, dopamine synthesized from tyrosine is transported into the vesicle by the vesicular monoamine transporter (VMAT). Inside the vesicle, dopamine is converted to norepinephrine by dopamine β-hydroxylase. Second, recycled NE is transported from the cytoplasm into the vesicle, also by VMAT (*not shown*). Neurotransmission is initiated by an action potential in the presynaptic neuron, which eventually causes synaptic vesicles to fuse with the plasma membrane in a Ca^{2+}-dependent manner. NE is removed from the synaptic cleft by a selective norepinephrine transporter (NET) as well as by nonselective reuptake transporters (*not shown*). NE can stimulate α_2-adrenergic autoreceptors to provide feedback inhibition. Cytoplasmic NE that is not sequestered in synaptic vesicles by VMAT is instead degraded to 3,4-dihydroxyphenylglycoaldehyde (DOPGAL) by monoamine oxidase (MAO) on the outer mitochondrial membrane.

as 5-HT. **Reserpine**, an indole alkaloid historically used to treat hypertension and certain psychiatric symptoms, binds irreversibly to VMAT and thereby inhibits the packaging of DA, NE, EPI, and 5-HT into vesicles.

Selective serotonin reuptake transporters recycle 5-HT from the extracellular space back into the presynaptic neuron. Selective monoamine reuptake transporters are 12-transmembrane-spanning proteins that couple neurotransmitter transport to the transmembrane sodium gradient. Unlike VMAT, which is a nonspecific monoamine transporter, the individual monoamine reuptake transporters show selectivity, high affinity, and low capacity for each individual monoamine. The selective monoamine transporters, which include the **serotonin transporter (SERT)**, **norepinephrine transporter (NET)**, and **dopamine transporter (DAT)**, are also capable of transporting the other monoamines, although less efficiently.

Once 5-HT is returned to the neuronal cytoplasm, the neurotransmitter is transported into vesicles via VMAT or degraded by the **monoamine oxidase (MAO)** system. MAOs are mitochondrial enzymes that regulate the levels of monoamines in neural tissues and inactivate circulating and dietary

monoamines (such as tyramine) in the liver and gut. The two isoforms, MAO-A and MAO-B, differ according to substrate specificity: MAO-A oxidizes 5-HT, NE, and DA, and MAO-B preferentially oxidizes DA. Monoamine oxidases inactivate monoamines by oxidative deamination, using a covalently attached flavin adenine dinucleotide (FAD) cofactor as an electron acceptor. **Catechol-O-methyltransferase (COMT)** in the extracellular space is another important degradation enzyme for monoamines.

Serotonin Receptors

Fifteen 5-HT receptors have been characterized, and all but one are G protein-coupled (Table 15-1). In general, the 5-HT$_1$ class of receptors inhibits cellular activity via the G$_i$ pathway (thus decreasing adenylyl cyclase activity and opening K$^+$ channels), the 5-HT$_2$ class increases signaling through the G$_q$ pathway to cause phosphatidylinositol turnover, and the 5-HT$_4$, 5-HT$_6$, and 5-HT$_7$ classes signal through the G$_s$ pathway to stimulate adenylyl cyclase. The only known ligand-gated ion channel is the 5-HT$_3$ receptor. 5-HT$_{1A}$ receptors are expressed both on serotonergic cell bodies in the raphe nuclei (autoreceptors) and on postsynaptic neurons in the hippocampus and act to hyperpolarize neurons via the G$_i$ pathway (as described above). Presynaptic 5-HT$_{1B}$ receptors are expressed on serotonergic nerve terminals, where they autoinhibit 5-HT neurotransmission. 5-HT$_{2A}$ and 5-HT$_{2C}$ signaling is excitatory and lowers the threshold for neuronal firing.

The various serotonin receptors are expressed differentially throughout the brain and are differentially innervated by raphe projections. For example, a subset of 5-HT projections to the cortex stimulates postsynaptic 5-HT$_{2A}$ receptors, while other projections to the limbic system stimulate postsynaptic 5-HT$_{1A}$ receptors. There is considerable overlap of receptor subtype expression, however, and the physiologic significance of this overlap is unclear.

The signaling mechanisms of norepinephrine (adrenergic) receptor subtypes are discussed in Chapter 11 and reviewed in Table 15-1.

TABLE 15-1 Signaling Mechanisms of Serotonin and Norepinephrine Receptor Subtypes

5-HT RECEPTOR SUBTYPE SIGNALING MECHANISMS	
5-HT$_{1A,B*,D,E,F}$	↓ cAMP, ↑ K$^+$ channel opening
5-HT$_{2A,B,C}$	↑ IP$_3$, DAG
5-HT$_3$	Ligand-gated ion channel
5-HT$_{4,6,7}$	↑ cAMP
NE RECEPTOR SUBTYPE	
α_1	↑ IP$_3$, DAG
α_2*	↓ cAMP
$\beta_{1,2}$	↑ cAMP

Abbreviations: cAMP, cyclic AMP; DAG, diacylglycerol; IP$_3$, inositol 1,4,5-trisphosphate
*5-HT$_{1B}$ serotonin receptors and α_2-adrenergic receptors are presynaptic autoreceptors important for feedback inhibition.

PATHOPHYSIOLOGY OF AFFECTIVE DISORDERS

Major depressive disorder (MDD) and bipolar disorder (BD) are characterized by mood dysregulation. MDD is typified by single or recurrent depressive episodes, whereas BD is defined by the presence of mania or hypomania as well as periods of depression.

The **monoamine hypothesis** proposes that decreased serotonin and/or norepinephrine levels cause mood disorders, based largely on the molecular mechanism of action of known antidepressants as well as animal models suggested to correspond to depression or mania. More current research suggests that these disorders reflect complex disturbances in neural circuit activity rather than a simple chemical imbalance. However, because the underlying etiologies of these disorders are still not well understood at a physiologic or molecular level, diagnostic criteria rely solely on clinical evaluation. To date, despite intriguing findings from neuroimaging and transcriptomic studies, no reliable biomarkers for these disorders have been identified. The American Psychiatric Association diagnostic criteria for MDD and BD are summarized in Boxes 15-1 and 15-2.

Clinical Characteristics of Affective Disorders

Major depressive disorder (MDD) is characterized by single or recurrent episodes of depressed mood, social isolation (including apathy, decreased ability to experience pleasure, and feelings of worthlessness), and characteristic somatic symptoms (decreased energy, changes in appetite and sleep, muscle pain, and slowing of movement with speech latency). Episodes are sometimes precipitated by major life events or stresses, although they may also occur spontaneously. A single depressive episode must last 2 weeks or longer and must interfere significantly with the patient's daily functions, such as work and personal relationships. An episode is not considered to be MDD if it is due to a general medical condition such as hypothyroidism or Cushing's disease.

In all depressed patients, it is crucial to determine whether there is any suicidality and whether there is evidence of psychosis. Although psychosis is more typical of BD, severely depressed patients may become psychotic, and either suicidality or psychosis is an indication for prompt psychiatric evaluation in a secure setting.

Psychotic depression is among the most severe and disabling forms of MDD. SSRIs and antipsychotics are considered first-line agents for this subtype of depression, but patients may require electroconvulsant therapy if the symptoms are refractory to first-line agents.

A **manic episode** is associated with irritable, elevated, or euphoric mood, as well as increased overall activity. Associated symptoms often include an inflated sense of self-worth (termed **grandiosity**) and distractibility. Rather than speech latency and soft speech, as seen in depression, there is increased, rapid, and loud speech that is often difficult to interrupt. Rather than the sense of fatigue and need for sleep seen in depression, there is often decreased need for sleep. At the extreme, patients may not sleep at all, and rather than feeling tired, they feel energized. Manic episodes are also characterized by disorganized, racing thoughts, often to point where

---

BOX 15-1 Criteria for Major Depressive Disorder (MDD), abbreviated from the Diagnostic and Statistical Manual of Mental Disorders, Fifth Edition (DSM-5)

A. Five (or more) of the following symptoms have been present during the same 2-week period and represent a change from previous functioning; at least one of the symptoms is either (1) depressed mood or (2) loss of interest or pleasure.

  1. Depressed mood most of the day, nearly every day, as indicated by either subjective report (e.g., feels sad, empty, hopeless) or observation made by others (e.g., appears tearful).
  2. Markedly diminished interest or pleasure in all, or almost all, activities most of the day, nearly every day (as indicated by either subjective account or observation).
  3. Significant weight loss when not dieting or weight gain (e.g., a change of more than 5% of body weight in a month), or a decrease or increase in appetite nearly every day.
  4. Insomnia or hypersomnia nearly every day.
  5. Psychomotor agitation or retardation nearly every day (observable by others, not merely subjective feelings of restlessness or being slowed down).
  6. Fatigue or loss of energy nearly every day.

  7. Feelings of worthlessness or excessive or inappropriate guilt (which may be delusional) nearly every day (not merely self-reproach or guilt about being sick).
  8. Diminished ability to think or concentrate, or indecisiveness, nearly every day (either by subjective account or as observed by others).
  9. Recurrent thoughts of death (not just fear of dying), recurrent suicidal ideation without a specific plan, or a suicide attempt or a specific plan for committing suicide.

B. The symptoms cause clinically significant distress or impairment in social, occupational, or other important area of functioning.
C. The episode is not attributable to the physiological effects of a substance or to another medical condition.
D. The occurrence of the major depressive episode is not better explained by schizoaffective disorder, schizophrenia, schizophreniform disorder, delusional disorder, or other specified and unspecified schizophrenia spectrum and other psychotic disorders.
E. There has never been a manic episode or a hypomanic episode. ■

BOX 15-2 Criteria for Bipolar Disorder (BD), abbreviated from the Diagnostic and Statistical Manual of Mental Disorders, Fifth Edition (DSM-5)

BIPOLAR I DISORDER

For a diagnosis of bipolar I disorder, it is necessary to meet the following criteria for a manic episode. The manic episode may have been preceded by and may be followed by hypomania or major depressive episodes.

Manic Episode:

A. A distinct period of abnormally and persistently elevated, expansive, or irritable mood and abnormality and persistently increased goal-directed activity or energy, lasting at least 1 week and present most of the day, nearly every day (or any duration of hospitalization is necessary).

B. During the period of mood disturbance and increased energy or activity, three (or more) of the following symptoms (four if the mood is only irritable) are present to a significant degree and represent a noticeable change from usual behavior:

1. Inflated self-esteem or grandiosity.
2. Decreased need for sleep (e.g., feels rested after only 3 hours of sleep).
3. More talkative than usual or pressure to keep talking.
4. Flight of ideas or subjective experience that thoughts are racing.
5. Distractibility (i.e., attention too easily drawn to unimportant or irrelevant external stimuli), as reported or observed.
6. Increase in goal-directed activity (either socially, at work or school, or sexually) or psychomotor agitation (i.e., purposeless non-goal-directed activity).
7. Excessive involvement in activities that have a high potential for painful consequences (e.g., engaging in unrestrained buying sprees, sexual indiscretion, or foolish business investments).

C. The mood disturbance is sufficiently severe to cause marked impairment in social or occupational functioning or to necessitate hospitalization to prevent harm to self or others, or there are psychotic features.

D. The episode is not attributable to the psychological effects of a substance (e.g., a drug of abuse, a medication, other treatment) or to another medical condition.

BIPOLAR II DISORDER

For a diagnosis of bipolar II disorder, it is necessary to meet the following criteria for a current or past hypomanic episode *and* the following criteria for a current or past depressive episode.

Hypomanic Episode:

A. A distinct period of abnormally and persistently elevated, expansive, or irritable mood and abnormality and persistently increased goal-directed activity or energy, lasting at least 4 consecutive days and present most of the day, nearly every day.

B. During the period of mood disturbance and increased energy or activity, three (or more) of the following symptoms (four if the mood is only irritable) represent a noticeable change from usual behavior and have been present to a significant degree:

1. Inflated self-esteem or grandiosity.
2. Decreased need for sleep (e.g., feels rested after only 3 hours of sleep).
3. More talkative than usual or pressure to keep talking.
4. Flight of ideas or subjective experience that thoughts are racing.
5. Distractibility (i.e., attention too easily drawn to unimportant or irrelevant external stimuli), as reported or observed.
6. Increase in goal-directed activity (either socially, at work or school, or sexually) or psychomotor agitation.
7. Excessive involvement in activities that have a high potential for painful consequences (e.g., engaging in unrestrained buying sprees, sexual indiscretion, or foolish business investments).

C. The episode is associated with an unequivocal change in functioning that is uncharacteristic of the individual when not symptomatic.

D. The disturbance in mood and the change in functioning are observable by others.

E. The episode is not severe enough to cause marked impairment in social or occupational functioning or to necessitate hospitalization. If there are psychotic features, the episode is, by definition, manic.

F. The episode is not attributable to the psychological effects of a substance (e.g., a drug of abuse, a medication, other treatment). ■

patients cannot stay on topic for more than a few seconds. While not core features of mania, these episodes may be associated with psychosis (delusions or hallucinations). Mania is associated with high risk for adverse outcomes (e.g., traffic accident, arrest, or psychiatric hospitalization), particularly in the absence of treatment. When some symptoms of a manic episode and a depressive episode are present simultaneously, the depressive or manic episode is said to have "mixed features."

If a patient has manic symptoms for at least 4 days without such an adverse outcome, and without causing significant distress to the patient, it is then by definition a **hypomanic episode** (literally, a "little mania"). In the introductory case, there is insufficient detail to determine whether Ms. R has experienced significant adverse consequences yet. If Dr. Lee had not intervened, her symptoms might be expected to worsen and her risk for such consequences would increase.

Although BD is characterized by manic symptoms (either mania or hypomania), the disorder is also notable for depression, which may be prolonged and debilitating. The depressive episodes may occur before any mania is experienced, and these patients are often mistakenly diagnosed with MDD. *Patients with BD sometimes experience rapid "switches" into mania when taking antidepressants (as in the case of Ms. R), or more frequent mood episodes referred to as rapid cycling.* The drug classes used to treat BD are discussed at the end of the pharmacology section and in the past were referred to as **mood stabilizers**. More recently, such drugs may be described in terms of their relative antidepressant or antimanic properties, or their ability to prevent such episodes. In many patients with BD, combinations of medications are required to achieve adequate control of mood symptoms and recurrences.

The Monoamine Theory of Depression

The biological basis for depression began to be understood in the 1940s and 1950s, when keen observers noticed that **imipramine**, **iproniazid**, and **reserpine** had unexpected effects on mood.

In the late 1940s, the tricyclic drug **imipramine** was developed for use in the treatment of psychotic patients, but it was subsequently noted to have strong antidepressant effects. Imipramine preferentially blocks the 5-HT transporter (SERT), and its active metabolite **desipramine** preferentially blocks the NE transporter (NET). By these mechanisms, imipramine allows 5-HT and NE to persist in the extracellular space at higher concentrations and for longer durations, yielding increased activation of 5-HT and NE receptors.

In 1951, the antituberculosis drug **iproniazid** was shown to have antidepressant effects. Iproniazid inhibits monoamine oxidase (MAO) and thereby prevents the degradation of 5-HT, NE, and DA. The resulting increase in cytosolic neurotransmitter leads to increased neurotransmitter uptake into vesicles and, consequently, to greater release of neurotransmitter after exocytosis.

In the 1950s, the antihypertensive agent **reserpine** was noted to induce depression in 10–15% of patients. Researchers then found that reserpine could induce depressive symptoms in animal models as well as in humans. Reserpine depletes 5-HT, NE, and DA in presynaptic neurons by inhibiting the transport of these neurotransmitters into synaptic vesicles. The drug binds irreversibly to VMAT and ultimately destroys the vesicles. The 5-HT, NE, and DA that accumulate in the cytoplasm are degraded by mitochondrial MAO. The resulting decrease in monoamine neurotransmission is thought to be responsible for inducing a depressed mood.

The findings described above strongly suggested that the central monoaminergic serotonin and norepinephrine systems are involved in the pathogenesis of depression. The **monoamine theory of depression** holds that depression results from pathologically decreased serotonin and/or norepinephrine neurotransmission. Based on this hypothesis, it follows that increasing serotonin and/or norepinephrine neurotransmission could ameliorate or reverse depression. As a biological disease related to long-term pathologic alterations in monoamine activity, MDD should thus be treatable by medications.

Limitations of the Monoamine Theory

Although nearly all of the antidepressants are pharmacologically active at their molecular and cellular sites of action almost immediately, their full antidepressant effects are generally not seen until the drugs have been administered for 6 or more weeks of continuous treatment. Similarly, although reserpine rapidly depletes neurotransmitter in monoaminergic systems, it takes several weeks of continuous treatment with reserpine to induce depression. The unexplained delay in the onset of full effect of these drugs remains a central conundrum and strong challenge to the monoamine theory.

In some patients, drugs that selectively increase 5-HT neurotransmission decrease depressive symptoms, while drugs that selectively increase NE neurotransmission have little or no effect. In other patients, drugs affecting the NE system are more beneficial than those affecting the 5-HT system. Overall, each individual drug is effective in about 70% of patients with depression, and drugs that have markedly different efficacies in blocking the reuptake of NE and/or 5-HT may have similar clinical effectiveness when tested in large populations. These clinical observations are not easily explained by the monoamine theory.

The time lag in the clinical effectiveness of antidepressants may reflect autoregulatory mechanisms in presynaptic monoaminergic neurons and/or in postsynaptic neural circuitry. Acute treatment with antidepressants actually produces a decrease in neuronal firing in the locus ceruleus and/or raphe nucleus (depending on the drug), due to acute feedback inhibition via 5-HT$_{1A}$ and α_2 autoreceptors on 5-HT- and NE-containing neurons, respectively. This causes a concomitant, acute decrease in the synthesis and release of 5-HT and NE.

In contrast, chronic use of antidepressants causes the inhibitory autoreceptors themselves to be down-regulated, leading to enhancement of neurotransmission. The change in autoreceptor sensitivity takes several weeks to occur, consistent with the time-course of the therapeutic response in patients. This could explain the lag in full therapeutic response; only after chronic antidepressant therapy does the gradual desensitization of autoreceptors allow increased neurotransmission (Fig. 15-4). Although speculative, this hypothesis regarding changes in monoamine receptor sensitivity offers an explanation for the delay in onset of the therapeutic action of fluoxetine experienced by Ms. R.

Recent research has also suggested that chronic, but not acute, antidepressant administration increases neurogenesis (i.e., the birth of new neurons) in the hippocampus and that some clinical effects of antidepressants may be mediated by neurogenesis. Other research has implicated effects on neurotrophic factors, such as brain-derived neurotrophic factor (BDNF). The role of neurogenesis and neurotrophic factors in mood disorders is currently an area of intense investigation.

▌ PHARMACOLOGIC CLASSES AND AGENTS

Serotonergic and central adrenergic neurotransmission are modulated by a broad range of agents that target storage, degradation, and reuptake of the neurotransmitters. Other agents target the neurotransmitter receptors. Because serotonin is involved in multiple physiologic processes, both centrally

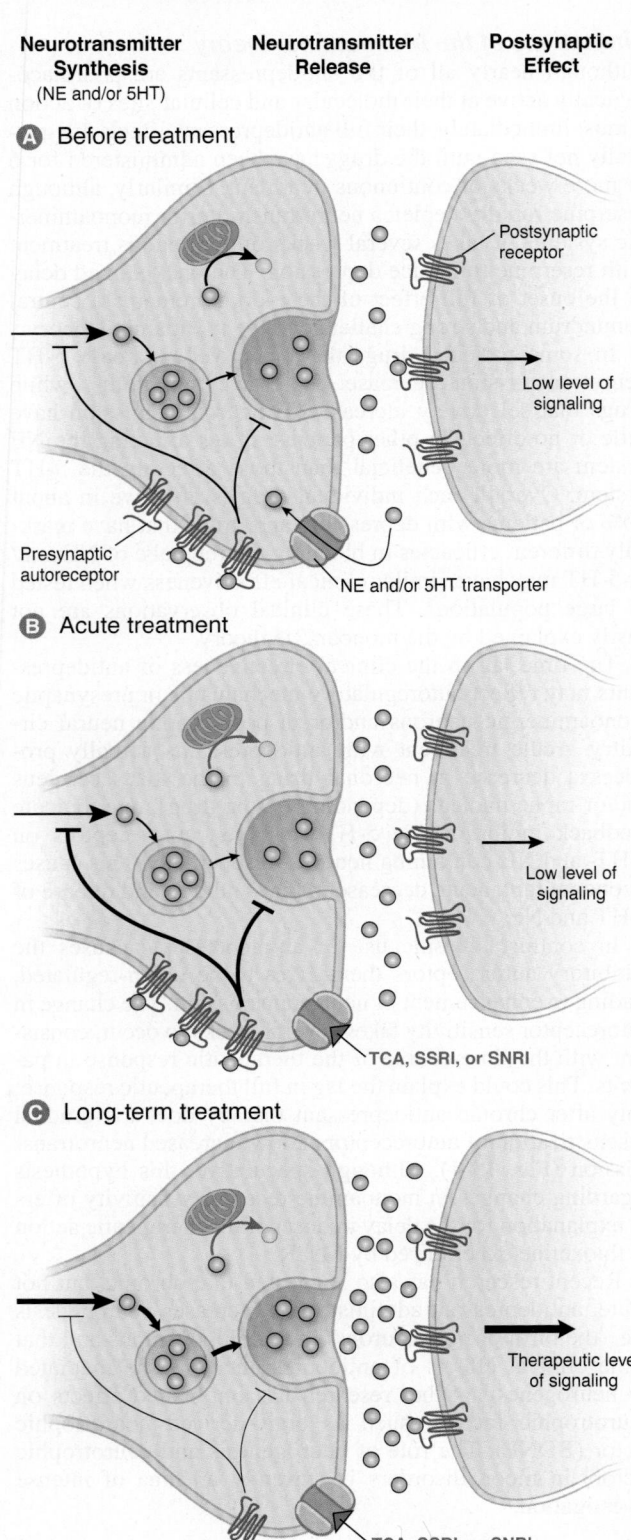

Neurotransmitter Synthesis (NE and/or 5HT)

Neurotransmitter Release

Postsynaptic Effect

A Before treatment

Postsynaptic receptor

Low level of signaling

Presynaptic autoreceptor

NE and/or 5HT transporter

B Acute treatment

Low level of signaling

TCA, SSRI, or SNRI

C Long-term treatment

Therapeutic level of signaling

TCA, SSRI, or SNRI

FIGURE 15-4. Postulated mechanism of the delay in onset of the therapeutic effect of antidepressant medications. A. Before treatment, neurotransmitters are released at pathologically low levels and exert steady-state levels of autoinhibitory feedback. The net effect is an abnormally low baseline level of postsynaptic receptor activity (signaling). **B.** Short-term use of antidepressant medication results in increased release of neurotransmitter and/or increased duration of neurotransmitter action in the synaptic cleft. Both effects cause increased stimulation of inhibitory autoreceptors, with increased inhibition of neurotransmitter synthesis and increased inhibition of exocytosis. The net effect is to dampen the initial effect of the medication, and postsynaptic receptor activity remains at pretreatment levels. **C.** Chronic use of antidepressant medication results in desensitization of the presynaptic autoreceptors. Thus, the inhibition of neurotransmitter synthesis and exocytosis is reduced. The net effect is enhanced postsynaptic receptor activity, leading to a therapeutic response. NE, norepinephrine; 5-HT, serotonin; TCA, tricyclic antidepressant; SSRI, selective serotonin reuptake inhibitor; SNRI, serotonin-norepinephrine reuptake inhibitor.

Inhibitors of Serotonin Storage

Amphetamine and related drugs interfere with the ability of synaptic vesicles to store monoamines such as serotonin (see Chapter 11). Thus, amphetamine, methamphetamine, and methylphenidate displace 5-HT, DA, and NE from their storage vesicles. For atypical depression and for depression in the elderly, stimulants such as **amphetamine**, **methylphenidate**, and **modafinil** have proved to be useful as second-line agents, in part because of their combined effects on serotonin, norepinephrine, and dopamine.

Amphetamine, methylphenidate, **dextroamphetamine**, and **lisdexamfetamine** are also widely used in the treatment of attention-deficit hyperactivity disorder (ADHD). Although it may seem counterintuitive that a hyperactivity disorder such as ADHD could be treated by drugs that increase catecholamine levels, this finding makes sense in light of the differing roles of central versus peripheral NE. In the prefrontal cortex, increased NE promotes attention and higher cognitive processes, while peripheral increases in NE increase heart rate and blood pressure and can induce tremors. These drugs have substantial potential for substance abuse; because the inactive prodrug lisdexamfetamine is converted relatively slowly to the active compound dextroamphetamine by rate-limiting hepatic metabolism, it may have less abuse potential than other amphetamine derivatives.

Fenfluramine and **dexfenfluramine** are halogenated amphetamine derivatives that are modestly selective for 5-HT storage vesicles. These drugs were used briefly in the United States for appetite suppression, but severe cardiac toxicity led to their withdrawal. Another amphetamine derivative, **methylenedioxymethamphetamine (MDMA)**, is both a selective serotonin storage inhibitor and a 5-HT receptor ligand. It is not approved for use in medical practice but is a significant drug clinically due to its illicit use (as "Ecstasy").

Inhibitors of Serotonin Degradation

The major pathway for serotonin degradation is mediated by MAO; accordingly, MAO inhibitors (MAOIs) have significant effects on serotonergic neurotransmission. The MAOIs are classified according to their specificity for the MAO-A and MAO-B isoenzymes and according to the reversibility or irreversibility of their binding. The older MAOIs are nonselective, and most older MAOIs, such as **iproniazid**, **phenelzine**, and **isocarboxazid**, are irreversible inhibitors. Newer

and peripherally, pharmacologic agents that alter serotonergic signaling have diverse actions on the brain (mood, sleep, migraines), on the gastrointestinal (GI) system, and on core temperature and hemodynamics (serotonin syndrome). Many of these biological effects are discussed as the pharmacologic agents are introduced, although the emphasis is on agents that regulate mood.

MAOIs, such as **moclobemide**, **befloxatone**, and **brofaromine**, are selective for MAO-A and bind reversibly. **Selegiline**, a selective MAO-B inhibitor at low doses (see Chapter 14, Pharmacology of Dopaminergic Neurotransmission), also inhibits MAO-A at higher doses.

MAOIs block the deamination of monoamines by binding to and inhibiting the FAD cofactor of MAO (Fig. 15-5). By inhibiting the degradation of monoamines, MAOIs increase the 5-HT and NE available in the cytoplasm of presynaptic neurons. The increase in cytoplasmic levels of these monoamines leads not only to increased uptake and storage of 5-HT and NE in synaptic vesicles but also to some constitutive leakage of the monoamines into the extracellular space.

As noted in Chapter 11, the most toxic adverse effect of MAOI use is systemic **tyramine toxicity**. Because GI and hepatic MAO metabolizes tyramine, consumption of foods that contain tyramine, such as processed meats, aged hard cheeses, and red wine, can lead to excess levels of circulating tyramine. Tyramine is an indirect sympathomimetic that can stimulate the release of large amounts of stored catecholamines by reversing the reuptake transporters. This uncontrolled catecholamine release can induce a *hypertensive crisis* characterized by headache, tachycardia, nausea, cardiac arrhythmia, and stroke. The older MAOIs are no longer considered first-line therapy for depression because of the potential for systemic tyramine toxicity; they should be prescribed only to patients able to commit to a tyramine-free diet.

The newer MAOIs (i.e., the reversible inhibitors of MAO-A [RIMAs] that bind reversibly to MAO) are displaced by high concentrations of tyramine, resulting in significantly more tyramine metabolism and hence less tyramine toxicity. **Selegiline** has been approved as a transdermal patch, thus bypassing the GI system. Transdermal selegiline can maximally inhibit brain MAO-A (and MAO-B) at doses that reduce gastrointestinal MAO-A activity by only 30–40%, thus reducing the risk of a tyramine-induced hypertensive crisis and allowing patients greater dietary freedom. *MAOIs, like other antidepressants, can precipitate manic or hypomanic episodes in some bipolar patients.*

All antidepressant drugs, including MAOIs, are hydrophobic and cross the blood–brain barrier. They are well absorbed orally and are metabolized to active metabolites by the liver. These metabolites are subsequently inactivated by acetylation, also in the liver. Excretion is primarily via renal clearance. The older, irreversibly binding MAOIs are cleared from the circulation as complexes with MAO and are effectively inactivated only when new enzyme is synthesized. Because of the extensive effects of MAOIs on cytochrome P450 enzymes in the liver, they can cause numerous drug–drug interactions. All members of a patient's medical team must prescribe other drugs with caution when a patient is taking an MAOI.

Reuptake Inhibitors

Serotonergic tone is maintained at steady state by the balance between transmitter release and reuptake. Thus, inhibitors of the serotonin reuptake transporter decrease the reuptake rate, resulting in a net increase in the concentration of 5-HT in the extracellular space. These drugs alleviate the symptoms of a variety of common psychiatric conditions, including depression, anxiety, and obsessive-compulsive

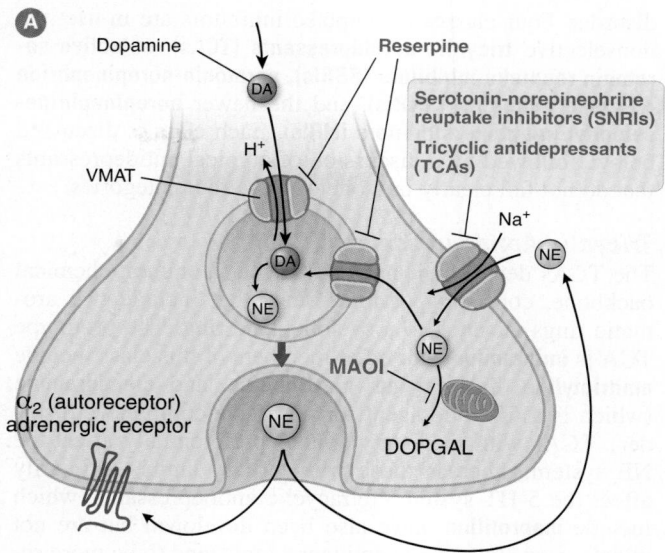

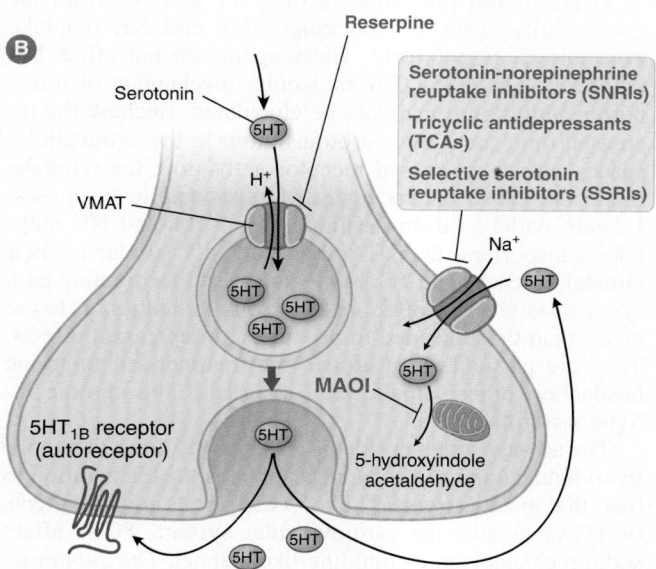

FIGURE 15-5. Sites and mechanisms of action of antidepressant drugs. The sites of action of antidepressant drugs and of reserpine (which can induce depression) are indicated in noradrenergic neurons (**A**) and serotonergic neurons (**B**). Monoamine oxidase inhibitors (MAOIs) inhibit the mitochondrial enzyme monoamine oxidase (MAO); the resulting increase in cytosolic monoamines leads to increased vesicular uptake of neurotransmitter and to increased release of neurotransmitter during exocytosis. Tricyclic antidepressants (TCAs) and serotonin-norepinephrine reuptake inhibitors (SNRIs) inhibit both the norepinephrine transporter (NET) and the serotonin transporter (SERT), thereby increasing the levels of both NE and 5-HT in the synaptic cleft. Selective serotonin reuptake inhibitors (SSRIs) specifically inhibit the SERT-mediated reuptake of 5-HT. TCAs, SNRIs, and SSRIs increase the duration of neurotransmitter action in the synaptic cleft, leading to increased downstream signaling. Reserpine, which can induce depression in humans and in animal models, blocks the VMAT-mediated uptake of monoamines into synaptic vesicles, which ultimately destroys the vesicles.

disorder. Four classes of reuptake inhibitors are in use: the nonselective **tricyclic antidepressants (TCAs)**, **selective serotonin reuptake inhibitors (SSRIs)**, **serotonin-norepinephrine reuptake inhibitors (SNRIs)**, and the newer **norepinephrine-selective reuptake inhibitors (NRIs)**. Each class is discussed below, followed by a discussion of atypical antidepressants that do not fall clearly into one of these four categories.

Tricyclic Antidepressants (TCAs)

The TCAs derive their name from their common chemical backbone, consisting of three rings that include two aromatic rings attached to a cycloheptane ring. The prototype TCA is **imipramine**, and other members of this class include **amitriptyline**, **desipramine**, **nortriptyline**, and **clomipramine** (which is a first-line agent for obsessive-compulsive disorder). TCAs with secondary amines preferentially affect the NE system, whereas those with tertiary amines primarily affect the 5-HT system. Tetracyclic antidepressants, which include **maprotiline**, have also been developed but are not widely used. Tetracyclic antidepressants tend to be more selective for the NE system.

TCAs inhibit the reuptake of 5-HT and NE from the extracellular space by blocking 5-HT and NE reuptake transporters, respectively. These agents do not affect DA reuptake (Fig. 15-5). The molecular mechanism of transporter inhibition remains to be elucidated. Because the increased time spent by neurotransmitter in the extracellular space leads to increased receptor activation, the reuptake inhibitors cause enhancement of postsynaptic responses. Despite widely varying affinities for 5-HT and NE reuptake transporters, the TCAs are markedly similar in their clinical efficacy. The TCAs are also useful for treating pain syndromes and are often used for this indication at lower doses than those needed to produce antidepressant effects. They are particularly useful in the treatment of migraine headaches, other somatic pain disorders, and chronic fatigue syndrome.

The adverse effect profile of TCAs results from their ability to bind a number of channels and receptors in addition to their therapeutic targets. The most dangerous adverse effects of TCAs involve the cardiovascular system. TCAs affect sodium channels in a quinidine-like manner. *The quinidine-like adverse effects of TCAs (and TCA overdose in particular) include potentially lethal conduction delays, such as first-degree atrioventricular and bundle branch blocks.* Therefore, TCAs should always be prescribed with caution in patients at risk of attempting suicide, and an electrocardiogram (ECG) should be examined to rule out conduction system disease prior to starting TCAs.

TCAs can also act as antagonists at muscarinic (cholinergic), histamine, adrenergic, and dopamine receptors. The *anticholinergic effects* are most prominent and include symptoms typical of muscarinic acetylcholine receptor blockade: nausea, vomiting, anorexia, dry mouth, blurred vision, confusion, constipation, tachycardia, and urinary retention. The *antihistaminergic effects* include sedation, weight gain, and confusion (in the elderly). The *antiadrenergic effects* include orthostatic hypotension, reflex tachycardia, drowsiness, and dizziness. Orthostatic hypotension is an especially significant risk for elderly patients, and TCA use must be monitored carefully in such patients. *Finally, TCAs may also precipitate mania in patients with BD.*

Selective Serotonin Reuptake Inhibitors (SSRIs)

In 1987, the treatment of depression was revolutionized with the introduction of **selective serotonin reuptake inhibitors (SSRIs)**. The first SSRI to be approved by the US Food and Drug Administration (FDA) was **fluoxetine**; this drug is still one of the most widely prescribed SSRIs. Other SSRIs include **citalopram**, its more active S-enantiomer **escitalopram**, **fluvoxamine**, **paroxetine**, and **sertraline**. Although the effectiveness of the SSRIs is similar to that of the TCAs for the treatment of depression, their greater safety in overdose and lower adverse effect profile has made them first-line agents for the treatment of depression, as well as for anxiety disorders. In particular, SSRI overdoses produce relatively benign effects compared to the potential lethality of TCA overdoses. SSRIs are also used in the treatment of panic disorder, generalized anxiety, obsessive-compulsive disorder, and posttraumatic stress disorder (PTSD). Because of their propensity to diminish or delay orgasm, they have also been used for the treatment of premature ejaculation.

The SSRIs are similar to the TCAs in their mechanism of action, except that the SSRIs are significantly more selective for 5-HT transporters (Fig. 15-5B). Inhibition of serotonin reuptake increases serotonin levels in the extracellular space, thereby increasing 5-HT receptor activation and enhancing postsynaptic responses. At low doses, SSRIs are believed to bind primarily to 5-HT transporters, whereas at higher doses, they can lose selectivity and also bind to NE transporters. Despite widely varying chemical structures, the SSRIs have clinical efficacies similar to the TCAs and to one another. Thus, the choice of drug often depends on issues such as cost and tolerability of adverse effects. In addition, because of the variability of individual patient responses to individual antidepressants, a patient may need to try more than one SSRI to find the most effective drug: despite their common mechanism, one SSRI may be effective after another one fails.

Because the SSRIs are more selective for serotonin reuptake than the TCAs at clinically effective doses, they have far fewer adverse effects. SSRIs lack significant cardiotoxicity (although one, citalopram, has rarely been associated with QTc prolongation at higher doses) and they do not bind as avidly to muscarinic (cholinergic), histamine, adrenergic, or dopamine receptors. As a consequence, SSRIs are generally better tolerated than TCAs. The enhanced selectivity of the SSRIs also means that these agents have a higher therapeutic index than the TCAs.

The SSRIs are not entirely without adverse effects, however. All SSRIs can cause some degree of sexual dysfunction, diminishing libido and/or delaying orgasm. Another common adverse effect is GI distress; sertraline is more often associated with diarrhea, while paroxetine is associated with constipation. A more serious adverse effect of the SSRIs is **serotonin syndrome**, a rare but dangerous elevation of 5-HT levels that can occur when both an SSRI and an MAOI are administered concurrently. *The clinical manifestations of serotonin syndrome include hyperthermia, muscle rigidity, myoclonus, and rapid fluctuations in mental status and vital signs.* SSRIs can also cause bleeding complications in a very small percentage of patients and have occasionally been associated with hyponatremia. Abrupt withdrawal from SSRIs can cause SSRI-discontinuation syndrome, which is characterized by anxiety, dysphoria, gastrointestinal flu-like symptoms, insomnia, depersonalization, and frank suicidality.

Finally, as with TCAs and MAOIs, SSRIs can sometimes cause a "switch" from depression to mania or hypomania in patients with BD. The fluoxetine that Ms. R was prescribed for MDD was likely responsible for her subsequent manic episode. The mechanism of the SSRI-induced switch from depression to mania or hypomania is unknown.

Serotonin-Norepinephrine Reuptake Inhibitors (SNRIs)

Although SSRIs are useful first-line agents for the treatment of depression, there is a significant patient population that does not respond, or responds only partially, to SSRIs. Also, although TCAs are often useful in cases in which somatic pain is a significant concern, the broad receptor profile of TCAs makes them difficult to prescribe in medically complicated or fragile patients.

A newer class of drugs, the serotonin-norepinephrine reuptake inhibitors (SNRIs), is proving to be useful in such patients. The SNRIs presently consist of **venlafaxine**, its active metabolite **desvenlafaxine**, **duloxetine**, and **milnacipran**. Venlafaxine and desvenlafaxine block the 5-HT reuptake transporter and the NE reuptake transporter in a concentration-dependent manner; at low doses, they behave as SSRIs, but at higher doses, they also increase extracellular NE levels. Duloxetine also inhibits NE and 5-HT reuptake specifically and has been approved for the treatment of depression as well as neuropathic pain and other pain syndromes. Milnacipran is a selective NE and 5-HT reuptake inhibitor that is approved for the treatment of fibromyalgia based on clinical trials in which it improved symptoms of pain and dysphoria.

Norepinephrine-Selective Reuptake Inhibitors (NRIs)

Atomoxetine is an NE-selective reuptake inhibitor that is used in the treatment of ADHD. It is thought to improve ADHD symptoms by blocking NE reuptake and thereby increasing NE levels in the prefrontal cortex. (Note that methylphenidate and amphetamines are also thought to improve ADHD symptoms by increasing NE levels in the prefrontal cortex, acting via increased NE release.) Atomoxetine has several advantages over the amphetamines, including a lower abuse/addiction potential and a longer plasma half-life that allows for once-daily dosing. Atomoxetine increases peripheral as well as central NE levels and thus increases heart rate and blood pressure.

Atypical Antidepressants

Several drugs that interact with multiple targets and are indicated for the treatment of depression are sometimes referred to as "atypical antidepressants." These agents include bupropion, mirtazapine, and trazodone; tianeptine and agomelatine are approved in Europe but not the U.S. Most recently, intravenous ketamine has been shown to have antidepressant effects. They are categorized together here only because they do not fit conveniently into other categories. These agents are newer than the TCAs and act by several different mechanisms, and some have unknown or incompletely characterized mechanisms of action.

Bupropion, an aminoketone, is particularly useful for the treatment of atypical depression. This drug appears to act mechanistically like the amphetamines, with weak occupancy of the dopamine transporter in the human brain. Its full mechanism of action is not well understood, however, in part because of its extensive metabolism to active metabolites that have effects on nicotinic acetylcholine (nACh) receptors. Bupropion is one of the antidepressants with the fewest sexual adverse effects. The principal contraindication to the use of bupropion is a predisposition to seizures, since it lowers the seizure threshold. Thus, bupropion is generally contraindicated in patients with seizure disorders, electrolyte abnormalities, or eating disorders (since these can cause electrolyte imbalances).

Mirtazapine, a tetracyclic molecule, blocks postsynaptic 5-HT$_{2A}$ and 5-HT$_{2C}$ receptors and the presynaptic α_2-adrenergic autoreceptor and presumably decreases neurotransmission at 5-HT$_2$ synapses while increasing NE neurotransmission. Mirtazapine is an effective anxiolytic and hypnotic, as well as an orexigenic (appetite stimulant), making it a particularly useful antidepressant for the elderly population (who often present with insomnia and weight loss) and for other patients with weight loss and depression.

Trazodone, a phenylpiperazine, blocks postsynaptic 5-HT$_{2A}$ and 5-HT$_{2C}$ receptors while also inhibiting the serotonin transporter. It is discussed in more detail below.

Tianeptine is a tricyclic antidepressant with anxiolytic effects. Despite its structure, this drug acts as a selective enhancer (rather than inhibitor) of serotonin reuptake. The mechanism of tianeptine's action as an antidepressant is poorly understood: possible mechanisms include effects on neuroplasticity through increasing BDNF, effects on glutamate receptors, and modulation of μ and δ opioid receptors. Tianeptine is currently approved for human use in Europe.

Agomelatine, a structural analogue of melatonin, is an agonist at the melatonin receptors 1 and 2 and an antagonist at the 5-HT$_{2C}$ receptor. It has no effect on the reuptake of monoamines and does not affect extracellular serotonin levels, although its antagonism of 5-HT$_{2C}$ receptors increases dopamine and norepinephrine release. Agomelatine is well tolerated and generally lacks sexual adverse effects. A distinguishing feature of agomelatine is its ability to modulate circadian rhythms and related physiologic effects through its actions at melatonin receptors.

Ketamine is an antagonist at glutamatergic *N*-methyl-D-aspartate (NMDA) receptors. This agent was originally developed as an anesthetic (see Chapter 17, General Anesthetic Pharmacology). It also has antidepressant effects with onset within hours but offset by 72 hours; such effects have been demonstrated even in patients who have failed to respond to standard antidepressants. The effectiveness of ketamine in treating depression challenges the monoamine theory of depression, as ketamine appears to lack a direct effect on the serotonergic system and, mechanistically, its actions are likely to involve regulation of mTOR-mediated translational control of synaptic proteins and regulation of GSK3β, one of the putative targets of the mood stabilizer lithium. While concerns exist regarding the abuse potential of this drug and its need for repeated IV administration, better understanding of the molecular pathways affected by ketamine may point the way to a new class of antidepressants.

Overall, the atypical antidepressants have relatively few adverse effects and demonstrate similar clinical efficacies despite their widely heterogeneous mechanisms of action and molecular targets. Indeed, such heterogeneity poses challenges for traditional monoaminergic models of antidepressant effect.

Serotonin Receptor Agonists

Ergots are naturally occurring serotonin receptor agonists. Several dozen structurally similar ergots are elaborated by the rye rust fungus *Claviceps purpurea*. Many naturally occurring **ergot alkaloids** produce intense vasoconstriction by acting as agonists at serotonin receptors in vascular smooth muscle. This action was responsible for ergotism—described during the Middle Ages as "St. Anthony's Fire"—in which consumers of fungus-infected grains experienced severe peripheral vasoconstriction leading to necrosis and gangrene. In modern times, several ergot alkaloids have been employed clinically. The semisynthetic ergot lysergic acid diethylamide (LSD) produces hallucinations and sensory dysfunction at doses as small as 50 μg in humans.

5-HT receptor subtype-selective agonists have become therapeutics of increasing interest in the past decade. These agents are used primarily to treat anxiety and migraine headaches. **Buspirone** is a nonbenzodiazepine anxiolytic that does not bind to GABA receptors but rather acts as a $5-HT_{1A}$-selective partial agonist. It is nonsedating with moderate anxiolytic properties. Although it is often not as clinically effective as other anxiety treatments such as a benzodiazepine, buspirone is nonetheless a useful option in some patients because it is nonaddictive, does not have abuse potential, and is nonsedating.

Vilazodone, a piperazine class antidepressant approved by the FDA in 2011, is an example of a newer generation of antidepressants designed to function as combined partial agonists at the $5-HT_{1A}$ receptor, which mediates negative feedback circuitry, and reuptake inhibitors at the 5-HT transporter (SERT). The dual activity at $5-HT_{1A}$ and SERT is expected to enhance endogenous adaptation mechanisms leading to increased serotonergic neurotransmission. Following a similar rationale, but more mixed in its actions, **vortioxetine**, a bisarylsulfanyl amine class antidepressant approved by the FDA in 2013, is a $5-HT_{1A}$ agonist; a $5-HT_{1B}$ partial agonist; an antagonist at $5-HT_3$, $5-HT_7$, and $5-HT_{1D}$ receptors; and a SERT inhibitor. Whether these two drugs represent agents with truly novel mechanisms or are simply additional SSRIs with similar or different adverse-effect profiles requires further evaluation.

Migraine headaches are believed to be precipitated by cerebral vasodilation with subsequent activation of small pain fibers. A class of selective serotonin agonists ($5-HT_1$ agonists) has been found to be particularly effective in the treatment of migraine headaches, presumably because of their potent vasoconstrictive effects. **Sumatriptan** is the prototype $5-HT_{1D}$ agonist in this group, known collectively as the **triptans**, which also includes **rizatriptan**, **almotriptan**, **frovatriptan**, **eletriptan**, and **zolmitriptan**. The triptans, as well as the less selective ergot alkaloid **ergotamine**, act on $5-HT_1$ receptors in the vasculature to alter intracranial blood flow. These agents are most useful for acute migraine attacks when taken at the onset of an episode rather than as prophylaxis. They must be taken early in a migraine (ideally, at the time of the aura) to effectively block the activation of pain receptors. The triptans are thought to activate both $5-HT_{1D}$ and $5-HT_{1B}$ receptors. In the CNS, both receptor subtypes are present on presynaptic endings of a variety of neurons in the vasculature.

Relatively few $5-HT_2$ agonists are used clinically. **Trazodone** is a prodrug used in the treatment of depression and insomnia that is converted into meta-chlorophenylpiperazine (mCPP), a selective $5-HT_{2A/2C}$ agonist. Trazodone is used principally as an anxiolytic and hypnotic (sleep-inducing) agent because the higher doses required for its antidepressant effect are usually oversedating. The ergot derivative methysergide is a partial agonist at $5-HT_2$ receptors that also has adrenergic and muscarinic effects; this agent is no longer available in the United States.

Serotonin and serotonin receptors are abundant in the GI tract. Serotonin is a critical regulator of GI motility, mediated in large part by $5-HT_4$ receptors. **Cisapride**, a $5-HT_4$ agonist that also enhances acetylcholine release from the myenteric plexus, induces gastric motility. However, cisapride has been withdrawn in the United States due to safety concerns; it can cause QT prolongation and cardiac arrhythmias as a consequence of hERG K^+ channel blockade.

Serotonin Receptor Antagonists

Serotonin receptor antagonists are increasingly important therapeutics. Like many receptor ligands, these drugs show varying degrees of receptor subtype selectivity and often cross-react with adrenergic, histamine, and muscarinic receptors. This property can limit their clinical utility because of intolerable adverse effects.

Ketanserin is a $5-HT_{2A/2C}$ antagonist with substantial α_1-adrenergic antagonist activity. It reduces blood pressure to a similar degree as β-blockers and has been used topically to reduce intraocular pressure in glaucoma. This drug is available in Europe.

Ondansetron is a $5-HT_3$ antagonist. This drug is of interest because, of all the currently identified monoamine receptors, only $5-HT_3$ is an ionotropic receptor belonging to the nicotinic acetylcholine superfamily of pentameric receptors. $5-HT_3$ receptors are expressed in the enteric nervous system, the nerve endings of the vagus, and the CNS, particularly the chemoreceptor trigger zone. Ondansetron is a potent antiemetic and is widely used as an adjunct to cancer chemotherapy and to treat refractory nausea. As predicted by its mechanism of action, it has little effect on nausea caused by vertigo.

Irritable bowel syndrome (IBS) is believed to be a disorder of GI motility, particularly in the colon. Patients experience episodes of diarrhea, constipation, or both, with significant GI cramping. The $5-HT_4$ antagonists **tegaserod** and **prucalopride** enhance GI motility and are effective in treating the constipation associated with IBS; tegaserod was withdrawn from the market in 2007 because of concerns about an increased risk of myocardial infarction and stroke. **Alosetron** is a $5-HT_3$ antagonist that decreases serotonergic tone in intestinal cells, thus reducing motility. It is particularly useful for diarrhea associated with IBS, although it carries a "black box" warning because it may cause severe ischemic colitis.

Mood Stabilizers

The discovery by the Australian psychiatrist John F.J. Cade of the therapeutic effect of lithium on "psychotic excitement" (corresponding to the modern concept of mania) in 1949 is often considered to be the founding event of modern psychopharmacology. However, historians now note that over half a century earlier, the Danish neurologist Carl Lange published studies on the treatment of "periodical depressions" with lithium, suggesting that he may more accurately be considered the founding father of lithium therapy for treatment of mood disorders.

Notwithstanding this debate, Cade's publication in 1949 led to the discovery (or rediscovery) of lithium's remarkable psychopharmacological effects, which continue to be investigated today. Pursuing an idea about the basis for psychiatric susceptibility that he had formulated as a prisoner of war during World War II, Cade sought to understand the basis for the elevated toxicity of urine samples from patients with mental disorders that he had observed when such samples were injected intraperitoneally into guinea pigs. Informed by the work of the English physician Sir Alfred B. Garrod, who had formally introduced lithium salts into the *materia medica* for the treatment of "gouty mania" in 1859 (apparently, independently of Lange's work), Cade fortuitously selected lithium urate, the most water-soluble form of uric acid, to determine whether the elevated urine toxicity was due to increased levels of uric acid. Having ruled out differences in urea levels, even though the administration of urea alone exhibited the same convulsant toxicity as whole urine, Cade observed less urea toxicity than expected after administering lithium urate. Subsequent investigation led him to determine that lithium had a protective effect on urea toxicity and that, administered alone, lithium was capable of causing a reversible lethargic and sedating response in guinea pigs. Next, in a medical leap of faith, based on the rationale that the sedating effects could be beneficial for treating psychosis, Cade went on to test lithium treatment in 10 patients with mania, 6 with dementia praecox (schizophrenia), and 3 with melancholia (depression). An eventual double-blind, placebo-controlled, discontinuation trial of lithium in BD patients by the Danish psychiatrists Poul C. Baastrup and Mogens Schou confirmed Cade's earlier findings; as they concluded in their published findings in 1970, "lithium is the first drug demonstrated as a clear-cut prophylactic agent against one of the major psychoses."

These founding discoveries in psychopharmacology sparked intense research on the biochemical effects of lithium and the mechanisms by which this drug exerts its antimanic effects. Although research on lithium has provided some insights, the mechanisms responsible for its psychiatric effects remain poorly understood.

In the 1970s, some researchers considered the possibility that mania could be related to epilepsy, because both disorders exhibit episodic patterns involving neural overactivity, grossly speaking. Subsequent research did not bear out this relationship, but certain antiepileptic drugs such as **carbamazepine** and **valproic acid** were found to have some efficacy in the treatment of BD. Carbamazepine and valproic acid (see Chapter 16, Pharmacology of Abnormal Electrical Neurotransmission in the Central Nervous System) are used to treat mania and to prevent future mood episodes, while **lamotrigine** is used to prevent subsequent depressive episodes. Traditionally, the term **mood stabilizer** has been used to refer to lithium, valproic acid, and carbamazepine; this term is now used less often in the setting of a broadening pharmacopeia for bipolar disorder.

In particular, antipsychotics have also been shown to be effective for the treatment of manic episodes. More recently, some second-generation antipsychotics have demonstrated efficacy in treating or preventing bipolar depressive episodes as well. (Some are also used in the treatment of MDD.)

Lithium

Lithium, commonly administered as lithium carbonate, is a monovalent cation that is similar in electrochemical properties to sodium and potassium. At therapeutic concentrations of 0.4 to 1.0 mEq/L, lithium enters cells via Na^+ channels. Because lithium can mimic other monovalent cations, as well as the divalent cation magnesium due to its water hydration shell, it has the potential to disrupt a number of proteins and transporters that require specific cation cofactors.

Lithium exerts numerous effects at the intracellular level. Its effect on the regeneration of inositol for second messenger signaling is particularly well studied, although this effect is not necessarily central to its therapeutic actions. In the inositol lipid pathway, G protein-coupled receptors (such as 5-HT_2 receptors) activate phospholipase C (PLC), which cleaves phosphatidylinositol 4,5-bisphosphate (PIP_2) to the signaling molecules diacylglycerol (DAG) and inositol 1,4,5-trisphosphate (IP_3). IP_3 signaling is terminated by conversion to inositol 4,5-bisphosphate (IP_2), either directly or via an IP_4 intermediate. Lithium inhibits both the inositol phosphatase that dephosphorylates IP_2 to inositol phosphate (IP_1) and the inositol phosphatase that dephosphorylates IP_1 to free inositol. Because free inositol is essential for the regeneration of PIP_2, lithium effectively blocks the phosphatidylinositol signaling cascade in the brain; this is the basis for the "inositol depletion hypothesis." Although inositol circulates freely in blood, it cannot cross the blood–brain barrier. The two mechanisms of inositol synthesis in CNS neurons—regeneration from IP_3 and de novo synthesis from glucose-6-phosphate—are both inhibited by lithium. By blocking the regeneration of PIP_2, lithium decreases central adrenergic, muscarinic, and serotonergic neurotransmission.

Disruption of the phosphatidylinositol signaling cascade was previously thought to be the primary mechanism of lithium's mood-stabilizing action. However, recent studies suggest that other actions of lithium may also be relevant. These actions include increasing 5-HT neurotransmission by enhancing neurotransmitter synthesis and release; decreasing NE and DA neurotransmission by inhibiting neurotransmitter synthesis, storage, release, and reuptake; inhibiting adenylyl cyclase by decoupling G proteins from neurotransmitter receptors; and altering electrochemical gradients across cell membranes by substituting for Na^+ and/or blocking K^+ channels. Possible neurotrophic effects of lithium are also under investigation. Recent studies indicate that lithium blocks glycogen synthase kinase 3 (GSK3) activity. GSK3 is a key enzyme involved in regulating the WNT signaling pathway, which controls adult neurogenesis and is a regulator of multiple neuroplasticity mechanisms. Growing pharmacologic and genetic evidence from preclinical models, as well as analysis of patient-derived samples, support the likelihood that GSK3 inhibition is involved in lithium's antimanic and antidepressant actions.

Immediately upon the introduction of lithium into clinical use for treating mood disorders, it was recognized that the drug has a narrow therapeutic window (desired range of 0.4 to 1.0 mEq/L, although the optimal level remains a subject of dispute). This recognition led patients such as Ms. R to be concerned about lithium's potential adverse effects. **Acute lithium intoxication**—a clinical syndrome characterized by nausea, vomiting, diarrhea, renal failure, neuromuscular dysfunction, ataxia, tremor, confusion, delirium, and seizures—is a medical emergency that may require dialysis for treatment. Hyponatremia or the administration of nonsteroidal anti-inflammatory drugs (NSAIDs) can lead to increased lithium reabsorption in the proximal tubule and can thereby elevate plasma lithium concentrations to toxic levels. Long-term lithium treatment has also been associated with increased risk for renal insufficiency.

Lithium's inhibition of K^+ entry into myocytes can lead to abnormalities in membrane repolarization, resulting in abnormal T waves on ECG. In addition, the transmembrane electrical potential is shifted because inhibition of K^+ entry into cells leads to extracellular hyperkalemia and intracellular hypokalemia. This shift in transmembrane potential exposes patients to a greater risk of sudden cardiac arrest from small changes in potassium balance.

Antidiuretic hormone and thyroid-stimulating hormone both activate adenylyl cyclase, which is inhibited by lithium. By this mechanism, lithium treatment can also lead to **nephrogenic diabetes insipidus**, hypothyroidism, and goiter.

Separate from the tremor associated with acute lithium intoxication, long-term lithium treatment can cause a tremor consisting of involuntary rhythmic oscillation (8–12 Hz), most often of the hands and upper limbs at rest, that is dose-dependent and nonprogressive. The pathophysiologic basis for this tremor remains to be elucidated; there is some evidence that it is both peripherally and centrally mediated. The central mechanisms may involve motor neurons in the cortex and serotonergic neurons in the brainstem.

Given the wide range of adverse effects that may accompany lithium treatment and the euphoria that may be associated with manic or hypomanic episodes, many patients are hesitant to begin treatment. Careful serum monitoring and lithium dose titration can help to avoid some, if not all, of the adverse effects discussed above, although this requires peripheral blood sampling on a regular basis. Despite its drawbacks, lithium remains one of the most effective agents for treating BD. Lithium and a limited number of other mood-stabilizing drugs (see Drug Summary Table) help to prevent depressive episodes as well as mania, and lithium remains the only drug demonstrated to reduce suicide risk in patients with bipolar disorder. Ongoing preclinical research aims to identify lithium "mimetics" with greater efficacy, higher therapeutic index, and reduced adverse effects through clarification of lithium's therapeutically relevant mechanism of action and identification of adjunctive therapeutic agents that can enhance lithium's mood-stabilizing activity.

▌ CONCLUSION AND FUTURE DIRECTIONS

This chapter discusses central monoamine neurotransmission—primarily serotonin pathways but also norepinephrine and, to a lesser extent, dopamine pathways. Serotonin is a critical mediator of mood and anxiety and is also involved in the pathophysiology of migraine headache and IBS. The focus of the chapter is on the antidepressant class of medications. The monoamine theory of depression has been an intellectual framework for conceptualizing the pathophysiology and treatment of MDD, although this theory is clearly an oversimplification. Therapy with drugs that increase synaptic concentrations of 5-HT and NE is still effective in many cases of MDD and forms the basis of treatment for this disorder. The delay between initiation of treatment and maximal clinical improvement may occur because of slow changes in presynaptic autoreceptor sensitivity and/or slow changes in postsynaptic neural circuitry. However, the necessity of directly modulating monoamine levels is being increasingly challenged by a subset of emerging drugs with antidepressant activity (e.g., tianeptine and agomelatine), and the monoamine theory is also challenged by agents with a more rapid albeit short-lived onset of therapeutic effect (e.g., ketamine).

TCAs, SSRIs, MAOIs, and other antidepressants have similar clinical efficacies when tested on groups of patients, although individual patients may respond to one drug and not to another. TCAs nonselectively inhibit 5-HT and NE reuptake transporters (in addition to other receptors); SSRIs selectively block 5-HT reuptake transporters; SNRIs selectively block 5-HT and NE reuptake transporters; and MAOIs inhibit the degradation of both 5-HT and NE. The choice of antidepressant medication for an individual patient depends on the two goals of finding an effective agent for that patient and minimizing adverse effects. SSRIs have become the most commonly prescribed antidepressants because of their favorable therapeutic index and are the first-line pharmacologic choice for treatment of MDD, anxiety, obsessive-compulsive disorder, and posttraumatic stress disorder.

The mechanisms underlying effective therapies in BD are even less well understood. Emerging research supports a role for common genetic variation in determining the risk for developing BD, although only a modest number of risk variants have been identified to date. Agents used to treat BD include lithium, some antiepileptics, and antipsychotics.

Recent advances in drug development for the treatment of MDD have focused on a deeper understanding of the mechanism of action of current drugs, the physiology of their molecular targets, and efforts to identify drugs with a more rapid onset of effect. Pharmacogenomic approaches have failed to convincingly implicate genetic variants that affect the likelihood of treatment response, though such efforts continue with the goal of better matching of drugs to patients by identifying patients who are particularly likely or particularly unlikely to respond to or tolerate a specific drug.

Drug targets beyond the monoamine systems are also showing promise, including agents targeting melatonergic and glutamatergic neurotransmission. Preclinical work in rodent models is beginning to elucidate novel targets with antidepressant-like activity, which further supports the notion of adaptive changes in neuroplasticity as key mediators of antidepressant effects. Some of this work involves pharmacologic agents targeting epigenetic mechanisms and glucocorticoid signaling. More generally, emerging understanding of the complex but ultimately tractable genetic liability, which may cross traditional diagnostic boundaries, is likely to point the way to entirely novel treatment targets.

Acknowledgment

We thank Mireya Nadal-Vicens, Jay H. Chyung, Timothy J. Turner, Miles Berger, and Bryan Roth for their valuable contributions to this chapter in the First, Second, and Third Editions of *Principles of Pharmacology: The Pathophysiologic Basis of Drug Therapy*.

Suggested Reading

Beaulieu JM, Caron MG. Looking at lithium: molecular moods and complex behaviour. *Mol Interv* 2008;8:230–241. (*Review of the likely mechanism[s] of action of lithium.*)

Berger M, Gray J, Roth BL. The expanded biology of serotonin. *Annu Rev Med* 2009;60:355–366. (*Broad review of the role of serotonin in modulating physiologic processes.*)

Dayan P, Huys QJ. Serotonin in affective control. *Annu Rev Neurosci* 2009;32:95–126. (*Review of serotonergic neurotransmission from the viewpoints of evolution and computational and systems neuroscience.*)

Insel T, Cuthbert B, Garvey M, et al. Research domain criteria (RDoC): toward a new classification framework for research on mental disorders. *Am J Psychiatry* 2010;167:748–751. (*Overview of a new framework for advancing research on MDD, BD, and other mental disorders that aims to revolutionize diagnosis and treatment; see also http://www.ted.com/talks /thomas_insel_toward_a_new_understanding_of_mental_illness.*)

Krishnan V, Nestler EJ. The molecular neurobiology of depression. *Nature* 2008;455:894–902. (*Current understanding of mood disorders and targets for new antidepressant drugs.*)

Nestler EJ. Epigenetic mechanisms of depression. *JAMA Psychiatry* 2014;71:454–456. (*Reviews possible epigenetic etiologies of depression.*)

Richelson E. Pharmacology of antidepressants. *Mayo Clin Proc* 2001; 76:511–527. (*Broad and thorough overview of the molecular mechanisms and cellular targets of first-generation antidepressant medications.*)

Schioldann J. *History of the introduction of lithium into medicine and psychiatry: birth of modern psychopharmacology 1949.* Adelaide: Adelaide Academic Press; 2009. (*Review of founding experiments on the psychopharmacology of lithium.*)

Schloesser RJ, Martinowich K, Manji HK. Mood-stabilizing drugs: mechanisms of action. *Trends Neurosci* 2012;35:36–46. (*Reviews primary targets of mood stabilizers and downstream molecular and cellular mechanisms of action.*)

Vialou V, Feng J, Robison AJ, Nestler EJ. Epigenetic mechanisms of depression and antidepressant action. *Annu Rev Pharmacol Toxicol* 2013;53: 59–87. (*Describes the emerging role for neuroepigenetic mechanisms and chromatin-mediated neuroplasticity in the pathophysiology and treatment of MDD.*)

DRUG SUMMARY TABLE: CHAPTER 15 Pharmacology of Serotonergic and Central Adrenergic Neurotransmission

DRUG	CLINICAL APPLICATIONS	SERIOUS AND COMMON ADVERSE EFFECTS	CONTRAINDICATIONS	THERAPEUTIC CONSIDERATIONS
INHIBITORS OF SEROTONIN STORAGE Mechanism—Interfere with the ability of synaptic vesicles to store monoamines; displace 5-HT, DA, and NE from their storage vesicles in presynaptic nerve terminals				
Amphetamine Methylphenidate	See Drug Summary Table: Chapter 11 Adrenergic Pharmacology			
Modafinil	Narcolepsy Obstructive sleep apnea Shift work sleep disorder	*Hypertension, Stevens-Johnson syndrome, toxic epidermal necrolysis, mania* Headache, anxiety, insomnia	Hypersensitivity to modafinil	Useful as second-line agent for atypical depression and for depression in the elderly. Can induce psychosis in susceptible patients, especially those with bipolar disorder.
Dextroamphetamine	ADHD Narcolepsy	*Tachycardia, myocardial infarction, peripheral vascular disease, decreased body growth, stroke, psychotic disorder, drug dependence*	Cardiovascular disease, agitation, concomitant or recent use of MAOIs, drug dependence, glaucoma, hypersensitivity, hypertension, hyperthyroidism	Dextroamphetamine has significant potential for substance abuse.
Lisdexamfetamine	ADHD	*Sudden death, myocardial infarction, ventricular hypertrophy, tachycardia, stroke, peripheral vascular disease, anaphylaxis, seizure* Rash, weight loss, gastrointestinal (GI) upset, dizziness, insomnia, irritability	Hypersensitivity to lisdexamfetamine Concomitant use of MAOIs	Lisdexamfetamine is a prodrug of dextroamphetamine and has less abuse potential.
INHIBITORS OF SEROTONIN DEGRADATION Mechanism—Block deamination of monoamines by inhibiting the flavin adenine dinucleotide (FAD) cofactor of MAO; increase the 5-HT and NE available in the cytoplasm of presynaptic neurons, which leads to increased uptake and storage of 5-HT and NE in synaptic vesicles and to some constitutive leakage of monoamines into the synaptic cleft				
Iproniazid Phenelzine Isocarboxazid	Depression	*Systemic tyramine toxicity from consumption of foods that contain tyramine (uncontrolled catecholamine release can induce a hypertensive crisis characterized by headache, tachycardia, nausea, cardiac arrhythmia, and stroke), fever associated with increased muscle tone, leukopenia, hepatic failure, drug-induced lupus, worsening depression (shared adverse effects); seizure, edema of glottis (phenelzine only)* Dizziness, somnolence, orthostatic hypotension, weight gain, increased liver aminotransferase level, orgasm disorder, GI upset	Hypersensitivity to drug Concomitant use of sympathomimetic drugs Concomitant use of bupropion, buspirone, guanethidine, other MAOIs, serotonergic drugs Concomitant use of methyldopa, L-DOPA, L-tryptophan, L-tyrosine, phenylalanine Concomitant use of CNS depressants, opioids, meperidine, dextromethorphan Concomitant, excessive coffee or chocolate intake Concomitant intake of foods with high tyramine content (cheese, beer, wine, pickled herring, yogurt, liver, yeast extract) Liver disease Pheochromocytoma Heart failure General anesthesia, local anesthesia with vasoconstrictors Renal disease	Due to the effects of MAOIs on P450 enzymes, MAOIs can cause extensive drug–drug interactions; extreme caution must be used when prescribing medications to patients concurrently taking an MAOI. Iproniazid, phenelzine, and isocarboxazid are irreversible, nonselective MAOIs. The most toxic effect of MAOI use is systemic tyramine toxicity; the older, nonselective MAOIs are no longer considered first-line therapy for depression because of their significant potential for systemic tyramine toxicity. MAOIs can precipitate manic or hypomanic episodes in some patients with bipolar disorder.

Drug	Indication	Adverse Effects	Contraindications	Notes
Moclobemide, Befloxatone, Brofaromine	Depression	*Same as iproniazid, except less tyramine toxicity*	Same as iproniazid	Moclobemide, befloxatone, and brofaromine are reversible inhibitors of monoamine oxidase A (RIMAs). These newer MAOIs are displaced by high concentrations of tyramine, resulting in significantly greater tyramine metabolism and thus less tyramine toxicity.
Selegiline	Depression	*Hypertensive crisis, suicidal thoughts*; Application site reaction, headache	Same as iproniazid except that patients have greater freedom with their diet	Selegiline is an MAO-B inhibitor that also inhibits MAO-A at higher doses. Transdermal selegiline reduces the risk of a tyramine-induced hypertensive crisis, allowing patients greater freedom with their diet.

TRICYCLIC ANTIDEPRESSANTS (TCAs)
Mechanism—Inhibit reuptake of 5-HT and NE from the synaptic cleft by respectively blocking 5-HT and NE reuptake transporters and thereby cause enhancement of postsynaptic responses

Drug	Indication	Adverse Effects	Contraindications	Notes
Amitriptyline, Clomipramine, Desipramine, Doxepin, Imipramine, Nortriptyline, Protriptyline, Trimipramine	Shared indication, except for clomipramine: Depression. Doxepin only: Anxiety, Pruritus. Imipramine only: Nocturnal enuresis. Clomipramine only: Obsessive-compulsive disorder	*Cardiac arrhythmia, orthostatic hypotension, myocardial infarction, bone marrow depression, worsening depression with suicidal thoughts (shared adverse effects); hepatotoxicity, seizure (shared except for doxepin); hyperglycemia, increased body temperature, serotonin syndrome (clomipramine only); nephrotoxicity (doxepin only); inappropriate antidiuretic hormone secretion, paralytic ileus, stroke, myoclonus, angioedema (nortriptyline only);* GI upset (shared adverse effect); dizziness, headache, somnolence, blurred vision (shared except for doxepin); diaphoresis, insomnia, tremor, impotence (clomipramine only); urinary retention (doxepin and imipramine only)	Shared contraindications: Hypersensitivity to drug; Concomitant use of MAOIs. Shared except for doxepin: Use in patients during acute recovery after myocardial infarction. Doxepin only: Glaucoma, Urinary retention	TCAs appear to affect cardiac sodium channels in a quinidine-like manner, leading to potentially lethal conduction delays; an ECG should be done to rule out conduction system disease prior to starting TCAs. Concomitant use of other agents that affect the cardiac conduction system requires careful monitoring. In patients taking TCAs, pressor response to IV epinephrine may be markedly enhanced. Orthostatic hypotension is a significant adverse effect for elderly patients. TCAs can precipitate mania in patients with bipolar disorder.

continues

DRUG SUMMARY TABLE: CHAPTER 15 Pharmacology of Serotonergic and Central Adrenergic Neurotransmission *continued*

DRUG	CLINICAL APPLICATIONS	SERIOUS AND COMMON ADVERSE EFFECTS	CONTRAINDICATIONS	THERAPEUTIC CONSIDERATIONS
SELECTIVE SEROTONIN REUPTAKE INHIBITORS (SSRIs)				
Mechanism—Selectively inhibit reuptake of serotonin and thereby increase synaptic serotonin levels, causing increased 5-HT receptor activation and enhanced postsynaptic responses; at high doses, also bind NE transporter				
Citalopram **Fluoxetine** **Fluvoxamine** **Paroxetine** **Sertraline**	Shared indication except for fluvoxamine: Depression Fluoxetine, fluvoxamine, paroxetine, and sertraline only: Obsessive-compulsive disorder Fluoxetine, paroxetine, and sertraline only: Pain disorder Premenstrual dysphoric disorder Fluoxetine only: Bulimia nervosa Paroxetine and sertraline only: Posttraumatic stress disorder Panic disorder Social phobia	*Serotonin syndrome from concomitant administration of MAOI (characterized by hyperthermia, muscle rigidity, myoclonus, and rapid fluctuations in mental status and vital signs), may precipitate mania in a bipolar patient (shared adverse effects); prolonged QT interval, erythema multiforme (fluoxetine, fluvoxamine, paroxetine, and sertraline only); hyponatremia, bleeding (fluoxetine, fluvoxamine, and sertraline only); GI hemorrhage, rhabdomyolysis (sertraline only)* Diaphoresis, headache, somnolence, tremor, anxiety, GI upset (shared adverse effects; sertraline is more often associated with diarrhea, and paroxetine is associated with constipation); sexual dysfunction (paroxetine and sertraline only)	Shared contraindications: Hypersensitivity to drug Concomitant use of MAOIs, pimozide, or thioridazine Sertraline only: Concomitant use of disulfiram	First-line agents for the treatment of depression, anxiety, and obsessive-compulsive disorder. SSRIs are significantly more selective than TCAs for 5-HT transporters; therefore, SSRIs have a higher therapeutic index and fewer adverse effects than TCAs.
SEROTONIN-NOREPINEPHRINE REUPTAKE INHIBITORS (SNRIs)				
Mechanism—Block 5-HT reuptake transporter and NE reuptake transporter in a concentration-dependent manner				
Venlafaxine **Duloxetine**	Shared indications: Depression Anxiety Venlafaxine only: Panic disorder with or without agoraphobia Social phobia Duloxetine only: Pain syndromes	*Serotonin syndrome, hepatotoxicity, bleeding, may exacerbate mania or depression in susceptible patients (shared adverse effects); hyponatremia, neuroleptic malignant syndrome, sustained hypertension (venlafaxine only)* Hypertension, sweating, GI upset, dizziness, headache, somnolence (shared adverse effects); blurred vision, nervousness, sexual dysfunction, asthenia, tremor (venlafaxine only)	Hypersensitivity to drug Concomitant use of MAOIs	Venlafaxine and duloxetine block the 5-HT and NE reuptake transporters in a concentration-dependent manner: at low concentrations, they act as SSRIs, but at high concentrations, they also increase NE levels.

Drug	Clinical Applications	Serious and Common Adverse Effects	Contraindications	Therapeutic Considerations
Desvenlafaxine	Major depressive disorder	*Hypertension, myocardial ischemia, hyponatremia, GI hemorrhage, abnormal bleeding, seizure, serotonin syndrome, suicidal thoughts, interstitial lung disease, pulmonary eosinophilia* Diaphoresis, increased serum cholesterol and triglycerides, GI upset, dizziness, insomnia, somnolence, erectile dysfunction, fatigue	Hypersensitivity to desvenlafaxine Concomitant or recent use of MAOIs	Desvenlafaxine is an active metabolite of venlafaxine.
Milnacipran	Fibromyalgia	*Hypertensive crisis, erythema multiforme, GI hemorrhage, abnormal bleeding, liver injury, serotonin syndrome, depression exacerbation* Increased blood pressure and heart rate, palpitations, diaphoresis, GI upset, headache	Concomitant or recent use of MAOIs Narrow-angle glaucoma	Milnacipran inhibits 5-HT and NE reuptake.

NOREPINEPHRINE-SELECTIVE REUPTAKE INHIBITORS (NRIs)
Mechanism—Selectively block norepinephrine transporter, leading to increased norepinephrine levels

Drug	Clinical Applications	Serious and Common Adverse Effects	Contraindications	Therapeutic Considerations
Atomoxetine	ADHD	*Myocardial infarction, prolonged QT interval, sudden cardiac death, liver injury, stroke, dyskinesia, seizure, psychotic disorder, suicidal thoughts, priapism, angioedema* Hypertension, tachycardia, weight loss, GI upset, headache, somnolence, urinary retention, dysmenorrhea, erectile dysfunction, hot flashes	Hypersensitivity to atomoxetine Concomitant use of MAOIs Narrow-angle glaucoma Cardiac or vascular disorders Pheochromocytoma	Atomoxetine has a lower abuse potential and a longer half-life than the amphetamines; the longer half-life allows for once-daily dosing.

OTHER ATYPICAL ANTIDEPRESSANTS
Mechanism—Bupropion is an aminoketone antidepressant that weakly inhibits neuronal uptake of 5-HT, dopamine, and NE. Mirtazapine blocks 5-HT$_{2A}$, 5-HT$_{2C}$, and the α_2-adrenergic autoreceptor and presumably decreases neurotransmission at 5-HT$_2$ synapses while increasing NE neurotransmission. Trazodone blocks postsynaptic 5-HT$_2$ receptors. Tianeptine affects neuroplasticity pathways and may target specific non-serotonergic receptors. Agomelatine is an agonist at the melatonin receptors 1 and 2 and an antagonist at 5-HT$_2$ receptors.

Drug	Clinical Applications	Serious and Common Adverse Effects	Contraindications	Therapeutic Considerations
Bupropion	Depression Smoking cessation	*Anaphylaxis, tachyarrhythmia, hypertension especially when combined with nicotine patch, seizure, may exacerbate mania in susceptible patients (the latter effect is less likely than with other antidepressants)* GI upset, pruritus, rash, dizziness, headache, insomnia, tremor, agitation	Hypersensitivity to bupropion Seizure Bulimia or anorexia Concomitant use of MAOIs Concomitant use of other bupropion products Patients undergoing abrupt discontinuation of alcohol or sedatives (including benzodiazepines)	Has the fewest sexual effects among antidepressant agents. Induces less mania than the other antidepressants.
Mirtazapine	Depression	*Agranulocytosis, seizure, may exacerbate depression or mania in susceptible patients, neuroleptic malignant syndrome* Somnolence, increased appetite, weight gain, hyperlipidemia, constipation, xerostomia, dizziness	Hypersensitivity to mirtazapine Concomitant use of MAOIs	Because mirtazapine is a potent anxiolytic and hypnotic (sleep-inducing agent) as well as an appetite stimulant, it is useful in the elderly population in whom insomnia and weight loss are frequent presentations.

continues

DRUG SUMMARY TABLE: CHAPTER 15 Pharmacology of Serotonergic and Central Adrenergic Neurotransmission *continued*

DRUG	CLINICAL APPLICATIONS	SERIOUS AND COMMON ADVERSE EFFECTS	CONTRAINDICATIONS	THERAPEUTIC CONSIDERATIONS
Trazodone	Depression Anxiety Insomnia	*Cardiac arrhythmia, hypotension, serotonin syndrome, suicidal thoughts, priapism* GI upset, dizziness, headache, somnolence, blurred vision, nervousness, fatigue	Hypersensitivity to trazodone Concomitant use of MAOIs Concomitant use of saquinavir or ritonavir	Trazodone is a prodrug used in the treatment of depression, anxiety, and insomnia that is converted into meta-chlorophenylpiperazine (mCPP), a selective 5-HT$_{2A/2C}$ agonist. Trazodone is used principally as an anxiolytic and hypnotic (sleep-inducing agent) because the higher doses required for antidepressant effects are usually oversedating.
Tianeptine	Depression	*Hepatitis (rare), dependency* Headache, fatigue, nausea, drowsiness, abdominal pain, muscle pain, joint pain, weight gain, insomnia, constipation, anxiety, irritability, vertigo, tremor, dry mouth	Hypersensitivity to tianeptine	Tianeptine functions as a selective enhancer of serotonin reuptake with the ability also to enhance neuroplasticity through effects mediated in part by elevating neurotrophic factors (e.g., BDNF) and affecting glutamate receptors and μ and δ opioid receptors. Lacks blood pressure and cardiovascular adverse effects. Additional anxiolytic effects may lead to dependence. Approved only in Europe.
Agomelatine	Depression	*Hepatotoxicity (rare)* GI upset, headache, fatigue, anxiety, insomnia, sweating	Hypersensitivity to agomelatine Hepatic impairment Concomitant use of CYP1A2 inhibitors such as fluvoxamine and ciprofloxacin	Agomelatine is the antidepressant with the most recently discovered mechanism of action. Exhibits agonist activity at melatonin receptors 1 and 2, leading to effects on circadian physiology, and antagonist activity at the 5-HT$_{2C}$ receptor. Lacks effects on extracellular serotonin levels but increases dopamine and norepinephrine release. Agomelatine is well tolerated, with infrequent sexual adverse effects.

SEROTONIN RECEPTOR AGONISTS

Mechanism—Buspirone is a 5-HT$_{1A}$-selective agonist. Vilazodone and vortioxetine are combined partial agonists at 5-HT$_1$ receptors and inhibitors of the 5-HT transporter (SERT). The vasoconstrictive therapeutic effect of triptans is mediated by 5-HT$_1$ receptors (both 5-HT$_{1D}$ and 5-HT$_{1B}$) expressed in the cerebral vasculature.

DRUG	CLINICAL APPLICATIONS	SERIOUS AND COMMON ADVERSE EFFECTS	CONTRAINDICATIONS	THERAPEUTIC CONSIDERATIONS
Buspirone	Anxiety	*Myocardial infarction, stroke* Dizziness, nausea, somnolence, headache, nervousness	Hypersensitivity to buspirone	Buspirone is nonsedating with moderate anxiolytic properties; although not as effective as benzodiazepines, it is a useful option in some patients because of its nonaddictive properties.
Vilazodone Vortioxetine	Depression	*Suicidal thoughts, serotonin syndrome (shared adverse effects); palpitations (vilazodone only); hyponatremia (vortioxetine only)* GI upset (shared adverse effect); insomnia (vilazodone only)	Hypersensitivity to drug Concomitant use of MAOIs	New class of agents for the treatment of depression that target adaptive mechanisms to facilitate serotonergic neurotransmission. Vilazodone, but not vortioxetine, lacks effects on sexual function, providing an advantage over TCAs and SSRIs.

Drug	Clinical Applications	Serious and Common Adverse Effects	Contraindications	Therapeutic Considerations
Sumatriptan Rizatriptan Almotriptan Frovatriptan Eletriptan Zolmitriptan	Migraine headache	*Myocardial infarction, vasospasm (shared adverse effects); serotonin syndrome (sumatriptan, rizatriptan, frovatriptan, and eletriptan only); hypertensive crisis (sumatriptan and rizatriptan only); vision loss (sumatriptan, frovatriptan, and zolmitriptan only); seizure (sumatriptan and eletriptan only); subarachnoid hemorrhage (sumatriptan and zolmitriptan only); analgesic overuse headache (rizatriptan and zolmitriptan only)* Chest pain, GI upset, dizziness	Shared contraindications: Hypersensitivity to drug; Ergot agent or serotonin 5-HT$_1$ agonist within 24 hours; Concomitant use of MAOIs; Ischemic cardiac, cerebrovascular, or peripheral vascular syndromes; Uncontrolled hypertension; Sumatriptan only: Hepatic impairment; Eletriptan only: Concomitant use of CYP3A4 inhibitors	Triptans are most useful for acute migraine attacks when taken at the onset of an episode rather than as prophylaxis.

SEROTONIN RECEPTOR ANTAGONISTS
Mechanism—Serotonin receptor antagonists show varying degrees of receptor subtype selectivity and often cross-react with adrenergic, histamine, and muscarinic receptors

Drug	Clinical Applications	Serious and Common Adverse Effects	Contraindications	Therapeutic Considerations
Ketanserin	Glaucoma Hypertension	*Orthostatic hypotension, ventricular tachycardia* Flushing, rash, fluid retention, dyspepsia, dizziness, sedation	Hypersensitivity to ketanserin	5-HT$_{2A/2C}$ antagonist. Primarily used topically to reduce intraocular pressure in glaucoma.
Ondansetron	Nausea	*Cardiac arrhythmia* Increased liver enzymes, constipation, diarrhea, fatigue, headache	Hypersensitivity to ondansetron; Concomitant use of apomorphine	5-HT$_3$ antagonist. A potent antiemetic that is frequently used as an adjunct to cancer chemotherapy or in cases of refractory nausea.
Tegaserod Prucalopride	Irritable bowel syndrome (IBS) with constipation predominance	*Stroke, chest pain, hypotension, hypovolemia, myocardial infarction, syncope, ischemic colitis, hypersensitivity reaction* Diarrhea, headache	Prucalopride only: Hypersensitivity to drug; History of bowel obstruction, abdominal adhesions, or symptomatic gallbladder disease; Severe renal impairment	5-HT$_4$ antagonists. Enhance GI motility to treat constipation associated with IBS. Tegaserod maleate was withdrawn from the market in 2007 due to increased risk of myocardial infarction and stroke.
Alosetron	Irritable bowel syndrome (IBS) with diarrhea predominance	*Severe constipation, acute ischemic colitis, toxic megacolon* Abdominal pain, nausea, headache	Preexisting constipation; Concurrent use of fluvoxamine or apomorphine; Crohn's disease, ulcerative colitis, diverticulitis; Severe hepatic impairment; History of hypercoagulable state; History of impaired intestinal circulation, intestinal stricture, ischemic colitis, or toxic megacolon	5-HT$_3$ antagonist. Decreases serotonergic tone in intestinal cells, thus reducing intestinal motility. Useful for diarrhea associated with IBS.

MOOD STABILIZERS

Drug				
Carbamazepine Valproic acid Lamotrigine	See Drug Summary Table: Chapter 16 Pharmacology of Abnormal Electrical Neurotransmission in the Central Nervous System			

continues

DRUG SUMMARY TABLE: CHAPTER 15 Pharmacology of Serotonergic and Central Adrenergic Neurotransmission *continued*

DRUG	CLINICAL APPLICATIONS	*SERIOUS* AND COMMON ADVERSE EFFECTS	CONTRAINDICATIONS	THERAPEUTIC CONSIDERATIONS
LITHIUM				
Mechanism—Lithium can mimic other monovalent cations and the divalent cation magnesium (Mg^{2+}) and thereby disrupt proteins and transporters that require cation cofactors. Lithium enters cells via Na^+ channels. Lithium inhibits both the inositol phosphatase that dephosphorylates IP_2 to inositol phosphate (IP_1) and the inositol phosphatase that dephosphorylates IP_1 to free inositol, thereby blocking the phosphatidylinositol signaling cascade in the brain. By blocking the regeneration of PIP_2, lithium inhibits central adrenergic, muscarinic, and serotonergic neurotransmission. Other mechanisms of action include increasing 5-HT neurotransmission, decreasing NE and DA neurotransmission, inhibiting adenylyl cyclase by decoupling G proteins from neurotransmitter receptors, altering electrochemical gradients across cell membranes by substituting for Na^+ and/or blocking K^+ channels, and inhibiting GSK3, a kinase critical to multiple neuroplasticity pathways.			
Lithium	Bipolar disorder	*Acute lithium intoxication (characterized by nausea, vomiting, diarrhea, renal failure, neuromuscular dysfunction, ataxia, tremor, confusion, delirium, seizures, giddiness, blurred vision, and tinnitus), severe bradyarrhythmia, hypotension, sinus node dysfunction, hyperkalemia, erythema multiforme, pseudotumor cerebri, increased intracranial pressure and papilledema, nephrotoxicity, angioedema* Acne, hypothyroidism, weight gain, GI upset, leukocytosis, tremor, hyperreflexia, polyuria, polydipsia	Severe debilitation, dehydration, or sodium depletion Significant cardiovascular disease Significant renal impairment Concomitant use of diuretics	Lithium has been shown to have antimanic activity and reduce suicide risk in patients with bipolar disorder. Lithium has a narrow therapeutic index and a wide range of adverse effects. Acute lithium intoxication is a medical emergency and may require dialysis for treatment. Nonsteroidal anti-inflammatory drugs (NSAIDs) or hyponatremia can lead to increased lithium reabsorption in the proximal tubule and elevation of plasma lithium concentrations. Lithium's inhibition of potassium entry into myocytes leads to abnormalities in myocyte repolarization, extracellular hyperkalemia, and intracellular hypokalemia. Chronic lithium treatment is also known to cause tremor and other neurological adverse effects.

Pharmacology of Abnormal Electrical Neurotransmission in the Central Nervous System

Susannah B. Cornes, Edmund A. Griffin, Jr., and Daniel H. Lowenstein

INTRODUCTION

With over 10 billion neurons and an estimated 10^{14} synaptic connections, the human brain boasts unparalleled electrical complexity. Unlike myocardial tissue, where electrical signals spread synchronously through a syncytium of cells, proper functioning of the brain requires distinct isolation of electrical signals and thus demands a far higher level of regulation. Control of this complex function begins at the level of the ion channel and is further maintained through the effects of these ion channels on the activity of highly organized neuronal networks. Abnormal function of ion channels and neural networks can result in rapid, synchronous, and uncontrolled spread of electrical activity, which is the basis of a **seizure**.

A seizure can present with a variety of symptoms and result from a variety of causes. A single seizure should be distinguished from **epilepsy**, which refers to the condition in which an individual has a tendency toward recurrent seizures (i.e., a patient who has had a single seizure does not necessarily have epilepsy). Seizure symptoms vary according to the location of seizure activity and may include prominent motor symptoms and loss of consciousness (as seen in tonic–clonic seizures), paroxysmal alterations in nonmotor functions (e.g., sensation, olfaction, vision), or changes in higher order functions (e.g., emotion, memory, language, insight).

This chapter explores the molecular mechanisms by which the brain maintains precise control over the spread of electrical activity and how various abnormalities can undermine these physiologic mechanisms and lead to seizures. The various classes of antiepileptic drugs are then discussed, with an emphasis on molecular mechanisms for restoring inhibitory function in the brain and suppressing seizure activity.

PHYSIOLOGY

The normal human brain, in the absence of any lesions or genetic abnormalities, is capable of undergoing a seizure. Acute changes in the availability of excitatory neurotransmitters

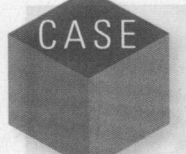

CASE

Jon arrives in the emergency department with his brother Rob at 9:12 PM. Because his brother is still too lethargic to speak, Jon relays most of the story to the attending physician. The two had been watching television when Jon noticed that his 40-year-old brother seemed to be daydreaming. Never missing an opportunity to tease, Jon began chiding his brother for "spacing out." But instead of the boisterous laugh that he was so used to, Jon observed only a confused, almost fearful stare.

Jon recalls that his brother's right hand suddenly began to bend into an awkward position and then to shake. The shaking grew worse, progressing gradually from the hand to the arm and then to the entire right side of the body. Jon then noticed that Rob's body stiffened, almost as if he were attempting to contract every muscle in his body. This sustained contraction lasted for about 15 seconds and was followed by shaking movements of all four limbs that lasted another 30 seconds or so. The frequency of the shaking slowed after several minutes, and Rob then became limp, began breathing very heavily, and remained unresponsive. Rob regained consciousness on the way to the emergency department.

At the hospital, a magnetic resonance imaging (MRI) scan shows a small neoplasm in Rob's left temporal lobe. Because the neoplasm appears to be benign, Rob, following the advice of his physician, decides not to undergo surgery. The potential benefits and risks of various antiepileptic drugs are discussed, including phenytoin, carbamazepine, valproic acid, and lamotrigine, and it is decided to start Rob on a regimen of carbamazepine to prevent further seizures.

Questions

1. By what mechanisms can a focal neoplasm result in a seizure?
2. Is there any clinical significance to the fearful, blank stare?
3. What is the significance of the order of spread of the seizure from the hand to the arm and then to the leg?
4. The generalized seizure that followed the right-sided shaking included a tonic phase (stiffening) followed by a clonic phase (shaking). What occurs at the molecular level to cause these symptoms?
5. Why was carbamazepine chosen as the antiepileptic treatment for Rob's seizures?

(e.g., caused by ingestion of the toxin **domoate**, which is a structural analogue of glutamate) or changes in the effect of inhibitory neurotransmitters (e.g., caused by injection of **penicillin**, a $GABA_A$ antagonist) can result in massive seizure activity in the otherwise healthy human brain. These examples demonstrate that the complex circuits within the brain exist in a balance between excitatory and inhibitory factors and that changes in either category of these control mechanisms can lead to major dysfunction.

In the CNS, two important elements normally involved in the fine-tuning of neuronal signaling also function to prevent the repetitious and synchronous firing characteristic of a seizure. At the cellular level, a "refractory period" induced by Na^+ channel inactivation and K^+ channel-mediated hyperpolarization prevents abnormal repetitive firing in neuronal cells. As discussed in Chapter 8, Principles of Cellular Excitability and Electrochemical Transmission, action potentials are propagated by voltage-sensitive ion channels. After initiation in the axon hillock, the action potential is propagated by alternating currents of depolarizing Na^+ influx and hyperpolarizing K^+ efflux. Throughout the course of an action potential (Fig. 16-1), the Na^+ channels exist in three distinct states: (1) a **closed state** before activation, (2) an **open state** during depolarization, and (3) an **inactivated state** shortly after the peak of depolarization.

Because Na^+ channels adopt the inactivated state in response to depolarization, action potentials are intrinsically self-limiting—Na^+ channels will not recover from the inactivated state until the membrane is sufficiently repolarized. K^+ channel opening repolarizes the cell, but the high K^+ efflux transiently hyperpolarizes the membrane beyond its resting potential, further increasing the time before a new action potential can be generated. Thus, *under physiologic*

conditions, the biochemical properties of Na^+ and K^+ channels impose a limit on the frequency of firing and help to prevent the repetitive firing characteristic of many seizure types.

Beyond the single-cell level, **neural networks** ensure the specificity of neuronal signaling by restricting the effects of a given action potential to a defined area. Even a strong train of action potentials, if contained within about 1,000 neurons, will not generate seizure activity. This is quite a remarkable feat, given the close proximity of neurons in the CNS and the fact that a single neuron in the neocortex may have more than 1,000 postsynaptic connections. As seen in the simplified neural network in Figure 16-2, the firing neuron activates immediately neighboring neurons in addition to interneurons that transmit inhibitory (**GABA**) signals to surrounding neurons. This contrast of local amplification and surrounding cell inhibition results in what is referred to as **surround inhibition**. Surround inhibition is essential to the normal function of the nervous system, because this phenomenon not only amplifies local signals but also provides insulation and protection against synchronicity in surrounding areas. Many seizure disorders appear to result from disruption of this intricate balance.

PATHOPHYSIOLOGY

Because the pathophysiologic mechanisms underlying seizure disorders are only beginning to be determined, seizures are in part classified according to their clinical manifestations. There has been a tendency to consider seizures as a dichotomous process involving the whole brain or part of the brain and referred to as **generalized** or **focal** accordingly. This is probably an oversimplification. In fact, a seizure can involve a neuronal network that is restricted to one

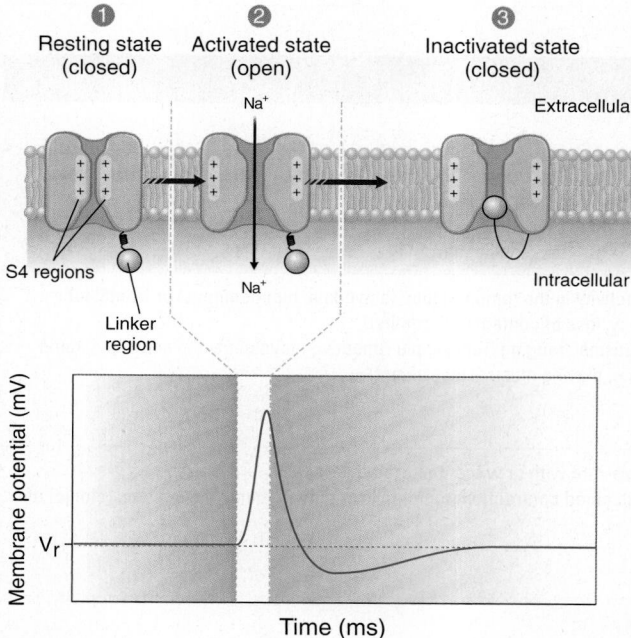

FIGURE 16-1. Duration and frequency of the action potential is limited by properties intrinsic to the sodium channel. The voltage-sensitive Na^+ channel exists in three different conformations during the course of an action potential. After opening transiently in response to membrane depolarization **(2)**, the Na^+ channel spontaneously inactivates **(3)**. This closure of the channel decreases the strength of the Na^+-mediated depolarization. Na^+ channels recover from inactivation only when the membrane potential is restored to its resting level (V_r). Membrane depolarization also has the effect of opening voltage-sensitive K^+ channels, which hyperpolarize the cell. Under hyperpolarizing conditions, the Na^+ channel adopts its resting (closed) conformation **(1)**. During these refractory periods of Na^+ channel inactivation and membrane hyperpolarization, the neuron is essentially insensitive to depolarizing signals (see also Fig. 12-7).

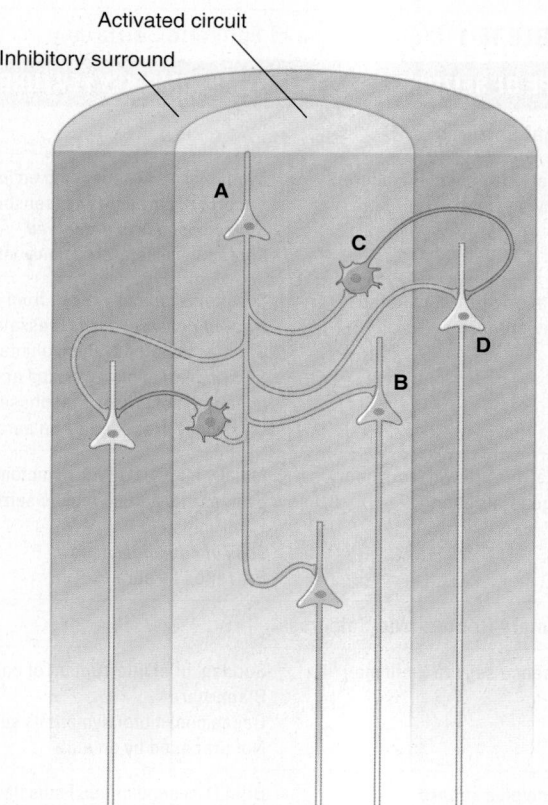

FIGURE 16-2. Surround inhibition prevents synchronization of adjacent neurons. In this simplified neuronal circuit, Neuron A sends excitatory projections (*light yellow*) to proximal neurons such as B. In addition to activating nearby neurons, Cell A also activates GABAergic interneurons (C) that send inhibitory projections (*dark yellow*) to surrounding neurons (D). This type of circuit creates an "inhibitory surround" (*light brown*), so that action potentials generated by Neuron A, even if rapid and robust, are unable to activate surrounding circuits.

hemisphere or that gradually or rapidly involves both hemispheres, and seizures involving both hemispheres may be asymmetric and may not involve the whole cortex. Thus, the term *generalized* should not be taken to mean "the whole brain" but rather to indicate that the involved neuronal network is bilaterally distributed.

When seizures involve part of the brain, they are said to be *focal*. Depending on the location and size of the seizure focus, there may be alteration in awareness, in which case the seizure is referred to as **focal dyscognitive** or "focal with alteration in awareness." (Note that this roughly corresponds to the previously termed *complex partial* seizure, a label that has been abandoned). In addition to helping the clinician define the underlying neuroanatomy, these associated symptoms have implications for the extent of disability and for defining appropriate treatments, including surgery (Table 16-1).

Whether a seizure involves one hemisphere or two, all seizures share the common characteristic of abnormal synchronous discharges. For this to occur, protective mechanisms must be compromised at the cellular and network levels. The direct causes of these changes can be primary (e.g., genetic abnormalities such as ion channel defects), secondary (e.g., changes in the neuronal environment induced by toxins, autoantibodies, or acquired lesions such as strokes or neoplasms), or a combination of the two (e.g., febrile seizures in children).

Pathophysiology of Focal Seizures

The focal seizure (Fig. 16-3A) occurs in three specific steps: (1) initiation at the cellular level by an increase in electrical activity, (2) synchronization of surrounding neurons, and (3) spread to adjacent regions of the brain. Seizures are initiated by a sudden depolarization within a group of neurons. This sudden change, called a **paroxysmal depolarizing shift (PDS)**, lasts up to 200 ms and results in the generation of an abnormally rapid train of action potentials. Changes in the extracellular milieu, attributable, for instance, to a space-occupying lesion (such as in the introductory case), can have major effects on neuronal burst activity. For example, the space-occupying lesion could cause an increase in extracellular K^+, which would blunt the effects of K^+-mediated after-hyperpolarization by decreasing the magnitude of the K^+ gradient between the outside and inside of the cell. Similarly, an increase in excitatory neurotransmitters or modulation of excitatory receptors by other exogenous molecules could increase burst activity. Increased burst activity could also result from properties intrinsic to the cell, such as abnormal channel conductance or altered membrane characteristics.

Because of surround inhibition, local discharges are often contained within a so-called **focus** and do not induce symptomatic pathology. These local discharges can be seen

TABLE 16-1 Classification of Epileptic Seizures

TYPE OF SEIZURE	SYMPTOMS/KEY FEATURES
Focal Seizures	
Focal seizure without altered awareness	Symptoms vary depending on location of abnormal activity in the brain: involuntary, repetitive movement (motor cortex), paresthesias (sensory cortex), flashing lights (visual cortex), etc. *Consciousness is preserved* Spread to ipsilateral regions within cortex (e.g., "Jacksonian march")
Focal seizure with altered awareness	Symptoms typically result from abnormal activity in the temporal lobe (amygdala, hippocampus) or frontal lobe *Altered consciousness* (cessation of activity, loss of contact with reality) Often associated with involuntary "automatisms" ranging from simple repetitive movements (lip smacking, hand wringing) to highly skilled activity (driving, playing musical instrument) Impaired memory of ictal phase Classically preceded by an aura
Focal seizure with secondary generalization	Initially manifests with symptoms of focal seizure with or without altered awareness Evolves into a tonic–clonic seizure with sustained contraction (tonic) followed by rhythmic movements (clonic) of all limbs *Loss of consciousness* Preceded by aura
Primary Generalized Seizures	
Absence seizure (petit mal)	Sudden, brief interruption of consciousness Blank stare Occasional motor symptoms such as lip smacking, rapid blinking Not preceded by an aura
Myoclonic seizure	Brief (1 second or less) muscle contraction; symptoms may occur in individual muscle or generalize to all muscle groups of the body (the latter can result in falling) Associated with systemic disease states such as uremia, hepatic failure, hereditary degenerative conditions, Creutzfeldt–Jakob disease
Tonic–clonic (grand mal) seizure	Symptoms as described above, but onset is abrupt and not preceded by symptoms of focal seizure

on an **electroencephalogram (EEG)** as sharp **interictal spikes**. Identification of these spikes can be useful in locating the seizure focus in a patient who is not actively undergoing a seizure. There are several pathways, however, whereby the seizure focus can override surround inhibition. Repetitive firing of neurons increases extracellular K^+. As described above, this weakens K^+-mediated hyperpolarization, allowing the seizure activity to spread. Rapidly firing neurons also open depolarization-sensitive NMDA channels (see Chapter 13, Pharmacology of GABAergic and Glutamatergic Neurotransmission) and accumulate Ca^{2+} in their synaptic terminals, both of which increase the likelihood of signal propagation and local synchronization. In many cases, it appears that the most important compromise of surround inhibition occurs at the level of GABAergic transmission. *Decreases in GABA-mediated inhibition—because of exogenous factors, degeneration of GABAergic neurons, or changes at the receptor level—are major factors that aid in the synchronization of a seizure focus.*

If the synchronizing focus is sufficiently strong, the abnormal, synchronized firing from a small neural network will begin to spread to neighboring regions of the cortex. During this spread to neighboring areas, the patient may experience an **aura**, a conscious "warning" of the spread of the seizure. In the introductory case, Rob's aura manifested as a blank, fearful stare. Although the aura is usually stereotypical for a given patient, a wide variety of auras exist. These include a sense of fear and confusion, disturbances of memory

(e.g., déjà vu) or language, altered sensations, or an olfactory hallucination. As the seizure continues to spread, it can lead to additional clinical manifestations; the specific manifestation depends on the brain regions that become involved. In the introductory case, the clinical symptoms initially started with shaking of the hand and progressed to the arm and then to the leg. This is a **Jacksonian march** (named after the English neurologist Hughlings Jackson, who first described the symptoms), where the clinical symptoms result from spread of synchronous activity across the motor homunculus.

Pathophysiology of Secondary Generalized Seizures

Focal seizures may become generalized by spreading along diffuse connections to involve both cerebral hemispheres. This is known as a **secondary (or secondarily) generalized seizure** (Fig. 16-3B). Typically, seizures spread to distant sites by following normal circuits, and this spread can occur through several pathways. **U fibers** connect various regions of the cortex; the **corpus callosum** allows for spread between hemispheres; and **thalamocortical projections** provide a pathway for diffuse synchronized spread throughout the brain. Once seizure activity spreads to involve both hemispheres, a patient usually loses consciousness.

Among the secondarily generalized seizures, the **tonic–clonic** subtype is the most common. In the introductory clinical case, Rob underwent a period where he appeared to

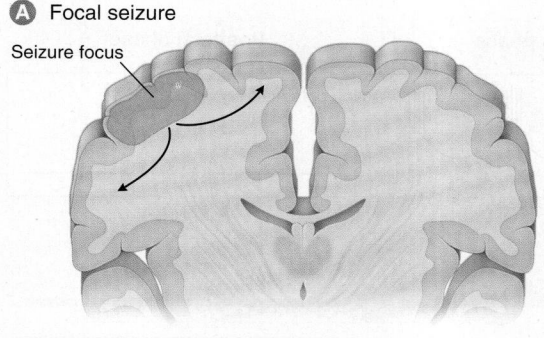

A Focal seizure

Seizure focus

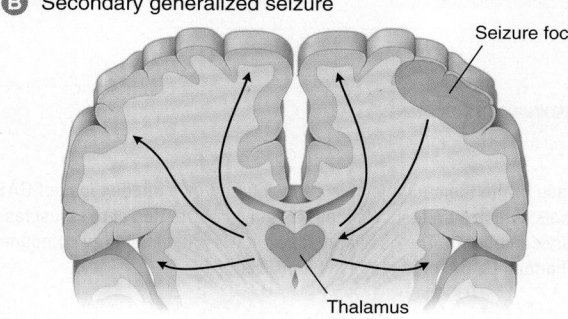

B Secondary generalized seizure

Seizure focus

Thalamus

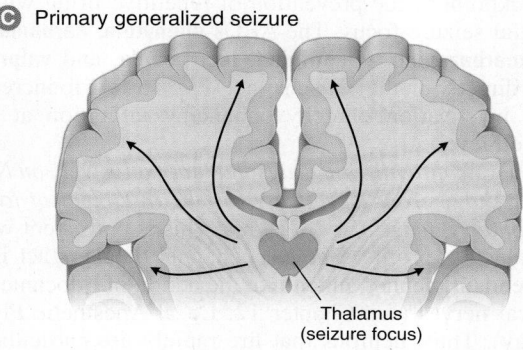

C Primary generalized seizure

Thalamus
(seizure focus)

FIGURE 16-3. Pathways of seizure propagation. A. In a focal seizure, paroxysmal activity begins in a seizure focus (*purple*) and spreads to adjacent areas via diffuse neuronal connections. When activity is confined to one region of the cortex that serves a basic function, such as motor movement or sensation, and there is no change in the patient's mental status, the seizure is referred to as a *focal seizure without altered awareness.* Seizures that involve brain regions serving more complex functions, such as language, memory, and emotions, are referred to as *focal seizures with altered awareness.* **B.** In a secondary generalized seizure, paroxysmal activity begins in a focus but then spreads to subcortical areas. Diffuse connections from the thalamus then synchronize the spread of activity to both hemispheres. **C.** Primary generalized seizures, such as the absence seizure, result from abnormal synchronization between thalamic and cortical cells (see Fig. 16-5B) or from neuronal networks that rapidly involve the bilateral hemispheres.

be contracting every muscle in his body, followed by an episode of uncontrolled shaking of all four limbs. These clinical symptoms can be understood at the level of abnormal channel activity (Fig. 16-4). The initial phase of the tonic–clonic seizure is associated with a sudden loss of GABA input, which leads to a long train of firing lasting for several seconds. This sustained, rapid firing manifests clinically as contraction of both agonist and antagonist muscles and is referred to as the **tonic** phase. Eventually, as GABA-mediated inhibition begins to be restored, AMPA-mediated and NMDA-mediated excitation starts to oscillate with the inhibitory component.

This oscillatory pattern (when involving the motor cortex) results in **clonic** or shaking movements of the body. With time, the GABA-mediated inhibition prevails, and the patient becomes flaccid and remains unconscious during the **postictal** period until normal brain function returns.

Pathophysiology of Primary Generalized Seizures

Primary generalized seizures differ from focal seizures in both pathophysiology and etiology (Fig. 16-3C). In contrast to the focal seizure, where synchronicity begins with sudden trains of action potentials within an aggregate of neurons and subsequently spreads to adjacent regions, the primary generalized seizure emanates from central brain regions and then spreads rapidly to both hemispheres. These seizures do not necessarily begin with an aura (which is an important method of clinically distinguishing primary generalized seizures from focal seizures that secondarily generalize).

Currently, the best understood of the primary generalized seizures is the **absence seizure** (also known as the **petit mal seizure**). Absence seizures are characterized by sudden interruptions in consciousness that are often accompanied by a blank stare and occasional motor symptoms, such as rapid blinking and lip smacking. Absence seizures are thought to result from abnormal synchronization of thalamocortical and cortical cells. The underlying pathophysiology of absence seizures is based on the observation that patients experiencing absence seizures have EEG readings somewhat similar to the patterns generated during **slow-wave (stage 3) sleep.**

Relay neurons connecting the thalamus to the cortex exist in two different states depending on the level of wakefulness (Fig. 16-5A). During the awake state, these neurons function in **transmission mode**, whereby incoming sensory signals are faithfully transmitted to the cortex. During sleep, however, the transient, bursting activity of a unique, dendritic **T-type calcium channel** alters incoming signals so that output signals to the cortex have an oscillatory firing rate, which, on an EEG, has a characteristic "spike and wave" readout. In this slow-wave sleep state, sensory information is not transmitted to the cortex.

For reasons not yet understood, absence seizures are associated with activation of the T-type calcium channel during the awake state (Fig. 16-5B). This channel is active only when the cell is hyperpolarized, and several mechanisms can mediate activation of the channel during the awake state. These mechanisms include an increase in intracellular K^+, an increase in GABAergic input from the reticular nucleus, or a loss of excitatory input. A variety of studies have shown that the activity of the T-type calcium channel in the relay neurons is essential to the 3-per-second spike-and-wave activity observed in absence seizures. Because of its important pathophysiologic role, the T-type calcium channel is a primary target in the pharmacologic treatment of absence seizures.

PHARMACOLOGIC CLASSES AND AGENTS

The current approach to treating a patient with epilepsy depends in part on the type of seizure(s) experienced by the patient. An appropriate antiepileptic drug regimen will take into account whether a patient is having focal seizures, with or without secondary generalization, or primary

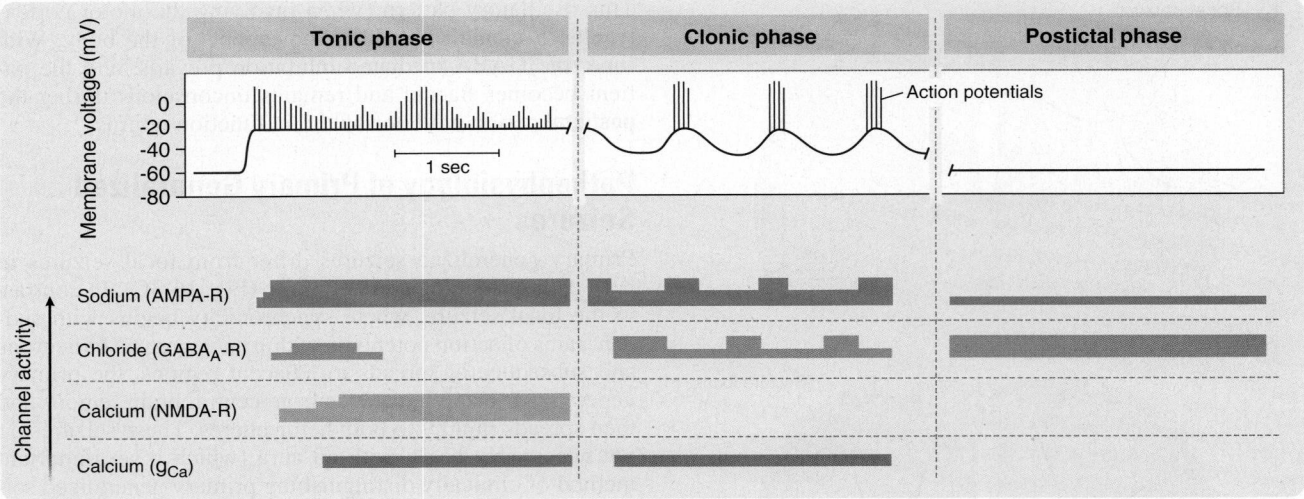

FIGURE 16-4. Abnormal channel activity in the tonic–clonic seizure. The tonic phase of the tonic–clonic seizure is initiated by a sudden loss of GABA-mediated surround inhibition. Loss of inhibition results in a rapid train of action potentials, which manifests clinically as tonic contraction of the muscles. As GABAergic innervation is restored, it begins to oscillate rhythmically with the excitatory component. The oscillation of excitatory and inhibitory components manifests clinically as clonic movements. The postictal phase is characterized by enhanced GABA-mediated inhibition.

generalized seizures. In addition, for patients with focal seizures, there is an attempt to determine whether the seizures are caused by an identifiable focal lesion that can be removed surgically or ablated by other means.

Mechanistically, the efficacy of antiepileptic drugs (AEDs) centers on manipulation of ion channel activity. As discussed above, physiologic protection against repetitive firing occurs via inhibition at two levels: the cellular level (e.g., Na^+ channel inactivation) and the network level (e.g., GABA-mediated inhibition). Accordingly, currently available AEDs fall into five main categories: (1) drugs that enhance Na^+ channel-mediated inhibition, (2) drugs that enhance K^+ channel-mediated inhibition, (3) drugs that inhibit calcium channels, (4) drugs that enhance GABA-mediated inhibition, and (5) drugs that inhibit glutamate receptors.

Although AEDs fall into several different mechanistic classes, it is important to keep in mind that *the therapeutic efficacy of many of the AEDs is only partially explained by the known mechanisms described below*, primarily because *the AEDs act pleiotropically.* Valproic acid, for example, stabilizes Na^+ channels, but the drug also has an effect on T-type calcium channels and may have effects on GABA metabolism as well. Thus, although in vitro studies may suggest that a drug is best suited for the treatment of one particular type of seizure, other seizure types may also respond to the drug. (One benefit of this pleiotropy is that many of the drugs are interchangeable, to the extent that minimization of adverse effects is often the main clinical criterion underlying the choice of AED.) The classification below is shown only for simplicity and is based on the primary target of the drug. A list of the drugs discussed here and their multiple mechanisms of action is provided in Table 16-2.

Drugs That Enhance Na⁺ Channel-Mediated Inhibition

Each neuron in the brain is equipped with the machinery to prevent rapid, repetitive firing. As discussed above, depolarization of the neuronal membrane results in sodium channel inactivation. This inactivation of the Na^+ channel provides a

key checkpoint in the prevention of repetitive firing within a potential seizure focus. The AEDs **phenytoin**, **carbamazepine**, **oxcarbazepine**, **lamotrigine**, **lacosamide**, and **valproic acid** act directly on the Na^+ channel (Fig. 16-6A) to increase channel inactivation, thereby enhancing inhibition at the single-cell level.

In general, *antiepileptic drugs that act exclusively on Na^+ channels show strong specificity for the treatment of focal and secondary generalized seizures.* This is consistent with their molecular profile. The Na^+ channel blockers act in a use-dependent manner, much like the action of lidocaine on peripheral nerves (see Chapter 12, Local Anesthetic Pharmacology). Thus, neurons that fire rapidly are particularly susceptible to inhibition by this class of drug. Conversely, many Na^+ channel blockers (particularly those that act only at the Na^+ channel, such as phenytoin) have little effect on absence seizures. Presumably, the thalamocortical cells activated during an absence seizure have a slow firing rate, such that Na^+ channel blockers do not have a use-dependent effect on the Na^+ channels in these cells.

Phenytoin

Phenytoin acts directly on the Na^+ channel to slow the rate of channel recovery from the inactivated state to the closed state. As described above, the Na^+ channel exists in three conformations—closed, open, and inactivated—and the probability of a channel existing in each state depends on the membrane potential (Fig. 16-1; see also Fig. 12-7). By slowing the rate of recovery from the inactivated state to the closed state, phenytoin increases the threshold for action potentials and prevents repetitive firing. This has the effect of stabilizing the seizure focus by preventing the paroxysmal depolarizing shift (PDS) that initiates the focal seizure. In addition, phenytoin prevents the rapid spread of seizure activity to other neurons, accounting for its efficacy in secondarily generalized seizures.

Importantly, phenytoin targets Na^+ channels in a use-dependent manner (see Fig. 12-8). Thus, only channels that are opened and closed at high frequency (i.e., those involved

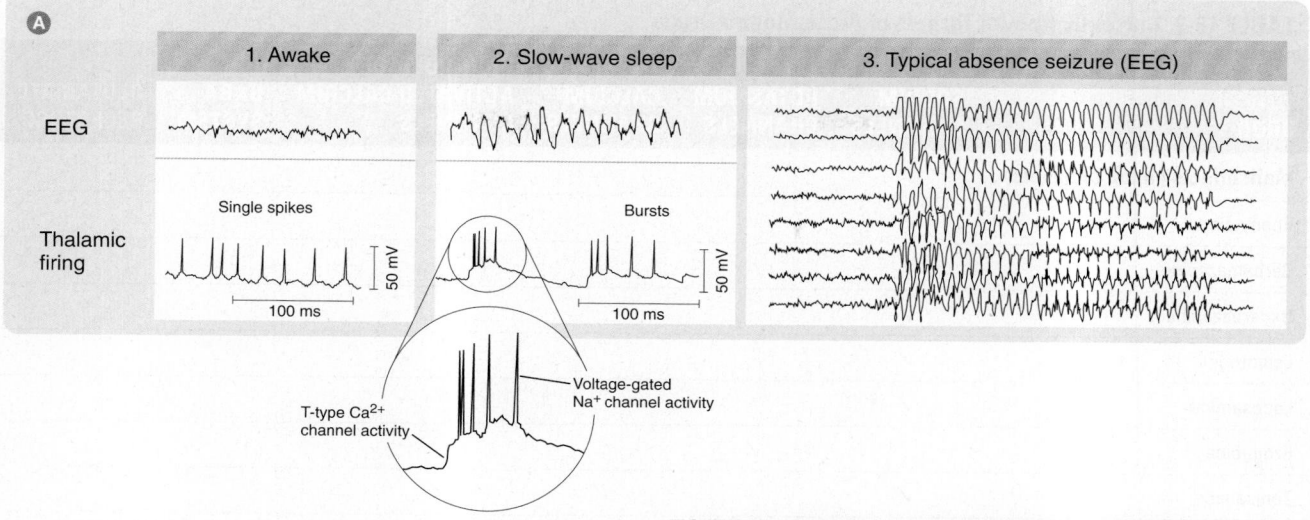

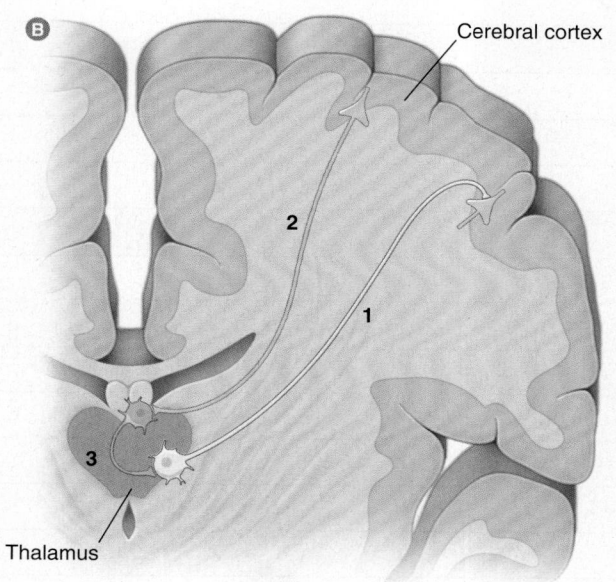

FIGURE 16-5. Mechanism of absence seizure. A. EEG recordings of patients experiencing absence seizures are similar to "sleep spindle" patterns generated during slow-wave sleep. The 3-per-second oscillatory pattern is generated by the burst activity of a dendritic T-type calcium channel in the thalamus. **1.** During the awake state, relay neurons of the thalamus are in "transmission mode," in which incoming signals are faithfully transmitted to the cortex as single spikes. These signals to the cortex register on the EEG as small, desynchronized, low-voltage waves. **2.** During slow-wave sleep, signals relayed through the thalamus are altered because of the bursting activity of a dendritic T-type calcium channel. During this stage, called *burst mode*, sensory information is not transmitted to the cortex. **3.** Absence seizures result from abnormal activation of the T-type calcium channel during the awake state, resulting in a similar spike-and-wave EEG pattern. **B.** The absence seizure is generated by a self-sustaining cycle of activity between the thalamus and the cortex. Synchronicity is initiated by hyperpolarization of the thalamic relay neurons (*white*). This occurs normally during slow-wave sleep and is caused by GABAergic input from the reticular thalamic nucleus (*purple*). The factors that cause hyperpolarization in relay neurons during an absence seizure are poorly understood. **1.** Hyperpolarization of relay neurons induces burst activity of the T-type calcium channel, resulting in synchronous depolarization in the cortex via excitatory connections. This large depolarization in the cortex registers as a spike-and-wave pattern on the EEG. **2.** Excitatory input from the cortex (*light yellow*) activates the reticular thalamic neurons (*dark yellow*). **3.** The activated GABAergic reticular neurons hyperpolarize the thalamic relay neurons and reinitiate the cycle.

in the PDS) are likely to be inhibited. This use-dependency lessens the effects of phenytoin on spontaneous neuronal activity and avoids many of the adverse effects observed with $GABA_A$ potentiators (which are not use-dependent).

Because of its use-dependent blockade, as well as its ability to prevent sudden rapid firing, phenytoin is a major drug of choice for focal seizures and tonic–clonic seizures. It is not used in absence seizures. The complex pharmacokinetics and drug interactions of phenytoin play a decisive role in the choice between phenytoin and similarly acting drugs such as carbamazepine.

Phenytoin is metabolized by the liver and, at typical doses, has a plasma half-life of about 24 hours. Phenytoin is also highly (95%) protein bound to albumin. Phenytoin metabolism shows properties of saturation kinetics, whereby small increases in doses above a certain level can cause large and often unpredictable increases in plasma drug concentration (see Chapter 3, Pharmacokinetics). These increases in plasma phenytoin concentration increase the risk of adverse

effects, including ataxia, nystagmus, incoordination, confusion, gingival hyperplasia, megaloblastic anemia, hirsutism, facial coarsening, and a systemic skin rash.

Phenytoin inactivation by the hepatic microsomal P450 enzyme system is susceptible to alteration by several drugs. Drugs that inhibit the P450 system, such as chloramphenicol, cimetidine, disulfiram, and isoniazid, increase phenytoin plasma concentration. Carbamazepine, an antiepileptic drug that induces the hepatic P450 system, increases the metabolism of phenytoin, thereby lowering phenytoin plasma concentration when these drugs are used concurrently. Similarly, phenytoin, because of its ability to induce the hepatic P450 system, increases the metabolism of drugs that are inactivated by this system. Some of these drugs include oral contraceptives, quinidine, doxycycline, cyclosporine, methadone, and levodopa.

Carbamazepine

Although structurally unrelated to phenytoin, **carbamazepine** appears to exert its antiseizure activity in a manner similar

TABLE 16-2 Currently Known Targets of Antiepileptic Drugs

DRUG	SODIUM CHANNELS	POTASSIUM CHANNELS	T-TYPE CALCIUM CHANNELS	HIGH-VOLTAGE-ACTIVATED CALCIUM CHANNELS	GABA SYSTEM	GLUTAMATE RECEPTORS
Main effects on ion channels						
Phenytoin	✓					
Carbamazepine	✓					
Oxcarbazepine	✓					
Lamotrigine	✓			✓		
Lacosamide	✓					
Ezogabine		✓				
Zonisamide	✓		✓			
Ethosuximide			✓			
Main effects on GABA mechanisms						
Benzodiazepines					✓	
Vigabatrin					✓	
Tiagabine					✓	
Main effects on glutamate mechanisms						
Perampanel						✓
Mixed actions						
Valproic acid	✓		✓		✓	
Gabapentin				✓	✓	
Pregabalin				✓	✓	
Levetiracetam				✓	✓	
Topiramate	✓			✓	✓	✓
Felbamate	✓			✓	✓	✓
Rufinamide	✓					✓
Phenobarbital				✓	✓	✓

to phenytoin. That is, carbamazepine is a Na^+ channel blocker that slows the rate of recovery of Na^+ channels from the inactivated state to the closed state. This has the effect of suppressing a seizure focus (by preventing the PDS) as well as preventing rapid spread of activity from the seizure focus. A metabolite of carbamazepine, 10,11-epoxycarbamazepine, also acts to slow Na^+ channel recovery and may be responsible for some of the therapeutic effects of the drug.

Carbamazepine is often the drug of choice for focal seizures because of its dual action in the suppression of seizure foci and the prevention of spread of activity. Carbamazepine was chosen for the treatment of Rob's seizures because his tumor was a specific focus for his seizure onset, and carbamazepine is likely the most effective drug for preventing spread of activity from that focus. The half-life of

carbamazepine is initially between 10 and 20 hours and is reduced with chronic treatment (because of P450 induction), requiring patients to take several doses daily or convert to an extended-release formulation, which remains twice daily. Metabolism of carbamazepine is linear (i.e., it exhibits first-order kinetics); this property makes carbamazepine a more attractive choice than phenytoin for patients with potential drug interactions. Individuals of Asian ancestry should be screened for HLA-B*1502 before starting carbamazepine, because the presence of HLA-B*1502 predicts a higher risk for the development of Stevens-Johnson syndrome.

Oxcarbazepine

Oxcarbazepine is structurally related to carbamazepine, also acts via the Na^+ channel, and has a similar clinical profile.

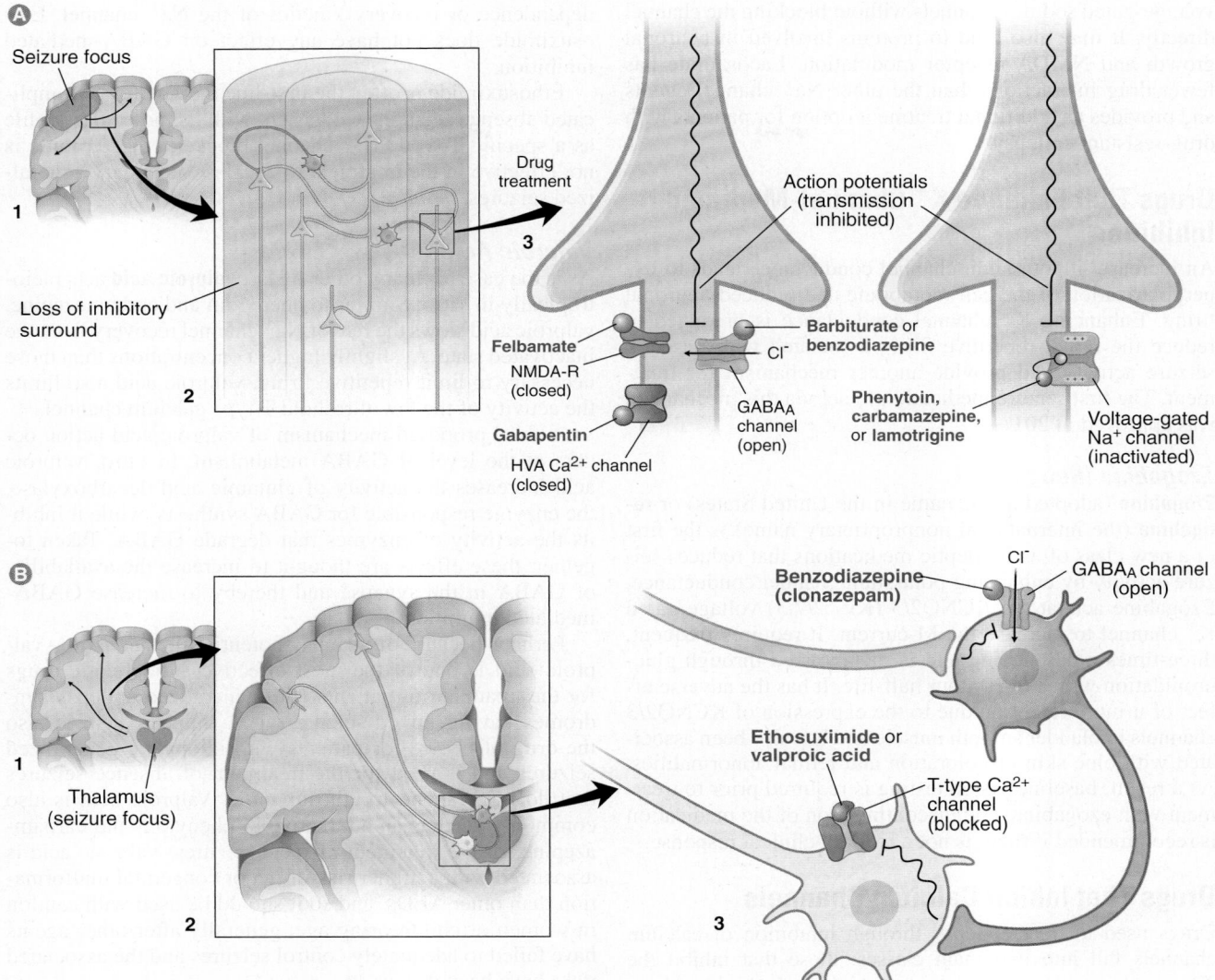

FIGURE 16-6. Mechanisms of pharmacotherapy for seizures. A. The focal seizure **(1)** results from rapid, uncontrolled neuronal firing and a loss of surround inhibition **(2)**. Antiepileptic drugs act at four molecular targets to enhance inhibition and prevent spread of synchronous activity **(3)**. Barbiturates and benzodiazepines prevent seizure spread by acting on the GABA$_A$ receptor to potentiate GABA-mediated inhibition. Na$^+$ channel inhibitors such as phenytoin, carbamazepine, and lamotrigine prevent rapid neuronal firing by selectively prolonging Na$^+$ channel inactivation in rapidly firing neurons (see Figs. 12-7 and 12-8). Felbamate suppresses seizure activity by inhibiting the NMDA receptor and thereby decreasing glutamate-mediated excitation. Gabapentin decreases release of excitatory neurotransmitter by inhibiting the high-voltage-activated (HVA) calcium channel. **B.** The absence seizure **(1)** is caused by a self-sustaining cycle of activity generated between thalamic and cortical cells **(2)**. Antiepileptic drugs prevent this synchronous thalamocortical cycle **(3)** by acting at two molecular targets. Clonazepam, a benzodiazepine, potentiates GABA$_A$ channels in the reticular thalamic nucleus, thus decreasing the activation of the inhibitory reticular neurons and decreasing the hyperpolarization of the thalamic relay neurons. T-type calcium channel inhibitors such as ethosuximide and valproic acid prevent the burst activity of thalamic relay neurons that is required for synchronous activation of cortical cells.

It is rapidly converted to an active metabolite, **eslicarbazepine**, which was recently approved as a separate drug. Oxcarbazepine distinguishes itself from carbamazepine by being a somewhat less potent P450 enzyme inducer, although clinically the same considerations apply. It has a somewhat lower risk for rash and a higher risk of clinically significant hyponatremia.

Lamotrigine

As with the other Na$^+$ channel agents, **lamotrigine** acts to stabilize the neuronal membrane by slowing Na$^+$ channel recovery from the inactivated state. It is hypothesized that lamotrigine may act by other undetermined mechanisms as well, because it appears to have broader clinical efficacy.

For example, in addition to treating focal and tonic–clonic seizures, lamotrigine is effective in the treatment of absence seizures along with ethosuximide and valproic acid (see below). Lamotrigine also distinguishes itself by having a relatively favorable adverse effect profile as evidenced by lower dropout rates among elderly patients taking lamotrigine in clinical trials. Slow titration (adjusted for P450 enzyme interactions) is required when starting lamotrigine to reduce the risk of Stevens-Johnson syndrome.

Lacosamide

Lacosamide is one of the newest antiepileptic medications that acts via sodium channel-mediated inhibition. In vitro studies show that lacosamide enhances slow inactivation of voltage-gated sodium channels without blocking the channel directly. It may also bind to proteins involved in neuronal growth and NMDA receptor modulation. Lacosamide has fewer drug interactions than the other Na^+ channel agents and provides an additional treatment option for patients with drug-resistant epilepsy.

Drugs That Enhance K^+ Channel-Mediated Inhibition

An increase in potassium channel conductance leads to hyperpolarization of the cell membrane and reduced neuronal firing. Enhancing K^+ channel conductance is predicted to reduce the rapid, repetitive firing associated with onset of seizure activity and provide another mechanism for treatment. The first seizure medication to act via this mechanism was approved in 2011.

Ezogabine (Retigabine)

Ezogabine (adopted as the name in the United States) or **retigabine** (the international nonproprietary name) is the first of a new class of antiepileptic medications that reduces seizure activity by enhancing potassium channel conductance. Ezogabine acts at the KCNQ2/3 (Kv7.2/7.3) voltage-gated K^+ channel to increase the M-current. It requires frequent, three-times-a-day dosing and is metabolized through glucuronidation with a 6–10-hour half-life. It has the adverse effect of urinary retention due to the expression of KCNQ2/3 channels in bladder smooth muscle and has also been associated with blue skin discoloration and retinal abnormalities. As a result, baseline vision testing is required prior to treatment with ezogabine, and discontinuation of the medication is recommended if there is not a marked clinical response.

Drugs That Inhibit Calcium Channels

Drugs used to treat epilepsy through inhibition of calcium channels fall into two main classes: those that inhibit the T-type calcium channel and those that inhibit the high-voltage-activated (HVA) calcium channel.

The T-type calcium channel is depolarized and inactive during the awake state (Fig. 16-5B). In absence (petit mal) seizures, paroxysmal hyperpolarization is thought to activate the channel during the awake state, initiating the spike-and-wave discharges characteristic of this seizure type. Thus, *drugs inhibiting the T-type calcium channel are specifically used to treat absence seizures.*

HVA calcium channels play an important role in controlling the entry of calcium into the presynaptic terminal and therefore help to regulate neurotransmitter release. The HVA calcium channel is formed by an α1 protein that assembles into the channel pore, and it has several auxiliary subunits. Drugs that inhibit HVA calcium channels tend to have pleiotropic effects; although they are used primarily for focal seizures with or without secondary generalization, they can also be used for generalized seizures other than absence seizures.

Ethosuximide

In vitro, **ethosuximide** has a highly specific molecular profile. In experiments on thalamocortical preparations from rats and hamsters, ethosuximide has been shown to reduce low-threshold T-type currents in a voltage-dependent manner. This inhibition occurs without altering the voltage dependence or recovery kinetics of the Na^+ channel. Ethosuximide does not have any effect on GABA-mediated inhibition.

Ethosuximide is often the first-line therapy for uncomplicated absence seizures. Consistent with its molecular profile as a specific T-type Ca^{2+} channel blocker, ethosuximide is not effective in the treatment of focal or secondary generalized seizures.

Valproic Acid

As is the case for many other AEDs, **valproic acid** acts pleiotropically in vitro. Similar to phenytoin and carbamazepine, valproic acid slows the rate of Na^+ channel recovery from the inactivated state. At slightly higher concentrations than those necessary to limit repetitive firing, valproic acid also limits the activity of the low-threshold T-type calcium channel.

A third proposed mechanism of valproic acid action occurs at the level of GABA metabolism. In vitro, valproic acid increases the activity of glutamic acid decarboxylase, the enzyme responsible for GABA synthesis, while it inhibits the activity of enzymes that degrade GABA. Taken together, these effects are thought to increase the availability of GABA in the synapse and thereby to increase GABA-mediated inhibition.

Perhaps because of its many potential sites of action, valproic acid is one of the most effective antiepileptic drugs for the treatment of patients with generalized epilepsy syndromes having mixed seizure types. Valproic acid is also the drug of choice for patients with idiopathic generalized seizures and is used for the treatment of absence seizures that do not respond to ethosuximide. Valproic acid is also commonly used as an alternative to phenytoin and carbamazepine for the treatment of focal seizures. Valproic acid is associated with a higher risk of major congenital malformation than other AEDs, and so it should be used with caution in women of childbearing age, generally after other agents have failed to adequately control seizures and the associated risks have been discussed.

Gabapentin

Gabapentin was one of the first AEDs developed using the concept of "rational drug design." That is, with the recognition that GABA receptors play an important role in the control of seizure spread, gabapentin was synthesized as a structural analogue of GABA and was predicted to enhance GABA-mediated inhibition. Consistent with this hypothesis, gabapentin has been shown to increase the content of GABA in neurons and glial cells in vitro. However, the main antiseizure effect of gabapentin appears to be through its inhibition of HVA calcium channels, which results in decreased neurotransmitter release. A main advantage of gabapentin is that, because its structure is similar to that of endogenous amino acids, it has few interactions with other drugs. On the other hand, gabapentin appears to be less effective than several other AEDs, and it is not generally used as a first-line agent.

Pregabalin

Like gabapentin, **pregabalin** is structurally related to GABA, but it exerts its main therapeutic effect through inhibition of HVA calcium channels, reducing the release of several neurotransmitters including glutamate and norepinephrine. It also has effects on substance P and calcitonin, which may contribute to its varied clinical uses. More potent than gabapentin, pregabalin is a reasonable adjunctive treatment for focal seizures. It is particularly useful in patients with hepatic dysfunction, since it is metabolized in the kidney and has few drug–drug interactions.

Drugs That Enhance GABA-Mediated Inhibition

In contrast to Na^+ channel blockers and calcium channel inhibitors, whose mechanistic properties correlate well with their clinical activity, the enhancers of GABA-mediated inhibition have more varied effects and tend not to be as interchangeable. This is largely because of the diversity of $GABA_A$ receptors in the brain. The $GABA_A$ receptor channel has five subunits, with at least two alternative splice variants of several of the subunits (see Chapter 13). There are at least 10 known subtypes of the $GABA_A$ receptor, with varying distributions of these subtypes throughout the brain. Barbiturates and benzodiazepines both increase Cl^- influx through $GABA_A$ channels, but benzodiazepines act on a specific subset of $GABA_A$ channels, whereas barbiturates appear to act on all $GABA_A$ channels. The recently approved drug **vigabatrin** enhances GABA-mediated activity indirectly via inhibition of GABA metabolism. These different mechanisms of action result in distinct clinical profiles. Drugs that nonspecifically increase GABA content (e.g., through enhancement of synthetic pathways or reduced metabolism of GABA) tend to have a profile similar to the barbiturates.

Benzodiazepines (Diazepam, Lorazepam, Midazolam, Clonazepam, Clobazam)

Benzodiazepines increase the affinity of GABA for the $GABA_A$ receptor and enhance $GABA_A$ channel gating in the presence of GABA, and thereby increase Cl^- influx through the channel (see Chapter 13). This action has the dual effect of suppressing the seizure focus (by raising the threshold of the action potential) and strengthening surround inhibition. Thus, benzodiazepines such as **diazepam**, **lorazepam**, and **midazolam** are well suited for the treatment of focal and tonic–clonic seizures. The benzodiazepines cause prominent adverse effects, however, including dizziness, ataxia, and drowsiness. Thus, these drugs are typically used only to abort seizures acutely.

Clonazepam is unique among the benzodiazepines in its ability to inhibit T-type Ca^{2+} channel currents in in vitro preparations of thalamocortical circuits. In vivo, clonazepam acts specifically at $GABA_A$ receptors in the reticular nucleus (Fig. 16-5B), augmenting inhibition in these neurons and essentially "turning off" the nucleus. By this action, clonazepam prevents GABA-mediated hyperpolarization of the thalamus and thereby indirectly inactivates the T-type Ca^{2+} channel, which is the channel thought to be responsible for generating absence seizures (see above). However, as with diazepam, clonazepam use is limited because of its extensive adverse effects. Clonazepam is the fourth drug of choice in the treatment of absence seizures after ethosuximide, valproic acid, and lamotrigine.

Clobazam is the most recently approved benzodiazepine, although it has been available for decades outside the United States. It is currently approved for adjunctive treatment of Lennox-Gastaut syndrome, a severe pediatric epilepsy syndrome with onset between 3 and 5 years of age that is characterized by developmental disability and refractory tonic, atonic, and atypical absence seizures. Like clonazepam, it has an elimination half-life of over 30 hours, so it is taken as a scheduled medication twice daily. Adverse effects are similar to other benzodiazepines except that clobazam is also associated with an increased risk of serious skin reactions, including Stevens-Johnson syndrome.

Barbiturates (Phenobarbital)

Phenobarbital binds to an allosteric site on the $GABA_A$ receptor and thereby potentiates the action of endogenous GABA by increasing the duration of Cl^- channel opening. In the presence of phenobarbital, there is a much greater influx of Cl^- ions for each activation of the channel (see Chapter 13). Barbiturates also display weak agonist activity at the $GABA_A$ channel, perhaps furthering the ability of this drug to increase Cl^- influx. This enhancement of GABA-mediated inhibition, similar to that of the benzodiazepines, may explain the effectiveness of phenobarbital in the treatment of focal seizures and tonic–clonic seizures.

In contrast to the benzodiazepines, which are sometimes useful in treating the spike-and-wave discharges of the absence seizure, the barbiturates may actually exacerbate this type of seizure. This exacerbation may be caused by two factors. First, barbiturates act at all $GABA_A$ receptors. Unlike benzodiazepines, which selectively augment GABA inhibition in the reticular nucleus, barbiturates potentiate $GABA_A$ receptors in both the reticular nucleus and the thalamic relay cells. Importantly, the latter effect enhances the T-type calcium currents that are responsible for the absence seizure (Fig. 16-5B). Second, unlike benzodiazepines, which are purely allosteric enhancers of endogenous GABA activity, barbiturates can also act on the $GABA_A$ channel in the absence of the endogenous ligand. The latter property may function to increase nonspecific activity of the barbiturates.

Phenobarbital is used primarily as an alternative drug in the treatment of focal seizures and tonic–clonic seizures. Because of the pronounced sedative effects of this drug, its clinical use has been decreasing as more effective antiepileptic medications have become available.

Vigabatrin

Vigabatrin is a structural analogue of GABA that irreversibly inhibits the enzyme GABA transaminase, thereby increasing levels of GABA in the brain (see Fig. 13-2). Serious adverse effects, most notably peripheral visual field defects, limit the clinical utility of vigabatrin. The drug is generally used for infantile spasms and refractory focal epilepsy. Patients treated with vigabatrin should undergo baseline and routine visual field testing and, even in the absence of visual changes, the drug should be discontinued within a few months if there is not a marked clinical benefit.

Drugs That Inhibit Glutamate Receptors

Glutamate is the principal excitatory neurotransmitter of the CNS (see Chapter 13). Not surprisingly, excessive activation of excitatory glutamatergic synapses is a key component of many forms of seizure activity. Numerous studies using animal models have shown that inhibition of the NMDA and AMPA subtypes of glutamate receptors can inhibit the generation of seizure activity and protect neurons from seizure-induced injury. However, none of the specific and potent glutamate receptor antagonists have been routinely used clinically for the treatment of seizures because of unacceptable behavioral adverse effects.

Felbamate

Felbamate has a variety of actions, including the inhibition of NMDA receptors. It appears to have some selectivity for NMDA receptors that include the NR2B subunit. Because this receptor subunit is not expressed ubiquitously throughout the brain, NMDA receptor antagonism by felbamate is not as widespread as that with other NMDA receptor antagonists. This relative selectivity may explain why felbamate lacks the behavioral adverse effects observed with the other agents. Benefits of felbamate include its potency as an antiepileptic drug and its lack of the sedative effects common to many other antiepileptic drugs. However, felbamate has been associated with a number of cases of fatal aplastic anemia and liver failure, and its use is now restricted primarily to patients with refractory epilepsy.

Rufinamide

Rufinamide is approved for the treatment of focal seizures and drop attacks in Lennox-Gastaut syndrome (described above). While rufinamide acts predominantly by prolonging sodium channel inactivation, it is structurally unrelated to the other antiepileptic agents with this mechanism of action. At higher doses, it may have an inhibitory effect on a subset of glutamate receptors (mGluR5 subtype), and it is included here based on that secondary mechanism and because its clinical profile is most similar to felbamate. Unlike felbamate, however, rufinamide has not been demonstrated to have serious adverse effects, and it may provide an alternative option for patients with refractory epilepsy.

Perampanel

Perampanel is a noncompetitive antagonist at the α-amino-3-hydroxy-5-methyl-4-isoxazole-propionic acid (AMPA) receptor, which is an excitatory glutamate receptor thought to play an important role in the generation and spread of seizure activity. While it was hoped that AMPA antagonists may have fewer psychomimetic adverse effects than NMDA antagonists, perampanel increases the risk of certain psychiatric symptoms, including irritability, aggression, hostility, and homicidal ideation. Perampanel is heavily protein bound and metabolized by the P450 system; it has a long elimination half-life, which allows for once-daily dosing.

Drugs with Mechanisms Under Investigation

Tiagabine, **topiramate**, **zonisamide**, and **levetiracetam** are additional seizure medications whose mechanisms of action are somewhat less certain. Tiagabine is thought to function by blocking GABA reuptake into presynaptic neurons, while topiramate and zonisamide likely block sodium channel activity but probably have other mechanisms as well given their broad application for focal and tonic–clonic seizures. Levetiracetam is believed to modulate vesicle exocytosis by binding to SV2A, a synaptic vesicle protein.

■ CONCLUSION AND FUTURE DIRECTIONS

In recent years, improved understanding of the physiology and pathophysiology of neuronal signaling in the CNS has led to a more thorough understanding of the current antiepileptic drugs (AEDs), as well as the design and discovery of novel agents. Under physiologic conditions, Na^+ channel inactivation and GABA-mediated surround inhibition prevent uncontrolled, rapid spread of electrical activity. There are, however, numerous potential alterations in the brain that can weaken these inhibitory forces, such as damage and degeneration of GABAergic neurons, abnormal ion gradients induced by space-occupying lesions, and gene mutations that alter channel function.

The AEDs described in this chapter restore the inherent inhibitory capacity of the brain. These include drugs such as phenytoin, which increases Na^+ channel inactivation, and clonazepam, which enhances GABA-mediated inhibition. Newer classes of AEDs extend this repertoire by acting through modulation of the Ca^{2+} channel required for neurotransmitter release, modulation of K^+ channel conductance to reduce rapid firing, and modulation of excitatory receptors such as the NMDA receptor.

Despite increased understanding of the mechanisms of certain seizure types, the efficacy of many of the antiepileptics is only partially explained by their known molecular profiles. Hence, current decisions about therapy are often driven by empirical example rather than by known molecular mechanisms. As a better understanding is gained of the role of genetics in not only simple inherited epilepsy but also complicated polygenic cases, the application of a more rational, mechanism-based pharmacology will become increasingly possible.

Suggested Reading

Lowenstein DH. Seizures and epilepsy. In: Kasper DL, Fauci AS, Hauser SL, Longo DL, Jameson JL, Loscalzo J, eds. *Harrison's principles of internal medicine.* 19th ed. New York: McGraw Hill; 2015:2542–2559. (*Discussion of seizure pathophysiology and extensive discussion of clinical uses of antiepileptic drugs.*)

Shorvon S. Drug treatment of epilepsy in the century of the ILAE: the second 50 years, 1959–2009. *Epilepsia* 2009;50(Suppl 3):93–130. (*A historical perspective cataloging the introduction of each therapeutic agent over time.*)

Westbrook GL. Seizures and epilepsy. In: Kandel ER, Schwartz JH, Jessell TM, Siegelbaum SA, Hudspeth AJ, eds. *Principles of neural science.* 5th ed. New York: McGraw-Hill; 2013:1116–1139. (*Detailed description of normal electrical signaling and seizure pathophysiology.*)

DRUG SUMMARY TABLE: CHAPTER 16 Pharmacology of Abnormal Electrical Neurotransmission in the Central Nervous System

DRUG	CLINICAL APPLICATIONS	SERIOUS AND COMMON ADVERSE EFFECTS	CONTRAINDICATIONS	THERAPEUTIC CONSIDERATIONS
SODIUM CHANNEL INHIBITORS Mechanism—Inhibit electrical neurotransmission by use-dependent block of neuronal voltage-gated sodium channel. Lacosamide may also bind to proteins involved in neuronal growth and NMDA receptor modulation.				
Phenytoin	Tonic–clonic seizures Focal seizures Status epilepticus	*Agranulocytosis, leukopenia, pancytopenia, thrombocytopenia, megaloblastic anemia, hepatitis, Stevens-Johnson syndrome, toxic epidermal necrolysis, bullous dermatosis, lupus erythematosus* Ataxia, nystagmus, incoordination, confusion, gingival hyperplasia, hirsutism, facial coarsening, morbilliform eruption, constipation, nausea	Hydantoin hypersensitivity Concomitant use with certain non-nucleoside reverse transcriptase inhibitors (NNRTIs) such as delavirdine and rilpivirine	Metabolized via P450 system; P450 enzyme inducer. At low doses, half-life is 24 hours; at higher doses, saturation of the P450 system leads to larger changes in plasma concentration per unit dose increase. Protein binding 90–95%. Elimination half-life ranges widely from person to person (7–42 hours).
Carbamazepine	Focal and tonic–clonic seizures Bipolar I disorder (see Box 15-2) Trigeminal neuralgia	*Aplastic anemia, agranulocytosis, thrombocytopenia, leukopenia, atrioventricular block, arrhythmia, Stevens-Johnson syndrome, toxic epidermal necrolysis, hyponatremia, hypocalcemia, SIADH, porphyria, hepatitis, nephrotoxicity, pancreatitis* Blood pressure lability, rash, confusion, dizziness, nystagmus, blurred vision, constipation, nausea	Concomitant use of monoamine oxidase inhibitors and NNRTIs History of bone marrow depression Prescreen for HLA-B*1502 in patients of Asian descent to avoid risk of Stevens-Johnson syndrome	Metabolized via P450 system; P450 enzyme inducer. Active metabolite, 10,11-epoxycarbamazepine, also slows sodium channel recovery. Protein binding 75–90%. Half-life is reduced (from 25–65 hours to 12–17 hours) with chronic treatment due to P450 auto-induction; further dose escalation after 1–2 months may be required to maintain stable levels.
Oxcarbazepine	Adjunctive or monotherapy for focal seizures	*Agranulocytosis, leukopenia, pancytopenia, Stevens-Johnson syndrome, toxic epidermal necrolysis, anaphylaxis, angioedema, clinically significant hyponatremia, status epilepticus* Dizziness, somnolence, diplopia, nystagmus, fatigue, nausea, vomiting, ataxia, abnormal vision, headache, tremor, dyspepsia, abnormal gait	Caution in patients with allergy to carbamazepine due to cross-reactivity in 25%–30%	Metabolized via P450 system; P450 enzyme inducer. Metabolized to active 10-monohydroxy metabolite (MHD) and then via glucuronidation to inactive 10,11-dihydroxy metabolite (DHD). MHD is 40% protein bound. Elimination half-life for parent drug is 2 hours and for MHD is 9 hours.
Lamotrigine	Focal and tonic–clonic seizures Atypical absence seizures Bipolar I disorder (see Box 15-2) Lennox-Gastaut syndrome	*Stevens-Johnson syndrome, toxic epidermal necrolysis, bone marrow suppression, anemia, disseminated intravascular coagulation, hepatic necrosis, amnesia, angioedema, aseptic meningitis* Rash, ataxia, somnolence, dizziness, headache, insomnia, tremor, blurred vision, diplopia, diarrhea, nausea, rhinitis	None known	Metabolized by glucuronic acid conjugation. Levels are affected by the P450 system; slower titration, lower target doses, and less frequent dosing required in the presence of valproic acid versus P450 enzyme inducers. Estrogen-containing oral contraceptive pills may reduce levels by 50%; doubling of the level may occur during the placebo week. Protein binding is 55%. Elimination half-life is 48–70 hours in the presence of valproic acid and 13–14 hours in the presence of P450 inducers.
Lacosamide	Focal seizures (adjunctive therapy)	*Atrial fibrillation, first-degree AV block* Dizziness, nausea, headache, fatigue, ataxia, nasopharyngitis, abnormal vision, diplopia, nystagmus	Caution in patients with known cardiac conduction problems or severe cardiac disease	No known drug interactions. Protein binding is <15%. Elimination half-life is 13 hours.

continues

DRUG SUMMARY TABLE: CHAPTER 16 Pharmacology of Abnormal Electrical Neurotransmission in the Central Nervous System *continued*

DRUG	CLINICAL APPLICATIONS	*SERIOUS* AND COMMON ADVERSE EFFECTS	CONTRAINDICATIONS	THERAPEUTIC CONSIDERATIONS
POTASSIUM CHANNEL POTENTIATORS Mechanism—Ezogabine (Retigabine) enhances the activity of voltage-gated K$^+$ channels, increasing the M-current and reducing neuronal excitability.				
Ezogabine (Retigabine)	Focal seizures (adjunctive therapy)	*Prolonged QT interval, amnesia, hallucinations, suicidal ideation, blue skin discoloration, retinal abnormalities, urinary retention* Dizziness, somnolence, fatigue, confusion, vertigo, tremor, blurred vision, gait disturbance, dysarthria, balance disorder	Patients should have baseline and periodic (every 6 months) ophthalmologic exam with visual acuity testing and funduscopy; discontinue for vision changes or lack of clinical response Consider avoiding in patients with urinary retention	Metabolized through glucuronidation to an N-acetyl active metabolite (NAMR). Plasma levels are reduced by P450 inducers. Protein binding 80% for parent drug and 45% for NAMR. Caution when combining with anticholinergics given risk of increased postvoid residual. Metabolites reduce the clearance of digoxin. Renally eliminated with 36% of drug unchanged in the urine and half-life of 7–11 hours.
CALCIUM CHANNEL INHIBITORS Mechanism—Ethosuximide and valproic acid inhibit the low-threshold T-type calcium channel; gabapentin and pregabalin inhibit the high-voltage-activated (HVA) calcium channel.				
Ethosuximide	Absence seizures	*Stevens-Johnson syndrome, bone marrow suppression, systemic lupus erythematosus, seizures* Gastrointestinal irritation, ataxia, somnolence, headache, dizziness	None known	Metabolized via the P450 system. Elimination half-life is 50–60 hours.
Valproic acid	Tonic–clonic seizures, absence seizures, atypical absence seizures, focal seizures Manic bipolar I disorder Migraine prophylaxis	*Palpitations, tachycardia, hematemesis, hepatotoxicity, pancreatitis, thrombocytopenia, hyperammonemia, ototoxicity* Alopecia, gastrointestinal irritation, weight gain, ataxia, asthenia, dizziness, headache, tremor, sedation, blurred vision, respiratory tract infection	Liver disease Urea cycle or mitochondrial disorders Caution in women of childbearing age due to higher rates of teratogenicity	Metabolized via P450 system, glucuronidation, and mitochondrial beta-oxidation. Mixed inhibition and induction of P450 enzymes leads to complex drug–drug interactions. Highly protein bound (80–90%) but free fraction increases at higher levels and in certain populations (elderly or renal/hepatic impairment). Extended-release formulation is slightly less (90%) bioavailable and conversion from immediate release may require commensurate dosage escalation. Elimination half-life is 9–16 hours.
Gabapentin	Focal seizures Postherpetic neuralgia	*Stevens-Johnson syndrome* Sedation, dizziness, ataxia, fatigue, gastrointestinal irritation, viral disease	None known	Few drug–drug interactions. Less than 3% protein bound. Renal elimination with half-life of 5–7 hours.
Pregabalin	Diabetic peripheral neuropathy Fibromyalgia Neuropathic pain (spinal cord injury) Focal seizures (adjunct) Postherpetic neuralgia	*Increased creatine kinase level, angioedema* Peripheral edema, weight gain, xerostomia, asthenia, ataxia, dizziness, somnolence, tremor, blurred vision, diplopia, euphoria	None known	Structurally similar to gabapentin but considered to be more effective. Renal elimination with half-life of 6 hours.

GABA CHANNEL POTENTIATORS
Mechanism—Potentiate GABA-mediated inhibition to increase chloride current through the channel

Benzodiazepines: Diazepam Lorazepam Midazolam Clonazepam Clobazam	Anxiety (shared indication) Status epilepticus (diazepam, lorazepam, and midazolam only) Focal and tonic–clonic seizures (shared indication) Absence seizures (clonazepam only) Lennox-Gastaut syndrome (clobazam only) Skeletal muscle spasm and alcohol withdrawal (diazepam only)	*Stevens-Johnson syndrome, toxic epidermal necrolysis (clobazam only); neutropenia (diazepam only); cardiac arrest (midazolam only)* Ataxia, dizziness, somnolence, fatigue (shared adverse effects); respiratory depression (diazepam only)	Shared contraindication: Acute narrow-angle glaucoma Untreated open-angle glaucoma Habit-forming; screen for history of substance abuse Diazepam only: Myasthenia gravis Diazepam and lorazepam only: Sleep apnea Clobazam only: Severe liver or respiratory disease	Hepatic metabolism with P450-mediated drug interactions in some cases.
Barbiturates: Phenobarbital	Focal and tonic–clonic seizures Insomnia Preoperative sedation	*Stevens-Johnson syndrome, bone marrow suppression, hepatotoxicity, osteopenia* Somnolence, ataxia, confusion, dizziness, depression, decreased libido	Porphyria Severe liver dysfunction Respiratory disease	Metabolized via P450 and glucuronide conjugation; P450 enzyme inducer. Sedative effects limit use; wean gradually to avoid withdrawal symptoms (agitation, seizure, or insomnia). Protein binding 20–45%. Elimination half-life is 53–140 hours in adults.
Vigabatrin	Focal epilepsy (refractory; adjunct) Infantile spasms	*Liver failure, vision loss, suicidal thoughts* Arthralgia, confusion, dizziness, insomnia, memory loss, sedation, tremor, blurred vision, diplopia, nystagmus, depression	None known	More elaborate consent process due to potential for vision loss. Weak P450 enzyme inducer. Elimination half-life is 10.5 hours.

GLUTAMATE RECEPTOR INHIBITORS
Mechanism—Felbamate inhibits the glycine binding site of the NMDA receptor, resulting in suppression of seizure activity. Rufinamide prolongs sodium channel inactivation and may inhibit mGluR5 glutamate receptors. Perampanel is a noncompetitive antagonist at the AMPA receptor, resulting in suppression of seizure activity.

Felbamate	Focal seizures Lennox-Gastaut syndrome	*Aplastic anemia, bone marrow depression, hepatic failure, Stevens-Johnson syndrome* Photosensitivity, purpuric disorder, gastrointestinal irritation, abnormal gait, dizziness	Blood dyscrasia Liver disease	Mixed inhibitor and inducer of P450 system. Lacks behavioral adverse effects observed with other NMDA receptor antagonists. Associated with fatal aplastic anemia and liver failure, and its use is restricted to patients with refractory epilepsy. Protein binding 22–55%. Elimination half-life is 13–23 hours; longer in renal impairment.

continues

DRUG SUMMARY TABLE: CHAPTER 16 Pharmacology of Abnormal Electrical Neurotransmission in the Central Nervous System *continued*

DRUG	CLINICAL APPLICATIONS	SERIOUS AND COMMON ADVERSE EFFECTS	CONTRAINDICATIONS	THERAPEUTIC CONSIDERATIONS
Rufinamide	Focal seizures Drop attacks associated with Lennox-Gastaut syndrome	*Status epilepticus* Shortened QT interval, dizziness, fatigue, headache, nausea, vomiting, diplopia, somnolence	Patients with familial short QT syndrome	Mild P450 enzyme inducer. Protein binding 34%. Elimination half-life is 6–10 hours.
Perampanel	Focal seizures (adjunctive therapy)	*Irritability, aggression, suicidal ideation* Dizziness, somnolence, fatigue, irritability, falls, headache, nausea, weight gain, vertigo, ataxia, balance disorder, gait disturbance	None known	Metabolized via P450 oxidation and glucuronidation; P450 enzyme inducer. Monitor for neuropsychiatric symptoms. Protein binding is 95%. Elimination half-life is 105 hours.
OTHER ANTIEPILEPTIC DRUGS **Mechanisms under investigation**				
Tiagabine	Focal and tonic–clonic seizures (adjunctive therapy)	*Unexplained sudden death* Confusion, sedation, dizziness, depression, psychosis, gastrointestinal irritation	None known	Metabolized via P450 system. Protein binding 96%. Elimination half-life is reduced from 7–9 hours to 2–5 hours in the presence of P450 inducers.
Topiramate	Focal and tonic–clonic seizures (adjunctive therapy) Migraine prophylaxis Lennox-Gastaut syndrome	*Stevens-Johnson syndrome, toxic epidermal necrolysis, hyperammonemia, hypohidrosis, acidosis, encephalopathy, glaucoma, myopia, nephrolithiasis* Sedation, psychomotor slowing, fatigue, speech or language problems, confusion, dizziness, memory impairment, paresthesia, abnormal serum bicarbonate levels, weight loss	Recent alcohol use (within 6 hours) Metabolic acidosis with concomitant metformin use Caution if history of renal calculi	Minor amounts metabolized via P450 system and glucuronidation; mixed inhibitor and inducer of the P450 enzymes. Largely excreted in the urine unchanged (70%). Elimination half-life is 21 hours.
Zonisamide	Focal and tonic–clonic seizures (adjunctive therapy)	*Stevens-Johnson syndrome, toxic epidermal necrolysis, agranulocytosis, status epilepticus, schizophreniform disorder* Sedation, dizziness, confusion, headache, anorexia, renal stones	Caution if history of renal calculi	Metabolized via P450 system with renal excretion (35% unchanged). Protein binding 40%–60%. Elimination half-life is 63 hours.
Levetiracetam	Focal seizures (adjunctive therapy) Myoclonic seizures Tonic–clonic seizures	*Stevens-Johnson syndrome, toxic epidermal necrolysis, anemia, leukopenia* Sedation, asthenia, fatigue, headaches, vomiting, nasopharyngitis, incoordination, psychosis; milder but significant psychiatric symptoms, such as anxiety and irritability, are often observed	None known	No known drug interactions. Not extensively metabolized, with 66% excreted unchanged in the urine. Protein binding 10%. Elimination half-life is 6–8 hours; longer in renal dysfunction.

17

General Anesthetic Pharmacology

Jacob Wouden and Keith W. Miller

▌ INTRODUCTION

Before the discovery of **general anesthetics**, pain and shock severely limited the possibilities for surgical intervention. Postoperative mortality dropped dramatically following the first public demonstration of **diethyl ether** at Massachusetts General Hospital in 1846. Since then, the administration of agents for the induction and maintenance of anesthesia has become a separate medical specialty. The modern anesthesiologist is responsible for all aspects of patient health during surgery. As part of this process, the anesthesiologist controls the depth of anesthesia and maintains homeostatic equilibrium with an arsenal of inhaled and intravenous anesthetics as well as many adjuvant drugs.

General anesthetics induce a generalized, reversible depression of the central nervous system (CNS). Under general anesthesia, there is a lack of perception of all sensations. The anesthetic state includes loss of consciousness, amnesia, and immobility (a lack of response to noxious stimuli) but not necessarily complete analgesia. Other desirable effects provided by anesthetics or adjuvants during surgery may include muscle relaxation, loss of autonomic reflexes, analgesia, and anxiolysis. All of these effects facilitate safe and painless completion of the procedure; some effects are more important in certain types of surgery than others.

For example, abdominal surgery necessitates near-complete relaxation of the abdominal muscles, whereas neurosurgery often requires light anesthesia that may be lifted rapidly when the neurosurgeon needs to judge the patient's ability to respond to commands.

This chapter provides a framework for understanding the pharmacodynamics and pharmacokinetics of general anesthetics in the context of physiologic and pathophysiologic variables. After discussing the pharmacology of specific agents and how a balanced anesthetic approach is achieved, the chapter considers what is currently known about the mechanism of action of general anesthetics.

▌ PHARMACODYNAMICS OF INHALED ANESTHETICS

General anesthetics distribute well to all parts of the body, becoming most concentrated in the fatty tissues. The CNS is the primary site of action of anesthetics. Most likely, loss of consciousness and amnesia ensue from supraspinal action (i.e., action in the brainstem, midbrain, and cerebral cortex), while immobility in response to noxious stimuli is caused by depression of both supraspinal and spinal sensory and motor pathways. Different sites in the CNS are

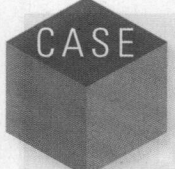

CASE

Matthew is a 7-year-old, 20-kg boy who has been undergoing multidrug chemotherapy for aggressive osteosarcoma of his right femur. The time has now come for a surgical resection.

- 8:00 PM (night before the operation): Dr. Snow, the anesthesiologist, provides reassurance and revisits the importance of fasting after midnight to prevent aspiration of gastric contents while under general anesthesia.
- 6:30 AM: Matthew clings to his mother and appears anxious, cachectic, and in some pain. His vital signs are stable with an elevated pulse of 120 and a blood pressure of 110/75. An oral dose of midazolam (a benzodiazepine; see Chapter 13, Pharmacology of GABAergic and Glutamatergic Neurotransmission) is given to relieve anxiety and to allow Matthew to separate from his parents.
- 7:00 AM: Dr. Snow injects a small amount of lidocaine subcutaneously (a local anesthetic; see Chapter 12, Local Anesthetic Pharmacology) before inserting an intravenous catheter (which he carefully conceals from Matthew until the last possible moment). Through the catheter, Dr. Snow delivers an infusion of morphine sulfate (an opioid; see Chapter 18, Pharmacology of Analgesia) for analgesia.
- 7:30 AM: Dr. Snow rapidly induces anesthesia with an intravenous bolus of 60 mg (3 mg/kg) of thiopental (a barbiturate; see Chapter 13). Within 45 seconds, Matthew is in a deep anesthetic state. The doctor adds a dose of intravenous succinylcholine (a depolarizing muscle relaxant; see Chapter 10, Cholinergic Pharmacology) to facilitate endotracheal intubation, and Matthew is placed on artificial respiration.
- 7:32 AM: A mixture of inhaled general anesthetics consisting of 2% isoflurane, 50% nitrous oxide,

and 48% oxygen is provided through the ventilator to maintain the anesthetic state.

- 7:50 AM: Matthew shows no response, either through movement or increased sympathetic tone (e.g., increased heart rate, increased blood pressure), to the first surgical incision.
- 8:20 AM: Dr. Snow notices with a start that Matthew's pulse has fallen to 55 and his blood pressure to 85/45. Berating himself for forgetting to turn down the inspired partial pressure of the anesthetic as its mixed venous partial pressure increased, Dr. Snow reduces the inspired isoflurane level to 0.8% while keeping the nitrous oxide level at 50%. Within 15 minutes, Matthew's pulse and blood pressure rebound.
- 12:35 PM: After a long surgery, Dr. Snow stops the isoflurane and nitrous oxide and turns on pure oxygen for a few minutes.
- 12:45 PM: In less than 10 minutes, Matthew is breathing spontaneously and is able to respond to questions, although he is still somewhat groggy. Matthew's parents are relieved to find him awake and alert after more than 5 hours of anesthesia.

Questions

1. What determines the rate of induction and recovery from anesthesia, and how does this differ for children as compared to adults?
2. Why is it necessary to reduce the inspired partial pressure of isoflurane some minutes into the procedure (as Dr. Snow initially neglected to do)?
3. Why did Dr. Snow give pure oxygen for a few minutes following the cessation of anesthetic administration?
4. What are the advantages of using a mixture of two anesthetics (in this example, nitrous oxide and isoflurane) instead of just one or the other?

differentially affected by general anesthetics, giving rise to the classical stages observed with increasing anesthetic depth (Fig. 17-1).

The Minimum Alveolar Concentration (MAC)

To control the depth of anesthesia, the anesthesiologist must control rather precisely the level of anesthetic in the CNS. This level is denoted by the partial pressure of anesthetic in the CNS, also called the **CNS partial pressure**, P_{CNS}. (See Box 17-1 for a discussion of partial pressures versus concentrations and Appendix A for a glossary of abbreviations and symbols.) The anesthesiologist maintains P_{CNS} within the desired range by varying the **inspired partial pressure**, P_I. Because the value of P_{CNS} cannot be monitored directly, it is commonly inferred from the **alveolar partial pressure**, P_{alv}. The alveolar partial pressure is a useful substitute for P_{CNS}, because P_{CNS} tracks P_{alv} with only a small time

lag (see below). P_{alv} may be measured directly as the partial pressure of anesthetic in the end-tidal exhaled gas, when the dead space no longer contributes to the exhaled gas.

The alveolar partial pressure that results in the lightest possible anesthesia is termed the **minimum alveolar concentration** (MAC). Specifically, MAC is the alveolar partial pressure that abolishes a movement response to a surgical incision in 50% of patients. The potency of an anesthetic is related inversely to its MAC. If the MAC is small, then the potency is high, and a relatively low partial pressure will be sufficient to cause anesthesia. For example, **isoflurane**—which has a MAC of 0.0114 atm—is much more potent than **nitrous oxide**—which has a MAC of 1.01 atm (Table 17-1).

Therapeutic and Analgesic Indices

Loss of response to extremely noxious stimuli, such as endotracheal intubation, requires a higher partial pressure of

Awake   Awake

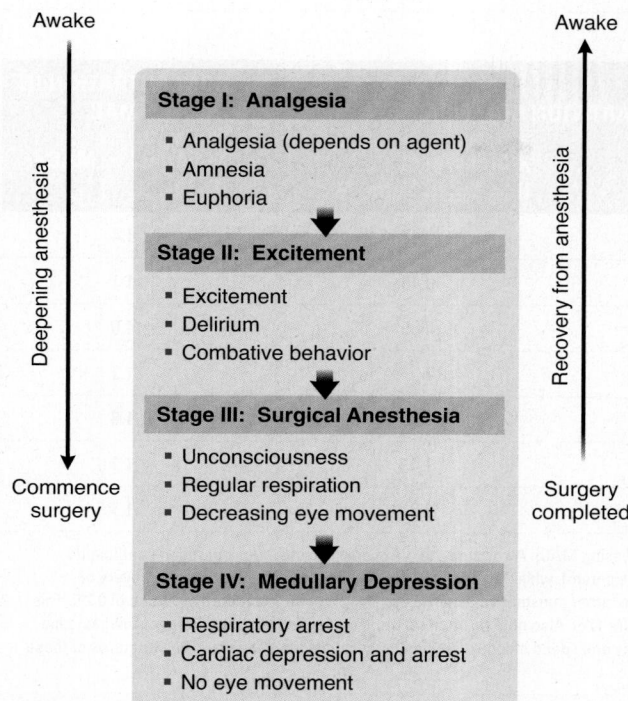

FIGURE 17-1. **The stages of anesthesia.** The deepening anesthetic state can be divided into four stages, based on observations with diethyl ether. The analgesia of stage I is variable and depends on the particular anesthetic agent. With fast induction, the patient passes rapidly through the undesirable "excitement" phase (stage II). Surgery is generally undertaken in stage III. The anesthesiologist must take care to avoid stage IV, which begins with respiratory arrest. Cardiac arrest occurs later in stage IV. During recovery from anesthesia, the patient progresses through the stages in reverse.

anesthetic than is required for loss of response to a surgical incision (Fig. 17-2). Still higher partial pressures of anesthetic cause medullary depression. In general, however, anesthetics have steep **dose–response curves** and low therapeutic indices, defined as the ratio of **LP_{50}** (the partial pressure that is lethal in 50% of subjects) to MAC (which is analogous to ED_{50}; see Chapter 2, Pharmacodynamics). Furthermore, the variability among patients in their response to a given dose of

anesthetic is small. Therefore, for all patients, the levels of anesthetic that cause respiratory and cardiac arrest are not much higher than the levels that cause general anesthesia. It should also be noted that no pharmacologic antagonists of general anesthetics exist to counteract inadvertently high levels of anesthetic. Although these disadvantages are partially offset by the ability to control P_{CNS} through control of P_I (i.e., the anesthetic can be breathed out), the combination of low therapeutic index and lack of antagonist means that anesthetics are dangerous drugs that demand specialty training for their proper and safe administration.

Pain relief (analgesia) may or may not occur at a partial pressure lower than that required for surgical anesthesia. The partial pressure at which 50% of persons lose nociception is the AP_{50} (partial pressure that results in analgesia in 50% of patients), and the **analgesic index** is the ratio of MAC to AP_{50}. A high analgesic index implies that analgesia is induced at a partial pressure of anesthetic significantly lower than that required for surgical anesthesia. For example, nitrous oxide has a high analgesic index and is a good analgesic, whereas **halothane** has a low analgesic index and is a poor analgesic.

The Meyer-Overton Rule

The potency of an anesthetic can be predicted from its physicochemical characteristics. The most reliable predictor has been the anesthetic's solubility in olive oil (or in another lipophilic solvent, such as octanol), as denoted by the **oil/gas partition coefficient**, λ**(oil/gas)** (Box 17-2). Specifically, *the potency of an anesthetic increases as its solubility in oil increases*. That is, *as λ(oil/gas) increases, MAC decreases*.

The relationship between MAC and λ(oil/gas) is such that MAC multiplied by λ(oil/gas) is nearly constant, independent of the identity of the anesthetic. Because multiplication of the partition coefficient by the partial pressure yields the concentration of anesthetic (Box 17-2), this is equivalent to saying that, at 1 MAC, the concentration of anesthetic in a lipophilic solvent (such as olive oil) is nearly constant for all anesthetics. Thus, the MAC, which varies with the identity of the anesthetic, is actually the partial pressure required to generate a particular concentration of anesthetic in a lipophilic medium, such as the lipid bilayers

---

BOX 17-1 Partial Pressure Versus Concentration

The **partial pressure** of Gas A in a mixture of gases is the portion of the total pressure that is supplied by Gas A. For ideal gases, the partial pressure of Gas A is obtained by multiplying the total pressure by the mole fraction of A in the mixture (i.e., the fraction of molecules in the mixture represented by Gas A). The concentration of Gas A in the mixture ($[A]_{mixture}$) is the number of moles of Gas A (n_A) divided by the volume (V); $[A]_{mixture}$ can also be obtained from the ideal gas equation by dividing the partial pressure of Gas A (P_A) by the temperature (T) and the universal gas constant (R):

$$[A]_{mixture} = n_A / V = P_A / RT$$

Inhaled anesthetics dissolve in the tissues of the body, such as the blood and the brain. The partial pressure of a gas dissolved in a liquid is equal to the partial pressure of free gas in equilibrium with that liquid. For gases, partial pressures are convenient because the partial pressures in all compartments are equal at equilibrium. This is true, independent of whether the compartments contain gas that is in the gaseous (alveoli) or the dissolved (tissues) form. In contrast, the concentrations within different compartments are not equal at equilibrium. To convert the partial pressure of a dissolved gas to its concentration within the solvent, the partial pressure is multiplied by a measure of solubility known as the **solvent/gas partition coefficient**. ∎

TABLE 17-1 Properties of Inhaled Anesthetics

| ANESTHETIC | MAC (atm) | SOLVENT/GAS PARTITION COEFFICIENTS | | CONCENTRATION IN OIL AT 1 MAC |
		λ(oil/gas) ($L_{gas}\ L_{tissue}^{-1}\ atm^{-1}$)	λ(blood/gas) ($L_{gas}\ L_{tissue}^{-1}\ atm^{-1}$)	λ(oil/gas) $\times$ MAC ($L_{gas}\ L_{tissue}^{-1}$)
Nitrous oxide	1.01	1.4	0.47	1.4
Desflurane	0.06	19	0.45	1.1
Sevoflurane	0.02	51	0.65	1.0
Diethyl ether	0.019	65	12	1.2
Enflurane	0.0168	98	1.8	1.6
Isoflurane	0.0114	98	1.4	1.1
Halothane	0.0077	224	2.3	1.7

The commonly used inhaled anesthetics are listed in order of increasing potency (or decreasing MAC). Also listed are the important solvent/gas partition coefficients λ(oil/gas) and λ(blood/gas). λ(oil/gas) defines the potency of the anesthetic (higher is more potent), while λ(blood/gas) defines the rate of induction and recovery of anesthesia (lower is faster). The product of λ(oil/gas) and MAC for these anesthetics has a rather constant value of 1.3 $L_{gas}\ L_{tissue}^{-1}$ (with a standard deviation of 0.27). This is an illustration of the Meyer-Overton Rule; another illustration of the rule is shown in Figure 17-3. Also note the general trend that anesthetics with larger λ(oil/gas) tend to have larger λ(blood/gas); this means that there is frequently a trade-off between potency and speed of induction among the inhaled anesthetics. The structures of these agents are shown in Figure 17-14.

in the CNS. This correlation, known as the **Meyer-Overton rule**, holds over at least five orders of magnitude of anesthetic potency (Fig. 17-3). The constant that represents the concentration of anesthetic at 1 MAC is 1.3 liters of gas per liter of oil (L_{gas} / L_{oil}), or 0.05 M after dividing by the volume of one mole (see Box 17-2). Thus, if one knows the oil/gas partition coefficient of an anesthetic, one can estimate its MAC from the following equation (see also Table 17-1):

$$MAC \approx 1.3/\lambda\,(oil/gas)$$ **Equation 17-1**

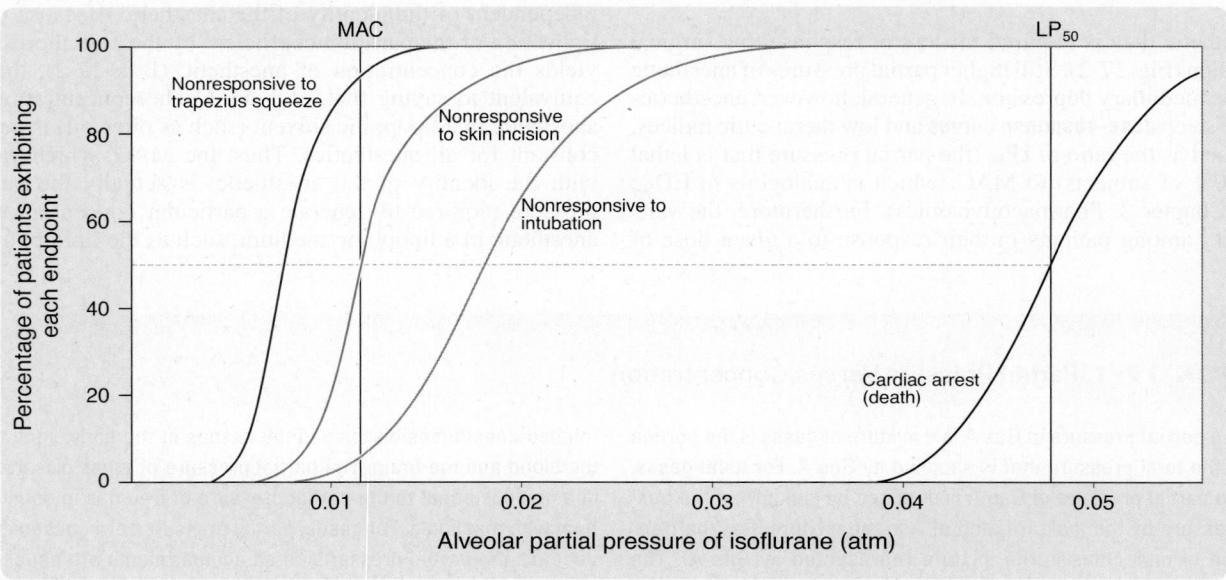

FIGURE 17-2. Isoflurane dose–response curves for various endpoints. These curves depict the percentage of patients exhibiting endpoints of nonresponsiveness to a set of stimuli and of cardiac arrest as the alveolar partial pressure of isoflurane is increased. Note that the dose–response curves are quite steep, especially for mild stimuli, and that higher partial pressures are required to achieve lack of response to stronger stimuli. In the example shown, lack of response to intubation in 50% of patients requires nearly 0.02 atm isoflurane, while lack of response to a squeeze of the trapezius muscle requires only 0.008 atm. The MAC is defined as the alveolar partial pressure at which 50% of patients do not respond to a skin incision. The therapeutic index is defined as the lethal pressure (LP_{50}) divided by the MAC. The theoretical curve for cardiac arrest is derived from a known therapeutic index of about 4 for isoflurane. Accordingly, the anesthesiologist must carefully monitor each individual patient to achieve the desired effect while avoiding cardiac depression.

BOX 17-2 Partition Coefficients

The **solvent/gas partition coefficient, λ(solvent/gas),** defines the solubility of a gas in a solvent or, in other words, the extent to which the gas "partitions" between its gaseous state and the solution. More specifically, λ(solvent/gas) is the ratio of the amount of gas dissolved in a given volume of solvent to the amount of free gas that would occupy the same volume of space, all at standard temperature (25°C) and pressure (1.0 atm) (STP). The solvent could be olive oil, blood, or brain tissue, for example.

Dissolved amounts of gas are typically given not in terms of moles but in terms of the volume that the gas would occupy at STP in a gaseous state. Recall that, to convert from moles to liters at STP, one multiplies by the volume of one mole of gas at 25°C and 1.0 atm (i.e., by 24.5 L/mol). Thus, λ(solvent/gas) is the number of liters of gas that will dissolve in one liter of solvent per atmosphere of partial pressure. [Note that the units of λ(solvent/gas) are $L_{gas} L_{solvent}^{-1} atm^{-1}$, or simply atm^{-1}.]

For a particular solvent, a gas with a larger λ(solvent/gas) is more soluble in that solvent. For example, diethyl ether has a λ(blood/gas) of about 12 $L_{diethyl\ ether} L_{blood}^{-1} atm^{-1}$, so diethyl ether is relatively soluble in blood. In contrast, nitrous oxide has a λ(blood/gas) of about 0.47 $L_{nitrous\ oxide} L_{blood}^{-1} atm^{-1}$, so nitrous oxide is relatively insoluble in blood (see Table 17-1 and Fig. 17-8 for examples).

Likewise, a gas may have different solubilities in different solvents. Solvents or tissues in which a gas has a high partition coefficient (high solubility) will dissolve large amounts of the gas at a given partial pressure, resulting in a high concentration of the gas in that solvent or tissue. Thus, large amounts of gas must be transferred to change the partial pressure by an appreciable amount. In contrast, solvents or tissues in which a gas has a low partition coefficient (low solubility) will dissolve only small amounts of the gas at a given partial pressure. In this case,

transferring a small amount of the gas will significantly change the partial pressure (Fig. 17-8).

For any given partial pressure, Henry's law for dilute solutions allows the concentration of Gas A in a solvent ($[A]_{solution}$) to be calculated from λ(solvent/gas). The partial pressure is multiplied by the partition coefficient to calculate the concentration in terms of L_{gas} per $L_{solvent}$. The result is divided by the volume of one mole of gas at 25°C at 1.0 atm (24.5 L/mol) to yield the molar concentration.

$$[A]_{solution} = P_{solvent} \times \lambda(solvent/gas)$$
$$\{in\ terms\ of\ L_{gas}/L_{solvent}\}$$
$$= P_{solvent} \times \lambda(solvent/gas)/(24.5\ L/mol)$$
$$\{in\ terms\ of\ mol_{gas}/L_{solvent}\}$$

For example, because the λ(blood/gas) of nitrous oxide is 0.47 $L_{nitrous\ oxide} L_{blood}^{-1} atm^{-1}$, if the partial pressure of nitrous oxide in the blood is 0.50 atm, then the concentration is 0.50 atm × 0.47 $L_{nitrous\ oxide} L_{blood}^{-1} atm^{-1}$ = 0.24 $L_{nitrous\ oxide} L_{blood}^{-1}$ or 9.6 mM (after dividing by 24.5 L/mol). Also note that doubling the partial pressure will double the concentration.

A partition coefficient can also be defined for the partitioning of a gas between two solvents. For example, the tissue/blood partition coefficient, λ(tissue/blood), is the ratio of the molar concentration of gas in the tissue ($[A]_{tissue}$) to the molar concentration of gas in the blood ($[A]_{blood}$) at equilibrium (note that this coefficient is unitless). From the previous equation defining concentration and the fact that partial pressures are equal at equilibrium, it follows that

$$\lambda(tissue/blood) = [A]_{tissue}/[A]_{blood}$$
$$= \lambda(tissue/gas)/\lambda(blood/gas)\ \blacksquare$$

PHARMACOKINETICS OF INHALED ANESTHETICS

A cardiopulmonary model of the **uptake** of anesthetic from the alveoli into the circulation and the **distribution** of anesthetic from the circulation to the tissues allows determination of the rate at which the partial pressure of anesthetic rises within the CNS. The anesthesiologist must navigate the small space between allowing a patient to awaken and causing medullary depression by predicting the effects of various physiologic responses and disease states on the depth of anesthesia. For example, an understanding of the distribution characteristics of anesthetics enabled Dr. Snow to respond appropriately to Matthew's hypotension by lowering the P_I of isoflurane without overcorrecting and causing him to awaken.

The anesthesiologist must also be aware of the differences in the pharmacokinetics of the various anesthetics. The pharmacokinetic characteristics of an ideal general anesthetic would be such that the anesthetic provides a rapid and pleasant induction of surgical anesthesia, followed by

a smooth and rapid recovery to a fully functional and conscious state. The pharmacokinetics of individual agents are discussed below; this section deals with general principles of the **uptake model**, which uses basic respiratory and cardiovascular physiology to predict the pharmacokinetics of the inhaled anesthetics. As discussed below, the uptake model depends on calculations of the time required for the equilibration of anesthetic partial pressures in the tissues with the inspired anesthetic partial pressure.

Concepts from Respiratory Physiology

Local Equilibration

During general anesthesia, the patient breathes, either spontaneously or via a ventilator, an anesthetic or mixture of anesthetics together with oxygen and/or normal air. Once the anesthetic gas reaches the alveoli, it must diffuse across the respiratory epithelium into the alveolar capillary bed. According to Fick's law, the rate of diffusion of gas through a sheet of tissue down its partial pressure gradient is proportional to the tissue area and the partial pressure difference

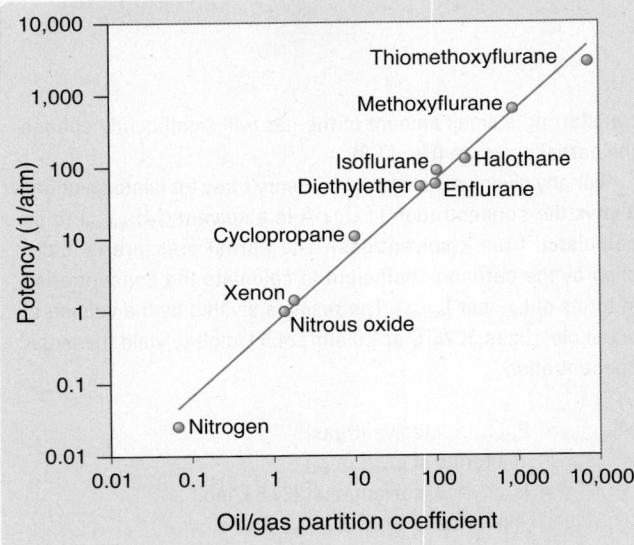

FIGURE 17-3. The Meyer-Overton rule. Molecules with a higher oil/gas partition coefficient [λ(oil/gas)] are more potent general anesthetics. This log–log plot shows the very tight correlation between lipid solubility [λ(oil/gas)] and anesthetic potency over five orders of magnitude. Note that even such gases as xenon and nitrogen can act as general anesthetics when breathed at sufficiently high partial pressures. The equation describing the line is: Potency = λ(oil/gas) / 1.3. Recall that Potency = 1/MAC.

between the two sides and is inversely proportional to the thickness of the sheet:

Diffusion rate = $D \times (A/l) \times \Delta P$ **Equation 17-2**

where D = diffusion constant; A = surface area; l = thickness; and ΔP = partial pressure difference.

One principle evident from Fick's law is that the equalization of the partial pressure of the gas, not its concentration, defines the approach to equilibrium across a boundary sheet. Thus, at equilibrium (i.e., when the net diffusion rate is zero), the partial pressure in the two compartments is the same, even though the concentration in the two compartments may be different.

With its enormous alveolar surface area (~75 m², or nearly half a tennis court) and thin epithelium (~0.3 μm, which is less than 1/20th the diameter of a red blood cell), the lung optimizes the rate of gas diffusion. Accordingly, the alveolar partial pressure P_{alv} and the systemic arterial partial pressure P_{art} are nearly the same at all times. (In normal individuals, small amounts of physiologic shunting keep P_{art} slightly lower than P_{alv}.) By using the lungs as an uptake system for inhaled anesthetics, anesthesiologists take advantage of the body's system for absorbing oxygen.

Similarly, the capillary beds in tissues have evolved to deliver oxygen rapidly to all cells in the body. The distances between arterioles are small, and diffusion pathways are on the order of one cell diameter. Consequently, the arterial partial pressure of a general anesthetic can equilibrate completely with tissues in the time required for blood to traverse the capillary bed. Likewise, the partial pressure in the postcapillary venules P_{venule} equals the partial pressure in the tissue P_{tissue}.

Another way of stating the above conclusion is that *the transfer of anesthetic in both the lungs and the tissues is limited by perfusion rather than diffusion.* Because perfusion is rate-limiting, increasing the rate of diffusion (e.g., by using a lower molecular weight anesthetic) will not, by itself, increase the rate of induction of anesthesia.

Global Equilibration

If an anesthetic is inspired for a sufficiently long period of time, all compartments in the body will equilibrate to the same partial pressure (equal to P_I). This global equilibration may be divided into a series of partial pressure equilibrations between each successive compartment and its incoming flow of anesthetic. In the case of the tissues, the incoming flow is the arterial blood flow, with partial pressure approximately equal to P_{alv}. In the case of the alveoli, the incoming flow is the alveolar ventilation with partial pressure P_I.

The **time constant** τ describes the rate of approach of a compartment's partial pressure to that of its incoming flow. Specifically, τ is the time required for equilibration to be 63% complete. This time constant is convenient because it can be calculated by dividing the compartment's **volume capacity** (relative to the delivering medium; see below) by the **flow rate**. In other words, once a volume of flow equal to the capacity of a compartment has gone through that compartment, the partial pressure of anesthetic in the compartment (i.e., in the tissues or alveoli) will be 63% of the partial pressure in the incoming flow (i.e., in the arterial blood flow or alveolar ventilation, respectively). Equilibration is 95% complete after three time constants.

τ = Volume Capacity/Flow Rate   **Equation 17-3**

$$P_{compartment} = P_{flow}[1 - e^{-(t/\tau)}]$$ **Equation 17-4**

where t = elapsed time.

These equations describe what should make intuitive sense: equilibration of the partial pressure of the compartment with the incoming flow takes place more quickly (i.e., the time constant is smaller) when the inflow is larger or the compartment capacity is smaller.

The Uptake Model

For simplicity, the model of anesthetic uptake and distribution organizes the tissues of the body into groups based on similar characteristics. Each group can be modeled as a container with a particular capacity for anesthetic and a particular level of blood flow delivering anesthetic. An adequate approximation groups the tissues into three main compartments that are perfused in parallel (Fig. 17-4). The **vessel-rich group (VRG)**, which consists of the CNS and visceral organs, has a low capacity and high flow. The **muscle group (MG)**, which consists of muscle and skin, has a high capacity and moderate flow. The **fat group (FG)** has a very high capacity and low flow. (A fourth group, the **vessel-poor group [VPG]**, which consists of bone, cartilage, and ligaments, has a negligible capacity and flow, and its omission does not significantly affect the model.)

The rate of increase of the partial pressure in the VRG (P_{VRG}) is of the greatest interest because the VRG includes the CNS. The overall equilibration of P_{VRG} with the inspired partial pressure occurs in two steps, either of which may be

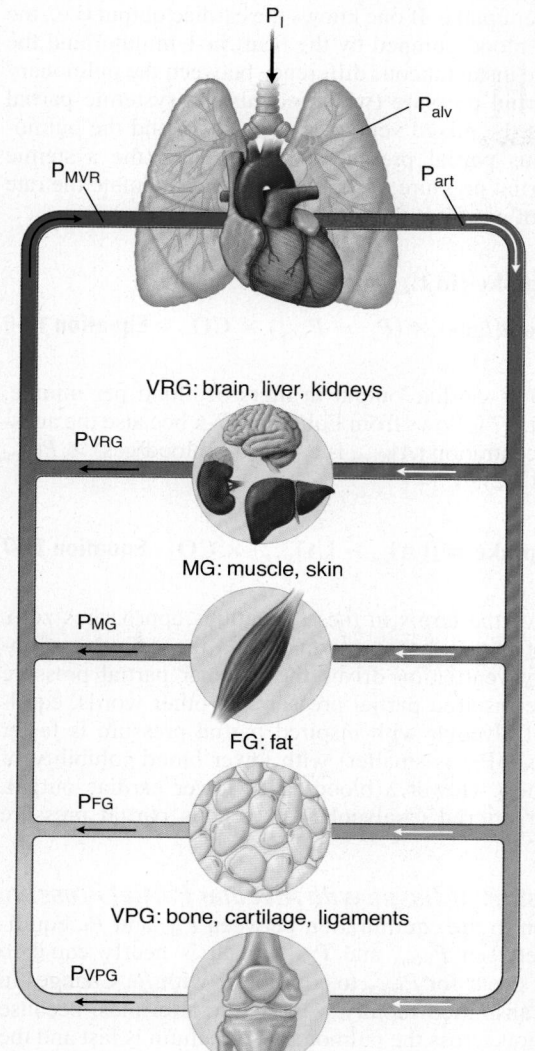

Tissue group	% Cardiac output	% Body weight	Vol. cap. for N_2O at P_{alv} = 0.8atm	Vol. cap. for halo. at P_{alv} = 0.01atm
VRG	75%	9%	2.6 L	0.30 L
MG	18%	50%	16 L	3.0 L
FG	5.5%	19%	12 L	17 L
VPG	1.5%	22%	7.0 L	1.3 L

FIGURE 17-4. Distribution of cardiac output and volume capacity for general anesthetics among the major tissue compartments. The tissues of the body can be divided into four groups based on their level of perfusion and their capacity to take up anesthetic. These include the vessel-rich group (VRG), muscle group (MG), fat group (FG), and vessel-poor group (VPG). (The contribution of the VPG is generally ignored in most pharmacokinetic models of anesthesia.) The VRG, which contains the internal organs including the brain, constitutes a small percentage of the total body weight (9%), has the lowest capacity for anesthetic, and receives most of the cardiac output (75%). The high perfusion and low capacity allow P_{VRG} to equilibrate rapidly with P_{art}. Also, the VRG makes the largest contribution to the mixed venous return partial pressure P_{MVR}, which is equal to (0.75 P_{VRG} + 0.18 P_{MG} + 0.055 P_{FG} + 0.015 P_{VPG}). N_2O, nitrous oxide; Halo., halothane; Vol. cap., volume capacity.

rate-limiting. First, the alveolar and inspired partial pressures equilibrate (P_{alv} approaches P_I, or $P_{alv} \rightarrow P_I$). Second, P_{VRG} (and specifically P_{CNS}) equilibrates with the arterial partial pressure (which is essentially equal to the alveolar partial pressure) ($P_{VRG} \rightarrow P_{art}$). The discussion will now consider the time constant for each of these two steps and define conditions under which one or the other is rate-limiting.

Equilibration of Alveolar with Inspired Partial Pressure

The equilibration of P_{alv} with P_I is conceptually the first step of the equilibration of P_{VRG} with P_I. During induction of anesthesia, P_{VRG} can never be higher than P_{alv}; if P_{alv} rises slowly, then P_{VRG} must also rise slowly.

To calculate the time constant for the approach of P_{alv} to P_I, $\tau\{P_{alv} \rightarrow P_I\}$, the flow rate and volume capacity must be defined. The delivering medium is free gas arriving through the airways, and the compartment is the lung and alveoli. The volume capacity is simply the volume of gas that remains in the lungs after normal exhalation, or the **functional residual capacity** (**FRC**, typically ~3 L for an average adult). Assume initially that the only component of the flow rate is the rate of **alveolar ventilation**, which delivers the anesthetic (V_{alv} = {Tidal Volume − Dead Space} × Respiratory Rate; for an average adult, V_{alv} = {0.5 L − 0.125 L} × 16 min^{-1} ≈ 6 L/min). Then, because

$$\tau\{P_{alv} \rightarrow P_I\} = FRC/V_{alv} \qquad \text{Equation 17-5}$$

a typical value for $\tau\{P_{alv} \rightarrow P_I\}$ is 3 L / 6 L/min, or 0.5 min—independent of the particular gas being inhaled. In children, the increased alveolar ventilation rate and decreased FRC (smaller lungs) both tend to shorten the time constant and to accelerate equilibration between the alveolar and inspired partial pressures.

The assumption to this point has been that no uptake of anesthetic into the bloodstream occurs, as would be the case if the solubility of the anesthetic in blood were zero. In practice, at the same time that alveolar ventilation is delivering anesthetic to the alveoli, anesthetic is also being removed from the alveoli by diffusion into the bloodstream. The balance between delivery and removal is analogous to adding water into a leaky bucket (Fig. 17-5). The level of water in the bucket (which represents the alveolar partial pressure) is determined both by the rate at which the water is added (the minute ventilation) and the size of the leak (the rate of anesthetic uptake from the alveoli into the bloodstream). Increasing anesthetic delivery (e.g., by using a higher ventilation rate or a higher inspired partial pressure) will increase the alveolar partial pressure of the gas, just as adding water faster will increase the level of water in the bucket. Conversely, increasing anesthetic removal (e.g., by increasing the perfusion rate or using a more blood-soluble anesthetic) will decrease the alveolar partial pressure of the gas; this is analogous to increasing the leakiness of the bucket. Thus, uptake of anesthetic from the alveoli into the bloodstream constitutes a negative component to the flow (i.e., a flow out of the lungs), which makes the time constant longer than the theoretical case where $\tau\{P_{alv} \rightarrow P_I\}$ equals FRC divided by V_{alv}.

The magnitude of the increase in the time constant compared to the limiting case depends on the rate of uptake of anesthetic by the blood, with longer $\tau\{P_{alv} \rightarrow P_I\}$ resulting

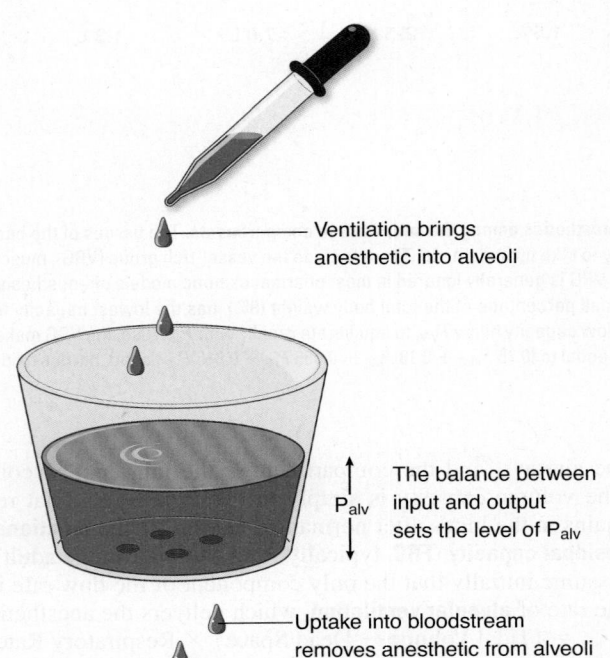

Ventilation brings anesthetic into alveoli

The balance between input and output sets the level of P_{alv}

P_{alv}

Uptake into bloodstream removes anesthetic from alveoli

FIGURE 17-5. Determinants of the alveolar partial pressure of an inhaled anesthetic. The alveolar partial pressure, represented by the depth of fluid in the bucket, results from the balance between delivery by ventilation and removal by uptake into the bloodstream. Increased delivery of anesthetic, resulting from either increased ventilation or an increased inspired partial pressure of anesthetic, raises P_{alv}. In contrast, increased uptake into the bloodstream, caused by a large λ(blood/gas) or increased cardiac output, lowers P_{alv}.

from greater uptake. If one knows the cardiac output (i.e., the volume of blood pumped by the heart in 1 minute) and the value of the instantaneous difference between the pulmonary arterial partial pressure (which equals the systemic partial pressure of the mixed venous return, P_{MVR}) and the pulmonary venous partial pressure (which equals the systemic arterial partial pressure, P_{art}), then one can calculate the rate of uptake of gas from the alveoli:

Rate of uptake {in L_{gas}/min}

$$= \lambda(\text{blood/gas}) \times (P_{art} - P_{MVR}) \times CO \quad \textbf{Equation 17-6}$$

where CO = cardiac output in liters of blood per minute. Equation 17-7 follows from Equation 17-6 because the anesthetic concentration $[A]_{blood}$ is equal to λ(blood/gas) $\times P_{blood}$ (see Box 17-2):

Rate of uptake $= ([A]_{art} - [A]_{MVR}) \times CO \quad \textbf{Equation 17-7}$

If any of the terms in these equations approaches zero, the rate of uptake becomes small, and the delivery of anesthetic by ventilation drives the alveolar partial pressure toward the inspired partial pressure. In other words, equilibration of alveolar with inspired partial pressure is faster (i.e., $\tau\{P_{alv} \rightarrow P_I\}$ is smaller) with lower blood solubility of the anesthetic [lower λ(blood/gas)], lower cardiac output, or smaller arterial ($\approx$alveolar) to venous partial pressure difference.

Equilibration of Tissue with Alveolar Partial Pressure

In addition to the equilibration between P_{alv} and P_I, equilibration between P_{tissue} and P_{art} (which is nearly equal to P_{alv}) must occur for P_{tissue} to equilibrate with P_I. Changes in P_{alv} are transmitted rapidly to systemic arterioles, because equilibration across the pulmonary epithelium is fast and the circulation time from pulmonary veins to tissue capillaries is generally less than 10 seconds. Thus, the time constant for equilibration between P_{tissue} and P_{alv} can be approximated as the time constant for equilibration between P_{tissue} and P_{art}. To calculate the time constant $\tau\{P_{tissue} \rightarrow P_{art}\}$, one must define the capacity of the compartment and the flow rate of the delivering medium. The flow rate is simply the rate at which blood perfuses the tissue. Recall that capacity is a volume capacity relative to the delivering medium. Specifically, *the capacity is the volume that the tissue would need to contain all of its gas if the solubility of the gas in the tissue were the same as that in the blood.* (This definition is similar to that of the volume of distribution of a drug; see Chapter 3, Pharmacokinetics):

Relative Volume Capacity of Tissue

$$= ([A]_{tissue} \times Vol_{tissue})/[A]_{blood} \quad \textbf{Equation 17-8}$$

where Vol_{tissue} is the volume of tissue. Equation 17-9 follows from Equation 17-8 because $[A]_{tissue}$ / $[A]_{blood}$ at equilibrium is equal to λ(tissue/blood) (see Box 17-2):

Relative Volume Capacity of Brain

$$= \lambda(\text{brain/blood}) \times Vol_{brain} \quad \textbf{Equation 17-9}$$

TABLE 17-2 Tissue/Blood Partition Coefficients

ANESTHETIC	TISSUE/BLOOD PARTITION COEFFICIENTS		
	λ(BRAIN/ BLOOD) (UNITLESS)	λ(MUSCLE/ BLOOD) (UNITLESS)	λ(FAT/ BLOOD) (UNITLESS)
Nitrous oxide	1.1	1.2	2.3
Diethyl ether	2.0	1.3	5
Desflurane	1.3	2.0	27
Enflurane	1.4	1.7	36
Isoflurane	1.6	2.9	45
Sevoflurane	1.7	3.1	48
Halothane	1.9	3.4	51

The tissue/blood partition coefficient describes the comparative solubility of an anesthetic in a tissue compared to blood. λ(tissue/blood) is obtained from the ratio of the concentration of anesthetic in the tissue to the concentration in the blood at equilibrium (i.e., when the partial pressure is the same in both tissues). Alternatively, one may calculate λ(tissue/blood) from the equation λ(tissue/blood) = λ(tissue/gas)/λ(blood/gas) (see Box 17-2). With very few minor exceptions, the general trend is λ(fat/blood) >> λ(muscle/blood) > λ(brain/blood). High values of λ(fat/blood) give the FG a very high capacity for the inhaled anesthetics.

Then, using Equation 17-3, we can write

$$\tau\{P_{tissue} \rightarrow P_{art}\} \approx \tau\{P_{tissue} \rightarrow P_{alv}\}$$

$$= \text{Relative Vol. Cap. of Tissue}/Q_{tissue} \qquad \textbf{Equation 17-10}$$

$$\tau\{P_{tissue} \rightarrow P_{art}\}$$

$$= \lambda(\text{tissue/blood}) \times \text{Vol}_{tissue}/Q_{tissue} \qquad \textbf{Equation 17-11}$$

where Q_{tissue} is tissue perfusion in L/min.

The tissue groups differ greatly in their capacities for anesthetic and in the time constants for their equilibration with arterial (and thus alveolar) partial pressure. With a low λ(tissue/blood) (Table 17-2) and a small volume (~6 L), the VRG has a low capacity for anesthetic. The combination of low capacity and high blood flow (75% of cardiac output) results in a very short equilibration time constant ($\tau\{P_{VRG} \rightarrow P_{alv}\}$) for the VRG. With a slightly higher λ(tissue/blood), a much larger volume (~33 L), and only moderate blood flow, the MG has a longer equilibration time constant ($\tau\{P_{MG} \rightarrow P_{art}\}$). Finally, with an extremely high λ(tissue/blood), a large volume, and low blood flow, the FG has an extremely long equilibration time constant ($\tau\{P_{FG} \rightarrow P_{art}\}$) (Table 17-3 and Fig. 17-6).

Because the anesthesiologist seeks to control P_{CNS}, the time constant for equilibration of the brain partial pressure P_{brain} with the arterial partial pressure P_{art} (which is nearly equal to P_{alv}) is of particular interest. The volume of the brain is approximately 1.4 L, the blood flow to the brain is about 0.9 L/min, and an average λ(brain/blood) for most anesthetics is about 1.6. Then, because

Relative Volume Capacity of Brain

$$= \lambda(\text{brain/blood}) \times \text{Vol}_{brain} \qquad \textbf{Equation 17-12}$$

$$\tau\{P_{brain} \rightarrow P_{art}\} = \lambda(\text{brain/blood}) \times \text{Vol}_{brain}/Q_{brain}$$

$$\tau\{P_{brain} \rightarrow P_{art}\} = (1.6 \times 1.4 \text{ L})/(0.9 \text{ L/min})$$

$$= 2.5 \text{ min} \qquad \textbf{Equation 17-13}$$

where Vol_{brain} is the volume of the brain and Q_{brain} is the blood flow to the brain.

Variations in λ(brain/blood) among the different anesthetic agents cause $\tau\{P_{brain} \rightarrow P_{art}\}$ to range from 1.5 min for nitrous oxide [λ(brain/blood) = 1.1] to 2.7 min for diethyl ether [λ(brain/blood) = 2.0] (Table 17-3). Of course, variability in blood flow to the brain also affects $\tau\{P_{brain} \rightarrow P_{art}\}$. In summary, *the time constant for equilibration of the CNS with the alveolar partial pressure is short and relatively independent of the particular anesthetic being used.*

The Rate-Limiting Step

As described above, the equilibration of the CNS with the inspired partial pressure occurs in two steps. Unlike $\tau\{P_{brain} \rightarrow P_{art}\}$, which is relatively independent of the particular anesthetic being used, $\tau\{P_{alv} \rightarrow P_I\}$ varies greatly among different anesthetics. On this basis, inhaled anesthetics can be divided into two broad categories:

- Ventilation-limited anesthetics, such as **diethyl ether, enflurane, isoflurane**, and **halothane**; and
- Perfusion-limited anesthetics, such as **nitrous oxide, desflurane**, and **sevoflurane**.

Ventilation-limited anesthetics have a long, rate-limiting $\tau\{P_{alv} \rightarrow P_I\}$ because of their high λ(blood/gas): the high rate of uptake of anesthetic into the bloodstream prevents P_{alv} from rising rapidly. Thus, the slow and rate-limiting equilibration of alveolar with inspired partial pressure results in slow induction of anesthesia and slow recovery

TABLE 17-3 Time Constants for Equilibration of Tissue with Arterial Partial Pressure

ANESTHETIC	TIME CONSTANT FOR EQUILIBRATION OF TISSUE WITH ARTERIAL PARTIAL PRESSURE, $\tau\{P_{tissue} \rightarrow P_{art}\}$		
	VRG (min)	MG (min)	FG (min)
Nitrous oxide	1.5	36	104
Diethyl ether	2.7	39	227
Desflurane	1.7	61	1,223
Enflurane	1.9	51	1,631
Isoflurane	2.1	88	2,039
Sevoflurane	2.3	94	2,175
Halothane	2.5	103	2,311

The time constants $\tau\{P_{tissue} \rightarrow P_{art}\}$ describe the time for 63% equilibration of the tissue with arterial (and therefore alveolar) partial pressure. Notice the very small time constants for equilibration of the VRG, in contrast to the large time constants for MG equilibration and very large time constants for FG equilibration. For all anesthetics except nitrous oxide, the partial pressure of the FG remains far below that of the alveolus for even the longest surgical procedures. Conversely, the VRG partial pressure is nearly in equilibrium with the alveolar partial pressure from almost the start of anesthetic administration. The values in this table were calculated from the equation $\tau\{P_{tissue} \rightarrow P_{art}\}$ = λ(tissue/blood) × Volume of tissue/Blood flow to tissue.

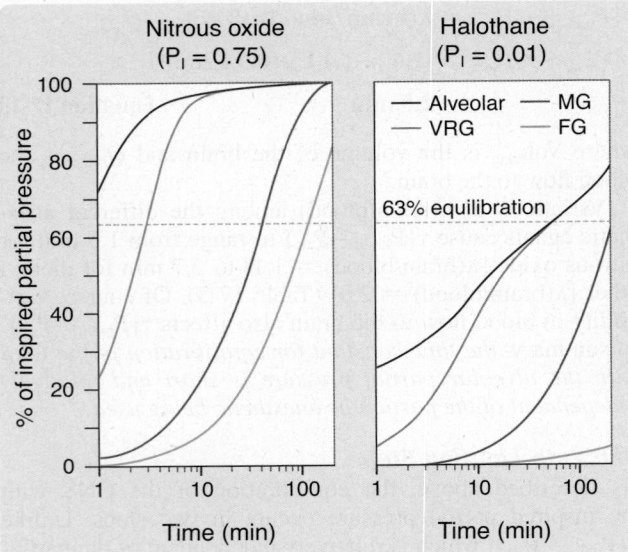

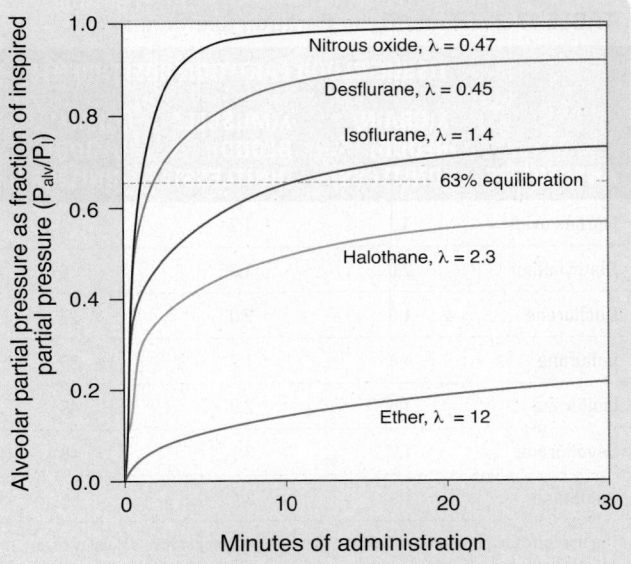

FIGURE 17-6. Equilibration of the tissue groups with the inspired partial pressure. These curves show, as a function of time, the approach of the partial pressures in the alveoli and in the three major tissue groups toward the inspired partial pressure. The partial pressure in the VRG equilibrates rapidly with the alveolar partial pressure, while the MG equilibrates more slowly, and the FG much more slowly. For a perfusion-limited anesthetic such as nitrous oxide, the alveolar partial pressure rises so quickly that the rate of rise of the VRG partial pressure is as much limited by its rise toward the alveolar partial pressure as by the rise of P_{alv} toward P_I. For a ventilation-limited anesthetic such as halothane, the rate at which the partial pressure in the VRG rises is limited not by its approach to the alveolar partial pressure but rather by the rise of the alveolar toward the inspired partial pressure. In other words, the rate-limiting step is the equilibration of the alveolar partial pressure with the inspired partial pressure. The *dashed line* shows the point at which the partial pressure is 63% of P_I, and the time constant for equilibration of each tissue group with P_I is approximated by the time at which each curve crosses this line.

FIGURE 17-7. Rate of approach of the alveolar toward the inspired partial pressure. For agents with lower λ(blood/gas), such as nitrous oxide, the alveolar partial pressure approaches the inspired partial pressure quickly, while for agents with higher λ(blood/gas), such as diethyl ether, the alveolar partial pressure approaches the inspired partial pressure much more slowly. The *dashed line* shows the point at which $P_{alv}/P_I = 0.63$; the time constant $\tau\{P_{alv} \rightarrow P_I\}$ is approximated by the time at which each curve crosses this line. $\lambda = \lambda$(blood/gas). Ether, diethyl ether.

from anesthesia. Accordingly, for these anesthetics, physiologic or pathologic changes that act to increase the rate of rise of the alveolar partial pressure will speed induction. Conversely, because equilibration of the tissue with the arterial partial pressure is not rate-limiting, physiologic or pathologic changes that shorten $\tau\{P_{VRG} \rightarrow P_{art}\}$ will have little effect on induction time (see below).

Perfusion-limited anesthetics have a $\tau\{P_{alv} \rightarrow P_I\}$ that is similar in magnitude to $\tau\{P_{VRG} \rightarrow P_{art}\}$ because their λ(blood/gas) is low. Induction and recovery occur quickly, and neither $\tau\{P_{alv} \rightarrow P_I\}$ nor $\tau\{P_{VRG} \rightarrow P_{art}\}$ may be clearly rate-limiting. Accordingly, induction time may be affected by changes in either the rate of rise of alveolar partial pressure or the rate at which P_{CNS} approaches P_{art} (e.g., see the discussion of hyperventilation below). Physiologic changes may alter the balance between $\tau\{P_{alv} \rightarrow P_I\}$ and $\tau\{P_{VRG} \rightarrow P_{art}\}$. See Figure 17-6 for a graphic comparison of the kinetics of ventilation-limited and perfusion-limited anesthetics.

The characteristic that distinguishes perfusion-limited from ventilation-limited anesthetics is the blood/gas partition coefficient, λ(blood/gas). With the lower λ(blood/gas) of perfusion-limited anesthetics, the bloodstream removes less anesthetic from the alveoli; thus, the alveolar partial pressure rises more quickly and induction is faster (Fig. 17-7). This is the key point, although the correlation may seem paradoxical at first: *agents that are less soluble in the blood induce anesthesia faster*.

To clarify, consider two hypothetical anesthetics that differ solely in λ(blood/gas) (Fig. 17-8): Anesthetic A has a low λ(blood/gas), while Anesthetic B has a high λ(blood/gas). Because Anesthetics A and B are identical in λ(oil/gas), they have the same MAC. They also have identical λ(brain/blood), so their $\tau\{P_{brain} \rightarrow P_{alv}\}$ is the same (see Equations 17-12 and 17-13). To cause anesthesia, both must achieve the same partial pressure in the CNS. At any particular partial pressure, however, the blood and CNS contain more moles of Anesthetic B than Anesthetic A because Anesthetic B is more soluble than Anesthetic A in the blood and CNS. The transfer of a larger number of moles of Anesthetic B out of the lungs slows the rate of rise of P_{alv}, so a longer period is necessary for Anesthetic B than for Anesthetic A to achieve the anesthetic partial pressure in the CNS (Fig. 17-8).[a]

---

[a]In this hypothetical model, one may correctly note that the *concentration* of Anesthetic B in the CNS *as a whole* will be higher than that of Anesthetic A at any particular time point. One may, therefore, wonder how Anesthetic B can have a slower induction, if anesthesia results when a particular concentration (0.05 M) is reached at the site of action (see "The Meyer-Overton Rule," above). At this point, one must recognize that the brain is primarily aqueous, but that anesthetics are likely to have a *hydrophobic* site of action, and that both Anesthetic A and Anesthetic B must have the same concentration (0.05 M) in the key hydrophobic portions of the brain at their anesthetic partial pressures. However, Anesthetic B, with its larger aqueous solubility [λ(blood/gas)], will partition relatively more than Anesthetic A into the aqueous portions of the brain. To provide the higher aqueous concentrations, many more moles of Anesthetic B than Anesthetic A must be transferred from the lungs.

The overall conclusion still holds if λ(oil/gas) and thus MAC differ for the two hypothetical anesthetics. P_{alv} for a less blood-soluble agent will rise proportionally faster toward its P_I than for a more blood-soluble agent, independent of what that P_I is (note that P_I will be larger for the less oil-soluble anesthetic). A larger λ(oil/gas) allows the anesthetic to cause anesthesia at a lower partial pressure but does not affect the proportional rate at which the partial pressure rises.

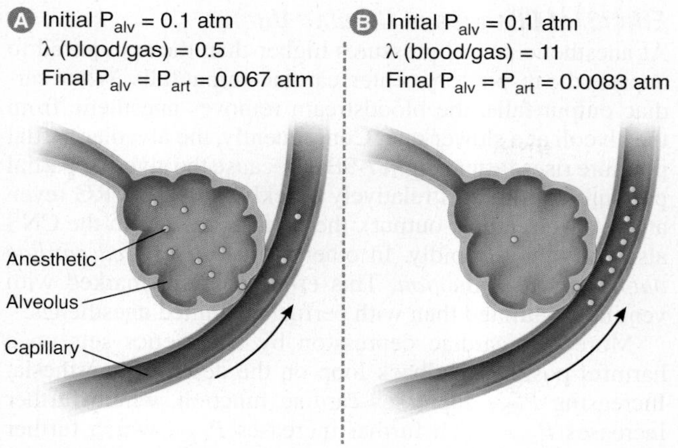

A Initial P_{alv} = 0.1 atm
λ (blood/gas) = 0.5
Final P_{alv} = P_{art} = 0.067 atm

B Initial P_{alv} = 0.1 atm
λ (blood/gas) = 11
Final P_{alv} = P_{art} = 0.0083 atm

Anesthetic

Alveolus

Capillary

FIGURE 17-8. Why do anesthetics with lower λ(blood/gas) have shorter induction times? Consider two equally potent anesthetics inspired at the same partial pressure, P_I. Before any anesthetic molecules have been taken up from the alveolus into the blood, the alveolar partial pressure, P_{alv}, of each anesthetic is 0.1 atm. This partial pressure would be represented in the diagram by 12 anesthetic "spheres" in each alveolus. For each anesthetic, equilibration of the partial pressures in the alveolus and the capillary then takes place. For a relatively blood-insoluble agent with λ(blood/gas) = 0.5 (**Anesthetic A**, which closely resembles nitrous oxide, desflurane, and sevoflurane), the transfer of a small amount of anesthetic from the alveolus significantly raises the partial pressure in the capillary. To illustrate, consider a time, t_v, when the volume of blood that has flowed past the alveolar wall is equal to the volume of the alveolus. At that time, the concentration in the alveolus will be twice that in the capillary (because λ(blood/gas) = 0.5; see Box 17-2), i.e., four of the "spheres" will have been transferred from the alveolus to the capillary and eight "spheres" will remain in the alveolus. The partial pressure in the alveolus will now have dropped to (8/12) × 0.1 = 0.067 atm. This is also the partial pressure in the capillary. In contrast, for a very blood-soluble agent with λ(blood/gas) = 11 (**Anesthetic B**, which closely resembles diethyl ether), much larger amounts of anesthetic must dissolve in the blood to raise the partial pressure in the capillary. Using the same illustration as above, at t_v, 11 of the 12 "spheres" will have been transferred from the alveolus to the capillary, and the remaining P_{alv} will be given by (1/12) × 0.1 = 0.0083 atm. Thus, although the inspired partial pressure of the two anesthetics is the same, at time t_v, the P_{alv} and P_{art} of Anesthetic A will be eight times higher than that of Anesthetic B. Within approximately 2 minutes (Table 17-3), P_{brain} will also reach these values. Thus, the brain partial pressure rises toward the inspired partial pressure much more rapidly for Anesthetic A than for Anesthetic B (i.e., the induction time for Anesthetic A is much shorter than that for Anesthetic B). If the reader is confused by the fact that more molecules of Anesthetic B are being carried to the brain, recall that λ(brain/blood) is ~1 for all of the commonly used anesthetics [that is, for each agent, λ(blood/gas) is approximately equal to λ(brain/gas); see Table 17-2]. Thus, proportionally, many more molecules of Anesthetic B than Anesthetic A must be delivered to the brain in order to raise the partial pressure of each anesthetic by an equivalent amount. See Boxes 17-1 and 17-2 and Appendix A for definitions.

Applications of the Uptake Model

Throughout the following discussion, it is critical to remember that the primary responsibility of the anesthesiologist is to keep the patient well oxygenated and the vital signs stable while manipulating the inspired partial pressure of anesthetic to maintain the desired depth of anesthesia.

Armed with the uptake model, the anesthesiologist can predict the effects of cardiopulmonary changes and pathologic states on the depth of anesthesia. Changes in ventilation and cardiac output may be caused by the general anesthetic itself, by the trauma of surgery, or by some other physiologic or pathophysiologic process.

The effects of changes in both ventilation and cardiac output on P_{CNS} are greatest when the difference between P_I and P_{alv} is greatest; that is, early in the course of anesthesia (Fig. 17-6). To understand this, consider the partial pressure in the mixed venous return (MVR), P_{MVR}, which is a weighted average of the partial pressures in each of the tissue groups, with P_{VRG} making the largest contribution because the VRG receives the majority of the cardiac output (Fig. 17-4). When P_{alv} (and thus P_{VRG}) is much less than P_I, P_{MVR} is low, and the bloodstream is capable of carrying large amounts of anesthetic away from the alveoli to the tissues. Under these conditions, the rate of uptake of anesthetic from the alveoli into the bloodstream can be greatly modified by cardiopulmonary changes, and P_{CNS} can be greatly affected by changes in ventilation and cardiac output. As each successive tissue group approaches saturation with anesthetic, P_{MVR} approaches P_I. When P_{MVR} is nearly equal to P_I, the bloodstream cannot remove much anesthetic from the lungs under any circumstances, and changes in ventilation or cardiac output have little effect on P_{CNS}.

Upon commencement of anesthetic administration, the length of time during which there is a significant difference between P_I and P_{alv} increases with λ(blood/gas). With ventilation-limited anesthetics, such as diethyl ether and halothane, the prolonged time during which P_{alv} lags behind P_I allows cardiopulmonary changes to modulate P_{alv} significantly, potentially leading to unexpected CNS partial pressures. With perfusion-limited anesthetics, such as nitrous oxide, the alveolar partial pressure rises so rapidly that P_{alv} is significantly less than P_I for only a short time, minimizing the time during which cardiopulmonary changes could have a significant effect on P_{CNS} (Fig. 17-7).

Effects of Changes in Ventilation

Hypoventilation decreases the delivery of anesthetic to the alveoli. Meanwhile, removal of anesthetic from the alveoli continues provided that cardiac output is maintained. Consequently, the alveolar partial pressure rises more slowly, and $\tau\{P_{alv}{\rightarrow}P_I\}$ is prolonged. In other words, *hypoventilation slows induction*. This effect is greater with ventilation-limited than with perfusion-limited anesthetics (Fig. 17-9A).

General anesthetics themselves can cause hypoventilation by depressing the medullary respiratory center. In this manner, anesthetic-induced hypoventilation sets up a beneficial negative feedback loop on the depth of anesthesia. Increasing anesthetic depth leads to medullary depression, which, in turn, depresses respiration. The beneficial effect of this physiologic response is that the depressed ventilation slows the rate of rise of the alveolar partial pressure, while perfusion continues to remove anesthetic from the lung at the same rate (Fig. 17-5). Thus, P_{alv} falls, and shortly thereafter, the partial pressure of anesthetic in the medulla falls as well. This decrease in P_{CNS} relieves the respiratory depression. In the extreme example of a respiratory arrest, there is no ventilation to deliver anesthetic to the alveoli, but cardiac output continues to distribute anesthetic from the alveoli and VRG to the MG and FG. In the case of diethyl ether, the decrease in P_{CNS} can be of a sufficient magnitude that spontaneous ventilation resumes.

Hyperventilation delivers anesthetic more quickly to the alveoli. This decreases the time constant for equilibration of the alveolar with the inspired partial pressure (recall that $\tau\{P_{alv}{\rightarrow}P_I\}$ = FRC / V_{alv}, in the limiting case). However, the

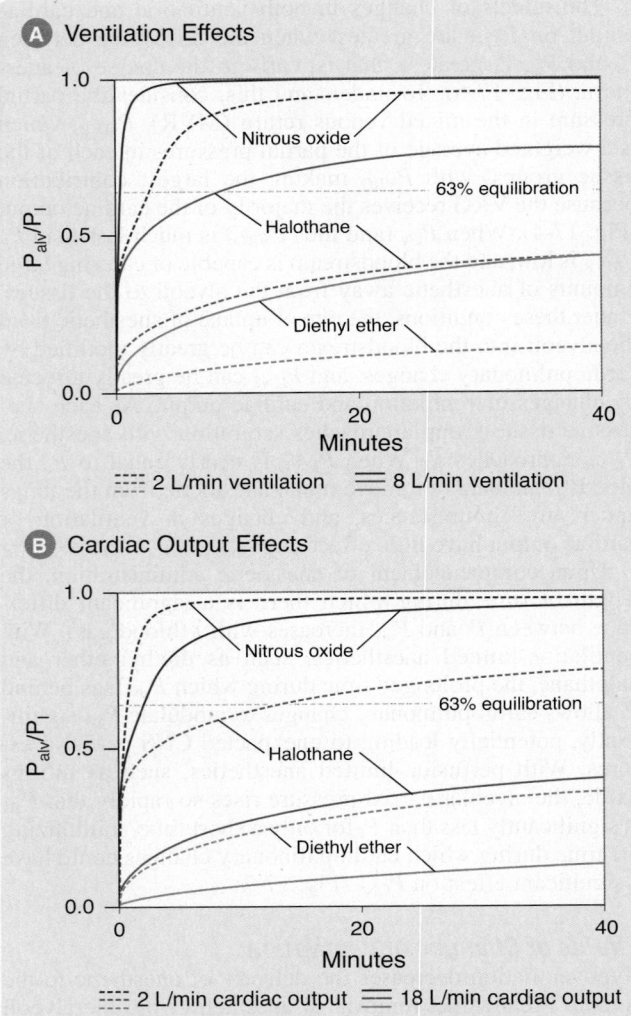

FIGURE 17-9. Effects of changes in ventilation and cardiac output on the rate at which alveolar partial pressure rises toward inspired partial pressure. The rate of equilibration of the alveolar partial pressure with the inspired partial pressure can be affected by changes in ventilation **(A)** and cardiac output **(B)**. Increasing ventilation from 2 L/min (*dashed lines*) to 8 L/min (*solid lines*) accelerates equilibration. On the other hand, increasing cardiac output from 2 L/min (*dashed lines*) to 18 L/min (*solid lines*) slows equilibration. Both effects are much larger for more blood-soluble gases, such as halothane and diethyl ether, which have rather slow induction times. For nitrous oxide, the rate of equilibration is so fast that any changes caused by hyperventilation or decreased cardiac output are small. The *dashed horizontal lines* represent 63% equilibration of P_{alv} with P_I, and the time required for each curve to cross this line represents $\tau\{P_{alv} \rightarrow P_I\}$.

hyperventilation-induced hypocapnia may concomitantly decrease cerebral blood flow, increasing $\tau\{P_{CNS} \rightarrow P_{art}\}$. Thus, while the partial pressure in the alveoli rises faster, the rate of equilibration between the CNS and the alveoli could be slower. The net effect depends on which of these two steps is rate-limiting. For perfusion-limited anesthetics such as nitrous oxide, the decrease in cerebral blood flow results in a slower induction. For the most soluble ventilation-limited anesthetics such as diethyl ether, the faster delivery of anesthetic to the alveoli speeds induction. For less soluble ventilation-limited anesthetics such as isoflurane, the effects roughly balance, and induction is not significantly affected.

Effects of Changes in Cardiac Output

At anesthetic partial pressures higher than those required to depress the respiratory center, cardiac output falls. When cardiac output falls, the bloodstream removes anesthetic from the alveoli at a slower rate. Consequently, the alveolar partial pressure rises faster (Fig. 17-9B). Because the alveolar partial pressure equilibrates relatively quickly with the VRG (even at the lower cardiac output), the partial pressure in the CNS also rises more rapidly. In other words, *decreased cardiac output speeds induction*. This effect is more marked with ventilation-limited than with perfusion-limited anesthetics.

Moreover, cardiac depression by anesthetics sets up a harmful positive feedback loop on the depth of anesthesia. Increasing P_{CNS} depresses cardiac function, which further increases P_{alv}, which further increases P_{CNS}, which further depresses cardiac function. If cardiac arrest occurs, then positive measures must be taken to restore the circulation (e.g., cardiopulmonary resuscitation [CPR]) while reducing the alveolar partial pressure through controlled breathing with oxygen.

Increased cardiac output increases perfusion to the lungs and accelerates equilibration between the alveoli and the tissues. However, because the increased blood flow to the lungs removes anesthetic from the alveoli at a faster rate, the rate of rise of the alveolar partial pressure is slowed. Thus, *increased cardiac output slows induction*. This effect is greater with ventilation-limited than with perfusion-limited agents.

Effects of Age

Relative to their body weight, young children such as Matthew have higher ventilation than do adults. This effect tends to speed induction. However, young children also have relatively higher cardiac output than do adults; this effect tends to slow induction. Although one might expect that these effects would cancel out, two additional factors cause the partial pressure of anesthetic in the mixed venous return to rise more rapidly in children. First, relative to adults, a greater proportion of the blood flow serves the VRG in children, resulting in a higher partial pressure of anesthetic in the mixed venous return early in the course of anesthesia. Second, the lower capacity of the tissues for anesthetic in children relative to adults accelerates the rate at which the tissues become saturated with anesthetic. Both effects lead to a decreased alveolar-to-venous partial pressure difference because P_{MVR} rises more rapidly, blunting the removal of anesthetic by the pulmonary circulation and moderating the extent to which cardiac output slows the rise in alveolar partial pressure.

Thus, proportional increases in ventilation and cardiac output result in an accelerated rise of alveolar partial pressure and faster induction in children than in adults (Fig. 17-10). Ventilation-limited anesthetics, which are most affected by cardiopulmonary changes, have a markedly faster induction in children. Therefore, care must be taken to guard against the attainment of unexpectedly high (toxic) levels of anesthetic during anesthesia induction in children.

Effects of Abnormal States

In hemorrhagic shock, perfusion to the CNS may be maintained in the face of decreased cardiac output and hyperventilation. The decreased cardiac output and hyperventilation both accelerate the rise in alveolar partial pressure of anesthetic. P_{MVR} also rises faster because of the relatively greater perfusion to the VRG, lowering the ability of the pulmonary circulation

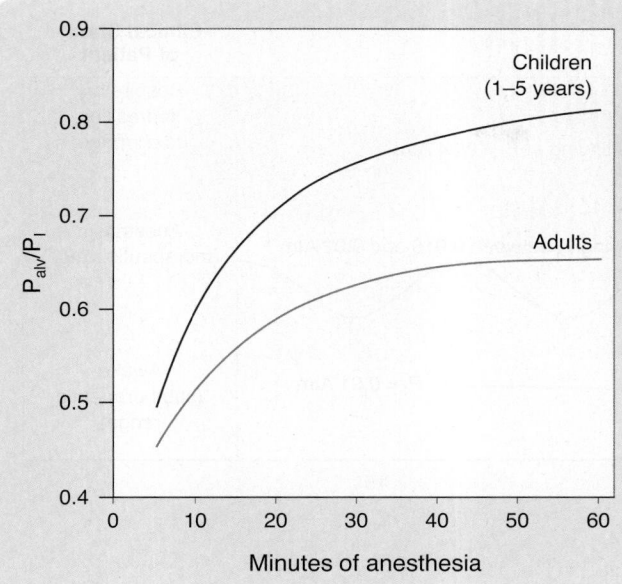

FIGURE 17-10. Anesthesia induction in children. Using halothane as an example, the alveolar partial pressure of anesthetic rises more quickly in children than in adults. The faster induction time in children results from a balance between children's increased respiration (favoring faster induction) and increased cardiac output (favoring slower induction). The time-dependent increase in the mixed venous partial pressure of anesthetic limits anesthetic uptake from the lungs, dampening the effect of increased cardiac output on induction time.

TABLE 17-4	Summary of the Effects of Physiologic, Pathophysiologic, and Clinical Variables on Rate of Induction of Anesthesia
CAUSE FASTER THAN USUAL INDUCTION	**CAUSE SLOWER THAN USUAL INDUCTION**
Hyperventilation (ventilation-limited anesthetics)	Hyperventilation (perfusion-limited anesthetics)
Decreased cardiac output	Hypoventilation
Young age (i.e., children)	Increased cardiac output
Shock	Chronic obstructive pulmonary disease
Thyrotoxicosis	Right-to-left shunt
Initial P_I higher than final desired P_{CNS}	—

Based on the uptake model for inhaled anesthetics, the effect of changes in physiologic variables on the rate of induction can be predicted. Entities in the column on the *left* speed induction, while entities on the *right* slow induction, as discussed in the text. Note that the effect of hyperventilation depends on whether a ventilation-limited or perfusion-limited anesthetic is being administered (see text).

to remove anesthetic from the alveoli and further accelerating the rise in the alveolar partial pressure. In patients with hemorrhagic shock, the additive combination of these effects can speed induction to a significant degree. In such cases, perfusion-limited anesthetics, whose kinetics are not greatly affected by cardiopulmonary changes, are preferred over ventilation-limited agents (Fig. 17-9).

In ventilation/perfusion (V/Q) mismatch (e.g., in chronic obstructive pulmonary disease [COPD]), some alveoli are underventilated and overperfused, while others may be adequately ventilated but underperfused. Because the alveolar partial pressure of anesthetic rises more slowly in the underventilated alveoli, the anesthetic partial pressure in the arterial blood leaving these alveoli is lower than normal. Conversely, the partial pressure of anesthetic leaving the adequately ventilated but underperfused alveoli is higher than normal. Because the former (overperfused) alveoli contribute a larger percentage to the overall perfusion, the weighted average partial pressure of anesthetic in the blood leaving the lung is decreased. Thus, P_{CNS} equilibrates with a lower than normal arterial partial pressure and may not achieve the level required to induce anesthesia. Therefore, higher inspired partial pressures are necessary to compensate for the effects of V/Q mismatch. This effect is mitigated somewhat with ventilation-limited anesthetics because the partial pressure in the underperfused but overventilated alveoli rises much faster than normal. For this reason, perfusion-limited anesthetics are most affected by V/Q mismatch.

Based on the principles and examples discussed above and summarized in Table 17-4, it should be possible to make reasonable predictions about the effect of other changes in cardiopulmonary function on anesthesia induction.

Control of Induction

An anesthesiologist can decrease induction time by setting the initial P_I higher than the final desired P_{CNS}. (This concept is similar to that of a loading dose, which is discussed in Chapter 3.) Because the time constant for equilibration of P_{CNS} with P_I does not depend on the absolute level of P_I, administration of anesthetic for a given amount of time always results in the same proportional equilibration of P_{CNS} with P_I. Consequently, a given absolute P_{CNS} is reached faster when P_I is higher because that P_{CNS} is a smaller fraction of the higher P_I. Dr. Snow took advantage of this concept by starting isoflurane at a P_I of 0.02 atm, even though the MAC of isoflurane is only 0.0114 atm. However, the anesthesiologist must remember to reduce P_I as P_{alv} approaches the target value, or, as demonstrated by Dr. Snow, P_{CNS} will equilibrate with this higher P_I and cause cardiopulmonary depression (Fig. 17-11).

Recovery

It is desirable that recovery from general anesthesia proceeds quickly, so that patients can maintain their own airways as soon as possible following surgery. In general, the stages of recovery from anesthesia occur in the opposite sequence from those of anesthesia induction, including the unpleasant excitement stage (Fig. 17-1). During recovery, the partial pressure of anesthetic in the mixed venous return (P_{MVR}) is the weighted average of the partial pressures in the VRG, MG, and FG, with the VRG making the largest contribution (see Fig. 17-4). Ventilation removes anesthetic from the bloodstream into the exhaled air, and therefore, increased ventilation always accelerates recovery. As is the case with induction, recovery from anesthesia with perfusion-limited agents is rapid, whereas recovery from ventilation-limited agents is more prolonged.

Recovery differs from induction in several important ways, however. First, the anesthesiologist can increase the inspired partial pressure of anesthetic to speed the process of induction, whereas during recovery, the inspired partial

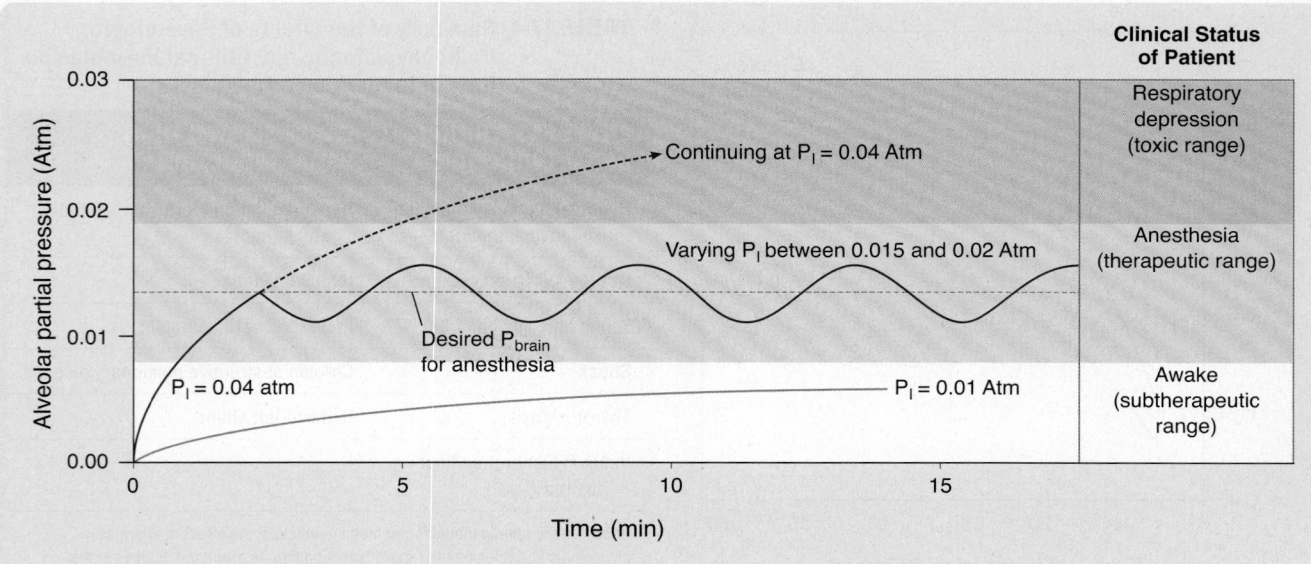

FIGURE 17-11. Applying overpressure to speed induction. Using halothane as an example, the anesthesiologist can use an initial P_I greater than the final desired P_{brain} to speed induction. If the desired partial pressure of anesthetic in the brain is about 0.013 atm, then the anesthesiologist could initially administer the inspired anesthetic at a higher partial pressure, for example, 0.04 atm. This method is effective because the time constant for $P_{alv} \rightarrow P_I$ is independent of the absolute value of P_I. In other words, if P_I is increased, then the ratio P_{alv}/P_I will increase proportionally at the same rate, resulting in a greater absolute rise in P_{alv} in a given amount of time. The anesthesiologist must be sure to decrease the inspired partial pressure in a timely manner, however, or the desired P_{brain} for anesthesia can be overshot and, instead, partial pressures capable of causing respiratory depression can be reached. On the other hand, if the inspired partial pressure is reduced too rapidly, the patient may awaken as P_{alv} is decreased because of uptake of anesthetic from the alveoli into the bloodstream (*not shown*).

pressure cannot be decreased below zero. Second, during induction, all of the tissue compartments start out at the same partial pressure (zero). In contrast, at the start of recovery, the compartments may have very different partial pressures depending on the duration of anesthesia and the characteristics of the anesthetic. The VRG quickly equilibrates with the alveolar partial pressure during most surgical procedures, but the MG may or may not equilibrate, and the FG equilibrates so slowly that, in all but the longest procedures, P_{FG} is far from equilibrium. Consequently, during recovery, perfusion **redistributes** anesthetic down its partial pressure gradient from the VRG to the MG and FG as well as to the lung. Because of this redistribution, the initial decrease in alveolar partial pressure during recovery is more rapid than the corresponding increase during induction. This initial decrease in alveolar partial pressure is dominated by the decrease in the VRG partial pressure. When the alveolar pressure falls to the level of the MG, then the decrease in the partial pressure of the MG becomes rate-limiting and likewise subsequently for the FG. If the MG or both the MG and FG are heavily saturated following prolonged administration of anesthetic, then recovery will also be prolonged (Fig. 17-12).

Third, although anesthetic is delivered by one route, ventilation, it can be eliminated by both ventilation and metabolism. In most cases, metabolism is not a significant route of anesthetic elimination. Halothane is an exception because metabolism may account for 20% of its elimination.

Finally, the outflow of high partial pressures of nitrous oxide into the lungs can cause an effect called **diffusion hypoxia**. To understand this, it is helpful first to understand an effect on anesthetic induction called the **concentration effect**. When high partial pressures of nitrous oxide are administered, the rate of anesthetic uptake by the blood may be quite large, on the order of 1 L/min for a 75% nitrous oxide mixture. The absorbed gas is rapidly replaced by inspired gas flowing into the lung, effectively increasing alveolar ventilation by 1 L/min above the normal minute ventilation and thereby accelerating induction.

Diffusion hypoxia is conceptually the opposite of the concentration effect. When anesthesia is terminated, nitrous oxide gas diffuses out of the blood into the alveoli at a high rate because of the high partial pressure difference between these two compartments (recall Fick's law). This volume of nitrous oxide displaces up to 1 L/min of air that would otherwise have been inhaled. Thus, the alveolar (and arterial) partial pressure of oxygen falls. The decrease is not significant for a healthy patient but may be threatening to a compromised patient. To counteract this effect, pure oxygen is routinely administered for a few minutes following anesthesia with nitrous oxide, as Dr. Snow did for Matthew.

PHARMACOLOGY OF GENERAL ANESTHETICS AND ADJUVANTS

Inhaled Anesthetic Agents

From the preceding analysis, we can distill two physicochemical properties of inhaled anesthetics that predict their behavior. First, the oil/gas partition coefficient predicts potency; *an anesthetic with a higher λ(oil/gas) is more potent and causes anesthesia at lower partial pressures.* Second, the blood/gas partition coefficient predicts the rate of induction; *an anesthetic with a lower λ(blood/gas) has a shorter induction time.* Typically, there is a trade-off between fast

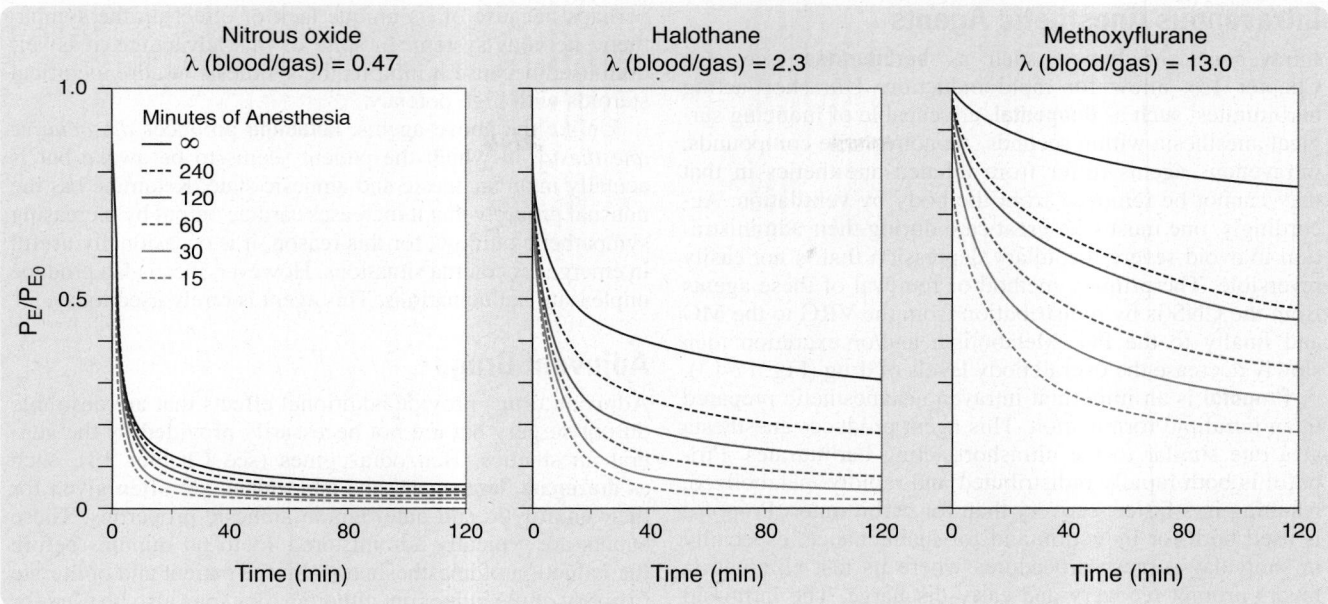

FIGURE 17-12. Recovery from inhaled anesthetics. These curves show, as a function of time, the exhaled partial pressure of anesthetic (P_E) as a fraction of the exhaled partial pressure at the moment administration of the anesthetic is stopped (P_{E0}). The rate of recovery is inversely proportional to the λ(blood/gas) of the anesthetic, because anesthetics with lower λ(blood/gas) values equilibrate faster between alveolar and inspired partial pressures (the latter being zero after anesthetic administration is stopped). The rate of recovery is also proportional to the duration of anesthesia because the partial pressures of anesthetic in the muscle group and fat group increase with duration. During recovery, anesthetic redistributes from these slowly equilibrating, high-capacity tissues to the vessel-rich group, thus slowing the rate of fall of P_{brain}. This effect occurs only with a long duration of anesthesia (see text).

induction and high potency. An anesthetic that has a rapid induction, as denoted by a low λ(blood/gas), typically has a low potency, represented by a low λ(oil/gas). Conversely, a very potent anesthetic with a high λ(oil/gas) typically has a high λ(blood/gas) and, thus, a long induction time (see Table 17-1).

Halothane has a high λ(oil/gas), providing high potency and, thus, low MAC; however, halothane also has a high λ(blood/gas), causing slow induction and recovery. The nonirritating smell of halothane makes it useful in pediatric anesthesia, but **sevoflurane** is increasingly replacing halothane for use in pediatric anesthesia (see below). One disadvantage of halothane is that toxic metabolites can result in fatal hepatotoxicity. The incidence of this serious adverse effect is approximately 1 in 35,000 in adult populations but much lower in pediatric populations; this is another reason for its continuing role in pediatric anesthesia. Another rare but potentially lethal adverse effect, seen most often with halothane but occasionally with the other halogenated anesthetics, is **malignant hyperthermia**. The susceptibility for this adverse reaction is inherited, typically as an autosomal dominant mutation in the sarcoplasmic reticulum Ca^{2+} channel (also known as the **ryanodine receptor**). In individuals expressing this mutation, halothane causes uncontrolled calcium efflux from the sarcoplasmic reticulum, with subsequent tetany and heat production. Malignant hyperthermia is treated with **dantrolene**, an agent that blocks calcium release from the sarcoplasmic reticulum.

Isoflurane and **enflurane** are somewhat less potent than halothane [they have a lower λ(oil/gas)], but they equilibrate faster because they have a lower λ(blood/gas). Enflurane is metabolically defluorinated to a greater extent than isoflurane and may thus have a higher risk of causing

renal toxicity. It also induces seizure-like activity in the EEG of some patients. Isoflurane is probably the most widely used general anesthetic today.

Although less potent than isoflurane and enflurane, **diethyl ether** is still quite potent, with a rather high λ(oil/gas). However, because of its flammability and very slow induction, attributable to its extremely high λ(blood/gas), this agent is no longer in common use in the United States and Europe. In developing countries, however, its low price and simplicity of application favor its continued use.

Nitrous oxide has a very low λ(blood/gas) and thus equilibrates extremely rapidly. However, its low λ(oil/gas) results in a very high MAC, close to one atmosphere. Thus, the need to maintain an acceptable partial pressure of oxygen (normally, greater than 0.21 atm) prevents the attainment of full anesthesia using nitrous oxide alone, and this agent is commonly employed in combination with other agents (see the section "Balanced Anesthesia").

Desflurane and **sevoflurane** are newer anesthetics that, by design, have low λ(blood/gas); times of equilibration between their alveolar and inspired partial pressures are nearly as short as that of nitrous oxide. Furthermore, they are much more potent than nitrous oxide because their oil/gas partition coefficients are higher. Thus, these agents offer great improvements over earlier agents. However, desflurane is a poor induction agent because its pungency irritates the airway, potentially causing cough or laryngospasm. Sevoflurane is sweet-tasting but can be chemically unstable when exposed to some carbon dioxide adsorbents in anesthetic machinery, degrading to an olefinic compound that is potentially nephrotoxic. These disadvantages have been overcome with improved machinery, and sevoflurane is gaining in popularity.

Intravenous Anesthetic Agents

Intravenous anesthetics, such as **barbiturates** (see also Chapter 13), allow for rapid induction. Ultrashort-acting barbiturates, such as **thiopental**, are capable of inducing surgical anesthesia within seconds. As nonvolatile compounds, intravenous agents differ from inhaled anesthetics in that they cannot be removed from the body by ventilation. Accordingly, one must take great care during their administration to avoid severe medullary depression that is not easily reversible. The primary method of removal of these agents from the CNS is by redistribution from the VRG to the MG and finally to the FG. Metabolism and/or excretion then slowly decrease the overall body levels of drug (Fig. 17-13).

Propofol is an important intravenous anesthetic prepared in an intralipid formulation. This agent produces anesthesia at a rate similar to the ultrashort-acting barbiturates. Propofol is both rapidly redistributed and rapidly metabolized, resulting in a faster recovery than for barbiturates. Propofol is used both for induction and for maintenance, especially in short day-surgery procedures where its fast elimination favors prompt recovery and early discharge. The intralipid preparation of propofol can rarely be a source of infection, and the lipid preparation provides a large caloric source; these considerations can be important in critically ill patients who may receive prolonged propofol infusions.

Etomidate is an imidazole that is used for induction of anesthesia because its kinetics are similar to those of propofol. This agent causes minimal cardiopulmonary depression, perhaps because of its unique lack of effect on the sympathetic nervous system. In spite of this advantage, it is seldom used because it inhibits the synthesis of adrenocortical steroids with high potency.

Unlike the above agents, **ketamine** produces *dissociative anesthesia*, in which the patient seems to be awake but is actually in an analgesic and amnesic state. Ketamine has the unusual property that it increases cardiac output by increasing sympathetic outflow; for this reason, it is occasionally useful in emergency trauma situations. However, it can also produce unpleasant hallucinations. This agent is rarely used today.

Adjuvant Drugs

Adjuvant drugs provide additional effects that are desirable during surgery but are not necessarily provided by the general anesthetics. Benzodiazepines (see Chapter 13), such as **diazepam**, **lorazepam**, and **midazolam**, are often given for their anxiolytic and anterograde amnesic properties. These agents are typically administered 15 to 60 minutes before the induction of anesthesia to calm the patient and obliterate memory of the induction, although they may also be used for intraoperative sedation. If necessary, benzodiazepine effects can be reversed with the antagonist **flumazenil**.

Opioids (see Chapter 18) such as **morphine** and **fentanyl** are used for their ability to produce analgesia. Their action can be reversed by an antagonist such as **naltrexone**. Opioids are poor amnesics, however, and are typically used in combination with a general anesthetic.

The combination of fentanyl and **droperidol** produces both analgesia and amnesia. Together with nitrous oxide, this combination is called *neuroleptanesthesia* (the prefix "neurolept" is added because droperidol is a butyrophenone antipsychotic related to haloperidol; see Chapter 14, Pharmacology of Dopaminergic Neurotransmission).

Nicotinic acetylcholine receptor blockers, such as the competitive antagonists **tubocurarine** and **pancuronium** or the depolarizing agonist **succinylcholine**, are commonly used to achieve muscle relaxation (see Chapter 10). The effects of the competitive antagonists can be reversed by an acetylcholinesterase inhibitor such as **neostigmine**.

Balanced Anesthesia

No single drug achieves all of the desired goals of anesthesia. Accordingly, in a method termed **balanced anesthesia**, several inhaled and/or intravenous drugs are used in combination to produce the anesthetic state. The anesthetic effects of simultaneously administered general anesthetics are additive. That is, 0.5 MAC of one inhaled anesthetic in combination with 0.5 MAC of another is equivalent in terms of potency to 1 MAC of either anesthetic as a single agent.

Using a mixture of inhaled anesthetics allows the two goals of potency and rapid recovery to be achieved. For example, although using nitrous oxide alone is generally impractical because the MAC of this gas is higher than atmospheric pressure, nitrous oxide is desirable for its fast induction and recovery characteristics and its high analgesic index. If nitrous oxide is part of the anesthetic mixture, then the nitrous oxide component of the anesthesia can be rapidly removed by ventilation during recovery or in an emergency situation. Matthew was able to awaken quickly from anesthesia because nitrous oxide was responsible for about half of his anesthetic state. He remained groggy because of the

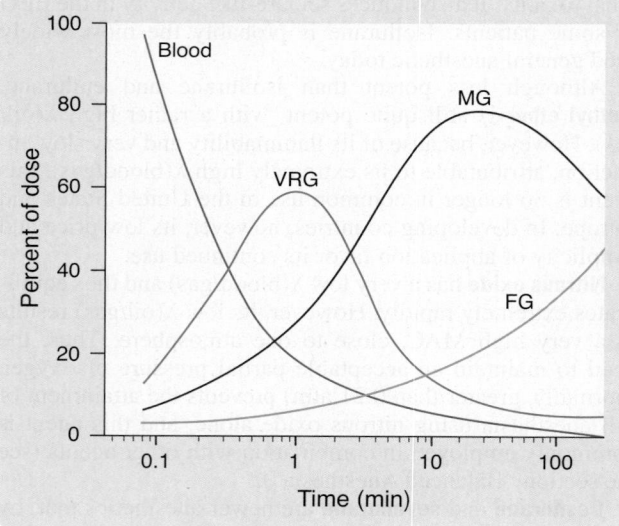

FIGURE 17-13. Distribution of a bolus of intravenous anesthetic. When a bolus of intravenous anesthetic is administered, it is initially transported through the vascular system to the heart and then distributed to the tissues. The vessel-rich group (VRG) receives the highest percentage of the cardiac output; its anesthetic concentration rises rapidly, reaching a peak within 1 minute. Redistribution of anesthetic to the muscle group (MG) then quickly decreases the anesthetic level in the VRG. Because of very low fat group (FG) perfusion, redistribution from the MG to the FG does not occur until much later. Note that rapid redistribution from the VRG to the MG does not occur if the MG has previously approached saturation through prolonged administration of anesthetic (*not shown*); this can lead to significant toxicity if intravenous barbiturates are administered continuously for long periods of time. Newer agents, such as propofol, are designed to be eliminated by rapid metabolism and, therefore, can be used safely for longer periods of time.

lingering isoflurane. The advantages of using isoflurane in combination with nitrous oxide include isoflurane's low cost and its relatively low incidence of adverse effects (especially hepatic and renal toxicity) as compared to other anesthetics.

Dr. Snow's use of the intravenous agent thiopental in combination with an inhaled anesthetic agent has a similar rationale. Short-acting intravenous agents can be used to induce stage III surgical anesthesia quickly, allowing the patient to pass through the undesirable excitement of stage II rapidly. Subsequently, the anesthetic depth can be maintained with inhaled anesthetics that could be removed by ventilation if necessary. Because intravenous agents act additively with inhaled anesthetics, less than 1 MAC of inhaled anesthetic will be required for as long as the intravenous agent is acting. As another example, the use of high concentrations of opioids in cardiac surgery allows the partial pressure of the inhaled anesthetic to be lowered significantly, reducing the risk of cardiovascular and respiratory depression.

Finally, balanced anesthesia is clinically useful because the anesthesiologist has more control if a different drug is used to mediate each desired effect. For example, if the surgeon requires more muscle relaxation, the anesthesiologist can administer more of a neuromuscular blocking agent without having to increase the depth of anesthesia and potentially cause cardiopulmonary depression. Similarly, a bolus of a short-acting opioid can be administered immediately before a particularly painful surgical maneuver.

MECHANISMS OF ACTION OF GENERAL ANESTHETICS

Despite intensive research, the exact mechanism of anesthetic action remains elusive. The **unitary hypothesis** states that a common mechanism accounts for the action of all anesthetics. Assuming the unitary hypothesis, it is difficult to imagine a specific binding site on a protein or receptor molecule capable of accommodating the molecules of disparate sizes and structures that are capable of causing anesthesia (Fig. 17-14). The traditional solution to this contradiction, which follows from the empirical Meyer-Overton rule (Fig. 17-3), is the **lipid solubility hypothesis**. This hypothesis postulates that the hydrophobic site of action of anesthetics is in the lipid bilayer of a cell membrane. According to this hypothesis, general anesthesia results when a sufficient amount of any anesthetic dissolves in the lipid bilayer and a critical ("anesthetic") concentration is reached. Various distinct lipid theories postulate that the dissolved anesthetics cause perturbations of different physical properties of the lipid bilayer, such as fluidity. A property that these lipid perturbation models share is that they all cause the bilayer to expand (this is called the **critical volume hypothesis**), a fact that is consistent with the observation that anesthetized animals can be aroused by raising the pressure, either hydrostatically in amphibians or with the nonanesthetic gas helium in mammals.

The lipid solubility hypothesis is remarkably successful at predicting potency for all the volatile agents and for some of the intravenous agents that have potencies less than 50 μM. However, for more potent agents, exceptions become increasingly common. For example, straight-chain alcohols increase in potency as each methylene group is added up to dodecanol, which has an anesthetic potency of 5 μM. Straight-chain alcohols with even longer chains lack any anesthetic activity, however, even though their λ(oil/gas) is higher than that of the shorter alcohols. Furthermore, R-etomidate, which is used clinically and causes anesthesia at 5 μM, is 10 times more potent than its enantiomer, S-etomidate. Such a degree of enantioselectivity is also seen in etomidate's action at the $GABA_A$ receptor, which points to action at a protein binding site. In a genetically engineered "knock-in" mouse, R-etomidate's potency was reduced tenfold by a single mutation in the β3-subunit of the $GABA_A$ receptor. The action of volatile and steroid anesthetics, which also act at $GABA_A$ receptors, was unaffected by this mutation. This finding suggests that $GABA_A$ receptors could have a number of allosteric anesthetic binding sites, each of which binds different structural classes of anesthetic.

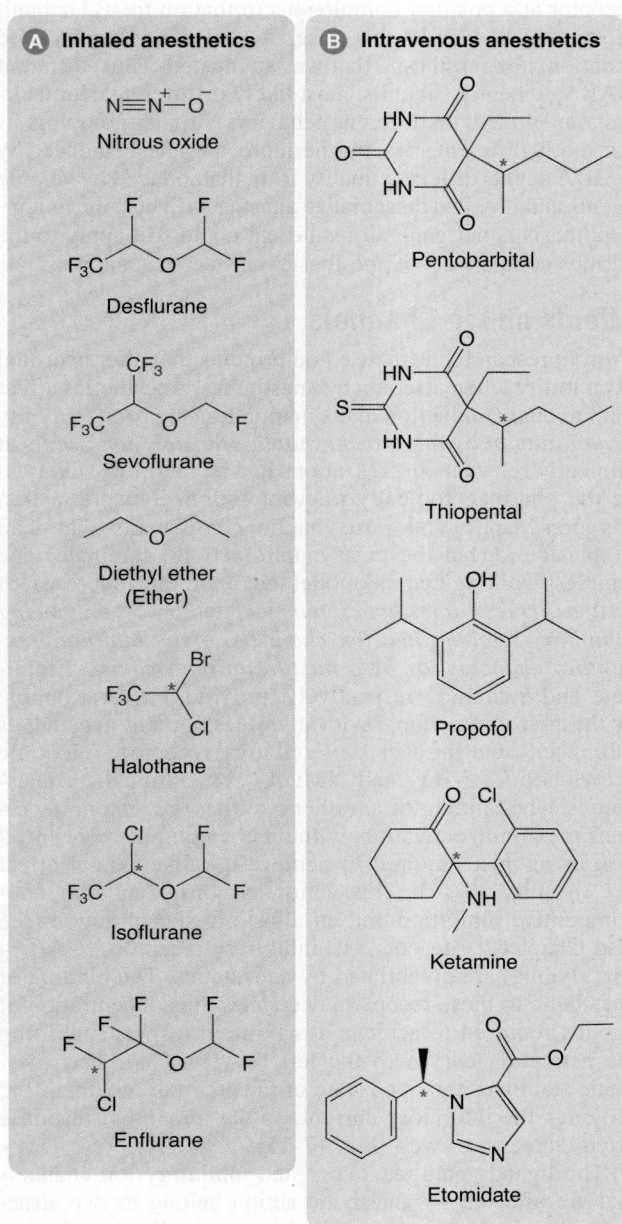

FIGURE 17-14. Structures of general anesthetics. A. Structures of some inhaled anesthetics. **B.** Structures of some intravenous anesthetics. The extreme variability in the structures of these molecules, all of which are capable of causing general anesthesia, suggests that not all general anesthetics interact with a single receptor site. *Indicates carbons where asymmetry results in enantiomeric structures.

If binding to any one of these sites could cause anesthesia, the unitary hypothesis would be satisfied without invoking lipids. On the other hand, nitrous oxide, cyclopropane, xenon, and ketamine, all of which have seen clinical use, have no action on GABA$_A$ receptors. Instead, they act on NMDA-type glutamate receptors. Thus, the anesthetic state may be induced by different mechanisms.

The anesthetic state incorporates many distinct actions of general anesthetics, including sedation, amnesia, antianxiety, and anticonvulsant actions. Do these actions share common sites? A clue to the answer to such questions is provided by another piece of research on knock-in mice. In this work, a mutation was introduced in the β2 subunit of the GABA$_A$ receptor at a position homologous to that on the β3 subunit mentioned above. In this case, it was etomidate-induced sedation, not anesthesia, that was attenuated. Thus, different GABA$_A$ receptor subunits, most likely in different neural circuits, may mediate different behaviors through homologous but subtly different sites. Furthermore, anesthesia induced by NMDA agents differs in quality from that induced by volatile agents and is called **dissociative anesthesia**. Thus, the unitary hypothesis is not generally valid but could still apply to the various components of anesthesia considered separately.

Effects on Ion Channels

Current research has focused on proteins that alter neuronal excitability when acted on by anesthetics. Anesthetics affect both axonal conduction and synaptic transmission, but only *modulation of ligand-gated synaptic transmission* occurs at clinically relevant concentrations and is, therefore, likely to be the pharmacologically relevant action. Synaptic action has presynaptic and postsynaptic components that lead to anesthesia, but the postsynaptic actions dominate. The simplest working general model that unites current research is that *general anesthetics may act either by enhancing inhibitory ligand-gated ion channels, or by inhibiting excitatory channels, or by a mixture of both effects.* Etomidate and ketamine, respectively, provide a clear example of the first two actions, with many less potent anesthetics falling into the third class. Excitatory receptors (nicotinic acetylcholine, 5-HT$_3$ and NMDA) are inhibited by anesthetics. The binding of anesthetic to these receptors lowers their maximum activation, without changing the concentration of agonist required to achieve a half-maximal effect (EC$_{50}$) (Fig. 17-15). This action is consistent with non-competitive inhibition and an allosteric site of action (see also Chapter 2). In contrast, inhibitory receptors (GABA$_A$ and glycine) are potentiated by anesthetics. The binding of anesthetic to these receptors decreases the concentration of agonist required to achieve a maximum response, shifting the activation curves to the left (lower EC$_{50}$). The anesthetic stabilizes the open state of the receptor and therefore prolongs the inhibitory current, so the maximum response often increases as well (Fig. 17-15).

The ligand-gated excitatory and inhibitory ion channels that are affected by anesthetic action belong to two structural classes. The first class is the structurally homologous *Cys-loop superfamily* of ligand-gated ion channels, which includes the inhibitory GABA$_A$ and glycine receptors as well as the excitatory nicotinic and 5-HT$_3$ receptors. The second structural class is the excitatory NMDA glutamate receptor family (compare Figs. 10-2 and 13-3 with Fig. 13-8). Most progress has been made with the mechanisms of action of

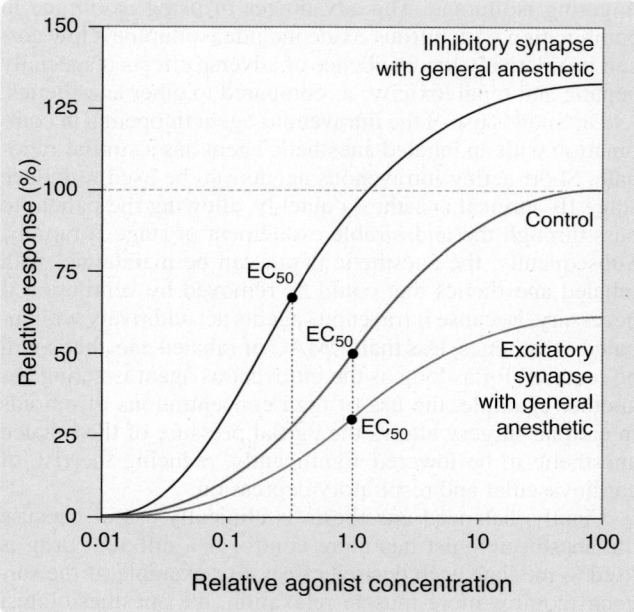

FIGURE 17-15. Actions of anesthetics on ligand-gated ion channels. Anesthetics potentiate the action of endogenous agonists at inhibitory receptors, such as GABA$_A$ and glycine receptors, and inhibit the action of endogenous agonists at excitatory receptors, such as nicotinic acetylcholine, 5-HT$_3$, and NMDA glutamate receptors. At GABA$_A$ receptors, anesthetics both decrease the EC$_{50}$ of GABA (i.e., GABA becomes more potent) and increase the maximum response (i.e., GABA becomes more efficacious). The latter effect is thought to be due to the ability of anesthetics to stabilize the open state of the receptor channel. At excitatory receptors, anesthetics decrease the maximum response while leaving the EC$_{50}$ unchanged; these are the pharmacologic hallmarks of noncompetitive inhibition.

anesthetics at the Cys-loop receptors. At the molecular level, *direct anesthetic–protein interactions are responsible for the effects of anesthetics on ligand-gated ion channels.* Site-directed mutagenesis, photolabeling, and kinetic studies suggest that inhibition of excitatory acetylcholine receptors occurs at a site in the pore of the ion channel that is on the central axis of symmetry and in contact with the channel-lining M2 helices of all five subunits (see Fig. 10-2 for terminology and structure). However, the site of anesthetic binding to inhibitory GABA$_A$ receptors (Fig. 13-3) cannot be in the ion pore because potentiation, not inhibition, is observed at therapeutic concentrations. Indeed, GABA$_A$ receptors lack a homologous stretch of hydrophobic amino acids in the M2 helices that line the ion pore in the excitatory receptors. The consensus view is that anesthetics bind in the transmembrane domain of the GABA$_A$ receptor to allosterically affect the channel's conformation (and, thus, the equilibria among its open, closed, and desensitized states). Early site-directed mutagenesis studies suggested that volatile anesthetics bind *within* the four transmembrane helices (intra-subunit sites) of each GABA$_A$ receptor subunit. In contrast, recent photolabeling with potent intravenous anesthetics places the binding site *between* the subunits (inter-subunit sites).

Members of the Cys-loop superfamily have five highly homologous subunits, each with four transmembrane helices. The *anesthetic sensitivity of ligand-gated ion channels may vary with their subunit composition.* Central GABA$_A$ receptors vary in subunit composition; some dozen combinations have been established to date (e.g., $\alpha_{1-6}\beta_{2-3}\gamma_2$, $\alpha_4\beta_{2-3}\delta$, $\alpha_6\beta_{2-3}\delta$, and ρ). Reading counterclockwise, the order in which the subunits are arranged around the center of symmetry of each pentameric receptor is $\beta\alpha\beta\alpha\gamma/\delta$. Thus, there are potentially three distinct intra-subunit anesthetic sites and four distinct inter-subunit anesthetic sites on each distinct GABA$_A$ receptor pentamer. Of the possible binding sites, only two are established on human GABA$_A$ receptors. Etomidate binds in the two β–α interfaces in the transmembrane domain, some 50 Å below the inter-subunit agonist sites in the same β–α interfaces in the extracellular domain. A derivative of mephobarbital photolabels the transmembrane domain in both the β–γ interface and the α–β interface but not in the etomidate site at the β–α interfaces. Propofol binds nonselectively to all four of these sites. Thus, subunit-dependent sequence variations within each of the homologous anesthetic binding pockets now provide an explanation for the diversity of general anesthetic structures, and for the selectivity of anesthetic binding, without invoking lipid solubility. Of potential clinical significance, this conclusion suggests the possibility of designing novel general anesthetics that bind selectively to only some subtypes of GABA$_A$ receptors.

CONCLUSION AND FUTURE DIRECTIONS

Inhaled and intravenous anesthetics are used to produce the clinical features of general anesthesia, including unconsciousness, immobility, and amnesia. The pharmacodynamics of general anesthetics are unique. Anesthetics have steep dose–response curves and low therapeutic indices, and they lack a pharmacologic antagonist. According to the Meyer-Overton rule, the potency of a general anesthetic can be predicted simply from its oil/gas partition coefficient.

The pharmacokinetics of inhaled anesthetics can be modeled assuming three principal tissue compartments that are perfused in parallel. Equilibration of the partial pressure of anesthetic in the CNS with the inspired partial pressure proceeds in two steps: (1) equilibration between the alveolar partial pressure and the inspired partial pressure and (2) equilibration between the CNS partial pressure and the alveolar partial pressure. With ventilation-limited anesthetics, which have a high blood/gas partition coefficient, the first of these steps is slow and rate-limiting. With perfusion-limited anesthetics, which have a low blood/gas partition coefficient,

both steps are rapid and neither is clearly rate-limiting; changes in either can affect induction time. Recovery from anesthesia occurs roughly as the reverse of induction, except that redistribution of anesthetic from the vessel-rich group to the muscle group and fat group can also occur.

The "ideal" inhaled anesthetic has not yet been found. Future researchers may attempt to identify a nonflammable anesthetic with high λ(oil/gas), low λ(blood/gas), high therapeutic index, good vapor pressure, and few or no significant adverse effects. Currently, the combined use of adjuvants and balanced anesthesia with multiple inhaled and/or intravenous anesthetics achieves all of the goals of general anesthesia, including fast induction and a state of analgesia, amnesia, and muscle relaxation.

The exact mechanism of action of general anesthetics remains a mystery. Although the site of action was formerly thought to reside in lipid bilayers, direct interactions with several ligand-gated ion channels—specifically, members of the Cys-loop superfamily and the NMDA glutamate receptor family—now seem to be more likely. More research is required to elucidate the mechanisms of action of general anesthetics. Once discovered, these mechanisms could shed light on such far-reaching issues as the generation of consciousness itself.

Suggested Reading

Campagna JA, Miller KW, Forman SA. The mechanisms of volatile anesthetic actions. *N Engl J Med* 2003;348:2110–2124. (*Reviews how general anesthetics act.*)

Eger EI. Uptake and distribution. In: Miller RD, ed. *Anesthesia*. Philadelphia: Churchill Livingstone; 2000:74–95. (*Pharmacokinetics and uptake of inhaled anesthetics.*)

Forman SA. Monod-Wyman-Changeux allosteric mechanisms of action and the pharmacology of etomidate. *Curr Opin Anaesthesiol* 2012;25:411–418. (*Reviews allosteric models of anesthetic action, with specific reference to etomidate.*)

Rudolph U, Antkowiak B. Molecular and neuronal substrates for general anesthetics. *Nat Rev Neurosci* 2004;5:709–720. (*A short review with good diagrams.*)

Various authors. Molecular and cellular mechanisms of anaesthesia. In: *Can J Anesth* 2011; Feb issue. (*This special issue is a compilation of detailed reviews relating to all major current theories on the mechanism of action of general anesthetics. An update will appear in mid-2016 in Anesth. Analg.*)

Wiklund RA, Rosenbaum SH. Anesthesiology. *N Engl J Med* 1997;337:1132–1151, 1215–1219. (*Two-part review covers many aspects of the modern practice of anesthesiology.*)

Winter PM, Miller JN. Anesthesiology. *Sci Am* 1985;252:124–131. (*A good account of the clinical approach of the anesthesiologist.*)

DRUG SUMMARY TABLE: CHAPTER 17 General Anesthetic Pharmacology

DRUG	CLINICAL APPLICATIONS	SERIOUS AND COMMON ADVERSE EFFECTS	CONTRAINDICATIONS	THERAPEUTIC CONSIDERATIONS
INHALED GENERAL ANESTHETICS **Mechanism—Modulation of ligand-gated ion channels (most likely)**				
Isoflurane **Enflurane**	General anesthesia Supplement to other anesthetic agents during obstetrical anesthesia	Cardiovascular and respiratory depression, arrhythmias, malignant hyperthermia, seizure (shared adverse effects); hyperkalemia (isoflurane only)	Susceptibility to malignant hyperthermia (shared contraindication) Seizure and epilepsy (enflurane only)	Less potent than halothane but faster induction. Pungency irritates respiratory tract. Malignant hyperthermia is treated with dantrolene. Enflurane has higher risk of causing renal toxicity than isoflurane.
Halothane	General anesthesia	Same as isoflurane Additionally, can cause hepatitis and fatal hepatic necrosis, blood coagulation disorder, carboxyhemoglobinemia	Obstetrical anesthesia Susceptibility to malignant hyperthermia History of hepatic damage from previous halothane exposure	Less pungent than isoflurane; useful in pediatric anesthesia due to its nonirritating smell. Toxic metabolites can result in fatal hepatotoxicity in adults. High potency but slow induction and recovery.
Diethyl ether	General anesthesia	Same as isoflurane	Susceptibility to malignant hyperthermia	Relatively high potency but very slow induction. Pungency irritates respiratory tract. Flammable; not in common use in the United States.
Nitrous oxide	General anesthesia (usually used in combination with other agents)	Can cause expansion of air cavities such as pneumothorax, obstructed middle ear, obstructed loop of bowel, and intracranial air; arrhythmias, cardiac depression, hypotension, pulmonary hypertension	Should not be administered without oxygen Should not be administered continuously for more than 24 hours Preexisting air cavity	Rapid induction and recovery but low potency. Analgesia in subhypnotic concentrations. The need to maintain an acceptable partial pressure of oxygen prevents the attainment of full anesthesia using nitrous oxide alone.
Desflurane **Sevoflurane**	General anesthesia	Same as isoflurane Additionally, desflurane can cause laryngeal spasm Additionally, sevoflurane can cause complete AV block, prolonged QT interval, torsades de pointes, and hepatic necrosis	Susceptibility to malignant hyperthermia	Newer anesthetic agents with relatively high potency as well as rapid induction and recovery. Desflurane irritates the airway. Sevoflurane can be chemically unstable when exposed to carbon dioxide adsorbents in older anesthetic machinery.
INTRAVENOUS GENERAL ANESTHETICS **Mechanism—Modulation of ligand-gated ion channels (most likely)**				
Propofol	Induction and maintenance of anesthesia Sedation of mechanically ventilated patients	Cardiovascular and respiratory depression, pancreatitis, seizure, priapism, bacterial septicemia Injection site reaction	Hypersensitivity to propofol	Induces anesthesia at a rate similar to the ultrashort-acting barbiturates and has a faster recovery than barbiturates; useful especially in short day-surgery procedures because of its rapid elimination.
Thiopental	Induction of anesthesia Narcoanalysis Elevated intracranial pressure Seizure	Same as propofol Additionally, can cause laryngeal spasm, hemolytic anemia, and radial neuropathy No injection site reaction	Acute intermittent porphyria or variegate porphyria Hypersensitivity to thiopental products	Ultrashort-acting barbiturate capable of inducing surgical anesthesia within seconds.

Drug	Uses	Adverse Effects	Contraindications	Notes
Etomidate	Induction of anesthesia Maintenance of general anesthesia	*Same as propofol* *Additionally, can cause myoclonus* *Inhibits the synthesis of adrenocortical steroids*	Hypersensitivity to etomidate	Binds in the interface between the β and α subunits of the $GABA_A$ receptor. Causes minimal cardiopulmonary depression, possibly due to lack of effect on the sympathetic nervous system.
Ketamine	Dissociative anesthesia/analgesia Sole anesthetic agent for procedures that do not require skeletal muscle relaxation	*Hypotension, cardiac arrhythmia, respiratory depression, pulmonary edema, apnea, laryngeal spasm* Hallucinations, vivid dreams, psychiatric symptoms	Hypersensitivity to ketamine Severe hypertension	Antagonizes NMDA receptor. Increases cardiac output by increasing sympathetic outflow.

BENZODIAZEPINES—Mechanism—Potentiation of $GABA_A$ receptors

Diazepam Lorazepam Midazolam	See Drug Summary Table: Chapter 13 Pharmacology of GABAergic and Glutamatergic Neurotransmission

OPIOIDS—Mechanism—Opioid receptor agonists

Morphine Meperidine Fentanyl Remifentanil	See Drug Summary Table: Chapter 18 Pharmacology of Analgesia

NEUROMUSCULAR BLOCKERS—Mechanism—Depolarizing or nondepolarizing inhibition of nicotinic acetylcholine receptors

Tubocurarine Pancuronium Vecuronium Cisatracurium Mivacurium Succinylcholine	See Drug Summary Table: Chapter 10 Cholinergic Pharmacology

Appendix A
Abbreviations and Symbols

P_I = inspired partial pressure

P_E = exhaled partial pressure

P_{alv} = alveolar partial pressure

P_{art} = arterial partial pressure

P_{tissue} = partial pressure in a tissue

P_{venule} = partial pressure in a venule

P_{MVR} = mixed venous partial pressure

$P_{solvent}$ = partial pressure in a solvent

P_{CNS} = partial pressure in the central nervous system

P_{VRG} = partial pressure in the vessel-rich group

λ(oil/gas) = partition coefficient defining solubility of a gas in a lipophilic solvent such as oil

λ(blood/gas) = partition coefficient defining solubility of a gas in blood

λ(tissue/gas) = partition coefficient defining solubility of a gas in a tissue

λ(tissue/blood) = partition coefficient describing ratio of solubility in tissue to solubility in blood = λ(tissue/gas) / λ(blood/gas)

τ = time constant for 63% equilibration

$\tau\{P_{alv} \rightarrow P_I\}$ = time constant for 63% equilibration of P_{alv} with P_I

$\tau\{P_{tissue} \rightarrow P_{alv}\}$ = time constant for 63% equilibration of P_{tissue} with P_{alv}

$[A]$ = concentration of gas A, in terms of either $L_{gas}/L_{solvent}$ or $mol/L_{solvent}$

CNS = central nervous system

VRG = vessel-rich group (includes CNS, liver, kidney)

MG = muscle group (includes muscle, skin)

FG = fat group (includes adipose tissue)

VPG = vessel-poor group (includes bone, cartilage, ligaments, tendons)

FRC = functional residual capacity of lung

V_{alv} = alveolar ventilation

CO = cardiac output

Q = perfusion rate

Vol_{tissue} = volume of tissue

MAC = minimum (or median) alveolar concentration

P_{50} = alveolar partial pressure sufficient for immobility in 50% of patients $\equiv$ MAC

AP_{50} = alveolar partial pressure sufficient to cause analgesia in 50% of patients

LP_{50} = alveolar partial pressure sufficient to cause death in 50% of subjects

EC_{50} = concentration of agonist required to activate 50% of channels

Appendix B
Equations

▶GAS CONCENTRATIONS

In an ideal gas mixture: $[A]_{\text{mixture}} = n_A / V = P_A / RT$
  {in terms of mol/L}
In solution (Henry's law):
$[A]_{\text{solution}} = P_{\text{solvent}} \times \lambda(\text{solvent/gas})$ {in terms of $L_{\text{gas}}/L_{\text{solvent}}$}
$[A]_{\text{solution}} = P_{\text{solvent}} \times \lambda(\text{solvent/gas}) / 24.5$ {in terms of mol/L_{solvent}}
{where n_A = moles of gas A, V = total volume, P_A = partial pressure of A, R = universal gas constant, T = temperature in degrees Kelvin}

▶MEYER-OVERTON RULE

$\text{MAC} \approx 1.3 / \lambda(\text{oil/gas})$

▶FICK'S LAW FOR DIFFUSION ACROSS A BOUNDARY

Rate of diffusion = $D \times (A / l) \times \Delta P$
{where D = Diffusion constant; A = Surface area; l = Thickness; ΔP = Partial pressure difference}

▶ALVEOLAR CAPILLARY RATE OF UPTAKE

Rate of uptake = $([A]_{\text{art}} - [A]_{\text{MVR}}) \times \text{CO}$ {in L_{gas}/min}
Rate of uptake = $\lambda(\text{blood/gas}) \times (P_{\text{art}} - P_{\text{MVR}}) \times \text{CO}$
{where CO = cardiac output}

▶EQUILIBRATION TIME CONSTANTS (FOR 63% EQUILIBRATION)

τ = Volume Capacity / Flow Rate
$\tau\{P_{\text{tissue}} \rightarrow P_{\text{alv}}\} \approx \tau\{P_{\text{tissue}} \rightarrow P_{\text{art}}\}$
  = Volume Capacity of Tissue / Tissue Blood Flow
  = $\lambda(\text{tissue/blood}) \times$ Volume of Tissue / Tissue Blood Flow
$\tau\{P_{\text{brain}} \rightarrow P_{\text{art}}\} = \lambda(\text{brain/blood}) \times$ Volume of Brain / Blood Flow to Brain
$P_{\text{container}} = P_{\text{flow}} [1 - e^{-(t/\tau)}]$

▶VOLUME CAPACITY

Volume Capacity = $([A]_{\text{compartment}} \times$ Volume of compartment) / $[A]_{\text{medium}}$ {at equilibrium}
  = $\lambda(\text{compartment/medium}) \times$ Volume of Compartment

▶MIXED VENOUS PARTIAL PRESSURE

$P_{\text{MVR}} = 0.75 P_{\text{VRG}} + 0.18 P_{\text{MG}} + 0.055 P_{\text{FG}} + 0.015 P_{\text{VPG}}$

18

Pharmacology of Analgesia

Robert S. Griffin and Clifford J. Woolf

INTRODUCTION

Everyone has experienced pain in response to an intense or noxious stimulus. This physiologic "ouch" pain helps us to avoid potential damage by acting as an early warning or protective signal. Pain can, however, also be incapacitating, as after trauma, during recovery from surgery, or in association with medical conditions that are characterized by inflammation, such as rheumatoid arthritis. Under circumstances where tissue injury and inflammation are present, noxious stimuli elicit more severe pain than normal because of increases in the excitability of the somatosensory system, and stimuli that would not normally cause pain become painful. In addition, nerve injury produced by disease or trauma—as in amputation, HIV infection, varicella-zoster (VZV) infection, cytotoxic treatment, and diabetes mellitus—evokes pain that persists long after the initiating cause has disappeared. In these conditions, pathologic and sometimes irreversible alterations in the structure and function of the nervous system lead to severe and intractable pain. For such patients, the pain is the pathology rather than a physiologic defense mechanism. Finally, there are patients who experience considerable pain in the absence of noxious stimuli, inflammation, or lesions to the nervous system. This dysfunctional pain, as in tension-type headache, fibromyalgia, or irritable bowel syndrome, results from an abnormal function of the nervous system.

These categories of pain—physiologic, inflammatory, neuropathic, and dysfunctional—are produced by different mechanisms. Ideally, treatment should be targeted at the specific mechanisms that produce pain rather than at suppressing the symptom of pain. That said, many of the currently available pharmacologic agents relieve pain by suppressing the symptom. The mechanisms of action of drugs that relieve pain involve interference with the response of primary sensory neurons to somatic or visceral sensory stimuli, inhibition of the relaying of pain information to the brain, and blockade of the perceptual response to a painful stimulus. In this chapter, the discussion of pain and analgesic pharmacology begins by describing the mechanisms by which noxious stimuli lead to the perception of pain. The chapter continues by considering the processes responsible for the heightened pain sensitivity that occurs in response to inflammation and lesions of the nervous system. The discussion concludes by describing the mechanisms of action of the major drug classes used for clinical pain relief.

PHYSIOLOGY

Pain is the end perceptual consequence of the neural processing of particular sensory information. The initial stimulus usually arises in the periphery and is transferred under

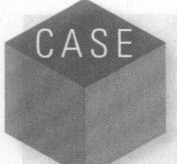

CASE

JD, a 15-year-old boy, is severely burned while escaping from a building fire. The extensive burns include first- and second-degree burns covering much of his body and a local, full-thickness burn on his right forearm. He reaches the emergency department in severe pain and is treated with intravenous morphine in increasing quantities until he reports that the pain has subsided. This dose of morphine is then maintained. The next day, he has surgical debridement of his burn wounds and a skin graft to his right forearm. During the operation, an anesthesiologist provides a continuous intravenous infusion of remifentanil, with a bolus dose of morphine added near the end of the operation. At the end of the operation, and for 4 days thereafter, JD receives intravenous morphine through a patient-controlled analgesia device. As the burns heal, the morphine dose is tapered and eventually replaced with an oral oxycodone/acetaminophen combination tablet. Three months later, JD reports severe loss of sensation to touch in the area of the skin graft. He also describes a persistent tingling sensation in this area, with occasional bursts of sharp, knife-like pain. After referral to a pain clinic, JD is prescribed oral gabapentin, which partially reduces his symptoms. However, he reports to the pain clinic again 2 months later, still in severe pain. At this time, amitriptyline is added to the gabapentin, and the pain is further relieved. Three years later, JD's lingering pain has resolved and he no longer requires medication, but the lack of forearm sensation persists.

Questions

1. What mechanisms produced and sustained the pain that lasted from JD's exposure to the fire until his initial treatment?
2. What was the rationale for the sequence of medications used during the skin debridement operation?
3. Explain the mechanisms that could produce spontaneous pain in the region of the full-thickness burn months to years after healing of the skin and the rationale for using gabapentin to treat JD's chronic pain.
4. Why was morphine tapered gradually and replaced with a combination oxycodone/acetaminophen tablet?

multiple controls through sensory relays in the central nervous system (CNS) to the cortex. This system can be usefully analyzed in terms of the sites of action at which drugs intervene to produce analgesia. First, transduction of intense external, noxious stimuli depolarizes the peripheral terminals of "high-threshold" primary sensory neurons. The primary sensory neurons, called **nociceptors** because they respond to noxious stimuli, are high-threshold because they require a strong, potentially tissue-damaging stimulus to depolarize their terminals. The resulting action potentials are conducted to the CNS by the axons of the primary afferent sensory neurons, running first in peripheral nerves and then in dorsal roots, which then synapse on neurons in the dorsal horn of the spinal cord. The secondary projection neurons transmit information to the brainstem and thalamus, which then relay signals to the cortex, hypothalamus, and limbic system. Transmission is modulated at all levels of the nervous system by remote and local circuit inhibitory and excitatory interneurons (Fig. 18-1).

Sensory Transduction: Excitation of Primary Afferent Neurons

The peripheral terminals of primary afferent somatic and visceral sensory nociceptor fibers respond to thermal, mechanical, and chemical stimuli (Fig. 18-2). Highly specialized ion channels/receptors undergo conformational changes

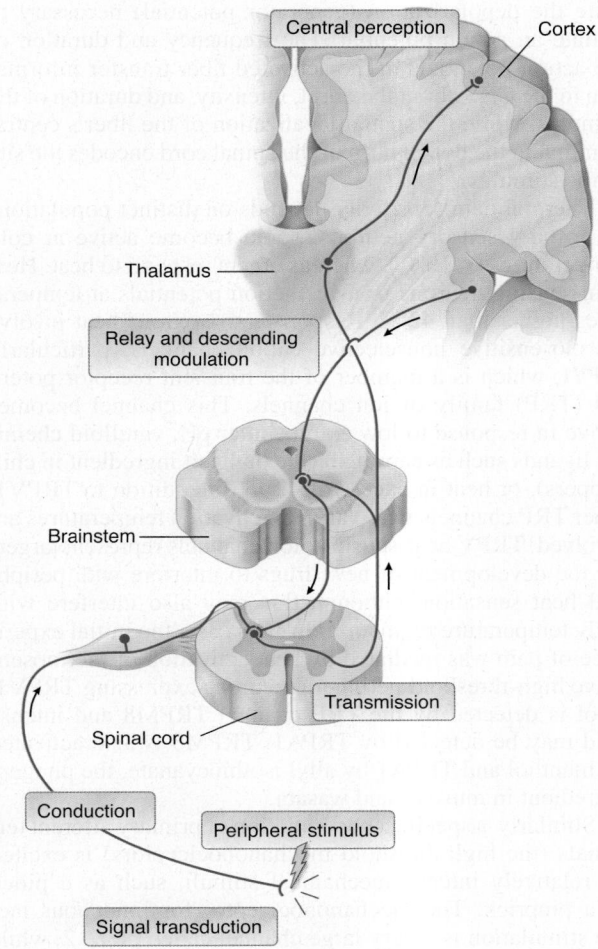

FIGURE 18-1. Overview of the nociceptive circuit. Activation of the peripheral terminal by a noxious stimulus leads to the generation of action potentials, which are conducted to the dorsal horn of the spinal cord. Neurotransmission in the dorsal horn relays the signal to CNS neurons, which send the signal to the brain. This circuit is also subject to descending modulatory control.

Central perception

Cortex

Thalamus

Relay and descending modulation

Brainstem

Transmission

Spinal cord

Conduction

Peripheral stimulus

Signal transduction

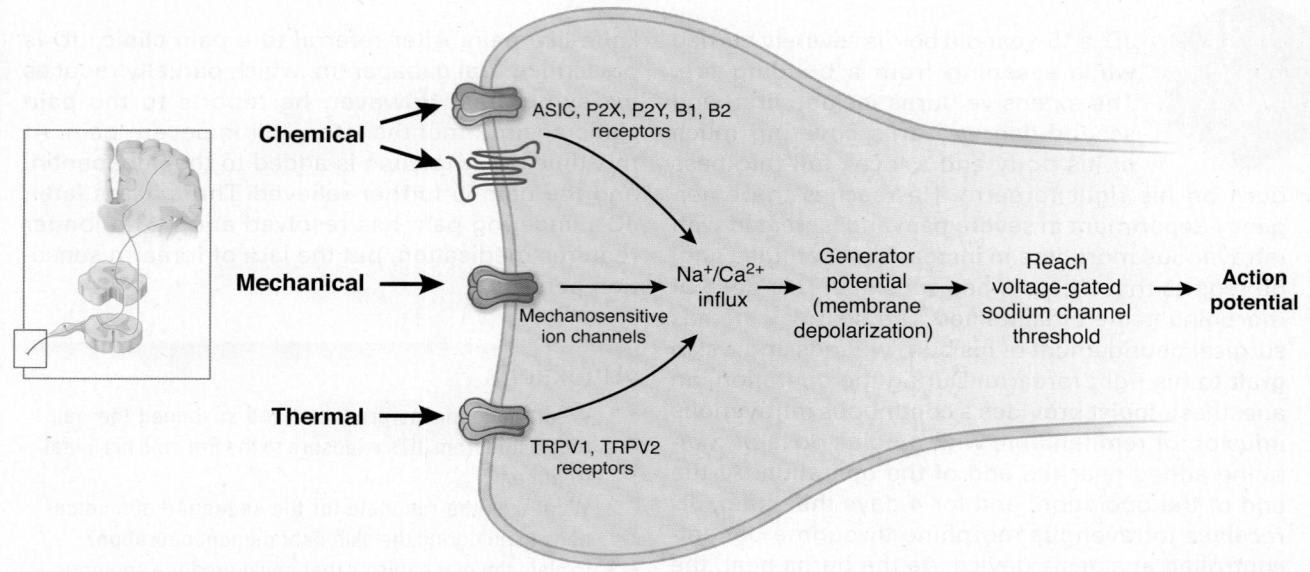

FIGURE 18-2. Peripheral transduction. A thermal, chemical, or mechanical sensory event activates a specific peripheral receptor, leading to ion influx and depolarization of the peripheral terminal. Thermal stimuli activate the transient receptor potential (TRP) vanilloid receptor 1 (TRPV1), or the TRP vanilloid receptor-like protein 1 (TRPV2), both of which are heat-sensitive cation channels. Chemical stimuli can activate acid-sensitive ion channels (ASIC), ATP-sensitive P2X or P2Y channels, or kinin-sensitive B1 or B2 receptors. Mechanical stimuli can also lead to ion influx and depolarization, but the molecular identity of the relevant channels is not certain. In each case, the generator potential induced by the nociceptive signal leads to action potential production if the threshold for activation of the voltage-gated sodium channel is reached.

in response to one or more of these stimuli and thereby mediate the depolarization (generator potential) necessary to initiate an action potential. The frequency and duration of the action potentials in the activated fiber transfer information to the CNS about the onset, intensity, and duration of the stimulus, while the spatial localization of the fiber's central terminal in the dorsal horn of the spinal cord encodes the site of the stimulus.

Thermal pain sensitivity depends on distinct populations of primary sensory neurons: some become active at cold temperatures (<16°C), whereas others respond to heat. Heat pain-sensing neurons produce action potentials at temperatures higher than 42°C. Responses to noxious heat involve thermosensitive nonselective cation channels, particularly **TRPV1**, which is a member of the transient receptor potential (TRP) family of ion channels. This channel becomes active in response to low extracellular pH, vanilloid chemical ligands such as capsaicin (the pungent ingredient in chili peppers), or heat in excess of 42°C. In addition to TRPV1, other TRP channels with varying activation temperatures are involved. TRPV heat-sensitive ion channels represent targets for the development of new drugs to interfere with peripheral heat sensation, although this may also interfere with body temperature regulation. In JD's case, the initial experience of pain was mediated by heat activation of thermosensitive high-threshold peripheral neurons expressing TRPV1. Cool is detected by the TRP channel TRPM8 and intense cold may be detected by TRPA1. TRPM8 is also activated by menthol and TRPA1 by allyl isothiocyanate, the pungent ingredient in mustard and wasabi.

Similarly, a specific subpopulation of primary afferent terminals (the high-threshold mechanonociceptors) is excited by relatively intense mechanical stimuli, such as a pinch or a pinprick. The mechanonociceptor for innocuous tactile stimulation is a very large channel called piezo 2, while

the transducer for noxious mechanotransduction has not yet been identified.

The peripheral terminals of **nociceptor neurons** respond not only to thermal and mechanical stimuli but also to multiple chemical signals. Some chemical agents directly excite peripheral terminals (**chemical activators**), whereas others increase the sensitivity of the peripheral terminals (**sensitizing agents**). Most known chemical ligands that evoke a somatosensory response are associated with cell injury or inflammation. These chemical ligands include protons, potassium ions, ATP, amines, prostanoids, cytokines, chemokines, nerve growth factor, and bradykinin. For example, cardiac angina is a nociceptive event that involves activation of visceral chemotransducers in nociceptor neurons innervating the heart. These chemotransducers are activated by protons that are released by inadequately perfused myocardial tissue.

Several different types of chemical stimuli can excite nociceptor neurons (Table 18-1). Low extracellular pH, which occurs in ischemia and inflammation, produces depolarizing cation influx through TRPV1 and likely also via **acid-sensitive ion channels (ASICs)**. Elevated extracellular ATP

TABLE 18-1 Chemosensitive Transduction Receptors Expressed by Nociceptor Neurons

NOCICEPTIVE STIMULUS	RECEPTORS	TYPE OF RECEPTOR
Low pH (H^+)	ASIC	pH-gated ion channel
ATP	P2X P2Y	Ligand-gated ion channel G protein-coupled receptor
Kinin peptides	B1 B2	G_q protein-coupled receptor G_q protein-coupled receptor

concentration also signals cell injury, because cell rupture releases millimolar concentrations of ATP into the extracellular space (where the ATP concentration is normally very low). Two major classes of ATP receptor include the **P2X** ligand-gated channels and the **P2Y** G protein-coupled ATP receptors.

Kinins are a third set of chemical stimuli that excite the peripheral terminals of sensory neurons. Kinin peptides are produced from kininogens by the action of kallikrein serine proteases; this process usually occurs in the setting of inflammation and tissue damage. Kinins act by stimulating **bradykinin B1** and **B2** receptors. The B2 receptor is constitutively expressed throughout the nervous system, while expression of the B1 receptor is induced in response to bacterial lipopolysaccharide, inflammatory cytokines, and peripheral nerve injury. Both kinin receptors are G protein-coupled and increase intracellular calcium by production of inositol 1,4,5-trisphosphate. Activation of the B2 receptor also leads to the formation of prostaglandins E_2 and I_2. In the introductory case, as the heat sensation was followed by burn injury, these chemical mediators likely further contributed to JD's pain. Bacterial pathogens can also directly activate nociceptors via formylated peptides acting on G protein-coupled receptors and via secretion of toxins such as alpha hemolysin, which is a channel-like protein that binds to certain nociceptors and thereby contributes to the pain of bacterial infection.

Conduction from the Periphery to the Spinal Cord

The axons of primary afferent neurons conduct information from the peripheral terminal to the CNS. These neurons can be classified into three major groups according to their conduction velocity and caliber; these groups also have distinct stimulus sensitivities and distinct central termination patterns. The first group (**Aβ**) consists of rapidly conducting fibers that respond with a low stimulus threshold to mechanical stimuli and are activated by light touch, vibration, or movement of hairs. Aβ-fibers synapse on CNS neurons located in the dorsal horn of the spinal cord and in dorsal column nuclei of the brainstem. The second population (**Aδ**) includes fibers that conduct with intermediate velocity and respond to cold, heat, or low- or high-intensity mechanical stimuli. The third group (**C-fibers**) conduct slowly, synapse in the spinal cord, and typically respond multimodally; they are capable of producing action potentials in response to heat, warmth, intense and innocuous mechanical stimuli, or chemical irritants (polymodal nociceptors, tactile detectors, and itch-provoking pruriceptors). Some C-fiber afferents (referred to as *silent* or *sleeping* nociceptor fibers) cannot be activated normally but become responsive only during inflammation. Aδ- and C-fibers terminate in the most superficial laminae of the dorsal horn (lamina I and II).

For conduction to occur, voltage-gated sodium channels must convert depolarization of the peripheral terminal into an action potential. Six types of voltage-gated sodium channels are expressed in primary afferent neurons, of which three, $Na_v1.7$, $Na_v1.8$, and $Na_v1.9$, are expressed uniquely in primary afferents. Gain-of-function mutations in $Na_v1.7$ produce hyperexcitability of nociceptors and thereby contribute to primary erythromelalgia, an inherited condition associated with severe burning pain that is either spontaneous or provoked in response to mild thermal stimuli. Loss-of-function mutations in $Na_v1.7$ result in congenital insensitivity to pain, highlighting the critical role of this channel in nociception and its potential attractiveness as a target for analgesics. $Na_v1.8$ and $Na_v1.9$ are selectively expressed in small-caliber neurons, most of which respond only to high-threshold peripheral stimuli (nociceptors). These two channel types also have higher activation thresholds and inactivate more slowly than other neuronal voltage-gated sodium channels. Because of their specific expression pattern in pain fibers, selective sodium channel blockers represent future pharmacologic targets of particular interest, especially if they produce a use-dependent block.

Currently, the topical or regional use of nonselective, sodium channel-blocking local anesthetic agents is a mainstay for the treatment of acute postoperative and procedural pain (see Chapter 12, Local Anesthetic Pharmacology). Sodium channel-blocking antiepileptic and antiarrhythmic drugs (see Chapter 16, Pharmacology of Abnormal Electrical Neurotransmission in the Central Nervous System, and Chapter 24, Pharmacology of Cardiac Rhythm, respectively) are also used for certain neuropathic pain conditions, particularly trigeminal neuralgia.

Transmission in the Dorsal Horn of the Spinal Cord

Action potentials generated in primary afferents induce neurotransmitter release upon reaching their central axon terminals in the dorsal horn of the spinal cord. **N-type voltage-gated calcium channels** have a substantial role in controlling neurotransmitter release from synaptic vesicles. **Gabapentin** and **pregabalin** are antiepileptic drugs that act on the alpha 2 delta calcium channel subunit. Via a mechanism that is not completely understood but involves disruption of calcium channel trafficking to the membrane, these agents likely modulate CNS transmission of nociceptive information. Although their effectiveness is limited, both agents are widely used in the treatment of chronic neuropathic pain because of their generally favorable adverse effect profile. A naturally occurring snail poison, omega-conotoxin, acts as a selective N-type calcium channel blocker; a synthetic mimic of this peptide, **ziconotide,** is currently used to treat severe pain conditions. However, such calcium channel blockers also alter the function of sympathetic neurons (producing hypotension) and many central neurons (affecting cognitive function). Thus, the use of ziconotide is limited to the highly specialized scenario of intrathecal administration because it is necessary to limit the drug's effects to the spinal cord.

Synaptic transmission takes place between C-fiber primary afferents and secondary projection neurons in the dorsal horn. This transmission has fast and slow components (Fig. 18-3). Acting on ionotropic AMPA and NMDA receptors, glutamate mediates fast excitatory transmission between primary and secondary sensory neurons. Acting on metabotropic mGluR receptors, glutamate also mediates a slow synaptic modulatory response. **Neuropeptides**, such as the tachykinins **substance P** and **calcitonin gene-related peptide (CGRP)**, as well as other **synaptic neuromodulators**, including the neurotrophin **brain-derived neurotrophic factor (BDNF)**, are co-released with glutamate and also produce slow synaptic effects by acting on metabotropic G protein-coupled receptors and receptor tyrosine kinases. The presence of these co-released peptides allows considerable use-dependent functional plasticity of

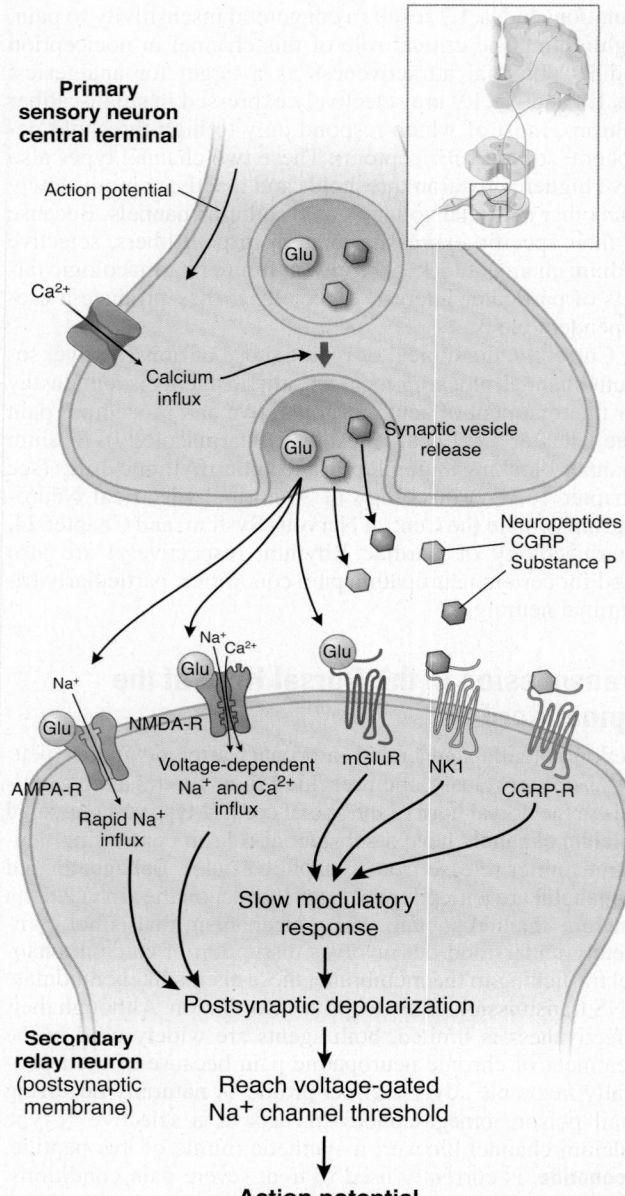

FIGURE 18-3. Neurotransmission in the spinal cord dorsal horn. An incoming action potential from the periphery activates presynaptic voltage-gated calcium channels, leading to calcium influx and subsequent synaptic vesicle release. The released neurotransmitters (i.e., glutamate and neuropeptides, such as calcitonin gene-related peptide [CGRP] and substance P) act on postsynaptic receptors. Stimulation of ionotropic glutamate receptors leads to fast postsynaptic depolarization, while activation of other modulatory receptors mediates slow depolarization. Postsynaptic depolarization, if sufficient, leads to action potential production (signal generation) in the secondary relay neuron.

pain transmission. The physiologic function of the neuropeptides in synaptic transmission involves signaling responses to stimuli of particularly high intensity, because release of neuropeptide-containing synaptic vesicles requires higher frequency and longer lasting action potential trains than release of glutamate-containing vesicles. New strategies to target CGRP and its actions are being developed, particularly for migraine.

Descending and Local Inhibitory Regulation in the Spinal Cord

Synaptic transmission in the spinal cord is regulated by the actions of both local inhibitory interneurons and projections that descend from the brainstem to the dorsal horn. Because these systems can limit transfer of incoming sensory information to the brain, they represent an important site for pharmacologic intervention. The major inhibitory neurotransmitters in the dorsal horn of the spinal cord are **opioid** peptides, **norepinephrine**, **serotonin (5-HT)**, **glycine**, and **GABA** (Fig. 18-4). The physiology of GABA receptors is discussed

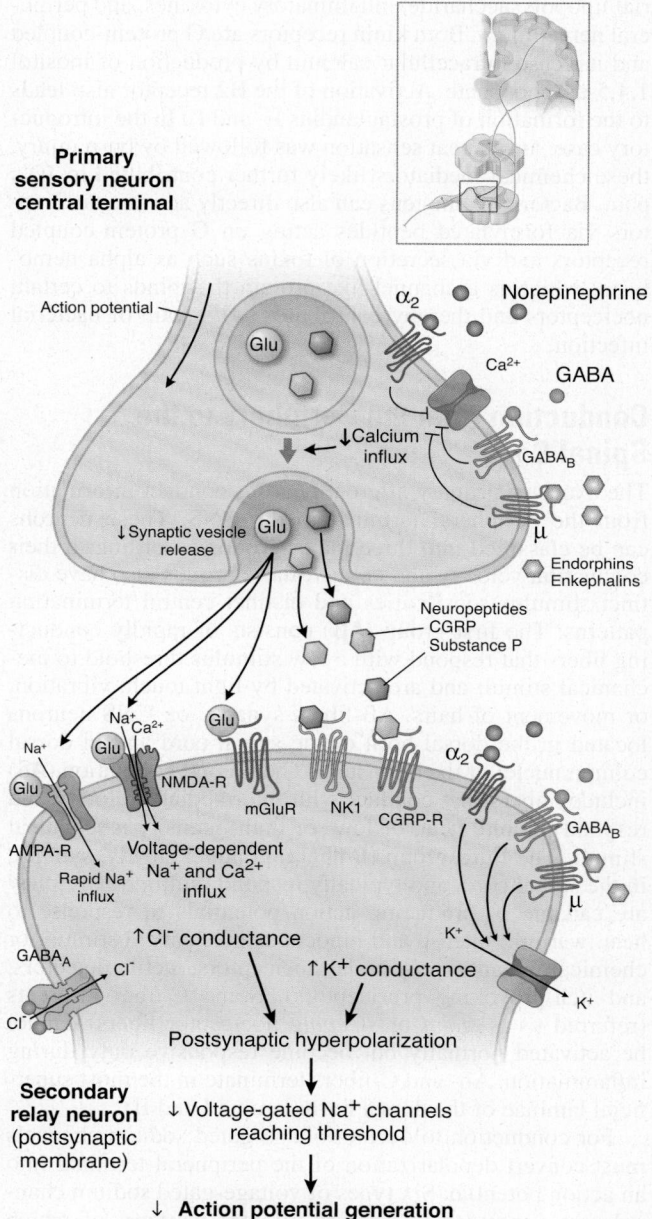

FIGURE 18-4. Inhibitory regulation of neurotransmission. Norepinephrine, GABA, and opioids, released by descending and/or local circuit inhibitory neurons, act both presynaptically and postsynaptically to inhibit neurotransmission. Presynaptic inhibition is mediated via reduced activity of voltage-gated calcium channels, whereas postsynaptic inhibition is mediated primarily by enhanced chloride influx and potassium efflux.

in Chapter 13, Pharmacology of GABAergic and Glutamatergic Neurotransmission.

The opioid peptides inhibit synaptic transmission and are released at several CNS sites in response to noxious stimuli. All endogenous opioid peptides, which include **β-endorphin**, the **enkephalins**, and the **dynorphins**, share the N-terminal sequence Tyr-Gly-Gly-Phe-Met/Leu. The opioids are proteolytically released from the larger precursor proteins proopiomelanocortin, proenkephalin, and prodynorphin. Opioid receptors fall into three classes, designated **μ**, **δ**, and **κ**, all of which are seven-transmembrane G protein-coupled receptors. The μ-opioid receptors mediate morphine-induced analgesia. This conclusion is based on the observation that the μ-opioid receptor knockout mouse exhibits neither analgesia nor adverse effects in response to **morphine** administration. The endogenous opioid peptides are receptor-selective: the dynorphins act primarily on κ receptors, while both enkephalins and β-endorphin act on μ and δ receptors. The physiologic role of the endogenous opioid peptides remains poorly understood, although they may mediate reward effects—for example, after sunburn. The effects of opioid receptor signaling include reduced presynaptic calcium conductance, enhanced postsynaptic potassium conductance, and reduced adenylyl cyclase activity. The first function impedes presynaptic neurotransmitter release; the second reduces postsynaptic neuronal responses to excitatory neurotransmitters; the physiologic role of the third remains unknown.

Opioids produce analgesia because of their action in the brain, brainstem, spinal cord, and peripheral terminals of primary afferent neurons. In the brain, opioids alter mood, produce sedation, and reduce the emotional reaction to pain. In the brainstem, opioids increase the activity of cells that provide descending inhibitory innervation to the spinal cord; here, opioids also produce nausea and respiratory depression. Spinal opioids inhibit synaptic vesicle release from primary afferents and hyperpolarize postsynaptic neurons (see above). Evidence also exists that peripheral opioid receptor stimulation reduces the activation of primary afferents and modulates immune cell activity. Action of opioids at these serially located sites is thought to have a synergistic effect to inhibit information flow from the periphery to the brain.

Norepinephrine is released by projections that descend from the brainstem to the spinal cord. The α_2-adrenergic receptor, a seven-transmembrane G protein-coupled receptor (see Chapter 11, Adrenergic Pharmacology), is the primary receptor for norepinephrine in the spinal cord. As with opioid receptor activation, α_2-adrenergic receptor activation inhibits presynaptic voltage-gated calcium channels, opens postsynaptic potassium channels, and inhibits adenylyl cyclase. Because α_2-adrenergic receptors are expressed both presynaptically and postsynaptically, spinal norepinephrine release can both reduce presynaptic vesicle release and decrease postsynaptic excitation. The α_2-adrenergic receptor agonist **clonidine** is sometimes used to treat pain, although this application is limited by adverse effects that include sedation and postural hypotension. Serotonin is also released in the spinal cord by projections descending from the brainstem. This neurotransmitter acts on several receptor subtypes that mediate both excitatory and inhibitory effects on nociception. The $5-HT_3$ ligand-gated channel may be responsible for the excitatory actions of serotonin in the spinal cord; several of the 5-HT G protein-coupled receptors may mediate the inhibitory actions of 5-HT. Given this complexity, the mechanism of the analgesic effect of serotonin is not fully understood. Selective serotonin reuptake inhibitors have been tested in the treatment of pain but have generally had little beneficial effect. Selective norepinephrine (NE) reuptake inhibitors do have analgesic action, as do dual NE/5-HT reuptake inhibitors such as **duloxetine**—this agent is used to treat many chronic pain conditions. **Tramadol**, a weak centrally acting opioid, also has monoaminergic actions and is widely used to treat mild pain. Its relatively weak efficacy as a single agent is increased when combined with acetaminophen, and its lack of abuse potential makes the drug attractive to prescribers. **Tapentadol** is a newer drug with similar dual action, although it is a more potent μ-opioid receptor agonist than tramadol.

Other compounds also have regulatory roles in the spinal cord. The **cannabinoid receptors** and the endogenous cannabinoids have recently become a focus for research on pain regulation. There are two cannabinoid receptors, both of which are G protein-coupled: CB_1, expressed in the brain, spinal cord, and sensory neurons; and CB_2, largely expressed in nonneural tissues, especially immune cells including microglia. Several endogenous cannabinoids have been identified, including members of the **anandamide** and **2-arachidonylglycerol (2AG)** families. A combination of anecdotal evidence and clinical trial data suggests that cannabinoids may have an analgesic effect in patients with AIDS neuropathy or multiple sclerosis. Selective cannabinoid pathway agents under development, such as CB_1 or CB_2 agonists or inhibitors of endocannabinoid metabolism, may prove useful for pain management.

PATHOPHYSIOLOGY

The pain processing circuit described above is responsible for producing acute **nociceptive pain**, a physiologic, adaptive sensation elicited only by noxious stimuli that acts as a warning or protective signal. There are some clinical situations, such as acute trauma, labor, or surgery, in which it is necessary to control nociceptive pain. In these cases, the pain pathway can be interrupted either by blocking transmission with local anesthetics (see Chapter 12) or by administering high-dose opioids. The opioids may be rapidly acting, such as **remifentanil** for intraoperative use, or more slowly acting, such as **morphine**; administered perioperatively, morphine retains activity for postoperative pain control.

Both peripheral inflammation and nervous system damage produce pain that is characterized by **hypersensitivity** to noxious and innocuous stimuli and by **spontaneous pain** that arises in the absence of any obvious stimulus. Understanding the mechanisms responsible for these types of clinical pain will facilitate both the appropriate use of currently available drugs and the development of novel therapeutic agents.

Clinical Nociceptive Pain

The ideal treatment of pain would be based on identifying and targeting the precise pain mechanisms operative in a particular patient and on normalizing abnormal pain sensitivity. Clinical pain syndromes may involve a combination of mechanisms, however, and there are few diagnostic tools to identify which specific mechanisms are responsible in a particular patient. Chronic pain conditions can be complicated to treat, and effective treatment usually demands multiple drugs (polypharmacy) to obtain the optimal therapeutic effect while reducing adverse effects. Chronic inflammatory pain conditions require the use of drugs that reduce the inflammatory response; such drugs may both correct the underlying inflammatory condition (disease-modifying therapy) and reduce the pain. For example, the **nonsteroidal anti-inflammatory drugs (NSAIDs)** (see Chapter 43, Pharmacology of Eicosanoids) are the first line of treatment for rheumatoid arthritis. By reducing inflammation, this intervention can decrease the release of chemical ligands that sensitize peripheral nerve terminals and thereby prevent peripheral sensitization (see below). Other disease-modifying anti-inflammatory treatments that may also reduce pain include cytokine inhibitors, sequestering agents such as TNF-α inhibitors, and immunosuppressants, as well as anti-nerve growth factor (NGF) monoclonal antibodies that are now under development.

The major agents used to treat most noninflammatory neuropathic or dysfunctional pain conditions are generally not disease-modifying because the underlying disease processes are either not known (e.g., fibromyalgia) or refractory to currently available treatments (e.g., neuropathic pain). Neuropathic pain associated with peripheral nervous tissue damage, spinal cord injury, or stroke commonly requires the use of several agents to alleviate pain symptoms. In nonmalignant pain, opioids have generally been used as a matter of last resort because of their adverse effects and because of the potential for the development of tolerance and physical dependence (see Chapter 19, Pharmacology of Drugs of Abuse). However, in recent years, opioids have increasingly been used for the management of chronic noncancer pain, albeit with the risks of producing drug-seeking behavior and creating opportunity for diversion of the drugs for illicit use. The U.S. Centers for Disease Control and Prevention (CDC) reported that opioid analgesics had a role in 71.3% of the 22,767 deaths due to prescription drug overdose occurring in the U.S. in 2013.

Severe acute pain due to trauma, surgery, or inflammation is usually treated with opioids and NSAIDs. The many available opioid agents permit a great deal of flexibility in both potency and duration of action. **Remifentanil**, a high-potency opioid, is cleared over the course of a few minutes, while **methadone** after prolonged use may be cleared over the course of days. Combinations of intermediate- and long-acting opioids may be used to tailor an analgesic regimen for pain that fluctuates in intensity over days, hours, or minutes. Remifentanil was administered during JD's surgical debridement for optimal control of intraoperative pain, followed by a morphine bolus and infusion for postoperative pain control. The nausea and sedation produced in many patients by opioids are potential problems when these agents are used for day-surgery cases. Acute inflammatory pain conditions, such as pancreatitis, are often treated with morphine. Gout, a second example of an acute inflammatory condition producing severe pain, is usually treated with indomethacin (an NSAID) to reduce the pain rapidly, and more specific disease-modifying agents are used to correct the underlying disorder over the longer term (see Chapter 49, Integrative Inflammation Pharmacology: Gout).

Peripheral Sensitization

Several peripheral stimuli can cause primary afferent neurons to lower their activation thresholds and increase their responsiveness (Fig. 18-5). These alterations, which constitute **peripheral sensitization**, can result in **allodynia**, in which normally innocuous stimuli are perceived as painful, and **hyperalgesia**,

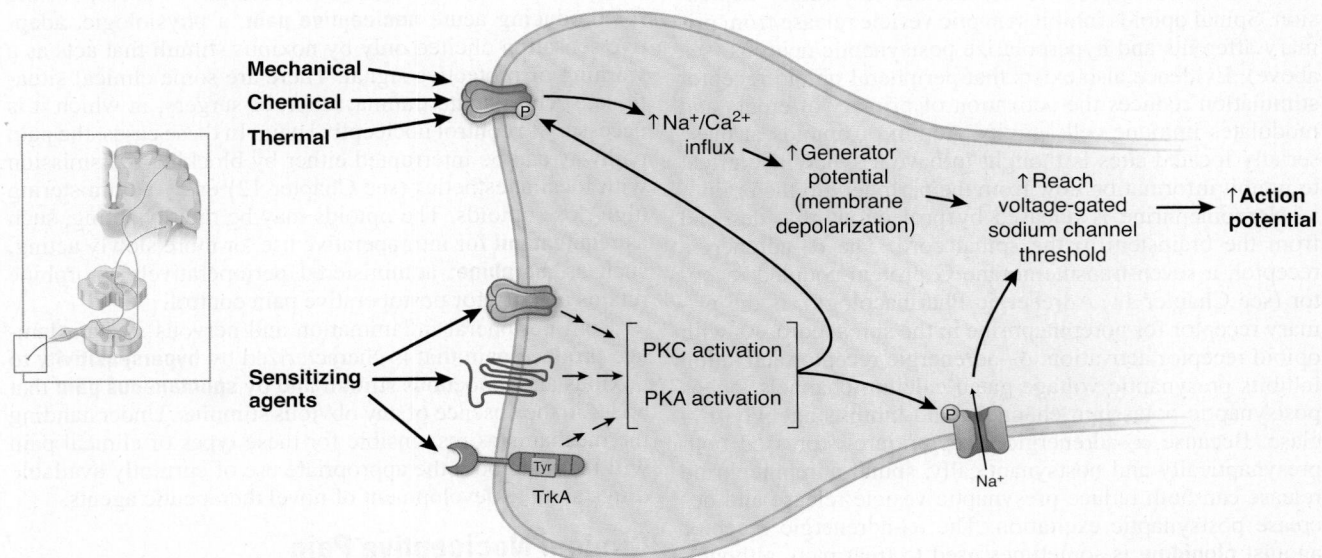

FIGURE 18-5. Peripheral sensitization. Peripherally released sensitizing agents activate signal transduction that can increase sensitivity of the peripheral nerve terminal. Mechanisms mediating increased sensitivity include (1) enhancement of ion influx in response to a noxious stimulus and (2) reduction of the activation threshold of the voltage-gated sodium channels responsible for initiating and propagating action potentials. In the example shown, a sensitizing agent activates one of three types of cell surface receptor, for example, a G protein-coupled receptor. This receptor initiates two parallel signaling cascades. One branch activates the phospholipase C (PLC) pathway, which results in increased release of calcium from intracellular stores and in activation of protein kinase C (PKC). Both of these effects increase ion influx—for example, through a TRPV1 receptor (*blue*)—in response to a nociceptive stimulus. The second branch of the signaling cascade activates adenylyl cyclase (AC), leading to increased formation of cAMP, activation of protein kinase A (PKA), and sodium channel phosphorylation. Both signaling cascades serve to increase the likelihood of action potential initiation and propagation. Nerve growth factor (NGF) is the ligand for the neurotrophic tyrosine kinase receptor family member TrkA. See text for further details.

in which high-intensity stimuli are perceived as more painful and longer lasting than usual at the site of injury (zone of primary hyperalgesia). Some inflammatory mediators released by injured (ATP) or immune (IL-1β) cells can directly activate nociceptors to signal to the CNS the presence of tissue injury and thereby evoke pain. The mechanisms responsible for primary hyperalgesia involve both direct changes in transduction and indirect changes induced by the release of effector molecules. An example of altered transduction is the change in heat activation of the TRPV1 receptor due to posttranslational modifications and altered membrane trafficking following activation of PKC and PI3K signaling pathways, which reduce the activation threshold of the receptor so that it can be activated by warm stimuli (38°–40°C) that are normally not painful. The major known effectors that produce peripheral sensitization are the inflammatory mediators bradykinin, the cytokine IL-1β, protons, histamine, prostaglandin E_2, and NGF. Prostaglandin E_2 acts on EP receptors, of which there are four types, while NGF acts on the neurotrophic tyrosine kinase receptor family member TrkA. The actions of histamine are more prominent on the subset of sensory neurons that contribute to itch.

Sensitizing chemical mediators act on G protein-coupled receptors or receptor tyrosine kinases expressed on the peripheral terminals of nociceptor neurons. Activation of phospholipase C, phospholipase A_2, and adenylyl cyclase occurs in response to the activation of G protein-coupled receptors, such as those for bradykinin, prostaglandin E_2, and adenosine. In turn, these signaling enzymes generate mediators that activate protein kinase A (PKA) or protein kinase C (PKC). Protein kinase A phosphorylates the voltage-gated sodium channel $Na_v1.8$, resulting in both a decrease in its activation threshold and an increase in the current passed when the channel opens. Protein kinase C phosphorylates TRPV1, thus reducing its activation threshold and thereby increasing the response of peripheral terminals to heat stimuli (see above).

In addition to the enhancement of peripheral response caused by an outside event that produces inflammation, the peripheral terminals themselves can contribute to inflammation (the neurogenic component of inflammation). Depolarization and chemical stimuli induce the release of neuropeptides, such as substance P and CGRP, from the peripheral terminals of primary afferents. The released neuropeptides produce vasodilation and increase capillary permeability, contributing to the wheal-and-flare response to tissue injury. In addition, neuropeptides can induce the release of histamine and TNF-α from inflammatory cells. The recruitment and activation of granulocytes, as well as the increase in local capillary diameter and permeability to plasma, result in a local inflammatory response at the site of the excited peripheral terminal. This response contributes to atopic dermatitis and psoriasis.

Peripheral sensitization is an important target for clinical pain pharmacology. The NSAIDs are the most widely used pain treatment. By inhibiting the activity of cyclooxygenase enzymes, NSAIDs reduce prostaglandin production and, hence, the local inflammatory response and peripheral sensitization. There are two isoforms of cyclooxygenase: COX-1 and COX-2 (see Chapter 43). The former is constitutively active and is important in a variety of physiologic functions, such as maintenance of gastric mucosal integrity and normal platelet function. COX-2 is selectively up-regulated at the site of inflammation, primarily in macrophages, in response to local secretion of cytokines, particularly IL-1β and TNF-α acting via the transcription factor NF-κB.

Selective inhibitors of COX-2, such as **celecoxib**, **rofecoxib**, and **valdecoxib**, were developed in an attempt to control inflammatory pain while decreasing some of the adverse effects of the nonselective NSAIDs, such as gastrointestinal bleeding. However, large postmarketing trials have revealed an increased incidence of serious cardiovascular effects associated with COX-2 inhibitor therapy, including an increased risk of myocardial infarction. This has led to the withdrawal of most COX-2 selective inhibitors, with celecoxib alone remaining on the market in the United States. In addition to the cyclooxygenases, the transduction molecules, signaling intermediates, and sodium channels expressed at peripheral terminals may all represent targets for the development of new analgesic drugs that reduce peripheral pain hypersensitivity.

In the case of JD, peripheral sensitization was induced at the burn site. The high-intensity stimulus led to neurogenic inflammation. The associated tissue damage further potentiated inflammatory mediator release, leading to the activation of second messenger cascades that heightened peripheral terminal excitability over time.

Central Sensitization

Hyperalgesia and allodynia frequently extend beyond the primary area of inflammation and tissue damage. Pain hypersensitivity in this region, described as the area of secondary hyperalgesia and/or allodynia, depends on alterations in sensory processing in the dorsal horn of the spinal cord. These alterations, which are a form of neuronal plasticity termed **central sensitization**, occur when repetitive, usually high-intensity, synaptic transmission activates intracellular signal transduction cascades in dorsal horn neurons that enhance the response to subsequent stimuli.

Several of the postsynaptic receptors expressed by dorsal horn neurons are involved in the induction of central sensitization (Fig. 18-6). These receptors include AMPA, NMDA, and metabotropic glutamate receptors, as well the substance P (neurokinin) receptor NK1 and the BDNF (neurotrophin) receptor TrkB. Upon activation of metabotropic receptors or calcium influx through NMDA channels, intracellular protein kinases are activated, such as PKC, calcium/calmodulin kinase (CAMK II), and extracellular signal-related protein kinase (ERK). In turn, these effectors can alter the function of existing membrane proteins by post-translational processing, usually by phosphorylation. For example, phosphorylated NMDA receptors open more rapidly and for longer periods in response to glutamate. Phosphorylation of AMPA receptors results in their translocation from cytosolic stores to the membrane, thus increasing synaptic efficacy. Activation of ERKs leads to a reduction in potassium channel activity in dorsal horn neurons; the decreased potassium current increases neuronal excitability. Most often, central sensitization slowly subsides after the inducing stimulus ceases. However, chronic injury or inflammation can produce a state of central sensitization that persists over time.

NMDA receptor blockade can prevent both the induction and maintenance of central sensitization. For example, NMDA receptor blockade instituted preoperatively has been shown to reduce pain experienced postoperatively. A component of postoperative pain is likely attributable to NMDA receptor-dependent central sensitization associated with the intense peripheral stimulation that occurs during surgery. The NMDA receptor blocker **ketamine** can be used to oppose

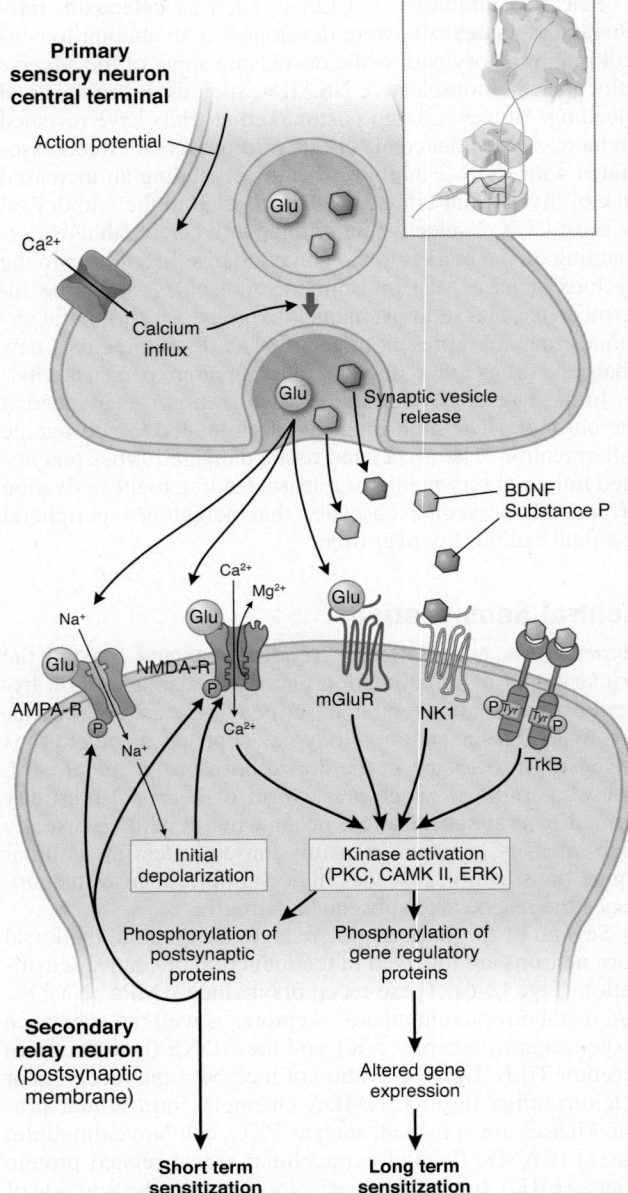

Primary sensory neuron central terminal

Action potential

Ca^{2+}

Calcium influx

Glu

Glu

Synaptic vesicle release

BDNF Substance P

Ca^{2+}

Mg^{2+}

Na^+

Glu

Glu

NMDA-R

mGluR

NK1

AMPA-R

Na^+

Ca^{2+}

Tyr

Tyr

TrkB

Initial depolarization

Kinase activation (PKC, CAMK II, ERK)

Phosphorylation of postsynaptic proteins

Phosphorylation of gene regulatory proteins

Secondary relay neuron (postsynaptic membrane)

Altered gene expression

Short term sensitization

Long term sensitization

FIGURE 18-6. Central sensitization. Sustained or intense activation of central transmission can lead to postsynaptic calcium influx, primarily through NMDA receptors. Together with a variety of neuromodulatory signals, calcium influx activates signal transduction cascades that can enhance both short-term and long-term excitability of the synapse.

activation of sensitized NMDA receptors. NMDA receptors are widely expressed, however, and NMDA blockers produce significant psychotropic effects, including amnesia and hallucinations. Protein kinase C or ERK is an alternative target. Although many of the signaling proteins involved in dorsal horn sensitization are expressed in all cells, it may be possible to target treatment to the spinal cord by intrathecal or epidural injection. **Pregabalin** and **gabapentin** reduce central sensitization by reducing transmitter release, as does **morphine**. **Duloxetine** enhances the inhibitor effects of amines on spinal cord neurons and also reduces central sensitization.

The intense peripheral activation produced by JD's burn injury also led to the development of central sensitization.

This effect further enhanced the lingering pain he felt at the burn site, and it produced pain surrounding the burn site, outside the primary area of tissue damage and inflammation.

Neuropathic Pain

The mechanisms responsible for the persistent pain that can occur following nerve injury involve both functional and structural alterations in the nervous system and occur in both primary afferent neurons and the CNS (Fig. 18-7). In the periphery, changes in the physiology and transcriptional profile of primary afferent sensory neurons occur after nerve damage, contributing to neuropathic pain. These alterations are induced by combinations of positive signals, such as inflammatory cytokines released by macrophages and Schwann cells, and negative signals, such as the loss of peripheral support from neurotrophic factors. In addition, the expression pattern of sodium channels changes in injured primary sensory neurons: $Na_v1.8$ and $Na_v1.9$ are down-regulated, while $Na_v1.3$, which is normally not detectable in primary sensory neurons, is up-regulated. $Na_v1.3$ channels exhibit accelerated recovery from inactivation and are thought to contribute to neuropathic pain by enhancing cellular excitability sufficiently to generate ectopic action potential activity. The contribution of sodium channels to some forms of neuropathic pain is supported by the effectiveness of sodium channel blockers, such as **carbamazepine** and **oxcarbazepine**, in treating trigeminal neuralgia.

Nerve damage also promotes reorganization of synaptic connection patterns within the dorsal horn of the spinal cord. Peripheral nerve injury leads to a regenerative response. Because primarily C-fibers are lost upon the withdrawal of peripheral trophic support, regenerating central terminals of Aβ-fibers are free to invade the area normally occupied by the central terminals of C-fibers. Another structural change is an excitotoxic loss of inhibitory neurons in the dorsal horn after peripheral nerve injury. The loss of inhibition (disinhibition) contributes to the heightened pain sensitivity, and augmenting GABAergic or glycinergic inhibition can be an effective strategy for treating neuropathic pain. A combination of these mechanisms would have been involved in maintaining JD's pain over the years following his operation. Neuroprotective treatment designed to prevent transsynaptic neurodegeneration could represent an opportunity for a disease-modifying approach to neuropathic pain, particularly when the time of nerve damage can be identified (e.g., after surgery). It may be possible to use neurotrophic factors to treat both the transcriptional changes and some of the structural alterations that contribute to neuropathic pain, as well as the changes in immune cells that occur locally at the site of nerve injury and in the CNS. A highly selective angiotensin II type 2 receptor antagonist has recently been shown to be effective in postherpetic neuralgia; the mechanism of action involves targeting abnormal excitability and sprouting in injured sensory neurons produced by activation of p38 MAPK.

Migraine

Migraine headache is a disorder consisting of headache attacks that last for up to 3 days, typically associated with light and sound avoidance and nausea. Some migraines are accompanied by aura, in which transient neurologic symptoms are associated with the migraine. It is thought that the pathophysiology of migraine comprises several events.

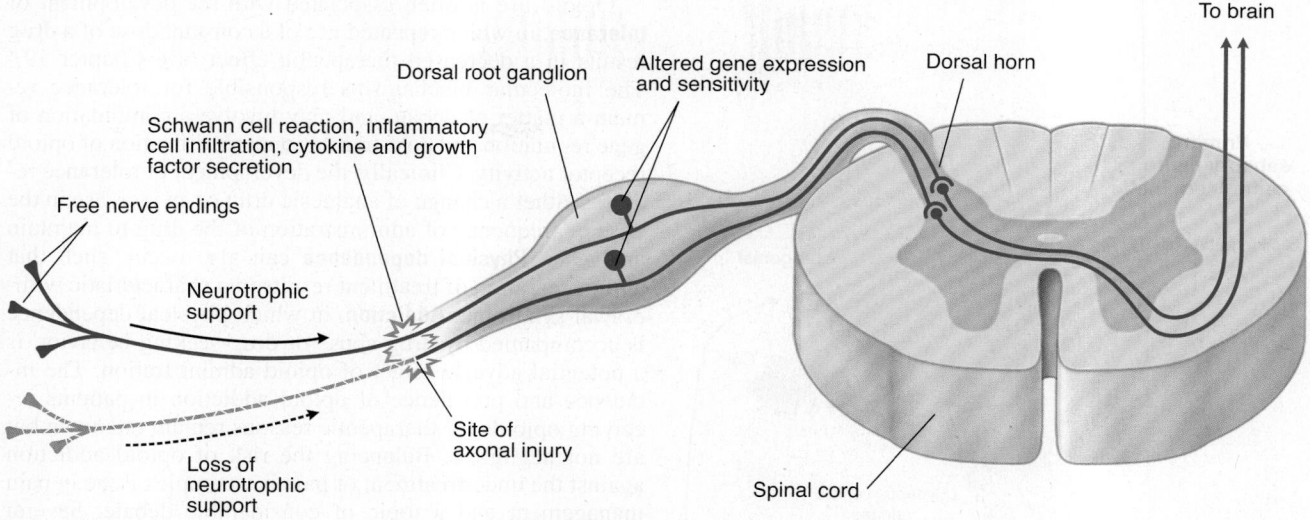

FIGURE 18-7. Schematization of neuropathic pain. Nerve injury results in a combination of negative signals and positive signals that alter the physiology of the nociceptive system. The loss of neurotrophic support alters gene expression in the injured nerve fiber, whereas the release of inflammatory cytokines alters gene expression in both the injured and adjacent uninjured nerve fibers. These changes in gene expression can lead to altered sensitivity and activity of nociceptive fibers and, thus, to the continued perception of injury that is characteristic of neuropathic pain.

First, before the headache occurs, a region of neural activation followed by inactivation travels across the cortex. This phenomenon is termed **cortical spreading depression** and is correlated with the sensory disturbances of the migraine aura such as scotoma (visual field disturbances). Second, release of multiple neuropeptides, possibly evoked by the cortical excitation, occurs in the dural vasculature. Third, trigeminal afferents from the dural vasculature are activated and sensitized by the local release of neuropeptides and inflammatory mediators. Fourth, the high degree of activity in trigeminal afferent high-threshold fibers produces central sensitization, leading to secondary hyperalgesia and tactile allodynia. Thus, a migraine attack can be considered the acute manifestation of abnormal intermittent peripheral and central excitability.

Evidence from a rare autosomal dominant disorder, familial hemiplegic migraine (FHM), may shed light on the mechanisms of migraine in general. This disorder consists of migraine attacks with a particular aura characterized by unilateral motor paralysis. Three genes have been associated with FHM: *CACNA1A*, *ATP1A2*, and *SCN1A*. *CACNA1A* encodes a $Ca_v2.1$ voltage-gated calcium channel subunit. In animal models, $Ca_v2.1$ gain-of-function mutations cause increased presynaptic calcium and increased glutamate release, which may help explain the trigger for cortical spreading depression. *ATP1A2* encodes a subunit of the Na^+/K^+ ATPase, which is critical for the maintenance of neuronal membrane potential and which produces the Na^+ gradient needed for glutamate transport. *SCN1A* encodes a voltage-gated sodium channel subunit that is involved in action potential conduction. Whether the more common forms of migraine are associated with similar changes in these genes remains unknown.

PHARMACOLOGIC CLASSES AND AGENTS

Several drug classes are widely used for pain relief. These include **opioid receptor agonists**, **NSAIDs** (see Chapter 43),

tricyclic antidepressants (see Chapter 15, Pharmacology of Serotonergic and Central Adrenergic Neurotransmission), **antiepileptic drugs** (sodium channel blockers) (see Chapter 16), **NMDA receptor antagonists** (see Chapter 13), and **adrenergic agonists**. In addition, **5-HT₁ receptor agonists** have specific applications in the acute treatment of migraine.

Opioid Receptor Agonists

Opioid receptor agonists are the primary drug class used in the acute management of moderate to severe pain. The naturally occurring opioid agonist **morphine** has the greatest historical importance and remains in wide use, but synthetic and semisynthetic opioids add pharmacokinetic versatility. Opioids have long been used to treat acute and cancer-related pain, but in recent years, they have become one component of the management of chronic noncancer pain as well.

Mechanism of Action and Major Adverse Effects

Opioid receptor agonists produce analgesia and other effects by acting on μ-opioid receptors (Fig. 18-8). Sites of analgesic action include the brain, brainstem, spinal cord, and primary afferent peripheral terminals, as described previously. The principal mechanism of opioid action, as discussed in greater detail above, is via G protein-coupled signaling that inhibits neurotransmission via decreased presynaptic calcium influx and/or increased postsynaptic potassium influx at either spinal or supraspinal sites.

Opioids produce a wide array of adverse effects. These effects are qualitatively similar across opioids but may vary in intensity. The major dose-limiting adverse effects are sedation and respiratory suppression. By acting on the medullary respiratory control center, opioids blunt the respiratory response to carbon dioxide and can cause periods of apnea. Importantly, the respiratory effects of opioids interact with other stimuli: painful or other arousing stimuli can promote ventilation, while natural sleep synergizes with opioids to

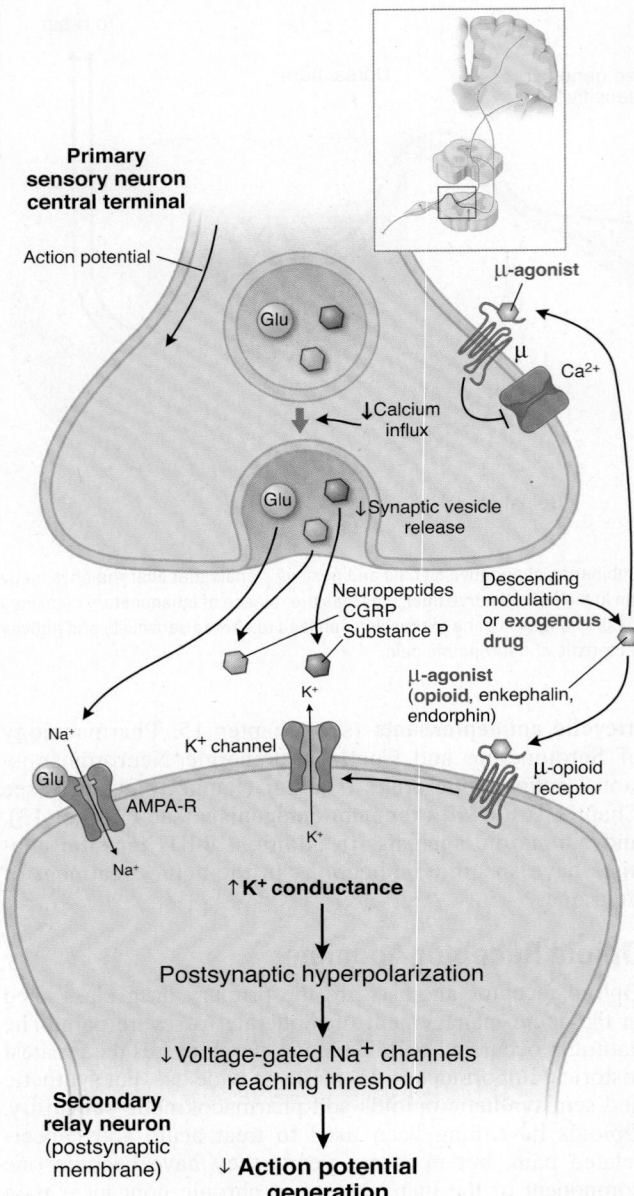

FIGURE 18-8. Mechanism of action of μ-opioid receptor agonists in the spinal cord. Activation of both presynaptic and postsynaptic μ-opioid receptors by descending and local circuit inhibitory neurons inhibits central relaying of nociceptive stimuli. In the presynaptic terminal, μ-opioid receptor activation decreases Ca^{2+} influx in response to an incoming action potential. Postsynaptic μ-opioid receptor activation increases K^+ conductance and thereby decreases the postsynaptic response to excitatory neurotransmission.

suppress ventilation. Opioids stimulate receptors in the medullary chemoreceptor zone and the gastrointestinal tract, leading to nausea, vomiting, and constipation. In the genitourinary system, opioids can cause urinary urgency and urinary retention. In the central nervous system, opioids can cause sedation, confusion, dizziness, euphoria, and myoclonus. It has recently become apparent that excessive use of opioids can lead to a paradoxical opioid-induced hyperalgesia. In the cardiovascular system, opioids can reduce sympathetic tone and lead to orthostatic hypotension. Opioids can also cause bradycardia. Respiratory effects are often the major, dose-limiting adverse effect of opioids.

Opioid use is often associated with the development of **tolerance**, in which repeated use of a constant dose of a drug results in a decreased therapeutic effect (see Chapter 19). The molecular mechanisms responsible for tolerance remain a matter of debate and may involve a combination of gene regulation and post-translational modification of opioid receptor activity. Clinically, the development of tolerance requires either a change of analgesic drug or an increase in the dose or frequency of administration of the drug to maintain analgesia. **Physical dependence** can also occur, such that abrupt cessation of treatment results in a characteristic withdrawal syndrome. **Addiction**, in which physical dependence is accompanied by drug abuse or drug-seeking behavior, is a potential adverse effect of opioid administration. The incidence and prevalence of opioid addiction in patients receiving opioids for therapeutic reasons remain unknown but are not negligible. Balancing the risk of opioid addiction against the undertreatment of pain is a complex issue in pain management and a topic of considerable debate. Several strategies are being investigated to reduce abuse potential, including mechanisms to prevent the disruption of slow-release opioid formulations (see next section), combinations that include both an opioid agonist and an opioid antagonist, and prodrugs that are slowly metabolized to the active opioid agonist. In JD's case, intravenous morphine was tapered and replaced with a combination oral analgesic to prevent the onset of opioid withdrawal symptoms.

Morphine, Codeine, and Derivatives

Morphine, **codeine (methylmorphine)**, and their semisynthetic derivatives are the most widely used opioids for control of pain outside of the context of anesthesia or procedural sedation. Morphine is metabolized in the liver, and its first-pass metabolism reduces its oral bioavailability. In the liver, morphine undergoes glucuronidation at either the 3 position (morphine-3-glucuronide; M3G) or the 6 position (M6G). While M3G is inactive, M6G has analgesic activity. M6G is excreted by the kidney, and its accumulation in patients with chronic kidney disease may contribute to opioid toxicity. Morphine does not undergo metabolism by the cytochrome P450 system and has relatively few interactions with other drugs. **Hydromorphone** is a widely used morphine derivative with similar properties to morphine but approximately 5 to 10 times higher potency. Like morphine, hydromorphone undergoes glucuronidation but not cytochrome P450-based metabolism and has few interactions with other drugs.

Codeine, like morphine, is a naturally occurring opioid receptor agonist. Codeine is commonly used for its antitussive (i.e., cough-suppressing) and antidiarrheal effects because it has considerably higher oral bioavailability than morphine; it is also used in conditions for which a low-potency oral opioid analgesic is preferred. The analgesic action of codeine results largely from its hepatic demethylation to morphine, which has substantially greater μ-agonist activity. Genetic polymorphisms in the cytochrome P450 enzymes CYP2D6 and CYP3A4, which are responsible for demethylation of codeine, may determine interindividual variation in response to codeine treatment. In some cases, most notably in children, ultrarapid metabolism of codeine to morphine has resulted in accidental death due to unanticipated opioid overdose.

The semisynthetic compounds **oxycodone** and **hydrocodone** are more potent analogues of codeine that are also orally available and are widely used, often in combination with acetaminophen. Oxycodone is hepatically metabolized via the cytochrome P450 system to the highly potent opioid agonist oxymorphone and the less potent metabolite noroxycodone. Hydrocodone is metabolized via the hepatic cytochrome P450 system to the active metabolite hydromorphone. For these two drugs, the primary drug is likely the agent responsible for the therapeutic effect, while metabolic products may affect drug interactions and interindividual variation in drug response.

Several different routes are available for administering morphine. Controlled-release oral preparations are marketed to reduce the number of daily doses required for analgesia. These formulations allow drug release over the course of 12–24 hours. Unfortunately, sustained-release formulations have been associated with a high abuse potential, especially when they are illegally reformulated to deliver the entire dose at once rather than over the course of hours. Abusers of these formulations seek a "high" from a rapid increase in plasma levels (see Chapter 19). As a result, several of the sustained-release opioids have been reformulated into abuse-deterrent pills that are difficult to crush or dissolve. Intravenous opioids, most commonly hydromorphone or morphine, may be administered in **patient-controlled analgesia** devices, which are now used to control a multitude of pain states, primarily in inpatient settings. Epidural or intrathecal morphine can produce highly effective analgesia by achieving locally high concentrations in the dorsal horn of the spinal cord. Neuraxial administration of the drug results in a much longer duration of action than does parenteral administration because of the time required for the relatively hydrophilic morphine to diffuse out of the CNS into the systemic circulation.

Synthetic Agonists

All of the opioids thus far discussed (morphine, codeine, hydromorphone, oxymorphone, oxycodone, and hydrocodone) are naturally occurring or semisynthetic and fall into the chemical class of phenanthrenes. The two major classes of synthetic μ-receptor agonists are the diphenylheptane (methadone) and phenylpiperidine (fentanyl, sufentanil, alfentanil, remifentanil, and meperidine) classes. Tramadol and tapentadol are classified separately and affect several biochemical pathways in addition to the μ-opioid pathway. Methadone is well known for its use in opioid addiction treatment but is also used for the treatment of pain.

Methadone has a half-life in the range of 25–35 hours, is more lipophilic than morphine, distributes highly into tissues, and binds to plasma proteins. Methadone undergoes extensive cytochrome P450-mediated metabolism and as a result is subject to numerous drug–drug interactions. Due to methadone's long duration of action, it is often used to achieve sustained relief of chronic pain. The half-life of methadone lengthens with repeated administration as its distribution and clearance mechanisms become progressively saturated. As a result, patients initiating methadone therapy are at risk for delayed respiratory depression after tolerating a starting drug regimen, and multiple daily dosing at a fixed dose rate can result in "dose stacking" and a progressively increasing drug level with time. Methadone also causes dose-related prolongation of the QT interval and has been associated with *torsades de pointes*, a form of ventricular tachycardia. In addition to its primary, high-potency action as a μ-opioid agonist, methadone has a low-potency effect

as an NMDA receptor antagonist. It is not clear whether the NMDA antagonism of methadone is a clinically important drug effect.

Fentanyl is a short-acting synthetic opioid agonist that is 75–100 times more potent than morphine and has an elimination half-life comparable to that of morphine. **Sufentanil**, which is even more potent than fentanyl, and **alfentanil**, which is less potent, are structurally related to fentanyl. Fentanyl is most widely used for intraoperative and periprocedural analgesia due to its high potency and rapid onset of action. Interestingly, fentanyl's analgesic effect is limited by redistribution to inactive tissue stores, which occurs over the course of minutes after a single, low-to-moderate bolus dose. With prolonged infusion, the effective analgesic (and respiratory suppressing) duration of action of fentanyl then progressively lengthens until the time required to eliminate fentanyl may be measured in hours rather than minutes. This prolonged duration of action is due to redistribution of fentanyl out of inactive tissue stores to active sites after the fentanyl infusion is terminated. The same phenomenon occurs with alfentanil and sufentanil, although there is less prolongation of the elimination time than with fentanyl.

Because of its high lipophilicity, fentanyl is bioavailable via several routes. For example, fentanyl has been formulated as a lozenge for buccal transmucosal administration, which is particularly valuable for avoiding parenteral treatment in pediatric patients. Fentanyl can also be administered transdermally in the form of a patch that releases the drug slowly over time to provide long-acting systemic analgesia.

Remifentanil, the most recently developed phenylpiperidine, exhibits distinct pharmacokinetic behavior. Remifentanil contains a methyl ester moiety that is essential for activity but that is also the substrate for the action of numerous nonspecific tissue esterases. Thus, it has unusually rapid metabolism and elimination, and the drug effect has an approximately 5-minute half-life. Administered as a continuous infusion during anesthesia, remifentanil permits precise matching of the drug dose to the clinical response (see Chapter 17, General Anesthetic Pharmacology). However, if any postoperative pain is anticipated, the rapid termination of action demands that the use of remifentanil during anesthesia be coupled with the administration of a longer acting drug to maintain analgesia postoperatively. In the introductory case, remifentanil was used for intraoperative analgesia during the skin debridement procedure to ensure that JD did not experience pain during surgery. Morphine was added before the end of the operation to provide postoperative pain coverage. Because of remifentanil's short half-life, pain associated with surgical tissue damage would have returned immediately after surgery if morphine had not been added.

Meperidine is a phenylpiperidine μ-agonist with analgesic efficacy similar to morphine, but lower potency: 75–100 mg of meperidine is equivalent to 10 mg of morphine. Unlike other opioids, meperidine causes mydriasis rather than miosis. The toxic meperidine metabolite normeperidine can cause increased CNS excitability and seizures. Normeperidine is excreted by the kidneys, and its elimination half-life is longer than that of meperidine; therefore, meperidine toxicity is a particular problem with repeated dosing of the drug or in patients with acute or chronic kidney disease. In addition, meperidine has a serotonergic effect and, in combination with MAO inhibitors or selective serotonin reuptake inhibitors, can precipitate serotonin syndrome.

Partial and Mixed Agonists

In addition to the full μ-opioid receptor agonists described earlier, several drugs have been developed as partial and mixed μ- or κ-agonists. These include buprenorphine, a partial μ-agonist, and nalbuphine, a κ-agonist with μ-antagonist activity.

Buprenorphine is widely used in opioid addiction treatment for either maintenance or detoxification and may also be used for pain treatment. Buprenorphine is highly potent (approximately 30-fold more potent than morphine) and has a prolonged duration of analgesic action (on the order of several hours). It is administered parenterally, sublingually, or transdermally. As a partial agonist, buprenorphine binds to the μ-opioid receptor with high binding affinity but only moderate receptor activation (see Chapter 2, Pharmacodynamics). As a result, there is a ceiling for both its analgesic and adverse opioid effects; as the buprenorphine dose increases, μ-opioid receptors eventually become saturated with bound but relatively inactive partial agonist. Because of buprenorphine's high μ-receptor binding affinity, patients treated with high-dose buprenorphine may be refractory to the effects of other opioids and to the effects of opioid reversal agents. Patients chronically exposed to other opioids should discontinue the other opioid prior to initiating buprenorphine therapy, because buprenorphine exposure can induce acute opioid withdrawal in opioid-dependent individuals.

Nalbuphine is an opioid agonist/antagonist with analgesic effects that are thought to be mediated through the κ-opioid receptor. Nalbuphine is commonly used in clinical practice to reverse the pruritus induced by neuraxial opioid administration.

Opioid Receptor Antagonists

μ-Opioid receptor antagonists are used to reverse life-threatening adverse effects of opioid administration, specifically respiratory depression. **Naloxone**, one such antagonist, is a synthetic derivative of oxymorphone that is administered parenterally. Because the half-life of naloxone is shorter than that of morphine, it is not safe to leave the patient unattended immediately after successful treatment of an episode of respiratory depression with naloxone; monitoring can be relaxed only when it is certain that morphine no longer remains in the system. The orally administered antagonist **naltrexone** is primarily used in outpatient settings, typically for detoxification of individuals addicted to opioids (see Chapter 19). Combinations of opioid agonists and antagonists are being developed to reduce illicit drug use. Antagonists restricted to the periphery, such as **alvimopan** and **methylnaltrexone**, have been developed to reduce postoperative ileus and to ameliorate the gastrointestinal effects of chronic opioid use.

Nonsteroidal Anti-Inflammatory Drugs and Nonopioid Analgesics

General Features

Nonsteroidal anti-inflammatory drugs (NSAIDs) inhibit the activity of **cyclooxygenase** enzymes (**COX-1** and **COX-2**) that are required for the production of prostaglandins (see Chapter 43). NSAIDs affect pain pathways in at least three different ways. First, prostaglandins reduce the activation threshold at the peripheral terminals of primary afferent nociceptor neurons (Fig. 18-9). By reducing prostaglandin synthesis, NSAIDs decrease inflammatory hyperalgesia and allodynia. Second, NSAIDs decrease the recruitment of

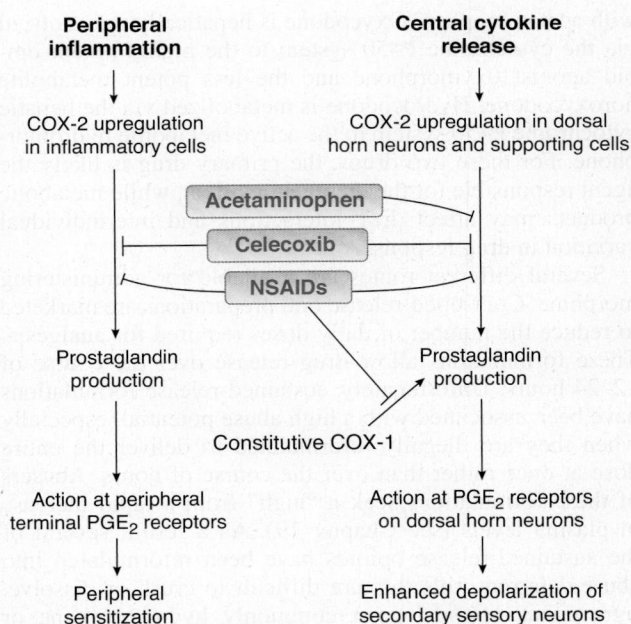

FIGURE 18-9. Mechanism of analgesic action of cyclooxygenase inhibitors. Inflammatory states are often associated with the production of prostaglandins, which are important mediators of both peripheral (*left*) and central (*right*) pain sensitization. In the periphery, prostaglandins produced by inflammatory cells sensitize peripheral nerve terminal prostaglandin (EP) receptors, making them more responsive to a painful stimulus. In central pain pathways, cytokines released in response to inflammation induce prostaglandin production in the dorsal horn of the spinal cord. These prostaglandins sensitize secondary nociceptive neurons and thereby increase the perception of pain. Nonsteroidal anti-inflammatory drugs (NSAIDs) block peripheral and central sensitization mediated by prostanoids that are released in inflammation; NSAIDs also reduce the extent of inflammation.

leukocytes and, thereby, the production of leukocyte-derived inflammatory mediators. Third, NSAIDs that cross the blood–brain barrier prevent the generation of prostaglandins that act as pain-producing neuromodulators in the spinal cord dorsal horn.

Acetaminophen and NSAIDs act through mechanisms that do not involve the μ-opioid receptor, and NSAID–opioid and acetaminophen–opioid combinations can act synergistically to reduce pain. NSAIDs and COX-2 inhibitors act both peripherally and centrally, whereas acetaminophen acts only centrally. Preclinical data suggest that, while the acute action of NSAIDs is peripheral, much of their analgesic effect derives from their central action to prevent a PGE_2-induced reduction in glycinergic inhibition. Like the opioids, nonselective COX-inhibiting NSAIDs have some deleterious adverse effects, particularly injury to the gastric mucosa and the kidneys. It had been thought that the anti-inflammatory and analgesic effects of the NSAIDs are primarily attributable to inhibition of COX-2, an inducible enzyme active in inflammatory states, whereas the adverse effects of the NSAIDs are primarily attributable to inhibition of COX-1, a constitutive enzyme responsible for the production of prostanoids involved in physiologic tissue maintenance and vascular regulation. However, this view may be an oversimplification, because COX-2 may be induced to support COX-1 activity in the setting of gastric mucosal injury, and COX-1 may produce prostaglandins in tandem with COX-2 in inflammatory states. There is also concern that COX-2 inhibition may promote thrombosis and reduce or delay wound healing.

Specific Agents

The major classes of NSAIDs include the salicylates (**aspirin** or **acetylsalicylate**), propionic acid derivatives (**ibuprofen**), indole acetic acid derivatives (**indomethacin**), phenylacetic acid derivatives (**diclofenac**), and oxicam derivatives (**piroxicam**) (see Fig. 43-8). The para-aminophenols (**acetaminophen**) are a related class of compounds with analgesic and antipyretic activity but not anti-inflammatory activity. The COX-2 selective inhibitors **celecoxib**, **rofecoxib**, and **valdecoxib** were designed to produce analgesia equivalent to that of the NSAIDs while decreasing the adverse effects associated with chronic NSAID use. However, both rofecoxib and valdecoxib have been withdrawn from the market because of an increased risk of adverse cardiovascular effects and skin reactions. Representative agents are discussed here; further information on their anti-inflammatory uses and adverse effects is discussed in Chapter 43.

Acetylsalicylic acid (aspirin) acts by covalently acetylating the cyclooxygenase active site in both COX-1 and COX-2. Aspirin is rapidly absorbed and distributed throughout the body. Chronic aspirin use can produce gastric irritation and erosion, hemorrhage, vomiting, and renal tubular necrosis. These concerns limit the usefulness of aspirin primarily to acute pain settings.

The coxibs are COX-2 selective enzyme inhibitors. Currently, only **celecoxib** remains in clinical use in the United States. This class of drugs was originally reserved for patients who required NSAIDs but were at high risk for developing gastrointestinal (GI), renal, or hematologic adverse effects, although there is no clinical evidence that celecoxib reduces the risk of adverse GI effects.

The widely used compound **ibuprofen** is a derivative of propionic acid. Used primarily for its analgesic and anti-inflammatory effects, ibuprofen is also an antipyretic, and it has a lower incidence of adverse effects than aspirin. Another common propionic acid derivative is **naproxen**. Compared to ibuprofen, naproxen is more potent and has a longer half-life; therefore, it can be administered less frequently with equivalent analgesic efficacy. Its adverse effect profile is similar to ibuprofen, and it is generally well tolerated. As with all NSAIDs, ibuprofen and naproxen can cause GI complications ranging from dyspepsia to gastric bleeding.

The phenylacetic acid derivatives **diclofenac** and **ketorolac** are used to treat moderate to severe pain. Ketorolac can be administered orally or parenterally, while diclofenac is available in oral formulations. Both agents carry a risk of severe adverse effects, including anaphylaxis, acute renal failure, Stevens-Johnson syndrome (a diffuse life-threatening rash involving the skin and mucous membranes), and gastrointestinal bleeding. Ketorolac is valuable for short-term pain control when avoidance of adverse opioid effects is desirable, for example, in day-surgery patients. Topical formulations of these drugs may have some utility.

Acetaminophen (paracetamol) preferentially reduces central prostaglandin synthesis by an uncertain mechanism; as a result, the drug produces analgesia and antipyresis but has little anti-inflammatory efficacy. Acetaminophen is frequently combined with weak opioids for the treatment of moderate pain, and preparations are available featuring acetaminophen combined with codeine, hydrocodone, oxycodone, pentazocine, or propoxyphene. After deacetylation to its primary amine, acetaminophen is conjugated to arachidonic acid by fatty acid amide hydrolase in the brain and spinal cord; the product of this reaction, N-arachidonoylphenolamine, may inhibit COX-1 and COX-2 in the CNS. N-arachidonoylphenolamine is an endogenous cannabinoid and an agonist at TRPV1 receptors, suggesting that direct or indirect activation of TRPV1 and/or cannabinoid CB_1 receptors could also be involved in the mechanism of acetaminophen action. A major concern with acetaminophen use is its low therapeutic index; overdose can result in liver failure (see Chapter 6, Drug Toxicity).

Antidepressants

Drugs originally developed to treat depression are widely used as adjuvant therapy in pain management, particularly for treatment of chronic pain conditions. Although patients with chronic pain commonly experience depression, and reducing depression may improve quality of life, antidepressants have an analgesic action distinct from their antidepressant effect. Based on results from animal models, the analgesic action appears to be mediated mainly in the spinal cord and to involve the reduction of central sensitization. It is thought that tricyclic antidepressants produce analgesia both by blocking sodium channels and by increasing the activity of antinociceptive noradrenergic and serotonergic projections descending from the brain to the spinal cord. In general, the least selective agents (i.e., those with the broadest neurochemical effects), such as the tricyclics **amitriptyline**, **nortriptyline**, and **imipramine**, have been more effective than the selective serotonin reuptake inhibitors (SSRIs) **paroxetine**, **fluoxetine**, and **citalopram**. The use of these drugs in mood disorders is discussed in Chapter 15.

Venlafaxine and **duloxetine** are dual norepinephrine/serotonin (NE/5-HT) reuptake inhibitors with actions as both antidepressants and analgesics. These agents are used in the treatment of neuropathic pain and fibromyalgia. Duloxetine has a balanced action on NE and 5-HT reuptake and a weak action on dopamine reuptake as well. Although SSRIs have minimal analgesic action by themselves, inhibition of the serotonin reuptake transporter appears to produce some analgesic effect when NE reuptake is also blocked.

Antiepileptic Drugs and Antiarrhythmics

Some therapeutic agents used to control the excessive cellular excitability that leads to seizures (see Chapter 16) or cardiac arrhythmias (see Chapter 24) can also be used to manage the symptoms of some chronic pain conditions. In the search for drugs that produce analgesia, several of these agents have been tested on the basis of their ability to reduce neuronal excitability. Of these, the most widely used are the antiepileptic drugs **gabapentin** and **pregabalin**.

Gabapentin is widely used for the management of chronic pain. It was originally developed as a structural analogue of GABA, but it does not bind to GABA receptors and does not affect the metabolism or reuptake of GABA. Gabapentin binds to the $\alpha 2\delta$ subunit of voltage-dependent calcium channels and reduces the trafficking of the channel to the membrane. Randomized clinical trials in diabetic neuropathy and trigeminal neuralgia show that gabapentin is superior to placebo in reducing subjectively reported pain.

Gabapentin also has some efficacy in reducing postoperative pain. Gabapentin is associated with several adverse effects, particularly dizziness, somnolence, confusion, and ataxia. In the introductory case, gabapentin reduced JD's spontaneous paroxysmal pain, probably by decreasing aberrant neuronal excitability and synaptic transmission.

One problem with gabapentin is that its oral bioavailability is not predictable or linear. Some patients require 10 times as much drug as others to achieve a similar effect; this may be related to variable GI absorption. A newer antiepileptic drug with a similar structure is **pregabalin**; this substituted GABA analogue is more potent, has a faster onset of action, and has more predictable bioavailability than gabapentin. Pregabalin produces an analgesic effect similar to that of gabapentin in patients with neuropathic pain and fibromyalgia, and the two drugs have similar adverse CNS effects. Pregabalin also produces a mild euphoric effect in some patients. Because of its increased potency, it is claimed that dose-related adverse effects may be lower with pregabalin than with gabapentin.

Carbamazepine acts to block sodium channels; the drug is used primarily to treat trigeminal neuralgia, but it has a relatively high adverse effect profile. **Oxcarbazepine** is a close structural derivative of carbamazepine with an additional oxygen atom decorating the benzylcarboxamide group. This difference alters metabolism of the drug in the liver. More importantly, it reduces the risk of aplastic anemia, which is a serious adverse effect occasionally associated with carbamazepine. **Lidocaine**, a use-dependent sodium channel blocker, is typically used as a local anesthetic for regional anesthesia (see Chapter 12); this drug is also used topically in patches for patients with cutaneous pain, for example, patients with postherpetic neuralgia. In some instances, lidocaine administered intravenously can be valuable for blunting the autonomic response to short-term, high-intensity painful stimuli, such as the placement of cranial pins for head positioning in neurosurgical procedures.

NMDA Receptor Antagonists

Because of the critical role of NMDA receptors in the induction and maintenance of central sensitization, NMDA receptor antagonists are currently under investigation for use in pain treatment. Two currently available analgesic drugs act as antagonists at the NMDA receptor: the anesthetic **ketamine** and the antitussive **dextromethorphan**. Ketamine is widely used at high doses as an anesthetic induction agent and at lower doses for procedural sedation and for periprocedural pain relief. It can also be of utility in the periprocedural management of highly opioid-tolerant patients. Since ketamine has no μ-agonist properties, it is not a respiratory depressant; as such, it may be useful in circumstances in which analgesia is needed without concomitant respiratory compromise. Ketamine use is severely limited by its psychomimetic effects, which contribute to its abuse liability; ketamine can also suppress cardiac contractility while stimulating sympathetic activity.

Adrenergic Agonists

Stimulation of α_2-adrenergic receptors in the dorsal horn of the spinal cord produces an anti-nociceptive state. Therefore, α_2-adrenergic agonists may have therapeutic utility as analgesics. The α_2-agonist **clonidine** has been used systemically,

epidurally, intrathecally, and topically, and appears to produce analgesia in both acute and chronic pain states. However, clonidine also causes postural hypotension, which limits its usefulness in pain control.

Migraine Therapy

The treatment of migraine pain has features distinct from the treatment of other pain conditions. In many but not all patients, an effective treatment for migraine is the **triptan** class of serotonin receptor agonists; the best-studied example is **sumatriptan**. The triptans are selective for the $5\text{-}HT_{1B}$ and $5\text{-}HT_{1D}$ receptor subtypes of the $5\text{-}HT_1$ family, one of the seven families of serotonin receptor (see Chapter 15). $5\text{-}HT_{1B}$ receptors are located on vascular endothelial cells, smooth muscle cells, and neurons, including trigeminal nerves. $5\text{-}HT_{1D}$ receptors are present on the trigeminal nerves that innervate meningeal blood vessels. Triptans reduce both sensory activation in the periphery and nociceptive transmission in the brainstem trigeminal nucleus, where they diminish central sensitization. The triptans also cause vasoconstriction, opposing the vasodilation thought to be involved in the pathophysiology of migraine attacks. It remains unclear whether the vasoconstriction is helpful in producing the antimigraine actions of these drugs, however. Furthermore, as a result of this vasoconstrictive effect, the triptans can be dangerous in patients with coronary heart disease. The triptans can reduce the pain and other symptoms associated with acute migraine attack and have replaced the vasoconstrictive agent **ergotamine** in the treatment of migraine. Sumatriptan can be administered subcutaneously, orally, or by nasal inhalation; the nasal formulation may have an improved therapeutic index. Several other orally administered agents in the triptan class are also available, including **zolmitriptan**, **naratriptan**, and **rizatriptan** (see Drug Summary Table).

NSAIDs, opioids, caffeine, and antiemetics also have activity and some utility for treatment of acute migraine headaches. For example, a combination of indomethacin, prochlorperazine, and caffeine may have effectiveness similar to triptans in the treatment of migraine attacks. During an attack, migraine patients often experience gastric stasis that can reduce the bioavailability of oral medications. CGRP receptor antagonists are promising candidates for migraine therapy.

Although the triptans are relatively effective in ameliorating the acute symptoms of migraine, other classes of drugs are used to reduce the frequency of attacks. Several drug classes are used for migraine prophylaxis, including β-adrenergic blockers, valproic acid, serotonin antagonists, and calcium channel blockers. These agents are generally chosen based on the severity and frequency of the migraine attacks, the cost of the drug, and the adverse effects of the drug in the context of the individual patient. None has been shown to have a high level of efficacy, and new drugs need to be developed for more effective migraine prophylaxis.

▌ CONCLUSION AND FUTURE DIRECTIONS

Because of the limited efficacy of any single drug, it is common in clinical practice to use a polypharmacy approach to manage pain. In combination, several drugs that are only moderately effective as single agents can have additive or supra-additive effects. This is largely a consequence of the multiple processing events and mechanisms responsible for producing pain; intervention at several steps may be required to achieve adequate analgesia (Fig. 18-10). Because many drugs used to treat pain are also active systemically and/or in parts of the nervous system that are not related to somatic sensation, analgesics can produce deleterious adverse effects. One approach to limiting toxicity is to use localized (nonsystemic) forms of drug delivery. In particular, epidural and topical delivery limit exposure to the drug to a local site of action. Many of the opioids are short-acting and must be administered frequently to patients in severe pain. Modes of drug delivery have also been developed to optimize the pharmacokinetics of the short-acting opioids; these methods include transdermal and buccal dosage forms, patient-controlled analgesia devices, and controlled-release oral preparations. Patient-controlled devices ensure that patients do not suffer pain because of waning drug effects, and instrumental controls can effectively prevent overdose. At the present time, however, patient-controlled technologies are suitable only for inpatient treatment.

Most of the currently available analgesics have been identified by empirical observation (opioids, NSAIDs, and local anesthetics) or serendipity (antiepileptic drugs). Now that the mechanisms responsible for pain are being explored at a molecular level, many new targets are being revealed that are likely to lead to new and different classes of analgesics. It is hoped that drugs active at these targets will achieve higher efficacy and have fewer adverse effects than current therapies. Effective pain management approaches must not rely only on pharmacologic intervention; physical therapy and rehabilitation and, in some situations, surgical approaches may also have a role. The growing complexity of pain management has spawned specialized pain services for inpatient pain control, as well as pain clinics and centers for the outpatient management of chronic pain.

Acknowledgment

The authors thank Salahadin Abdi, Rami Burstein, and Carl Rosow for their valuable comments.

Suggested Reading

Chou R, Turner JA, Devine EB, et al. The effectiveness and risks of long term opioid therapy for chronic pain: a systemic review for a National Institutes of Health Pathways to Prevention Workshop. *Ann Intern Med* 2015;162:276–286. (*A systematic review of randomized controlled trials using opioids to treat chronic pain.*)

Costigan M, Scholz J, Woolf CJ. Neuropathic pain: a maladaptive response of the nervous system to damage. *Annu Rev Neurosci* 2009;32:1–32. (*Overview of mechanisms of neuropathic pain.*)

Finnerup NB, Attal N, Haroutounian S, et al. Pharmacotherapy for neuropathic pain in adults: a systematic review and meta-analysis. *Lancet Neurol* 2015;14:162–173. (*Clinical approach to management of neuropathic pain.*)

Rosow CE, Dershwitz M. Pharmacology of opioid analgesics. In: Longnecker D, Brown DL, Newman MF, Zapol WM, eds. *Anesthesiology.* New York: McGraw Hill; 2008. (*Detailed review of opioid pharmacology.*)

von Hehn CA, Baron R, Woolf CJ. Deconstructing the neuropathic pain phenotype to reveal neural mechanisms. *Neuron* 2012;73:638–652.

Waxman SG, Merkles IS, Gerrits MM, et al. Sodium channel genes in pain-related disorders: phenotype-genotype associations and recommendations for clinical use. *Lancet Neurol* 2014;13:1152–1160. (*Reviews channelopathies that produce pain and their treatment.*)

Woolf CJ. Central sensitization: implications for the diagnosis and treatment of pain. *Pain* 2011;152(3)(Suppl):S2–S15.

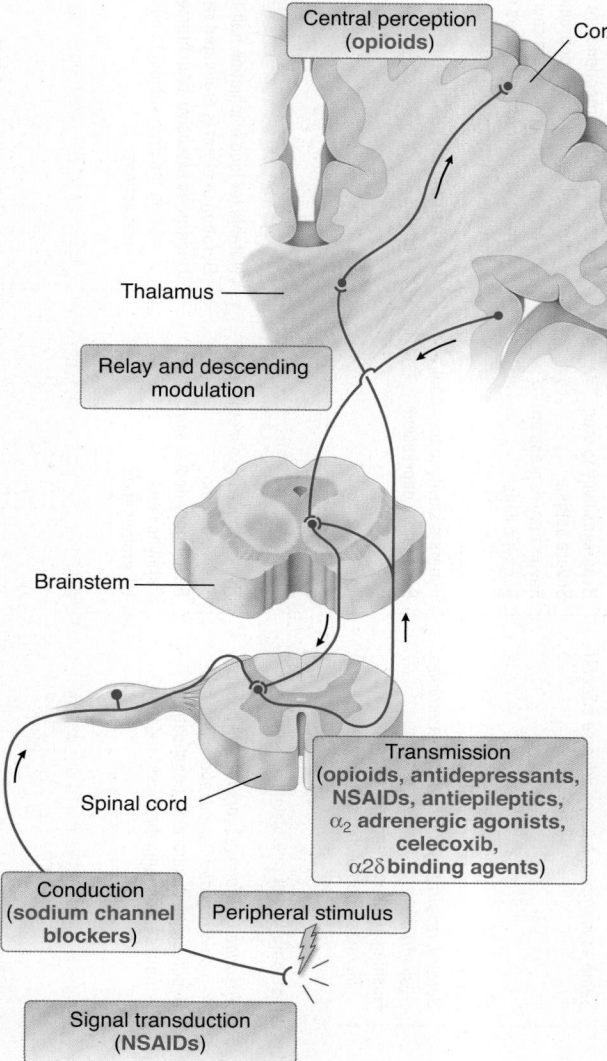

FIGURE 18-10. Summary of the sites of action of the major drug classes used for pain management. Analgesics target various steps in pain perception, from the initiation of a pain stimulus to the central perception of that pain. NSAIDs modulate the initial membrane depolarization (signal transduction) in response to a peripheral stimulus. Sodium channel blockers decrease action potential conduction in nociceptive fibers. Opioids, antidepressants, NSAIDs, antiepileptic drugs (anticonvulsants), and α_2-adrenergic agonists all modulate transmission of pain sensation in the spinal cord by decreasing the signal relayed from peripheral to central pain pathways. Opioids also modulate the central perception of painful stimuli. The multiple sites of action of analgesics allow a combination drug approach to be used in pain management. For example, moderate pain is often treated with combinations of opioids and NSAIDs. Because these drugs have different mechanisms and sites of action, the combination of the drugs is more effective than one drug alone.

DRUG SUMMARY TABLE: CHAPTER 18 Pharmacology of Analgesia

DRUG	CLINICAL APPLICATIONS	SERIOUS AND COMMON ADVERSE EFFECTS	CONTRAINDICATIONS	THERAPEUTIC CONSIDERATIONS
μ-OPIOID RECEPTOR AGONISTS				
Morphine, Codeine, and Semisynthetic Derivatives				
Mechanism—Natural or semisynthetic agonists at the μ-opioid receptor that result in inhibition of neurotransmission				
Morphine **Hydromorphone**	Pain (moderate to severe)	*Anaphylactoid reaction, respiratory depression, abuse potential* Pruritus, constipation, nausea, vomiting, dizziness, headache, sedation, urinary retention, miosis	Hypersensitivity to drug Paralytic ileus Severe asthma Respiratory depression Acute alcoholism and delirium tremens Cardiovascular disease CNS depression	Morphine is metabolized in the liver, and its active metabolite M6G is excreted by the kidneys; dose adjustment may be required in patients with renal disease. Controlled-release oral preparations reduce the number of daily doses, but these formulations are associated with abuse potential. Intravenous or subcutaneous morphine is commonly used in patient-controlled analgesia devices. Epidural or intrathecal morphine can produce highly effective analgesia by achieving locally high concentrations in the dorsal horn of the spinal cord.
Codeine	Pain (mild to moderate)	*Same as morphine*	Hypersensitivity to codeine Use in children is controversial Severe asthma Respiratory depression Paralytic ileus	Much less effective than morphine in pain treatment. Used for its antitussive and antidiarrheal effects. High variability among individuals in potency.
Oxycodone **Hydrocodone**	Pain (moderate to severe)	*Same as morphine (shared adverse effects)*	Hypersensitivity to drug Severe asthma Respiratory depression Paralytic ileus	Oxycodone and hydrocodone are hepatically metabolized via the cytochrome P450 system. The primary drug is likely the source of the therapeutic effect, while drug metabolites may be involved in drug interactions and variations in drug response.
Tramadol	Pain (moderate to severe)	*Seizure, respiratory depression, serotonin syndrome* Flushing, nausea, vomiting, constipation, dizziness, headache, somnolence	Hypersensitivity to tramadol Respiratory depression	May interact with SSRIs and other serotonergic agents.
Synthetic Agonists				
Mechanism—Synthetic agonists at the μ-opioid receptor that result in inhibition of neurotransmission				
Methadone	Detoxification of patients with opioid addiction Severe pain	*Prolonged QT interval, torsades de pointes, respiratory depression, abuse potential* Hypotension, diaphoresis, constipation, nausea, vomiting, dizziness, sedation	Hypersensitivity to methadone Severe asthma Respiratory depression Paralytic ileus QT prolongation	Notable for long elimination half-life. Duration of effect is prolonged with repeat dosing. Undergoes extensive cytochrome P450 metabolism, making the drug subject to numerous drug–drug interactions.

Drug	Indications	Contraindications	Adverse Effects	Notes
Fentanyl **Alfentanil** **Sufentanil**	Pain (moderate to severe)	Hypersensitivity to drug Severe asthma Respiratory depression Paralytic ileus	*Bradycardia, respiratory depression, paralytic ileus, coma, abuse potential, seizure (shared adverse effects)* Constipation, nausea, vomiting, somnolence, pruritus (shared adverse effects)	Fentanyl is more potent than morphine and is bioavailable via several routes. Fentanyl's analgesic effect is limited by redistribution to inactive tissue stores. Transmucosal administration of fentanyl (as lozenge) is useful in pediatric patients; a transdermal (patch) formulation releases the drug slowly over time. Alfentanil and sufentanil are structurally related to fentanyl; alfentanil is less potent than fentanyl, whereas sufentanil is more potent than fentanyl.
Remifentanil	Pain (moderate to severe) Primarily used for anesthesia or sedation	Hypersensitivity to remifentanil	*Respiratory depression, anaphylaxis, bradycardia* Pruritus, nausea, vomiting, myoclonus, headache	Remifentanil has unusually rapid metabolism and elimination, requiring co-administration of a longer acting drug to maintain analgesia postoperatively. Remifentanil permits precise matching of the drug dose to the clinical response.
Meperidine	Pain (moderate to severe)	Hypersensitivity to meperidine Recent or concomitant use of MAOIs Respiratory depression	*Cardiac arrest, hypotension, anaphylaxis, myoclonus, raised intracranial pressure, seizure, respiratory depression* Sweating, nausea, vomiting, dizziness, sedation, mydriasis	The toxic metabolite normeperidine can cause increased CNS excitability and seizures. Renal excretion of normeperidine makes toxicity a problem in repeat-dosing regimens and in patients with kidney disease. Unlike other opioids, meperidine causes mydriasis rather than miosis. Recent or concomitant MAOI use is an absolute contraindication due to the risk of life-threatening serotonin syndrome. Co-administration with selegiline or sibutramine is usually avoided due to the theoretical risk of serotonin syndrome.

Partial and Mixed Agonists

Mechanism—Partial μ-receptor agonist (buprenorphine) and κ-agonist with partial μ-antagonist activity (nalbuphine)

Drug	Indications	Contraindications	Adverse Effects	Notes
Buprenorphine	Pain (moderate to severe) Opioid dependence	Hypersensitivity to buprenorphine Severe asthma Respiratory depression Paralytic ileus	*Hypotension, prolonged QT interval, severe application site reaction, hepatotoxicity, anaphylaxis, coma, respiratory depression, abuse potential* Constipation, nausea, vomiting, dizziness, headache, somnolence	Long elimination half-life; ceiling effect for both therapeutic and adverse effects due to partial agonist activity. Patients chronically exposed to other opioids should discontinue the other opioid prior to initiating buprenorphine to avoid acute opioid withdrawal.
Nalbuphine	Pain (moderate to severe)	Hypersensitivity to nalbuphine	*Hypersensitivity reaction, seizure, respiratory depression* Diaphoresis, nausea, vomiting, dizziness, headache, sedation	Commonly used to reverse the pruritus induced by neuraxial opioid administration.

continues

DRUG SUMMARY TABLE: CHAPTER 18 Pharmacology of Analgesia *continued*

DRUG	CLINICAL APPLICATIONS	*SERIOUS* AND COMMON ADVERSE EFFECTS	CONTRAINDICATIONS	THERAPEUTIC CONSIDERATIONS
OPIOID RECEPTOR ANTAGONISTS **Mechanism**—Antagonists at μ-opioid receptor that block endogenous or exogenous opioid effects				
Naloxone **Naltrexone**	Acute opioid toxicity Opioid and alcohol addiction (naltrexone only)	*Cardiac arrhythmia, hypertension, hypotension, hepatotoxicity, pulmonary edema, opioid withdrawal (shared adverse effects)* Nausea, vomiting, acute opioid withdrawal (shared adverse effects)	Hypersensitivity to drug	Naltrexone is primarily used in outpatient settings. Naloxone has short half-life
Methylnaltrexone	Postoperative ileus, opioid-induced bowel dysfunction	*Gastrointestinal perforation* Diaphoresis, abdominal pain, flatulence, nausea, dizziness	Gastrointestinal obstruction	Antagonist at *peripheral* μ-opioid receptors; prevents morphine-induced constipation but has no effect on morphine analgesia
NONSTEROIDAL ANALGESICS **Mechanism**—Affect prostaglandin synthetic pathway				
Acetaminophen **Aspirin** **Naproxen** **Ibuprofen** **Indomethacin** **Diclofenac** **Piroxicam** **Celecoxib** **Diclofenac** **Ketorolac**	See Drug Summary Table: Chapter 43 Pharmacology of Eicosanoids			
TRICYCLIC ANTIDEPRESSANTS AND SEROTONIN-NOREPINEPHRINE REUPTAKE INHIBITORS **Mechanism**—Promote serotonergic and noradrenergic neurotransmission by inhibiting neurotransmitter reuptake				
Amitriptyline **Nortriptyline** **Imipramine** **Desipramine** **Duloxetine** **Venlafaxine**	See Drug Summary Table: Chapter 15 Pharmacology of Serotonergic and Central Adrenergic Neurotransmission			

ANTIEPILEPTIC DRUGS AND ANTIARRHYTHMICS
Mechanism—Inhibit action potential initiation or conduction

Carbamazepine
Oxcarbazepine
Gabapentin
Pregabalin
Lamotrigine

See Drug Summary Table: Chapter 16 Pharmacology of Abnormal Electrical Neurotransmission in the Central Nervous System

Mexiletine

See Drug Summary Table: Chapter 24 Pharmacology of Cardiac Rhythm

NMDA RECEPTOR ANTAGONISTS
Mechanism—Block NMDA receptor-dependent postsynaptic depolarization

Ketamine	*Cardiac arrhythmia, hypotension, anaphylaxis, laryngeal spasm, respiratory depression* Hypertension, tachycardia, psychiatric symptoms	Hypersensitivity to ketamine Severe hypertension	Minimal risk of respiratory depression. Wider application of ketamine is limited by its psychomimetic effects.
Analgesia Anesthesia			

5-HT$_{1D}$ SEROTONIN RECEPTOR AGONISTS
Mechanism—Induce cerebrovascular vasoconstriction, reduce nociceptive transmission

Sumatriptan
Rizatriptan
Naratriptan
Zolmitriptan
Almotriptan
Eletriptan

See Drug Summary Table: Chapter 15 Pharmacology of Serotonergic and Central Adrenergic Neurotransmission

19

Pharmacology of Drugs of Abuse

Peter R. Martin and Sachin Patel

INTRODUCTION

This chapter considers pharmacologic agents implicated in substance use disorders and the relevant brain processes involved in the clinical progression of these disorders. While the pharmacology of these agents is important to understanding their effects on behavior and their abuse liability, personality characteristics, as well as the presence of co-occurring psychiatric and medical conditions, may also contribute to the risk of developing substance use disorders. Understanding substance use disorders as biopsychosocial syndromes, rather than simply the pharmacologic consequences of chronic alcohol/drug use, has led to recognition of the central role that learning plays in substance use disorders and the potential for an integrated pharmacopsychosocial approach to treatment.

Most individuals with substance use disorders also have a second diagnosable psychiatric condition, but it is not easy to determine whether psychiatric symptoms are a cause or consequence of alcohol/drug use. For example, although alcohol is widely used to self-medicate depression and/or anxiety, it may be difficult to determine whether such psychiatric symptoms in alcoholics are the cause of drinking or its effect, because the actions of alcohol per se, as well as alcohol withdrawal and dependence, can also result in significant anxiety or depression.

Genetic determinants of the psychopharmacologic actions of abused drugs are increasingly recognized. Nonetheless, environmental variables have a significant influence on the development of substance use. For example, societal attitudes toward substance use often influence the likelihood that a substance will be taken in the first place. The availability and cost of a substance are also affected by its legal and tax status. The availability of other, nondrug alternatives may be a key factor in determining the likelihood that substance use disorders emerge for a given agent.

This chapter describes the mechanisms of action of selected representative substances of abuse, and the mechanisms of other important substances of abuse are summarized in Table 19-1. Since addiction is a disorder of brain reward pathways, learning, and motivated behavior, the use of medications in an *integrated* pharmacopsychosocial approach to treat substance use disorders is also discussed.

DEFINITIONS

The empirically based nomenclature promulgated by the American Psychiatric Association (APA) in the Diagnostic and Statistical Manual (DSM, Box 19-1) defines **substance use disorder** (used interchangeably in this chapter with **addiction**) as "a problematic pattern of use" leading to "significant impairment or distress." This definition avoids value judgment and is generalizable across cultures. Psychosocial features of substance use disorders are similar for diverse psychopharmacologic agents with abuse liability and are likely more important in the development and maintenance of pathologic drug use than the unique pharmacologic profile

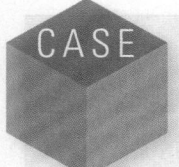

CASE

CA, a 33-year-old man, is brought to the emergency department with chills, severe nausea, vomiting, diarrhea, muscle aches, and anxiety. Mr. A explains that he is currently shooting morphine or heroin about 3 days per week and using marijuana or cocaine "whenever." He feels he wants to die. On examination, he has enlarged pupils, temperature is 103°F, blood pressure is 170/95 mm Hg, and heart rate is 108 beats/min. He is irritable and has abdominal cramping, hyperalgesia, and photophobia. Mr. A is given clonidine, with loperamide, ibuprofen, and promethazine as needed for diarrhea, pain, and nausea/vomiting, respectively. The severity of withdrawal does not diminish significantly until he is given sublingual buprenorphine/naloxone every 8 hours. Over the next week, Mr. A's buprenorphine/naloxone is titrated to a once-daily dose, with progressive diminution of withdrawal symptoms and drug craving.

Mr. A is discharged to a 28-day intensive outpatient treatment program during which he continues buprenorphine/naloxone. He agrees to attend daily mutual support self-help meetings (Alcoholics or Narcotics Anonymous), where he tells the tale of his addiction. *He began diet pills in his teens for weight control and drinking as a response to physical abuse by his alcoholic father. He was prescribed acetaminophen and codeine for pain after minor surgery; thereafter, he started "street" pain pills and "doctor shopping" for back pain and depression, and he even had healthy teeth extracted to get opioids from the dentist. He was distraught when a close relative died, and he switched to intravenous opioids, including fentanyl patches that he ate or injected. He had three inpatient treatments, always relapsing after discharge to increasingly higher drug doses. He also tried methadone maintenance treatment for 6 months with some benefit but was unable to completely stop using "street drugs" and "never felt normal on methadone."*

Mr. A continues to be abstinent from illicit opioids after 10 years on sublingual buprenorphine/naloxone. He visits his psychiatrist monthly for psychotherapy and adheres to his treatment contract of monthly attendance at group therapy and weekly Narcotics Anonymous (NA) or Alcoholics Anonymous (AA) meetings. He consistently provides drug-free urine tests. He has been promoted at work, has negotiated a loan for purchase of a house, and seems relatively content having gained considerable understanding about management of his drug use disorder. Recently, he has begun discussing tapering and eventually discontinuing buprenorphine/naloxone maintenance.

Questions

1. What caused Mr. A's physical symptoms and signs (i.e., chills, nausea, vomiting, fever, enlarged pupils, and hypertension) on his initial visit to the emergency department?
2. How could Mr. A's pain be managed if he were to need surgery while taking buprenorphine/naloxone?
3. How can mutual support programs such as AA or NA help treat addiction, and how should such programs be complemented by medical oversight?
4. What was the rationale for initiating clonidine treatment for Mr. A?
5. Why did Mr. A's initial symptoms and long-term opioid craving abate with the combination of buprenorphine/naloxone? How long should maintenance be continued?

of any given drug. Diagnostic features are conceptualized as clinical clusters "of cognitive, behavioral, and physiological symptoms indicating that the individual continues using the substance despite significant substance-related problems:" loss of control, salience to the behavioral repertoire, and neuroadaptation. However, the fundamental element is **drug-seeking**, the sine qua non of addiction. In the introductory case, Mr. A felt that he had little else than drugs in his life and could not stop using without help, and it is likely that he was addicted to opioids (and to the other drugs he was using).

The terms *tolerance*, *dependence*, and *withdrawal* may be defined based on clinically apparent physiologic changes as well as more subtle alterations in brain reward neurocircuitry. **Tolerance** refers to the decreased effect of a substance that develops with continued use, in other words, the dose–response curve shifts to the right as *larger doses are needed to produce the same response*, as happened in the case of Mr. A. The drug toxicity profile and the drug lethality profile often do not shift in the same way or to the same degree as the psychopharmacologic effect(s) for which the drug is primarily self-administered. Thus, when taking heroin, it is likely that Mr. A experienced adverse effects of constipation and pupillary

constriction at a dose insufficient to get "high." Additionally, since the brain respiratory centers often do not develop tolerance to increased doses of heroin, a lethal overdose is more likely as a person takes higher doses of this drug. The opposite effect, termed **sensitization** (also called **inverse tolerance**), refers to a shift of the dose–response curve to the left, so that *repeated administrations of a drug result in a greater effect of a given dose*, and a lower dose is required to achieve the same effect. Interestingly, tolerance and sensitization to different pharmacologic actions of a drug may occur concurrently. Thus, upon repeated administration of central nervous system (CNS) depressants like alcohol, stimulant effects (e.g., disinhibition) demonstrate sensitization, whereas depressant actions (e.g., sleep) acquire tolerance.

Dependence can be defined only *indirectly* by (1) tolerance, (2) the emergence of a withdrawal syndrome upon drug discontinuation or administration of a specific antagonist, (3) drug "craving," or (4) drug-seeking behavior manifested as a result of conditioned stimuli after withdrawal has abated. In Mr. A's case, his initial symptoms in the emergency department were caused by heroin withdrawal, a manifestation of **physical dependence** that could be alleviated by any

TABLE 19-1 Major Drugs of Abuse

DRUG CLASS	EXAMPLES	RECEPTOR (ACTION)	CLINICAL SIGNS	NOTES
Opioids	Morphine Heroin Codeine Oxycodone	μ-Opioid (agonist)	Euphoria, followed by sedation, respiratory depression	Used therapeutically as analgesics (except for heroin) Prescription opioid abuse is rapidly increasing
Benzodiazepines	Triazolam Lorazepam Diazepam	GABA$_A$ (modulator)	Sedation, respiratory depression	Used therapeutically as anxiolytics, sedatives; risk of overdose death in combination with alcohol or opioids
Barbiturates	Phenobarbital Pentobarbital	GABA$_A$ (modulator, weak agonist)	Sedation, respiratory depression	Used therapeutically as anxiolytics and sedatives; greater danger of death from overdose than benzodiazepines
Alcohol	Ethanol	GABA$_A$ (modulator), NMDA (antagonist)	Intoxication, sedation, memory loss	Legal in many countries and often used in conjunction with other psychoactive agents
Nicotine	Tobacco	Nicotinic ACh (agonist)	Alertness, muscle relaxation	Legal in many countries and often complicates other drug use disorders
Psychostimulants	Cocaine Amphetamine	Dopamine, adrenergic, serotonin (reuptake inhibitor)	Euphoria, alertness, hypertension, paranoia	Amphetamines also reverse the reuptake transporter and release neurotransmitter from synaptic vesicles into the cytoplasm
Caffeine	Coffee Soft drinks	Adenosine (antagonist)	Alertness, tremulousness	Generally legal, addiction rare
Cannabinoids	Cannabis	CB$_1$, CB$_2$ (agonist)	Changes in mood, hunger, giddiness	Controversial recent legalization in many states of US
Phencyclidine (PCP)	N/A	NMDA (antagonist)	Hallucinations, hostile behavior	Effects may be confused with psychosis
Phenylethylamines	MDMA (Ecstasy), MDA	Serotonin, dopamine, adrenergic (reuptake inhibitors, multiple actions)	Euphoria, alertness, hypertension, hallucinations	Structurally related to amphetamines, effects similar to psychedelic agents, may cause lasting injury to serotonergic neurons
Psychedelic agents	LSD DMT Psilocybin	5-HT$_2$ (partial agonist)	Hallucinations	Flashbacks may relate to overlearning of traumatic experience with intoxication
Inhalants	Toluene Amyl nitrate Nitrous oxide	Unknown	Dizziness, intoxication	May result in lasting brain damage

MDMA, methylenedioxymethamphetamine; MDA, methylenedioxyamphetamine; LSD, lysergic acid diethylamide; DMT, dimethyltryptamine; GABA, γ-aminobutyric acid; ACh, acetylcholine; CB, cannabinoid; 5-HT, serotonin; NMDA, N-methyl-D-aspartate.

μ-opioid receptor agonist. Physical dependence is sometimes distinguished from **psychological dependence**, or the continued craving for drug and proclivity to return to out-of-control opioid use even after acute withdrawal symptoms have abated. Physical dependence results from many of the same mechanisms that produce tolerance. As with tolerance, homeostatic set-points are altered to compensate for the presence of the drug. If drug use is discontinued, the altered set-points produce effects opposite to those manifested in the presence of the drug. The altered set-points also activate autonomic nervous system stress responses, which partially explains the benefits of drugs such as clonidine in treating withdrawal. For example, abrupt withdrawal from a CNS depressant involves hyperarousal, whereas withdrawal from a stimulant involves depression and lethargy; discontinuing a drug of either class results in a nonspecific increase in autonomic activity. Psychological dependence involves resetting the **reward system** of the brain as a result of repeated drug use. Thus, even after

drug use has ceased, brain reward mechanisms may be altered so that affective and neuroendocrine disturbances and drug craving persist and the individual is prone to relapse. There is significant neurobiological overlap between "psychological" and "physical" components of dependence, and some have questioned the real utility of such a distinction. In any event, the recently published DSM-5 eschews the term "dependence" because the clinical and pharmacologic meanings of this term can be confusing. The newly adopted diagnostic term is "substance use disorder," which is meant unequivocally to serve as a clinical construct, whereas dependence retains its pharmacologic meaning only (Box 19-1).

Tolerance and dependence typically coexist, but the presence of either does not necessarily imply pathologic drug use. For example, a patient given an opioid for surgical pain will likely develop tolerance to the drug and require progressively larger doses for analgesia; moreover, should drug administration cease or an opioid antagonist be given,

BOX 19-1 Criteria for Substance Use Disorders (Addiction) from the Diagnostic and Statistical Manual of Mental Disorders, Fifth Edition (DSM-5)

A problematic pattern of substance use leading to clinically significant impairment or distress, as manifested by at least two of the following, occurring within a 12-month period:

1. The substance is often taken in larger amounts or over a longer period than was intended.
2. There is a persistent desire or unsuccessful efforts to cut down or control substance use.
3. A great deal of time is spent in activities necessary to obtain the substance (e.g., visiting multiple doctors or driving long distances), to use the substance (e.g., chain-smoking), or to recover from its effects.
4. Craving, or a strong desire or urge to use the substance.
5. Recurrent substance use resulting in a failure to fulfill major role obligations at work, school, or home.
6. Continued substance use despite having persistent or recurrent social or interpersonal problems caused or exacerbated by the effects of the substance.
7. Important social, occupational, or recreational activities are given up or reduced because of substance use.
8. Recurrent substance use in situations in which it is physically hazardous.
9. Substance use is continued despite knowledge of having a persistent or recurrent physical or psychological problem that is likely to have been caused or exacerbated by the substance (e.g., current cocaine use despite recognition of cocaine-induced depression, or continued drinking despite recognition that an ulcer was made worse by alcohol consumption).
10. Tolerance, as defined by either of the following:
    a. A need for markedly increased amounts of the substance to achieve intoxication or desired effect.
    b. A markedly diminished effect with continued use of the same amount of substance.
11. Withdrawal, as manifested by either of the following:
    a. The characteristic withdrawal syndrome for the substance (as defined by the APA criteria for withdrawal for a specific substance).
    b. The same (or closely related) substance is taken to relieve or avoid withdrawal symptoms. ■

The presence of 2–3 of the above symptoms is specified as "Mild" substance use disorder; 4–5 symptoms, "Moderate" substance use disorder; and 6 or more symptoms, "Severe" substance use disorder.
Reprinted with permission from the American Psychiatric Association. *Diagnostic and statistical manual of mental disorders.* 5th ed. Arlington, VA: American Psychiatric Association; 2013

the patient will likely develop a withdrawal syndrome. However, it will likely be possible to taper and eventually eliminate the analgesic once the surgical basis of pain abates. In this case, if the patient does not manifest drug-seeking behavior, a pathologic condition (substance use disorder) is not present despite the presence of tolerance and dependence. This point underlines the vital role of physicians in (1) effectively treating postsurgical pain without providing open-ended opioid prescriptions and (2) directly addressing drug-seeking should it arise.

MECHANISMS OF TOLERANCE, DEPENDENCE, AND WITHDRAWAL

Tolerance

Acquired tolerance results when repeated administration of a drug shifts the dose–response curve of the drug to the right, so that a larger dose of the drug is required to produce the same effect. **Innate tolerance** refers to preexisting interindividual variations in sensitivity to the drug (i.e., variations that are present before the first administration of the drug). Innate differences in sensitivity can arise from genetic variation of receptors at which the drug acts or differences among individuals in drug absorption, metabolism, or excretion. As with any multifactorial trait, genetic variability is strongly influenced by the environment. An example of innate tolerance is observed with alcohol: those with low innate sensitivity as young adults are at higher risk for alcoholism later in life.

Acquired tolerance includes pharmacokinetic, pharmacodynamic, and learned components. **Pharmacokinetic tolerance**

develops when the capacity to metabolize or excrete the drug increases as a result of drug exposure. Increased metabolism is typically attributable to induction of metabolic enzymes such as the cytochrome P450s (see Chapter 4, Drug Metabolism). In such cases, pharmacokinetic tolerance results in a *lower concentration* of drug at its site of action for any given dose.

Pharmacodynamic tolerance is caused by neuronal adaptations resulting in *reduced response* to the same concentration of drug at its site of action in the nervous system. Short-term exposure to a drug can induce neuroadaptive changes in neurotransmitter release and clearance from the synapse, a decrease in the number of neurotransmitter receptors, altered conductance of ion channels, or modified signal transduction (Fig. 19-1). Longer term administration of the drug can cause neuroadaptive changes in the expression of genes relevant to the pharmacologic action of the drug; these changes are closely linked with adaptations in the brain that are thought to be involved in learning and memory formation (Fig. 19-2). Indeed, persistent adaptations to drug use both modify existing synapses and create new synapses, effectively "rewiring" the brain. Such long-lasting molecular and cellular adaptations are likely to explain the cravings and relapses that can occur long after drug use has been discontinued.

Pharmacodynamic tolerance is closely related to another form of tolerance, termed **learned tolerance**. In **behavioral tolerance**, a form of learned tolerance, drug use results in compensatory changes in behavior that are not directly related to the pharmacologic action of the drug but rather to accommodation to drug effects through learning acquired while the person is in the intoxicated "state" or in the environment in which the intoxication occurred. **Conditioned tolerance**

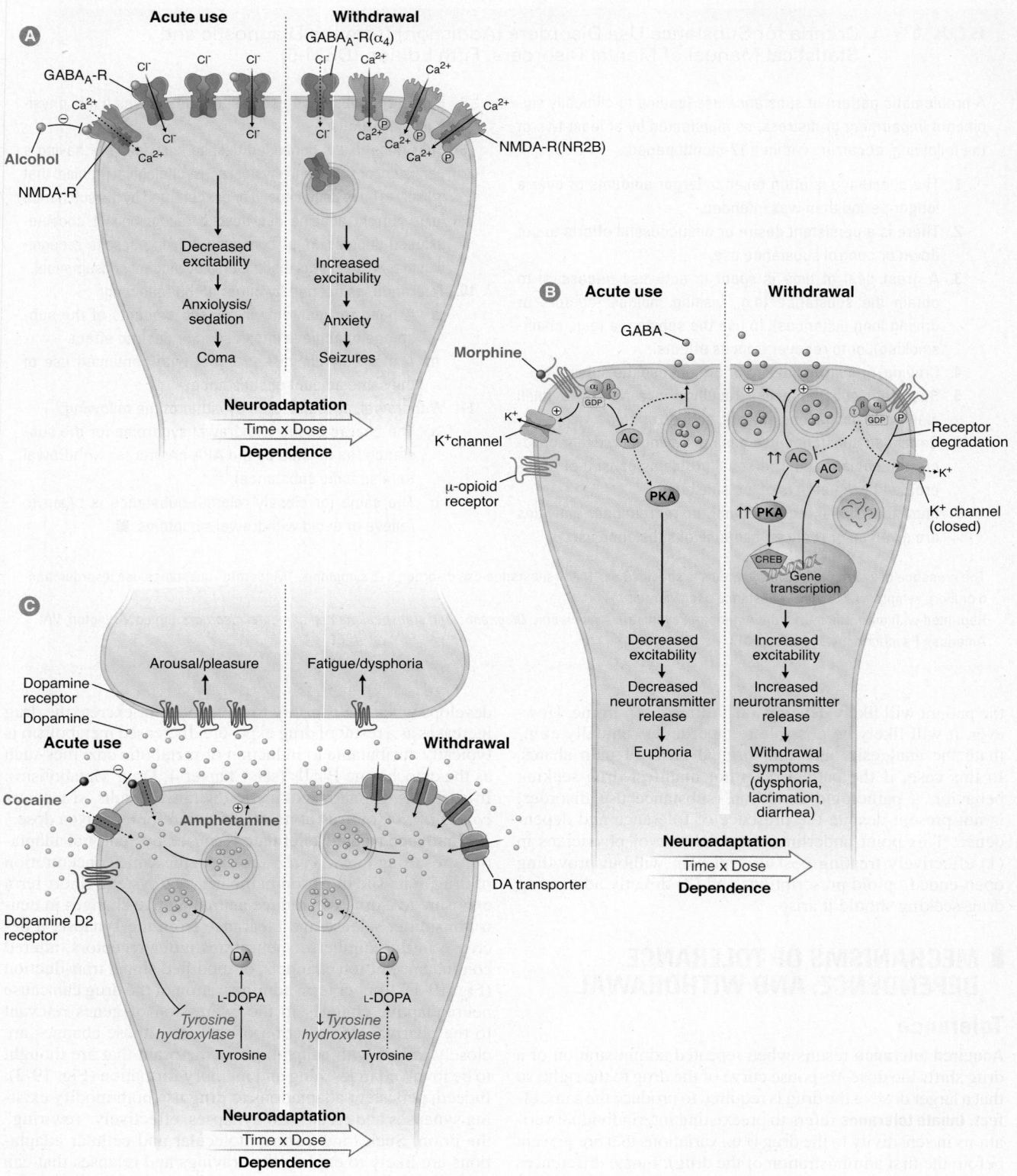

FIGURE 19-1. **Mechanisms of acute drug action for depressants, opioids, and psychostimulants and development of neuroadaptation and dependence in response to chronic drug use. A.** Alcohol modulates the major inhibitory and excitatory neurotransmitter systems of the brain via effects on $GABA_A$ and NMDA receptors ($GABA_A$-R and NMDA-R), respectively. Alcohol is a positive allosteric modulator of $GABA_A$ receptors. Alcohol increases chloride conductance through $GABA_A$ receptors, resulting in cellular hyperpolarization. Alcohol also decreases calcium conductance through NMDA receptors, further decreasing cellular excitation. These dual actions on $GABA_A$ and NMDA receptors contribute to alcohol's anxiolytic, sedative, and CNS-depressant effects. Molecular adaptations to chronic alcohol exposure include (1) internalization and decreased surface expression of "normal" $\alpha 1$ subunit-containing $GABA_A$ receptors, (2) increased surface expression of "low alcohol sensitivity" $\alpha 4$ subunit-containing $GABA_A$ receptors, and (3) increased phosphorylation of NMDA receptors containing "high conductance" NR2B subunits. Thus, neuroadaptation results in tolerance to the acute depressant effects of alcohol and occurs concomitantly with dependence. During withdrawal (i.e., in the dependent state but in the absence of alcohol), these adaptations result in generalized hyperexcitability of neurons. CNS excitation is expressed as anxiety, insomnia, delirium, and potentially seizures. **B.** Opioids activate μ-opioid receptors located on synaptic nerve terminals. Acute activation of μ-opioid receptors results in G protein-dependent activation of potassium channels and inhibition of adenylyl cyclase activity. These effects result in cellular hyperpolarization and decreased GABA release from the nerve terminal; the decreased GABA release results in disinhibition of ventral tegmental area (VTA) dopamine neurons. Molecular adaptations to chronic μ-opioid receptor stimulation include (1) increased μ-opioid receptor phosphorylation, resulting in receptor internalization and degradation; (2) decreased efficacy of μ-opioid signal transduction; and (3) hyperactivation of adenylyl cyclase signaling, leading to enhanced GABA release and to increased gene transcription via activation of transcription factors including cyclic AMP response element binding protein (CREB). Thus, neuroadaptation results in tolerance to the euphoric effects of opioids. During withdrawal (i.e., in the dependent state but in the absence of opioid), the enhanced GABA release from inhibitory interneurons results in inhibition of VTA dopamine neurons, dysphoria, and anhedonia. **C.** Acute cocaine exposure inhibits dopamine reuptake transporters (DAT), resulting in increased synaptic dopamine levels and increased postsynaptic dopamine receptor activation at synapses in the nucleus accumbens; in turn, these effects cause feelings of euphoria and increased energy. Increased extrasynaptic dopamine also results in D_2 autoreceptor activation, which decreases dopamine synthesis. Amphetamine both releases vesicular transmitter stores into the cytoplasm and inhibits neurotransmitter reuptake into vesicles; these combined actions cause neurotransmitter concentrations to increase in the synaptic cleft. During chronic psychostimulant exposure, DAT expression increases, the number of postsynaptic dopamine receptors decreases, and presynaptic dopamine is depleted. Thus, neuroadaptation results in tolerance to the euphoric effects of psychostimulants. During withdrawal (i.e., in the dependent state but in the absence of psychostimulant), the decreased synaptic levels of dopamine that result from reduced dopamine synthesis and increased clearance through DAT cause decreased activation of postsynaptic dopamine receptors and feelings of dysphoria, fatigue, and anhedonia.

occurs when environmental cues associated with exposure to a drug induce preemptive, reflexive compensatory changes, called a **conditioned opponent response**. This mechanism of conditioning is an unconscious phenomenon but is often the basis for relapse in addicts. For example, seeing paraphernalia associated with use of a drug such as cocaine (which produces tachycardia) may elicit preemptive bradycardia and, thus, craving for the drug.

Dependence and Withdrawal

Dependence is typically associated with tolerance, and it results from mechanisms closely related to those that produce pharmacodynamic and learned tolerance. Substance use disorders are clinical manifestations of dependence and result from the need for the drug to be present in the brain to maintain "near-normal" functioning. If the drug is eliminated from the body so that it no longer occupies its site of action, the adaptations that produced dependence are unmasked and manifested as an **acute withdrawal syndrome** that lasts until the system re-equilibrates to the absence of drug (days). Subsequently, a **protracted withdrawal syndrome**, characterized by **craving** for the drug (i.e., an intense preoccupation with obtaining the drug), may emerge and continue indefinitely (years). Protracted withdrawal is also associated with subtle dysregulation of learning, drives/motivations, reward, and the potential for relapse. This syndrome should be distinguished from premorbid risk factors for addiction that do not resolve with abstinence and from brain injury that is sustained as a result of drug use.

Like tolerance, dependence is associated with changes in cellular signaling pathways (Fig. 19-1). For example, up-regulation of the cAMP pathway by a drug contributes to acute withdrawal upon discontinuation of the drug because up-regulated adenylyl cyclase causes a "supranormal" response in neurons when physiologic levels of neurotransmitter stimulate the cAMP-coupled receptor. Conversely, a drug

that produces dependence by decreasing receptor number or receptor sensitivity renders the down-regulated receptors understimulated by physiologic levels of neurotransmitter after drug discontinuation.

The effects of alcohol illustrate that excitatory and inhibitory mechanisms can act in a synergistic fashion on opposing neurotransmitter systems. Acute alcohol intake causes sedation by facilitating the inhibitory activity of GABA at its receptors and inhibiting the excitatory activity of glutamate at its receptors. Over time, the GABA receptors are down-regulated and their subunit structure is modified through a variety of molecular mechanisms, thus decreasing the level of inhibition to counter the sedative effects of alcohol. Simultaneously, the NMDA receptors are up-regulated, also decreasing the level of inhibition due to alcohol. If the alcohol is abruptly removed, the decreased GABAergic inhibition and enhanced glutamatergic excitation result in a state of central nervous system hyperactivity, which causes the signs and symptoms of alcohol withdrawal. The balance between these inhibitory (GABAergic) and excitatory (glutamatergic) pathways may explain the alternating sedation and hyperactivity characteristic of alcohol intoxication and withdrawal, respectively.

Because dependence can occur without tolerance and vice versa, it is clear that learning-related changes, not necessarily due to the pharmacologic actions of a drug, are also involved. In the 1950s, Olds and Milner implanted electrodes in various regions of the rat brain to systematically determine which neuroanatomic areas could reinforce self-stimulation. (Self-stimulation consisted of a short pulse of nondestructive electric current that was delivered in the brain at the site of the electrode upon the animal's pressing of a lever.) The **medial forebrain bundle** and **ventral tegmental area (VTA)** in the midbrain were found to be particularly effective sites. These sites have been termed *pleasure centers*, or the foci of reward in the brain. A subset of dopaminergic neurons projects directly from the VTA to the **nucleus accumbens (NAc)** via the

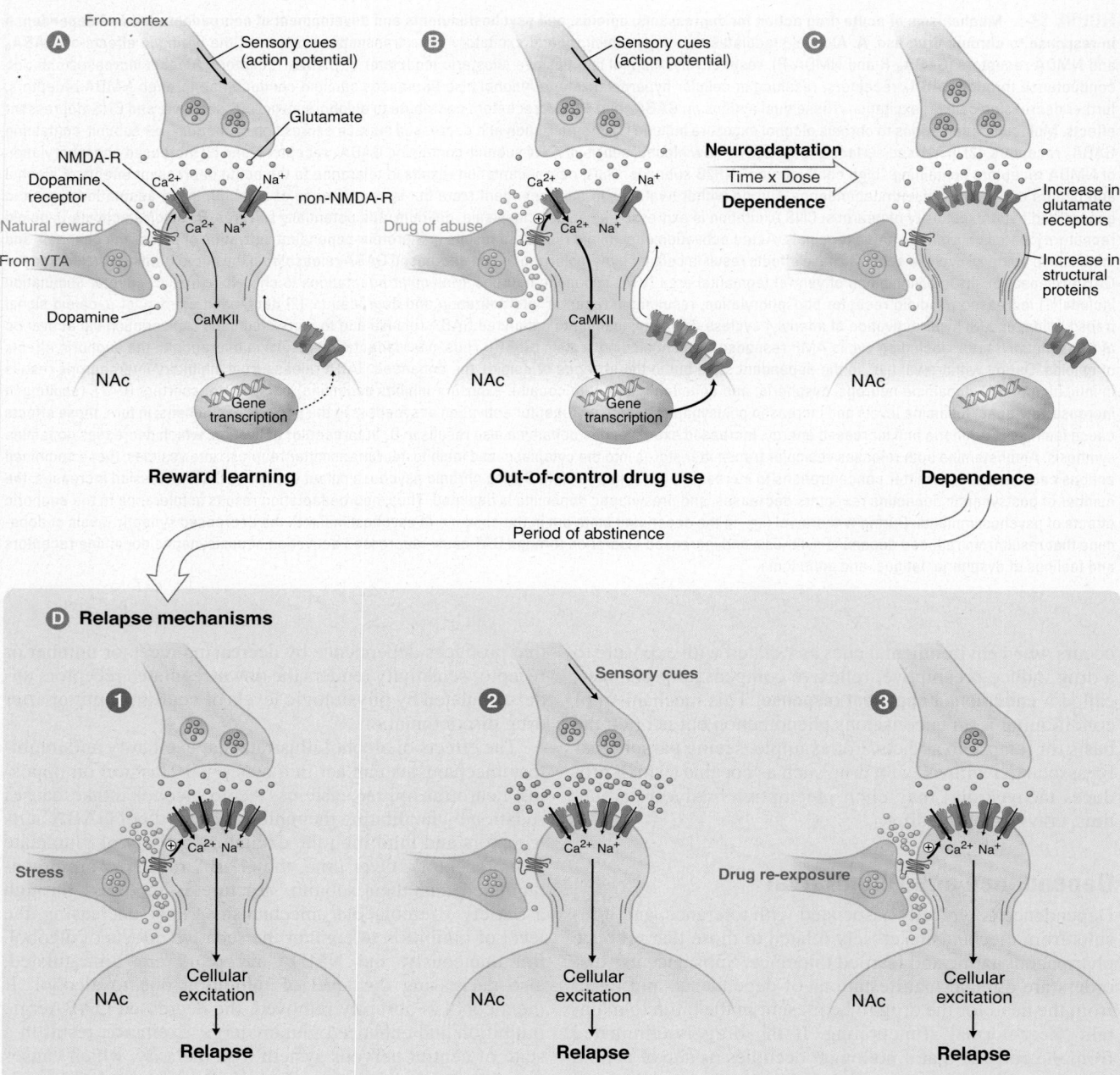

FIGURE 19-2. Synaptic changes linking environmental stimuli, drug effects, and reward learning in drug dependence and mechanisms of relapse after abstinence. A. Natural rewards such as food or sex increase dopamine release in the nucleus accumbens (NAc) and give rise to reward learning that links relevant environmental stimuli (sensory cues) with concurrent rewarding elements by altering neural circuitry in associative areas of the brain. Spiny neurons within the NAc receive glutamatergic inputs from the cortex that relay sensory cue information and dopaminergic inputs from the ventral tegmental area (VTA). The glutamatergic inputs act via NMDA receptors (permeable to calcium) and non-NMDA receptors (permeable to sodium). Coincident release of dopamine and glutamate results in potentiation of NMDA signaling, activation of calcium-calmodulin dependent kinase (CaMKII), and ultimately alterations in transcription of structural protein genes and glutamate receptor genes. These synaptic changes are thought to underlie reward learning. **B.** Drugs of abuse induce amplified dopamine release and activate the same synaptic adaptations as natural reinforcers. Thus, drugs of abuse are thought to "hijack" evolutionary brain reward learning systems in a manner that leads to out-of-control drug use. **C.** After chronic drug use, synaptic adaptations result in "potentiated synapses." This potentiation is mediated via increased dendritic spine size, increased structural protein expression, and increased glutamate receptor surface expression; all of these adaptations occur in response to long-term transcriptional changes. **D.** After a period of abstinence from drug use, multiple mechanisms can induce relapse to drug-taking behavior. **1.** Stress can trigger relapse by increased dopamine release. In this potentiated state, dopamine can trigger cellular excitation and trigger relapse behaviors. **2.** Exposure to drug-related sensory cues can trigger relapse via increased glutamate release, and the increased surface expression of glutamate receptors can lead to cellular excitation and relapse. **3.** Exposure to small amounts of drug can reactivate relapse to drug self-administration in this potentiated state, since the amplified dopamine release can trigger cellular excitation.

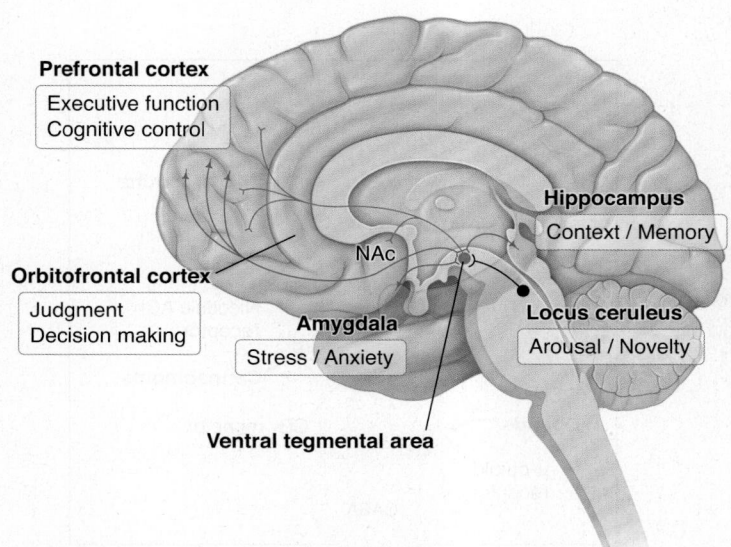

FIGURE 19-3. Integration of brain behavioral systems via connections to the mesolimbic dopamine pathway. Noradrenergic neurons originating in the locus ceruleus (*black*) relay information regarding novelty and arousal to dopaminergic neurons in the ventral tegmental area (VTA). The VTA projects to the nucleus accumbens (NAc) and cortex (*red*). Multiple inputs from the brain modify VTA output: glutamatergic input from the prefrontal cortex relays executive function and cognitive control; excitatory input from the amygdala signals stress and anxiety; and glutamatergic input from the hippocampus conveys contextual information and past experiences (*blue*). Together, these multiple inputs modify signaling in the mesolimbic dopamine pathway and modulate the perception of pleasure.

Prefrontal cortex
Executive function
Cognitive control

Orbitofrontal cortex
Judgment
Decision making

NAc

Amygdala
Stress / Anxiety

Ventral tegmental area

Hippocampus
Context / Memory

Locus ceruleus
Arousal / Novelty

medial forebrain bundle. It is believed that these neurons are crucial for the brain reward pathway, which reinforces motivated behavior and facilitates learning and memory via links to the hippocampus, amygdala, and prefrontal cortex. Severing this pathway, or blocking dopamine receptors in the NAc with a dopamine receptor antagonist (such as haloperidol; see Chapter 14, Pharmacology of Dopaminergic Neurotransmission), decreases electrical self-stimulation of the VTA. Moreover, release of dopamine in the NAc can be detected in vivo using the technique of microdialysis, whereby a cannula is inserted into a specific brain region in order to determine the concentrations of neurotransmitters. These measurements show that increases in concentrations of dopamine are associated with drug self-administration by laboratory animals and that dopaminergic synapses in the NAc are active during electrical stimulation of the brain reward pathway, supporting the hypothesis that NAc dopamine is necessary for reward. Drugs capable of causing dependence are readily self-administered by animals directly into the VTA, NAc, or the cortical or subcortical areas that innervate these two areas, often at the cost even of eating food (Fig. 19-3).

Although the dopaminergic pathway mediates reward, dopamine may also increase the salience of stimuli, alert the organism to the importance of stimuli, and guide motor activity to seek rewarding stimuli. As discussed above, *the dopamine pathway is activated by all drugs of abuse.* Importantly, behaviors that are necessary for survival of the species (e.g., feeding, reproduction, and exploration) also result in dopamine release in the NAc but to a much smaller degree, suggesting that drugs of abuse may pharmacologically "hijack" the normal evolutionary functions of reward pathways. With repeated experiences via conditioning (i.e., the association of an element of the environment with the reward through rewiring of brain circuits), this dopamine pathway is also activated during *anticipation* of the reward, as can be demonstrated in humans using functional neuroimaging techniques such as positron emission tomography (PET) and functional magnetic resonance imaging (fMRI) when addicts are exposed to drug-related sensory cues. Although the dopaminergic neurons that link the VTA and the NAc serve as the final common pathway of reward, these neurons receive inputs from

a number of brain regions (cortex, hippocampus, thalamus, amygdala, and raphe nuclei) that modify reward and thereby mediate reward-associated learning (Figs. 19-3 and 19-4).

Since withdrawal from certain drugs of abuse can be aversive, avoiding acute withdrawal was for many years thought to be the primary motivation for continued abuse. However, this explanation is not consistent with the observations that the effects of addiction are felt long after the physical symptoms of withdrawal have abated; withdrawal can occur without concomitant drug-seeking, as is often the case after treatment for acute pain; and drugs such as stimulants, hallucinogens, and cannabinoids cause significant dependence without a striking acute withdrawal syndrome. Years after an addict has discontinued use of a substance, he or she can experience intense cravings and, thus, is prone to **relapse**. The likelihood of relapse is especially strong in situations in which individuals simultaneously encounter both stress and the context in which the drug was previously used. In part, this is due to the interplay between reward and memory circuitry in the brain that, under normal circumstances, assigns emotional value to certain memories. Hence, the motivational underpinnings of drug-seeking are tied to both socioenvironmental stimuli and subjective effects of the drug, each of which can have both rewarding and aversive linkages with previous experiences via learning. This is a more complex explanation than the "simple" avoidance of acute withdrawal.

MECHANISMS OF SUBSTANCE USE DISORDERS

The drug-seeking activity characteristic of substance use disorders results from the interplay of learning, reward mechanisms, and individual propensity toward the development of addiction.

Learning and Development of Substance Use Disorders

Recognition that chronic drug self-administration results in long-lasting changes in the experience of reward has led to

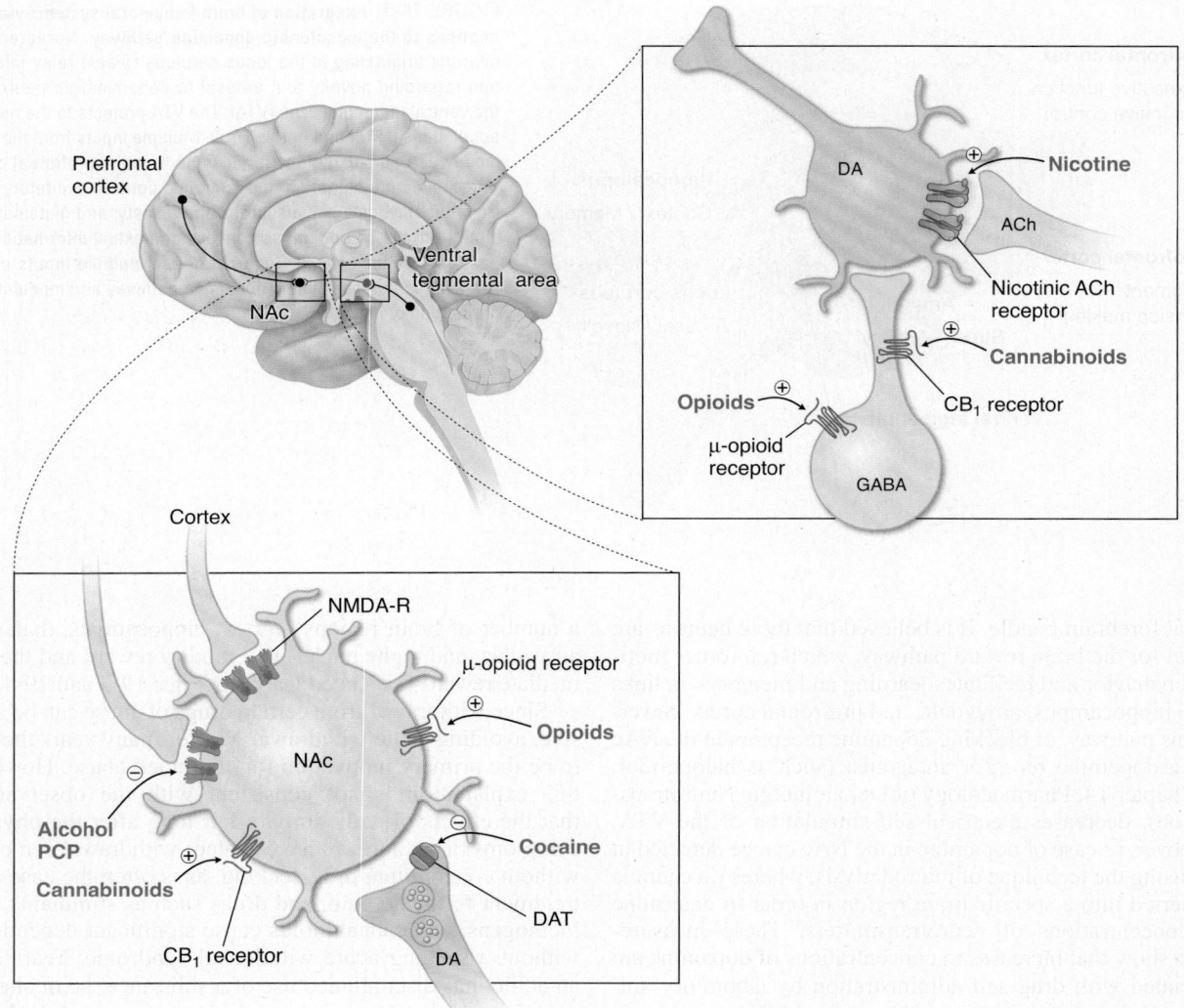

FIGURE 19-4. The mesolimbic dopamine pathway: a final common substrate for the rewarding actions of drugs. All drugs of abuse activate the mesolimbic dopamine pathway, which comprises ventral tegmental area (VTA) dopamine neurons that project to the nucleus accumbens (NAc). Different interneurons interact with VTA neurons and NAc neurons to modulate mesolimbic neurotransmission. **Nicotine** interacts with excitatory nicotinic cholinergic receptors located on VTA dopamine neuron cell bodies to enhance dopamine release in the NAc. **Cocaine** acts predominantly at the dopamine nerve terminal to inhibit reuptake of dopamine via the dopamine transporter (DAT), thus increasing synaptic levels of dopamine that can impinge on the NAc. **Amphetamine** also acts at the dopamine nerve terminal to facilitate release of dopamine-containing vesicles and possibly to enhance reverse transport of dopamine through DAT (*not shown*). Both **cannabinoids** and **opioids** decrease GABA release from local inhibitory interneurons in the VTA, resulting in disinhibition of dopamine neuron activity and increased dopaminergic neurotransmission. Cannabinoids and opioids can also act within the NAc. **Alcohol**, other **CNS depressants**, and **phencyclidine [PCP]** act on NMDA receptors (NMDA-R) to reduce glutamatergic neurotransmission in the NAc. The effects of alcohol on dopaminergic neurons in the VTA appear to be both excitatory and inhibitory and are the subject of active investigation (*not shown*).

our understanding that the relevant neural circuits can never return to their predrug state. The term **allostasis** describes this enduring, progressively evolving adaptive process in brain reward pathways upon repeated exposure to abused drugs. Allostasis means that the baseline to which the brain returns upon discontinuing drug use can change even after acute withdrawal has abated. (This is in contrast to homeostasis, which is defined as the process whereby a system repeatedly re-equilibrates to the *same* baseline.) Accordingly, even when the drug is no longer present in the brain, the addict cannot experience positive emotions in the way he or she did prior to beginning drug use (termed **anhedonia**); the unsuccessful attempt to recapture the previous "near-normal"

state fuels drug-seeking. Human and animal studies have found evidence for long-term neuroadaptation in altered neurotransmitter levels (e.g., dopamine and serotonin depletion after chronic alcohol or stimulant use), changes in neurotransmitter receptors, altered signal transduction pathways, changes in gene expression, and altered synaptic configuration and function. Clinically, abstinent patients report not only craving but also dysphoria, sleep disturbances, and increased stress reactivity (e.g., panic attacks), which can last for weeks, months, or years after detoxification.

A common misconception is that addicts are pleasure seekers and that their focus on drugs represents withdrawal from life into irresponsible hedonism. Current thinking about addiction recognizes the heterogeneity of the addictive process. For some individuals, reward factors (**positive reinforcement**) may predominate, and getting high or feeling euphoric motivates drug use. For others, relief factors (**negative reinforcement**) predominate, such as drinking to reduce stress or to reduce the dysphoria of protracted withdrawal. A large proportion of addicts self-medicate to reduce distress associated with co-occurring psychiatric and medical disorders. Furthermore, the motivations to use early in the course of substance use disorder may differ substantially from motivations as the illness progresses (Fig. 19-5). As a result of allostasis, positive reinforcement is rare in the later stages of the illness. For example, drinking in one's teens to relieve shyness may progress to drinking for euphoria and disinhibition. Ultimately, after years of drinking to intoxication, the middle-aged person may drink to prevent withdrawal-associated depression and anxiety, or perhaps to alleviate chronic pain. Drug use in each of these situations is linked via learning to elements of the environment associated with drug use or to memories and emotions, each of which can trigger craving and drug-seeking.

The essence of substance use disorder is drug-seeking behavior, whereby an individual cannot control the urge to obtain and use a psychoactive substance despite recognized negative consequences and at the exclusion of other needs that typi-

cally constitute a balanced life. Studies in laboratory animals suggest that drug-seeking behavior is the result of dysfunctional "reward learning" (i.e., the processes that guide the organism to fulfill needs or goals have gone awry). Thus, if the organism initiates an action that results in a goal or "reward" (e.g., self-administration of a psychoactive agent), and if the organism "learns" that its action resulted in the reward, the likelihood of engaging in that behavior is enhanced. For example, if a person uses cocaine for the first time and finds it pleasurable or that it alleviates depressive symptoms from which the individual is suffering, obtaining and using cocaine are reinforced. The intense experience of cocaine, relative to natural rewards such as food and sex, results in a preferential expenditure of energy to obtain cocaine over other rewards. Thus, cocaine has effectively "hijacked" reward-learning systems, biasing future behavior in favor of obtaining cocaine over natural rewards. Reexposure to environmental or affective states that are associated with cocaine use serve as cues to increase drug-seeking behavior. For example, reexposure to drug paraphernalia can induce intense craving, drug-seeking behavior, and relapse in cocaine addicts.

Variables Affecting the Development of Substance Use Disorders

The development of substance use disorder is dependent on the nature of the drug; genetic, acquired, psychological, and social traits of the drug user; and environmental factors.

The ability of a drug to activate reward mechanisms is strongly correlated with its ability to cause addiction. Pharmacokinetic properties of the drug can significantly influence its effects on the brain. In general, the more rapid the rise in drug concentrations at the target neurons, the greater the activation of reward pathways. For example, many drugs of abuse are highly lipophilic and can easily permeate the blood–brain barrier. In addition, direct injection or rapid absorption of drug through a large surface area (e.g., through the lungs via smoking) is more highly reinforcing than slower absorption through the intestinal or nasal mucosa. Furthermore, rapidly eliminated drugs are more addictive than slowly eliminated drugs, since slow clearance of a drug maintains the drug concentration at the site of action for a longer duration, diminishing the severity of acute withdrawal.

The importance of pharmacokinetic effects is demonstrated by the potential for abuse of various forms of cocaine (Fig. 19-6), and these principles are readily applicable to other drugs of abuse. The use of coca leaves as a chew or in teas is widely practiced among people living in the Andean mountains: this has a relatively low potential for addiction because of the slow rate of rise and low peak concentration of drug attained by absorption through the buccal or intestinal mucosa. The rapid absorption of extracted cocaine through the nasal mucosa is substantially more reinforcing. The most reinforcing and addictive forms of cocaine are intravenous injections and inhalation of smoked freebase (crack cocaine), both of which result in a very rapid rise in plasma concentration and a high peak concentration of drug.

Different people react differently to drugs. Some individuals use a drug once and never use it again; others use a drug repeatedly in moderate amounts without developing a drug use disorder; in others, the first use of a drug produces such an intense effect that the likelihood of addiction

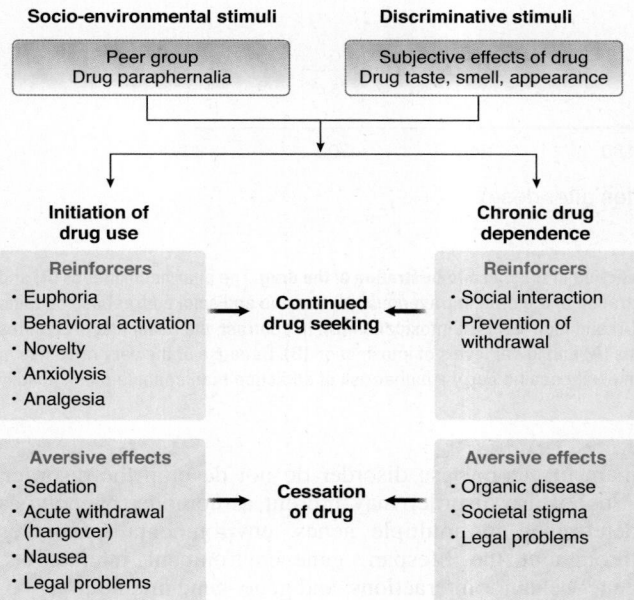

FIGURE 19-5. Clinical determinants of drug-seeking change throughout the life course of addiction. The motivational underpinnings of drug-seeking are determined by socioenvironmental stimuli paired with subjective effects of the drug. Reinforcers of drug self-administration result in continued drug use, whereas aversive drug effects contribute to cessation of drug self-administration: whether an individual continues to use is a function of whether reinforcing or aversive effects predominate under the circumstances. Brain reward pathways are modified during the course of repeated drug self-administration, such that reinforcing and aversive effects are often different when drug use first begins compared to later in the course when drug self-administration may have become repetitive and out-of-control. Ultimately, whether addiction progresses or the addictive disorder can be successfully arrested is determined by learning-related modification of reinforcing and aversive effects of drugs using pharmacopsychosocial interventions.

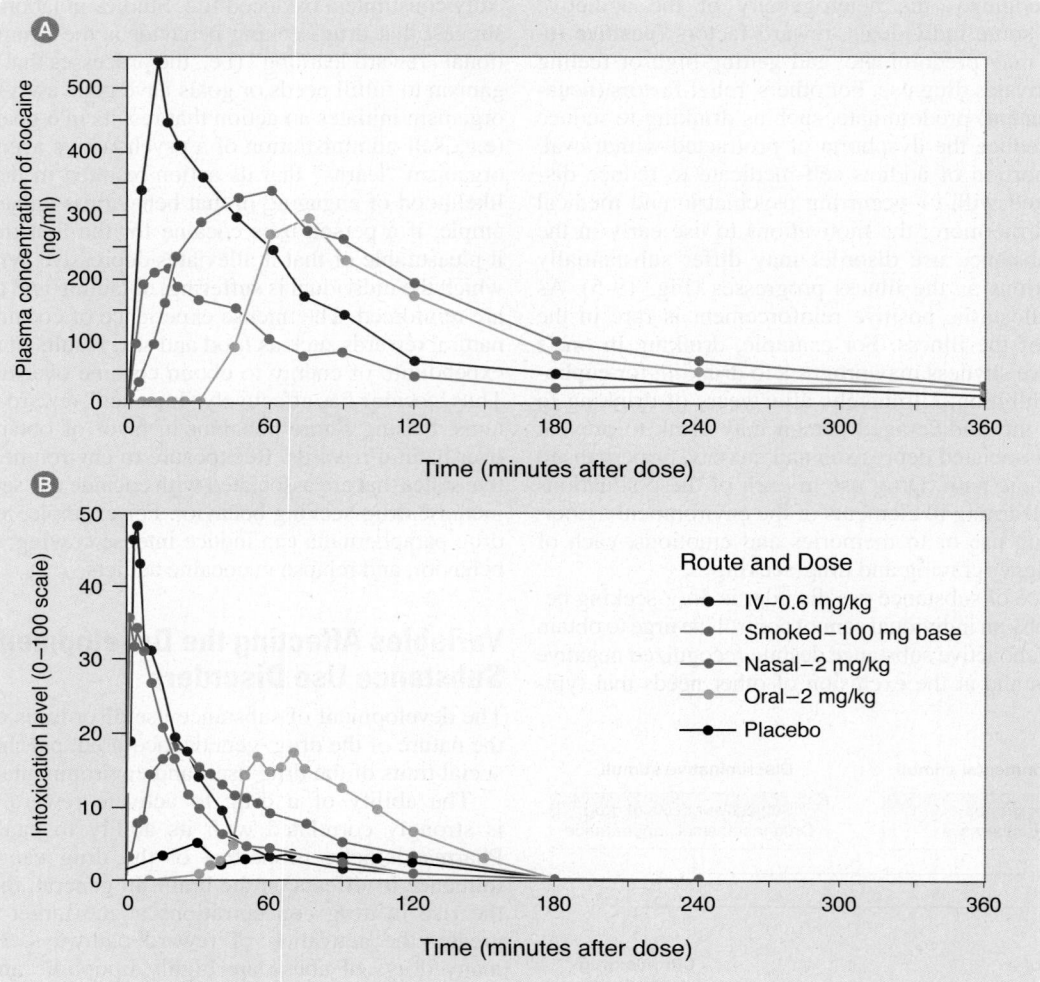

FIGURE 19-6. Plasma cocaine concentrations and levels of intoxication as a function of route of administration of the drug. The pharmacokinetics **(A)** and pharmacodynamics **(B)** of cocaine are highly dependent on the route of administration of the drug. Intravenous (IV) cocaine and smoked freebase cocaine are associated with very rapid attainment of peak plasma drug concentrations **(A)** and high levels of intoxication **(B)**. In contrast, the nasal and oral routes of administration are associated with a slower rise in plasma drug concentrations **(A)** and lower levels of intoxication **(B)**. Because of the very rapid rise in plasma drug concentration and very high intoxication levels, intravenous and smoked cocaine carry a higher risk of addiction than cocaine taken nasally or orally.

is high. The factors that make individuals more or less vulnerable to addiction upon exposure to a given drug are of continued research interest. A variety of predisposing or protective genetic, acquired, psychosocial, and environmental factors have been identified, but—as expected in a complex, multifactorial illness—*individually* each can explain only a relatively small component of the risk for addiction. Individual factors include (1) resistance or sensitivity to the acute effects of a given drug, (2) differences in drug metabolism, (3) the potential for neuroadaptive changes with chronic drug exposure, (4) personality traits and co-occurring psychiatric and medical disorders that incline an individual to drug use, and (5) susceptibility of the individual to brain injury associated with drug use that may modify drug effects.

Genetic influences have been best studied in individuals with alcohol use disorder. Heritability estimates suggest that genetic factors account for 50–60% of the variance associated with alcohol use disorder, but the specific determinant(s) that lead to alcoholism in an individual are not known. In fact, many individuals whose family history highly predisposes

them to alcohol use disorder do not develop the disorder. Alcohol use disorder may present as complex phenotypes determined by multiple genes, environmental exposures throughout the lifespan, gene–environment interactions, gene–behavior interactions, and gene–gene interactions.

The best known examples of candidate genes that alter risk for alcohol use disorder are the alcohol metabolism genes, including those encoding the alcohol dehydrogenases ADH1B*2, ADH2, and ADH3 that metabolize alcohol more rapidly and those encoding certain aldehyde dehydrogenases (particularly ALDH2*2). Polymorphisms in these genes alter enzymatic activity and increase the levels of acetaldehyde, which causes aversive symptoms that may act as a deterrent to drinking alcohol and to the development of alcohol use disorder.

Sensitivity to alcohol is also a physiologically based trait influenced by genetic inheritance. Low sensitivity to alcohol (**high innate tolerance**) is associated with an increased risk for developing alcoholism. Schuckit and colleagues have found evidence for genetic linkage of the "low level of response" phenotype to the same region on chromosome 1 that is linked to the "alcohol use disorder" phenotype. However, subjective response to alcohol is a complex trait affected by several neurotransmitter systems. For example, individuals with the alcohol dependence-associated *GABRA2* allele have a blunted subjective response to alcohol, and individuals carrying the Asp40 variant of the μ-opioid receptor or those with a certain single nucleotide polymorphism of the cannabinoid receptor appear to have an enhanced euphoric response to alcohol.

Role of Personality Characteristics and Co-Occurring Disorders in Substance Use Disorders

The clinical characterization of individuals who develop a substance use disorder has been most extensively studied for alcoholism. The Cloninger classification of alcohol use disorder subtypes relates genetic and neurobiological differences to the age of alcoholism onset and to personality traits. Type 1 ("late" onset) alcohol use disorder is characterized by alcohol-related problems beginning after 25 years of age, less antisocial behavior, infrequent spontaneous drinking or loss of control, and guilt and concern about one's alcoholism. Type 1 alcoholics are low in thrill-seeking, are harm-avoidant, and are dependent on approval from others. In contrast, type 2 alcohol use disorder is characterized by early onset of alcohol-related problems (before age 25), antisocial behavior, frequent spontaneous alcohol-seeking and loss of control, and little concern about the consequences of one's drinking or its effects on others. Genetic predispositions to late-onset alcohol use disorder are significantly influenced by precipitating environmental factors, whereas genetic predispositions to early-onset alcohol use disorder are less influenced by the environment. The Lesch classification envisions four alcoholism subtypes: type 1 exhibits withdrawal symptoms, including alcohol-related delirium and seizures, relatively early in the drinking history; type 2 exhibits anxiety related to premorbid conflicts; type 3 is characterized by associated mood disorders; and type 4 has premorbid cerebral injuries and associated social problems. Alcohol use disorder subtypes are now being examined as predictors of response to medications used for the treatment of alcoholism. For example, early-onset alcoholics may worsen their drinking and impulsive behavior in response to a selective serotonin reuptake inhibitor (SSRI), whereas late-onset alcoholics may improve with an SSRI.

According to a major epidemiologic survey in the United States, the odds of having a mental disorder are three times greater if an individual also has a drug use disorder than if the individual has no drug use disorder. In decreasing order of association, these psychiatric diagnoses include bipolar disorder, antisocial personality disorder, schizophrenia, major depressive disorder, and anxiety disorders. Drug use disorders occur at higher rates in those with alcohol use disorder, and alcoholism is more prevalent among individuals with addiction to other drugs. The association between psychiatric disorders and drug use disorders has led to theories of common pathogenesis and treatment strategies. For example, individuals with major depressive disorder are two to three times more likely to have a drug use disorder throughout their lifetime than those without depression, and exacerbations of mood symptoms are prime precipitants of relapse to drug use (and vice versa). Of note, these associations seem to be generic with respect to which drugs are abused, suggesting that such abuse is related more to availability than to a specific pharmacologic mechanism of action.

Physical disability and pain associated with medical illness or traumatic injury can greatly enhance the risk of a co-occurring drug use disorder. Moreover, drug use not only complicates certain medical conditions, but for many of these illnesses (e.g., cirrhosis or traumatic brain injury due to motor vehicle accidents), alcohol and drug use should also be considered a significant causal factor. Similarly, *increased* pain perception is now understood to be a frequent complication of chronic opioid administration (**opioid hyperalgesia**). Thus, many pain physicians no longer advise long-term use of opioid analgesics for treatment of chronic (nonterminal) pain, recognizing that detoxifying a patient from chronic opioid use can often result in a preferable outcome to continuing to increase the opioid dose. In conclusion, substance use disorders are not only illnesses in their own right but also common consequences of many psychiatric and medical conditions that, in turn, are further exacerbated by continued substance use.

■ DRUGS OF ABUSE

Many psychoactive substances have abuse potential through their activation of inputs in brain reward pathways. It is vital to understand the unique pharmacology of each agent to appropriately address overdose complications, metabolic consequences, and organ toxicity associated with a specific substance use disorder. Several drugs with the potential to cause addiction are readily available and widely used, and they exact an enormous toll on public health (e.g., alcohol, nicotine). Other drugs are commonly prescribed for accepted medical purposes, and their mechanisms of action have been discussed in detail in previous chapters (e.g., opioids, barbiturates, benzodiazepines, stimulants). These drugs represent a significant cause of iatrogenic dependence in patients, and prescription drug abuse represents perhaps the fastest growing US drug problem. In recent years, deaths associated with prescription drug use have surpassed deaths due to motor vehicle accidents in many parts of the country. Other commonly abused drugs are not generally prescribed in medical practice and are typically available only from illicit sources (e.g., cocaine, heroin). Finally, some drugs affect receptors that are actively being pursued as potential targets for therapeutic intervention, and it is controversial whether or how they should be regulated (e.g., cannabis, nicotine).

Opioids

Opioid alkaloids have been used medically for centuries for analgesia, treatment of diarrhea and cough, and sleep induction. Central effects of opioids are biphasic, with behavioral activation at low doses and sedation at higher doses. These drugs depress respiration, and death from opioid overdose is invariably due to respiratory arrest. The μ-opioid receptor appears to be the most important subtype for the reinforcing actions of opioids. Addicts describe an intense euphoric feeling ("rush") that lasts for less than a minute upon the intravenous injection of heroin and that seems to be the reason for abuse.

There appear to be two pathways by which opioids interact with the brain reward system. One site of action lies in the ventral tegmental area, where GABAergic interneurons tonically inhibit the dopaminergic neurons responsible for activating the brain reward pathway in the nucleus accumbens.

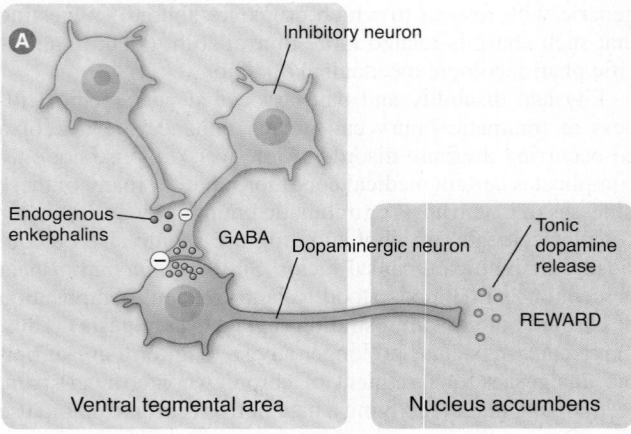

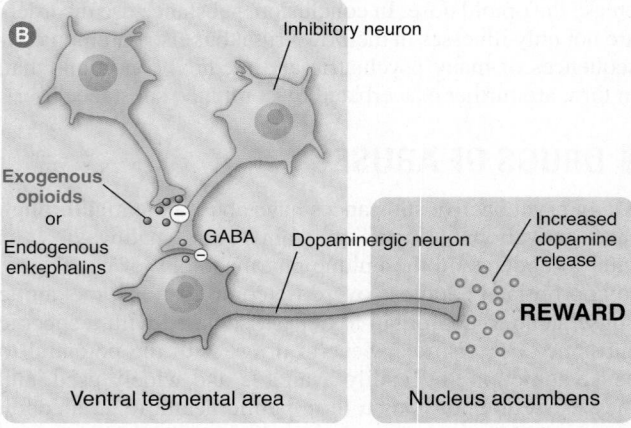

FIGURE 19-7. Role of opioids in the brain reward pathway. A. GABAergic neurons tonically inhibit the dopaminergic neurons that originate in the ventral tegmental area and are responsible for reward. These GABAergic neurons can be inhibited by endogenous enkephalins, which locally modulate the release of neurotransmitter at the GABAergic nerve terminal. **B.** Administration of exogenous opioids results in decreased GABA release and disinhibition of the dopaminergic reward neurons. The increased release of dopamine in the nucleus accumbens signals a strong reward.

These GABAergic interneurons can be inhibited by endogenous enkephalins, which bind to μ-opioid receptors on the GABAergic terminals. Because exogenous opioids such as morphine also bind to and activate μ-opioid receptors (see Chapter 18, Pharmacology of Analgesia), exogenously administered opioids can activate the brain reward pathway by disinhibiting dopaminergic neurons in the ventral tegmental area (Fig. 19-4, Fig. 19-7). The second pathway is localized in the nucleus accumbens. Opioids acting in this region may inhibit GABAergic neurons that project back to the ventral tegmental area, perhaps as part of an inhibitory feedback loop. The relative importance of these two pathways is still being debated. As the case of Mr. A illustrates, opioid use disorder can lead to significant alterations in these reward pathways that manifest as opioid craving and a high probability of relapse long after the physical symptoms of withdrawal have abated. The partial agonist buprenorphine binds to and modulates activation of μ-opioid receptor-mediated reward circuits and can greatly diminish craving for opioids, as the case of Mr. A demonstrates (Fig. 19-8).

The multiple inputs into brain reward circuits underline the potential for co-occurrence of addiction to opioids and to other pharmacologically disparate drugs of abuse (**cross-dependence**). For example, self-administration of opioids together with other psychoactive drugs, such as the cocaine/heroin combination "speedball," is used to enhance reward (Fig. 19-4); this combination also augments the risk of abuse and death due to overdose. In addition, open-ended opioid prescriptions after surgery may precipitate relapse to another drug of abuse to which the person was previously addicted and from which abstinence has been achieved, even if the individual has never previously had an opioid use disorder. However, the potential for addiction should not deter physicians from prescribing a medication for legitimate medical purposes.

Unfortunately, opioids are often under-prescribed for the treatment of pain because tolerance—manifested as a request for increasingly higher doses of drug—is mistaken for an opioid use disorder. Tolerance is an expected effect of the drug, and physicians should be prepared to increase the dose, if necessary, to control the patient's pain. Because of the high potential for withdrawal symptoms upon discontinuation of an opioid, physicians should also be careful to taper the opioid dose and to explain to the patient the rationale for the taper. Finally, drug-addicted patients who must undergo surgery or require analgesia for other reasons should be treated with sufficient medication to attain analgesia, and they may need considerably higher doses due to preexisting tolerance to opioids. This can be a common problem when patients are chronically taking buprenorphine. Buprenorphine may partially block the effects of opioid analgesics because it is a partial agonist at opioid receptors, and a patient may require much higher opioid doses than usual to attain adequate analgesia. Nevertheless, whenever opioids are used, there needs to be a clear understanding of exactly how the decision to discontinue the medication will be made, and treatment should be determined by the physiologic basis of the expected pain rather than allowed to continue indefinitely.

Although all opioids have the potential to cause tolerance and dependence, certain opioids are more reinforcing and more likely to cause drug-seeking. Opioids associated with the fastest rise in brain concentration of drug, including those injected intravenously, have the highest likelihood for abuse. Abuse of the drug oxycodone (sold as slow-release OxyContin®), which is commonly prescribed for moderate or severe pain, has received much publicity because of misuse and cases of iatrogenic addiction when patients take the medication "as prescribed." Experienced addicts have learned that the oral tablets of oxycodone can be broken up, dissolved, and injected. This form of administration results in a much more rapid rise in plasma (and hence brain) concentration of drug, a more intense feeling of euphoria, and a greater abuse liability compared to the prescribed, slow-release oral form of the drug. Analogously, although heroin and morphine are close structural analogues (heroin is deacetylated to 6-monoacetylmorphine, and morphine is acetylated to the same compound), heroin is significantly more hydrophobic than morphine. Because of this property, intravenously administered heroin crosses the blood–brain barrier more rapidly than morphine. The more rapid increase in brain concentration of heroin produces a sharper "high," which explains why heroin is typically preferred over morphine as a drug of abuse. The rapid rise in brain concentration of heroin, together with the uncertain dose and potentially toxic impurities in heroin preparations available "on the street," account for the substantial mortality by respiratory arrest due to heroin overdose.

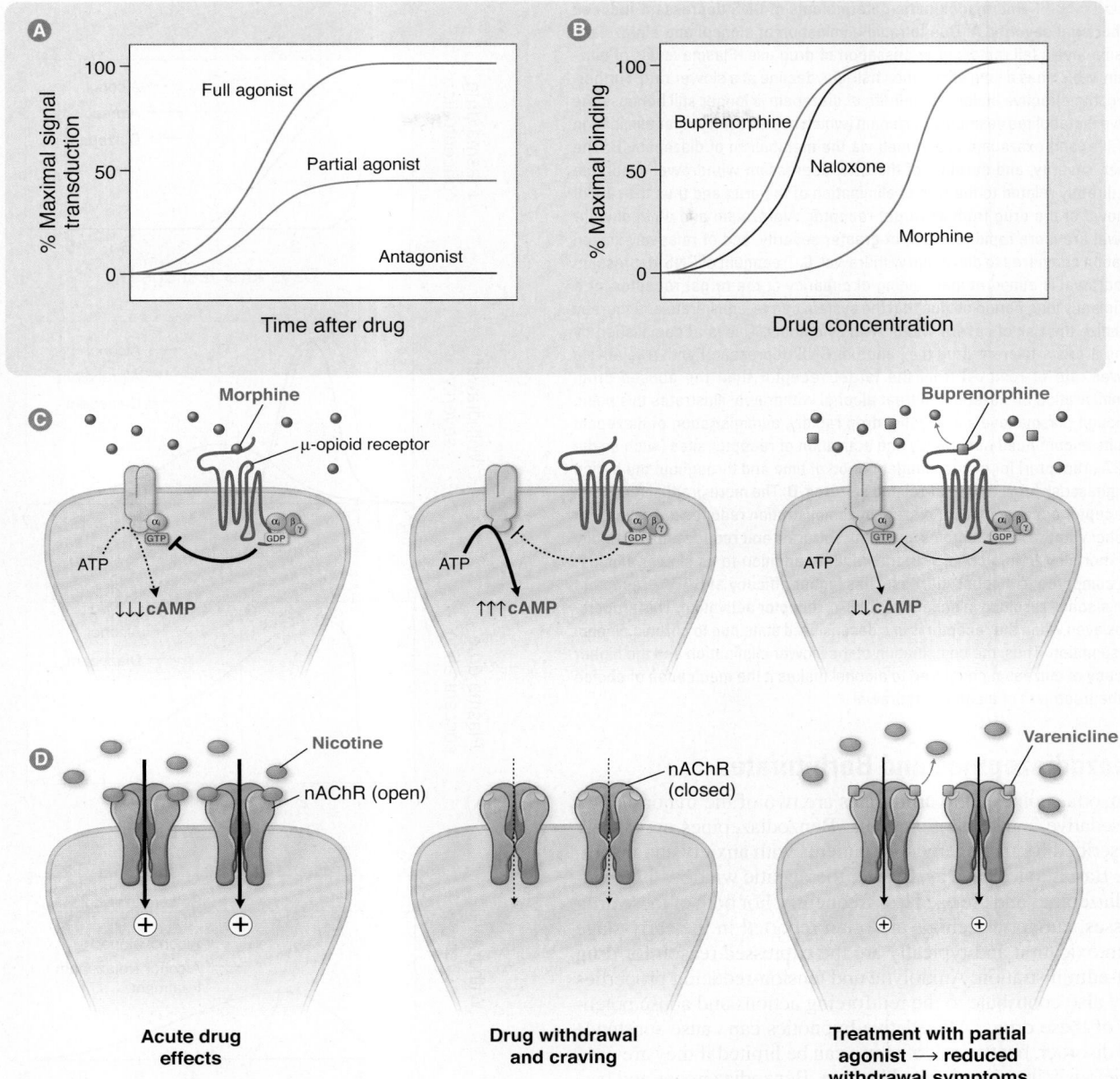

FIGURE 19-8. **Partial agonists in the treatment of addiction. A.** Full agonists at μ-opioid receptors, such as morphine, produce maximal signal transduction (100%). Partial agonists, such as buprenorphine, produce reduced signal transduction (~50% of a full agonist). Antagonists, such as naloxone, do not stimulate signal transduction. **B.** Both buprenorphine and naloxone have very high binding affinities for μ-opioid receptors compared to morphine. Consequently, when μ-opioid receptors are fully occupied by an agonist like morphine, both naloxone and buprenorphine displace morphine from the receptor and lead to withdrawal. **C.** Upon morphine binding to μ-opioid receptors, intracellular signaling leads to inhibition of adenylyl cyclase activity and a decrease in cyclic AMP (cAMP) production. Upon removal of morphine from μ-opioid receptors, either by discontinuing morphine or by administration of an antagonist or partial agonist (withdrawal), the inhibition of adenylyl cyclase is released. The resulting large increase in cAMP production causes withdrawal symptoms, such as diarrhea, hyperalgesia, tachypnea, and photophobia. The use of a partial agonist, buprenorphine, can alleviate these withdrawal symptoms by "partial" activation of μ-opioid receptors. In addition, binding of the high-affinity buprenorphine molecule to μ-opioid receptors prevents lower affinity full agonists, such as morphine, from binding to and activating the receptor. Thus, the antagonist property of buprenorphine prevents the "high" associated with morphine use but also alleviates craving and drug-seeking behavior. **D.** Nicotine activates nicotinic acetylcholine receptors (nAChR), causing neuronal excitation. Nicotine withdrawal causes a rapid decrease in nAChR activity and a withdrawal syndrome associated with intense craving. Treatment with the partial nAChR agonist varenicline results in partial activation of nAChR and alleviation of withdrawal symptoms, but this activation is insufficient to cause dependence or a "high." Importantly, binding of the high-affinity varenicline molecule to nAChRs prevents the lower affinity nicotine molecule from binding to and activating the receptor. Thus, varenicline can prevent the subjective "high" associated with nicotine use.

FIGURE 19-9. Pharmacokinetic determinants of CNS depressant-induced withdrawal severity. A. Due to rapid elimination of alcohol and alprazolam, plasma levels fall rapidly after cessation of drug use. Plasma levels of diazepam, which has a long elimination half-life, decline at a slower rate. Furthermore, the effective biological half-life of diazepam is longer still because the active metabolites desmethyldiazepam (which has an even longer elimination half-life) and oxazepam are formed via the metabolism of diazepam. **B.** The onset, severity, and duration of the CNS-depressant withdrawal syndrome are directly related to the rate of elimination of the drug and thus the rate of removal of the drug from its target receptor. Alprazolam and alcohol withdrawal are more rapid in onset, of greater severity, and of relatively limited duration compared to diazepam withdrawal. **C.** Treatment of CNS-depressant withdrawal is aimed at maintaining occupancy of the target receptor for a sufficiently long period of time that the system can re-equilibrate and thereby minimize the risk of severe withdrawal symptoms. This is accomplished by using a cross-tolerant drug (i.e., another CNS depressant) with a relatively slower rate of removal from the target receptor than the abused drug. Administration of diazepam to treat alcohol withdrawal illustrates this point. Although plasma levels of alcohol drop rapidly, administration of diazepam results in continued occupancy and activation of receptor sites (such as the GABA_A receptor) for a much longer period of time and throughout the period of highest risk for withdrawal-related seizures. **D.** The more gradual reduction in receptor occupancy after diazepam administration reduces the severity of alcohol withdrawal symptoms, prevents seizures, and reduces the morbidity and mortality from alcohol withdrawal. **E.** In addition to its slower elimination compared to alcohol, diazepam has higher efficacy at GABA_A receptors than alcohol, resulting in enhanced GABA_A receptor activation. This property holds even when the receptor is in a desensitized state due to chronic alcohol consumption. Thus, the combination of the slower elimination and the higher efficacy of diazepam compared to alcohol makes it the medication of choice for the treatment of alcohol withdrawal.

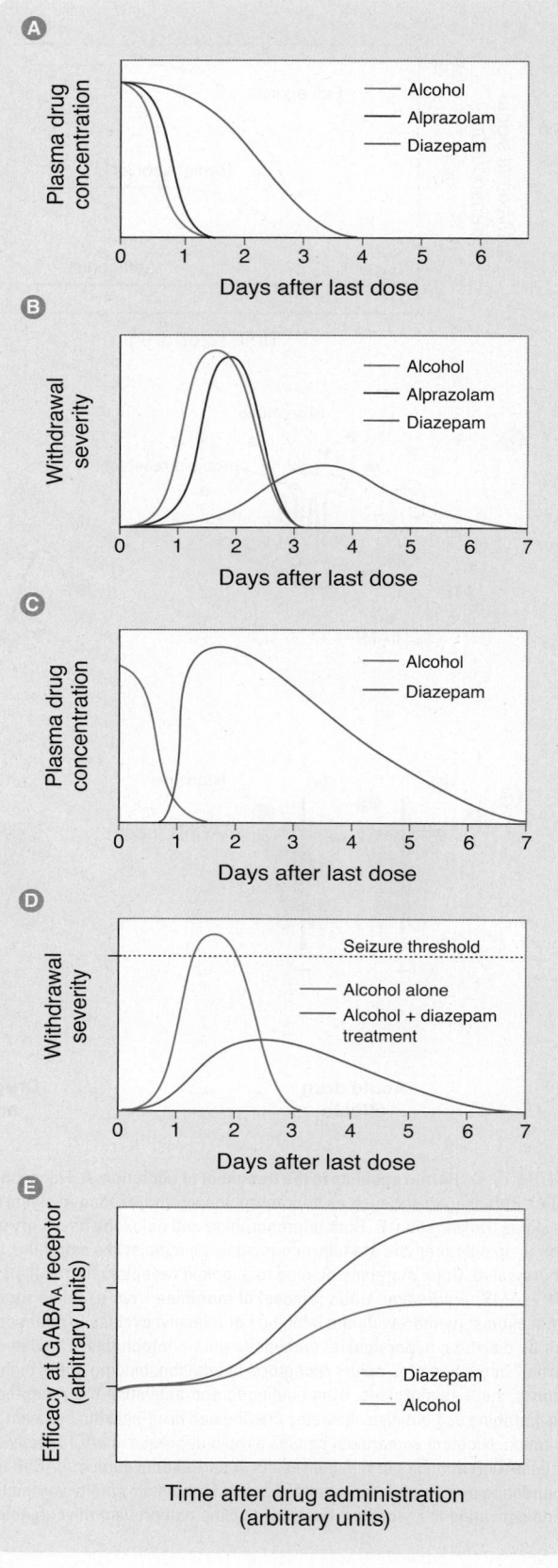

Benzodiazepines and Barbiturates

Benzodiazepines and barbiturates are two of the major classes of sedative and hypnotic agents. Benzodiazepines are widely prescribed for management of patients with anxiety and insomnia. Barbiturates have a narrower therapeutic window than benzodiazepines and are used less frequently. For both of these drug classes, euphoric feelings are often reported in the early stage of intoxication and typically are the expressed reason for drug self-administration. Anxiolytic and tension-reducing properties may also contribute to the reinforcing actions and abuse potential of these drugs. All sedative-hypnotics can cause substance use disorder, but the risk of abuse can be limited if they are used judiciously in a time-limited fashion. Benzodiazepines and barbiturates increase the efficiency of GABAergic pathways, and chronic use can induce down-regulation of these pathways by neuroadaptation. One possible mechanism of down-regulation is uncoupling of the benzodiazepine site from the GABA site on **GABA_A receptors** (see Chapter 13, Pharmacology of GABAergic and Glutamatergic Neurotransmission). Thus, the binding of benzodiazepines to GABA_A receptors would remain unchanged, but the drug would have little or no potentiating effect on the binding of GABA to the receptor. Down-regulation of inhibitory GABAergic pathways would be expected to leave the brain "underinhibited," increasing the possibility of seizures and delirium upon abrupt withdrawal of the benzodiazepine or barbiturate (see Chapter 16, Pharmacology of Abnormal Electrical Neurotransmission in the Central Nervous System). Associated central sympathetic hyperactivity can lead to physical symptoms such as anxiety, sleep disturbance, and dizziness and to emotional concomitants such as fear and panic. Because the central nervous system depressant actions of barbiturates are more widespread than those of the GABA_A-specific benzodiazepines (Fig. 19-9), barbiturate dependence is associated with a more severe and potentially dangerous withdrawal syndrome than benzodiazepine dependence. Within a given class of sedative-hypnotics, the onset, amplitude, and duration of the withdrawal syndrome are determined by the rate of elimination of the drug and its active metabolites. For example, among the barbiturates and benzodiazepines, withdrawal usually begins within 12 hours after drug discontinuation and is most severe for rapidly eliminated compounds (e.g., amobarbital and alprazolam); withdrawal may be delayed for several days and is less severe for slowly eliminated compounds (e.g., phenobarbital, diazepam, and clonazepam) (Fig. 19-9).

Co-occurring benzodiazepine and/or barbiturate use disorder and alcohol use disorder are particularly prevalent due to the similarity of these drugs' effects on GABAergic neurotransmission (Fig. 19-9). Benzodiazepines (not barbiturates) are the accepted treatment for alcohol withdrawal; these drugs are efficacious in alleviating "rough spots" when alcoholics cannot drink, and the effects of alcohol are greatly accentuated by benzodiazepines (or barbiturates). Benzodiazepines are almost never associated with mortality due to overdose when used alone; combined with alcohol, however, they can be fatal because of synergistic depression of cardiorespiratory centers.

Benzodiazepines and opioids can sometimes be co-prescribed under conditions when pain is associated with significant anxiety. This combination can also be fatal due to synergistic effects on respiration; in fact, even the relatively safe partial agonist buprenorphine can cause respiratory arrest when combined with benzodiazepines. Physicians may try to limit use of these dangerous combinations, but some drug-seeking patients may resort to obtaining prescriptions from multiple physicians or even forging prescriptions, especially in cases where the underlying condition has been suboptimally managed. Nonetheless, under-medication of pain must be avoided, and benzodiazepines should only be used over the short term for treatment of alcohol withdrawal or significant anxiety.

Another serious concern is the misuse of prescription opioids (or, less commonly, benzodiazepines or barbiturates) by health professionals. For at least two reasons, health professionals who misuse prescription medication are at greater risk for developing substance use disorder. First, they have more ready access to prescription medication. Second, they may mistakenly believe that, because they understand a drug's effects, they will be able to control its use more easily.

Alcohol

Alcoholic beverages are readily available at affordable cost with minimal legal restriction. Alcohol use disorder stands as the most prevalent drug problem in the United States. Early in intoxication, CNS stimulation and euphoria result from depression of inhibitory control, and aspects of discrimination, memory, and insight are impaired. As blood levels rise, judgment, emotional control, and motor coordination suffer. Traumatic injuries sustained while intoxicated are likely the most common public health problem associated with alcohol abuse. Respiratory depression and death can result from overdose, and the most serious consequences occur when alcohol is combined with other psychoactive agents.

Ethanol affects GABA$_A$ receptors, NMDA glutamate receptors, and cannabinoid receptors. Although the specific sites of action are unknown, **GABA$_A$ channels** are believed to mediate the anxiolytic and sedative effects of alcohol, as well as the effects of alcohol on motor coordination, tolerance, dependence, and self-administration. Alcohol increases

GABA-mediated chloride conductance and enhances hyperpolarization of the neuron. Its mechanisms of dependence are likely similar to those of other sedative-hypnotic drugs affecting GABA neurotransmission. In severity and time course, the symptoms of alcohol withdrawal lie between those of short-acting barbiturates and intermediate-acting benzodiazepines.

Evidence also points to a role for **NMDA receptors** in the development of tolerance and dependence to alcohol, and NMDA receptors also have a role in the alcohol withdrawal syndrome. Specifically, alcohol inhibits subtypes of NMDA receptors that seem to be capable of long-term potentiation. The rewarding effects of alcohol may also be mediated in part by indirect activation of **cannabinoid receptors**. Endogenous cannabinoids are "retrograde" neuromodulators that act as a feedback mechanism to enhance dopaminergic activity in the mesolimbic reward pathway (Fig. 19-10; see also Fig. 19-4). Endocannabinoid signaling has been implicated in reward learning, appetite regulation, mood regulation, pain modulation, and cognition. Thus, although GABA$_A$ receptors have a vital role in mediating the effects of alcohol, the ability of alcohol to interact with a number of different receptor types suggests that our understanding of its mechanisms of action remains incomplete.

Nicotine and Tobacco

Smoking, or the combustion of tobacco for the purpose of nicotine self-administration, represents a major source of preventable medical morbidity and mortality. Nicotine activates nicotinic acetylcholine receptors that are located centrally, peripherally, and at the neuromuscular junction. Cholinergic neurons arising from the **laterodorsal tegmental area** (near the border of the midbrain and pons) activate nicotinic and muscarinic acetylcholine receptors on dopaminergic neurons in the ventral tegmental area; stimulation of these nicotinic receptors by nicotine activates the dopaminergic brain reward pathway (Fig. 19-4). In addition, activation of presynaptic nicotinic receptors on dopaminergic axon terminals facilitates the release of dopamine. These strong and direct effects on the mesolimbic reward pathway, combined with the inhalational route of administration and short half-life of nicotine, explain the high addiction potential of nicotine and hence of cigarettes and other forms of tobacco. Activation of central nicotinic receptors also produces anxiolytic effects, increases arousal, and suppresses appetite, while activation of peripheral nicotinic receptors increases blood pressure and stimulates smooth muscle contraction.

A strong and spontaneous withdrawal syndrome is associated with the decreases in plasma levels of nicotine that occur upon cessation of smoking. The major symptoms include irritability, anxiety, autonomic arousal, and intense craving and associated drug-seeking behavior. These symptoms are readily relieved by smoking, and given the widespread availability of tobacco products, it is easy to see why smoking is so recalcitrant to treatment. Because smoking can alleviate a number of symptoms associated with depression and anxiety, it is commonly associated with the use of other drugs and with mental disorders.

Cocaine and Amphetamine

Cocaine is isolated from the South American shrub *Erythroxylon coca* and has been used as a local anesthetic since 1884.

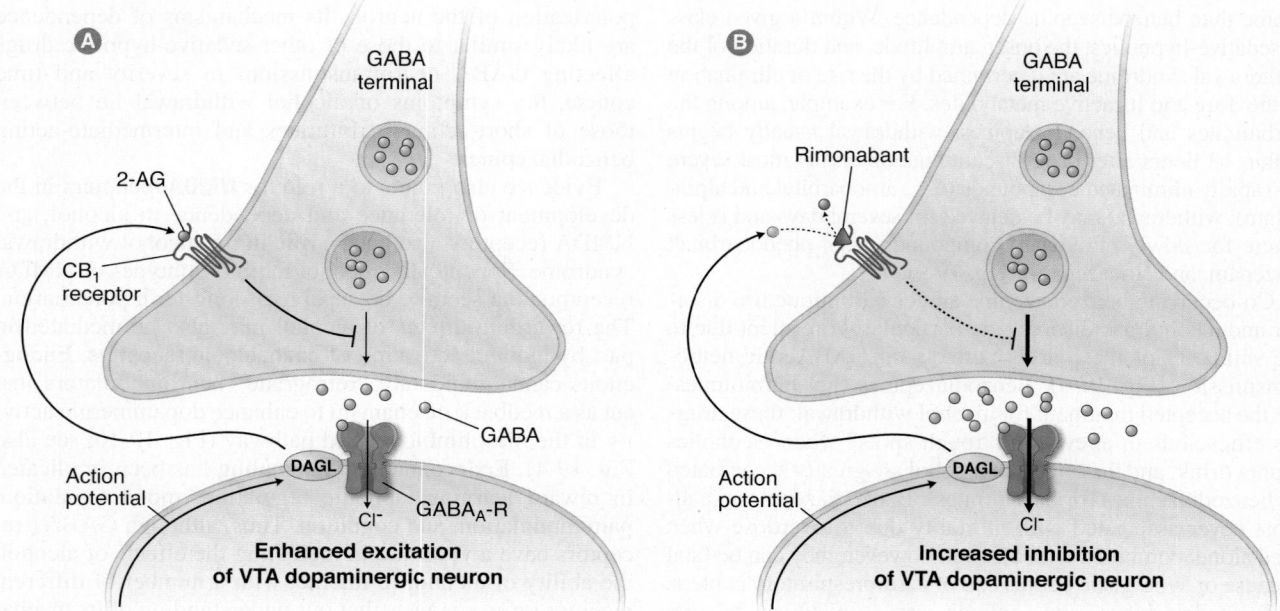

FIGURE 19-10. Endogenous cannabinoid neurotransmission in the mesolimbic dopamine pathway. A. Endogenous cannabinoids are a class of lipid neurotransmitters that act as "retrograde signals" to inhibit release of other neurotransmitters. Here, activation of dopaminergic neurons in the ventral tegmental area (VTA) results in rapid synthesis of the endocannabinoid 2-arachidonoylglycerol (2-AG) via the activity of diacylglycerol lipase (DAGL). 2-AG then activates CB$_1$ cannabinoid receptors located on presynaptic GABAergic terminals. Activation of CB$_1$ receptors causes a transient decrease in vesicular release of GABA on a time scale of seconds to minutes. This results in "feed-forward" enhancement of VTA dopaminergic neuron activity and could contribute to drug-seeking behavior. Thus, endocannabinoids can modulate VTA dopaminergic neuronal activity by inhibiting GABAergic (inhibitory) inputs to the VTA. Activation of VTA dopaminergic neurons in response to environmental cues associated with drug use can often trigger relapse (see Fig. 19-2). **B.** The CB$_1$ receptor antagonist rimonabant has been shown to inhibit cue-induced relapse in preclinical studies. A putative mechanism of action of rimonabant involves blockade of CB$_1$ receptors on presynaptic GABAergic terminals in the VTA, which would sustain high levels of GABA and thus inhibit VTA dopaminergic neuron activity in response to drug-associated cues, and possibly reduce relapse.

Amphetamine and congeners are used clinically as nasal decongestants, analeptics, antidepressants, and diet pills and for treatment of attention-deficit hyperactivity disorder (ADHD). Cocaine and many amphetamine-related drugs have substantial abuse liability; hence, other medications with lower risk profiles have taken their place for many of their uses. Nevertheless, these drugs are widely available by prescription and through illicit sources. They are highly reinforcing because of the profound sense of well-being, energy, and optimism associated with stimulant intoxication; however, this state can rapidly progress to psychomotor agitation, severe paranoia, and even psychosis due to augmented dopamine neurotransmission. The initial euphoric effects of cocaine appear to be more pronounced than those of amphetamine, while amphetamine intoxication far outlasts that of cocaine. Elevated mood is often followed by listlessness, drowsiness, and depressed mood upon the withdrawal of stimulants. Appetite suppression can be followed by ravenous hunger. Stimulants are almost always taken with another drug of abuse, most commonly alcohol, since the other drug accentuates the "high" and alleviates the sleeplessness and sense of being "wired" (Fig. 19-4).

By blocking or reversing the direction of the neurotransmitter transporters that mediate reuptake of the monoamines dopamine, norepinephrine, and serotonin into presynaptic terminals, cocaine and amphetamine potentiate dopaminergic, adrenergic, and serotonergic neurotransmission. Cocaine is most potent at blocking the **dopamine transporter**

(DAT), although higher concentrations block the serotonin and norepinephrine transporters as well (SERT and NET, respectively). Recall that the tricyclic antidepressants (TCAs), serotonin-norepinephrine reuptake inhibitors (SNRIs), and selective serotonin reuptake inhibitors (SSRIs) function in a similar manner, blocking reuptake of norepinephrine and serotonin (TCAs and SNRIs) or serotonin alone (SSRIs) into presynaptic neurons. Amphetamine reverses the direction of all three monoamine transporters, although this drug is more effective at the **norepinephrine transporter**. Amphetamine also releases vesicular transmitter stores into the cytoplasm; these combined actions cause the catecholamine neurotransmitter to be transported into, rather than out of, the extracellular space. By these actions, cocaine and amphetamine increase the concentration of monoamine neurotransmitters in the extracellular space, potentiating neurotransmission (Fig. 19-1).

Although cocaine and amphetamine act on monoaminergic neurons throughout the body, it is the action of these drugs on neurons in two major centers in the brain that likely governs their potential for abuse. The first set of neurons, in the **locus ceruleus** in the pons, sends ascending adrenergic projections throughout the hypothalamus, thalamus, cerebral cortex, and cerebellum and descending projections to the medulla and spinal cord. These projections maintain alertness and responsiveness to unexpected stimuli (see Chapter 11, Adrenergic Pharmacology). Thus, drugs such as cocaine and amphetamine, which potentiate the actions of norepinephrine by inhibiting neurotransmitter reuptake, produce enhanced arousal and vigilance and are called **psychostimulants**. The second major site at which cocaine and amphetamine act is on midbrain dopaminergic neurons, the axons of which terminate in the nucleus accumbens, striatum, and cortex (Fig. 19-4). As discussed above, these dopaminergic terminals in the nucleus accumbens are a critical component of the brain's reward pathway.

It was long believed that the psychostimulants do not cause significant withdrawal and that behaviors to seek these drugs rarely attain levels that are out of control. However, cocaine use can be associated with withdrawal symptoms such as bradycardia, sleepiness, and fatigue. Withdrawal from cocaine or amphetamine also produces psychological symptoms, such as dysphoria and anhedonia (an inability to experience pleasure), that are opposite to the euphoria experienced immediately after administration of the drug. Many of these symptoms are not strictly attributable to withdrawal because they cannot be alleviated by the administration of more cocaine or amphetamine. In fact, symptoms of withdrawal can appear even when psychostimulant levels in the plasma are high. This phenomenon occurs both because of allostasis of reward pathways (discussed earlier) and because these drugs cause **tachyphylaxis**, an acute process in which the target tissue becomes less and less responsive to constant concentrations of a drug. In the case of cocaine and amphetamine, tachyphylaxis may be caused by depletion of the neurotransmitter. Because the drugs block presynaptic neurotransmitter reuptake, the elevated levels of neurotransmitter in the extracellular space feed back to inhibit its synthesis, and neurotransmitter stores in the presynaptic terminal are progressively depleted. The combination of tachyphylaxis and allostasis makes discontinuation of stimulants particularly difficult for addicts, both in the short and long term.

Marijuana

Cannabinoids are compounds derived from *Cannabis sativa* (marijuana). The primary psychoactive component of marijuana is Δ^9-**tetrahydrocannabinol (THC)**, which is a partial agonist at the G protein-coupled type-1 **cannabinoid receptor (CB$_1$)**. The endogenous ligand of the CB$_1$ receptor is the arachidonic acid derivative **anandamide**, which is representative of a class of endocannabinoid "retrograde" neuromodulators that act as a feedback mechanism to reduce neuronal excitation (Fig. 19-10). Since blockade of CB$_1$ receptors by the antagonist **rimonabant** eliminates the effects of smoked marijuana in humans, the subjective effects of marijuana are thought to be mediated by the CB$_1$ receptor. The CB$_1$ receptor is widely distributed within the prefrontal cortex, hippocampus, amygdala, basal ganglia, and cerebellum. In rats, the administration of natural and synthetic cannabinoids causes dopamine release in the nucleus accumbens of the brain reward pathway.

Endogenous cannabinoids appear to modulate a variety of appetitive (reinforcing and consumptive) behaviors including eating, smoking, and alcohol drinking. Cannabinoid use causes a prompt and generalized "high" characterized by euphoria, laughter, giddiness, and depersonalization. After 1–2 hours, cognitive functions such as memory, reaction time, coordination, and alertness are compromised, and the user has difficulty concentrating. This effect corresponds to a "mellowing" phase, which results in relaxation and even sleep. High doses of marijuana can cause anxiety, overt panic reactions, perceptual distortions, impairments in

reality testing, and, rarely, overt psychosis in susceptible individuals. Synthetic cannabinoids (colloquially, *K2* or *Spice*) that have recently become available "on the street" seem particularly prone to present with florid manifestations, which are potentially misdiagnosed as primary psychotic disorders. Overt panic reactions are the most common reason cited for stopping marijuana use.

Tolerance to marijuana occurs via down-regulation of CB$_1$ receptor expression and post-translational modifications that reduce signal transduction efficiency. Withdrawal from marijuana is generally mild due to its high volume of distribution and long elimination half-life. Withdrawal symptoms can include insomnia, loss of appetite, irritability, and anxiety, perhaps due to activation of central corticotropin-releasing factor (CRF) systems, particularly in the amygdala. Blockade of CB$_1$ receptors by rimonabant can precipitate a withdrawal syndrome in chronic users.

Other Abused Drugs

Phencyclidine (PCP) was developed as a dissociative anesthetic but is no longer used because of behavioral toxicity. PCP blocks NMDA glutamate receptors, which mediate excitatory synaptic transmission and are involved in synaptic plasticity and memory. By interfering with these processes, PCP produces complex effects such as anesthesia, delirium, hallucinations, intense paranoia, and amnesia.

Methylenedioxymethamphetamine (MDMA), known colloquially as *Ecstasy*, is one in the class of phenylethylamine hallucinogenics that unfortunately has been falsely advertised by some as a "safe" drug. Although it is chemically related to methamphetamine and has similar dopaminergic effects, the primary effect of MDMA is on serotonergic neurotransmission. MDMA causes serotonin release into the extracellular space, inhibition of serotonin synthesis, and block of serotonin reuptake. Together, these complex actions of MDMA increase serotonin in the extracellular space while depleting presynaptic stores of the neurotransmitter. The drug causes a central stimulant effect like cocaine and amphetamine but, unlike those drugs, it also has hallucinogenic properties. Like cocaine and amphetamine, MDMA affects the brain reward pathway through dopaminergic stimulation. MDMA may be neurotoxic to a subpopulation of serotonergic neurons when the drug is administered repeatedly or in large amounts.

Caffeine and the related methylxanthines theophylline and theobromine are ubiquitous drugs found in coffee, tea, cola, "energy" drinks, chocolate, and many prescribed and over-the-counter medications. Methylxanthines act by blocking adenosine receptors that are expressed presynaptically on many neurons, including dopaminergic and adrenergic neurons. Because activation of adenosine receptors inhibits dopamine and norepinephrine release, competitive antagonism of the receptors by caffeine increases dopamine and norepinephrine release and, thus, acts as a stimulant. Caffeine may also block adenosine receptors on cortical neurons and thereby disinhibit these neurons. Because CNS adenosine is a natural promoter of sleep and drowsiness, caffeine's blocking of adenosine receptors has alerting effects and improves performance in a variety of circumstances but can also produce insomnia. Symptoms of withdrawal from caffeine can include lethargy, irritability, and a characteristic headache, but addiction, although documented, is rare. Caffeine withdrawal symptoms are commonly observed in even low to moderate users of caffeine, but these typically resolve without treatment.

Inhalants are volatile organic compounds that are inhaled (sometimes called *huffing*) for their psychoactive effects. The typical user of inhalants is a male teenager. Inhalants include organic solvents such as gasoline, toluene, ethyl ether, fluorocarbons, and volatile nitrates, including nitrous oxide and butyl nitrate. Inhalants are readily available in many households and workplaces. At low doses, inhalants produce mood changes and ataxia; at high doses, they may produce dissociative states and hallucinations. Dangers of organic solvent use include suffocation and organ damage, especially hepatotoxicity and neurotoxicity in the central and peripheral nervous systems. Cardiac arrhythmias and sudden death can occur. Inhaled nitrates can produce hypotension and methemoglobinemia. Hydrocarbon inhalants do not appear to act at a specific receptor but rather to disrupt cell functions by binding nonspecifically to hydrophobic sites on receptors, signal transduction proteins, and other macromolecules. Nitrates, however, act at specific receptors for nitric oxide, a small-molecule neuromodulator (see Chapter 22, Pharmacology of Vascular Tone).

MEDICAL COMPLICATIONS OF SUBSTANCE USE DISORDERS

Individuals with substance use disorders typically present to a physician complaining of the *indirect* effects of drug/alcohol self-administration. These can include family disruptions and emotional trauma, legal problems and physical injury, self-neglect (e.g., malnutrition, harm from adulterants mixed with drugs, infection from needle administration), inappropriate use of prescribed medication (e.g., analgesics, anxiolytics), and lack of adherence with medical regimens for coexisting illnesses. These effects are clearly not specific to the pharmacologic actions of any given drug but are the consequence of out-of-control, often self-destructive behaviors that interfere with a balanced life because the reward and salience of drug use supersede that of other elements of the environment. Less commonly, patients seek medical care for acute and chronic *direct* pharmacologic and toxic actions of the substance(s) of abuse. Given the multiplicity of drugs, the means by which they are obtained, and the variety of routes of administration, complications may also be secondary to tissue toxicity and induced metabolic changes. Adequate treatment of the medical complications related to substance use disorders requires knowledge of a given substance's pharmacologic actions.

Many patients with substance use disorder use more than one drug or alcohol. Pharmacodynamic and pharmacokinetic effects of having more than one substance use disorder are often difficult to predict from the actions of each individual agent. For example, research has revealed a potentially dangerous interaction between cocaine and alcohol. When taken together, the two drugs are converted to **cocaethylene**. Cocaethylene has a longer duration of action in the brain and is more toxic than either drug alone. The vast majority of individuals with substance use disorders also smoke cigarettes and, despite attaining abstinence from their "drug of choice," the eventual cause of death is often related to complications of cigarettes (e.g., cancer, cardiovascular disease).

Alcohol use disorder is associated with widespread toxicity. Alcoholic cardiomyopathy can result in a life-threatening decrease in left ventricular function. Ethanol is directly toxic to heart muscle cells, affecting contractility of the myocytes and inhibiting the repair of injury to these cells. The mechanism of myocyte damage may relate to the overproduction of oxygen-containing molecules (reactive oxygen species) secondary to alcohol metabolism, with damage to the plasma membrane of the myocyte. Nutritional deficiencies of water-soluble vitamins such as thiamine may also be involved. With moderate drinking, there is typically an increase in systolic blood pressure. Alcohol withdrawal also plays a role in hypertension because sympathetic activity is increased during withdrawal. Stress appears to cause a greater rise in blood pressure in drinkers than in nondrinkers. There appears to be a protective effect of drinking on coronary artery disease, at least in older individuals and those otherwise at risk for coronary disease. The so-called J-shaped mortality curve shows that these populations have decreased mortality with low to moderate drinking (generally 0.5–2 drinks/day) and increased mortality with heavy drinking. The mechanism of this protection involves beneficial effects of ethanol on lipoprotein metabolism and thrombosis: ethanol increases high-density lipoprotein (HDL) levels in a dose-dependent manner in low to moderate drinkers, and ethanol inhibits platelet aggregation and lowers plasma fibrinogen levels.

Chronic alcoholism has other significant medical complications. Metabolic consequences of alcohol use disorder include gout, hyperlipidemia and fatty liver, and hypoglycemia. Chronic alcoholics can develop obesity when the high caloric content of alcohol is added to normal food intake; when food intake is limited and/or malabsorption is present, weight loss with mineral and electrolyte imbalances and vitamin deficiencies can result. Alcohol toxicity can lead to pancreatic insufficiency and diabetes. The gastrointestinal system is frequently affected by chronic alcohol consumption, resulting in esophagitis, gastritis or ulcer, pancreatitis, and alcoholic hepatitis and cirrhosis. Effects of alcohol on the cytochrome P450 system alter drug and carcinogen metabolism, accounting for significant drug interactions and increased cancer incidence in chronic alcoholics. Alcohol increases the release of ACTH, glucocorticoids, and catecholamines and inhibits testosterone synthesis and the release of ADH and oxytocin. Neurologic complications of chronic alcoholism include dementia, amnestic disorder, cerebellar degeneration, and neuropathy, due to both direct neurotoxicity and thiamine deficiency. Finally, alcohol consumption during pregnancy has widespread teratogenic consequences, termed **fetal alcohol spectrum disorder**.

Pharmacologic consequences of psychostimulant abuse relate to specific effects of these drugs on the nervous and cardiovascular systems. Potentiation of norepinephrine neurotransmission increases heart rate and blood pressure. Cocaine, in particular, can cause vasospasm leading to stroke, cerebrovasculitis, myocardial infarction, and aortic dissection. The inhibition of cardiac and CNS sodium channels by cocaine can cause arrhythmias and seizures. Psychostimulants can reset temperature regulation, causing hyperpyrexia and associated rhabdomyolysis. Cocaine and amphetamine can also cause involuntary movements through their action on the basal ganglia.

TREATMENTS FOR SUBSTANCE USE DISORDERS

Despite the high prevalence of alcohol and drug problems in medical practice (10–15% in ambulatory care, 30–50% in emergency departments, and 30–60% in general hospital settings), the diagnosis is often overlooked. As is the case with other stigmatized diseases, specialized services are often inaccessible. Recent health legislation in the United States promises parity for medical and mental disorders (including alcohol and drug problems) and more widespread availability of addiction treatment.

Treatments for substance use disorders can be divided into two broad approaches: pharmacologic and psychosocial. Traditionally, pharmacologic treatments for substance use disorder have focused on acute detoxification to relieve the withdrawal symptoms that accompany the cessation of drug use. It has been increasingly recognized, however, that detoxification alone does not affect the long-term course of substance use disorder. Based on this understanding, new pharmacologic agents are being developed to specifically treat the chronic condition of substance use disorder by diminishing craving, to prevent relapse when the patient has attained abstinence, and to reduce harmful alcohol and drug use. These agents are summarized in the Drug Summary Table at the end of this chapter. Attention is also being directed toward treatment of co-occurring psychiatric disorders that may contribute to drug relapse.

Thus, substance use disorder is now considered a chronic medical condition, and treatment must include lifelong management. Psychosocial treatment approaches—for example, counseling techniques such as cognitive-behavioral therapy and an emphasis on wellness such as exercise and mindfulness/relaxation techniques—have been effective when used alone or in combination with pharmacologic treatment. Often, the integrated use of both pharmacologic and psychosocial approaches increases the positive outcomes of treatment. In addition, participation in mutual support self-help programs (e.g., Alcoholics Anonymous) often improves outcomes, either utilized alone or when self-help messages are incorporated into psychiatric treatment programs. These psychosocial strategies specifically address the role of social learning and motivation in the pathogenesis of substance use disorders.

Although counseling typically focuses on an individual patient's psychological needs, effective treatment must also address the underlying social factors that impede long-term recovery, such as unemployment, housing, family disruption, and lack of access to health care.

Treatment outcomes in substance use disorders are comparable to those in other chronic diseases, such as diabetes, hypertension, and asthma. Although some treatments are more effective in some patients than in others, the best predictor of positive outcomes is participation in treatment.

Detoxification

The first step in the treatment of substance use disorder is **detoxification**. The goals of detoxification are to allow the body to adapt to the absence of drug or alcohol, to diagnose and manage medical and psychiatric complications of substance use disorder, and to prepare the patient for long-term rehabilitation. Although detoxification may be achieved technically within a few days, protracted withdrawal symptoms such as anxiety and insomnia may persist and require prolonged attention. Psychosocial counseling should begin early in detoxification and proceed with more intensity after detoxification. For example, Mr. A completed a 28-day intensive outpatient rehabilitation program after acute detoxification.

The manifestations of drug withdrawal depend on the class of drug abused and can range from mild dysphoria to life-threatening seizures. The most commonly employed strategies for alleviating withdrawal are to taper the dose of the drug slowly or to use a long-acting drug in the same class that demonstrates **cross-tolerance**. For example, a common treatment for nicotine withdrawal is the administration of nicotine via a sustained-release transdermal patch or via a chewing gum. The dose is tapered slowly to allow the patient to avoid many of the unpleasant effects of nicotine withdrawal. Another example is the administration and tapering of the long-acting opioid **methadone** for the treatment of opioid withdrawal. Buprenorphine can also be used for opioid withdrawal treatment; however, care must be taken to ensure that the patient is actually in withdrawal prior to starting buprenorphine, because administration of this partial agonist can precipitate or worsen withdrawal if μ-opioid receptors are still occupied by the opioid of abuse (Fig. 19-8). Withdrawal symptoms from alcohol, benzodiazepines, and barbiturates can be severe and, in some cases, even life-threatening. In alcohol withdrawal, administration of a long-acting benzodiazepine (such as **diazepam**) is indicated to prevent withdrawal seizures (Fig. 19-9). Withdrawal from benzodiazepines is accomplished with either a loading dose of phenobarbital, which has a very long elimination half-life, or tapering doses of a longer acting benzodiazepine. Withdrawal from barbiturates should be managed only with phenobarbital. Other antiepileptic medications also suppress CNS hyperactivity due to withdrawal from CNS depressants and can be efficacious in alcohol and benzodiazepine withdrawal (but not barbiturate withdrawal).

Detoxification can also be accomplished by using medications from a different class to block the signs and symptoms of withdrawal. For example, α2-adrenergic agonists such as **clonidine** and **lofexidine** can block sympathetic hyperactivity, which is a manifestation of withdrawal from all drugs of abuse. α2-Receptors inhibit noradrenergic outflow from neurons in the brain to the periphery and modulate the activity of cells in the gut responsible for fluid absorption and intestinal motility; by these two mechanisms, α2-agonists partially block opioid withdrawal symptoms. Clonidine also diminishes symptoms of withdrawal from nicotine and several other drugs. However, such a strategy is not recommended to treat withdrawal from central nervous system depressants because it does not adequately prevent withdrawal seizures.

Self-Help and Mutual Support Programs

As the case of Mr. A illustrates, the risk of relapse after detoxification is high, and long-term management of addiction is needed to achieve continued sobriety. While not acceptable or helpful to all patients, self-help and mutual support programs have played a prominent role in successful recovery for millions of individuals. These approaches are modeled after **Alcoholics Anonymous (AA)**. Foremost is the understanding that the problem is drinking and, therefore, the focus is on acquiring strategies to prevent a relapse. AA and related programs such as Narcotics Anonymous (NA) and Cocaine Anonymous (CA) provide community support groups and mentoring. The presence of such help mitigates the sense of alienation and loneliness often felt by addicts. Participation is free and readily available. Related mutual support groups such as Al-Anon for spouses and Alateen for teenage family members provide important support for recovery. The mechanisms by which AA-related programs provide benefit are not fully understood but may reside in powerful social learning effects that can modify the incentive salience of drugs of abuse. Most physicians now recognize that these programs can be useful and complementary to the medical treatment of substance use disorders.

Moderation management, another therapeutic stance toward alcoholism, emphasizes moderation rather than abstinence. This strategy is ineffective in individuals with alcohol use disorder, who (by definition) can no longer control their drinking, and thus is recommended only in "problem drinkers"—patients who sometimes overindulge but have not yet lost control over their drinking.

Pharmacologic Treatment of Substance Use Disorders

The recognition that addiction is caused by fundamental changes in brain reward pathways indicates that pharmacotherapy could have an important role in the management of substance use disorders. To date, several pharmacologic strategies have been employed.

The first of these strategies is the chronic administration of an agent that causes aversive effects when the drug of abuse is used. For example, **disulfiram** inhibits aldehyde dehydrogenase, a critical enzyme in the alcohol metabolism pathway. In an individual who ingests ethanol while taking disulfiram, alcohol dehydrogenase oxidizes the ethanol to acetaldehyde, but disulfiram prevents aldehyde dehydrogenase from metabolizing the acetaldehyde. Therefore, this toxic metabolite accumulates in the blood. Acetaldehyde causes a number of aversive symptoms, including facial flushing, headache, nausea, vomiting, weakness, orthostatic hypotension, and respiratory difficulty. These symptoms can last from 30 minutes to several hours and are followed by exhaustion and fatigue. The aversive effects of alcohol consumption in the presence of disulfiram are intended as a deterrent to further drinking. Unfortunately, the effectiveness of disulfiram is limited by failures in adherence and by substantial toxicity.

A second strategy used to treat addiction is to block the effects of the drug of abuse. **Naltrexone** is an opioid antagonist that competitively blocks the binding of opioids to the opioid receptor. Thus, a patient who injects an opioid, such as heroin, while taking naltrexone will not experience the "high" that normally accompanies drug use. Studies have shown that naltrexone also acts as an opioid inhibitor in the brain reward pathway. Thus, the effects of a drug such as ethanol, which releases endogenous opioids that cause disinhibition (or stimulation) of mesolimbic dopamine, share a final common reward pathway involving the opioid receptor and dopamine and are therefore also inhibited by naltrexone. For this reason, naltrexone has been used to treat alcohol use disorder. Placebo-controlled clinical trials have generally shown efficacy of naltrexone compared to placebo, particularly in reducing relapse to heavy drinking. Naltrexone should not be administered when there are traces of exogenous opioids in the system, because antagonism of remaining drug by naltrexone can lead to the development or exacerbation of opioid withdrawal symptoms. Although naltrexone can effectively prevent the "high" associated with opioids, it does not alleviate cravings or withdrawal effects, and there is a relatively high likelihood of nonadherence. Therefore, naltrexone has been effective only in individuals addicted to opioids or alcohol who have a high motivation to stay drug-free or who have supervised administration. An injectable long-acting naltrexone preparation has been approved by the US Food and Drug Administration (FDA) for the treatment of alcohol use disorder. Sustained-release naltrexone is injected intramuscularly once a month, and it has been demonstrated to reduce heavy alcohol consumption and increase alcohol abstinence. This formulation is also beneficial in opioid use disorder, especially in those with low adherence to treatment.

A third pharmacologic approach is the use of a long-acting agonist for medication maintenance. **Methadone**, as discussed earlier, is a long-acting opioid agonist. Because it is taken orally, it is less likely to produce the sharp increases in plasma levels required to elicit a "high" such as that accompanying the injection of heroin or other opioids. Methadone also has a long half-life compared to heroin or morphine. Thus, once-daily administration of methadone produces plasma opioid levels that remain relatively constant over time and, therefore, mitigate cravings and prevent the emergence of withdrawal signs and symptoms. Moreover, methadone produces cross-tolerance to other opioids, so that a patient who injects heroin or another opioid while taking methadone experiences a reduced effect of the injected drug. However, methadone has significant abuse liability, and there is a risk of death by overdose when methadone is combined with another opioid or CNS depressant. For these reasons, methadone should be dispensed for opioid maintenance treatment only under controlled circumstances in government-licensed programs.

Conceptually similar to substitution treatments for opioid use disorder, **nicotine replacement therapy** is often the first line of treatment for nicotine use disorder. Nicotine replacement is available in the form of chewable gum, lozenge, transdermal patch, smokeless inhaler, or the recently popularized electronic nicotine delivery system ("e-cigarettes"). These forms of nicotine replacement curb cravings and withdrawal symptoms caused by decreases in plasma nicotine levels after cessation of smoking. All forms of nicotine replacement therapy are more effective than placebo for smoking cessation, with the important benefit of avoiding exposure to toxic products of tobacco pyrolysis.

Based on the observations that antagonist (e.g., naltrexone)-based treatment of opioid use disorder suffers from poor adherence and that full agonists with advantageous pharmacokinetic properties (e.g., methadone) can nevertheless be diverted from medical care and abused, partial agonist medications have been developed for the treatment of opioid use disorder. The partial agonist action of **buprenorphine** at μ-opioid receptors alleviates withdrawal symptoms associated with decreases in plasma levels of abused opioids, and reduces opioid cravings by increasing mesolimbic dopaminergic neurotransmission (Fig. 19-8). Thus, buprenorphine not only facilitates opioid detoxification but also can be employed for maintenance treatment. Since it is not a full agonist, buprenorphine carries a low risk of overdose; since it antagonizes the reinforcing effects of full opioid agonists such as heroin, it reduces the likelihood of relapse. Because of its partial agonist properties and relatively long half-life (compared to most abused opioids), withdrawal from buprenorphine per se is mild. To minimize abuse in the outpatient setting, buprenorphine is usually administered daily or on alternate days as a sublingual preparation (**Suboxone®**) that also contains the opioid antagonist naloxone. If Suboxone® is diverted and administered parenterally, the naloxone antagonizes the agonist effects of buprenorphine; when administered sublingually, the naloxone is not bioavailable and the full effects of buprenorphine are experienced. Outpatient use of buprenorphine will likely replace methadone-based treatment programs for opioid use disorder in all but the most severely addicted patients.

The nicotinic receptor partial agonist **varenicline** has recently been demonstrated to facilitate smoking cessation in large-scale clinical trials. Varenicline is a partial agonist at the $\alpha_4\beta_2$ nicotinic acetylcholine receptor subtype; hence, this agent has an analogous mechanism of action for treatment of nicotine dependence as that of buprenorphine for opioid dependence (Fig. 19-8). The partial agonist effect of varenicline increases mesolimbic dopaminergic neurotransmission and thus both reduces withdrawal symptoms and diminishes the nicotine cravings that can lead to relapse. Varenicline also acts as a pharmacologic antagonist at nicotinic receptors in the presence of the full agonist nicotine, thus mitigating the dopamine-enhancing effects (and addictive potential) of nicotine. Importantly, varenicline administration has been associated with neuropsychiatric adverse effects including emotional lability and acute psychosis, leading to an FDA warning regarding the use of varenicline in patients with psychiatric disorders; however, most recent evidence has not supported these concerns.

A fourth approach is to utilize medications to prevent the long-term dysphoria and dysfunctional reward mechanisms (allostasis) that are common in addicts who are newly abstinent. For example, one of the consequences of long-term alcohol consumption is a hyperactive glutamatergic system that persists even after alcohol consumption ceases. **Acamprosate**, which modulates glutamate hyperactivity to reestablish a more normal state, has been efficacious in preventing relapse to alcohol drinking in some but not all studies and has been approved for the treatment of alcohol use disorder. Recent comparisons of naltrexone and acamprosate with and without cognitive therapy have shown only naltrexone to be significantly more efficacious than placebo, however. The antiepileptic medication **topiramate**, which inhibits the AMPA/kainate class of glutamate receptors, significantly reduced alcohol drinking in a double-blind, placebo-controlled study. Importantly, topiramate treatment response in patients with alcohol use disorder has recently been found to be moderated by a polymorphism in *GRIK1*, which encodes the kainate GluK1 receptor subunit. Together with other antiepileptic drugs, topiramate is being studied in larger clinical trials, but none of these drugs is currently FDA-approved for the treatment of alcohol use disorder. The antidepressant **bupropion** inhibits reuptake of dopamine and norepinephrine and has demonstrated efficacy in smoking cessation. The mechanism of action of bupropion may be related to increased dopaminergic neurotransmission in the mesolimbic reward pathway, thus buffering nicotine withdrawal-induced cravings. Bupropion lowers the seizure threshold, suggesting that this treatment may not be appropriate for patients with underlying seizure disorders or those who abuse drugs that are associated with intoxication- or withdrawal-induced seizures.

A fifth approach is to specifically treat co-occurring psychiatric symptoms that are highly prevalent in individuals diagnosed with substance use disorders. Depressed and anxious mood, mood instability, and psychotic symptoms are often observed in abstinent patients. A meta-analysis of antidepressant treatment of patients with substance use disorders found that these medications are not effective unless the patients are diagnosed with a co-occurring major depression. In fact, there is some evidence that selective serotonin reuptake inhibitors (SSRIs) may cause early-onset, antisocial alcoholics to become worse and drink more alcohol than those receiving a placebo. Also, the high co-occurrence of bipolar spectrum disorders in those with substance use disorders suggests that depressive symptoms in these patients often do not warrant antidepressant treatment but rather mood stabilization. Treatment of abstinent addicts with bipolar or psychotic disorders, using mood stabilizers and antipsychotics, is generally viewed as beneficial. Nevertheless, most clinicians recognize that it may be difficult to accurately diagnose and treat co-occurring psychiatric disorders if individuals are actively using alcohol or other drugs.

In contrast to the various pharmacologic treatments available for alcohol and opioid use disorders, there is a paucity of current treatments for cocaine and amphetamine use disorders, and none is approved by the FDA. Several trials have attempted to use antidepressants, such as the tricyclic antidepressant **desipramine** or the selective serotonin reuptake inhibitor **fluoxetine**. Desipramine acts by blocking monoamine reuptake (especially norepinephrine reuptake), whereas fluoxetine inhibits serotonin reuptake. Both agents have been shown to reduce drug craving, but unfortunately, neither has been shown to prevent cocaine use. There is recent evidence that disulfiram (see above) may have some effectiveness in the treatment of cocaine dependence. In addition to its inhibition of aldehyde dehydrogenase, disulfiram inhibits dopamine β-hydroxylase and can increase brain dopamine levels, possibly counteracting the dopamine-depleting effects of chronic cocaine use. Because cocaine sensitization involves glutamate, antiepileptics (e.g., carbamazepine, oxcarbazepine, and topiramate) are also being studied for efficacy in the treatment of cocaine dependence.

CONCLUSION AND FUTURE DIRECTIONS

This chapter has discussed the major causes of substance use disorders. Substance use disorder is defined as a problematic pattern of drug use associated with context-induced craving and drug-seeking, especially under situations of stress, that leads to clinically significant impairment or distress. Substance use disorder is caused by an allostatic adaptation to the presence of the drug in brain reward pathways. Although each drug has its own molecular and cellular mechanism of action that may account for drug toxicity, all abused drugs specifically affect the mesolimbic dopamine brain reward pathway. This chapter has also discussed the major treatments for substance use disorders, including the pharmacologic prevention and treatment of withdrawal symptoms, the long-term psychosocial management of addiction, and newer pharmacologic treatments that, when integrated with psychosocial approaches, promote long-lasting sobriety. Together, these addiction treatments achieve outcomes approximating those of other long-term chronic medical disorders, such as atherosclerosis, hypertension, and diabetes.

New directions in addiction research are focused on the pharmacologic modulation of brain reward, stress responses, and learning-related neural processes. In addition, these approaches are complemented by basic and clinical studies of the neurobiology of learning and memory and the

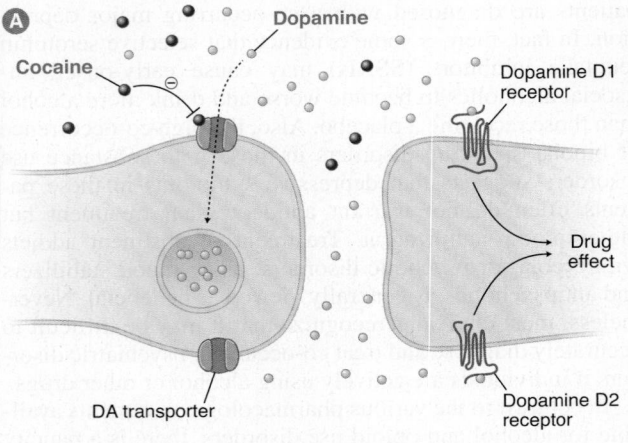

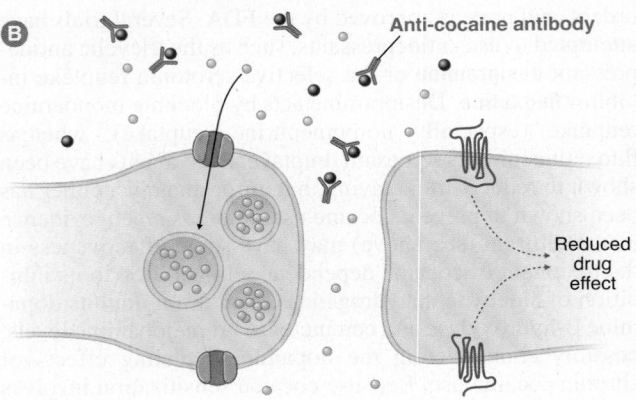

FIGURE 19-11. Vaccine approach to treat cocaine use disorder. A. Cocaine inhibits the dopamine transporter (DAT), thereby preventing dopamine reuptake and allowing excessive stimulation of postsynaptic dopamine receptors (D1 and D2). **B.** After treatment with a "cocaine vaccine," antibodies are generated that bind to exogenous cocaine once it enters the bloodstream. The antibody-bound cocaine is incapable of binding to and inhibiting DAT, and the rewarding effects of the drug are reduced.

modification of these processes through psychosocial treatments. Current approaches to cocaine use disorder provide two specific examples. First, drugs that specifically interact with different dopamine receptor subtypes have been explored, investigating the hypotheses that a D1-specific agonist or D4-specific antagonist could suppress drug cravings, and that a D2-specific antagonist could prevent the reinforcing effects of cocaine. Second, researchers have recently completed clinical trials of a cocaine vaccine, under the theory that cocaine will be less reinforcing in vaccinated persons who are exposed to the drug (Fig. 19-11). If successful, this approach could be extended to other drugs of abuse. (Trials of an analogous anti-nicotine vaccine are also forthcoming.) However, vaccinated individuals may switch to other drugs of abuse for which they have not produced antibodies, and hence, this is not likely to be a totally satisfactory approach.

Broader and more promising are efforts to develop pharmacologic treatments for addiction aimed at (1) modulating the chemical mediators of synaptic plasticity that underlie reward learning and memory (Fig. 19-2) and (2) modifying the negative affective states and stress responses, the previously mentioned "allostatic load," associated with chronic drug abuse. These approaches address *shared brain mechanisms* of addiction to all drugs of abuse. For example, a failure of the prefrontal cortex to control drug-seeking behaviors has been linked to glutamatergic dysfunction in reward pathways, which may be amenable to new glutamate- and neuroplasticity-based pharmacotherapies. Another approach targets neural systems mediating behavioral stress responses; for example, an antagonist at the neurokinin-1 receptor, which is expressed in brain areas involved in stress responses and drug reward, has been shown in preliminary studies to suppress alcohol cravings, improve well-being, and attenuate the cortisol stress response in abstinent alcoholics. Preclinical studies have shown that CRF antagonists may block stress-induced reinstatement of drug use in animal models of substance use disorder (Fig. 19-12). Endocannabinoid signaling has also been implicated in a variety of physiologic

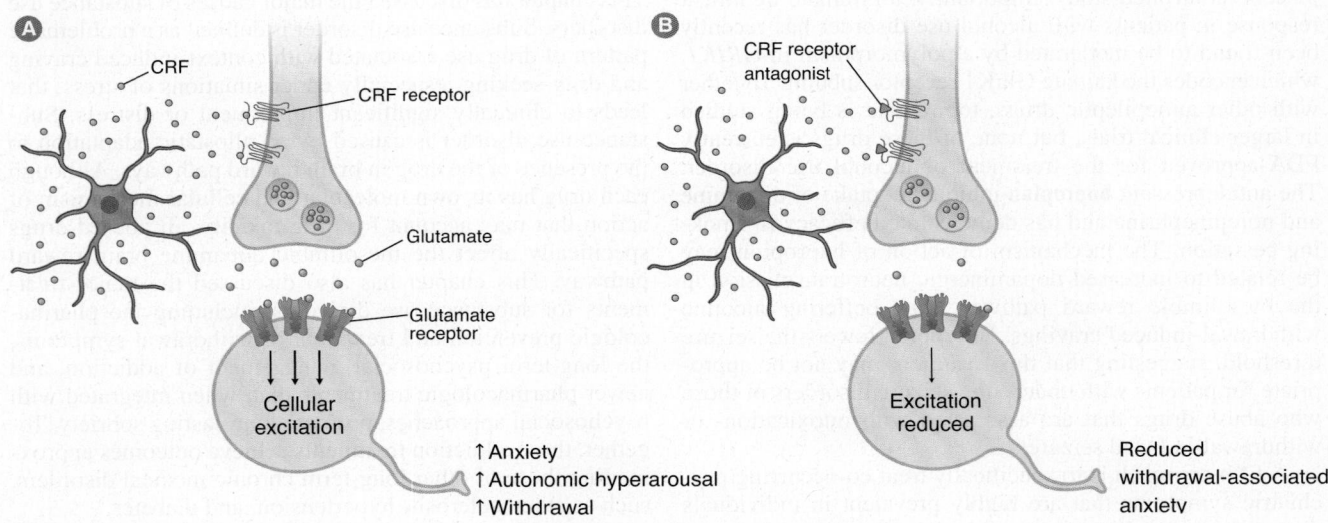

Figure 19-12. Corticotropin-releasing factor (CRF) antagonist approach to reduce alcohol/drug withdrawal and relapse. A. As a result of allostatic changes associated with chronic alcohol/drug use, when use is discontinued, a small subset of extended amygdala neurons (*red*) locally release CRF, which activates glutamatergic neurotransmission via stimulation of CRF receptors on nearby amygdala neurons, contributing to anxiety and negative affect. This state is important in driving continued drug-seeking behavior (relapse). **B.** CRF receptor antagonist blocks CRF activation of extended amygdala neurons during alcohol/drug discontinuation. This approach has been suggested to mitigate aversive affective concomitants of drug withdrawal that lead to relapse-associated behaviors.

functions including reward learning, appetite, mood, pain, and cognition (Fig. 19-10). Elucidation of endocannabinoid signaling as a pro-hedonic system involving CB_1 receptor activation led to findings that the CB_1 cannabinoid receptor antagonist rimonabant was effective in obesity treatment, and this drug is now being investigated as a treatment for drug addiction. Rimonabant has not received FDA approval because it is associated with significant psychiatric adverse effects, but this approach remains a promising direction for future research.

Acknowledgment

We thank David C. Lewis, Robert M. Swift, Joshua M. Galanter, and Alan A. Wartenberg for their valuable contributions to this chapter in the First, Second, and Third Editions of *Principles of Pharmacology: The Pathophysiologic Basis of Drug Therapy*.

Suggested Reading

Alcoholics Anonymous. www.aa.org. (*Excellent information on Alcoholics Anonymous.*)

Camí J, Farré M. Mechanisms of disease: drug addiction. *N Engl J Med* 2003;349:975–986. (*Current understanding of neural mechanisms leading to addiction.*)

Dani JA, Harris RA. Nicotine addiction and comorbidity with alcohol abuse and mental illness. *Nat Neurosci* 2005;8:1465–1470. (*Examines the interface between the neuropharmacologic underpinnings of nicotine addiction and psychiatric disorders, especially alcoholism.*)

Goldman D, Oroszi G, Ducci F. The genetics of addictions: uncovering the genes. *Nat Rev Genet* 2005;6:521–532. (*A review that examines how heritable factors operate in causation of drug use disorders.*)

Goldstein RZ, Craig AD, Bechara A, et al. The neurocircuitry of impaired insight in drug addiction. *Trends Cogn Sci* 2009;13:372–380. (*Discusses current understanding of lack of insight and awareness in addiction.*)

Kalivas PW. The glutamate homeostasis hypothesis of addiction. *Nat Rev Neurosci* 2009;10:561–572. (*Review that links learning mechanisms to reward through the glutamatergic system.*)

Koob GF, Le Moal M. Neurobiological mechanisms for opponent motivational processes in addiction. *Philos Trans R Soc B Biol Sci* 2008;363:3113–3123. (*Reviews relationships between stress and reward pathways.*)

McLellan AT, Lewis DC, O'Brien CP, Kleber HD. Drug dependence, a chronic medical illness: implications for treatment, insurance, and outcomes evaluation. *JAMA* 2000;284:1689–1695. (*Seminal analysis of the status of drug use disorders in the health care system.*)

Nestler EJ. Transcriptional mechanisms of addiction: role of delta-FosB. *Philos Trans R Soc B Biol Sci* 2008;363:3245–3255. (*Reviews the role of gene regulation as a unitary neurobiological mechanism in reward and stress responses.*)

Substance Abuse and Mental Health Services Administration. www.samhsa.gov. (*Contains a wealth of information about prevention and treatment and co-occurring diagnoses; also access to listings of evidence-based treatment practices.*)

Volkow ND, Baler RD, Goldstein RZ. Addiction: pulling at the neural threads of social behaviors. *Neuron* 2011;69:599–602. (*Review of interface between medical and societal/legal aspects of addiction.*)

DRUG SUMMARY TABLE: CHAPTER 19   Pharmacology of Drugs of Abuse

DRUG	CLINICAL APPLICATIONS	SERIOUS AND COMMON ADVERSE EFFECTS	CONTRAINDICATIONS	THERAPEUTIC CONSIDERATIONS
INHIBITOR OF ALCOHOL METABOLISM Mechanism—Ethanol is oxidized by alcohol dehydrogenase to acetaldehyde, and acetaldehyde is metabolized by aldehyde dehydrogenase. Disulfiram inhibits aldehyde dehydrogenase and thereby prevents metabolism of acetaldehyde. Accumulation of serum acetaldehyde causes aversive symptoms.				
Disulfiram	Alcoholism	Hepatitis, peripheral neuropathy, optic neuritis, psychotic disorder Metallic or garlic-like aftertaste, dermatitis	Concomitant use of paraldehyde, metronidazole, ethanol, or ethanol-containing products Coronary occlusion, severe myocardial disease Psychoses	Acetaldehyde accumulation causes facial flushing, headache, nausea, vomiting, weakness, orthostatic hypotension, and respiratory difficulty; these symptoms last from 30 minutes to several hours. Disulfiram's effectiveness is limited by failures in adherence. Co-administration with isoniazid may result in adverse CNS effects. Disulfiram increases anticoagulant effects of warfarin.
OPIOID ANTAGONISTS Mechanism—Competitively block binding of opioids to the μ-opioid receptor				
Naloxone	Opioid overdose Rapid reversal of opioid action	Cardiac arrhythmia, hypertension, hypotension, coma, encephalopathy, seizure, pulmonary edema, opioid withdrawal	Hypersensitivity to naloxone	Interacts with opioid analgesics. Short half-life.
Naltrexone	Opioid use disorder Alcoholism	Injection site necrosis, deep vein thrombosis, hepatotoxicity, eosinophilic pneumonia, pulmonary embolism, retinal artery occlusion Abdominal pain, constipation, nausea, headache, anxiety	Concomitant opioid analgesics Hypersensitivity to naltrexone	Naltrexone prevents the "high" associated with opioid use, but it does not alleviate cravings or withdrawal effects. High likelihood of nonadherence with naltrexone; only effective in motivated individuals. An injectable, sustained-release naltrexone formulation is approved for treatment of alcohol and opioid use disorders.
LONG-ACTING OPIOID AGONISTS Mechanism—Synthetic opioid agonist that binds and activates the μ-opioid receptor				
Methadone	Opioid detoxification, maintenance Severe pain	Prolonged QT interval, torsades de pointes, shock, respiratory acidosis, hypotension, respiratory arrest Diaphoresis, constipation, nausea, asthenia, dizziness, somnolence	Hypersensitivity to methadone Acute or severe asthma in an unmonitored setting or in the absence of resuscitative equipment Hypercarbia Paralytic ileus Significant respiratory depression	Suppresses symptoms of withdrawal in individuals with opioid use disorder due to slow absorption and long half-life. Produces plasma opioid levels that remain fairly constant over time and thereby mitigate cravings and prevent withdrawal symptoms. Produces cross-tolerance to other opioids. May decrease the metabolism of CYP2B6, CYP2D6, and CYP3A4 substrates, e.g., zidovudine. May increase the metabolism of CYP3A4 substrates and may undergo increased metabolism when co-administered with other CYP3A4 substrates; for example, co-administration with carbamazepine, phenytoin, or rifampin may decrease serum methadone concentration, resulting in methadone withdrawal symptoms. Methadone interacts with antiretrovirals in multiple ways. Methadone has significant abuse liability. There is risk of death if combined with another CNS depressant.

OPIOID PARTIAL AGONISTS
Mechanism—Partial μ-opioid receptor agonist and κ-opioid receptor antagonist

Drug	Indication	Serious and Common Adverse Effects	Contraindications	Therapeutic Considerations
Buprenorphine	Moderate to severe pain	*Prolonged QT interval, hypotension, hepatic insufficiency, liver failure, coma, respiratory depression, drug dependence, neonatal abstinence syndrome* Somnolence, headache, dizziness, nausea, constipation	Hypersensitivity to buprenorphine Acute or severe asthma in an unmonitored setting or in the absence of resuscitative equipment Paralytic ileus Respiratory depression	Alleviates opioid cravings and withdrawal symptoms; carries low risk of overdose. The withdrawal effects of buprenorphine are mild compared to those of full opioid agonists. Buprenorphine is usually administered as Suboxone®, a sublingual preparation that also contains naloxone; if Suboxone® is abused and administered parenterally, the naloxone antagonizes the effects of buprenorphine; when administered sublingually, the naloxone is inactivated and the full effects of buprenorphine are experienced. May precipitate or worsen withdrawal if μ-opioid receptors are still occupied by the opioid of abuse; should be administered only in patients who are already in withdrawal. Can be used for detoxification as well as maintenance treatment.

GABAergic AGONISTS
Mechanism—Analogue of homotaurine, a GABAergic agonist. Stimulates inhibitory GABAergic neurotransmission in the brain and antagonizes the effects of glutamate; active at postsynaptic GABA$_B$ receptors but not at GABA$_A$ receptors in vitro

Drug	Indication	Serious and Common Adverse Effects	Contraindications	Therapeutic Considerations
Acamprosate	Maintenance of abstinence in alcoholism	*Cardiomyopathy, heart failure, arterial and venous thrombosis, shock, anxiety, depression, suicidal ideation* Dizziness, insomnia, diarrhea, nausea	Severe renal impairment Hypersensitivity to acamprosate	Modulates glutamate hyperactivity to reestablish a more normal state for the treatment of alcohol use disorder. Decreases spontaneous alcohol consumption in animal studies. Acamprosate has little or no abuse potential and does not induce dependence.

SODIUM CHANNEL INHIBITORS
Mechanism—Inhibit electrical neurotransmission by use-dependent block of neuronal voltage-gated sodium channel

Drug				
Carbamazepine	See Drug Summary Table: Chapter 16 Pharmacology of Abnormal Electrical Neurotransmission in the Central Nervous System			

CALCIUM CHANNEL INHIBITORS
Mechanism—Inhibit the high-voltage-activated (HVA) calcium channel

Drug				
Gabapentin	See Drug Summary Table: Chapter 16 Pharmacology of Abnormal Electrical Neurotransmission in the Central Nervous System			

GABA CHANNEL POTENTIATORS
Mechanism—Potentiate GABA-mediated inhibition to increase chloride current through the channel

Drug				
Diazepam	See Drug Summary Table: Chapter 16 Pharmacology of Abnormal Electrical Neurotransmission in the Central Nervous System			
Phenobarbital	See Drug Summary Table: Chapter 16 Pharmacology of Abnormal Electrical Neurotransmission in the Central Nervous System			

OTHER ANTIEPILEPTIC DRUGS
Mechanisms under investigation

Drug				
Topiramate	See Drug Summary Table: Chapter 16 Pharmacology of Abnormal Electrical Neurotransmission in the Central Nervous System			

continues

DRUG SUMMARY TABLE: CHAPTER 19 Pharmacology of Drugs of Abuse *continued*

DRUG	CLINICAL APPLICATIONS	*SERIOUS* AND COMMON ADVERSE EFFECTS	CONTRAINDICATIONS	THERAPEUTIC CONSIDERATIONS
PARTIAL NICOTINE AGONISTS Mechanism—Partial neuronal $\alpha_4 \beta_2$ nicotinic receptor agonist that prevents nicotine stimulation of mesolimbic dopamine system				
Varenicline	Smoking cessation aid	*Suicidal thoughts, erratic/aggressive behavior, exacerbation of underlying psychiatric illness, sedation with impairment of physical or mental abilities, angina, myocardial infarction, stroke* Insomnia, headache, abnormal dreams, nausea	Exercise caution with preexisting psychiatric illnesses (e.g., bipolar disorder, major severe depression, schizophrenia) because patients with these illnesses were not included in clinical trials History of serious hypersensitivity reactions to varenicline	Alleviates nicotine cravings and withdrawal symptoms. The withdrawal effects are mild compared to nicotine. Should be started 1 week before target quit date and titrated to maintenance dose over that week.
TRICYCLIC ANTIDEPRESSANTS Mechanism—Inhibit reuptake of serotonin (5-HT) and norepinephrine (NE) from the synaptic cleft				
Desipramine	See Drug Summary Table: Chapter 15 Pharmacology of Serotonergic and Central Adrenergic Neurotransmission			
SELECTIVE SEROTONIN REUPTAKE INHIBITORS Mechanism—Selectively inhibit reuptake of 5-HT from the synaptic cleft				
Fluoxetine	See Drug Summary Table: Chapter 15 Pharmacology of Serotonergic and Central Adrenergic Neurotransmission			
OTHER ATYPICAL ANTIDEPRESSANTS Mechanism—Bupropion is an aminoketone antidepressant that weakly inhibits neuronal uptake of 5-HT, dopamine, and NE				
Bupropion	See Drug Summary Table: Chapter 15 Pharmacology of Serotonergic and Central Adrenergic Neurotransmission			

myocardial O₂ demand

$\uparrow$

Ventricular wall stress

$\uparrow$

Preload

$\uparrow$

Venous tone

Heart
(pump)

Arteriolar t

Veins

III

Principles of
Cardiovascular Pharmacology

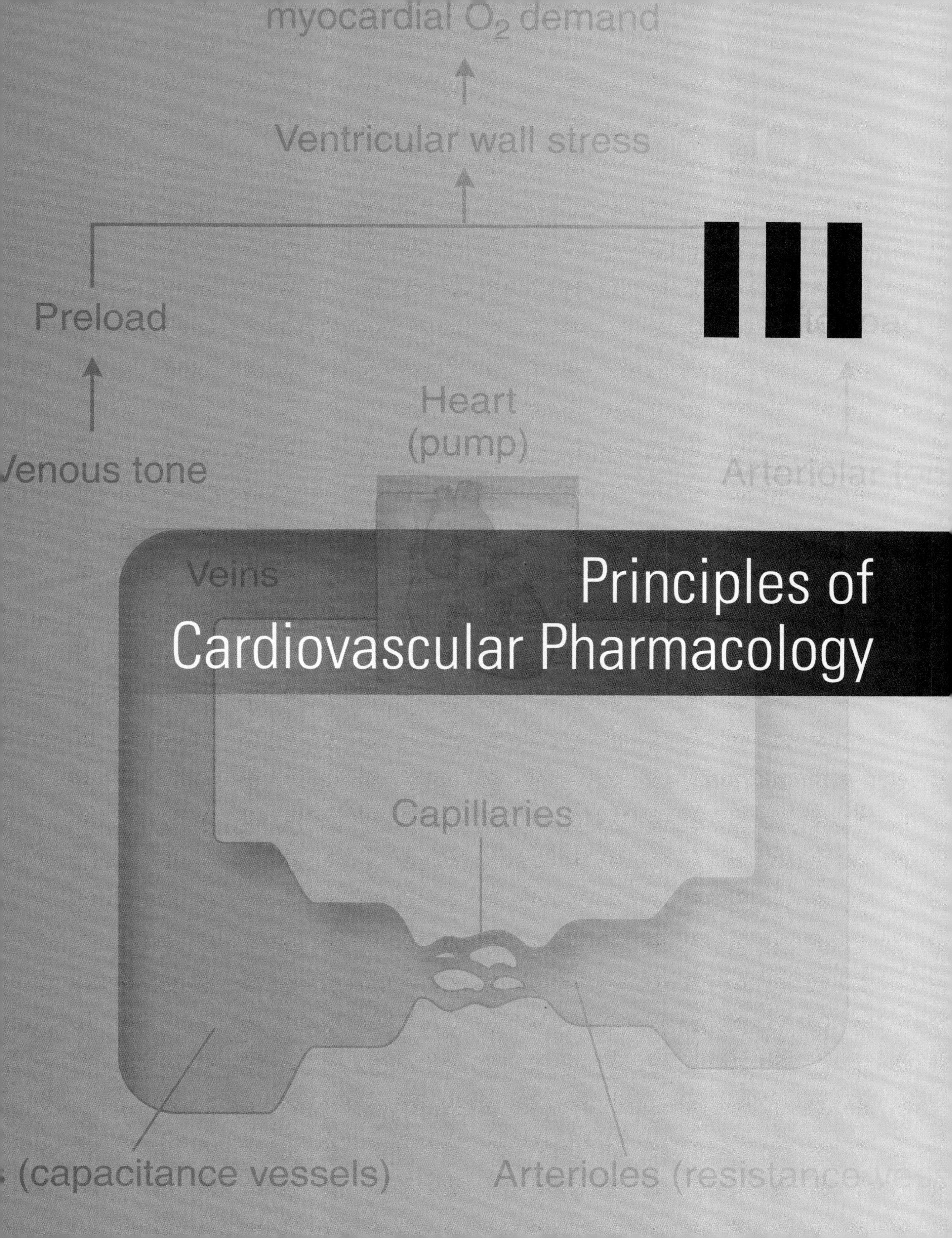

Capillaries

: (capacitance vessels)   Arterioles (resistance v

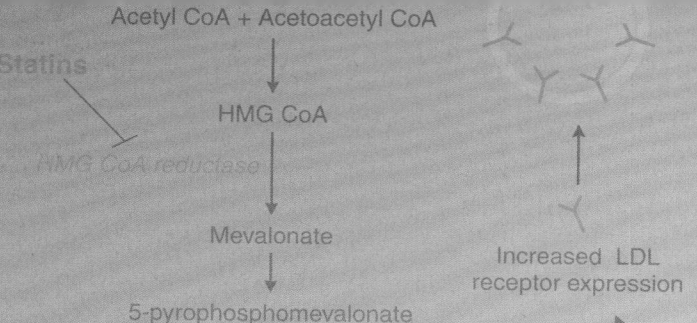

20

Pharmacology of Cholesterol and Lipoprotein Metabolism

Tibor I. Krisko, Ehrin J. Armstrong, and David E. Cohen

INTRODUCTION

Lipids are insoluble or sparingly soluble molecules that are essential for membrane biogenesis and maintenance of membrane integrity. They also serve as energy sources, hormone precursors, and signaling molecules. In order to facilitate transport through the relatively aqueous environment of the blood, nonpolar lipids, such as cholesteryl esters and triglycerides, are packaged within lipoproteins.

Increased concentrations of certain lipoproteins in the circulation are associated strongly with atherosclerosis. Much of the prevalence of cardiovascular disease (CVD), the leading cause of death in the United States and most Western countries, can be attributed to elevated blood concentrations of cholesterol-rich low-density lipoprotein (LDL) particles as well as lipoproteins that are rich in triglycerides. Epidemiologically, decreased concentrations of high-density lipoproteins (HDL) also predispose to atherosclerotic disease. The major contributors to lipoprotein abnormalities appear to be Western diets combined with sedentary lifestyles, but a limited number of genetic causes of hyperlipidemia have also been identified. The role of genetics in common forms of hyperlipidemia is the subject of intense study utilizing cutting-edge genomic

approaches. It is apparent that genes modify both the sensitivity of individuals to adverse dietary habits and lifestyles and the response of individuals to lipid-lowering therapies.

This chapter highlights the biochemistry and physiology of cholesterol and lipoproteins, with an emphasis on the role of lipoproteins in atherogenesis, and the pharmacologic interventions that can ameliorate hyperlipidemia. Abundant clinical outcomes data have proven that morbidity and mortality from cardiovascular disease can be reduced by the use of lipid-lowering drugs.

BIOCHEMISTRY AND PHYSIOLOGY OF CHOLESTEROL AND LIPOPROTEIN METABOLISM

Lipoproteins are macromolecular aggregates that transport triglycerides and cholesterol in the blood. Circulating lipoproteins can be differentiated on the basis of density, size, and protein content (Table 20-1). As a general rule, larger, less dense lipoproteins have a higher percentage composition of lipids; **chylomicrons** are the largest and least dense lipoprotein subclass, whereas HDLs are the smallest lipoproteins, containing the lowest lipid content and the highest proportion of protein.

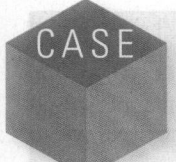

CASE

Jake P., a 29-year-old construction worker, makes an appointment to see Dr. Cush. Jake complains of hard, elevated swellings around his Achilles tendon that seem to rub constantly against his construction boots. Jake had been hesitant to see the doctor (his last appointment was 10 years ago), but he remembers that his dad, who died at age 42 of a heart attack, had similar swellings. On examination, Dr. Cush recognizes the Achilles swellings as xanthomas (lipid deposits); the physical exam is otherwise within normal limits. Jake comments that his diet is quite "fatty," including three to four donuts each day and frequent hamburgers. Dr. Cush explains that the xanthomas on Jake's feet are the result of cholesteryl ester deposition, probably from high cholesterol levels in his blood. Dr. Cush orders a fasting plasma cholesterol level and recommends that Jake reduce his intake of foods high in saturated fat and cholesterol and increase his intake of poultry, fish, whole cereal grains, fruits, and vegetables. Jake has gained about 15 pounds since he was 19 and has a small paunch. Dr. Cush recommends regular exercise and weight loss.

Results of the blood test reveal a total plasma cholesterol concentration of 315 mg/dL (normal, <200), with elevated LDL cholesterol of 250 mg/dL (desirable, <100), low HDL of 35 mg/dL (normal, 35 to 100), and normal concentrations of triglycerides and very-low-density lipoprotein (VLDL). Based on these test results, his age, the Achilles heel xanthomas, and a positive family history for an early myocardial infarction, Dr. Cush tells Jake that he likely has an inherited disorder of cholesterol metabolism known as heterozygous familial hypercholesterolemia. This disease puts Jake at very high risk for early atherosclerosis and myocardial infarction. The low HDL cholesterol level also contributes to his increased risk of cardiovascular disease.

Dr. Cush tells Jake that aggressive lowering of cholesterol levels can ameliorate many of the disease sequelae. In addition to the dietary changes, Dr. Cush prescribes a statin to help reduce Jake's cholesterol. A starting dose of a statin reduces his LDL by 45% to 138 mg/dL, while his HDL increases slightly. Dr. Cush then increases the statin dose, and this produces an additional 12% reduction in LDL. Because LDL has still not reached <100 mg/dL, and HDL remains low, Dr. Cush adds the cholesterol absorption inhibitor ezetimibe as well as extended-release niacin. After these modifications, Jake's LDL drops below 100, and his HDL increases to 45 mg/dL. Jake experiences cutaneous flushing during the first few months of niacin treatment, but after that period, he has only occasional flushing episodes.

Questions

1. How do high cholesterol levels predispose to cardiovascular disease?

2. What is the etiology of familial hypercholesterolemia?

3. How do statins, ezetimibe, niacin, lomitapide, mipomersen, and PCSK9 inhibitors act pharmacologically?

4. What are the major adverse effects of concomitant statin and niacin therapy about which Jake should be aware?

TABLE 20-1 Characteristics of Plasma Lipoproteins

	CM	VLDL	IDL	LDL	HDL
Density (g/mL)	<0.95	0.95–1.006	1.006–1.019	1.019–1.063	1.063–1.210
Diameter (nm)	75–1,200	30–80	25–35	18–25	5–12
Total lipid (% wt)	98	90	82	75	67
Composition, % dry weight					
Protein	2	10	18	25	33
Triglycerides	83	50	31	9	8
Unesterified cholesterol and cholesteryl esters	8	22	29	45	30
Phospholipids (% wt lipid)	7	18	22	21	29
Electrophoretic mobility[a]	None	Pre-β	β	β	α or Pre-β
Plasma half-life	<1 hour	30–60 minutes	<30 minutes	2–4 days	2–5 days
Major apolipoproteins	B48, AI, AIV, E, CI, CII, CIII	B100, E, CI, CII, CIII	B100, E, CI, CII, CIII	B100	AI, AII, CI, CII, CIII, E

[a]Electrophoretic mobility of lipoprotein particles is designated relative to migration of plasma α- and β-globulins.
CM, chylomicron; VLDL, very-low-density lipoprotein; IDL, intermediate-density lipoprotein; LDL, low-density lipoprotein; HDL, high-density lipoprotein

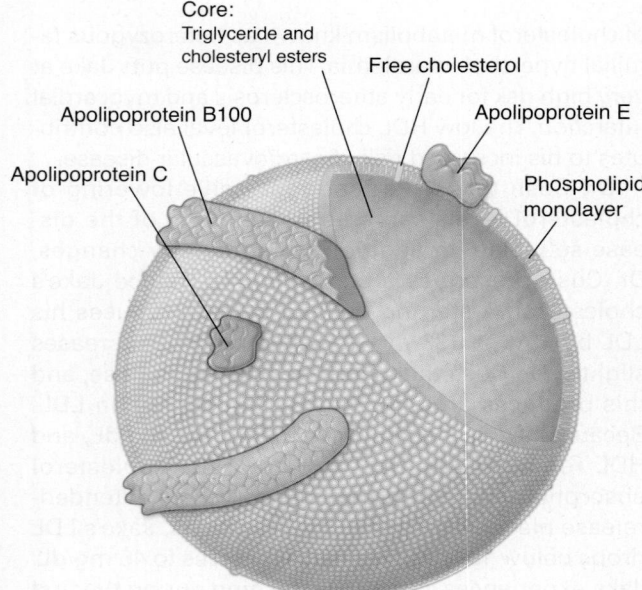

FIGURE 20-1. Structure of lipoprotein particles. Lipoproteins are spherical particles (5–>1,000 nm in diameter) that transport hydrophobic molecules, principally cholesterol and triglycerides, as well as fat-soluble vitamins. The surface of the particle is composed of a monolayer of phospholipid and unesterified cholesterol molecules. These polar lipids form a coating that shields a hydrophobic core of nonpolar triglyceride and cholesteryl esters from interacting with the aqueous environment of plasma. Lipoproteins contain amphipathic apolipoproteins (also called *apoproteins*) that associate with the surface lipids and hydrophobic core. Apolipoproteins provide structural stability to the lipoprotein particle and act as ligands for specific cell surface receptors or as cofactors for enzymatic reactions. In the example shown, a very-low-density lipoprotein (VLDL) particle contains apolipoprotein E, apolipoprotein B100, and apolipoproteins CI, CII, and CIII (*shown here as apolipoprotein C*).

Structurally, lipoproteins are microscopic spherical particles ranging from 5 to >1,000 nm in diameter. Each lipoprotein particle consists of a monolayer of polar, amphipathic lipids that surrounds a hydrophobic core. Each lipoprotein particle also contains one or more types of apolipoprotein (Fig. 20-1). The polar lipids that comprise the surface coat are unesterified cholesterol and phospholipid molecules arranged in a monolayer. The hydrophobic core of a lipoprotein contains cholesteryl esters (cholesterol molecules linked by an ester bond to a fatty acid) and triglycerides (three fatty acids esterified to a glycerol molecule). Apolipoproteins (also referred to as *apoproteins*) are amphipathic proteins that intercalate into the surface coat of lipoproteins. In addition to stabilizing the structure of lipoproteins, apolipoproteins engage in biological functions. They may act as ligands for lipoprotein receptors or may activate enzymatic activities in the plasma. The apolipoprotein composition determines the metabolic fate of the lipoprotein. For example, each **LDL** particle contains one apolipoprotein B (**apoB**) 100 molecule, which is a ligand for the low-density lipoprotein receptor (discussed below); in turn, binding of LDL to the LDL receptor promotes cholesterol uptake into cells.

From a metabolic perspective, lipoprotein particles can be divided into lipoproteins that participate in the delivery of triglyceride molecules to muscle and fat tissue (the apoB-containing lipoproteins, chylomicrons, and **VLDL**)

and lipoproteins that are involved primarily in cholesterol transport (**HDL** and the remnants of apoB-containing lipoproteins). HDL also serves as a reservoir for exchangeable apolipoproteins in the plasma, including apoAI, apoCII, and apoE. The following discussion presents each lipoprotein class in the context of its function.

Metabolism of ApoB-Containing Lipoproteins

The primary function of apoB-containing lipoproteins is to deliver fatty acids in the form of **triglycerides** to muscle tissue for use in ATP biogenesis and to adipose tissue for storage. Chylomicrons are formed in the intestine and transport dietary triglycerides, whereas VLDL particles are formed in the liver and transport triglycerides that are synthesized endogenously. The metabolic lifespan of apoB-containing lipoproteins can be divided into three phases: assembly, intravascular metabolism, and receptor-mediated clearance. This is a convenient categorization because pharmacologic agents are available that influence each phase.

Assembly of ApoB-Containing Lipoproteins

The cellular mechanisms by which chylomicrons and VLDL are assembled are quite similar. Regulation of the assembly process depends on the availability of apoB and triglycerides, as well as the activity of **microsomal triglyceride-transfer protein (MTP)**.

The gene that encodes apoB is transcribed principally in the intestine and the liver. Apart from this tissue-specific expression, there is little transcriptional regulation of the apoB gene. In contrast, a key regulatory event that differentiates chylomicron metabolism from VLDL metabolism is the editing of apoB mRNA (Fig. 20-2). Within enterocytes but not hepatocytes, a protein named **apoB editing complex-1 (apobec-1)** is expressed. This protein constitutes the catalytic subunit of the apoB editing complex, which deaminates a cytosine at position 6666 of the apoB mRNA molecule. Deamination converts the cytosine

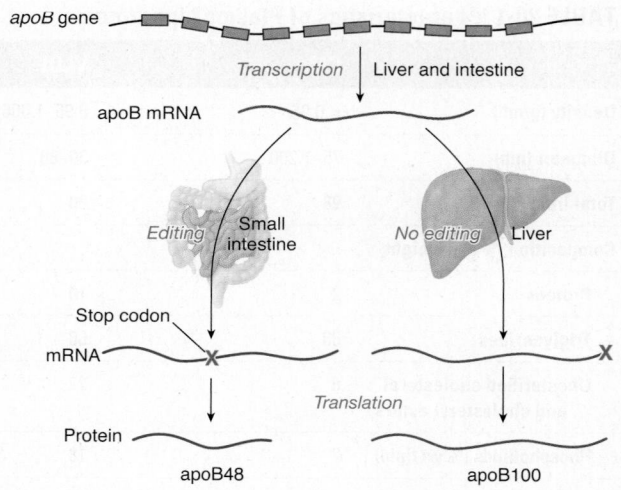

FIGURE 20-2. Editing of apoB mRNA. The *apoB* gene, with exons represented by *rectangles* and introns by *lines*, is transcribed in both the intestine and the liver. In the intestine, but not the liver, a protein complex containing apobec-1 modifies a single nucleotide in the apoB mRNA. As a result, the codon containing this nucleotide is converted to a premature stop codon, as indicated by the *red X*. The protein that is synthesized in the intestine (apoB48) is only 48% as long as the full-length protein that is synthesized in the liver (apoB100).

to uridine. As a result, the codon containing this nucleotide is converted from glutamine to a premature stop codon. When translated, the intestinal form **apoB48** is 48% as long as the full-length protein that is expressed in the liver and referred to as **apoB100**. As a consequence, chylomicrons, the apoB-containing lipoprotein produced by the intestine, contain apoB48, whereas VLDL particles produced by the liver contain apoB100.

Figure 20-3 illustrates the cellular mechanisms by which apoB-containing lipoproteins are assembled and secreted. As the apoB protein is synthesized by ribosomes, it crosses into the endoplasmic reticulum. Within the endoplasmic reticulum, triglyceride molecules are added co-translationally to the elongating apoB protein (i.e., apoB is lipidated) by the action of a cofactor protein, MTP. Once apoB has been fully synthesized, the nascent lipoprotein is enlarged in the Golgi apparatus; during this process, MTP adds additional triglycerides to the core of the particle. By unclear mechanisms, cholesteryl esters are also added to the core. Each lipoprotein particle assembled by this process contains a single molecule of apoB.

Because the triglyceride component of chylomicrons originates primarily from the diet (Fig. 20-4), the assembly, secretion, and metabolism of chylomicrons are collectively referred to as the *exogenous* pathway of lipoprotein metabolism. During digestion, cholesteryl esters and triglycerides in food are hydrolyzed to form unesterified cholesterol, free fatty acids, and monoglycerides. Bile acids, phospholipids, and cholesterol are secreted by the liver into bile and stored in the gallbladder during fasting as micelles and vesicles, which are macromolecular lipid aggregates that form due to the detergent properties of bile acid molecules. The stimulus of eating a meal promotes

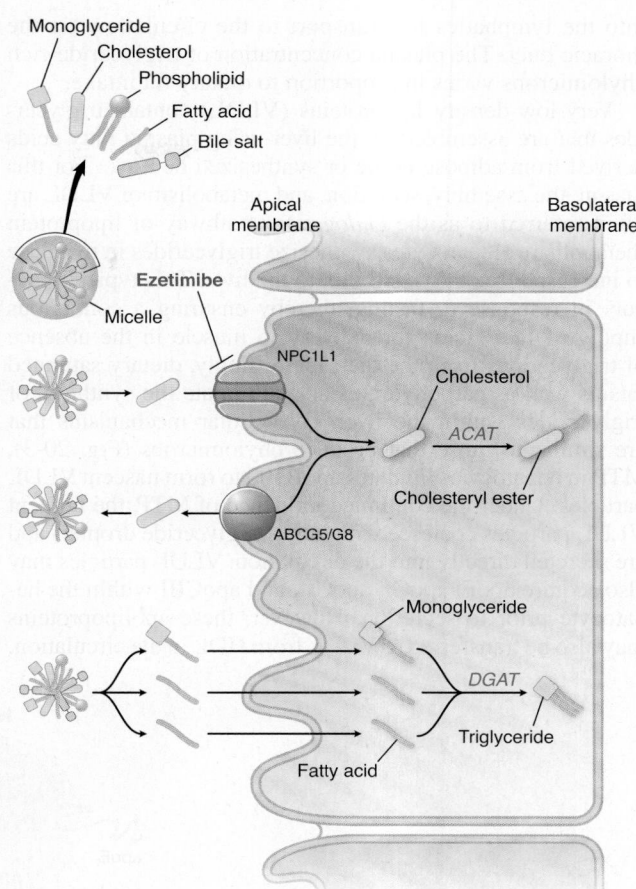

FIGURE 20-4. **Absorption of cholesterol and triglycerides.** Exogenous cholesterol and triglycerides are simultaneously absorbed from the intestinal lumen by different mechanisms. Cholesterol is taken up from micelles through a regulatory channel named **NPC1L1**. A fraction of the cholesterol is pumped back into the lumen by ABCG5/G8, a heterodimeric ATP-dependent plasma membrane protein. The remainder of the cholesterol is converted to cholesteryl esters by ACAT. Triglycerides are taken up as fatty acids and monoglycerides, which are re-esterified to triglycerides by DGAT. Ezetimibe inhibits cholesterol uptake through NPC1L1.

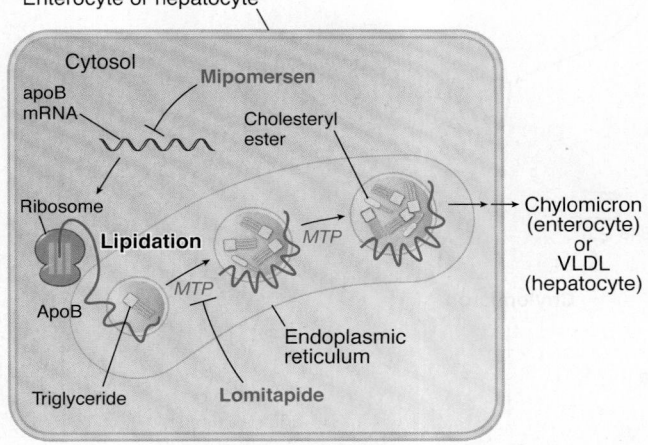

FIGURE 20-3. **Assembly and secretion of apolipoprotein B-containing lipoproteins.** Chylomicrons and VLDL particles are assembled and secreted by similar mechanisms in the enterocyte and hepatocyte, respectively. The apoB mRNA (i.e., apoB48 or apoB100 mRNA) is translated by ribosomes to yield a protein that enters the lumen of the endoplasmic reticulum. If triglycerides are available, the apoB protein is lipidated by the action of microsomal triglyceride-transfer protein (MTP) in two distinct steps, accumulating triglyceride as well as cholesteryl ester molecules. The resulting chylomicron or VLDL particle is secreted by exocytosis into the lymphatics by enterocytes or into the plasma by hepatocytes. In the absence of triglycerides, the apoB protein is degraded (*not shown*). Sortilin (*not shown*) regulates the intracellular trafficking of VLDL particles and can direct apoB to lysosomal-dependent degradation, thereby decreasing its secretion. Mipomersen inhibits translation of apoB by binding to apoB mRNA. Lomitapide inhibits lipidation of apoB by binding to MTP.

emptying of gallbladder bile into the small intestine, where the micelles and vesicles solubilize the digested lipids.

Lipid absorption into enterocytes of the duodenum and jejunum is facilitated mainly by micelles. Long-chain fatty acids and monoglycerides are taken up separately into the enterocyte by carrier-mediated transport and then re-esterified to form triglycerides by the enzyme **diacylglycerol acyltransferase (DGAT)**. By contrast, medium-chain fatty acids are absorbed directly into the portal blood and metabolized by the liver. Dietary and biliary cholesterol from micelles enter the enterocyte via a protein channel named **Niemann-Pick C1-like 1 protein (NPC1L1)**. Some of this cholesterol is immediately pumped back into the intestinal lumen by the ATP-dependent action of a heterodimeric protein, ABCG5/ABCG8 (ABCG5/G8). The fraction of cholesterol that remains is esterified to a long-chain fatty acid by **acetyl-CoA:cholesterol acyltransferase (ACAT)**. Once triglycerides and cholesteryl esters are packaged together with apoB48, apoA1 is added as an additional structural apolipoprotein and the chylomicron particle is exocytosed into the lymphatics for transport to the circulation via the thoracic duct. The plasma concentration of triglyceride-rich chylomicrons varies in proportion to dietary fat intake.

Very-low-density lipoproteins (VLDL) contain triglycerides that are assembled by the liver using plasma fatty acids derived from adipose tissue or synthesized de novo. For this reason, the assembly, secretion, and metabolism of VLDL are often referred to as the *endogenous* pathway of lipoprotein metabolism. Hepatocytes synthesize triglycerides in response to increased free fatty acid flux to the liver. This typically occurs in response to fasting, thereby ensuring a continuous supply of fatty acids for delivery to muscle in the absence of triglycerides from the diet. Interestingly, dietary saturated fats as well as carbohydrates also stimulate the synthesis of triglycerides within the liver. By cellular mechanisms that are similar to those that produce chylomicrons (Fig. 20-3), MTP in hepatocytes lipidates apoB100 to form nascent VLDL particles. Under the continued influence of MTP, the nascent VLDL particles coalesce with larger triglyceride droplets and are secreted directly into the circulation. VLDL particles may also acquire apoE, apoCI, apoCII, and apoCIII within the hepatocyte prior to secretion. However, these apolipoproteins may also be transferred to VLDL from HDL in the circulation.

The synthesis of apoB48 in the intestine and apoB100 in the liver is constitutive. This permits the immediate production of chylomicrons and VLDL particles when triglyceride molecules are available. In the absence of triglycerides, such as in enterocytes during fasting, apoB is degraded by a variety of cellular mechanisms. Recent studies have revealed a role for **sortilin** in the cellular trafficking of VLDL particles. Sortilin is encoded by the *Sort1* gene, and genome-wide association studies (GWAS) have shown that *Sort1* is associated with reduced levels of LDL cholesterol (LDL-C). Sortilin facilitates the post-translational degradation of apoB by a lysosome-dependent mechanism.

Intravascular Metabolism of ApoB-Containing Lipoproteins

Within the circulation, chylomicrons and VLDL particles must be activated in order to target triglyceride delivery to muscle and adipose tissue (Fig. 20-5). Activation requires the addition of an optimal complement of apoCII molecules, which occurs by aqueous transfer of apoCII from HDL particles. Because there is an inherent delay in the transfer of apoCII to chylomicrons and VLDL particles, there is time for widespread circulation of triglyceride-rich particles throughout the body.

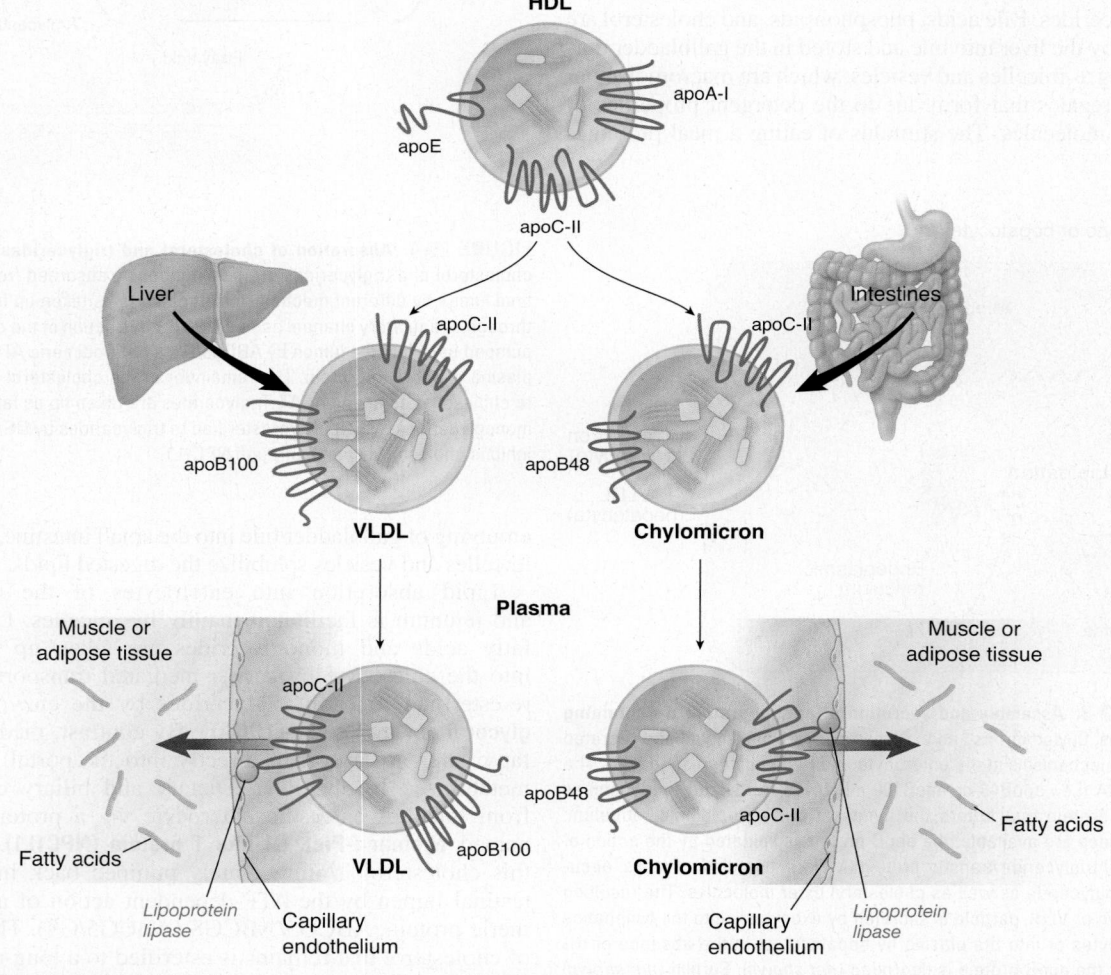

FIGURE 20-5. Intravascular metabolism of apoB-containing lipoproteins. After secretion, chylomicrons and VLDL particles are activated for lipolysis when they encounter HDL particles in the plasma and acquire the exchangeable apolipoprotein apoCII. When chylomicrons and VLDL circulate into capillaries of muscle or adipose tissue, apoCII promotes binding of the particle to lipoprotein lipase, which is bound to the surface of endothelial cells. Lipoprotein lipase mediates hydrolysis of triglycerides, but not cholesteryl esters, from the core of the lipoprotein particle. The resulting fatty acids are taken up into muscle or adipose tissue.

Lipoprotein lipase (LPL) is a lipolytic enzyme expressed on the endothelial surface of capillaries in muscle and fat tissue. LPL is a glycoprotein that is synthesized by myocytes and adipocytes and transported to the endothelial cell surface by a specific glycosylphosphatidylinositol (GPI)-linked protein, GPIHBP1. On the endothelial cell membrane, GPIHBP1 also serves to anchor LPL in place. Once chylomicrons and VLDL particles acquire apoCII, they can bind to LPL, which hydrolyzes triglycerides from the core of the lipoprotein (Fig. 20-5). LPL-mediated lipolysis liberates free fatty acids and glycerol. The free fatty acids are then taken up by the neighboring parenchymal cells. The expression level and intrinsic activity of LPL in muscle and adipose tissue are regulated according to the fed/fasting state, allowing the body to direct the delivery of fatty acids preferentially to muscle during fasting and to adipose after a meal. The rate of lipolysis of chylomicron and VLDL triglycerides is also controlled by apoCIII, which is an inhibitor of LPL activity. LPL inhibition by apoCIII may be

an additional mechanism promoting widespread distribution of triglyceride-rich particles in the circulation.

Receptor-Mediated Clearance of ApoB-Containing Lipoproteins

As LPL continues to hydrolyze triglycerides from chylomicrons and VLDL, the particles become progressively depleted of triglycerides and relatively enriched in cholesterol. Once approximately 50% of the triglycerides have been removed, the particles lose their affinity for LPL and dissociate from the enzyme. The exchangeable apolipoproteins apoAI and apoCII (as well as apoCI and apoCIII) are then transferred to HDL in exchange for **apoE** (Fig. 20-6A), which serves as a high-affinity ligand for receptor-mediated clearance of the particles. Upon acquiring apoE, the particles are termed **chylomicron** or **VLDL remnants**.

Remnants of chylomicrons and VLDL are taken up by the liver in a three-step process (Fig. 20-6B). The first step is

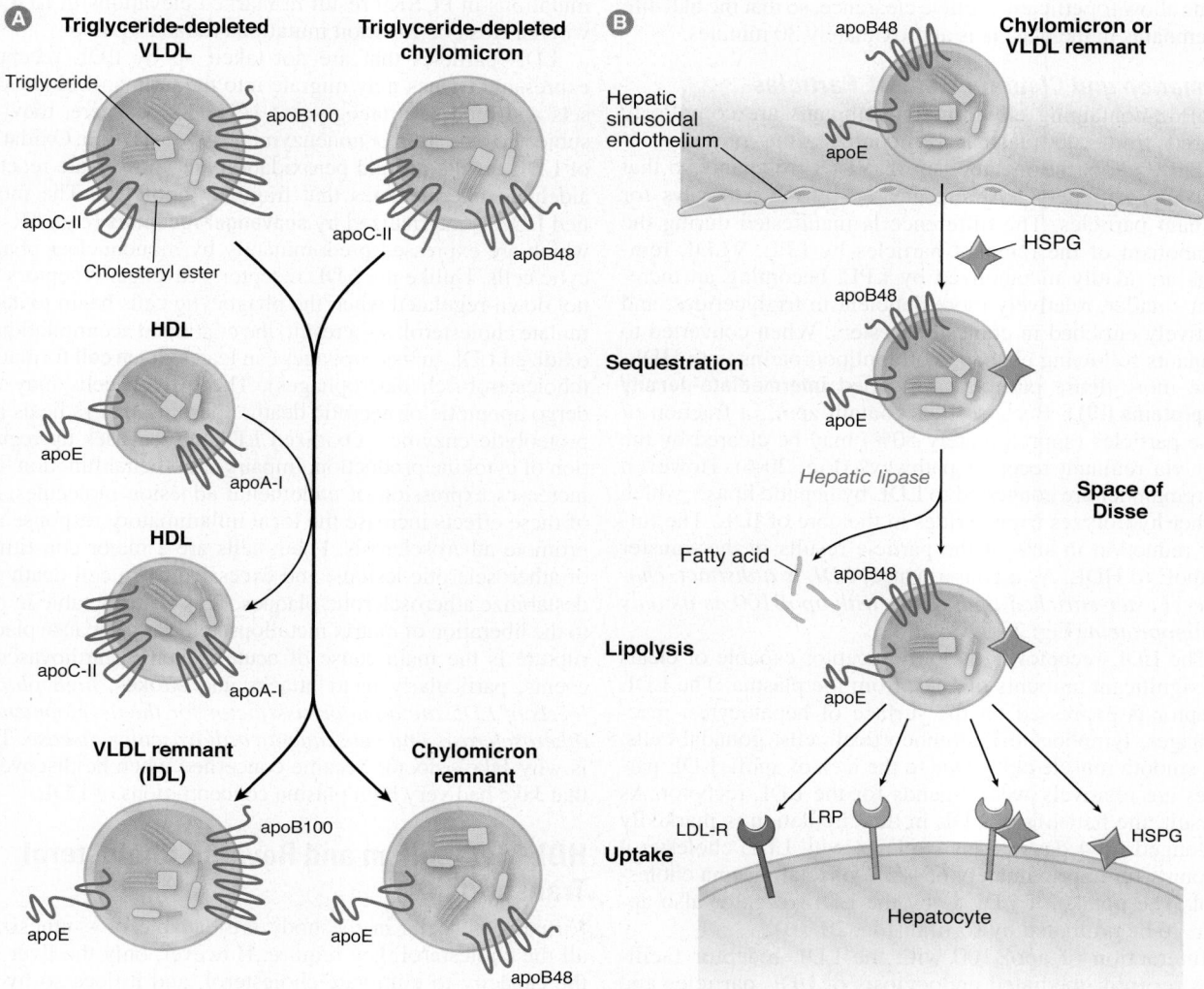

FIGURE 20-6. Formation and hepatic uptake of remnant particles. A. Upon completion of hydrolysis, chylomicrons and VLDL lose affinity for lipoprotein lipase. When an HDL particle is encountered, apoCII is transferred back to HDL particles in exchange for apoE. The resulting particles are chylomicron and VLDL remnants. **B.** The activity of lipoprotein lipase results in remnant lipoprotein particles that are small enough to enter the space of Disse. Remnant lipoproteins are sequestered in the space of Disse by binding to high-molecular-weight heparan sulfate proteoglycan (HSPG) molecules. This is followed by the action of hepatic lipase, which promotes lipolysis of some residual triglycerides in the core of the remnant lipoproteins and the release of fatty acids. Uptake of remnant lipoprotein particles into hepatocytes is mediated by the LDL receptor (LDL-R), the LDL receptor-related protein (LRP), a complex formed between LRP and HSPG, or HSPG alone.

sequestration of the particles within the **space of Disse** between the fenestrated endothelium of the liver sinusoids and the sinusoidal (basolateral) plasma membrane of the hepatocytes. Sequestration requires that the remnant particles become small enough during lipolysis to fit between the endothelial cells. Once in the space of Disse, remnants are bound and sequestered by large **heparan sulfate proteoglycans**. The next step is particle remodeling within the space of Disse by the action of **hepatic lipase**, a lipolytic enzyme that is similar to LPL but is expressed by hepatocytes. Hepatic lipase appears to optimize the triglyceride content of remnant particles so that they can be cleared efficiently by receptor-mediated mechanisms. The final phase of remnant clearance is receptor-mediated particle uptake. This is accomplished by one of four pathways. At the sinusoidal hepatocyte plasma membrane, remnant particles may be bound and taken up by the **LDL receptor**, the **LDL receptor-related protein (LRP)**, or heparan sulfate proteoglycans. A fourth pathway is mediated by the combined activities of LRP and heparan sulfate proteoglycans. These redundant mechanisms allow for efficient particle clearance, so that the half-life of remnants in the plasma is approximately 30 minutes.

Formation and Clearance of LDL Particles

ApoB48-containing chylomicron remnants are completely cleared from the plasma. By contrast, the presence of apoB100 alters the metabolism of VLDL remnants so that only approximately 50% are cleared by the pathways for remnant particles. The difference is manifested during the metabolism of the remnant particles by LPL. VLDL remnants are avidly metabolized by LPL, becoming an increment smaller, relatively more deficient in triglycerides, and relatively enriched in cholesteryl esters. When converted to remnants following exchange of apolipoproteins with HDL, these more dense particles are called **intermediate-density lipoproteins (IDL)**. Because IDL contain apoE, a fraction of these particles (approximately 50%) may be cleared by the liver via remnant receptor pathways (Fig. 20-6). However, the remainder are converted to LDL by hepatic lipase, which further hydrolyzes triglycerides in the core of IDL. The further reduction in size of the particle results in the transfer of apoE to HDL. As a consequence, *LDL is a distinct, cholesteryl ester-enriched lipoprotein with apoB100 as its only apolipoprotein* (Fig. 20-7A).

The LDL receptor is the only receptor capable of clearing significant amounts of LDL from the plasma. The LDL receptor is expressed on the surface of hepatocytes, macrophages, lymphocytes, adrenocortical cells, gonadal cells, and smooth muscle cells. Due to the lack of apoE, LDL particles are relatively weak ligands for the LDL receptor. As a result, the half-life of LDL in the circulation is markedly prolonged (2–4 days). This explains why LDL cholesterol accounts for approximately 65–75% of total plasma cholesterol. The uptake of LDL-C by the LDL receptor also appears to be promoted by sortilin (Fig. 20-7B).

Interaction of apoB100 with the LDL receptor facilitates receptor-mediated endocytosis of LDL particles and subsequent vesicle fusion with lysosomes (Fig. 20-7B). The LDL receptor is recycled to the cell surface, while the cholesteryl esters and triglycerides within the LDL particle are hydrolyzed by **lysosomal acid lipase (LAL)** to release unesterified cholesterol and fatty acids. These hydrolysis products affect three major homeostatic pathways. First, intracellular cholesterol inhibits HMG-CoA reductase, the enzyme that catalyzes the rate-limiting step in de novo cholesterol synthesis. Second, cholesterol activates ACAT to increase esterification and storage of cholesterol in the cell. Third, LDL receptor expression is down-regulated, reducing further uptake of cholesterol into the cells. The majority of LDL receptors (70%) are expressed on the surface of hepatocytes. As a result, the liver is primarily responsible for the removal of LDL particles from the circulation.

Proprotein convertase subtilisin-like kexin type 9 (PCSK9) is a plasma protein that regulates LDL receptor activity. PCSK9 is synthesized as a 72-kDa proPCSK9 proprotein that is autocatalytically cleaved in the endoplasmic reticulum to form the mature protein. It then enters the secretory pathway, and with the assistance of sortilin in the *trans*-Golgi network, it is secreted into the plasma. PCSK9 then binds to the epidermal growth factor-like repeat A (EGF-A) motif of the LDL receptor. This complex is targeted to lysosomes for degradation (Fig. 20-7B). Gain-of-function mutations in PCSK9 result in marked elevations in LDL-C, whereas loss-of-function mutations reduce LDL-C.

LDL particles that are not taken up by LDL receptor-expressing tissues may migrate into the intima of blood vessels and bind to proteoglycans (Fig. 20-8). There, they are subject to oxidation or nonenzymatic glycosylation. Oxidation of LDL results in lipid peroxidation and may create reactive aldehyde intermediates that fragment apoB100. The modified LDL is internalized by **scavenger receptors** (e.g., SR-A), which are expressed predominantly by mononuclear phagocytic cells. Unlike the LDL receptor, scavenger receptors are not down-regulated when the phagocytic cells begin to accumulate cholesterol. As a result, the continued accumulation of oxidized LDL in macrophages can lead to **foam cell** formation (cholesterol-rich macrophages). These foam cells may undergo apoptotic or necrotic death, releasing free radicals and proteolytic enzymes. Oxidized LDL also causes up-regulation of cytokine production, impairs endothelial function, and increases expression of endothelial adhesion molecules. All of these effects increase the local inflammatory response and promote atherosclerosis. Foam cells are a major constituent of atherosclerotic lesions, and excessive foam cell death can destabilize atherosclerotic plaques. This is attributable in part to the liberation of matrix metalloproteinases. Because plaque rupture is the main cause of acute ischemic cardiovascular events, particularly heart attacks and strokes, *high plasma levels of LDL are a major risk factor for the development of atherosclerosis and subsequent cardiovascular disease*. This is why Jake's doctor became concerned when he discovered that Jake had very high plasma concentrations of LDL.

HDL Metabolism and Reverse Cholesterol Transport

Virtually all cells in the body are capable of synthesizing all the cholesterol they require. However, only the liver has the capacity to eliminate cholesterol, and it does so by secreting unesterified cholesterol into the bile or by converting cholesterol to bile acids. As noted above, HDL serves as a reservoir for exchangeable apolipoproteins for the metabolism of apoB-containing lipoproteins. HDL also plays a key role in cholesterol homeostasis by removing excess cholesterol from cells and transporting it in plasma to the liver. This process is often referred to as **reverse cholesterol**

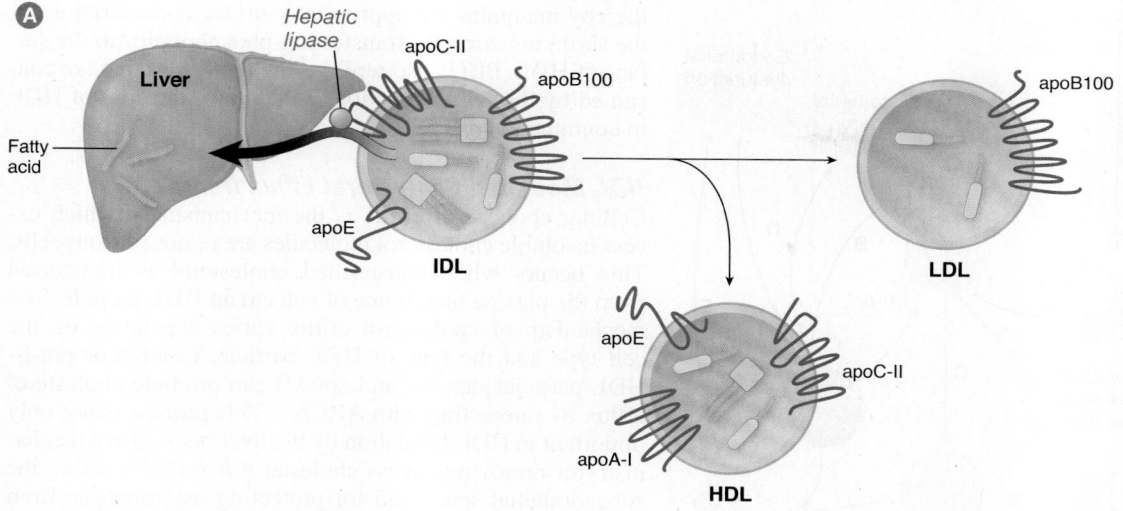

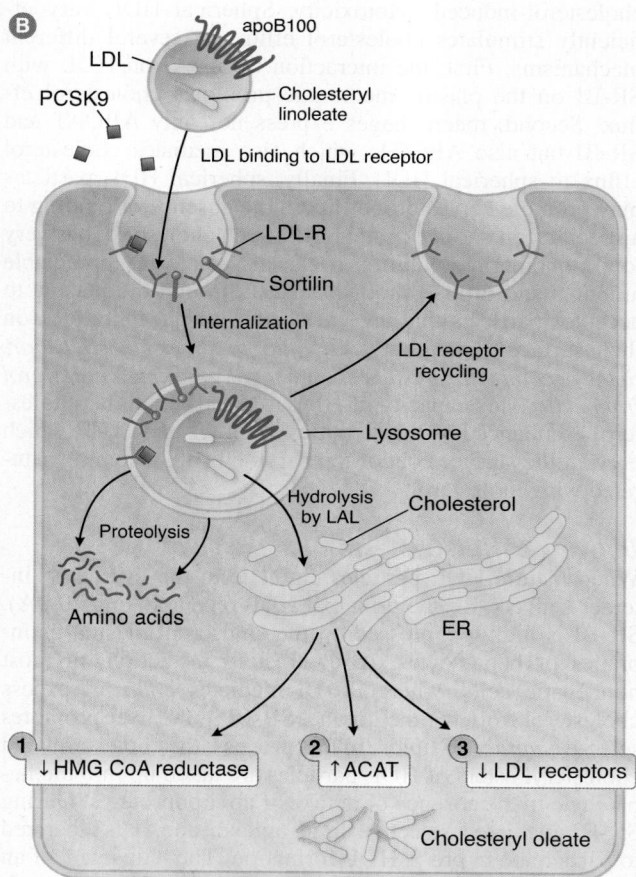

FIGURE 20-7. Formation and clearance of LDL particles. A. Formation of LDL occurs when IDL particles interact with hepatic lipase to become denser and cholesteryl ester-enriched. As a result, both apoE and apoCII lose affinity for the particle and are transferred to HDL, leaving only apoB100. **B.** Binding of apolipoprotein B100 to the LDL receptor (LDL-R) sortilin complex on hepatocytes or other cell types promotes LDL internalization into endocytic vesicles and fusion of the vesicles with lysosomes. LDL receptors are recycled to the cell surface unless bound to PCSK9, whereas lipoprotein particles are proteolyzed to amino acids (from apoB100 and PCSK9-bound LDL-R) and free cholesterol and fatty acids (from the action of lysosomal acid lipase [LAL] on cholesteryl esters and triglycerides). Intracellular free cholesterol has three regulatory effects on the cell. First, cholesterol decreases the activity of HMG-CoA reductase, the rate-limiting enzyme in cholesterol biosynthesis. Second, cholesterol activates acetyl-CoA:cholesterol acyltransferase (ACAT), an enzyme that esterifies free cholesterol into cholesteryl esters for intracellular storage or export. Third, cholesterol inhibits the transcription of the gene encoding the LDL receptor and thereby decreases further uptake of cholesterol by the cell.

transport (Fig. 20-9A). The major apolipoproteins of HDL are apoAI and apoAII. ApoAI, the main structural determinant of HDL, participates in the formation of the particle and its interaction with its receptor, **scavenger receptor class B, type I** (SR-BI). The function of apoAII is not well understood—it appears to play a role in maintaining the structural integrity of HDL.

HDL Formation

HDL formation occurs mainly in the liver, although a small percentage is contributed by the small intestine. The earliest events occur when lipid-poor apoAI is secreted by the liver or intestine or dissociates from lipoprotein particles in the plasma. These amphipathic apoAI molecules interact with **ABCA1**, which is localized in the sinusoidal membrane of the hepatocyte or the basolateral membrane of the enterocyte. ABCA1 incorporates a small amount of membrane phospholipid and unesterified cholesterol into the apoAI molecule. The resulting small, disk-shaped particle, which consists mainly of phospholipid and apolipoprotein AI, is referred to as nascent or **pre-β-HDL**, due to its characteristic migration on agarose gels.

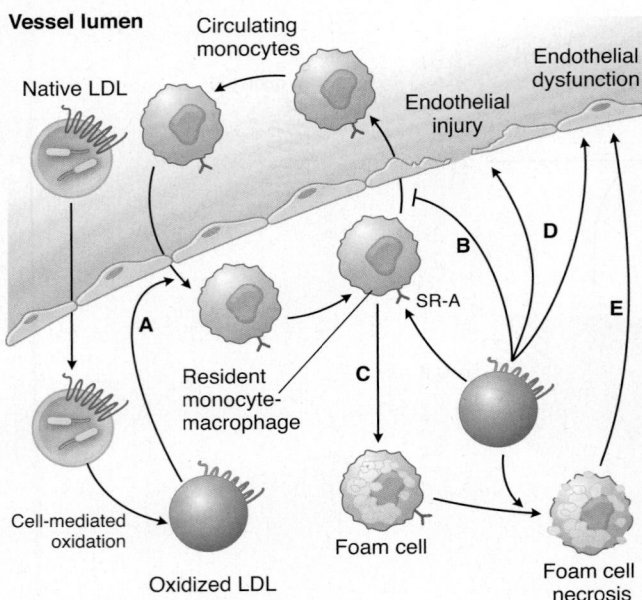

FIGURE 20-8. LDL and atherosclerosis. Elevated LDL is a major factor for the development of atherosclerosis. Native LDL that migrates into the subendothelial space can undergo chemical transformation to oxidized LDL via lipid peroxidation and fragmentation of apoB100. Oxidized LDL has a number of deleterious effects on vascular function. Oxidized LDL promotes monocyte chemotaxis into the subendothelial space **(A)** and inhibits monocyte egress from that space **(B)**. Resident monocyte–macrophages bind to oxidized LDL via a scavenger receptor (SR-A), resulting in the formation of lipid-laden foam cells **(C)**. Oxidized LDL can directly injure endothelial cells and cause endothelial dysfunction **(D)**. Continued accumulation of oxidized LDL in foam cells can also cause foam cell necrosis, with release of numerous proteolytic enzymes that can damage the intima **(E)**.

Intravascular Maturation of HDL

Because disk-shaped pre-β-HDL particles are relatively inefficient at removing excess cholesterol from cell membranes, these particles must mature into spherical particles in the plasma. HDL maturation occurs as a result of the activity of two distinct circulating proteins (Fig. 20-9A, B). **Lecithin:cholesterol acyltransferase (LCAT)** binds preferentially to disk-shaped HDL and converts cholesterol molecules within the particle to cholesteryl esters. This is accomplished by transesterification of a fatty acid from a phosphatidylcholine molecule on the surface of the HDL to the hydroxyl group of a cholesterol molecule. The reaction also creates a lysophosphatidylcholine molecule, which dissociates from the particle and binds to serum albumin. Because they are highly insoluble, cholesteryl esters migrate into the core of the HDL particle. The development of a hydrophobic core converts the pre-β-HDL to a spherical **α-HDL** particle.

The second important protein that contributes to HDL maturation in the plasma is **phospholipid transfer protein (PLTP)**. PLTP transfers phospholipids from the surface coat of apoB-containing remnant particles to the surface coat of HDL. During LPL-mediated lipolysis of apoB-containing lipoproteins, the particles become smaller as triglycerides are removed from the core. This leaves a relative excess of phospholipids on the surface of the particle. Because phospholipids are highly insoluble and cannot otherwise dissociate from a particle, PLTP removes excess phospholipids and

thereby maintains the appropriate surface concentration for the shrinking core. By transferring phospholipids to the surface of HDL, PLTP also replaces the molecules that are consumed by the LCAT reaction. This allows the core of HDL to continue to enlarge.

HDL-Mediated Cholesterol Efflux from Cells

Cellular cholesterol efflux is the mechanism by which excess insoluble cholesterol molecules are removed from cells. This occurs when unesterified cholesterol is transferred from the plasma membrane of cells to an HDL particle. The mechanism of cholesterol efflux varies depending on the cell type and the type of HDL particle. Lipid-poor pre-β-HDL particles, apoAI, and apoAII can promote cholesterol efflux by interacting with ABCA1. This process is not only important in HDL formation by the liver but is also a mechanism for removing excess cholesterol from cells within the subendothelial space and for protecting macrophages from cholesterol-induced cytotoxicity. Spherical HDL very efficiently stimulates cholesterol efflux by several different mechanisms. First, the interaction of apoAI on HDL with SR-BI on the plasma membrane promotes cholesterol efflux. Second, macrophages express not only ABCA1 and SR-BI but also ABCG1, which also mediates cholesterol efflux to spherical HDL. Finally, spherical HDL particles may promote cholesterol efflux in the absence of binding to a specific cell surface protein. Although cholesterol has very low monomeric solubility, it can dissociate in appreciable amounts and diffuse short distances through the plasma to acceptor particles that are enriched with phospholipids on their surfaces. Quantitatively, *efflux to spherical HDL particles accounts for most of the removal of excess cholesterol from cells*. This capacity of HDL to remove cellular cholesterol is enhanced by the activities of LCAT and PLTP, which prevent the surface coat of the particle from becoming saturated with cholesterol.

Delivery of HDL Cholesterol to the Liver

When mature HDL particles circulate to the liver, they interact with SR-BI, the principal HDL receptor (Fig. 20-9A). SR-BI is highly expressed on the sinusoidal plasma membranes of hepatocytes. In contrast to its action on most nonhepatic cells, where SR-BI mediates *efflux* of excess cholesterol from the membrane, SR-BI in the liver promotes selective *uptake* of lipids. In this process, the cholesterol and cholesteryl esters of HDL particles are taken up into the hepatocyte in the absence of uptake of apolipoproteins. During SR-BI–mediated selective lipid uptake, apoAI is liberated to participate in pre-β-HDL formation. The "lifespan" of an HDL particle is 2–5 days, suggesting that each apoAI molecule can participate in many cycles of reverse cholesterol transport. Among the nonhepatic tissues that express high levels of SR-BI are the adrenal glands and gonads, presumably reflecting the requirement of these organs for cholesterol to support steroidogenesis.

Delivery of cholesterol from extrahepatic tissues to the liver is optimized by two additional proteins: **cholesterol ester transfer protein (CETP)** and hepatic lipase. CETP is a plasma protein that transfers cholesteryl esters from mature spherical HDL to the cores of remnant lipoproteins in exchange for a triglyceride molecule, which is inserted into the core of the HDL particle (Fig. 20-9B). This process allows the body to utilize remnant particles that have completed

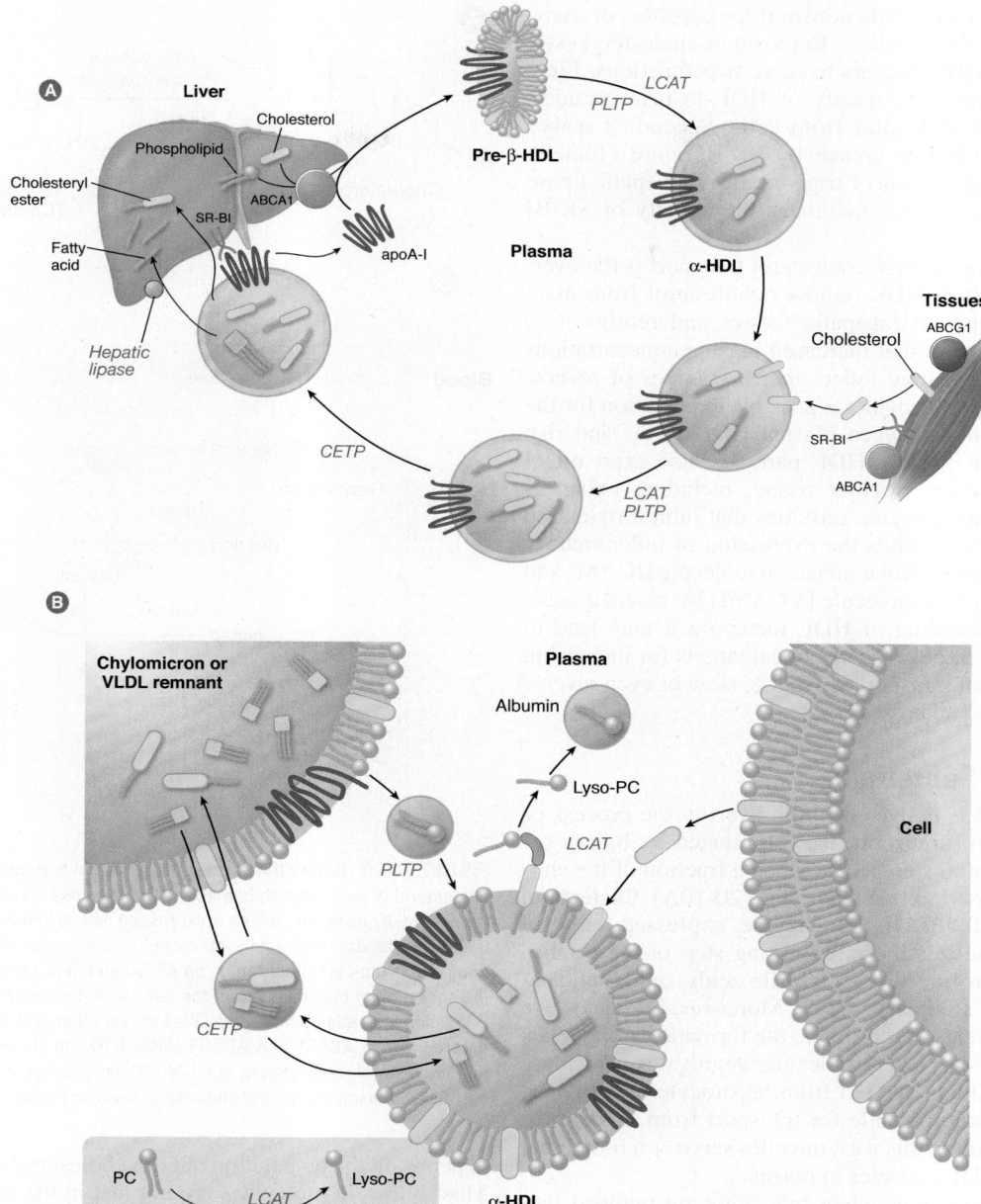

FIGURE 20-9. Reverse cholesterol transport. A. The process of reverse cholesterol transport begins when apoAI is secreted from the liver. ApoAI in plasma interacts with ATP binding cassette protein AI (ABCA1), which incorporates a small amount of phospholipid and unesterified cholesterol from hepatocyte plasma membranes to form a discoidal-shaped pre-β-HDL particle. Due to the activity of lecithin:cholesterol acyltransferase (LCAT) in plasma, pre-β-HDL particles mature to form spherical α-HDL. Spherical α-HDL particles function to accept excess unesterified cholesterol from the plasma membranes of cells in a wide variety of tissues. The unesterified cholesterol is transferred from the cell to nearby HDL particles by interactions with ABCA1, ABCG1, and SR-BI, as well as by aqueous diffusion through the plasma. As explained in panel B, LCAT and phospholipid transfer protein (PLTP) increase the capacity of HDL to accept unesterified cholesterol molecules from cells by allowing for expansion of the core and the surface coat of the particle. Cholesteryl ester transfer protein (CETP) removes cholesteryl ester molecules from HDL and replaces them with triglycerides from remnant particles. HDL particles interact with scavenger receptor, class B type I (SR-BI), which mediates selective hepatic uptake of cholesterol and cholesteryl esters, but not apoAI. This process is facilitated when hepatic lipase hydrolyzes triglycerides from the core of the particle. The remaining apoAI molecules may begin the cycle of reverse cholesterol transport again. **B.** LCAT, PLTP, and CETP promote the removal of excess cholesterol from the plasma membranes of cells. LCAT removes a fatty acid from a phosphatidylcholine molecule in the surface coat of α- (or pre-β-) HDL and esterifies an unesterified cholesterol molecule on the surface of the particle. The resulting lysophosphatidylcholine (lyso-PC) becomes bound to albumin in the plasma, whereas the cholesteryl ester migrates spontaneously into the core of the lipoprotein particle. The unesterified cholesterol molecules that are consumed by LCAT are replaced by unesterified cholesterol from cells. HDL phospholipids that are consumed by LCAT action are replaced with excess phospholipids from remnant particles by the activity of PLTP. As described in panel A, CETP increases the efficiency of cholesterol transport to the liver by exchanging cholesteryl ester molecules in α-HDL for triglycerides in VLDL remnants. Unlike phospholipids, triglycerides, and cholesteryl esters (which require transport proteins), unesterified cholesterol and lyso-PC can diffuse over short distances in the plasma.

their function of triglyceride transport for purposes of transporting cholesterol to the liver. Removal of cholesteryl ester molecules from HDL appears to serve two functions. First, it further increases the capacity of HDL to take on additional cholesterol molecules from cells. Second, it makes the process of selective uptake by SR-BI more efficient. This is because hydrolysis of triglycerides by hepatic lipase on the hepatocyte surface facilitates the activity of SR-BI (Fig. 20-9A).

As noted above, reverse cholesterol transport is the overall process by which HDL removes cholesterol from macrophages and other extrahepatic tissues and returns it to the liver. The concept that increased plasma concentrations of HDL cholesterol may reflect increased rates of reverse cholesterol transport provides a possible explanation for the inverse relationship between plasma HDL levels and risk of cardiovascular disease. HDL particles also exert direct beneficial effects on vascular tissue, including enhancement of antioxidant enzyme activities that inhibit oxidation of LDL. HDL also inhibits the expression of inflammatory mediators (e.g., intercellular adhesion molecule [ICAM] and vascular cell adhesion molecule [VCAM]) by vascular cells. Increased understanding of HDL metabolism may lead to the development of novel biochemical targets for increasing reverse cholesterol transport in order to slow or even reverse the progression of atherosclerosis.

Biliary Lipid Secretion

Once cholesterol is delivered to the liver by the process of reverse cholesterol transport, it is eliminated by biliary secretion. An essential step occurs when a fraction of the cholesterol is converted to bile acids (Fig. 20-10A). **Cholesterol 7α-hydroxylase (CYP7A1)**, an enzyme expressed only in hepatocytes, catalyzes the rate-limiting step in the catabolism of cholesterol to bile acids. Bile acids, unlike cholesterol, are highly soluble in water. Moreover, bile acids are biological detergents that promote the formation of micelles (Fig. 20-10B). These macromolecular aggregates, which are rich in phospholipids derived from hepatocyte membranes, solubilize cholesterol in bile for transport from the liver to the small intestine. In this way, micelles serve as a functional counterpart to HDL particles in plasma.

Bile formation begins when bile acids are pumped into bile by the action of a canalicular membrane transport pump known as *ABCB11* (Fig. 20-10B). In turn, these bile acids stimulate the biliary secretion of phospholipids and cholesterol. Phospholipid and cholesterol secretion are mediated by two additional transporters: ABCB4 for phospholipids and a heterodimer of ABCG5 and ABCG8 for cholesterol. Large amounts of bile acids, phospholipids, and cholesterol are secreted into bile at approximate rates of 24, 11, and 1.2 grams each day, respectively. These molecules comprise the biliary lipids, which are stored in the gallbladder during fasting. The stimulus of a fatty meal leads to gallbladder contraction, which propels its contents into the small intestine. As described above, bile facilitates the digestion and absorption of fats, in addition to promoting the elimination of endogenous cholesterol.

Cholesterol Balance

Because cholesterol is converted by the liver to bile acids and secreted unmodified into bile, overall cholesterol balance

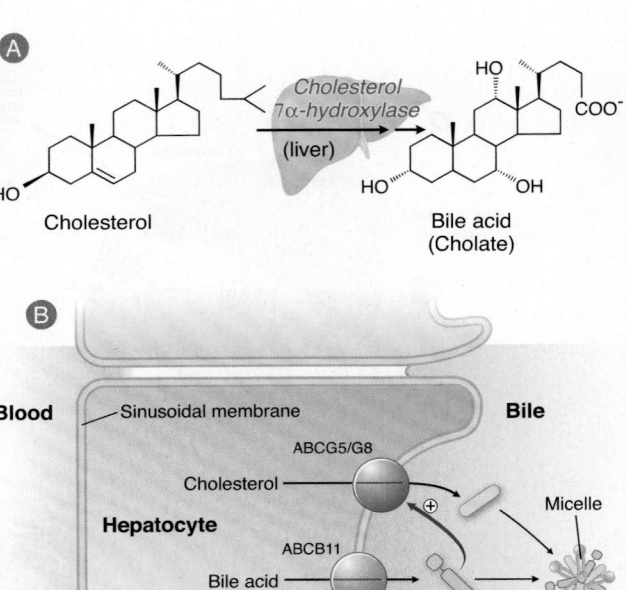

FIGURE 20-10. Biliary lipid secretion. A. Within hepatocytes, a portion of cholesterol is converted to bile acids. This process is rate-limited by cholesterol 7α-hydroxylase, which is expressed only in hepatocytes. Cholate is the most abundant bile acid synthesized by the human liver. **B.** Within the canalicular (apical) membranes, an ATP-dependent pump ABCB11 drives the secretion of bile acids out of the cell against a concentration gradient. Bile acids then stimulate the activities of two other proteins, ABCB4 and a heterodimer of ABCG5 and ABCG8 (ABCG5/G8), to secrete phospholipids and cholesterol, respectively, into bile. Within bile, the interactions among bile acids, phospholipids, and cholesterol result in the formation of micelles.

depends on the disposition of both cholesterol and bile acids. Most bile acid molecules are not lost in the feces after participating in cholesterol transport and fat digestion; instead, they are taken up and recycled by high-affinity transport proteins in the distal ileum. Bile acids enter the portal circulation and are transported back to the liver, where they are cleared from the blood by hepatocytes with high first-pass efficiency. Bile acids are then re-secreted into bile. The process of recycling bile acids between the liver and intestine is referred to as **enterohepatic circulation**.

The enterohepatic circulation is highly efficient, allowing <5% of secreted bile acids to be lost in the feces. However, because bile acids are secreted in such large amounts, the small fractional loss of bile acids amounts to about 0.4 grams per day. Considering that cholesterol is the substrate for bile acid synthesis, fecal bile acids represent a source of cholesterol loss from the body. Sensitive nuclear hormone receptors within the liver are capable of detecting the rate of loss of bile acids into the feces. These receptors tightly regulate transcription of bile acid synthetic genes. As a result, the liver synthesizes precisely the amount of bile acids that is sufficient to replace what is lost in the feces.

In addition to the 1.2 grams of cholesterol that are secreted into bile each day, the average American diet contributes approximately 0.4 grams each day to intestinal cholesterol. Therefore, dietary cholesterol represents only a minor fraction (25%) of the total (i.e., biliary and dietary) cholesterol that passes through the intestine. The extent to which intestinal cholesterol is absorbed appears to be genetically regulated. Each individual absorbs a fixed percentage of intestinal cholesterol. In the population, percentages range from as low as 20% to more than 80%. For example, when an average individual absorbs 50% of intestinal cholesterol, this will amount to half of the 1.6 grams (i.e., 1.2 grams of biliary cholesterol plus 0.4 grams of dietary cholesterol), and the other half (0.8 grams) will be lost in the feces. Combined with a loss of 0.4 grams per day of cholesterol in the form of fecal bile acids, this yields a total cholesterol loss from the body of 1.2 grams each day. Taking into account intestinal absorption of dietary cholesterol and reabsorption of biliary cholesterol, total body cholesterol synthesis is approximately 0.8 grams per day (i.e., cholesterol synthesis = fecal loss of cholesterol + bile acids − dietary cholesterol intake). Thus, the amount of endogenous cholesterol synthesis is about twofold greater than the amount consumed in the average diet.

▌PATHOPHYSIOLOGY

Numerous studies have demonstrated a definitive link between elevated plasma lipid concentrations and the risk of cardiovascular disease. Increased risk of cardiovascular mortality is most closely linked to elevated levels of LDL cholesterol and decreased levels of HDL cholesterol. In addition, hypertriglyceridemia represents an independent risk factor. The risk is further increased when hypertriglyceridemia is associated with low HDL-cholesterol concentrations, even if LDL-cholesterol concentrations are normal. From a clinical perspective, the dyslipidemias can be divided into hypercholesterolemia, hypertriglyceridemia, mixed hyperlipidemia, and disorders of HDL metabolism.

The causes of hyperlipidemia are multifactorial. These include well-defined monogenic diseases and the contributions of genetic polymorphisms, as well as less well-defined gene–environment interactions. For many individuals, elevated cholesterol may be the consequence of a diet high in saturated fat and cholesterol superimposed on a susceptible genetic profile. The following section describes the major genetic predispositions for hyperlipidemia. This is followed by a brief overview of the secondary causes of hyperlipidemia. It is important to appreciate that the decision to treat elevated cholesterol concentrations is based on estimations of the risk of cardiovascular disease. Current clinical practice does not incorporate genetic causes of hyperlipidemia into these calculations. As common genetic predispositions to dyslipidemia and the contributions of these predispositions to cardiovascular disease become better understood, lipid-lowering therapies may one day be tailored toward individual genetic susceptibilities.

Hypercholesterolemia

Isolated hypercholesterolemia is characterized by elevated levels of total plasma cholesterol and LDL cholesterol, with normal concentrations of triglycerides. The causes of primary hypercholesterolemia are familial hypercholesterolemia, familial defective apoB100, gain-of-function mutations in PCSK9, familial combined hyperlipidemia (FCHL), and, most commonly, polygenic hypercholesterolemia.

Familial hypercholesterolemia (FH) is an autosomal dominant disease involving defects in the LDL receptor. Mutations in the gene encoding the LDL receptor result in one of four molecular defects: lack of receptor synthesis, failure to reach the plasma membrane, defective LDL binding, and failure to internalize bound LDL particles. Heterozygous individuals (1 in 500 in the United States) have elevated total plasma cholesterol concentrations from birth throughout life, with adult levels averaging 275–500 mg/dL (normal, <200 mg/dL). Clinical features include tendon xanthomas (caused by intracellular and extracellular accumulation of cholesterol) and arcus corneae (deposition of cholesterol in the cornea). Homozygous FH is a much more severe but rare disorder (1 in 1 million in the United States) that is characterized by the absence of functional LDL receptors. This leads to very high plasma cholesterol concentrations (700–1,200 mg/dL) and cardiovascular disease that presents clinically prior to the age of 20. Heterozygotes for FH respond well to statins and other LDL-lowering drugs that up-regulate LDL receptor density on the cell surface. In the introductory case, Jake was most likely heterozygous for FH. Because homozygotes lack functional LDL receptors, until recently, the only effective treatment has been plasmapheresis with immunoadsorption of LDL particles. However, the development of molecules that inhibit PCSK9, MTP, or apoB synthesis now show promise toward a complementary treatment to reduce the severe elevations in LDL-C observed in patients with homozygous FH. An autosomal recessive form of hypercholesterolemia has also been described in which a defective molecular adaptor protein that participates in LDL receptor internalization leads to a phenotype similar to that of FH.

Familial defective apoB100 is an autosomal dominant disorder in which mutations in the apoB100 protein lead to decreased affinity of the LDL particle for LDL receptors. Due to decreased catabolism of LDL, cholesterol concentrations in familial defective apoB100 can be similar to those in patients with FH. Gain-of-function mutations in PCSK9 have been identified in families with clinical features similar to FH; the pathophysiology of this disorder reflects increased PCSK9 function and decreased LDL receptor expression on cell surfaces. Familial combined hyperlipidemia is characterized by different combinations of hyperlipidemia in different families (see below); one presentation is elevated LDL cholesterol.

Polygenic hypercholesterolemia is a general term that has been used to categorize the majority of patients with hypercholesterolemia who have no defined genetic cause for the disorder. Polygenic hypercholesterolemia may be the result of complex gene–environment interactions, multiple uncharacterized genetic susceptibilities, or variant LDL particles such as small dense LDL and lipoprotein(a) [Lp(a)]. Further research into genetic predispositions for hypercholesterolemia will be necessary in order to identify clear etiologies for the majority of patients with hypercholesterolemia.

Hypertriglyceridemia

Primary hypertriglyceridemia is characterized by high plasma triglyceride concentrations (200–500 mg/dL or higher; normal, <150 mg/dL), when measured following an overnight fast. Three major etiologies of hypertriglyceridemia have been identified: familial hypertriglyceridemia, familial lipoprotein lipase (LPL) deficiency, and apoCII deficiency. Familial combined hyperlipidemia can also present with isolated hypertriglyceridemia. More commonly, hypertriglyceridemia develops with age, weight gain, obesity, and diabetes and is an important component of the metabolic syndrome.

Familial hypertriglyceridemia is a common autosomal dominant disorder characterized by hypertriglyceridemia with normal LDL-cholesterol concentrations. HDL cholesterol is often reduced. Although the underlying defect in this disorder is unknown, it is hypothesized to be a defect in bile acid metabolism, leading to increased hepatic production of triglyceride-rich VLDL. A strong family history of premature coronary heart disease is usually absent. Management is generally with exercise and diet. If that approach is unsuccessful at reducing triglyceride concentrations below 500 mg/dL, a fibrate should be considered. Drug therapy should be initiated if triglycerides exceed 1,000 mg/dL.

Familial lipoprotein lipase deficiency is an autosomal recessive disorder caused by the absence of active LPL. This condition may be diagnosed by testing the plasma for lipase activity following an infusion of heparin, which competes for binding sites on endothelial cells and dislodges LPL molecules into the plasma. Patients with LPL deficiency exhibit profound hypertriglyceridemia, which is characterized by elevated chylomicrons during infancy and impaired removal of VLDL later in life. Infants or young adults may present with pancreatitis, eruptive xanthomas, hepatomegaly, and splenomegaly attributable to the accumulation of lipid-laden foam cells. Treatment consists of a fat-free diet and avoidance of substances that increase VLDL production by the liver, such as alcohol and glucocorticoids.

ApoCII deficiency is a rare genetic disorder with presentation and treatment similar to familial lipoprotein lipase deficiency. It is caused by deficiency of apoCII, a cofactor protein of LPL. It may be distinguished from LPL deficiency by demonstrating that the triglyceride levels of patients are reduced following infusion of plasma that contains normal apoCII; this does not occur in patients with familial LPL deficiency. It is now appreciated that mutations in apoAV can present with chylomicronemia and severe hypertriglyceridemia, consistent with an apparent role for apoAV in facilitating the interaction between apoCII and LPL.

Mixed Hyperlipidemia

Patients with mixed hyperlipidemia exhibit complex lipid profiles that may consist of elevated total cholesterol, LDL cholesterol, and triglyceride concentrations. HDL cholesterol is often reduced. Etiologies of mixed hyperlipidemia include **familial combined hyperlipidemia (FCHL)**, **dysbetalipoproteinemia**, and **lysosomal acid lipase deficiency (LAL-D)**.

FCHL is a common disease associated with moderately elevated concentrations of fasting triglycerides and total cholesterol and reduced concentrations of HDL cholesterol. These patients often present with other features of the **metabolic syndrome**, including abdominal obesity, glucose intolerance, and hypertension. The molecular defects are still under investigation. Current hypotheses focus on insulin resistance, which leads to increased lipolysis in fat tissue. Fatty acids liberated from fat tissue return to the liver, where they are reassembled into triglycerides. The increase in triglycerides increases the production of VLDL particles, which leads to an increase in apoB-containing lipoproteins in the plasma. In part because of the complex phenotypes of FCHL, the underlying genetic defects have remained elusive. Faithful adherence to dietary modification may be an effective means of controlling FCHL. However, drug treatment is often required, and statins are commonly utilized. Combination therapy that includes addition of a fibrate or niacin may be

necessary to normalize triglyceride and LDL-cholesterol concentrations, as well as to increase HDL cholesterol.

Dysbetalipoproteinemia is a disorder characterized by increased cholesterol-rich chylomicrons and IDL-like particles. These findings are the result of accumulated chylomicron and VLDL remnants, leading to both hypertriglyceridemia and hypercholesterolemia. ApoE has three isoforms (E2, E3, and E4) in humans, and apoE2 has been implicated in the disease. Chylomicrons and VLDL particles in patients with the homozygous apoE2/apoE2 phenotype have reduced affinity for their lipoprotein receptors, leading to accumulation of remnant particles in the plasma. Although the apoE isoform is present at birth, symptoms generally present in adult males and in postmenopausal females. The mechanism underlying this delay in expression of the phenotype is unknown, and additional metabolic factors (e.g., obesity, diabetes, or hypothyroidism) may be required to unmask the disorder. Dysbetalipoproteinemia can be managed by decreased intake of fat and cholesterol, along with weight reduction and omission of alcohol intake. In addition, niacin and fibrates are effective pharmacologic therapies.

Lysosomal acid lipase deficiency (LAL-D) is a rare lysosomal storage disorder caused by mutations in the *LIPA* gene, which encodes lysosomal acid lipase. This mutation leads to deficiency of the enzyme, with a corresponding reduction in the ability of LDL-C to be processed normally by hepatocytes. The result is hepatic steatosis and dyslipidemia, with elevated LDL-C, elevated triglycerides, and reduced HDL-C. Clinically, LAL-D is referred to as Wolman disease in infants and children or as cholesterol ester storage disease (CESD) in adults. Patients with LAL-D develop early atherosclerosis and progressive liver disease, with associated high rates of mortality at a young age.

Disorders of HDL Metabolism

Decreased HDL cholesterol is an independent risk factor for development of atherosclerosis and cardiovascular disease. Numerous rare genetic defects in HDL metabolism have been identified, including defects in apoAI, ABCA1, and LCAT. Each of these defects results in decreased levels of HDL, for which no effective treatments are currently available. More commonly, low HDL is associated with visceral obesity and insulin resistance.

Elevated concentrations of HDL occur in the setting of aerobic activity, alcohol consumption, estrogen use, and corticosteroid therapy. Recently, reductions in CETP activity have been characterized as a relatively common genetic cause of increased HDL levels. The increased plasma HDL concentration associated with decreased CETP activity has been attributed to a decrease in the transfer of cholesterol from HDL to remnant particles. Although it might be assumed that the increased HDL levels would be cardioprotective, this is not always observed. Decreased CETP activity may increase the risk of atherogenesis in some cases, whereas in others, it appears to be cardioprotective. Additional research will be necessary before the role of CETP polymorphisms in lipid metabolism and cardiovascular disease risk can be identified. Genetic variations in hepatic lipase and endothelial lipase can also lead to increased HDL.

Secondary Hyperlipidemia

In addition to the genetic causes of primary dyslipidemia described above, a number of secondary factors can lead to

TABLE 20-2 Secondary Causes of Hyperlipidemia

HYPERTRIGLYCERIDEMIA	HYPERCHOLESTEROLEMIA
Diabetes mellitus	Hypothyroidism
Chronic renal failure	Nephrotic syndrome
Hypothyroidism	Anorexia nervosa
Glycogen storage disease	Acute intermittent porphyria
Stress	Cholestasis
Sepsis	Obstructive liver disease
Alcohol excess	Corticosteroid treatment
Lipodystrophy	Protease inhibitor therapy
Pregnancy	
Oral estrogen replacement therapy	
Antihypertensive drugs: beta-blockers, diuretics	
Glucocorticoid treatment	
Protease inhibitor therapy	
Acute hepatitis	
Systemic lupus erythematosus	

Numerous secondary causes of hyperlipidemia exist; screening for the presence of these underlying factors should be performed before initiating pharmacologic therapy for a dyslipidemia. These lists are not exhaustive.

hyperlipidemia (Table 20-2). For example, alcohol intake increases the synthesis of fatty acids, which are then esterified to glycerol to form triglycerides. Therefore, excess alcohol consumption can result in increased VLDL production. Hypertriglyceridemia in type 2 diabetes mellitus results from increased VLDL synthesis and secretion and from reduced chylomicron and VLDL catabolism by LPL. Furthermore, apoCIII levels are increased in association with insulin resistance, and this reduces the catabolism of chylomicrons and VLDL particles. Hypothyroidism is an important and common cause of secondary hyperlipidemia. Any patient with a lipid disorder should be screened for hypothyroidism.

PHARMACOLOGIC CLASSES AND AGENTS

The decision to treat dyslipidemia is largely dependent on the calculated cardiovascular risk. A number of clinical algorithms exist for determining initiation of therapy. Goals for lipid lowering were established in the 2001 National Cholesterol Education Program Adult Treatment Panel III (ATP III) guidelines, which were updated in 2004 based on the results of several additional large, randomized clinical trials. These guidelines provide target LDL levels based on 10-year risk of death from cardiovascular disease (Table 20-3) and have been generally adopted in clinical practice. In 2013, the American College of Cardiology and American Heart Association (ACC/AHA) published new guidelines on the treatment of cholesterol. These guidelines no longer utilize baseline LDL-C as an indication to initiate treatment, nor do they establish LDL-C goals of treatment. Instead, the new guidelines define four discrete "statin benefit groups" (Table 20-4). Both sets of guidelines emphasize the importance of therapeutic lifestyle changes (TLCs), which include reduction of dietary saturated fat and cholesterol intake, weight reduction, increased physical activity, avoidance of tobacco products, and, possibly, stress reduction.

Successful dietary therapy can reduce total cholesterol by up to about 25%, depending on adherence and the metabolic basis for elevated cholesterol concentrations. If this approach is unsuccessful or insufficient to normalize lipid levels, drug therapy is generally recommended. Five well-established classes of drugs are available for pharmacologic modification of lipid metabolism. Three of these classes (inhibitors

TABLE 20-3 Updated National Cholesterol Education Program Adult Treatment Panel III Guidelines

ATP 2004 UPDATE: LDL-C THERAPY BY RISK CATEGORIES BASED ON RECENT CLINICAL TRIAL EVIDENCE

RISK CATEGORY	LDL-C GOAL	INITIATE THERAPEUTIC LIFESTYLE CHANGES	CONSIDER DRUG THERAPY
High risk: CHD or CHD risk equivalents (10-year risk >20%)	<100 mg/dL; *optional goal <70 mg/dL*	≥100 mg/dL	≥100 mg/dL
Moderately high risk: 2+ risk factors (10-year risk 10–20%)	<130 mg/dL	≥130 mg/dL	≥130 mg/dL (consider drug options if 100–129 mg/dL)
Moderate risk: 2+ risk factors (10-year risk <10%)	<130 mg/dL	≥130 mg/dL	>160 mg/dL
Low risk: 0–1 risk factor	<160 mg/dL	≥160 mg/dL	≥190 mg/dL (consider drug options if 160–189 mg/dL)

Adapted with permission from Grundy SM, Cleeman JI, Merz CN, et al. Implications of recent clinical trials for the National Cholesterol Education Program Adult Treatment Panel III Guidelines. *J Am Coll Cardiol* 2004;44:720–732.
More information about lipid management guidelines and details about calculation of cardiovascular risk are available at: https://www.nhlbi.nih.gov/health-pro/guidelines/in-develop/cholesterol-in-adults.
LDL-C, low-density lipoprotein cholesterol; CHD, coronary heart disease.

TABLE 20-4 2013 American College of Cardiology/American Heart Association Guideline on the Treatment of Blood Cholesterol to Reduce Atherosclerotic Cardiovascular Risk in Adults

Statin Therapy for Individuals at Increased ASCVD Risk Based on Recent Clinical Trial Evidence	
STEP 1: For adults, check baseline fasting lipids, counsel on therapeutic lifestyle changes, and assign to a statin benefit group:	
Clinical ASCVD	Initiate statin therapy at moderate intensity (age ≤75) or high intensity (age >75).
LDL ≥190 mg/dL	Initiate statin therapy at high intensity.
Diabetes type I/II	Initiate statin therapy at moderate intensity (high intensity if 10-year ASCVD risk ≥7.5%).
≥7.5% estimated 10-year ASCVD risk	Moderate- to high-intensity statin therapy.
STEP 2: Reassess for adherence, response to treatment; consider checking LDL-C and other biomarkers as indicated.	

Adapted with permission from Stone NJ, Robinson JG, Lichtenstein AH, et al. 2013 ACC/AHA guideline on the treatment of blood cholesterol to reduce atherosclerotic cardiovascular risk in adults. *Circulation* 2014;129:S1–S45. (*New clinical guidelines for cholesterol-lowering therapy based on the definition of four "statin benefit groups."*) More information about lipid management guidelines and details about calculation of cardiovascular risk are available at https://my.americanheart.org/professional/StatementsGuidelines/PreventionGuidelines/Prevention-Guidelines_UCM_457698_SubHomePage.jsp.
Moderate-intensity statin therapy: daily dose lowers LDL-C by ~30% to <50%.
High-intensity statin therapy: daily dose lowers LDL-C by ~50% or greater.
ASCVD, atherosclerotic cardiovascular disease; LDL-C, low-density lipoprotein cholesterol.

of cholesterol synthesis, bile acid sequestrants, and cholesterol absorption inhibitors) have relatively well-defined effects on lipid metabolism. While the overall effects of the other two classes (fibrates and niacin) are clear, their molecular mechanisms of actions are diverse and remain subjects of active investigation. The inhibitors of cholesterol synthesis (i.e., HMG-CoA reductase inhibitors, also known as *statins*) are the most important class due to their well-demonstrated efficacy in reducing cardiovascular morbidity and mortality. However, agents in each of the other classes act as important adjunctive therapies and may be the agents of choice for patients with certain specific causes of dyslipidemia. The newest therapies for treating rare diseases and individuals with inadequate response to maximum medical management include VLDL secretion inhibitors and PCSK9 inhibitors.

Inhibitors of Cholesterol Synthesis

Statins competitively inhibit the activity of HMG-CoA reductase, the rate-limiting enzyme in cholesterol synthesis. Inhibition of this enzyme results in a transient, modest decrease in cellular cholesterol concentration (Fig. 20-11). The decrease in cholesterol concentration activates a cellular signaling cascade culminating in the activation of **sterol regulatory element binding protein 2 (SREBP2)**, a transcription factor that up-regulates expression of the gene encoding the LDL receptor. Increased LDL receptor expression causes increased uptake of plasma LDL and consequently decreases plasma LDL-cholesterol concentration. Approximately 70% of LDL receptors are expressed by hepatocytes, with the remainder expressed by a variety of cell types in the body.

Statins have been shown in numerous clinical trials to reduce mortality significantly after a myocardial infarction. This is referred to as **secondary prevention**. Recent studies have also concluded that lowering of LDL with statins can decrease mortality even in the absence of overt cardiovascular disease, which is called **primary prevention**. Despite these convincing percentage risk reductions in both secondary and primary prevention trials, it should be noted that statin use is associated with a greater absolute risk reduction in secondary prevention; the reason may be that patients in this treatment group have a higher absolute risk of death and therefore display the greatest benefit from statins. It is also important to note that statins have proven to be effective in reducing cardiovascular disease risk for high-risk patients (e.g., diabetic patients) with average, or even below average, LDL-cholesterol levels.

The magnitude of LDL-cholesterol lowering depends on the efficacy and dose of the statin that is administered. In general, statins reduce LDL-cholesterol concentrations by up to about 60%. Statins increase HDL-cholesterol concentrations by an average of 10% and reduce triglyceride concentrations by up to about 40%, depending on statin dose and degree of hypertriglyceridemia. The effect of statins on triglyceride levels is mediated by decreased VLDL production and increased clearance of remnant lipoproteins by the liver. The dose–response relationship of statins is nonlinear: the largest effect occurs with the starting dose. Each subsequent doubling of the dose produces, on average, an additional 6% LDL reduction. This is sometimes referred to as the "rule of 6s."

In addition to reducing LDL-cholesterol concentrations, statins have a number of other pharmacologic consequences. These are collectively referred to as *pleiotropic effects*, which include decreased inflammation, reversal of endothelial dysfunction, decreased thrombosis, and improved stability of atherosclerotic plaques. Evidence for diminished inflammation with statin therapy includes decreases in acute-phase reactants, which are plasma proteins that are increased during inflammatory states and may play a role in the destabilization of atherosclerotic plaques. The best characterized acute-phase reactant is C-reactive protein (CRP). Importantly, a recent large randomized clinical trial has shown that, among patients with a moderate risk of developing cardiovascular

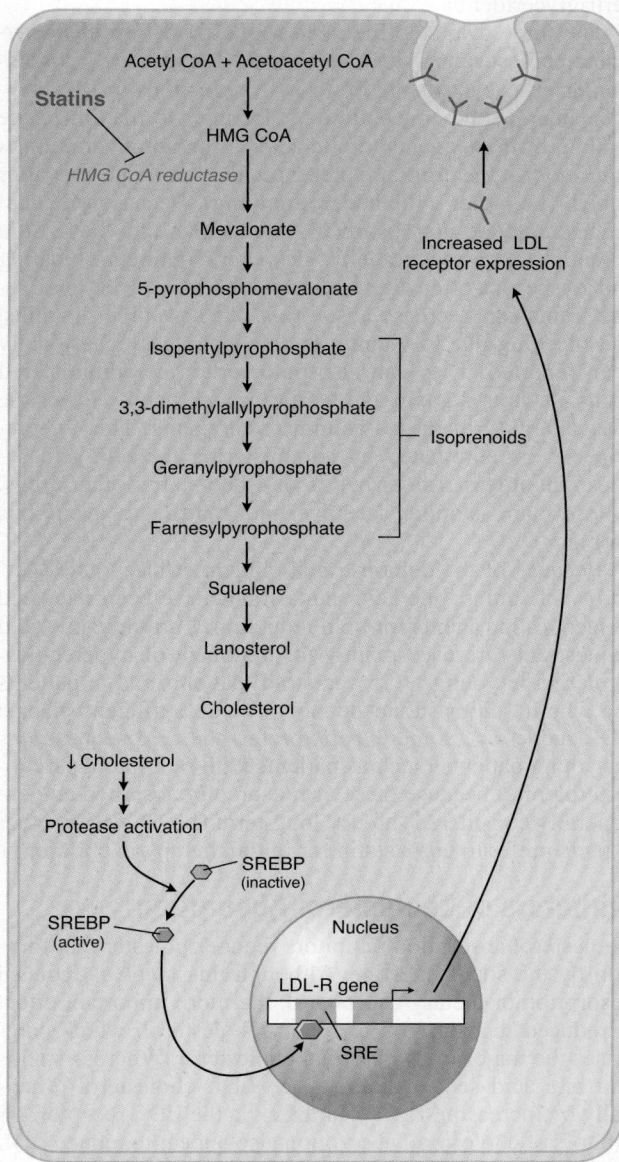

Increased
LDL-R expression
and uptake of
plasma LDL

FIGURE 20-11. Mechanism of LDL lowering by statins. Statins competitively inhibit HMG-CoA reductase, the enzyme that catalyzes the rate-limiting step in cholesterol biosynthesis. Decreased cellular cholesterol concentrations lead to protease activation and cleavage of the sterol regulatory element binding protein (SREBP), which is a transcription factor that normally resides in the cytoplasm. The cleaved SREBP diffuses into the nucleus, where it binds to sterol response elements (SRE), leading to up-regulation of LDL receptor gene transcription. This leads to increased cellular LDL receptor expression. This promotes uptake of LDL particles and results in reduced LDL-cholesterol concentrations in the plasma.

disease and with elevated baseline CRP levels, use of a statin reduces cardiovascular morbidity and mortality, even when the patients do not have elevated LDL-cholesterol concentrations.

Evidence for reversal of endothelial dysfunction with statin therapy includes an improved vasodilatory response of endothelium to nitric oxide. Improved vasodilation could

help prevent ischemia. Evidence for decreased thrombosis with statin therapy includes a decrease in prothrombin activation and a decrease in tissue factor production. Because thrombosis is at the root of most acute coronary syndromes, its reduction could contribute to the survival benefit of statins. Finally, plaque stability is enhanced with statin therapy because the fibrous cap that overlies the lipid-rich plaque becomes thicker. This effect may be attributable to decreased macrophage infiltration and inhibition of vascular smooth muscle proliferation. It is important to emphasize that most of these pleiotropic effects of statins have been demonstrated only in vitro or in animal models, and their relevance in humans is unclear. Clinical data indicate that the reductions in cardiovascular morbidity and mortality due to statins are primarily attributable to the lowering of LDL-cholesterol concentrations in the plasma.

Seven statins—**lovastatin**, **pravastatin**, **simvastatin**, **fluvastatin**, **atorvastatin**, **rosuvastatin**, and **pitavastatin**—are currently approved for use in hypercholesterolemia and mixed hyperlipidemia. They are considered first-line therapy for increased LDL levels, and their use is supported by numerous trials showing that statins decrease both cardiovascular-related and total mortality. Stroke is also reduced. All of the statins are believed to act by the same mechanism. The main differences are attributable to potency and pharmacokinetic parameters. Among the statins, fluvastatin is the least potent, and atorvastatin and rosuvastatin are the most potent. Beyond their capacity to reduce LDL-cholesterol concentrations, the clinical relevance of these potency differences has not been determined. The pharmacokinetic differences among the statins result from differential cytochrome P450 metabolism. Lovastatin, simvastatin, and atorvastatin are metabolized by CYP3A4, whereas other cytochrome P450-mediated pathways metabolize fluvastatin and pitavastatin. Pravastatin and rosuvastatin are not metabolized via the cytochrome P450 pathway. As explained below, the pathways of statin metabolism have important implications for drug interactions.

Statins are generally well tolerated; the incidence of adverse effects is lower with statins than with any of the other lipid-lowering drug classes. The main adverse effect is myopathy and/or myositis with rhabdomyolysis. The latter is a very rare complication that occurs primarily at high doses of the most potent statins. Therefore, plasma creatine kinase levels (a marker of muscle injury) are not useful for routine monitoring of statin-treated patients. Certain patients who have inherited a molecular variant of an organic anion transporter responsible for statin uptake may be at higher risk of developing statin-induced myopathy (see Chapter 7, Pharmacogenomics).

High-potency statins can also cause increases in serum transaminase levels (i.e., alanine transaminase [ALT] and aspartate transaminase [AST]). In the vast majority of cases, these commonly observed elevations in ALT and AST most likely reflect an adaptive response of the liver to changes in cholesterol homeostasis. True hepatotoxicity is indicated by ALT and AST elevations that are accompanied by elevations in serum bilirubin concentrations.

If a statin alone is insufficient to lower LDL to target levels, the statin can be used effectively in combination with other agents. The combination of a statin with a bile acid sequestrant or cholesterol absorption inhibitor results in additive LDL decreases and is not associated with significant drug interactions. The combination of niacin and a statin may be most useful in patients with high levels of LDL cholesterol and low levels of HDL cholesterol. However, because co-administration of niacin and a statin could slightly increase the risk of myopathy, such patients should be closely monitored for the development of adverse effects.

Fibrates and statins have also been reported to be efficacious in combination. However, certain fibrates inhibit both the transport of statins into the liver and the glucuronidation of statins in the liver, thereby decreasing statin clearance. These agents may therefore raise the plasma statin concentration and increase the risk of rhabdomyolysis. This effect has been documented for **gemfibrozil** but does not occur with **fenofibrate**. Finally, in patients who require LDL lowering and are taking drugs that are metabolized by cytochrome P450—such as certain antibiotics, calcium channel blockers, warfarin, and protease inhibitors (see Chapter 4, Drug Metabolism)—a statin that is not metabolized by P450 enzymes is preferable.

Inhibitors of VLDL Secretion

Currently approved inhibitors of VLDL secretion act by two different mechanisms (Fig. 20-3). **Lomitapide** is a small molecule that inhibits lipid transfer by binding to MTP, while **mipomersen** is a synthetic single-strand antisense oligonucleotide that binds to the apoB100 mRNA and thereby reduces apoB protein levels. The net effect of each drug is to reduce VLDL secretion.

Lomitapide is approved for use in patients with homozygous familial hypercholesterolemia (HoFH). At therapeutic doses, lomitapide reduces LDL-C by 30–50% in these patients. Adverse effects include gastrointestinal distress due to fat malabsorption, reductions in plasma vitamin E levels, and transaminase elevations that are correlated with increased hepatic fat content. Transaminase elevations have not been associated with parallel increases in plasma bilirubin concentrations and generally normalize with continued lomitapide treatment.

Mipomersen is indicated for the treatment of patients with homozygous FH who are already prescribed maximal medical therapy. Adverse effects may include injection site reactions, flu-like symptoms, increases in C-reactive protein, and increased transaminases. Similar to lomitapide, the liver test abnormalities likely correspond to an increase in liver fat content. This increased fat content appears to remain stable over 1 year of treatment and is reversible with cessation of therapy.

Inhibitors of Bile Acid Absorption

The bile acid sequestrants are cationic polymer resins that bind noncovalently to negatively charged bile acids in the small intestine. The resin–bile acid complex cannot be reabsorbed in the distal ileum and is excreted in the stool. Decreased bile acid reabsorption by the ileum partially interrupts enterohepatic bile acid circulation, causing hepatocytes to up-regulate 7α-hydroxylase, the rate-limiting enzyme in bile acid synthesis (Fig. 20-10A). The increase in bile acid synthesis decreases hepatocyte cholesterol concentration, leading to increased expression of the LDL receptor and enhanced LDL clearance from the circulation. The effectiveness of bile acid sequestrants in clearing LDL from the plasma is partially offset by concomitant up-regulation of hepatic cholesterol and triglyceride synthesis, which

stimulates the production of VLDL particles by the liver. As a result, bile acid sequestrants may also raise triglyceride levels and should be used with caution in patients with hypertriglyceridemia.

The three available bile acid sequestrants are **cholestyramine**, **colesevelam**, and **colestipol**. These drugs possess similar efficacy, causing up to 28% reductions in LDL levels at therapeutic concentrations. In order to maximize the binding of these agents to bile acids, drug administration is timed so that the drugs are present in the small intestine after a meal (i.e., after gallbladder emptying). Because bile acid sequestrants are not absorbed systemically, they have little potential for serious toxicity. However, significant bloating and dyspepsia often limit patient adherence. Bile acid sequestrants can decrease absorption of fat-soluble vitamins, and bleeding due to vitamin K deficiency has occasionally been reported. They can also bind certain co-administered drugs, such as digoxin and warfarin, and thereby lower the bioavailability of the co-administered agents. This interaction can be eliminated by administering the bile acid sequestrant at least 1 hour before or 4 hours after other drugs. Colesevelam is more selective and appears to avoid this problem.

Because of the demonstrated clinical efficacy and tolerability of statins, bile acid sequestrants have been relegated to second-line agents for lipid reduction. Currently, bile acid sequestrants are used mainly for treatment of hypercholesterolemia in young (<25 years old) patients and in patients for whom statins alone do not provide sufficient plasma LDL reduction. Some experts prefer bile acid sequestrants for young patients (such as patients with familial hypercholesterolemia) because these agents are not absorbed and are generally considered safe for long-term use. However, other experts prefer to use a statin for initial therapy in children.

Inhibitors of Cholesterol Absorption

Cholesterol absorption inhibitors reduce cholesterol absorption by the small intestine. Although this involves reduced absorption of dietary cholesterol, the more important effect is reduced reabsorption of biliary cholesterol, which comprises the majority of intestinal cholesterol. Whereas statins and bile acid sequestrants reduce LDL cholesterol principally by increasing LDL clearance via the LDL receptor, inhibitors of cholesterol absorption also appear to reduce LDL cholesterol by inhibiting hepatic production of VLDL.

The two available cholesterol absorption inhibitors are **plant sterols** and **ezetimibe**. Plant sterols and stanols are naturally present in vegetables and fruits, and they may be consumed in larger amounts from nutritional supplements. Plant sterols and stanols are similar in molecular structure to cholesterol but are substantially more hydrophobic. As a result, plant sterols and stanols displace cholesterol from micelles, increasing the excretion of cholesterol in the stool. The plant sterols and stanols are themselves poorly absorbed. Based on their mechanism of action, gram quantities of plant sterols and stanols are required to reduce plasma LDL-cholesterol concentrations by approximately 15%. Because an average diet contains 200–400 mg of plant sterols and stanols, these molecules must be highly enriched in dietary supplements (to approximately 2 grams) in order to be effective.

Ezetimibe decreases cholesterol transport from micelles into enterocytes by selectively inhibiting cholesterol uptake through the brush border protein NPC1L1 (Fig. 20-4).

At therapeutic concentrations, ezetimibe reduces intestinal cholesterol absorption by about 50%, without reducing the absorption of triglycerides or fat-soluble vitamins.

The end result of reduced cholesterol absorption, achieved by either plant sterols and stanols or ezetimibe, is a decrease in LDL-cholesterol concentrations in the plasma. A reduction in cholesterol absorption presumably decreases the cholesterol content of chylomicrons and therefore decreases the transport of cholesterol from the intestine to the liver. Within the liver, cholesterol derived from chylomicron remnants contributes to the cholesterol that is packaged into VLDL particles. Therefore, inhibiting cholesterol absorption can reduce cholesterol incorporation into VLDL and decrease LDL-cholesterol concentrations in the plasma. Importantly, reduced hepatic cholesterol content also leads to up-regulation of the LDL receptor, which contributes to the mechanism of LDL lowering by cholesterol absorption inhibitors.

A single daily dose of ezetimibe lowers LDL-cholesterol concentrations by up to about 20%. Ezetimibe also lowers triglyceride concentrations by about 8% and elevates HDL cholesterol to a small extent (approximately 3%). Ezetimibe is particularly effective in combination with a statin, for the following reason. The reduction in hepatic cholesterol content due to inhibition of cholesterol absorption leads to a compensatory increase in hepatic cholesterol synthesis that partially offsets the benefits of reducing absorption. By combining ezetimibe with a statin, the compensatory increase in hepatic cholesterol synthesis is prevented. This approach reduces LDL-cholesterol concentrations by an additional 15% compared with the effect of the statin alone. The effect is similar throughout the statin dose range. Unlike bile acid sequestrants (which are not absorbed), ezetimibe is rapidly absorbed by the enterocyte and extensively glucuronidated, so that systemic concentrations of both unmodified and glucuronidated forms can be measured. Ezetimibe undergoes enterohepatic circulation up to several times each day in conjunction with meals. Cholesterol absorption inhibitors have exhibited good safety profiles, with few if any adverse effects. Ezetimibe can increase plasma concentrations of cyclosporine, which should be monitored whenever these two drugs are co-administered.

Fibrates

Fibrates bind to and activate peroxisome proliferator-activated receptor α (PPARα), a nuclear receptor expressed in hepatocytes, skeletal muscle, macrophages, and the heart. Upon binding of fibrate, PPARα heterodimerizes with the retinoid X receptor (RXR). This heterodimer binds to peroxisome proliferator response elements (PPREs) in the promoter regions of specific genes, activating transcription of these genes and thereby increasing protein expression.

Activation of PPARα by fibrates results in numerous changes in lipid metabolism that act collectively to decrease plasma triglyceride levels and increase plasma HDL (Fig. 20-12). The decrease in plasma triglyceride levels is caused in part by increased muscle expression of lipoprotein lipase, decreased hepatic expression of apolipoprotein CIII, and increased hepatic oxidation of fatty acids. The increased muscle expression of LPL results in increased uptake of triglyceride-rich lipoproteins, with a resultant decrease in plasma triglyceride levels. Because apoCIII normally functions to inhibit interaction of triglyceride-rich lipoproteins with their receptors, the decrease in hepatic production of apoCIII may potentiate the increased LPL activity.

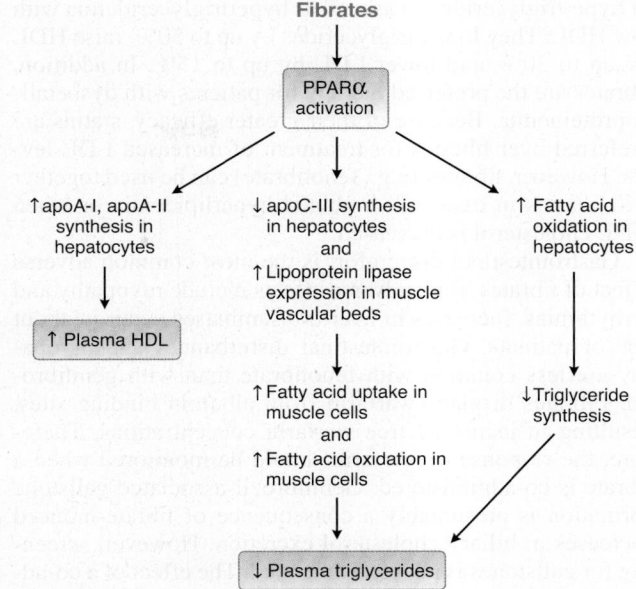

FIGURE 20-12. Influence of fibrates on lipid metabolism. Fibrates have several beneficial effects on lipid metabolism, all of which appear to be secondary to the activation of the transcription factor PPARα. PPARα activation by fibrates increases hepatic synthesis of apoAI and apoAII, which leads to increased plasma HDL-cholesterol concentrations. PPARα activation also down-regulates hepatic synthesis of apoCIII and increases lipoprotein lipase expression in muscle vascular beds. The decrease in apoCIII, an inhibitor of lipoprotein lipase, combines with the increase in lipoprotein lipase expression to increase fatty acid uptake and fatty acid oxidation in muscle cells. PPARα also increases fatty acid oxidation in hepatocytes. The combined effects of these metabolic changes are decreased plasma triglyceride concentrations and increased plasma HDL cholesterol. Because of decreased hepatic fatty acid and triglyceride synthesis (*not shown*), LDL-cholesterol concentrations also decrease modestly.

The mechanisms by which fibrate-mediated PPARα activation raises plasma HDL depend at least in part on increased hepatic production of apolipoprotein AI. This would be expected to contribute directly to increased plasma HDL. Up-regulation of ABCA1 in macrophages presumably promotes cholesterol efflux from these cells in vivo. Hepatocytes also increase expression of SR-B1 in response to PPARα activation, providing a pathway for increased reverse cholesterol transport, with subsequent cholesterol excretion into bile.

Fibrates also lower LDL levels modestly. The lower LDL levels result from a PPARα-induced shift in hepatocyte metabolism toward fatty acid oxidation. PPARα increases the expression of numerous enzymes involved in fatty acid transport and oxidation, thereby increasing fatty acid catabolism and decreasing triglyceride synthesis and VLDL production. PPARα activation also results in LDL particles of larger size, which appear to be taken up more efficiently by LDL receptors. Many of the effects of PPARα on lipid metabolism remain the subject of basic and clinical investigation, which may lead to the development of more selective PPARα agonists that are capable of targeting selective aspects of lipid metabolism. Finally, fibrates have a beneficial anti-inflammatory effect, decreasing the vulnerability of atherosclerotic plaques to rupture.

Gemfibrozil and **fenofibrate** are the available fibrates in the United States. Two other fibrates, **bezafibrate** and **ciprofibrate**, are available in Europe. Fibrates are indicated for treatment of hypertriglyceridemia as well as hypertriglyceridemia with low HDL. They lower triglycerides by up to 50%, raise HDL by up to 20%, and lower LDL by up to 15%. In addition, fibrates are the preferred therapy for patients with dysbetalipoproteinemia. Because of their greater efficacy, statins are preferred over fibrates for treatment of increased LDL levels. However, fibrates (e.g., fenofibrate) can be used together with statins in cases of combined hyperlipidemia or when HDL cholesterol is decreased.

Gastrointestinal discomfort is the most common adverse effect of fibrates. Rare adverse effects include myopathy and arrhythmias. Increases in liver transaminases occur in about 5% of patients. Gastrointestinal disturbances and myopathy are less common with fenofibrate than with gemfibrozil. Fibrates displace warfarin from albumin binding sites, resulting in increased free warfarin concentrations. Therefore, the response to warfarin should be monitored when a fibrate is co-administered. Gemfibrozil-associated gallstone formation is presumably a consequence of fibrate-induced increases in biliary cholesterol excretion. However, screening for gallstones is not recommended. The effect of a co-administered statin on fibrate metabolism is described above.

Niacin

Niacin (nicotinic acid, vitamin B_3) is a water-soluble vitamin. At physiologic concentrations, it is a substrate in the synthesis of nicotinamide adenine dinucleotide (NAD) and nicotinamide adenine dinucleotide phosphate (NADP), which are important cofactors in intermediary metabolism.

The pharmacologic use of niacin necessitates large doses (1,500–3,000 mg/day) and is independent of the conversion of nicotinic acid to NAD or NADP (Fig. 20-13). Niacin decreases plasma LDL-cholesterol and triglyceride concentrations and increases HDL cholesterol. Studies have identified a G protein-coupled receptor on adipocytes that appears to mediate the metabolic changes associated with niacin administration. Stimulation of this receptor by niacin decreases adipocyte hormone-sensitive lipase activity, leading to reduced peripheral tissue triglyceride catabolism and therefore decreased flux of free fatty acids to the liver. This decreases

the rate of hepatic triglyceride synthesis and VLDL production, leading to decreases in triglycerides (by up to 45%) and LDL (by up to 20%). Niacin also increases the half-life of apoAI, the major apolipoprotein in HDL. The increase in plasma apoAI increases plasma HDL concentrations by up to 30% and presumably augments reverse cholesterol transport.

Pharmacologic doses of niacin are available as oral agents for daily administration. The major adverse effects of niacin are cutaneous flushing and pruritus (itching). The flushing is mediated by the G protein-coupled niacin receptor and involves the release of prostaglandins D_2 and E_2 within the skin. It can be mitigated by pretreatment with aspirin or another nonsteroidal anti-inflammatory drug (NSAID). These adverse effects usually disappear after several weeks of niacin use. Timed-release formulations of niacin are associated with less cutaneous flushing than the immediate-release dosage form.

In addition to flushing and pruritus, important adverse effects of niacin include hyperuricemia, impaired insulin sensitivity, hepatotoxicity, and the potentiation of statin-induced myopathy. Hyperuricemia may precipitate gout. Impaired insulin sensitivity may precipitate diabetes in patients at risk, and niacin should be used with caution in diabetic patients. Rarely, niacin may cause myopathy. Concurrent administration of niacin with a statin slightly increases the risk of myopathy.

Niacin is indicated for patients with elevations of both triglycerides and cholesterol, usually in combination with a statin. Because niacin is currently the most effective agent available for raising HDL, it may also be the drug of choice for patients with modestly elevated LDL and decreased HDL. It is not clear whether both the LDL-lowering and HDL-raising effects of niacin contribute to improved clinical outcomes.

Omega-3 Fatty Acids

The omega-3 fatty acids **eicosapentaenoic acid (EPA)** and **docosahexaenoic acid (DHA)**, also referred to as fish oils, are effective at reducing plasma triglycerides by up to 50% in patients with hypertriglyceridemia. The likely mechanism

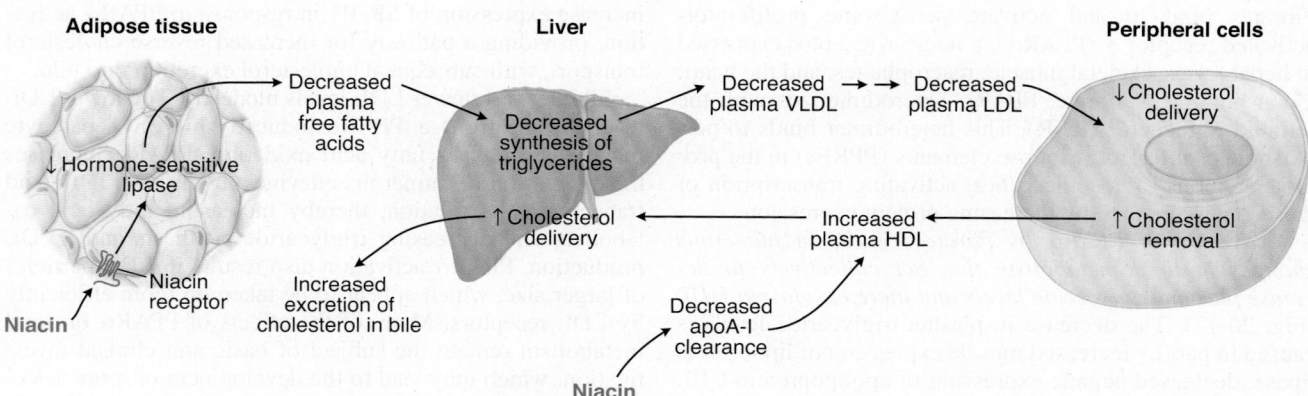

FIGURE 20-13. Influence of niacin on lipid metabolism. Niacin lowers triglyceride and LDL levels while increasing HDL. Activation by niacin of a G protein-coupled receptor on adipocytes results in decreased hormone-sensitive lipase activity in adipose tissue, which decreases the flux of free fatty acids to the liver. The decreased free fatty acid flux reduces hepatic triglyceride synthesis and limits VLDL synthesis. Because LDL is derived from VLDL, the decreased VLDL synthesis decreases plasma concentrations of LDL cholesterol. Niacin also increases the half-life of apoAI, an important apolipoprotein in HDL. The increased apoAI levels directly increase levels of plasma HDL and may also augment reverse cholesterol transport, delivery of cholesterol from HDL to the liver, and excretion of cholesterol in the bile.

of triglyceride lowering involves regulation of nuclear transcription factors, including SREBP-1c and PPARα, to cause reduced triglyceride biosynthesis and increased fatty acid oxidation in the liver. Omega-3 fatty acids are available over the counter as nutritional supplements in the form of fatty acid ethyl esters. **Lovaza®**, a prescription-strength form of omega-3 fatty acids, has also become available. Lovaza® is enriched (84%) in EPA and DHA, whereas most dietary supplements contain 13–63% fish oils. The recommended dose of Lovaza® is 4 grams once a day. Omega-3 fatty acids are generally added to therapy when plasma triglyceride concentrations exceed 500 mg/dL. The influence of omega-3 fatty acid use on clinical outcomes is uncertain.

PCSK9 Inhibitors

When LDL-R degradation is reduced by genetic loss-of-function mutations in PCSK9, cardiovascular disease incidence is dramatically reduced by 88%. This observation has led to aggressive interest in PCSK9 as a therapeutic target. Monoclonal antibodies that target the LDL-R—interacting domain of PCSK9 are newly approved by the FDA for the treatment of patients with heterozygous FH or clinical atherosclerotic cardiovascular disease (ASCVD) who require additional therapy beyond diet and maximal statin therapy. These include **evolocumab** and **alirocumab**, which are administered subcutaneously and can lower LDL-C by 50–72%. These drugs have been well tolerated in short-term clinical trials and in post-marketing surveillance, with no major reported adverse effects. The half-life of these antibodies is long, and the LDL-C lowering effects persist for up to 2–4 weeks. Interestingly, PCSK9 degrades many receptor targets (LDL-R, apoE-R2, VLDL-R, and LRP1) that are also receptors for viruses, such as human rhinovirus and hepatitis C virus. This suggests that the incidence of viral infection will need to be monitored closely in ongoing large-scale clinical trials of PCSK9 inhibitors.

■ CONCLUSION AND FUTURE DIRECTIONS

LDL reduction by available lipid-lowering drugs—particularly statins—represents an important advance in reducing cardiovascular disease mortality. The recent FDA approval of inhibitors of VLDL secretion has provided valuable new therapies for the treatment of patients with homozygous and severe heterozygous FH. PCSK9 inhibitors will now offer options for patients who require additional LDL-C reduction despite maximal medical therapy. Future research will evaluate the long-term safety of these new medications, clarify the biology of sortilin, and examine the possible benefits on cardiovascular disease of therapies that raise HDL-C (e.g., CETP inhibitors) and lower triglyceride levels.

Suggested Reading

Ballantyne CM, ed. *Clinical lipidology: a companion to Braunwald's heart disease*. 2nd ed. Philadelphia: Saunders/Elsevier; 2015;550 pp. (*Concise chapters cover all aspects of lipoprotein metabolism and pharmacology*.)

Degoma EM, Rader DJ. Novel HDL-directed pharmacotherapeutic strategies. *Nat Rev Cardiol* 2011;8:266–277. (*Review of treatments targeting HDL pathways*.)

Lukasova M, Malaval C, Gille A, Kero J, Offermanns S. Nicotinic acid inhibits progression of atherosclerosis in mice through its receptor GPR109A expressed by immune cells. *J Clin Invest* 2011;121:1163–1173. (*Recent developments in biology of niacin and its therapeutic potential*.)

Rader D, Kastelein J. Lomitapide and mipomersen: two first-in-class drugs for reducing low-density lipoprotein cholesterol in patients with homozygous familial hypercholesterolemia. *Circulation* 2014;129:1022–1032. (*Summary of the role of VLDL synthesis inhibition therapies, including clinical trial data*.)

Shimada YJ, Cannon CP. PCSK9 (Proprotein convertase subtilisin/kexin type 9) inhibitors: past, present, and the future. *Eur Heart J* 2015;36:2415–2424. (*A comprehensive review of PCSK9 biology and pharmacology*.)

Strong A, Rader D. Sortilin as a regulator of lipoprotein metabolism. *Curr Atheroscler Rep* 2012;14:211–218. (*Review of sortilin's role in lipoprotein biology*.)

DRUG SUMMARY TABLE: CHAPTER 20 Pharmacology of Cholesterol and Lipoprotein Metabolism

DRUG	CLINICAL APPLICATIONS	SERIOUS AND COMMON ADVERSE EFFECTS	CONTRAINDICATIONS	THERAPEUTIC CONSIDERATIONS
INHIBITORS OF CHOLESTEROL SYNTHESIS				
Mechanism—Inhibit HMG-CoA reductase, the rate-limiting enzyme in cholesterol synthesis → LDL decreases up to 60%, HDL increases ~10%, triglycerides decrease up to 40%				
Lovastatin **Pravastatin** **Simvastatin** **Fluvastatin** **Atorvastatin** **Rosuvastatin** **Pitavastatin**	Shared indications: Hypercholesterolemia Familial hypercholesterolemia Coronary atherosclerosis Prophylaxis for coronary atherosclerosis Pravastatin and simvastatin only: Stroke Atorvastatin only: Diabetes mellitus type 2	*Myopathy, rhabdomyolysis, hepatotoxicity, dermatomyositis, systemic lupus erythematosus (shared adverse effects); pancreatitis (pravastatin and rosuvastatin only); hemorrhagic cerebral infarction (atorvastatin only); acute renal failure (rosuvastatin only)* Abdominal pain, constipation, arthralgia (shared adverse effects); musculoskeletal pain, upper respiratory infection (pravastatin only)	Shared contraindications: Active liver disease Pregnancy and lactation Serum transaminase elevations Hypersensitivity to drug Pitavastatin only: Concomitant use of cyclosporine	Statins are drugs of choice for lowering LDL. Atorvastatin and rosuvastatin are the most potent; fluvastatin is the least potent. Lovastatin, simvastatin, and atorvastatin are metabolized by CYP3A4; inhibitors of CYP3A4 increase risk of myopathy; fluvastatin and pitavastatin are metabolized via a different cytochrome P450-mediated pathway; pravastatin and rosuvastatin are not metabolized by cytochrome P450s; consider choosing a statin not metabolized via P450s in patients who are concurrently taking drugs that are metabolized by cytochrome P450s. Combination with a bile acid sequestrant or cholesterol absorption inhibitor results in additive decrease in LDL. Combination with niacin may be useful in patients with high LDL and low HDL; however, co-administration with niacin increases the risk of myopathy. Co-administration with gemfibrozil decreases statin clearance and raises plasma concentration of statins, which can induce rhabdomyolysis.
INHIBITORS OF VLDL SECRETION				
Mechanism—Inhibit apoB mRNA translation (mipomersen) or apoB lipidation by MTP (lomitapide) to decrease VLDL secretion → at least 25–35% decrease in LDL (both agents) and 15% increase in HDL (mipomersen)				
Mipomersen **Lomitapide**	Homozygous familial hypercholesterolemia (HoFH)	*Steatosis of liver, anti-glomerular basement membrane tubulointerstitial nephritis, angioedema, cancer* Mild increase in liver transaminases, increased hepatic fat, injection site reaction, flu-like symptoms, headache, fatigue, mild gastrointestinal distress, reduced vitamin E levels (shared adverse effects); chest pain, weight loss (lomitapide only)	Shared contraindications: FDA approved for HoFH and requires physician certification and risk evaluation and mitigation strategy (REMS) Hepatic impairment Serum transaminase elevations Lomitapide only: Use of CYP3A4 inhibitors	Mipomersen is administered as a weekly subcutaneous injection and lomitapide as a daily oral regimen. Both agents are co-administered in addition to standard medical therapy, including a statin. Lomitapide may be co-administered with oral vitamin E supplementation.
INHIBITORS OF BILE ACID ABSORPTION				
Mechanism—Bind to bile acids, preventing enterohepatic circulation → LDL decreases up to 28%, HDL increases ~5%				
Cholestyramine **Colesevelam** **Colestipol**	Hypercholesterolemia (shared indication) Pruritus (cholestyramine only) Diabetes mellitus type 2 (colesevelam only)	*Pancreatitis, heart disease (colesevelam only)* Increase in triglyceride levels, bloating, dyspepsia, flatulence, bleeding diathesis secondary to vitamin K deficiency	Shared contraindications: Hypersensitivity to drug Hypertriglyceridemia Cholestyramine and colesevelam only: Complete biliary obstruction	Lowering of LDL levels is dose-dependent. Increase HDL modestly. Second-line agents for lipid reduction; used mainly to treat hypercholesterolemia in young patients and patients for whom statins alone do not provide sufficient LDL reduction. Increase triglyceride levels. Significant bloating and dyspepsia limit patient adherence. Decrease absorption of fat-soluble vitamins; bleeding may result due to vitamin K deficiency; bind certain drugs, such as digoxin and warfarin.

INHIBITORS OF CHOLESTEROL ABSORPTION

Mechanism—Decrease cholesterol transport from micelles into enterocytes by inhibiting uptake through brush border protein NPC1L1 → LDL decreases up to 20%, HDL increases ~3%, TG decrease ~8%

Drug	Indications	Adverse Effects	Contraindications	Notes
Ezetimibe	Primary hypercholesterolemia; Familial hypercholesterolemia; Sitosterolemia (very rare); Mixed hyperlipidemia	*Hepatitis, myopathy, rhabdomyolysis;* Arthralgia, myalgia	Hypersensitivity to ezetimibe; Concomitant use with a statin in pregnancy or while nursing; Active liver disease; Unexplained hepatic transaminase elevations	Modest LDL reduction; small effect on HDL and triglycerides (TG). Often combined with a statin to prevent a compensatory increase in hepatic cholesterol synthesis. Ezetimibe is rapidly absorbed by enterocytes and circulates enterohepatically. Ezetimibe levels are increased by cyclosporine and fibrates. Ezetimibe can increase plasma concentrations of cyclosporine.

FIBRATES

Mechanism—Agonists of peroxisome proliferator-activated receptor α (PPARα) → triglycerides decrease up to 50%, HDL increases up to 20%, LDL decreases up to 15%

Drug	Indications	Adverse Effects	Contraindications	Notes
Gemfibrozil Fenofibrate	Isolated hypertriglyceridemia; Hypertriglyceridemia with low HDL; Dysbetalipoproteinemia	*Elevated liver function tests, myopathy when co-administered with a statin (shared adverse effects); pancreatitis, serum creatinine elevation (fenofibrate only)* Abdominal discomfort	Shared contraindications: Preexisting gallbladder disease; Hepatic dysfunction; Severe renal impairment; Nursing mothers; Hypersensitivity to drug. Gemfibrozil only: Concomitant use with repaglinide or simvastatin	Drugs of choice for hypertriglyceridemia. Bezafibrate and ciprofibrate are available in Europe. Used in combination with statins for combined hyperlipidemia or when HDL cholesterol is decreased; however, there is an increased risk of myopathy when combined with statins. Fenofibrate has fewer GI and myopathy adverse effects than gemfibrozil. Fibrates increase warfarin levels.

NIACIN

Mechanism—Reduces free fatty acid release from adipose tissue and increases plasma residence time for apoAI → triglycerides decrease up to 45%, LDL decreases up to 20%, HDL increases up to 30%

Drug	Indications	Adverse Effects	Contraindications	Notes
Niacin	Isolated low HDL; Low HDL with mildly elevated LDL or TG; Familial combined hyperlipidemia	*Hepatotoxicity, rhabdomyolysis;* Flushing, abdominal discomfort	Active liver disease; Active peptic ulcer; Arterial bleeding; Hypersensitivity to niacin	Decreases LDL and triglyceride; increases HDL. Flushing occurs during first few weeks of use and can be prevented by pretreatment with NSAID; flushing limits use. Hyperuricemia may precipitate gout. Niacin use is associated with impaired insulin sensitivity.

OMEGA-3 FATTY ACIDS

Mechanism—Regulate nuclear transcription factors including SREBP-1c and PPARα to reduce triglyceride biosynthesis and increase fatty acid oxidation → reduce plasma triglycerides by up to 50%

Drug	Indications	Adverse Effects	Contraindications	Notes
EPA DHA	Hypertriglyceridemia	*Increased low-density lipoprotein cholesterol;* GI discomfort	Hypersensitivity to omega-3 fatty acids	Lovaza® is a prescription-strength formulation of eicosapentaenoic acid (EPA) and docosahexaenoic acid (DHA).

PCSK9 INHIBITORS

Mechanism—Bind to PCSK9 in plasma, thereby promoting antibody complex-mediated degradation; reduced PCSK9 levels decrease the rate of LDL-R degradation, leading to net increase in the rate of LDL-C clearance and a 50–72% decrease in LDL-C levels

Drug	Indications	Adverse Effects	Contraindications	Notes
Evolocumab Alirocumab	Shared indication: Heterozygous familial hypercholesterolemia (HeFH) or clinical ASCVD requiring additional lowering of LDL-C. Evolocumab only: Homozygous FH (HoFH)	*Hypersensitivity reaction (including vasculitis);* Nasopharyngitis, upper respiratory tract infection, injection site reaction, influenza, back pain, myalgia, diarrhea (shared adverse effects); dizziness, hypertension (evolocumab only); elevated liver enzymes (alirocumab only)	Hypersensitivity to any component of drug	Subcutaneous injection every 2 weeks (every 4 weeks for evolocumab in HoFH). Discontinue treatment for serious hypersensitivity reactions.

21

Pharmacology of Volume Regulation

Hakan R. Toka and Seth L. Alper[+]

INTRODUCTION

Coordinated regulation of volume homeostasis and vascular tone maintains adequate tissue perfusion in response to varying environmental stimuli. This chapter discusses the pharmacologically relevant physiology of volume regulation, with emphasis on the hormonal pathways and renal mechanisms that modulate systemic volume. (Control of vascular tone is discussed in Chapter 22, Pharmacology of Vascular Tone.) Dysregulation of volume homeostasis can result in edema, the pathologic accumulation of fluid in the extravascular space. Pharmacologic modulation of volume is targeted at reducing volume excess; this is an effective treatment for hypertension and heart failure (HF), as well as for cirrhosis and the nephrotic syndrome. The two broad classes of pharmacologic agents used to modify volume status are modulators of neurohormonal regulators (such as angiotensin converting enzyme [ACE] inhibitors) and diuretics (agents that increase renal Na+ excretion). Drugs that modify volume regulation also have many other clinically important effects on the body, because these volume regulators act as diverse hormonal modulators in multiple physiologic pathways. Many of the clinical applications of these agents are discussed further in Chapter 26, Integrative Cardiovascular Pharmacology: Hypertension, Ischemic Heart Disease, and Heart Failure.

PHYSIOLOGY OF VOLUME REGULATION

An intricate set of mechanisms sense, signal, and modulate changes in plasma volume. Volume sensors are located throughout the vascular tree, including in the atria and in the kidneys. Many of the volume regulators activated by these sensors include systemic and autocrine hormones, while others involve neural circuits. The integrated result of these signaling mechanisms is to alter vascular tone and to regulate renal Na+ reabsorption and excretion. Vascular tone maintains end-organ tissue perfusion; changes in renal Na+ excretion alter total volume status.

Determinants of Intravascular Volume

Intravascular volume is a small proportion of total body water, but the amount of fluid in the vascular compartment critically determines the extent of tissue perfusion. Approximately 2/3 of total body water is intracellular, while 1/3 is extracellular. Of the extracellular fluid (ECF), approximately 3/4 resides in the interstitial space, while 1/4 of ECF is plasma.

Fluid exchange between plasma and interstitial compartments occurs as a result of changes in capillary permeability, oncotic pressure, and hydrostatic pressure. Capillary permeability is determined largely by the junctions between

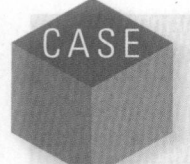

CASE

Mr. R, a 70-year-old male, is taken by ambulance to the emergency department at 1:00 AM after waking up with shortness of breath for the fourth night in a row. Each time, he "felt tight in the chest" and "couldn't get a breath"; this discomfort was relieved somewhat by sitting up in bed. He also recalls previous episodes of shortness of breath while climbing stairs.

Physical exam reveals tachycardia (heart rate, 112/min), mild hypertension (blood pressure, 155/95 mm Hg), decreased oxygen saturation (90% on room air), increased respiratory rate (28/min), bilateral pulmonary crackles on inspiration, and 1–2+ edema of the feet. Serum troponin T level (a marker of cardiomyocyte injury) is normal, but serum creatinine (1.5 mg/dL) and blood urea nitrogen (BUN, 30 mg/dL) are mildly elevated. Urinalysis is normal. Electrocardiogram shows evidence of an old myocardial infarction (Q wave in leads II, III, and V4–V6). Echocardiography reveals diminished left ventricular ejection fraction (LVEF, 35%; the fraction of blood in the ventricle at the end of diastole that is ejected when the ventricle contracts) without ventricular dilatation.

Based on the clinical findings of decreased cardiac output, pulmonary congestion, and peripheral edema, Mr. R is diagnosed with acute heart failure. His increased creatinine and BUN also indicate an element of renal insufficiency. Pharmacologic therapy is started, including a coronary vasodilator, an antihypertensive calcium channel blocker, and a loop diuretic. After Mr. R's condition stabilizes over the course of 3 days, the dose of the loop diuretic is decreased and then discontinued. Elective coronary angiography reveals significant stenosis of the left anterior descending coronary artery. Mr. R undergoes balloon angioplasty and stent placement and remains stable. Mr. R is discharged on a regimen that includes an ACE inhibitor and spironolactone.

Questions

1. What mechanisms led to Mr. R's pulmonary congestion and pedal edema?

2. Why was Mr. R given a loop diuretic?

3. How do ACE inhibitors improve cardiovascular hemodynamics?

4. Why was Mr. R prescribed spironolactone?

---

individual endothelial cells lining a vascular space. The capillary beds of some organs are more permeable than those of others and, as a result, allow larger intercompartmental fluid shifts. In the context of inflammation and other pathologic conditions (see below), increased capillary permeability allows proteins to shift, along with "oncotically obligated water," between intravascular and perivascular compartments under the influence of the plasma oncotic pressure gradient. Oncotic pressure is determined by the molecular solute components of a fluid space that are differentially partitioned between adjacent compartments (such constituents are said to be *osmotically active*). Because albumin, globulins, and other large plasma proteins are normally confined to the plasma space, these oncotically active proteins serve to retain water in the vascular space. The hydrostatic pressure gradient across the capillary barrier between compartments is another force for water movement. An elevated intracapillary pressure favors increased transudation of fluid from plasma into the interstitial space.

The relationship between fluid filtration and capillary permeability, oncotic pressure, and hydrostatic pressure is represented by the following equation

Fluid Filtration $= K_f (P_c - P_{if}) - (\Pi_c - \Pi_{if})$ **Equation 21-1**

where K_f is the capillary permeability coefficient, P_c is capillary hydrostatic pressure, P_{if} is interstitial fluid hydrostatic pressure, Π_c is capillary oncotic pressure, and Π_{if} is interstitial fluid oncotic pressure. This equation emphasizes that transcapillary fluid movement is governed by intercompartmental gradients rather than by the absolute value of each

compartmental pressure. Note that *the hydrostatic and oncotic gradient terms have opposing vectors* and therefore favor fluid movement in opposite directions. ΔP_c normally favors transudation from the capillary lumen to the interstitium, whereas $\Delta \Pi_c$ normally favors fluid retention within the capillary lumen.

The extent of fluid filtration that occurs along the length of the capillary differs for each tissue's capillary bed and is determined by cellular and junctional permeability properties of tissue-specific capillary endothelial cells. In the example shown in Figure 21-1, liver capillaries filter fluid into the interstitium along their entire length. At the arterial end of the capillary bed, $(P_c + \Pi_{if})$ exceeds $(P_{if} + \Pi_c)$, thus favoring plasma filtration from the capillary into the interstitial space. P_c gradually decreases along the length of the capillary, and the rate of fluid filtration into the interstitium decreases. At the venous end of the capillary, hydrostatic fluid filtration and oncotic fluid absorption are almost balanced. Liver sinusoids, which transfer fluid into the interstitial space during perfusion, return this fluid to the circulation via lymphatic flow. In capillary beds of other tissues, the integrated oncotic pressure gradient favoring fluid flow into the capillary balances the integrated hydrostatic pressure gradient, resulting in no net volume change between the vascular and interstitial spaces. Thus, the physiologic steady state of extracellular fluid represents a balance of driving forces between fluids of the intravascular and interstitial compartments. Pathologic alterations in the determinants of transcapillary fluid shifts, coupled with changes in renal Na^+ handling, can result in the formation of edema, as discussed below.

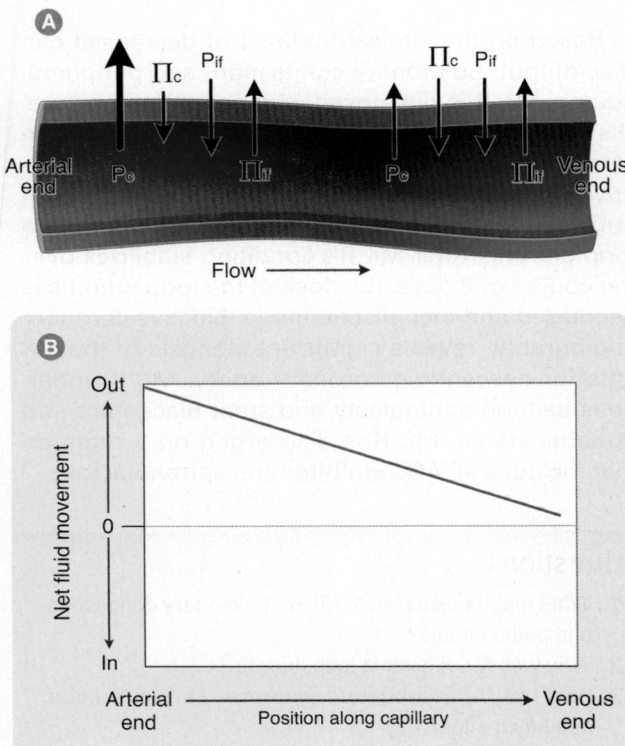

FIGURE 21-1. Capillary fluid filtration. The balance of hydrostatic pressure and oncotic pressure determines fluid filtration along the capillary. The example shown here is for a capillary in the liver in which fluid filtration exceeds fluid reabsorption. **A.** At the arterial end of the capillary, the capillary hydrostatic pressure (P_c) is high (*largest arrow*), and the sum of P_c and interstitial oncotic pressure (Π_{if}) exceeds the sum of interstitial hydrostatic pressure (P_{if}) and capillary oncotic pressure (Π_c). Therefore, fluid moves out of the capillary into the interstitial space. As fluid continues to filter along the length of the capillary, the increased fluid filtration results in decreased P_c and increased Π_c, thus decreasing the driving force for fluid filtration from the capillary to the interstitium. Throughout the length of the capillary, P_{if} and Π_{if} remain relatively constant. **B.** A graphic representation of net fluid movement along the capillary length shows the decreasing driving force for fluid filtration into the interstitium. In the capillary shown here, fluid is filtered into the interstitium along the entire capillary length; lymphatic vessels eventually return the excess interstitial fluid to the systemic circulation (*not shown*).

Volume Sensors

Vascular volume sensors can be divided into low-pressure and high-pressure feedback systems. The low-pressure system consists of the atria and pulmonary vasculature. In response to decreased wall stress (e.g., caused by decreased intravascular volume), peripheral nervous system cells lining the atria and pulmonary vasculature transmit a signal to noradrenergic neurons in the medulla of the central nervous system (CNS). This signal is relayed to the hypothalamus, resulting in increased secretion by the posterior pituitary gland of **antidiuretic hormone** (**ADH**, also known as **arginine vasopressin, AVP**). ADH promotes vasoconstriction and antidiuresis (increased renal water reabsorption). Together with increased peripheral sympathetic tone, this maintains distal tissue perfusion. In response to increased wall stress (e.g., caused by increased intravascular volume), cells of the atria produce and secrete natriuretic peptide, which promotes vasodilation and **natriuresis** (increased renal Na^+ excretion).

The high-pressure system consists of specialized baroreceptors in the aortic arch, carotid sinus, and juxtaglomerular apparatus. These sensors modulate hypothalamic control of ADH secretion and sympathetic outflow from the brainstem. In addition, sympathetic input stimulates the juxtaglomerular apparatus to secrete **renin**, a proteolytic enzyme that activates the renin-angiotensin-aldosterone system (see below).

Volume Regulators

Together, the low-pressure and high-pressure feedback systems integrate neurohumoral volume signals to maintain volume homeostasis in the face of volume perturbations. The neurohormonal response to a change in volume status is controlled by four main systems: the renin-angiotensin-aldosterone system (RAAS), natriuretic peptides, ADH, and renal sympathetic nerves. The RAAS, ADH, and renal sympathetic nerves are active in situations of intravascular volume depletion, while natriuretic peptides are released in response to intravascular volume overload.

Renin-Angiotensin-Aldosterone System

Renin is an aspartyl protease that activates the RAAS by cleavage of the circulating prohormone **angiotensinogen** to generate **angiotensin I**. Renin is produced and secreted by the **juxtaglomerular apparatus (JGA)**, a specialized set of granule-containing smooth muscle cells derived from the afferent arteriole that line the afferent and efferent arterioles of the renal glomerulus. The JGA is also adjacent to the macula densa, a nephron segment between the end of the thick ascending limb of the loop of Henle and the distal convoluted tubule, containing specialized tubular epithelial cells capable of sensing distal chloride (and/or sodium) delivery. The JGA in the renal cortex represents the major structural component of the RAAS and one of the most important regulatory sites of renal volume conservation and blood pressure maintenance. The ultimate result of renin secretion is *vasoconstriction and Na^+ retention, actions that maintain tissue perfusion and increase extracellular fluid volume* (Fig. 21-2).

At least three mechanisms are thought to control juxtaglomerular cell renin release (Fig. 21-3). First, a direct pressure-sensing mechanism of the afferent arteriole, equivalent to an intrarenal baroreceptor, responds to changes in renal perfusion pressure (arteriolar wall tension) to increase juxtaglomerular cell release of renin. The detailed molecular mechanism of this sensory transduction is unknown in humans; in rodents, it involves autocrine prostaglandin and purinergic signaling. Second, sympathetic innervation of juxtaglomerular cells promotes renin release via β_1-adrenoceptor stimulation. Third, the autoregulatory mechanism known as **tubuloglomerular feedback** senses distal nephron delivery of chloride (and/or sodium) to modulate renin release. Nephron anatomy is organized such that the distal end of the cortical thick ascending limb (TAL) of each nephron is closely apposed to the juxtaglomerular mesangium of the same nephron. This spatial proximity allows rapid integrative regulation of afferent arteriolar diameter and glomerular mesangial contractility by distal nephron electrolyte concentration and/or salt load. **Macula densa** cells of the cortical thick ascending limb respond to increased luminal NaCl delivery by increasing extracellular adenosine in the juxtaglomerular interstitium, thereby activating A_1 receptors on the juxtaglomerular mesangial cells to decrease renin release. Conversely, decreased luminal NaCl delivery

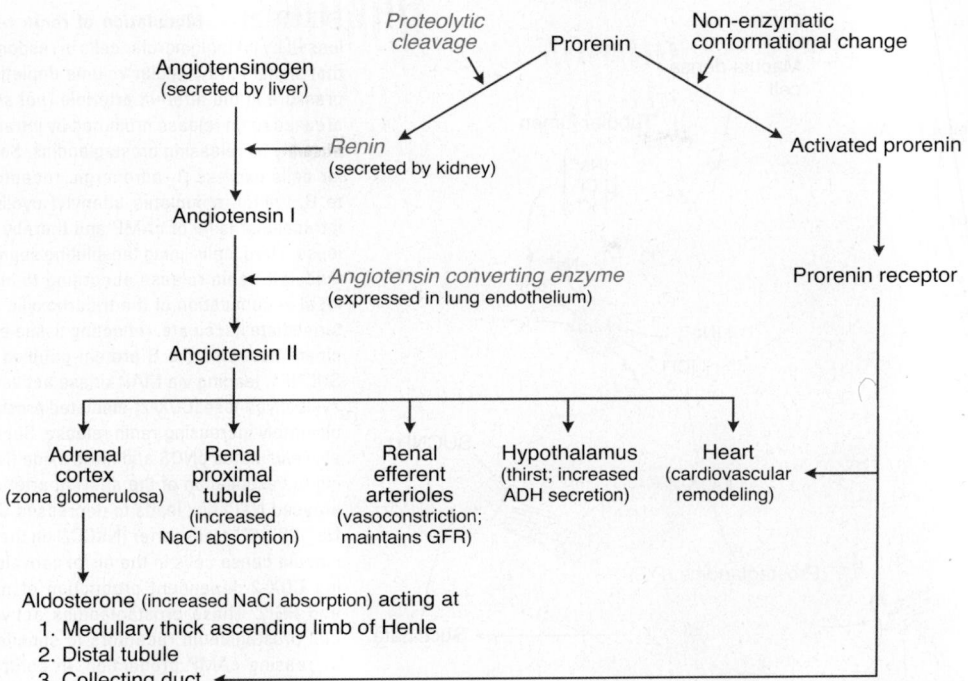

FIGURE 21-2. The renin-angiotensin-aldosterone axis. Angiotensinogen is a prohormone secreted into the circulation by hepatocytes. Renin, an aspartyl protease secreted by juxtaglomerular cells of the kidney, cleaves angiotensinogen to the decapeptide angiotensin I, which has no known intrinsic biological activity. Prorenin, the proenzyme of renin, may have additional biologic effects by signaling through the prorenin receptor. Angiotensin converting enzyme (ACE), a protease expressed on pulmonary capillary endothelium (and elsewhere in tissues), cleaves angiotensin I to the octapeptide angiotensin II. Angiotensin II has at least four actions via the angiotensin II type 1 receptor (AT_1R) that increase intravascular volume and maintain tissue perfusion. First, angiotensin II stimulates zona glomerulosa cells of the adrenal cortex to secrete aldosterone, a hormone that increases renal NaCl reabsorption at multiple segments along the nephron. Second, angiotensin II directly stimulates renal proximal tubule reabsorption of NaCl. Third, angiotensin II causes efferent arteriolar vasoconstriction, an action that increases intraglomerular pressure and thereby increases GFR. Fourth, angiotensin II stimulates hypothalamic thirst centers and promotes ADH secretion. Angiotensin II has additional tissue-specific and cellular effects that can activate the sympathetic nervous system and promote cardiovascular remodeling. Aldosterone (via the mineralocorticoid receptor; *not shown*) and prorenin (via the prorenin receptor) can have similar effects on the cardiovascular system.

activates a mesangial prostaglandin signaling cascade that culminates in increased renin release. Macula densa cells sense luminal NaCl delivery by monitoring both luminal NaCl concentration and luminal fluid flow rate as sensed by shear stress. NaCl delivery may be sensed directly by receptors in the apical sensory monocilia of macula densa cells; fluid flow may be sensed by direct bending of the monocilia. Molecular components in the extraciliary apical membrane likely also contribute to these signal transduction processes.

Prorenin, the renin proenzyme, was for many years considered an inactive precursor of renin lacking any intrinsic function. It now seems, however, that prorenin can be activated either by proteolytic cleavage to renin or by nonenzymatic conformational change induced by acid pH or elevated temperature. Renin activation typically occurs before its release from juxtaglomerular cells. Proconvertase I and cathepsin B are among the several enzymes that have been proposed to mediate proteolytic activation of renin; the potential roles of plasma and tissue kallikrein in renin cleavage have been disputed.

Recent studies have suggested that prorenin has cleavage-independent functions mediated through its binding to the (pro)renin receptor (PRR). Reversible binding of prorenin to PRR in tissues promotes a nonenzymatic conformational change that allows the uncleaved prorenin to act as an angiotensinogen convertase, thereby converting

angiotensinogen to angiotensin I (Ang I; see below). In addition, binding of prorenin to PRR triggers downstream activation of the MAP kinase ERK1/2 signaling pathway, leading to up-regulation of profibrotic and cyclooxygenase-2 genes and to regulation of the vacuolar H^+ ATPase in the collecting duct (see below). Interestingly, circulating plasma levels of prorenin are higher than those of renin, particularly in the setting of diabetic kidney disease. Transgenic mice overexpressing PRR develop hypertension and glomerulosclerosis, whereas genetic engineering of PRR loss-of-function leads to embryonic lethality, suggesting that essential cellular functions of PRR are not yet understood.

Secreted renin (produced by cleavage of prorenin) acts as a protease to cleave the first 10 amino acids of the circulating prohormone **angiotensinogen**, generating **angiotensin I (Ang I)**. Ang I (Ang 1-10) is then cleaved to the active octapeptide angiotensin II (Ang II, AT II, or Ang 1-8) by the carboxypeptidase angiotensin converting enzyme (ACE) located on the endothelial cell surface. Although ACE is expressed primarily in the pulmonary vascular endothelium and coronary circulation, ACE activity regulates local production of AT II in all vascular beds. Indeed, an incompletely understood "local" renin-angiotensin system is also expressed in the vasculature, producing these substances as autocrine factors independently of the kidney and liver. ACE has a broad proteolytic substrate specificity that includes

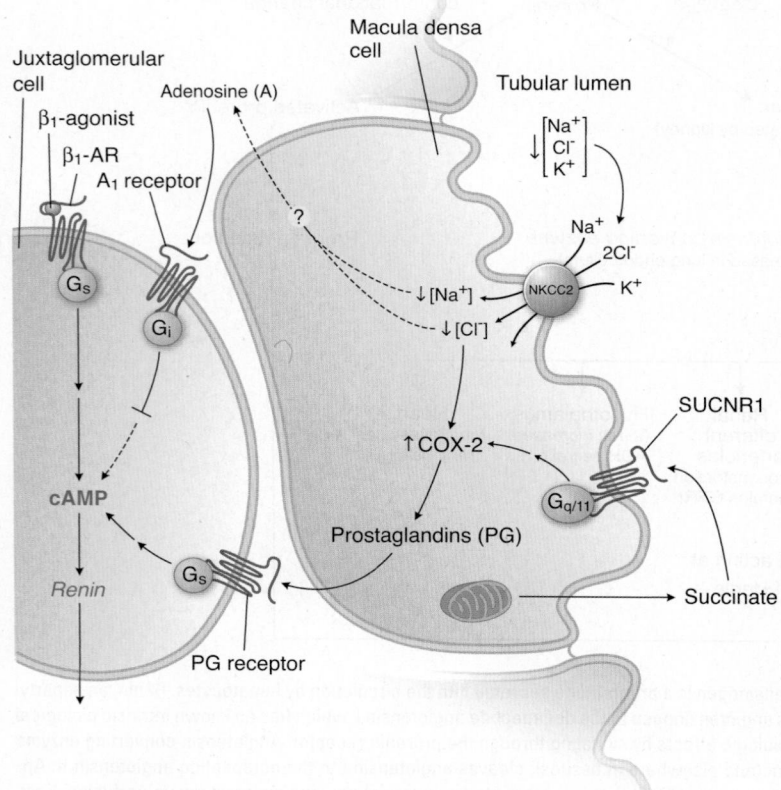

FIGURE 21-3. Modulation of renin release. Renin is released by juxtaglomerular cells in response to diverse stimuli that signal intravascular volume depletion. First, decreased pressure in the afferent arteriole (*not shown*) stimulates increased renin release promoted by intrarenal baroreceptors, possibly by releasing prostaglandins. Second, juxtaglomerular cells express β_1-adrenergic receptors (β_1-AR) coupled to G_s, which stimulates adenylyl cyclase to increase the intracellular level of cAMP and thereby stimulates renin release. Third, cells lining the diluting segments of the nephron modulate renin release according to luminal NaCl flux and local accumulation of the tricarboxylic acid (TCA) cycle intermediate succinate, reflecting tissue energy balance. Succinate activates the G protein-coupled succinate receptor SUCNR1, leading via MAP kinase activation to stimulation of cyclooxygenase (COX-2)-mediated prostaglandin production, ultimately increasing renin release. Succinate accumulation also stimulates eNOS and nitric oxide (NO) production, leading to vasodilation of the afferent arteriole (*not shown*). Decreased NaCl flux leads to decreased Cl^- entry through the $Na^+/2Cl^-/K^+$ transporter (NKCC2) on the apical membrane of macula densa cells in the distal convoluted tubule, increasing COX-2-dependent production of prostaglandins PGE2 and PGI2. These prostaglandins activate juxtaglomerular cell prostaglandin receptors to stimulate renin release by increasing cAMP production. In contrast, increased NaCl delivery to the cortical thick ascending limb (TAL) leads, through still-debated mechanisms, to increased generation of adenosine in the juxtaglomerular mesangial interstitium. Activation of G_i-coupled A_1 adenosine receptors of the juxtaglomerular cell decreases intracellular cAMP, which leads to decreased renin release.

many other substrates such as neuropeptides and kinins (e.g., bradykinin) that are venodilatory autacoids released in response to inflammation. For this reason, ACE is also known as **kininase II**. Kininase activity has important pharmacologic consequences, as discussed below.

The recently identified ACE homolog ACE2 is highly expressed in the kidney, where it is localized predominantly in tubular epithelial cells and less prominently in glomeruli and the renal vasculature. ACE2 degrades both Ang I and Ang II to the heptapeptide Ang 1-7. In contrast to the vasoconstrictor and pro-proliferative peptide Ang II, Ang 1-7 is considered an antiproliferative vasodilator that counteracts the cardiovascular and baroreflex actions of Ang II. Ang 1-7 binds to the G protein-coupled receptor MAS rather than to the angiotensin II (AT II) receptor (see below). ACE2 activity is altered in diabetic kidney disease and hypertensive renal disease and in experimental models of kidney injury. Dissociation between tubular and glomerular ACE2 expression can occur in diabetic kidney disease, in which ACE2 expression is increased in tubular epithelial cells but decreased in glomeruli. In addition to Ang I (Ang 1-10), Ang II (Ang 1-8), and Ang 1-7, angiotensin III (Ang 2-8) and angiotensin IV (Ang 3-8) have been identified. Ang 2-8 is a less potent vasopressor than Ang II but retains 100% of its aldosterone-stimulating activity. The vasopressor activity of Ang 3-8 resembles that of Ang 2-8.

Ang II (AT II) binding to the **AT II receptor subtype 1** (G protein-coupled **AT₁ receptor**, **AT₁R**) produces at least four stimulatory physiologic responses: (1) stimulation of

aldosterone secretion by zona glomerulosa cells of the adrenal glands, (2) increased reabsorption of NaCl from the proximal tubule and other nephron segments, (3) arteriolar vasoconstriction, and (4) central stimulation of thirst and ADH secretion. All four of these actions increase intravascular volume and therefore help to maintain perfusion pressure: aldosterone secretion increases distal tubule Na^+ reabsorption; proximal tubule NaCl reabsorption increases the fraction of filtered Na^+ that is reabsorbed; arteriolar vasoconstriction maintains blood pressure; stimulation of thirst increases free water absorbed into the vasculature; and secretion of ADH increases collecting duct free water absorption. Ang II also negatively regulates renin secretion through binding to AT_1R on juxtaglomerular cells. Ang II has many other AT_1R-mediated tissue- and cell type-specific effects, leading to sympathetic nervous system activation, generation of reactive oxygen species (ROS), and cell growth. Conversion of Ang I to Ang II by tissue-specific ACE (chymase) of cardiac myocytes can promote cardiac remodeling, hypertrophy, and fibrosis. Similar cardiovascular effects are also potentiated through aldosterone activation of extrarenal mineralocorticoid receptors.

The actions of Ang II are best understood in vascular smooth muscle cells, where AT_1R activates phospholipase C, leading to release of Ca^{2+} from intracellular stores, activation of protein kinase C, and vasoconstriction. Inhibition of AT_1R decreases vascular smooth muscle cell contractility and thereby decreases systemic vascular resistance and blood pressure (see the following discussion). The related

G protein-coupled AT II receptor AT_2R has a vasodilator role, in part by increasing nitric oxide production. AT_2R is highly expressed in fetal kidney and intestine, whereas high expression in adults is restricted to myometrium, with lower levels in adrenals and oviducts. AT_2R action has recently been implicated in some types of refractory pain syndromes.

Natriuretic Peptides

Natriuretic peptides are hormones released by atria, ventricles, and vascular endothelium in response to volume overload. The classical natriuretic peptides are A-type, B-type, and C-type natriuretic peptides. **A-type natriuretic peptide (ANP)** is released primarily by the atria, while **B-type natriuretic peptide (BNP)** is released mainly by the ventricles. **C-type natriuretic peptide (CNP)** is released by vascular endothelial cells. The natriuretic peptide **uroguanylin (UGN)** is released by enterocytes in response to dietary ingestion of salt.

Vascular natriuretic peptides are released in response to increased intravascular volume, an effect that may be signaled by increased stretch of natriuretic peptide-secreting cells. Circulating natriuretic peptides bind to one of three receptors, termed **NPR-A**, **NPR-B**, and **NPR-C**. NPR-A and NPR-B are transmembrane proteins with cytoplasmic **guanylyl cyclase** domains (see Chapter 1, Drug–Receptor Interactions); activation of these receptors increases intracellular cGMP levels. NPR-C lacks an intracellular guanylyl cyclase domain and may serve as a "decoy" or "buffer" receptor to reduce the level of circulating natriuretic peptides available to bind to the two signaling receptors. Both ANP and BNP bind with high affinity to NPR-A, while only CNP binds to NPR-B. All three natriuretic peptides bind to NPR-C (Fig. 21-4A). Deletion of the ANP gene (*Nppa*) in mice causes salt-sensitive hypertension. Common human allelic gene variants in the ANP (*NPPA*) and BNP (*NPPB*) genes have been associated with higher levels of ANP and BNP, higher blood pressure, and risk of hypertension. In mice, UGN binds and activates transmembrane guanylyl cyclase C in both enterocytes (promoting enteric Cl^- secretion) and renal proximal tubule cells (reducing renal Na^+ and Cl^- reabsorption). UGN also promotes natriuresis in the renal collecting duct by additional, less well characterized mechanisms.

Natriuretic peptides affect the cardiovascular system, the kidney, and the central nervous system. Integration of natriuretic peptide-derived signals serves to decrease volume overload and its sequelae. ANP relaxes vascular smooth muscle by increasing intracellular cGMP, which causes dephosphorylation of myosin light chain and subsequent vasorelaxation (see Chapter 22). ANP also increases capillary endothelial permeability, which reduces blood pressure by favoring fluid filtration from the plasma into the interstitium (see Equation 21-1).

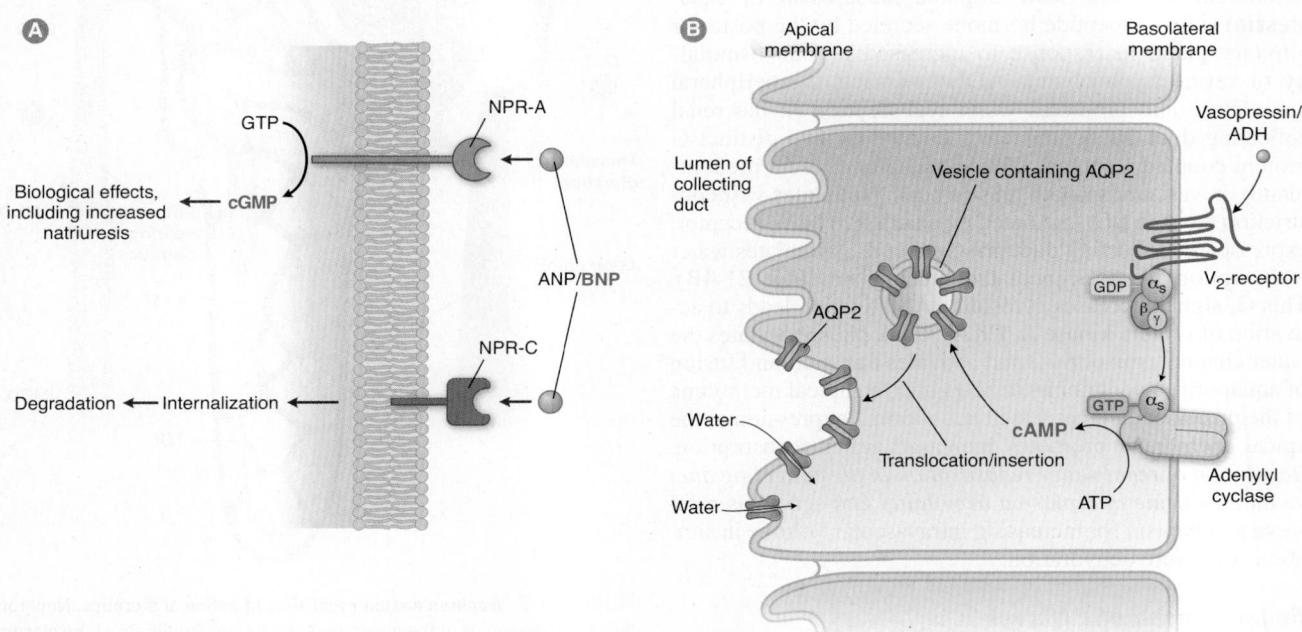

FIGURE 21-4. Natriuretic peptide and antidiuretic hormone signaling pathways. A. A-type and B-type natriuretic peptides (ANP and BNP) are hormones secreted in response to volume overload. These peptides bind to natriuretic peptide receptor-A (NPR-A) and natriuretic peptide receptor-C (NPR-C). NPR-A is a transmembrane receptor with intrinsic guanylyl cyclase activity associated with its cytoplasmic domain. Increased intracellular cGMP levels mediate the effects of natriuretic peptides, including increased natriuresis. NPR-C is believed to be a "decoy receptor" because the protein lacks the intracellular catalytic domain. Binding of natriuretic peptide to NPR-C may result in internalization and degradation of the receptor together with its bound natriuretic peptide. A third natriuretic peptide, CNP, is expressed by vascular endothelial cells and binds exclusively to NPR-B (*not shown*). **B.** Antidiuretic hormone (ADH), also known as *vasopressin*, is secreted by the hypothalamus in response to increased osmolality and volume depletion. ADH mediates renal collecting duct water reabsorption by activating the G_s-coupled V_2 vasopressin receptor. Activation of G_s leads to increased adenylyl cyclase activity and increased cAMP levels. cAMP increases collecting duct water reabsorption by promoting the translocation and insertion of aquaporin 2 water channel (AQP2)-containing vesicles into the collecting duct apical membrane. The increased expression of apical-membrane AQP2 results in increased water flux across the collecting duct and therefore increased reabsorption of filtered water. Hydrolysis of cAMP by phosphodiesterase leads to removal of AQP2 from the luminal membrane by endocytosis of AQP2-containing vesicles (*not shown*).

In the kidney, natriuretic peptides promote both increased glomerular filtration rate (GFR) and natriuresis. GFR is increased because of constriction of the efferent arteriole and dilation of the afferent arteriole, resulting in higher intraglomerular pressure and therefore increased plasma filtration. The natriuretic effects on the kidney result from antagonism of ADH action in the collecting ducts and antagonism of Na^+ reabsorption in multiple nephron segments.

The central effects of natriuretic peptides are less well understood, but they include decreased perception of thirst (and therefore decreased fluid intake), decreased release of antidiuretic hormone, and decreased sympathetic tone. The signaling mechanisms mediating these actions are uncertain, but may be via CNP, as this natriuretic peptide is expressed at high levels in the brain.

Although many of the effects of natriuretic peptides remain incompletely understood, these hormones appear to play an important role in regulating the pathophysiology of volume excess. Much interest has recently focused on the relationship between natriuretic peptides and heart failure. In particular, BNP and N-terminal proBNP (NT-proBNP) have emerged as promising markers for heart failure diagnosis, prognosis, and treatment. The physiology and pharmacology of natriuretic peptides and their receptors remain subjects for active investigation.

Antidiuretic Hormone

Antidiuretic hormone (ADH, arginine vasopressin, or **vasopressin)** is a nonapeptide hormone secreted by the posterior pituitary gland in response to increased plasma osmolality or severe hypovolemia. ADH constricts the peripheral vasculature and promotes water reabsorption in the renal collecting duct. Its actions are mediated by two distinct G protein-coupled receptors. The V_1 receptor, present predominantly in vascular smooth muscle cells, stimulates vasoconstriction through a G_q-mediated mechanism. The V_2 receptor, expressed in collecting duct principal cells, stimulates water reabsorption by a G_s-mediated mechanism (Fig. 21-4B). This G_s signal increases cytosolic cAMP, which leads to activation of protein kinase A (PKA). PKA phosphorylates the water channel aquaporin 2 and activates transport and fusion of aquaporin 2-containing vesicles into the apical membrane of the principal cell. Increased aquaporin 2 expression at the apical membrane promotes increased water reabsorption. *Regulation of renal water reabsorption in the collecting duct modulates urine and plasma osmolality* and serves as a reserve mechanism for increasing intravascular volume in situations of severe dehydration.

Renal Sympathetic Nerves

Renal sympathetic nerves innervate both afferent and efferent arterioles. In response to a decrease in intravascular volume, the renal sympathetic nerves decrease GFR by stimulating constriction of the afferent arteriole to a greater degree than the efferent arteriole. The decreased GFR resulting from preferential constriction of the afferent arteriole ultimately leads to decreased natriuresis. Renal sympathetic nerves also increase renin production by stimulation of β_1-adrenergic receptors on juxtaglomerular mesangial cells and increase proximal tubule NaCl reabsorption. Since transplanted kidneys function normally in the initial absence of sympathetic nerve input, renal innervation is not required for clinically normal kidney function.

Renal Control of Na^+ Excretion

Over the course of 24 hours, the kidneys filter approximately 180 L of fluid. To increase or decrease body fluid volume, the kidneys must increase or decrease renal Na^+ reabsorption from the large daily volume of glomerular filtrate. For this reason, the neurohormonal mechanisms controlling extracellular volume status have important actions on the kidney. An understanding of the renal control of Na^+ excretion is crucial to understanding the role of the kidney in regulation of body fluid volume.

The renal glomerulus produces an ultrafiltrate of plasma that flows through and is processed by renal tubules of the nephron, the functional unit of the kidney (Fig. 21-5). The postglomerular nephron is responsible for solute and water reabsorption from the filtrate, as well as for excretion of

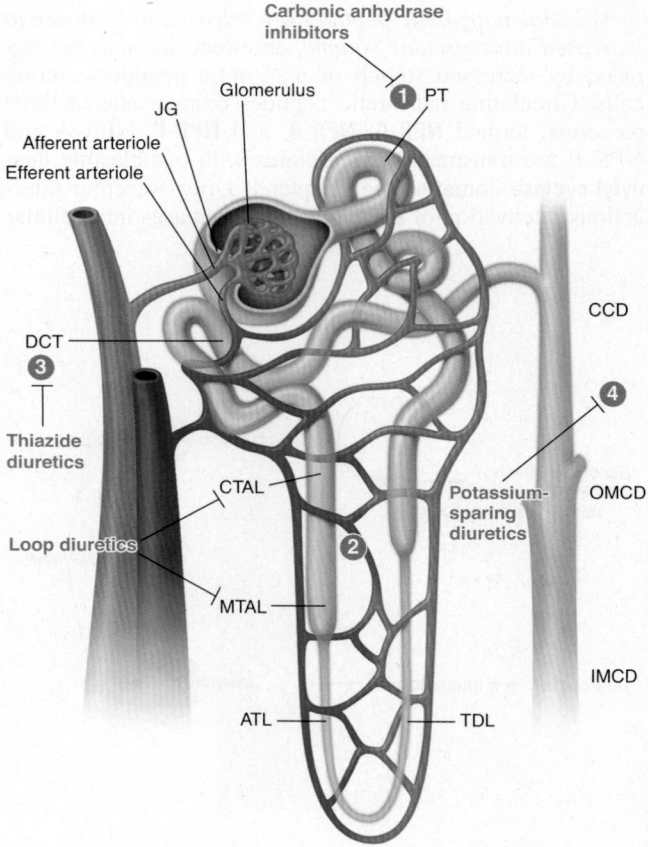

FIGURE 21-5. Nephron anatomy and sites of action of diuretics. Nephron fluid filtration begins at the glomerulus, where an ultrafiltrate of the plasma enters the renal epithelial (urinary) space. This ultrafiltrate then flows sequentially through four axially distinct nephron segments (**1–4**). From the glomerulus, ultrafiltrate travels to the proximal tubule (*PT*) (**1**), then to the loop of Henle (**2**), which includes the thin descending limb (*TDL*), ascending thin limb (*ATL*), medullary thick ascending limb (*MTAL*), and cortical thick ascending limb (*CTAL*) of Henle. The distal convoluted tubule (*DCT*) (**3**) includes the macula densa and juxtaglomerular (*JG*) apparatus. The collecting duct (**4**) consists of the cortical collecting duct (*CCD*), outer medullary collecting duct (*OMCD*), and inner medullary collecting duct (*IMCD*). Pharmacologic agents inhibit specific solute transporters within each segment of the nephron. Carbonic anhydrase inhibitors act primarily at the proximal tubule; loop diuretics act at the medullary and cortical thick ascending limbs; thiazide diuretics inhibit solute transport in the distal convoluted tubule; and potassium-sparing diuretics inhibit collecting-duct Na^+ reabsorption.

metabolic waste products and xenobiotics, including drugs. The renal tubular epithelial cells of the postglomerular nephron enclose a lengthy tubular lumen, the "urinary space," which leads to the ureters, urinary bladder, and urethra. The initial glomerular ultrafiltrate contains solutes of low molecular weight at concentrations similar to those in the plasma. As the ultrafiltrate passes through the nephron, substrate-specific transporters and channels in the luminal (apical) membrane of polarized renal tubular epithelial cells sequentially alter the solute concentrations of the tubular fluid. The function of these transporters and channels is, in turn, influenced by changes in solute concentrations in the cells themselves, as regulated in part by channels and transporters on the contraluminal (basolateral) side of the cells. Systemic volume regulation by the kidney is accomplished by tubular solute reabsorption through integrated action of ion channels and ion transporters in the apical and basolateral membranes of tubular epithelial cells and by the accompanying reabsorption of water.

The postglomerular nephron exhibits remarkable heterogeneity along its length. Four segments of the nephron are especially relevant to the pharmacology of systemic volume regulation (Fig. 21-5). These are the **proximal tubule**, the **thick ascending limb (TAL)** of the loop of Henle, the **distal convoluted tubule (DCT)**, and the **cortical collecting duct (CCD)**. In each tubular segment, a complex but tightly choreographed group of segment-specific ion transporters and channels collaborate in the reabsorption of NaCl from the lumen across the cellular monolayer of tubular epithelium into the interstitial space. NaCl reabsorption is key for systemic water retention. Solute and water transport across each segment requires coordination of transporter function in the luminal and basolateral membranes. In addition, paracellular transport of ions across the tight junctions between cells requires regulated communication between adjacent cells of the tubular epithelium. Integration of the transcellular and paracellular components of transepithelial transport requires integration of signals transmitted by sensors of extracellular and intracellular ion concentrations and of intracellular, local extracellular, and systemic volume. Alteration of ion transport by drugs in any nephron segment can induce compensatory regulation locally and in more distally located nephron segments.

Proximal Tubule

The proximal tubule (PT) is the first reabsorptive site in the nephron. It is responsible for approximately two-thirds of sodium reabsorption, 85–90% of bicarbonate reabsorption, and approximately 60% of chloride reabsorption (Fig. 21-6). Specific sodium-coupled symporters in the proximal tubule apical membrane drive renal reabsorption of all glucose, amino acids, phosphate, and sulfate from the glomerular filtrate. The proximal tubule also mediates secretion and reabsorption of weak organic acids and weak organic bases; these are coupled to processes of sodium or proton symport or antiport or to anion exchange mechanisms. Among these weak acids and bases are many of the drugs used to regulate systemic volume (see below).

Bicarbonate reabsorption requires the coordinated action of apical and basolateral ion transporters together with apical and intracellular enzymatic activities (Fig. 21-6). At the luminal surface of the proximal tubule, filtered bicarbonate encounters active proton secretion across the proximal tubule

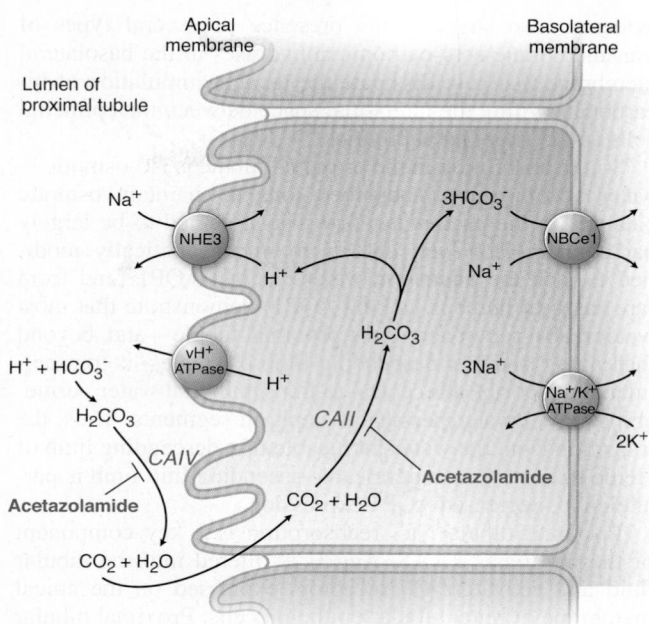

FIGURE 21-6. Proximal tubule cell. A significant percentage of filtered Na^+ in the proximal tubular lumen is reabsorbed via the NHE3 Na^+/H^+ exchanger. The activity of NHE3, together with that of an apical membrane vacuolar ATPase (vH$^+$ ATPase), results in significant H$^+$ extrusion into the proximal tubule urinary space. H$^+$ extrusion is coupled to HCO_3^- reabsorption by the action of apical membrane carbonic anhydrase IV (CAIV), which catalyzes the cleavage of HCO_3^- into OH$^-$ and CO_2. OH$^-$ combines with H$^+$ to form water, while CO_2 diffuses into the cytoplasm of the epithelial cell. The cytoplasmic enzyme carbonic anhydrase II (CAII) catalyzes the formation of HCO_3^- from CO_2 and OH$^-$; the HCO_3^- is then transported into the interstitium together with Na^+. The net result of this process is reabsorption of HCO_3^- and Na^+ by the basolateral co-transporter NBCe1. Acetazolamide inhibits both isoforms of carbonic anhydrase; the decreased carbonic anhydrase activity results in decreased Na^+ and HCO_3^- absorption.

brush-border microvilli. Two-thirds of the proton efflux is in exchange for influx of Na^+, largely via the **NHE3 Na^+/H^+ exchanger**. The remaining third of proton efflux is mediated by the **vacuolar H$^+$ ATPase (vH$^+$ ATPase)**.

The HCO_3^- permeability of the luminal membrane of the proximal tubular cell is low. However, the outer leaflet of the luminal membrane harbors the glycosylphosphatidylinositol-linked exoenzyme **carbonic anhydrase IV (CAIV)**. CAIV converts luminal HCO_3^- to CO_2 and OH$^-$. The OH$^-$ is rapidly hydrated to water by the abundance of local protons, and the CO_2 freely diffuses into the cytoplasm of the proximal tubular epithelial cell. The intracellular CO_2 is rapidly rehydrated to HCO_3^- by cytoplasmic **carbonic anhydrase II (CAII)**; this reaction consumes the intracellular OH$^-$ accumulated as a result of the H$^+$-extruding activities of apical NHE3 and vH$^+$ ATPase. The HCO_3^- produced by the CAII reaction is then co-transported with Na^+ across the basolateral membrane of the epithelial cell, accounting for the net reabsorption of sodium and bicarbonate. The Na^+/HCO_3^- co-transporter **NBCe1** mediates electrogenic basolateral efflux of three HCO_3^- ions with each co-transported Na^+ ion. Basolateral K$^+$ channels maintain an inside-negative membrane potential to enhance the driving force for net efflux of two negative charges per NBCe1 transport cycle. Emerging evidence also suggests the presence of several types of transmembrane ecto-carbonic anhydrases in the basolateral membrane that help dissipate the local accumulation of bicarbonate within the interstitial space between the epithelial cells and peritubular capillaries.

Solute absorption in the proximal tubule is iso-osmotic—water accompanies reabsorbed ions to maintain osmotic balance. In the past, water flow was assumed to be largely paracellular. However, data from mice genetically modified to lack the **aquaporin** water channel AQP1 (and from rare cases of humans lacking AQP1) demonstrate that most water reabsorption across the proximal tubule—and, beyond that, across the thin descending limb of Henle—is transcellular. Aquaporins are central to transepithelial water permeability in all water-permeable nephron segments. Thus, the transition from the water-permeable thin descending limb of Henle to the water-impermeable ascending thin limb is paralleled by decreased AQP1 expression.

Proximal tubule Na^+ reabsorption is a key component of the intrarenal RAAS. Ang II is filtered into the tubular fluid and activates AT_1 receptors expressed on the apical membrane of renal tubular epithelial cells. Proximal tubular lumen concentrations of Ang I and Ang II have been found to be higher than their corresponding plasma concentrations, leading to the discovery that proximal tubular epithelial cells express angiotensinogen that is converted to Ang I and Ang II through intrarenal (pro)renin and ACE activity. Elevated Ang II levels sustain or up-regulate tubular epithelial cell AT_1R but downregulate vascular AT_1R. The critical importance of kidney AT_1R has been demonstrated by using proximal tubule-specific AT_1R knockout mice (with intact expression of AT_1R in all other tissues). Infusion of Ang II into these mice failed to increase blood pressure to the same degree as in control mice. The reduced positive Na^+ balance observed in these mice was consistent with facilitated natriuresis as a mechanism for resistance to hypertension.

Thick Ascending Limb of the Loop of Henle

The tubular fluid emerging from the ascending thin limb is hypertonic and has an elevated NaCl concentration. The three nephron segments into which this fluid flows, the thick ascending limb (TAL), the distal convoluted tubule (DCT), and the connecting tubule or segment (CNT), together constitute "the diluting segment." The apical membrane of the thick ascending limb of Henle is devoid of aquaporins, as is the apical membrane of the rest of the diluting segment; therefore, these nephron segments reabsorb NaCl and urea without accompanying water (Fig. 21-7), thus diluting the solutes of the tubular fluid. Reabsorption of NaCl and urea across the TAL provides the interstitial solute that generates and maintains the corticomedullary osmotic gradient of the kidney, allowing operation of the "countercurrent multiplier" that can concentrate the urine of humans to 1,200 mOsM and that of desert rodents to 4,000 mOsM.

The TAL reabsorbs between 25% and 35% of the filtered Na^+ load by means of the luminal membrane Na^+-K^+-$2Cl^-$ co-transporter, **NKCC2**. The Cl^- imported by NKCC2 exits the basolateral side of the cell via **CLC-K2** chloride channels. CLC-K2's β-subunit, Barttin, which colocalizes with CLC-K2 at the basolateral membrane, is essential for intracellular trafficking and function of CLC-K2. (Barttin also serves as the β-subunit for a related Cl^- channel, CLC-K1, in potassium-secreting stria vascularis epithelial cells of the

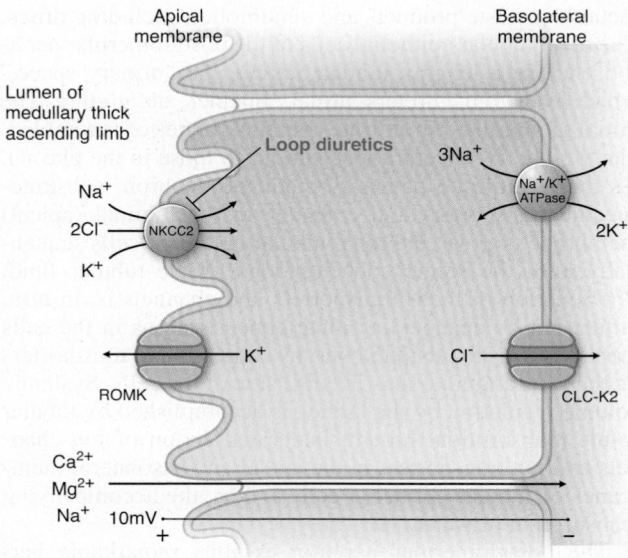

FIGURE 21-7. Medullary thick ascending limb cell. The medullary ascending limb of the loop of Henle absorbs Na^+ through an apical membrane Na^+/K^+/$2Cl^-$ (NKCC2) transporter. The Na^+/K^+ ATPase pumps sodium from the cytoplasm into the interstitium, and a basolateral Cl^- channel (CLC-K2) transports Cl^- into the interstitium. K^+ is primarily recycled back into the urinary space via a luminal K^+ channel (ROMK). The combined activities of apical ROMK and basolateral CLC-K2 result in a lumen-positive transepithelial potential difference (approximately 10 mV) that drives paracellular absorption of cations, including Ca^{2+} and Mg^{2+}. Loop diuretics inhibit NKCC2, resulting in significantly increased renal sodium excretion. Attenuation of the positive transepithelial potential by loop diuretics also increases the excretion of Ca^{2+} and Mg^{2+}.

inner ear.) The Na^+ imported from the lumen via NKCC2 leaves the basolateral side of the cell via the Na^+/K^+ ATPase. Because Cl^- carries a negative charge, exit of unaccompanied Cl^- through basolateral CLC-K2 depolarizes the cell. The stoichiometry of the Na^+/K^+ ATPase, $3Na^+$ outward per $2 K^+$ inward, partly counters this depolarization; additional repolarization of the cell is accomplished by the apical K^+ channel **ROMK**, which recycles back into the lumen the K^+ imported into the cell via NKCC2.

Reduced function of any one of these transporters or channels, secondary either to pharmacologic inhibition (e.g., with loop diuretics, inhibiting NKCC2 function) or to loss-of-function mutation, is associated with renal salt wasting. Several TAL transporter gene defects cause Bartter syndrome, which is characterized by renal salt wasting, possible hypotension, hypokalemia, metabolic alkalosis, and, in some patients, hypercalciuria (Table 21-1).

The coordinated operation of these apical and basolateral transporters and channels generates a lumen-positive electrical potential across the TAL. The transepithelial potential difference in the TAL constitutes the electrical driving force favoring paracellular reabsorption of additional Na^+ from lumen to interstitium. The paracellular component of Na^+ reabsorption reduces the energetic cost to TAL epithelial cells (measured as ATP consumption), because Na^+/K^+ transport consumes most of the ATP in the TAL cell. Even with the energy conserved by the paracellular Na^+ absorptive pathway, the TAL working at maximal capacity can consume up to 25% of the body's total ATP production, or approximately

TABLE 21-1 Bartter Syndrome: Renal Salt Wasting in the Thick Ascending Limb (TAL) Associated with Hypercalciuria

SYNDROME	INHERITANCE	K⁺	pH	RENIN	ALDOSTERONE	TREATMENT	GENE LOCUS	GENE
Bartter	AR	↓	↑	↑	↑	Increase salt intake (for all types)	15q21	*SLC12A1* (type 1, neonatal)
	AR	↓	↑	↑	↑		11q24	*KCNJ1* (type 2, neonatal)
	AR	↓	↑	↑	↑		1p36	*CLCNKB* (type 3, classic)
	AR	↓	↑	↑	↑		1p32	*BSND* (type 4, associated with deafness)
	AD	↓	↑	↑	↑		3q21	*CASR* (type 5 or autosomal dominant hypocalcemia)

SLC12A1 (NKCC2) and KCNJ1 (ROMK) are located at the apical membrane of the TAL epithelial cells, whereas CLCNKB (CLC-K2), BSND (Barttin), and CASR (calcium-sensing receptor) are located at the basolateral membrane. AR, autosomal recessive; AD, autosomal dominant.

65 moles per day at rest. The lumen-positive transepithelial potential of the TAL also drives paracellular reabsorption of luminal calcium and magnesium ions. This paracellular transport is now known to be mediated by *claudins 16 and 19*, which form tight junctional, heteromeric, cation-selective channels comprised of the ectodomains of claudin polypeptides from adjacent TAL epithelial cells. Recent studies have demonstrated that claudins, in addition to their barrier function, regulate paracellular transport across epithelia by interacting with multiple intra- and extracellular signaling pathways. For example, the extracellular calcium-sensing receptor (CaSR), a widely expressed G protein-coupled receptor, responds to changes in basolateral (serum) $[Ca^{2+}]$ by modifying claudin expression in TAL cells, thereby modulating TAL permeability to paracellular calcium.

Distal Convoluted Tubule

This continuation of the diluting segment actively reabsorbs between 2% and 10% of the filtered NaCl load, while remaining impermeable to luminal water (Fig. 21-8). Luminal Na^+ enters the epithelial cells of the distal convoluted tubule (DCT) via the electroneutral, K^+-independent **NCC** Na^+-Cl^- co-transporter. Basolateral exit of Na^+ is mediated by Na^+/ K^+ ATPase in coordination with basolateral K^+ recycling by the heterotetrameric K^+ channel Kir4.1/5.1 (KCNJ10/ KCNJ16). The Cl^- imported across the apical membrane exits via basolateral anion pathways that include both electrogenic Cl^- channels and (at least in the mouse) electroneutral K^+-Cl^- co-transport. Pharmacologic inhibition of the NCC sodium channel with thiazide diuretics leads to increased Na^+ excretion accompanied by hypokalemia and other electrolyte and acid–base changes. Genetic loss of function of NCC underlies Gitelman syndrome, which is characterized by salt wasting much milder than that with Bartter syndrome. Genetic loss of function of Kir4.1 underlies SeSAME syndrome (also known as *EAST syndrome*), in which hypokalemia, hypomagnesemia, and metabolic alkalosis is accompanied by epilepsy, ataxia, sensorineural deafness, and intellectual dysfunction; the latter manifestations reflect loss of Kir4.1 expression in the brain (Table 21-2). Mutations in WNK protein kinases of the distal convoluted tubule and collecting duct (WNK4 and WNK1), as well as in

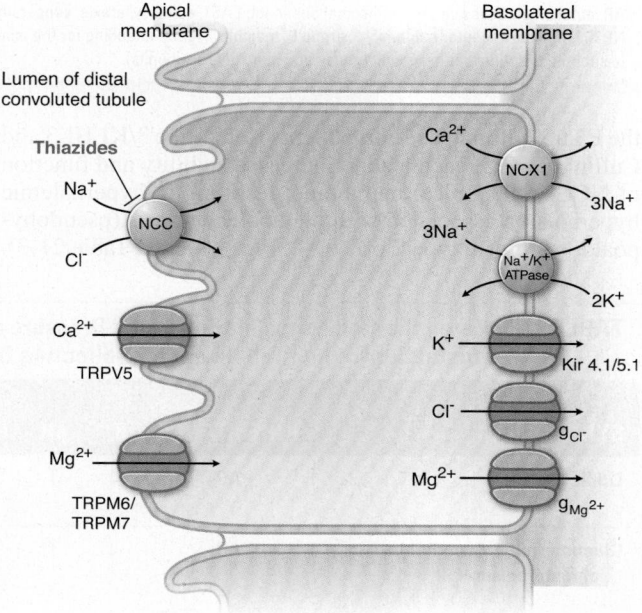

FIGURE 21-8. Distal convoluted tubule cell. Distal convoluted tubule (DCT) cells absorb Na^+ via the NaCl co-transporter (NCC) at the apical membrane. NCC abundance is up-regulated by activation of the mineralocorticoid receptor through aldosterone (*not shown*). NCC activation by phosphorylation is mediated by SPAK, under the influence of "upstream" WNK and other kinases (*not shown*). Positive and negative regulation of NCC may arise from antagonistic actions of the different WNK kinases and their interactions with the Cullin3-KLHL3 E3 ligase ubiquitination system (*not shown*). Na^+ is transported across the basolateral membrane into the interstitium via the Na^+/K^+ ATPase, aided by basolateral K^+ recycling via the heterotetrameric K^+ channel Kir4.1/5.1. Cl^- exits the cell across the basolateral membrane via Cl^- channels (g_{Cl^-}) and likely also via K^+-Cl^- co-transporters (*not shown*). DCT epithelial cells absorb Ca^{2+} via apical membrane Ca^{2+} channels (TRPV5), and Ca^{2+} is transported across the basolateral membrane into the interstitium by the Na^+/Ca^{2+} exchanger NCX1 and by the Ca^{2+} ATPase PMCA (*not shown*). Mg^{2+} is absorbed by magnesium-selective heteromeric TRPM6/TRPM7 channels at the apical membrane and transported across the basolateral membrane via pathways that are incompletely characterized ($g_{Mg^{2+}}$). Thiazides inhibit NCC, resulting in increased Na^+ excretion. Thiazides also increase epithelial cell absorption of Ca^{2+} and Mg^{2+} by an unknown mechanism (*not shown*).

TABLE 21-2 Syndromes of Renal Salt Wasting Associated with Low Blood Pressure Caused by Defects in the Distal Nephron

SYNDROME	INHERITANCE	K⁺	pH	RENIN	ALDOSTERONE	TREATMENT	GENE LOCUS	GENE
Gitelman	AR	↓	↑	↑	↑	Increase salt intake	16q13	*SLC12A3* (NCC)
EAST (also known as SeSAME)	AR	↓	↑	↑	↑	Increase salt intake	1q23	*KCNJ10* (Kir4.1)
Pseudohypoaldosteronism type 1 (PHA type I)	AD AR AR AR	↑	↓	↑	↑	Increase salt intake	4q31 12p13 16p13 16p13	*NR3C2* (type 1A) *SCNN1A* (type 1B) *SCNN1B* (type 1B) *SCNN1G* (type 1B)
Renal tubular dysgenesis (RTD)	AR	↑	↓	↑ or ↓	↓	Vasopressors	1q32 1q42 3q24 17q23	*REN* (renin) *AGT* (angiotensinogen) *ACE* (angiotensin converting enzyme) *AGT1R* (angiotensin II type 1 receptor)

AR, autosomal recessive; AD, autosomal dominant; EAST, epilepsy, ataxia, sensorineural deafness, tubulopathy; Kir 4.1, inward rectifier-type K⁺-channel, member 4.1; NR3C2, nuclear receptor subfamily 3, group C, member 2 (gene encoding for the mineralocorticoid receptor); SCNN1A, 1B, or 1G, Na⁺ channel, non-voltage-gated 1, α-subunit, β-subunit, or γ-subunit (genes encoding ENaC subunits).

the E3 ubiquitin ligase components Kelch-like 3/KLHL3 and Cullin 3/CUL3, each lead to increased stability and function of NCC in the apical membrane, resulting in hyperkalemic hypertension associated with metabolic acidosis (pseudohypoaldosteronism type 2 or PHA2; Fig. 21-8 and Table 21-3).

The DCT also mediates transepithelial reabsorption of luminal calcium and magnesium ions via calcium-specific TRPV5 channels and magnesium-specific TRPM6/TRPM7 channels in the apical membrane. The reabsorbed calcium is transported across the DCT cell basolateral membrane

TABLE 21-3 Rare Inherited Forms of High Blood Pressure due to Increased Salt Reabsorption in the Distal Nephron (Distal Convoluted Tubule and/or Collecting Duct)

SYNDROME	INHERITANCE	K⁺	pH	RENIN	ALDO	TREATMENT	GENE LOCUS	DISEASE GENE(S)
Liddle	AD	↓	↑	↓	↓	ENaC inhibitors	16p12	*ENaC* (epithelial Na channel)
Glucocorticoid-remediable aldosteronism	AD	↓	↑	↓	N (↑)	Corticosteroid therapy	8q24	Chimeric gene: *11-β-hydroxylase/aldosterone synthase*
Apparent mineralocorticoid excess	AR	↓	↑	↓	↓	Spironolactone (ENaC inhibitors)	16q22	*11-β-hydroxysteroid dehydrogenase*
Aldosterone-producing adrenal adenomas	de novo* de novo de novo de novo	↓	↑	↓	↑	Spironolactone (adrenal adenomectomy)	11q24 3p21 1p13 Xq28	*KCNJ5* *CACNA1D* *ATP1A1* *ATP2B3*
Congenital adrenal hyperplasia	AR	↓	↑	↓	↓	Corticosteroid therapy	10q24 8q24	*17-α-hydroxylase* *11-β-hydroxylase*
Pseudohypoaldosteronism type 2 (Gordon syndrome)	AD	↑	↓	↓	N (↑)	Thiazide diuretics	12p13 17q21 5q31 2q36	*WNK1* *WNK4* *Kelch-like3* *Cullin3*

These syndromes feature intravascular volume expansion associated with acid–base and electrolyte abnormalities.
Aldo, aldosterone; AD, autosomal dominant; AR, autosomal recessive; N, normal; *KCNJ5*, K⁺ inwardly-rectifying channel, subfamily J, member 5; *CACNA1D*, calcium channel, voltage-dependent L type, α-1D subunit; *ATP1A1*, Na⁺/K⁺ ATPase α-1 subunit; *ATP2B3*, PMCA3 (plasmalemmal Ca²⁺ ATPase 3).
*Rarely, can also be inherited in Mendelian (autosomal dominant) fashion.

via specific NCX Na^+/Ca^{2+} exchangers and Ca^{2+} ATPases. The still undefined basolateral exit pathway(s) for DCT cell Mg^{2+} may include the magnesium transporter polypeptides SLC41A3 and CNNM2, with additional required basolateral function of FXYD2 (the $\gamma 1$ subunit of the basolateral Na^+/K^+ ATPase) and the heterotetrameric K^+ channel Kir4.1/5.1.

Collecting Duct

This terminal portion of the nephron is divided into **cortical, outer medullary,** and **inner medullary** collecting duct (CD) segments (Fig. 21-9). The cortical and outer medullary CD segments consist of two cell types: **principal cells** and **intercalated cells**. Principal cells reabsorb between 1% and 5% of the filtered sodium load, depending on plasma aldosterone levels (aldosterone increases sodium reabsorption and water retention, see below). Luminal Na^+ enters the principal cells at the apical membrane of the cortical collecting duct via heterotrimeric epithelial Na^+ channels, **ENaC**, consisting of α-, β-, and γ-subunits. Loss-of-function mutations in each of the three ENaC subunits cause a syndrome of low blood pressure associated with hyperkalemia and metabolic acidosis (pseudohypoaldosteronism type 1B; Table 21-2). In contrast, ENaC gain-of-function mutations in β- or γ-subunits cause severe hypertension associated with hypokalemia and metabolic alkalosis (Liddle syndrome; Table 21-3). Several other gene defects can increase ENaC activity by enhancing activation of the mineralocorticoid receptor. WNK kinase regulation of NCC and (likely also) ENaC contributes to the ability of aldosterone to increase Na^+ reabsorption by DCT and CCD cells in response to hypovolemia. WNK kinase regulation of ROMK contributes to the ability of aldosterone to increase K^+ secretion by CCD cells in response to hyperkalemia.

ENaC activity at the apical cell surface is regulated by the serum/glucocorticoid regulated kinase 1 (SGK1). SGK1

phosphorylates and sequesters ENaC's ubiquitin ligase Nedd4-2, thereby preventing endocytosis of ENaC from the apical cell surface and increasing ENaC activity. Serine proteases also activate ENaC under physiologic and pathophysiologic conditions by excision of amino acids from extracellular loops of its α- and γ-subunits, thereby increasing the probability of ion channel opening. The protease furin mediates intracellular cleavage, whereas the channel-activating protease prostasin (CAP-1), anchored to the apical cell surface, mediates important extracellular cleavage. Soluble protease activity is very low in urine under physiologic conditions but can rise in proteinuric conditions. In nephrotic syndrome (proteinuria >3.5 g/day), the dominant soluble protease activity is plasmin, which is generated from filtered plasminogen by the action of urokinase-type plasminogen activator. Plasmin activates ENaC directly at high concentrations and through CAP-1 activation at lower concentrations. This filtered protease activity may thus contribute to the edema that accompanies nephrotic-range proteinuria.

Intracellular Na^+ exits the basolateral side of the cell via the Na^+/K^+ ATPase. Principal cells also secrete K^+ into the

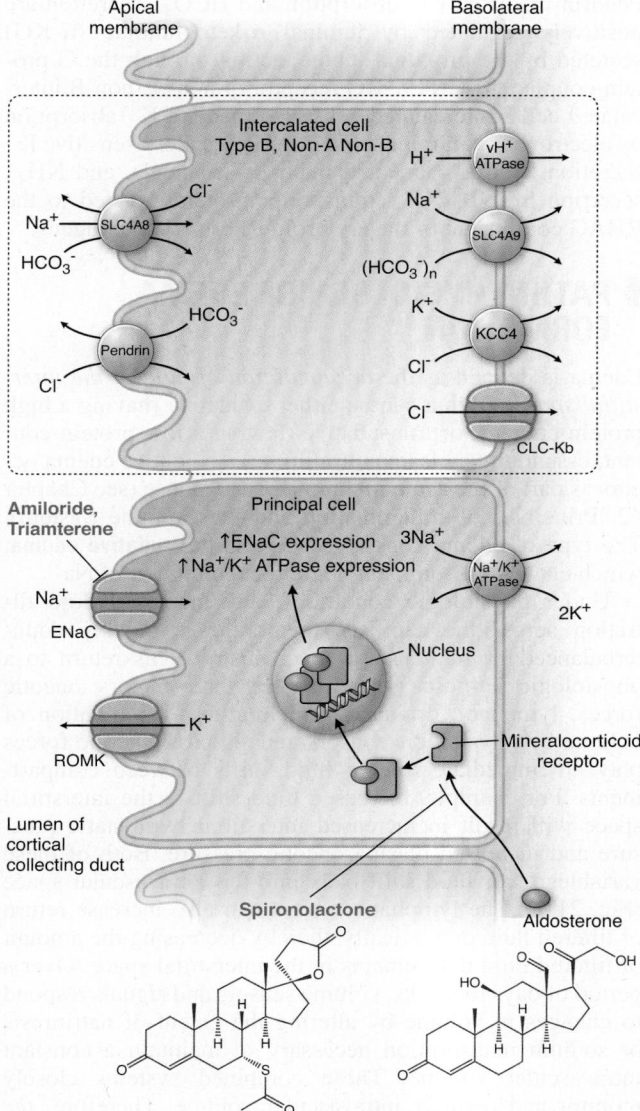

FIGURE 21-9. Cortical collecting duct. Cortical collecting duct principal cells (**lower cell**) absorb Na^+ via an apical membrane Na^+ channel (ENaC). Cytoplasmic Na^+ is transported across the basolateral membrane via the Na^+/K^+ ATPase. In addition, collecting duct cells express apical membrane K^+ channels (especially ROMK) that allow K^+ to exit into the urinary space. ENaC expression and apical surface localization is modulated by aldosterone. The kinase SGK1 increases membrane expression of ENaC via phosphorylation and sequestration of the E3 ubiquitin ligase Nedd4-2, which otherwise promotes ENaC endocytosis (*not shown*). The WNK/SPAK-OSR1 kinase cascade likely regulates SGK1 and Nedd4-2 in the cortical collecting duct, as well as ENaC and ROMK, by mechanisms that are still being elucidated. Aldosterone binds to the mineralocorticoid receptor, which then increases transcription of the gene encoding ENaC as well as genes encoding other proteins involved in Na^+ reabsorption (such as Na^+/K^+ ATPase). The collecting duct principal cell is the site of action of the two classes of potassium-sparing diuretics. Mineralocorticoid receptor antagonists such as spironolactone and eplerenone (*not shown*) competitively inhibit the interaction of aldosterone with the mineralocorticoid receptor and thereby decrease expression of ENaC. Direct inhibitors of ENaC, such as amiloride and triamterene, inhibit Na^+ influx through ENaC channels at the apical plasma membrane. Cortical collecting duct intercalated cells of type B or of "non-A, non-B" type (**upper cell,** *within dashed box*) have been proposed to mediate electroneutral reabsorption of NaCl. Based on studies with knockout mice, apical NaCl uptake via parallel operation of pendrin and SLC4A8 is coupled to basolateral NaCl efflux via SLC4A9 in parallel with KCC4 and CLC-Kb. Transepithelial NaCl transport by this cell type appears to be energized by basolateral vH^+ ATPase rather than by Na^+/K^+ ATPase. Note that this proposed mechanism of distal nephron electroneutral NaCl reabsorption is still under investigation.

lumen to maintain tight control of plasma [K^+], as well as to minimize the transepithelial potential difference resulting from Na^+ reabsorption. In addition, cortical and outer medullary principal cells, as well as cells of the inner medullary collecting duct, express vasopressin (ADH)-responsive water channels. ADH activates water reabsorption by stimulating a G_s protein-coupled V_2 receptor in the basolateral membrane; in turn, G_s protein signaling promotes the reversible insertion into the apical membrane of intracellular vesicles containing aquaporin 2 (AQP2) water channels (Fig. 21-4B).

At least two subtypes of intercalated cells (IC) contribute to systemic acid–base balance through cell type-specific polarized expression of the vacuolar H^+ ATPase (vH^+ ATPase). Type A IC secrete protons via the apical H^+ ATPase and reabsorb bicarbonate through the basolateral Cl^-/HCO_3^- exchanger (also known as *kidney AE1*). Type B IC secrete HCO_3^- through the apical Cl^-/HCO_3^- exchanger pendrin and reabsorb protons via the basolateral H^+ ATPase. Pendrin likely also mediates apical Cl^- reabsorption via a third IC type, the "non-A, non-B" IC. In rodents, pendrin-mediated electroneutral NaCl reabsorption may be equivalent in magnitude to ENaC-mediated electrogenic Na^+ absorption accompanied by paracellular Cl^- absorption across the CCD. Pendrin-mediated Cl^- absorption and HCO_3^- secretion are positively regulated by luminal α-ketoglutarate (α-KG) secreted by the proximal tubule, acting through the G protein-coupled OXGR1 α-KG receptor of non-A, non-B intercalated cells. Intercalated cells also mediate K^+ absorption by electroneutral luminal H^+/K^+ ATPases, flow-sensitive K^+ secretion by Ca^{2+}-activated maxi-K^+ channels, and NH_4^+ secretion by NH_3/NH_4^+ transporter proteins related to the RHAG component of the erythroid Rhesus (Rh) antigens.

■ PATHOPHYSIOLOGY OF EDEMA FORMATION

Edema is defined as the *accumulation of fluid in the interstitial space*. Edema can be either exudative (having a high protein content) or transudative (having a low protein content, essentially a plasma ultrafiltrate). Exudative edema occurs as part of the acute inflammatory response (see Chapter 42, Principles of Inflammation and the Immune System). The type of edema considered here is **transudative edema**, which can result from pathologic renal retention of Na^+.

Under physiologic conditions, any increased fluid filtration across the capillary membrane is quickly counterbalanced by homeostatic mechanisms. This return to a physiologic set-point is mediated by three factors: oncotic forces, lymphatic drainage, and long-term modulation of volume by physiologic sensors and signals. Oncotic forces play an immediate role in fluid shifts between compartments. For example, increased fluid shift to the interstitial space will result in increased interstitial hydrostatic pressure and increased plasma oncotic pressure. Both of these variables favor fluid shift back into the intravascular space (Fig. 21-1). The lymphatic system can also increase return of filtered fluid dramatically, thereby decreasing the amount of filtered fluid that remains in the interstitial space. Over a period of days to weeks, volume sensors and signals respond to changes in volume by altering the extent of natriuresis or sodium reabsorption necessary to maintain a constant intravascular volume. These combined systems closely monitor and regulate intravascular volume. Therefore, the *pathophysiology of transudative edema formation almost always requires an element of pathologic renal Na^+ retention.*

The three most common clinical situations resulting in edema formation are heart failure, cirrhosis, and nephrotic syndrome. All of these diseases manifest deranged Na^+ reabsorption caused by pathologic alterations in volume regulation. Understanding the pathophysiology of edema formation in these diseases provides a rationale for the therapeutic use of natriuretic agents.

Heart Failure

Heart failure (HF) is defined by the inability of the heart to perfuse tissues and organs adequately. Insufficient cardiac output and subsequent decreased blood flow through the arterial vascular bed leads to congestion in the venous "capacitance" vessels. The resulting increase in capillary hydrostatic pressure favors fluid transudation into tissue interstitial spaces. Right heart failure leads initially to peripheral edema, whereas left heart failure can lead first to pulmonary edema. In the introductory case, Mr. R's compromised cardiac function caused pulmonary venous congestion and peripheral edema; the pulmonary congestion was responsible for his sensation of dyspnea. The pathophysiology of heart failure is discussed in further detail in Chapter 26; the current discussion is restricted to the pathophysiology of edema formation.

The fundamental cause of Na^+ retention in HF is *perceived volume depletion* (Fig. 21-10). The inadequate arterial blood flow is perceived by high-pressure volume receptors, including the juxtaglomerular apparatus, as a decrease in intravascular volume. The kidney therefore increases renin production, leading to increased angiotensin II (AT II) production and secretion of aldosterone by the adrenal cortex. AT II and aldosterone both increase renal Na^+ absorption. Other important mediators of increased renal Na^+ reabsorption may include renal sympathetic innervation and autacoids such as endothelin and prostaglandins; these pathways act to maintain renal perfusion pressure and glomerular filtration fraction in the presence of (renally) perceived volume depletion.

Under physiologic conditions, low-pressure systems such as neural responses and natriuretic peptides sense the increased pressure resulting from venous congestion and therefore promote natriuresis. This response limits the extent of renal Na^+ reabsorption and prevents pathologic extracellular fluid volume expansion. However, both neural and natriuretic peptide signaling pathways are disrupted in heart failure. Heart failure activates excessive sympathetic responses, in part to increase ventricular inotropy through the action of norepinephrine, thus augmenting ejection fraction and maintaining cardiac output. Plasma natriuretic peptide is significantly increased in heart failure, but coexisting end-organ resistance may blunt the natriuretic response to the increased concentration of circulating hormone.

Diuretics and ACE inhibitors have found significant application in the interruption of heart failure pathophysiology. As discussed below, diuretics decrease renal Na^+ reabsorption and thereby reduce the extracellular volume expansion that favors edema formation. As demonstrated in the introductory case, diuretics can be used in an acute setting to reduce pulmonary edema. Over the longer term, decreased Na^+ retention also affects afterload by reducing intravascular volume, which can lower ventricular systolic pressure and systemic blood pressure. ACE inhibitors may interrupt

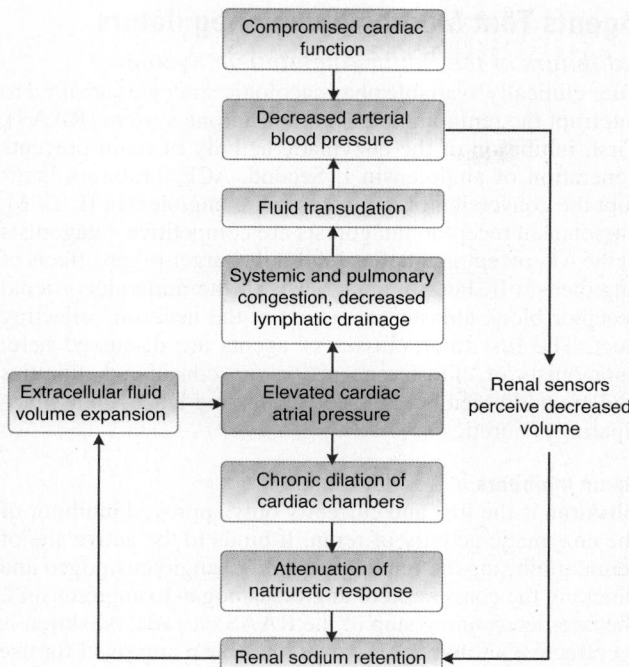

FIGURE 21-10. Mechanisms of Na⁺ retention in heart failure. In heart failure, compromised cardiac function leads to decreased arterial blood pressure and subsequent activation of renal volume sensors. These sensors activate renal sodium retention to expand extracellular volume and thereby correct the decreased arterial blood pressure. The expansion of extracellular volume increases cardiac atrial pressure. In the failing heart, the increased atrial pressure leads to increased hydrostatic pressure in the pulmonary and systemic circuits, leading to fluid transudation and edema. In addition, evidence suggests that chronic dilation of the cardiac chambers leads to local resistance to stimulation by natriuretic peptide; in the absence of an appropriate natriuretic response, the kidney continues reabsorbing Na⁺ despite the increased extracellular volume.

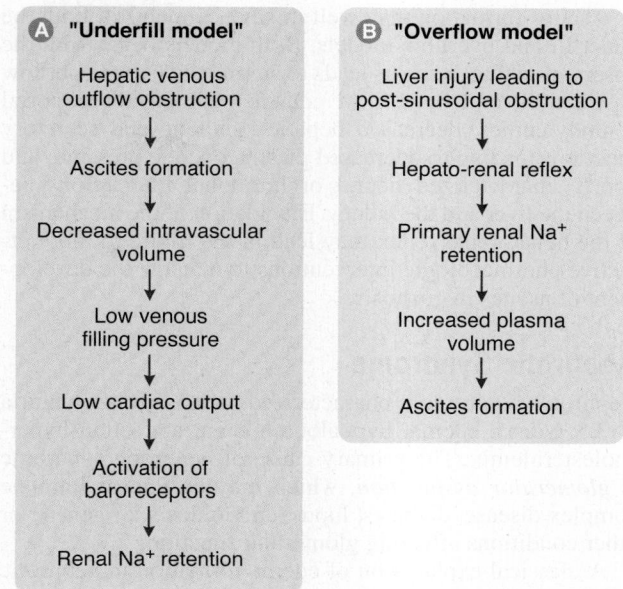

FIGURE 21-11. Proposed mechanisms of Na⁺ retention in cirrhosis. The postsinusoidal obstruction in cirrhosis is associated with renal Na⁺ retention as well as the accumulation of ascites fluid. Two models have been proposed to explain the mechanisms of these effects. **A.** Hepatic venous outflow obstruction causes increased hydrostatic pressure, which initiates ascites formation. The accumulation of ascites fluid decreases intravascular volume, leading to low venous filling pressure, decreased cardiac output, and subsequent activation of arterial baroreceptors that initiate renal Na⁺ retention. **B.** Postsinusoidal obstruction activates the hepatorenal reflex, an autonomic response involving the liver and kidney that initiates renal Na⁺ reabsorption by a poorly understood mechanism. The renal Na⁺ retention leads to an expansion of plasma volume, increased hydrostatic pressure in the portal circuit, and the formation of ascites.

pathologic paracrine signaling pathways that otherwise lead to deterioration of cardiac tissue and worsening of HF (see below).

Cirrhosis

Cirrhosis is caused by hepatic parenchymal fibrosis resulting from chronic inflammation or hepatotoxic insult. The fibrotic changes alter hepatic hemodynamics by obstructing venous outflow from the liver and increasing hydrostatic pressure in the portal vein. The obstruction to flow causes portosystemic shunting of blood away from the liver and into the systemic circulation. Hepatocellular injury disrupts the synthetic and metabolic functions of the liver, leading to decreased production of albumin and of other important macromolecular contributors to plasma oncotic pressure. Liver dysfunction decreases biosynthesis and secretion of peptide hormones, serum hormone-binding proteins, and coagulation factors (thereby increasing the risk for bruising and bleeding).

The mechanism of renal Na⁺ retention in cirrhosis remains controversial, as reflected in two proposed models (Fig. 21-11). The **underfill model** (Fig. 21-11A) suggests that obstruction of hepatic venous outflow leads to an increase in intrahepatic hydrostatic pressure. The increased hydrostatic pressure causes increased fluid transudation across the hepatic sinusoids, increasing lymphatic flow through the thoracic duct. Under physiologic conditions, the lymphatic

system is able to increase its flow dramatically and thereby limit the extent of interstitial fluid accumulation. In cirrhosis, however, lymphatic flow can exceed 20 L/day, overwhelming the ability of the lymphatic system to return transudate to the systemic circulation and leading to the formation of **ascites** (an accumulation of serous fluid in the abdominal cavity). Ascites formation decreases intravascular volume, because fluid is shunted from the plasma into the abdominal cavity. The decreased intravascular volume leads to a decrease in cardiac output, with subsequent activation of baroreceptors that increase renal Na⁺ retention. Thus, the underfill model is conceptually similar to the mechanism of edema formation in heart failure, in that the kidney initiates Na⁺ reabsorption in response to a *perceived* decrease in intravascular volume.

The **overflow model** postulates that ascites formation involves an element of *primary* renal Na⁺ retention (Fig. 21-11B). In this model, postsinusoidal obstruction activates the **hepatorenal reflex**, an incompletely characterized autonomic response that increases renal Na⁺ retention. This pathologic Na⁺ retention leads to intravascular volume expansion, increased portal hydrostatic pressure, and formation of ascites. Although not well understood, this mechanism is consistent with a number of experimental model systems demonstrating that renal Na⁺ retention in cirrhosis occurs before the development of ascites.

Ascites formation may well involve elements of both the underfill and overflow models. Both models begin with the observation that cirrhosis leads to significant hepatic outflow obstruction, and both must consider compromised portal hemodynamics, decreased hepatic synthetic and secretory functions leading to decreased plasma oncotic pressure, and poorly characterized neural or hormonal interactions between the liver and the kidney. Elucidation of the mechanism of the hepatorenal reflex may lead in the future to more effective pharmacologic interventions to manage the development of ascites in cirrhosis.

Nephrotic Syndrome

Nephrotic syndrome is characterized by massive proteinuria (>3.5 g/day), edema, hypoalbuminemia, and often hypercholesterolemia. The primary cause of nephrotic syndrome is *glomerular dysfunction*, which may be due to immune complex disease, diabetes, lupus, amyloidosis, or genetic or other conditions affecting glomerular function.

A classical explanation of edema formation in nephrotic syndrome follows this sequence. First, massive proteinuria leads to decreased plasma oncotic pressure, reducing the forces favoring fluid retention in the capillary and leading to fluid transudation into the interstitium. The increased net fluid transudation decreases intravascular volume, activating volume sensors to enhance renal Na^+ retention. The resulting expansion in fluid volume, in the absence of adequate compensatory albumin synthesis, maintains low plasma oncotic pressure and continued edema formation. In this view, renal Na^+ retention is secondary to decreased renal arterial perfusion. However, the edema of nephrotic syndrome may also be caused by intrinsic changes in capillary junctional permeability and/or by primary renal Na^+ retention. The postulated primary Na^+ retention of nephrotic syndrome may be localized to the distal nephron, arising from resistance to natriuretic peptides, increased sympathetic nervous system activity, or increased ENaC activation by filtered luminal proteases, as described above.

Although treatment of nephrotic syndrome can include diuretics to counter renal Na^+ retention, correction of edema typically requires correction of the underlying glomerular disorder, eventually leading to decreased proteinuria and correction of the edema. The glucocorticoids and immunosuppressants used to treat some forms of nephrotic syndrome can themselves promote further sodium retention. Diuretics are used in the short term to minimize edema formation.

■ PHARMACOLOGIC CLASSES AND AGENTS

Pharmacologic modulators of extracellular fluid volume can be divided into agents that modify neurohormonal volume regulators and agents that act directly on the nephron segments to alter renal Na^+ handling. The former category includes agents that interrupt the renin-angiotensin axis, alter circulating levels of natriuretic peptides, or interrupt ADH signaling. The latter category includes the various classes of diuretics, which directly target renal ion transporter or channel function or expression to increase renal Na^+ excretion. Neurohormonal volume regulators may also act directly on Na^+ reabsorption through mechanisms less well understood than those of the diuretics.

Agents That Modify Volume Regulators

Inhibitors of the Renin-Angiotensin System

Four clinically available pharmacologic strategies are used to interrupt the renin-angiotensin-aldosterone system (RAAS). First, inhibition of the enzymatic activity of renin prevents generation of angiotensin I. Second, ACE inhibitors interrupt the conversion of angiotensin I to angiotensin II. Third, angiotensin receptor antagonists are competitive antagonists at the AT_1 receptor and thus inhibit the target-organ effects of angiotensin II. Fourth, antagonists of the mineralocorticoid receptor block aldosterone action at the nephron collecting duct. The first three classes of agents are discussed here; antagonists of aldosterone action are considered diuretics and are addressed below (see "Collecting Duct [Potassium-Sparing] Diuretics").

Renin Inhibitors

Aliskiren is the first and currently only approved inhibitor of the enzymatic activity of renin. It binds to the active site of renin, inhibiting the binding of renin to angiotensinogen and blocking the conversion of angiotensinogen to angiotensin I, the rate-determining step of the RAAS cascade. Aliskiren is an effective antihypertensive and has been approved for use in hypertensive patients with renal insufficiency. Aliskiren is approved for use with thiazide diuretics, which improve the efficacy of drugs targeting the RAAS. Aliskiren may also be useful in slowing the progression of heart failure and chronic kidney disease (Fig. 21-12). Aliskiren should not be combined with ACE inhibitors or angiotensin receptor blockers (ARBs) in patients with diabetes or chronic kidney disease of stage 3 (GFR <60 mL/min) or higher. The risks include worsening of kidney function, hypotension, and hyperkalemia. Aliskiren is contraindicated in pregnancy, since drugs that act directly on the renin-angiotensin system are teratogenic.

Angiotensin Converting Enzyme Inhibitors

Pharmacologic interruption of the renin-angiotensin axis is achieved most commonly via inhibition of angiotensin converting enzyme (ACE). Because angiotensin II is the primary mediator of the activity of the renin-angiotensin-aldosterone system, decreased conversion of angiotensin I to angiotensin II inhibits arteriolar vasoconstriction, decreases aldosterone synthesis, inhibits renal proximal tubule NaCl reabsorption, and decreases ADH release. All of these actions result in decreased blood pressure and increased natriuresis. In addition, because ACE proteolytically cleaves bradykinin (among other substrates), ACE inhibitors also increase levels of bradykinin and other kinins. Bradykinin causes vascular smooth muscle relaxation by binding to bradykinin receptors on endothelial cell surfaces, leading to intracellular Ca^{2+} mobilization, eNOS activation, and increased NO production (see Chapter 22). Thus, ACE inhibitors decrease blood pressure both by decreasing angiotensin II levels and by increasing bradykinin levels (Fig. 21-12).

The contribution of reduced plasma aldosterone levels to the antihypertensive effects of ACE inhibitors remains unclear. This uncertainty is related to the observation that the renal vasoconstrictive effects of angiotensin II occur primarily at the efferent arteriole of the glomerulus. A preferential decrease in efferent relative to afferent arteriolar tone reduces intraglomerular pressure, resulting in decreased GFR. This reduction in GFR may counterbalance the anticipated reduction

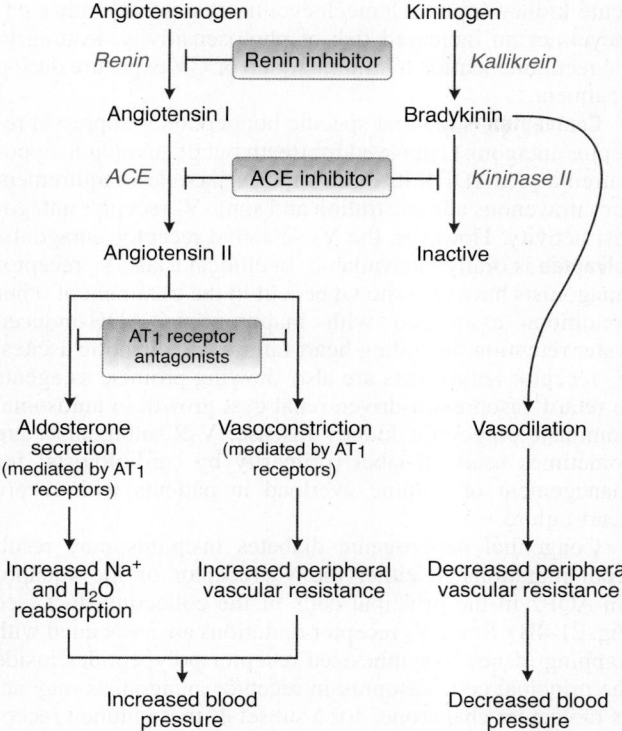

FIGURE 21-12. Effects of renin-angiotensin system inhibitors on blood pressure. Renin inhibitors prevent the conversion of angiotensinogen to angiotensin I. ACE inhibitors prevent the conversion of angiotensin I to angiotensin II (both in the lung and locally in blood vessels and tissues) and inhibit the inactivation of bradykinin. Both actions of ACE inhibitors lead to vasodilation. The inhibition of angiotensin I conversion decreases AT_1-mediated vasoconstriction and decreases aldosterone secretion; both of these effects act to decrease blood pressure. The inhibition of kininase II activity results in higher bradykinin levels, which promote vasodilation. The increased vasodilation decreases peripheral vascular resistance, which decreases blood pressure. AT_1 antagonists (also known as *angiotensin receptor blockers*, or *ARBs*) similarly decrease aldosterone synthesis and interrupt AT_1-mediated vasoconstriction, but do not alter bradykinin levels. Note that bradykinin-induced cough is a major adverse effect of ACE inhibitors but not of AT_1 antagonists.

in Na^+ and H_2O retention that should occur as a result of the reduced aldosterone levels.

ACE inhibitors exhibit three patterns of metabolism. The prototypical ACE inhibitor, **captopril**, represents the first pattern: it is active as administered but is also biotransformed to an active metabolite. The second and most common pattern, exemplified by **enalapril** and **ramipril**, is that of an ester prodrug converted in the plasma to an active metabolite. The active forms of each of these drugs are denoted by the letters "-at" added to the drug name; thus, enalaprilat and ramiprilat are the active forms of enalapril and ramipril, respectively. **Lisinopril** exemplifies the third pattern, in which the drug is administered in active form and excreted unchanged by the kidneys. Captopril, enalapril, ramipril, and lisinopril have all been studied in large-scale clinical trials and are among the ACE inhibitors in clinical use (see Drug Summary Table). Fosinopril is unique among approved ACE inhibitors in its excretion by both renal and hepatic pathways rather than only via the kidneys. This characteristic makes fosinopril a safer drug choice than other ACE inhibitors for heart failure

patients with decreased renal function resulting from poor perfusion.

Although ACE inhibitors are generally well tolerated, important adverse effects of these agents include **cough** and **angioedema** caused by potentiation of bradykinin action. The cough, occurring in up to 20% of patients taking captopril, is usually dry and nonproductive. While not causing serious physiologic effects, the cough may cause discomfort, impair voice quality, and limit patient adherence. Angioedema (rapid swelling/edema of the dermis, subcutaneous tissue, mucosa, and submucosal tissues), which can occur in 0.1–0.2% of patients, is a potentially life-threatening cause of airway obstruction. Lisinopril-induced angioedema that is isolated to the small intestine can present with abdominal pain. These adverse effects usually occur during the first week of therapy and may require emergent intervention.

ACE inhibitors can precipitate first-dose **hypotension** and/or **acute renal failure** and thus are administered at a low initial dose. These adverse effects are more common in patients with bilateral renal artery stenosis. In such patients, renal function can depend on increased angiotensin II activity, because elevated angiotensin II maintains GFR by preferential constriction of the efferent arteriole. For this reason, bilateral renal artery stenosis is a relative contraindication to ACE inhibitor therapy. ACE inhibitors reduce aldosterone synthesis and so can produce **hyperkalemia**. Hyperkalemia is more commonly observed when ACE inhibitors are used in conjunction with potassium-sparing diuretics such as spironolactone, amiloride, and triamterene (see below).

ACE inhibitors are widely used to treat hypertension, heart failure, acute myocardial infarction, and chronic kidney disease. In many cases, ACE inhibitors are increasingly considered first-line agents for hypertension, especially when a patient has concomitant left ventricular wall dysfunction or diabetes (see Chapter 26). ACE inhibitors have broad applicability to all forms of hypertension, including hypertension in which there is no clear increase in plasma renin levels. By incompletely understood mechanisms that may involve inhibition of paracrine growth factors and hormones that stimulate pathologic tissue hypertrophy and fibrosis, long-term use of ACE inhibitors retards progression of the cardiac contractile dysfunction observed in heart failure and after myocardial infarction. ACE inhibitors can also delay progression of diabetic nephropathy, likely through attenuation of renal paracrine signaling pathways, with consequent improvement in renal hemodynamics. As noted above, worsened clinical outcomes have led to discontinuation of the combined use of ACE inhibitors and aliskiren. Combined administration of ACE inhibitors and angiotensin receptor blockers (ARBs) is similarly no longer recommended, as it increases the risks of hyperkalemia and acute kidney injury compared to monotherapy.

Like aliskiren, ACE inhibitors are teratogenic and are therefore contraindicated in pregnancy.

Angiotensin Receptor Antagonists

AT_1 receptor antagonists, such as **losartan** and **valsartan**, inhibit the action of angiotensin II at its receptor (Fig. 21-12). Compared to ACE inhibitors, AT_1 receptor antagonists may allow more complete inhibition of the actions of angiotensin II, because ACE is not the only enzyme that can generate angiotensin II. In addition, because AT_1 receptor antagonists have no effect on bradykinin metabolism, their use may minimize the incidence of drug-induced cough and angioedema. However, the inability of AT_1 receptor antagonists to potentiate the vasodilatory effects of bradykinin may result in less effective vasodilation. Unlike ACE inhibitors, AT_1 receptor antagonists may indirectly increase vasorelaxant AT_2 receptor activity. Both ACE inhibitors and AT_1 antagonists induce increased renin release as a compensatory mechanism; in the case of AT_1 blockade, the increased angiotensin II that results could lead to increased interaction of angiotensin II with AT_2 receptors.

AT_1 receptor antagonists are approved for the treatment of hypertension. Although these agents were initially prescribed only for patients with intolerable adverse reactions to ACE inhibitors, they are now considered first-line treatments for hypertension. AT_1 receptor antagonists are also under study for the treatment of heart failure. Recent trials have suggested that the combination of an AT_1 receptor antagonist and an ACE inhibitor may have some clinical benefit in severe heart failure, and studies testing such combinations in the treatment of chronic kidney disease and cardiac disease progression are currently underway. Combined therapy using AT_1 receptor antagonists and aliskiren is also under investigation for treatment of hypertension, heart failure, and renal failure. AT_1 receptor antagonists may protect against stroke, not only by controlling hypertension but also through beneficial secondary effects. These include reduced platelet aggregation, decreased serum uric acid levels, decreased incidence of atrial fibrillation, and antidiabetic effects. The mechanisms of these secondary effects remain to be elucidated.

B-Type Natriuretic Peptide

Nesiritide, a recombinant human-sequence B-type natriuretic peptide (BNP), can be used for short-term management of decompensated heart failure. Because nesiritide is a peptide, it is ineffective when given orally. In clinical trials of nesiritide in acute heart failure, the drug decreased pulmonary capillary wedge pressure (a measure of hydrostatic pressure in the pulmonary system), decreased systemic vascular resistance, and improved cardiac hemodynamic parameters such as stroke volume. Although nesiritide was not more efficacious in these trials than the more commonly used dobutamine (see Chapter 26), nesiritide may be associated with a lower incidence of arrhythmias than dobutamine. At low doses, nesiritide appears to promote water excretion to a greater degree than sodium excretion.

Hypotension is a major adverse effect of nesiritide, reflecting the vasorelaxant properties of the natriuretic peptides. The risk of hypotension is increased by co-administration of nesiritide with an ACE inhibitor. Nesiritide treatment is also associated with an increased risk of renal dysfunction. These adverse effects have not been reported in preliminary clinical trials of an investigational peptide related to ANP, which exhibits powerful natriuretic as well as diuretic properties.

Vasopressin Receptor Antagonists and Agonists

The tetracycline analogue **demeclocycline** has long been used in the treatment of syndromes of inappropriate ADH secretion (SIADH), when dietary water restriction is not feasible or sufficient. Its mechanism of action is uncertain, although vasopressin receptor type 2 (V_2R) blockade has been suggested. Demeclocycline use in the setting of chronic kidney disease has been associated with precipitation of

acute kidney injury. Demeclocycline shares with other tetracyclines an increased risk of photosensitivity, leading to the recommendation to minimize sun or UV exposure during treatment.

Conivaptan is the first specific nonpeptide vasopressin receptor antagonist approved for treatment of euvolemic hyponatremias (SIADH). Its disadvantages include a requirement for intravenous administration and some V_1 receptor antagonist activity. However, the V_2-selective receptor antagonist **tolvaptan** is orally bioavailable. In clinical trials, V_2 receptor antagonists have also shown benefit in the treatment of other conditions associated with inappropriate ADH-induced water retention, including heart failure and cirrhotic ascites. V_2 receptor antagonists are also showing promise as agents to retard vasopressin-driven renal cyst growth in autosomal dominant polycystic kidney disease. V_2R antagonists are sometimes used off-label (primarily by cardiologists) for management of volume overload in patients with severe heart failure.

Congenital nephrogenic diabetes insipidus may result from mutations in either the V_2 receptor or the aquaporin AQP2 in the principal cells of the collecting duct (see Fig. 21-4B). Some V_2 receptor mutations are associated with trapping of newly synthesized receptor polypeptides inside the principal cell. Vasopressin receptor antagonists may act as molecular chaperones for a subset of these mutant receptors; in these cases, antagonist binding presumably promotes a receptor conformation that allows insertion of the mutant protein into the apical membrane of the cell. Cell-permeant, vasopressin-mimetic small molecules have also been shown to activate mutant V_2 receptors inside cells, generating sufficient cAMP to mobilize aquaporin 2 water channels to the apical surface. This strategy is thus far the most promising approach to the treatment of V_2 receptor-linked nephrogenic diabetes insipidus. Similar strategies are being adopted for many hereditary diseases of G protein-coupled receptors.

Terlipressin is an investigational vasopressin analog with moderate V_1 receptor agonist activity and specificity. It may have potential clinical application in reducing portal hypertension and improving renal hemodynamics in liver failure and ascites.

Agents That Decrease Renal Na^+ Reabsorption

As discussed above, the kidney modifies the ionic composition of the glomerular filtrate by the concerted action of ion transporters and channels in both apical and basolateral membranes of renal tubular epithelial cells. This transepithelial ion transport can be modulated pharmacologically by the actions of diuretic drugs to regulate urinary volume and composition. Pharmacologic inhibition of ion reabsorption leads to reduction of the osmotic driving force that favors water reabsorption in the water-permeable segments of the nephron. Diuretics target sodium reabsorption along four segments of the nephron: the proximal tubule, medullary thick ascending limb, distal convoluted tubule, and collecting duct. The kidney concentrates and secretes these drugs into the tubule lumen, allowing diuretics to reach higher concentrations in the tubule than in the blood. Because of this concentrating effect, therapeutic diuretic doses are often accompanied by low blood levels of diuretics and by mild extrarenal adverse effects.

Carbonic Anhydrase Inhibitors

Carbonic anhydrase inhibitors, exemplified by **acetazolamide**, inhibit sodium reabsorption by noncompetitively and reversibly inhibiting cytoplasmic carbonic anhydrase II and luminal carbonic anhydrase IV in proximal tubule cells (Fig. 21-6). Inhibition of carbonic anhydrase leads to increased delivery of sodium bicarbonate to more distal segments of the nephron. Much of this sodium bicarbonate is initially excreted, resulting in an acute decrease in plasma volume (diuresis). However, over the course of several days of therapy, the diuretic effect of the drug is diminished by compensatory up-regulation of $NaHCO_3$ reabsorption and compensatory increased NaCl reabsorption across more distal nephron segments (by incompletely understood mechanisms).

Use of carbonic anhydrase inhibitors is often associated with mild to moderate metabolic acidosis, arising not only from inhibition of proximal tubular H^+ secretion but also from inhibition of carbonic anhydrase in acid-secreting intercalated cells of the collecting duct. The alkalinized urine resulting from carbonic anhydrase inhibition increases the urinary excretion of organic acid anions, including aspirin.

The clinical use of carbonic anhydrase inhibitors is primarily restricted to several carbonic anhydrase-dependent conditions (see below). In addition, carbonic anhydrase inhibitors are occasionally used to restore acid–base balance in heart failure patients with metabolic alkalosis due to treatment with loop diuretics.

Carbonic anhydrase inhibitors have ophthalmologic applications. The ciliary process epithelium of the anterior chamber of the eye secretes sodium chloride into the aqueous humor. This NaCl secretion requires carbonic anhydrase activity, because a portion of the basolateral Cl^- uptake by the ciliary epithelium requires coupled Cl^--HCO_3^- and Na^+-H^+ exchange as well as Na^+-HCO_3^- symport. The basolateral membrane Na^+-K^+-$2Cl^-$ co-transporter NKCC1 mediates most of the remaining Cl^- uptake by ciliary epithelial cells. **Glaucoma** is characterized by increased pressure in the anterior chamber of the eye. This is usually attributed to partially obstructed outflow of aqueous humor, but in some cases, overproduction of aqueous humor may also contribute. Inhibition of carbonic anhydrase in the ciliary process epithelium reduces secretion of aqueous humor and may thereby reduce elevated intraocular pressure. Topical lipophilic carbonic anhydrase inhibitors such as **brinzolamide** are often used in concert with topical β-adrenergic antagonists in the treatment of glaucoma (see Chapter 11, Adrenergic Pharmacology).

Ascent to altitudes higher than 3,000 m above sea level predisposes several body organs, including the brain, to edema and ionic disequilibria. Symptoms of **acute mountain sickness** can include nausea, headache, dizziness, insomnia, pulmonary edema, and confusion. Carbonic anhydrase is involved in the secretion of chloride and bicarbonate into the cerebrospinal fluid by the choroid plexus of the cerebral ventricles, and inhibition of carbonic anhydrase can be used prophylactically against acute mountain sickness. The still-controversial mechanism(s) of action include effects on the choroid plexus and ependyma, on the respiratory control centers of the brain, and on the blood–brain barrier. Carbonic anhydrase inhibitors are also used in the treatment of epilepsy, although the antiepileptic mechanism of some of these drugs may not require inhibition of carbonic anhydrase. One such antiepileptic drug, **topiramate**, can produce mild to moderate acidosis due to impaired renal acidification of the urine.

The treatment of hyperuricemia or **gout** (see Chapter 49, Integrative Inflammation Pharmacology: Gout) may involve alkalinization of the urine to increase the urinary solubility of uric acid. Increased uric acid solubility prevents uric acid precipitation in the urine and consequent uric acid nephropathy and nephrolithiasis (kidney stones). Urinary alkalinization can be achieved by oral bicarbonate, supplemented as needed by a carbonic anhydrase inhibitor to reduce renal reabsorption of the filtered bicarbonate.

Osmotic Diuretics

Osmotic diuretics, such as **mannitol**, are small molecules that are filtered at the glomerulus but not subsequently reabsorbed in the nephron. Thus, they constitute an intraluminal osmotic force that limits reabsorption of water across water-permeable nephron segments. The effect of osmotic agents is greatest in the proximal tubule, where most iso-osmotic reabsorption of water takes place. By causing water loss in excess of sodium excretion, osmotic diuresis can sometimes lead to unintended hypernatremia. Alternatively, the increased urine volume associated with osmotic diuresis can also promote vigorous natriuresis. Therefore, careful monitoring of clinical volume status and serum electrolytes is warranted. Mannitol is used primarily for rapid (emergent) treatment of **increased intracranial pressure**. In the setting of head trauma, brain hemorrhage, or a symptomatic cerebral mass, the increased intracranial pressure can be relieved, at least transiently, by the acute reduction in cerebral intravascular volume that follows the mannitol-induced reduction in systemic vascular volume.

Osmotic diuresis can also occur as a result of pathologic states. Two common examples of this phenomenon are hyperglycemia and the use of radiocontrast dyes. In diabetic hyperglycemia, the filtered glucose load exceeds the reabsorptive capacity of the proximal tubule for glucose. As a result, significant quantities of glucose remain in the lumen of the nephron and act as an osmotic agent to increase fluid retention in the tubular lumen, thereby decreasing fluid reabsorption. Radiocontrast agents used for radiologic imaging studies are filtered at the glomerulus but not reabsorbed by the tubular epithelium. Thus, these dyes constitute an osmotic load and can produce osmotic diuresis. In patients with borderline cardiovascular status, the consequent reduction in intravascular volume can lead to hypotension or to renal and/or cardiac insufficiency secondary to reduced organ perfusion.

Loop Diuretics

The so-called loop diuretics act at the TAL of the loop of Henle. These agents reversibly and competitively inhibit the Na^+-K^+-$2Cl^-$ co-transporter NKCC2 in the apical (luminal) membrane of TAL epithelial cells (Fig. 21-7). In addition to the primary effect of inhibiting Na^+ reabsorption across the TAL, inhibition of transcellular NaCl transport secondarily reduces or abolishes the lumen-positive transepithelial potential difference across the TAL. Consequently, paracellular reabsorption of divalent cations, particularly calcium and magnesium, is also inhibited. The increased delivery of luminal calcium and magnesium to downstream reabsorptive sites in the distal convoluted tubule can lead to increased urinary excretion of calcium and magnesium. The resultant hypocalcemia and/or hypomagnesemia can be clinically significant in some patients who require prolonged administration of loop agents. Furthermore, increased downstream delivery of sodium increases the Na^+ load presented to principal cells of the collecting duct. The increased Na^+ load stimulates increased secretion of K^+ and protons, predisposing to hypokalemia and metabolic alkalosis. Together, the clinical consequences of loop diuretic treatment are often described as **volume-contraction alkalosis**. Diuretic-associated hypokalemia can predispose to cardiac arrhythmias in the setting of coronary or cardiac insufficiency.

The prototypical loop diuretic is **furosemide**. Other drugs in this class include **bumetanide**, **torsemide**, and **ethacrynic acid**. All of these agents are generally well tolerated. Apart from their effects on renal electrolyte handling, loop diuretics are associated with dose-related **ototoxicity**, presumably because of altered electrolyte handling in the endolymph. For this reason, co-administration of loop diuretics with aminoglycosides (which are also ototoxic; see Chapter 34, Pharmacology of Bacterial Infections: DNA Replication, Transcription, and Translation) should be avoided. The major differences among the loop diuretics are in potency and incidence of allergies. Bumetanide is approximately 40 times more potent than the other loop diuretics. Furosemide, bumetanide, and torsemide are all **sulfonamide derivatives**, while ethacrynic acid is not of this structural class. Therefore, ethacrynic acid is a therapeutic option for patients who are allergic to "sulfa" drugs.

The high sodium reabsorption capacity of the TAL makes loop diuretics a first-line therapy for acute relief of pulmonary and peripheral edema in the context of heart failure. Loop diuretics are capable of reducing intravascular volume to the extent that filling pressures are decreased below the threshold for pulmonary and peripheral edema. This was the rationale for the intravenous furosemide used to treat Mr. R's pulmonary edema and peripheral edema in the introductory case. Hypoalbuminemia, resulting from decreased synthesis of albumin (liver disease) or increased clearance of the protein (nephrotic proteinuria), can diminish intravascular oncotic pressure and cause edema. These **edematous states** can also be treated with low-dose loop diuretics.

Loop agents can be used therapeutically to increase calcium diuresis, and thereby provide acute relief of **hypercalcemia**, in states such as hyperparathyroidism or malignancy-associated hypercalcemia caused by tumor secretion of parathyroid hormone-related protein or other calciotropic hormones (see Chapter 32, Pharmacology of Bone Mineral Homeostasis). Loop agents are also used to counteract **hyperkalemia** caused by potassium-retaining adverse effects of other drugs or by renal insufficiency with impaired urinary K^+ excretion in the context of normal or elevated dietary K^+ intake.

In **acute renal failure**, the increased urine flow elicited by loop diuretics can facilitate clinical management of fluid balance in the face of decreased glomerular filtration. However, there is no evidence to support the oft-repeated claim that increased urine output itself intrinsically enhances renal tubular epithelial cell recovery from the ischemic or toxic event that precipitated the acute renal failure.

Thiazides

Thiazide diuretics inhibit sodium chloride reabsorption in the distal convoluted tubule (Fig. 21-8). These agents act from the apical (luminal) side as competitive antagonists of the NCC Na^+-Cl^- co-transporter in the luminal membrane of distal convoluted tubule cells. The modest natriuresis produced by thiazides stems from the fact that 90% of sodium reabsorption occurs upstream of their site of action in the nephron; nonetheless, thiazides do cause a modest reduction in intravascular volume. The decrease in intravascular volume, possibly combined with a poorly understood direct vasodilatory effect, decreases systemic blood pressure.

The distal tubule is also a site of parathyroid hormone-regulated reabsorption of calcium via voltage-independent TRPV5 Ca^{2+} channels. Thiazides promote increased transcellular calcium reabsorption in the distal convoluted tubule. Thiazides have been used to decrease urinary Ca^{2+} wasting in **osteoporosis** (although this is no longer common practice in the absence of hypercalciuria) and to diminish hypercalciuria in patients at risk for **nephrolithiasis**. The mechanism by which inhibition of NaCl uptake enhances apical Ca^{2+} entry remains incompletely understood, but part of the response is mediated by increased expression of the apical membrane TRPV5 Ca^{2+} channel and the basolateral membrane Na^+/Ca^{2+} exchanger. Additionally (and more speculatively), the decreased intracellular Cl^- concentration that results from thiazide inhibition of apical Na^+-Cl^- co-transport may favor Cl^- entry via basolateral Cl^- channels, and the consequent membrane hyperpolarization may favor apical Ca^{2+} entry. In mice, the inhibitory action of thiazide diuretics on distal tubular Na^+ reabsorption and the stimulatory influence of thiazides on Ca^{2+} reabsorption both require expression of the small intracellular Ca^{2+}-binding protein parvalbumin, but the mechanism connecting these processes remains undefined.

Hydrochlorothiazide is the prototypical thiazide diuretic. In addition to its effects on renal electrolyte handling, hydrochlorothiazide decreases glucose tolerance and may unmask diabetes in patients at risk for impaired glucose metabolism. The mechanism of this effect is unknown but may be attributable to drug-induced impairment of insulin secretion and/or decreased peripheral insulin sensitivity. Thiazide diuretics should not be administered concurrently with antiarrhythmic agents that prolong the QT interval (e.g., quinidine, sotalol), since co-administration of these drugs predisposes patients to torsades de pointes (polymorphic ventricular tachycardia; see Chapter 24, Pharmacology of Cardiac Rhythm). The mechanism of this adverse effect may be related to thiazide-induced hypokalemia, which increases the potential for cardiac arrhythmias (see Chapter 24).

Thiazide diuretics are first-line agents for treatment of hypertension (see Chapter 26). In numerous randomized clinical trials, these drugs have been shown to reduce both cardiovascular-related and total mortality. In addition, thiazide diuretics are often used together with loop agents for their synergistic diuretic effects in heart failure. This synergism arises because the increased Na^+ load, delivered from the loop diuretic-blocked TAL to the thiazide diuretic-blocked DCT, proceeds further downstream to the collecting duct, which has only a limited ability to up-regulate compensatory Na^+ reabsorption. The dose of thiazide must be carefully considered in this setting, for as with loop diuretics, thiazides can increase K^+ and H^+ secretion by increasing Na^+ presentation to the collecting duct, thus leading to hypokalemic metabolic alkalosis.

Hydrochlorothiazide should be taken several times a day. A longer acting thiazide, **chlorthalidone**, can be taken once a day and may better prevent the nocturnal blood pressure elevation that correlates, over time, with end-organ damage. The majority of the clinical trials that documented beneficial effects of thiazide diuretics for treatment of hypertension were based on chlorthalidone.

Patients with impaired secretion of vasopressin by the posterior pituitary gland, or with impaired signaling by the V_2 vasopressin receptor in collecting duct principal cells, fail to reabsorb water in the terminal nephron. These patients generate large volumes of hypotonic urine. **Central diabetes insipidus** (defective pituitary secretion of vasopressin) can be treated with the exogenous vasopressin agonist **desmopressin** (see Chapter 27, Pharmacology of the Hypothalamus and Pituitary Gland). Patients with **nephrogenic diabetes insipidus** do not respond to desmopressin; paradoxically, however, thiazide diuretics can produce a modest *decrease* in urine flow in this setting. It is thought that, by reducing intravascular volume and decreasing glomerular filtration rate, thiazides reduce the volume of tubular fluid delivered to the collecting duct and thereby decrease urine volume. For nephrogenic diabetes insipidus associated with chronic lithium therapy, traditional treatment with thiazides will likely be supplanted by treatment with amiloride (see below) and, possibly, with acetazolamide.

Collecting Duct (Potassium-Sparing) Diuretics
In contrast to all other diuretic classes, potassium-sparing diuretics increase nephron reabsorption of potassium. Agents in this class interrupt Na^+ reabsorption by principal cells of the collecting duct by one of two mechanisms. Spironolactone and eplerenone inhibit biosynthesis of new Na^+ channels in principal cells, while amiloride and triamterene block the activity of Na^+ channels in the luminal membranes of these cells (Fig. 21-9).

The epithelial sodium channel (ENaC) of collecting duct principal cells comprises a complex of partly homologous α, β, and γ subunits. Control of sodium channel expression is regulated primarily by aldosterone, which is secreted by the adrenal cortical zona glomerulosa under the regulation of angiotensin II and plasma potassium. Circulating aldosterone diffuses into collecting duct principal cells and binds to an intracellular mineralocorticoid receptor. Activation of the mineralocorticoid receptor increases transcription of mRNAs that encode proteins involved in Na^+ handling, including ENaC expressed in the apical membrane and Na^+/K^+ ATPase expressed in the basolateral membrane. Increased ENaC expression allows increased Na^+ influx across the luminal membrane, while increased Na^+/K^+ ATPase activity allows increased Na^+ efflux from the cytoplasm across the basolateral membrane into the interstitium. These two actions of aldosterone, mediated by complex, multistep signaling pathways, increase transepithelial Na^+ reabsorption and hence increase both the Na^+ content of the extracellular space and the intravascular volume.

Spironolactone and **eplerenone** inhibit aldosterone action by binding to and preventing nuclear translocation of the mineralocorticoid receptor. Recent studies suggest that up to 20% of patients with essential hypertension have elevated aldosterone levels. Mineralocorticoid receptor antagonists are used to treat hypertension, and they seem to have greater efficacy in obesity-associated hypertension. This increased sensitivity of obese individuals has been attributed to increased adrenal aldosterone synthesis secondary to factors released by the increased mass of adipocytes. Unlike most diuretics, which must reach their luminal sites of action

through glomerular filtration of the albumin-unbound fraction, spironolactone requires neither albumin-binding nor glomerular filtration to reach its target receptor and thus can exhibit greater efficacy in the settings of liver failure and nephrotic syndrome. The ability of spironolactone to cross-react with and inhibit the androgen receptor can cause male impotence and gynecomastia, but the more selective eplerenone, primarily used for the treatment of chronic heart failure, has a lower incidence of these adverse effects.

Amiloride and **triamterene** are competitive inhibitors of the ENaC Na^+ channel in the apical membrane of collecting duct principal cells. These agents are also used to treat hypertension. Both types of potassium-sparing diuretics can cause **hyperkalemia**, because inhibition of electrogenic Na^+ uptake by either mechanism decreases the normal transepithelial lumen-negative potential and thus decreases the driving force for potassium secretion from collecting duct cells. Decreased Na^+ uptake through ENaC may also diminish H^+ secretion, leading to **metabolic acidosis**. The longer half-life of amiloride may be preferable in the treatment of some patients. Triamterene occasionally induces crystalluria and, more rarely, triamterene stone formation, sometimes with reversible acute kidney injury.

Used in isolation, potassium-sparing diuretics are mild diuretics because the collecting duct reabsorbs only 1–5% of filtered sodium. However, they can be strong potentiators of more proximally acting diuretics, including loop diuretics. Potassium-sparing diuretics are occasionally used to counteract the potassium-wasting effects of the thiazides. Amiloride and triamterene are drugs of choice to treat Liddle's syndrome, a rare, Mendelian form of hypertension resulting from gain-of-function mutations in β- or γ-subunits of the ENaC Na^+ channel of the principal cell (Table 21-3). The antidepressant **lithium** (Li^+) is reabsorbed by ENaC in an amiloride-sensitive manner. In experimental animals, amiloride attenuates or prevents both acute and chronic impairment of urinary concentrating ability by Li^+. Amiloride may thus also serve to reduce the elevated risk of renal cancer potentially associated with long-term Li^+ use.

Potassium-sparing diuretics are used clinically to treat hypokalemic alkalosis secondary to the mineralocorticoid excess that can accompany heart failure, liver failure, and other disease processes associated with diminished aldosterone metabolism. The mild diuretic action of spironolactone or eplerenone minimizes the risk of cardiovascular compromise from excessively rapid or extensive diuresis when diminished oncotic pressure impairs the mobilization of extravascular fluid into the vasculature. Therefore, mineralocorticoid receptor antagonists are the diuretics of choice for treatment of ascites and edema associated with impaired plasma protein biosynthesis secondary to liver failure.

Studies have suggested that mineralocorticoid receptor antagonists preserve cardiac function in the setting of coronary ischemia and that these agents retard the development of heart failure. Both spironolactone and eplerenone reduce mortality in patients with heart failure and in patients with significant cardiac dysfunction (ejection fraction <40%) after myocardial infarction. This is why Mr. R was prescribed spironolactone in the introductory case. In addition, as in Mr. R's case, patients with heart failure are often prescribed ACE inhibitors in combination with spironolactone or eplerenone. Because both of these drug classes also decrease K^+ excretion, plasma K^+ levels should be monitored carefully.

The mechanism by which mineralocorticoid receptor antagonists preserve cardiac function may be related to inhibition of cardiac fibrosis resulting, in part, from a paracrine aldosterone signaling pathway involving mineralocorticoid receptor action in macrophages. Mineralocorticoid antagonists also minimize the aldosterone-dependent decrease in the activity of glucose-6-phosphate dehydrogenase, an important cellular defense against oxidant stress in endothelial and epithelial cells. Mineralocorticoid antagonists have similar effects in slowing the progression of chronic kidney disease and the development of renal fibrosis.

■ CONCLUSION AND FUTURE DIRECTIONS

This chapter has reviewed the physiology and pathophysiology of extracellular volume regulation. Control of intravascular volume maintains adequate perfusion pressure to organs and ensures that the kidney is able to filter waste products from the plasma. Regulation of extracellular volume is accomplished by integrated neurohormonal mechanisms that respond to changes in arterial and atrial wall stress. These hormones modulate numerous steps in renal Na^+ handling and thereby maintain a homeostatic balance between dietary Na^+ intake and Na^+ excretion. Edema can develop when the capillary hydrostatic pressure gradient favoring fluid filtration exceeds the opposing oncotic forces favoring fluid entry into the intravascular space. Pharmacologic treatment of dysregulated extracellular volume involves modification of neurohormonal signaling and direct inhibition of renal Na^+ reabsorption. ACE inhibitors prevent the conversion of angiotensin I to angiotensin II; drugs in this class have important vasodilatory actions. Angiotensin receptor antagonists and renin inhibitors are also useful in interrupting the angiotensin-aldosterone axis. Both ACE inhibitors and angiotensin receptor antagonists have beneficial effects in slowing the progression of hypertrophy and fibrosis in the heart, the kidney, and the vasculature. B-type natriuretic peptide (nesiritide) is used in the treatment of decompensated heart failure, and terlipressin is under investigation for the treatment of portal hypertension.

Diuretics are agents that alter nephron Na^+ reabsorption and secondarily alter the reabsorption and secretion of other ions. Essential to understanding diuretic mechanisms is an appreciation of the functional organization of the nephron. With the exception of osmotic diuretics, which increase urinary flow by osmotic retention of water throughout the nephron, specific classes of diuretic drugs target each of the four segments of the nephron. Carbonic anhydrase inhibitors such as acetazolamide decrease sodium and bicarbonate reabsorption in the proximal tubule; loop agents such as furosemide decrease sodium and chloride reabsorption by the apical Na^+-K^+-$2Cl^-$ (NKCC2) pump in the thick ascending limb of the loop of Henle; thiazides such as hydrochlorothiazide inhibit the apical Na^+-Cl^- co-transporter (NCC) in the distal convoluted tubule; and potassium-sparing diuretics such as spironolactone and amiloride inhibit, respectively, the aldosterone receptor and the ENaC apical Na^+ channel in the collecting duct. The most important use of diuretics is in the treatment of hypertension; the second most important use is to treat edema of any cause.

Future developments in the pharmacology of extracellular volume regulation will likely focus on interrupting or enhancing the hormonal pathways implicated in the disruption of volume homeostasis, as well as on the solute and water transporters themselves. New drugs to interrupt the renin-angiotensin-aldosterone axis may include neutral endopeptidase inhibitors, (pro)renin receptor antagonists, AT_2 receptor agonists, selective endothelin receptor antagonists, and natriuretic peptides of increased potency and selectivity. The latter will likely play an increasingly important role in the management of decompensated heart failure and possibly the ascites of liver failure. Drugs acting on the renin-angiotensin-aldosterone axis will also likely be useful in slowing the rate of renal and cardiac fibrosis, reinforcing or improving on the actions of ACE inhibitors, AT_1 receptor antagonists, and mineralocorticoid receptor blockers. These drugs also have general and cell type-specific trophic actions. One example is provided by the role of the AT_1 receptor in promoting proliferation of epidermal growth factor receptor ERBB2-negative mammary tumor cells in culture and in xenografts. AT_1 receptor blockers have slowed mammary cell tumor growth in xenograft models. Thus, AT_1 blockade is a reasonable candidate adjunct therapy for breast tumors that may not respond to more conventional therapy.

Promising inhibitors of the renal outer medullary potassium channel ROMK are in late-stage development. Inhibitors of the intercalated cell NaCl reabsorption pathway, targeting the apical Cl^-/HCO_3^- exchanger pendrin or the Na^+-dependent exchanger SLC4A8, are in early-stage development. These will most likely take the form of inhibitors of the transport proteins themselves, but inhibitors of OXGR1 or the proximal tubular α-KG secretory pathway are also potential drug candidates. Drug therapies targeting the WNK and SPAK kinases are in early stages of development. The extrarenal WNK and SPAK kinases are also potential targets for treatment of cystic fibrosis and central nervous system diseases, including autism, epilepsy, and stroke. "Gliflozin" inhibitors of proximal tubular Na^+-glucose co-transporter SGLT2, although not approved for treatment of hypertension, have some antihypertensive effects and may be useful additions to drug regimens targeting more distal tubular segments, especially if current safety concerns are addressed. Specific V_2 vasopressin receptor antagonists such as tolvaptan will be used increasingly in hypervolemic conditions accompanied by elevated ADH levels or action. V_2 receptor antagonists have also shown promise in retarding progression of cyst growth in autosomal dominant polycystic kidney disease. The synthetic A-type natriuretic peptide carperitide, currently approved in Japan to treat heart failure through its diuretic effects and direct vasodilation, could be used in combination with loop diuretics and tolvaptan. Aquaporin blockers (aquaretics) and urea transporter inhibitors (uraretics) are under development for regulation of fluid homeostasis, and aquaglyceroporin blockers are under investigation as treatments for skin conditions and as modulators of lipid metabolism. Chloride channel blockers and potassium channel blockers are under development to treat the volume depletion of severe toxigenic and infectious diarrhea as well as rare congenital diarrheas. Chloride channel activators and potassium channel activators are being developed to treat the pulmonary, gastrointestinal, and genitourinary hyposecretion disorders of cystic fibrosis, sicca syndromes, and inflammatory biliary cirrhosis. Carbonic anhydrase II has recently been shown to act as a nitrite reductase and thereby to generate nitric oxide at the acidic pH of ischemic or hypoxic tissue. Surprisingly, this nitrite reductase activity is activated by sulfonamide carbonic anhydrase inhibitors even as they inhibit carbonic anhydrase activity. This property may explain the vasodilation associated with use of carbonic anhydrase inhibitors and encourages consideration of new uses for this old drug class.

Suggested Reading

Christova M, Alper SL. Core curriculum in nephrology. Tubular transport: core curriculum 2010. *Am J Kidney Dis* 2010;56:1202–1217. (*Annotated review of transport by renal tubular epithelial cells.*)

Danziger J, Zeidel M. Osmotic homeostasis. *Clin J Am Soc Nephrol* 2015;10:852–862. (*Reviews mechanisms of water homeostasis and disorders of water balance.*)

Ellison EH. Physiology and pathophysiology of diuretic action. In: Alpern RJ, Hebert SC, eds. *The kidney: physiology and pathophysiology.* 5th ed. Philadelphia: Lippincott Williams & Wilkins; 2013:1353–1404. (*Full discussion of the physiology and pathophysiology of diuretics.*)

Ernst ME, Moser M. Drug therapy: use of diuretics in patients with hypertension. *N Engl J Med* 2009;361:2153–2164. (*Clinical pharmacology of diuretics.*)

Palmer L, Schnermann J. Integrated control of sodium transport along the nephron. *Clin J Am Soc Nephrol* 2015;10:676–687. (*Reviews renal mechanisms that integrate control of Na$^+$ reabsorption, Na$^+$ excretion, and K$^+$ excretion.*)

Seva Pessoa B, van der Lubbe N, Verdonk K, Roks AJ, Hoorn EJ, Danser AH. Key developments in renin-angiotensin-aldosterone system inhibition. *Nat Rev Nephrol* 2013;9:26–36. (*Recent advances in renin-angiotensin physiology.*)

Townsend RR, Peixoto AJ. Hypertension. *NephSAP (Am Soc Nephrol)* 2014;13:57–131. (*Updated nephrology board review summary and questions about hypertension and antihypertensive therapy.*)

Verbalis JG, Goldsmith SR, Greenberg A, et al. Diagnosis, evaluation, and treatment of hyponatremia: expert panel recommendations. *Am J Med* 2013;126(suppl 1):S1–S42. (*Includes update on clinical physiology of and indications for use of vasopressin receptor antagonists.*)

Vongpatanasin W. Resistant hypertension: a review of diagnosis and management. *JAMA* 2014;311:2216–2224. (*Clinical review of resistant hypertension.*)

Zois NE, Bartels ED, Hunter I, Kousholt BS, Olsen LH, Goetze JP. Natriuretic peptides in cardiometabolic regulation and disease. *Nat Rev Cardiol* 2014;11:403–412. (*Overview of natriuretic peptide physiology in volume regulation.*)

DRUG SUMMARY TABLE: CHAPTER 21 Pharmacology of Volume Regulation

DRUG	CLINICAL APPLICATIONS	SERIOUS AND COMMON ADVERSE EFFECTS	CONTRAINDICATIONS	THERAPEUTIC CONSIDERATIONS
RENIN INHIBITORS Mechanism—Inhibition of renin decreases conversion of angiotensinogen to angiotensin I, thereby reducing the substrate for ACE and decreasing subsequent arteriolar vasoconstriction, aldosterone synthesis, renal proximal tubule NaCl reabsorption, and ADH release				
Aliskiren	Hypertension	Hypotension, torsades de pointes, hyperkalemia, stroke, seizure, acute renal failure, angioedema Diarrhea, dizziness, headache	Pregnancy Concomitant use of ARBs or ACE inhibitors in patients with diabetes mellitus or GFR <60 mL/min	Hepatobiliary excretion with minimal hepatic metabolism by CYP3A4. Minimal hyperkalemia observed to date with monotherapy. Increased risk of renal impairment, hypotension, and severe hyperkalemia in combination therapy with ACE inhibitors and ARBs. Plasma concentrations and half-life increased by atorvastatin and ketoconazole, decreased by furosemide. May reduce proteinuria in chronic kidney disease.
ANGIOTENSIN CONVERTING ENZYME (ACE) INHIBITORS Mechanism—Inhibition of ACE decreases conversion of angiotensin (AT) I to AT II and thereby decreases arteriolar vasoconstriction, aldosterone synthesis, renal proximal tubule NaCl reabsorption, and ADH release; ACE inhibitors also inhibit the degradation of bradykinin and thereby increase vasodilation				
Captopril **Enalapril** **Ramipril** **Benazepril** **Fosinopril** **Moexipril** **Perindopril** **Quinapril** **Trandolapril** **Lisinopril** **Zofenopril** **Imidapril** **Cilazapril**	Shared indication: Hypertension Captopril, enalapril, ramipril, fosinopril, quinapril, trandolapril, and lisinopril only: Heart failure Captopril and lisinopril only: Myocardial infarction Captopril only: Diabetic nephropathy	Angioedema (more frequent in black patients), agranulocytosis, neutropenia (shared adverse effects); cardiac arrest (perindopril and trandolapril only); Stevens-Johnson syndrome (captopril, ramipril, benazepril only); hepatotoxicity (enalapril, ramipril, perindopril, and benazepril only); renal impairment (enalapril, benazepril, moexipril, perindopril, lisinopril, and fosinopril only) Hyperkalemia, cough (shared adverse effect); hypotension, rash (captopril only); dizziness (trandolapril and lisinopril only)	Shared contraindications: Hypersensitivity to drug History of angioedema Pregnancy Enalapril, benazepril, moexipril, perindopril, quinapril, lisinopril, and ramipril only: Concomitant aliskiren use in patients with diabetes Quinapril only: Renal failure Diabetic patients with end-organ damage Severe heart failure with hypotension	ACE inhibitors exhibit three patterns of metabolism: (1) administered as active drug and processed to active metabolite (e.g., captopril); (2) ester prodrugs converted to active metabolites in plasma (e.g., enalapril and ramipril); and (3) administered as active drug and excreted unchanged (lisinopril). Fosinopril is the only phosphonate-containing ACE inhibitor; in addition, it is partially metabolized in the liver and may be therefore safer in patients with advanced kidney disease. Cough and angioedema are caused by bradykinin action; angioedema occurs within the first week of therapy in 0.1–0.2% of patients and can be potentially life-threatening. First-dose hypotension and/or acute renal failure are more common in patients with bilateral renal artery stenosis; hyperkalemia is more common when ACE inhibitors are used in combination with potassium-sparing diuretics. ACE inhibitors delay progression of cardiac contractile dysfunction in heart failure and after myocardial infarction and delay progression of diabetic nephropathy. A few case reports suggest that co-administration with allopurinol may predispose to hypersensitivity reactions including Stevens-Johnson syndrome and anaphylaxis. Most clinical trials show that the blood pressure–lowering effect of ACE inhibitors is increased when combined with thiazide diuretics.

ANGIOTENSIN II RECEPTOR ANTAGONISTS

Mechanism—Antagonize action of angiotensin II at AT_1 receptor; may also indirectly increase vasorelaxant AT_2 receptor activity

Drugs	Indications	Contraindications	Adverse / Notes

Candesartan
Irbesartan
Losartan
Telmisartan
Valsartan
Azilsartan
Olmesartan
	Shared indication:
	  Hypertension
	Irbesartan and losartan only:
	  Diabetic nephropathy
	Losartan and telmisartan only:
	  Prevention of stroke
	Valsartan only:
	  Heart failure
	  Myocardial infarction
		Rhabdomyolysis, angioedema,
		hepatotoxicity, renal failure (shared
		adverse effects); thrombocytopenia
		(irbesartan only)
		Diarrhea (shared adverse effect);
		headache, upper respiratory infection,
		fatigue (irbesartan only); cough
		(telmisartan and valsartan only);
		hypotension, dizziness (valsartan)
			Hypersensitivity to drug
			Pregnancy
			Concomitant aliskiren use in diabetic patients
				Also called *angiotensin receptor blockers (ARBs)*.
				ARBs generally do not cause cough as adverse effect but rarely can occur.
				Small risk of cross-reactivity in patients having experienced angioedema with ACE inhibitor therapy.
				AT_1 receptor antagonists may also protect against stroke.
				Initially prescribed only for patients with intolerable reactions to ACE inhibitors but now accepted potential first-line treatments for hypertension.
				Combination therapy with ACE inhibitors is no longer recommended for patients with diabetes-related kidney disease due to increased risk for renal impairment, hypotension, and hyperkalemia.
				ARBs may be beneficial in migraine prophylaxis and retard cognitive decline.
				ARBs are thought to have no relevant adverse effects on male sexual function compared with other antihypertensive medications.

B-TYPE NATRIURETIC PEPTIDE (BNP)

Mechanism—BNP increases intracellular concentrations of cGMP by binding to the particulate guanylyl cyclase receptor NPR-A of vascular smooth muscle and endothelial cells, resulting in smooth muscle relaxation; it also acts directly on cardiocytes

Drug	Indications	Contraindications	Adverse / Notes
Nesiritide (BNP)	Acutely decompensated heart failure	*Hypersensitivity reaction, renal dysfunction* Hypotension, nausea, dizziness, headache	Hypersensitivity to drug Cardiogenic shock Systolic blood pressure <100 mm Hg	Nesiritide decreases pulmonary capillary wedge pressure, decreases systemic vascular resistance, and improves cardiac hemodynamic parameters such as stroke volume. Nesiritide may be associated with a lower incidence of arrhythmias than dobutamine. Hypotension and renal dysfunction more common in setting of acute heart failure. Risk of hypotension is increased by co-administration with ACE inhibitors. Nesiritide lowers plasma levels of aldosterone and endothelin-1.

VASOPRESSIN RECEPTOR 2 (V_2) ANTAGONISTS

Mechanism—Conivaptan: antagonist at V_1 and V_2 receptors; tolvaptan: selective V_2 receptor antagonist; both drugs prevent vasopressin-stimulated water reabsorption via V_2-coupled aquaporin channels in apical membrane of collecting duct cells

Drugs			
Conivaptan Tolvaptan	See Drug Summary Table: Chapter 27 Pharmacology of the Hypothalamus and Pituitary Gland		

continues

DRUG SUMMARY TABLE: CHAPTER 21 Pharmacology of Volume Regulation *continued*

DRUG	CLINICAL APPLICATIONS	*SERIOUS* AND COMMON ADVERSE EFFECTS	CONTRAINDICATIONS	THERAPEUTIC CONSIDERATIONS
CARBONIC ANHYDRASE INHIBITORS Mechanism—Inhibit sodium and bicarbonate reabsorption by noncompetitively and reversibly inhibiting proximal tubule cytoplasmic carbonic anhydrase II and luminal carbonic anhydrase IV, leading to increased delivery of sodium bicarbonate to more distal segments of the nephron				
Acetazolamide	Acute mountain sickness Edema Epilepsy Glaucoma Metabolic alkalosis	*Metabolic acidosis, sulfonamide adverse reactions (including anaphylaxis, blood dyscrasias, erythema multiforme, fulminant hepatic necrosis, Stevens-Johnson syndrome, toxic epidermal necrolysis)*	Hypersensitivity to acetazolamide Hypersensitivity to sulfonamides Adrenal gland failure Chronic angle-closure glaucoma Cirrhosis Hyponatremia/ hypokalemia Hyperchloremic acidosis Severe hepatic or renal disease	Clinical use is associated with mild to moderate metabolic acidosis. Used occasionally in heart failure to restore acid–base balance. Carbonic anhydrase inhibition in ciliary process of the eye reduces secretion of aqueous humor and may thereby reduce elevated intraocular pressure in glaucoma. Can be used prophylactically against acute mountain sickness, presumably owing to the drug's effects on choroid plexus and ependyma, respiratory control centers of brain, and blood–brain barrier. Carbonic anhydrase inhibitors alkalinize urine and increase urinary excretion of endogenous (uric acid) and exogenous (aspirin) organic anions; can be used in the treatment of hyperuricemia or gout. Aspirin increases plasma concentration of acetazolamide, potentially leading to CNS toxicity.
OSMOTIC DIURETICS Mechanism—Act as an osmole, filtered at the glomerulus but not subsequently reabsorbed in the nephron; exert an intraluminal osmotic force and limit reabsorption of water across water-permeable nephron segments				
Mannitol	Cerebral edema Increased intraocular pressure Prophylaxis of oliguria in acute renal failure Inhalation bronchial challenge testing Irrigation of urinary bladder Measurement of renal clearance	*Thrombophlebitis, acidosis, seizure, urinary retention, pulmonary edema, hyperkalemia* Chest discomfort, gastrointestinal upset, dizziness, headache, fluid and/or electrolyte imbalance, cough, rhinitis, throat irritation	Hypersensitivity to mannitol Anuria Severe dehydration Heart failure, pulmonary congestion, or renal dysfunction after initiation of mannitol Active intracranial bleeding Renal dysfunction Pulmonary edema	*Promotes vigorous natriuresis; requires careful monitoring of volume status.* Water loss in excess of sodium excretion can lead to unintended hypernatremia. Used primarily for rapid (emergent) reduction of intracranial pressure in the setting of head trauma, brain hemorrhage, or symptomatic cerebral mass; also used rarely in treatment of compartment syndrome.

LOOP DIURETICS

Mechanism—Inhibit sodium reabsorption by reversibly and competitively inhibiting sodium-potassium-chloride co-transporter NKCC2 in apical (luminal) membrane of cells in thick ascending limb of loop of Henle; also reduce or abolish the lumen-positive transepithelial potential difference

Drugs	Therapeutic Considerations	Adverse Effects	Contraindications
Furosemide Bumetanide Torsemide Ethacrynic acid	Shared indications: Edema associated with heart failure, hepatic cirrhosis, or renal dysfunction Furosemide and torsemide only: Hypertension Furosemide only: Acute pulmonary edema	Stevens-Johnson syndrome (furosemide, bumetanide, and torsemide only); thrombocytopenia (furosemide, ethacrynic acid, and bumetanide only); toxic epidermal necrolysis (furosemide and torsemide only); erythema multiforme, aplastic anemia (furosemide only); pancreatitis, agranulocytosis, (furosemide and ethacrynic acid only); encephalopathy (bumetanide only); ototoxicity (torsemide and ethacrynic acid only); ventricular tachycardia (torsemide only); gastrointestinal perforation, thromboembolic disorder, hepatotoxicity (ethacrynic acid only) Electrolyte imbalance (ethacrynic acid, furosemide, and bumetanide only); hypotension, loss of appetite, bladder spasm (furosemide only); gastrointestinal upset, dizziness, headache, azotemia (bumetanide only); polyuria, rhinitis (torsemide only)	Shared contraindications: Hypersensitivity to drug Anuria Bumetanide only: Hepatic coma Electrolyte depletion Ethacrynic acid only: Diarrhea Infancy Renal disease	Bumetanide is ~40 times more potent than the other loop diuretics. Furosemide, bumetanide, and torsemide are sulfonamides, while ethacrynic acid has a different chemical structure. First-line therapy for acute relief of pulmonary and peripheral edema in heart failure; edematous states secondary to diminished oncotic pressure of hypoalbuminemia (as in nephrotic proteinuria or liver disease) can be treated with low-dose loop diuretics. Also used to counteract hypercalcemic and hyperkalemic states. Ethacrynic acid used in patients with sulfonamide allergy. Loop diuretics reduce uric acid excretion by increased net uric acid reabsorption and can induce gout.

THIAZIDE DIURETICS

Mechanism—Inhibit sodium chloride reabsorption by acting as competitive antagonists at NCC sodium-chloride co-transporter in apical (luminal) membrane of distal convoluted tubule cells; promote increased transcellular calcium reabsorption in distal convoluted tubule

Drugs	Therapeutic Considerations	Adverse Effects	Contraindications
Hydrochlorothiazide Chlorothiazide Bendroflumethiazide Hydroflumethiazide Polythiazide Chlorthalidone Metolazone Indapamide	Hypertension Adjunct in edema states associated with heart failure, hepatic cirrhosis, renal dysfunction, corticosteroid, and estrogen therapy Gordon syndrome (PHA2; pseudohypoaldosteronism type 2)	Cardiac arrhythmia, Stevens-Johnson syndrome, toxic epidermal necrolysis, pancreatitis, hepatotoxicity (shared adverse effects); hyponatremia, hypokalemic metabolic alkalosis, glaucoma, renal impairment (hydrochlorothiazide only); systemic lupus erythematosus, coma (chlorothiazide and bendroflumethiazide only); agranulocytosis, aplastic or hemolytic anemia (chlorothiazide, bendroflumethiazide, indapamide, and metolazone only); pulmonary edema (chlorothiazide only); seizure, venous thrombosis (metolazone only) Hypotension, vasculitis, rash, photosensitivity, hyperglycemia, hyperuricemia, gastrointestinal upset, headache, blurred vision, fatigue	Shared contraindications: Anuria Hypersensitivity to sulfonamides Metolazone only: Hepatic coma	First-line agents for treatment of hypertension; also used in combination with loop agents for synergistic diuretic effect in heart failure. Used to diminish hypercalciuria in patients at risk for nephrolithiasis and (rarely) to decrease urinary calcium wasting in osteoporosis. Hydrochlorothiazide decreases glucose tolerance and may unmask diabetes in patients at risk for impaired glucose metabolism. Should not be administered concurrently with antiarrhythmic agents that prolong the QT interval. In patients with nephrogenic diabetes insipidus, thiazide diuretics can paradoxically produce a modest decrease in urine flow. Thiazides reduce uric acid excretion by increased net uric acid reabsorption and can induce gout attacks.

continues

DRUG SUMMARY TABLE: CHAPTER 21 Pharmacology of Volume Regulation *continued*

COLLECTING DUCT (POTASSIUM-SPARING) DIURETICS

Mechanism—Spironolactone and eplerenone inhibit aldosterone action by binding to and preventing nuclear translocation of the mineralocorticoid receptor. Amiloride and triamterene are competitive inhibitors of the ENaC sodium channel in the apical membrane of the principal cell.

DRUG	CLINICAL APPLICATIONS	*SERIOUS* AND COMMON ADVERSE EFFECTS	CONTRAINDICATIONS	THERAPEUTIC CONSIDERATIONS
Spironolactone **Eplerenone**	Shared indications: Hypertension Edema associated with heart failure, liver cirrhosis (with or without ascites), or nephrotic syndrome Spironolactone only: Hypokalemia Primary aldosteronism	*Stevens-Johnson syndrome, toxic epidermal necrolysis, hyperkalemic metabolic acidosis, gastrointestinal hemorrhage, agranulocytosis, systemic lupus erythematosus, breast cancer (not established)* Gastrointestinal upset (shared adverse effect); gynecomastia, somnolence, abnormal menstruation, impotence (spironolactone only)	Shared contraindications: Anuria Hyperkalemia Acute renal insufficiency Eplerenone only: Concomitant use with strong CYP3A4 inhibitors Concomitant use with potassium supplements or potassium-sparing diuretics Serum potassium >5.5 mEq/L Type 2 diabetes with microalbuminuria	Potassium-sparing diuretics are mild diuretics when used in isolation but can potentiate the action of more proximally acting loop diuretics. Occasionally used in combination with thiazides to counteract potassium-wasting effect of thiazide. Spironolactone also antagonizes the androgen receptor; this cross-reactivity can cause impotence and gynecomastia in men but confers therapeutic advantage in women with acne and hirsutism; eplerenone has less antiandrogenic activity. Used to treat hypokalemic alkalotic states secondary to mineralocorticoid excess in heart failure, hepatic failure, and other disease states associated with diminished aldosterone metabolism. Both spironolactone and eplerenone reduce mortality in patients with heart failure; the mechanism may be related to inhibition of cardiac fibrosis resulting from a paracrine aldosterone-signaling pathway.
Amiloride **Triamterene**	Amiloride only: Hypertension Heart failure Triamterene only: Edema	*Diseases of the hematopoietic system, hyperkalemic metabolic acidosis (shared adverse effects); nephrotoxicity (triamterene only)* Electrolyte imbalance, dyspepsia, headache	Shared contraindications: Hypersensitivity to drug Anuria Concomitant use with potassium-sparing agents or potassium supplementation Hyperkalemia Diabetic nephropathy Renal insufficiency Triamterene only: Liver disease	Amiloride and triamterene are drugs of choice for treatment of Liddle syndrome, a rare, Mendelian form of hypertension resulting from gain-of-function mutations in ENaC β- or γ-subunits.

22

Pharmacology of Vascular Tone

William M. Oldham and Joseph Loscalzo

INTRODUCTION

While the heart provides cardiac output, the blood vessels play a critical role in the distribution of oxygen and nutrients to metabolically active tissues. Blood flow to these tissues is exquisitely controlled by a variety of stimuli that act on vascular smooth muscle cells to regulate **vascular tone** (i.e., the degree of contraction of vascular smooth muscle). Dysregulation of vascular tone contributes to the pathogenesis of a variety of diseases, including hypertension, coronary artery disease, Raynaud's phenomenon, and migraine headache. Multiple signal transduction pathways converge on the vascular smooth muscle contractile apparatus, offering numerous targets for pharmacologic intervention. Many successful therapies have already been developed based on a molecular understanding of the regulation of vascular tone. New targets continue to be identified, offering hope that, in the future, even better therapies will be available to treat patients with vascular disease.

PHYSIOLOGY OF VASCULAR TONE

Vascular tone is a key regulator of tissue perfusion, which determines whether tissues receive sufficient oxygen and nutrients to meet their metabolic demands. Blood flow distribution and circulating blood volume are tightly controlled by the tone of resistance arterioles and capacitance veins, respectively. Vascular smooth muscle cells are the functional regulatory unit of vessel tone in these regions, integrating a variety of signals to optimize their contractile state. In general, these regulatory units act through the signal transduction pathways discussed in this chapter, many of which are targets for therapeutic intervention.

Blood Vessel Physiology

Poiseuille's law approximates flow through blood vessels:

$$\text{Flow} = \frac{\Delta P \cdot r^4}{\eta \cdot L} \qquad \textbf{Equation 22-1}$$

where ΔP is the pressure drop across a length (L) of vessel, r is the vessel radius, and η is blood viscosity. This relationship demonstrates that small changes in the tone of circumferential layers of vascular smooth muscle cells, and thus vessel diameter, can have a significant impact on blood flow. The tone of the arterial portion of the circulation and the tone of the venous portion of the circulation have important yet distinctive effects on the cardiovascular system. Arterial tone directly controls systemic vascular resistance (*SVR*)

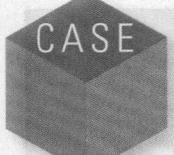

CASE

GF, a 63-year-old man with a history of hypertension, diabetes, and hyper-cholesterolemia, begins to develop episodes of chest pain with exertion. One week after his first episode, a bout of chest pain occurs while he is mowing the lawn. Twenty minutes after the onset of his pain, GF takes two of his wife's sublingual nitroglycerin tablets. Within a few minutes, he feels much better. GF feels so well that he decides to take one of the sildenafil (Viagra®) pills that a friend had previously offered to him. A few minutes after taking sildenafil, he feels flushed, develops a throbbing headache, and senses his heart racing. Upon standing, GF becomes light-headed and faints. He is taken immediately to the emergency department, where he is found to have severe hypotension. He is quickly placed in a supine position with his legs raised and monitored until he regains consciousness. The physician considers administering an α-adrenergic agonist, such as phenylephrine, but the rapid improvement in GF's blood pressure after he is placed in a supine position suggests that pharmacologic intervention is unnec-essary. After GF recovers, his physician discusses with him the dangers of taking medications without a prescription and, specifically, the risk of concurrent administration of organic nitrates and sildenafil.

Questions

1. What is the mechanism by which sublingual nitroglycerin acts so quickly to relieve chest pain?
2. What are the common adverse effects of nitroglycerin?
3. How can sildenafil and organic nitrates interact to pre-cipitate severe hypotension?
4. Are non-nitrate antihypertensives, such as calcium chan-nel blockers, also contraindicated for men taking sildenafil?
5. How can the mechanisms of action of drugs be used to pre-dict possible drug–drug interactions or lack of interactions?

and, with cardiac output (*CO*), is an important determinant of mean arterial blood pressure (*MAP*):

$$MAP = SVR \times CO$$ **Equation 22-2**

Perhaps more importantly, these changes in arteriolar resistance regulate blood flow into tissue capillary beds, where increased smooth muscle cell contraction increases vascular resistance and decreases distal perfusion. At the organismal level, a coordinated response of resistance vessels is absolutely required to redirect oxygen and nutrients to the tissues most in need.

Venous tone, by contrast, plays an important role in determining circulating blood volume. Veins are highly compliant (i.e., can accommodate large changes in volume with little change in pressure) and contain approximately 70% of blood volume during rest. Venoconstriction mobilizes these stores to increase the effective circulating blood volume, allowing perfusion of additional vascular beds (i.e., venoconstriction can be thought of as an "autotransfusion").

The heart and blood vessels form an integrated and interdependent system, and physiologic or pathophysiologic changes in vascular tone can have a significant impact on tissue perfusion as well as cardiac output. Vasoconstriction and the resulting increase in vascular resistance increases ventricular afterload, or the systolic ventricular wall stress. The volume and thickness of the left ventricle also contribute to the net stress experienced by the contracting ventricle. Venoconstriction and the resulting increase in blood return to the heart increases ventricular preload, defined as end-diastolic ventricular wall stress. These changes directly affect cardiac stroke volume through the Frank-Starling mechanism and indicate the close coupling between vascular and cardiac physiology (Fig. 22-1).

Vascular Smooth Muscle Contraction and Relaxation

As in cardiac and skeletal muscle cells, vascular smooth muscle cells use cyclic interactions between actin and myosin to generate force. This process is regulated by the **intracellular calcium (Ca^{2+})** concentration, which is normally 10,000 times lower than the extracellular concentration (2 mM). The steep transmembrane Ca^{2+} gradient is maintained by the relative impermeability of the plasma membrane to Ca^{2+} and by the actions of membrane pumps that actively export Ca^{2+}

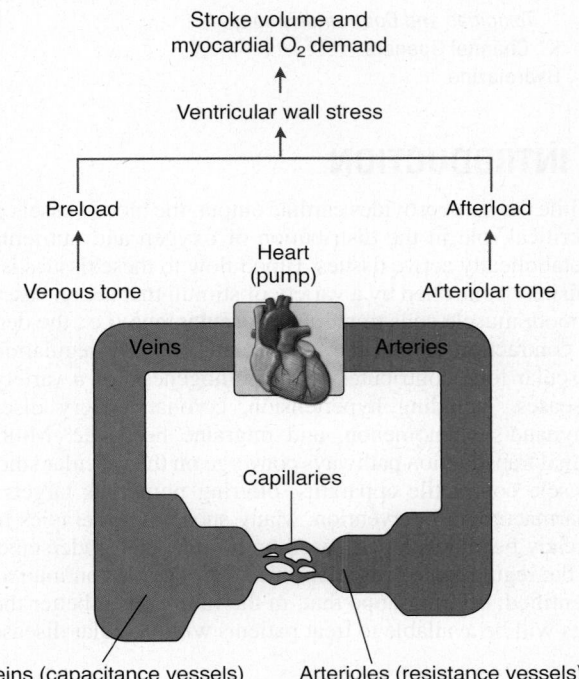

FIGURE 22-1. Coupling of vascular tone and cardiac output. Cardiac stroke volume and myocardial oxygen demand are determined, in part, by ventricular wall stress, which is a function of ventricular preload, afterload, volume, and thickness. Changes in vascular tone are coupled to cardiac output through their effects on preload and afterload. Contraction of resistance arterioles increases ventricular afterload while contraction of capacitance veins increases ventricular preload.

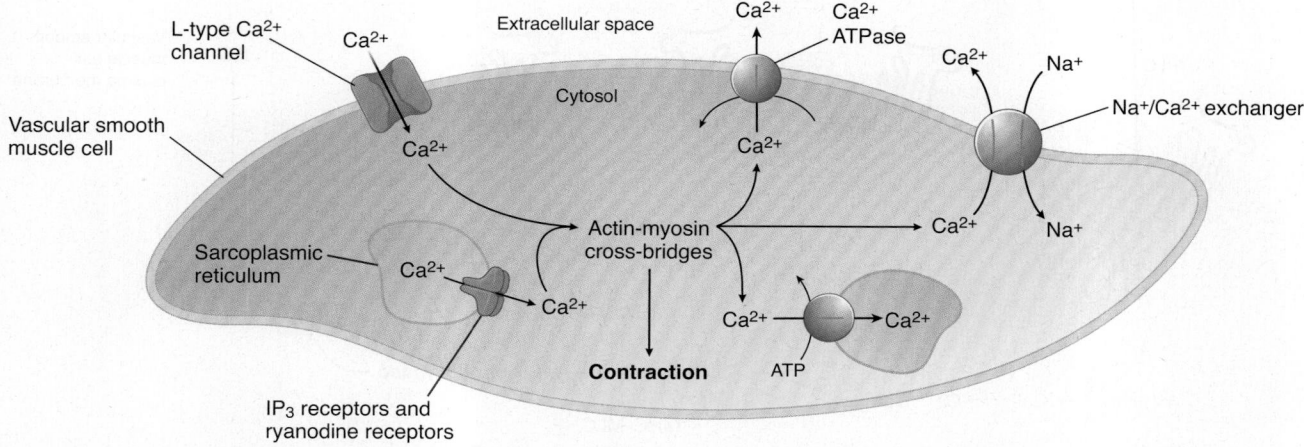

FIGURE 22-2. Regulation of intracellular Ca²⁺ in vascular smooth muscle cells. Cytosolic Ca^{2+} concentration is ~100 nM, while the extracellular and sarcoplasmic reticulum Ca^{2+} concentration is ~2 mM. Upon activation by contractile stimuli, Ca^{2+} diffuses into the cytoplasm down its concentration gradient through L-type Ca^{2+} channels in the plasma membrane and IP_3 or ryanodine receptors in the sarcoplasmic reticulum. Increased cytoplasmic Ca^{2+} triggers actin–myosin cross-bridge formation and cell contraction. Ca^{2+} is cleared from the cytoplasm by Ca^{2+} ATPases in the plasma membrane and sarcoplasmic reticulum and Na^+/Ca^{2+} exchangers in the plasma membrane.

from the cell. Contractile stimuli serve to increase intracellular Ca^{2+} through two mechanisms. First, Ca^{2+} can diffuse down its concentration gradient into the cell through Ca^{2+}-selective channels in the plasma membrane that can be opened by the activation of cell surface receptors (receptor-operated Ca^{2+} channels), by mechanical stretch, or by membrane depolarization (voltage-dependent or L-type Ca^{2+} channels). Second, Ca^{2+} can be released from intracellular stores by activation of inositol 1,4,5-trisphosphate (IP_3) receptors and Ca^{2+}-induced Ca^{2+} release through ryanodine receptors located in the sarcoplasmic reticulum. Upon termination of the contractile stimulus, Ca^{2+} is removed from the cytoplasm through active transport by Ca^{2+} ATPases in the plasma membrane and sarcoplasmic reticulum and Na^+/Ca^{2+} exchangers in the plasma membrane (Fig. 22-2).

Increases in intracellular Ca^{2+} are tightly coupled to vasoconstriction. Ca^{2+} binds to **calmodulin (CaM)**, and the Ca^{2+}/CaM complex binds to and activates **myosin light chain kinase (MLCK)**. Active MLCK phosphorylates myosin light chain (MLC), permitting myosin interactions with actin filaments, leading to cross-bridge cycling and smooth muscle contraction. Vasodilation occurs as a consequence of decreasing intracellular Ca^{2+} and dephosphorylation of MLC by MLC phosphatase (Fig. 22-3).

Regulation of Vascular Tone

Vascular smooth muscle cells integrate a variety of signals to regulate vascular tone, including local environmental factors, endothelium-derived signaling molecules, neurotransmitters, and hormones. Extracellular stimuli generally converge on shared intracellular signal transduction pathways that regulate the smooth muscle contractile apparatus. These signaling cascades are targeted by the drugs discussed in this chapter and, thus, provide the framework for understanding the mechanisms of drug action.

Signal Transduction Pathways

Intracellular signaling pathways are often shared among a variety of extracellular stimuli. These intracellular pathways will be reviewed in this section, and the extracellular

signals that activate them will be discussed in subsequent sections (Fig. 22-4).

Vasoconstriction is potentiated by three signaling pathways. First, activation of G protein-coupled receptors (GPCR) associated with heterotrimeric G_q proteins activates phospholipase C (PLC) to produce IP_3 and diacylglycerol (DAG). IP_3 stimulates Ca^{2+} release from intracellular stores by activating IP_3 receptors in the sarcoplasmic reticulum. DAG activates protein kinase C, which also promotes contraction through a variety of phosphorylation events. Second, GPCRs coupled to heterotrimeric $G_{12/13}$ proteins stimulate nucleotide exchange on the small G protein RhoA. RhoA activates Rho-kinase to phosphorylate and inactivate MLC phosphatase, thereby maintaining MLC phosphorylation. This pathway provides a mechanism to sustain smooth muscle contraction beyond transient increases in intracellular Ca^{2+}. Third, activation of G_i-coupled receptors inhibits adenylyl cyclase and thereby

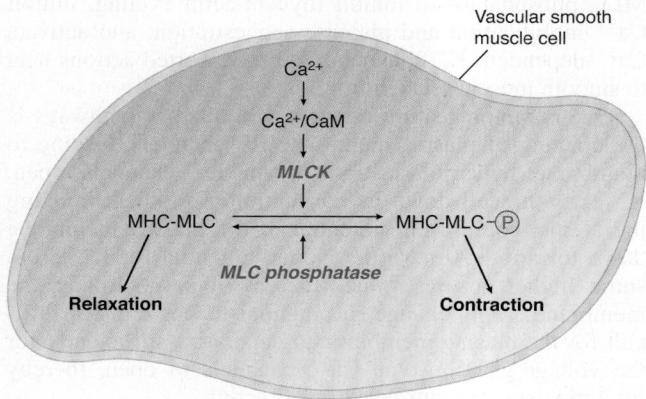

FIGURE 22-3. Vascular smooth muscle cell contractile apparatus. Increased cytoplasmic Ca^{2+} binds and activates calmodulin (CaM). The Ca^{2+}/CaM complex stimulates myosin light chain kinase (MLCK) to phosphorylate myosin light chain (MLC), which permits myosin heavy chain (MHC) binding to actin, forming actin–myosin cross-bridges. Actin and myosin filaments slide past one another as a consequence of ATP hydrolysis by myosin. Contraction ceases with the dephosphorylation of MLC by MLC phosphatase.

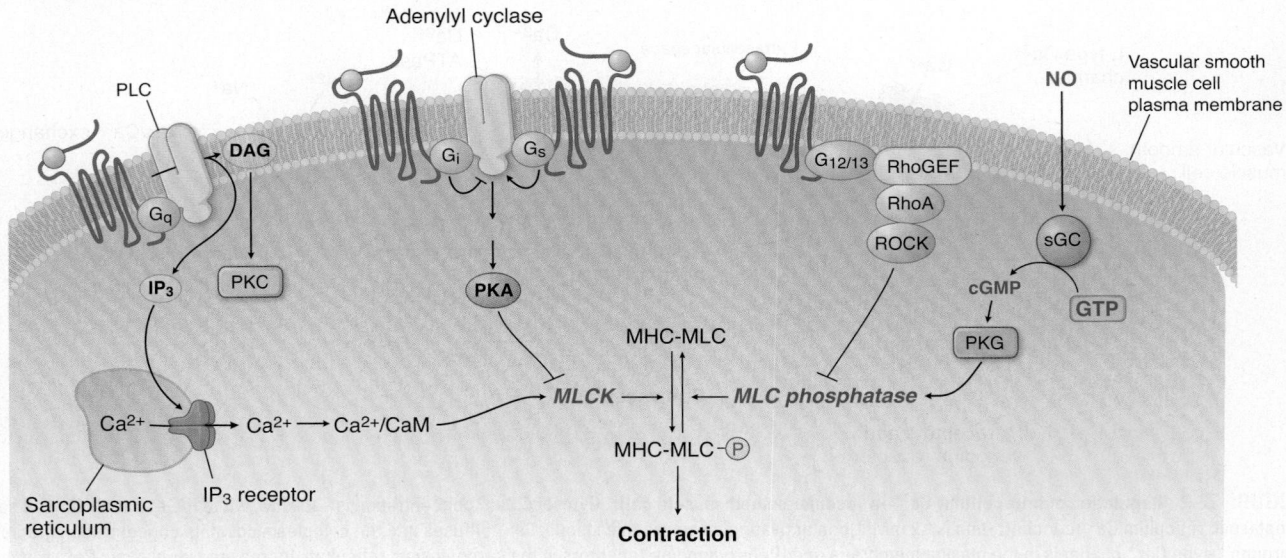

FIGURE 22-4. Intracellular signaling in vascular smooth muscle cells. Activation of G_q-coupled receptors stimulates phospholipase C (PLC) to hydrolyze membrane-bound phosphatidylinositol 4,5-bisphosphate (PIP_2) to inositol 1,4,5-trisphosphate (IP_3) and diacylglycerol (DAG). IP_3 activates receptors in the sarcoplasmic reticulum to release stored Ca^{2+}, while DAG activates protein kinase C (PKC). PKC phosphorylates Ca^{2+} channels and components of the contractile apparatus to promote smooth muscle contraction (*not shown*). Production of cAMP by adenylyl cyclase is regulated by G_i (inhibitory)- and G_s (stimulatory)-coupled receptors. Cytosolic cAMP activates protein kinase A (PKA), which phosphorylates and inactivates MLCK. Thus, G_s-coupled receptors that increase cAMP cause smooth muscle relaxation, while G_i-coupled receptors that decrease cAMP cause contraction. $G_{12/13}$-coupled receptors activate Rho kinase (ROCK) by stimulating nucleotide exchange (mediated by Rho guanine nucleotide exhange factor [RhoGEF]) on the small G protein RhoA. ROCK inhibits myosin light chain (MLC) phosphatase, thereby potentiating smooth muscle contraction. Nitric oxide (NO) stimulates cGMP production by soluble guanylyl cyclase (sGC), leading to protein kinase G (PKG) activation. PKG activates MLC phosphatase to induce smooth muscle relaxation. MHC, myosin heavy chain.

decreases production of cyclic adenosine monophosphate (cAMP). Reduced cAMP decreases protein kinase A (PKA) activity, thereby relieving inhibition of MLCK.

Vasodilation is potentiated by two signaling pathways. First, G_s-coupled receptors stimulate cAMP formation, PKA activation, MLCK inhibition, and ATP-regulated K^+ channel (K^+_{ATP}) opening. Second, nitric oxide (NO) activates soluble guanylyl cyclase (sGC) to produce cyclic guanosine monophosphate (cGMP). This second messenger activates protein kinase G (i.e., cGMP-dependent protein kinase), which phosphorylates a variety of downstream targets that activate MLC phosphatase to inhibit myosin-actin cycling, inhibit Ca^{2+} mobilization and increase sequestration, and activate Ca^{2+}-dependent K^+ channels. These concerted actions lead to smooth muscle relaxation.

One common feature of these vasodilatory pathways is the opening of plasma membrane K^+ channels, leading to membrane hyperpolarization. When K^+ channels open, K^+ exits the cell down its concentration gradient, moving the Nernst equilibrium potential of the plasma membrane down toward −90 mV (the Nernst potential for K^+) from some higher resting value (thereby hyperpolarizing the membrane). This change in potential makes it more difficult for the plasma membrane to depolarize sufficiently for the voltage-gated L-type Ca^{2+} channels to open, thereby inhibiting smooth muscle cell contraction.

Environmental Factors

Arteriolar smooth muscle cells coordinate blood flow into the capillary beds of metabolically active tissues. In regions where tissue metabolic demand exceeds supply, increases in H^+ (as lactic acid), CO_2, K^+, and adenosine (from ATP utilization) all lead to vasodilation and increased blood flow. The cerebral

circulation is particularly sensitive to fluctuations in pH and CO_2, which is why acute hyperventilation (which decreases pH and CO_2, leading to vasoconstriction and decreased cerebral blood flow) is one therapy for intracranial hypertension. Increases in extracellular K^+ activate inward rectifier K^+ channels, thereby causing hyperpolarization of the plasma membrane and inhibiting voltage-gated Ca^{2+} channel opening. Adenosine activates A_2 G_s-coupled receptors. Systemic vessels also respond to decreased O_2 by vasodilation, in contrast to pulmonary vessels that vasoconstrict (i.e., hypoxic vasoconstriction) to preserve ventilation–perfusion matching in the lung. The molecular mechanisms mediating these disparate responses remain active areas of research.

In addition to metabolic factors, vascular smooth muscle cells contract in response to stretch through the opening of stretch-activated Ca^{2+} channels in the cell membrane. This myogenic reflex protects distal capillary beds from high pressures by increasing vascular resistance. In combination with local control by metabolic factors, the myogenic reflex is an important mechanism of vascular autoregulation where the vessels adjust resistance in an attempt to maintain steady blood flow over a range of perfusion pressures (recall that Flow = Pressure/Resistance). Autoregulation is particularly evident in vascular beds that are sensitive to ischemia, such as the brain, heart, and kidneys.

Endothelial Factors

Vascular endothelial cells play a critical role in regulating vascular smooth muscle tone through direct cellular contacts and the elaboration of signaling molecules. Among these signaling molecules, NO, endothelium-derived hyperpolarizing factors, prostacyclin, and endothelin are the most relevant pharmacologically.

The obligatory role of endothelial cells in regulating vascular tone was first recognized with the observation that acetylcholine causes vasoconstriction when applied directly to de-endothelialized blood vessels but causes vasodilation when applied to normally endothelialized vessels. This finding suggested that endothelial cells produce a vasodilatory compound, initially termed endothelium-derived relaxing factor (EDRF) and subsequently proven to be NO.

Nitric oxide is a membrane-permeable gas that reacts with a variety of biomolecules to elicit cellular responses, particularly activation of sGC in vascular smooth muscle cells, leading to cGMP production. Vascular endothelial cells synthesize NO in response to a variety of stimuli, including shear stress, acetylcholine, histamine, bradykinin, sphingosine-1-phosphate, serotonin, substance P, and ATP. These factors increase intracellular Ca^{2+}, thereby stimulating the Ca^{2+}/CaM-activated endothelial NO synthase (eNOS). Endothelial eNOS produces NO from arginine, and NO subsequently diffuses to the vascular smooth muscle cell to initiate downstream signaling events and vasorelaxation (Figs. 22-4 and 22-5).

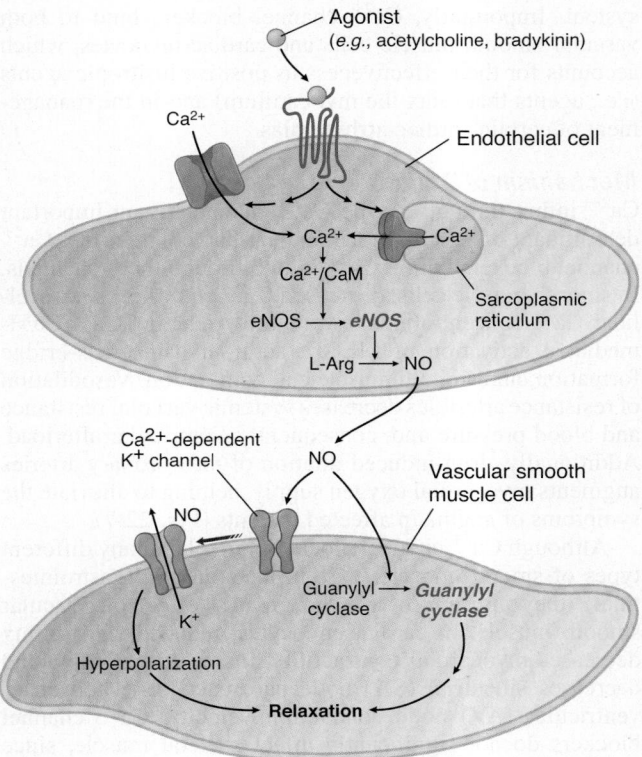

Interestingly, measured levels of NO cannot explain all of the endothelium-dependent responses of vascular smooth muscle cells. Indeed, endothelium-dependent vasodilation can be caused by smooth muscle cell hyperpolarization that is not due to NO. Several molecules have been implicated as *endothelium-derived hyperpolarizing factors* (EDHFs), including epoxyeicosatrienoic acids (arachidonic acid metabolites), hydrogen peroxide, carbon monoxide, hydrogen sulfide, C-natriuretic peptide, and K^+ itself. These mediators open a variety of K^+ channels on smooth muscle cells, leading to membrane hyperpolarization and smooth muscle cell relaxation. Hydrogen sulfide has a variety of additional effects that lead to smooth muscle relaxation, largely mediated by covalent S-sulfhydration of target proteins, including not only K^+ channels but also Ca^{2+} channels, and by stimulating release of other EDHFs.

Prostacyclin is also a vasodilatory molecule produced in endothelial cells from arachidonic acid in reactions that involve the cyclooxygenase (COX) enzymes. Prostacyclin activates G_s-coupled receptors on the vascular smooth muscle cells, leading to vasodilation. Since the COX enzymes are inhibited by nonsteroidal anti-inflammatory drugs, such drugs should be used with caution in patients with hypertension because they decrease prostacyclin production.

In contrast to the potent vasodilating effects of the molecules described above, endothelial cells also produce the most potent endogenous vasoconstrictor known, **endothelin-1** (ET-1). ET-1 is a 21-amino acid peptide synthesized as preproendothelin, which is cleaved to big endothelin and subsequently to ET-1 by endothelin converting enzyme. ET-1 is released by endothelial cells in response to mechanical stress and vasoactive agents (e.g., vasopressin, angiotensin II), while its release is inhibited by prostacyclin, NO, and atrial natriuretic peptide. ET-1 binds to two receptor subtypes, ET_A and ET_B, and both are G_q-coupled receptors. Both subtypes are located on vascular smooth muscle cells and mediate vasoconstriction. Interestingly, endothelial cells express ET_B receptors, which, when occupied by ET-1, activate eNOS and COX, leading to NO and prostacyclin release. This negative feedback pathway is one mechanism by which endothelial cells assist in modulating vascular tone (Fig. 22-6).

Autonomic Nervous System

Vascular smooth muscle cells receive input from the sympathetic nervous system, which is an important determinant of vascular tone. Sympathetic nerves innervate vascular smooth muscle cells in both arteries and veins, and sympathetic activation leads to both vasoconstriction and venoconstriction. Sympathetic postganglionic neurons release norepinephrine, which binds to postsynaptic α_1- and α_2-adrenergic receptors coupled to G_q and G_i, respectively, leading to contraction of the smooth muscle cell (Fig. 22-4). The presynaptic nerve terminal also expresses α_2-adrenergic autoreceptors, which inhibit further release of norepinephrine in a negative feedback loop.

Sympathetic activation also induces epinephrine release from the adrenal medulla. In contrast to norepinephrine, epinephrine activates both α- and β_2-adrenergic receptors on vascular smooth muscle cells. The β_2 receptors activate the G_s signaling pathway, leading to smooth muscle cell relaxation (Fig. 22-4). Thus, the effects of epinephrine on a given vascular bed depend on the dose (β_2 receptors have a higher affinity for epinephrine and, thus, are activated at lower epinephrine

FIGURE 22-5. Endothelial regulation of nitric oxide-mediated vascular smooth muscle relaxation. Endothelial cell production of nitric oxide (NO) controls the extent of vascular smooth muscle cell relaxation. Production of NO is stimulated by agonists such as acetylcholine or bradykinin. Stimulation of receptors by these agonists activates Ca^{2+} second messenger systems and promotes direct entry of Ca^{2+} into the cytosol. The increased cytosolic Ca^{2+} activates a Ca^{2+}/calmodulin (Ca^{2+}/CaM) complex that stimulates endothelial nitric oxide synthase (eNOS), an enzyme that catalyzes the formation of NO from L-arginine (L-Arg, an amino acid). Nitric oxide diffuses from the endothelial cell into subjacent vascular smooth muscle cells, where it activates guanylyl cyclase, promoting smooth muscle cell relaxation. NO can also directly activate Ca^{2+}-dependent K^+ channels. This parallel signaling pathway contributes to relaxation by hyperpolarizing the smooth muscle cell. The active form of each enzyme is shown in *italicized blue*.

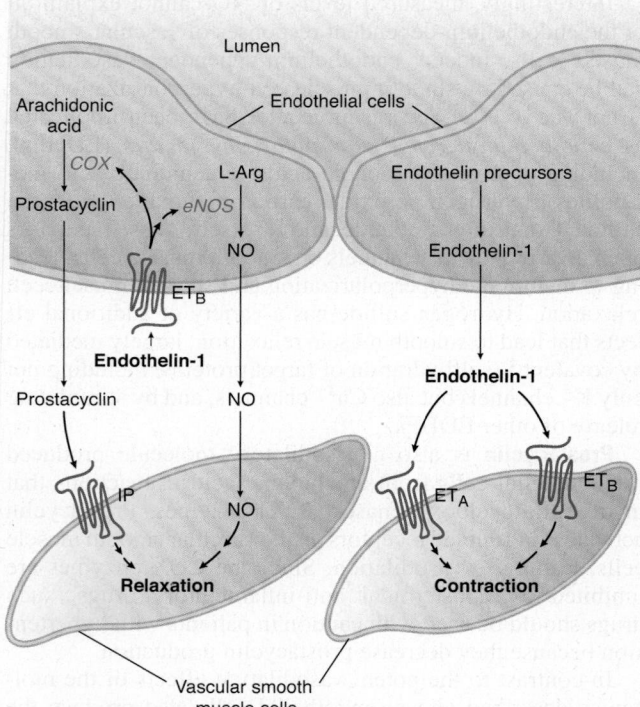

FIGURE 22-6. Effects of endothelin on the blood vessel wall. Endothelin mediates both contraction and relaxation of vascular smooth muscle cells. Endothelin precursors in endothelial cells are processed to ET-1. ET-1 is secreted on the basal side of the endothelial cell, where it interacts with G_q-coupled ET_A and ET_B receptors on vascular smooth muscle cells to stimulate vasoconstriction. ET_B receptors are also expressed on endothelial cells. Endothelial cell ET_B activation stimulates cyclooxygenase (COX), which catalyzes the formation of prostacyclin from arachidonic acid. Prostacyclin diffuses from the endothelial cell to the vascular smooth muscle cell membrane, where it binds to and activates the prostacyclin (IP) receptor. ET_B activation also stimulates endothelial nitric oxide synthase (eNOS), which catalyzes the formation of NO from arginine (L-Arg). Both prostacyclin and NO stimulate vascular smooth muscle cell relaxation.

concentrations than α receptors) and the relative composition of receptors expressed on the target cells. For example, during a "fight or flight" response, blood flow is diverted away from skin and viscera, where $\alpha > \beta_2$, and toward skeletal muscle, where $\beta_2 > \alpha$.

While most blood vessels lack parasympathetic innervation, acetylcholine does cause vasodilation through M_3-muscarinic receptor-mediated NO release from vascular endothelial cells (Fig. 22-5).

Humoral Regulators

In addition to the autonomic nervous system, several humoral mediators contribute to the regulation of vascular tone and integrate renal and cardiovascular function. Among these, angiotensin II and vasopressin are potent vasoconstrictors through their activation of G_q-coupled AT_1 and V_1 receptors, respectively (Fig. 22-4). These mediators act to increase both vascular resistance and intravascular volume in response to hypovolemia (i.e., hemorrhagic shock) through coordinated actions in the blood vessels and kidney. Atrial and brain natriuretic peptides are released in response to hypervolemia and induce vasodilation through the activation of membrane-bound guanylyl cyclase receptors and

production of cGMP. Histamine and bradykinin also act as vasodilators. Histamine activates G_s-coupled H_2 receptors on vascular smooth muscle cells to cause vasodilation (Fig. 22-4) and G_q-coupled H_1 receptors on endothelial cells to cause NO generation (Fig. 22-5). Bradykinin also stimulates NO production through the β_2 receptor on endothelial cells (Fig. 22-5).

■ PHARMACOLOGIC CLASSES AND AGENTS

The pharmacologic agents considered in this chapter are all vasodilators, that is, drugs that act on vascular smooth muscle cells or endothelial cells to decrease vascular tone. This effect can be accomplished either by inhibiting components of contractile signal transduction pathways or by potentiating effects of relaxing signal transduction pathways.

Ca²⁺ Channel Blockers

Ca^{2+} channel blockers are among the most prescribed agents for the management of hypertension and angina owing to their effectiveness and ease of use. These agents are primarily arterial vasodilators, having little impact on the venous system. Importantly, Ca^{2+} channel blockers bind to both vascular smooth muscle cells and cardiac myocytes, which accounts for their effectiveness as positive lusitropic agents (i.e., agents that relax the myocardium) and in the management of certain cardiac arrhythmias.

Mechanism of Action

Ca^{2+} influx through L-type Ca^{2+} channels is an important determinant of vascular tone and cardiac contractility. Ca^{2+} channel blockers inhibit Ca^{2+} influx through these channels. In smooth muscle cells, decreased Ca^{2+} entry keeps intracellular Ca^{2+} concentrations low, thereby reducing Ca^{2+}/CaM-mediated activation of MLCK, actin–myosin cross-bridge formation, and smooth muscle cell contraction. Vasodilation of resistance arterioles decreases systemic vascular resistance and blood pressure and, consequently, ventricular afterload. Additionally, drug-induced dilation of the coronary arteries augments myocardial oxygen supply, helping to alleviate the symptoms of angina in affected patients (Fig. 22-7).

Although Ca^{2+} channel blockers can relax many different types of smooth muscle (e.g., bronchiolar and gastrointestinal), they appear to have the greatest effect on vascular smooth muscle. In cardiac myocytes, reduced Ca^{2+} influx decreases myocardial contractility, increases lusitropy, and decreases sinoatrial (SA) node pacemaker rate and atrioventricular (AV) node conduction velocity. Ca^{2+} channel blockers do not significantly affect skeletal muscle, since these cells depend mainly on intracellular Ca^{2+} stores in the sarcoplasmic reticulum to support excitation–contraction coupling and do not rely on transmembrane Ca^{2+} influx.

Chemical Classes

Three chemical classes of Ca^{2+} channel blockers are currently in clinical use: dihydropyridines (e.g., **nifedipine**, **amlodipine**, and **felodipine**), benzothiazepines (e.g., **diltiazem**), and phenylalkylamines (e.g., **verapamil**). All three classes inhibit L-type Ca^{2+} channels, but each class has distinctive pharmacologic effects owing to differences in drug binding sites on the channels, different affinities for particular channel conformations (e.g., closed, open, or inactivated), and different affinities for the subtypes of L-type Ca^{2+} channels.

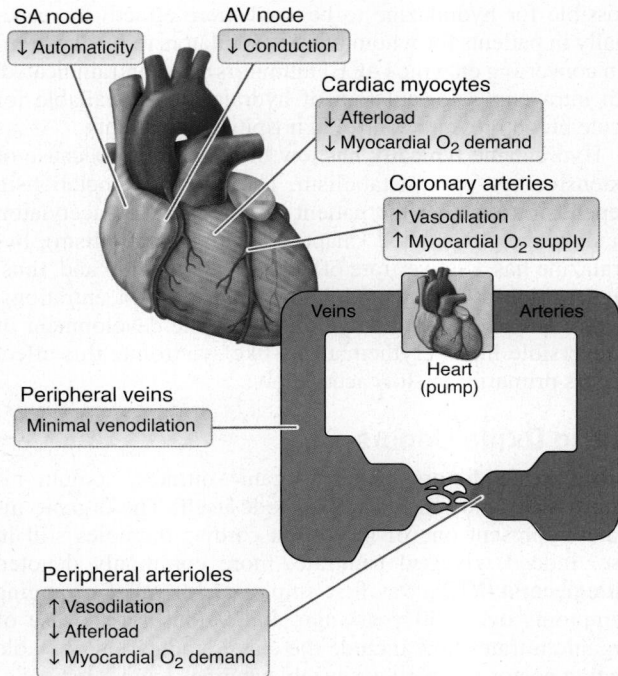

FIGURE 22-7. Sites of action of Ca²⁺ channel blockers. Ca²⁺ channel blockers dilate coronary arteries and peripheral arterioles, but not veins. They also decrease cardiac contractility, automaticity at the SA node, and conduction at the AV node. Dilation of the coronary arteries increases myocardial O₂ supply. Dilation of systemic (peripheral) arterioles decreases afterload and thereby decreases myocardial O₂ demand. However, some Ca²⁺ channel blockers (especially dihydropyridines) cause reflex tachycardia, which can paradoxically increase myocardial O₂ demand. Decreased cardiac contractility and decreased SA node automaticity also decrease myocardial O₂ demand. The inhibition of AV node conduction by some Ca²⁺ channel blockers makes them useful as antiarrhythmic agents. Note that the effects diagrammed here are representative effects of the class of drugs; individual agents are more or less selective for each of these effects.

All three classes of Ca²⁺ channel blockers bind to separate but allosterically connected binding sites on the α₁ ion pore-forming subunit of the channel. Dihydropyridines inhibit the Ca²⁺ channel from the extracellular space through a binding site buried in the lipid bilayer. Diltiazem binds the ion pore from the extracellular side of the channel, while verapamil is thought to enter the cell and block the cytoplasmic opening of the pore.

Dihydropyridines exhibit much greater arterial vasodilation than non-dihydropyridines, while having relatively little impact on cardiac tissue (i.e., there is less depression of myocardial contractility, less impairment of SA node automaticity, and less slowing of AV node conduction velocity). These differential effects are due, in part, to the preference of dihydropyridines to bind to inactivated channels. Since smooth muscle cells have a relatively depolarized resting membrane potential (-70 mV) compared to cardiac myocytes (-100 mV), their calcium channels are more likely to be in the inactive conformation and are, therefore, inhibited by lower concentrations of dihydropyridine agents. By contrast, non-dihydropyridines bind to the open conformation and prolong the channel refractory period (i.e., increase the channel recovery time), thereby decreasing the number of conducting channels as depolarizations occur more frequently.

Thus, non-dihydropyridines are more effective in tissue with frequent channel openings (i.e., SA node, AV node, and cardiac myocytes), and channel inhibition increases in proportion to heart rate. The negative chronotropic and inotropic effects of non-dihydropyridine agents appear greater for verapamil than diltiazem.

L-type Ca²⁺ channels are a family of four different multimeric protein complexes defined by the gene encoding the pore-forming α₁ subunit ($Ca_V1.1–1.4$). $Ca_V1.2$ and $Ca_V1.3$ are the isoforms found on cardiac myocytes and vascular smooth muscle cells. Alternate splicing of the $Ca_V1.2$ gene in heart and vascular smooth muscle cells also contributes to preferential inhibition of smooth muscle by dihydropyridines.

Pharmacokinetics

Ca²⁺ channel blockers are typically administered in oral dosage forms, although intravenous formulations of diltiazem and verapamil are available. **Clevidipine** is a dihydropyridine agent that is available only as an intravenous formulation. Three pharmacokinetic properties of most Ca²⁺ channel blockers are suboptimal. First, orally administered Ca²⁺ channel blockers undergo significant first-pass metabolism in the gut and liver, significantly reducing bioavailability to 10–30%. Second, most of these drugs have a rapid onset of action, between 20 minutes and 2 hours. In the case of nifedipine, oral administration can lead to a rapid and precipitous fall in blood pressure, resulting in severe reflex tachycardia. This worsens myocardial ischemia by increasing myocardial O₂ demand and it also decreases O₂ supply as a result of shortened diastole. Third, these agents typically have short elimination half-lives (2–10 hours), necessitating short dosing intervals or extended-release preparations (available for all commonly administered Ca²⁺ channel blockers).

Amlodipine was developed in an attempt to overcome the pharmacokinetic limitations of nifedipine. This drug has an increased oral bioavailability of 60%, a long time to onset of 6 hours, and a long elimination half-life of 40 hours. These kinetic properties are likely due, in part, to its lipophilic character and its positive charge at physiologic pH, which lead to increased association with negatively charged plasma membranes.

All Ca²⁺ channel blockers are metabolized by the liver. Diltiazem is primarily excreted by the liver, while dihydropyridines and verapamil are primarily excreted in the urine.

Toxicities and Contraindications

The toxicities of Ca²⁺ channel blockers are mainly a consequence of the mechanism of action. Like all vasodilators, Ca²⁺ channel blockers can cause headache, dizziness, lightheadedness, and flushing. Constipation is a common adverse effect of verapamil that is likely caused by excessive smooth muscle relaxation in the gastrointestinal tract. These agents also cause peripheral edema by increasing the transcapillary hydrostatic pressure. Venodilating agents can mitigate this effect, while diuretics are less efficacious with this class of agents.

When taken at doses that lead to drug concentrations higher than the therapeutic window, the negative chronotropic and inotropic effects of verapamil and diltiazem can lead to bradycardia, AV block, and heart failure. Patients taking β-adrenergic blockers (which are also negative inotropes) are often advised not to use diltiazem or verapamil concomitantly because of the increased likelihood of excessive cardiac depression. Some studies have suggested that Ca^{2+} channel blockers increase the risk of mortality in patients with heart failure, and Ca^{2+} channel blockers are contraindicated in the management of heart failure. Some reports also suggest that the short-acting agents, such as nifedipine, are associated with an increased risk of myocardial ischemia and infarction due to impairment of myocardial O_2 supply (see above).

K^+ Channel Openers

K^+ channel openers cause direct arterial vasodilation by opening K^+_{ATP} channels in the plasma membrane of vascular smooth muscle cells, leading to membrane hyperpolarization and preventing Ca^{2+} channel opening (see above). While not commonly employed as first-line agents owing to the multiple adverse effects described below, K^+ channel openers represent a useful family of drugs for refractory hypertension because of this unique mechanism of action.

The K^+_{ATP} channel openers include **minoxidil** and **nicorandil**. These drugs act primarily on arterial smooth muscle cells and therefore decrease arterial blood pressure. Adverse effects of K^+ channel openers include headache and flushing, caused by excessive dilation of cerebral and cutaneous arteries, respectively. Similar to Ca^{2+} channel blockers, these agents can cause peripheral edema, necessitating the use of diuretics. When arterial vasodilators are used as monotherapy, the decrease in arterial pressure often elicits sympathetic activation, reflex tachycardia, and increased myocardial O_2 demand. Use of β-adrenergic blockers can mitigate these adverse effects and preserve the therapeutic utility of arterial vasodilators. Minoxidil can also cause hypertrichosis; as a result, it is more commonly prescribed as a therapy for male pattern baldness.

Hydralazine

Hydralazine is an arteriolar vasodilator that is sometimes used in the treatment of hypertension and, in combination with isosorbide dinitrate, in the treatment of heart failure. The mechanism of action of hydralazine remains unclear; current evidence suggests that hydralazine may cause membrane hyperpolarization by opening K^+_{ATP} channels and inhibiting IP_3-induced Ca^{2+} release from the sarcoplasmic reticulum in vascular smooth muscle cells. More recently, hydralazine has been shown to decrease the promoter methylation and, thereby, increase the gene expression of *SERCA2a*, which is the Ca^{2+} pump that transports cytoplasmic Ca^{2+} back into the sarcoplasmic reticulum. While this mechanism would not account for the acute effects of hydralazine, it may play an important role in patients on chronic therapy. Hydralazine appears to prevent the development of nitrate tolerance, perhaps by inhibiting vascular superoxide production and by scavenging peroxynitrite formed from superoxide and NO. The combination of hydralazine and nitrates has a demonstrated mortality benefit in patients with persistent symptoms of advanced systolic heart failure despite optimal medical therapy. The data suggest that this effect is stronger in black Americans, possibly because of decreased NO bioavailability or NO signaling in this population.

Hydralazine is not first-line therapy for hypertension owing to the requirement for frequent dosing and the rapid development of tachyphylaxis to its antihypertensive effects. As the benefits of combination therapy for hypertension and heart failure are becoming better appreciated, it may be possible for hydralazine to be used more effectively, especially in patients for whom other vasodilators (e.g., angiotensin converting enzyme [ACE] inhibitors) are contraindicated. An intravenous formulation of hydralazine is available for acute blood pressure control in hospitalized patients.

Hydralazine typically has low bioavailability because of extensive first-pass metabolism. The rate of its metabolism depends on whether the patient is a slow or fast acetylator. In slow acetylators (see Chapter 4, Drug Metabolism), hydralazine has a slower rate of hepatic degradation and, thus, higher bioavailability and higher plasma concentrations. A rare adverse effect of hydralazine is the development of a reversible lupus erythematosus-like syndrome; this effect occurs primarily in slow acetylators.

Nitric Oxide Donors

Nitric oxide donors include organic nitrates, sodium nitroprusside, and inhaled nitric oxide itself. The organic nitrates represent one of the oldest cardiac therapies still in use. Indeed, glyceryl trinitrate, more commonly denoted **nitroglycerin (NTG)**, was first employed for relief of angina symptoms over 100 years ago. Indications for the use of organic nitrates now include the classic indication of stable angina pectoris as well as unstable angina, acute myocardial infarction, hypertension, and heart failure.

Mechanism of Action

Within the body, nitric oxide donors are chemically reduced to release NO, the first described *gasotransmitter*, or gaseous signaling molecule. Nitric oxide reacts with a variety of biomolecules; however, soluble guanylyl cyclase is recognized as its primary physiologic receptor. Activation of guanylyl cyclase by NO induces smooth muscle relaxation as described above (Fig. 22-4).

Although NO can dilate both arteries and veins, venous dilation predominates at therapeutic doses. This effect contrasts with Ca^{2+} channel blockers and K^+ channel openers, which cause primarily arteriolar vasodilation. Venodilation increases venous capacitance, leading to a decrease in blood return to the right ventricle and, consequently, to decreased right and left ventricular end-diastolic pressure and volume. Decreased preload decreases myocardial O_2 demand while facilitating subendocardial perfusion owing to decreased diastolic wall stress. Mild effects on arterial vasodilation decrease afterload and improve blood flow through coronary arteries, all contributing to improved myocardial O_2 supply/demand matching. Moreover, this hemodynamic profile is beneficial in patients with congestive heart failure, since decreases in ventricular preload minimize the development of pulmonary edema while decreases in afterload improve ventricular stroke volume (Fig. 22-8).

In the coronary circulation, NTG predominantly dilates large epicardial coronary arteries with only minimal effects on the coronary resistance vessels. This preferential action minimizes the development of the coronary steal phenomenon, where vasodilators, by decreasing the resistance of normal arteries, can divert ("steal") blood flow away from regions of the heart with stenotic coronary arteries that are already maximally dilated.

The generation of NO from organic nitrates can also cause relaxation of other types of smooth muscle, including esophageal, bronchial, biliary, intestinal, and genitourinary. Indeed, the ability of NTG to relieve the angina-like chest

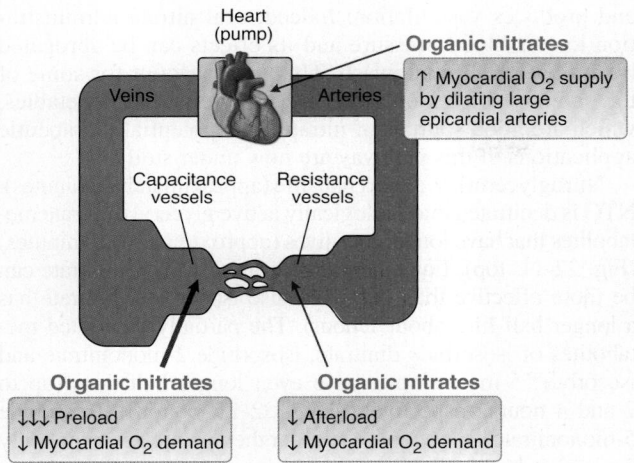

FIGURE 22-8. Sites of action of organic nitrates. Organic nitrates exert the majority of their vasodilator action on venous capacitance vessels. This selectivity results in greatly decreased preload, with resulting decreased myocardial O_2 demand. Organic nitrates also mildly dilate arteriolar resistance vessels, with resulting decreased afterload and decreased myocardial O_2 demand. Myocardial O_2 supply is mildly increased by dilation of large epicardial arteries.

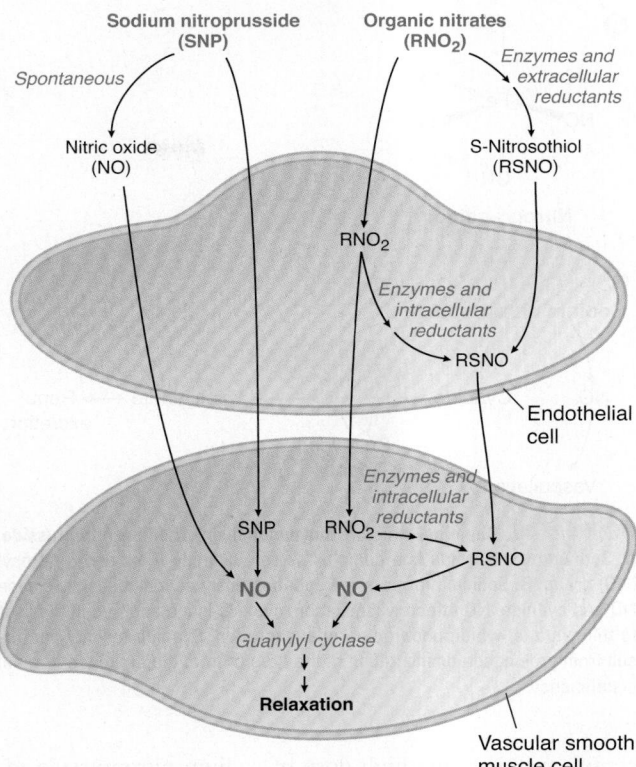

FIGURE 22-9. Biotransformation of organic nitrates and sodium nitroprusside. Organic nitrates and sodium nitroprusside increase local levels of nitric oxide (NO) by different mechanisms. Organic nitrates have the chemical structure RNO_2. The nitro group is reduced to form NO in the presence of specific enzymes and extracellular or intracellular reductants (e.g., thiols). In comparison, sodium nitroprusside releases NO spontaneously without enzymatic aid. Both agents effect relaxation via the formation of NO. However, the requirement of organic nitrates for specific cellular enzymes or reductants may result in tissue selectivity. Because sodium nitroprusside spontaneously converts to NO, it does not dilate vascular beds selectively.

pain of esophageal spasm can occasionally result in a misdiagnosis of coronary artery disease. These actions of nitrates on nonvascular smooth muscle are usually of limited clinical significance.

Nitric oxide generated from organic nitrates also functions as an antiplatelet agent. Nitric oxide-mediated increases in platelet cGMP inhibit platelet aggregation. Together with the vasodilatory effect of nitrates, this antiplatelet effect may decrease the likelihood of coronary artery thrombosis. Nitrate-induced inhibition of platelet aggregation may be especially important in the treatment of rest angina (i.e., chest pain that occurs spontaneously at rest) because rest angina frequently results from the formation of occlusive platelet aggregates at the site of atherosclerotic coronary artery lesions. Rest angina is also known as unstable angina because the thrombotic occlusions that cause rest angina can evolve into complete occlusion, resulting in myocardial infarction.

Chemical Classes

Organic nitrates do not release NO directly but are chemically or enzymatically reduced to form S-nitrosothiols with available sulfhydryl groups on proteins or glutathione (Fig. 22-9). The S-nitrosothiols are subsequently reduced to generate free NO, which then activates sGC. The reduction of organic nitrates can be catalyzed in tissues expressing specific enzymes, such as mitochondrial aldehyde dehydrogenase, suggesting one mechanism by which their effects may be "targeted" to specific vascular tissues. (In contrast, the inorganic nitrate sodium nitroprusside does not manifest tissue-specific effects; see below). Interestingly, S-nitrosylation itself is becoming increasingly recognized as an important post-translational modification of proteins, with a variety of effects on protein structure and function, and has been implicated in the pathogenesis of a variety of diseases (e.g., Alzheimer's disease).

Several different preparations of organic nitrates are available. The most commonly used organic nitrates include NTG, **isosorbide dinitrate**, and **isosorbide 5-mononitrate**. Although these drugs share a common mechanism of action, they differ in their routes of administration and pharmacokinetics, leading to important differences in therapeutic utility.

Sodium nitroprusside is an inorganic compound in which one nitrosyl group and five cyanide groups are coordinated to an iron atom (Fig. 22-10). Upon infusion, sodium nitroprusside is reduced by oxyhemoglobin and subsequently releases NO and five cyanide molecules. As a result of the nonenzymatic release of NO, sodium nitroprusside's action does not appear to be targeted to specific vessels, and, consequently, the drug dilates both arteries and veins. This agent is used intravenously for effective hemodynamic control in hypertensive emergencies and severe heart failure. Owing to its rapid onset of action, short duration of action, and high efficacy, sodium nitroprusside must be infused with continuous blood pressure monitoring and careful titration of dose to effect. In addition to NO release, decomposition of sodium nitroprusside releases cyanide, which is metabolized to thiocyanate by thiosulfate sulfotransferase (rhodanese) in the liver. Thiocyanate is subsequently excreted by the kidneys (Fig. 22-10). Excessive cyanide accumulation can lead to acid–base disturbances, cardiac arrhythmias, and death. Thiocyanate toxicity can occur in patients with impaired renal function, causing disorientation, psychosis, muscle spasms, and seizures. The accumulation of methemoglobin is usually not clinically

A

NO

NC⟋⟋⟋ Fe^{+2} ⟍⟍⟍ CN
NC ⟍ ⟍ CN

CN

Nitroprusside

B

Sodium nitroprusside

NO   Cyanide → Liver → Thiocyanate → Renal excretion

Sulfhydryl donor

Vasodilation

FIGURE 22-10. Chemical structure and metabolism of sodium nitroprusside. **A.** Sodium nitroprusside is a complex of iron, cyanide (CN), and a nitrosyl (NO) group. **B.** Sodium nitroprusside spontaneously decomposes to release NO and cyanide. NO effects vasodilation; cyanide is metabolized in the liver to thiocyanate, which undergoes renal excretion. Cyanide toxicity can result from prolonged administration of the drug or from the presence of renal insufficiency.

significant given the high dose of sodium nitroprusside required to generate significant amounts of methemoglobin.

Inhaled NO gas can be used to dilate the pulmonary vasculature selectively. Because NO is rapidly inactivated by binding to blood hemoglobin, NO gas has little effect on systemic blood pressure when administered by inhalation. Therapy with inhaled NO has established efficacy in the treatment of primary pulmonary hypertension of the newborn. In adults with severe acute respiratory distress syndrome, inhaled NO improves ventilation–perfusion matching and oxygenation by vasodilating vessels adjacent to ventilated alveoli but has not been shown to improve mortality.

Pharmacokinetics

The pharmacokinetics of the different nitrate formulations provide a basis for the preferential use of specific agents and dosage forms in certain settings. For example, the rapid onset of action of sublingual nitrate preparations is desirable for rapid relief of acute angina attacks, while longer acting nitrates are more valuable for angina prophylaxis in the long-term management of coronary artery disease. Orally administered NTG and isosorbide dinitrate have low bioavailability because organic nitrate reductases in the liver rapidly metabolize these drugs. NTG or isosorbide dinitrate can be administered sublingually to circumvent the first-pass effect and to attain therapeutic blood levels within minutes. Intravenous administration of NTG is indicated when continuous titration of drug effect is necessary, for example, in the treatment of unstable angina or acute heart failure. Slow-release transdermal and buccal preparations of NTG provide therapeutic steady-state levels of NTG that can be useful for angina prevention in patients with stable coronary artery disease.

Interestingly, nitrate from dietary sources also plays an important role in blood pressure regulation. Facultative anaerobes on the tongue utilize nitrate as an electron acceptor, releasing nitrite into the saliva. In the acidic environment of the stomach, some nitrite is reduced to NO, which is absorbed

and produces vasodilation. Indeed, oral nitrate administration lowers blood pressure and its effects can be abrogated by antibacterial mouthwash. This may account for some of the salutary effects of a diet rich in fruits and vegetables, which are good sources of nitrate. The potential therapeutic applications of this pathway are now under study.

Nitroglycerin has a short half-life (approximately 5 minutes). NTG is denitrated into biologically active glyceryl dinitrate metabolites that have longer half-lives (approximately 40 minutes) (Fig. 22-11, top). Equivalent doses of isosorbide dinitrate can be more effective than NTG because isosorbide dinitrate has a longer half-life (about 1 hour). The partially denitrated metabolites of isosorbide dinitrate, isosorbide 2-mononitrate and isosorbide 5-mononitrate, have even longer half-lives (up to 2 and 4 hours, respectively) (Fig. 22-11, bottom). Isosorbide 5-mononitrate has become a popular therapeutic agent, not only because it has prolonged therapeutic effects but also because it is well absorbed from the gastrointestinal tract and is not susceptible to extensive first-pass metabolism in the liver. The bioavailability of orally administered isosorbide 5-mononitrate

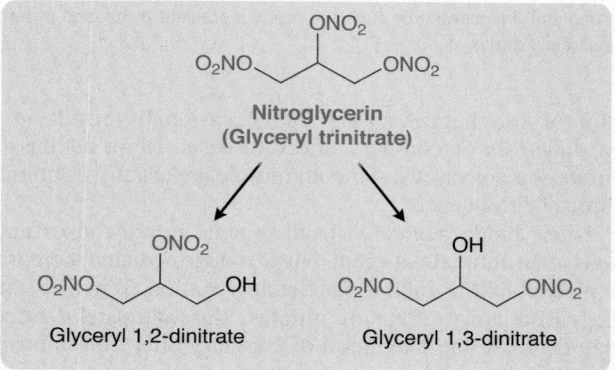

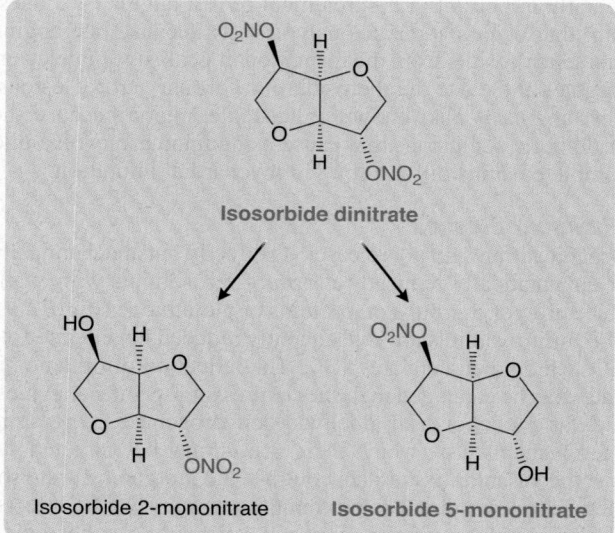

FIGURE 22-11. Chemical structures and metabolism of nitroglycerin and isosorbide dinitrate. Nitroglycerin and isosorbide dinitrate are biologically active nitrates that are metabolized into active molecules with longer half-lives than their parent compounds. Nitroglycerin is denitrated into glyceryl 1,2-dinitrate and glyceryl 1,3-dinitrate; these active metabolites have a half-life of approximately 40 minutes. Isosorbide dinitrate is denitrated into isosorbide 2-mononitrate and isosorbide 5-mononitrate; these active metabolites have half-lives of 2 and 4 hours, respectively.

is nearly 100%, allowing it to be significantly more effective than equivalent amounts of isosorbide dinitrate. After denitration, organic nitrates are typically glucuronidated in the liver and excreted renally.

Pharmacologic Tolerance

The desirable effects of nitrates can, unfortunately, be offset by compensatory sympathetic nervous system responses (e.g., a reflex increase in sympathetic vascular tone) and compensatory renal responses (e.g., increased salt and water retention). In addition to these mechanisms of physiologic tolerance, pharmacologic tolerance to organic nitrates is an important and clinically relevant phenomenon that significantly limits the efficacy of this class of vasodilators. Pharmacologic tolerance was first documented in munitions workers exposed to volatile organic nitrates in the workplace. These workers suffered headaches at the start of the workweek, but as the week progressed, the headaches tended to disappear and remain absent for the rest of the week. Upon returning to work after a weekend without nitrate exposure, the headaches returned. These "Monday morning headaches" were initially ascribed to weekend intemperance, but it later became clear that the vasodilatory effect of NTG was responsible. Development of tolerance to NTG as the workweek progressed allowed relief from the headaches, and loss of tolerance to NTG over the weekend allowed the headaches to recur upon the workers' return to work.

Although tolerance to adverse effects such as headaches can be desirable, tolerance to the antianginal effects of nitrates diminishes their clinical efficacy. Tolerance to NTG does not appear to depend on the route of administration. Importantly, it is possible to minimize the development of tolerance by modulating the dosing schedule to include daily "nitrate-free intervals." For transdermal NTG, simple removal of the NTG patch each night can minimize the development of tolerance. In cases of severe angina that require uninterrupted nitrate therapy to manage symptoms adequately, however, patients may experience rebound angina during periods that are completely nitrate free. The pharmacokinetic properties of oral isosorbide 5-mononitrate make this preparation an attractive solution to the dilemma of balancing nitrate tolerance and angina rebound: its high bioavailability and long half-life produce periods of high-therapeutic plasma concentrations followed by periods of low-therapeutic (rather than zero) nitrate concentrations. The examples of transdermal NTG and oral isosorbide 5-mononitrate illustrate how the pharmacokinetic properties of two mechanistically similar drugs can have a significant impact on their therapeutic utility.

The cellular and molecular mechanisms that underlie the development of pharmacologic tolerance to organic nitrates remain unclear. There are currently two major hypotheses. First, the so-called classic (sulfhydryl) hypothesis suggests that tolerance results mainly from the intracellular depletion of sulfhydryl-containing groups, such as glutathione or other cysteine-bearing species, that are involved in the formation of NO from organic nitrates. According to the sulfhydryl hypothesis, tolerance could be attenuated or reversed by administering reduced thiol-containing compounds, such as N-acetylcysteine. Second, the free radical (superoxide) hypothesis posits that cellular tolerance results from the formation of peroxynitrite, a highly reactive metabolite of NO that appears to inhibit sGC. According to the superoxide hypothesis, tolerance could be attenuated or reversed by agents that inhibit free radical formation. Because the specific mechanisms of nitrate tolerance remain uncertain, the most effective means of preventing tolerance is the use of a dosing strategy that includes an interval of low plasma nitrate levels every day.

Toxicities and Contraindications

Nitrates are contraindicated in patients with hypotension. Nitrates are also contraindicated in patients with elevated intracranial pressure because NO-mediated vasodilation of cerebral arteries could further elevate intracranial pressure. Nitrates are not advised for the angina pain associated with hypertrophic cardiomyopathy because the outflow obstruction can be exacerbated by reductions in preload. Nitrates should also be used with caution in patients with diastolic heart failure who depend on elevated ventricular preload for optimal cardiac output. These medications should also be avoided in patients taking phosphodiesterase type V inhibitors. GF's case provides an example of the deleterious effects of concurrently administering organic nitrates and sildenafil (see below).

cGMP Potentiators

Three other classes of medications act on the NO signaling pathway to enhance smooth muscle relaxation. These agents inhibit phosphodiesterase type V or stimulate cGMP production, thereby potentiating vasodilation.

Phosphodiesterase Type V Inhibitors

The phosphodiesterase type V (PDE5) inhibitors **sildenafil**, **vardenafil**, **tadalafil**, and **avanafil** prevent the hydrolysis of cGMP to 5'-GMP, thereby potentiating the effects of sGC-induced cGMP production on smooth muscle relaxation. PDE5 is mainly expressed in the smooth muscle of the corpus cavernosum but is also expressed in the retina and vascular smooth muscle cells. PDE5 inhibitors are most commonly prescribed for erectile dysfunction, a relatively common condition in men, such as GF, who have vascular disease. Normally, NO release from penile nerve terminals activates sGC in the smooth muscle of the corpus cavernosum, leading to increased cellular cGMP, smooth muscle relaxation, inflow of blood, and penile erection. Through inhibition of PDE5, these drugs potentiate the effects of endogenous NO signaling. Although PDE5 is predominantly expressed in erectile smooth muscle tissue, it is also expressed in the pulmonary vasculature, and PDE5 inhibitors at high doses have demonstrated efficacy in the management of pulmonary hypertension.

The adverse effects of PDE5 inhibitors primarily result from drug-induced vasodilation in the systemic vasculature. Headache and flushing are likely caused by vasodilation of cerebral and cutaneous vascular beds, respectively. Sildenafil-related myocardial infarction and sudden cardiac death may also be related to its vasodilatory effects. PDE5 inhibitors have only a nominal effect on blood pressure, and the adverse effects described above are relatively rare because of the small amounts of PDE5 in the systemic vasculature. However, in the presence of excess NO (e.g., when organic nitrates are used concomitantly with PDE5 inhibitors), the inhibition of cGMP degradation can markedly amplify the vasodilatory effect of NO. Excessive vasodilation can lead to severe, refractory hypotension, as GF experienced after taking NTG and sildenafil at the same time. Therefore, all PDE5 inhibitors are contraindicated for patients taking organic nitrate vasodilators. Sildenafil, vardenafil, tadalafil, and avanafil all have significant and potentially dangerous drug–drug interactions with nitrates. Similarly, patients taking α-blockers should be monitored carefully upon the addition of PDE5 inhibitors to their medical regimen. Co-administration of PDE5 inhibitors with other antihypertensive medications (e.g., Ca^{2+} channel blockers) is generally considered safe; however, such patients require close monitoring. Sudden sensorineural hearing loss has been reported in a small number of patients taking PDE5 inhibitors, and medication use appears to increase the risk of hearing loss twofold. Cases of vision loss due to nonarteritic ischemic optic neuropathy have been reported with PDE5 inhibitor use; however, larger studies have failed to demonstrate an increased risk compared to placebo.

The PDE5 inhibitors are metabolized by hepatic cytochrome P450 3A4.

Riociguat

Riociguat is a stimulator of sGC that has recently been approved for the treatment of chronic thromboembolic pulmonary hypertension and pulmonary arterial hypertension. Similar to PDE5 inhibitors, riociguat potentiates NO signaling and smooth muscle relaxation, but by two different mechanisms. First, riociguat stabilizes the interaction between NO and sGC. Second, riociguat directly stimulates sGC production of cGMP independently of NO. In contrast to the PDE5 inhibitors, riociguat has more commonly been associated with systemic hypotension and should be used with caution in patients at risk for ischemia or who are taking antihypertensive medications. Given this concern for systemic hypotension, riociguat use is contraindicated in patients taking either organic nitrates or PDE5 inhibitors. Riociguat is metabolized by cytochrome P450s 2C8 and 3A4.

Nesiritide

Nesiritide is a recombinant form of B-type natriuretic peptide that stimulates membrane-bound receptor guanylyl cyclases in the plasma membrane, providing an alternative route for vascular smooth muscle cell cGMP production. Nesiritide must be administered as a continuous intravenous infusion. Its primary indication is the treatment of decompensated heart failure; recent clinical studies, however, failed to show a change in mortality or rehospitalization rates in patients treated with nesiritide compared to controls. Nesiritide is discussed in more detail in Chapter 21, Pharmacology of Volume Regulation.

Prostacyclin Analogues

Prostacyclin is a potent vasodilator through its activation of G_s-coupled IP receptors on vascular smooth muscle cells. Three prostanoids have been developed and used primarily for the treatment of pulmonary arterial hypertension: **epoprostenol** (a stable prostacyclin preparation), **treprostinil**, and **iloprost**. Prostacyclin not only relaxes vascular smooth muscle but also decreases smooth muscle cell proliferation, platelet aggregation, thrombosis, and extracellular matrix elaboration, all of which contribute to the pathogenesis of pulmonary arterial hypertension.

Epoprostenol was the first drug in this class and is the only drug to demonstrate a mortality benefit in patients with pulmonary arterial hypertension. Epoprostenol is administered as a continuous infusion through an indwelling central venous catheter, limiting its use to patients with severe, lifestyle-limiting symptoms. An inhaled formulation is also available, the use of which is limited to critically ill patients with pulmonary hypertension or severe lung disease (similar to the use of inhaled NO). Epoprostenol has a half-life of 6 minutes; abrupt discontinuation can result in rebound pulmonary hypertension and a rapid clinical decline.

Treprostinil is available in oral, subcutaneous, intravenous, and inhaled formulations. The subcutaneous form is delivered via continuous infusion; this modality alleviates the disadvantages associated with a chronic indwelling catheter, although there is a small risk of abscess formation at the infusion site. Treprostinil also has a longer half-life than epoprostenol (4 hours), which may mitigate the adverse consequences associated with abrupt discontinuation (caused, for example, by malfunction of the infusion pump). However, clinically evident increases in pulmonary arterial pressures are seen within 1 hour of discontinuation. Intravenous treprostinil has similar efficacy to intravenous epoprostenol. Inhaled treprostinil requires less frequent dosing than inhaled iloprost due to its longer half-life. The oral dosage form appears to be less effective than inhaled or parenteral therapy. Treprostinil requires dose reduction in patients with liver disease, and the oral dosage form is contraindicated in patients with severe impairment.

Iloprost is available only as an inhaled formulation. Again, this formulation avoids the risks of central venous catheterization. Additionally, inhalation therapy is theoretically more specific for the pulmonary vasculature. Indeed, inhaled iloprost has been shown to increase arterial O_2 saturation, which is not observed in patients receiving parenteral therapies. This is likely a consequence of selective vasodilation of ventilated alveoli and improved ventilation–perfusion matching.

The adverse effects of all prostanoids include flushing, headache, nausea, leg edema, hypotension, and syncope. Jaw pain and diarrhea are also common complaints. These symptoms tend to abate as therapy is continued. Subcutaneous iloprost can cause intense infusion site reactions and pain, which limit its administration by that route. Inhaled medications are, not surprisingly, associated with cough and throat irritation. Complications from the intravenous delivery system can be life-threatening and include local soft-tissue infections, bloodstream infections, catheter-associated thrombosis, and paradoxical embolism.

Endothelin Receptor Antagonists

Bosentan is a competitive antagonist at the ET_A and ET_B endothelin receptors that is approved for use in the treatment of pulmonary arterial hypertension. In clinical trials involving patients with severe dyspnea related to pulmonary hypertension, bosentan significantly improved 6-minute walk distance (i.e., the distance a patient can walk in 6 minutes) and decreased pulmonary vascular resistance relative to placebo. The major adverse effect of bosentan is an elevation of serum transaminase levels, with approximately 10% of patients having elevations that exceed three times the upper limit of normal. It is, therefore, necessary to monitor serum transaminase levels monthly in patients taking bosentan.

Ambrisentan is an ET_A receptor selective antagonist. As with bosentan, patients with pulmonary hypertension have improved 6-minute walk distance and increased functional status when taking this medication. Ambrisentan may be less hepatotoxic than bosentan. **Macitentan** is a recently approved nonselective ET receptor antagonist with a safety profile similar to that of ambrisentan.

Sympathetic Nervous System Antagonists

α_1-Adrenergic Antagonists

Epinephrine and norepinephrine stimulate G_q-coupled α_1-adrenergic receptors on vascular smooth muscle cells to induce vasoconstriction. α_1-Adrenergic antagonists, such as **prazosin**, block receptor activation and cause vasodilation. The effect of these agents is greater in arterioles than in venules. These agents cause a significant reduction in arterial pressure and are useful in the treatment of hypertension. Initiation of therapy with α_1-blockers can be associated with orthostatic hypotension. These agents are also associated with fluid retention that can be mitigated by co-administration of a diuretic. Some α_1-adrenergic antagonists, such as **terazosin**, are used principally to inhibit the contraction of nonvascular smooth muscle (e.g., prostatic smooth muscle), but these agents also have some effects on the vasculature. α_1-Adrenergic antagonists are discussed in greater detail in Chapter 11, Adrenergic Pharmacology.

β-Adrenergic Antagonists

While activation of G_s-coupled β_2-adrenergic receptors on vascular smooth muscle cells leads to vasodilation, β-adrenergic receptor *antagonists* are of major clinical importance in the treatment of hypertension, angina, cardiac arrhythmias, and other conditions through inhibition of cardiac β_1-adrenergic receptors. Inhibition of β_1-receptors has negative inotropic and chronotropic effects on the heart; these actions reduce cardiac output, which is an important determinant of both myocardial O_2 demand and blood pressure. Systemic inhibition of β_2-adrenergic receptors on vascular smooth muscle cells can lead to unopposed vasoconstriction through α_1-adrenergic stimulation and, consequently, to increased systemic vascular resistance. Over time, however, the net effect is a decrease in blood pressure owing to the cardiac effects of these medications as well as inhibition of renin secretion and effects of β-blockers on the central nervous system. β-Adrenergic antagonists are discussed in greater detail in Chapter 11.

Renin-Angiotensin-Aldosterone System Blockers

Inhibition of the renin-angiotensin-aldosterone system results in significant vasodilation (see Chapter 21). The hypotensive effect of ACE inhibitors may be caused, in part, by decreased catabolism of bradykinin, a vasorelaxant released in response to inflammatory stimuli, as well as decreased stimulation of AT_1 angiotensin receptors that are coupled to G_q and G_i. Antagonists of the AT_1 receptor have a more direct effect by inhibiting angiotensin II-mediated stimulation of these receptors. The direct renin inhibitor **aliskiren** has recently been approved for the treatment of hypertension. Mineralocorticoid receptor antagonists, such as **spironolactone** and **eplerenone**, are also effective in the treatment of hypertension and heart failure.

■ CONCLUSION AND FUTURE DIRECTIONS

Vascular tone is subject to exquisite control, as would be expected for a system that must regulate blood flow to all tissues in the body. Vascular tone represents a balance between vascular smooth muscle relaxation and contraction that is ultimately determined by the intracellular Ca^{2+} concentration. Increases in cytoplasmic Ca^{2+} stimulate Ca^{2+}/CaM-dependent MLCK phosphorylation, permitting actin–myosin cross-bridge formation and cellular contraction. The vascular smooth muscle cell relaxes when intracellular Ca^{2+} concentrations decrease. Vascular smooth muscle cells integrate a variety of stimuli from the local environment, adjacent endothelial cells, sympathetic nervous system, and humoral mediators to optimize vessel caliber. A molecular understanding of the critical signaling pathways involved in vascular smooth muscle cell biology has enabled the development of numerous targeted pharmacologic therapies for disorders of vascular tone, including systemic and pulmonary hypertension, angina, coronary artery disease, and congestive heart failure.

Indeed, new insights into novel regulators of vascular smooth muscle cell tone have identified novel therapeutic targets. One of these, fasudil, is a RhoA-kinase (ROCK) inhibitor. In vascular smooth muscle cells, ROCK phosphorylates myosin light chain phosphatase, inhibiting its ability to dephosphorylate and inactivate myosin light chain. ROCK signaling thus potentiates vascular smooth muscle contraction, and ROCK inhibitors block this signaling pathway. In clinical studies, fasudil has shown promise for treatment of pulmonary hypertension and cerebral vasospasm.

Lipid signaling molecules, such as those that constitute the endothelial-derived hyperpolarizing factors and sphingosine-1-phosphate, likely represent additional targets for therapeutic intervention. These compounds are known to bind G protein-coupled receptors in the plasma membrane and stimulate signal transduction pathways leading to changes in vascular smooth muscle tone. Additional research is necessary, however, to identify and characterize the ligands, receptors, signaling pathways, and relevant tissue distributions, prior to clinical trials.

These examples demonstrate how continued elucidation of the complex signaling pathways regulating vascular smooth muscle cell tone will lead to the identification of new targets for pharmacologic intervention in the cellular milieu of the vascular wall and will help to integrate the pharmacology of vascular tone across the spectrum of cardiovascular diseases.

Acknowledgment

We thank Deborah Yeh Chong and Thomas Michel for their valuable contributions to this chapter in the First, Second, and Third Editions of *Principles of Pharmacology: The Pathophysiologic Basis of Drug Therapy*.

Suggested Reading

Abrams J. Chronic stable angina. *N Engl J Med* 2005;352:2524–2533. (*Informative case vignette and review of the pathophysiology and pharmacotherapy of angina pectoris.*)

Flynn JT, Pasko DA. Calcium channel blockers: pharmacology and place in therapy of pediatric hypertension. *Pediatr Nephrol* 2000;15:302–316. (*Overview of Ca^{2+} channel blocker pharmacology with pharmacokinetic data, including Ca^{2+} channel structure and function, with data from adults extrapolated for pediatric care.*)

Frumkin LR. The pharmacological treatment of pulmonary arterial hypertension. *Pharmacol Rev* 2012;64:583–620. (*Comprehensive review of the current pharmacologic management of pulmonary arterial hypertension.*)

Gilchrist M, Shore AC, Benjamin N. Inorganic nitrate and nitrite and control of blood pressure. *Cardiovasc Res* 2011;89:492–498. (*Detailed review of nitrate and nitrite metabolism and the role of dietary nitrate in blood pressure control.*)

Giles TD, Sander GE, Nossaman BD, Kadowitz PJ. Impaired vasodilation in the pathogenesis of hypertension: focus on nitric oxide, endothelial-derived hyperpolarizing factors, and prostaglandins. *J Clin Hypertens* 2012;14:198–205. (*Review of endothelial-derived factors regulating vascular smooth muscle tone.*)

Loirand G, Guérin P, Pacaud P. Rho kinases in cardiovascular physiology and pathophysiology. *Circ Res* 2006;98:322–334. (*This review explores the functional role of Rho kinases in vascular biology and their therapeutic implications.*)

DRUG SUMMARY TABLE: CHAPTER 22 Pharmacology of Vascular Tone

CALCIUM CHANNEL BLOCKERS

Mechanism—Block voltage-gated L-type calcium channels and prevent the influx of calcium that promotes actin–myosin cross-bridge formation. Different classes of calcium channel blockers have unique binding sites on the calcium channel and different affinities for the various conformational states of the channel.

DRUG	CLINICAL APPLICATIONS	SERIOUS AND COMMON ADVERSE EFFECTS	CONTRAINDICATIONS	THERAPEUTIC CONSIDERATIONS
Dihydropyridines: **Nifedipine** **Amlodipine** **Nicardipine** **Isradipine** **Nimodipine** **Nisoldipine** **Felodipine** **Clevidipine**	Shared indication, except for nimodipine: Hypertension Nifedipine, amlodipine, and nicardipine only: Exertional angina Unstable angina Coronary spasm Nimodipine only: Subarachnoid hemorrhage	*Increased angina, myocardial infarction (shared adverse effects); aplastic anemia (nifedipine only); angioedema (amlodipine only); hepatitis (nicardipine only); stroke (felodipine only)* Hypotension, palpitations, peripheral edema, flushing, gastrointestinal upset, dizziness, headache	Shared contraindication: Hypersensitivity to drug Nifedipine only: Cardiogenic shock Concomitant use of strong CYP450 inducers Nicardipine and clevidipine only: Aortic stenosis Clevidipine only: Defective lipid metabolism Nimodipine only: Concomitant use with strong CYP3A4 inhibitors	Arteriolar dilation greater than venous dilation. High vascular-to-cardiac selectivity; compared to diltiazem and verapamil, less depression of myocardial contractility and minimal effects on SA-node automaticity and AV-node conduction velocity. Oral nifedipine has a rapid onset of action and can cause a brisk, precipitous fall in blood pressure, which can trigger severe reflex tachycardia. Compared to nifedipine, amlodipine has higher bioavailability, longer time to peak plasma concentration, and slower hepatic metabolism. Co-administration with nafcillin results in large decrease in plasma nifedipine level. Clevidipine is administered as an intravenous infusion for management of hypertensive urgency and emergency.
Benzothiazepine: **Diltiazem**	Prinzmetal's or variant angina Chronic stable angina Hypertension Atrial fibrillation or flutter, paroxysmal supraventricular tachycardia	*Atrioventricular block, myocardial infarction, bradyarrhythmia, hepatotoxicity* Peripheral edema, headache, dizziness, cough, fatigue	Hypersensitivity to diltiazem Sick sinus syndrome or second- or third-degree AV block Supraventricular tachycardia associated with a bypass tract (see Fig. 24-8) Hypotension (systolic blood pressure <90 mm Hg) Acute myocardial infarction (MI) with x-ray-documented pulmonary congestion Administration of IV β-blockers within a few hours of IV diltiazem Cardiogenic shock	Low ratio of vascular-to-cardiac selectivity. Depresses both SA-node automaticity and AV-node conduction velocity. Raises serum carbamazepine levels, which may result in carbamazepine toxicity. Avoid concomitant use of β-adrenergic blockers.
Phenylalkylamine: **Verapamil**	Same as diltiazem	*Atrioventricular block, myocardial infarction, pulmonary edema* Edema, hypotension, constipation, dizziness, headache, pharyngitis, sinusitis	Same as diltiazem Additionally, left ventricular dysfunction	Same therapeutic considerations as diltiazem. Additionally, verapamil has a greater suppressive effect on cardiac contractility than diltiazem. Alcohol consumption with chronic verapamil therapy may result in higher serum alcohol concentrations. Co-administration with pimozide may result in higher pimozide concentrations and cardiac arrhythmias. Co-administration with simvastatin markedly increases simvastatin concentrations.

POTASSIUM CHANNEL OPENERS
Mechanism—Open ATP-modulated potassium channels and hyperpolarize the plasma membrane, thereby inhibiting influx of calcium through voltage-gated calcium channels

Drug	Clinical Applications	Adverse Effects	Contraindications	Therapeutic Considerations
Minoxidil Nicorandil	Severe or refractory hypertension Male pattern alopecia (topical minoxidil)	Angina, pericardial effusion, reflex tachycardia, Stevens-Johnson syndrome, leukopenia, thrombocytopenia Hypotension, edema, hirsutism, hypernatremia	Hypersensitivity to minoxidil or nicorandil Pheochromocytoma (minoxidil only)	Arteriolar dilation greater than venous dilation. Typically used in combination with a β-blocker and a diuretic. Use with caution in patients with impaired renal function or dissecting aortic aneurysm or after acute MI.

HYDRALAZINE
Mechanism—Arteriolar vasodilator. Mechanism of action is unclear; proposed mechanisms include membrane hyperpolarization, potassium channel activation, and inhibition of IP_3-induced calcium release from sarcoplasmic reticulum in vascular smooth muscle

Drug	Clinical Applications	Adverse Effects	Contraindications	Therapeutic Considerations
Hydralazine	Moderate to severe hypertension	Agranulocytosis, leukopenia, hepatotoxicity, systemic lupus erythematosus Headache, palpitations, tachycardia, chest pain, gastrointestinal upset	Hypersensitivity to hydralazine Coronary artery disease Mitral valvular rheumatic heart disease	Arteriolar dilation greater than venous dilation. Typically used in combination with a β-blocker and a diuretic in the treatment of hypertension. Used in combination with isosorbide dinitrate for heart failure; combination formulation with isosorbide dinitrate may have morbidity and mortality benefits in black Americans with advanced heart failure.

NITRIC OXIDE DONORS
Mechanism—Nitrates and nitroprusside: donate NO, which activates guanylyl cyclase and increases dephosphorylation of myosin light chain in vascular smooth muscle, causing vasodilation. Inhaled nitric oxide gas: selectively dilates the pulmonary vasculature

Drug	Clinical Applications	Adverse Effects	Contraindications	Therapeutic Considerations
Isosorbide dinitrate	Prophylaxis and treatment of acute anginal attacks	Syncope, methemoglobinemia Hypotension, headache	Hypersensitivity to organic nitrates	Venous dilation greater than arteriolar dilation. Continuous therapy leads to tolerance; tolerance can be avoided by providing nitrate-free interval.
Isosorbide 5-mononitrate	Prophylaxis of angina	Bradyarrhythmia, heart failure Dizziness, headache	Same as isosorbide dinitrate	Same therapeutic considerations as isosorbide dinitrate. Additionally, isosorbide 5-mononitrate is preferred over isosorbide dinitrate due to longer half-life, better absorption from the GI tract, nonsusceptibility to extensive first-pass metabolism in the liver, less rebound angina, and greater efficacy at equivalent doses.
Nitroglycerin	*Short-acting (sublingual, spray):* Short-term treatment of acute anginal attacks *Long-acting (oral, buccal, transdermal patch):* Prophylaxis of angina Treatment of chronic ischemic heart disease *Intravenous:* Unstable angina Acute heart failure	Anaphylaxis, methemoglobinemia, increased intracranial pressure Hypertension, flushing, dizziness, headache	Hypersensitivity to nitroglycerin Concomitant use with phosphodiesterase type 5 (PDE5) inhibitors Constrictive pericarditis, pericardial tamponade, and restrictive cardiomyopathy Early myocardial infarction Increased intracranial pressure Severe anemia	Same therapeutic considerations as isosorbide dinitrate. Additionally, equivalent doses of nitroglycerin may be less effective than isosorbide dinitrate due to shorter half-life of nitroglycerin. Ergotamine may oppose coronary vasodilation of nitrates.

continues

DRUG SUMMARY TABLE: CHAPTER 22 Pharmacology of Vascular Tone *continued*

DRUG	CLINICAL APPLICATIONS	SERIOUS AND COMMON ADVERSE EFFECTS	CONTRAINDICATIONS	THERAPEUTIC CONSIDERATIONS
Sodium nitroprusside	Hypertensive emergencies Severe cardiac failure Induction and maintenance of hypotension for surgical procedure	*Cyanide toxicity, cardiac arrhythmia, excessive bleeding, excessive hypotension, metabolic acidosis, toxic epidermal necrolysis, bowel obstruction, methemoglobinemia, increased intracranial pressure* Palpitations, rash, excessive sweating, muscle twitching, confusion, dizziness, headache, somnolence, anxiety, increased serum creatinine	Preexisting hypotension, obstructive valvular disease, heart failure associated with reduced peripheral vascular resistance Hepatic or renal failure Optic atrophy Surgery patients with inadequate cerebral circulation Tobacco amblyopia	Venous dilation equal to arteriolar dilation. Thiocyanate toxicity becomes life-threatening at serum concentrations of 200 mg/L. Co-administration of sodium thiosulfate may reduce the risk of cyanide toxicity, but this interaction is not well studied.
Inhaled nitric oxide gas	Neonatal respiratory failure Perinatal hypoxia Pulmonary hypertension	*Hypotension, methemoglobinemia, hypoxemia, withdrawal syndrome*	Neonates with dependence on right-to-left shunting	Inhaled nitric oxide gas has a short half-life and is rapidly reversible. Inhaled NO selectively dilates the pulmonary vasculature because NO in the blood is rapidly inactivated by binding to hemoglobin.

cGMP POTENTIATORS
Mechanism—All increase cellular cGMP, which stimulates MLC phosphatase through phosphorylation by PKG, leading to vasorelaxation. PDE5 inhibitors: Block degradation of cGMP by PDE5. Riociguat: stimulates soluble guanylyl cyclase to produce cGMP. Nesiritide: recombinant B-type natriuretic peptide that activates membrane-bound guanylyl cyclase receptors

PDE5 Inhibitors: **Sildenafil** **Vardenafil** **Tadalafil** **Avanafil**	Shared indication: Erectile dysfunction Sildenafil and tadalafil only: Pulmonary hypertension Tadalafil only: Benign prostatic hyperplasia	*Myocardial infarction, nonarteritic ischemic optic neuropathy, sudden hearing loss, priapism (shared adverse effects); vasoocclusive crisis in sickle cell anemia (sildenafil only); seizure (vardenafil and tadalafil only); Stevens-Johnson syndrome, cerebral hemorrhage, stroke (tadalafil only)* Flushing, dizziness, headache, rhinitis (shared adverse effects); gastrointestinal upset (sildenafil and tadalafil only)	Shared contraindications: Hypersensitivity to drug Concomitant use of organic nitrate vasodilators Sildenafil only: Concomitant use with HIV protease inhibitors or elvitegravir, cobicistat, tenofovir, or emtricitabine	PDE5 inhibitors promote systemic vasodilation at doses much higher than those used to treat erectile dysfunction. High doses are efficacious in treatment of pulmonary hypertension. Patients with prior episodes of vision loss may be at increased risk for nonarteritic ischemic optic neuropathy. Tadalafil has longer elimination half-life than sildenafil and vardenafil.
Riociguat	Pulmonary arterial hypertension Chronic thromboembolic pulmonary hypertension	*Hemorrhage* Hypotension, gastrointestinal upset, anemia, dizziness, headache	Pregnancy Co-administration with NO donors or PDE5 inhibitors	Plasma drug concentrations are 50–60% lower in smokers.
Nesiritide	Acute decompensated heart failure	*Anaphylaxis* Hypotension, nausea, dizziness, headache, increased serum creatinine	Hypersensitivity to nesiritide Cardiogenic shock (as primary therapy) Systolic blood pressure < 100 mm Hg prior to therapy	Ask about hypersensitivity to other recombinant proteins. Avoid in patients with low filling pressures or patients who are preload dependent.

PROSTACYCLIN ANALOGUES
Mechanism—Stimulate G$_s$-coupled IP receptors on smooth muscle cells, activate PKA, and cause vasorelaxation through inhibition of MLCK

Drug	Clinical Applications	Adverse Effects	Contraindications	Therapeutic Considerations
Epoprostenol (IV, inhaled) Iloprost (inhaled) Treprostinil (oral, SQ, IV, inhaled)	Pulmonary hypertension	*Hemorrhage, sepsis (epoprostenol and treprostinil only); splenomegaly (epoprostenol only); bronchospasm (iloprost only)* Flushing, gastrointestinal upset, headache, musculoskeletal pain (shared adverse effects); hypotension, dizziness, bradyarrhythmia, arthralgia, anxiety (epoprostenol only); rash, injection site reaction (treprostinil only)	Shared contraindications: Hypersensitivity to drug Chronic use in patients with LV systolic dysfunction Epoprostenol only: Development of pulmonary edema during dose initiation	Epoprostenol for severe disease; only medication to show mortality benefit. Mild inhibitors of platelet aggregation, although hemorrhage not reported as an adverse event. Treprostinil requires dose reduction in patients with liver disease. Route of administration is an important consideration since IV therapy requires indwelling catheter placement for chronic therapy.

ENDOTHELIN RECEPTOR ANTAGONISTS
Mechanism—Block activation of endothelin receptors ET$_A$ and ET$_B$ by endogenous endothelin. Ambrisentan has greater selectivity for ET$_A$ than bosentan.

Drug	Clinical Applications	Adverse Effects	Contraindications	Therapeutic Considerations
Bosentan Ambrisentan Macitentan	Severe pulmonary hypertension	*Anemia (shared adverse effect); hepatotoxicity, angioedema (bosentan and ambrisentan only)* Headache (shared adverse effect); edema, flushing (bosentan and ambrisentan only); urinary tract infection, bronchitis, nasopharyngitis (macitentan only)	Shared contraindications: Hypersensitivity to drug Pregnancy Bosentan only: Concomitant use of cyclosporine A or glyburide Ambrisentan only: Idiopathic pulmonary fibrosis	Do not use in pregnant women. Monitor liver function tests monthly. Generally avoid use in patients with moderate to severe hepatic impairment. Use with caution in patients with hypovolemia, hypotension, heart failure, or anemia. Potential for interactions with other drugs metabolized by CYP2C9 or CYP3A4 (e.g., hormonal contraceptives, simvastatin, warfarin, ketoconazole). Ambrisentan may have less hepatotoxicity than bosentan.

α$_1$-ADRENERGIC ANTAGONISTS
Mechanism—Block activation of α$_1$-adrenergic receptors by endogenous receptor agonists

Drug				
Prazosin Doxazosin Terazosin	See Drug Summary Table: Chapter 11 Adrenergic Pharmacology			

β-ADRENERGIC ANTAGONISTS
Mechanism—Block activation of β-adrenergic receptors by endogenous receptor agonists

Drug				
Propranolol (nonselective) Atenolol, metoprolol (β$_1$-selective)	See Drug Summary Table: Chapter 11 Adrenergic Pharmacology			

continues

DRUG SUMMARY TABLE: CHAPTER 22 Pharmacology of Vascular Tone *continued*

DRUG	CLINICAL APPLICATIONS	*SERIOUS* AND COMMON ADVERSE EFFECTS	CONTRAINDICATIONS	THERAPEUTIC CONSIDERATIONS
RENIN INHIBITOR Mechanism—Inhibits cleavage of angiotensin (AT) to AT I by renin				
Aliskiren	See Drug Summary Table: Chapter 21 Pharmacology of Volume Regulation			
ACE INHIBITORS Mechanism—Inhibit cleavage of angiotensin (AT) I to AT II by angiotensin converting enzyme (ACE); inhibit degradation of bradykinin by kininase II				
Captopril Enalapril Lisinopril	See Drug Summary Table: Chapter 21 Pharmacology of Volume Regulation			
AT₁ RECEPTOR ANTAGONISTS Mechanism—Block activation of AT₁ receptors by endogenous AT II				
Losartan Valsartan	See Drug Summary Table: Chapter 21 Pharmacology of Volume Regulation			

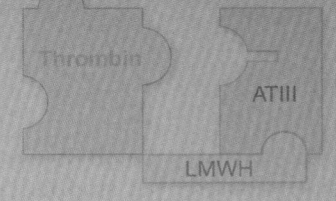

Low molecular weight (LMW) heparins

(about 15 saccharide units, MW ~ 4,500)

Binds to antithrombin III (ATIII) but not to thrombin (poorly inactivates thrombin)

Binds to via penta (sufficient

Selective factor Xa inhibitors

No effect on thrombin

23

Pharmacology of Hemostasis and Thrombosis

Ehrin J. Armstrong and David E. Golan

Binds to antithrombin III (ATIII) via pentasaccharide (sufficient to inactivate Xa)

INTRODUCTION

Blood carries oxygen and nutrients to tissues and takes metabolic waste products away from tissues. Humans have developed a well-regulated system of **hemostasis** to keep the blood fluid and clot-free in normal vessels and to form a localized plug rapidly in injured vessels. **Thrombosis** describes a pathologic state in which normal hemostatic processes are activated inappropriately. For example, a blood clot (thrombus) may form as the result of a relatively minor vessel injury and occlude a branch of the vascular tree. This chapter presents the normal physiology of hemostasis, the pathophysiology of thrombosis, and the pharmacology of drugs that can be used to prevent or reverse a thrombotic state. Drugs introduced in this chapter are used to treat a variety of cardiovascular diseases, such as deep vein thrombosis, stroke, and myocardial infarction.

PHYSIOLOGY OF HEMOSTASIS

An injured blood vessel must induce the formation of a blood clot to prevent blood loss and to allow healing. Clot formation must also remain localized to prevent widespread clotting within intact vessels. The formation of a localized clot at the site of vessel injury is accomplished in four temporally overlapping stages (Fig. 23-1). First, **localized vasoconstriction** occurs as a response to a reflex neurogenic mechanism and to the secretion of endothelium-derived vasoconstrictors such as endothelin. Immediately following vasoconstriction, **primary hemostasis** occurs. During this stage, platelets are activated and adhere to the exposed subendothelial matrix. **Platelet activation** involves both a change in shape of the platelet and the release of secretory granule contents from the platelet. The secreted granule substances recruit other platelets, causing more platelets to adhere to the subendothelial matrix and to aggregate with one another at the site of vascular injury. Primary hemostasis ultimately results in the formation of a **primary hemostatic plug**.

The goal of the final two stages of hemostasis is to form a stable, permanent plug. During **secondary hemostasis**, also known as the **coagulation cascade**, the activated endothelium and other nearby cells (see below) express a membrane-bound procoagulant factor called **tissue factor**, which complexes

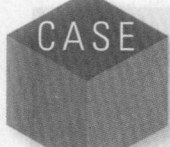

CASE

Mr. S, a 55-year-old man with a history of hypertension and cigarette smoking, is awakened in the middle of the night with substernal chest pressure, sweating, and shortness of breath. He calls 911 and is taken to the emergency department. An electrocardiogram shows deep T-wave inversions in leads V2 to V5. A cardiac biomarker panel shows a troponin T level of 3.2 μg/L (normal, <0.01 μg/L), consistent with myocardial infarction. He is treated with intravenous nitroglycerin, aspirin, unfractionated heparin, and eptifibatide, but his chest pain persists. He is taken to the cardiac catheterization laboratory, where he is found to have a 90% mid-LAD (left anterior descending artery) thrombus with sluggish distal flow. He undergoes successful angioplasty and stent placement. At the time of stent placement, an oral loading dose of clopidogrel is administered. The heparin is stopped, intravenous eptifibatide is continued for 18 more hours, and he is transferred to the telemetry ward. Six hours later, Mr. S is noted to have an expanding hematoma (an area of localized hemorrhage) in his right thigh below the arterial access site. The eptifibatide is stopped and pressure is applied to the access site, and the hematoma ceases to expand. He is discharged 2 days later with prescriptions that include clopidogrel and aspirin, which are administered to prevent thrombosis of the stent.

Questions

1. How did a blood clot arise in Mr. S's coronary artery?
2. How do aspirin, heparin, clopidogrel, and eptifibatide act in the attempt to treat Mr. S's blood clot and to prevent recurrent thrombus formation?
3. What accounts for the efficacy of eptifibatide (a platelet GPIIb–IIIa antagonist) in inhibiting platelet aggregation?
4. When the expanding hematoma was observed, could any measure other than stopping the eptifibatide have been used to reverse the effect of this agent?
5. If low-molecular-weight heparin had been used instead of unfractionated heparin, how would the monitoring of the patient's coagulation status during the procedure have been affected?

with coagulation factor VII to initiate the coagulation cascade. The end result of this cascade is the activation of thrombin, a critical enzyme. Thrombin serves two pivotal functions in hemostasis: (1) it converts soluble fibrinogen to an insoluble fibrin polymer that forms the matrix of the clot and (2) it induces more platelet recruitment and activation. Evidence indicates that fibrin clot formation (secondary hemostasis) overlaps temporally with platelet plug formation (primary hemostasis), and that each process reinforces the other. During the final stage, platelet aggregation and fibrin polymerization lead to the formation of a stable, **permanent plug**. In addition, **antithrombotic mechanisms** restrict the permanent plug to the site of vessel injury, ensuring that the permanent plug does not inappropriately extend to occlude the vascular tree.

Vasoconstriction

Transient arteriolar vasoconstriction occurs immediately after vascular injury. This vasoconstriction is mediated by a poorly understood reflex neurogenic mechanism. Local endothelial secretion of **endothelin**, a potent vasoconstrictor, potentiates the reflex vasoconstriction. Because the vasoconstriction is transient, bleeding would resume if primary hemostasis were not activated.

Primary Hemostasis

The goal of primary hemostasis is to form a platelet plug that rapidly stabilizes vascular injury. Platelets play a pivotal role in primary hemostasis. **Platelets** are cell fragments that arise by budding from megakaryocytes in the bone marrow; these small, membrane-bound discs contain cytoplasm but lack nuclei. Glycoprotein receptors in the platelet plasma membrane are the primary mediators by which platelets are activated. Primary hemostasis involves the transformation of platelets into a hemostatic plug through three reactions: (1) adhesion, (2) the granule release reaction, and (3) aggregation and consolidation.

Platelet Adhesion

In the first reaction, platelets adhere to subendothelial collagen that is exposed after vascular injury (Fig. 23-2). This adhesion is mediated initially by two molecular interactions. First, **von Willebrand factor (vWF)**, a large multimeric protein that is secreted by both activated platelets and the injured endothelium, binds both to surface receptors (especially glycoprotein Ib [GPIb]) on the platelet membrane and to the exposed collagen. This "bridging" action mediates adhesion of platelets to the collagen. Second, platelet **glycoprotein VI (GPVI)** interacts directly with collagen in the exposed vessel wall. Both the GPIb:vWF:collagen interaction and the GPVI:collagen interaction are required for initiation of primary hemostasis.

Platelet Granule Release Reaction

Adherent platelets undergo a process of **activation** (Fig. 23-3) during which the cells' granule contents are released. The release reaction is initiated by agonist binding to cell surface receptors, which activates intracellular protein phosphorylation cascades and ultimately causes release of granule contents. Specifically, stimulation by adenosine diphosphate (ADP), epinephrine, and collagen leads to activation of platelet membrane phospholipase A_2 (PLA$_2$). PLA$_2$ cleaves membrane phospholipids and liberates **arachidonic acid**, which is converted into a **cyclic endoperoxide** by platelet cyclooxygenase. Thromboxane synthase subsequently converts the cyclic endoperoxide into **thromboxane A2 (TxA2)**. TxA$_2$, via a G protein-coupled receptor, causes vasoconstriction at the site of vascular injury by inducing a decrease in cAMP levels within vascular smooth muscle cells. TxA$_2$ also stimulates the granule **release**

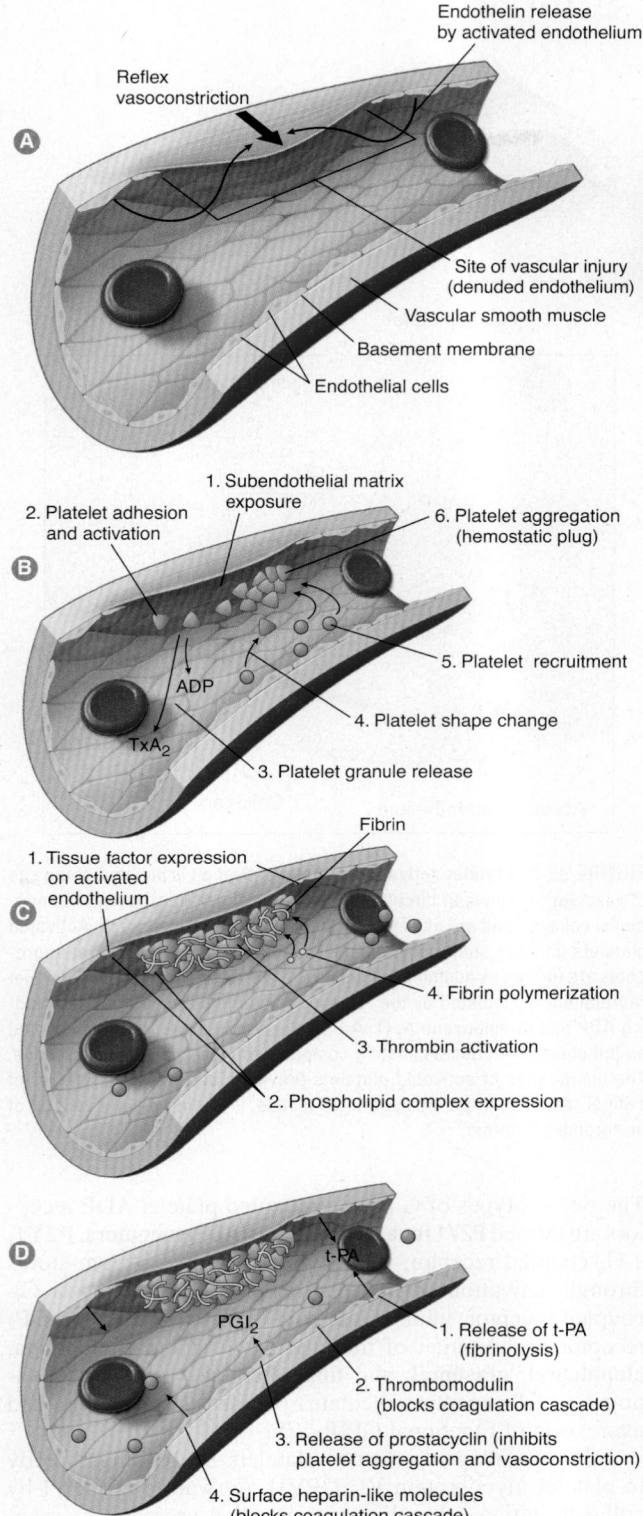

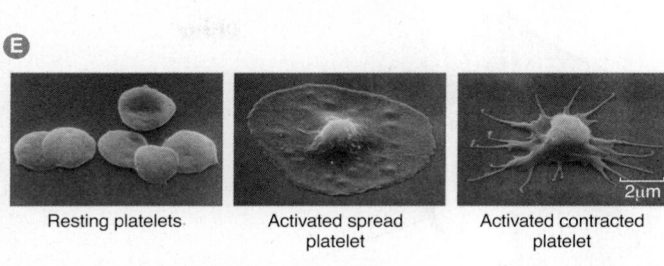

Resting platelets | Activated spread platelet | Activated contracted platelet

FIGURE 23-1. Sequence of events in hemostasis. The hemostatic process can be divided conceptually into four stages—vasoconstriction, primary hemostasis, secondary hemostasis, and resolution—although recent evidence suggests that these stages are temporally overlapping and may be nearly simultaneous. **A.** Vascular injury causes endothelial denudation. Endothelin, released by activated endothelium, and neurohumoral factor(s) induce transient vasoconstriction. **B.** Injury-induced exposure of the subendothelial matrix (*1*) provides a substrate for platelet adhesion and activation (*2*). In the granule release reaction, activated platelets secrete thromboxane A₂ (TxA₂) and ADP (*3*). TxA₂ and ADP released by activated platelets cause nearby platelets to become activated; these newly activated platelets undergo shape change (*4*) and are recruited to the site of injury (*5*). The aggregation of activated platelets at the site of injury forms a primary hemostatic plug (*6*). **C.** Tissue factor expressed on activated endothelial cells (*1*) and leukocyte microparticles (*not shown*), together with acidic phospholipids expressed on activated platelets and activated endothelial cells (*2*), initiate the steps of the coagulation cascade, culminating in the activation of thrombin (*3*). Thrombin proteolytically activates fibrinogen to form fibrin, which polymerizes around the site of injury, resulting in the formation of a definitive (secondary) hemostatic plug (*4*). **D.** Natural anticoagulant and thrombolytic factors limit the hemostatic process to the site of vascular injury. These factors include tissue plasminogen activator (t-PA), which activates the fibrinolytic system (*1*); thrombomodulin, which activates inhibitors of the coagulation cascade (*2*); prostacyclin, which inhibits both platelet activation and vasoconstriction (*3*); and surface heparin-like molecules, which catalyze the inactivation of coagulation factors (*4*). **E.** Scanning electron micrographs of resting platelets (*1*), a platelet undergoing cell spreading shortly after cell activation (*2*), and a fully activated platelet after actin filament bundling and cross-linking and myosin contraction (*3*).

reaction within platelets, thereby propagating the cascade of platelet activation and vasoconstriction.

During the release reaction, large amounts of ADP, Ca²⁺, adenosine triphosphate (ATP), serotonin, vWF, and platelet factor 4 are *actively secreted* from platelet granules. *ADP is particularly important in mediating platelet aggregation,* causing platelets to become "sticky" and adhere to one another (see below).

Although strong agonists (such as thrombin and collagen) can trigger granule secretion even when aggregation is prevented, ADP can trigger granule secretion only in the presence of platelet aggregation. Presumably, this difference is due to the set of intracellular effectors that are coupled to the various agonist receptors. Release of Ca²⁺ ions is also important for the coagulation cascade, as discussed below.

Although platelet activation can be initiated via exposure of subendothelial collagen, a separate and parallel process of platelet activation occurs without disruption of the endothelium and without the involvement of von Willebrand factor. This second pathway of platelet activation is initiated by **tissue factor**, a lipoprotein expressed by activated endothelial cells, activated leukocytes, and microparticles derived from activated leukocytes (see below). As in the coagulation cascade, tissue factor forms a complex with factor VIIa, and the tissue factor–factor VIIa complex activates factor IX. Factor IX activation leads to a proteolytic cascade that results in the generation of **thrombin** (factor IIa), a multifunctional enzyme that plays a critical role in the coagulation cascade (see below). In the tissue factor-initiated pathway of platelet activation, thrombin cleaves **protease-activated receptor 1 (PAR-1)** and

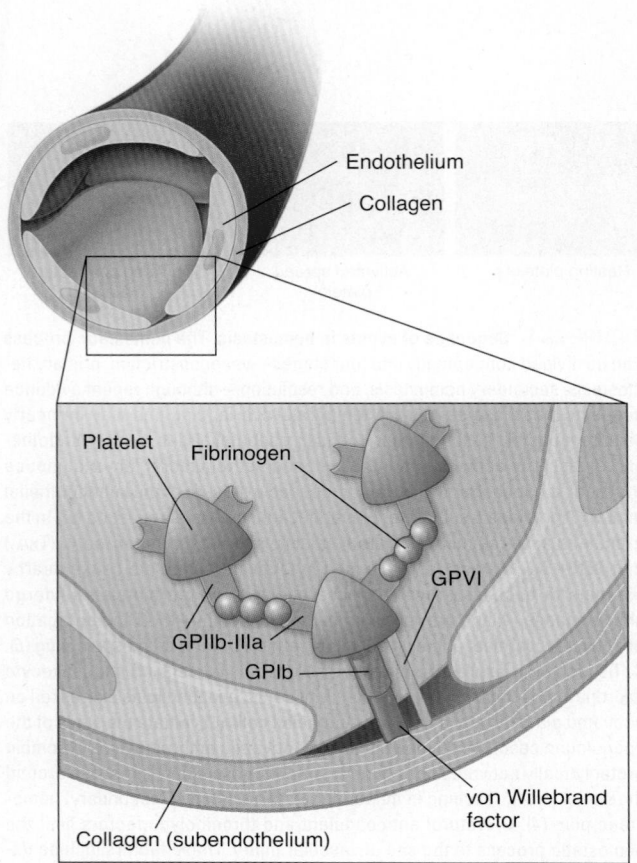

FIGURE 23-2. Platelet adhesion and aggregation. von Willebrand factor mediates platelet adhesion to the subendothelium by binding both to platelet membrane glycoprotein GPIb and to exposed subendothelial collagen. Platelet adhesion to the subendothelial matrix also requires a direct binding interaction between platelet membrane glycoprotein GPVI and subendothelial collagen. During platelet aggregation, fibrinogen cross-links platelets to one another by binding to GPIIb–IIIa receptors on platelet membranes. GPIb exists in the platelet membrane in a complex with glycoproteins GPIX and GPV (*not shown*).

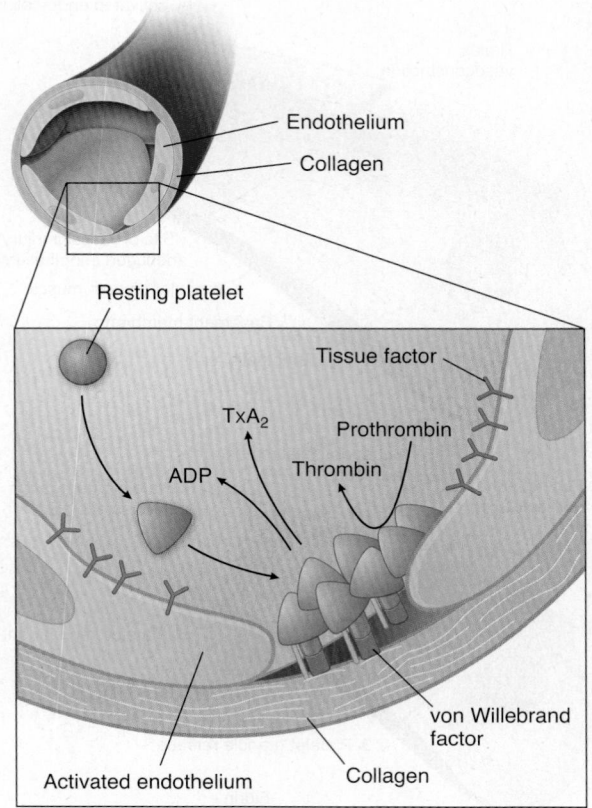

FIGURE 23-3. Platelet activation. Platelet activation is initiated at the site of vascular injury when circulating platelets adhere to exposed subendothelial collagen and are activated by locally generated mediators. Activated platelets undergo shape change and granule release, and platelet aggregates are formed as additional platelets are recruited and activated. Platelet recruitment is mediated by the release of soluble platelet factors, including ADP and thromboxane A_2 (TxA$_2$). Tissue factor, expressed on activated endothelium, is a critical initiating component in the coagulation cascade. The membranes of activated platelets provide a surface for a number of critical reactions in the coagulation cascade, including the conversion of prothrombin to thrombin.

protease-activated receptor 4 (PAR-4) on the platelet surface and thereby causes the platelets to release ADP, serotonin, and TxA$_2$. By activating other nearby platelets, these agonists amplify the signal for thrombus formation.

Platelet Aggregation and Consolidation

TxA$_2$, ADP, and fibrous collagen are all potent mediators of platelet aggregation. TxA$_2$ promotes platelet aggregation through stimulation of G protein-coupled TxA$_2$ receptors in the platelet membrane (Fig. 23-4). Binding of TxA$_2$ to platelet TxA$_2$ receptors leads to activation of phospholipase C (PLC), which hydrolyzes phosphatidylinositol 4,5-bisphosphate (PI[4,5]P$_2$) to yield inositol 1,4,5-trisphosphate (IP$_3$) and diacylglycerol (DAG). IP$_3$ raises the cytosolic Ca^{2+} concentration, and DAG activates protein kinase C (PKC), which in turn promotes the activation of PLA$_2$. Through an incompletely understood mechanism, PLA$_2$ activation induces the expression of functional GPIIb–IIIa, the membrane integrin that mediates platelet aggregation.

ADP triggers platelet activation by binding to G protein-coupled ADP receptors on the platelet surface (Fig. 23-5).

The two subtypes of G protein-coupled platelet ADP receptors are termed **P2Y1 receptors** and **P2Y(ADP) receptors**. P2Y1, a G$_q$-coupled receptor, releases intracellular calcium stores through activation of phospholipase C. P2Y(ADP), a G$_i$-coupled receptor, inhibits adenylyl cyclase. The P2Y(ADP) receptor is the target of the antiplatelet agents **ticlopidine, clopidogrel, prasugrel,** and **ticagrelor** (see below). Activation of ADP receptors mediates platelet shape change and expression of functional GPIIb–IIIa.

Fibrous collagen activates platelets by binding directly to platelet glycoprotein VI (GPVI). Activation of GPVI by collagen initiates signaling cascades that promote the granule release reaction and that induce conformational changes in cell surface integrins (especially GPIIb–IIIa and $\alpha_2\beta_1$) that promote the direct or indirect binding of these integrins to collagen. These additional binding interactions further strengthen the adhesion of activated platelets to the subendothelial matrix.

Platelets aggregate with one another through a bridging molecule, **fibrinogen**, which has multiple binding sites for functional GPIIb–IIIa (Fig. 23-2). *Just as the vWF:GPIb*

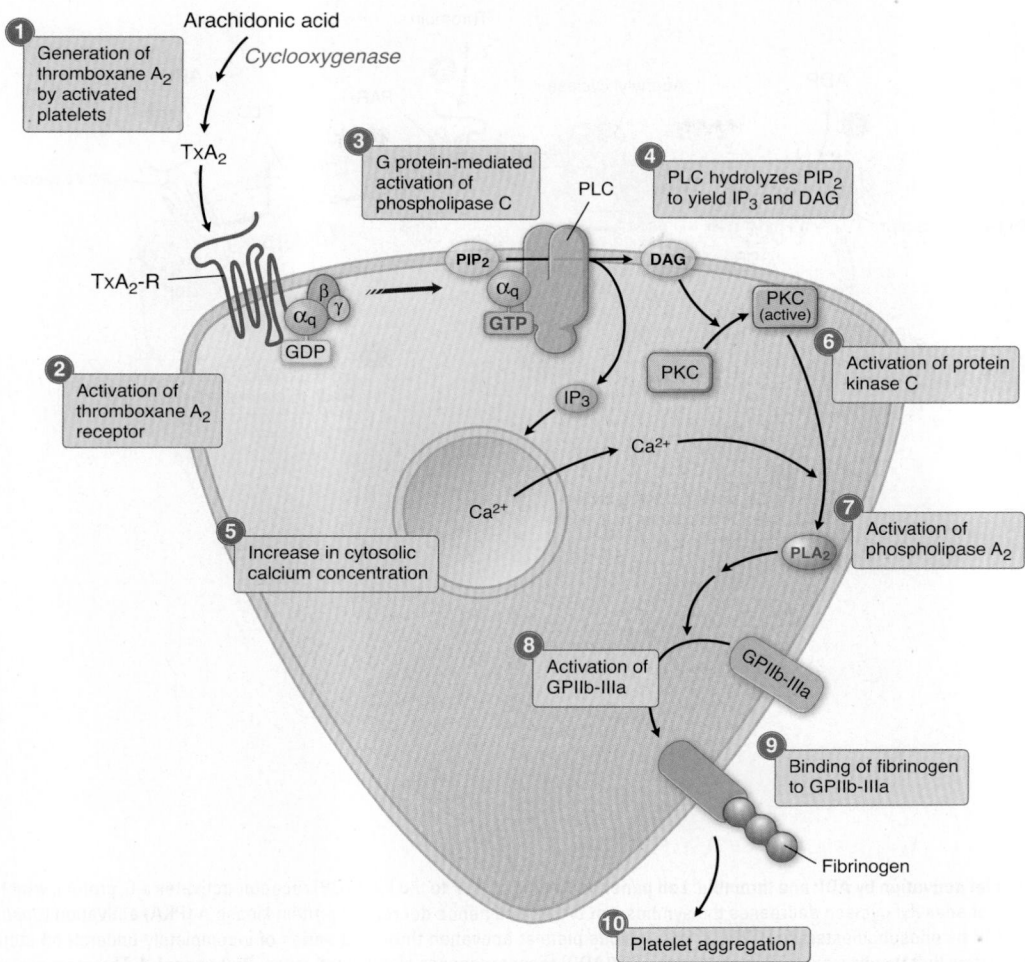

FIGURE 23-4. Platelet activation by thromboxane A$_2$. 1. Thromboxane A$_2$ (TxA$_2$) is generated from arachidonic acid in activated platelets; cyclooxygenase catalyzes the committed step in this process. **2.** Secreted TxA$_2$ binds to the cell surface TxA$_2$ receptor (TxA$_2$-R), a G protein-coupled receptor. **3.** The Gα isoform Gα_q activates phospholipase C (PLC). **4.** PLC hydrolyzes phosphatidylinositol 4,5-bisphosphate (PIP$_2$) to yield inositol 1,4,5-trisphosphate (IP$_3$) and diacylglycerol (DAG). **5.** IP$_3$ increases the cytosolic Ca^{2+} concentration by promoting vesicular release of Ca^{2+} into the cytosol. **6.** DAG activates protein kinase C (PKC). **7.** PKC activates phospholipase A$_2$ (PLA$_2$). **8.** Through an incompletely understood mechanism, activation of PLA$_2$ leads to the activation of GPIIb–IIIa. **9.** Activated GPIIb–IIIa binds to fibrinogen. **10.** Fibrinogen cross-links platelets by binding to GPIIb–IIIa receptors on other platelets. This cross-linking leads to platelet aggregation and formation of a primary hemostatic plug.

interaction is important for platelet adhesion to exposed subendothelial collagen, *the fibrinogen:GPIIb–IIIa interaction is critical for platelet aggregation*. Platelet aggregation ultimately leads to the formation of a reversible clot, or a **primary hemostatic plug**.

Activation of the **coagulation cascade** proceeds nearly simultaneously with the formation of the primary hemostatic plug, as described below. Activation of the coagulation cascade leads to the generation of fibrin, initially at the periphery of the primary hemostatic plug. Platelet pseudopods attach to the fibrin strands at the periphery of the plug and *contract* (Fig. 23-1E). Platelet contraction yields a compact, solid, irreversible clot, or a **secondary hemostatic plug**.

Secondary Hemostasis: The Coagulation Cascade

Secondary hemostasis is also termed the **coagulation cascade**. The goal of this cascade is to form a stable fibrin clot at the site of vascular injury. Details of the coagulation

cascade are presented schematically in Figure 23-6. Several general principles should be noted.

First, the coagulation cascade is a sequence of enzymatic events. Most plasma coagulation factors circulate as inactive *proenzymes*, which are synthesized by the liver. These proenzymes are proteolytically cleaved, and thereby activated, by the activated factors that precede them in the cascade. The activation reaction is catalytic and not stoichiometric. For example, one "unit" of activated factor X can potentially generate 40 "units" of thrombin. This robust amplification process rapidly generates large amounts of fibrin at a site of vascular injury.

Second, the major activation reactions in the cascade occur at sites where a *phospholipid-based protein–protein complex* has formed (Fig. 23-7). This complex is composed of a membrane surface (provided by activated platelets, activated endothelial cells, and possibly activated leukocyte microparticles [see below]), an enzyme (an activated coagulation factor), a substrate (the proenzyme form of the downstream coagulation factor), and a cofactor. The presence of

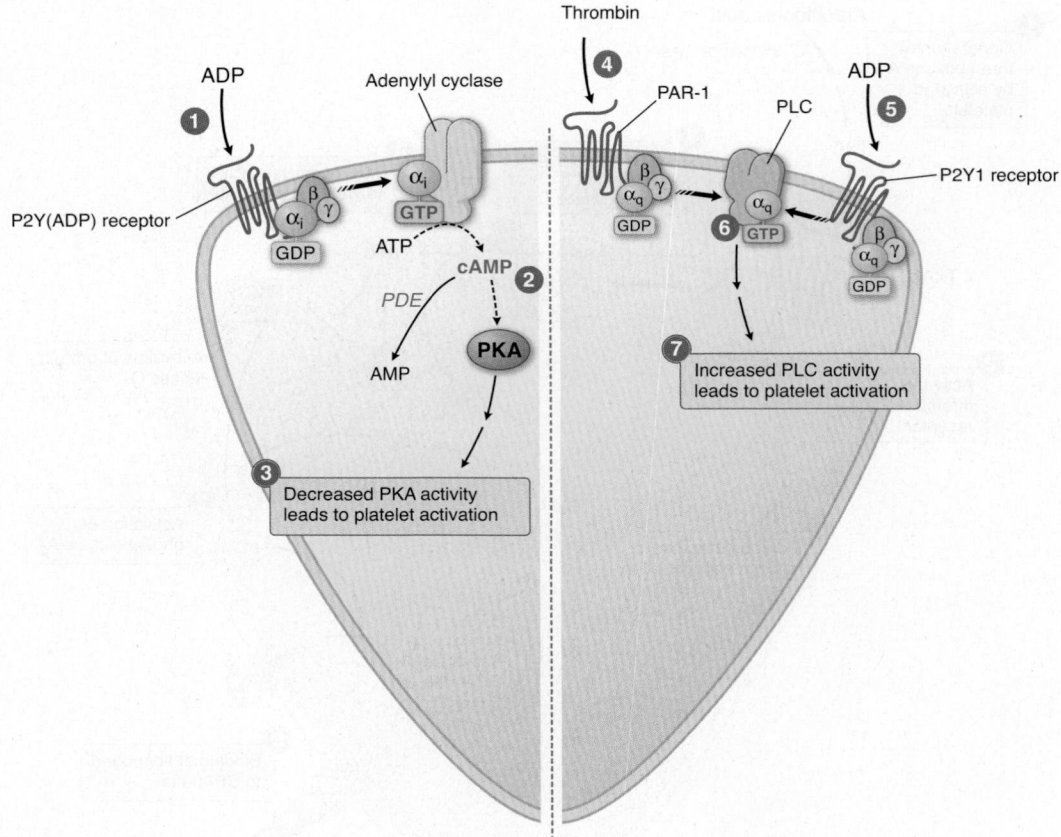

FIGURE 23-5. Platelet activation by ADP and thrombin. Left panel: 1. Binding of ADP to the P2Y(ADP) receptor activates a G_i protein, which inhibits adenylyl cyclase. **2.** Inhibition of adenylyl cyclase decreases the synthesis of cAMP and hence decreases protein kinase A (PKA) activation (*dashed arrow*). cAMP is metabolized to AMP by phosphodiesterase (PDE). **3.** PKA inhibits platelet activation through a series of incompletely understood steps. Therefore, the decreased PKA activation that results from ADP binding to the P2Y(ADP) receptor causes platelet activation. **Right panel: 4.** Thrombin proteolytically cleaves the extracellular domain of protease-activated receptor 1 (PAR-1). This cleavage creates a new N-terminus, which binds to an activation site on PAR-1 to activate a G_q protein. **5.** ADP also activates G_q by binding to the P2Y1 receptor. **6.** G_q activation (by either thrombin or ADP) activates phospholipase C (PLC). **7.** PLC activation leads to platelet activation, as shown in Figure 23-4. Note that ADP can activate platelets by binding to either the P2Y(ADP) receptor or the P2Y1 receptor, although evidence suggests that full platelet activation requires the participation of both receptors. High concentrations of thrombin can also activate platelets via proteolytic cleavage of PAR-4 on platelet surfaces (*not shown*).

negatively charged phospholipids, especially phosphatidylserine, is critical for assembly of the complex. Phosphatidylserine, which is normally sequestered in the inner leaflet of the plasma membrane, translocates to the outer leaflet of the membrane in response to agonist stimulation of platelets, endothelial cells, or leukocytes. Calcium is required for the enzyme, substrate, and cofactor to adopt the proper conformation for the proteolytic cleavage of a coagulation factor proenzyme to its activated form.

Third, the coagulation cascade has been divided traditionally into the **intrinsic** and **extrinsic pathways** (Fig. 23-6). This division is a result of in vitro testing and is essentially arbitrary. The intrinsic pathway is activated in vitro by factor XII (Hageman factor), while the extrinsic pathway is initiated in vivo by *tissue factor*, activated endothelial cells, subendothelial smooth muscle cells, and subendothelial fibroblasts at the site of vascular injury. Although these two pathways converge at the activation of factor X, there is also much interconnection between the two pathways. Because factor VII (activated by the extrinsic pathway) can proteolytically activate factor IX (a key factor in the intrinsic pathway), the

extrinsic pathway is regarded as the primary pathway for the initiation of coagulation in vivo.

Fourth, both the intrinsic and extrinsic coagulation pathways lead to the activation of factor X. In an important reaction that requires factor V, activated factor X proteolytically cleaves prothrombin (factor II) to *thrombin* (factor IIa) (Fig. 23-8). Thrombin acts in the coagulation cascade in four important ways: (1) it converts the soluble plasma protein fibrinogen into fibrin, which then forms long, insoluble polymer fibers; (2) it activates factor XIII, which cross-links the fibrin polymers into a highly stable meshwork or clot; (3) it amplifies the clotting cascade by catalyzing the feedback activation of factors VIII and V; and (4) it strongly activates platelets, causing granule release, platelet aggregation, and platelet-derived microparticle generation. In addition to its procoagulant properties, thrombin acts to modulate the coagulation response. Thrombin activates protease-activated receptors (PARs) on the *intact* vascular endothelial cells adjacent to the area of vascular injury and stimulates these cells to release the platelet inhibitors prostacyclin (PGI_2) and nitric oxide (NO), the profibrinolytic protein tissue plasminogen

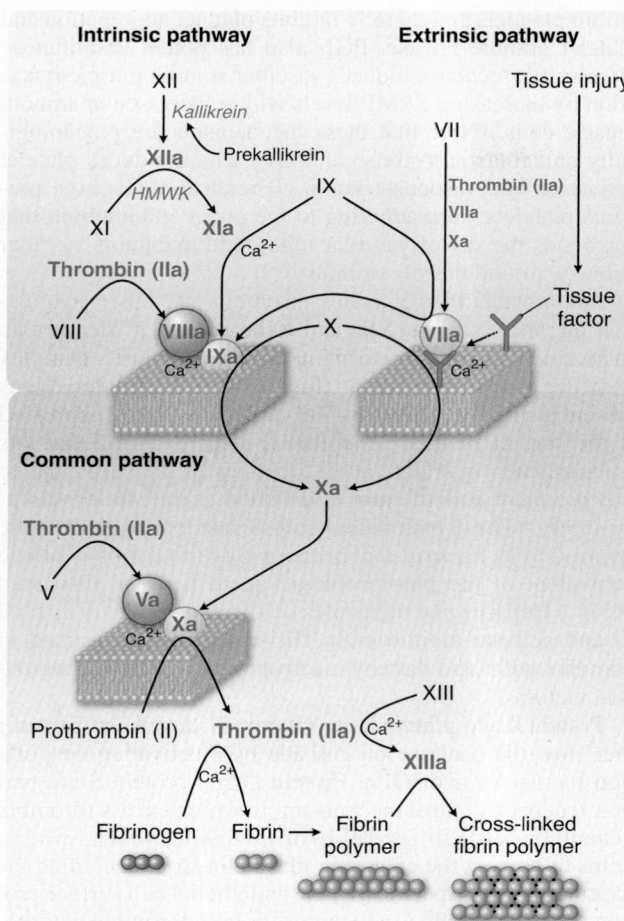

Intrinsic pathway

Extrinsic pathway

Common pathway

FIGURE 23-6. Coagulation cascade. The coagulation cascade is arbitrarily divided into the intrinsic pathway, the extrinsic pathway, and the common pathway. The intrinsic and extrinsic pathways converge at the level of factor X activation. The intrinsic pathway is largely an in vitro pathway, while the extrinsic pathway accounts for the majority of in vivo coagulation. The extrinsic pathway is initiated at sites of vascular injury by the expression of tissue factor on several different cell types, including activated endothelial cells, activated leukocytes (and leukocyte microparticles), subendothelial vascular smooth muscle cells, and subendothelial fibroblasts. Note that Ca^{2+} is a cofactor in many of the steps, and that a number of the steps occur on phospholipid surfaces provided by activated platelets, activated endothelial cells, and activated leukocytes (and leukocyte microparticles). Activated coagulation factors are shown in *blue* and indicated with a lower case "a." HMWK, high-molecular-weight kininogen.

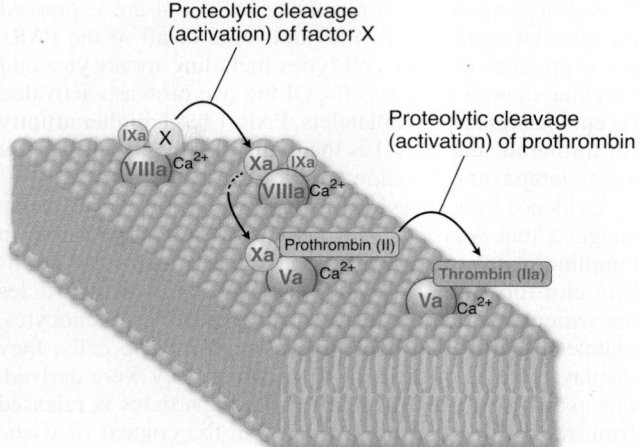

FIGURE 23-7. Coagulation factor activation on phospholipid surfaces. Surface catalysis is critical for a number of the activation reactions in the coagulation cascade. Each activation reaction consists of an enzyme (e.g., factor IXa), a substrate (e.g., factor X), and a cofactor or reaction accelerator (e.g., factor VIIIa), all of which are assembled on the phospholipid surface of activated platelets, endothelial cells, and leukocytes. Ca^{2+} allows the enzyme and substrate to adopt the proper conformation in each activation reaction. In the example shown, factor VIIIa and Ca^{2+} act as cofactors in the factor IXa-mediated cleavage of factor X to factor Xa. Factor Va and Ca^{2+} then act as cofactors in the factor Xa-mediated cleavage of prothrombin to thrombin.

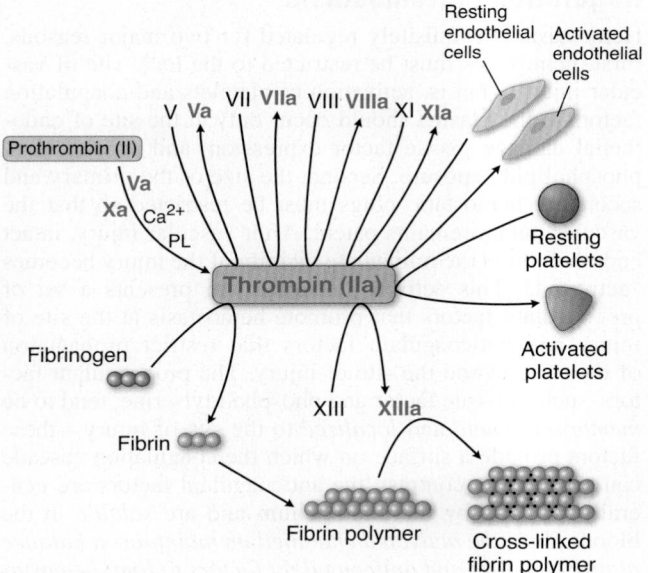

FIGURE 23-8. Central role of thrombin in the coagulation cascade. In the coagulation cascade, prothrombin is cleaved to thrombin by factor Xa; factor Va and Ca^{2+} act as cofactors in this reaction, and the reaction takes place on an activated (phosphatidylserine-expressing) phospholipid surface (PL). Thrombin converts the soluble plasma protein fibrinogen to fibrin, which spontaneously polymerizes. Thrombin also activates factor XIII, a transglutaminase that cross-links the fibrin polymers into a highly stable meshwork or clot. Thrombin also activates cofactors V and VIII, as well as coagulation factors VII and XI. In addition, thrombin activates both platelets and endothelial cells. Finally, thrombin stimulates the release of several antithrombotic factors—including PGI_2, NO, and t-PA—from resting (intact) endothelial cells near the site of vascular injury; these factors limit primary and secondary hemostasis to the injured site (*not shown*).

activator (t-PA), and the endogenous t-PA modulator plasminogen activator inhibitor 1 (PAI-1) (see below).

Thrombin binds to **protease-activated receptors (PARs)**, which are G protein-coupled receptors expressed in the plasma membrane of platelets, vascular endothelial cells, monocytes, vascular smooth muscle cells, and fibroblasts. Activation of PARs involves proteolytic *cleavage* of an extracellular domain of the receptor by thrombin. The new NH_2-terminal-tethered ligand binds intramolecularly to a discrete site within the receptor and initiates intracellular signaling. Activation of PAR-1 results in G protein-mediated activation of PLC (Fig. 23-5) and inhibition of adenylyl cyclase. Four different PARs have been identified (PARs 1–4). PAR-1 and

PAR-4 are expressed on platelets; PARs 1–4 are expressed on vascular endothelial cells; and some or all of the PARs are expressed on other cell types including monocytes and vascular smooth muscle cells. Of the two protease-activated receptors expressed on platelets, PAR-1 has a higher affinity for thrombin, and PAR-1 is the target of the new antiplatelet agent **vorapaxar** (see below).

Evidence from intravital (in vivo) microscopy experiments suggests that *microparticles* also have an important role in coupling platelet plug formation (primary hemostasis) to fibrin clot formation (secondary hemostasis). Microparticles are vesicular structures derived from leukocytes, monocytes, platelets, endothelial cells, and smooth muscle cells; they display proteins of the cells from which they were derived. For example, a subpopulation of microparticles is released from monocytes that are activated in the context of tissue injury and inflammation. These microparticles express both tissue factor and P-selectin glycoprotein ligand-1 (PSGL-1). In turn, PSGL-1 on the microparticles binds to the P-selectin adhesion receptor expressed on activated platelets. By recruiting tissue factor-bearing microparticles throughout the developing platelet plug (primary hemostasis), thrombin generation and fibrin clot formation (secondary hemostasis) could be greatly accelerated within the plug itself. Indeed, both vessel-wall tissue factor (expressed by activated endothelial cells, subendothelial fibroblasts, and smooth muscle cells) and microparticle tissue factor are important for the formation of a stable clot.

Regulation of Hemostasis

Hemostasis is exquisitely regulated for two major reasons. First, hemostasis must be restricted to the local site of vascular injury. That is, activation of platelets and coagulation factors in the plasma should occur only at the site of endothelial damage, tissue factor expression, and procoagulant phospholipid exposure. Second, the size of the primary and secondary hemostatic plugs must be restricted so that the vascular lumen remains patent. After vascular injury, intact endothelium in the immediate vicinity of the injury becomes "activated." This activated endothelium presents a set of procoagulant factors that promote hemostasis at the site of injury and anticoagulant factors that restrict propagation of the clot beyond the site of injury. The procoagulant factors, such as tissue factor and phosphatidylserine, tend to be *membrane-bound* and *localized* to the site of injury—these factors provide a surface on which the coagulation cascade can proceed. In contrast, the anticoagulant factors are generally *secreted* by the endothelium and are *soluble* in the blood. Thus, *the activated endothelium maintains a balance of procoagulant and anticoagulant factors to limit hemostasis to the site of vascular injury.*

After vascular injury, the endothelium surrounding the injured area participates in five separate mechanisms that limit the initiation and propagation of the hemostatic process to the immediate vicinity of the injury. These mechanisms involve prostacyclin (PGI_2), antithrombin III, proteins C and S, tissue factor pathway inhibitor (TFPI), and tissue-type plasminogen activator (t-PA).

Prostacyclin (PGI_2) is an eicosanoid (i.e., a metabolite of arachidonic acid) that is synthesized and secreted by the endothelium. By acting through G_s protein-coupled platelet-surface PGI_2 receptors, this metabolite increases cAMP levels within platelets and thereby inhibits platelet aggregation and platelet granule release. PGI_2 also has potent vasodilatory effects; this mediator induces vascular smooth muscle relaxation by increasing cAMP levels within the vascular smooth muscle cells. (Note that these mechanisms are physiologically antagonistic to those of TxA_2, which induces platelet activation and vasoconstriction.) Therefore, PGI_2 both prevents platelets from adhering to the intact endothelium that surrounds the site of vascular injury and maintains vascular patency around the site of injury.

Antithrombin III inactivates thrombin and other coagulation factors (IXa, Xa, XIa, and XIIa, where "a" denotes an "activated" factor) by forming a stoichiometric complex with the coagulation factor (Fig. 23-9). These interactions are enhanced by a heparin-like molecule that is expressed at the surface of intact endothelial cells, ensuring that this mechanism is operative at all locations in the vascular tree *except* where endothelium is denuded at the site of vascular injury. (These endothelial cell surface proteoglycans are referred to as *heparin-like* because they are the physiologic equivalent of the pharmacologic agent heparin, discussed below.) Heparin-like molecules on the endothelial cells bind to and activate antithrombin III, which is then primed to complex with (and thereby inactivate) the activated coagulation factors.

Protein C and **protein S** are vitamin K-dependent proteins that slow the coagulation cascade by inactivating coagulation factors Va and VIIIa. Protein C and protein S are part of a feedback control mechanism, in which excess thrombin generation leads to activation of protein C, which, in turn, helps to prevent the enlarging fibrin clot from occluding the vascular lumen. Specifically, the endothelial cell surface protein **thrombomodulin** is a receptor for both thrombin and protein C in the blood. Thrombomodulin binds these proteins in such a way that thrombomodulin-bound thrombin cleaves protein C to activated protein C (also known as *protein Ca*). In a reaction that requires the cofactor protein S, activated protein C then inhibits clotting by cleaving (and thereby inactivating) factors Va and VIIIa.

Tissue factor pathway inhibitor (TFPI), as its name indicates, limits the action of tissue factor (TF). The coagulation cascade is initiated when factor VIIa complexes with TF at the site of vascular injury (Fig. 23-6). The resulting VIIa:TF complex catalyzes the activation of factors IX and X. After limited quantities of factors IXa and Xa are generated, the VIIa:TF complex is feedback inhibited by TFPI in a two-step reaction. First, TFPI binds to factor Xa and neutralizes its activity in a Ca^{2+}-independent reaction. Subsequently, the TFPI:Xa complex interacts with the VIIa:TF complex via a second domain on TFPI, so that a quaternary Xa:TFPI:VIIa:TF complex is formed. The molecular "knots" of the TFPI molecule hold the quaternary complex tightly together and thereby inactivate the VIIa:TF complex. In this manner, TFPI prevents excessive TF-mediated activation of factors IX and X.

Plasmin exerts its anticoagulant effect by proteolytically cleaving fibrin into fibrin degradation products. Because plasmin has powerful antithrombotic effects, the *formation* of plasmin has intrigued researchers for many years, and a number of pharmacologic agents have been developed to target the plasmin formation pathway (Fig. 23-10). Plasmin is generated by the proteolytic cleavage of plasminogen, a plasma protein that is synthesized in the liver. The proteolytic cleavage is catalyzed by **tissue plasminogen activator (t-PA)**,

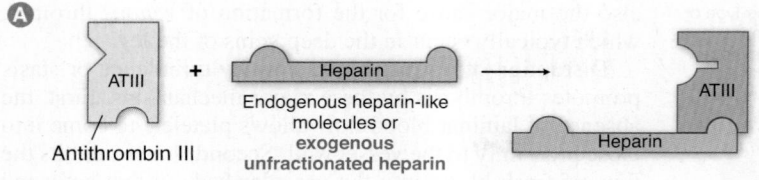

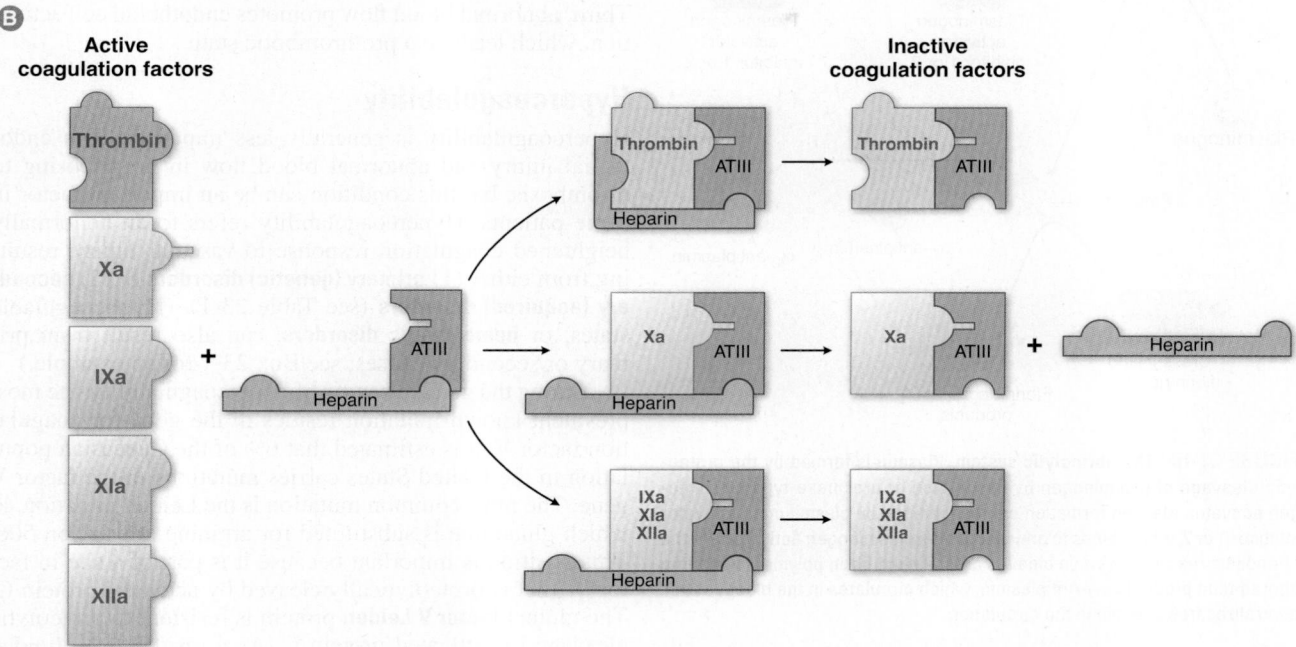

FIGURE 23-9. Antithrombin III action. Antithrombin III (ATIII) inactivates thrombin and factors IXa, Xa, XIa, and XIIa by forming a stoichiometric complex with these coagulation factors. These reactions are catalyzed physiologically by heparin-like molecules expressed on healthy endothelial cells; sites of vascular injury do not express heparin-like molecules because the endothelium is denuded or damaged. Pharmacologically, these reactions are catalyzed by exogenously administered heparin. In more detail, the binding of heparin to ATIII induces a conformational change in ATIII **(A)** that allows the ATIII to bind thrombin or coagulation factors IXa, Xa, XIa, or XIIa. The stoichiometric complex between ATIII and the coagulation factor is highly stable, allowing heparin to dissociate without breaking up the complex **(B)**.

which is synthesized and secreted by the endothelium. Plasmin activity is carefully modulated by three regulatory mechanisms in order to restrict plasmin action to the site of clot formation. First, t-PA is most effective when it is bound to a fibrin meshwork. Second, t-PA activity can be inhibited by **plasminogen activator inhibitor (PAI)**. When local concentrations of thrombin and inflammatory cytokines (such as IL-1 and TNF-α) are *high*, endothelial cells *increase* the release of PAI, preventing t-PA from activating plasmin. This ensures that a stable fibrin clot forms at the site of vascular injury. Third, α_2-**antiplasmin** is a plasma protein that neutralizes free plasmin in the circulation and thereby prevents systemic degradation of plasma fibrinogen. Plasma fibrinogen is important for platelet aggregation in primary hemostasis (see above), and it is also the precursor for the fibrin polymer that is required to form a stable clot.

PATHOGENESIS OF THROMBOSIS

Thrombosis is the pathologic extension of hemostasis. In thrombosis, coagulation reactions are inappropriately regulated so that a clot uncontrollably enlarges and occludes the lumen of a blood vessel. The pathologic clot is now termed a **thrombus**. Three major factors predispose to thrombus formation—endothelial injury, abnormal blood flow, and hypercoagulability. These three factors influence one another and are collectively known as **Virchow's triad** (Fig. 23-11).

Endothelial Injury

Endothelial injury is the dominant influence on thrombus formation in the *heart* and the *arterial circulation*. There are many possible causes of endothelial injury, including changes in shear stress associated with hypertension or turbulent flow, hyperlipidemia, elevated blood glucose in diabetes mellitus, traumatic vascular injury, and some infections. (Recall that Mr. S developed coronary artery thrombosis, which was probably attributable to endothelial injury secondary to hypertension and cigarette smoking.)

Endothelial injury predisposes the vascular lumen to thrombus formation through three mechanisms. First, platelet activators, such as exposed subendothelial collagen, promote platelet adhesion to the injured site. Second, exposure of tissue factor on injured endothelium initiates the coagulation cascade. Third, natural antithrombotics, such as t-PA and PGI$_2$, become depleted at the site of vascular injury because these mechanisms rely on the functioning of an intact endothelial cell layer.

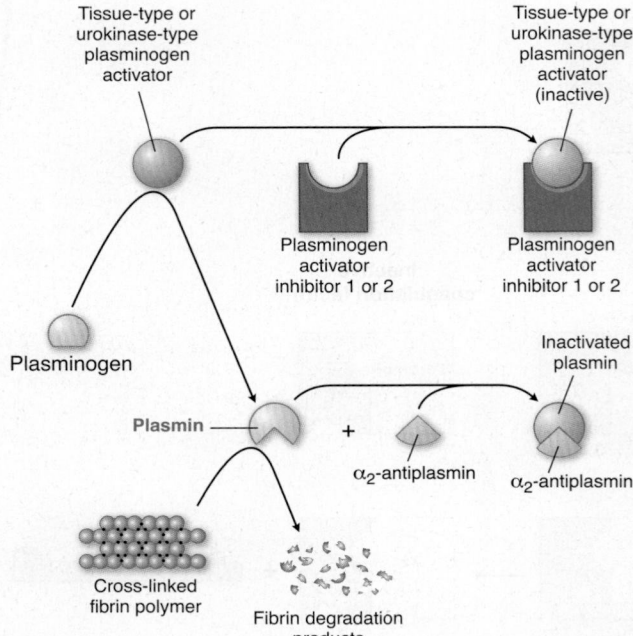

FIGURE 23-10. The fibrinolytic system. Plasmin is formed by the proteolytic cleavage of plasminogen by tissue-type or urokinase-type plasminogen activator. Plasmin formation can be inhibited by plasminogen activator inhibitor 1 or 2, which binds to and inactivates plasminogen activators. In the fibrinolytic reaction, plasmin cleaves cross-linked fibrin polymers into fibrin degradation products. α_2-Antiplasmin, which circulates in the bloodstream, neutralizes free plasmin in the circulation.

Abnormal Blood Flow

Abnormal blood flow refers to a state of **turbulence** or **stasis** rather than laminar flow. Atherosclerotic plaques commonly predispose to turbulent blood flow in the vicinity of the plaque. Bifurcations of blood vessels can also create areas of turbulent flow. Turbulent blood flow causes endothelial injury, forms countercurrents, and creates local pockets of stasis. Local stasis can also result from formation of an aneurysm (a focal outpouching of a vessel or a cardiac chamber) and from myocardial infarction. In the latter condition, a region of noncontractile (infarcted) myocardium serves as a favored site for stasis. Cardiac arrhythmias, such as atrial fibrillation, can also generate areas of local stasis. Stasis is

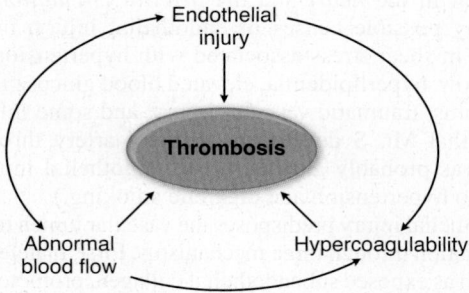

FIGURE 23-11. Virchow's triad. Endothelial injury, abnormal blood flow, and hypercoagulability are three factors that predispose to thrombus formation. These three factors are interrelated; endothelial injury predisposes to abnormal blood flow and hypercoagulability, while abnormal blood flow can cause both endothelial injury and hypercoagulability.

also the major cause for the formation of *venous* thrombi, which typically occur in the deep veins of the leg.

Disruption of normal blood flow by turbulence or stasis promotes thrombosis by three major mechanisms. First, the absence of laminar blood flow allows platelets to come into close proximity to the vessel wall. Second, stasis inhibits the flow of fresh blood into the vascular bed, so that activated coagulation factors in the region are not removed or diluted. Third, abnormal blood flow promotes endothelial cell activation, which leads to a prothrombotic state.

Hypercoagulability

Hypercoagulability is generally less important than endothelial injury and abnormal blood flow in predisposing to thrombosis, but this condition can be an important factor in some patients. Hypercoagulability refers to an abnormally heightened coagulation response to vascular injury, resulting from either (1) **primary (genetic) disorders** or (2) **secondary (acquired) disorders** (see Table 23-1). (Hypocoagulable states, or **hemorrhagic disorders**, can also result from primary or secondary causes; see Box 23-1 for an example.)

Among the genetic causes of hypercoagulability, the most prevalent known mutation resides in the gene for coagulation factor V. It is estimated that 6% of the Caucasian population in the United States carries mutations in the factor V gene. The most common mutation is the Leiden mutation, in which glutamine is substituted for arginine at position 506. This position is important because it is part of a site in factor Va that is proteolytically cleaved by activated protein C. The mutant **factor V Leiden** protein is resistant to proteolytic cleavage by activated protein C. As a result of the Leiden mutation, factor Va is allowed to accumulate and thereby to promote coagulation.

A second common mutation (2% incidence) is the **prothrombin G20210A mutation**, in which adenine (A) is substituted for guanine (G) in the 3'-untranslated region of the prothrombin gene. This mutation leads to a 30% increase in plasma prothrombin levels. Both the factor V Leiden mutation and the prothrombin G20210A mutation are associated with a significantly increased risk of venous thrombosis and a modestly increased risk of arterial thrombosis. Other genetic disorders that predispose some individuals to thrombosis include mutations in the fibrinogen, protein C, protein S, and antithrombin III genes. Although the latter disorders are relatively uncommon (less than 1% incidence), patients with a genetic deficiency of protein C, protein S, or antithrombin III often present with spontaneous venous thrombosis.

Hypercoagulability can sometimes be acquired (secondary) rather than genetic. An example of acquired hypercoagulability is the **heparin-induced thrombocytopenia** syndrome. In some patients, administration of the anticoagulant heparin stimulates the immune system to generate circulating antibodies directed against a complex consisting of heparin and platelet factor 4. Because platelet factor 4 is present on platelet and endothelial cell surfaces, antibody binding to the heparin:platelet factor 4 complex results in antibody-mediated removal of platelets from the circulation; that is, in thrombocytopenia. In some patients, however, antibody binding also causes platelet activation, endothelial injury, and a prothrombotic state. Although both unfractionated and low-molecular-weight heparin (see below) can cause thrombocytopenia, low-molecular-weight heparin is associated with a lower incidence of thrombocytopenia than unfractionated heparin.

TABLE 23-1 Major Causes of Hypercoagulability

CONDITION	MECHANISM OF HYPERCOAGULABILITY
Primary (Genetic)	
Factor V Leiden mutation (factor V R506Q) (common)	Resistance to activated protein C → excess factor Va
Hyperhomocysteinemia (common)	Endothelial damage due to accumulation of homocysteine
Prothrombin G20210A mutation (common)	Increased prothrombin level and activity
Antithrombin III deficiency (less common)	Decreased inactivation of factors IIa, IXa, and Xa
Protein C or S deficiency (less common)	Decreased proteolytic inactivation of factors VIIIa and Va
Secondary (Acquired)	
Antiphospholipid syndrome	Autoantibodies to negatively charged phospholipids → ↑ platelet adhesion
Heparin-induced thrombocytopenia	Antibodies to platelet factor 4 → platelet activation
Malignancy	Tumor cell induction of tissue factor expression
Myeloproliferative syndromes	Elevated blood viscosity, altered platelets
Nephrotic syndrome	Loss of antithrombin III in urine, ↑ fibrinogen, ↑ platelet activation
Oral contraceptive use, estrogen replacement therapy	↑ Hepatic synthesis of coagulation factors and/or effects of estrogen on endothelium (effect may be more prominent in patients with underlying primary hypercoagulability)
Paroxysmal nocturnal hemoglobinuria	Lack of glycosylphosphatidylinositol-linked proteins on red blood cells, white blood cells, and platelets, leading to complement-mediated intravascular hemolysis, nitric oxide scavenging by plasma free hemoglobin, formation of procoagulant microvesicles, and potential disorders of fibrinolysis and tissue factor pathway inhibitor function
Postpartum period	Venous stasis, increased coagulation factors, tissue trauma
Surgery/trauma	Venous stasis, immobilization, tissue injury

BOX 23-1 Hemorrhagic Disorders

When the vascular endothelium is injured, the hemostatic process ensures localized, stable clot formation without obstruction of the vascular lumen. Just as thrombosis constitutes a pathologic variation on this otherwise orchestrated physiologic process, disorders involving insufficient levels of functional platelets or coagulation factors can lead to a hypocoagulable state characterized clinically by episodes of uncontrolled hemorrhage. Hemorrhagic disorders result from a multitude of causes, including disorders of the vasculature, vitamin K deficiency, and disorders or deficiencies of platelets, coagulation factors, and von Willebrand factor. Hemophilia A serves as an example of a hemorrhagic disorder in which hypocoagulability is the underlying pathology.

Hemophilia A is the most common genetic disorder of serious bleeding. The hallmark of the disorder is a reduction in the amount or activity of coagulation factor VIII. The syndrome has an X-linked mode of transmission, and the majority of patients are males or homozygous females. Thirty percent of patients have no family history of hemophilia A and presumably represent spontaneous mutations. The severity of the disease depends on the type of mutation in the factor VIII gene. Patients with 6–50% of normal factor VIII activity manifest a mild form of the disease; those with 2–5% activity

manifest moderate disease; patients with less than 1% activity develop severe disease. All symptomatic patients demonstrate easy bruisability and can develop massive hemorrhage after trauma or surgery. Spontaneous hemorrhage can occur in body areas that are normally subjected to minor trauma, including joint spaces, where spontaneous hemorrhage leads to the formation of hemarthroses. Petechiae (microhemorrhages involving capillaries and small vessels, especially in mucocutaneous areas), which are usually an indication of platelet disorders, are absent in patients with hemophilia.

Patients with hemophilia A are currently treated with infusions of factor VIII that is either recombinant or derived from human plasma. Factor VIII infusion therapy is sometimes complicated in patients who develop antibodies against factor VIII. HIV infection was a serious complication of infusion therapy in patients who received factor VIII products before the institution of routine screening of blood for HIV infection (before the mid-1980s). Some sources suggest that the entire cohort of hemophiliacs who received factor VIII concentrates (factor VIII concentrated from the blood of many individuals) between 1981 and 1985 has been infected with HIV. With current blood screening practices and the development of recombinant factor VIII, the risk of contracting HIV through factor VIII infusions is now virtually zero. ■

Microparticles bearing tissue-factor *protein* have been demonstrated in the blood of healthy individuals, but no detectable tissue-factor *activity* is present in normal blood. This observation has led to the hypothesis that such microparticles contain inactive tissue factor (in "encrypted" form) and that the tissue factor is activated only upon recruitment of the particles to a site of vascular injury (see above). In pathologic states, circulating microparticles may contain activated tissue factor, which could predispose to the development of thrombotic events. High levels of circulating microparticles have been implicated in the thrombosis associated with a variety of disorders, such as cancer-related thrombosis, atherothrombosis, and paroxysmal nocturnal hemoglobinuria.

PHARMACOLOGIC CLASSES AND AGENTS

Multiple classes of drugs have been developed to prevent and/or reverse thrombus formation. These classes consist of antiplatelet agents, anticoagulants, and thrombolytic agents. Hemostatic agents, discussed at the end of the chapter, are occasionally used to reverse the effects of anticoagulants or to inhibit endogenous fibrinolysis.

Antiplatelet Agents

As described above, formation of a localized platelet plug in response to endothelial injury is the initial step in arterial thrombosis. Therefore, inhibition of platelet function is a useful prophylactic and therapeutic strategy against myocardial infarction and stroke caused by thrombosis in coronary and cerebral arteries, respectively. The classes of antiplatelet agents in current clinical use include cyclooxygenase (COX) inhibitors, phosphodiesterase inhibitors, ADP receptor pathway inhibitors, GPIIb–IIIa antagonists, and thrombin receptor (PAR-1) antagonists.

Cyclooxygenase Inhibitors

Aspirin inhibits the synthesis of prostaglandins, thereby inhibiting the platelet granule release reaction and interfering with normal platelet aggregation.

The biochemistry of prostaglandin synthesis in platelets and endothelial cells provides a basis for understanding the mechanism of action of aspirin as an antiplatelet agent. Figure 23-12 depicts the prostaglandin synthesis pathway, which is discussed in more detail in Chapter 43, Pharmacology of Eicosanoids. Briefly, activation of both platelets and endothelial cells induces phospholipase A_2 (PLA_2) to cleave membrane phospholipids and release arachidonic acid. Arachidonic acid is then transformed into a cyclic endoperoxide (also known as **prostaglandin G_2** or **PGG_2**) by the enzyme COX. In platelets, the cyclic endoperoxide is converted into thromboxane A_2 (TxA_2). Acting through cell surface TxA_2 receptors, TxA_2 causes localized vasoconstriction and is a potent inducer of platelet aggregation and the platelet granule release reaction. In endothelial cells, the cyclic endoperoxide is converted into prostacyclin (PGI_2). PGI_2, in turn, causes localized vasodilation and inhibits platelet aggregation and the platelet granule release reaction.

Aspirin acts by *covalently* acetylating a serine residue near the active site of the COX enzyme, thereby inhibiting the synthesis of the cyclic endoperoxide and the various metabolites of the cyclic endoperoxide. In the absence of TxA_2, there is a marked decrease in platelet aggregation and the platelet granule release reaction (Fig. 23-13A). *Because platelets do not contain DNA or RNA, these cells cannot regenerate new COX enzyme once aspirin has permanently inactivated all of the available COX enzyme.* That is, the platelets become irreversibly "poisoned" for the lifetime of these cells (7–10 days). Although aspirin also inhibits the COX enzyme in endothelial cells, its action is not permanent in endothelial cells because these cells are able to synthesize new COX molecules. Thus, the endothelial cell production of prostacyclin is relatively unaffected by aspirin at pharmacologically low doses (see below).

Aspirin is most often used as an antiplatelet agent to prevent arterial thrombosis leading to transient ischemic attack, stroke, and myocardial infarction. Because the action of aspirin on platelets is permanent, it is most effective as a selective antiplatelet agent when taken *in low doses and/or at infrequent intervals*. For example, aspirin is often used as an antiplatelet agent at a dose of 81 mg once daily, while a typical anti-inflammatory dose of this agent could be 650 mg three to four times daily. When taken at high doses, aspirin can inhibit prostacyclin production without increasing the effectiveness of the drug as an antiplatelet agent. A more extended discussion of the uses and toxicities of aspirin is found in Chapter 43. Compared with aspirin, other nonsteroidal anti-inflammatory drugs (NSAIDs) are not as widely used in the prevention of arterial thrombosis because the inhibitory action of these drugs on cyclooxygenase is not permanent.

COX-1 is the predominant COX isoform in platelets, but endothelial cells express both COX-1 and COX-2 under physiologic conditions. Because aspirin inhibits COX-1 and COX-2 nonselectively, this drug serves as an effective antiplatelet agent. In contrast, selective COX-2 inhibitors cannot be used as antiplatelet agents because they are poor inhibitors of COX-1. Furthermore, use of the selective COX-2 inhibitors appears to be associated with increased cardiovascular risk, which has resulted in the withdrawal of most of these agents from the market (see Chapter 43).

Phosphodiesterase Inhibitors

In platelets, an *increase* in the concentration of intracellular cAMP leads to a *decrease* in platelet aggregability. Platelet cAMP levels are regulated physiologically by TxA_2 and PGI_2, among other mediators (see above). The mechanism by which increased intracellular cAMP concentration leads to decreased platelet aggregability is not well understood. cAMP activates protein kinase A, which, through incompletely elucidated mechanisms, decreases availability of the intracellular Ca^{2+} necessary for platelet aggregation (Fig. 23-13B). Inhibitors of platelet phosphodiesterase decrease platelet aggregability by inhibiting cAMP degradation, while activators of platelet adenylyl cyclase decrease platelet aggregability by increasing cAMP synthesis. (There are currently no direct adenylyl cyclase activators in clinical use.)

Dipyridamole is an inhibitor of platelet phosphodiesterase that decreases platelet aggregability (Fig. 23-13B). Dipyridamole by itself has only weak antiplatelet effects and is therefore usually administered in combination with warfarin or aspirin. The combination of dipyridamole and warfarin can be used to inhibit thrombus formation on prosthetic heart valves, while the combination of dipyridamole and aspirin

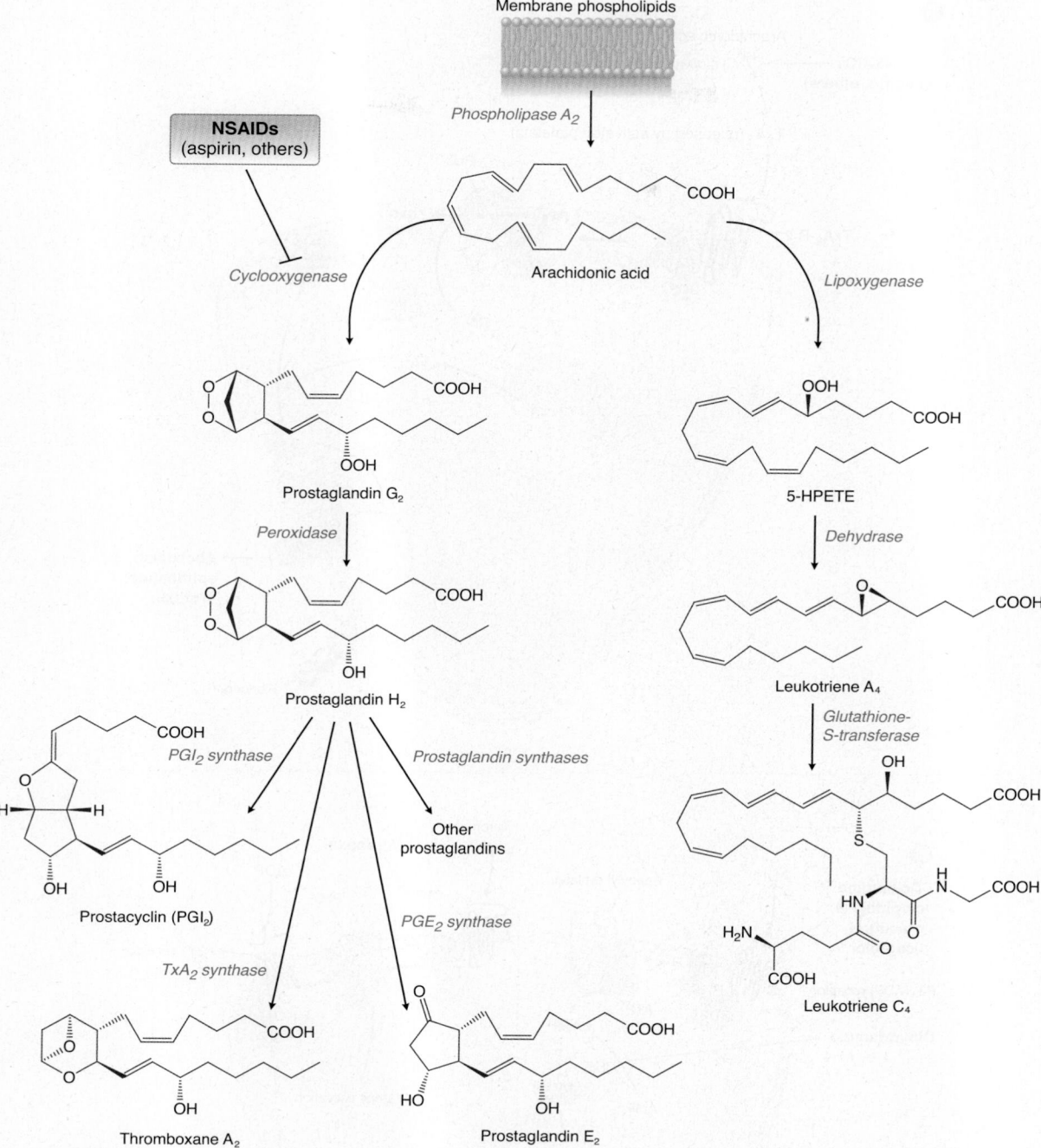

FIGURE 23-12. Overview of prostaglandin synthesis. Membrane phospholipids are cleaved by phospholipase A_2 to release free arachidonic acid. Arachidonic acid can be metabolized through either of two major pathways: the cyclooxygenase pathway or the lipoxygenase pathway. The cyclooxygenase pathway, which is inhibited by aspirin and other nonsteroidal anti-inflammatory drugs (NSAIDs), converts arachidonic acid into prostaglandins and thromboxanes. Platelets express TxA_2 synthase and synthesize the pro-aggregatory mediator thromboxane A_2; endothelial cells express PGI_2 synthase and synthesize the anti-aggregatory mediator prostacyclin. The lipoxygenase pathway converts arachidonic acid into leukotrienes, which are potent inflammatory mediators. (See Chapter 43, Pharmacology of Eicosanoids, for a detailed discussion of the lipoxygenase and cyclooxygenase pathways.) Aspirin inhibits cyclooxygenase by covalent acetylation of the enzyme near its active site. Because platelets lack the capability to synthesize new proteins, aspirin inhibits thromboxane synthesis for the life of the platelet.

can be used to reduce the likelihood of thrombosis in patients with a thrombotic diathesis. Dipyridamole also has vasodilatory properties. It may paradoxically induce angina in patients with coronary artery disease by causing the coronary artery steal, which involves intense dilation of coronary arterioles (see Chapter 22, Pharmacology of Vascular Tone).

ADP Receptor Pathway Inhibitors

Ticlopidine, **clopidogrel**, and **prasugrel** are derivatives of thienopyridine. These agents, which irreversibly inhibit the ADP-dependent pathway of platelet activation, have antiplatelet effects in vitro and in vivo. Ticlopidine, clopidogrel, and prasugrel act by covalently modifying and inactivating

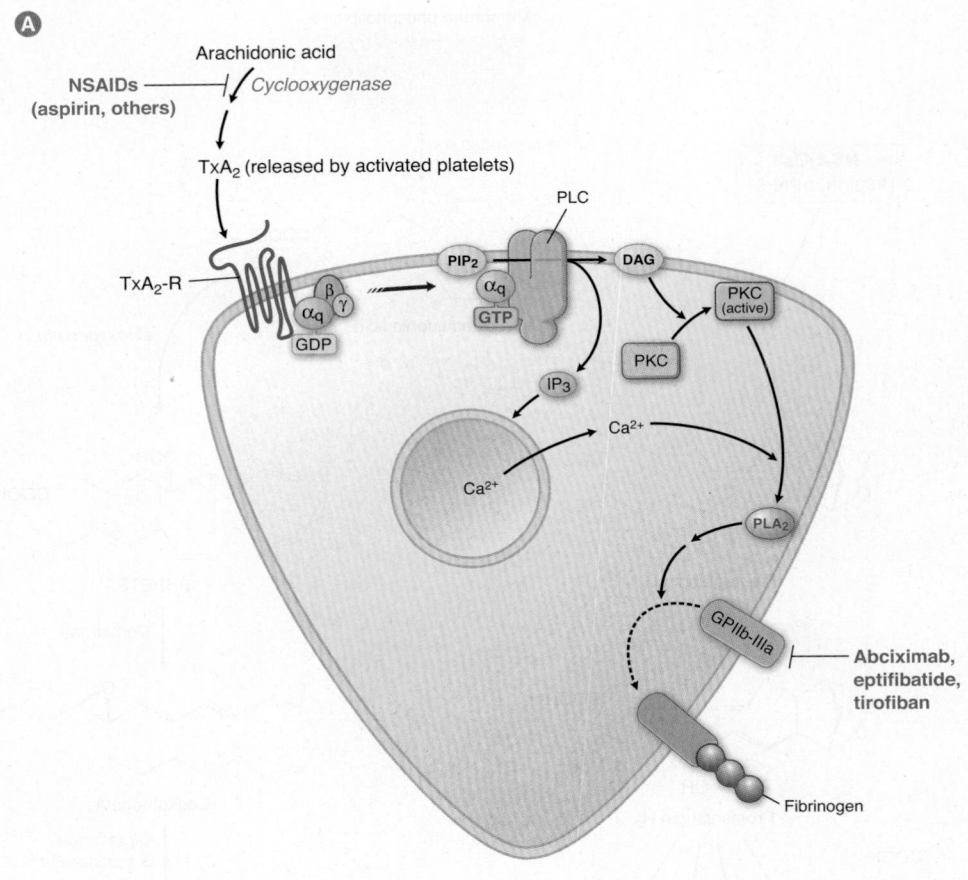

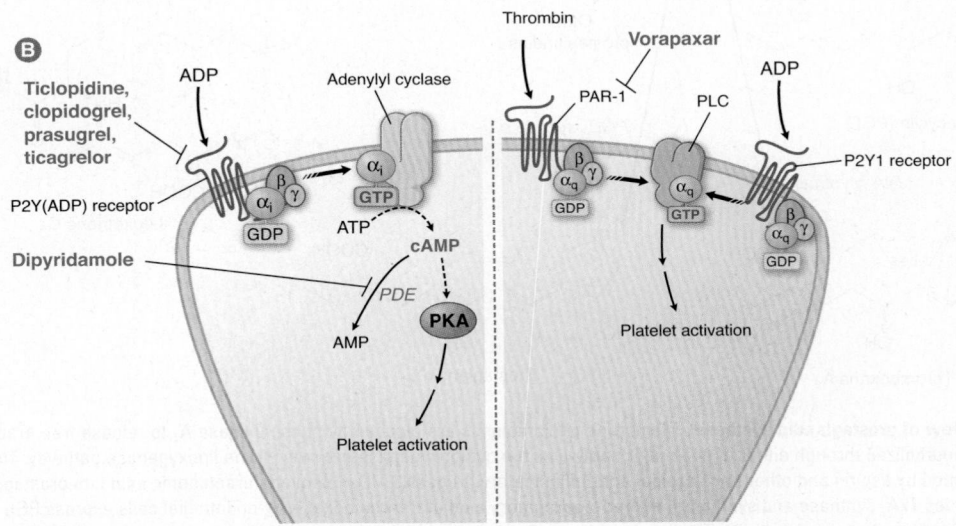

FIGURE 23-13. Mechanism of action of antiplatelet agents. A. NSAIDs and GPIIb–IIIa antagonists inhibit steps in thromboxane A_2 (TxA_2)-mediated plate-let activation. Aspirin inhibits cyclooxygenase by covalent acetylation of the enzyme near its active site, leading to decreased TxA_2 production. The effect is profound because platelets lack the ability to synthesize new enzyme molecules. GPIIb–IIIa antagonists, such as the monoclonal antibody abciximab and the small-molecule antagonists eptifibatide and tirofiban, inhibit platelet aggregation by preventing activation of GpIIb–IIIa (*dashed line*), leading to decreased platelet cross-linking by fibrinogen. **B.** Ticlopidine, clopidogrel, prasugrel, ticagrelor, and dipyridamole inhibit steps in ADP-mediated platelet activation. Ticlopidine, clopidogrel, prasugrel, and ticagrelor are antagonists of the P2Y(ADP) receptor. Dipyridamole inhibits phosphodiesterase (PDE), thereby preventing the breakdown of cAMP and increasing cytoplasmic cAMP concentration. Vorapaxar inhibits PAR-1, thereby decreasing phospholipase C (PLC)-mediated platelet activation.

the platelet P2Y(ADP) receptor (also called $P2Y_{12}$), which is physiologically coupled to the inhibition of adenylyl cyclase (Fig. 23-13B).

Ticlopidine, a first-generation thienopyridine, is a prodrug that requires conversion to active thiol metabolites in the liver. Maximal platelet inhibition is observed 8–11 days after initiating therapy with the drug; when used in combination with aspirin, 4–7 days are needed to achieve maximal platelet inhibition. Administration of a loading dose can produce a more rapid antiplatelet response. Ticlopidine is approved in the United States for two indications: (1) secondary prevention of thrombotic strokes in patients intolerant of aspirin, and (2) in combination with aspirin, prevention of stent thrombosis after placement of coronary artery stents. The use of ticlopidine has occasionally been associated with neutropenia, thrombocytopenia, and thrombotic thrombocytopenic purpura (TTP); for this reason, blood counts must be monitored frequently when using ticlopidine. Ticlopidine has largely been replaced by clopidogrel because of the latter drug's more favorable adverse effect profile and more rapid onset of action.

Clopidogrel, a second-generation thienopyridine closely related to ticlopidine, has been used widely *in combination with aspirin* for improved platelet inhibition during and after percutaneous coronary intervention. Clopidogrel is a prodrug that must undergo oxidation by hepatic P450 enzymes to the active drug form; it may therefore interact with statins, proton pump inhibitors, and other drugs metabolized by these P450 isoforms (see Chapter 4, Drug Metabolism). Clopidogrel is approved for secondary prevention in patients with recent myocardial infarction, stroke, or peripheral vascular disease. It is also approved for use in acute coronary syndromes that are treated with either percutaneous coronary intervention or coronary artery bypass grafting. Like ticlopidine, clopidogrel requires a loading dose to achieve a maximal antiplatelet effect rapidly. For this reason, Mr. S was given an oral loading dose of clopidogrel in the context of his myocardial infarction. The adverse effect profile of clopidogrel is more acceptable than that of ticlopidine: the gastrointestinal effects of clopidogrel are similar to those of aspirin, and clopidogrel lacks the significant bone marrow toxicity associated with ticlopidine.

Prasugrel, a third-generation thienopyridine, is an irreversible antagonist of the $P2Y_{12}$ ADP receptor. This drug is approved for use in acute coronary syndromes treated with percutaneous coronary intervention. Like clopidogrel, prasugrel is a prodrug and is used in combination with aspirin. Prasugrel is more efficiently metabolized than clopidogrel, resulting in higher concentrations of the active drug and more complete inhibition of the $P2Y_{12}$ ADP receptor. Because of its more complete platelet inhibition, prasugrel may increase the risk of bleeding relative to clopidogrel, especially in patients over 75 years of age or weighing less than 60 kilograms. It is also contraindicated for use in patients with a prior history of stroke or transient ischemic attack because of an increased risk of intracranial hemorrhage.

Ticagrelor is a competitive antagonist at the $P2Y_{12}$ ADP receptor. Unlike the other agents in this class, ticagrelor is a cyclopentyltriazolopyrimidine. Ticagrelor is approved for use in patients with acute coronary syndromes. It is an orally active drug that does not require hepatic activation. Compared to other agents in its class, ticagrelor inhibits platelet activation more than clopidogrel but slightly less than prasugrel. Adverse effects specific to ticagrelor may include dyspnea and bradycardia. Similar to prasugrel, ticagrelor is

contraindicated for use in patients with a history of intracranial hemorrhage.

GPIIb–IIIa Antagonists

As noted above, platelet membrane GPIIb–IIIa receptors constitute the final common pathway of platelet aggregation, serving to bind fibrinogen molecules that bridge platelets to one another. A variety of stimuli (e.g., TxA_2, ADP, epinephrine, collagen, and thrombin), acting through diverse signaling pathways, are capable of inducing the expression of functional GPIIb–IIIa on the platelet surface. It could therefore be predicted that antagonists of GPIIb–IIIa would serve as powerful inhibitors of platelet aggregation by preventing fibrinogen binding to the GPIIb–IIIa receptor (Fig. 23-13A). **Eptifibatide**, the GPIIb–IIIa receptor antagonist used in the opening case, is a highly efficacious inhibitor of platelet aggregation. A synthetic peptide, eptifibatide antagonizes the platelet GPIIb–IIIa receptor with high affinity. This drug is used to reduce ischemic events in patients undergoing percutaneous coronary intervention and to treat unstable angina and non-ST elevation myocardial infarction.

Abciximab is a chimeric mouse–human monoclonal antibody directed against the human GPIIb–IIIa receptor. Experiments in vitro have shown that occupation of 50% of platelet GPIIb–IIIa receptors by abciximab significantly reduces platelet aggregation. The binding of abciximab to GPIIb–IIIa is essentially *irreversible*, with a dissociation half-time of 18–24 hours. In clinical trials, adding abciximab to conventional antithrombotic therapy reduces both long-term and short-term ischemic events in patients undergoing high-risk percutaneous coronary intervention.

Tirofiban is a nonpeptide tyrosine analogue that reversibly antagonizes fibrinogen binding to the platelet GPIIb–IIIa receptor. Both in vitro and in vivo studies have demonstrated the ability of tirofiban to inhibit platelet aggregation. Tirofiban has been approved for use in patients with acute coronary syndromes.

Because of their mechanism of action as antiplatelet agents, all of the GPIIb–IIIa antagonists can cause bleeding as an adverse effect. In the opening case, Mr. S developed a hematoma in his right thigh near the arterial access site. The expanding hematoma was caused by the excessive antiplatelet effect of eptifibatide. Importantly, the ability to reverse the effect of GPIIb–IIIa receptor antagonists differs for the different agents. Because abciximab is an irreversible inhibitor of platelet function, and all the abciximab previously infused is already bound to platelets, infusion of fresh platelets after the drug has been stopped can reverse the antiplatelet effect. In contrast, because the two small-molecule antagonists (eptifibatide and tirofiban) bind the receptor reversibly and are infused in great stoichiometric excess of receptor number, infusion of fresh platelets simply offers new sites to which the drug can bind, and it is not practical to deliver a sufficient number of platelets to overwhelm the vast excess of drug present. Therefore, one must stop the drug infusion and wait for platelet function to return to normal as the drug is cleared. In the case of Mr. S, no other measure could have been taken to reverse the effect of eptifibatide at the time his hematoma was recognized.

Thrombin Receptor (PAR-1) Antagonists

Vorapaxar is a reversible antagonist of protease-activated receptor 1 (PAR-1), one of two major thrombin receptors expressed on platelets (Fig. 23-13B). Inhibition of PAR-1 inhibits platelet activation with minimal effect on the coagulation cascade. Vorapaxar is approved for secondary prevention of myocardial infarction, death, and stroke in patients with a prior myocardial infarction or with peripheral artery disease. It is orally available and metabolized by hepatic CYP3A4 enzymes, with primarily hepatic clearance. Vorapaxar should not be administered to patients with a prior history of stroke, transient ischemic attack, or intracranial hemorrhage.

Anticoagulants

As with antiplatelet agents, anticoagulants are used both to prevent and treat thrombotic disease. There are four classes of anticoagulants: warfarin, unfractionated and low-molecular-weight heparins, selective factor Xa inhibitors, and direct thrombin inhibitors. Anticoagulants target various factors in the coagulation cascade, thereby interrupting the cascade and preventing the formation of a stable fibrin meshwork (secondary hemostatic plug). In this section, the four classes of anticoagulants are discussed in order of selectivity, from the least selective agents (warfarin and unfractionated heparin) to the most selective agents (selective factor Xa inhibitors and direct thrombin inhibitors). Recombinant activated protein C also has anticoagulant activity, although its clinical indication is severe sepsis. Because of the mechanisms of action of these drugs, bleeding is an adverse effect common to all anticoagulants.

Warfarin

In the early 1900s, farmers in Canada and the North Dakota plains adopted the practice of planting sweet clover instead of corn for fodder. In the winter months of 1921 to 1922, a fatal hemorrhagic disease was reported in cattle that had foraged on the sweet clover. In almost every case, it was found that the affected cattle had foraged on sweet clover that had been spoiled by the curing process. After an intensive investigation, scientist K. P. Link reported that the spoiled clover contained the natural anticoagulant 3,3'-methylene-bis-(4-hydroxycoumarin) or *dicumarol.* Dicumarol and **warfarin** (a potent synthetic congener) were introduced during the 1940s as rodenticides and as oral anticoagulants. Because the oral anticoagulants act by affecting vitamin K-dependent reactions, it is important to understand how vitamin K functions.

Mechanism of Action of Vitamin K

Vitamin K ("K" is derived from the German word "Koagulation") is required for the normal hepatic synthesis of four coagulation factors (II, VII, IX, and X), protein C, and protein S. The coagulation factors, protein C, and protein S are biologically inactive as unmodified polypeptides following protein synthesis on ribosomes. These proteins gain biological activity by post-translational carboxylation of their 9 to 12 amino-terminal glutamic acid residues. The γ-carboxylated glutamate residues (but not the unmodified glutamate residues) are capable of binding Ca^{2+} ions. Ca^{2+} binding induces a conformational change in these proteins that is required for efficient binding of the proteins to phospholipid surfaces. The binding of Ca^{2+} to the γ-carboxylated molecules increases the enzymatic activity of coagulation factors IIa, VIIa, IXa, Xa, and protein Ca by approximately 1,000-fold. Thus, vitamin K-dependent carboxylation is crucial for the enzymatic activity of the four coagulation factors and protein C and for the cofactor function of protein S.

The carboxylation reaction requires (1) a precursor form of the target protein with its 9 to 12 amino-terminal glutamic acid residues, (2) carbon dioxide, (3) molecular oxygen, and (4) *reduced* vitamin K. The carboxylation reaction is schematically presented in Figure 23-14. During this reaction, vitamin K is oxidized to the inactive 2,3-epoxide. An enzyme, vitamin K epoxide reductase (also called *VKORC1*), is then required to convert the inactive 2,3-epoxide into the active, reduced form of vitamin K. *Thus, the regeneration of reduced vitamin K is essential for the sustained synthesis of biologically functional clotting factors II, VII, IX, and X, all of which are critical components of the coagulation cascade.*

Mechanism of Action of Warfarin

Warfarin acts on the carboxylation pathway, not by inhibiting the carboxylase directly but by blocking the epoxide reductase that mediates the regeneration of reduced vitamin K (Fig. 23-14). Because depletion of reduced vitamin K in the liver prevents the γ-carboxylation reaction that is required for the synthesis of biologically active coagulation factors, the onset of action of the oral anticoagulants parallels the half-life of these coagulation factors in the circulation. Of the four affected clotting factors (II, VII, IX, and X), factor VII has the shortest half-life (6 hours). Thus, the pharmacologic effect of a single dose of warfarin is not manifested for approximately 18–24 hours (i.e., 3–4 factor VII half-lives). This *delayed action* is one pharmacologic property that distinguishes the warfarin class of anticoagulants from all the other classes of anticoagulants.

Evidence from studies of long-term rodenticide use and of anticoagulant use supports the hypothesis that the epoxide reductase is the molecular target of oral anticoagulant action. The use of oral anticoagulants as rodenticides has been a widespread practice in farming communities. In some areas of the United States, heavy rodenticide use has selected for a population of wild rodents that is resistant to 4-hydroxycoumarins. In vitro studies of tissues from these rodents have demonstrated a mutation in the rodent epoxide reductase that renders the enzyme resistant to inhibition by the anticoagulant. Similarly, a small population of patients is genetically resistant to warfarin because of mutations in their epoxide reductase gene. These patients require 10–20 times the usual dose of warfarin to achieve the desired anticoagulant effect. More generally, genetic variation in the *VKORC1* gene has been associated with approximately 25–30% of the variance in warfarin maintenance dose in patients taking this drug (see Chapter 7, Pharmacogenomics).

Clinical Uses of Warfarin

Warfarin is often administered to complete a course of anticoagulation that has been initiated with heparin (see below) and to prevent thrombosis in predisposed patients. Orally administered warfarin is nearly 100% bioavailable, and its levels in the blood peak at 0.5–4 hours after administration. *In the plasma, 99% of racemic warfarin is bound to plasma protein (albumin).* Warfarin has a relatively long elimination half-life (approximately 36 hours). The drug is hydroxylated by the cytochrome P450 system in the liver to inactive metabolites that are subsequently eliminated in the urine (see Table 4-3).

Drug–drug interactions must be carefully considered in patients taking warfarin. Because warfarin is highly albumin-bound in the plasma, co-administration of warfarin with other albumin-bound drugs can increase the free

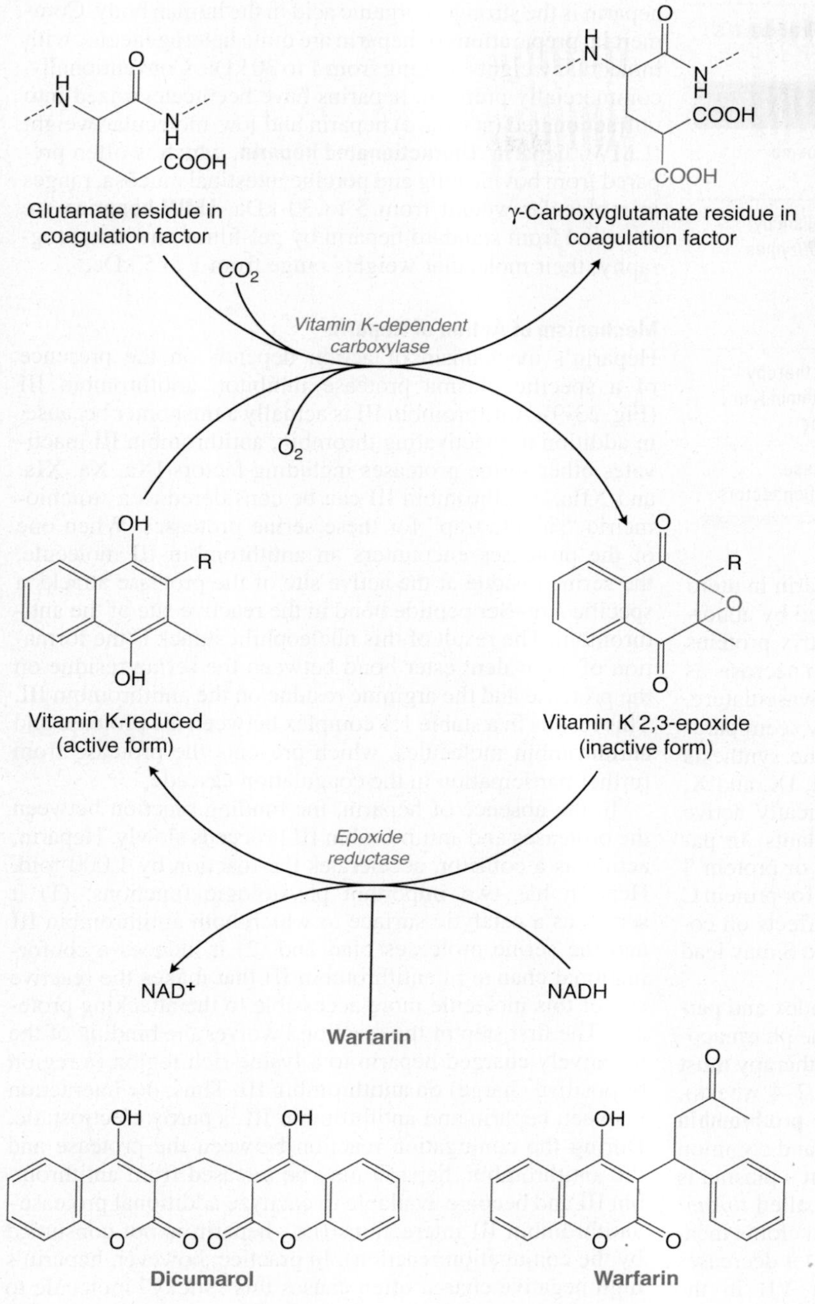

Glutamate residue in coagulation factor

γ-Carboxyglutamate residue in coagulation factor

CO_2

Vitamin K-dependent carboxylase

O_2

Vitamin K-reduced (active form)

Vitamin K 2,3-epoxide (inactive form)

Epoxide reductase

NAD^+

NADH

Warfarin

Dicumarol

Warfarin

FIGURE 23-14. Mechanism of action of warfarin. Vitamin K is a necessary cofactor in the post-translational carboxylation of glutamate residues on factors II, VII, IX, and X. During the carboxylation reaction, vitamin K is oxidized to the inactive 2,3-epoxide. The enzyme vitamin K epoxide reductase (also called *VKORC1*) converts the inactive vitamin K 2,3-epoxide into the active, reduced form of vitamin K. The regeneration of reduced vitamin K is essential for the sustained synthesis of biologically functional coagulation factors II, VII, IX, and X. Warfarin acts on the carboxylation pathway by inhibiting the epoxide reductase that is required for the regeneration of reduced (active) vitamin K. Dicumarol is the natural anticoagulant formed in spoiled clover. Both warfarin and dicumarol are orally bioavailable.

(unbound) plasma concentrations of both drugs. In addition, because warfarin is metabolized by P450 enzymes in the liver, co-administration of warfarin with drugs that induce and/or compete for P450 metabolism can affect the plasma concentrations of both drugs. Tables 23-2 and 23-3 list some of the major interactions between warfarin and other drugs.

Among the adverse effects of warfarin, bleeding is the most serious and predictable toxicity. Withdrawal of the drug may be recommended for patients who suffer from repeated bleeding episodes at otherwise therapeutic drug concentrations. For severe hemorrhage, patients should promptly receive fresh frozen plasma, which contains biologically functional clotting factors II, VII, IX, and X. *Warfarin should never be administered to pregnant women* because it can cross the placenta and cause a hemorrhagic disorder in

TABLE 23-2 Examples of Drugs That Diminish Warfarin's Anticoagulant Effect

DRUG OR DRUG CLASS	MECHANISM
Cholestyramine	Inhibits warfarin absorption in the gastrointestinal tract
Barbiturates, carbamazepine, phenytoin, rifampin	Accelerate warfarin metabolism by inducing hepatic P450 enzymes (especially P450 2C9)
Vitamin K (reduced)	Bypasses warfarin's inhibition of epoxide reductase

TABLE 23-3 Examples of Drugs That Enhance Warfarin's Anticoagulant Effect

DRUG OR DRUG CLASS	MECHANISM
Chloral hydrate	Displaces warfarin from plasma albumin
Amiodarone, clopidogrel, ethanol (intoxicating dose), fluconazole, fluoxetine, metronidazole, sulfamethoxazole	Decrease warfarin metabolism by inhibiting hepatic P450 enzymes (especially P450 2C9)
Broad-spectrum antibiotics	Eliminate gut bacteria and thereby reduce availability of vitamin K in the gastrointestinal tract
Anabolic steroids (testosterone)	Inhibit synthesis and increase degradation of coagulation factors

the fetus. In addition, newborns exposed to warfarin in utero may have serious congenital defects characterized by abnormal bone formation (note that certain bone matrix proteins are γ-carboxylated). Rarely, warfarin causes skin necrosis as a result of widespread thrombosis in the microvasculature. The fact that warfarin can cause thrombosis may seem paradoxical. Recall that, in addition to inhibiting the synthesis of biologically active coagulation factors II, VII, IX, and X, warfarin also prevents the synthesis of biologically active proteins C and S, which are natural anticoagulants. In patients who are genetically deficient in protein C or protein S (most commonly, patients who are heterozygous for protein C deficiency), an imbalance between warfarin's effects on coagulation factors and its effects on proteins C and S may lead to microvascular thrombosis and skin necrosis.

Because warfarin has a narrow therapeutic index and participates in numerous drug–drug interactions, the pharmacodynamic (functional) effect of chronic warfarin therapy must be monitored regularly (on the order of every 2–4 weeks). Monitoring is most easily performed using the **prothrombin time (PT)**, which is a simple test of the extrinsic and common pathways of coagulation. In this test, the patient's plasma is added to a crude preparation of tissue factor (called *thromboplastin*), and the time for formation of a fibrin clot is measured. Warfarin prolongs the PT mainly because it decreases the amount of biologically functional factor VII in the plasma. (Recall that factor VII is the vitamin K-dependent coagulation factor with the shortest half-life.) Measurement of the PT has been standardized worldwide and is expressed as the **international normalized ratio (INR)** of the prothrombin time in the patient sample to that in a control sample, normalized for the international sensitivity index (ISI) of the laboratory's thromboplastin preparation compared to the World Health Organization's reference thromboplastin preparation. The formula used to calculate the INR is as follows: $INR = [PT_{patient} / PT_{control}]^{ISI}$.

Unfractionated and Low-Molecular-Weight Heparins
Structure of Heparin
Heparin is a sulfated mucopolysaccharide stored in the secretory granules of mast cells. It is a highly sulfated polymer of alternating uronic acid and D-glucosamine. Heparin molecules are highly negatively charged; indeed, endogenous

heparin is the strongest organic acid in the human body. Commercial preparations of heparin are quite heterogeneous, with molecular weights ranging from 1 to 30 kDa. Conventionally, commercially prepared heparins have been categorized into unfractionated (standard) heparin and low-molecular-weight (LMW) heparin. **Unfractionated heparin**, which is often prepared from bovine lung and porcine intestinal mucosa, ranges in molecular weight from 5 to 30 kDa. **LMW heparins** are prepared from standard heparin by gel-filtration chromatography; their molecular weights range from 1 to 5 kDa.

Mechanism of Action of Heparin
Heparin's mechanism of action depends on the presence of a specific plasma protease inhibitor, antithrombin III (Fig. 23-9). Antithrombin III is actually a misnomer because, in addition to inactivating thrombin, antithrombin III inactivates other serine proteases including factors IXa, Xa, XIa, and XIIa. Antithrombin III can be considered as a stoichiometric "suicide trap" for these serine proteases. When one of the proteases encounters an antithrombin III molecule, the serine residue at the active site of the protease attacks a specific Arg–Ser peptide bond in the reactive site of the antithrombin. The result of this nucleophilic attack is the formation of a covalent ester bond between the serine residue on the protease and the arginine residue on the antithrombin III. This results in a stable 1:1 complex between the protease and antithrombin molecules, which prevents the protease from further participation in the coagulation cascade.

In the absence of heparin, the binding reaction between the proteases and antithrombin III proceeds slowly. Heparin, acting as a cofactor, accelerates the reaction by 1,000-fold. Heparin has two important physiologic functions: (1) it serves as a catalytic surface to which both antithrombin III and the serine proteases bind and (2) it induces a conformational change in antithrombin III that makes the reactive site of this molecule more accessible to the attacking protease. The first step of the reaction involves the binding of the negatively charged heparin to a lysine-rich region (a region of positive charge) on antithrombin III. Thus, the interaction between heparin and antithrombin III is partly electrostatic. During the conjugation reaction between the protease and the antithrombin, heparin may be released from antithrombin III and become available to catalyze additional protease–antithrombin III interactions (i.e., heparin is not consumed by the conjugation reaction). In practice, however, heparin's high negative charge often causes this "sticky" molecule to remain electrostatically bound to protease, antithrombin, or another nearby molecule in the vicinity of a thrombus.

Interestingly, heparins of different molecular weights have divergent anticoagulant activities. These divergent activities derive from the differential requirements for heparin binding exhibited by the inactivation of thrombin and factor Xa by antithrombin III (Fig. 23-15). To catalyze most efficiently the inactivation of thrombin by antithrombin III, a single molecule of heparin must bind simultaneously to both thrombin and antithrombin. This "scaffolding" function is required in addition to the heparin-induced conformational change in antithrombin III that renders the antithrombin susceptible to conjugation with thrombin. In contrast, to catalyze the inactivation of factor Xa by antithrombin III, the heparin molecule must bind only to the antithrombin, because the conformational change in antithrombin III induced by heparin binding is sufficient by itself to render the antithrombin susceptible

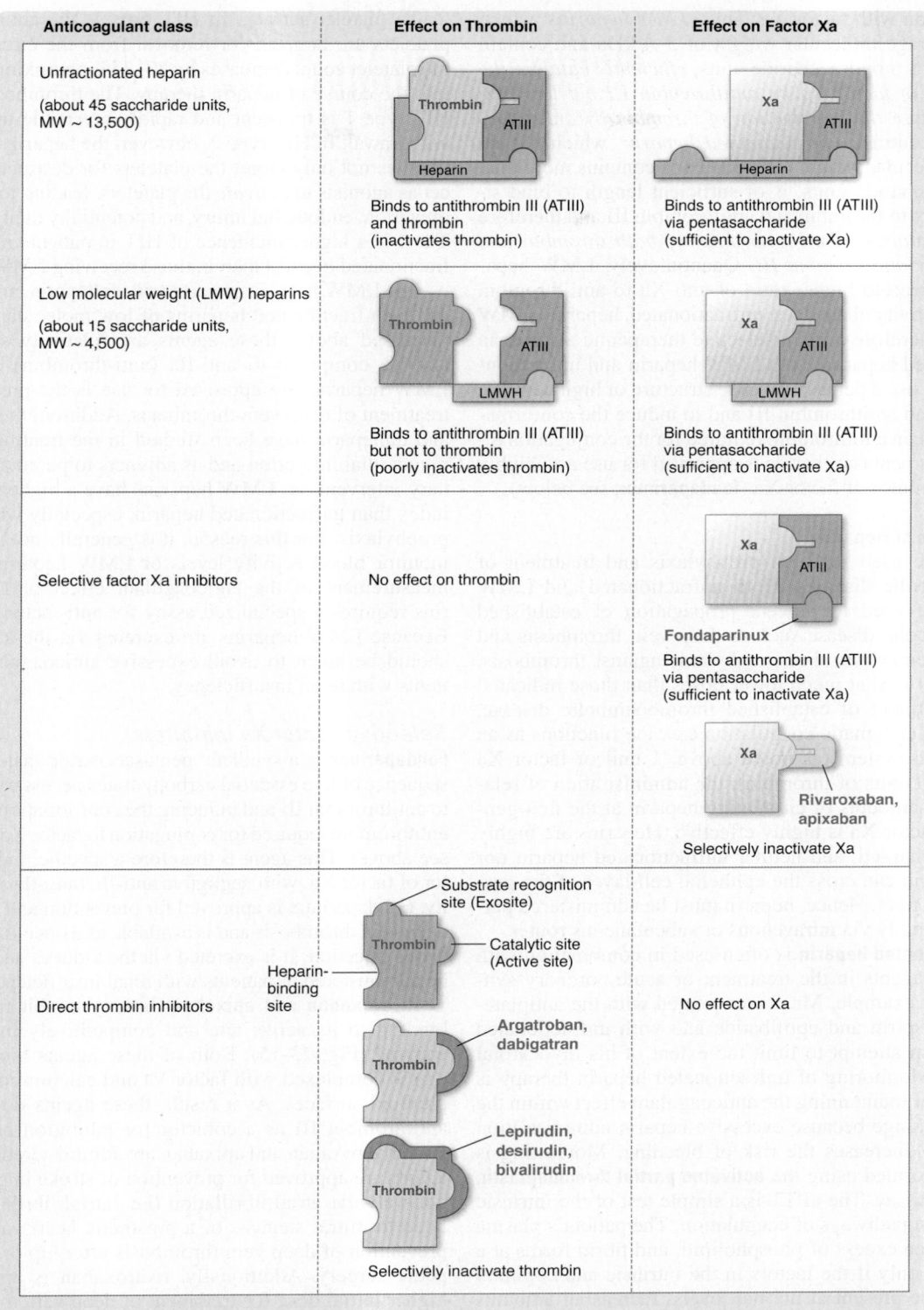

Anticoagulant class	Effect on Thrombin	Effect on Factor Xa
Unfractionated heparin (about 45 saccharide units, MW ~ 13,500)	Binds to antithrombin III (ATIII) and thrombin (inactivates thrombin)	Binds to antithrombin III (ATIII) via pentasaccharide (sufficient to inactivate Xa)
Low molecular weight (LMW) heparins (about 15 saccharide units, MW ~ 4,500)	Binds to antithrombin III (ATIII) but not to thrombin (poorly inactivates thrombin)	Binds to antithrombin III (ATIII) via pentasaccharide (sufficient to inactivate Xa)
Selective factor Xa inhibitors	No effect on thrombin	**Fondaparinux** Binds to antithrombin III (ATIII) via pentasaccharide (sufficient to inactivate Xa) / **Rivaroxaban, apixaban** Selectively inactivate Xa
Direct thrombin inhibitors	**Argatroban, dabigatran** / **Lepirudin, desirudin, bivalirudin** Selectively inactivate thrombin	No effect on Xa

FIGURE 23-15. Differential effects of unfractionated heparin, low-molecular-weight heparins, selective factor Xa inhibitors, and direct thrombin inhibitors on coagulation factor inactivation. Effect on thrombin: To catalyze the inactivation of thrombin, heparin must bind both to antithrombin III via a high-affinity pentasaccharide unit and to thrombin via an additional 13-saccharide unit. Low-molecular-weight heparin (LMWH) does not contain a sufficient number of saccharide units to bind thrombin and therefore is a poor catalyst for thrombin inactivation. Selective factor Xa inhibitors do not inactivate thrombin, while direct thrombin inhibitors selectively inactivate thrombin. Argatroban and dabigatran bind only to the active (catalytic) site of thrombin, while lepirudin, desirudin, and bivalirudin bind to both the active site and the substrate-recognition site of thrombin. **Effect on factor Xa:** Inactivation of factor Xa requires only the binding of antithrombin III to the high-affinity pentasaccharide unit. Since unfractionated heparin, low-molecular-weight heparin, and fondaparinux all contain this pentasaccharide, these agents are all able to catalyze the inactivation of factor Xa. Rivaroxaban and apixaban competitively inhibit factor Xa by binding to the active site of the enzyme; these agents bind factor Xa that is complexed with factor Va and Ca^{2+} on phospholipid surfaces, as shown in Figure 23-7. Direct thrombin inhibitors have no effect on factor Xa.

to conjugation with factor Xa. Thus, *LMW heparins*, which have an average molecular weight of 3–4 kDa and contain fewer than 18 monosaccharide units, *efficiently catalyze the inactivation of factor Xa by antithrombin III but less efficiently catalyze the inactivation of thrombin by antithrombin III*. In contrast, *unfractionated heparin*, which has an average molecular weight of 20 kDa and contains more than 18 monosaccharide units, is of sufficient length to bind simultaneously to thrombin and antithrombin III and therefore *efficiently catalyzes the inactivation of both thrombin and factor Xa by antithrombin III*. Quantitatively, LMW heparin has a threefold higher ratio of anti-Xa to anti-thrombin (anti-IIa) activity than does unfractionated heparin. LMW heparin is therefore a more selective therapeutic agent than unfractionated heparin. Both LMW heparin and unfractionated heparin use a pentasaccharide structure of high negative charge to bind antithrombin III and to induce the conformational change in antithrombin required for the conjugation reactions. This pentasaccharide is approved for use as a highly selective inhibitor of factor Xa (**fondaparinux**; see below).

Clinical Uses of Heparins

Heparins are used for both prophylaxis and treatment of thromboembolic diseases. Both unfractionated and LMW heparins are used to prevent propagation of established thromboembolic disease such as deep vein thrombosis and pulmonary embolism. For prophylaxis against thrombosis, heparins are used at much lower doses than those indicated for the treatment of established thromboembolic disease. Because the enzymatic coagulation cascade functions as an amplification system (as noted above, 1 unit of factor Xa generates 40 units of thrombin), the administration of relatively small amounts of circulating heparin at the first generation of factor Xa is highly effective. Heparins are highly negatively charged, and neither unfractionated heparin nor LMW heparin can cross the epithelial cell layer of the gastrointestinal tract. Hence, heparin must be administered parenterally, usually via intravenous or subcutaneous routes.

Unfractionated heparin is often used in combination with antiplatelet agents in the treatment of acute coronary syndromes. For example, Mr. S was treated with the antiplatelet agents aspirin and eptifibatide and with unfractionated heparin in an attempt to limit the extent of his myocardial infarction. Monitoring of unfractionated heparin therapy is important for maintaining the anticoagulant effect within the therapeutic range because excessive heparin administration significantly increases the risk of bleeding. Monitoring is usually performed using the **activated partial thromboplastin time (aPTT)** assay. The aPTT is a simple test of the intrinsic and common pathways of coagulation. The patient's plasma is added to an excess of phospholipid, and fibrin forms at a normal rate only if the factors in the intrinsic and common pathways are present at normal levels. Increasing amounts of unfractionated heparin in the plasma prolong the time required for the formation of a fibrin clot.

As is true of the other anticoagulants, the major adverse effect of heparin is bleeding. Thus, it is critical to maintain the anticoagulant effect of unfractionated heparin within the therapeutic range in order to prevent the rare, devastating adverse effect of intracranial hemorrhage. As discussed above, a small fraction of patients taking heparin develop **heparin-induced thrombocytopenia (HIT)**. In this syndrome, patients develop antibodies to a hapten created when heparin molecules bind

to the platelet surface. In HIT type 1, the antibody-coated platelets are targeted for removal from the circulation, and the platelet count decreases by 50–75% approximately 5 days into the course of heparin therapy. The thrombocytopenia in HIT type 1 is transient and rapidly reversible upon heparin withdrawal. In HIT type 2, however, the heparin-induced antibodies not only target the platelets for destruction but also act as agonists to *activate* the platelets, leading to platelet aggregation, endothelial injury, and potentially fatal thrombosis. There is a higher incidence of HIT in patients receiving unfractionated heparin than in those receiving LMW heparin.

The LMW heparins **enoxaparin**, **dalteparin**, and **tinzaparin** are each fractionated heparins of low molecular weight. As discussed above, these agents are relatively selective for anti-Xa compared to anti-IIa (anti-thrombin) activity. All LMW heparins are approved for use in the prevention and treatment of deep vein thrombosis. Additionally, enoxaparin and dalteparin have been studied in the treatment of acute myocardial infarction and as adjuncts to percutaneous coronary intervention. LMW heparins have a higher therapeutic index than unfractionated heparin, especially when used for prophylaxis. For this reason, it is generally not necessary to monitor blood activity levels of LMW heparins. Accurate measurement of the anticoagulant effect of LMW heparins requires a specialized assay for anti-factor Xa activity. Because LMW heparins are excreted via the kidneys, care should be taken to avoid excessive anticoagulation in patients with renal insufficiency.

Selective Factor Xa Inhibitors

Fondaparinux is a synthetic pentasaccharide that contains the sequence of five essential carbohydrates necessary for binding to antithrombin III and inducing the conformational change in antithrombin required for conjugation to factor Xa (Fig. 23-15; see above). This agent is therefore a specific, indirect inhibitor of factor Xa, with negligible anti-IIa (anti-thrombin) activity. Fondaparinux is approved for prevention and treatment of deep vein thrombosis and is available as a once-daily subcutaneous injection. It is excreted via the kidneys and should not be administered to patients with renal insufficiency.

Rivaroxaban and **apixaban** directly inhibit factor Xa by binding to its active site and competitively inhibiting the enzyme (Fig. 23-15). Both of these agents bind factor Xa that is complexed with factor Va and calcium ions on phospholipid surfaces. As a result, these agents do not require antithrombin III as a cofactor for inhibition of factor Xa. Both rivaroxaban and apixaban are administered orally. Both agents are approved for prevention of stroke in patients with non-valvular atrial fibrillation (i.e., atrial fibrillation not related to mitral stenosis or a prosthetic heart valve) and for prevention of deep vein thrombosis after hip or knee orthopedic surgery. Additionally, rivaroxaban is approved at a higher initial dose for treatment of deep vein thrombosis or pulmonary embolism. Rivaroxaban and apixaban are cleared by both metabolism in the liver and excretion in the kidney and should be administered at reduced doses in patients with renal impairment.

Direct Thrombin Inhibitors

As discussed above, thrombin has a number of critical roles in the hemostatic process (Fig. 23-8). Among other effects, this clotting factor (1) proteolytically converts fibrinogen to fibrin; (2) activates factor XIII, which cross-links fibrin polymers to form a stable clot; (3) activates platelets; and (4) induces endothelial release of PGI_2, t-PA, and PAI-1. Thus, direct thrombin inhibitors would be expected to have profound effects on coagulation. The currently approved direct thrombin inhibitors include lepirudin, desirudin, bivalirudin, argatroban, and dabigatran. These agents are specific inhibitors of thrombin, with negligible anti-factor Xa activity (Fig. 23-15).

Lepirudin, a recombinant 65-amino-acid polypeptide derived from the medicinal leech protein **hirudin**, is the prototypical direct thrombin inhibitor. For years, surgeons have used medicinal leeches to prevent thrombosis in the fine vessels of reattached digits. Lepirudin binds with high affinity to two sites on the thrombin molecule—the enzymatic active site and the "exosite," a region of the thrombin protein that orients substrate proteins. Lepirudin binding to thrombin prevents the thrombin-mediated activation of fibrinogen and factor XIII. Lepirudin is a highly effective anticoagulant because it can inhibit both free and *fibrin-bound* thrombin in developing clots and because lepirudin binding to thrombin is essentially irreversible. It is approved for use in the treatment of heparin-induced thrombocytopenia. Lepirudin has a short half-life, is available parenterally, and is renally excreted. It can be administered with relative safety to patients with hepatic insufficiency. As with all direct thrombin inhibitors, bleeding is the major adverse effect of lepirudin, and clotting times must be monitored closely. A small percentage of patients may develop anti-hirudin antibodies, limiting the long-term effectiveness of this agent as an anticoagulant. Another recombinant formulation of hirudin, **desirudin**, has been approved for prophylaxis against deep vein thrombosis in patients undergoing hip replacement.

Bivalirudin is a synthetic 20-amino-acid peptide that, like lepirudin and desirudin, binds to both the active site and exosite of thrombin and thereby inhibits thrombin activity. Thrombin slowly cleaves an arginine–proline bond in bivalirudin, leading to reactivation of the thrombin. Bivalirudin is approved for anticoagulation in patients undergoing coronary angiography and angioplasty and may reduce rates of bleeding relative to heparin for this indication. The drug is excreted renally and has a short half-life (25 minutes).

Argatroban is a small-molecule inhibitor of thrombin that is approved for the treatment of patients with heparin-induced thrombocytopenia. Unlike the polypeptide-based direct thrombin inhibitors (i.e., lepirudin, desirudin, and bivalirudin), argatroban binds only to the active site of thrombin (i.e., it does not interact with the exosite). Also unlike the polypeptide-based direct thrombin inhibitors, argatroban is excreted by biliary secretion and can therefore be administered with relative safety to patients with renal insufficiency. Argatroban has a short half-life and is administered by continuous intravenous infusion.

Dabigatran is an orally available direct thrombin inhibitor that is approved for prevention of thromboembolism in patients with non-valvular atrial fibrillation. It is also indicated for the treatment of established deep vein thrombosis and pulmonary embolism. Dabigatran is a prodrug that is metabolized to an active species that, like argatroban, binds competitively to the active site of thrombin. Like other anticoagulants, dabigatran may cause significant bleeding. One advantage relative to warfarin is that plasma levels of dabigatran do not need to be monitored. Dabigatran should not be administered as an alternative to warfarin in patients with a mechanical heart valve, because such patients have been found to have an increased risk of valve thrombosis.

Recombinant Activated Protein C (r-APC)

As described above, endogenously activated protein C (APC) exerts an anticoagulant effect by proteolytically cleaving factors Va and VIIIa. APC also reduces the amount of circulating plasminogen activator inhibitor 1, thereby enhancing fibrinolysis. Finally, APC reduces inflammation by inhibiting the release of tumor necrosis factor α (TNF-α) by monocytes. Because enhanced coagulability and inflammation are both hallmarks of septic shock, APC has been tested both in animal models of this disorder and in humans. **Recombinant activated protein C (r-APC)** has been found to significantly reduce mortality in patients at high risk of death from septic shock, and the US Food and Drug Administration (FDA) has approved r-APC for the treatment of patients with severe sepsis who demonstrate evidence of acute organ dysfunction, shock, oliguria, acidosis, and hypoxemia. r-APC is not indicated for the treatment of patients with severe sepsis and a lower risk of death, however. As is the case with other anticoagulants, r-APC increases the risk of bleeding. This agent is therefore contraindicated in patients who have recently undergone a surgical procedure and in those with chronic liver failure, kidney failure, or thrombocytopenia.

Thrombolytic Agents

Although warfarin, unfractionated and low-molecular-weight heparins, selective factor Xa inhibitors, and direct thrombin inhibitors are effective in preventing the formation and propagation of thrombi, these agents are generally ineffective against preexisting clots. Thrombolytic agents are used to lyse already-formed clots and thereby to restore the patency of an obstructed vessel before distal tissue necrosis occurs. Thrombolytic agents act by converting the inactive zymogen plasminogen to the active protease plasmin (Fig. 23-10). As noted above, plasmin is a relatively nonspecific protease that digests fibrin to fibrin degradation products. Unfortunately, thrombolytic therapy has the potential to dissolve not only pathologic thrombi but also physiologically appropriate fibrin clots that have formed in response to vascular injury (systemic fibrinolysis). Thus, the use of thrombolytic agents can lead to hemorrhage of varying severity.

Streptokinase

Streptokinase is a protein produced by β-hemolytic streptococci as a component of that organism's tissue-destroying machinery. The pharmacologic action of streptokinase involves two steps—complexation and cleavage. In the complexation reaction, streptokinase forms a stable, noncovalent 1:1 complex with plasminogen. The complexation reaction produces a conformational change in plasminogen that exposes this protein's proteolytically active site. Streptokinase-complexed plasminogen, with its active site exposed and available, can then proteolytically cleave *other* plasminogen molecules to plasmin. In fact, the thermodynamically stable streptokinase:plasminogen complex is the most catalytically efficient plasminogen activator in vitro.

Although streptokinase exerts its most dramatic and potentially beneficial effects in fresh thrombi, its use has been limited by two factors. First, streptokinase is a foreign protein that is capable of eliciting antigenic responses in humans upon repeated administration. Previous administration of streptokinase is a contraindication to its use because of the risk of anaphylaxis. Second, the thrombolytic actions of streptokinase are relatively nonspecific and can result in systemic fibrinolysis. Streptokinase is approved for treatment of ST elevation myocardial infarction and for treatment of life-threatening pulmonary embolism.

Recombinant Tissue Plasminogen Activator (t-PA)

An ideal thrombolytic agent would be nonantigenic and would cause local fibrinolysis only at the site of a pathologic thrombus. Tissue plasminogen activator (t-PA) approximates these goals. t-PA is a serine protease produced by human endothelial cells; therefore, t-PA is not antigenic. t-PA binds to newly formed (fresh) thrombi with high affinity, causing fibrinolysis at the site of a thrombus. Once bound to the fresh thrombus, t-PA undergoes a conformational change that renders it a potent activator of plasminogen. In contrast, t-PA is a poor activator of plasminogen in the absence of fibrin-binding.

Recombinant DNA technology has allowed the production of **recombinant t-PA**, generically referred to as **alteplase**. Recombinant t-PA is effective at recanalizing occluded coronary arteries, limiting cardiac dysfunction, and reducing mortality following an ST elevation myocardial infarction. At pharmacologic doses, however, recombinant t-PA can generate a systemic lytic state and (as with other thrombolytic agents) cause unwanted bleeding, including cerebral hemorrhage. Thus, its use is contraindicated in patients who have had a recent hemorrhagic stroke. Like streptokinase, t-PA is approved for use in the treatment of patients with ST elevation myocardial infarction or life-threatening pulmonary embolism. It is also approved for the treatment of acute ischemic stroke.

Tenecteplase

Tenecteplase is a genetically engineered variant of t-PA. The molecular modifications in tenecteplase increase its fibrin specificity relative to t-PA and make tenecteplase more resistant to plasminogen activator inhibitor 1. Large trials have shown that tenecteplase is identical in efficacy to t-PA, with similar (and possibly decreased) risk of bleeding. Additionally, tenecteplase has a longer half-life than t-PA. This pharmacokinetic property allows tenecteplase to be administered as a single weight-based bolus, thus simplifying administration.

Reteplase

Similar to tenecteplase, **reteplase** is a genetically engineered variant of t-PA with longer half-life and increased specificity for fibrin. Its efficacy and adverse-effect profile are similar to those of streptokinase and t-PA. Because of its longer half-life, reteplase can be administered as a "double bolus" (two boluses, 30 minutes apart).

Inhibitors of Anticoagulation and Fibrinolysis

Protamine

Protamine, a low-molecular-weight polycationic protein, is a chemical antagonist of heparin. This agent rapidly forms a stable complex with the negatively charged heparin molecule through multiple electrostatic interactions. Protamine is administered intravenously to reverse the effects of heparin in situations of life-threatening hemorrhage or great heparin excess (e.g., at the conclusion of coronary artery bypass graft surgery). Protamine is most active against the large heparin molecules in unfractionated heparin and it can partially reverse the anticoagulant effects of low-molecular-weight heparins, but it is inactive against fondaparinux.

Serine-Protease Inhibitors

Aprotinin, a naturally occurring polypeptide, is an inhibitor of the serine proteases plasmin, t-PA, and thrombin. By inhibiting fibrinolysis, aprotinin promotes clot stabilization. Inhibition of thrombin may also promote platelet activity by preventing platelet hyperstimulation. At higher doses, aprotinin may also inhibit kallikrein and thereby (paradoxically) inhibit the coagulation cascade. Although clinical trials demonstrated decreased perioperative bleeding and erythrocyte transfusion requirement in patients treated with aprotinin during cardiac surgery, these positive findings were tempered by evidence suggesting that, compared to other antifibrinolytic agents, aprotinin may increase the risk of postoperative acute renal failure. Aprotinin has also been associated with fatal anaphylactic reactions. Aprotinin was removed from the US market in 2008 because of an increased risk of mortality.

Lysine Analogues

Aminocaproic acid and **tranexamic acid** are analogues of lysine that bind to and inhibit plasminogen and plasmin. These agents are used to promote hemostasis in situations where fibrinolysis contributes to bleeding. Like aprotinin, these agents are also used to reduce perioperative bleeding during coronary artery bypass grafting. Unlike aprotinin, these agents may not increase the risk of postoperative acute renal failure.

▌ CONCLUSION AND FUTURE DIRECTIONS

Hemostasis is a highly regulated process that maintains the fluidity of blood in normal vessels and initiates rapid formation of a stable fibrin-based clot in response to vascular injury. Pathologic thrombosis results from endothelial injury, abnormal blood flow, and hypercoagulability. Antiplatelet agents, anticoagulants, and thrombolytic agents target different stages of thrombosis and thrombolysis. Antiplatelet agents interfere with platelet adhesion, the platelet release reaction, and platelet aggregation; these agents can provide powerful prophylaxis against thrombosis in susceptible individuals. Anticoagulants primarily target plasma coagulation factors and disrupt the coagulation cascade by inhibiting crucial intermediates. After a fibrin clot has been established, thrombolytic agents mediate dissolution of the clot by promoting the conversion of plasminogen to plasmin. These classes of pharmacologic agents can be administered, individually or in combination, to prevent or disrupt thrombosis and to restore the patency of blood vessels occluded by thrombus.

Future development of new antiplatelet, anticoagulant, and thrombolytic agents will be forced to contend with two major constraints. First, for many clinical indications in this field, highly effective, orally bioavailable, and inexpensive therapeutic agents are already available: these include the antiplatelet drug aspirin and the anticoagulant warfarin. Second, virtually every antithrombotic and thrombolytic agent is associated with the mechanism-based toxicity of bleeding, and this adverse effect is likely to plague new agents under development. Nonetheless, opportunities remain for the development of safer and more effective therapies. It is likely that pharmacogenomic techniques (see Chapter 7) will be capable of identifying individuals in the population who carry an increased genetic risk of thrombosis, and such individuals may benefit from long-term antithrombotic treatment. Combinations of antiplatelet agents, low-molecular-weight heparins, orally bioavailable direct thrombin inhibitors, and new agents that target currently unexploited components of hemostasis (such as inhibitors of the factor VIIa/tissue factor pathway) could all be useful in these settings. At the other end of the spectrum, there remains a great need for new agents that can achieve rapid, noninvasive, convenient, and selective lysis of acute thromboses associated with life-threatening emergencies such as ST elevation myocardial infarction and stroke. Carefully designed clinical trials will be critical to optimize the indications, dose, and duration of treatment for such drugs and drug combinations.

Acknowledgment

We thank April W. Armstrong for her valuable contributions to this chapter in the First, Second, and Third Editions of *Principles of Pharmacology: The Pathophysiologic Basis of Drug Therapy.*

Suggested Reading

Abrams CS, Plow EF. Molecular basis for platelet function. In: Hoffman R, Benz EJ Jr, Silberstein LE, Heslop H, Weitz J, Anastasi J, eds. *Hematology: basic principles and practice.* 6th ed. Philadelphia: Churchill Livingstone; 2012:1809–1820. (*Detailed and mechanistic description of platelet activation.*)

Angiolillo DJ. The evolution of antiplatelet therapy in the treatment of acute coronary syndromes: from aspirin to the present day. *Drugs* 2012;72:2087–2116. (*Reviews the clinical evidence supporting the use of antiplatelet agents.*)

Furie B, Furie BC. Mechanisms of thrombus formation. *N Engl J Med* 2008;359:938–949. (*Reviews mechanisms of hemostasis and thrombosis, with an emphasis on in vivo coagulation.*)

Owens AP III, Mackman N. Microparticles in hemostasis and thrombosis. *Circ Res* 2011;108:1284–1297. (*Reviews biology of microparticles in regulating thrombosis.*)

Perzborn E, Roehrig S, Straub A, Kubitza D, Misselwitz F. The discovery and development of rivaroxaban, an oral, direct factor Xa inhibitor. *Nat Rev Drug Discov* 2011;10:61–75. (*Reviews the development of anticoagulants with a focus on rivaroxaban.*)

Yeh CH, Hogg K, Weitz JI. Overview of the new oral anticoagulants: opportunities and challenges. *Arterioscler Thromb Vasc Biol* 2015;35:1056–1065. (*Reviews mechanisms of action and clinical indications for direct thrombin inhibitors and factor Xa inhibitors.*)

DRUG SUMMARY TABLE: CHAPTER 23 Pharmacology of Hemostasis and Thrombosis

DRUG	CLINICAL APPLICATIONS	SERIOUS AND COMMON ADVERSE EFFECTS	CONTRAINDICATIONS	THERAPEUTIC CONSIDERATIONS
ANTIPLATELET AGENTS **Cyclooxygenase Inhibitors** Mechanism—Inhibit platelet cyclooxygenase, thereby blocking thromboxane A_2 generation and inhibiting platelet granule release reaction and platelet aggregation				
Aspirin	Prophylaxis against transient ischemic attack, myocardial infarction, and thromboembolic disorders Treatment of acute coronary syndromes Prevention of reocclusion in coronary revascularization procedures and stent implantation Arthritis, juvenile arthritis, rheumatic fever Systemic lupus erythematosus Mild pain or fever	*Gastrointestinal ulcer, major bleeding, macular degeneration, tinnitus, bronchospasm, angioedema, Reye's syndrome*	NSAID-induced sensitivity reactions Children with chickenpox or flu-like syndromes Bleeding disorders such as hemophilia, von Willebrand's disease, or immune thrombocytopenia Syndrome of asthma, rhinitis, and nasal polyps	Inhibits COX-1 and COX-2 nonselectively. Use cautiously in patients with GI lesions, impaired renal function, hypoprothrombinemia, vitamin K deficiency, thrombotic thrombocytopenic purpura, or hepatic impairment. Co-administration with aminoglycosides, bumetanide, capreomycin, cisplatin, erythromycin, ethacrynic acid, furosemide, or vancomycin may potentiate ototoxic effects. Co-administration with ammonium chloride or other urine acidifiers may lead to aspirin toxicity. Aspirin antagonizes uricosuric effects of phenylbutazone, probenecid, and sulfinpyrazone; avoid co-administration with these agents.
Phosphodiesterase Inhibitors Mechanism—Inhibit platelet cAMP degradation and thereby decrease platelet aggregability				
Dipyridamole	Prophylaxis against thromboembolic disorders Alternative to exercise in thallium myocardial perfusion imaging	*Exacerbation of angina (IV route), rare myocardial infarction, rare ventricular arrhythmia, liver failure, immune hypersensitivity reaction, stroke, seizure, rare bronchospasm* Abnormal ECG, chest pain, flushing, rash, abdominal discomfort (oral route), dizziness, headache, dyspnea	Hypersensitivity to dipyridamole	Weak antiplatelet effect. Usually administered in combination with warfarin or aspirin. Has vasodilatory properties; may paradoxically induce angina by causing coronary artery steal.
ADP Receptor Pathway Inhibitors Mechanism—Inhibit platelet ADP receptor, thereby preventing receptor signaling and inhibiting ADP-dependent platelet activation pathway. Ticlopidine, clopidogrel, and prasugrel covalently modify the receptor, while ticagrelor is a reversible inhibitor.				
Ticlopidine	Secondary prevention of thrombotic stroke in patients intolerant of aspirin Prevention of stent thrombosis (in combination with aspirin)	*Aplastic anemia, neutropenia, thrombotic thrombocytopenic purpura, hemorrhage* Rash, gastrointestinal upset, abnormal liver function tests, dizziness	Hypersensitivity to ticlopidine Active bleeding disorder Neutropenia, thrombocytopenia, thrombotic thrombocytopenic purpura Severe liver dysfunction	Use is limited by associated myelotoxicity. Requires a loading dose to achieve immediate antiplatelet effect. Has largely been replaced by clopidogrel.

Drug	Clinical Applications	Serious and Common Adverse Effects	Contraindications	Therapeutic Considerations
Clopidogrel	Secondary prevention of atherosclerotic events in patients with recent myocardial infarction, stroke, or peripheral vascular disease Acute coronary syndromes Prevention of stent thrombosis (in combination with aspirin)	*Gastrointestinal hemorrhage (in combination with aspirin), pancytopenia, thrombotic thrombocytopenic purpura, immune thrombocytopenic purpura, rare intracranial hemorrhage* Bleeding	Hypersensitivity to clopidogrel Active bleeding disorder	More favorable adverse effect profile than ticlopidine; significantly less myelotoxic than ticlopidine. Requires a loading dose to achieve immediate antiplatelet effect.
Prasugrel	Acute coronary syndromes with percutaneous coronary intervention	*Atrial fibrillation, bradycardia, major bleeding, leukopenia, thrombotic thrombocytopenic purpura, angioedema, neoplasm of colon* Hypertension, hyperlipidemia, back pain, headache, epistaxis	Hypersensitivity to prasugrel Active bleeding disorder Transient ischemic attack Stroke	Used in combination with aspirin. Compared with clopidogrel, prasugrel is more efficiently metabolized and achieves more complete platelet inhibition but also increases the risk of bleeding.
Ticagrelor	Acute coronary syndromes Percutaneous coronary intervention	*Atrial fibrillation, syncope, major bleeding* Headache, increased serum creatinine, cough, dyspnea	Hypersensitivity to ticagrelor Prior intracranial hemorrhage Active bleeding disorder Severe hepatic impairment	Ticagrelor is a reversible inhibitor of the $P2Y_{12}$ ADP receptor. Administered as a twice-daily dose. Any co-administered aspirin must be low-dose ($\leq$100 mg).

GPIIb–IIIa Antagonists
Mechanism—Bind to platelet receptor GPIIb–IIIa and thereby prevent binding of fibrinogen and other adhesion ligands

Drug	Clinical Applications	Serious and Common Adverse Effects	Contraindications	Therapeutic Considerations
Eptifibatide	Acute coronary syndromes Percutaneous coronary intervention	*Major bleeding, intracerebral hemorrhage, thrombocytopenia, anaphylaxis* Hypotension, bleeding	Hypersensitivity to eptifibatide History of bleeding diathesis or recent abnormal bleeding Concomitant administration of a second GPIIb–IIIa antagonist Recent major surgery Recent stroke or history of hemorrhagic stroke Intracranial hemorrhage, mass, or arteriovenous malformation Severe uncontrolled hypertension Renal dialysis	Avoid co-administration with a second GPIIb–IIIa antagonist. Minimize use of arterial and venous punctures, urinary catheters, and nasotracheal and nasogastric tubes. Eptifibatide is a synthetic peptide delivered via parenteral administration.
Abciximab	Adjunct to percutaneous coronary intervention or atherectomy to prevent acute cardiac ischemic complications Unstable angina not responding to conventional therapy in patients scheduled for percutaneous coronary intervention	*Thrombocytopenia, anaphylaxis, stroke, intracranial or pulmonary hemorrhage* Chest pain, hypotension, gastrointestinal upset, bleeding	Hypersensitivity to abciximab History of stroke Concomitant use of IV dextran History of gastrointestinal or genitourinary bleeding Uncontrolled hypertension Intracranial neoplasm Recent surgery Thrombocytopenia Vasculitis	Same therapeutic considerations as eptifibatide, except abciximab is a chimeric mouse–human monoclonal antibody. Adding abciximab to conventional antithrombotic therapy reduces both long-term and short-term ischemic events in patients undergoing high-risk coronary angioplasty.

continues

DRUG SUMMARY TABLE: CHAPTER 23 Pharmacology of Hemostasis and Thrombosis *continued*

DRUG	CLINICAL APPLICATIONS	*SERIOUS* AND COMMON ADVERSE EFFECTS	CONTRAINDICATIONS	THERAPEUTIC CONSIDERATIONS
Tirofiban	Acute coronary syndromes in patients undergoing angioplasty or atherectomy or managed medically	*Dissection aneurysm of coronary artery, major bleeding, thrombocytopenia, anaphylaxis, intracranial or pulmonary hemorrhage* Bradyarrhythmia, pelvic pain	Hypersensitivity to tirofiban Active or history of bleeding Recent surgery or severe trauma History of thrombocytopenia after administration of tirofiban	Same therapeutic considerations as eptifibatide, except tirofiban is a nonpeptide tyrosine analogue.

Thrombin Receptor (PAR-1) Antagonists
Warfarin
Mechanism—Competitive inhibitor of protease-activated receptor 1 (PAR-1), one of the major thrombin receptors expressed on platelets

DRUG	CLINICAL APPLICATIONS	*SERIOUS* AND COMMON ADVERSE EFFECTS	CONTRAINDICATIONS	THERAPEUTIC CONSIDERATIONS
Vorapaxar	Prevention of myocardial infarction, stroke, and cardiovascular death in patients with prior myocardial infarction or peripheral artery disease	*Major bleeding, gastrointestinal or intracranial hemorrhage, anemia*	Prior stroke or intracranial hemorrhage Active bleeding	Recently approved by the FDA Studied primarily in conjunction with aspirin and clopidogrel co-administration

ANTICOAGULANTS
Warfarin
Mechanism—Inhibits hepatic epoxide reductase that catalyzes the regeneration of reduced vitamin K, which is required for synthesis of biologically active coagulation factors II, VII, IX, and X and anticoagulant proteins C and S

DRUG	CLINICAL APPLICATIONS	*SERIOUS* AND COMMON ADVERSE EFFECTS	CONTRAINDICATIONS	THERAPEUTIC CONSIDERATIONS
Warfarin	Prophylaxis and treatment of pulmonary embolism, deep vein thrombosis, systemic embolism after myocardial infarction, or systemic embolism associated with atrial fibrillation; rheumatic heart disease with heart valve damage, or prosthetic mechanical heart valve	*Cholesterol embolization syndrome, skin and other tissue necrosis, hemorrhage, hypersensitivity reaction, compartment syndrome* Alopecia	Hypersensitivity to warfarin Pregnancy Hemorrhagic tendency or blood dyscrasia Bleeding tendency associated with active ulceration or bleeding due to mucosal lesions, cerebrovascular hemorrhage, cerebral or aortic aneurysm, pericarditis and pericardial effusion, bacterial endocarditis Recent eye, brain, or spinal surgery Severe uncontrolled hypertension Threatened abortion, eclampsia, preeclampsia Regional or lumbar block anesthesia Unsupervised patients with psychosis, dementia, alcoholism, or lack of cooperation, and especially those with risk of falling	Monitoring is required by using the prothrombin time (PT), expressed as the international normalized ratio (INR). Drug–drug interactions must be carefully considered with warfarin (refer to Tables 23-2 and 23-3 for examples of important interactions); co-administration of warfarin with other albumin-bound drugs can increase the free (unbound) plasma concentrations of both drugs; co-administration of drugs that induce and/or compete for P450 metabolism can affect the plasma concentrations of both drugs. Warfarin should never be given to pregnant women because it can cause a hemorrhagic disorder and/or congenital defects in the fetus. Warfarin can cause skin necrosis as a result of widespread thrombosis in the microvasculature. For severe hemorrhage due to warfarin, patients should promptly receive fresh frozen plasma.

Unfractionated Heparin and Low-Molecular-Weight (LMW) Heparins
Mechanism—Unfractionated heparin: combines with antithrombin III and inhibits secondary hemostasis via nonselective inactivation of thrombin (factor IIa), factor Xa, factor IXa, factor XIa, and factor XIIa.
LMW heparins: combine with antithrombin III and inhibit secondary hemostasis via relatively (threefold) selective inactivation of factor Xa

Drug	Clinical Applications	Serious and Common Adverse Effects	Contraindications	Therapeutic Considerations
Unfractionated heparin	Prevention and treatment of pulmonary embolism, deep vein thrombosis, cerebral thrombosis, or left ventricular thrombus Prevention of systemic embolism associated with myocardial infarction Open-heart surgery Disseminated intravascular coagulation Maintain patency of IV catheters	*Hemorrhage, heparin-induced thrombocytopenia, hypersensitivity reactions including anaphylactoid reactions, non-traumatic spinal subdural hematoma* Increased liver aminotransferase level	Instances where blood coagulation tests cannot be performed at necessary intervals Active major bleeding Bleeding tendencies such as hemophilia, thrombocytopenia, or hepatic disease with hypo-prothrombinemia Neonates or infants Pregnant or nursing women	There is a higher incidence of heparin-induced thrombocytopenia in patients receiving unfractionated heparin than in those receiving LMW heparin. Antihistamines, cardiac glycosides, nicotine, and tetracyclines may partially counteract anticoagulant effect. Cephalosporins, penicillins, oral anticoagulants, and platelet inhibitors may increase anticoagulant effect. Discourage concomitant use of herbs such as dong quai, garlic, ginger, ginkgo, motherwort, and red clover due to increased risk of bleeding.
LMW heparins: **Enoxaparin** **Dalteparin** **Tinzaparin**	Prevention and treatment of deep vein thrombosis (shared indications) Treatment of acute coronary syndromes and adjunct to percutaneous coronary intervention (enoxaparin and dalteparin only)	*Hematoma, hemorrhage, paraplegia (shared adverse effects); atrial fibrillation, heart failure, skin necrosis, pneumonia (enoxaparin only)* Increased liver function tests (enoxaparin and tinzaparin only); gastrointestinal upset, anemia, fever (enoxaparin only); erythema (tinzaparin only)	Shared contraindications: Hypersensitivity to heparin or pork products Active major bleeding Thrombocytopenia Dalteparin only: Patients undergoing epidural/neuraxial anesthesia	Administered as weight-based subcutaneous injection. Avoid excessive anticoagulation in patients with renal insufficiency.

Selective Factor Xa Inhibitors
Mechanism—Fondaparinux: combines with antithrombin III and inhibits secondary hemostasis via highly selective inactivation of factor Xa. Apixaban and rivaroxaban: competitively inhibit factor Xa by binding to the active site of the enzyme

Drug	Clinical Applications	Serious and Common Adverse Effects	Contraindications	Therapeutic Considerations
Fondaparinux	Prophylaxis and treatment of deep vein thrombosis Prophylaxis and treatment of pulmonary embolism	*Anemia, hemorrhage, thrombocytopenia, anaphylactoid reaction* Rash, fever	Hypersensitivity to fondaparinux Active major bleeding Severe renal impairment Bacterial endocarditis Body weight < 50 kg Thrombocytopenia	Fondaparinux is a pentasaccharide composed of the essential five carbohydrates necessary for binding to antithrombin III; it is a specific indirect inhibitor of factor Xa, with negligible anti-thrombin (anti-IIa) activity. Avoid excessive anticoagulation in patients with renal insufficiency. Fondaparinux has not been associated with heparin-induced thrombocytopenia.

continues

DRUG SUMMARY TABLE: CHAPTER 23 Pharmacology of Hemostasis and Thrombosis *continued*

DRUG	CLINICAL APPLICATIONS	SERIOUS AND COMMON ADVERSE EFFECTS	CONTRAINDICATIONS	THERAPEUTIC CONSIDERATIONS
Apixaban **Rivaroxaban**	Prevention of thromboembolism in non-valvular atrial fibrillation Prevention of deep vein thrombosis and pulmonary embolism after hip or knee replacement surgery Treatment of deep vein thrombosis and pulmonary embolism (rivaroxaban only)	*Hematoma, hemorrhage, severe hypersensitivity reaction (shared adverse effects); abnormal liver function tests (apixaban only); syncope (rivaroxaban only)*	Hypersensitivity to drug Active major bleeding	Both apixaban and rivaroxaban are orally available. Apixaban is administered twice daily, while rivaroxaban is administered once daily. Apixaban and rivaroxaban are cleared by both hepatic metabolism and renal excretion and should be administered at reduced doses in patients with renal impairment.
Direct Thrombin Inhibitors **Mechanism—Bind directly to thrombin and thereby inhibit secondary hemostasis**				
Hirudin-related agents: **Lepirudin** **Desirudin** **Bivalirudin**	Heparin-induced thrombocytopenia (lepirudin and bivalirudin only) Prophylaxis against deep vein thrombosis (desirudin only) Anticoagulation in patients undergoing coronary angiography and angioplasty (bivalirudin only)	*Hemorrhage, cerebral ischemia, peripheral nerve paralysis, facial nerve paralysis, hematuria, renal failure, extrinsic allergic respiratory disease, pneumonia, sepsis* Cutaneous hypersensitivity, anemia, hypotension, nausea, headache, fever	Hypersensitivity to drug Active major bleeding	Recombinant polypeptides based on the medicinal leech protein hirudin; bind to both active site and exosite of thrombin. Lepirudin inhibits both free and fibrin-bound thrombin. After bivalirudin binds to thrombin, the thrombin slowly cleaves an arginine–proline bond in bivalirudin, leading to reactivation of thrombin. Dose adjustment is required in patients with renal insufficiency because these agents are excreted via the kidneys.
Argatroban	Coronary artery thrombosis Prophylaxis in percutaneous coronary intervention Heparin-induced thrombocytopenia	*Cardiac arrest; gastrointestinal, intracranial, genitourinary tract, or retroperitoneal hemorrhage; pulmonary edema* Bradyarrhythmia, chest pain, gastrointestinal upset, fever	Hypersensitivity to argatroban Active major bleeding	Binds to active site but not exosite of thrombin. Dose adjustment is required in patients with liver disease because argatroban is excreted in the bile.
Dabigatran	Prevention of thromboembolism in non-valvular atrial fibrillation Treatment of deep vein thrombosis and pulmonary embolism	*Hemorrhage, severe hypersensitivity reaction*	Active major bleeding Mechanical prosthetic heart valve	Orally available prodrug; active metabolite binds to active site but not exosite of thrombin. Avoid co-administration with rifampin, which induces P-glycoprotein and increases hepatic elimination of dabigatran.
Recombinant Activated Protein C (r-APC) **Mechanism—Proteolytically inactivates factors Va and VIIIa; may also exert anti-inflammatory effect by inhibiting tumor necrosis factor production and blocking leukocyte adhesion to selectins**				
Recombinant activated protein C (r-APC)	Severe sepsis with organ dysfunction and high risk of death	*Hemorrhage*	Active internal bleeding Intracranial mass Hemorrhagic stroke within 3 months Recent intracranial or intraspinal surgery or severe head trauma within 2 months Presence of an epidural catheter Major trauma with an increased risk of life-threatening bleeding	Prolongs activated partial thromboplastin time (aPTT) but has little effect on prothrombin time (PT).

THROMBOLYTIC AGENTS
Mechanism—Proteolytically activate plasminogen to form plasmin, which digests fibrin to fibrin degradation products

Drug	Clinical Applications	Serious and Common Adverse Effects	Contraindications	Therapeutic Considerations
Streptokinase	ST elevation myocardial infarction; Arterial thrombosis; Deep vein thrombosis; Pulmonary embolism; Intra-arterial or intravenous catheter occlusion	Cardiac arrhythmia, myocardial infarction, non-traumatic splenic rupture, major bleeding, cholesterol embolus syndrome, anaphylactoid reaction, intracranial hemorrhage, acute respiratory distress syndrome; Hypotension, fever	Hypersensitivity to streptokinase; Active internal bleeding or known bleeding diathesis; Intracranial or intraspinal surgery or trauma within 2 months; Stroke within 2 months; Intracranial mass; Severe uncontrolled hypertension	Streptokinase is a foreign bacterial protein that can elicit antigenic responses in humans upon repeated administration; prior administration of streptokinase is a contraindication to use due to the risk of anaphylaxis. Thrombolytic actions of streptokinase are relatively nonspecific and can result in systemic fibrinolysis.
Recombinant tissue plasminogen activator (t-PA) (Alteplase)	Acute myocardial infarction; Acute cerebrovascular thrombosis; Pulmonary embolism; Central venous catheter occlusion	Cardiac arrhythmia, cholesterol embolus syndrome, gastrointestinal hemorrhage, rare allergic reaction, intracranial hemorrhage, sepsis	Same as streptokinase	Binds to newly formed (fresh) thrombi with high affinity, causing fibrinolysis at the site of a thrombus. As with other thrombolytic agents, t-PA can generate a systemic lytic state and cause unwanted bleeding.
Tenecteplase Reteplase	Acute myocardial infarction	Gastrointestinal and intracranial hemorrhage, anaphylactoid reaction (shared adverse effects); cardiac arrhythmia, cholesterol embolus syndrome, hematoma, renal artery hemorrhage, stroke (tenecteplase only); anemia (reteplase only)	Same as streptokinase	Genetically engineered variants of t-PA with increased specificity for fibrin. Longer half-life than t-PA; tenecteplase is administered as a single weight-based bolus; reteplase is administered as a double bolus.

INHIBITORS OF ANTICOAGULATION AND FIBRINOLYSIS
Protamine
Mechanism—Inactivates heparin by forming a stable 1:1 protamine:heparin complex

Drug	Clinical Applications	Serious and Common Adverse Effects	Contraindications	Therapeutic Considerations
Protamine	Heparin overdose	Bradyarrhythmia, hypotension, anaphylactoid reaction, circulatory collapse, capillary leak, noncardiogenic pulmonary edema; Flushing, nausea, vomiting, dyspepsia	Hypersensitivity to protamine	Protamine can also partially reverse the anticoagulant effect of low-molecular-weight heparin, but it cannot reverse the anticoagulant effect of fondaparinux.

Serine-Protease Inhibitor
Mechanism—Inhibits serine proteases, including plasmin, t-PA, and thrombin

| Aprotinin | Reduce perioperative bleeding during coronary artery bypass graft surgery | Heart failure, myocardial infarction, shock, thrombotic disorder, anaphylaxis with reexposure, cerebral artery occlusion, renal failure | Hypersensitivity to aprotinin; Known or suspected aprotinin exposure within the last 12 months | At higher doses, aprotinin may also inhibit kallikrein and thereby paradoxically inhibit the coagulation cascade. Aprotinin may increase the risk of postoperative acute renal failure relative to other antifibrinolytic agents. Removed from US market in 2008 because of increased risk of mortality. |

continues

DRUG SUMMARY TABLE: CHAPTER 23 Pharmacology of Hemostasis and Thrombosis *continued*

Lysine Analogues
Mechanism—Analogues of lysine that bind to and inhibit plasminogen and plasmin

DRUG	CLINICAL APPLICATIONS	*SERIOUS* AND COMMON ADVERSE EFFECTS	CONTRAINDICATIONS	THERAPEUTIC CONSIDERATIONS
Aminocaproic acid **Tranexamic acid**	Hemorrhage from increased fibrinolysis (shared indication) Hematuria (aminocaproic acid only) Menorrhagia (tranexamic acid only)	*Thromboembolic disorder, anaphylaxis, renal toxicity (shared adverse effects); myocardial necrosis, hemorrhage, muscle necrosis, intracranial hypertension, seizure (aminocaproic acid only); visual disturbance (tranexamic acid only)* Abdominal pain, anemia, arthralgia, musculoskeletal pain, headache, fatigue (tranexamic acid only)	Shared contraindication: Disseminated intravascular coagulation Tranexamic acid only: Hypersensitivity to tranexamic acid Acquired defective color vision Concomitant use with hormonal contraceptives Subarachnoid hemorrhage	May cause less acute renal failure relative to aprotinin.

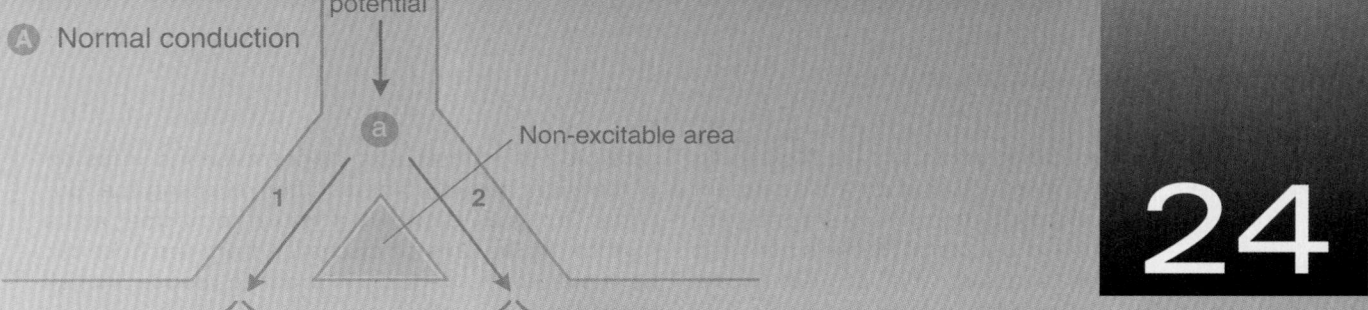

24

Pharmacology of Cardiac Rhythm

Ehrin J. Armstrong and David E. Clapham

INTRODUCTION

The human heart is both a mechanical and an electrical organ. To perfuse the body adequately with blood, the mechanical and electrical components of the heart must work in precise concert with each other. The mechanical component pumps the blood; the electrical component controls the rhythm of the pump. When the mechanical component fails despite a normal rhythm, heart failure can result (see Chapter 26, Integrative Cardiovascular Pharmacology: Hypertension, Ischemic Heart Disease, and Heart Failure). When the electrical component goes awry (called an *arrhythmia*), cardiac myocytes fail to contract in synchrony, and effective pumping is compromised. Changes in the membrane potential of cardiac cells directly affect cardiac rhythm, and most antiarrhythmic drugs act by modulating the activity of ion channels in the plasma membrane. This chapter discusses the ionic basis of electric rhythm formation and conduction in the heart, the pathophysiology of electrical dysfunction, and the pharmacologic agents used to restore a normal cardiac rhythm.

ELECTRICAL PHYSIOLOGY OF THE HEART

Electrical activity in the heart, leading to rhythmic cardiac contraction, is a manifestation of the heart's exquisite control of cell depolarization and impulse conduction. Once initiated, a cardiac action potential is a spontaneous event that proceeds based on the characteristic responses of ion channels to changes in membrane voltage. At the completion of a cycle, the spontaneous depolarization of pacemaker cells ensures that the process repeats without interruption.

Pacemaker and Nonpacemaker Cells

The heart contains cardiac myocytes that can spontaneously initiate action potentials and myocytes that cannot. Cells possessing the ability to initiate spontaneous action potentials are termed **pacemaker cells**. All pacemaker cells possess **automaticity**, the ability to depolarize above a threshold voltage in a rhythmic fashion. Automaticity results in the generation of spontaneous action potentials. Pacemaker cells are found in the sinoatrial node (SA node), the atrioventricular node (AV node), and the ventricular conducting system (bundle of His, bundle branches, and Purkinje fibers). Together, the pacemaker cells constitute the specialized conducting system that governs the electrical activity of the heart. The second type of cardiac cells, the **nonpacemaker cells**, includes the atrial and ventricular myocytes. The nonpacemaker cells contract in response to depolarization and are responsible for the majority of cardiac contraction. In *pathologic* conditions, these nonpacemaker cells can acquire automaticity and thereby also act as pacemaker cells.

Cardiac Action Potentials

Ions are not distributed equally across cell membranes. Transporters (pumps) drive K^+ into cells while pumping Na^+ and Ca^{2+} out, giving rise to electrical and chemical gradients across the membrane. These gradients ultimately determine the membrane potential of a cardiac cell. The **Nernst equilibrium**

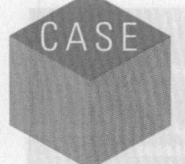

CASE

One winter morning, Dr. J, a 74-year-old professor, is lecturing on the treatment of cardiomyopathies to the second-year medical school class. He feels his heart beating irregularly and becomes nauseated. He is able to finish his lecture, but he continues to feel significantly short of breath throughout the morning. His persistent symptoms prompt him to walk down the street to the local emergency department.

Physical examination reveals an irregular heartbeat ranging from 120 to 140 beats/min. Dr. J's blood pressure is stable (132/76 mm Hg), and his oxygen saturation is 100% on room air. An electrocardiogram (ECG) confirms that Dr. J has atrial fibrillation, without any evidence of ischemia. Several intravenous boluses of diltiazem are administered, and his heart rate decreases to 80–100 beats/min, but his rhythm remains irregular. Further laboratory studies, an echocardiogram, and a chest x-ray do not reveal an underlying cause for Dr. J's atrial fibrillation.

During observation over the next 12 hours, Dr. J remains in atrial fibrillation. Although his heart rate is under better control, he continues to experience palpitations. Under continuous ECG monitoring, a cardiologist administers an intravenous infusion of ibutilide. Twenty minutes after receiving the ibutilide, Dr. J's ECG shows a return to normal sinus rhythm. At the time of discharge from the hospital, he is started on warfarin in order to reduce his risk of stroke.

Dr. J feels fine at first, but he develops recurrent palpitations within 3 weeks of his initial event. After discussion with his cardiologist, he elects to start amiodarone at a maintenance dose of 200 mg/day, in addition to continuing his warfarin. Dr. J tolerates the amiodarone well and reports no difficulty breathing. He remains symptom-free during the rest of his cardiology lectures.

Questions

1. Why were ibutilide and amiodarone effective in converting Dr. J's heart rhythm to normal sinus rhythm?
2. Why should ibutilide be administered only under carefully monitored circumstances?
3. What adverse effects of amiodarone could develop at higher daily doses?
4. Why did diltiazem slow Dr. J's heart rate without affecting his underlying heart rhythm, atrial fibrillation?

potential for each ion ($E_{Na} = +70$ mV, $E_K = -94$ mV, and $E_{Ca} = +150$ mV) depends on the relative concentrations of ions inside and outside the cell. The difference between an ion's Nernst potential and the cell's membrane potential determines the driving force for ions into or out of the cell. Refer to Chapter 8, Principles of Cellular Excitability and Electrochemical Transmission, for a detailed discussion of the Nernst equilibrium potential.

When an ion-selective channel opens, the membrane potential approaches the equilibrium potential for that ion. For example, opening a K^+-selective channel drives the membrane potential toward E_K (-94 mV). When a Na^+-selective channel opens, the membrane potential is driven toward E_{Na} ($+70$ mV), and opening a Ca^{2+}-selective channel drives the membrane potential toward E_{Ca} ($+150$ mV). Note that the reversal potential for a nonselective ion channel (e.g., a channel that passes all cations nonselectively) is 0 mV. The final membrane potential depends on the number of channels of each type, their conductances (i.e., the ability of each channel to pass ions), and the duration for which each channel remains open. *The resting membrane of the cardiac myocyte is relatively permeable to K^+ (because some types of K^+-selective channels are open) but not to Na^+ or Ca^{2+}*; hence, the **resting membrane potential** is close to the equilibrium potential for K^+. (The actual cardiac myocyte membrane potential is a bit more positive than the equilibrium potential for K^+, due to the contribution of other ion channels to the resting membrane potential.)

Changing the membrane potential requires the movement of relatively few ions across the membrane. Therefore, despite the opening and closing of ion channels, the ionic concentration gradients across the membrane remain relatively stable, and the Nernst potential for each ion remains relatively constant.

Cardiac action potentials are strikingly longer than those of nerve or skeletal muscle, lasting for almost half a second. Prolonged cardiac action potentials provide the sustained depolarization and contraction needed to empty the heart's chambers. Sinoatrial (SA) nodal cells pace the heart at normal resting heart rates between 60 and 100 beats/min, while ventricular muscle cells orchestrate the contraction that ejects blood from the heart (Fig. 24-1).

SA nodal cells fire spontaneously in a cycle defined by three phases, referred to as *phase 4*, *phase 0*, and *phase 3* (Fig. 24-2 and Table 24-1). **Phase 4** consists of a slow, spontaneous depolarization that is caused by an inward pacemaker current (I_f –encoded by *HCN*). This spontaneous depolarization accounts for the automaticity of the SA node. The channels that carry the I_f current are activated during the repolarization phase of the previous action potential. The I_f channels are relatively nonselective cation channels. **Phase 0** consists of a more rapid depolarization mediated by highly selective voltage-gated Ca^{2+} channels that, upon opening, drive the membrane potential toward E_{Ca} ($+150$ mV). In **phase 3**, the Ca^{2+} channels slowly close and K^+-selective channels open, resulting in membrane repolarization. Once the membrane potential repolarizes to approximately -60 mV, the opening of I_f channels is triggered and the cycle begins again.

Although the I_f (inward pacemaker) current is responsible for the slow spontaneous depolarization in phase 4 of the SA-node action potential, the kinetics of this depolarization are modulated by voltage-gated Na^+ channels that are also expressed in the SA node. There are gradients of expression

The five phases of the ventricular myocyte action potential result from an intricately woven cascade of channel openings and closings; the phases are numbered from 0 to 4 (Fig. 24-3 and Table 24-1).

In **phase 0**, an action potential upstroke of very rapid depolarization is caused by a transient increase in inward

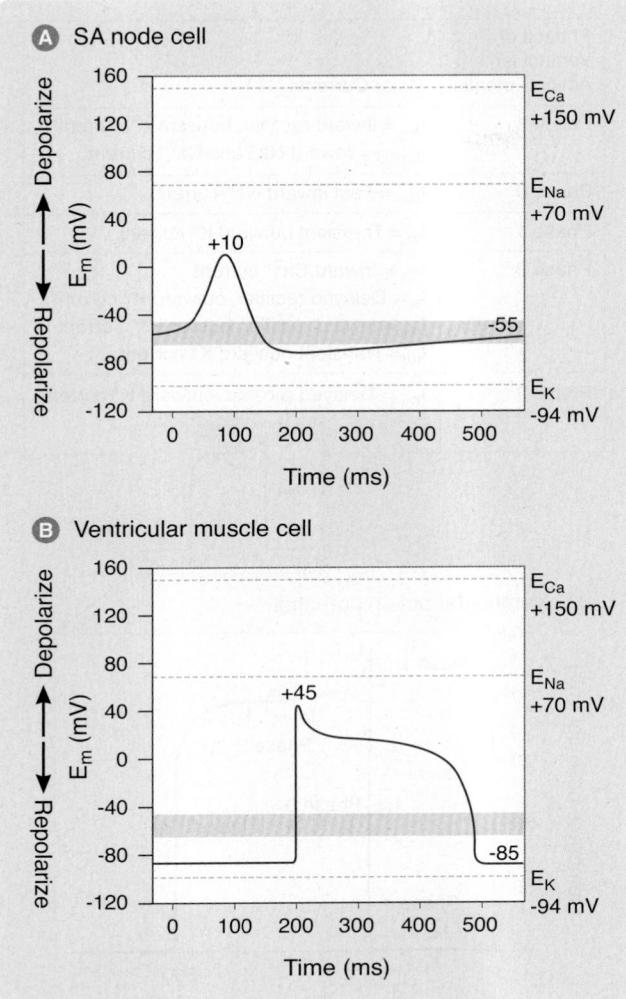

FIGURE 24-1. SA node and ventricular muscle cell action potentials. The resting membrane potential of a sinoatrial (SA) node cell is approximately −55 mV, while that of a ventricular muscle cell is −85 mV. The shaded areas represent the approximate depolarization required to trigger an action potential in each cell type. Together, the cardiac action potentials last for approximately half a second. SA node cells **(A)** depolarize to a peak of +10 mV, and ventricular muscle cells **(B)** depolarize to a peak of +45 mV. Note that the ventricular action potential has a much longer plateau phase. This long plateau ensures that ventricular myocytes have adequate time to contract before the onset of the next action potential. The Nernst equilibrium potentials of the major ions (E_{Ca}, E_{Na}, E_K) are shown as *dashed horizontal lines*. E_m, membrane potential.

Phases of SA Node Action Potential	Major Currents
Phase 4	I_f = Pacemaker current, relatively nonselective. I_{K_1} = Inward rectifier, outward K⁺ current
Phase 0	I_{Ca} = Inward Ca²⁺ current
Phase 3	I_K = Delayed rectifier, outward K⁺ current

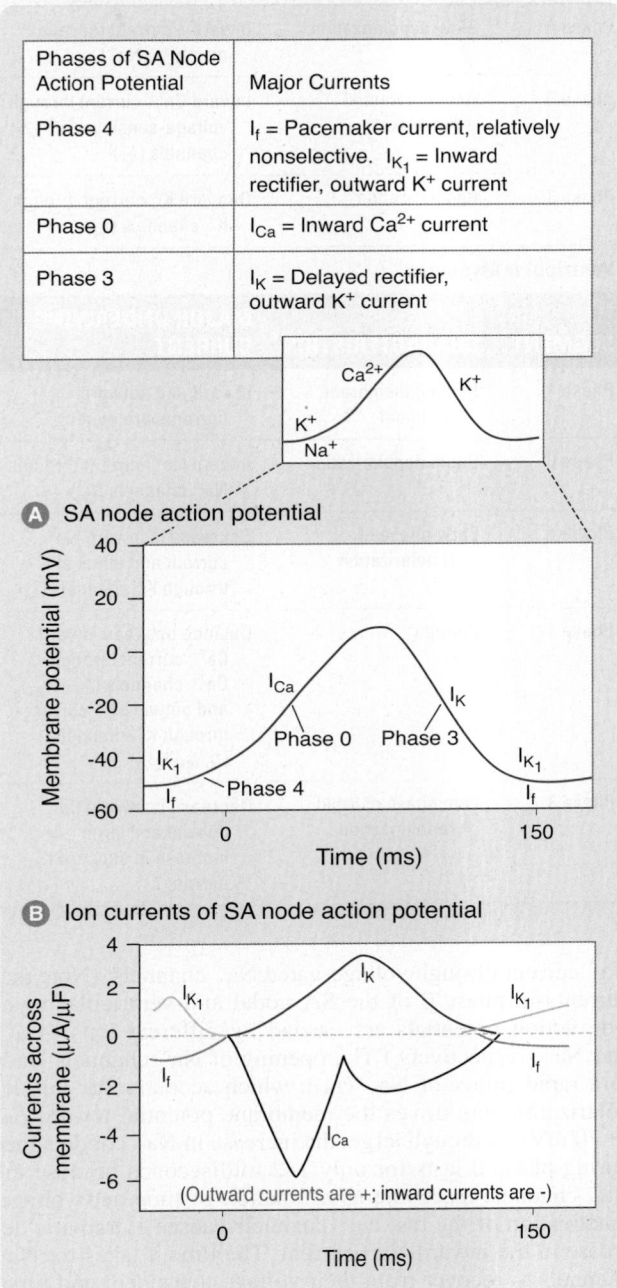

FIGURE 24-2. SA-node action potential and ion currents. A. SA nodal cells are depolarized slowly by the pacemaker current (I_f) (phase 4), which consists of an inward flow of sodium (mostly) and calcium ions. Depolarization to the threshold potential opens highly selective voltage-gated calcium channels, which drive the membrane potential toward E_{Ca} (phase 0). As the calcium channels close and potassium channels open (phase 3), the membrane potential repolarizes. **B.** The flux of each ion species correlates roughly with each phase of the action potential. Positive currents indicate an outward flow of ions (*blue and purple*), while negative currents are inward (*gray and black*).

of I_f channels and of the more selective voltage-gated Na⁺ and Ca²⁺ channels within the SA node, such that cells at the border of the node express relatively more voltage-gated Na⁺ channels and cells in the center of the node express relatively more I_f and voltage-gated Ca²⁺ channels. The expression of voltage-gated Na⁺ channels in the SA node is partly responsible for the effect of certain antiarrhythmics on the automaticity of SA nodal cells (see below).

Unlike SA nodal cells, ventricular myocytes do not depolarize spontaneously under physiologic conditions. As a result, the membrane potential of the resting ventricular myocyte remains near E_K until the cell is stimulated by a wave of depolarization that is initiated by nearby pacemaker cells.

TABLE 24-1 Major Characteristics of Action Potential Phases for SA Nodal Cells and Ventricular Myocytes

SA Nodal Cells

SEGMENT	CHARACTERISTICS	MAJOR UNDERLYING CURRENT
Phase 4	Slow depolarization	Inward I_f current (carried mainly by Na^+)
Phase 0	Action potential upstroke	Inward Ca^{2+} current through voltage-sensitive Ca^{2+} channels (I_{Ca})
Phase 3	Repolarization	Outward K^+ current through K^+ channels (I_K)

Ventricular Myocytes

SEGMENT	CHARACTERISTICS	MAJOR UNDERLYING CURRENT
Phase 4	Resting membrane potential	Inward and outward currents are equal
Phase 0	Rapid depolarization	Inward Na^+ current through Na^+ channels (I_{Na})
Phase 1	Early phase of repolarization	Decrease in inward Na^+ current and efflux of K^+ through K^+ channels (I_{to})
Phase 2	Plateau	Balance between inward Ca^{2+} current through Ca^{2+} channels ($I_{Ca,T}$, $I_{Ca,L}$) and outward K^+ current through K^+ channels (I_K, I_{K1}, I_{to})
Phase 3	Late phase of rapid repolarization	Decrease in inward Ca^{2+} current and large increase in outward K^+ current

Phases of Ventricular Action Potential	Major Currents
Phase 4	I_{K_1} = Inward rectifier, outward K^+ current $I_{Na/Ca}$ = Inward Na^+ and Ca^{2+} current
Phase 0	I_{Na} = Fast inward Na^+ current
Phase 1	I_{to} = Transient outward K^+ current
Phase 2	I_{Ca} = Inward Ca^{2+} current I_K = Delayed rectifier, outward K^+ current I_{K_1} = Inward rectifier, outward K^+ current I_{to} = Transient outward K^+ current
Phase 3	I_K = Delayed rectifier, outward K^+ current

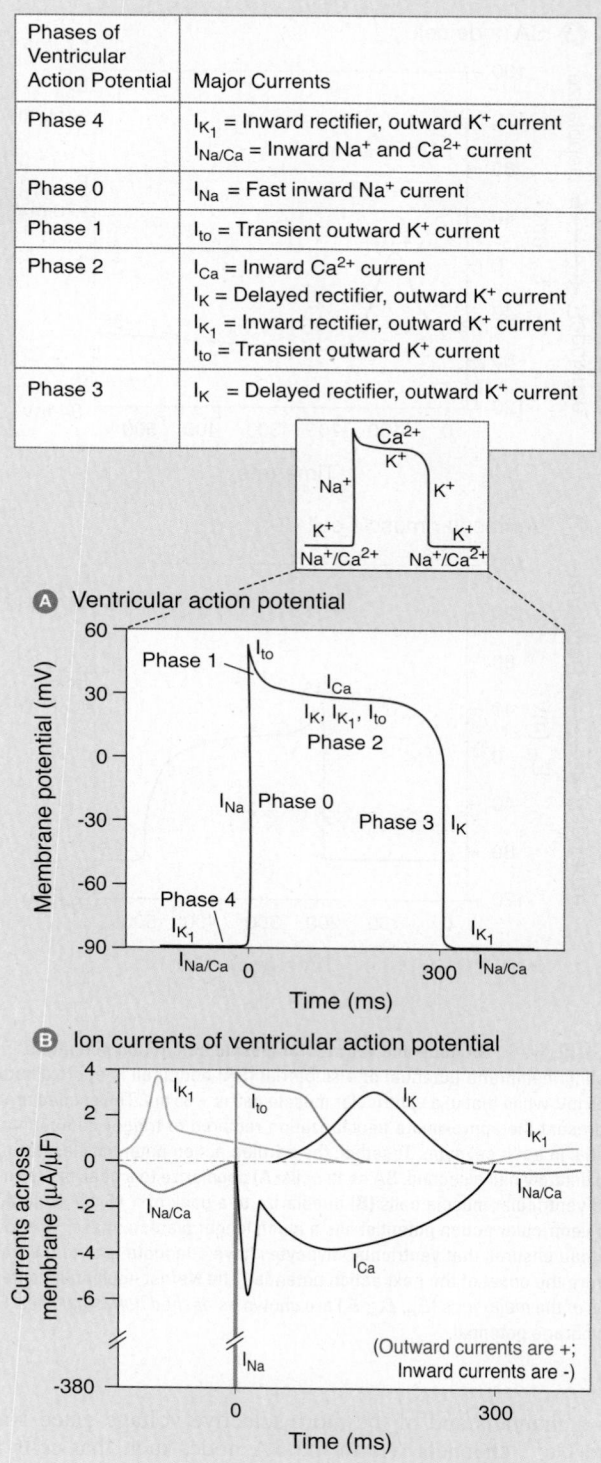

FIGURE 24-3. Ventricular action potential and ion currents. A. At the resting membrane potential (phase 4), the inward and outward currents are equal and the membrane potential approaches the K^+ equilibrium potential (E_K). During the action potential upstroke (phase 0), a large transient increase in Na^+ conductance occurs. This event is followed by a brief period of initial repolarization (phase 1), which is mediated by a transient outward K^+ current. The plateau of the action potential (phase 2) results from the opposition of an inward Ca^{2+} current and an outward K^+ current. The membrane repolarizes (phase 3) when the inward Ca^{2+} current decreases and the outward K^+ current predominates. **B.** The ion fluxes that give rise to the ventricular action potential consist of a complex pattern of changing ion permeabilities that are separated in time. Note especially that the Na^+ current in phase 0 is very large but extremely brief.

Na^+ current through voltage-gated Na^+ channels. (Note that currents in phase 0 of the SA nodal and ventricular myocyte action potentials are carried by different ions—Ca^{2+} and Na^+, respectively.) The opening of Na^+ channels leads to a rapid influx of Na^+ (I_{Na}), which accounts for the depolarization and drives the membrane potential toward E_{Na} (+70 mV). Although large, the increase in Na^+ conductance during phase 0 lasts for only 1–2 milliseconds because the Na^+ channels inactivate as a function of time and voltage. Inactivation of the fast Na^+ channels causes a dramatic decrease in the inward Na^+ current. The time it takes for Na^+ channels to recover from their voltage-dependent and time-dependent inactivation determines the *refractory period* of the myocyte. The refractory period is the time during which another action potential cannot fire. This serves as a protective mechanism to ensure that the heart has sufficient time to eject blood from its chambers. The refractory period lasts from the initiation of the action potential upstroke until the repolarization phase. I_{Na} is the major determinant of the velocity of impulse conduction throughout the ventricle.

The threshold-dependent activation of I_{Na} quickly depolarizes the membrane. The upstroke terminates before

BOX 24-1 The Electrocardiogram

The electrocardiogram (ECG or EKG) is used to infer changes in cardiac impulses by recording electrical potentials at various locations on the surface of the body. An ECG recording reflects changes in the excitation of the myocardium. A basic understanding of the ECG is useful for discussions of the clinical applications of the various antiarrhythmic agents.

A normal electrocardiogram contains three electrical waveforms: the P wave, the QRS complex, and the T wave (Fig. 24-4). The **P wave** represents *atrial depolarization*; the **QRS complex** represents *ventricular depolarization*; and the **T wave** represents *ventricular repolarization*. The ECG does not show atrial repolarization explicitly because the atrial repolarization is "drowned out" by the QRS complex. The ECG also contains two intervals and one segment: the PR interval, the QT interval, and the ST segment. The **PR interval** spans from the beginning of the P wave (initial depolarization of the atria) to the beginning of the Q wave (initial depolarization of the ventricles). Hence, the length of the PR interval varies with conduction velocity through the AV node. For example, if a patient has an electrical block in the AV node, then the conduction velocity through the AV node decreases and the PR interval increases. The **QT interval** spans from the beginning of the Q wave to the end of the T wave, representing the entire sequence of ventricular depolarization and repolarization. The **ST segment** extends from the end of the S wave to the beginning of the T wave; this segment, which represents the period during which the ventricles are depolarized, corresponds to the plateau phase of the ventricular action potential. ∎

reaching E_{Na}, however, and is followed by an early phase of rapid repolarization to about $+20$ mV. This **phase 1** repolarization is a consequence of two events: (1) the rapid voltage-dependent inactivation of I_{Na} and (2) the activation of transient K^+ currents (transient outward; I_{to}).

Phase 2, the plateau phase of the ventricular action potential, is unique to cardiac cell electrophysiology. The plateau is maintained by a finely tuned balance between an inward Ca^{2+} current through two types of Ca^{2+} channels ($I_{Ca.T}$, $I_{Ca.L}$) and an outward K^+ current through several types of K^+ channels (I_K, I_{K1}, I_{to}). Remarkably, only a few hundred channels per cell are used to maintain this fine balance. Because only a small number of channels are open, the total membrane conductance is low. The high membrane resistance during the plateau phase insulates the cardiac cells electrically, allowing rapid propagation of the action potential with little current dissipation.

During the plateau phase, two distinct Ca^{2+} currents—the transient Ca^{2+} current, $I_{Ca.T}$, and the long-lasting Ca^{2+} current, $I_{Ca.L}$—mediate the influx of Ca^{2+} needed to initiate cardiac myocyte contraction. T-type Ca^{2+} channels inactivate with time and are insensitive to block by dihydropyridines such as nifedipine. Current through the L-type Ca^{2+} channels ($I_{Ca.L}$) provides the dominant Ca^{2+} current in virtually all cardiac cells. $I_{Ca.L}$ is activated at -30 mV and inactivates slowly (hundreds of milliseconds). It is sensitive to block by dihydropyridines (**nifedipine**), benzothiazepines (**diltiazem**), and phenylalkylamines (**verapamil**), as discussed below. L-type Ca^{2+} channels carry inward current throughout the plateau phase; because Ca^{2+} stimulates the contraction of cardiac myocytes, these channels are crucial for coupling membrane excitability to myocardial contraction.

Opposing the inward Ca^{2+} currents are outward currents through the K^+ channels that are activated during the plateau phase. As the time-dependent inward Ca^{2+} currents inactivate, the outward K^+ currents (mostly I_K) rapidly drive the membrane potential toward E_K, thus repolarizing the cell in **phase 3**. However, these channels are unable to drive the membrane potential all the way to E_K because they deactivate at -40 mV. In **phase 4**, the resting membrane potential is reestablished by the activation of time-independent K^+ currents (I_{K1}), which drive the membrane potential close to the K^+ equilibrium potential.

In clinical practice, the overall electrical activity of the heart is measured rather than the ionic changes that occur at a single-cell level. This overall activity is reported in the electrocardiogram, or ECG (Box 24-1 and Fig. 24-4).

Determination of Firing Rate

The specialized conduction system of the heart consists of the SA node, AV node, bundle of His, and Purkinje system. These different populations of cells have different intrinsic rates of firing. Three factors determine the firing rate. First, as the rate of spontaneous depolarization in phase 4 increases, the rate of firing increases because the threshold potential (the minimum potential necessary to trigger an action potential) is reached more quickly at the end of phase 4. Second, if the threshold potential becomes more negative,

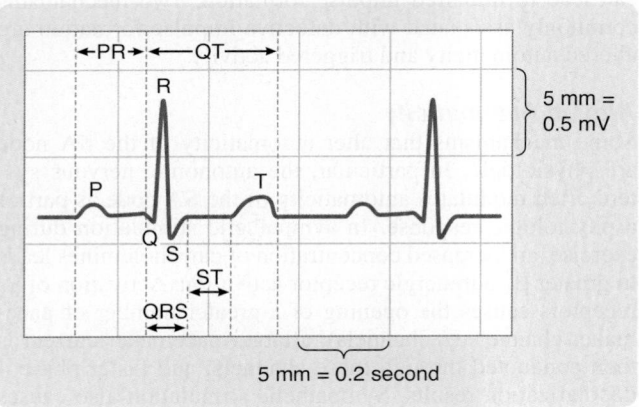

FIGURE 24-4. Electrocardiogram. The electrocardiogram (ECG or EKG) measures the body surface potentials induced by cardiac electrical activity. The **P wave** reflects *atrial depolarization*, the **QRS complex** represents *ventricular depolarization*, and the **T wave** indicates *ventricular repolarization*. The **PR interval** spans from the beginning of the P wave (initial depolarization of the atria) to the beginning of the Q wave (initial depolarization of the ventricles). The QT interval spans from the beginning of the Q wave to the end of the T wave, representing the entire interval of ventricular depolarization and repolarization. The **ST segment** extends from the end of the S wave to the beginning of the T wave, representing the period during which the ventricles are depolarized (i.e., the plateau phase of the action potential).

the rate of firing increases because the threshold potential is reached more quickly at the end of phase 4. Third, if the maximum diastolic potential (the resting membrane potential) becomes more positive, the rate of firing increases because less time is needed to repolarize the membrane fully at the end of phase 3.

Because the various populations of pacemaker cells possess different intrinsic rates of firing, the pacemaker population with the fastest firing rate sets the heart rate. The SA node possesses the fastest intrinsic firing rate (60–100 times per minute) and is the **native pacemaker** of the heart. The cells of the atrioventricular (AV) node and bundle of His fire intrinsically between 50 and 60 times per minute, and the cells of the Purkinje system have the slowest intrinsic firing rate at 30–40 times per minute. The cells of the AV node, bundle of His, and Purkinje system are termed **latent pacemakers** because their intrinsic rhythm is overridden by the faster SA-node automaticity. In a mechanism termed **overdrive suppression**, the SA node suppresses the intrinsic rhythm of the other pacemaker populations and entrains them to fire at the SA nodal firing rate.

■ PATHOPHYSIOLOGY OF ELECTRICAL DYSFUNCTION

Causes of electrical dysfunction in the heart can be divided into defects in impulse formation and defects in impulse conduction. In the former case, SA-node automaticity is interrupted or altered, leading to missed beats or ectopic beats, respectively. In the latter case, impulse conduction is altered (e.g., in the case of reentrant rhythms), and sustained arrhythmias can result.

Defects in Impulse Formation (SA Node)

As the native pacemaker of the heart, the SA node has a pivotal role in normal impulse formation. Electrical events that alter SA nodal function or disturb overdrive suppression can lead to impaired impulse formation. Two mechanisms commonly associated with defective impulse formation are altered automaticity and triggered activity.

Altered Automaticity

Some mechanisms that alter automaticity of the SA node are physiologic. In particular, the autonomic nervous system often modulates automaticity of the SA node as part of a physiologic response. In sympathetic stimulation during exercise, an increased concentration of catecholamines leads to greater β_1-adrenergic receptor activation. Activation of β_1 receptors causes the opening of a greater number of pacemaker channels (I_f channels); a larger pacemaker current is then conducted through these channels; and faster phase 4 depolarization results. Sympathetic stimulation also causes the opening of a greater number of Ca^{2+} channels and thereby shifts the threshold to more negative potentials. Both of these mechanisms increase heart rate. The parasympathetic vagus nerve affects the SA node by a number of mechanisms that oppose the sympathetic regulation of heart rate. Vagus nerve release of acetylcholine initiates an intracellular signaling cascade that (1) reduces the pacemaker current by decreasing pacemaker channel opening, (2) shifts the threshold to more positive potentials by reducing Ca^{2+} channel opening, and (3) makes the maximum diastolic potential (analogous

to the resting membrane potential in these spontaneously firing cells) more negative by increasing K^+ channel opening. The SA node, atria, and AV node are highly innervated and are thus more sensitive than the ventricular conducting system to the effects of vagal stimulation.

In pathologic conditions, automaticity can be altered when latent pacemaker cells take over the SA node's role as the pacemaker of the heart. *When the SA nodal firing rate becomes pathologically slow* or when conduction of the SA impulse is impaired, an **escape beat** may occur as a latent pacemaker initiates an impulse. A series of escape beats, known as an **escape rhythm**, may result from prolonged SA nodal dysfunction. On the other hand, an **ectopic beat** occurs *when latent pacemaker cells develop an intrinsic rate of firing that is faster than the SA nodal rate*, in some cases despite the presence of a normally functioning SA node. A series of ectopic beats, termed an **ectopic rhythm**, can result from ischemia, electrolyte abnormalities, or heightened sympathetic tone.

Direct tissue damage (such as can occur after a myocardial infarction) also results in altered automaticity. Tissue injury can cause structural disruption of the cell membrane. Disrupted membranes are unable to maintain ion gradients, which are critical for maintaining appropriate membrane potentials. If the resting membrane potential becomes sufficiently positive (more positive than −60 mV), nonpacemaker cells may begin to depolarize spontaneously. Another mechanism by which tissue damage leads to altered automaticity is through the loss of gap junction connectivity. Direct electrical connectivity is important for the effective delivery of overdrive suppression from the SA node to the rest of the cardiac myocytes. When connectivity is disrupted due to tissue injury, overdrive suppression is not efficiently relayed, and the unsuppressed cells can initiate their own rhythm. This abnormal rhythm can lead to cardiac arrhythmia.

Triggered Activity

Afterdepolarizations occur when a *normal* action potential triggers extra *abnormal* depolarizations. That is, the first (normal) action potential triggers additional oscillations of membrane potential, which may lead to arrhythmia. There are two types of afterdepolarizations—early afterdepolarizations and delayed afterdepolarizations.

If the afterdepolarization occurs *during the inciting action potential*, it is termed an **early afterdepolarization** (Fig. 24-5). *Conditions that prolong the action potential (e.g., drugs that prolong the QT interval, such as procainamide and ibutilide) tend to trigger early afterdepolarizations.* Specifically, an early afterdepolarization can occur during the plateau phase (phase 2) or the rapid repolarization phase (phase 3). During the plateau phase, because most of the Na^+ channels are inactivated, an inward Ca^{2+} current is responsible for the early afterdepolarization. On the other hand, during the rapid repolarization phase, partially recovered Na^+ channels can conduct an inward Na^+ current that contributes to the early afterdepolarization. If an early afterdepolarization is sustained, it can lead to a type of ventricular arrhythmia termed **torsades de pointes**. Torsades de pointes, French for "twisting of the points," is characterized by QRS complexes of varying amplitudes as they "twist" along the baseline; this rhythm is a medical emergency that can lead to death if not treated immediately.

In contrast to early afterdepolarizations, **delayed afterdepolarizations** occur shortly *after the completion of repolarization*

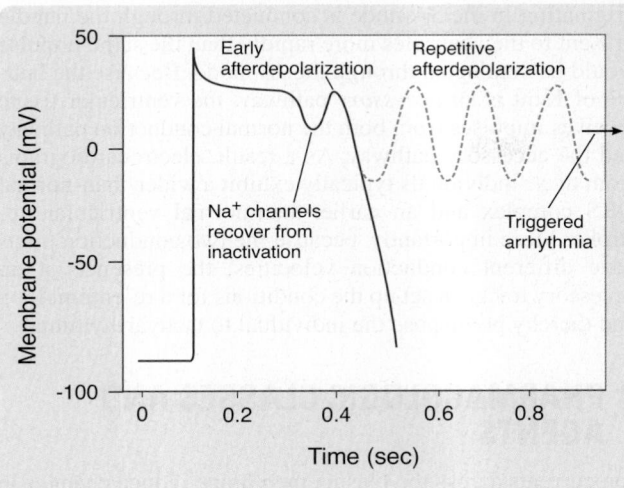

FIGURE 24-5. Early afterdepolarization. Early afterdepolarizations generally occur during the repolarizing phase of the action potential, although they can also occur during the plateau phase. Repetitive afterdepolarizations can trigger an arrhythmia.

(Fig. 24-6). The mechanism of delayed afterdepolarizations is not well understood; it has been proposed that high intracellular Ca^{2+} concentrations (such as in digoxin toxicity) lead to an inward Na^+ current, which, in turn, triggers the delayed afterdepolarization.

Defects in Impulse Conduction

The second type of electrical disturbance of the heart involves defects in impulse conduction. Normal cardiac function requires unobstructed and timely propagation of an electrical impulse through the cardiac myocytes. In pathologic conditions, altered impulse conduction can result from one or a combination of three mechanisms: re-entry, conduction block, and accessory tract pathways.

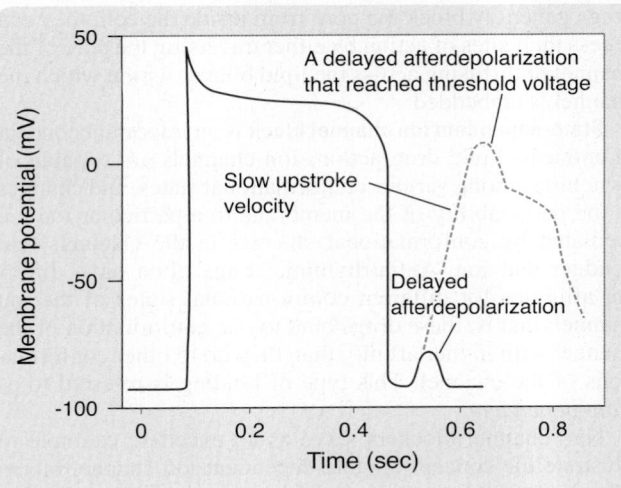

FIGURE 24-6. Delayed afterdepolarization. Delayed afterdepolarizations occur shortly after repolarization. Although the mechanism has not been firmly elucidated, it appears that intracellular Ca^{2+} accumulation activates the Na^+/Ca^{2+} exchanger, and the resulting electrogenic influx of 3 Na^+ for each extruded Ca^{2+} depolarizes the cell.

Re-entry

Normal cardiac conduction is initiated at the SA node and propagated to the AV node, bundle of His, Purkinje system, and myocardium in an orderly fashion. The cellular refractory period ensures that stimulated regions of the myocardium depolarize only once during propagation of an impulse. Figure 24-7A depicts normal impulse conduction, in which an impulse arriving at point *a* travels synchronously down two parallel pathways, 1 and 2.

Re-entry of an electrical impulse occurs when a self-sustaining electrical circuit stimulates an area of the myocardium repeatedly and rapidly. Two conditions must be present for a re-entrant electrical circuit to occur: (1) *unidirectional block* (anterograde conduction is prohibited, but retrograde conduction is permitted) and (2) *slowed retrograde conduction velocity*. Figure 24-7B shows a re-entrant electrical circuit. As the impulse arrives at point *a*, it can travel only down pathway 1 (the left branch) because pathway 2 (the right branch) is blocked *unidirectionally* in the anterograde direction. The impulse

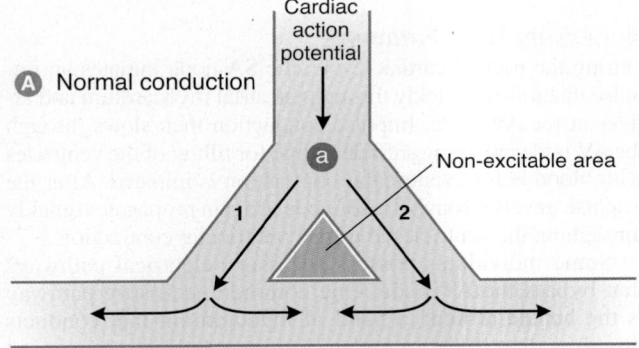

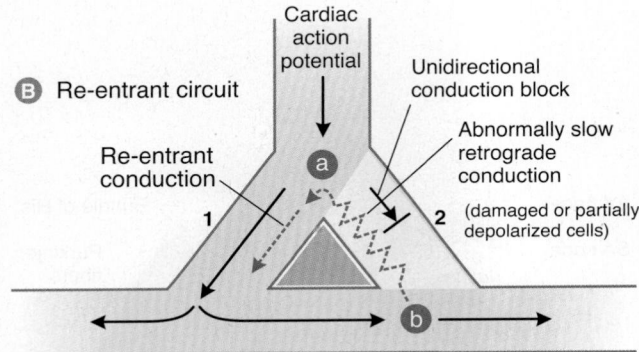

FIGURE 24-7. Normal and re-entrant electrical pathways. A. In normal impulse conduction, an impulse traveling down a pathway arrives at point *a*, where it is able to travel down two alternate pathways, 1 and 2. In the absence of re-entry, the impulses continue on and depolarize different areas of the ventricle. **B.** A re-entrant circuit can develop if one of the branch pathways is pathologically disrupted. When the impulse arrives at point *a*, it can travel only down pathway 1 because pathway 2 is blocked *unidirectionally* (i.e., the effective refractory period of the cells in pathway 2 is prolonged to such an extent that anterograde conduction is prohibited). The impulse conducts through pathway 1 and proceeds to point *b*. At this point, the cells in pathway 2 are no longer refractory, and the impulse conducts in a retrograde fashion up pathway 2 toward point *a*. When the retrograde impulse arrives at point *a*, it can initiate re-entry. Re-entry can result in a sustained pattern of rapid depolarizations that trigger tachyarrhythmias. This mechanism can occur over small or large regions of the heart.

conducts through pathway 1 and travels to point *b*. At this junction, the impulse travels in a *retrograde* fashion up pathway 2 toward point *a*. The conduction time from point *b* to point *a* is slowed because of cell damage or the presence of cells that are still in the refractory state. By the time the impulse reaches point *a*, the cells in pathway 1 have had adequate time to repolarize, and these cells are stimulated to continue conducting the action potential toward point *b*. In this manner, tachyarrhythmias result from the combination of unidirectional block and decreased conduction velocity in the abnormal pathway.

Conduction Block

Conduction block occurs when an impulse fails to propagate because of the presence of an area of inexcitable cardiac tissue. This area of inexcitable tissue could consist of normal tissue that is still refractory, or it could represent tissue that has been damaged by trauma, ischemia, or scarring. In either case, the myocardium is unable to conduct an impulse. Because conduction block removes overdrive suppression by the SA node, the cardiac myocytes are free to beat at their intrinsically slower frequency. For this reason, conduction block can be manifested clinically as bradycardia.

Accessory Tract Pathways

During the normal cardiac cycle, the SA node initiates an impulse that travels quickly through the atrial myocardium and arrives at the AV node. Impulse conduction then slows through the AV node, allowing sufficient time for filling of the ventricles with blood before ventricular contraction is initiated. After the impulse travels through the AV node, it again propagates quickly throughout the ventricles to trigger ventricular contraction.

Some individuals possess accessory electrical pathways that bypass the AV node. One common accessory pathway is the **bundle of Kent**, a band of myocardium that conducts impulses directly from the atria to the ventricles, bypassing the AV node (Fig. 24-8). In these individuals, an impulse

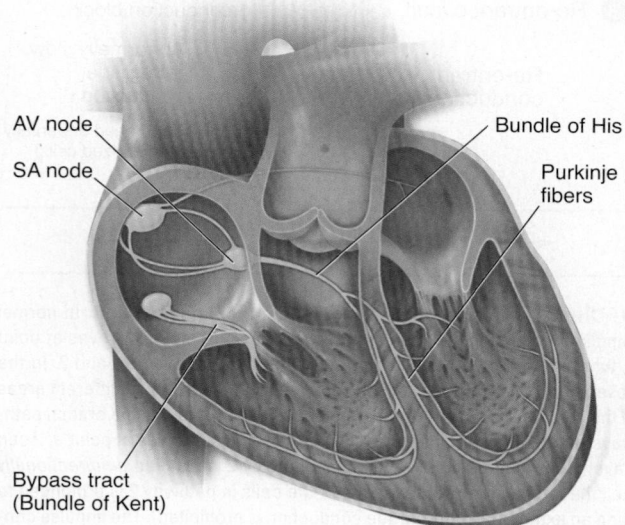

FIGURE 24-8. Bundle of Kent. The bundle of Kent is an accessory electrical pathway that conducts impulses directly from the atria to the ventricles, bypassing the AV node. Impulse conduction through this accessory tract is more rapid than conduction through the AV node, setting up the conditions for re-entrant tachyarrhythmias.

AV node

SA node

Bundle of His

Purkinje fibers

Bypass tract (Bundle of Kent)

originating in the SA node is conducted through the bundle of Kent to the ventricles more rapidly than the same impulse would be conducted through the AV node. Because the bundle of Kent is an *accessory* pathway, the ventricular tissue receives impulses from both the normal conduction pathway and the accessory pathway. As a result, electrocardiograms from these individuals typically exhibit a wider-than-normal QRS complex and an earlier-than-normal ventricular upstroke. More importantly, because the two conduction tracts have different conduction velocities, the presence of an accessory tract can set up the conditions for a re-entrant loop and thereby predispose the individual to tachyarrhythmias.

PHARMACOLOGIC CLASSES AND AGENTS

Ion currents across the plasma membrane induce changes in the membrane potential of cells. Changes in the membrane potential of cardiac pacemaker cells underlie the timely contraction of cardiac myocytes. Defects in impulse formation and altered impulse conduction can lead to disturbances in cardiac rhythm. Antiarrhythmic agents are used to restore normal cardiac rhythm by targeting proarrhythmic regions of the heart.

General Mechanisms of Action of Antiarrhythmic Agents

Although there are many different antiarrhythmic agents, there are surprisingly few mechanisms of antiarrhythmic action. In general, drugs that affect cardiac rhythm act by altering (1) the maximum diastolic potential in pacemaker cells (and/or the resting membrane potential in ventricular cells), (2) the rate of phase 4 depolarization, (3) the threshold potential, or (4) the action potential duration. The specific effect of a particular channel blocker follows directly from the role of the current carried by that channel in the cardiac action potential. For example, Na^+ and Ca^{2+} channel blockers typically alter the threshold potential, while K^+ channel blockers tend to prolong action potential duration. These drugs generally block the pore from inside the cell; they can access their sites of action by either traversing the pore of the channel or diffusing across the lipid bilayer within which the channel is embedded.

State-dependent ion channel block is an important concept in antiarrhythmic drug action. Ion channels are capable of switching among various conformational states, and changes in the permeability of the membrane to a particular ion are mediated by conformational changes in the channels that conduct that ion. Antiarrhythmic drugs often have different affinities for different conformational states of the ion channel; that is, these drugs bind to one conformation of the channel with higher affinity than they do to other conformations of the channel. This type of binding is referred to as *state-dependent*.

Na^+ channel blockers serve as an excellent example to illustrate the concept of state-dependent ion channel block. The Na^+ channel undergoes three major state changes (open–closed–inactivated) throughout the course of an action potential. During the upstroke, the channel is in the open conformation. The channel becomes inactivated during the plateau phase, and it changes again to the resting (closed) conformation as the membrane is repolarized to its resting potential. Most Na^+ channel blockers bind preferentially to the open and inactivated states of the Na^+ channel, not to the resting (closed) state of the channel. In this way, the drugs tend to block the channels during the action potential (cardiac systole) and to dissociate from the channels during diastole.

The unblocking rate (dissociation rate) of the various Na^+ channel blockers is an important determinant of the steady-state block of Na^+ channels. For example, when heart rate increases, the time available for unblocking (dissociation of the drug from its binding site on the channel) decreases and the degree of steady-state Na^+ channel block increases. The action of Na^+ channel blockers on ischemic tissue illustrates the therapeutic utility of state-dependent block. It has been observed that Na^+ channel blockers depress Na^+ conduction in ischemic tissue to a much greater extent than in normal tissue. In ischemic tissue, cardiac myocytes are depolarized for a longer period of time. This increase in action potential duration prolongs the inactivation state of the Na^+ channels, thereby making the inactivated Na^+ channels accessible to Na^+ channel blockers for a longer period of time. The rate of channel recovery from block is also decreased in depolarized ischemic myocytes because of the prolonged action potential. Thus, *the higher affinity of Na^+ channel blockers for open and inactivated states of the channel allows these agents to act preferentially on ischemic tissue and thereby to block an arrhythmogenic focus at its source.* See Chapter 12, Local Anesthetic Pharmacology, for more discussion on the concept of state-dependent Na^+ channel block.

Developing and using effective antiarrhythmic treatments is often complicated by the possibility that the antiarrhythmic agent can also cause arrhythmias. For example, many efforts have been directed at the treatment of re-entry, a mechanism responsible for a large proportion of arrhythmias. One way to treat re-entry is to block action potential propagation. If the retrograde impulse in the re-entrant circuit is *completely extinguished* by an antiarrhythmic agent, then the impulse will be unable to repeatedly depolarize the cardiac tissue in the re-entrant circuit. If the impulse is not completely extinguished, however, then the antiarrhythmic-induced slowing of conduction can actually promote re-entry arrhythmia. The "surviving" impulse may use the original re-entrant pathway to propagate the arrhythmia, or it may find other pathways and create new re-entrant circuits.

Classes of Antiarrhythmic Agents

Antiarrhythmic agents have traditionally been organized into four classes based on their mechanism of action (known as the *Vaughn-Williams classification*). Class I antiarrhythmics are Na^+ channel blockers; class II antiarrhythmics are β-adrenergic receptor antagonists; class III antiarrhythmics are K^+ channel blockers; and class IV antiarrhythmics are Ca^{2+} channel blockers. *It is important to realize, however, that many antiarrhythmic agents are not entirely selective blockers of Na^+, K^+, or Ca^{2+} channels; rather, many of these agents block more than one channel type.* This section presents some useful definitions of common cardiac electrical disturbances (Box 24-2) and describes the mechanism of drug action for each class of antiarrhythmic agent.

Class I Antiarrhythmic Agents: Fast Na^+ Channel Blockers

Na^+ channel blockers decrease automaticity in SA nodal cells by (1) shifting the threshold to more positive potentials and (2) decreasing the slope of phase 4 depolarization (Fig. 24-9). The block of Na^+ channels leaves fewer channels available to open in response to membrane depolarization, thereby raising the threshold for action potential firing and slowing the rate of depolarization. Both of these effects

---

BOX 24-2 Definitions of Common Cardiac Electrical Disturbances

To appreciate the clinical applications of the various antiarrhythmic agents, it is helpful to understand the basic definitions of terms that describe common electrical abnormalities of the heart.

Effective refractory period: The period during which a region of cardiac tissue cannot be excited by an electrical impulse.

Sinus tachycardia: The SA node fires between 100 and 180 times per minute, and the ECG shows normal P waves and QRS complexes. Sinus tachycardia can be a normal physiologic response (e.g., during exercise) or a pathologic condition that results from altered SA-node automaticity.

Paroxysmal supraventricular tachycardia (PSVT): PSVT is characterized by atrial firing rates of 140–250 beats per minute, but it is usually transient and self-limited. In 90% of cases, PSVT is caused by re-entry involving the AV node, SA node, or atrial tissue.

Atrial flutter: The atrial rate is between 280 and 300 beats per minute, and the ECG shows a rapid, "saw-tooth" appearance of atrial electrical activity. Because the pace of atrial firing is so rapid, some impulses from the atria reach the AV node during its refractory period. These impulses are not transmitted to the ventricles and, therefore, the ventricular rate is slower than the atrial rate. The ratio of atrial to ventricular firing rate is typically 2:1.

Atrial or ventricular fibrillation: These arrhythmias are characterized by chaotic, re-entrant impulse conduction through the atrium or ventricle. Ventricular fibrillation (VF) is invariably fatal if the arrhythmia is not converted, while atrial fibrillation (AF) can be tolerated for many years.

Ventricular tachycardia (VT): A series of three or more ventricular extrasystoles at rates between 100 and 250 beats per minute.

Torsades de pointes: This arrhythmia is often generated by afterdepolarizations in individuals with prolonged QT syndrome. The varying amplitudes of the QRS complex are described as a "twisting of points" along the baseline of an ECG tracing. Torsades is often transient and self-limited but can lead to more life-threatening arrhythmias. ∎

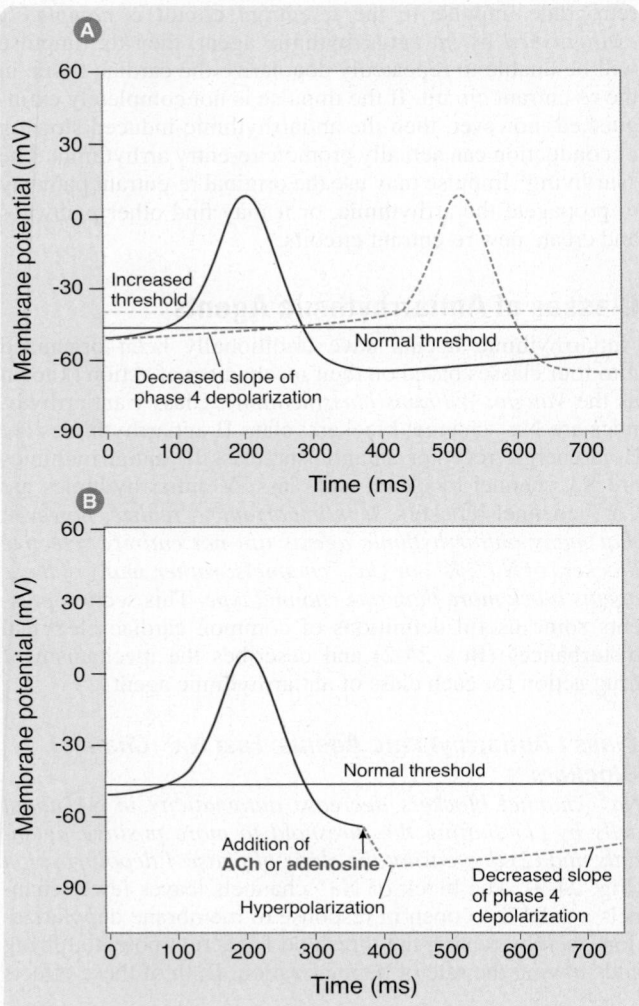

FIGURE 24-9. Effects of class I antiarrhythmics and natural agonists on the SA-node action potential. A. The normal SA-node action potential is shown as a *solid curve*. Class I antiarrhythmics (Na^+ channel blockers) alter SA-node automaticity by affecting two aspects of the SA nodal action potential: (1) the threshold is shifted to more positive potentials and (2) the slope of phase 4 depolarization is decreased. **B.** Acetylcholine (ACh) and adenosine slow the SA nodal firing rate by opening K^+ channels that hyperpolarize the cell and decrease the slope of phase 4 depolarization.

extend the duration of phase 4 and thereby decrease heart rate. Furthermore, the shift in threshold potential means that, in patients with implanted defibrillators who are treated with Na^+ channel blockers, a higher voltage is needed to defibrillate the heart. Therefore, it is important to take into account the effect of Na^+ channel blockers when choosing appropriate settings for implanted defibrillators.

In addition to decreasing SA-node automaticity, Na^+ channel blockers act on ventricular myocytes to decrease re-entry. This is achieved mainly by decreasing the upstroke velocity of phase 0 and, for some Na^+ channel blockers, by prolonging repolarization (Fig. 24-10). By decreasing phase 0 upstroke velocity, Na^+ channel blockers decrease the conduction velocity through cardiac tissue. Ideally, conduction velocity is reduced to such an extent that the propagating wavefront is extinguished before it is able to restimulate

myocytes in a re-entrant pathway. However, if conduction velocity is not sufficiently decreased, and the impulse is not extinguished, then the slowed impulse can support re-entry as it reaches cells that are no longer refractory (see above) and thereby precipitate an arrhythmia. In addition to decreasing phase 0 upstroke velocity, class IA Na^+ channel blockers prolong repolarization. Prolonged repolarization increases the effective refractory period, so that cells in a re-entrant circuit cannot be depolarized by the re-entrant action potential. In summary, *Na^+ channel blockers decrease the likelihood of re-entry, and thereby prevent arrhythmia, by (1) decreasing conduction velocity and (2) increasing the refractory period of ventricular myocytes.*

Although the three subclasses of class I antiarrhythmics (class IA, IB, and IC) have similar effects on the action potential in the SA node, there are important differences in their effects on the ventricular action potential.

Class IA Antiarrhythmics

Class IA antiarrhythmics exert a moderate block on Na^+ channels and prolong the repolarization of both SA nodal cells and ventricular myocytes. By blocking Na^+ channels, these agents decrease the phase 0 upstroke velocity, which decreases conduction velocity through the myocardium. Class IA antiarrhythmics also block K^+ channels and thereby reduce the outward K^+ current responsible for repolarization of the membrane. This prolongation of repolarization increases the effective refractory period of the cells. Together, the decreased conduction velocity and increased effective refractory period decrease re-entry.

Quinidine is often considered the prototypical drug among the class IA antiarrhythmics, but it is becoming less frequently used due to its adverse effects. In addition to the pharmacologic actions described above for all class IA antiarrhythmics, quinidine exerts an anticholinergic (vagolytic) effect, most likely by blocking the K^+ channels that are opened upon vagal stimulation of M_2 muscarinic receptors in the AV node (see Fig. 24-9B, Fig. 10-1). *The anticholinergic effect is significant clinically because it can increase conduction velocity through the AV node.* For this reason, an agent that slows AV nodal conduction—such as a β-adrenergic antagonist or verapamil (a Ca^{2+} channel blocker)—should be used in conjunction with quinidine to prevent an excessively rapid ventricular response in patients with atrial flutter or other supraventricular tachycardias.

The most common adverse effects of quinidine are diarrhea, nausea, headache, and dizziness. These effects make it difficult for patients to tolerate chronic therapy with quinidine. Quinidine is contraindicated in patients with QT prolongation and in patients who are taking medications that predispose to QT prolongation because of the increased risk of torsades de pointes. Relative contraindications to quinidine use include sick sinus syndrome, bundle branch block, myasthenia gravis (because of quinidine's anticholinergic action), and liver failure.

Quinidine is administered orally and metabolized by cytochrome P450 enzymes in the liver. Quinidine increases plasma levels of digoxin (an inotropic agent), most likely by competing for the P450 enzymes that are responsible for digoxin metabolism. Because digoxin has a narrow therapeutic index (see Chapter 25, Pharmacology of Cardiac Contractility), quinidine-induced digoxin toxicity occurs in a significant fraction of patients. The plasma potassium

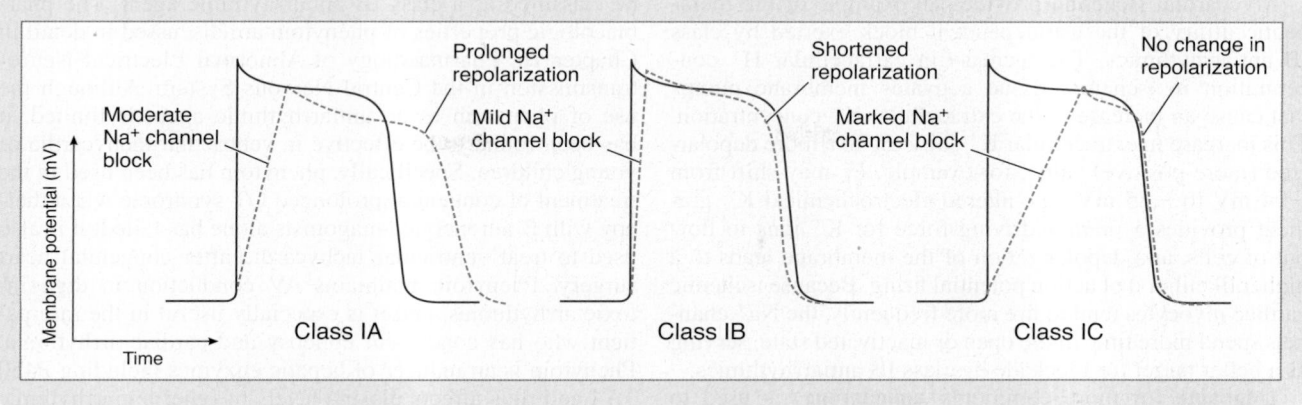

FIGURE 24-10. Effects of class IA, IB, and IC antiarrhythmics on the ventricular action potential. Class I antiarrhythmics (Na⁺ channel blockers) act on ventricular myocytes to decrease re-entry. All subclasses of the class I antiarrhythmics block the Na⁺ channel to some degree: class IA agents exhibit moderate Na⁺ channel block, class IB agents rapidly bind to (block) and dissociate from (unblock) Na⁺ channels, and class IC agents produce marked Na⁺ channel block. Class IA, IB, and IC agents also differ in the degree to which they affect the duration of the ventricular action potential.

level must be carefully monitored in patients treated with quinidine because hypokalemia decreases quinidine efficacy, exacerbates QT prolongation, and, most importantly, predisposes to torsades de pointes. *It is hypothesized that torsades de pointes is the mechanism most likely responsible for quinidine-induced syncope.* Because of quinidine's numerous adverse effects and contraindications, this drug has largely been replaced by class III agents—such as ibutilide and amiodarone—for the pharmacologic conversion of atrial flutter or atrial fibrillation to normal sinus rhythm.

Procainamide is a class IA antiarrhythmic agent that is effective in the treatment of many types of supraventricular and ventricular arrhythmias. Procainamide can be used in the pharmacologic conversion of new-onset atrial fibrillation to normal sinus rhythm, although with lower efficacy than intravenous ibutilide. Procainamide can also be used safely to decrease the likelihood of re-entrant arrhythmias in the setting of acute myocardial infarction, even in the presence of decreased cardiac output. Procainamide can be administered by slow intravenous infusion to treat acute ventricular tachycardia.

Unlike quinidine, procainamide has few anticholinergic effects and does not alter plasma levels of digoxin. Procainamide can cause peripheral vasodilation via inhibition of neurotransmission at sympathetic ganglia. With chronic therapy, almost all patients develop a lupus-like syndrome and positive antinuclear antibodies; the precise mechanism of this reaction is not known, but it remits if the drug is discontinued. Procainamide is acetylated in the liver to N-acetyl-procainamide (NAPA); this active metabolite produces the pure class III antiarrhythmic effects of prolonging the refractory period and lengthening the QT interval. NAPA does not appear to cause the lupus-like adverse effects of procainamide.

Disopyramide is similar to quinidine in its electrophysiologic and antiarrhythmic effects; the difference between the two drugs lies in their adverse effects. Disopyramide causes fewer gastrointestinal problems but has even more profound anticholinergic effects than quinidine, producing such adverse effects as urinary retention and dry mouth. The profound anticholinergic effects of disopyramide appear to be related to the drug's action as an antagonist at muscarinic

acetylcholine receptors. Disopyramide is contraindicated in patients with obstructive uropathy or glaucoma. Disopyramide is also contraindicated in patients with conduction block between the atria and ventricles and in patients with sinus-node dysfunction. Disopyramide has the prominent but unexplained effect that it depresses cardiac contractility, which has led to its use in the treatment of hypertrophic obstructive cardiomyopathy and neurocardiogenic syncope. Because of its negative inotropic effects, disopyramide is absolutely contraindicated in patients with decompensated heart failure. Oral disopyramide is approved only for the treatment of life-threatening ventricular arrhythmias; oral or intravenous disopyramide is sometimes used to convert supraventricular tachycardia to normal sinus rhythm. The current trend in the treatment of life-threatening arrhythmias, however, is away from class I antiarrhythmic agents and toward class III agents and electrical devices such as implantable defibrillators.

Class IB Antiarrhythmics

Class IB antiarrhythmics include **lidocaine**, **mexiletine**, and **phenytoin**. Lidocaine is the prototypical class IB agent. These drugs alter the ventricular action potential by blocking Na⁺ channels and sometimes by shortening repolarization; the latter effect may be mediated by the drugs' ability to block the few Na⁺ channels that inactivate late during phase 2 of the cardiac action potential (Fig. 24-10). In comparison to class IA antiarrhythmics, which preferentially bind to open Na⁺ channels, *class IB drugs bind to both open and inactivated Na⁺ channels.* Therefore, the more time Na⁺ channels spend in the open or inactivated state, the more blockade the class IB antiarrhythmics can exert. The major distinguishing characteristic of the class IB antiarrhythmics is their *fast dissociation* from Na⁺ channels. Because Na⁺ channels recover quickly from class IB blockade, these drugs are most effective in blocking depolarized or rapidly driven tissues, where there is a higher likelihood of the Na⁺ channels being in the open or inactivated state. Thus, class IB antiarrhythmics exhibit *use-dependent block* in diseased myocardium, where the cells have a tendency to fire more frequently; these antiarrhythmics have relatively little effect on normal cardiac tissue.

Myocardial ischemia provides an example of the therapeutic utility of the use-dependent block exerted by class IB antiarrhythmics. The increase in extracellular H^+ concentration in ischemic tissue activates membrane pumps that cause an increase in the extracellular K^+ concentration. This increase in extracellular K^+ shifts E_K to a more depolarized (more positive) value; for example, E_K may shift from -94 mV to -85 mV. The altered electrochemical K^+ gradient provides a *smaller* driving force for K^+ ions to flow out of cells, and depolarization of the membrane leads to a higher likelihood of action potential firing. Because ischemic cardiac myocytes tend to fire more frequently, the Na^+ channels spend more time in the open or inactivated state, serving as a better target for blockade by class IB antiarrhythmics.

Lidocaine (or more commonly **amiodarone**) is used to treat ventricular arrhythmias in emergency situations. This drug is not effective in treating supraventricular arrhythmias. In hemodynamically stable patients, lidocaine is reserved for treatment of ventricular tachyarrhythmias or frequent premature ventricular contractions (PVCs) that are bothersome or hemodynamically significant.

Lidocaine has a short plasma half-life (approximately 20 minutes), and it is metabolically de-ethylated in the liver. Its metabolism is governed by two factors: liver blood flow and liver cytochrome P450 activity. For patients whose liver blood flow is decreased by old age or heart failure, or whose P450 enzymes are acutely inhibited, for example, by cimetidine (see Chapter 4, Drug Metabolism), a lower dose of lidocaine should be considered. For patients whose P450 enzymes are induced by drugs such as barbiturates, phenytoin, or rifampin, the dose of lidocaine should be increased.

Because lidocaine shortens repolarization, possibly by blocking the few Na^+ channels that inactivate late during phase 2 of the cardiac action potential, it does not prolong the QT interval. Therefore, the drug is safe for use in patients with long QT syndrome. However, because lidocaine also blocks Na^+ channels in the central nervous system (CNS), it can produce CNS adverse effects such as confusion, dizziness, and seizures. In addition to its use as an acute intravenous therapy for ventricular arrhythmias, lidocaine is used as a local anesthetic (see Chapter 12).

Mexiletine, an analogue of lidocaine, is available in oral formulation. While the efficacy of mexiletine is similar to that of quinidine, mexiletine does not prolong the QT interval and it lacks vagolytic effects. In addition, little hemodynamic depression has been reported with the use of mexiletine. The primary indication for mexiletine is life-threatening ventricular arrhythmia. In practice, however, mexiletine is often used as an adjunct to other antiarrhythmic agents. For example, mexiletine is used in combination with **amiodarone** in patients with implantable cardioverter-defibrillators (ICDs) and in patients with recurrent ventricular tachycardia. Mexiletine is also used in combination with **quinidine** or **sotalol** to increase antiarrhythmic efficacy while reducing adverse effects. There are no data supporting reduced mortality with the use of mexiletine or any of the other class IB antiarrhythmic agents. Major adverse effects of mexiletine include dose-related nausea and tremor, which can be ameliorated when the drug is taken with food. Mexiletine undergoes hepatic metabolism, and its plasma levels may be altered by inducers of hepatic P450 enzymes such as phenytoin and rifampin.

While **phenytoin** is usually considered an antiepileptic medication, its effects on the myocardium also allow it to be classified as a class IB antiarrhythmic agent. The pharmacologic properties of phenytoin are discussed in detail in Chapter 16, Pharmacology of Abnormal Electrical Neurotransmission in the Central Nervous System. Although the use of phenytoin as an antiarrhythmic agent is limited, it has been found to be effective in ventricular tachycardia of young children. Specifically, phenytoin has been used in the treatment of congenital prolonged QT syndrome when therapy with β-adrenergic antagonists alone has failed; it is also used to treat ventricular tachycardia after congenital heart surgery. Phenytoin maintains AV conduction in digoxin-toxic arrhythmias, and it is especially useful in the rare patient who has concurrent epilepsy and cardiac arrhythmia. Phenytoin is an inducer of hepatic enzymes including P450 3A4 and thus affects plasma levels of other antiarrhythmic agents such as mexiletine, lidocaine, and quinidine.

Class IC Antiarrhythmics

Class IC antiarrhythmics are the most potent Na^+ channel blockers, and they have little or no effect on action potential duration (Fig. 24-10). By markedly decreasing the rate of phase 0 upstroke of ventricular cells, these drugs suppress premature ventricular contractions. Class IC antiarrhythmics also prevent paroxysmal supraventricular tachycardia and atrial fibrillation. However, these drugs have marked depressive effects on cardiac function and, thus, must be used with discretion. In addition, the CAST (Cardiac Arrhythmia Suppression Trial) and other studies have brought attention to the proarrhythmic effects of these agents.

Flecainide is the prototypical class IC drug; other members of this class include **encainide**, **moricizine**, and **propafenone**. Flecainide illustrates the principle that antiarrhythmic agents can also cause arrhythmia. When flecainide is administered to patients with preexisting ventricular tachyarrhythmias and to those with a history of myocardial infarction, it can worsen the arrhythmia even at normal doses. Because flecainide is pro-arrhythmic in patients with ischemic or structural heart disease, its major use is for prevention of atrial arrhythmias (e.g., atrial fibrillation) in patients with structurally normal hearts. Flecainide is eliminated very slowly from the body; it has a plasma half-life of 12–30 hours. Because of its marked blockade of Na^+ channels and its suppressive effects on cardiac function, flecainide use is associated with adverse effects that include sinus-node dysfunction, a marked decrease in conduction velocity, and conduction block.

Class II Antiarrhythmic Agents: β-Adrenergic Antagonists

Class II antiarrhythmic agents are β-adrenergic antagonists (also called *β-blockers*). These agents act by inhibiting sympathetic input to the pacing regions of the heart. (β-Adrenergic antagonists are more extensively discussed in Chapter 11, Adrenergic Pharmacology.) Although the heart is capable of beating on its own without innervation from the autonomic nervous system, both sympathetic and parasympathetic fibers innervate the SA node and the AV node and thereby alter the rate of automaticity. Sympathetic stimulation releases norepinephrine, which binds to β_1-adrenergic receptors in the nodal tissues. (β_1-Adrenergic receptors are the adrenergic subtype preferentially expressed in cardiac tissue.) Activation of β_1-adrenergic receptors in the SA node triggers an increase in the pacemaker current (I_f), which increases the rate of phase 4 depolarization and, consequently,

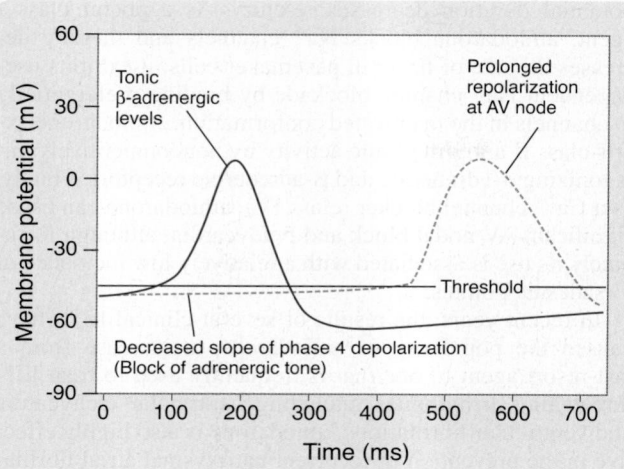

FIGURE 24-11. Effects of class II antiarrhythmics on pacemaker cell action potentials. Class II antiarrhythmics (β-antagonists) reverse the tonic sympathetic stimulation of cardiac β₁-adrenergic receptors. By blocking the adrenergic effects on the SA and AV nodal action potentials, these agents decrease the slope of phase 4 depolarization (especially important at the SA node) and prolong repolarization (especially important at the AV node). These agents are useful in the treatment of supraventricular and ventricular arrhythmias that are precipitated by sympathetic stimulation.

leads to more frequent firing of the node. Stimulation of β_1-adrenergic receptors in the AV node increases Ca^{2+} and K^+ currents, thereby increasing the conduction velocity and decreasing the refractory period of the node.

β_1-Antagonists block the sympathetic stimulation of β_1-adrenergic receptors in the SA and AV nodes (Fig. 24-11). The AV node is more sensitive than the SA node to the effects of β_1-antagonists. β_1-Antagonists affect the action potentials of SA and AV nodal cells by (1) decreasing the rate of phase 4 depolarization and (2) prolonging repolarization. Decreasing the rate of phase 4 depolarization results in decreased automaticity, and this, in turn, reduces myocardial oxygen demand. Prolonged repolarization at the AV node increases the effective refractory period, which decreases the incidence of re-entry.

β_1-Antagonists are the most frequently used agents in the treatment of supraventricular and ventricular arrhythmias precipitated by sympathetic stimulation. β_1-Adrenergic antagonists have been shown to reduce mortality after myocardial infarction, even in patients with relative contraindications to this therapy such as severe diabetes mellitus or asthma. Because of their wide spectrum of clinical application and established safety record, β-adrenergic antagonists are the most useful antiarrhythmic agents currently available.

There are several generations of β-antagonists, each characterized by slightly different pharmacologic properties. First-generation β-antagonists, such as **propranolol**, are nonselective β-adrenergic antagonists that antagonize both β_1-adrenergic and β_2-adrenergic receptors. They are widely used to treat tachyarrhythmias caused by catecholamine stimulation during exercise or emotional stress. Because propranolol does not prolong repolarization in ventricular tissue, it can be used in patients with long QT syndrome. Second-generation agents, including **atenolol**, **metoprolol**, **acebutolol**, and **bisoprolol**, are relatively selective for β_1-adrenergic receptors when administered in low doses.

Third-generation β-antagonists cause vasodilation in addition to β_1-receptor antagonism. **Labetalol** and **carvedilol** induce vasodilation by antagonizing α-adrenergic receptor-mediated vasoconstriction; **pindolol** is a partial agonist at the β_2-adrenergic receptor; and **nebivolol** stimulates endothelial production of nitric oxide.

The different generations of β-antagonists produce varying degrees of adverse effects. Three general mechanisms are responsible for the adverse effects of β-blockers. First, antagonism at β_2-adrenergic receptors causes smooth muscle spasm, leading to bronchospasm, cold extremities, and impotence. These effects are more commonly caused by the nonselective first-generation β-antagonists. Second, exaggeration of the therapeutic effects of β_1-receptor antagonism can lead to excessive negative inotropic effects, heart block, and bradycardia. Third, drug penetration into the CNS can produce insomnia and depression.

Class III Antiarrhythmic Agents: Inhibitors of Repolarization

Class III antiarrhythmic agents block K^+ channels. Two types of currents determine the duration of the plateau phase of the cardiac action potential: inward, depolarizing Ca^{2+} currents, and outward, hyperpolarizing K^+ currents. During a normal action potential, the hyperpolarizing K^+ currents eventually dominate, returning the membrane potential to more hyperpolarized values. Larger hyperpolarizing K^+ currents shorten plateau duration, returning the membrane potential to its resting value more rapidly, while smaller hyperpolarizing K^+ currents lengthen plateau duration and delay return of the membrane potential to its resting value.

When K^+ channels are blocked, a smaller hyperpolarizing K^+ current is generated. Therefore, K^+ channel blockers cause a longer plateau and prolong repolarization (Fig. 24-12). The ability of K^+ channel blockers to lengthen plateau duration is responsible for both their pharmacologic uses and their adverse effects. On the beneficial side, prolongation of the plateau duration increases the effective

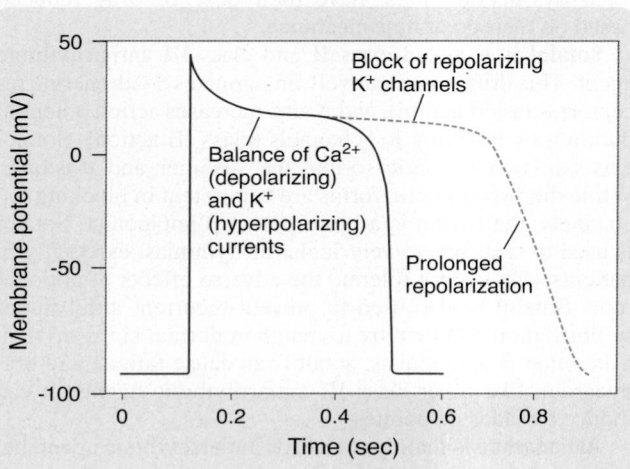

FIGURE 24-12. Effects of class III antiarrhythmics on the ventricular action potential. Class III antiarrhythmics (K^+ channel blockers) decrease the magnitude of the repolarizing K^+ currents during phase 2 of the action potential and thereby prolong action potential duration. This prolongation of the plateau phase decreases re-entry, but it can also predispose to early afterdepolarizations.

refractory period, which, in turn, decreases the incidence of re-entry. On the toxic side, prolongation of the plateau duration increases the likelihood of developing early afterdepolarizations and torsades de pointes. With the exception of amiodarone, K^+ channel blockers also exhibit the undesirable property of "reverse use-dependency": action potential prolongation is most pronounced at slow rates (undesirable) and least pronounced at fast rates (desirable). K^+ channel blockers have little or no effect on the upstroke phase or conduction velocity of the impulse.

Ibutilide is a class III agent that prolongs repolarization by inhibiting the delayed rectifier K^+ current. This agent also enhances a slow inward Na^+ current that further prolongs repolarization. Ibutilide is used to terminate atrial fibrillation and flutter, as exemplified in the introductory case. The major adverse effect of ibutilide results from its prolongation of the QT interval; the serious arrhythmia torsades de pointes may result, requiring electrical cardioversion (delivery of an electrical shock to resynchronize the heart) in almost 2% of patients taking the drug. For this reason, Dr. J was closely monitored by a cardiologist during his ibutilide infusion. Ibutilide is generally not administered to patients with preexisting long QT syndrome.

Dofetilide is a class III agent that is only available orally. It inhibits exclusively the rapid component of the delayed rectifier K^+ current and has no effect on the inward Na^+ current. Dofetilide increases the action potential duration and prolongs the QT interval in a dose-dependent manner. Because dofetilide has the potential of inducing ventricular arrhythmias, it is reserved for patients with highly symptomatic atrial fibrillation and/or atrial flutter. Dofetilide is used in the cardioversion of atrial fibrillation and atrial flutter to normal sinus rhythm, and it is effective in the maintenance of sinus rhythm in such patients after cardioversion. Because dofetilide has no negative inotropic effects, it can be used in patients with depressed ejection function. Similar to ibutilide, the major adverse effect of dofetilide is torsades de pointes, which occurs in 1–3% of patients taking the drug. Because dofetilide is excreted by the kidneys, patients with renal dysfunction must have their dose of drug reduced based on their creatinine clearance.

Sotalol is a mixed class II and class III antiarrhythmic agent. This drug nonselectively antagonizes β-adrenergic receptors (class II action), and it also increases action potential duration by blocking K^+ channels (class III action). Sotalol exists in two isomeric forms: the *l*-isomer and *d*-isomer. While the two isomeric forms are equipotent in blocking K^+ channels, the *l*-form is a more potent β-antagonist. Sotalol is used to treat severe ventricular arrhythmias, especially in patients who cannot tolerate the adverse effects of amiodarone. Sotalol is also used to prevent recurrent atrial flutter or fibrillation and thereby to maintain normal sinus rhythm. Like other β-antagonists, sotalol can cause fatigue and bradycardia; like other class III antiarrhythmic agents, it can induce torsades de pointes.

Amiodarone is mainly a class III antiarrhythmic agent, but it also acts as a class I, class II, and class IV antiarrhythmic. The ability of amiodarone to exert such a diverse range of effects can be explained by its mechanism of action: *alteration of the lipid membrane in which ion channels and receptors are located*. In all cardiac tissues, amiodarone lengthens the effective refractory period by inhibiting the K^+ channels responsible for repolarization; this prolongation of action potential duration decreases re-entry. As a potent class I agent, amiodarone blocks Na^+ channels and thereby decreases the rate of firing in pacemaker cells; it exhibits use-dependent Na^+ channel blockade by binding preferentially to channels in the inactivated conformation. Amiodarone exerts class II antiarrhythmic activity by noncompetitively antagonizing α-adrenergic and β-adrenergic receptors. Finally, as a Ca^{2+} channel blocker (class IV), amiodarone can cause significant AV nodal block and bradycardia, although fortunately its use is associated with a relatively low incidence of torsades de pointes.

In recent years, the results of several clinical trials have caused the popularity of amiodarone to increase from a last-resort agent to one that is frequently used to treat life-threatening arrhythmias, including ventricular tachycardia and ventricular fibrillation. Amiodarone is also highly effective in the prevention of recurrent paroxysmal atrial fibrillation or flutter, as exemplified in the introductory case.

The wide spectrum of action of amiodarone is accompanied by a panoply of serious adverse effects when the drug is used for long periods or in high doses. These effects include cardiac, pulmonary, thyroid, hepatic, neurological, and idiosyncratic complications (Table 24-2). In the heart, amiodarone can decrease AV- or SA-node function by blocking Ca^{2+} channels. Amiodarone can exert a negative inotropic effect by inhibiting β-adrenergic receptors, especially when the drug is used chronically. As an α-adrenergic antagonist, amiodarone can cause hypotension. Severe pulmonary complications can occur in patients taking high doses of amiodarone (400 mg daily or higher). Pneumonitis leading to pulmonary fibrosis is the most dreaded of all complications associated with amiodarone use. Fortunately, such complications occur rarely in patients taking prophylactic doses (200 mg daily) for prevention of ventricular or atrial arrhythmias. Because of its structural similarity to thyroxine, amiodarone affects thyroid hormone metabolism by inhibiting peripheral conversion of thyroxine (T4) to triiodothyronine (T3). Either hyperthyroidism or hypothyroidism can occur as a consequence of this dysregulation of thyroid hormone metabolism (see Chapter 28, Pharmacology of the Thyroid Gland). Of patients taking amiodarone, 10–20% manifest an abnormal increase in liver enzymes, although this effect is reversible when the dose of the drug is reduced.

TABLE 24-2 Major Adverse Effects of Amiodarone, Particularly at High Doses

CATEGORY	ADVERSE EFFECT
Cardiovascular	↓ AV- or SA-node function ↓ Cardiac contractility Hypotension
Pulmonary	Pneumonitis leading to pulmonary fibrosis
Thyroid	Hyperthyroidism or hypothyroidism
Hepatic	Elevated liver enzymes
Neurological	Peripheral neuropathy, headache, ataxia, tremors
Other	Corneal microdeposits Testicular dysfunction Skin discoloration

Neurological symptoms can include peripheral neuropathy, headache, ataxia, and tremors. Patients taking amiodarone should be monitored for abnormal pulmonary, thyroid, and liver function. Amiodarone is contraindicated in patients with cardiogenic shock, second-degree or third-degree heart block, or severe SA-node dysfunction with marked sinus bradycardia or syncope.

Dronedarone is a class III agent that is structurally similar to amiodarone. It was developed in an attempt to create a drug with the antiarrhythmic effects of amiodarone, while limiting the adverse effects. Compared to amiodarone, dronedarone is less lipophilic (resulting in a shorter half-life) and lacks iodine moieties in its structure (thereby reducing the incidence of thyroid toxicity). In clinical studies of patients with atrial fibrillation, dronedarone reduced the incidence of recurrent atrial fibrillation when compared with placebo, with relatively few adverse effects. However, a separate study suggested that dronedarone is associated with increased mortality in a subgroup of patients with systolic heart failure. Thus, dronedarone should be used with caution, if at all, in patients with systolic heart failure. Dronedarone is also contraindicated in patients with permanent atrial fibrillation (i.e., atrial fibrillation that cannot be cardioverted to normal sinus rhythm), due to increased mortality. Recent reports have suggested an association between dronedarone and rare but severe hepatotoxicity. Liver function tests should therefore be monitored periodically.

Class IV Antiarrhythmic Agents: Ca^{2+} Channel Blockers

Drugs that block cardiac Ca^{2+} channels act preferentially on *SA and AV nodal tissues* because these pacemaker tissues depend on Ca^{2+} currents for the depolarization phase of the action potential (Fig. 24-2). In contrast, Ca^{2+} channel blockers have little effect on fast Na^+ channel-dependent tissues, such as Purkinje fibers and atrial and ventricular muscle. *The major therapeutic action of the class IV antiarrhythmics is to slow the action potential upstroke in AV nodal cells, leading to slowed conduction velocity through the AV node* (Fig. 24-13). This also blocks re-entrant arrhythmias in which the AV node is part of the re-entry circuit. In the introductory case, however, the re-entry circuit responsible for atrial fibrillation was isolated to the atria. This is why diltiazem, a Ca^{2+} channel blocker, slowed Dr. J's heart rate but did not change his underlying heart rhythm. (Refer to Chapter 22, Pharmacology of Vascular Tone, for a more extended discussion of Ca^{2+} channel blockers.)

Because different tissues express different subtypes of Ca^{2+} channels, and different subclasses of Ca^{2+} channel blockers interact preferentially with different Ca^{2+} channel subtypes, the various Ca^{2+} channel blockers have differential effects in different tissues. Dihydropyridines (such as **nifedipine**) have a relatively greater effect on the Ca^{2+} current in *vascular smooth muscle*, while **verapamil** and **diltiazem** are relatively more selective for *cardiac tissues*. Verapamil and diltiazem are used to treat re-entrant paroxysmal supraventricular tachycardias because these are often re-entrant arrhythmias that involve the AV node. Verapamil and diltiazem are *rarely* used in ventricular tachycardia. In fact, the only indications for these agents in ventricular arrhythmias are idiopathic right ventricular outflow tract tachycardia and fascicular tachycardias. Verapamil is also used to treat hypertension and vasospastic (Prinzmetal's) angina. Class IV

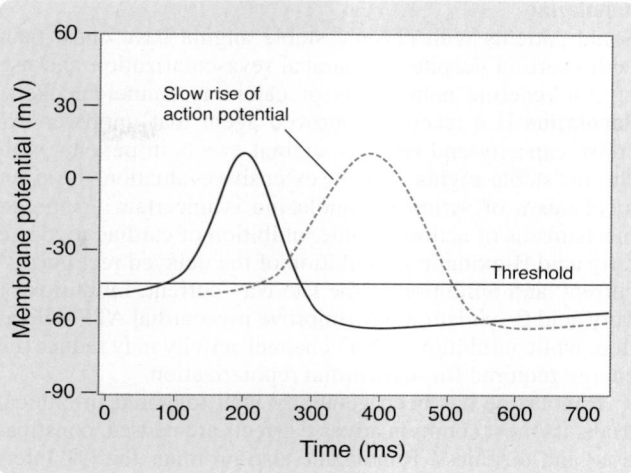

FIGURE 24-13. Effects of class IV antiarrhythmics on pacemaker cell action potentials. Class IV antiarrhythmics (Ca^{2+} channel blockers) decrease excitability of SA nodal cells and prolong AV nodal conduction, primarily by slowing the action potential upstroke in nodal tissue. Class IV antiarrhythmics are useful in the treatment of arrhythmias that involve re-entry through the AV node, but high doses of Ca^{2+} channel blockers can prolong AV nodal conduction to such an extent that heart block results.

agents can cause AV nodal block by reducing the conduction velocity excessively. Administration of intravenous verapamil to patients taking β-blockers can precipitate severe heart failure and lead to irreversible electromechanical dissociation. Verapamil and diltiazem increase plasma digoxin levels by competing with digoxin for renal excretion.

Other Agents That Modulate Cardiac Rhythm or Ion Channels

Adenosine, while not considered a classical antiarrhythmic agent, has important effects on cardiac electrophysiology. **Ranolazine** is a recently approved agent for the treatment of chronic stable angina; its mechanism of action appears to involve inhibition of the late Na^+ current. **Ivabradine** is an investigational agent that slows the heart rate by modulating the I_f current.

Adenosine

The nucleoside **adenosine** is naturally present throughout the body. By stimulating the P1 class of purinergic receptors, adenosine opens a G protein-coupled K^+ channel (I_{KACh}) and thereby inhibits SA nodal, atrial, and AV nodal conduction (Fig. 24-9B). The AV node is more sensitive than the SA node to the effects of adenosine. Adenosine also inhibits the potentiation of Ca^{2+} channel activity by cAMP and thereby suppresses Ca^{2+}-dependent action potentials. Adenosine has a plasma half-life of less than 10 seconds and is often used as the first-line agent for converting narrow-complex paroxysmal supraventricular tachycardia to normal sinus rhythm. For this indication, it is efficacious in 90% of cases. Most adverse effects of adenosine are transient, including headache, flushing, chest pain, and excessive AV or SA nodal inhibition. Adenosine can also cause bronchoconstriction lasting for up to 30 minutes in patients with asthma. In many patients, a *transient* new arrhythmia occurs at the onset of adenosine administration.

Ranolazine

Some patients with chronic stable angina have chest pain with exertion despite mechanical revascularization and use of β-adrenergic antagonists or calcium channel blockers. **Ranolazine** is a recently approved agent that improves exercise capacity and reduces anginal events in patients with chronic stable angina. Despite extensive evaluation, the exact mechanism of action of ranolazine is uncertain. Proposed mechanisms of action include inhibition of cardiac myocyte fatty acid β-oxidation, inhibition of the delayed rectifier K^+ current, and inhibition of the late Na^+ current. Inhibition of fatty acid β-oxidation may improve myocardial ATP utilization, while inhibition of Na^+ channel activity may reduce the energy required for myocardial repolarization.

Ranolazine has been generally well tolerated in clinical trials; its most common adverse effects are nausea, constipation, and dizziness. Ranolazine also prolongs the QT interval. It is currently approved as a second-line treatment for patients with chronic stable angina.

Ivabradine

Ivabradine inhibits the I_f current responsible for phase 4 depolarization in SA nodal cells. By inhibiting phase 4 depolarization, ivabradine slows the heart rate, thereby decreasing myocardial oxygen demand. Ivabradine is currently approved in Europe for use in patients with chronic stable angina but remains investigational in the United States. It is also occasionally used to treat inappropriate sinus tachycardia, a syndrome where the pacemaker cells fire more than 100 times per minute without any secondary cause. Ivabradine is contraindicated in patients with preexisting bradycardia.

▌ CONCLUSION AND FUTURE DIRECTIONS

Cardiac arrhythmias arise from defects in impulse formation, defects in impulse conduction, or a combination of the two mechanisms. Because derangements in ion conductance lead to arrhythmias, antiarrhythmic agents act directly or indirectly to alter the conformational states of ion channels and thereby change the membrane permeability to ions. The pharmacologic property of use-dependent ion channel blockade allows many antiarrhythmic agents to target diseased cardiac tissues preferentially based on the altered electrophysiology of these tissues. In general, class I antiarrhythmics block Na^+ channels; class II antiarrhythmics (β-blockers) inhibit sympathetic stimulation and thereby decrease automaticity; class III agents block K^+ channels; and class IV agents block Ca^{2+} channels. Despite continuing developments in antiarrhythmic drugs, the paradox still exists that antiarrhythmic drugs can also generate arrhythmias. Nonetheless, judicious use of antiarrhythmic agents can reduce mortality in certain clinical circumstances, and careful tailoring of a drug regimen to the individual patient's clinical status can reduce the adverse effects of these agents.

The most important new directions in the pharmacology of cardiac rhythm involve identifying specific genes for ion channels in the human heart (Table 24-3). Currently, animal models are used for the majority of ion channel research; comparatively little is known about the clinical pharmacology of ion channels expressed in humans. With the mouse and human genomes now completely sequenced, researchers will be able to investigate the possibility that newly identified gene products can serve as selective targets for new therapeutic agents. The identification of ion channel gene expression in the various tissues of the human heart (SA node, AV node, atrial conduction pathways, endocardium, ventricular conduction pathways, etc.), both during development and in response to injury, may provide new targets that are not now known. Many of the genes are likely to encode channels that form heteromultimers, and there are likely to be many genetic variants within the population. This enormous complexity will likely represent a boon to drug development because it will allow more tailored strategies to be employed. For example, current research in atrial fibrillation has focused on the development of antiarrhythmics selective for ion channels that are expressed selectively in the atria. In parallel, the development of implantable computers, stimulators, and defibrillators will constitute an alternative strategy to prevent or terminate arrhythmias.

TABLE 24-3 Molecular Identity of Known Cardiac Ion Currents

ION CURRENT	CHANNEL PROTEIN
I_{Na}	$Na_V1.5$
$I_{Ca.L}$ (dihydropyridine-sensitive)	$Ca_V1.2$
$I_{Ca.T}$	$Ca_V3.1$
I_f	HCN2, HCN4
I_{to}	$K_V4.3$
I_{Ks}*	$K_V7.1$ (KvLQT1)
I_{Kr}*	K_V11, HERG
I_{K1}	Kir2.1 (inward rectifier)
I_{KACh}	Kir3.1 + Kir3.4 (G protein-gated)

*Collectively referred to as I_K.

Suggested Reading

Ackerman MJ, Clapham DE. Ion channels—basic science and clinical disease. *N Engl J Med* 1997;336:1575–1586. (*Broad review of ion channels.*)

Dobrev D, Nattel S. New antiarrhythmic drugs for treatment of atrial fibrillation. *Lancet* 2010;375:1212–1223. (*Future directions in drug development for treatment of atrial fibrillation.*)

Link MS. Clinical practice. Evaluation and initial management of supraventricular tachycardia. *N Engl J Med* 2012;367:1438–1448. (*Discussion of the clinical uses of antiarrhythmic agents in treating supraventricular tachycardia.*)

Rudy Y, Silva JR. Computational biology in the study of cardiac ion channels and cell electrophysiology. *Q Rev Biophys* 2006;39:57–116. (*Summarizes the known cardiac ion channels in models of cardiac action potentials.*)

Swedberg K, Komajda M, Böhm M, et al. Ivabradine and outcomes in chronic heart failure (SHIFT): a randomised placebo-controlled study. *Lancet* 2010;376:875–885. (*Large trial suggesting that ivabradine may benefit patients with heart failure.*)

DRUG SUMMARY TABLE: CHAPTER 24 Pharmacology of Cardiac Rhythm

CLASS IA ANTIARRHYTHMICS

Mechanism—Moderate block of voltage-gated Na⁺ channels and block of K⁺ channels in ventricular myocytes (decreases phase 0 upstroke velocity and prolongs repolarization) and SA nodal cells (shifts threshold to more positive potentials and decreases slope of phase 4 depolarization); quinidine also blocks K⁺ channels that are opened upon vagal stimulation of muscarinic receptors in the AV node (vagolytic effect)

DRUG	CLINICAL APPLICATIONS	SERIOUS AND COMMON ADVERSE EFFECTS	CONTRAINDICATIONS	THERAPEUTIC CONSIDERATIONS
Quinidine	Conversion of atrial flutter or fibrillation and maintenance of normal sinus rhythm Paroxysmal supraventricular tachycardia Premature atrial or ventricular contractions Paroxysmal AV junctional rhythm or atrial or ventricular tachycardia	*Torsades de pointes, complete AV block, ventricular tachycardia, agranulocytosis, thrombocytopenia, hepatotoxicity, acute asthma attack, respiratory arrest, angioedema, rare occurrence of systemic lupus* Fatigue, headache, light-headedness, widening of QRS complex and lengthening of QT and PR intervals, hypotension, premature ventricular contractions (PVCs), tachycardia, diarrhea, cinchonism	History of torsades de pointes or prolonged QT interval Concurrent use of drugs that prolong QT interval Conduction defects Myasthenia gravis	Co-administration of other drugs known to prolong QT interval (such as thioridazine, ziprasidone) is contraindicated. Quinidine inhibits conversion of codeine to morphine, thereby reducing codeine's analgesic effect. Quinidine-induced digoxin toxicity occurs in a significant fraction of patients. Amiodarone, amprenavir, azole antifungals, cimetidine, and ritonavir increase quinidine levels. Co-administration of anticholinergics results in additive anticholinergic effects. An agent that slows AV nodal conduction (a β-adrenergic blocker or a Ca²⁺ channel blocker) should be used in conjunction with quinidine to prevent an excessively rapid ventricular response in patients with atrial flutter or other supraventricular tachycardias.
Procainamide	Symptomatic premature ventricular contractions (PVCs) Life-threatening ventricular tachycardia Maintenance of normal sinus rhythm after conversion of atrial flutter Malignant hyperthermia	*Same as quinidine, except fewer anticholinergic effects; additionally, lupus-like syndrome may occur after prolonged use*	Same as quinidine Additional contraindications include systemic lupus erythematosus	Co-administration of drugs known to prolong QT interval is contraindicated. Procainamide does not alter plasma levels of digoxin. Ventricular rate may accelerate due to vagolytic effects on AV node; consider pretreatment with a cardiac glycoside. Baseline and periodic determination of anti-nuclear antibodies (ANA), and monitor for development of lupus-like syndrome.
Disopyramide	PVCs Ventricular tachycardia Conversion of atrial fibrillation, atrial flutter, and paroxysmal atrial tachycardia to normal sinus rhythm	*Same as quinidine, except more profound anticholinergic effects and fewer gastrointestinal effects*	Same as quinidine Additionally, cardiogenic shock and hypersensitivity to disopyramide	Co-administration of drugs known to prolong QT interval is contraindicated. Rifampin impairs antiarrhythmic activity of disopyramide. Ventricular rate may accelerate due to vagolytic effects on AV node; consider pretreatment with a cardiac glycoside. Disopyramide is commonly prescribed for patients who cannot tolerate quinidine or procainamide.

continues

DRUG SUMMARY TABLE: CHAPTER 24 Pharmacology of Cardiac Rhythm *continued*

DRUG	CLINICAL APPLICATIONS	*SERIOUS* AND COMMON ADVERSE EFFECTS	CONTRAINDICATIONS	THERAPEUTIC CONSIDERATIONS
CLASS IB ANTIARRHYTHMICS Mechanism—Use-dependent block of voltage-gated Na$^+$ channels in ventricular myocytes (decreases phase 0 upstroke velocity); may also shorten repolarization				
Lidocaine Mexiletine	Ventricular arrhythmias in the context of myocardial infarction (MI), cardiac manipulation, or cardiac glycosides Lidocaine only: Local anesthesia of skin or mucous membranes Pain, burning, or itching Postherpetic neuralgia	*Seizures, asystole, bradycardia, cardiac arrest, new or worsened arrhythmias, hepatotoxicity, anaphylaxis (shared adverse effects); methemoglobinemia (lidocaine only)* Restlessness, stupor, tremor, hypotension, gastrointestinal upset, blurred or double vision, dizziness, tinnitus, nervousness	Stokes-Adams syndrome Wolff-Parkinson-White syndrome Severe SA, AV, or intraventricular block Contraindications for spinal or epidural block (lidocaine only) include inflammation or infection in puncture region, septicemia, severe hypertension, spinal deformities, neurologic disorders Hypersensitivity to amide local anesthetics	Dosage of both lidocaine and mexiletine should be adjusted when co-administered with P450 inhibitors (such as cimetidine) and inducers (such as barbiturates, phenytoin, or rifampin). In severely ill patients, seizures may be the first sign of toxicity. Intramuscular injection of lidocaine can cause large increase in serum creatine kinase (CK).
Phenytoin	Tonic–clonic seizures, focal seizures, status epilepticus Seizures related to eclampsia	*Agranulocytosis, leukopenia, pancytopenia, thrombocytopenia, megaloblastic anemia, hepatitis, Stevens–Johnson syndrome, toxic epidermal necrolysis, bullous dermatosis, lupus erythematosus, nephrotoxicity, suicidal ideation* Ataxia, nystagmus, incoordination, confusion, diplopia, hirsutism, facial coarsening, gingival hyperplasia, morbilliform eruption, constipation, nausea	Hydantoin hypersensitivity Sinus bradycardia, SA node block, second- or third-degree AV block Stokes-Adams syndrome Concomitant use with delavirdine or rilpivirine	Phenytoin interacts with numerous drugs due to its hepatic metabolism. Phenytoin is metabolized by P450 2C9/10 and P450 2C19. Other drugs that are metabolized by these enzymes can increase plasma concentration of phenytoin. Phenytoin can also induce various P450s, such as P450 3A4, which can lead to increased metabolism of oral contraceptives and other drugs.
CLASS IC ANTIARRHYTHMICS Mechanism—Marked block of voltage-gated Na$^+$ channels in ventricular myocytes (decreases phase 0 upstroke velocity)				
Encainide Flecainide Moricizine Propafenone	Sustained ventricular tachycardia Paroxysmal supraventricular tachycardia, paroxysmal atrial fibrillation unresponsive to other measures	*Cardiac arrest, heart failure, new or worsened arrhythmia, sinus-node dysfunction, marked decrease in conduction velocity, conduction block (shared adverse effects); agranulocytosis, thrombosis, hepatomegaly, lupus erythematosus, anemia, stroke, renal failure, impotence, respiratory failure (propafenone only)* Dizziness, headache, syncope, nausea, visual disturbances, dyspnea	Shared contraindications: Cardiogenic shock Second- or third-degree AV block, right bundle branch block with left hemiblock Proarrhythmic effects in patients with atrial fibrillation or flutter Hypersensitivity to encainide, flecainide, moricizine Propafenone only: Bradycardia, bronchospastic disorder, severe obstructive pulmonary disease, Brugada syndrome, electrolyte imbalance, hypotension	Associated with excessive mortality and nonfatal cardiac arrest; restrict use to patients who have failed other measures. Can worsen arrhythmia in patients with preexisting ventricular tachyarrhythmias and in those with a history of myocardial infarction. May increase acute and chronic endocardial pacing threshold and suppress ventricular escape rhythms. Monitor levels in patients with significant hepatic impairment.

CLASS II ANTIARRHYTHMICS: β-ADRENERGIC ANTAGONISTS

Mechanism—Antagonize sympathetic stimulation of β₁-adrenergic receptors in SA and AV nodal cells, thereby decreasing slope of phase 4 depolarization (important at SA node) and prolonging repolarization (important at AV node)

Propranolol	See Drug Summary Table: Chapter 11 Adrenergic Pharmacology
Atenolol	
Metoprolol	
Acebutolol	
Bisoprolol	
Nebivolol	
Labetalol	
Carvedilol	
Pindolol	

CLASS III ANTIARRHYTHMIC AGENTS: INHIBITORS OF REPOLARIZATION

Mechanism—Block K⁺ channels, resulting in longer action potential plateau and prolonged repolarization

Ibutilide	Conversion of atrial fibrillation or atrial flutter to normal sinus rhythm	*AV block, bradycardia, sustained ventricular tachycardia, 2% develop torsades de pointes requiring electrical cardioversion*	Class IA and class III antiarrhythmic agents may increase potential for prolonged refractoriness. Drugs that prolong QT interval (such as antihistamines, phenothiazines, and tricyclic antidepressants) increase the risk of arrhythmia. Monitor QT interval during ibutilide administration.	History of polymorphic ventricular tachycardia, such as torsades de pointes Preexisting long QT syndrome Hypersensitivity to ibutilide
Dofetilide	Conversion of atrial fibrillation or atrial flutter to normal sinus rhythm Maintenance of normal sinus rhythm in patients with symptomatic atrial fibrillation or atrial flutter	*Same as ibutilide*	Only available orally. Due to its potential for inducing ventricular arrhythmias, dofetilide is reserved for patients with highly symptomatic atrial fibrillation and/or atrial flutter. Reduction in dosage in patients with renal dysfunction.	Same as ibutilide Additionally, creatinine clearance less than 20 mL/min as well as concomitant use of cimetidine, dolutegravir, hydrochlorothiazide, ketoconazole, megestrol, prochlorperazine, trimethoprim, or verapamil
Sotalol	Life-threatening ventricular arrhythmias Maintenance of normal sinus rhythm in patients with symptomatic atrial fibrillation or flutter	*Heart failure, prolonged QT interval, torsades de pointes, stroke* Bradyarrhythmia, chest pain, light-headedness, palpitations, nausea, dizziness, headache, dyspnea, fatigue	Sotalol is a mixed class II and class III antiarrhythmic agent that nonselectively antagonizes β-adrenergic receptors and prolongs action potential duration by blocking potassium channels. Used frequently in patients who cannot tolerate adverse effects of amiodarone. Use with caution in patients with impaired renal function or diabetes mellitus. Avoid co-administration with ziprasidone and sparfloxacin, which can prolong QT interval.	Severe sinus-node dysfunction, sinus bradycardia, second- or third-degree AV block Long QT syndrome Cardiogenic shock, uncontrolled heart failure Asthma Creatinine clearance less than 40 mL/min Hypersensitivity to sotalol Hypokalemia

continues

DRUG SUMMARY TABLE: CHAPTER 24 Pharmacology of Cardiac Rhythm *continued*

DRUG	CLINICAL APPLICATIONS	*SERIOUS* AND COMMON ADVERSE EFFECTS	CONTRAINDICATIONS	THERAPEUTIC CONSIDERATIONS
CLASS III ANTIARRHYTHMIC AGENTS: INHIBITORS OF REPOLARIZATION Mechanism—Block K$^+$ channels, resulting in longer action potential plateau and prolonged repolarization				
Amiodarone	Recurrent ventricular fibrillation, unstable ventricular tachycardia Supraventricular arrhythmias	*Arrhythmias, asystole, bradycardia, heart block, heart failure, prolonged QT interval, vasculitis, hypotension, sinus arrest, Stevens-Johnson syndrome, toxic epidermal necrolysis, thrombocytopenia, hepatic failure, lupus erythematosus, rhabdomyolysis, severe pulmonary toxicity (pneumonitis, alveolitis, fibrosis), thyroid dysfunction, pseudotumor cerebri, elevated intracranial pressure, blindness, renal impairment* Fatigue, corneal microdeposits, blue-gray skin pigmentation, photosensitivity, gastrointestinal upset	Patients receiving ritonavir Severe SA-node disease Second- or third-degree AV block Bradycardia with syncope Cardiogenic shock Hypersensitivity to amiodarone	IV formulation (Cordarone®) contains benzyl alcohol, which has caused gasping respiration and cardiovascular collapse ("gasping syndrome") in neonates. Pulmonary toxicity is more common at high doses. Co-administration of β-blockers or calcium channel blockers may increase risk of sinus bradycardia, sinus arrest, and AV block. Co-administration of cholestyramine increases amiodarone elimination. Co-administration of cyclosporine, digoxin, flecainide, lidocaine, phenytoin, procainamide, quinidine, or theophylline may lead to increased levels of these drugs. Co-administration of drugs that prolong QT interval, such as disopyramide, thioridazine, phenothiazine, pimozide, quinidine, sparfloxacin, or tricyclic antidepressants, may lead to prolonged QT interval and induce torsades de pointes. Co-administration of phenytoin may decrease amiodarone levels.
Dronedarone	Atrial fibrillation	*Heart failure, prolonged QT interval, hepatic failure, stroke, acute renal failure* Gastrointestinal upset, asthenia, elevated serum creatinine	Bradycardia, prolonged QTc or PR interval, atrioventricular block Heart failure Permanent atrial fibrillation Hepatic impairment Pregnancy Concomitant use of QT-prolonging drugs Concomitant use of P450 3A inhibitors Hypersensitivity to dronedarone Sick sinus syndrome	Dronedarone is similar to amiodarone but has a shorter half-life and decreased incidence of thyroid toxicity. Increases creatinine without affecting the glomerular filtration rate.
CLASS IV ANTIARRHYTHMIC AGENTS: CALCIUM CHANNEL BLOCKERS Mechanism—Preferentially block cardiac Ca^{2+} channels; slow action potential upstroke in SA and AV nodal tissues				
Verapamil **Diltiazem**	See Drug Summary Table: Chapter 22 Pharmacology of Vascular Tone			

OTHER AGENTS THAT MODULATE CARDIAC RHYTHM OR ION CHANNELS
Mechanism—See specific drug

Drug			
Adenosine	Conversion of paroxysmal supraventricular tachycardia to normal sinus rhythm	*Cardiac arrest, cardiac dysrhythmia, complete AV block, ventricular arrhythmias, bronchospasm* Facial flushing, chest pressure, gastrointestinal upset, pain of head and neck region, dizziness, headache, dyspnea	Second- or third-degree AV block Do not use adenosine for atrial fibrillation or atrial flutter Bronchoconstrictive or bronchospastic lung disease Hypersensitivity to adenosine Sinus node disease	Opens G protein-coupled K^+ channel and suppresses Ca^{2+}-dependent action potential, thereby inhibiting SA nodal, atrial, and AV nodal conduction. Co-administration of carbamazepine may increase the degree of heart block. Transient arrhythmia may occur at the onset of adenosine infusion.
Ranolazine	Chronic angina pectoris	*Prolongs QT interval* Syncope, constipation, dizziness, headache	Concurrent use of drugs that prolong QT interval Preexisting long QT syndrome Concurrent use of moderately potent P450 3A inhibitors or inducers Hepatic dysfunction	Mechanism of action unclear—may inhibit fatty acid oxidation, delayed rectifier potassium current, or late sodium current. Frequently used in combination with β-blockers, amlodipine, or nitrates in patients who have not achieved adequate response with other anti-anginal agents. Avoid concurrent use of moderately potent P450 3A inhibitors or drugs that prolong QT interval. Avoid use in patients with severe renal impairment.
Ivabradine	Investigational (United States) Chronic stable angina (Europe)	Bradycardia	Preexisting bradycardia Sick sinus syndrome Unstable angina Third-degree AV block Cardiogenic shock Hypotension Myocardial infarction Pacemaker dependency Sinoatrial block Pregnancy Concomitant use with CYP3A4 inhibitors Heart failure Hypersensitivity to ivabradine Hepatic insufficiency	Inhibits the I_f channel, thereby slowing phase 4 depolarization. Also occasionally used to treat inappropriate sinus tachycardia. Avoid concurrent use of P450 3A inhibitors.

25

Pharmacology of Cardiac Contractility

Ehrin J. Armstrong

INTRODUCTION

In 1785, Dr. William Withering described the cardiovascular benefits of a preparation from the foxglove plant called *digitalis*. He used this preparation to treat patients suffering from "dropsy," a condition in which accumulation of extravascular fluid leads to dyspnea (difficulty breathing) and peripheral edema. These symptoms are now recognized as characteristic manifestations of **heart failure (HF)**, a clinical syndrome most commonly caused by systolic dysfunction of the left ventricle (LV). In this condition, the LV is unable to maintain adequate stroke volume despite normal filling volumes, and the LV end-diastolic volume increases in an effort to preserve stroke output. However, beyond a certain end-diastolic volume, LV diastolic pressures begin to increase, often precipitously. This increase in LV diastolic pressure results in increased left atrial and pulmonary capillary pressures, which, in turn, lead to interstitial and alveolar pulmonary edema and to increased right heart and pulmonary artery pressures. The elevated right heart pressures result in systemic venous hypertension and peripheral edema.

Dr. Withering's use of digitalis presaged the current use of **digoxin**, a member of the cardiac glycoside family of drugs, to treat conditions in which myocardial contractility is impaired. Cardiac glycosides are **positive inotropes**, defined as *agents that increase the contractile force of cardiac myocytes*. Since the advent of digitalis, elucidation of the cellular mechanism of cardiac contraction has facilitated the development of other inotropic agents. After reviewing the physiology of

cardiac contraction and the cellular pathophysiology of contractile dysfunction, this chapter describes four classes of positive inotropic drugs that are either approved for use or under investigation in clinical trials. An integrated discussion of therapeutic strategies for HF can be found in Chapter 26, Integrative Cardiovascular Pharmacology: Hypertension, Ischemic Heart Disease, and Heart Failure.

PHYSIOLOGY OF CARDIAC CONTRACTION

The heart is responsible for receiving deoxygenated blood from the periphery, propelling this blood through the pulmonary circulation (where the hemoglobin is reoxygenated), and ultimately distributing the oxygenated blood to peripheral tissues. To accomplish the latter task, the left ventricle (LV) must develop sufficient tension to overcome the impedance to ejection that resides in the peripheral circulation. The relationship between the tension generated during the systolic phase of the cardiac cycle and the extent of LV filling during diastole is referred to as the **contractile state** of the myocardium. Together with **preload** (intraventricular blood volume), **afterload** (the resistance against which the left ventricle ejects), and **heart rate**, myocardial contractility is a primary determinant of cardiac output. Cardiac pump performance at the organ level has been studied by cardiac physiologists for many years, but now the major cellular and molecular mechanisms of cardiac contraction are understood as well.

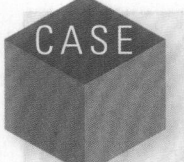

CASE

GW, a 68-year-old man with known systolic dysfunction and heart failure, is admitted to the hospital with shortness of breath and nausea. GW's cardiac history is notable for two prior myocardial infarctions, the more recent occurring about 2 years ago. Since the second infarction, he has had significant limitation of his exercise capacity. A two-dimensional echocardiogram is notable for an LV ejection fraction of 25% (normal, >55%) and moderate mitral valve regurgitation. GW has been treated with aspirin, carvedilol (a β-adrenergic receptor antagonist), captopril (an angiotensin converting enzyme inhibitor), digoxin (a cardiac glycoside), furosemide (a loop diuretic), and spironolactone (an aldosterone receptor antagonist). He has also had an automatic internal cardioverter-defibrillator (AICD) placed to prevent sustained ventricular arrhythmia and sudden cardiac death.

Physical examination in the emergency department is notable for a blood pressure of 90/50 mm Hg and an irregular heart rate of 120 beats/min. An electrocardiogram indicates that the underlying cardiac rhythm is atrial fibrillation. GW is started on amiodarone (a class III antiarrhythmic), and his heart rate decreases to approximately 80 beats/min. Laboratory tests are notable for serum Na^+ 148 mEq/L (normal, 135–145), BUN 56 mg/dL (normal, 7–19), K^+ 2.9 mEq/L (normal, 3.5–5.1), and creatinine

4.8 mg/dL (normal, 0.6–1.2). The serum digoxin level is 3.2 ng/mL (therapeutic concentration, typically ~1 ng/mL).

Based on these findings, GW is admitted to the cardiology intensive care unit (ICU). His oral digoxin dose is held, and he is given intravenous K^+ to increase his serum potassium concentration. Based on the severity of this clinical decompensation, a pulmonary artery (PA) catheter is placed to monitor cardiac pressures. GW is also started on dobutamine, and his carvedilol is held. After initiation of intravenous dobutamine, he has increased urine output and begins to feel symptomatically improved. He remains in the cardiology ICU for 7 days, and his digoxin level decreases to the therapeutic range.

Questions

1. What are the major cellular mechanisms that contribute to the pathophysiology of systolic heart failure?
2. What is the mechanism of action of digoxin?
3. What factors (including drug interactions) have contributed to digoxin toxicity in this patient?
4. Why is GW being treated with a β-adrenergic receptor antagonist and a positive inotrope (digoxin) at the same time?
5. What is the mechanism of action of dobutamine?

Myocyte Anatomy

Like skeletal muscle, cardiac muscle contracts when action potentials depolarize the plasma membranes of cardiac muscle cells. The process of **excitation–contraction (EC) coupling**, in which the intracellular machinery transduces an electrochemical signal into mechanical force, involves the following cascade of events: voltage-gated calcium channels open, intracellular calcium increases, contractile proteins are activated, and actin–myosin interactions shorten the contractile elements.

The cellular anatomy of ventricular myocytes is well suited to the excitation and regulation of cardiac contraction (Fig. 25-1). Specialized components of the ventricular myocyte include the sarcolemma, or myocyte plasma membrane; the sarcoplasmic reticulum (SR), a large internal membrane system that encircles the myofibrils; and the myofibrils themselves. Myofibrils are rope-like units containing precisely organized contractile proteins; the coordinated interaction of these proteins is responsible for the physical shortening of the cardiac muscle. These anatomic specializations are illustrated in Figures 25-1 and 25-2, and summarized in Table 25-1.

Myocyte Contraction

Increased cytosolic Ca^{2+} is the link between excitation and contraction. During the ventricular action potential (see Chapter 24, Pharmacology of Cardiac Rhythm), Ca^{2+} influx through L-type Ca^{2+} channels in the sarcolemma causes an

increase in the cytosolic Ca^{2+} concentration. This "trigger calcium" stimulates the ryanodine receptor in the SR membrane, causing release of stored Ca^{2+} from the SR into the cytosol. When the Ca^{2+} concentration in the cytoplasm reaches approximately 10^{-5} M, calcium binds to troponin C and induces a conformational change in tropomyosin that releases the inhibitory protein troponin I. This release of troponin I exposes an interaction site for myosin on the actin filament, and the binding of myosin to actin initiates the contraction cycle.

Figure 25-2 illustrates the cycle by which actin–myosin interactions physically shorten the sarcomere. Each myosin filament is studded with protruding flexible heads that form reversible cross-bridges with actin filaments. Formation of actin–myosin cross-bridges, bending of the myosin heads at their flexible hinges, and detachment of the cross-bridges together allow the myosin filament to "walk up" the actin filament in both directions and thereby to pull the two ends of the sarcomere together.

The normal function of the sarcomeric cross-bridge cycle is critically dependent on adenosine triphosphate (ATP). The ATP hydrolase (ATPase) activity of myosin provides the energy used both to drive contraction and to reset the contractile proteins, leading to relaxation. If an insufficient amount of ATP is available for cross-bridge cycling, myosin and actin remain "locked" in the associated state and the myocardium is unable to relax. This ATP dependence explains the profound impact of ischemia on both systolic

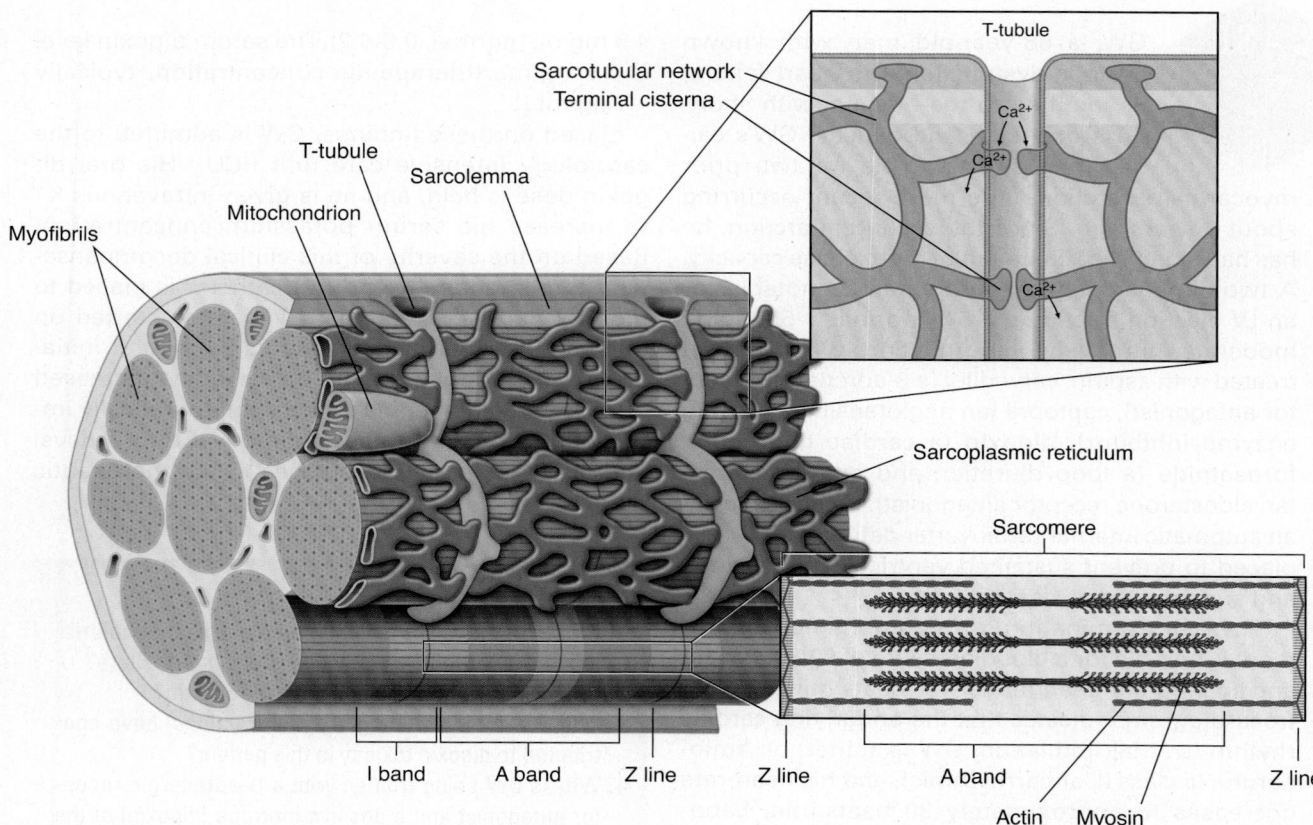

FIGURE 25-1. Cardiac myocyte structure. Each cardiac myocyte contains myofibrils and mitochondria surrounded by a specialized plasma membrane termed the *sarcolemma*. Invaginations of the sarcolemma, called *T-tubules*, provide conduits for Ca^{2+} influx. Within the cell, an extensive sarcoplasmic reticulum stores Ca^{2+} for use in contraction. Extracellular Ca^{2+} enters through the sarcolemma and its T-tubules during phase 2 of the action potential. This trigger Ca^{2+} binds to channels on the sarcoplasmic reticulum membrane, causing release into the cytosol of a large pool of so-called activation Ca^{2+}. Increased cytosolic Ca^{2+} initiates myofibril contraction. The *sarcomere* is the functional unit of the myofibril. Each sarcomere consists of interdigitating bands of actin and myosin. These bands form distinctive structures that can be visualized using an electron microscope. The *A* bands correspond to regions of overlapping actin and myosin. The *Z* lines demarcate the borders of each sarcomere. The *I* bands span neighboring sarcomeres and correspond to regions of actin without overlapping myosin. During cardiac myocyte contraction, the *I* bands become shorter (i.e., the *Z* lines move closer to one another), but the *A* bands maintain a constant length.

contraction (the contraction cycle cannot proceed) and diastolic relaxation (actin and myosin cannot dissociate) of the myocardium.

The organization of the sarcomere and the physical mechanism of contraction explain the fundamental relationship between muscle length and tension development. Increased stretch (length) of the muscle exposes additional sites for calcium binding and for actin–myosin interaction; increased stretch also effects greater release of calcium from the SR. These cellular events provide the mechanistic explanation for the **Frank-Starling law**: *an increase in the end-diastolic volume of the left ventricle leads to an increase in ventricular stroke volume during systole.* Chapter 26 describes the organ-level implications of the Frank-Starling law in more detail.

Regulation of Contractility

Three major control mechanisms regulate calcium cycling and myocardial contractility in cardiac myocytes. At the sarcolemma, calcium flux is mediated by interactions between the sodium pump and sodium–calcium exchanger. At the sarcoplasmic reticulum, calcium channels and pumps regulate the extent of calcium release and reuptake. Neurohumoral influences, especially the β-adrenergic signaling pathway,

further modulate calcium cycling through these channels and transporters.

The Sodium Pump and Sodium–Calcium Exchange
In the sarcolemma, three key proteins are involved in calcium regulation: the Na^+/K^+-ATPase, hereafter referred to as the **sodium pump**; the **sodium–calcium exchanger**; and the calcium–ATPase or **calcium pump** (Fig. 25-3). The activity of the sodium pump is crucial to maintain both the resting membrane potential and the concentration gradients of sodium and potassium across the sarcolemma ($[Na^+]_{out} = 145$ mM, $[Na^+]_{in} = 15$ mM, $[K^+]_{out} = 5$ mM, $[K^+]_{in} = 150$ mM). Sodium pump activity is closely linked to the intracellular calcium concentration via the sodium–calcium exchanger; this antiporter exchanges sodium and calcium in both directions across the sarcolemma. Changes in the concentration of either sodium or calcium ions inside or outside the cell affect the direction and magnitude of sodium–calcium exchange. Under normal conditions, the low intracellular sodium concentration favors sodium influx and calcium efflux. Some drugs take advantage of the functional coupling between the sodium pump and the sodium–calcium exchanger to exert their effect as positive inotropes. **Digoxin**, discussed in the

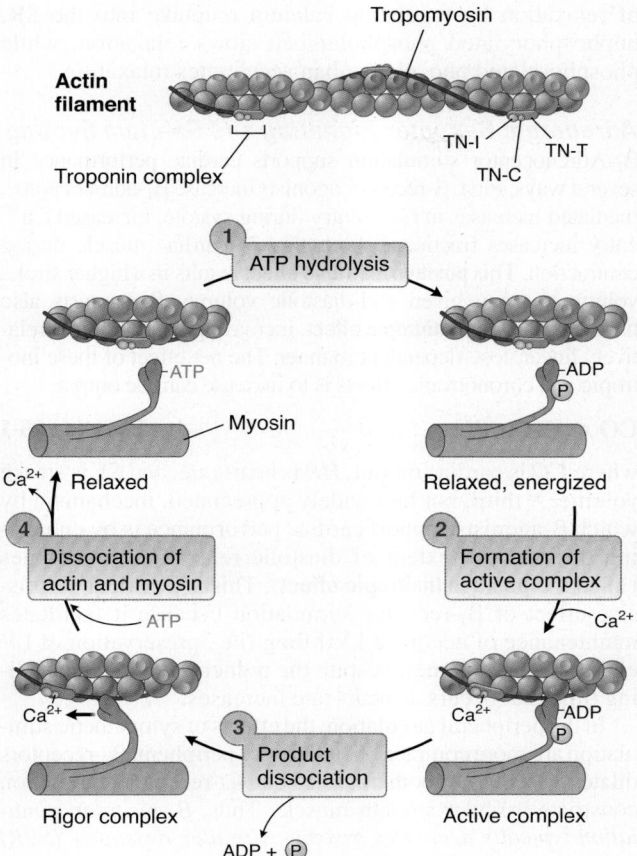

FIGURE 25-2. Cardiac contractile proteins and the contraction cycle. During contraction, myosin ratchets along actin filaments, resulting in an overall shortening of sarcomere length. Actin filaments **(top panel)** consist of two actin polymers wound around one another, three troponin proteins (TN-I, TN-C, and TN-T), and tropomyosin. In the absence of Ca^{2+}, tropomyosin is oriented on actin so that it inhibits the interaction of actin with myosin. The contraction cycle **(bottom panel)** occurs in a four-step process. **1.** Cardiac myocyte contraction begins with hydrolysis of ATP to ADP by myosin; this reaction energizes the myosin head. **2.** Ca^{2+} released from the sarcoplasmic reticulum binds to TN-C; this reaction causes a conformational change in tropomyosin that allows myosin to form an active complex with actin. **3.** Dissociation of ADP from myosin allows the myosin head to bend; this bending pulls the Z lines closer together and thus shortens the I band (*not shown*). This contracted state is often referred to as a *rigor complex* because muscle remains in the contracted state until there is sufficient ATP available to displace the myosin heads from actin. **4.** Binding of a new ATP molecule to myosin allows the actin–myosin complex to dissociate. Ca^{2+} also dissociates from TN-C, and the contraction cycle is repeated.

introductory case and described in detail below, is the prototype of an inotropic agent that acts by inhibiting the sodium pump. A sarcolemmal calcium pump also helps to maintain calcium homeostasis by actively extruding calcium from the cytoplasm after cardiac contraction. A high concentration of ATP favors calcium removal (relaxation), both directly via the calcium pump and indirectly via the sodium pump.

Calcium Storage and Release

As described above, Ca^{2+} signaling is central to both cardiac contraction and relaxation. As such, the cardiac myocyte has well-developed systems to regulate Ca^{2+} flux during the cardiac cycle. In the SR, the calcium release channel (**ryanodine**

receptor) and the calcium pump (**sarcoendoplasmic reticulum calcium ATPase, SERCA**) are critical to the regulation of contractility (Fig. 25-3). Proper contraction requires both that Ca^{2+} release into the cytoplasm is adequate to stimulate contraction and that Ca^{2+} reuptake into the SR is sufficient to permit relaxation and to replenish calcium stores. Cytoplasmic concentrations of both calcium and ATP regulate the activity of both the ryanodine receptor and SERCA.

As noted above, trigger calcium opens the ryanodine receptor. Cytoplasmic calcium concentration is directly related to the number of receptors that open. A safety mechanism also exists whereby high calcium levels lead to calcium–calmodulin complex formation: this complex inhibits calcium release by decreasing the open time of the ryanodine receptor. High concentrations of ATP favor the open channel conformation and thereby facilitate SR calcium release into the cytosol.

In addition to opening the ryanodine receptor, cytoplasmic calcium also stimulates SERCA, which pumps calcium back into the SR. This pump provides another control mechanism to prevent a positive feedback cycle that could irreversibly deplete the SR of calcium. As calcium pumps refill the SR, the rate of Ca^{2+} reuptake slows because of the declining cytoplasmic calcium concentration. ATP also favors SERCA activity; conversely, decreased ATP impairs calcium reuptake. The latter mechanism causes the rate and extent of diastolic relaxation to decrease in ischemic myocardium.

TABLE 25-1 Functional Anatomy of Cardiac Myocyte Contraction

Sarcolemma	
T-tubules	Invaginations of sarcolemma, facilitate ion flux across the cell membrane
Voltage-gated L-type Ca^{2+} channels	Mediate influx of trigger Ca^{2+} ions when sarcolemma is depolarized
Sarcoplasmic Reticulum (SR)	
Ca^{2+} release channels	Stimulated by trigger Ca^{2+}, release internal Ca^{2+} stores
Ca^{2+}-ATPase pumps	Sequester intracellular Ca^{2+} in SR to terminate contraction
Terminal cisternae	Sacs at distal branches of SR that store Ca^{2+}
Myofibril	
Sarcomere	Basic contractile unit of the myofibril
Myosin	Thick filament, hydrolyzes ATP for energy
Actin	Thin filament, provides scaffolding for myosin binding
Tropomyosin	Coils around actin, preventing actin–myosin binding at rest
Troponin complex:	Complex of three proteins that regulate actin–myosin binding:
Troponin T	Binds troponin complex to tropomyosin
Troponin I	Inhibits actin–myosin binding at rest
Troponin C	Binds Ca^{2+}, displacing troponin I from actin–myosin binding site

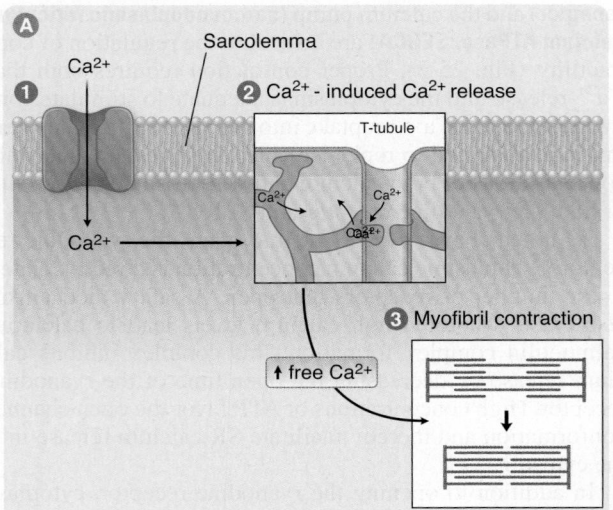

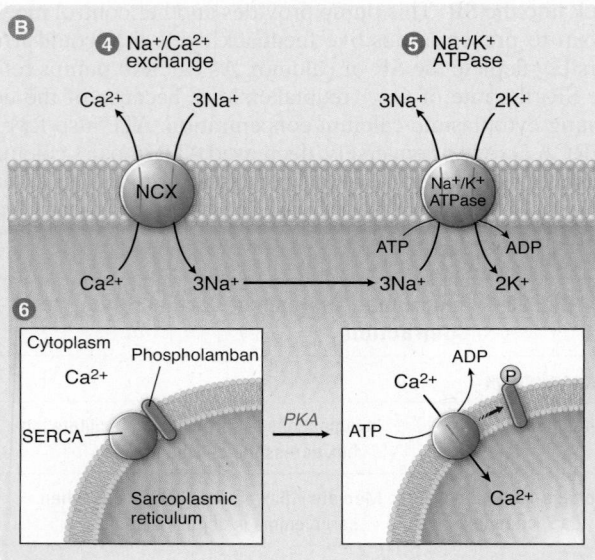

FIGURE 25-3. Regulation of cardiac myocyte Ca²⁺ flux. A. During contraction: **1.** Extracellular Ca²⁺ enters the cardiac myocyte through Ca²⁺ channels in the sarcolemma. **2.** This trigger Ca²⁺ induces release of Ca²⁺ from the sarcoplasmic reticulum into the cytosol (so-called Ca²⁺-induced Ca²⁺ release). **3.** The increased cytosolic Ca²⁺ facilitates myofibril contraction. **B.** During relaxation: **4.** The Na⁺/Ca²⁺ exchanger (NCX) extrudes Ca²⁺ from the cytosol, using the Na⁺ gradient as a driving force. **5.** The Na⁺/K⁺ ATPase (sodium pump) maintains the Na⁺ gradient, thus keeping the cardiac myocyte hyperpolarized. The sodium pump is tonically inhibited by phospholemman; phosphorylation of phospholemman by protein kinase A (PKA) disinhibits the pump, thereby increasing sodium extrusion and indirectly enhancing Na⁺/Ca²⁺ exchange (*not shown*). **6.** The sarcoendoplasmic reticulum Ca²⁺ ATPase (SERCA) in the sarcoplasmic reticulum membrane is tonically inhibited by phospholamban. Phosphorylation of phospholamban by PKA disinhibits the Ca²⁺ ATPase, allowing sequestration of cytosolic Ca²⁺ in the sarcoplasmic reticulum. A sarcolemmal Ca²⁺ ATPase (calcium pump) also helps to maintain calcium homeostasis by actively extruding calcium from the cytoplasm (*not shown*).

A third mediator of SERCA activity is **phospholamban**, an SR membrane protein that inhibits SERCA. High levels of intracellular **cAMP** stimulate **protein kinase A** to phosphorylate phospholamban, which reverses its inhibition of SERCA (Fig. 25-3). Phospholamban thus controls the rate

of relaxation by regulating calcium reuptake into the SR: unphosphorylated phospholamban slows relaxation, while phosphorylated phospholamban accelerates relaxation.

Adrenergic Receptor Signaling and Calcium Cycling

β₁-Adrenoceptor stimulation supports cardiac performance in several ways. First, β-receptor agonists increase β₁-adrenoceptor-mediated increases in Ca²⁺ entry during systole; increased Ca²⁺ entry increases fractional shortening of cardiac muscle during contraction. This **positive inotropic effect** results in a higher stroke volume for any given end-diastolic volume. β-Agonists also have a **positive chronotropic effect**, increasing heart rate in a relatively linear dose-dependent manner. The net effect of these inotropic and chronotropic effects is to increase cardiac output:

$$CO = HR \times SV \qquad \text{Equation 25-1}$$

where *CO* is cardiac output, *HR* is heart rate, and *SV* is stroke volume. A third, but less widely appreciated, mechanism by which β-agonists support cardiac performance is by enhancing the rate and extent of diastolic relaxation (sometimes called the **positive lusitropic effect**). This is a critical permissive effect of β₁-receptor stimulation because it facilitates maintenance of adequate LV filling (i.e., preservation of LV end-diastolic volume), despite the reduction in diastolic filling time that occurs as heart rate increases.

In the peripheral circulation, the effects of sympathetic stimulation are more complex. Activation of peripheral β₂-receptors dilates vascular smooth muscle, but α₁-receptor stimulation constricts vascular smooth muscle. Thus, *β₂-receptor stimulation typically decreases systemic vascular resistance (SVR) and afterload, while α₁-receptor stimulation increases SVR and afterload.* Dopamine receptors in the splanchnic and renal circulations also modulate the resistance vessels in these vascular beds, as discussed below.

As noted above, the cardiostimulatory actions of the sympathetic nervous system are mediated by activation of β₁-, β₂-, and α₁-adrenergic receptor subtypes located in the heart and peripheral vasculature. Stimulation of these **G protein-coupled receptors** induces conformational changes in the receptors and their associated G proteins that activate **adenylyl cyclase** and thereby elevate intracellular cAMP levels (Fig. 25-4). Higher levels of cAMP activate protein kinase A, which phosphorylates multiple targets in the cell. These targets include L-type calcium channels in the sarcolemma and phospholamban in the SR membrane. As discussed above, the phosphorylation of phospholamban releases its inhibition of SERCA, allowing calcium to be pumped from the cytosol back into the SR; this is one of the molecular mechanisms of enhanced diastolic relaxation induced by β₁-adrenoceptor stimulation.

Sensitivity of Contractile Proteins to Calcium

As mentioned above, the tension developed by cardiac myocytes during contraction is directly related to the precontraction length of the sarcomere units. Increased stretch of the sarcomeres exposes more calcium binding sites on troponin C, making more sites available for actin–myosin cross-bridge formation and thereby increasing the *sensitivity* of the contractile proteins to calcium. Several other mechanisms also regulate contractile protein sensitivity. Phosphorylation of troponin I by protein kinase A (a process that, like phospholamban phosphorylation, depends on cAMP levels) decreases contractile protein sensitivity to calcium. Expression of various isoforms of the contractile proteins, particularly troponin T, has also been linked to altered calcium sensitivity. Pharmacologic agents that sensitize contractile proteins to calcium are under investigation.

PATHOPHYSIOLOGY

Many disease processes can lead to myocyte dysfunction or death, causing replacement of myocardium with fibrous tissue and leading to impaired contractility. The most common etiology of contractile dysfunction in the United States is coronary artery disease (CAD) resulting in myocardial infarction; other common etiologies of contractile dysfunction include systemic hypertension and valvular heart disease. In each of the aforementioned disease states, dysfunction of the cardiac myocyte occurs as a consequence of a nonmyocardial disease process. A less common cause of LV dysfunction is idiopathic cardiomyopathy, in which the principal abnormality occurs at the level of the cardiac myocyte.

Irrespective of underlying etiology, progressive contractile dysfunction of the myocardium leads ultimately to the syndrome of **systolic heart failure (HF)**. It is important to note, however, that HF can occur in the absence of contractile dysfunction. For example, several common cardiovascular disease states—such as acute myocardial ischemia and restrictive cardiomyopathy—are associated with abnormalities of LV relaxation and/or filling, leading to decreased chamber compliance and elevated LV diastolic pressure. This abnormal elevation of intraventricular pressure can occur even in the presence of normal systolic function, leading to a syndrome referred to as **diastolic heart failure** (also known as *heart failure with preserved ejection fraction*). The organ-level pathology and treatment of HF are discussed in detail in Chapter 26. Here, we focus on the salient cellular and molecular aspects of normal and abnormal contractile function.

The clinical expression of HF often reflects the impact of neurohumoral systems that are activated by inadequate forward cardiac output. In advanced stages of the disease, it may be difficult to determine whether the cellular abnormalities observed in failing cardiac myocytes reflect primary cellular defects or secondary responses to extracardiac stimuli (such as circulating cytokines and neuroendocrine peptides). Nonetheless, the cellular and molecular alterations in the failing myocardium can be contrasted with the events of normal contraction in an effort to obtain mechanistic insight, and many of these changes are active areas of investigation. Study of these alterations also promises to identify potential new molecular targets for pharmacologic intervention.

Cellular Pathophysiology of Contractile Dysfunction

At the cellular level, pathophysiologic mechanisms associated with decreased cardiac contractility include dysregulation of calcium homeostasis, changes in the regulation and expression pattern of contractile proteins, and alterations in β-adrenoceptor signal transduction pathways (Fig. 25-5). As noted above, some of these alterations may result from local myocardial pathology, whereas others likely represent responses to circulating hormonal and inflammatory signals.

Altered calcium homeostasis in failing cardiac myocytes results in prolongation of the action potential and of the Ca^{2+} transient associated with each contraction. Mechanisms that increase the cytosolic concentration of Ca^{2+} and deplete

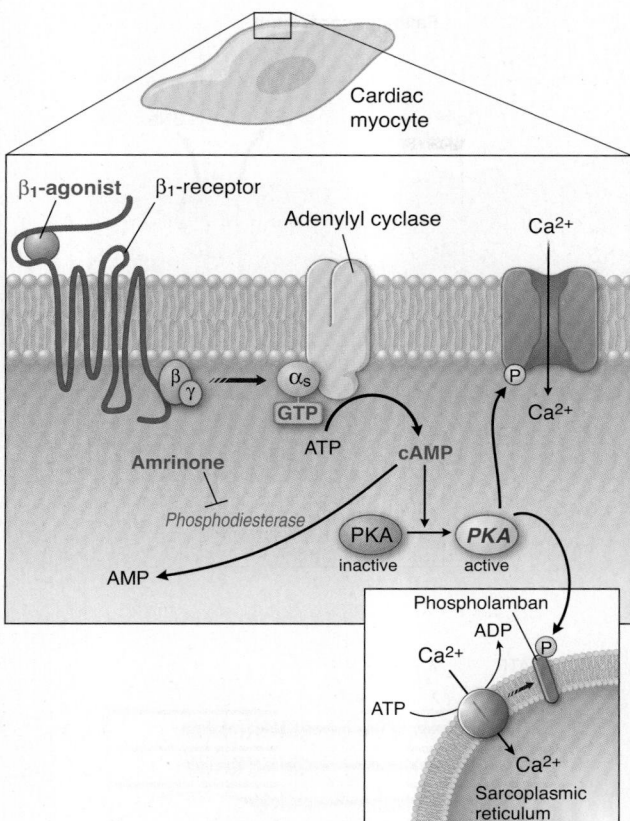

FIGURE 25-4. Regulation of cardiac contractility by β-adrenergic receptors. β-Adrenergic receptors both increase cardiac myocyte contractility and enhance relaxation. Binding of an endogenous or exogenous agonist to β1-adrenergic receptors on the surface of cardiac myocytes causes $G\alpha_s$ proteins to activate adenylyl cyclase, which in turn catalyzes the conversion of ATP to cAMP. cAMP activates multiple protein kinases, including protein kinase A (PKA). PKA phosphorylates and activates sarcolemmal Ca^{2+} channels and thereby increases cardiac myocyte contractility. PKA also phosphorylates phospholamban and thereby disinhibits the SERCA pump, which pumps Ca^{2+} into the sarcoplasmic reticulum; the increased rate of Ca^{2+} sequestration enhances cardiac myocyte relaxation. Finally, PKA phosphorylates phospholemman, thereby disinhibiting the sarcolemmal sodium pump and enhancing sarcolemmal Na^+/Ca^{2+} exchange (*not shown*). The conversion of cAMP to AMP by phosphodiesterase terminates β1-adrenergic receptor-mediated actions. Phosphodiesterase is inhibited by amrinone (also known as *inamrinone*), a drug that can be used in the treatment of heart failure.

TABLE 25-2 Effects of Increased Intracellular cAMP in Cardiac Cells

Sarcolemma	↑ Phosphorylation of voltage-gated Ca^{2+} channel → ↑ contractility, heart rate, and AV conduction ↑ Phosphorylation of phospholemman → ↑ Ca^{2+} efflux from cytoplasm via Na^+/Ca^{2+} exchange
Sarcoplasmic reticulum	↑ Phosphorylation of phospholamban → ↑ Ca^{2+} uptake and release
Contractile proteins	↑ Phosphorylation of troponin I → ↓ Ca^{2+} sensitivity
Energy production	↑ Glycogenolysis → ↑ ATP availability

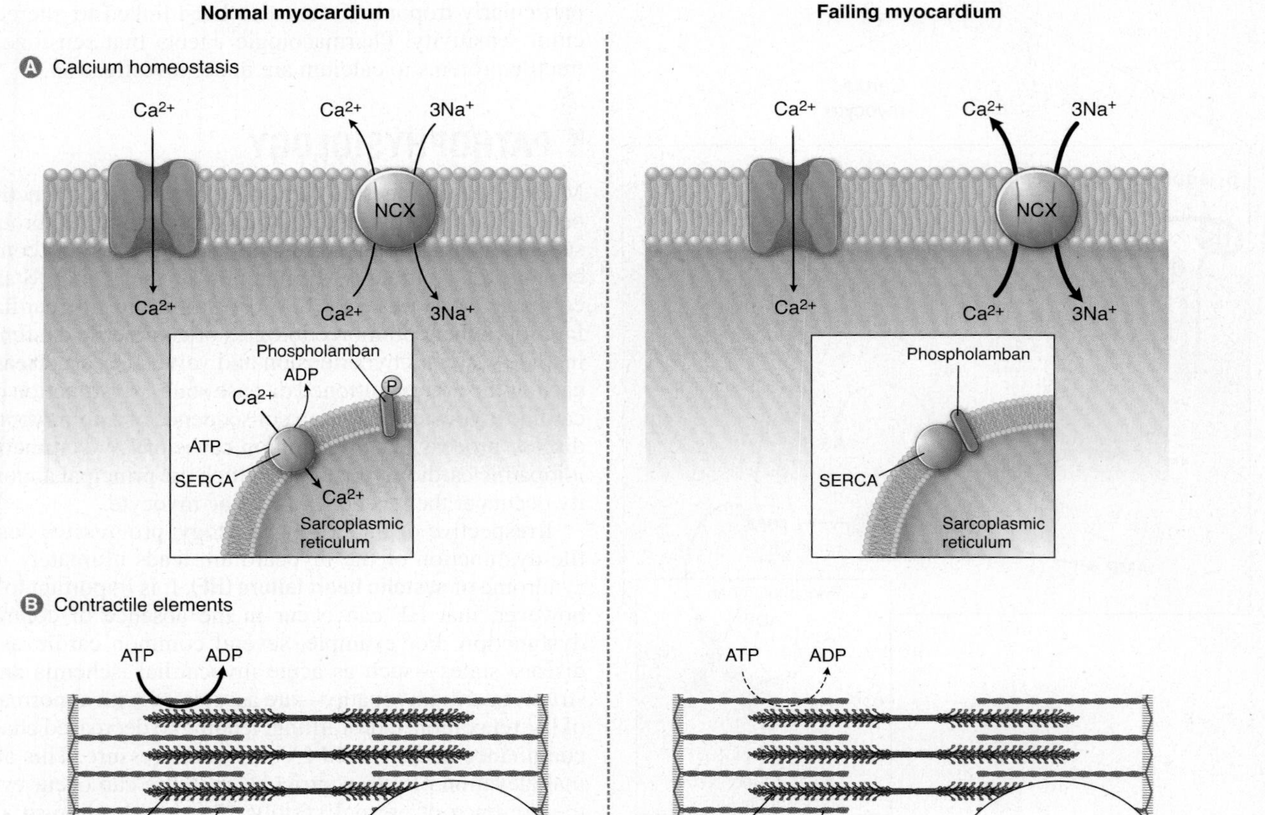

FIGURE 25-5. Cellular mechanisms of contractile pathophysiology. The failing myocardium exhibits derangements in Ca^{2+} homeostasis, the contractile elements, and the adenylyl cyclase signaling pathway. In each panel (*A*, *B*, and *C*), normal myocardium is shown on the *left* and failing myocardium on the *right*. **A.** In the normal myocardium, Ca^{2+} homeostasis is tightly controlled by Ca^{2+} pumps and channels, including the Na^+/Ca^{2+} exchanger (NCX) and the Ca^{2+} ATPase (SERCA). Operation of these pathways allows the myocardium to relax during diastole. In the failing myocardium, diastolic Ca^{2+} remains elevated because phospholamban is not phosphorylated and therefore tonically inhibits SERCA. Also, the expression of NCX increases (*thick arrows*), so that cytosolic Ca^{2+} is extruded from the cardiac myocyte rather than stored in the sarcoplasmic reticulum. **B.** In the normal myocardium, phosphorylation of troponin-I (TN-I) exposes the actin–myosin interaction site, and myosin effectively hydrolyzes ATP during each contraction cycle. In the failing myocardium, there is decreased phosphorylation of TN-I, resulting in less efficient actin–myosin cross-linking. Myosin does not hydrolyze ATP as efficiently (*dashed arrow*), further reducing the effectiveness of each contraction cycle. The failing myocardium also exhibits increased expression of the fetal isoform of TN-T; the significance of this alteration is uncertain. **C.** In the normal myocardium, β-agonists stimulate cAMP formation and subsequent activation of protein kinase A (PKA) (*arrows*). In the failing myocardium, β-arrestin binds to and inhibits the activity of β-adrenergic receptors (β-AR), leading to decreased stimulation of adenylyl cyclase (*dashed arrows*). Expression of the inhibitory Gα isoform $G\alpha_i$ is also induced in the failing myocardium (*not shown*).

SR Ca^{2+} stores include reduced SR Ca^{2+} reuptake and an increased number of sodium–calcium exchangers in the sarcolemma. As described above, efficient sequestration of calcium by the SR is essential for the termination of contraction. Thus, the inability of the myocyte to regulate intracellular calcium impairs both systolic contraction and diastolic relaxation.

Changes in the transcription of various genes in failing cardiac myocytes result in the synthesis of dysfunctional contractile proteins. The available data suggest that myocytes enter a maladaptive growth phase, reverting to production of the fetal isoforms of some proteins. For example, failing myocytes exhibit increased expression of the fetal isoform of troponin T, which is potentially a more efficient contractile protein. Other contractile protein alterations identified in heart failure include a reduction in phosphorylation of troponin I and diminished ATP hydrolysis by myosin; each of these changes results in a slower rate of cross-bridge cycling. In addition, activation of collagenase and matrix metalloproteinases may disrupt the stromal framework that maintains the structural and functional integrity of the myocardium.

Desensitization of the β-adrenergic receptor–G protein–adenylyl cyclase signaling pathway is the third major abnormal finding in cardiac myocytes of patients with systolic HF. Failing myocytes down-regulate the number of β-adrenergic receptors expressed at the cell surface, possibly as an adaptive response to the presence of increased neurohormonal stimulation. Sympathetic stimulation of the remaining receptors results in a smaller increase in cAMP than would occur in the presence of a normal number of receptors. The reduction in β-adrenergic signaling may also reflect increased expression of both **β-adrenergic receptor kinase** (which phosphorylates and thereby inhibits β-adrenoceptors) and the **inhibitory G protein ($G\alpha_i$)**. Another contributor to the reduction of β-adrenergic signaling may be **inducible nitric oxide synthase (iNOS)**, the expression of which is increased in HF. The diminished response of failing myocytes to adrenergic stimulation causes decreased phosphorylation of phospholamban, which impairs SR Ca^{2+} uptake capacity. Decreased cAMP levels also result in a decreased ability to produce and use ATP. Together, the impaired calcium regulation, altered contractile elements, and decreased cAMP levels in failing cardiac myocytes attenuate many of the steps of myocyte contraction and relaxation.

PHARMACOLOGIC CLASSES AND AGENTS

The central roles of intracellular calcium and cAMP in cardiac myocyte contraction provide a basis for the classification of inotropic agents. The **cardiac glycosides** elevate intracellular Ca^{2+} concentration via inhibition of the sarcolemmal Na^+/K^+-ATPase (sodium pump), while **β-agonists** and **phosphodiesterase inhibitors** increase intracellular levels of cAMP. **Calcium-sensitizing agents**, a class of drugs under active investigation, are also discussed briefly.

Cardiac Glycosides

The cardiac glycosides include the digitalis derivatives **digoxin** and **digitoxin** and nondigitalis agents such as **ouabain**. Glycosides are defined by a common chemical scaffold that includes a steroid nucleus, an unsaturated lactone ring, and one or more sugar residues. This common structural substrate underlies the common mechanism of action of these agents. In clinical practice, digoxin is both the most frequently used cardiac glycoside and the most widely used inotropic agent, although its overall use in the treatment of heart failure has declined in recent years.

Digoxin

Digoxin is a selective inhibitor of the plasma membrane sodium pump (Fig. 25-6). Cardiac myocytes exposed to digoxin extrude less sodium, leading to a rise in intracellular sodium concentration. In turn, the increase in intracellular sodium concentration alters the equilibrium of the sodium–calcium exchanger: calcium efflux is decreased because the gradient for sodium entry is decreased, while calcium influx is increased because the gradient for sodium efflux is increased. The net result is an increase in the intracellular calcium concentration. In response to this increase, the SR of the digoxin-treated cell sequesters more calcium. When the digoxin-treated cell depolarizes in response to an action potential, more Ca^{2+} is available to bind troponin C, and tension development during contraction is facilitated.

In addition to its effects on myocardial contractility, digoxin exerts autonomic effects through its binding to sodium pumps in the plasma membranes of neurons in the central and peripheral nervous systems. These effects include inhibition of sympathetic nervous outflow, sensitization of baroreceptors, and increased parasympathetic (vagal) tone. Digoxin also alters the electrophysiologic properties of the heart by a direct action on the cardiac conduction system. At therapeutic doses, digoxin decreases automaticity at the atrioventricular (AV) node, prolonging the effective refractory period

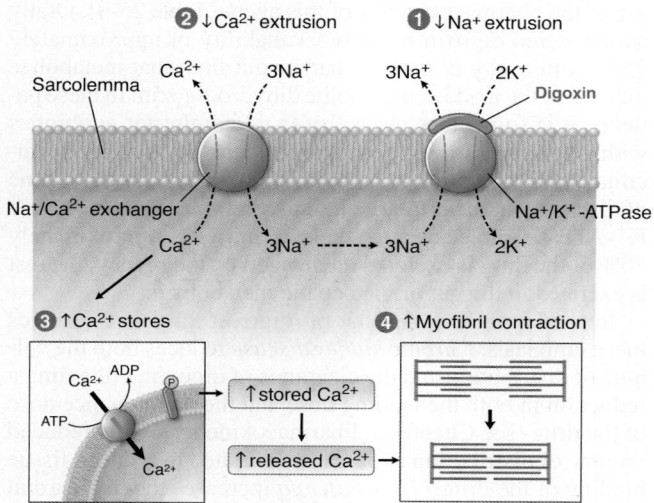

FIGURE 25-6. Positive inotropic mechanism of digoxin. 1. Digoxin selectively binds to and inhibits the Na^+/K^+-ATPase. Decreased Na^+ extrusion (*dashed arrows*) leads to an increased concentration of cytosolic Na^+. **2.** The increased intracellular Na^+ decreases the driving force for the Na^+/Ca^{2+} exchanger (*dashed arrows*), leading to decreased extrusion of Ca^{2+} from the cardiac myocyte into the extracellular space and to increased cytosolic Ca^{2+}. **3.** The increased cytosolic Ca^{2+} is pumped by the SERCA Ca^{2+}-ATPase into the sarcoplasmic reticulum (*thick arrow*), increasing the Ca^{2+} that is available for release from the SR during subsequent contractions. **4.** During each contraction, the increased Ca^{2+} released from the sarcoplasmic reticulum leads to increased myofibril contraction and therefore to increased cardiac inotropy.

TABLE 25-3 Pharmacokinetics of Digoxin

Oral bioavailability	~75%
Onset of action (intravenous)	~30 minutes
Peak effect (intravenous)	1–5 hours
Half-life	36 hours
Elimination	~70% renal excretion, proportional to glomerular filtration rate
Volume of distribution	Large (~640 L/70 kg): binds to skeletal muscle

of AV nodal tissue and slowing conduction velocity through the node. These combined vagotonic and electrophysiologic properties underlie the use of digoxin in the treatment of patients with atrial fibrillation and rapid ventricular response rates; both the decreased automaticity of AV nodal tissue and the decreased conduction velocity through the node increase the degree of AV block and thereby decrease the ventricular response rate.

In contrast to its effects at the AV node, digoxin enhances automaticity of the infranodal (His–Purkinje) conduction system. These divergent effects at the AV node and His–Purkinje system explain the characteristic electrophysiologic disturbance of complete heart block with accelerated junctional or accelerated idioventricular escape rhythm (referred to as *regularized* atrial fibrillation) in patients with atrial fibrillation and digoxin toxicity.

Digoxin has a *narrow therapeutic window*, and prevention of digoxin toxicity depends on a complete understanding of the pharmacokinetics of this agent (Table 25-3). Orally administered digoxin has a bioavailability of approximately 75%. A minority of patients harbor gut flora that metabolize digoxin to the inactive metabolite dihydrodigoxin. In these patients, it is sometimes necessary to co-administer antibiotics with digoxin in order to decontaminate the gut and thereby facilitate oral absorption of digoxin. Digoxin has a large volume of distribution; the primary binding reservoir consists of Na^+/K^+-ATPase molecules in skeletal muscle. Approximately 70% of the drug is excreted unchanged by the kidney; the rest is excreted in the gut or via hepatic metabolism.

Several specific aspects of digoxin pharmacokinetics merit emphasis. *Chronic kidney disease* reduces both the volume of distribution and the clearance of digoxin, obligating a reduction in both the loading dose and the maintenance dose of the drug (see Chapter 3, Pharmacokinetics). (The reduced volume of distribution appears to be related to reduced tissue binding of the drug.) *Hypokalemia* increases the myocardial localization of digoxin. Reductions in extracellular K^+ concentration appear to result in increased phosphorylation of the sodium pump and/or its regulator phospholemman, and digoxin may have a higher binding affinity for the phosphorylated forms of these proteins than for the dephosphorylated forms. (Note that increasing plasma K^+ concentration can help to relieve symptoms of digoxin toxicity by promoting dephosphorylation of these proteins.)

Digoxin also *interacts* with many drugs. These interactions can be divided into pharmacodynamic and pharmacokinetic interactions. Co-administration of digoxin with β-adrenergic

antagonists, Ca^{2+} channel blockers, or K^+-wasting diuretics can result in pharmacodynamic drug–drug interactions. β-Adrenergic antagonists decrease AV nodal conduction, and the combined use of β-antagonists and digoxin can increase the risk of developing high-grade AV block. Both β-antagonists and Ca^{2+} channel blockers can decrease cardiac contractility and potentially attenuate the inotropic effects of digoxin. K^+-wasting diuretics (e.g., furosemide) can decrease plasma potassium concentration, which can increase the affinity of digoxin for the Na^+/K^+-ATPase and thereby predispose to digoxin toxicity (see above).

Pharmacokinetic interactions can result from changes in the absorption, volume of distribution, or renal clearance of digoxin (Table 25-3). Many antibiotics, such as erythromycin, can increase digoxin absorption by killing the enteric bacteria that would ordinarily metabolize a fraction of orally administered digoxin before its absorption. Co-administration of digoxin with verapamil (a calcium channel blocker), quinidine (a class IA antiarrhythmic), or amiodarone (a class III antiarrhythmic) can increase digoxin levels because of the impact of these drugs on the volume of distribution and/or renal clearance of digoxin.

In the introductory case, multiple factors likely contributed to the marked increase in GW's serum digoxin level. The glomerular filtration rate (GFR) was reduced (indicated by the elevated creatinine), resulting in decreased digoxin clearance. Administration of a loop diuretic likely contributed to the reduction in GFR. This reduction of GFR could have been exacerbated by co-administration of an angiotensin converting enzyme inhibitor via interference with angiotensin II-mediated autoregulation of glomerular hydrostatic pressure. Together, these factors likely contributed to the elevated serum digoxin concentration (3.2 ng/mL). To put this value into perspective, toxic effects, such as ventricular ectopy, begin to appear at digoxin concentrations of 2–3 ng/mL.

Treatment of digoxin toxicity relies on normalizing plasma K^+ levels and minimizing the potential for ventricular arrhythmias. In addition, life-threatening digoxin toxicity can be treated with **antidigoxin antibodies**. These polyclonal antibodies form 1:1 complexes with digoxin that are rapidly cleared from the body. Fab fragments of these antibodies (i.e., the portion of the antibody that interacts with antigen) have been shown to be less immunogenic than antidigoxin IgG and to have a larger volume of distribution, more rapid onset of action, and higher clearance than the intact IgG.

It may seem counterintuitive to co-administer digoxin (a positive inotrope) with the β-antagonist carvedilol (a negative inotrope). However, both agents have been shown to provide benefit in patients with HF. β-Antagonists reduce mortality by 30% or more in patients with HF. It is postulated that β-receptor antagonists counteract the cardiotoxic effects of the chronic sympathetic stimulation that can occur in patients with contractile dysfunction. β-Antagonists have been shown to effect changes in cellular morphology and chamber remodeling. The mechanism underlying the benefit of digoxin in HF is not fully understood; it is thought to be related to both digoxin's positive effect on contractile function and its neurohumoral effects. This issue is discussed in greater detail in Chapter 26.

Several large randomized trials provide a consistent picture of the clinical efficacy and limitations of digoxin. These trials indicate that withdrawal of digoxin in patients with HF leads to a decline in clinical status compared to patients who continue digoxin therapy. For example, withdrawal of digoxin is associated with deterioration in exercise capacity and increased frequency of hospitalization for worsening heart failure. However, the use of digoxin in patients with heart failure does not have a significant impact on survival. In short, while digoxin has not been shown to improve survival, it does palliate symptoms, improve functional status, and reduce hospitalization rates. These clinical benefits can provide significant improvement in quality of life for patients with HF; in all such patients, the circulating levels of digoxin should be monitored closely.

Digoxin is also used to control ventricular rate in patients with long-standing atrial fibrillation. The combined bradycardic and inotropic effects of digoxin make it an especially useful agent for patients with both HF and atrial fibrillation.

Digitoxin

Digitoxin is a less frequently used digitalis preparation that may be preferable to digoxin in selected clinical circumstances. Digitoxin is structurally identical to digoxin except for the presence (digoxin) or absence (digitoxin) of a hydroxyl group at position 12 of the steroid nucleus. This structural modification renders digitoxin less hydrophilic than digoxin and significantly alters the pharmacokinetics of the drug—in particular, digitoxin is metabolized and excreted primarily by the liver. The fact that its clearance does not depend on renal excretion makes digitoxin a suitable alternative to digoxin for the treatment of patients with HF and chronic kidney disease. Dosing regimens need to account for the very long half-life of digitoxin (approximately 7 days) compared to digoxin (approximately 36 hours).

β-Adrenergic Receptor Agonists

β-Adrenoceptor agonists are a heterogeneous group of drugs that have differential specificity for adrenergic receptor subtypes. Inhaled formulations of these medications are also used frequently in the treatment of asthma, as discussed in Chapter 48, Integrative Inflammation Pharmacology: Asthma. For all these agents, it merits emphasis that *the differential activation of receptor subtypes is influenced both by the agent selected and by the dose at which that agent is administered*. For example, dopamine administered at low infusion rates (2–5 μg/kg/min) has an overall cardiostimulatory effect (caused by increased contractility and decreased systemic vascular resistance), while the same drug infused at higher rates (>10 μg/kg/min) has an overall impact that is largely related to α$_1$-receptor activation.

Thus, the pharmacodynamic effects of the agent (Table 25-4) must be considered in the context of the patient's overall hemodynamic profile; this often requires placement of hemodynamic monitoring catheters to quantify intracardiac filling pressures, systemic vascular resistance (SVR), and cardiac output. For this reason, in the introductory case, GW's physicians placed a PA catheter before starting the dobutamine infusion.

The clinical use of sympathomimetic inotropes is generally reserved for short-term support of the failing circulation. This is attributable to the adverse effect profile of these agents and to their pharmacodynamic and pharmacokinetic properties. In general, sympathomimetic agents that stimulate myocardial β-adrenergic receptors share the adverse effect profile of tachycardia, arrhythmia, and increased myocardial oxygen consumption. These agents also induce tolerance via rapid down-regulation and desensitization of adrenergic receptors. In addition, the sympathomimetic amines have low oral bioavailability and must typically be administered by continuous intravenous infusion.

Dopamine

Dopamine (**DA**) is an endogenous sympathomimetic amine that functions as a neurotransmitter; it is also a biosynthetic precursor of norepinephrine and epinephrine (see Chapter 11, Adrenergic Pharmacology). At low doses, dopamine has a vasodilatory effect in the periphery by stimulating dopaminergic D1 receptors in the renal and mesenteric vascular beds. This regional vascular dilation reduces the impedance to left ventricular ejection (afterload). At intermediate doses, DA causes vasodilation via stimulation of β$_2$-adrenergic receptors; at these doses, DA also activates β$_1$-receptors, thereby increasing contractility and heart rate. At higher doses, activation of α$_1$-receptors predominates in the periphery, leading to generalized vasoconstriction and increased afterload.

Dopamine must be administered intravenously in a closely monitored setting. It is metabolized rapidly by monoamine oxidase (MAO) and dopamine β-hydroxylase to inactive metabolites that are excreted by the kidney. Patients receiving dopamine and MAO inhibitors concomitantly have decreased metabolism of dopamine; in these patients, dopamine can cause significant tachycardia, arrhythmia, and increased myocardial oxygen consumption.

Despite its complex pharmacology, DA finds wide clinical application in patients with sepsis and anaphylaxis, syndromes in which peripheral vasodilation is a major contributor to circulatory failure. At low and intermediate doses, DA is

TABLE 25-4 Receptor Selectivity of Sympathomimetics

AGENT	RECEPTOR TYPE				
	α$_1$	α$_2$	β$_1$	β$_2$	D1
	VASOCONSTRICTS PERIPHERAL VESSELS	PRESYNAPTIC INHIBITION AT NE SYNAPSE	INCREASES HEART RATE, CONTRACTILITY, DIASTOLIC RELAXATION	VASODILATES PERIPHERAL VESSELS	LOW DOSES VASODILATE RENAL VESSELS
Dopamine	+		++	+	++
Dobutamine	+/−		++	+	
Epinephrine	++	++	++	++	
Norepinephrine	++	++	++		

used occasionally in patients with cardiogenic shock or HF. However, its use in cardiogenic circulatory failure has largely been supplanted by alternative agents (such as dobutamine and the phosphodiesterase inhibitors) that have a more predictable vasodilator effect in the periphery and/or are less likely to induce tachycardia and ventricular arrhythmia.

Dobutamine

Dobutamine is a synthetic sympathomimetic amine that was developed in an attempt to optimize the overall hemodynamic benefits of β-adrenergic receptor activation for patients with acute cardiogenic circulatory failure. Overall, dobutamine approximates the desirable hemodynamic profile of a "pure" β₁ agonist. However, this profile is *not* the result of selective activation of β₁-receptors but rather derives from the fact that the clinically available formulation is a racemic mixture of enantiomers that have differential effects on adrenergic receptor subtypes. Both the (+) and (−) enantiomers stimulate β₁-receptors and, to a lesser degree, β₂-receptors, but the (+) enantiomer acts as an α₁ antagonist, whereas the (−) enantiomer is an α₁ agonist. Because the clinical formulation includes both enantiomers, the opposing hemodynamic responses produced by these enantiomers at the α₁-receptor effectively negate one another. The predominant overall effect is that of an agonist at cardiac β₁-receptors, with modest peripheral vasodilation mediated by agonist action at peripheral β₂-receptors.

Dobutamine is administered by continuous intravenous infusion and titrated to achieve the desired clinical effect. Catechol-O-methyl transferase rapidly metabolizes dobutamine, so that the circulating half-life is only about 2.5 minutes. As with all sympathomimetic amines with β-agonist effects, dobutamine has the potential to induce cardiac arrhythmias. In clinical practice, supraventricular tachycardia and high-grade ventricular arrhythmia occur less frequently with dobutamine than with dopamine. On the basis of this constellation of clinical effects, dobutamine has become the sympathomimetic inotrope of choice for patients with acute cardiogenic circulatory failure.

Epinephrine

Epinephrine (**Epi**) is a nonselective adrenergic agonist that is endogenously released by the adrenal glands to support the circulation. Exogenously administered Epi stimulates β₁-, β₂-, α₁-, and α₂-receptors; the net effect depends on the dose. At all dose levels, Epi is a potent β₁ agonist with positive inotropic, chronotropic, and lusitropic effects. Low-dose Epi predominantly stimulates peripheral β₂-receptors, causing vasodilation. At higher Epi doses, however, stimulation of α₁-receptors causes vasoconstriction and increased afterload. These effects make high-dose Epi a suboptimal agent for patients with HF.

As with other adrenergic agonists, epinephrine is primarily administered intravenously, although it can also be administered as an inhaled agent (for treatment of asthma) or subcutaneously (for treatment of anaphylaxis). Epinephrine is rapidly metabolized to metabolites that are excreted by the kidney. At high doses, epinephrine can cause tachycardia and life-threatening ventricular arrhythmias.

The primary clinical application of Epi is in the setting of resuscitation from cardiac arrest, a situation in which rapid restoration of spontaneous circulatory function is the immediate treatment goal. In this clinical setting, the potent inotropic

and chronotropic effects of Epi supersede concerns related to its adverse peripheral vasomotor effects. Noncardiovascular indications for Epi include relief of bronchospasm (via β₂-mediated bronchial relaxation), potentiation of the effect of local anesthetics (via local α₁-mediated vasoconstriction), and treatment of allergic hypersensitivity reactions.

Norepinephrine

Norepinephrine (**NE**) is the endogenous neurotransmitter released at sympathetic nerve terminals. NE is a potent β₁-receptor agonist, and therefore, it supports both systolic and diastolic cardiac performance. NE is also a potent α₁-receptor agonist in the peripheral vessels, and thus, it increases systemic vascular resistance. During exercise, the release of NE increases heart rate and contractility, enhances diastolic relaxation, and, via its α₁ agonist-mediated vasoconstriction, supports redistribution of the cardiac output away from noncritical vascular beds.

Intravenous NE is rapidly metabolized by the liver to inactive metabolites. At therapeutic doses, NE may precipitate tachycardia, arrhythmia, and increased myocardial oxygen consumption. When administered to patients with contractile dysfunction, NE has a tendency to cause tachycardias involving both the sinoatrial (SA) node and ectopic sites in the atria and ventricles. Furthermore, the peripheral vasoconstriction induced by NE increases afterload and thereby limits the inotropic benefit of this agent. The increase in afterload occurs most frequently in patients who have already recruited compensatory vasoconstrictive responses via sympathoadrenal and renin-angiotensin-aldosterone system activation. NE is, however, frequently used for acute hemodynamic support in patients with distributive shock (e.g., Gram-negative bacterial sepsis) in the absence of underlying heart disease.

Isoproterenol

Isoproterenol is a synthetic β-adrenergic agonist with relative selectivity for β₁-receptors. The hemodynamic effects of isoproterenol are dominated by a significant chronotropic response. The β₂ effects of isoproterenol can cause peripheral vasodilation and hypotension. Isoproterenol should not be administered to patients with active coronary artery disease, as it can worsen ischemia. Isoproterenol is used infrequently, but it may be indicated in patients with refractory bradycardia not responsive to atropine. It may also be administered in the treatment of β-antagonist overdose.

Phosphodiesterase (PDE) Inhibitors

Like β-adrenergic receptor agonists, phosphodiesterase (PDE) inhibitors increase cardiac contractility by raising intracellular cAMP levels (Fig. 25-4). PDE inhibitors inhibit the enzyme that hydrolyzes cAMP, thereby increasing intracellular cAMP and indirectly increasing intracellular calcium concentration. There are multiple isoforms of PDE, each of which is linked to a distinct signal transduction pathway. Nonspecific PDE inhibitors, such as **theophylline**, have been studied since the 1960s. Theophylline was initially used to treat asthma (see Chapter 48) but was later observed to have possible inotropic benefits.

Although cardiac muscle expresses multiple PDE isoenzymes, selective inhibition of PDE3 has been shown to have beneficial cardiovascular effects. The relatively selective PDE3 inhibitors **inamrinone** (also known as *amrinone*) and **milrinone** increase contractility and enhance the rate and extent of diastolic relaxation. PDE3 inhibitors also have important vasoactive effects in the peripheral circulation. These peripheral actions occur through cAMP-mediated effects on intracellular calcium handling in vascular smooth muscle and result in decreased arterial and venous tone. In the systemic arterial circulation, vasodilation leads to a decrease in systemic vascular resistance (decreased afterload); in the systemic venous circulation, an increase in venous capacitance results in a decrease in venous return to the heart (decreased preload). The combination of positive inotropy and mixed arterial and venous dilation has led to the designation of PDE inhibitors as "ino-dilators."

Similar to β-agonists, PDE inhibitors have found clinical utility in short-term support of the severely failing circulation. Widespread application of inamrinone has been limited by the adverse effect of clinically significant thrombocytopenia in about 10% of patients. Both intravenous and oral formulations of PDE3 inhibitors have been developed. Unfortunately, long-term use of these agents has been limited by data demonstrating increased mortality.

Calcium-Sensitizing Agents

Calcium-sensitizing drugs, such as **levosimendan**, are a novel class of positive inotropes that are under investigation as possible therapeutic agents. Calcium sensitizers, which have the same "ino-dilator" actions as PDE inhibitors, augment myocardial contractility by enhancing the sensitivity of troponin C to calcium. This potentiating effect increases the extent of actin–myosin interactions at any given concentration of intracellular calcium, without a substantial increase in myocardial oxygen consumption. In the peripheral circulation, levosimendan activates ATP-sensitive K^+ channels, leading to peripheral vasodilation. Preliminary clinical trial data suggest that levosimendan improves cardiac hemodynamics in severe systolic HF and may reduce short-term mortality. Levosimendan is available in some European countries but is not currently approved for use in the United States.

▌ CONCLUSION AND FUTURE DIRECTIONS

Knowledge of the cellular and molecular bases for myocardial contraction has provided several pharmacologic strategies designed to increase myocardial contractility in patients with heart failure attributable to left ventricular systolic dysfunction. By inhibiting the sodium pump, *digoxin* raises intracellular calcium levels and thereby increases contractile force. This drug is the only oral inotropic agent in wide clinical use today. Although digoxin has no demonstrable impact on the mortality of patients with heart failure, it helps alleviate symptoms and improves functional capacity. Digoxin also slows AV nodal conduction, an effect that is useful in treating patients with atrial fibrillation and rapid ventricular response rates. The *β-adrenergic receptor agonists*—including the endogenous amines *dopamine*, *norepinephrine*, and *epinephrine* and the synthetic agents *dobutamine* and *isoproterenol*—act through G protein-mediated elevation of intracellular cAMP to enhance both myocardial contractility and diastolic relaxation. The latter effect allows the left ventricle to fill adequately during diastole, despite the increase in heart rate that is stimulated by these agents. β-Agonists are administered intravenously, and they provide short-term hemodynamic support to patients with cardiogenic circulatory failure. The longer term utility of these agents has been limited both by the lack of an oral formulation with acceptable bioavailability and by the adverse effect profile of these drugs. *PDE inhibitors*, including *inamrinone* and *milrinone*, act as positive inotropes and as mixed arterial and venous dilators by increasing the levels of cyclic AMP in the heart and vascular smooth muscle. The increased mortality associated with longer term use of these agents has similarly restricted their role to the short-term management of severe HF.

New classes of pharmacologic agents are under investigation for their ability to augment myocardial contractility. These agents are directed at a variety of biochemical targets, including the efficiency of actin–myosin interactions (e.g., **cardiac myosin activators**) and the synthesis of contractile proteins (e.g., **cardiac neuregulins**). These approaches may improve cardiac contractility without increasing myocardial oxygen demand or significantly altering calcium signaling. Alternative strategies attempt to preserve myocardial contractility by inhibiting the effects of proinflammatory cytokines associated with HF, but recent trials of these agents, such as endothelin receptor antagonists, have met with limited success. Finally, **gene therapy** methods are being investigated to increase contractility, including the delivery of genes with cardiac-specific promoters that alter the production of contractile proteins, pumps, channels, and regulators in the heart. At the present time, the most promising candidates for gene therapy include the SR calcium pump, phospholamban, and cardiac troponin I.

Acknowledgment

We thank Thomas P. Rocco for his valuable contributions to this chapter in the First, Second, and Third Editions of *Principles of Pharmacology: The Pathophysiologic Basis of Drug Therapy.*

Suggested Reading

Aronson D, Krum H. Novel therapies in acute and chronic heart failure. *Pharmacol Ther* 2013;135:1–17. (*Pathophysiology of acute and chronic heart failure, with a focus on emerging treatment strategies.*)

Endoh M. Cardiac calcium signaling and calcium sensitizers. *Circ J* 2008;72:1915–1925. (*Physiology of excitation–contraction coupling and pharmacology of investigational agents for treatment of heart failure.*)

Gheorghiade M, Adams KF, Colucci WS. Digoxin in the management of cardiovascular disorders. *Circulation* 2004;109:2959–2964. (*Reviews the clinical pharmacology of digoxin.*)

Hasenfuss G, Teerlink JR. Cardiac inotropes: current agents and future directions. *Eur Heart J* 2011;32:1838–1845. (*Excellent review of contractile physiology and inotrope pharmacology.*)

Teerlink JR. A novel approach to improve cardiac performance: cardiac myosin activators. *Heart Fail Rev* 2009;14:289–298. (*One of the possible future approaches to treatment of acute heart failure.*)

DRUG SUMMARY TABLE: CHAPTER 25 Pharmacology of Cardiac Contractility

DRUG	CLINICAL APPLICATIONS	SERIOUS AND COMMON ADVERSE EFFECTS	CONTRAINDICATIONS	THERAPEUTIC CONSIDERATIONS
CARDIAC GLYCOSIDES				
Mechanism—(1) In myocardium, inhibit plasma membrane Na^+/K^+-ATPase, leading to increased cytoplasmic Ca^{2+} concentration, which results in positive inotropy; (2) in autonomic nervous system, inhibit sympathetic outflow and increase parasympathetic (vagal) tone; (3) at AV node, prolong effective refractory period and slow conduction velocity. Digoxin immune Fab is an antibody fragment that binds to and neutralizes digoxin.				
Digoxin **Digitoxin**	Systolic heart failure Supraventricular arrhythmias including atrial fibrillation, atrial flutter, and paroxysmal atrial tachycardia	*Arrhythmias (especially conduction disturbances with or without AV block, premature ventricular contractions [PVCs], and supraventricular tachycardias)* Agitation, fatigue, muscle weakness, blurred vision, yellow-green halo around visual images, anorexia, nausea, vomiting	Hypersensitivity to drug Ventricular fibrillation	Digoxin has many significant drug interactions. Co-administration with β-blockers increases the risk of developing high-grade AV block. β-Blockers and calcium channel blockers counteract positive inotropic effects of digoxin. Potassium-wasting diuretics and hypokalemia predispose to digoxin toxicity. Some antibiotics, such as erythromycin, increase digoxin absorption. Co-administration with verapamil, quinidine, or amiodarone can increase digoxin levels. Treat digoxin toxicity by normalizing plasma potassium level or, in severe cases, using digoxin antibodies. Chronic kidney disease requires reduction in loading dose and maintenance dose of digoxin. Digoxin has not been shown to improve survival; it palliates symptoms and improves functional status. Digitoxin undergoes hepatic metabolism and biliary excretion.
Digoxin Immune Fab	Potentially life-threatening digitalis toxicity Acute digoxin toxicity in which ingested amount or serum digoxin level is unknown	*Heart failure, anaphylaxis*	No known contraindications Use with caution in patients allergic to ovine proteins	Keep resuscitation equipment available during administration of digoxin immune Fab.
β-ADRENERGIC AGONISTS				
Mechanism—Increase cAMP by activating G protein-coupled adrenergic receptors; acting at cardiac β₁-adrenergic receptors, agonists have positive inotropic, chronotropic, and lusitropic effects				
Dopamine	In distributive or cardiogenic shock, used as adjunct to increase cardiac output, blood pressure, and urine flow Short-term treatment of severe, refractory, chronic heart failure	*Widening of QRS complex, cardiac arrhythmias, gangrenous disorder* Angina, hypertension, injection site reaction, nausea, vomiting, headache, mydriasis, anxiety, oliguria, dyspnea	Hypersensitivity to dopamine Pheochromocytoma Uncorrected tachyarrhythmia Ventricular fibrillation	Low doses cause vasodilation in the periphery via stimulation of dopaminergic D1 receptors in renal and mesenteric vascular beds. Intermediate doses cause vasodilation via stimulation of β₂-receptors and increased contractility and heart rate via activation of β₁-receptors. High doses cause generalized vasoconstriction via stimulation of α₁-receptors. Co-administration with MAO inhibitors results in decreased metabolism of dopamine, which can lead to significant tachycardia and arrhythmia.

Drug	Indications	Adverse Effects	Contraindications	Comments
Dobutamine	Short-term treatment of cardiac decompensation secondary to depressed contractility (cardiogenic shock)	*Cardiac arrhythmias* Syncope, dyspnea, angina, hypertension, headache	Hypersensitivity to dobutamine Idiopathic hypertrophic subaortic stenosis	A racemic mixture of enantiomers that have differential effects on adrenergic receptor subtypes; overall effect is predominantly β_1, and modest β_2. Sympathomimetic inotrope of choice for patients with acute cardiogenic circulatory failure Dobutamine induces less supraventricular tachycardia and high-grade ventricular arrhythmia than dopamine.
Epinephrine	Bronchospasm Hypersensitivity reaction, anaphylactic shock Cardiac resuscitation Hemostasis (topical use) Prolong local anesthetic effect (local use) Open-angle glaucoma Inhibit uterine contractions	*Arrhythmias including ventricular fibrillation, cerebral hemorrhage, severe hypertension, pulmonary edema* Angina, sweating, nausea, vomiting, asthenia, dizziness, headache, nervousness, tremor, palpitations, dyspnea	Hypersensitivity to epinephrine Active labor Angle-closure glaucoma Shock (other than anaphylaxis) Organic brain damage Cardiac arrhythmias Coronary insufficiency Severe hypertension Cerebral atherosclerosis Concurrent use with halogenated hydrocarbon anesthetics Concurrent use with local anesthetics for injection into fingers, toes, or ears due to increased risk of vasoconstriction Concomitant MAOI use within 2 weeks	Nonselective agonist at β_1-, β_2-, α_1-, and α_2-receptors. High doses can cause tachycardia and life-threatening ventricular arrhythmias.
Norepinephrine	Blood pressure support in acute hypotensive states (shock)	*Cardiac arrhythmias* Hypertension, nausea, vomiting, confusion, headache, tremor, anxiety, restlessness, urinary retention	Hypotension from loss of blood volume	Nonselective agonist at β_1-, α_1-, and α_2-receptors. May cause tachycardias involving the SA node or ectopic atrial or ventricular sites in patients with contractile dysfunction. Avoid co-administration with MAO inhibitors or amitriptyline or imipramine-type antidepressants due to risk of severe hypertension.
Isoproterenol	Emergency treatment of arrhythmias (IV) Atropine-resistant hemodynamically significant bradycardia (IV) Heart block and shock (IV) Bronchospasm (inhalation)	*Cardiac arrhythmias* Syncope, confusion, headache, tremor	Hypersensitivity to isoproterenol Tachyarrhythmia Angina pectoris	Nonselective β-agonist at β_1- and β_2-receptors. Isoproterenol may be useful in treating patients with refractory bradycardia not responsive to atropine and in treating patients with β-antagonist overdose. Do not administer to patients with active coronary artery disease.

continues

DRUG SUMMARY TABLE: CHAPTER 25 Pharmacology of Cardiac Contractility *continued*

DRUG	CLINICAL APPLICATIONS	SERIOUS AND COMMON ADVERSE EFFECTS	CONTRAINDICATIONS	THERAPEUTIC CONSIDERATIONS
PHOSPHODIESTERASE (PDE) INHIBITORS Mechanism—Increase cAMP by inhibiting the PDE enzymes that hydrolyze it; in cardiac myocytes, PDE inhibitors have positive inotropic and lusitropic effects; PDE inhibitors also relax vascular smooth muscle and thereby decrease preload (venodilation) and afterload (arteriodilation)				
Theophylline	See Drug Summary Table: Chapter 48 Integrative Inflammation Pharmacology: Asthma			
Inamrinone Milrinone Vesnarinone	Short-term treatment of severely failing circulation in patients refractory to conventional therapy	*Ventricular arrhythmias, thrombocytopenia (greater incidence with inamrinone than with milrinone) (shared adverse effects); atrial fibrillation, abnormal liver function tests (milrinone only); reversible neutropenia and agranulocytosis (vesnarinone only)*	Hypersensitivity to drug (shared contraindication) Stenotic valvular heart disease (vesnarinone only)	Co-administration with disopyramide may cause severe hypotension. Use of inamrinone is limited by 10% occurrence of thrombocytopenia. Oral formulation of milrinone is available; milrinone use is associated with statistically significant increase in mortality in patients with HF. Survival benefit of vesnarinone is controversial. PDE inhibitors are useful for short-term support, but long-term use is linked to increased mortality.
CALCIUM-SENSITIZING AGENT Mechanism—Enhances the sensitivity of troponin C to calcium, which increases the extent of actin–myosin interactions without a substantial increase in myocardial oxygen consumption				
Levosimendan	Not approved for use in the United States	*Dose-related hypotension and reflex tachycardia* Nausea, headache	Hypersensitivity to levosimendan or racemic simendan	Preliminary data suggest that levosimendan improves cardiac hemodynamics in severe systolic HF and may reduce short-term mortality.

26

Integrative Cardiovascular Pharmacology: Hypertension, Ischemic Heart Disease, and Heart Failure

James M. McCabe and Ehrin J. Armstrong

469

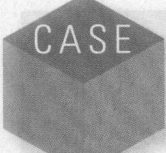

CASE

PART I: HYPERTENSION

Thomas N, a 45-year-old manager at a telecommunications company, presents to the cardiology clinic for evaluation of exertional shortness of breath. Mr. N had always been zealous in maintaining aerobic fitness, but about 6 months before his cardiology clinic visit, he began to note severe breathlessness as he approached the completion of his daily run, which concludes with a long but gentle uphill climb. During the intervening 6 months, the patient reports a progression in his symptoms to the point that, now, he rarely completes the first half of his daily run without resting. He denies chest discomfort at rest or with exercise. His family history is notable for hypertension and premature atherosclerosis. Mr. N has never used tobacco products.

On examination, the patient is hypertensive (blood pressure, 160/102 mm Hg), and a prominent presystolic S4 is heard at the left ventricular apex. The exam is otherwise unremarkable. The chest x-ray is reported as normal. The electrocardiogram (ECG) reveals normal sinus rhythm with voltage criteria for left ventricular hypertrophy. Mr. N is referred for noninvasive cardiac evaluation, including a treadmill exercise test (ETT) and a transthoracic echocardiogram. On the ETT, he reaches a peak heart rate of 170 beats/min during exercise and has to terminate the test because of severe dyspnea at a workload of 7 METS. (METS are metabolic equivalents, a measure of energy consumption; a value of 7 METS is below normal for this patient's age.) His blood pressure at peak exercise is 240/120 mm Hg. There is no evidence of myocardial ischemia by ECG criteria. The two-dimensional echocardiogram reveals concentric-pattern left ventricular hypertrophy, an enlarged left atrium, and normal aortic and mitral valves. Global and regional left ventricular systolic function are normal. Left ventricular diastolic filling is abnormal, with a reduced rate of early rapid filling and a significant increase in the extent of filling during atrial systole.

Questions

1. What are the current recommendations for initiation of antihypertensive drug therapy, and what are the therapeutic goals?

2. Thiazide diuretics have been used for many years as first-line therapy in patients with hypertension. What specific clinical circumstances might favor use of another agent, such as an angiotensin converting enzyme inhibitor?

3. Given the severity of hypertension in this case, Mr. N will likely require at least two drugs to achieve adequate control of his blood pressure. When is multidrug therapy required?

■ INTRODUCTION

In Chapters 20–25, cardiovascular pharmacology is considered in the context of individual physiologic systems. For example, diuretics are discussed in the context of volume regulation, while inhibitors of angiotensin converting enzyme (ACE) are discussed in the context of vascular tone. However, the clinical presentation of cardiovascular diseases often involves interactions among these individual systems. As a result, pharmacologic management often necessitates the use of agents from several drug classes. This chapter presents three common cardiovascular disease states—hypertension, ischemic heart disease, and heart failure—in a single, longitudinal clinical case. For each disease, an understanding of the disease pathophysiology underscores the rationale for pharmacologic interventions and may also highlight the potential for adverse effects (such as serious drug–drug interactions). This chapter aims to integrate pathophysiology with pharmacology to provide a thorough and mechanistic understanding of the contemporary management of these common cardiovascular disease states.

■ PATHOPHYSIOLOGY OF HYPERTENSION

Hypertension is a widely prevalent disease and a major risk factor for adverse cardiovascular events including stroke, coronary artery disease, peripheral vascular disease, heart failure, and chronic kidney disease. In primary prevention studies, there is a continuous relationship between blood pressure and adverse cardiovascular outcomes including death. Although elevated diastolic blood pressure had long been the main indication for initiating antihypertensive treatment, it is now appreciated that elevated systolic blood pressure alone (**isolated systolic hypertension**) is also sufficient indication for treatment, particularly in elderly patients. Recommendations for treatment of hypertension have recently undergone revision, with differential treatment thresholds based on age and presence of chronic kidney disease or diabetes (Fig. 26-1). The current recommendations reflect the results of recent randomized trials, which did not show a benefit of intensive blood pressure control in some populations and which also found that patients with chronic kidney disease or diabetes are at higher risk of cardiovascular events.

One of the main obstacles in the treatment of hypertension is the largely asymptomatic nature of the disease, even in patients with marked elevation in systemic blood pressure. This disconnect between symptoms and long-term adverse consequences has earned hypertension the designation "silent killer." For example, Mr. N began to exhibit symptoms only after exercising. Nonetheless, the severity of his hypertension puts him at major risk for developing coronary artery disease, stroke, and heart failure. Thus, effective strategies for detection and management of hypertension are critical elements in the primary and secondary prevention of cardiovascular disease.

Fortunately, the number and spectrum of agents available to treat patients with hypertension have expanded dramatically over the past two decades. These drugs can be administered

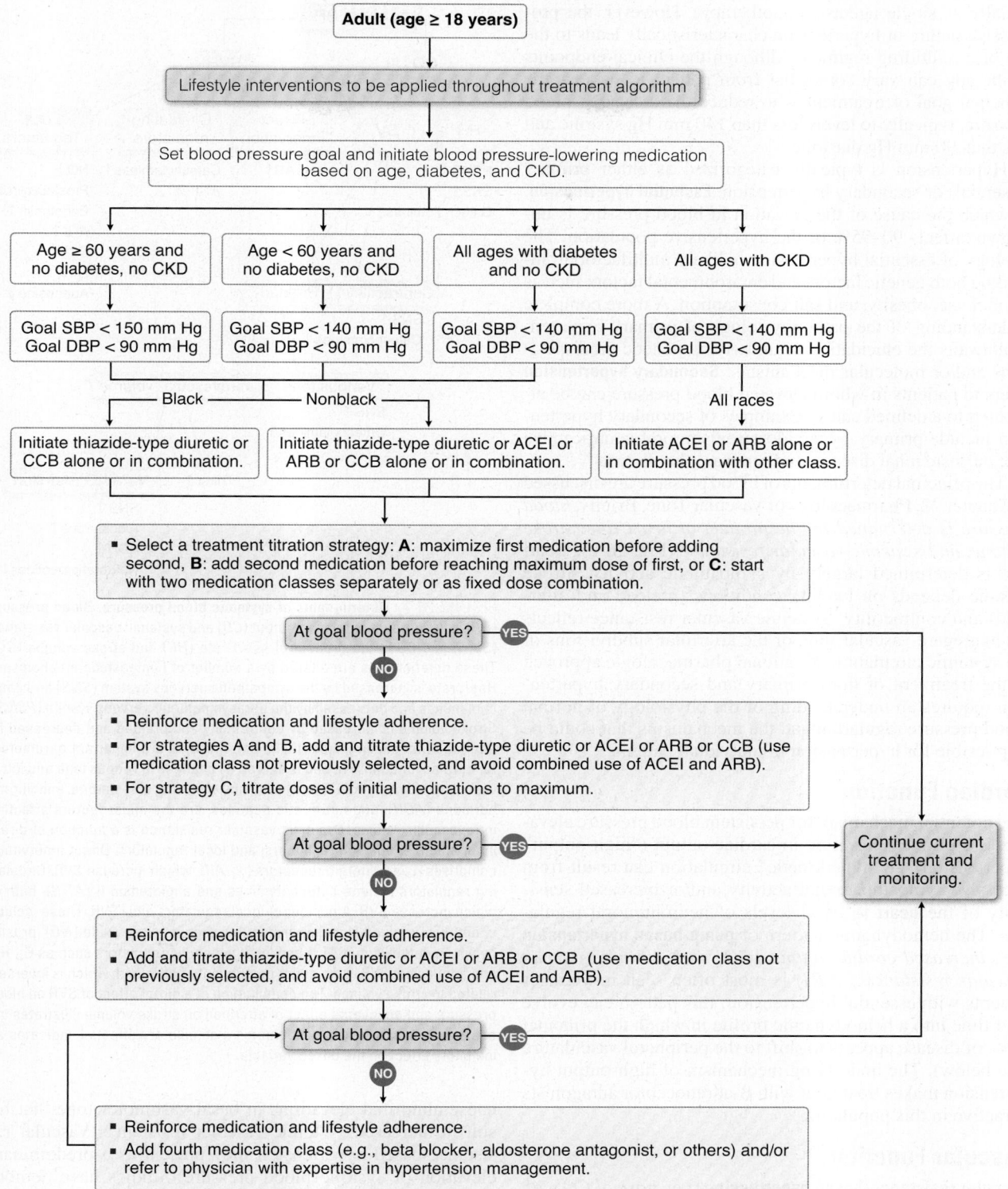

FIGURE 26-1. Current recommendations for treatment of hypertension. Current treatment guidelines have incorporated different treatment thresholds and blood pressure goals based on the patient's age and presence of chronic kidney disease (CKD) or diabetes. Patients over the age of 60 who do not have diabetes or chronic kidney disease can be treated with a more liberal blood pressure threshold of 150/90 mm Hg. Patients under the age of 60 without diabetes or chronic kidney disease should be treated to a target blood pressure of 140/90 mm Hg. All patients with diabetes or chronic kidney disease should be treated to a target blood pressure of 140/90 mm Hg, regardless of age. Among patients without chronic kidney disease, initial treatment should consist of a thiazide-type diuretic or calcium channel blocker (CCB); angiotensin converting enzyme inhibitors (ACEI) or angiotensin receptor blockers (ARB) may also be considered as initial therapy in nonblack patients. The subsequent treatment algorithm emphasizes continued lifestyle modification and addition of multiple agents to achieve the goal systolic and diastolic blood pressure (SBP and DBP, respectively). (Adapted, with permission, from James PA, Oparil S, Carter BL, et al. 2014 evidence-based guidelines for the management of high blood pressure in adults. *JAMA* 2014;311:507–520.)

initially as single agents (monotherapy). However, the progressive nature of hypertension characteristically leads to the use of a multidrug regimen. Although the clinical endpoints of therapy can vary somewhat from patient to patient, the principal goal of treatment is to reduce the measured blood pressure, typically to levels less than 140 mm Hg systolic and less than 90 mm Hg diastolic.

Hypertension is typically categorized as either primary (essential) or secondary hypertension. **Essential hypertension**, in which the cause of the elevation in blood pressure is unknown, affects 90–95% of the hypertensive population. The etiology of essential hypertension is likely multifactorial, including both genetic factors and environmental factors such as alcohol use, obesity, and salt consumption. A more complete understanding of the pathophysiology of primary hypertension awaits the elucidation of underlying genetic predispositions and/or molecular mechanisms. **Secondary hypertension** refers to patients in whom elevated blood pressure can be attributed to a defined cause. Examples of secondary hypertension include primary hyperaldosteronism, oral contraceptive use, intrinsic renal disease, and renovascular disease.

The principal determinants of blood pressure are discussed in Chapter 22, Pharmacology of Vascular Tone. Briefly, *blood pressure is determined by the product of heart rate, stroke volume, and systemic vascular resistance* (Fig. 26-2). Heart rate is determined largely by sympathetic activity. Stroke volume depends on loading conditions (preload and afterload) and contractility. Systemic vascular resistance reflects the aggregate vascular tone of the arteriolar subdivisions of the systemic circulation. A rational pharmacologic approach to the treatment of both primary and secondary hypertension requires an understanding of the physiology of normal blood pressure regulation and the mechanisms that could be responsible for hypertension in individual patients.

Cardiac Function

One potential mechanism for persistent blood pressure elevation is a primary elevation in cardiac output ("high-output" hypertension). A "hyperkinetic" circulation can result from excessive sympathoadrenal activity and/or increased sensitivity of the heart to basal levels of neurohumoral regulators. The hemodynamic pattern of **pump-based hypertension** (i.e., *increased cardiac output [CO] with normal systemic vascular resistance [SVR]*) is most often seen in younger patients with essential hypertension; this pattern can evolve over time into a hemodynamic profile in which the principal locus of disease appears to shift to the peripheral vasculature (see below). The underlying mechanism of high-output hypertension makes treatment with β-adrenoceptor antagonists attractive in this population.

Vascular Function

Vascular resistance-based hypertension (i.e., *normal CO with increased SVR*) is a common mechanism underlying hypertension in the elderly. In individuals with this form of hypertension, it is hypothesized that the vasculature is abnormally responsive to sympathetic stimulation, circulating factors, or local regulators of vascular tone. The abnormal responsiveness of the vasculature may be mediated in part by endothelial damage or dysfunction, which is known to disrupt the normal equilibrium between local vasodilatory (e.g., nitric oxide) and vasoconstrictive (e.g., endothelin) factors. In addition, ion channel defects in vascular smooth muscle can

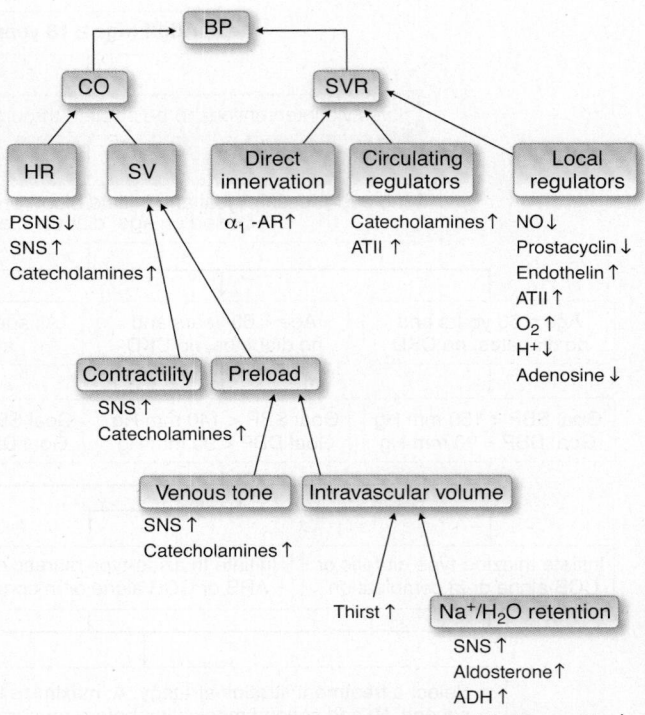

FIGURE 26-2. Determinants of systemic blood pressure. Blood pressure (*BP*) is the product of cardiac output (*CO*) and systemic vascular resistance (*SVR*), and CO is the product of heart rate (*HR*) and stroke volume (*SV*). These determinants are altered by a number of homeostatic mechanisms. Heart rate is increased by the sympathetic nervous system (*SNS*) and catecholamines and decreased by the parasympathetic nervous system (*PSNS*). Stroke volume is increased by contractility and preload and decreased by afterload (*not shown*); all of these determinants are important parameters for cardiac function. Preload is altered by changes in venous tone and intravascular volume. The SNS and hormones, including aldosterone, antidiuretic hormone (*ADH*), and natriuretic peptides, are the major factors affecting intravascular volume. Systemic vascular resistance is a function of direct innervation, circulating regulators, and local regulators. Direct innervation comprises α_1-adrenergic receptors (α_1-*AR*), which increase SVR. Circulating regulators include catecholamines and angiotensin II (*AT II*), both of which increase SVR. A number of local regulators alter SVR. These include endothelial-derived signaling molecules such as nitric oxide (*NO*), prostacyclin, endothelin, and AT II and local metabolic regulators such as O_2, H^+, and adenosine. SVR is the major component of afterload, which is inversely related to stroke volume. The combination of a direct effect of SVR on blood pressure and an inverse effect of afterload on stroke volume illustrates the complexity of the system. ↑ indicates a stimulatory effect; ↓ indicates an inhibitory effect on the boxed variable.

cause abnormal elevations in basal vasomotor tone that result in increased systemic vascular resistance. Vascular resistance-based hypertension may present as a predominant elevation of systolic blood pressure. Studies have demonstrated the effectiveness of thiazide diuretics in this population, making such agents the preferred initial treatment.

Renal Function

Abnormalities of renal function can also contribute to the development of systemic hypertension. Excessive Na^+ and H_2O retention by the kidney is responsible for **volume-based hypertension**. *Renal parenchymal disease*, caused by glomerular injury with reduction of functional nephron mass and/or excessive secretion of renin, can lead to an abnormal

TABLE 26-1 Major Classes of Antihypertensive Agents

DIURETICS	SYMPATHOLYTICS	VASODILATORS	RENIN–ANGIOTENSIN SYSTEM BLOCKERS

Thiazide diuretics
Loop diuretics
K^+-sparing diuretics
	CNS sympathetic outflow blockers
	Ganglionic blockers
	Postganglionic adrenergic nerve terminal antagonists
	    α_1-Adrenergic antagonists
	    β_1-Adrenergic antagonists
	    Mixed α-adrenergic/β-adrenergic antagonists
		Calcium channel
		  blockers
		Minoxidil
		Hydralazine
		Sodium nitroprusside
			Renin inhibitors
			ACE inhibitors
			AT_1 antagonists
			Aldosterone antagonists

increase in intravascular volume. Alternatively, ion channel mutations can impair normal Na^+ excretion. *Renovascular disease* (e.g., renal artery stenosis caused by atherosclerotic plaques, fibromuscular dysplasia, emboli, vasculitis, or external compression) can result in decreased renal blood flow. In response to this decrease in perfusion pressure, juxtaglomerular cells increase the secretion of renin, which in turn leads to increased production of angiotensin II and aldosterone. The latter mediators increase both vasomotor tone and Na^+ and H_2O retention, leading to a hemodynamic profile in which *both CO and SVR are elevated.*

Neuroendocrine Function

Dysfunction of the neuroendocrine system—including abnormal central regulation of basal sympathetic tone, atypical stress responses, abnormal responses to signals from baroreceptors and intravascular volume receptors, and excessive production of hormones that act to regulate the circulation—can alter cardiac, vascular, and/or renal function, leading to increased systemic blood pressure. Examples of endocrine abnormalities associated with systemic hypertension include excessive secretion of catecholamines (pheochromocytoma), excessive secretion of aldosterone by the adrenal cortex (primary aldosteronism), and excessive production of thyroid hormones (hyperthyroidism).

■ CLINICAL MANAGEMENT OF HYPERTENSION

As discussed above, hypertension presents a complex clinical challenge, since blood pressure elevation may be asymptomatic for many years even as substantial end-organ damage occurs. As a result, the effective treatment of hypertension requires strategies to identify asymptomatic patients, especially those at high risk for the adverse end-organ effects of the disease. Because antihypertensive drugs can add inconvenience to the life of a patient who is asymptomatic, long-term treatment of the hypertensive patient requires the use of drug regimens that are individualized for optimal adherence and efficacy. This requires consideration of safety profile, dosing schedule, and cost.

The first line in hypertension treatment is counseling regarding the importance of lifestyle modifications. Lifestyle modifications associated with favorable results in hypertensive patients include weight loss, increased physical activity, smoking cessation, and a low-fat, low-sodium diet. Reduction or elimination of exogenous agents that can induce hypertension—such as ethanol, oral contraceptives, glucocorticoids, and stimulant drugs—can also have demonstrable clinical benefit. While nonpharmacologic therapies alone

may not achieve a sufficient reduction in blood pressure, they remain critical adjuncts to pharmacologic treatment.

An extensive armamentarium of drugs is used to treat systemic hypertension. Ultimately, though, these agents all exert their effects on blood pressure through a reduction in cardiac output and/or systemic vascular resistance. Strategies currently used to treat hypertension include reduction of intravascular volume with concomitant vasodilation (diuretics), down-regulation of sympathetic tone (β-antagonists, α_1-antagonists, central sympatholytics), modulation of vascular smooth muscle tone (calcium channel blockers, K^+ channel openers), and inhibition of the neurohumoral regulators of the circulation (renin inhibitors, ACE inhibitors, AT_1 antagonists [angiotensin II type 1 receptor antagonists]) (Table 26-1 and Fig. 26-3). The reduction in blood

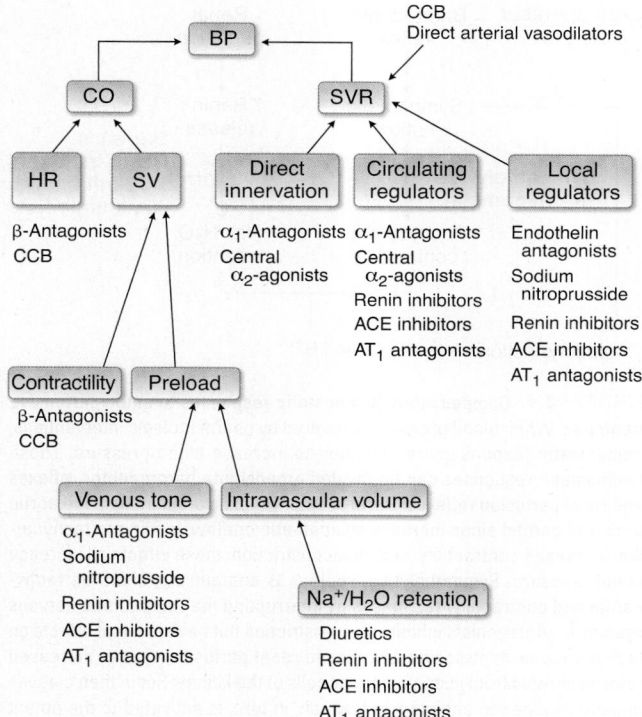

FIGURE 26-3. Pharmacologic effects of commonly used antihypertensive agents. Antihypertensive agents modulate blood pressure by interfering with the determinants of blood pressure. Many of these antihypertensive drugs have multiple actions. For example, renin-angiotensin system blockers, such as ACE inhibitors and AT_1 antagonists, alter the levels of local regulators and circulating regulators and affect renal Na^+ retention and venous tone. BP, blood pressure; CO, cardiac output; SVR, systemic vascular resistance; HR, heart rate; SV, stroke volume; CCB, Ca^{2+} channel blockers; ACE, angiotensin converting enzyme.

pressure caused by these agents is sensed by baroreceptors and renal juxtaglomerular cells, which can activate counter-regulatory responses that attenuate the magnitude of blood pressure reduction. These compensatory responses can be substantial, necessitating dose adjustments and/or the use of more than one agent to achieve long-term blood pressure control (Fig. 26-4).

Reduction of Intravascular Volume

Diuretics

Although diuretics have long been a cornerstone of antihypertensive therapy, the mechanism of action of diuretics in hypertension is incompletely understood. As discussed in Chapter 21, Pharmacology of Volume Regulation, diuretics decrease intravascular volume by increasing renal excretion of Na^+ and H_2O. However, volume depletion alone is unlikely to fully explain the antihypertensive effect of diuretics.

Thiazide diuretics (e.g., **hydrochlorothiazide**) are the natriuretic drugs most commonly prescribed for the treatment of hypertension (Table 26-2). The pharmacokinetic

TABLE 26-2 Diuretics Used in the Treatment of Hypertension	
DRUG	**DURATION OF ACTION (HOURS)**
Thiazide Diuretics	
Chlorothiazide	6–12
Chlorthalidone	48–72
Hydrochlorothiazide	16–24
Indapamide	24
Metolazone	24
Loop Diuretics	
Bumetanide	4–5
Ethacrynic acid	4–5
Furosemide	4–5
Torsemide	6–8
Potassium-Sparing Diuretics	
Amiloride	6–24
Eplerenone	24
Spironolactone	72–96
Triamterene	8–12

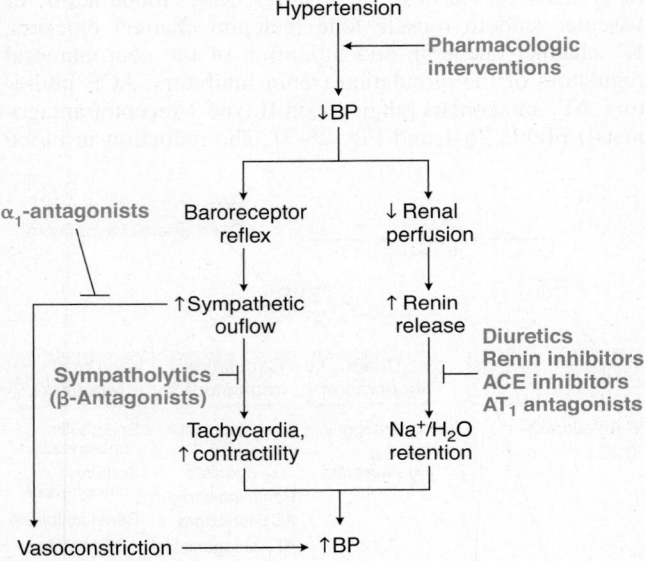

FIGURE 26-4. Compensatory homeostatic responses to antihypertensive treatment. When blood pressure is lowered by pharmacologic interventions, homeostatic responses are activated to increase blood pressure. These homeostatic responses can be divided broadly into baroreceptor reflexes and renal perfusion reflexes. Baroreceptor reflexes originating in the aortic arch and carotid sinus increase sympathetic outflow, leading to tachycardia, increased contractility, and vasoconstriction; these effects all increase blood pressure. Sympatholytics, such as β-antagonists, blunt the tachycardia and contractility responses by interrupting the sympathetic nervous system. α₁-Antagonists inhibit vasoconstriction but have minimal effects on tachycardia or contractility. Decreased renal perfusion causes increased release of renin from juxtaglomerular cells of the kidney. Renin then cleaves angiotensinogen to angiotensin I, which, in turn, is activated to the potent vasoconstrictor angiotensin II (*not shown*). Angiotensin II increases adrenal secretion of aldosterone, which acts on principal cells of the collecting duct to increase Na^+ (and, therefore, water) reabsorption. The increased Na^+ reabsorption increases intravascular volume and thereby results in increased blood pressure. Diuretics interrupt this homeostatic response by decreasing Na^+ reabsorption from the nephron; renin inhibitors prevent the generation of angiotensin I; angiotensin converting enzyme (*ACE*) inhibitors interrupt the formation of angiotensin II; and AT₁ antagonists prevent the target-organ signaling of angiotensin II.

and pharmacodynamic characteristics of the thiazides make them especially useful agents in the treatment of chronic hypertension. Thiazides have high oral availability and long duration of action. The initial antihypertensive effect seems to be mediated by decreasing intravascular volume. Therefore, *thiazides are particularly effective in patients with volume-based hypertension, such as patients with primary renal disease and African American patients.* Thiazides induce an initial decrease in intravascular volume that decreases blood pressure by lowering cardiac output. However, the decrease in cardiac output stimulates the renin-angiotensin system, which leads to volume retention and attenuation of the effect of the thiazide on volume status. It is hypothesized that a vasodilatory effect of the thiazides complements the compensated volume depletion, leading to a sustained decrease in blood pressure. This hypothesis is supported by the observation that the maximal antihypertensive effect of the thiazides is frequently achieved at doses lower than those needed to achieve a maximal diuretic effect. Therefore, thiazides achieve their blood pressure effect by influencing both cardiac output and systemic vascular resistance.

The Joint National Commission (JNC) treatment algorithm suggests thiazide diuretics as a potential first-line agent for many patients and a preferred first-line agent for African American patients (Fig. 26-1). This recommendation arises from the results of large-scale trials, which found favorable outcomes and decreased cost associated with thiazide therapy. The practice at present is to initiate thiazide therapy at low doses (e.g., 12.5–25 mg/day).

Loop diuretics (e.g., **furosemide**) are infrequently prescribed for the treatment of mild or moderate hypertension. These agents typically have a relatively short duration of action (4–6 hours), and despite the brisk diuresis that follows their administration, their antihypertensive efficacy is often modest. It is thought that this modest impact on blood pressure is due to activation of compensatory responses involving the neurohumoral regulators of intravascular volume and systemic vascular resistance. *There are, however, several well-recognized clinical situations in which loop diuretics are preferable to thiazides, including malignant hypertension* (see below) *and volume-based hypertension in patients with advanced chronic kidney disease.*

K^+-sparing diuretics (e.g., **spironolactone**, **triamterene**, **amiloride**) are less efficacious than thiazide and loop diuretics and are used primarily in combination with other diuretics to attenuate or correct drug-induced kaliuresis (K^+ excretion) and the resultant hypokalemia. An exception is *spironolactone, an aldosterone receptor antagonist that is especially effective in the treatment of secondary hypertension caused by hyperaldosteronism.* Hypokalemia is a common metabolic adverse effect of the thiazide and loop diuretics, which inhibit Na^+ reabsorption in proximal segments of the nephron and thereby increase delivery of Na^+ and water to distal segments of the nephron. Increased distal Na^+ delivery results in a compensatory increase in Na^+ reabsorption in the distal tubule, which is coupled to an increase in K^+ excretion. Because the latter effect is mediated by aldosterone (see Chapter 21), the K^+-sparing diuretics attenuate this effect and thereby help to maintain normal serum potassium levels. It should be emphasized that both ACE inhibitors (which decrease aldosterone activity and K^+ excretion) and K^+ supplements may need to be decreased or eliminated in patients taking K^+-sparing diuretics, because life-threatening hyperkalemia has been reported in association with clinical use of the K^+-sparing agents. Use of these agents should be undertaken with great caution in patients with even mild degrees of renal insufficiency.

Down-Regulation of Sympathetic Tone

Drugs that modulate adrenergic activity are discussed in detail in Chapter 11, Adrenergic Pharmacology; refer to that chapter for descriptions of the tissue distribution of α- and β-adrenergic receptors and the cardiovascular effects mediated by these receptors. *Sympatholytic drugs treat hypertension via two major mechanisms: reduction of systemic vascular resistance and/or reduction of cardiac output.* Clinically, these agents are broadly divided into β-adrenoceptor antagonists, α-adrenoceptor antagonists, and central sympatholytics.

β-Adrenoceptor Antagonists

β-Adrenoceptor antagonists (e.g., **propranolol, metoprolol, atenolol, nebivolol**) are commonly prescribed agents in the treatment of hypertension. The negative chronotropic and inotropic effects of these agents (and the reductions in heart rate, stroke volume, and cardiac output that follow) account for the initial antihypertensive effect of the β-antagonists. Decreased vasomotor tone, with a consequent decrease in systemic vascular resistance, has also been reported with longer term therapy.

The β-antagonist-induced reduction in vasomotor tone may seem paradoxical, given that β_2-adrenergic receptors

in the peripheral vasculature mediate vasodilation. However, antagonism of β_1-adrenergic receptors in the kidney decreases secretion of renin and thereby decreases production of the potent vasoconstrictor, angiotensin II. The latter effect likely predominates, even when nonselective β-receptor antagonists are administered. Although β-antagonists effectively reduce blood pressure in hypertensive patients, these agents typically do not cause hypotension in individuals with normal blood pressure. Increased baseline sympathetic activity in hypertensive patients may in part explain the efficacy of β-antagonists in lowering blood pressure in these individuals. In contrast, basal activation of β-receptors in normal individuals may be sufficiently low that receptor antagonists have little hemodynamic effect. β-Antagonist therapy has been associated with both elevation of serum triglyceride levels and reduction of high-density lipoprotein (HDL) levels; the clinical significance of these potentially harmful metabolic effects remains unclear. Noncardiac adverse effects of β-antagonist therapy may include exacerbation of glucose intolerance (hyperglycemia), sedation, impotence, depression, and bronchoconstriction.

Mixed α–β antagonists (e.g., **labetalol**) are available in both oral and parenteral formulations. Intravenous administration of labetalol causes a substantial reduction in blood pressure and has found wide use in the treatment of hypertensive emergencies. Oral labetalol is also used in the long-term treatment of hypertension. One potential advantage of this drug is that the decrease in blood pressure achieved by reduction of systemic vascular resistance (because labetalol antagonizes α_1-receptors) is not associated with the reflex increase in heart rate or cardiac output that can occur when pure vasodilator drugs are used as monotherapy (because labetalol also antagonizes cardiac β_1-receptors).

In recent years, β-adrenoceptor antagonists have been used less frequently in the initial treatment of hypertension, due to clinical data suggesting that they may not be as efficacious as diuretics or inhibitors of the renin-angiotensin-aldosterone system. However, these agents are still important in the treatment of hypertension when there are other clinical indications for a β-adrenoceptor antagonist, such as coronary artery disease or heart failure. β-Receptor antagonists are generally efficacious in the treatment of hypertension in younger patients.

α-Adrenoceptor Antagonists

α_1-Adrenergic antagonists (e.g., **prazosin, terazosin, doxazosin**) are also used in the treatment of high blood pressure. α_1-Adrenergic antagonists inhibit peripheral vasomotor tone, reducing vasoconstriction and decreasing systemic vascular resistance. The absence of adverse effects on the serum lipid profile during long-term treatment with α_1-adrenergic antagonists is often cited as a distinctive advantage of these agents relative to other antihypertensive medications. However, the long-term benefit of this advantage, if any, remains to be determined in randomized clinical trials. Furthermore, in a large trial comparing different antihypertensives, an increased incidence of heart failure was observed in the group randomized to doxazosin.

Nonselective α-adrenergic antagonists (e.g., **phenoxybenzamine, phentolamine**) are not employed in the long-term treatment of hypertension because excessive compensatory responses can result from their long-term use. For example, antagonism of central α_2-adrenergic receptors disinhibits sympathetic outflow, resulting in unopposed reflex tachycardia. However, *these agents are indicated for the medical treatment of pheochromocytoma.*

Central Sympatholytics

The α_2-adrenergic agonists **methyldopa**, **clonidine**, and **guanabenz** reduce sympathetic outflow from the medulla, leading to decreases in heart rate, contractility, and vasomotor tone. These drugs are available in oral formulations (clonidine is also available as a transdermal patch) and were widely used in the past despite their unfavorable adverse effect profile. The availability of multiple alternative agents, as well as the current trend toward the use of multidrug regimens at submaximal doses, have substantially diminished the clinical role of α_2-agonists in the treatment of hypertension.

Ganglionic blockers (e.g., **trimethaphan**, **hexamethonium**) inhibit nicotinic cholinergic activity at sympathetic ganglia. These agents are extremely effective at lowering blood pressure. However, the severe adverse effects of combined parasympathetic and sympathetic blockade (e.g., constipation, blurred vision, sexual dysfunction, and orthostatic hypotension) have made ganglionic blockers of historic interest only.

Some sympatholytic agents (e.g., **reserpine**, **guanethidine**) are taken up into the terminals of postganglionic adrenergic neurons, where they induce long-term depletion of neurotransmitter from norepinephrine-containing synaptic vesicles (see Chapter 11). These agents lower blood pressure by decreasing the activity of the sympathetic nervous system. However, reserpine and guanethidine have little role in the contemporary treatment of hypertension because of their significant adverse-effect profiles, which include severe depression (reserpine) and orthostatic hypotension and sexual dysfunction (guanethidine).

Modulation of Vascular Smooth Muscle Tone

As discussed in Chapter 22, vascular tone is dependent on the degree of vascular smooth muscle contraction. Vasodilators reduce systemic vascular resistance by acting on arteriolar smooth muscle and/or the vascular endothelium. The major mechanisms of action of the arterial vasodilators include blockade of Ca^{2+} channels and opening of metabotropic K^+ channels.

Ca^{2+} Channel Blockers

Ca^{2+} channel blockers (e.g., **verapamil**, **diltiazem**, **nifedipine**, **amlodipine**) are oral agents that are widely used in the long-term treatment of hypertension. Calcium channel blockers (CCBs) have a variety of hemodynamic effects, reflecting the multiple sites at which calcium is involved in the electrical and mechanical events of the cardiac cycle and in vascular regulation. These agents can act as arterial vasodilators, negative inotropes, and/or negative chronotropes. The dihydropyridine agents nifedipine and amlodipine act primarily as vasodilators. In contrast, the nondihydropyridine drugs verapamil and diltiazem act principally as negative inotropes and chronotropes, thereby decreasing myocardial contractility, heart rate, and impulse conduction. Thus, *CCBs can lower blood pressure through reduction of both systemic vascular resistance and cardiac output.* CCBs are often used in combination with other cardioactive drugs, either as components of a multidrug antihypertensive regimen or for combined antihypertensive and antianginal treatment in patients with ischemic heart disease (IHD).

Given the distinctive pharmacodynamic effects of the different CCBs, the potential adverse effects of CCB therapy (including adverse interactions with other cardiovascular therapies) are agent specific. The nondihydropyridine agents verapamil and diltiazem should be used with caution in patients who have impaired left ventricular (LV) systolic function, as these agents can exacerbate systolic heart failure (see below). These agents should also be used with caution in patients with conduction system disease, as these drugs can potentiate functional abnormalities of the sinoatrial (SA) and atrioventricular (AV) nodes. Both of these cautions are particularly relevant in patients receiving concomitant β-antagonist therapy.

K^+ Channel Openers

Minoxidil and **hydralazine** are orally available arterial vasodilators that are occasionally used in the long-term treatment of hypertension. Minoxidil is a metabotropic K^+ channel opener that hyperpolarizes vascular smooth muscle cells and thereby attenuates the cellular response to depolarizing stimuli. Hydralazine is a less powerful vasodilator with an uncertain mechanism of action. Both minoxidil and hydralazine can cause compensatory retention of Na^+ and H_2O as well as reflex tachycardia; these adverse effects are more frequent and more severe with minoxidil than with hydralazine. Concomitant use of a β-antagonist and a diuretic can mitigate these adverse effects. The use of hydralazine is limited by the frequent occurrence of tolerance and tachyphylaxis to the drug. In addition, increases in the total daily dose of hydralazine can be associated with a drug-induced lupus syndrome. Given the more favorable safety profile of the Ca^{2+} channel blockers, the use of minoxidil is now largely restricted to patients with severe hypertension that is refractory to other pharmacologic therapies. Of note, hydralazine (in combination with isosorbide dinitrate) has now emerged as an adjunctive therapy (i.e., in patients who are already receiving an ACE inhibitor and a β-antagonist) in the treatment of systolic heart failure in African American patients.

Modulation of the Renin-Angiotensin-Aldosterone System

Renin-angiotensin-aldosterone system blockers include the renin inhibitor **aliskiren**, the ACE inhibitors (e.g., **captopril**, **enalapril**, **lisinopril**), and the angiotensin receptor (AT_1) antagonists (e.g., **losartan**, **valsartan**). These agents are increasingly used in the treatment of hypertension.

Renin Inhibitors

Aliskiren is a competitive inhibitor of renin, the enzyme that cleaves angiotensinogen to angiotensin I. This early-stage blockade of the renin-angiotensin-aldosterone system may theoretically result in more effective reduction of blood pressure and regression of left ventricular hypertrophy than that achieved by angiotensin converting enzyme inhibitors or angiotensin receptor blockers. Recent clinical trials have suggested that increased renal failure and hypotension may occur when aliskiren is prescribed in combination with ACE inhibitors or ARBs. For this reason, aliskiren is less commonly used in the treatment of hypertension.

Angiotensin Converting Enzyme Inhibitors

ACE inhibitors prevent the ACE-mediated conversion of angiotensin I to angiotensin II, leading to decreased circulating levels of angiotensin II and aldosterone. By decreasing angiotensin II levels, ACE inhibitors decrease systemic vascular resistance and thereby decrease the impedance to LV ejection. By decreasing aldosterone levels, these agents promote natriuresis and thereby reduce intravascular volume. ACE inhibitors also decrease bradykinin degradation, and the resulting increase in circulating bradykinin causes vasodilation. *ACE inhibitors are effective in patients with hyperreninemic hypertension, but these agents also reduce blood pressure in patients with low-to-normal circulating renin levels.* The antihypertensive effectiveness of ACE inhibitors in patients with low-to-normal plasma renin activity may be due to potentiation of the vasodilatory effects of bradykinin, although this hypothesis is unproven.

Therapy with ACE inhibitors is as effective as therapy with thiazide diuretics or β-antagonists in the treatment of hypertension. ACE inhibitors are attractive antihypertensive agents because these drugs seem to have unique benefits (e.g., a decrease in the loss of renal function in patients with chronic kidney disease) and relatively few adverse effects (ACE inhibitors do not increase the risk of hypokalemia or cause elevated serum glucose or lipid levels). Despite these attractive features, it merits emphasis that, in at least one large comparison trial, thiazide diuretics were more cardioprotective than ACE inhibitors.

ACE inhibitors should be administered with caution in patients with intravascular volume depletion. Such patients may have reduced renal perfusion at baseline, leading to a compensatory increase in renin and angiotensin II; this increase in angiotensin II is one of the physiologic mechanisms by which glomerular filtration rate (GFR) is maintained in the face of relative renal hypoperfusion. Administration of ACE inhibitors to such patients can disrupt this autoregulatory mechanism, leading to renal insufficiency. The same autoregulatory mechanism is the basis for the contraindication to ACE inhibitors in patients with bilateral renal artery stenosis (or unilateral stenosis in patients with a single kidney). Despite these cautionary notes, it should be emphasized that *ACE inhibitors are considered the preferred therapy in the hypertensive diabetic patient*, as these agents have been shown to delay the onset and progression of diabetic glomerular disease through favorable effects on intraglomerular pressure.

AT₁ Antagonists (Angiotensin Receptor Blockers)

Angiotensin II receptor (AT_1) antagonists (also known as **angiotensin receptor blockers**, or **ARBs**) are oral antihypertensive agents that competitively antagonize the binding of angiotensin II to its cognate AT_1 receptors; examples include losartan, valsartan, and irbesartan. In addition to their antihypertensive effect, these agents may also reduce reactive arteriolar intimal proliferation. Like ACE inhibitors, AT_1 antagonists are effective in lowering blood pressure and are sometimes substituted for ACE inhibitors in patients with ACE inhibitor-induced cough. Cough, a common adverse effect of ACE inhibitor therapy, results from drug-induced increases in bradykinin levels; this effect often leads to nonadherence or discontinuation of the drug. Because AT_1 antagonists do not affect the activity of the converting enzyme responsible for bradykinin degradation, cough is not an adverse effect of therapy with ARBs.

Monotherapy and Stepped Care

Monotherapy (treatment with a single drug) is often sufficient to normalize blood pressure in patients with mild hypertension; this approach may improve patient adherence and avoid the risk of potential drug interactions. Controversy exists as to which antihypertensive agents are preferred as initial therapy. Thiazide diuretics, ACE inhibitors, AT_1 antagonists, and calcium channel blockers (CCBs) are similar in terms of efficacy in lowering blood pressure (each effectively lowers blood pressure in 30–50% of patients). Ultimately, the ideal agent is that which reduces a patient's blood pressure to the optimal range with the least severe adverse effects. Drug toxicities are often related to drug dose, and therefore, the clinician must also consider the use of a combination of "synergistic" agents at lower doses, especially if blood pressure control is marginal or inadequate.

Certain clinical circumstances favor initiating a specific class of antihypertensive medication (Table 26-3). β-Antagonists are the agents of choice in patients with a

TABLE 26-3 Relative Indications and Contraindications for Antihypertensive Agents

DRUG CLASS	INDICATIONS	CONTRAINDICATIONS
Diuretics	Heart failure Systolic hypertension	Gout
β-Antagonists	Coronary artery disease Heart failure Migraine Tachyarrhythmias	Asthma Heart block
α-Antagonists	Prostatic hypertrophy	Heart failure
Calcium channel blockers	Systolic hypertension	Heart block
ACE inhibitors	Diabetic or other nephropathy Heart failure Previous myocardial infarction	Bilateral renal artery stenosis Hyperkalemia Pregnancy
AT₁ antagonists	ACE inhibitor-associated cough Diabetic or other nephropathy Heart failure	Bilateral renal artery stenosis Hyperkalemia Pregnancy

history of myocardial infarction (MI). ACE inhibitors are recommended in patients with left ventricular dysfunction, diabetes, and/or chronic kidney disease. Diuretics are effective in treating hypertension associated with volume retention in nephrotic syndrome. ACE inhibitors are also used in nephrotic syndrome to attenuate the degree of proteinuria.

Stepped care refers to the progressive, step-by-step addition of drugs to a therapeutic regimen for hypertension. Combination therapy is based on the use of agents with distinct mechanisms of action; it also emphasizes the use of submaximal doses of drugs in an attempt to minimize potential adverse effects and toxicities.

Two examples of combination therapy are the use of an ACE inhibitor with either a diuretic or a calcium channel blocker. These combinations have several potential mechanistic advantages. By inducing a mild degree of volume depletion, thiazide diuretics activate the renin-angiotensin system. If this response is blocked by an ACE inhibitor, then the antihypertensive effect of the thiazide is potentiated. Furthermore, inhibition of the renin-angiotensin system by itself promotes natriuresis. Finally, the combination of a thiazide and an ACE inhibitor decreases systemic vascular resistance.

When an ACE inhibitor is used with a calcium channel blocker, the combination may have an additive effect on regression of left ventricular hypertrophy. The addition of a calcium channel blocker may also potentiate ACE inhibitor-mediated peripheral vasodilation. A recent study (ACCOMPLISH trial) has suggested that the combination of an ACE inhibitor with a calcium channel blocker may reduce the incidence of cardiovascular events more than the combination of an ACE inhibitor with a thiazide diuretic, despite similar reductions in blood pressure.

Possible Demographic Factors

Certain classes of antihypertensive drugs have been reported to be more effective than others in special populations. Some data also suggest that distinct etiologies of hypertension may be more or less prevalent in different populations.

Elderly patients tend to respond more favorably to diuretics and dihydropyridine Ca^{2+} channel blockers than to other antihypertensive agents. β-Antagonists are more likely to cause SA or AV node dysfunction or to impair myocardial function in elderly patients; these effects are likely related to the higher prevalence of conduction system disease and LV systolic dysfunction in such patients. Elderly patients also tend to have decreased circulating levels of renin and have been reported to be less responsive to ACE inhibitors.

Hypertension in patients of African descent seems to be more responsive to diuretics and Ca^{2+} channel blockers than to β-antagonists and ACE inhibitors. (A notable exception is the favorable response of young African Americans to β-antagonist therapy.) Reports indicate that some African Americans may have lower circulating renin levels, and this could account for the observation that ACE inhibitors are less effective in these patients. Reports have also suggested that the prevalence of Na^+ sensitivity is substantially increased in some African Americans, including both the hypertensive and the normotensive cohort. Although less well studied, there is some evidence of differential responsiveness to the various classes of antihypertensive agents in hypertensive Asian and Hispanic cohorts.

Despite these demographic observations, the clinical benefit of drug selection on the basis of differential responsiveness to specific drug classes has not been evaluated systematically. For example, although elderly patients are reportedly less responsive to β-antagonists, the results of the Systolic Hypertension in the Elderly Project (SHEP Trial) indicate that both β-antagonists and diuretics are, in fact, associated with mortality reduction, and this favorable treatment effect is demonstrated within several years of treatment initiation. Similarly, although reports have suggested that African Americans are less responsive to β-antagonists and ACE inhibitors, it would be difficult to apply these observations to the treatment of a hypertensive, diabetic African American with chronic kidney disease or to advocate for the use of a thiazide diuretic in a hypertensive African American with a history of previous MI. Finally, it should again be emphasized that the risk of disease complications related to hypertension cannot be explained by the degree of blood pressure elevation alone. Conversely, the full spectrum of treatment benefits cannot be explained by the degree of blood pressure reduction alone. For these reasons, the empirical observation that some antihypertensive agents do not lower blood pressure as effectively in some patients does not necessarily mean that these drugs will be less effective in preventing future cardiovascular disease morbidity and mortality in these patients. These questions remain the focus of active research.

Hypertensive Crisis

The term **hypertensive crisis** refers to clinical syndromes characterized by severe (typically acute) elevations in blood pressure. This abrupt increase in blood pressure can cause acute vascular injury and derivative end-organ damage. Although most cases of severe hypertension were, at one time, designated as "hypertensive crisis" or "malignant hypertension," current practice attempts to distinguish those patients in whom the blood pressure elevation and vascular injury are acute (**hypertensive emergency**) from the patient cohort in which the temporal course of blood pressure elevation is more gradual and the end-organ damage is chronic and slowly progressive.

A true hypertensive emergency is a life-threatening condition in which severe and acute blood pressure elevation is associated with acute vascular injury. The vascular injury can manifest clinically as retinal hemorrhages, papilledema, encephalopathy, and acute (or acute superimposed on chronic) renal insufficiency; this syndrome is often associated with acute left ventricular failure. The pathogenesis of malignant hypertension remains unclear. However, it is likely that **fibrinoid arteriolar necrosis** contributes to the signs and symptoms of this syndrome. Fibrinoid arteriolar necrosis of specific vascular beds can result in acute vascular injury and end-organ hypoperfusion (e.g., renal failure, stroke). Fibrinoid arteriolar necrosis can also lead to microangiopathic hemolytic anemia.

Treatment of patients with hypertensive emergency necessitates rapid reduction of blood pressure to prevent end-organ damage. Drug classes used to treat this condition include parenteral vasodilators (e.g., clevidipine, nitroprusside, fenoldopam, nicardipine), diuretics (e.g., furosemide), and/or β-antagonists (e.g., labetalol). Because of the acuity of the syndrome and the need to titrate these powerful antihypertensive agents carefully, patients are hospitalized for treatment. After the acute episode has been controlled, subsequent lowering of blood pressure to the normal range of the patient is then attempted more cautiously over a longer

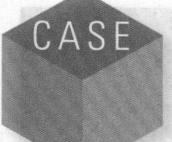

CASE — PART II: ISCHEMIC HEART DISEASE

Mr. N is treated for hypertension with low-dose hydrochlorothiazide and an ACE inhibitor. He returns for follow-up visits at 1 month and 6 months, and reports that he is doing well. He faithfully adheres to his prescribed medical regimen and notes a definite improvement in exercise capacity. His regular blood pressure measurements now show readings of 130 to 150/86 to 90 mm Hg. A serum lipid profile is notable for increased total cholesterol, with a moderately elevated LDL. Low-dose aspirin is added to his regimen. Treatment with a lipid-lowering agent is also advised, but Mr. N declines, instead requesting that his lipid profile be rechecked after a period of diet and lifestyle modifications.

An exercise tolerance test 1 year after his initial visit is notable for improved exercise capacity (10 MET workload), with blunting of the heart rate and reduction of the blood pressure at peak exercise compared to the original study (120/min and 190/90 mm Hg, respectively); there is no evidence of myocardial ischemia by ECG criteria. A repeat LDL cholesterol determination is within the normal range (128 mg/dL). His medications (aspirin, hydrochlorothiazide, and ACE inhibitor) are continued, and routine follow-up is established.

One week later, Mr. N experiences the abrupt onset of severe retrosternal chest pressure. He is visibly diaphoretic and dyspneic. He calls 911 and is transported to the local emergency department, where an ECG shows sinus tachycardia and ST segment elevation in the inferior leads. Emergency cardiac catheterization is performed, confirming total occlusion of a dominant right coronary artery, and percutaneous coronary intervention (PCI) is performed with placement of a coronary stent. The procedure is successful, and he remains free of chest pain and is hemodynamically stable. ECG and serum enzyme changes (peak creatine kinase [CK], 2,400 IU/L [normal, 60–400 IU/L]; cardiac isoform [MB] fraction, positive) are consistent with an evolving myocardial infarction. A repeat echocardiogram immediately before Mr. N's discharge from the hospital demonstrates concentric left ventricular hypertrophy with a left ventricular ejection fraction of 40% (normal, >55%); the inferior wall from the base to the apex is akinetic, with thinning of the myocardium in this akinetic region.

Questions

4. Which class of lipid-lowering agent is appropriate for this patient?
5. Which pharmacologic interventions are appropriate during the interval between the patient's emergency department evaluation and his cardiac catheterization?
6. What are the critical drug components of a postmyocardial infarction treatment regimen in the setting of left ventricular dysfunction?

---

period of time (12–24 hours), in an effort to decrease the risk of critical-organ hypoperfusion and extension of vascular injury.

Although malignant hypertension is a life-threatening medical emergency, it is an uncommon expression of hypertensive disease that occurs in far less than 1% of hypertensive patients. More common are cases of **hypertensive urgency**, in which the blood pressure elevation is less acute and the target organ disease has been present for some time. Conditions illustrative of hypertensive urgency include a stroke or MI that is accompanied by severe blood pressure elevation or acute left heart failure with severe hypertension.

▌ PATHOPHYSIOLOGY OF ISCHEMIC HEART DISEASE

Ischemic heart disease (IHD), the leading cause of mortality in the United States, accounts for more than 500,000 deaths each year. Since the advent of cardiac intensive care units in the early 1960s, an improved understanding of the biology of IHD has resulted in a spectrum of diagnostic and therapeutic advances. These advances, coupled with increased public awareness, healthier lifestyles, and sustained efforts to improve both primary and secondary prevention strategies, have resulted in significant mortality reduction for patients with IHD.

With respect to pharmacotherapy, IHD can be considered in two broad categories: **chronic coronary artery disease** (**CAD**) and **acute coronary syndromes** (**ACS**). Each of these clinical presentations of IHD has a distinct pathogenesis, and as a result, the pharmacologic strategies employed to treat these distinct clinical entities differ in emphasis. The therapeutic goal in patients with chronic CAD is to *maintain the balance between myocardial oxygen supply and demand*; in patients with ACS, the goal is to *restore and/or maintain patency of the coronary artery lumen* (Fig. 26-5).

Chronic Coronary Artery Disease

Chronic CAD is characterized by impaired coronary vasodilator reserve. Under conditions of hyperemic stress (i.e., stress requiring increased coronary blood flow), this can result in an imbalance between myocardial oxygen supply and demand, leading to functional cardiac abnormalities (poor contraction of the ischemic portion of the myocardium) as well as clinical symptoms of CAD. The basic physiology of myocardial oxygen supply and demand is discussed in Chapter 22. Imbalances in myocardial oxygen supply and demand occur mainly as a result of coronary flow reduction and endothelial dysfunction.

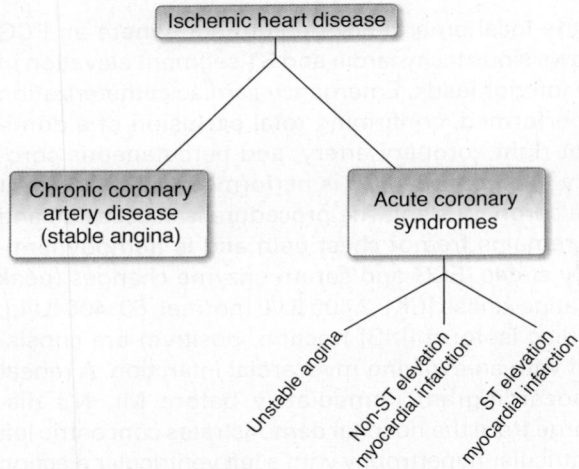

FIGURE 26-5. Classification of ischemic heart disease. Ischemic heart disease is divided into two broad categories: chronic coronary artery disease and acute coronary syndromes. Stable angina is the prototypical manifestation of chronic coronary artery disease. Acute coronary syndromes constitute a series (not necessarily a linear progression) of clinical presentations, including unstable angina, non-ST elevation myocardial infarction, and ST elevation myocardial infarction.

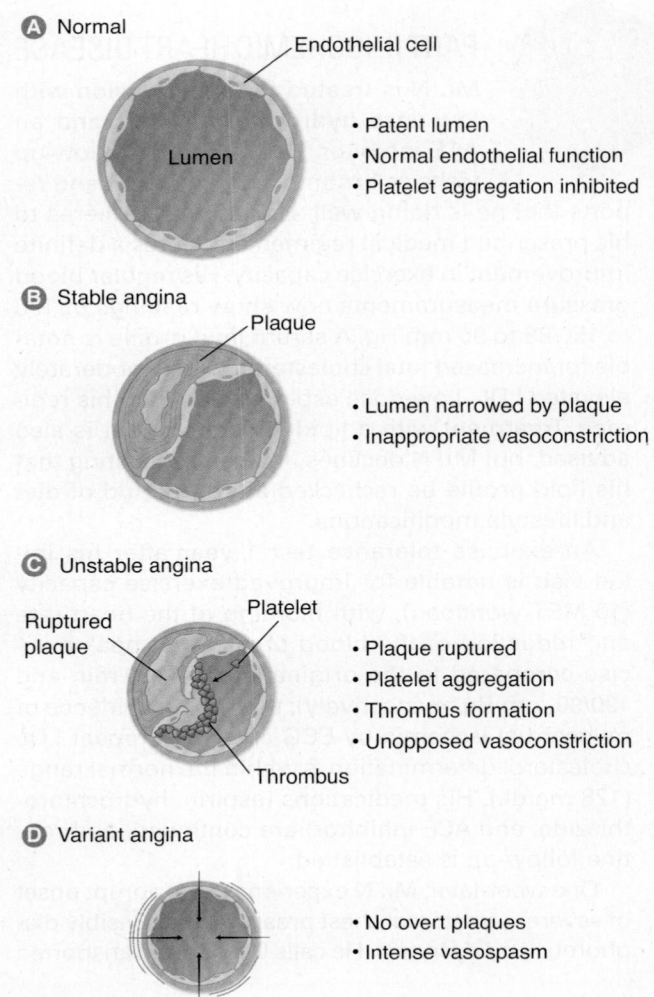

FIGURE 26-6. Pathophysiology of anginal syndromes. A. Normal coronary arteries are widely patent, the endothelium functions normally, and platelet aggregation is inhibited. **B.** In stable angina, atherosclerotic plaque and inappropriate vasoconstriction (caused by endothelial damage) reduce the vessel lumen diameter and hence decrease coronary blood flow. **C.** In unstable angina, rupture of the plaque triggers platelet aggregation, thrombus formation, and vasoconstriction. Depending on the anatomic site of plaque rupture, this process can progress to non-Q wave (non-ST elevation) or Q wave (ST elevation) myocardial infarction. **D.** In variant angina, atherosclerotic plaques are absent, and ischemia is caused by intense vasospasm.

Coronary Flow Reduction

The coronary vasculature is composed of two types of vessels: large, proximal epicardial vessels and small, distal endocardial vessels. The epicardial vessels are the more frequent sites of atheroma formation; in disease states, total coronary artery blood flow is limited by the extent of epicardial vessel stenosis. In comparison, endocardial vessels regulate intrinsic coronary vascular resistance in response to local metabolic changes. When myocardial oxygen demand is increased, endocardial vessels dilate in response to local metabolic factors, resulting in a regional increase in myocardial blood flow and thereby providing increased oxygen to these metabolically active tissues.

Angina pectoris (Fig. 26-6) is the principal clinical manifestation of chronic CAD. This symptom is characterized by precordial pressure-like discomfort resulting from myocardial ischemia. Most patients with chronic CAD experience **stable angina**, a clinical syndrome in which *ischemic chest pain occurs at characteristic and reproducible workloads* (e.g., walking up a flight of stairs). Pathologically, chronic CAD is associated with subintimal deposition of atheroma in the epicardial coronary arteries. In general, atherosclerotic plaques in patients with chronic stable angina are characterized by an overlying fibrous cap that is thick and resistant to disruption.

The immediate cause of angina pectoris is *an imbalance between myocardial oxygen supply and demand*. Under normal physiologic conditions, coronary blood flow is modulated carefully to ensure adequate tissue perfusion in response to varying levels of myocardial oxygen demand. This ability to modulate blood flow is referred to as the **coronary flow reserve**:

$$\text{CFR} = \text{maximal CBF/resting CBF}$$

where CFR is coronary flow reserve and CBF is coronary blood flow. In healthy individuals, the maximal CBF is approximately fivefold greater than the resting CBF.

Because of this wide safety margin, the resting CBF does not decrease until an epicardial stenosis exceeds 80–90% of the original arterial diameter. Changes in maximal CBF can be observed more readily with exercise, as maximal CBF begins to decrease during exercise when an epicardial stenosis exceeds 50–70% of the original arterial diameter. In patients with chronic CAD, the decrease in CFR is directly related to the severity of epicardial artery stenosis; the coronary flow reserve may be further impaired as a consequence of endothelial dysfunction (discussed below), resulting in a further reduction in CBF. Demand-related ischemia occurs during periods in which myocardial oxygen demand exceeds myocardial oxygen delivery, and the patient experiences angina pectoris.

The degree of epicardial artery stenosis and the degree of compensatory endocardial artery dilation determine the hemodynamic consequence of an atherosclerotic plaque (Fig. 26-7). If the endocardial arteries are normal, an epicardial stenosis that narrows the diameter of the arterial lumen by less than 50% does not significantly reduce maximal coronary blood flow. However, if the stenosis narrows the arterial lumen diameter by more than 80%, then the endocardial vessels must dilate to provide adequate perfusion to the myocardium, even at rest. The need for endocardial vessels to dilate at rest attenuates coronary flow reserve, because the endocardial vessels cannot then dilate further during exercise. This reduction in coronary flow reserve leads to inadequate myocardial blood flow during hyperemic stress. Myocardial ischemia can occur at rest when the epicardial artery stenosis exceeds 90% of the lumen diameter: under these conditions, endocardial vessels cannot maintain adequate myocardial perfusion even at maximal dilation.

Endothelial Dysfunction

Endothelial dysfunction is a general term for pathologic endothelial cell regulation. Clinically, endothelial dysfunction is manifested by abnormal vascular tone and prothrombotic properties.

Abnormal vascular tone is a result of dysregulated endothelial control of smooth muscle contraction: arterial beds with endothelial dysfunction cannot dilate in response to hyperemic stimuli. For example, when mental stress or physical exertion triggers activation of the sympathetic nervous system (SNS), two opposing forces act on the coronary vascular endothelium: catecholamine-mediated vasoconstriction and nitric oxide (NO)-mediated vasodilation. Normally, endothelial release of NO is stimulated by the shear stress on the

coronary vascular endothelium that results from increased blood flow. Eventually, the vasodilator effects of NO predominate over the vasoconstrictor effects of SNS activation, and the overall effect is coronary vasodilation. However, when the vascular endothelium is damaged, the production of endothelial vasodilators is decreased and catecholamine-mediated vasoconstriction predominates.

Because the endothelium also plays a crucial role in regulating platelet activation and the coagulation cascade, endothelial dysfunction can promote blood coagulation (thrombosis) at the site of endothelial injury. Endothelial-derived NO and prostacyclin exert significant antiplatelet effects, and molecules on the surface of healthy endothelial cells have significant anticoagulant properties (see Chapter 23, Pharmacology of Hemostasis and Thrombosis). Endothelial damage decreases the ability of the endothelium to utilize these endogenous antiplatelet and anticoagulant mechanisms, leading to a local predominance of procoagulant factors and increasing the likelihood of platelet and coagulation factor activation.

Acute Coronary Syndromes

Acute coronary syndromes (ACS) are most often caused by the fissuring or rupture of atherosclerotic plaques. These so-called **unstable** or **vulnerable plaques** are characterized by thin fibrous caps that are prone to rupture. Plaque rupture results in the exposure of procoagulant factors, such as subendothelial collagen (Fig. 26-8), that activate platelets and the coagulation cascade. Under physiologic circumstances, hemostasis at a site of vascular injury is self-limited by endogenous anticoagulant mechanisms (see Chapter 23). However, the dysfunctional endothelium overlying the atherosclerotic plaque cannot elaborate sufficient anticoagulant factors to control the extent of clot formation. Dysregulated coagulation can then result in intraluminal thrombus formation, which leads to myocardial ischemia and potentially to irreversible myocardial injury.

The three subtypes of acute coronary syndromes are unstable angina, non-ST elevation MI, and ST elevation MI. In **unstable angina**, patients experience either acceleration in the frequency or severity of chest pain, new-onset anginal pain, or characteristic anginal chest pain that abruptly occurs at rest. Enzymatic evidence of tissue infarction (e.g., elevated troponin levels) is absent in unstable angina, but patients are at high risk for MI because of the presence of an active prothrombotic surface at the site of plaque rupture.

Non-ST elevation myocardial infarction occurs when an unstable plaque abruptly ruptures and significantly compromises (but does not completely occlude) the lumen of an epicardial coronary artery. Because the artery is partially occluded and there is a persistent prothrombotic surface at the site of plaque rupture, patients with non-ST elevation MI are at high risk for recurrence of ischemia. The pathophysiology and clinical management of unstable angina and non-ST elevation MI are very similar, and these two syndromes are often referred to by the combined acronym **unstable angina/non-ST elevation MI** (**UA/NSTEMI**).

If the intraluminal thrombus completely occludes the epicardial coronary artery at the site of plaque rupture, then blood flow ceases downstream from the locus of obstruction. Persistent, total epicardial artery occlusion provides the substrate for acute myocardial injury (**ST elevation myocardial infarction**; **STEMI**), which progresses inexorably to transmural

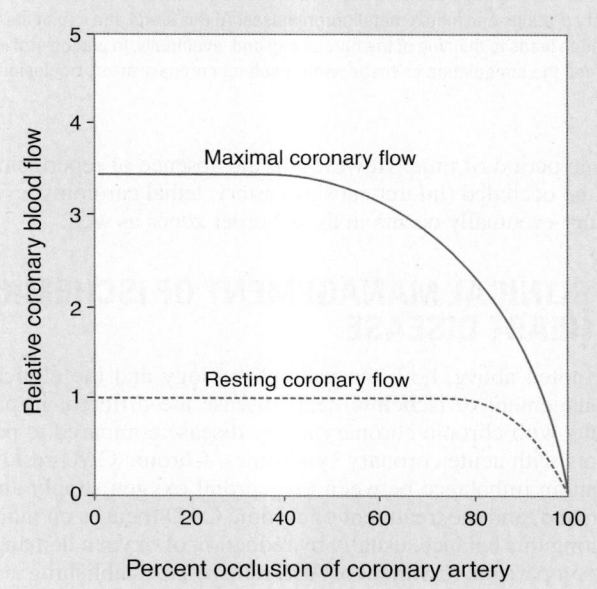

FIGURE 26-7. Effect of coronary artery occlusion on resting and maximal coronary blood flow. The *dotted line* depicts resting coronary blood flow, and the *solid line* represents maximal blood flow when there is full dilation of distal coronary arteries. Comparison of these two lines shows that maximal coronary blood flow is compromised when the lesion occludes more than about 50% of the arterial lumen, whereas resting coronary blood flow is relatively unaffected until the lesion exceeds about 80% of the arterial diameter. The y-axis represents coronary artery blood flow relative to the flow in a resting coronary artery with 0% occlusion.

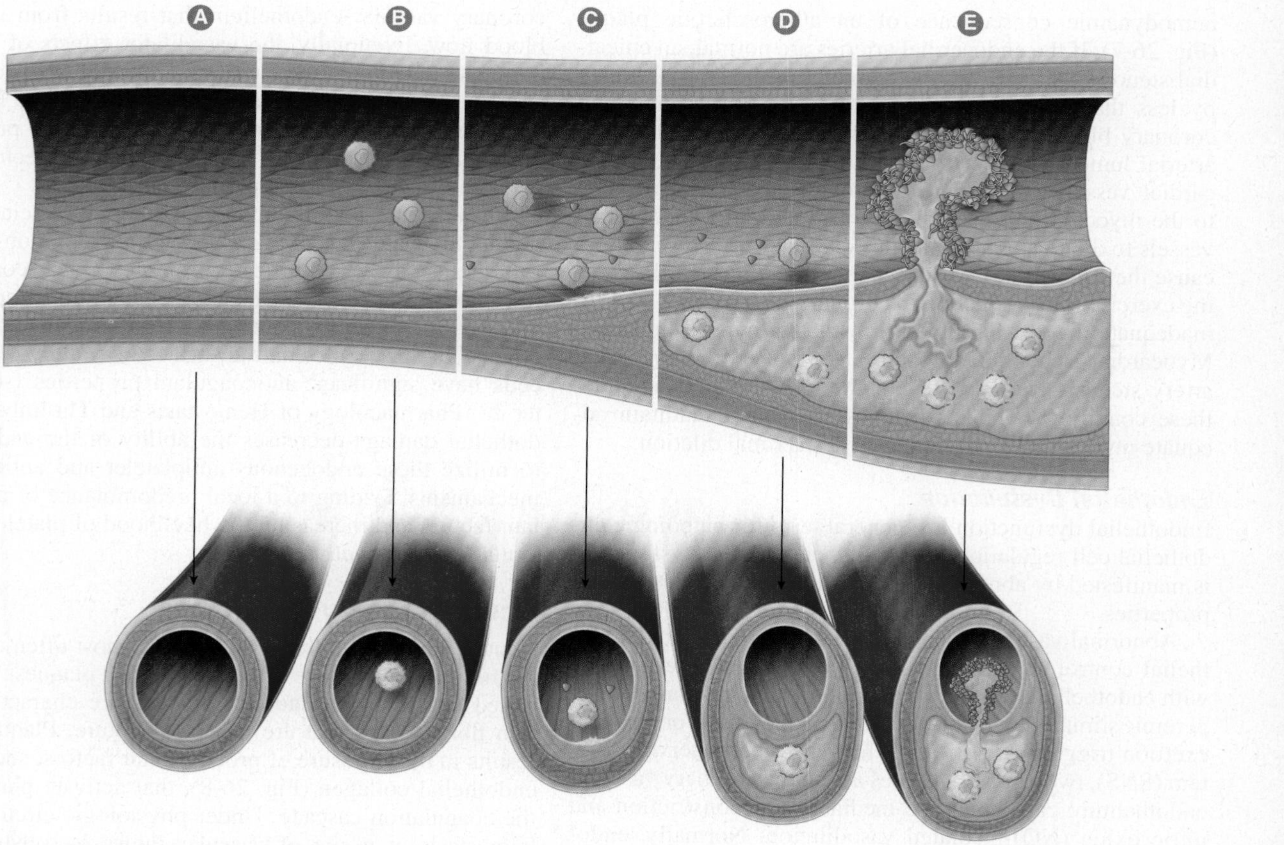

FIGURE 26-8. Pathogenesis of acute coronary syndromes. A. A normal coronary artery has an intact endothelium surrounded by smooth muscle cells. **B.** Endothelial cell activation or injury recruits monocytes and T lymphocytes to the site of injury, leading to development of a fatty streak. **C.** Continued oxidative stress within a fatty streak leads to development of an atherosclerotic plaque. **D.** Macrophage apoptosis and continued cholesterol deposition cause further plaque organization and may induce the expression of additional inflammatory proteins and matrix metalloproteinases. At this stage, the cap of the fibroatheroma remains intact. **E.** Continued inflammation within an atherosclerotic plaque leads to thinning of the fibrous cap and, eventually, to plaque erosion or rupture. Exposure of plaque constituents to the bloodstream activates platelets and the coagulation cascade, with resulting coronary artery occlusion.

infarction unless perfusion is reestablished. This clinical syndrome can also present as out-of-hospital **sudden cardiac death** (~30% of patients); in these cases, death is usually caused by ischemia-induced electrical instability of the myocardium. In the absence of fatal electrical instability, ST elevation MI typically presents with unremitting chest pain that is often accompanied by dyspnea and ischemic left heart failure. *Mortality in STEMI is significantly reduced by prompt relief of the complete epicardial obstruction. Therefore, the principal management goal in STEMI is expeditious reperfusion of the occluded artery.*

The extent of myocardial necrosis after ischemic injury depends on the mass of myocardium supplied by the occluded artery, the amount of time over which the artery is totally occluded, and the degree of collateral circulation. Regions of the myocardium that are supplied directly and exclusively by the occluded artery sustain extensive ischemic injury. Cell death occurs in a "wavefront" that progresses both spatially and temporally from the subendocardial region to the epicardial surface of the myocardium. As a result, the extent of "transmurality" of an MI bears a direct relationship to the duration of coronary artery occlusion. Adjacent to the region of transmural necrosis, a border zone of myocardium receives nutrients and oxygen from collateral vessels; this collateral perfusion can maintain the viability of border zone cells for

some period of time. However, in the absence of reperfusion of the occluded (infarct-causing) artery, lethal cardiomyocyte injury eventually occurs in these border zones as well.

CLINICAL MANAGEMENT OF ISCHEMIC HEART DISEASE

As noted above, both the pathophysiology and the clinical management of ischemic heart disease are different in patients with chronic coronary artery disease compared to patients with acute coronary syndromes. Chronic CAD results from an imbalance between myocardial oxygen supply and demand, and the treatment of chronic CAD focuses on modulating this balance, usually by reduction of oxygen demand. In comparison, treatment of ACS relies on reestablishing and maintaining the patency of the occluded epicardial coronary artery as rapidly as possible. All patients with CAD, irrespective of clinical presentation, also require modification of underlying risk factors, including aggressive lipid-lowering therapy and blood pressure control.

Chronic Coronary Artery Disease

The treatment goal in chronic CAD is to restore the balance between myocardial oxygen supply (coronary artery blood flow) and myocardial oxygen demand (myocardial oxygen consumption). *Pharmacologic therapies concentrate on the reduction of myocardial oxygen demand*, which is governed by heart rate, contractility, and ventricular wall stress (see Chapter 22). Antianginal drugs can be categorized on the basis of their impact on these parameters.

β-Adrenoceptor Antagonists

Activation of β_1-adrenergic receptors by the sympathoadrenal system leads to an increase in heart rate, contractility, and conduction through the AV node. It follows that antagonists acting at β_1-adrenergic receptors decrease sinus rate, reduce inotropic state, and slow AV nodal conduction.

β_1-Adrenoceptor antagonists (also referred to as *β-blockers*) are the cornerstone of medical treatment regimens in patients with chronic stable angina. *β-Antagonists reduce myocardial oxygen demand by decreasing heart rate and contractility*, and the drug-induced decrease in heart rate may also increase myocardial perfusion via prolongation of the diastolic filling time. When used in chronic angina, β-antagonists decrease both the resting heart rate and the peak heart rate achieved during exercise and delay the time to onset of angina. Dosing regimens for β-antagonists are drug-specific, reflecting the characteristic pharmacokinetics of each individual agent. As a general rule, the dose of drug is calibrated to maintain the resting heart rate at approximately 50 beats/min and to maintain the peak heart rate during exertion at approximately 110 to 120 beats/min.

β-Antagonists are frequently co-administered with organic nitrates in patients with stable angina. This combination is often more effective than either agent used alone. β-Antagonists are also frequently combined with CCBs—typically, with agents of the dihydropyridine class (see below). (In early clinical trials, short-acting formulations of the dihydropyridine CCB nifedipine were associated with reflex tachycardia when administered as monotherapy; this tachycardia was attenuated when nifedipine was co-administered with a β-antagonist. In current practice, the availability of long-acting dihydropyridine agents has effectively diminished this adverse effect.)

Although β-antagonists are generally well tolerated in patients with stable angina, certain clinical scenarios require caution. Combining β-antagonists with CCBs of the nondihydropyridine classes (e.g., diltiazem or verapamil) can result in synergistic suppression of SA-node automaticity (leading to extreme sinus bradycardia) and/or AV-node conduction (leading to high-grade AV conduction block). Likewise, because of their depressant effects on nodal tissues, β-antagonists may exacerbate preexisting bradycardia and/or high-grade AV block. However, given the clear and consistent mortality benefit associated with β-antagonists in secondary prevention trials, it is currently standard clinical practice to implant a permanent transvenous pacing device if such rhythm abnormalities are the major contraindication to the use of β-antagonists and then to administer the β-antagonist. (**Secondary prevention trials** test the efficacy of pharmacologic interventions to reduce adverse cardiovascular events *in patients with known CAD*.)

β-Antagonists are now also used in patients with clinically stable heart failure (see the following discussion). It must be emphasized that the survival benefit demonstrated in HF treatment trials occurred when these agents were initiated during periods of clinical stability. *β-Antagonists must not be administered to patients with decompensated HF.*

When used in an attempt to treat the rare patient with pure vasospastic or **variant angina** (i.e., angina in the absence of epicardial artery obstruction; see Fig. 26-6), β-antagonists can *induce coronary vasospasm* as a consequence of unopposed α-receptor-mediated vasoconstriction. β-Antagonists can also exacerbate bronchospasm in patients with asthma and chronic airway obstruction. However, in such patients, the decision to avoid β-antagonists should be based on objective documentation of exacerbation of airflow obstruction during β-antagonist therapy. Peripheral vascular disease is another relative contraindication to β-antagonist therapy; the concern in this circumstance is the potential for antagonism of the β_2-adrenergic receptors that mediate dilation of peripheral vessels. In clinical practice, however, this concern is rarely justified. Furthermore, patients with peripheral arterial disease have an extremely high risk of concomitant CAD and are therefore likely to benefit significantly from β-antagonist therapy.

Common adverse effects of β-antagonists include fatigue, lethargy, insomnia, and impotence. Although the precise mechanism of fatigue is unclear, decreased exercise capacity is directly related to drug-induced blunting of the physiologic tachycardia of exertion. The impotence reported by 1% of patients treated with β-antagonists is due to inhibition of β_2-adrenoceptor-mediated peripheral vasodilation.

Ca²⁺ Channel Blockers

Calcium channel blockers (CCBs) decrease the influx of calcium through voltage-gated L-type calcium channels in the plasma membrane. The resulting decrease in intracellular calcium concentration leads to reduced contraction of both cardiac myocytes and vascular smooth muscle cells (see Chapter 22).

Calcium channel blockers decrease myocardial oxygen demand and may also increase myocardial oxygen supply. *Calcium channel blockers decrease myocardial oxygen demand by decreasing systemic vascular resistance and by decreasing cardiac contractility.* In the periphery, calcium entry into vascular smooth muscle cells is required for contraction of the cells and is therefore a central determinant of resting vasomotor tone. By blocking calcium entry, CCBs cause relaxation of vascular smooth muscle and thereby reduce systemic vascular resistance. Calcium channel blockers can theoretically increase myocardial oxygen supply by blocking calcium-mediated increases in coronary vasomotor tone; the resulting dilation of epicardial vessels and arteriolar resistance vessels would, in theory, increase coronary blood flow. However, the contribution of this coronary vasodilator mechanism to the clinical effects of the CCBs is controversial, because regional metabolic abnormalities that result from myocardial ischemia should effect a maximal vasodilator response in the absence of pharmacologic modulation.

The various classes of calcium channel blockers have distinctive inotropic effects on cardiac myocytes. Compared to verapamil and diltiazem, dihydropyridines (such as nifedipine) are more selective for calcium channels in the peripheral vasculature. Nonetheless, all CCBs do have the potential to impair contractile function by reducing intracellular calcium levels in cardiac myocytes. Therefore, decompensated heart failure is a contraindication to the use of certain CCBs because of their negative inotropic effects. However, newer generation vasoselective dihydropyridines, such as amlodipine and felodipine, are typically tolerated by patients with reduced LV ejection fractions and can therefore be administered to patients with LV dysfunction and refractory angina.

Calcium channel blockers are reported to be as effective as β-antagonists in the treatment of chronic stable angina. If the initial treatment of angina with β-antagonists alone is not successful, CCBs can be used either in combination with β-antagonists or as monotherapy. Calcium channel blockers appear to produce a greater antianginal effect when co-administered with β-antagonists than when administered alone, although combination therapy can induce bradyarrhythmias (see above). Despite the proven efficacy of CCBs in reducing symptoms in patients with chronic CAD, there are no data to support a mortality benefit associated with CCB therapy in either primary or secondary prevention in patients with CAD.

Unlike β-antagonists, *CCBs can be effective in the treatment of vasospastic angina.* Calcium channel blockers relieve the vasospasm of coronary vessels by dilating both epicardial coronary arteries and arteriolar resistance vessels. It is common practice to use nitrates in combination with CCBs when treating vasospastic angina.

Nitrates

Organic nitrates exert their principal therapeutic effect by dilation of peripheral capacitance veins, thereby decreasing preload and reducing myocardial oxygen demand (see Chapter 22). Some investigators argue that nitrates also increase myocardial blood flow by reducing coronary vasomotor tone, although the magnitude of the incremental vasodilator effect is debated in patients with regional myocardial ischemia. Nitrates do have a coronary vasodilator effect in patients with vasospastic angina. Nitrates also have anti-aggregatory effects on platelets.

In patients with *stable exertional angina*, nitrates improve exercise tolerance when used as monotherapy and act synergistically with β-antagonists or CCBs. Sublingual nitroglycerin tablets or nitroglycerin sprays are effective for immediate relief of exertional angina. Provided that sufficient nitrate-free intervals are allowed to attenuate the development of tolerance, long-acting nitrates (e.g., isosorbide dinitrate and mononitrate) are also effective for prophylaxis and treatment of exertional angina.

Nitrates are also effective in the treatment of both acute and chronic LV failure. This treatment effect is related to the powerful venodilator action of the nitrates, which causes peripheral redistribution of intravascular volume and marked reduction of preload. The anti-ischemic effect of nitrates may be of particular benefit in patients with ischemia-related diastolic dysfunction. In this clinical setting, nitrates may effect both preload reduction and restoration of normal diastolic chamber compliance and filling.

The development of tolerance is the major obstacle to long-term use of nitrates. Through uncertain mechanisms (see Chapter 22), tolerance develops to both vasodilator and antiplatelet effects of these drugs. Dosing regimens that are punctuated by sufficiently long nitrate-free intervals (8–12 hours) may prevent nitrate tolerance. Headache, the most common adverse effect of nitrate therapy, can develop as a result of cerebral vessel dilation.

Aspirin

Platelet activation is critically important in the initiation of thrombus formation (see Chapter 23), and antiplatelet agents play a central role in the treatment of patients with CAD. Aspirin irreversibly inhibits platelet cyclooxygenase, an enzyme required for generation of the pro-aggregatory compound thromboxane A_2 (TxA_2). Therefore, the platelet inhibition that follows aspirin administration persists for the lifespan of the platelet (approximately 10 days).

Unless specific contraindications are present, aspirin is an essential therapy for patients with chronic CAD. Aspirin is used to prevent arterial thrombosis leading to MI, transient ischemic attack, and stroke. *Aspirin is most effective as a selective antiplatelet agent when taken at low doses and/ or infrequent intervals* (see Chapter 23). Clinical data have demonstrated a significant treatment benefit for aspirin in patients with unstable angina (~50% reduction in death and nonfatal MI). Aspirin is contraindicated in patients with a known allergy to the drug; in this setting, clopidogrel is indicated as an alternative. Aspirin and other antiplatelet agents should be used cautiously in patients with compromised liver function, because such patients may have a bleeding diathesis due to decreased circulating levels of hepatically synthesized coagulation factors. Aspirin use also predisposes to gastrointestinal adverse effects such as gastritis and peptic ulcer disease; these effects can often be alleviated by co-administration of agents that decrease gastric acid production (see Chapter 47, Integrative Inflammation Pharmacology: Peptic Ulcer Disease).

Lipid-Lowering Agents

Clinical studies indicate that, in patients with known CAD, the administration of drugs that lower serum LDL cholesterol decreases the risk of ischemic cardiovascular events. (Refer to Chapter 20, Pharmacology of Cholesterol and Lipoprotein Metabolism, for a detailed discussion of lipid-lowering agents.) The selection of a specific lipid-lowering agent is based on both clinical trial data and the patient's lipid phenotype.

HMG-CoA reductase inhibitors (statins) are the most frequently used and best-studied lipid-lowering agents. Because HMG-CoA reductase mediates the first committed step in sterol biosynthesis, inhibitors of HMG-CoA reductase dramatically reduce the extent of hepatic cholesterol synthesis. This reduction in cholesterol synthesis results in increased hepatic LDL receptor expression and thereby increases clearance of cholesterol-containing lipoprotein particles from the bloodstream. Clinical trials (e.g., the Scandinavian Simvastatin Survival Study and the Cholesterol and Recurrent Events Study) demonstrate that lipid-lowering therapy reduces cardiovascular event rates in patients with CAD. All patients with a myocardial infarction should be treated with a statin, with goal LDL cholesterol targets of 70 mg/dL or lower (note that current guidelines do not specify exact target values). Dietary and other lifestyle modifications should also be included as part of a comprehensive approach to primary and secondary prevention. HMG-CoA reductase inhibitors are contraindicated in women who are or may become pregnant or who are nursing.

Metabolic Modulators

Some patients with stable angina continue to experience frequent angina despite maximal attempts at medical management and revascularization. In these cases, metabolic modulators that increase the efficiency of ATP utilization may be clinically useful. In this class of drugs, **ranolazine** is approved for the second-line treatment of refractory angina (i.e., angina that occurs despite otherwise maximal therapy).

Clinical trials of ranolazine in stable angina have demonstrated improved effort tolerance and decreased frequency of anginal symptoms relative to placebo. There may also be gender-specific effects, with women deriving greater benefit from ranolazine than men. Other metabolic modulators remain an active area of investigation and drug development.

Unstable Angina and Non-ST Elevation Myocardial Infarction

Unstable angina (UA) and non-ST elevation myocardial infarction (NSTEMI) may occur as the first presentation of CAD or in patients with a history of stable CAD. (In the latter circumstance, management strategies appropriate for unstable angina take precedence over those for stable CAD.) It is estimated that, in the absence of treatment, patients with

UA have a 15–20% risk of progression to acute MI over a period of 4–6 weeks. Aggressive treatment can reduce this risk by more than 50%. Patients with UA have no overt evidence of myocardial damage, whereas patients with NSTEMI have elevated biomarkers that reflect cardiomyocte necrosis. Untreated UA may progress to NSTEMI, or NSTEMI may be the initial result of plaque rupture with extensive inflammation and coagulation at the rupture site.

Goals of treatment in UA/NSTEMI are to relieve ischemic symptoms and to prevent additional thrombus formation at the site of plaque rupture. UA/NSTEMI is typically treated with aspirin, heparin, and β-antagonists. Other antiplatelet agents (GPIIb–IIIa antagonists and ADP receptor antagonists) and/or direct thrombin inhibitors (bivalirudin) are indicated in high-risk patients to prevent additional thrombus formation (Fig. 26-9). Although conventional

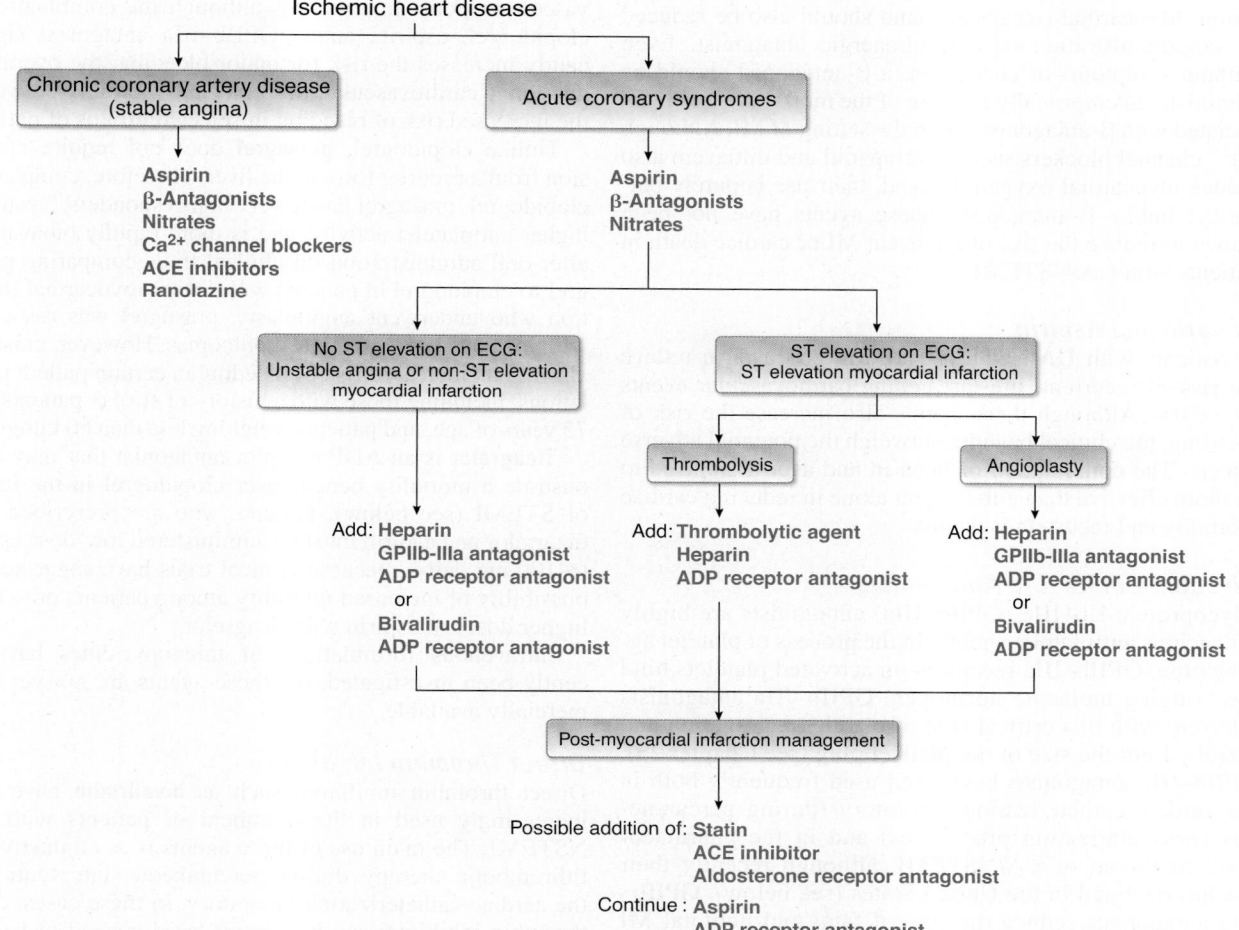

FIGURE 26-9. Pharmacologic management of acute coronary syndromes. All patients with chronic coronary artery disease are given aspirin unless a life-threatening contraindication is present. β-Antagonists, nitrates, calcium channel blockers, ACE inhibitors, and ranolazine are primarily used to reduce myocardial oxygen demand. All patients with symptoms that raise concerns about a possible acute coronary syndrome are given aspirin and, if tolerated, a β-antagonist. Sublingual or intravenous nitrates can also be administered to relieve chest discomfort and minimize ischemia. Electrocardiographic (ECG) findings of ST elevation should prompt emergency measures to open the occluded artery, either with a thrombolytic agent (thrombolysis) or mechanical revascularization (angioplasty). Additional adjunctive pharmacologic therapies for ST elevation myocardial infarction may include aspirin, β-antagonists, nitrates, heparin, ADP receptor antagonists, and GPIIb–IIIa antagonists or bivalirudin. For patients with acute coronary syndrome but no ST elevation on the electrocardiogram, laboratory assays of myocyte damage (e.g., troponin I or troponin T) determine whether the patient is classified as experiencing unstable angina or non-ST elevation myocardial infarction. In either case, management generally includes administration of aspirin, β-antagonists, nitrates, ADP receptor antagonists, and bivalirudin or heparin with GPIIb–IIIa antagonists. For all patients with acute coronary syndrome, postmyocardial infarction management should include modification of risk factors; possible addition of lipid-lowering agents (statins), ACE inhibitors, and aldosterone receptor antagonists; and continuation of aspirin and ADP receptor antagonists.

antianginal drugs have no demonstrable impact on mortality in UA/NSTEMI, these "demand-based" agents are also used empirically for symptom relief.

Thrombolytic agents are contraindicated in patients with UA/NSTEMI: use of these agents in UA/NSTEMI has been associated with a significant increase in morbidity and a trend toward increased mortality. If ischemic chest discomfort recurs after initiation of treatment, or if a patient presents with certain high-risk features, urgent coronary angiography is warranted (with revascularization guided by the angiographic data).

Antianginal Drugs

Intravenous nitroglycerin is often administered for the first 24 hours after the onset of UA/NSTEMI. The intravenous formulation is used to achieve and maintain predictable blood levels of the drug. After 24 hours, the asymptomatic patient can be switched to a long-acting oral nitrate preparation. Myocardial oxygen demand should also be reduced by co-administration of a β-adrenergic antagonist. Even without symptoms of chest pain, a β-antagonist should be administered empirically because of the mortality benefit associated with β-antagonist use in the setting of MI. Although Ca^{2+} channel blockers such as verapamil and diltiazem also reduce myocardial oxygen demand, their use is purely palliative; unlike β-antagonists, these agents have not been shown to reduce the risk of recurrent MI or cardiac death in patients with UA/NSTEMI.

Heparin and Aspirin

In patients with UA/NSTEMI, heparin and aspirin reduce the risk of recurrent, life-threatening cardiovascular events by ~50%. Although these agents also increase the risk of bleeding, the clinical benefits outweigh the potential adverse effects. The combination of heparin and aspirin appears to be more effective than either agent alone in reducing cardiac mortality and recurrent ischemia.

Glycoprotein IIb–IIIa Antagonists

Glycoprotein IIb–IIIa (GPIIb–IIIa) antagonists are highly efficacious antiplatelet agents. In the process of platelet aggregation, GPIIb–IIIa receptors on activated platelets bind the bridging molecule fibrinogen. GPIIb–IIIa antagonists interfere with this critical step of platelet aggregation and thereby limit the size of the platelet plug (see Chapter 23). GPIIb–IIIa antagonists have been used frequently both in the cardiac catheterization laboratory (during percutaneous revascularization procedures) and in the pharmacologic treatment of UA/NSTEMI, although recently their use has declined in the United States (see below). GPIIb–IIIa antagonists reduce the risk of fatal and nonfatal MI in patients with UA, and these agents reduce the risk of recurrent MI and urgent revascularization in patients with NSTEMI. In UA/NSTEMI patients with ongoing ischemia or certain high-risk features, a GPIIb–IIIa antagonist may be administered in addition to aspirin and heparin; both eptifibatide and tirofiban have been approved for this use. The use of abciximab has been restricted largely to the periprocedural setting (i.e., in preparation for and immediately following percutaneous coronary intervention). Studies have shown that GPIIb–IIIa antagonist use is associated with increased bleeding outcomes compared to the use of direct thrombin inhibitors such as bivalirudin; consequently, the use of the GPIIb–IIIa antagonists has waned recently.

ADP Receptor Antagonists

Antagonists at the platelet ADP receptor P2Y$_{12}$ are used in the treatment of many patients with ACS. The thienopyridines **clopidogrel**, **prasugrel**, and the rarely used **ticlopidine** are irreversible ADP receptor antagonists. **Ticagrelor** is a reversible P2Y$_{12}$ antagonist that is also used in the treatment of patients with acute coronary syndromes. Because these are all powerful antiplatelet agents, ADP receptor antagonists are routinely used in the setting of ACS. **Clopidogrel** is indicated in all patients with ACS who have true aspirin allergy. Clopidogrel reduces recurrent coronary events in patients with UA/NSTEMI who undergo percutaneous coronary intervention and in patients with UA/NSTEMI who are treated with a noninvasive approach (e.g., patients who do not undergo cardiac catheterization and target-vessel revascularization). Importantly, although the combination of clopidogrel, aspirin, and a GPIIb–IIIa antagonist significantly increases the risk for major bleeding, the overall reduction in cardiovascular morbidity and mortality outweighs the increased risk of bleeding in selected groups of patients.

Unlike clopidogrel, **prasugrel** does not require conversion from a prodrug form in the liver. Therefore, compared to clopidogrel, prasugrel has fewer "non-responders," results in higher antiplatelet activity, and is more rapidly bioavailable after oral administration. In clinical trials comparing prasugrel to clopidogrel in patients with recent myocardial infarction who underwent angioplasty, prasugrel was associated with improved overall clinical outcomes. However, prasugrel also has an increased risk of bleeding in certain patient populations, including those with a history of stroke, patients over 75 years of age, and patients weighing less than 60 kilograms.

Ticagrelor is an ADP receptor antagonist that may demonstrate a mortality benefit over clopidogrel in the setting of STEMI (see below). Patients who are prescribed both ticagrelor and aspirin must be administered low-dose aspirin (≤100 mg daily), because clinical trials have suggested the possibility of increased mortality among patients prescribed higher doses of aspirin with ticagrelor.

Intravenous formulations of thienopyridines have recently been investigated, but these agents are not yet commercially available.

Direct Thrombin Inhibitors

Direct thrombin inhibitors such as **bivalirudin** have been increasingly used in the treatment of patients with UA/NSTEMI. The main use of these agents is as adjunctive antithrombotic therapy during percutaneous intervention in the cardiac catheterization laboratory. In these cases, direct thrombin inhibitors can be administered instead of heparin and a GPIIb–IIIa antagonist. Compared to the dual use of heparin and a GPIIb–IIIa antagonist, the administration of a direct thrombin inhibitor for this indication may result in fewer adverse bleeding events, although compared to heparin alone, there may be clinical equipoise.

ST Elevation Myocardial Infarction

The treatment of STEMI is aimed at expeditious reperfusion of the occluded epicardial coronary artery. As with UA/NSTEMI, aspirin and heparin are standards of care for STEMI; used alone, however, these agents are often not sufficient to recanalize an occluded coronary artery (Fig. 26-9). Two approaches are used to open an occluded coronary artery: pharmacologic (thrombolysis) and mechanical (angioplasty or emergency coronary artery bypass). When thrombolysis is used, clopidogrel co-administration increases the likelihood that the infarct vessel will remain patent. GPIIb–IIIa antagonists are not utilized with thrombolytics because this combination confers a significantly increased risk of bleeding, including hemorrhagic stroke. When angioplasty is performed, a GPIIb–IIIa antagonist may be employed together with clopidogrel as adjunctive treatment.

Thrombolytics

Four thrombolytic agents are currently used in the pharmacologic management of STEMI: streptokinase, alteplase, tenecteplase, and reteplase. (All are discussed in greater detail in Chapter 23.) The timeliness of administration is a crucial factor in determining the success of thrombolytic therapy in acute MI. *Patients who receive thrombolytic therapy within 2 hours of the onset of symptoms have a twofold improvement in survival rate compared to patients who receive thrombolytic therapy more than 6 hours after the onset of symptoms.* This observation is consistent with the known relationship between the duration of vessel occlusion and the extent of infarction. Several important contraindications to thrombolysis, primarily related to increased bleeding risk, may also limit use of this intervention.

Streptokinase

The pharmacologic action of streptokinase involves two steps: complexation and cleavage. In the complexation reaction, streptokinase forms a stable, noncovalent 1:1 complex with plasminogen (either free plasminogen or fibrin-bound plasminogen). The complexation reaction produces a conformational change that exposes the active site on plasminogen. Plasminogen, now with its active site exposed, can effect proteolytic cleavage of *other* plasminogen molecules (again, either free plasminogen or fibrin-bound plasminogen) to plasmin and thereby initiate thrombolysis.

In the treatment of STEMI, streptokinase is administered as an intravenous loading dose followed by a continuous intravenous infusion. After 90 minutes of administration, streptokinase produces reperfusion in 60% of acutely occluded vessels. However, the usefulness of streptokinase is limited by two factors. First, streptokinase is a foreign protein that is capable of eliciting antigenic reactions upon repeated administration. Patients with antibodies against streptokinase (from either a previous streptococcal infection or previous treatment with streptokinase) can develop an allergic reaction and fever. Second, because the streptokinase:plasminogen complex activates both fibrin-bound and free plasminogen molecules, its relatively nonspecific antithrombotic activity can result in systemic fibrinolysis.

Alteplase

Alteplase is the generic name for recombinant tissue plasminogen activator (t-PA). Alteplase is effective in restoring the patency of occluded coronary arteries, limiting cardiac dysfunction, and reducing mortality following STEMI. As with endogenously produced t-PA, recombinant t-PA binds to newly formed thrombi with high affinity, causing fibrinolysis at the site of a thrombus. Once bound to the nascent thrombus, t-PA undergoes a conformational change that enhances plasminogen activation. t-PA is a poor activator of plasminogen in the absence of fibrin binding.

Recombinant t-PA is typically administered intravenously at a high dose rate for 1 hour and then at a lower dose rate for the next 2 hours. Despite its high affinity for fibrin-bound plasminogen, recombinant t-PA at pharmacologic doses can generate a systemic lytic state (as can other thrombolytic agents) and cause undesirable bleeding, including cerebral hemorrhage. Thus, this agent is contraindicated in patients who have had a recent stroke or other major bleeding event.

Tenecteplase

Tenecteplase is a genetically engineered variant of t-PA. The molecular modifications in tenecteplase increase its fibrin specificity relative to t-PA and make it more resistant to plasminogen activator inhibitor 1. Large trials have shown that tenecteplase is identical in efficacy to t-PA, with similar (and possibly decreased) risk of bleeding. Additionally, tenecteplase has a longer half-life than t-PA. This pharmacokinetic property allows tenecteplase to be administered as a single, weight-based bolus, thus simplifying administration.

Reteplase

Similar to tenecteplase, **reteplase** is a genetically engineered variant of t-PA with increased half-life and increased specificity for fibrin relative to t-PA. Its efficacy and adverse effect profile are similar to those of t-PA. Because of its longer half-life, reteplase can be administered as a "double bolus" (two boluses, 30 minutes apart).

Primary Percutaneous Intervention

In the United States, the majority of patients with STEMI are treated with thrombolytics. Multiple studies have shown, however, that primary angioplasty, if performed within 90 minutes of presentation to the emergency department, yields a mortality benefit compared to thrombolysis. Increasingly, primary angioplasty includes placement of a **drug-eluting stent**. The four currently approved devices consist of a stainless steel or cobalt chromium alloy stent coated with **sirolimus**, **everolimus**, **zotarolimus**, or **paclitaxel**. Each of these agents decreases early restenosis by interrupting cell cycle progression (see Chapter 46, Pharmacology of Immunosuppression). Although drug-eluting stents were originally approved for the treatment of stable coronary artery disease, these devices are now often used in the treatment of acute coronary syndromes. Recent evidence has suggested that patients with drug-eluting stents may be at increased risk for late stent thrombosis (i.e., thrombosis occurring within the stent more than 30 days after initial stent placement), and dual antiplatelet therapy with aspirin and an ADP receptor antagonist for up to 1 year is indicated to prevent this complication in such patients.

Postmyocardial Infarction Management

Patients must be carefully managed after an MI to prevent reinfarction. The goals of any post-MI medical regimen are twofold: (1) to prevent and treat residual ischemia and (2) to identify and treat major risk factors such as hypertension, smoking, hyperlipidemia, and diabetes. Because the extent of the MI and its functional consequences vary greatly among patients, the medical regimen must be individualized. The American College of Cardiology and the American

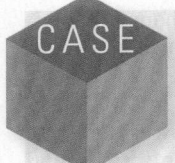

PART III: HEART FAILURE

Mr. N is discharged from the hospital on a multidrug regimen that includes aspirin, clopidogrel, metoprolol, atorvastatin, lisinopril, and eplerenone. He does well as he increases his activity level during the first 4–6 weeks after the infarction. At that point, however, he once again experiences breathlessness at moderate levels of exertion. He initially attributes this to deconditioning, but he becomes concerned early one morning when he awakens from sleep with severe breathlessness. He schedules an appointment with his physician for later that day.

On examination in the physician's office, Mr. N appears comfortable seated in the upright position. His heart rate is 64 beats/min, and his blood pressure is 168/100 mm Hg. The pulmonic component of S2 is prominent (representing a change from his previous exams), and the apical S4 is again noted; there is a grade III/VI apical holosystolic murmur with radiation to the left axilla. An echocardiogram reveals akinesis of the basal segment of the inferior wall of the left ventricle, with prominent thinning and aneurysmal remodeling of the segment. The LV ejection fraction is again quantified at 40%. Although the mitral valve leaflets and the supporting structures of the valve appear structurally normal, there is a degree of posterior leaflet prolapse (LV → LA) during ventricular systole. A Doppler study confirms the presence of mitral regurgitation

that is at least moderate in severity. The right ventricle is dilated and hypertrophic, with relative preservation of systolic function. Repeat catheterization is performed to assess the etiology of the patient's new biventricular heart failure. Angiography shows wide patency of the right coronary artery at the site of the previous percutaneous coronary intervention, and the left coronary system is free of obstruction. Hemodynamic data demonstrate increased pulmonary artery and right ventricular pressures as well as an elevated pulmonary capillary wedge pressure.

Mr. N is prescribed oral furosemide at a sufficient dose that he loses approximately 5 pounds in the next 3 days. Because his blood pressure remains elevated despite near maximal doses of lisinopril and metoprolol, he is also prescribed candesartan. Over the course of the next week, Mr. N notes an improvement in his exercise tolerance. He checks his weight frequently and, if it increases by more than 2 pounds above his usual level, he takes an extra dose of furosemide.

Questions

7. How does the addition of furosemide improve Mr. N's symptoms?

8. Which drug interactions are of concern when Mr. N adds candesartan to his regimen?

9. Which parenteral inotropic agents would be available if Mr. N's heart failure were to decompensate acutely?

Heart Association have made the following general recommendations for the management of post-MI patients:

1. Aspirin (75–325 mg/d), in the absence of contraindications, or clopidogrel for patients with a contraindication to aspirin
2. β-Antagonists
3. Lipid-lowering agents (targeting reductions in LDL cholesterol)
4. ACE inhibitors for patients with heart failure, left ventricular dysfunction (ejection fraction, <40%), hypertension, or diabetes
5. Spironolactone or eplerenone for patients with left ventricular dysfunction (ejection fraction, <40%)
6. Clopidogrel, prasugrel, or ticagrelor in addition to aspirin, for a designated period, in patients who have undergone percutaneous coronary intervention

In addition to designing an individualized drug regimen, the physician must also educate the patient about risk factors for the recurrence of MI. A useful mnemonic for guiding overall treatment in post-MI patients is **ABCDE**: **A**ntiplatelet agents, ACE inhibitors, antianginals, and aldosterone antagonists; **B**eta-antagonists and blood pressure control; **C**holesterol-lowering and quitting cigarettes; **D**iet and diabetes control; **E**ducation and exercise.

PATHOPHYSIOLOGY OF HEART FAILURE

Heart failure is a common clinical problem. As many as 5 million patients in the United States carry this diagnosis, with approximately 500,000 new cases diagnosed each year. The syndrome of HF has a grave prognosis: the mortality rate at 5 years approximates 50%, and in the subset of patients with the most severe clinical symptoms, the annual mortality is as high as 30–50%.

Because the impairment of cardiac function that underlies this syndrome is often irreversible, HF is typically a chronic illness with intercurrent episodes of acute decompensation. Acute exacerbations are often multifactorial in etiology, with contributions from dietary indiscretion (excess sodium or fluid intake), nonadherence to prescribed medications, and concomitant noncardiac illness. Myocardial ischemia, progression of the proximate cause of cardiac disease, and activation of neurohumoral regulatory systems may also lead to clinical decompensation. The management of HF requires the clinician to construct, evaluate, and periodically modify a treatment regimen that includes multiple drugs, some of which may carry significant risk for adverse interactions.

Although the discussion that follows emphasizes cardiogenic circulatory failure, it should be noted that circulatory failure can occur in the absence of contractile

TABLE 26-4 Causes of Circulatory Failure in the Absence of Cardiac Pump Dysfunction

CAUSE OF CIRCULATORY FAILURE	MECHANISM
Abnormal cardiac filling	Hypovolemia (e.g., hemorrhage) Cardiac tamponade (compression by pericardial fluid prevents normal diastolic filling)
Abnormal cardiac rhythm	Bradycardia (↓ rate → ↓ forward output) Tachycardia (↑ rate → ↓ duration of diastolic filling interval)
Abnormal peripheral circulation	Hypertensive crisis (↑ SVR → ↑ impedance to LV ejection → ↓ stroke volume) Distributive shock (↓ SVR → ↓ MAP → organ hypoperfusion)

SVR, systemic vascular resistance; MAP, mean arterial pressure.

dysfunction (Table 26-4). Common examples include abnormalities of cardiac filling (e.g., hypovolemia), cardiac rhythm (e.g., bradycardia or tachycardia), or the peripheral circulation (e.g., distributive shock related to sepsis). As always, treatment should be tailored to the pathophysiology in each individual case.

Etiologies of Contractile Dysfunction

Left ventricular contractile dysfunction (**systolic heart failure**) is the primary cause of heart failure. Although multiple disease states can result in contractile dysfunction, the majority of cases of left HF (~70%) are attributed to CAD. Additional causes of systolic HF include chronic abnormalities of the loading conditions imposed on the heart, such as systemic arterial hypertension (pressure loading) and valvular heart disease (volume loading from mitral regurgitation or aortic insufficiency; pressure loading from aortic stenosis). The contractile performance of the myocardium is initially preserved in disease states associated with abnormal loading conditions, but cardiomyocyte injury and whole-organ contractile dysfunction supervene if the abnormal loading conditions are not corrected. The latter phase of cardiac pump dysfunction has been referred to as *cardiomyopathy of chronic overload*. Systolic dysfunction can also result from diverse conditions in which the proximate pathologic abnormality is cardiomyocyte injury or dysfunction. These conditions are referred to as **dilated cardiomyopathies**, because the heart characteristically remodels to produce LV chamber dilation (with or without wall thinning) in states of primary myocyte dysfunction.

Symptomatic HF can also occur in patients with normal or near-normal LV systolic function (i.e., preserved LV ejection fraction). In such cases, the symptoms of left HF are caused by abnormalities of LV relaxation and/or filling (**diastolic heart failure**). Impaired relaxation results in the elevation of LV diastolic pressure at any given filling volume. This elevation of LV diastolic pressure causes elevation of left atrial and pulmonary capillary pressures, leading to transudation of fluid into the pulmonary interstitium (as well as secondary, or passive, elevation of pulmonary artery

and right heart pressures). The most common acute cause of isolated diastolic HF is acute myocardial ischemia. In the setting of acute reversible ischemia (i.e., ischemia not associated with MI), LV diastolic pressures increase as a consequence of incomplete LV relaxation. (Recall from the discussion in Chapter 25, Pharmacology of Cardiac Contractility, that both contraction and relaxation of cardiomyocytes depend on adequate levels of intracellular ATP.)

Both systolic and diastolic HF can be understood by considering the determinants of cardiac performance and the pathophysiologic conditions that affect these parameters. Although diastolic dysfunction is now appreciated as a common cause of clinical heart failure, the balance of this section will deal principally with heart failure due to systolic dysfunction. Each of the major factors affecting stroke volume—preload, afterload, and contractility—can be described by its effect on cardiac function curves. Figure 26-10 illustrates a normal LV pressure-volume loop. In the normal cycle, LV volume increases when the mitral valve opens during diastole. Isovolumetric contraction begins when LV pressure exceeds left atrial pressure and the mitral valve closes; during this segment of the cardiac cycle, intraventricular pressure increases while intracavitary volume remains constant. Ejection begins when the impedance to LV ejection is exceeded and the aortic valve opens; ejected blood is then transmitted to the systemic circulation by the elastic properties of the aorta. The aortic valve closes when LV pressure falls below aortic pressure; at this point, intraventricular pressure decreases rapidly (isovolumetric relaxation), up to (and perhaps beyond) the point at which the mitral valve opens, and the cycle is repeated.

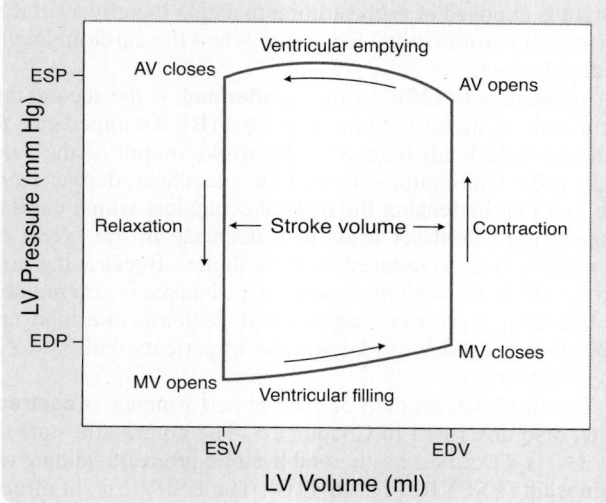

FIGURE 26-10. Normal left ventricular pressure-volume loop. Mitral valve (*MV*) opening allows the left ventricular (*LV*) volume to increase as the chamber fills with blood during diastole. When ventricular pressure exceeds left atrial pressure, the mitral valve closes. During the isovolumetric phase of systolic contraction, the left ventricle generates a high pressure, which eventually forces open the aortic valve (*AV*). Ejection of the stroke volume ensues, and the aortic valve closes when aortic pressure exceeds LV pressure. Isovolumetric relaxation returns the ventricle to its lowest pressure state, and the cycle is repeated. Stroke volume (i.e., the volume of blood ejected with each contraction cycle) is the difference between end-diastolic volume (*EDV*) and end-systolic volume (*ESV*). EDP, end-diastolic pressure; ESP, end-systolic pressure.

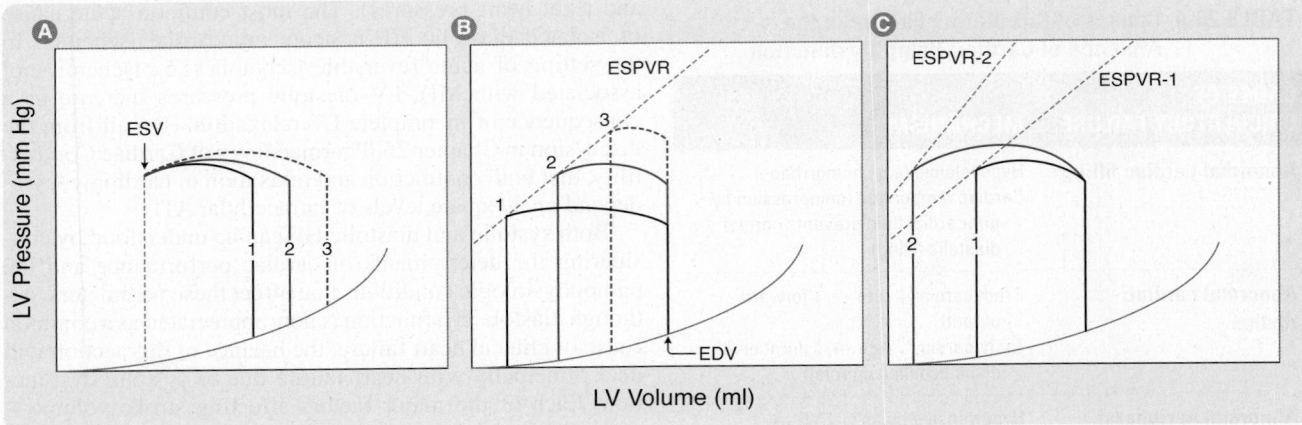

FIGURE 26-11. Determinants of cardiac output. Changes in preload, afterload, and myocardial contractility alter the pressure-volume relationship of the cardiac cycle. **A.** Increases in preload (*lines 1, 2, 3*) result in greater stretch of ventricular myocytes, development of greater ventricular end-diastolic pressure, and ejection of greater stroke volume (the Frank-Starling mechanism). Note that the end-systolic volume (*ESV*) is the same in each case, because the contractility of the heart has not changed. **B.** Increases in afterload (*points 1, 2, 3*) create greater impedance to left ventricular output and result in proportionately decreased stroke volume (the difference between end-diastolic volume [*EDV*] and ESV). The end-systolic pressure is linearly related to ESV; this linear relationship is called the *end-systolic pressure-volume relationship* (*ESPVR*). **C.** Increases in myocardial contractility (*lines 1, 2*), as occurs after administration of a positive inotrope, shift the ESPVR up and to the left, resulting in increased stroke volume.

As illustrated in Figure 26-11A, the forward stroke volume ejected by the LV depends on the degree of LV filling during diastole, or **preload**. This fundamental relationship between preload and stroke volume is the **Frank-Starling law**; it derives from the relationship between muscle length and degree of muscle shortening, as described in Chapter 25. In brief, increased diastolic volume increases myocardial fiber length. As a result, a higher fraction of the actin filament length is exposed in each sarcomere and is thereby available for myosin cross-bridge formation when the cardiomyocyte is depolarized.

Impedance to LV ejection, or **afterload**, is the second determinant of stroke volume (Fig. 26-11B). As impedance to ejection (afterload) increases, the stroke output of the ventricle falls. This characteristic of the intact heart derives from the fact that increasing the resistance against which cardiac muscle must contract leads to a decrease in the extent of shortening (i.e., to reduced stroke volume). Because the sensitivity of stroke volume to outflow resistance is accentuated in the failing ventricle, agents that decrease afterload are able to increase LV stroke volume in patients with systolic HF (see below).

The third determinant of cardiac performance is **contractility**, also described in Chapter 25. The contractile state of the LV is described by the **end-systolic pressure-volume relationship** (**ESPVR**, Fig. 26-11C). The ESPVR is, in effect, a variant of the Frank-Starling law. While the Frank-Starling law defines the relationship between LV diastolic volume (or preload) and LV stroke volume (or cardiac output), the ESPVR describes the relationship between diastolic filling volume and LV tension development during isovolumetric contraction. As shown in Figure 26-11C, an increase in the contractile state of the LV, reflected by an upward shift of the ESPVR, results in a greater degree of tension development for any given end-diastolic volume. In the presence of a fixed afterload, increased contractility results in a greater degree of muscle shortening and an increase in LV stroke volume.

The final determinant of cardiac pump performance is **heart rate**. Heart rate can be an important determinant of cardiac output in patients with systolic contractile dysfunction. However, if LV contractile performance is preserved, then impairment of cardiac output occurs as a consequence of abnormal heart rate only at extreme rates outside the physiologic range.

Cardiac Compensation

As the ability of the myocardium to maintain normal forward output fails, compensatory mechanisms are activated to preserve circulatory function. The Frank-Starling mechanism increases stroke volume in direct response to increased preload. This recruitment of preload reserve is the first response of the system to hemodynamic stress. Hemodynamic stress that cannot be fully compensated by the Frank-Starling mechanism stimulates signaling systems that initiate structural changes at the cellular level, a process referred to as **remodeling** of the myocardium. Although the underlying stimuli for remodeling remain an active area of investigation, it has been noted that the specific pattern of remodeling is determined by the nature of the applied stress. If the Frank-Starling mechanism and remodeling mechanisms are unable to reestablish adequate forward cardiac output, neurohumoral systems are then activated. These systems modulate intravascular volume and vasomotor tone to maintain oxygen delivery to critical organs. Although each of these compensatory mechanisms contributes to the maintenance of circulatory function, each may also contribute to the development and progression of pump dysfunction and circulatory failure, as described below.

Frank-Starling Mechanism

In the intact heart, increased preload leads to increased stroke volume via the Frank-Starling mechanism. This mechanism remains operative in the failing heart; importantly, though, the relationship between end-diastolic volume and stroke

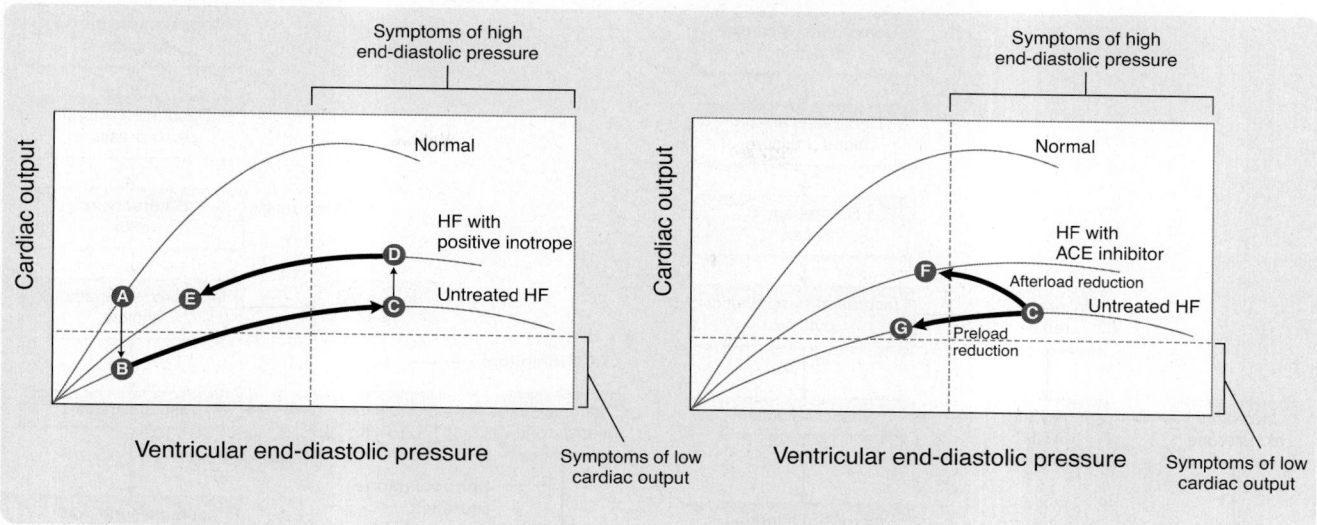

FIGURE 26-12. The Frank-Starling relationship in heart failure (HF). Left panel: The normal Frank-Starling relationship shows a steep increase in cardiac output with increasing ventricular end-diastolic pressure (preload). **Point A** describes the end-diastolic pressure and cardiac output of a normal heart under resting conditions. With contractile dysfunction (untreated HF), cardiac output falls (**B**) and the Frank-Starling curve flattens, so that increasing preload translates to only a modest increase in cardiac output (**C**). This increase in cardiac output is accompanied by symptoms of high end-diastolic pressure, such as dyspnea. Treatment with a positive inotrope, such as digitalis, shifts the Frank-Starling curve upward, and cardiac output increases (**D**). The improvement in myocardial contractility supports a sufficient reduction in preload that the venous congestion is relieved (**E**). **Right panel:** Two of the principal pharmacologic treatments of HF are afterload reduction (e.g., ACE inhibitors) and preload reduction (e.g., diuretics). Afterload reduction (**F**) increases cardiac output at any given preload and thereby elevates the Frank-Starling relationship. Preload reduction (**G**) alleviates congestive symptoms by decreasing ventricular end-diastolic pressure along the same Frank-Starling curve.

volume is altered. *In patients with systolic dysfunction, the relationship between end-diastolic volume and stroke volume is characterized by a flatter plateau* (Fig. 26-12). Therefore, unlike normal individuals who are operating on the ascending limb of the Frank-Starling curve, where volume expansion can be a useful strategy for increasing stroke volume, the majority of patients with heart failure operate with *elevated* intravascular volume. This increased intravascular volume reflects the end result of neurohumoral activation (i.e., the sympathoadrenal axis and the renin-angiotensin-aldosterone system; see below). Thus, *the treatment of cardiogenic circulatory failure rarely involves volume expansion.* It also merits emphasis that preload expansion can result in significant LV dilation, thereby increasing LV systolic and diastolic wall stress and exacerbating pulmonary congestion.

Cardiac Remodeling and Hypertrophy

In the setting of increased myocardial wall stress, cardiac hypertrophy develops in order to maintain ventricular systolic performance. Because LV ejection fraction is inversely proportional to wall stress, adaptations that decrease systolic wall stress increase LV ejection fraction. **Laplace's law** states that wall stress (σ) is directly proportional to the pressure (P) and radius (R) of a chamber and inversely proportional to wall thickness (h):

$$\sigma = P \times R/2h \qquad \text{\textbf{Equation 26-1}}$$

In cases of chronic pressure overload, such as aortic stenosis or systemic hypertension, the LV develops a concentric pattern of hypertrophy as contractile proteins and new sarcomeres are added in *parallel* to the existing myofilaments. **Concentric hypertrophy** simultaneously increases wall thickness (h) and decreases cavity size (R), resulting in

a net reduction in systolic wall stress and thereby preserving systolic performance. The disadvantage of concentric remodeling derives from the *decrease in LV compliance* that occurs as a consequence of this pattern of hypertrophy. In a ventricle with reduced compliance, diastolic pressure in the chamber is increased at any given filling volume. This in turn leads to elevation of LA and pulmonary capillary pressures, thereby predisposing to congestive symptoms.

In conditions of chronic volume overload, such as mitral or aortic regurgitation, the LV develops an eccentric pattern of hypertrophy as contractile proteins and new sarcomeres are added in *series* to the existing myofilaments. **Eccentric hypertrophy** helps to maintain cardiac performance via modulation of diastolic wall stress. In contrast to the situation that occurs after concentric remodeling, eccentric hypertrophy is associated with *increased LV compliance*. The increase in compliance allows LV end-diastolic volume to increase without a significant elevation in left ventricular and left atrial diastolic pressures. This attenuation of the rise in chamber pressure allows the system to maintain forward cardiac output by a volume-driven increase in total stroke volume. During the compensated phase of eccentric hypertrophy, LV wall thickness increases in approximate proportion to the increase in chamber radius.

Neurohumoral Activation

Failure of the heart to provide adequate forward output activates several neurohumoral systems, often with deleterious consequences (Fig. 26-13). Decreased arterial pressure activates the baroreceptor reflex, stimulating release of catecholamines; in turn, the catecholamines produce *tachycardia* (via β_1-receptors) and *vasoconstriction* (via peripheral α_1-receptors). Stimulation of β_1-receptors on renal

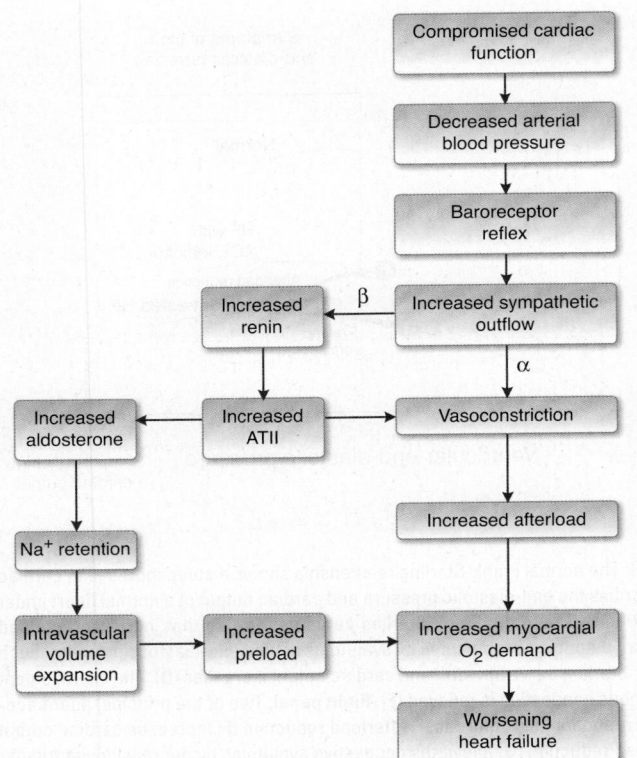

FIGURE 26-13. Neurohumoral effects of heart failure. Compromised cardiac function leads to decreased arterial blood pressure, which activates baroreceptors that increase sympathetic outflow. α-Adrenergic sympathetic outflow (α) causes vasoconstriction, which increases afterload. The increased afterload creates a greater pressure against which the heart must contract and thereby increases myocardial O_2 demand. β-Adrenergic sympathetic outflow (β) increases juxtaglomerular cell release of renin. Renin cleaves angiotensinogen to angiotensin I, and angiotensin I is then converted to the active hormone angiotensin II (AT II). AT II has a direct vasoconstrictor action; it also increases aldosterone synthesis and secretion. Aldosterone increases collecting duct Na^+ reabsorption, leading to intravascular volume expansion and increased preload. Together, the increased afterload and preload increase myocardial O_2 demand. In the already compromised heart, these increased stresses can lead to worsening heart failure.

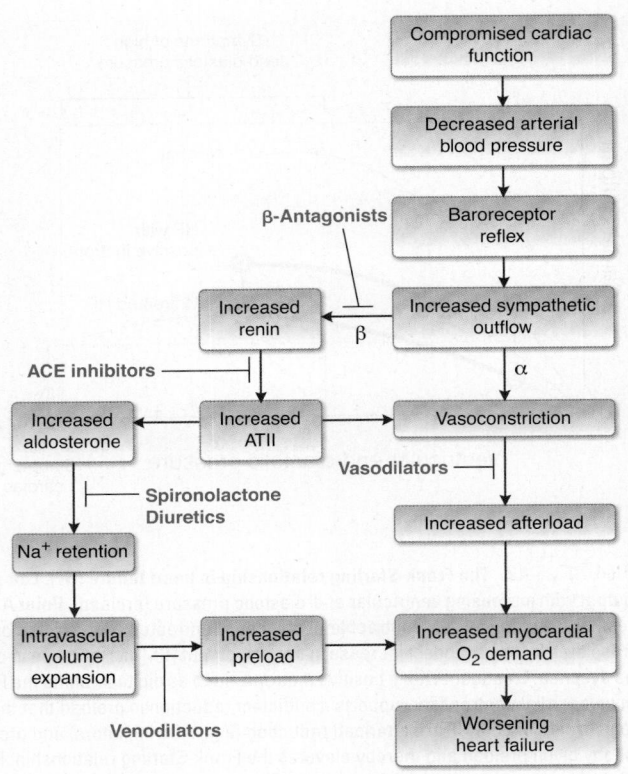

FIGURE 26-14. Pharmacologic modulation of the neurohumoral effects of heart failure. Many therapeutic agents used in the management of heart failure modulate the neurohumoral systems that are activated by compromised cardiac function. The renin-angiotensin-aldosterone system can be inhibited by (1) β-adrenergic antagonists, which inhibit renin release by the juxtaglomerular cells of the kidney; (2) ACE inhibitors, which prevent the conversion of angiotensin I to the active hormone angiotensin II; and (3) spironolactone, which competitively antagonizes aldosterone binding to the mineralocorticoid receptor. Diuretics promote Na^+ excretion and thereby counteract the Na^+ retention stimulated by activation of the renin-angiotensin-aldosterone system. Venodilators counteract the effect of intravascular volume expansion by increasing peripheral venous capacitance and thereby decreasing preload. Direct arterial vasodilators alleviate the α-adrenergic receptor-mediated and angiotensin II receptor-mediated vasoconstriction induced by increased sympathetic outflow. Cardiac glycosides, β-adrenergic agonists, and cardiac phosphodiesterase inhibitors are also used in HF to increase myocardial contractility (*not shown*).

juxtaglomerular (JG) cells promotes the release of renin. JG cells also release renin in response to the decreased renal perfusion that accompanies decreased cardiac output. Renin cleaves circulating angiotensinogen to angiotensin I, which is subsequently converted by angiotensin converting enzyme (ACE) to angiotensin II (AT II). AT II acts through AT_1 receptors to *increase arterial vasomotor tone*. AT II also activates several physiologic mechanisms that *increase intravascular volume*, including aldosterone release from the adrenal glands (thus promoting salt and water retention), vasopressin (ADH) release from the posterior pituitary gland, and thirst center activation in the hypothalamus. In addition, AT II appears to be an important mediator of vascular and myocardial hypertrophy.

The tachycardia and increased intravascular volume that accompany activation of these neurohumoral mechanisms help to maintain forward cardiac output, and the systemic vasoconstriction provides a mechanism by which central regulatory centers can override local autoregulation of blood

flow. Together, these mechanisms allow the cardiovascular system to maintain perfusion of critical organs in the setting of reduced cardiac output. However, sympathetic stimulation of the heart also increases myocardial oxygen demand by increasing both afterload (arteriolar constriction) and preload (retention of sodium and water). Continued sympathetic stimulation eventually results in down-regulation of β-adrenergic receptors, further impairing the ability of the system to maintain forward output. *The central aim of the current pharmacologic management of HF is to modulate the action of these neurohumoral effectors* (Fig. 26-14).

CLINICAL MANAGEMENT OF HEART FAILURE

The pharmacologic treatment of HF has expanded dramatically over the past three decades. Numerous large-scale clinical trials have demonstrated that the new, "load-active" therapies are associated with statistically significant reductions in morbidity and mortality in patients with HF. In addition, improvements in the detection and treatment of hypertension and the management of complex multivessel CAD have dramatically altered the clinical course of patients with contractile dysfunction. It is helpful to organize the treatment strategies for contractile dysfunction in patients who exhibit or are at risk to develop symptomatic heart failure according to the following physiologic goals: preload reduction, afterload reduction, and contractility enhancement (increased inotropy). Table 26-5 provides a summary of the hemodynamic effects and mechanisms of action of the drug classes that are commonly used to treat heart failure.

Preload Reduction

Diuretics

Diuretics have long been cornerstones of the pharmacologic management of patients with left ventricular failure and remain integral components of the treatment of patients with congestive symptoms and/or intravascular volume overload.

However, despite the efficacy of these agents at reducing congestive symptoms, there is no evidence of a mortality benefit from treatment with either loop diuretics or thiazide diuretics.

The natriuretic agents most commonly used in HF are the loop diuretics furosemide and bumetanide. These drugs inhibit the Na^+-K^+-$2Cl^-$ co-transporter (NKCC2) in the thick ascending limb of Henle, resulting in increased excretion of sodium, potassium, and water. Thiazide diuretics such as hydrochlorothiazide are also used to treat congestive symptoms, particularly in patients with hypertensive heart disease and LV systolic dysfunction. Thiazides inhibit sodium and chloride reabsorption via the Na^+-Cl^- co-transporter (NCC) in the distal convoluted tubule. Thiazides are less efficacious natriuretic agents than loop diuretics and are often ineffective as monotherapy for congestive symptoms in patients with chronic kidney disease. Thiazides are sometimes co-administered with loop diuretics in patients with reduced GFR and refractory volume overload and in selected patients with HF in whom treatment with loop diuretics alone does not achieve adequate diuresis. (Refer to Chapter 21 for an

TABLE 26-5 Pharmacologic Agents Used in the Treatment of Heart Failure

DRUG OR DRUG CLASS	MECHANISM OF ACTION	HEMODYNAMIC EFFECT	CLINICAL NOTES
Drugs with Proven Mortality Reduction			
ACE inhibitors	Inhibit AT II generation → ↓ AT_1 receptor activation	Decreased afterload Decreased preload	May cause hyperkalemia
β-Antagonists	Competitive antagonists at β-adrenergic receptor → ↓ renin release	Decreased afterload Decreased preload	May be relatively contraindicated in severely decompensated heart failure
Spironolactone	Competitive antagonist at aldosterone receptor	Decreased preload	Mortality benefit may be independent of hemodynamic effects; may cause hyperkalemia
Drugs or Treatments Used to Improve Symptoms			
Na^+/H_2O restriction	Decreases intravascular volume	Decreased preload	May help limit edema formation
Diuretics	Inhibit renal Na^+ reabsorption	Decreased preload	Furosemide most effective for treating congestive symptoms
Aquaretics	Competitive antagonists at vasopressin V_2 receptor → ↓ renal aquaporin expression and membrane trafficking → ↓ free water reabsorption	Decreased preload	Increased output of solute-free urine; increased serum sodium
Digoxin	Inhibits Na^+/K^+ ATPase → ↑ intracellular Ca^{2+} → ↑ contractility	Increased contractility	Delays atrioventricular nodal conduction
Organic nitrates	Increase NO → venous smooth muscle relaxation → ↑ venous capacitance	Decreased preload	Reduces myocardial O_2 demand
Dobutamine	Stimulates β-adrenergic receptors	Increased contractility ($β_1$ effect) Decreased afterload ($β_2$ effect)	Used in the acute setting only
Inamrinone, milrinone	Inhibit phosphodiesterase → ↑ β-adrenergic effect	Increased contractility Decreased afterload Decreased preload	Used in the acute setting only

extended discussion of diuretics.) In the introductory case, the decrease in intravascular volume achieved with furosemide significantly improves Mr. N's congestive symptoms, and he may require long-term administration of oral furosemide to stabilize these symptoms.

Aquaretics

Patients with heart failure have increased circulating levels of vasopressin, and the extent of vasopressin elevation correlates with the severity of heart failure. Selective antagonism of the vasopressin V_2 receptor results in increased output of solute-free urine and increased serum sodium levels in patients with heart failure. The clinical application of vasopressin antagonists (so-called aquaretics) in heart failure remains controversial, but both **conivaptan** and **tolvaptan** are approved for use in patients with heart failure. Conivaptan is available as an intravenous infusion for the treatment of hypervolemic hyponatremia. In patients with acute decompensated heart failure requiring hospitalization, addition of oral tolvaptan to a standard therapy regimen increases weight loss and decreases edema over the first seven days but has no significant long-term effect on recurrent hospitalizations or mortality (EVEREST trial).

Aldosterone Receptor Antagonists

Spironolactone is a potassium-sparing diuretic that acts as a competitive antagonist at the aldosterone receptor, thus decreasing sodium–potassium exchange in the distal tubule and collecting duct of the nephron. A clinical trial of this agent in patients with systolic HF has received much attention (RALES trial). In this study, patients with severe HF were treated with low-dose spironolactone (25–50 mg daily); enrolled patients were free of significant renal impairment and were concomitantly receiving standard therapy for heart failure (ACE inhibitor, β-blocker, loop diuretic ± digoxin). In patients treated with spironolactone, all-cause mortality (including sudden cardiac death and death from progressive heart failure) was reduced by approximately 30%, as were hospital admissions for exacerbations of HF. A subsequent trial with a similar agent, eplerenone, confirmed these findings in patients with HF after MI (EPHESUS trial). Spironolactone is often administered in combination with an ACE inhibitor and/or angiotensin receptor blocker (see below). Because spironolactone, ACE inhibitors, and angiotensin receptor blockers all decrease K^+ excretion, plasma K^+ levels must be monitored carefully, and potassium supplementation must be undertaken with caution.

Venodilators

Venodilator agents are often co-administered with diuretics in patients with congestive symptoms. The prototypical venodilator is nitroglycerin (NTG). This drug increases venous capacitance and thereby decreases venous return to the heart. The decrease in venous return results in reduced LV chamber volume and reduced LV diastolic pressure. These effects of the nitrates decrease myocardial oxygen demand, which may be especially beneficial in patients with coexisting angina and LV dysfunction.

Nitrates may also be particularly effective in cases where left HF results from acute myocardial ischemia. In this condition, LV relaxation is impaired, LV compliance is decreased, and LV diastolic pressure is typically elevated. By increasing venous capacitance, nitrates reduce venous return to the heart and decrease LV diastolic volume. In turn, the decrease in diastolic volume leads to a decrease in myocardial oxygen consumption. In addition, nitrates may alleviate ischemia, thereby improving diastolic relaxation. Thus, the beneficial effects of nitrate administration in this setting include both preload reduction and improvement in LV compliance.

Afterload Reduction

ACE Inhibitors

ACE inhibitors reversibly inhibit angiotensin converting enzyme (ACE). The resulting decrease in angiotensin II (AT II) leads to several potential benefits. AT II is an important component of the neurohumoral regulation of the failing circulation. In response to renal hypoperfusion, the kidney increases renin secretion, which results in increased production of AT II, as noted above (also see Chapter 21). In turn, AT II stimulates the adrenal gland to secrete aldosterone. Overall, activation of the renin-angiotensin-aldosterone system increases vasomotor tone as well as sodium and water retention. These hemodynamic alterations result in increased intravascular volume (leading, ultimately, to increased LV diastolic filling and increased LV stroke volume) and peripheral redistribution of the cardiac output (mediated by the vasoconstrictor effects of AT II).

Administration of an ACE inhibitor reverses the vasoconstriction and volume retention that characterize renin-angiotensin-aldosterone system activation. The reduction in afterload decreases the impedance to LV ejection and thereby increases LV stroke volume. The reversal of aldosterone-related volume retention decreases preload. These effects are synergistic in patients with HF: as stroke volume increases, GFR is also increased, leading to increased delivery of sodium and water to the distal nephron, where (in the absence of renin-stimulated elevation of aldosterone levels) natriuresis and diuresis occur. ACE inhibition can also increase venous capacitance (and thereby reduce preload) by decreasing degradation of the endogenous vasodilator bradykinin. By altering the myocardial remodeling that occurs after ST elevation myocardial infarction, ACE inhibitors can provide further benefit in patients with concomitant HF and CAD.

ACE inhibitors have a statistically significant impact on survival in patients with heart failure. This mortality benefit was first demonstrated in patients with severe heart failure in the CONSENSUS trial: the mortality reduction approximated 40% at 6 months and 31% at 1 year. The mortality benefit of the ACE inhibitors was confirmed in a broader spectrum of patients in the SOLVD Treatment trial (16% reduction in mortality) and the V-Heft II trial (28% reduction in mortality), as well as in patients in the convalescent phase following MI (SAVE trial, 19% reduction in mortality).

AT_1 antagonists (sometimes called *angiotensin receptor blockers* or *ARBs*) are a class of agents that inhibit the renin-angiotensin-aldosterone axis at the level of the angiotensin II receptor. The hemodynamic profile of these agents is similar to that of the converting enzyme inhibitors. Recent clinical trials have demonstrated a mortality benefit for AT_1 antagonists in patients with severe systolic HF (LV ejection fraction, <40%) who are unable to take ACE inhibitors. In patients with HF who are already taking an ACE inhibitor, the addition of an AT_1 antagonist reduces hospital readmissions for HF but does not reduce mortality (CHARM-Added trial).

Recent data suggest that combining blockade of the renin-angiotensin system with up-regulation of the natriuretic peptides bradykinin and adrenomedullin may improve clinical outcomes. Up-regulation of the natriuretic peptides can be achieved through inhibition of neprilysin, an endopeptidase that degrades bradykinin and adrenomedullin. In a recent clinical trial, combination therapy with an ACE inhibitor and a neprilysin inhibitor resulted in a 20% reduction in cardiovascular death and a 21% reduction in heart failure hospitalization compared to therapy with an ACE inhibitor alone in patients with severe systolic HF. These data, published in the PARADIGM-HF trial, may represent a new therapeutic modality for patients with heart failure and reduced systolic function.

β-Adrenoceptor Antagonists

Much recent attention has been directed at the use of β-adrenoceptor antagonists in the treatment of patients with HF. Although the use of β-antagonists might seem counterintuitive, clinical trials have now established that these agents increase survival in heart failure patients. The benefits of β-antagonists in patients with heart failure have been variably attributed to (1) inhibition of renin release, (2) attenuation of the cytotoxic and signaling effects of elevated circulating catecholamines, and, more generally, (3) prevention of myocardial ischemia. Thus, β-antagonists, like ACE inhibitors, may attenuate the adverse effects of neurohumoral regulators in patients with heart failure. Furthermore, because β-antagonists and ACE inhibitors act via distinct mechanisms and have non-overlapping toxicities, it is reasonable to co-administer these classes of drugs to HF patients.

Vasodilators

Hydralazine is a direct-acting vasodilator that decreases systemic vascular resistance and thereby reduces afterload. The mechanism of action of hydralazine remains to be determined. The arterial vasodilation produced by hydralazine is particularly pronounced when the drug is administered intravenously. The clinical use of hydralazine has been limited by several factors, including the induction of reflex tachycardia during intravenous administration, the development of tachyphylaxis, and the occurrence of a drug-induced lupus syndrome during chronic administration. This agent has demonstrated a mortality benefit in HF when co-administered with organic nitrates (AHEFT Trial). The nitrate–hydralazine combination is typically reserved for patients who cannot tolerate therapy with an ACE inhibitor, although in certain populations, particularly African Americans, the addition of nitrates and hydralazine to standard therapy may be superior.

Inotropic Agents

Cardiac Glycosides

Digitalis glycosides inhibit the sarcolemmal Na^+/K^+ ATPase in cardiac myocytes. This action increases intracellular Na^+, activates the Na^+/Ca^{2+} exchanger, and increases intracellular Ca^{2+}, including the Ca^{2+} stores in the sarcoplasmic reticulum. This, in turn, leads to increased calcium release upon myocyte stimulation, resulting in increased myocardial contractility (i.e., upward/leftward shift of the ESPVR). Although patients with HF often experience relief of congestive symptoms during treatment with the cardiac glycosides, these drugs have not been shown to decrease mortality.

Sympathomimetic Amines

Dobutamine is the parenteral sympathomimetic amine used most commonly in the treatment of decompensated systolic HF (pulmonary congestion accompanied by reduced forward cardiac output). This agent is a synthetic congener of epinephrine that stimulates β_1-receptors and, to a lesser extent, β_2-receptors and α_1-receptors. The stimulation of β_1-receptors predominates at therapeutic infusion rates, leading ultimately to an increase in the contractility of cardiac myocytes. Stimulation of vascular β_2-receptors causes arterial vasodilation and a reduction in afterload. The combined effects of increased contractility and decreased afterload lead to improvement in overall cardiac performance. Dobutamine is typically used in the acute setting (i.e., intensive care unit). In the introductory case, if Mr. N were to become hypotensive due to decreased cardiac output or to develop evidence of decreased end-organ perfusion such as a rise in serum creatinine, dobutamine could be administered acutely to stabilize his hemodynamic status.

Phosphodiesterase Inhibitors

Phosphodiesterase inhibitors (such as **inamrinone** and **milrinone**) inhibit the degradation of cAMP in cardiac myocytes and thereby increase intracellular calcium and enhance contractility (inotropy). In the systemic vasculature, these agents cause dilation of both arteriolar resistance vessels and venous capacitance vessels, thereby decreasing afterload and preload. As a result of these aggregate effects, phosphodiesterase inhibitors have been referred to as *ino-dilators*. Despite these positive actions, both phosphodiesterase inhibitors and sympathomimetic amines are reserved for short-term treatment of patients with acute decompensation of heart failure. Indeed, long-term treatment with oral phosphodiesterase inhibitors has been shown to *increase* mortality.

Combination Therapy

The drugs described in this chapter offer a number of approaches to the pharmacotherapy of heart failure. Some agents, most notably ACE inhibitors and β-antagonists, have demonstrated significant mortality benefit in randomized clinical trials and should probably be viewed as the new cornerstones of therapy. Other drugs, such as digoxin and diuretics, have been mainstays of symptomatic relief despite a lack of mortality benefit.

Use of combination therapies must be approached cautiously in HF patients to avoid adverse effects such as hypotension, arrhythmias, electrolyte imbalances, and renal insufficiency. Nonetheless, it is typical for these patients to require multidrug regimens to optimize their functional status.

▋ CONCLUSION AND FUTURE DIRECTIONS

Hypertension, ischemic heart disease, and HF are common cardiovascular diseases that occur singly and in combination. Therapeutic strategies target the cellular and molecular pathways that are dysfunctional in these disease states. Combination therapy with drugs from multiple classes is often required to address the complex pathophysiology of these conditions and achieve the desired therapeutic result.

Current research in cardiovascular genomics and neurohumoral pathways promises to provide new understanding of the pathophysiology of cardiovascular disease. For example, the pathophysiology of essential hypertension may, in many cases, involve mutations or polymorphisms in the genes that code for angiotensinogen, renin, the angiotensin II receptor (AT_1), endothelin, the glucocorticoid receptor, the insulin receptor, endothelial nitric oxide synthase, and the epithelial Na^+ channel (ENaC). As the genetic determinants of cardiovascular regulation are clarified, it may be possible to identify high-risk patients prospectively and to develop targeted therapies that exert their therapeutic effects on the molecular and cellular mechanisms predicted to drive the disease in these patients.

In recent years, agents targeting neurohumoral pathways—such as ACE inhibitors and β-antagonists—have become cornerstones of therapy for all cardiovascular diseases. Large clinical trials have consistently demonstrated that these drugs reduce adverse cardiovascular events, including mortality, in patients with hypertension, patients with coronary artery disease and prior MI, and patients with systolic HF. Over the past 25 years, increased understanding of basic disease mechanisms has improved the physician's ability to alter both the clinical expression and progression of cardiovascular diseases: examples include recent advances in the primary prevention of coronary artery disease and the positive impact of neurohumoral modulation on the progression of HF. Current research aims to identify and characterize new drug targets, including a host of signaling molecules that are abnormal in the failing heart. Elevated levels of inflammatory mediators—such as tumor necrosis factor-α (TNF-α), interleukin-6 (IL-6), and endothelin-1—and enzymes—such as inducible nitric oxide synthase, collagenases, and matrix metalloproteinases—have all been reported to contribute in some way to the detrimental structural and functional changes that occur in the failing heart.

Acknowledgment

We thank April W. Armstrong and Thomas P. Rocco for their valuable contributions to this chapter in the First, Second, and Third Editions of *Principles of Pharmacology: The Pathophysiologic Basis of Drug Therapy*.

Suggested Reading

Hypertension

ALLHAT Officers and Coordinators for the ALLHAT Collaborative Research Group. Major outcomes in high-risk hypertensive patients randomized to angiotensin-converting enzyme inhibitor or calcium channel blocker vs. diuretic: the Antihypertensive and Lipid-Lowering Treatment to Prevent Heart Attack Trial (ALLHAT). *JAMA* 2002;288:2981–2997. (*Results of a major trial comparing agents for initial treatment of hypertension.*)

Jamerson K, Weber MA, Bakris GL, et al. Benazepril plus amlodipine or hydrochlorothiazide for hypertension in high-risk patients. *N Engl J Med* 2008;359:2417–2428. (*Clinical trial suggesting benefit of combination therapy with ACE inhibitor and calcium channel blocker.*)

James PA, Oparil S, Carter BL, et al. 2014 evidence-based guidelines for the management of high blood pressure in adults. *JAMA* 2014;311:507–520. (*Current guidelines for classifying and treating hypertension.*)

Ischemic Heart Disease

Abrams J. Chronic stable angina. *N Engl J Med* 2005;352:2524–2533. (*Clinical pharmacology of chronic coronary artery disease treatments.*)

Anderson JL, Adams CD, Antman EM, et al. ACC/AHA 2007 guidelines for the management of patients with unstable angina and non-ST elevation myocardial infarction. Summary article: a report of the American College of Cardiology/American Heart Association Task Force on practice guidelines. *J Am Coll Cardiol* 2007;50:652–726. (*Current guidelines for evaluating and treating patients with unstable angina and non-ST elevation myocardial infarction.*)

Armstrong EJ, Morrow DA, Sabatine MS. Inflammatory biomarkers in acute coronary syndromes. Part I: introduction and cytokines. Part II: acute-phase reactants and biomarkers of endothelial cell activation. Part III: biomarkers of oxidative stress and angiogenic growth factors. Part IV: matrix metalloproteinases and biomarkers of platelet activation. *Circulation* 2006;113:72–75, 152–155, 289–292, 382–385. (*Four-part series reviewing pathophysiology and clinical evidence concerning the role of inflammatory mediators in acute coronary syndromes.*)

Cannon CP, Braunwald E, McCabe CH, et al. Intensive versus moderate lipid lowering with statins after acute coronary syndromes. *N Engl J Med* 2004;350:1495–1504. (*Trial demonstrating clinical benefit for aggressive statin therapy after acute coronary syndrome.*)

Libby P. The molecular mechanisms of the thrombotic complications of atherosclerosis. *J Intern Med* 2008;263:517–527. (*Molecular basis of coronary artery atherosclerosis.*)

Heart Failure

ACCF/AHA 2009 focused update: guidelines for the diagnosis and management of heart failure in adults. *J Am Coll Cardiol* 2009;53:e1–e90. (*Consensus guidelines for management of heart failure.*)

Jessup M, Brozena S. Heart failure. *N Engl J Med* 2003;348:2007–2018. (*Clinical approach to heart failure.*)

McMurray JJV, Packer M, Desai AS, et al. Angiotensin-neprilysin inhibition versus enalapril in heart failure. *N Engl J Med* 2014;371:993–1004. (*Trial showing mortality benefit to inhibition of neprilysin in addition to ACE inhibition.*)

Opie LH. Cellular basis for therapeutic choices in heart failure. *Circulation* 2004;110:2559–2561. (*Molecular basis of heart failure therapeutics.*)

Taylor AL, Ziesche S, Yancy C, et al. Combination of isosorbide dinitrate and hydralazine in blacks with heart failure. *N Engl J Med* 2004;351:2049–2057. (*Trial showing mortality benefit in self-identified black patients.*)

IV

Principles of Endocrine Pharmacology

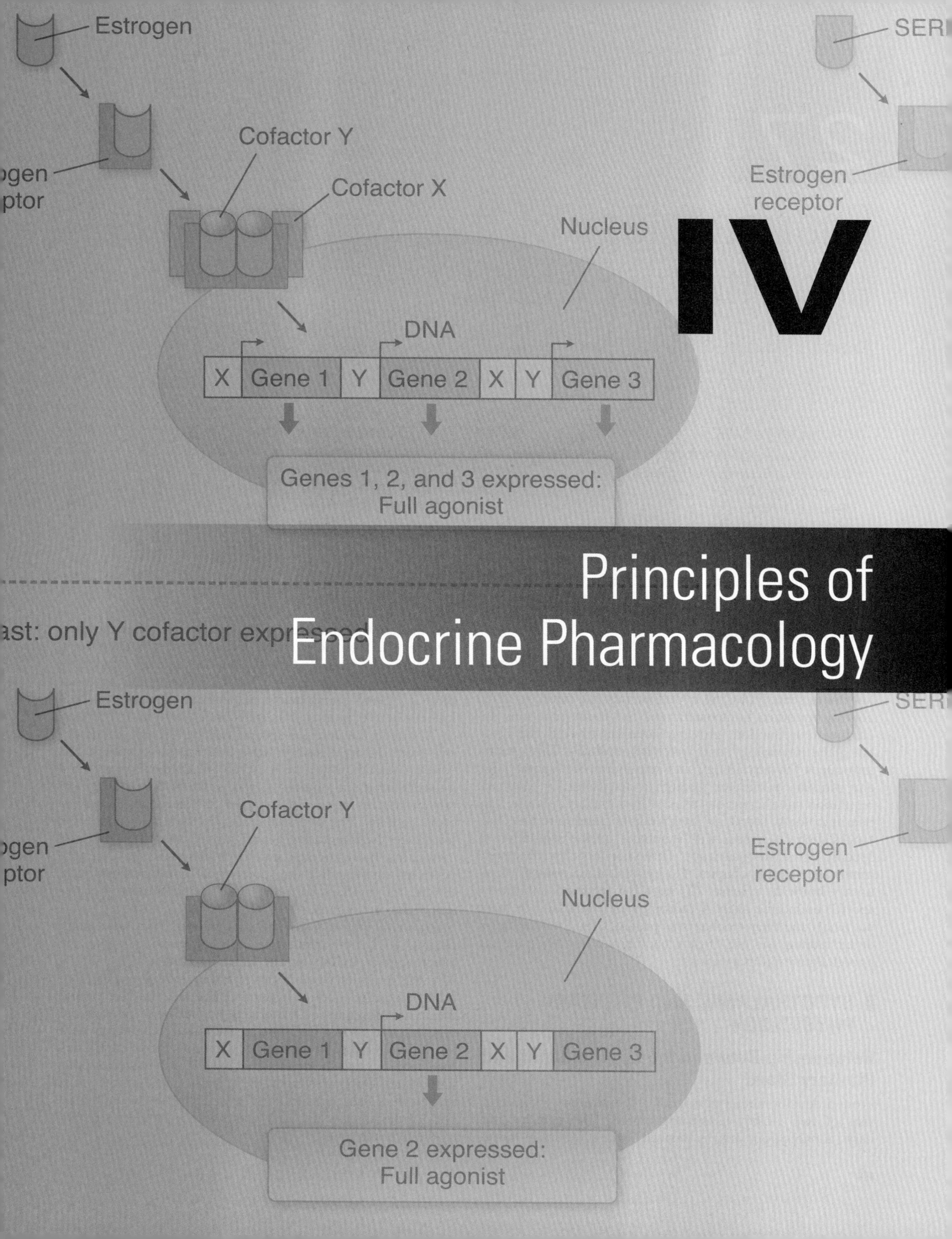

27

Pharmacology of the Hypothalamus and Pituitary Gland

Anand Vaidya and Ursula B. Kaiser

INTRODUCTION

The hypothalamus and pituitary gland function cooperatively as master regulators of the endocrine system. Together, hormones secreted by the hypothalamus and pituitary gland control important homeostatic and metabolic functions, including reproduction, growth, lactation, thyroid and adrenal gland physiology, and water homeostasis. This chapter introduces the physiology and regulation of hypothalamic and pituitary hormones through a discussion of feedback regulation and the various axes of hormonal regulation. The pharmacologic utility of hypothalamic and pituitary factors is then discussed, with emphasis on the regulation of specific endocrine pathways. Three concepts are of special importance in this chapter: (1) hypothalamic control of pituitary hormone release, (2) negative feedback inhibition, and (3) endocrine axes. A thorough understanding of these pathways and their mechanisms provides the foundation for understanding the use of pharmacotherapy to modulate the hypothalamic-pituitary axes.

HYPOTHALAMIC AND PITUITARY PHYSIOLOGY

Relationship Between the Hypothalamus and Pituitary Gland

From a developmental perspective, the pituitary gland consists of two closely associated organs. The **anterior pituitary** (adenohypophysis) is derived from ectodermal tissue.

The **posterior pituitary** (neurohypophysis) is a neural structure derived from the ventral surface of the diencephalon. The prefixes adeno- and neuro- denote the oral ectodermal and neural ectodermal origin of the anterior and posterior pituitary gland components, respectively. An intermediate lobe also exists in most mammals but is vestigial in humans.

Although the anterior and posterior pituitary glands derive from different embryologic origins, the hypothalamus controls the activity of both lobes. The connection between hypothalamus and pituitary gland is one of the most important points of interaction between the nervous and endocrine systems. The hypothalamus acts as a neuroendocrine transducer by integrating neural signals from the brain and converting those signals into chemical messages (largely peptides) that regulate the secretion of pituitary hormones. In turn, the pituitary hormones alter the activities of peripheral endocrine organs.

Hypothalamic control of the anterior pituitary gland occurs via hypothalamic secretion of hormones into the **hypothalamic-pituitary portal vascular system** (Fig. 27-1). The initial capillary bed of this portal system is formed from branches of the superior hypophyseal artery that fan around the axon terminals of hypothalamic neurons. Endothelial fenestrations in this capillary bed allow hypothalamic factors to be released into the bloodstream. These capillaries then coalesce into short veins that extend to the anterior pituitary gland. Upon arriving at the anterior pituitary, the veins branch into a second capillary bed and bathe the endocrine cells of the anterior pituitary gland with hormones secreted by the hypothalamus.

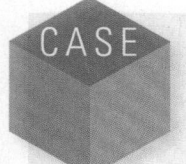
CASE

GR is a 42-year-old sales executive. She travels constantly and prides herself on being energetic and surpassing sales projections each quarter. Three years ago, she developed irregular menses, and she then completely stopped menstruating. Over the past 2 years, she has begun to feel increasingly fatigued, has difficulty rushing the length of airport terminals, and is bothered by frequent headaches. She has always had a firm handshake, but lately, she has also noticed that her wedding ring is excessively tight. GR is also frustrated that she has recently had to replace her entire shoe collection because her shoe size has increased from 7½ to 9, with a need for increased width as well. Additionally, she has noticed increased perspiration, even when she is not exerting herself, and increased spacing between her teeth. Concerned about her progressive cosmetic changes and her lack of menses, GR turns to Internet searches for more information and comes across a condition called *acromegaly*.

Struck by the uncanny resemblances between her complaints and those she has read about on the Internet, GR arranges to see her doctor for further evaluation. A serum insulin-like growth factor (IGF-1) level is significantly elevated after correction for GR's age and gender, and her serum growth hormone level is 10 ng/mL (normal, <1 ng/mL) after an oral glucose load of 75 mg. A magnetic resonance imaging (MRI) study of her head reveals a pituitary adenoma with maximal diameter of 1.5 cm. These findings are consistent with a diagnosis of acromegaly due to a growth hormone-secreting adenoma. After referral to an endocrinologist and neurosurgeon, GR elects to undergo transsphenoidal pituitary surgery. GR tolerates the surgery well, but her postoperative growth hormone and IGF-1 levels remain elevated.

Based on the continued elevation in serum growth hormone and IGF-1 levels, GR's endocrinologist recommends medical treatment with octreotide. GR tolerates the thrice-daily injections well, except for occasional mild nausea. After 2 weeks of frequent injections, GR switches to a long-acting, depot form of octreotide that is injected once a month. GR is much happier with the reduced frequency of drug administration, although she continues to experience mild nausea and bloating as adverse effects of this medication.

After 6 months of depot octreotide injections, GR's growth hormone and IGF-1 levels remain elevated. GR is frustrated at the lack of improvement of her biochemical assays but does feel that she has more energy than before treatment, and her menses have resumed. GR's endocrinologist recommends treatment with pegvisomant as an alternative medical approach to treating the effects of her elevated growth hormone levels. GR begins daily injections with pegvisomant. Six months later, GR's IGF-1 level is in the normal range. GR is again flying around the nation in pursuit of increased sales, and she stops in town just long enough to complete her yearly head MRI and liver function tests.

Questions

1. Why was it necessary for GR to receive injections of octreotide and pegvisomant rather than taking the drugs orally?
2. Why are serum levels of IGF-1 a more appropriate screening test for acromegaly than growth hormone levels?
3. What anatomical and hormonal considerations are raised by the abrupt cessation of normal menstruation?
4. How do octreotide and pegvisomant act to lower IGF-1 levels?

In contrast to the indirect vascular connection between the hypothalamus and the anterior pituitary gland, a direct neural connection exists between the hypothalamus and the posterior pituitary gland. Neurons synthesize hormones, destined for storage in the posterior pituitary gland, in cell bodies of the hypothalamic supraoptic and paraventricular nuclei. These hormones are then transported down axons to the posterior pituitary gland, where they are stored in neuronal terminals until a release stimulus occurs. The posterior pituitary gland can, therefore, be thought of as an extension of the hypothalamus. As with the anterior pituitary gland, the fenestrated endothelial cells in a capillary bed surrounding the posterior pituitary gland, in this case arising from the inferior hypophyseal artery, facilitate release of hormones into the systemic circulation.

During development and proliferation, the fate of anterior pituitary gland cells is determined by a network of transcription factors that shepherd the terminal differentiation of these cells into thyrotrophs, corticotrophs, lactotrophs,

somatotrophs, and gonadotrophs. Three examples of transcription factors that are instrumental in anterior pituitary cell development are Pit-1, T-Pit, and Prophet of Pit-1 (Prop-1).

The anterior pituitary gland is a heterogeneous collection of numerous cell types, each of which has the capacity to respond to specific stimuli and to release specific hormones into the systemic circulation. Each of the several hypothalamic releasing or inhibiting factors alters the hormone secretion pattern of one or more anterior pituitary gland cell types (Table 27-1). Releasing factors also modify other cellular processes in the anterior pituitary gland, including hormone synthesis and pituitary cell growth. Interestingly, *the relationship between hypothalamic releasing factors and pituitary gland hormones is not always 1:1, nor is the interaction always stimulatory*. Somatostatin, for example, primarily inhibits the release of growth hormone (GH), but it can also inhibit release of thyroid-stimulating hormone (TSH) and prolactin. Conversely, thyrotropin-releasing hormone (TRH)

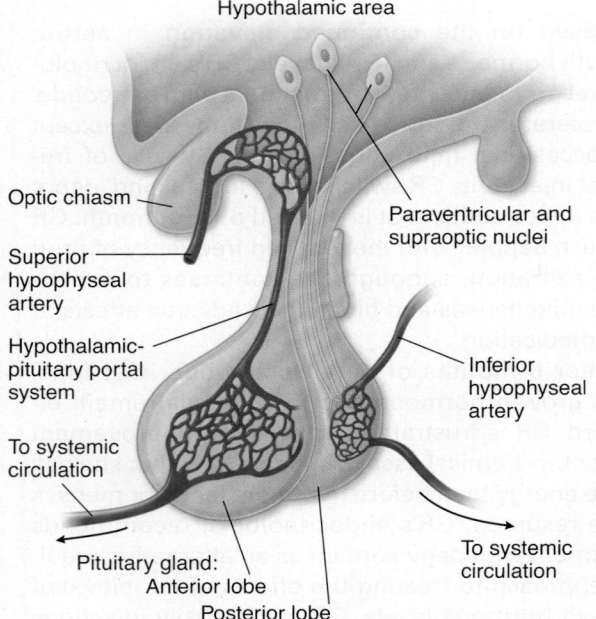

Hypothalamic area

Optic chiasm

Superior
hypophyseal
artery

Hypothalamic-
pituitary portal
system

To systemic
circulation

Paraventricular and
supraoptic nuclei

Inferior
hypophyseal
artery

Pituitary gland:
Anterior lobe
Posterior lobe

To systemic
circulation

FIGURE 27-1. The hypothalamic-pituitary portal system. Neurons in the hypothalamus release regulatory factors that are carried by the hypothalamic-pituitary portal system to the anterior pituitary gland, where they control the release of anterior pituitary hormones. Posterior pituitary hormones are synthesized in cell bodies of the supraoptic and paraventricular neurons in the hypothalamus and then transported down axonal pathways to terminals in the posterior pituitary gland. These hormones are stored in the posterior pituitary gland from which they are released into the systemic circulation. Note the separate vascular supplies to the anterior and posterior lobes of the pituitary gland.

primarily stimulates the release of TSH, but it can also cause release of prolactin. The overlapping activities of some releasing factors and release-inhibiting factors, together with the antagonistic actions of some stimulatory and inhibitory hypothalamic factors, provide a mechanism for the precise regulation of secretory pathways.

With the exception of dopamine, all known hypothalamic releasing factors are peptides. The anterior pituitary gland hormones are proteins and glycoproteins. Anterior pituitary gland hormones fall into three groups. Somatotropic hormones—**growth hormone (GH)** and **prolactin**—are 191 and 198 amino acids long, respectively, and exist as monomeric proteins that share significant structural homology. Glycoprotein hormones—**luteinizing hormone (LH)**, **follicle-stimulating hormone (FSH)**, and **thyroid-stimulating hormone (TSH)**—are heterodimeric proteins with carbohydrates attached to certain residues. These three hormones share the

same homologous α subunit, which is also shared by the human chorionic gonadotropin (hCG) hormone, but each has a unique β subunit that confers biological specificity. **Adrenocorticotropic hormone (ACTH)** belongs to a separate class, as it is processed by proteolysis from a larger precursor protein. Of importance, intact peptides and proteins are not absorbed across the intestinal lumen; local proteases digest them into their constituent amino acids. For this reason, therapeutic administration of a peptide hormone or hormone antagonist must be accomplished by a non-oral route—this is why, in the introductory case, it was necessary for GR to take octreotide and pegvisomant by injection.

The response of an anterior pituitary gland cell to a hypothalamic factor is initiated when the hypothalamic factor binds to specific G protein-coupled receptors located on the plasma membrane of the appropriate anterior pituitary cell type. Most of these receptors alter the levels of either intracellular

TABLE 27-1 Anterior Pituitary Gland Cell Types, Hypothalamic Control Factors, and Hormonal Targets

ANTERIOR PITUITARY GLAND CELL TYPE	STIMULATORY HYPOTHALAMIC FACTORS	INHIBITORY HYPOTHALAMIC FACTORS	PITUITARY HORMONES RELEASED	MAJOR TARGET ORGAN OF HORMONE	HORMONES PRODUCED BY TARGET ORGAN
Somatotroph	GHRH, ghrelin	Somatostatin	GH	Liver, cartilage	Insulin-like growth factors
Lactotroph	TRH	Dopamine, somatostatin	Prolactin	Mammary gland	None
Thyrotroph	TRH	Somatostatin	TSH	Thyroid gland	Thyroxine, triiodothyronine
Corticotroph	CRH	None known	ACTH	Adrenal cortex	Cortisol, aldosterone, adrenal androgens
Gonadotroph	GnRH	None known	LH and FSH	Gonads	Estrogen, progesterone, testosterone, inhibin

Each anterior pituitary gland cell type responds to multiple hypothalamic stimulatory and inhibitory factors. Integration of these signals determines the relative extent of hormone release by the anterior pituitary gland. Each hormone has one or more specific target organs, which are, in turn, stimulated to release their own hormones. These target hormones cause feedback inhibition at the hypothalamus and anterior pituitary gland. ACTH, adrenocorticotropic hormone; CRH, corticotropin-releasing hormone; FSH, follicle-stimulating hormone; GH, growth hormone; GHRH, growth hormone-releasing hormone; GnRH, gonadotropin-releasing hormone; LH, luteinizing hormone; TRH, thyrotropin-releasing hormone; TSH, thyroid-stimulating hormone.

cyclic adenosine monophosphate (cAMP), or inositol 1,4,5-trisphosphate (IP_3) and calcium (Ca^{2+}) (see Chapter 1, Drug–Receptor Interactions). The molecular details of receptor signaling provide a basis for understanding hypothalamic factor action. For example, **growth hormone-releasing hormone (GHRH)** binding to its receptors on somatotrophs increases intracellular cAMP and Ca^{2+} levels, whereas somatostatin binding to its receptors on somatotrophs decreases intracellular cAMP and Ca^{2+}. These signaling pathways provide a biochemical explanation for the opposing activities of GHRH and somatostatin on somatotroph release of GH.

The timing and pattern of hypothalamic factor release are important determinants of anterior pituitary cell response. *Most hypothalamic releasing factors are secreted in a cyclical or pulsatile, rather than continuous, manner.* For example, the hypothalamus releases pulses of **gonadotropin-releasing hormone (GnRH)** with a periodicity of a few hours. The frequency and magnitude of GnRH release determine the extent of pituitary gonadotropin release as well as the ratio of LH secretion to FSH secretion. Interestingly, continuous administration of GnRH suppresses rather than stimulates pituitary gonadotroph activity. These different pharmacologic effects of GnRH—depending on the frequency and pattern of administration—have important clinical consequences, as discussed below. Although not studied in as much detail, the majority of the other hypothalamic releasing factors are also thought to be secreted in a pulsatile manner.

Feedback Inhibition

End-product inhibition tightly controls hypothalamic and pituitary gland hormone release. For each hypothalamic-pituitary-target organ system, an integrated picture can be constructed of how each set of hormones affects the system. Each pathway, including one or more hypothalamic factors, its pituitary gland target cell type, and the ultimate target gland(s), is referred to as an **endocrine axis**; the term *axis* is used to connote one of multiple homeostatic systems that the hypothalamus and pituitary gland control. A simplified model consists of five endocrine axes, with a single type of anterior pituitary gland cell at the center of each axis (see Table 27–1 for anterior pituitary gland cell types).

Each axis regulates an important aspect of endocrine homeostasis and is, therefore, subject to close regulation. Feedback inhibition is usually discussed in terms of loops, because the regulatory connection between a given hormone and its target creates a "loop" that alters the subsequent extent of hormone release. These feedback loops closely regulate the hypothalamic-pituitary axes by providing levels of control at each stage of action (Fig. 27-2). *In general, systemic hormones produced by target organs negatively regulate the pituitary and hypothalamus to maintain an equilibrium level of hormone release.*

Just as regulatory loops are referred to based on a hormone's relationship to its target organ, many endocrine diseases are described based on whether the disease etiology is a disorder of the hypothalamus, pituitary gland, or target organ. The disease is referred to as *primary, secondary,* or *tertiary,* depending on whether the underlying abnormality is in the target organ, pituitary gland, or hypothalamus, respectively. *Therefore, a primary endocrine disorder is caused by target organ pathology, a secondary disorder reflects pituitary disease, and a tertiary endocrine disorder results from hypothalamic pathology.* Whether the underlying disease cause is primary, secondary, or tertiary can have important consequences for disease diagnosis and treatment, as discussed below.

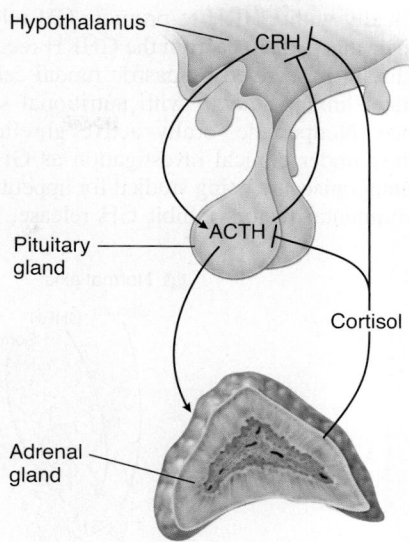

FIGURE 27-2. Hypothalamic-pituitary-target organ feedback. The general mechanism of hypothalamic-pituitary-target organ feedback is depicted here, using the hypothalamic-pituitary-adrenal axis as an example. Stimulatory hypothalamic factors (CRH in this case) stimulate the release of pituitary hormones (ACTH in this case). In response to pituitary hormone signals, the target organ (the adrenal gland in this case) produces a hormone (cortisol in this case). In addition to its systemic physiologic actions (*not shown*), cortisol negatively regulates the hypothalamic-pituitary-adrenal axis by inhibiting CRH and ACTH. ACTH also negatively regulates CRH, providing more sensitive control of the axis.

PHYSIOLOGY, PATHOPHYSIOLOGY, AND PHARMACOLOGY OF INDIVIDUAL AXES

Anterior Pituitary Gland

Hypothalamic-Pituitary-Growth Hormone Axis

The hypothalamic-pituitary-growth hormone axis regulates general processes that promote growth. Somatotrophs of the anterior pituitary gland produce and secrete growth hormone. GH is first expressed at high concentrations during puberty; it is secreted in a striking pulsatile manner, with the largest pulses usually occurring at night during sleep. Most of the anabolic effects of GH are mediated by insulin-like growth factors, especially **insulin-like growth factor 1 (IGF-1)**, a hormone released into the circulation by hepatocytes in response to stimulation by GH. Although several cell types are capable of producing IGF-1, hepatocytes contribute the overwhelming majority of detectable IGF-1 in the circulation. Unlike GH, which has a short circulating half-life and a pulsatile pattern of secretion, IGF-1 is protein-bound and stable in the circulation for longer periods of time at steady concentrations. Thus, IGF-1 measurements represent an integrated surrogate for GH activity that is stable throughout the day, and IGF-1 levels are a more appropriate tool than GH levels in screening for acromegaly (as in the introductory case).

Several environmental and biological stimuli regulate GH secretion. Environmental factors such as hypoglycemia, sleep, exercise, and adequate nutritional status can all increase GH secretion. Endogenous biological inputs that promote GH release include hypothalamic GHRH, sex steroids (most notably during puberty), dopamine, and **ghrelin**. Ghrelin is an important endogenous growth hormone-releasing peptide that has been identified and well characterized in the last decade. Ghrelin acts synergistically with GHRH to promote GH release, acting on a receptor that is distinct from the GHRH receptor. The majority of ghrelin is secreted by gastric fundal cells during the fasting state, linking growth with nutritional status and energy balance. Nonpeptide, orally active ghrelin mimetics are currently under clinical investigation as GH secretagogues, and antagonists are being studied for appetite control. Several environmental factors inhibit GH release, including hyperglycemia, sleep deprivation, and poor nutritional status. The most significant endogenous biological factors that inhibit GH secretion are somatostatin, IGF-1, and GH.

Pathophysiology and Pharmacology of Growth Hormone Deficiency

Failure to secrete growth hormone or to enhance IGF-1 secretion during puberty results in growth retardation (Fig. 27-3A–D). GH deficiency most commonly results

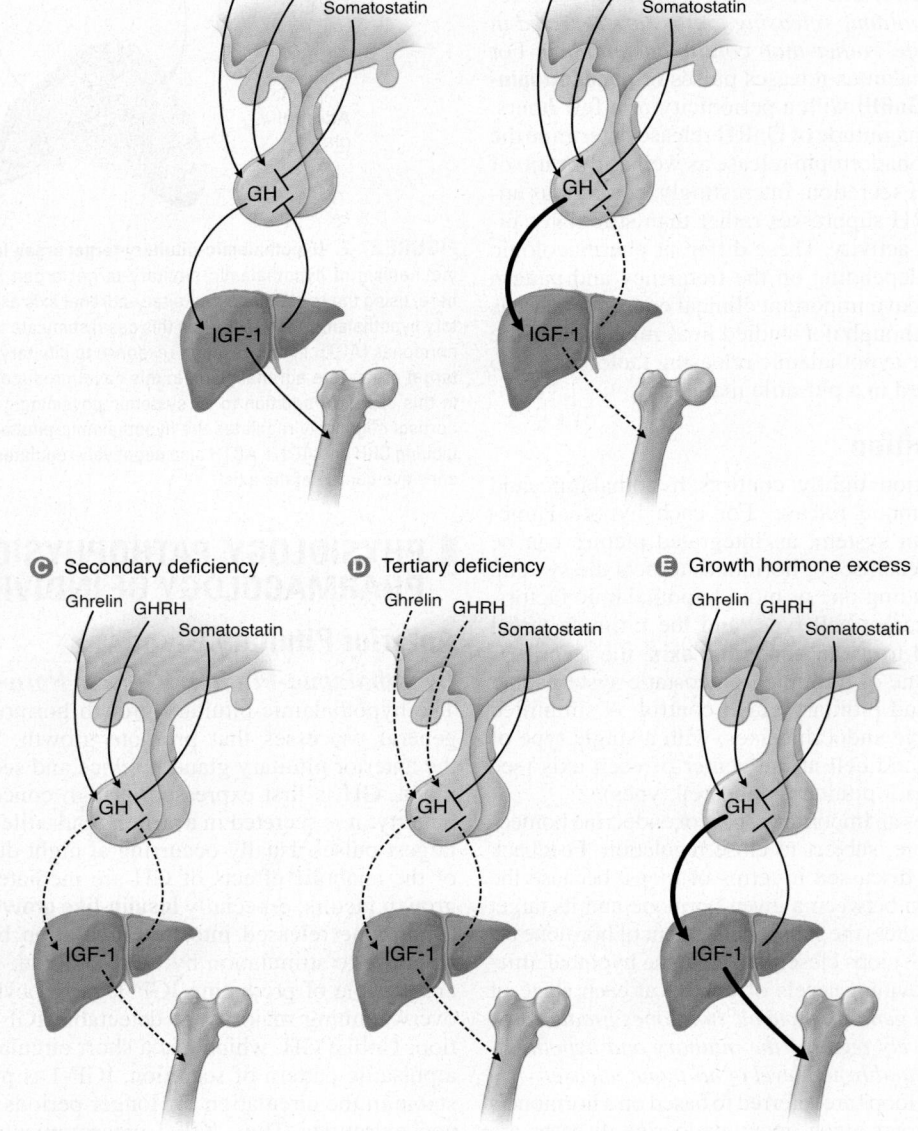

FIGURE 27-3. Hypothalamic-pituitary-growth hormone axis in health and disease. A. In the normal hypothalamic-pituitary-growth hormone axis, hypothalamic secretion of growth hormone-releasing hormone (GHRH) or ghrelin stimulates release of growth hormone (GH), while somatostatin inhibits release of GH. Secreted GH then stimulates the liver to synthesize and secrete insulin-like growth factor 1 (IGF-1), which promotes systemic growth. IGF-1 also inhibits GH release from the anterior pituitary gland. **B.** In GH insensitivity, the anterior pituitary gland secretes GH, but the liver is unresponsive to stimulation by GH. As a result, IGF-1 secretion is reduced (indicated by *dashed lines*). The decreased feedback inhibition of GH release results in higher plasma levels of GH (*thick line*). **C.** In secondary deficiency, the pathology lies in an unresponsive anterior pituitary gland, which secretes reduced amounts of GH. Because GH levels are low, the liver is not stimulated to produce IGF-1. **D.** In tertiary deficiency, the hypothalamus fails to secrete GHRH appropriately (*dashed line*); the role of ghrelin in this condition is unknown. Lack of sufficient GHRH results in lack of adequate stimulation of GH secretion by the anterior pituitary gland and, therefore, diminished production of IGF-1. **E.** In GH excess, GH is most commonly hypersecreted from an anterior pituitary adenoma. Elevated, and unregulated, GH levels result in increased hepatic production of IGF-1 and thus in systemic trophic effects. Because GH secretion occurs via an autonomous adenoma in the pituitary, negative feedback by IGF-1 is usually less effective.

from defective hypothalamic release of GHRH (tertiary deficiency, Fig. 27-3D) or from pituitary insufficiency (secondary deficiency, Fig. 27-3C). Importantly, however, failure of IGF-1 secretion in response to GH (Laron dwarfism or primary deficiency, Fig. 27-3B) is one etiology of short stature that is not amenable to treatment with GH. **Sermorelin** (synthetic GHRH) can be administered parenterally to help determine the disease etiology. **Tesamorelin**, a novel GHRH analogue, has also been shown to augment basal and pulsatile GH secretion and has been used in the treatment of HIV-associated lipodystrophy. If a patient possesses defective hypothalamic release of GHRH but has normally functioning anterior pituitary gland somatotrophs, administration of exogenous GHRH results in increased GH release. As of 2008, sermorelin has become unavailable in the United States due to discontinuation of industrial manufacturing. Alternative exogenous agents currently used to stimulate GH release include **glucagon**, **arginine**, **clonidine**, and **insulin**-induced hypoglycemia.

Most cases of growth hormone-dependent growth retardation are treated with replacement **recombinant human growth hormone**, referred to by the generic name **somatropin**. Typical dosing schedules involve daily subcutaneous or intramuscular injection. Newer GH analogues with longer half-lives, which would allow less frequent dosing, are currently in development. Somatropin therapy is costly and thus approved for use in the United States only for specific indications. In adults, either *confirmed GH deficiency* or *panhypopituitarism* (at least three hormonal axes affected) is required for approval, although unapproved use in competitive sports is prevalent. Some pediatric indications for GH use include idiopathic short stature, chronic kidney disease, Turner's syndrome, and Prader-Willi syndrome. The use of somatropin in AIDS cachexia and in critical illness is an area of active study, although not yet approved for use. Orally bioavailable peptidomimetics of growth hormone are an active area of research.

Recombinant IGF-1, known by the generic name **mecasermin**, is an effective treatment for patients with GH insensitivity (so-called Laron dwarfism). Mecasermin is also approved for use in patients with GH deficiency and antibodies against growth hormone. Mecasermin administration can be associated with adverse effects, including hypoglycemia and rare intracranial hypertension.

Pathophysiology and Pharmacology of Growth Hormone Excess

GH excess usually results from a somatotroph adenoma (Fig. 27-3E). Rarer syndromes of GH excess include ectopic production of GH or GHRH but are beyond the scope of this chapter. This entity has two differing disease presentations, depending on whether the GH excess occurs before or after closure of the bone epiphyses. Gigantism occurs if GH is secreted at abnormally high levels in children before closure of the epiphyses because increased IGF-1 levels promote excessive longitudinal bone growth. After the epiphyses close, abnormally high levels of GH result in **acromegaly**, as illustrated in the introductory case. This condition occurs because IGF-1, although it can no longer stimulate long bone growth, can still promote growth of organs and cartilaginous tissue. Typical manifestations include the nonspecific symptoms that GR initially experienced, such as increased hand thickness, enlarging shoe size, hyperhidrosis, and fatigue. Other frequent findings include large facial structures,

macroglossia, and organomegaly. Consequences of a pituitary mass lesion (adenoma) may also be evident, including headache, loss of other pituitary hormone functions (as manifested by cessation of menstruation, in the case of GR), and visual field loss.

Available management options for a somatotroph adenoma are surgical resection, medical therapy, and radiation therapy. Transsphenoidal surgical resection of the adenoma is the current standard of care. As seen in the case of GR, surgical treatment has variable success, especially when the adenoma exceeds 1 centimeter in size, and adjuvant medical therapy is frequently required. Medical options include somatostatin receptor agonists (also known as *somatostatin receptor ligands [SRLs]* or *somatostatin analogues*), dopamine analogues, and GH receptor antagonists.

Somatostatin receptor ligands (SRLs) are the mainstay of medical therapy. Somatostatin physiologically inhibits growth hormone secretion, making it a logical treatment for somatotroph adenomas. Somatostatin itself is rarely used clinically because it has a half-life of only a few minutes. **Octreotide** and **lanreotide** are synthetic, longer acting peptide analogues of somatostatin that have been used with extensive experience. **Pasireotide** is a somatostatin analogue first approved for the treatment of Cushing's disease; it has also shown clinical efficacy in the treatment of acromegaly and is now approved for this indication. In addition, trials are underway to evaluate the efficacy of an orally active octreotide in acromegaly. Somatostatin receptors are distributed widely, and somatostatin and its analogues affect many secretory processes. Therefore, octreotide can be used for several indications, including treatment of esophageal varices and certain hormone-secreting tumors. However, systemic administration of SRLs can lead to diverse adverse effects, including nausea, diarrhea, gallstones, and glucose dysregulation. Sustained-release formulations of SRLs, as exemplified in the introductory case, allow less frequent dosing but do not appear to alter the adverse effect profile. The efficacy of SRLs lies in their ability to normalize GH and IGF-1 levels in approximately 60–80% of acromegalic patients and to decrease pituitary adenoma size in 40–50% of affected patients.

Dopamine is a hypothalamic factor that acts mainly on lactotrophs to physiologically inhibit prolactin release. Dopamine also stimulates somatotrophs to release GH under physiologic conditions, but patients with acromegaly can have a paradoxical decrease in growth hormone secretion in response to dopamine. This effect may be due, in part, to the shared embryonic lineage of lactotrophs and somatotrophs; in fact, 20–30% of somatotroph adenomas also secrete excess prolactin. Based on this observation, the dopamine analogues **bromocriptine** and **cabergoline** are sometimes used as adjunctive agents in the treatment of acromegaly. Although these agents are much less expensive than SRLs and can be administered orally, dopamine receptor agonists are generally much less effective than SRLs and are thus typically used as second-line agents in the medical management of acromegaly. These agents are discussed below in relation to the hypothalamic-pituitary-prolactin axis.

The GH molecule has two binding sites, each of which is capable of binding one GH receptor monomer. GH action requires dimerization of the receptor after GH binding in order to initiate receptor activation and intracellular signaling. **Pegvisomant** is a GH analogue that has been modified such that one of the sites binds to the GH receptor with higher affinity than the native molecule, but the other binding site is inactive. Therefore, although pegvisomant binds tightly to the monomeric GH receptor, it prevents the receptor dimerization required for subsequent receptor activation and intracellular signaling. In effect, therefore, the drug acts as a competitive antagonist of GH activity. Pegvisomant also contains multiple polyethylene glycol (PEG) residues, which prolong the half-life of the drug and thereby allow once-daily dosing.

Of the available medical therapies, pegvisomant has the most potent IGF-1 reducing potential, but it also increases GH levels by decreasing IGF-1-mediated feedback inhibition of GH secretion. Concerns have arisen regarding increased tumorigenesis and accelerated somatotroph adenoma growth in the setting of the elevated GH levels induced by pegvisomant use; however, to date, no convincing data have emerged to support these concerns. Current practice suggests the performance of an annual pituitary MRI scan to monitor pituitary adenoma growth in patients taking pegvisomant. Despite its effectiveness at achieving biochemical control of IGF-1 excess, pegvisomant has several major limitations, including limited experience with its use, expensive cost, and liver function abnormalities. As seen in the case of GR, pegvisomant is currently used as a second- or third-line medical agent after SRL therapy has been attempted. In the future, the use of pegvisomant may become more prevalent if its overall safety profile remains favorable.

Hypothalamic-Pituitary-Prolactin Axis

Lactotrophs of the anterior pituitary gland produce and secrete prolactin. Their activity is inhibited by hypothalamic secretion of **dopamine**. TRH can enhance prolactin release, in addition to stimulating anterior pituitary thyrotrophs. Estrogen and breast feeding also enhance prolactin release, as described below.

Unlike other cells of the anterior pituitary gland, lactotrophs are under tonic *inhibition* by the hypothalamus, presumably mediated by hypothalamic release of dopamine (Fig. 27-4). *Therefore, a disease condition that interrupts the hypothalamic-pituitary portal system results in decreased secretion of most anterior pituitary gland hormones but causes increased prolactin release.* In patients taking phenothiazine antipsychotics or metoclopramide (see Chapter 14, Pharmacology of Dopaminergic Neurotransmission), increased levels of prolactin are frequently observed because these agents are dopamine receptor antagonists. Prolactin secretion does not appear to be regulated by any identified negative feedback system.

The physiologic actions of prolactin involve regulation of mammary gland development and milk protein biosynthesis and secretion. Prolactin levels are normally low in men and nonpregnant women. Increased estrogen levels during pregnancy stimulate lactotrophs to secrete increasing quantities of prolactin. During pregnancy, however, estrogen antagonizes prolactin action in the breast; this prevents lactation until after parturition. Suckling provides a powerful neural stimulus for prolactin release; prolactin levels increase as much as 100-fold within 30 minutes after the initiation of breast feeding. The positive feedback of breast feeding on prolactin secretion ensures continued replenishment of milk reserves. If a mother does not breast feed, prolactin levels decrease over the course of several weeks.

Interestingly, increased prolactin levels suppress estrogen synthesis, both by antagonizing hypothalamic release of

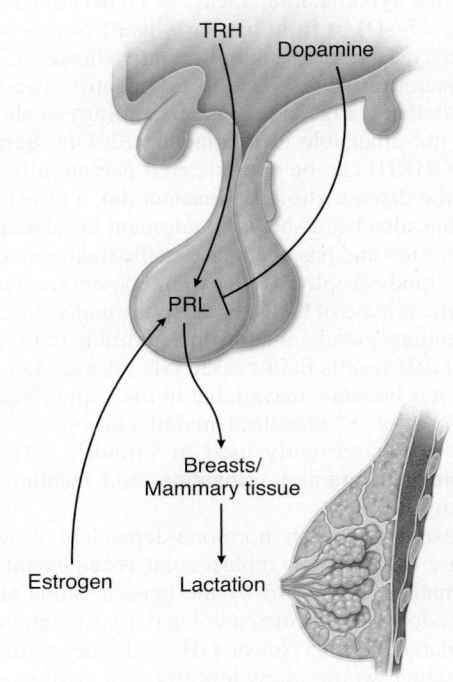

FIGURE 27-4. Regulation of the hypothalamic-pituitary-prolactin axis. Secretion of prolactin by anterior pituitary gland lactotrophs is tonically inhibited by hypothalamic dopamine. Hypothalamic TRH and circulating estrogens stimulate prolactin release. These stimulatory and inhibitory inputs on lactotrophs result in a baseline equilibrium of prolactin production. Disruption of this equilibrium results in an imbalance of prolactin production; for example, interruption of the pituitary stalk diminishes hypothalamic dopamine delivery to lactotrophs, resulting in increased prolactin secretion.

GnRH and by decreasing gonadotroph sensitivity to GnRH. The resulting decrease in LH and FSH release decreases end-organ stimulation of the hypothalamic-pituitary-gonadal axis, resulting in both decreased estrogen synthesis and suppression of ovulation while a woman is breast feeding. *Chronically high secretion of prolactin, such as by a prolactinoma, also suppresses the hypothalamic-pituitary-gonadal axis.* For this reason, prolactinomas are a common cause of infertility, especially in women, who may present with oligomenorrhea or amenorrhea.

Bromocriptine is a synthetic dopamine receptor agonist that inhibits lactotroph cell growth and prolactin secretion and is an established medical therapy for prolactinoma. Bromocriptine is orally bioavailable. As with octreotide, many of the adverse effects of bromocriptine result from systemic actions of the drug. The adverse effects of bromocriptine include nausea and vomiting, presumably because the area postrema in the medulla, which stimulates nausea and lies outside the blood–brain barrier, possesses dopamine receptors. The adverse effect profile of dopamine receptor agonists is dependent on their relative specificity for the various dopamine receptor subtypes (see Chapter 14).

Cabergoline and **quinagolide** are two other dopamine receptor agonists used to treat prolactinoma; the former is commonly used in the United States and the latter is available only in Europe. The advantages of cabergoline include a weekly or bi-weekly dosing interval and less frequent gastrointestinal adverse effects. Although both cabergoline and bromocriptine are considered category B for pregnancy (i.e., inadequate well-controlled safety data in pregnancy or adverse effects in animal studies), most practitioners typically use bromocriptine over cabergoline in pregnancy because of its significantly longer track record of experience and safety.

Recent reports have shown a link between the use of cabergoline and valvular heart disease. Comparative studies have correlated this risk with the higher dose cabergoline therapy used in Parkinson's disease, while the smaller doses frequently used to treat prolactinoma have not to date shown a significant link to valvular heart disease.

Hypothalamic-Pituitary-Thyroid Axis

The hypothalamus secretes **thyrotropin-releasing hormone (TRH)**, which stimulates thyrotrophs in the anterior pituitary gland to produce and secrete TSH. In turn, TSH promotes biosynthesis and secretion of thyroid hormone by the thyroid gland. Thyroid hormone regulates overall body energy homeostasis. Thyroid hormone negatively controls hypothalamic and pituitary release of TRH and TSH, respectively (see Fig. 28-4).

Because thyroid hormone replacement is an effective therapy for hypothyroidism, TRH and TSH are used mainly for diagnosis of disease etiology. If hypothyroidism is caused by an unresponsive thyroid gland (primary deficiency), serum TSH levels will be high because of decreased negative feedback from thyroid hormone. *For this reason, serum TSH is the main test used in screening for primary thyroid disease.* TRH administration would produce an exaggerated increase in TSH, although this test is no longer used regularly in clinical practice. Conversely, if hypothyroidism is caused by a defect in pituitary TSH production (secondary deficiency), the TSH level will not be high despite the presence of low thyroid hormone levels. In this scenario, if TRH were to be administered, the normally expected rise in TSH would be absent or significantly reduced.

Most cases of hyperthyroidism are primary, resulting from excessive thyroid hormone production or release from the thyroid gland; in this setting, thyroid hormone levels are high and TSH levels are low (see Chapter 28, Pharmacology of the Thyroid Gland). Rarely, hyperthyroidism can result from TSH-secreting pituitary adenomas (secondary hyperthyroidism), with inappropriately nonsuppressed (high or normal) TSH levels in the face of high thyroid hormone levels. Surgical resection is the recommended therapy for TSH-secreting pituitary tumors. If surgery is not curative or is contraindicated, medical therapy with octreotide or lanreotide can be effective in inhibiting TSH secretion, controlling hyperthyroidism, and reducing tumor volume.

Recombinant TSH (**thyrotropin**) is commonly used in conjunction with radioactive iodine treatment of thyroid cancer. Thyrotropin is administered before radioactive iodine therapy to maximize uptake of radiolabeled ^{131}I isotope into thyroid tissue in patients with thyroid cancer. This approach enables the administration of smaller quantities of radioisotope, maintaining maximum radiation exposure specifically to thyroid tissue with less radiation exposure to other tissues. Other aspects of thyroid gland pharmacology are discussed in Chapter 28.

Hypothalamic-Pituitary-Adrenal Axis

Neurons from the paraventricular nucleus of the hypothalamus synthesize and secrete **corticotropin-releasing hormone (CRH)**. CRH binds to cell surface receptors on corticotrophs of the anterior pituitary gland and stimulates corticotrophs to synthesize and release adrenocorticotropic hormone (ACTH; also called *corticotropin*). ACTH is synthesized as part of proopiomelanocortin (POMC), a precursor polypeptide that is cleaved into multiple effector molecules. In addition to ACTH, cleavage of POMC yields **melanocyte-stimulating hormone** (**MSH**), **lipotropin**, and **β-endorphin**. MSH has effects on skin pigmentation. ACTH is structurally similar to MSH, and high concentrations of ACTH can bind to and activate MSH receptors. In primary hypoadrenalism, increased ACTH levels result in enhanced skin pigmentation.

ACTH stimulates the synthesis and secretion of adrenocortical steroid hormones, including glucocorticoids, androgens, and mineralocorticoids (Fig. 27-5A). ACTH is required for secretion of glucocorticoids and adrenal androgens. Mineralocorticoid production is also regulated by potassium balance and volume status, and ACTH has a relatively minor role in regulating mineralocorticoids. ACTH also has a trophic effect on the zona fasciculata and zona reticularis of the adrenal cortex (see Fig. 29-1); excessive ACTH secretion causes adrenal hyperplasia, while ACTH deficiency ultimately causes adrenal atrophy. Among the several steroid hormone products of adrenal biosynthesis, cortisol is arguably the most crucial. In addition to serving as the main feedback inhibitor of pituitary ACTH release, cortisol functions as a "stress hormone" and is involved in vascular tone, electrolyte balance, and glucose homeostasis. Deficiency of cortisol can rapidly lead to critical illness or death, while cortisol excess results in Cushing's syndrome (Fig. 27-5B).

A synthetic form of ACTH, known as **cosyntropin**, can be used to diagnose suspected cases of adrenal insufficiency and also to assist in ascertaining whether the insufficiency is primary or secondary. Administration of cosyntropin to a patient with primary adrenal insufficiency will fail to increase plasma cortisol concentration due to the inherent dysfunction of adrenal biosynthesis. Conversely, administration of cosyntropin to a patient with new-onset secondary adrenal insufficiency will result in a robust increase in plasma cortisol. However, patients with long-standing secondary adrenal insufficiency may have a blunted cortisol response to cosyntropin, owing mainly to progressive adrenal cortical atrophy in the absence of the trophic effects of ACTH. Conditions requiring physiologic replacement of glucocorticoids are usually treated with synthetic analogues of cortisol, rather than ACTH, because use of the target hormone generally allows for more precise physiologic control. Cortisol physiology and pharmacology are discussed in greater detail in Chapter 29, Pharmacology of the Adrenal Cortex.

CRH is used as a diagnostic tool in petrosal sinus sampling for ACTH. CRH can be used to distinguish whether excessive cortisol secretion results from an ACTH-secreting pituitary adenoma or from an ectopic ACTH-secreting tumor (Fig. 27-5). If the hypercortisolism derives from a pituitary corticotroph adenoma (Cushing's disease), administration of CRH will usually increase blood ACTH levels (Fig. 27-5C). This response is not seen in the case of an ectopic ACTH-secreting tumor, which secretes ACTH at a constant autonomous rate (Fig. 27-5D).

Cushing's syndrome resulting from a primary adrenal tumor is often treated with surgical resection; however, several medical therapies also exist. **Metyrapone, ketoconazole**, and **mitotane** all have potent inhibitory effects on adrenal steroidogenesis and can be used to reduce cortisol production, while **mifepristone** antagonizes peripheral cortisol receptor

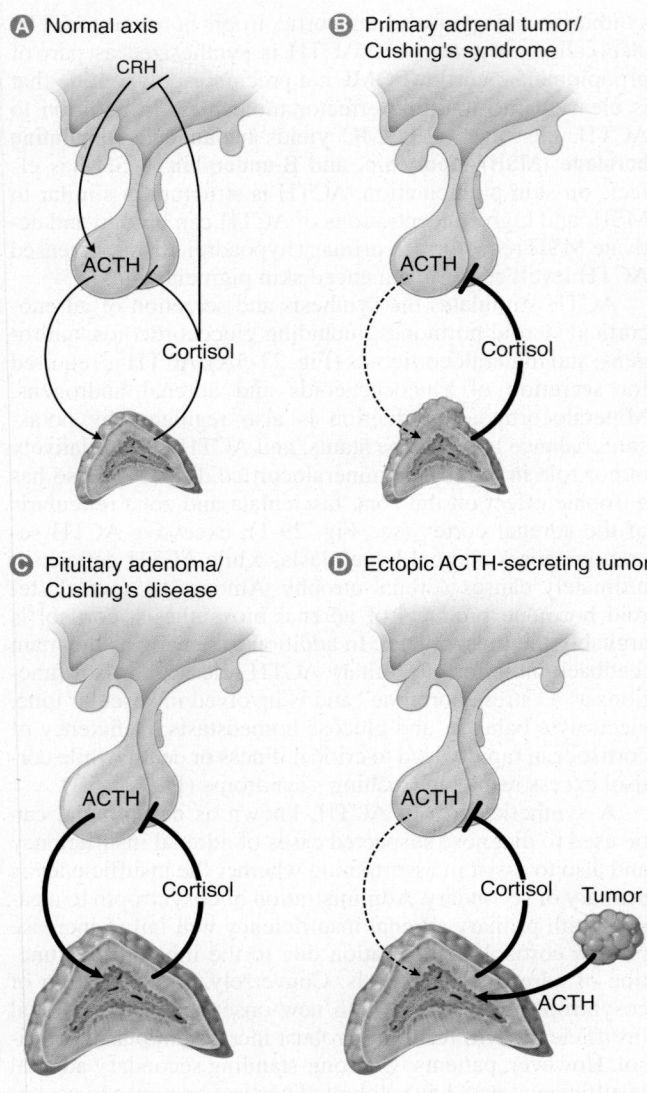

FIGURE 27-5. Hypothalamic-pituitary-adrenal axis in health and disease.
A. In the normal hypothalamic-pituitary-adrenal axis, hypothalamic secretion of corticotropin-releasing hormone (CRH) stimulates release of adrenocorticotropic hormone (ACTH). ACTH, in turn, stimulates synthesis and
secretion of cortisol by the adrenal cortex. Cortisol inhibits further release
of CRH and ACTH. **B.** A primary adrenal tumor causes Cushing's syndrome
by autonomously producing cortisol (*thick line*), independent of regulation
by ACTH. The excessive cortisol production suppresses ACTH production
(*dashed line*). **C.** An ACTH-producing pituitary adenoma causes Cushing's
disease by autonomously secreting excessive levels of ACTH (*thick line*),
which stimulate the adrenal gland to produce increased levels of cortisol
(*thick line*). ACTH secretion by the tumor has a blunted sensitivity to feedback inhibition by cortisol. **D.** An ectopic ACTH-secreting tumor (such as a
small cell carcinoma of the lung) also stimulates the adrenal gland to produce increased levels of cortisol, which suppress pituitary ACTH production.
However, circulating ACTH levels remain elevated due to the ectopic-source
production of the hormone.

binding (see Chapter 29). These therapies can also be used
in patients with Cushing's disease, although they are not targeted at the pituitary tumor itself. To date, there have been
few effective treatments targeted at the level of the pituitary
to reduce ACTH secretion in Cushing's disease.

Pasireotide was recently approved for therapy of Cushing's
disease. Pasireotide is a somatostatin analogue that targets

somatostatin receptors, with the highest affinity for somatostatin receptor subtype 5. In clinical trials, increased cortisol
levels in patients with Cushing's disease were significantly reduced during treatment with pasireotide. Hyperglycemia was
a common adverse effect even though cortisol levels were
reduced.

Hypothalamic-Pituitary-Gonadal Axis
Gonadotrophs are unique among anterior pituitary gland
cells because they secrete two glycoprotein hormones—LH
and FSH. Together, these hormones are referred to as *gonadotropins*. LH and FSH are both heterodimers composed of α
and β subunits. LH and FSH share the same α subunit with
TSH and hCG but possess unique β subunits. Gonadotrophs
regulate the secretion of LH and FSH independently. This
axis is diagrammed in Figure 27-6.

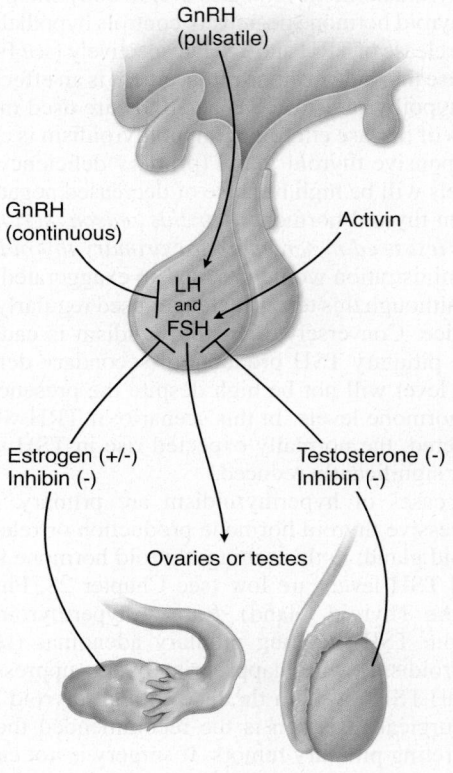

FIGURE 27-6. Hypothalamic-pituitary-gonadal axis. Gonadotropin-releasing
hormone (GnRH) is secreted by the hypothalamus in a pulsatile fashion, stimulating gonadotroph cells of the anterior pituitary gland to secrete luteinizing
hormone (LH) and follicle-stimulating hormone (FSH). LH and FSH stimulate
the ovaries or testes to produce the sex hormones estrogen or testosterone,
respectively, which inhibit further release of LH and FSH. Paradoxically, however, the increasing estrogen levels that are secreted from developing follicles
during the follicular phase of the menstrual cycle induce a positive feedback,
midcycle ovulatory surge of LH and FSH secretion. Inhibin is also produced by
the gonads in response to FSH and exerts negative feedback on gonadotrophs
to inhibit further release of FSH. Locally produced pituitary activin acts in a
paracrine fashion to stimulate FSH secretion. Exogenous pulsatile GnRH can
be used to induce ovulation in women with infertility of hypothalamic origin.
However, continuous administration of GnRH suppresses the gonadotroph
response to endogenous GnRH and thereby causes decreased production
of sex hormones. Analogues of GnRH with increased metabolic stability and
prolonged half-lives take advantage of this effect and are used to suppress
sex hormone production in clinical conditions such as precocious puberty
and prostate cancer.

Gonadotropins control hormone production by the gonads, promoting the synthesis of androgens and estrogens. The effects of estrogen and other reproductive hormones on the anterior pituitary gland are complex. In males, gonadotropins are inhibited via negative feedback by testosterone. In contrast, in females, depending on the rate of change and absolute concentration of estrogen, as well as the stage of the menstrual cycle, estrogen can exert both inhibitory and excitatory effects on gonadotropins. **Inhibin** is a hormone produced in the gonads that has inhibitory effects primarily on FSH secretion, with little effect on LH secretion. **Activin** is a paracrine factor that is produced and acts locally both in the pituitary and in the gonads and functions in the pituitary gland to stimulate primarily FSH secretion (Fig. 27-6). Endocrine control of the reproductive process is discussed in greater detail in Chapter 30, Pharmacology of Reproduction.

Native GnRH, which has a short half-life, can be administered in a pulsatile fashion to stimulate patterned gonadotropin release, while GnRH analogues with longer half-lives are used to suppress production of sex hormones by desensitizing the pituitary gland to the stimulating activity of the native releasing factor (Fig. 27-6). The main pharmacologic difference among the currently approved GnRH agonists is the route of administration. **Leuprolide** is the most commonly used GnRH agonist and can be administered as a daily subcutaneous injection or as a monthly depot injection. Osmotic pump implants (see Chapter 55, Drug Delivery Modalities) are also available that deliver leuprolide acetate at a controlled rate for up to 12 months. Long-acting agonists are utilized therapeutically to suppress gonadotropins in several clinical conditions, including in vitro fertilization, endometriosis, uterine fibroids, precocious puberty, and androgen-dependent prostate cancer. Their main drawback is that gonadotroph suppression does not occur immediately; instead, there is a transient (several days) increase ("flare") in sex hormone levels, followed by a lasting suppression of hormone synthesis and secretion.

FSH is used to stimulate ovulation for in vitro fertilization. Two US Food and Drug Administration (FDA)-approved formulations are available. **Urofollitropin** is purified FSH isolated from the urine of postmenopausal women, and **follitropin** is a recombinant form of FSH. Both agents effectively stimulate ovulation but may cause **ovarian hyperstimulation syndrome**. Interestingly, a rare form of ovarian hyperstimulation syndrome that occurs during pregnancy (familial gestational ovarian hyperstimulation syndrome) is caused by an inherited mutation in the FSH receptor. This mutation allows human chorionic gonadotropin (hCG), a hormone present in high concentrations during the early stages of pregnancy, to stimulate the FSH receptor. The resulting overstimulation of the FSH receptor is thought to cause the follicular enlargement and other sequelae characteristic of this syndrome. Whether similar mutations in the FSH receptor could be associated with cases of drug-induced ovarian hyperstimulation syndrome is an area of active investigation.

The GnRH receptor antagonists **cetrorelix** and **ganirelix** are sometimes used in assisted reproduction; they suppress premature surges in LH in the early to mid-follicular phase of the menstrual cycle, resulting in improved rates of implantation and pregnancy (see Chapter 30). GnRH antagonists also have applications for palliation of metastatic prostate cancer. In this situation, a direct GnRH antagonist has the advantage of avoiding the initial surge in testosterone caused by treatment with GnRH agonists.

Posterior Pituitary Gland

The anterior lobe of the pituitary gland secretes numerous hormones, while the posterior lobe of the pituitary gland (neurohypophysis) secretes only two hormones: antidiuretic hormone (ADH) and oxytocin. ADH is an important regulator of plasma volume and osmolality, while oxytocin has physiologic effects on uterine contraction and lactation.

Antidiuretic Hormone (ADH)

ADH is a peptide hormone produced by magnocellular cells of the hypothalamus. Cells in this region possess osmoreceptors that sense changes in extracellular osmolality. Increased osmolality stimulates ADH secretion from nerve terminals in the posterior pituitary gland. ADH binds to two types of receptors: V_1 and V_2. V_1 receptors, located in systemic arterioles, mediate vasoconstriction. This property gives ADH its alternative name, **vasopressin**. V_2 receptors, located in the nephron, stimulate the cell surface expression of water channels in order to increase water reabsorption in the collecting duct, as discussed in Chapter 21, Pharmacology of Volume Regulation. These two actions of ADH combine to maintain vascular tone by (1) increasing blood pressure and (2) increasing water reabsorption.

Disruption of ADH homeostasis results in two important pathophysiologic conditions. Excessive secretion of ADH causes the **syndrome of inappropriate ADH (SIADH)**; deficient secretion of ADH or decreased responsiveness to ADH causes **diabetes insipidus**. In SIADH, ADH secretion occurs irrespective of plasma volume status or osmolality. One of the most common causes of SIADH is the ectopic secretion of ADH by small cell carcinoma of the lung, but SIADH may also be caused by a medication effect or result from almost any pulmonary process, central nervous system insult, or pituitary surgery. Excessive ADH secretion results in persistent stimulation of V_1 and V_2 receptors, causing hypertension and excessive water retention. The inappropriate water retention can result in low extracellular sodium concentration. Until recently, if the source of excess ADH could not be removed, the only effective therapy for SIADH was restriction of fluid intake or administration of hypertonic saline. Over the past decade, the discovery and clinical use of vasopressin receptor antagonists has provided more therapeutic options for the treatment of SIADH.

Conivaptan and **tolvaptan** are vasopressin receptor antagonists that have recently been approved by the FDA for SIADH-induced hyponatremia. Tolvaptan is a specific V_2 receptor antagonist approved for use in heart failure, while conivaptan is a mixed V_{1a} and V_2 receptor antagonist approved for use in euvolemic and hypervolemic hyponatremia. Both are available as oral agents. **Demeclocycline** (a tetracycline antibiotic; see Chapter 34, Pharmacology of Bacterial Infections: DNA Replication, Transcription, and Translation) and **lithium** (see Chapter 15, Pharmacology of Serotonergic and Central Adrenergic Neurotransmission) are two other pharmacologic treatments that can also be used to treat SIADH.

Both diabetes insipidus and diabetes mellitus are characterized by symptoms of thirst, polydipsia, and polyuria. Despite their phenotypic similarities, however, the etiologies of diabetes mellitus and diabetes insipidus are unrelated. Diabetes insipidus is a disorder of vasopressin deficiency or resistance, whereas diabetes mellitus is caused by deficient production of insulin or target tissue insensitivity to insulin (see Chapter 31, Pharmacology of the Endocrine Pancreas and Glucose Homeostasis). Diabetes insipidus is characterized by polyuria and polydipsia secondary to an inability to concentrate urine and retain free water at the level of the renal collecting duct. A distinction is made between two types of diabetes insipidus. **Neurogenic diabetes insipidus** results from an inability of hypothalamic neurons to synthesize or secrete ADH. In this condition, administration of the exogenous ADH analogue, **desmopressin**, results in stimulation of V_2 receptors and a robust concentration of urine and decrease in thirst (Fig. 27-7). **Nephrogenic diabetes insipidus** results from an inability of renal collecting duct cells to respond to ADH (or, in other words, resistance to ADH). Nephrogenic diabetes insipidus can be caused by a mutation in the V_2 receptor, such that ADH is unable to bind the receptor

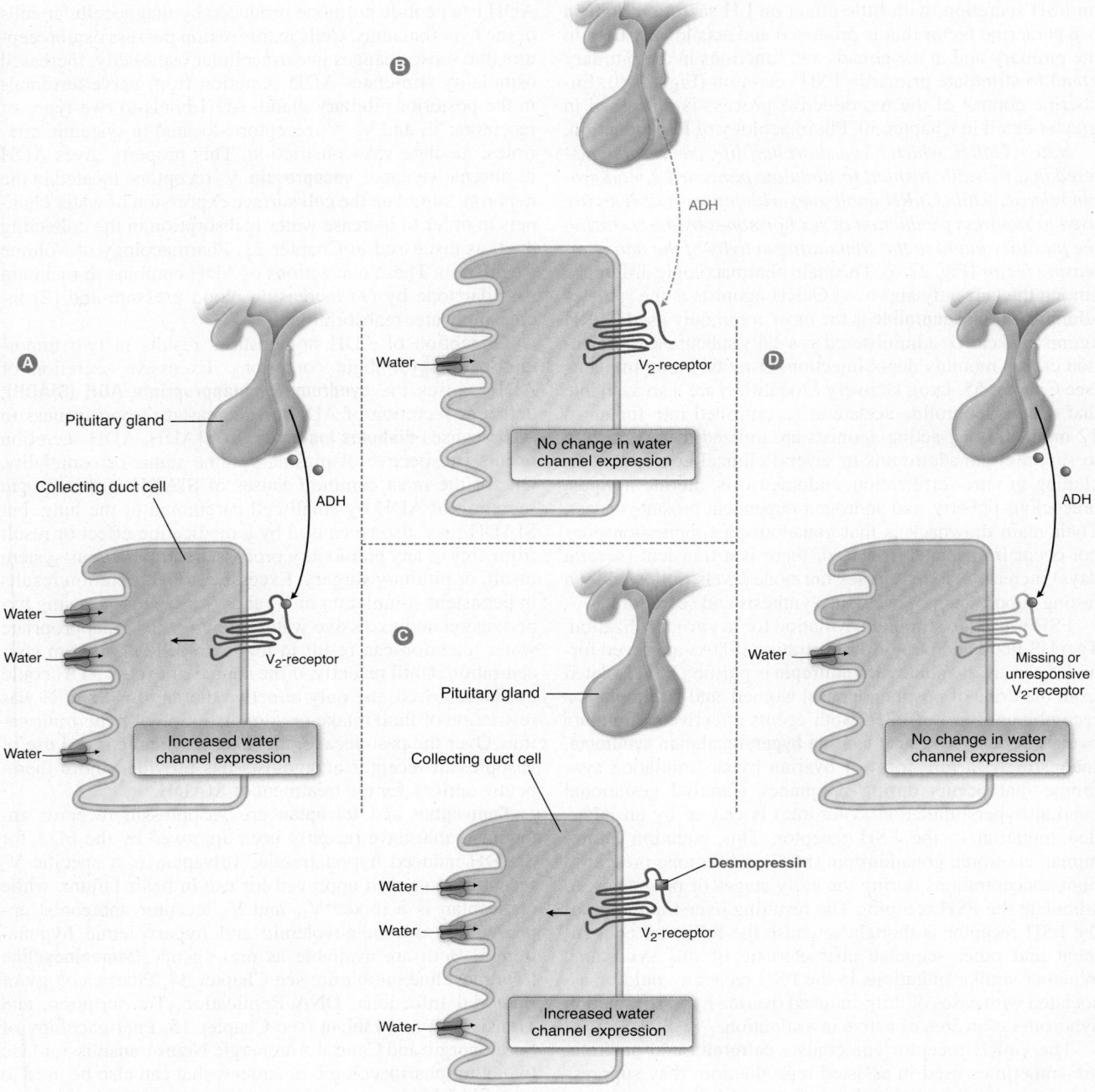

FIGURE 27-7. Comparison of neurogenic and nephrogenic diabetes insipidus. A. Antidiuretic hormone (ADH), released by nerve terminals in the posterior pituitary gland, stimulates V_2 receptors on renal collecting duct cells and thereby increases expression of water channels in the apical membrane of these cells. Increased water channel expression increases water flux through the cell. **B.** In neurogenic diabetes insipidus, the posterior pituitary gland is unable to secrete ADH. Consequently, there is no stimulation of renal V_2 receptors by ADH, and the collecting duct cells do not increase water channel expression. **C.** Exogenous administration of desmopressin, an ADH analogue, can replace the deficiency of posterior pituitary gland-derived ADH and thereby treat neurogenic diabetes insipidus. **D.** In nephrogenic diabetes insipidus, the V_2 receptor is either missing or unresponsive to stimulation by ADH. The lack of functional V_2 receptors prevents the cell from responding to ADH with an increase in water channel expression.

or stimulate receptor signaling, or by medication-induced resistance; lithium is one such medication.

In nephrogenic diabetes insipidus, administration of desmopressin results in little or no change in urine concentration or thirst because the V_2 receptor is insensitive to ADH and its analogues. Patients with nephrogenic diabetes insipidus can be treated with diuretics such as **amiloride** or **hydrochlorothiazide**. The proposed mechanism by which these diuretics prevent excessive loss of free water is paradoxical: they induce a volume-contracted state, which promotes enhanced absorption of water in the proximal tubule and thereby decreases delivery of water to the site of ADH resistance, the collecting ducts.

Oxytocin

Oxytocin is a peptide hormone produced by paraventricular cells of the hypothalamus. Many of the known physiologic roles of oxytocin involve muscle contraction; two such effects are milk release during lactation and uterine contraction. In the milk letdown response, stimuli to the hypothalamus cause oxytocin release into the blood from nerve terminals in the posterior pituitary gland. Oxytocin causes contraction of myoepithelial cells surrounding the mammary gland alveoli. This is an important physiologic action during breast feeding. In addition, it has long been known that administration of oxytocin causes uterine contraction. Oxytocin release is probably not the physiologic stimulus for initiation of labor during pregnancy; however, oxytocin is used pharmacologically to induce labor exogenously.

▌CONCLUSION AND FUTURE DIRECTIONS

Hormones of the hypothalamus and pituitary gland can be used as pharmacologic agents to modify the respective endocrine axes of each hormone. Recognizing the relationships and effects of primary, secondary, and tertiary disorders of any hypothalamic-pituitary axis is of paramount importance in understanding the appropriate diagnostic and treatment choices. Hypothalamic hormones can be used as diagnostics to determine the causes of underlying endocrine pathology (CRH, GHRH, TRH) or as therapeutics to suppress an axis (GnRH, somatostatin, dopamine). Hormones of the anterior pituitary gland can be given as replacement therapy in cases of deficiency (GH) or used diagnostically (ACTH). The posterior pituitary gland produces two hormones, ADH and oxytocin, which can be used to treat neurogenic diabetes insipidus and to induce labor, respectively. Recent advances have led to new medical therapies that extend the ability to treat pituitary hormone hypersecretion due to Cushing's disease. Future directions in hypothalamic and pituitary gland pharmacology will include design of new drug delivery systems; synthesis of orally active, nonpeptide analogues of hormones; and investigations to better understand hormone receptor mechanisms and signaling to assist in the design of new pharmacotherapies.

Acknowledgment
We thank Ehrin J. Armstrong and the late Armen H. Tashjian, Jr. for their valuable contributions to this chapter in the First and Second Editions of *Principles of Pharmacology: The Pathophysiologic Basis of Drug Therapy*.

Suggested Reading
Colao A, Petersenn S, Newell-Price J, et al. A 12-month phase 3 study of pasireotide in Cushing's disease. *N Engl J Med* 2012;366:914–924. (*Recent clinical trial of pasireotide.*)

Gadelha MR, Bronstein MD, Brue T, et al. Pasireotide C2402 Study Group. Pasireotide versus continued treatment with octreotide or lanreotide in patients with inadequately controlled acromegaly (PAOLA): a randomised, phase 3 trial. *Lancet Diabetes Endocrinol* 2014;2:875–884. (*Clinical trial of pasireotide for acromegaly.*)

Hays R. Vasopressin antagonists—progress and promise. *N Engl J Med* 2006;355:2146–2148. (*Perspective on SIADH and the future of vasopressin antagonists.*)

Melmed S. Acromegaly. *N Engl J Med* 2006;355:2558–2273. (*Review of growth hormone pathophysiology and treatment for acromegaly.*)

Verhelst J, Abs R. Hyperprolactinemia. *Treat Endocrinol* 2003;2:23–32. (*Review of the pathophysiology and management of hyperprolactinemia.*)

DRUG SUMMARY TABLE: CHAPTER 27   Pharmacology of the Hypothalamus and Pituitary Gland

DRUG	CLINICAL APPLICATIONS	SERIOUS AND COMMON ADVERSE EFFECTS	CONTRAINDICATIONS	THERAPEUTIC CONSIDERATIONS
GROWTH HORMONE AND INSULIN-LIKE GROWTH FACTOR REPLACEMENT Mechanism—Replace or stimulate release of growth hormone or insulin-like growth factor				
Somatropin (growth hormone [GH]) Somatrem	Growth failure in children with GH deficiency, Turner's syndrome, Prader-Willi syndrome, or chronic kidney disease Idiopathic short stature Replacement of endogenous GH in adults with GH deficiency	*Increased intracranial pressure, hypothyroidism, pancreatitis, scoliosis, slipped upper femoral epiphysis, intracranial tumor, pseudotumor cerebri, otitis media, rapid growth of nevi* Hyperglycemia, peripheral edema, injection site reaction, arthralgia, myalgia, paresthesia, headache, flu-like symptoms	Hypersensitivity to drug Patients with closed epiphyses Active underlying intracranial lesion Active malignancy Proliferative diabetic retinopathy Acute respiratory failure Acute critical illness due to complications following open heart surgery, abdominal surgery, or multiple accidental trauma Prader-Willi syndrome in patients who are severely obese, have a history of upper airway obstruction, or sleep apnea	Use with caution in patients with diabetes and in children whose GH deficiency results from an intracranial lesion. Available as depot injection. Glucocorticoids inhibit growth-promoting effect of somatropin.
Sermorelin (growth hormone-releasing hormone [GHRH]) Tesamorelin	Diagnostic evaluation of ↓ plasma growth hormone (sermorelin only) HIV lipodystrophy (tesamorelin only)	Injection site reaction (shared adverse effect); transient flushing, antibody development (sermorelin only); arthralgia, peripheral edema, myalgia (tesamorelin only)	Shared contraindication: Hypersensitivity to drug Tesamorelin only: Active malignancy Pregnancy Disruption of the hypothalamic-pituitary axis	As of 2008, sermorelin is no longer available in the United States. Monitor IGF-1 and glucose levels during therapy (tesamorelin only).
Mecasermin	Primary IGF-1 deficiency	*Hypoglycemia, increased intracranial pressure, seizure* Tonsillar hypertrophy, injection site reaction, lipohypertrophy	Hypersensitivity to mecasermin Growth promotion in patients with closed epiphyses Suspected or active neoplasm	Recombinant IGF-1. Available as twice-daily and once-daily injections.
AGENTS THAT DECREASE GROWTH HORMONE SECRETION OR ACTION Mechanism—Inhibit GH release (somatostatin receptor ligands: octreotide, lanreotide), antagonize GH receptor (pegvisomant)				
Octreotide Lanreotide	Shared indication: Acromegaly Octreotide only: Carcinoid syndrome Diarrhea from vasoactive intestinal peptide-secreting tumors	*Hyperglycemia, hypoglycemia, hypothyroidism (shared adverse effects); arrhythmias, bradycardia, ascending cholangitis (octreotide only)* Abdominal upset (shared adverse effect); backache, headache, dizziness, fatigue (octreotide only)	Hypersensitivity to drug	Also used to control GI bleeding and to reduce secretory diarrhea. Octreotide and lanreotide are available in a monthly depot formulation.
Pegvisomant	Acromegaly	*Chest pain, hepatitis, anaphylactoid reaction* Diarrhea, nausea, infectious disease, flu-like illness	Specific contraindications have not been determined	Patients should have yearly MRI to exclude enlarging adenoma. Effective at achieving biochemical control but also costly. Ongoing concern for GH-induced tumorigenesis and accelerated somatotroph adenoma growth.

AGENTS THAT DECREASE PROLACTIN LEVELS
Mechanism—Inhibit pituitary prolactin release

Bromocriptine	Hyperprolactinemia Acromegaly Parkinson's disease Diabetes mellitus type 2 Non-pregnancy related amenorrhea-galactorrhea syndrome	*Coronary artery thrombosis, heart valve disorder, pericardial effusion, gastrointestinal ulcer, hallucinations, psychotic disorder, pleural effusion, pulmonary fibrosis* Gastrointestinal upset, asthenia, dizziness, headache, rhinitis, fatigue	Hypersensitivity to drug Breast feeding Postpartum period in women with a history of coronary artery disease or severe cardiovascular condition Syncopal migraine Uncontrolled hypertension	Ergot alkaloid; dose twice a day. Intravaginal administration may reduce gastrointestinal adverse effects. Alcohol intolerance may occur. First-dose phenomenon occurs in 1% of patients and may result in syncope. Co-administration with amitriptyline, butyrophenones, imipramine, methyldopa, phenothiazines, or reserpine increases prolactin levels. Co-administration with antihypertensives may potentiate hypotension. Use of bromocriptine to suppress lactation in postpartum women is not recommended.
Cabergoline	Hyperprolactinemia	*Heart failure, disorder of pericardium, heart valve disorder, retroperitoneal fibrosis, pulmonary fibrosis, pleural effusion* Nausea, dizziness, headache	Hypersensitivity to drug Heart valve disorder Uncontrolled hypertension History of pulmonary, pericardial, or retroperitoneal fibrotic disorders	Use cautiously in patients prone to arrhythmias and with underlying psychiatric disorders. Use cautiously in patients with history of pleuritis, pleural effusion, pleural fibrosis, pericarditis, cardiac valvulopathy, or retroperitoneal fibrosis. CNS depressants have additive effects. Cabergoline produces less nausea than bromocriptine.

AGENTS THAT TEST THYROID FUNCTION OR STIMULATE IODIDE UPTAKE
Mechanism—TRH stimulates TSH release from pituitary; TSH stimulates thyroid gland to take up iodide

Protirelin (TRH)	Diagnosis of thyroid or pituitary function	*Seizure, amaurosis fugax in patients with pituitary tumors* Hypertension, hypotension, flushing, abdominal discomfort, nausea, xerostomia, headache, urinary urgency	Hypersensitivity to drug	Rarely used clinically. Transient changes in blood pressure can occur immediately following administration. Cyproheptadine and thioridazine decrease protirelin-induced TSH response.
Thyrotropin (TSH)	Adjunctive treatment of malignant tumor of thyroid gland	*Atrial arrhythmia, hyperthyroidism, hypersensitivity reaction, stroke* Nausea, vomiting, paresthesia, headache	Specific contraindications have not been determined	Used to stimulate radioactive iodine uptake in the treatment of thyroid cancer.

continues

DRUG SUMMARY TABLE: CHAPTER 27 Pharmacology of the Hypothalamus and Pituitary Gland *continued*

DRUG	CLINICAL APPLICATIONS	SERIOUS AND COMMON ADVERSE EFFECTS	CONTRAINDICATIONS	THERAPEUTIC CONSIDERATIONS
AGENTS THAT TEST ADRENAL FUNCTION **Mechanism—Stimulates adrenal cortisol and androgen production**				
Cosyntropin (ACTH 1-24)	Diagnosis of adrenocortical function	*Bradyarrhythmia, hypertension, tachycardia, anaphylaxis*	Hypersensitivity to cosyntropin	Can help differentiate primary from secondary adrenal insufficiency. Cosyntropin (contains first 24 amino acid residues of ACTH) is less antigenic and less likely to cause allergic reactions than corticotropin (contains all 39 amino acid residues of ACTH).
AGENTS THAT DECREASE CORTISOL SECRETION **Mechanism—Inhibit secretion of ACTH from corticotroph tumors**				
Pasireotide	Adult patients with Cushing's disease in whom pituitary surgery has not been curative or is contraindicated	*Hypocortisolism, hyperglycemia, diabetes mellitus, bradyarrhythmia, abnormal liver function tests, cholelithiasis* Abdominal pain, diarrhea, nausea, vomiting, headache	None	Hyperglycemia-related adverse events are common, the result of inhibition of insulin secretion and reduced incretin hormone responses, and frequently require initiation of a glucose-lowering medication.
AGENTS THAT ALTER GONADOTROPIN EXPRESSION AND INHIBIT OR STIMULATE GONADAL MATURATION AND STEROID PRODUCTION **Mechanism (GnRH and analogues)—Continuous: inhibit LH and FSH release; pulsatile: stimulate LH and FSH release. Mechanism (ganirelix, cetrorelix)—GnRH receptor antagonists. Mechanism (FSH)—Stimulate gonadal maturation and steroid production**				
Gonadorelin (GnRH)	Diagnosis of hypogonadism	*Anaphylaxis with multiple administrations* Light-headedness, flushing, injection site reaction, pruritus, abdominal discomfort, nausea, headache	Hypersensitivity to GnRH or GnRH analogues	Normal response to gonadorelin testing indicates the presence of functional pituitary gonadotrophs. Pulsatile form for stimulation of ovulation.
GnRH analogues: **Goserelin** **Histrelin** **Leuprolide** **Nafarelin**	Prostate cancer (goserelin, histrelin, and leuprolide only) Breast cancer (goserelin only) Endometriosis (goserelin, leuprolide, and nafarelin only) Precocious puberty (histrelin, leuprolide, and nafarelin only) Anemia associated with uterine leiomyoma (leuprolide only)	*Heart failure (goserelin and leuprolide only); diabetes mellitus, tumor flare, stroke, renal impairment, chronic obstructive pulmonary disease (goserelin only); pituitary apoplexy, seizure (histrelin and leuprolide only); liver injury, vertebral fracture, suicidal thoughts (leuprolide only); pulmonary embolism (leuprolide and nafarelin only); deep vein thrombosis, stroke (nafarelin only)* Sexual dysfunction, sweating (shared adverse effects); headache (goserelin and nafarelin only); peripheral edema, acne, seborrhea, breast atrophy, depression, mood swings, vaginitis (goserelin only); implant site reaction, amenorrhea (histrelin only); hot sweats, vaginal dryness, decreased bone mineral density (nafarelin only)	Shared contraindications: Hypersensitivity to GnRH or GnRH analogues Pregnancy Leuprolide and nafarelin only: Breastfeeding Vaginal bleeding	Depot formulations that result in gonadotropin suppression and consequent decrease in gonadal steroid production. Can initially increase testosterone and estrogen levels.

Drug	Clinical Applications	Adverse Effects	Contraindications	Therapeutic Considerations
Ganirelix Cetrorelix	Inhibition of premature LH surges in women undergoing controlled ovarian hyperstimulation	*Immune hypersensitivity reaction, ovarian hyperstimulation syndrome (shared adverse effects); spontaneous abortion (ganirelix only)* Abdominal pain (ganirelix only); swelling, bruising (cetrorelix only)	Hypersensitivity to drug Pregnancy Renal impairment	These drugs are GnRH receptor antagonists.
Follitropin (rFSH) Urofollitropin (FSH)	Ovulation induction Male hypogonadotropic hypogonadism	*Embolism and thrombosis, acute respiratory distress syndrome, ovarian hyperstimulation syndrome* Ovarian cysts and hypertrophy, upper respiratory infection (shared adverse effects); multiple births (urofollitropin only)	Hypersensitivity to drug Any endocrine disorder other than anovulation: abnormal uterine bleeding, primary gonadal failure, pituitary tumor, ovarian cyst or enlargement of unknown origin, pregnancy, sex hormone-dependent tumors, thyroid or adrenal dysfunction	May result in multiple fetuses.

VASOPRESSIN RECEPTOR ANTAGONISTS
Mechanism—Conivaptan: antagonist at V_1 and V_2 receptors; tolvaptan: selective V_2 receptor antagonist; both drugs prevent vasopressin-stimulated water reabsorption via V_2-coupled aquaporin channels in apical membrane of renal collecting duct cells (also, see Chapter 21)

Drug	Clinical Applications	Adverse Effects	Contraindications	Therapeutic Considerations
Conivaptan Tolvaptan	Euvolemic and hypervolemic hyponatremia (shared indications) Heart failure (tolvaptan only)	*Atrial fibrillation (conivaptan only); hypovolemia, gastrointestinal hemorrhage, liver injury, anaphylaxis, demyelinating disease (tolvaptan only)* Gastrointestinal upset, thirst, polyuria (shared adverse effects); phlebitis, injection site reaction, orthostatic hypotension, hypokalemia (conivaptan only); hyperglycemia, xerostomia, dizziness (tolvaptan only)	Shared contraindications: Hypersensitivity to drug Concurrent use of potent P450 3A4 inhibitors Hypovolemic hyponatremia Anuria Tolvaptan only: Inability to autoregulate fluid balance Urgent need to raise serum sodium acutely	Conivaptan is relatively nonselective for V_2 and V_1 receptors and must be administered IV. Tolvaptan is an orally bioavailable, V_2-selective agent. Requires careful titration to avoid overcorrection of hyponatremia. Conivaptan is a P450 3A4 substrate, and it is contraindicated to use this drug concurrently with P450 3A4 inhibitors such as ketoconazole, itraconazole, ritonavir, clarithromycin, and indinavir.

VASOPRESSIN ANALOGUE
Mechanism—Synthetic analogue of 8-arginine vasopressin (ADH)

Drug	Clinical Applications	Adverse Effects	Contraindications	Therapeutic Considerations
Desmopressin	Hemophilia A Neurohypophyseal diabetes insipidus Primary nocturnal enuresis Von Willebrand disease type I	*Myocardial infarction, hyponatremia, anaphylaxis, seizure*	Hypersensitivity to desmopressin History of or existing hyponatremia Renal impairment	Desmopressin stimulates V_2 receptors, resulting in concentrated urine and thirst.

28

Pharmacology of the Thyroid Gland

Anthony Hollenberg and William W. Chin

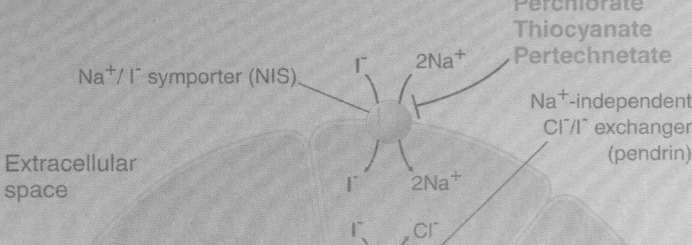

INTRODUCTION

The thyroid gland has diverse and important effects on many aspects of metabolic homeostasis. **Follicular thyroid cells** constitute the majority of thyroid tissue; these cells produce and secrete the classical thyroid hormones: thyroxine (T4), triiodothyronine (T3), and reverse triiodothyronine (rT3). Thyroid hormones regulate growth, metabolism, and energy expenditure, from oxygen consumption to cardiac contractility. **Parafollicular C cells** of the thyroid gland secrete **calcitonin**, a regulator of bone mineral homeostasis. Calcitonin is discussed in Chapter 32, Pharmacology of Bone Mineral Homeostasis.

The major diseases of the thyroid gland involve disruption of the normal hypothalamic-pituitary-thyroid axis (see Chapter 27, Pharmacology of the Hypothalamus and Pituitary Gland). Replacement of deficient thyroid hormone is an effective and established therapy for hypothyroidism. Treatment of hyperthyroidism is more complex, with options including antithyroid drugs, radioactive iodine, and surgical excision of abnormal tissue. Understanding the pathways and mechanisms of feedback regulation of thyroid hormone synthesis and thyroid hormone actions serves to explain the rationale for effective drug treatment of thyroid diseases.

THYROID GLAND PHYSIOLOGY

Synthesis and Secretion of Thyroid Hormones

The thyroid is an endocrine gland located in the neck inferior to the larynx and spanning the ventral surface of the trachea. The main function of the thyroid gland is to produce the thyroid hormones, T3 and T4. Structurally, the thyroid hormones are built on a backbone of two tyrosine molecules that are iodinated and connected by an ether linkage (Fig. 28-1). An important structural feature of thyroid hormones is the placement of iodines on this backbone. The position and relative orientation of iodines attached to the tyrosine residues determine the specific form of thyroid hormone. **3,5,3′,5′-Tetraiodothyronine (thyroxine, T4)** has four iodines attached to the tyrosine backbones and is the major form of thyroid hormone secreted by the thyroid gland. **3,5,3′-Triiodothyronine (T3)** has three iodines. Most T3 is produced by peripheral or extra-thyroidal 5′ deiodination of T4 (see below). A biologically inactive form of thyroid hormone is 3,3′,5′-triiodothyronine, also referred to as **reverse triiodothyronine (rT3)** because the single iodine is on the opposite tyrosine in the backbone relative to T3. In a normal individual, circulating thyroid hormone consists of about 90% T4, 9% T3, and 1% rT3, and most of the hormone is bound to plasma proteins (both specific binding proteins and albumin).

Iodine is a trace element that is a crucial component of thyroid hormone structure. Thyroid follicular cells, which synthesize and secrete thyroid hormones, selectively concentrate iodide (I^-) via a Na^+/I^- symporter (NIS) located on the basolateral membrane of the cell (Fig. 28-2). This active transport mechanism has the ability to concentrate iodide to intracellular concentrations up to 500 times that of plasma; most individuals have thyroid gland to plasma iodide ratios of approximately 30.

Once inside thyroid gland follicular cells, iodide is transported across the apical membrane of the cell via a Na^+-independent Cl^-/I^- exchanger (one is known as *pendrin*) into the colloid space (Fig. 28-2). Iodide is then oxidized

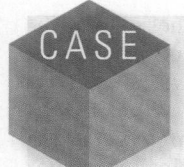

CASE

Over the course of a few months, Diana L, 45 years old, notices a number of disconcerting changes in the way she feels and in her general appearance. Ms. L feels nervous all the time; small events make her jumpy. She also keeps the temperature unusually cold in her house, to the point where her husband and children begin to complain. Because of these symptoms and the occasional feeling that her heart "skips a beat," Ms. L goes to see her doctor. After some questioning, he palpates her neck and notes that her thyroid gland is diffusely enlarged. He also notes that Ms. L's eyes are more prominent than normal. Tests for thyroid hormone levels reveal high serum free triiodothyronine (T3) and low thyrotropin (TSH). In addition, a test for TSH receptor antibody is positive. Ms. L is diagnosed with Graves' disease, a form of hyperthyroidism, and treated with methimazole. Although initially comforted by the fact that her doctor can explain her symptoms, she soon becomes discouraged because she does not notice any improvement for a couple of weeks. After a month, however, her symptoms begin to subside. Repeat tests confirm that her thyroid hormone levels are normalized. One year after starting treatment with methimazole, however, she begins to reexperience palpitations and feels

anxious. Her doctor confirms that her thyroid hormone levels are again elevated, despite methimazole therapy. After discussion with her doctor, Ms. L elects to undergo treatment with radioactive iodine. She tolerates the treatment well, and testing over the next 3 years shows that she has normal thyroid hormone levels. However, 4 years after radioactive iodine treatment, she develops symptoms that are the opposite of her original problems: she feels tired and cold all the time, and she gains 30 pounds over the course of 6 months. Her doctor confirms that Ms. L has developed hypothyroidism. He prescribes thyroxine (T4), which she now takes once a day, and she feels well again.

Questions

1. Why was Ms. L's serum thyrotropin level low but her triiodothyronine level high?
2. Which features of the thyroid gland make radioactive iodine a generally safe and specific therapy for hyperthyroidism?
3. Why did Ms. L develop hypothyroidism after treatment with radioactive iodine?
4. What is the mechanism of action of methimazole? Why did methimazole eventually stop working?

by the enzyme **thyroid peroxidase** (Fig. 28-2). This oxidation reaction creates a reactive iodide intermediate that couples to specific tyrosine residues on **thyroglobulin**. Thyroglobulin is a protein synthesized by thyroid follicular cells and secreted at the apical surface into the colloid space. Thyroid peroxidase is also concentrated at the apical surface,

and it is thought that generation of oxidized iodide at this surface allows the iodide to react with tyrosine residues in the newly secreted thyroglobulin molecules. The process of thyroglobulin iodination is known as **organification**. Organification results in thyroglobulin molecules containing **monoiodotyrosine** (MIT) and **diiodotyrosine** (DIT) residues; these tyrosine residues have one or two covalently attached iodines, respectively.

After MITs and DITs are generated within thyroglobulin, thyroid peroxidase also catalyzes **coupling** between these residues. An MIT joined to DIT generates T3, while the joining of two DITs creates T4. Note again that the majority of plasma T3 is produced by metabolism of T4 in the circulation (also see the following section, "Metabolism of Thyroid Hormones")

Thyroxine (T4)

Outer ring deiodination   *Inner ring deiodination*

3,5,3'-Triiodothyronine (T3)
(biologically active)

3,3',5'-Triiodothyronine (rT3)
(biologically inactive)

FIGURE 28-1. Structure and peripheral metabolism of thyroid hormones. Thyroid hormones are synthesized from two derivatized tyrosine molecules that are attached by an ether linkage. The outer ring is hydroxylated, whereas the inner ring is linked covalently to thyroglobulin during thyroid hormone synthesis. Iodine is attached to three or four positions of the tyrosine backbone, creating several different substitution patterns. Thyroxine (T4) has four iodines attached, two on each ring. Thyroxine is the predominant thyroid hormone produced by the thyroid gland. Triiodothyronine (T3) has two iodines attached to the inner ring but only one iodine attached to the outer ring. In contrast, reverse triiodothyronine (rT3) has two iodines on the outer ring but only one iodine on the inner ring. During peripheral metabolism, thyroxine is deiodinated by deiodinases present in target tissues and in the liver. The pattern of deiodination produces either T3 or rT3. If the iodine is removed from the outer ring by 5'-deiodinase, the biologically active T3 is produced. If the iodine is removed from the inner ring, the biologically inactive rT3 is produced.

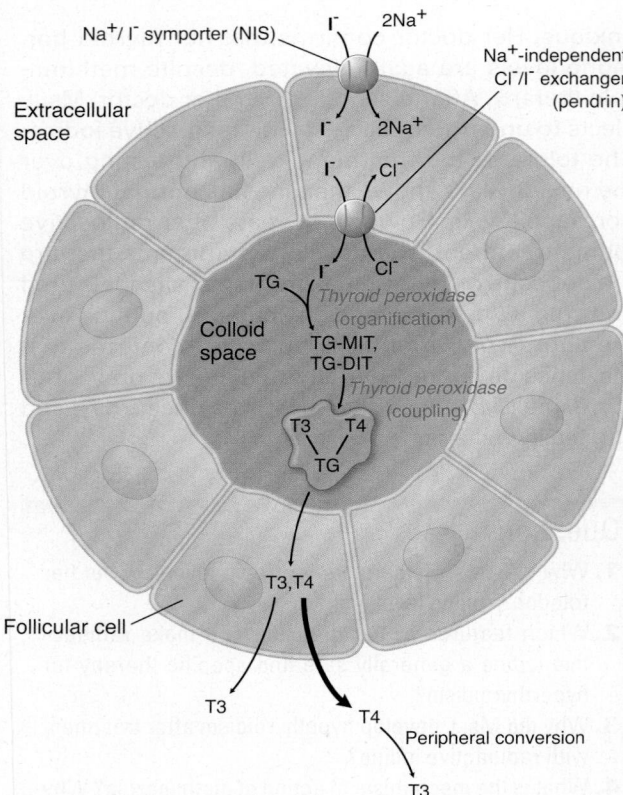

FIGURE 28-2. Thyroid hormone synthesis, storage, and release. Follicular cells of the thyroid gland concentrate iodide (I⁻) from plasma via a basolateral membrane Na⁺/I⁻ symporter (NIS). Iodide is further transported to the colloid space via the sodium-independent Cl⁻/I⁻ exchanger (pendrin). In a reaction (called *organification*) catalyzed by thyroid peroxidase, iodide reacts covalently with tyrosine residues on thyroglobulin (TG) molecules at the apical membrane of the follicular cell. Addition of one I⁻ to tyrosine results in the formation of monoiodinated tyrosine (MIT); addition of two I⁻ to tyrosine results in the formation of diiodinated tyrosine (DIT). MIT and DIT associate covalently on thyroglobulin via a mechanism known as *coupling*, which is also catalyzed by thyroid peroxidase. The derivatized thyroglobulin is stored as colloid within follicles in the thyroid gland. Upon stimulation by TSH, thyroid follicular cells endocytose colloid into lysosomal compartments, where the thyroglobulin is degraded to yield free T4, free T3, and uncoupled MIT and DIT. T3 and T4 are secreted into the plasma, and MIT and DIT are deiodinated intracellularly to yield free iodide for use in new thyroid hormone synthesis (*not shown*). The thyroid gland secretes more T4 than T3, although T4 is converted to T3 in peripheral tissues. The monocarboxylate 8 transporter (MCT8) is localized at the basolateral membrane of thyroid follicular cells and is one of the transporters involved in secretion of thyroid hormones from the thyroid gland (*not shown*).

and that nascent T3 and T4 are covalently part of the thyroglobulin protein at this point. These thyroglobulin molecules are then stored in the lumen of the follicle as **colloid**.

When thyroid-stimulating hormone (discussed below) stimulates the thyroid gland to secrete thyroid hormone, the follicular cells endocytose colloid. The ingested thyroglobulin enters lysosomes, where proteases digest the thyroglobulin. Proteolytic digestion releases free T3, T4, MIT, and DIT. T3 and T4 are transported across the follicular cell basolateral membrane and into the blood. Free MIT and DIT are rapidly deiodinated within the cell, allowing the iodide to be recycled for new thyroid hormone synthesis.

Most endocrine organs concurrently synthesize and release new hormone when activated rather than storing large quantities of precursor hormone. *The thyroid gland is unusual among endocrine glands in that it stores large quantities of thyroid prohormone in the form of thyroglobulin.* It is not understood why the thyroid gland maintains this elaborate pathway for hormone synthesis and release, but doing so makes it possible to maintain plasma thyroid hormone at a constant level despite fluctuations in the availability of dietary iodide.

Metabolism of Thyroid Hormones

Thyroid hormone circulates mostly bound to plasma proteins, notably **thyroid-binding globulin (TBG)** and transthyretin. Although T4 is the predominant thyroid hormone found in the blood, the physiologic activity of T3 is fourfold higher than that of T4 on target tissues. Some serum T4 is inactivated by deamination, decarboxylation, or conjugation and excretion by the liver. Most T4, however, is deiodinated to the more active T3 form in several locations in the body. This deiodination reaction is catalyzed by the enzyme **iodothyronine 5′-deiodinase** (Fig. 28-1).

There are three subtypes of deiodinase. **Type I 5′-deiodinase**, expressed in the liver and kidneys, is important for converting T4 to the majority of serum T3. **Type II 5′-deiodinase** is expressed primarily in the pituitary gland, brain, and brown fat. This enzyme is located intracellularly and converts T4 to T3 locally. **Type III 5-deiodinase** is responsible largely for conversion of T4 to the biologically inactive rT3.

The presence of T4 in the blood provides a buffer, or reservoir, for thyroid hormone effects. Most T4 to T3 conversion occurs in the liver, and many pharmacologic agents that increase hepatic cytochrome P450 enzyme activity also increase T4 to T3 conversion. In addition, T4 has a half-life in the plasma of approximately 6 days, whereas plasma T3 has a half-life of only 1 day. *Because T4 has a long plasma half-life, changes in thyroid hormone-regulated functions caused by pharmacologic intervention are generally not observed for a period of 1 to 2 weeks,* as seen with Ms. L in the introductory case.

Effects of Thyroid Hormones on Target Tissues

Thyroid hormones have effects on virtually every cell of the body. While the majority of the effects of thyroid hormones likely occur at the level of gene transcription, there is growing evidence that these hormones also act at the plasma membrane and/or in the cytoplasm. Both modes of action are mediated by hormone binding to thyroid hormone receptors (TRs).

Free hormone enters the cell by both passive diffusion and active transport, the latter mediated by hormone-specific and nonspecific carriers such as organic anion and monocarboxylate transporters that are located in the plasma membrane. The best described of these is the monocarboxylate 8 transporter (MCT8), although other transporters likely also contribute to thyroid hormone transport. Once inside the cell, thyroid hormone binds to thyroid hormone receptors. These TRs are proteins containing thyroid hormone-binding, DNA-binding, and dimerization domains. There are two classes of thyroid hormone receptor, termed **TRα** and **TRβ**. In addition, both TRα and TRβ can be expressed as multiple isoforms. TR monomers can interact in a dimerization reaction to form homodimers or with another transcription factor, **retinoid**

X receptor (RXR), to form heterodimers. These TR dimers bind to gene regulatory regions and are activated by binding of thyroid hormones. Together, the multiple different combinations of TRs and the variability in their tissue distributions create tissue specificity for thyroid hormone effects.

In the absence of hormone, thyroid hormone receptor dimers associate with corepressor molecules and constitutively bind to (and thereby inactivate) thyroid hormone-stimulated genes. Binding of thyroid hormone to TR:RXR or TR:TR dimers promotes dissociation of the corepressors and recruitment of coactivators to the DNA. Thus, thyroid hormone binding to TR dimers serves as a molecular switch from inhibition to activation of gene transcription (Fig. 28-3). Thyroid hormone also acts to down-regulate gene expression by a TR-dependent mechanism, the exact nature of which is not fully understood. For example, thyroid hormone is able to down-regulate TSH subunit gene expression, causing negative feedback of thyroid hormone on the hypothalamic-pituitary-thyroid axis (see Chapter 27). Increasing evidence suggests that thyroid hormone also has nongenomic effects on mitochondrial metabolism and that it interacts with plasma membrane receptors to stimulate intracellular signal transduction.

Thyroid hormone is important in infancy for growth and development of the nervous system. Congenital deficiency of thyroid hormone results in **cretinism**, a severe but preventable form of mental retardation. Genetic mutations in the MCT8 transporter are associated with **Allan-Herndon-Dudley syndrome**, a neurologic disease that presents in male children with a constellation of motor, cognitive, and developmental problems. These children also have abnormalities in thyroid

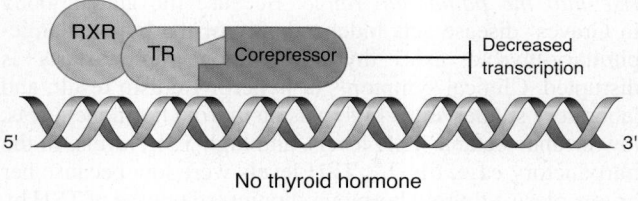
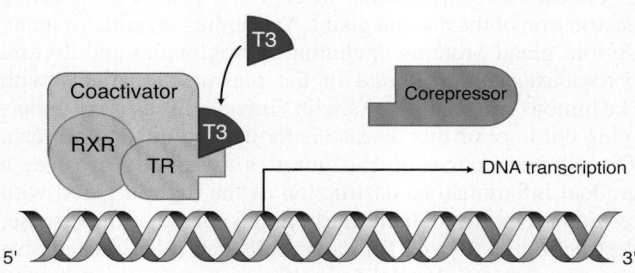

FIGURE 28-3. Thyroid hormone receptor actions. In the absence of thyroid hormone, the thyroid hormone receptor (TR):retinoid X receptor (RXR) heterodimer associates with a corepressor complex, which binds to promoter regions of DNA and inhibits gene expression. In the presence of thyroid hormone (T3), the corepressor complex dissociates from the TR:RXR heterodimer, coactivators are recruited, and gene transcription occurs. This example demonstrates the action of T3 on a TR:RXR heterodimer, but similar mechanisms are probable for TR:TR homodimers. A useful therapeutic strategy in the future may involve pharmacologic targeting of tissue-specific corepressors or coactivators.

function, with normal TSH levels in the setting of elevated circulating T3 levels and low T4 levels. Thus, MCT8 mutations appear to impair central feedback of thyroid hormones (see below), leading to elevated levels of T3 in the presence of a normal level of TSH. The low T4 level appears to be multifactorial; one factor is that MCT8 is involved in secretion of T4 from the thyroid gland. MCT8 mutations might lead to severe neurologic disease because of the lack of transport of thyroid hormone into key areas of the brain during development. It is also possible, however, that MCT8 transports other factors that are key to normal neurologic development.

In the adult, thyroid hormone regulates general body metabolism and energy expenditure. Enzymes regulated by thyroid hormone include the Na^+/K^+ ATPase and many of the enzymes of intermediary metabolism, both anabolic and catabolic. At high levels of thyroid hormone, this effect can result in futile cycling and a consequent increase in body temperature—this is why Ms. L started turning down the heat in her home. Many of the effects of thyroid hormone resemble the effects of sympathetic neural stimulation, including increased cardiac contractility and heart rate, excitability, nervousness, and diaphoresis (sweating). These symptoms were also seen in Ms. L—she was nervous all the time and was startled by slight provocations. Conversely, low levels of thyroid hormone result in **myxedema**, a hypometabolic state characterized by lethargy, dry skin, coarse voice, and cold intolerance.

Hypothalamic-Pituitary-Thyroid Axis

Thyroid hormone secretion follows a negative regulatory feedback scheme similar to that of the other hypothalamic-pituitary-target organ axes (Fig. 28-4). **Thyrotropin-releasing hormone (TRH)** is a tripeptide secreted by the hypothalamus that travels via the hypothalamic-pituitary portal circulation to the anterior pituitary gland (see Chapter 27). TRH binds to a G protein-coupled receptor located in the plasma membrane of anterior pituitary gland thyrotropes, or TSH-producing cells. This stimulates a signal transduction cascade that ultimately promotes the synthesis and release of **thyroid-stimulating hormone (TSH)**. TSH is the most important direct regulator of thyroid gland function. TSH stimulates every known aspect of thyroid hormone production, including iodide uptake, organification, coupling, thyroglobulin internalization, and secretion of thyroid hormone. In addition, TSH promotes increased vascularization and growth of the thyroid gland. In pathologic conditions where TSH or a TSH mimic (see below) is secreted at high levels, the thyroid gland can enlarge to several times its normal size, resulting in the characteristic diffusely hypertrophied thyroid gland referred to as a **goiter**, which Ms. L's doctor noted when he palpated her neck.

Negative feedback of the hypothalamic-pituitary-thyroid axis occurs through regulatory actions of thyroid hormone on both the hypothalamus and pituitary gland. Secreted thyroid hormone diffuses and is transported into the thyrotropes of the anterior pituitary gland, where it binds and activates nuclear thyroid hormone receptors. These bound receptors inhibit TSH gene transcription and, hence, TSH synthesis. Thyroid hormone also has important regulatory effects on the hypothalamus; thyroid hormone binding to receptors in hypothalamic cells inhibits transcription of the gene that codes for the TRH precursor protein.

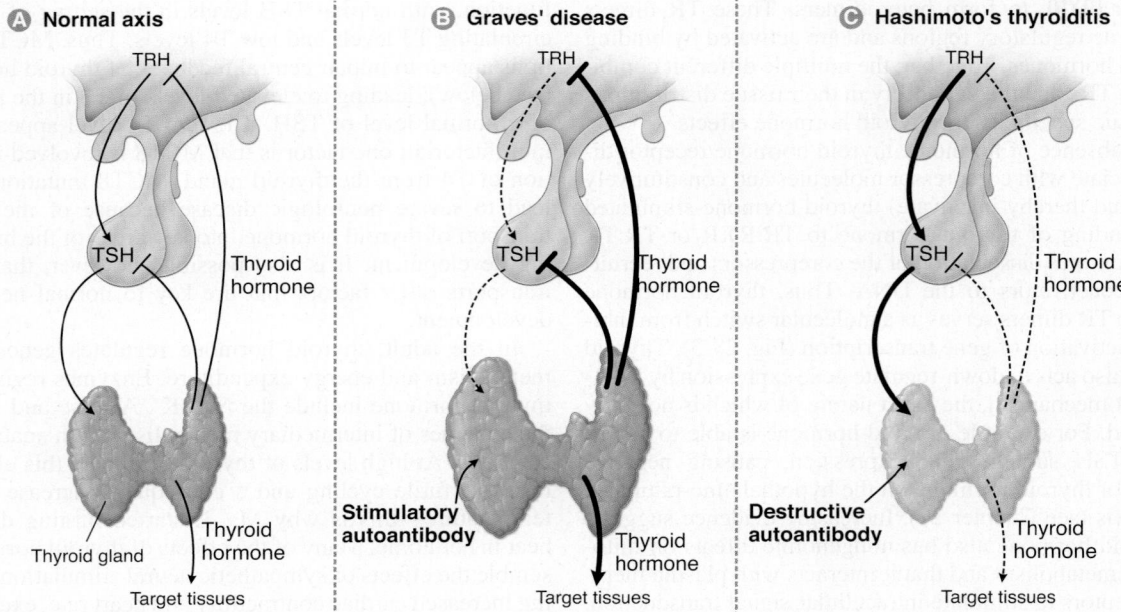

FIGURE 28-4. The hypothalamic-pituitary-thyroid axis in health and disease. A. In the normal axis, thyrotropin-releasing hormone (TRH) stimulates thyrotropes of the anterior pituitary gland to release thyroid-stimulating hormone (TSH). TSH stimulates synthesis and release of thyroid hormone by the thyroid gland. Thyroid hormone, in addition to its effects on target tissues, inhibits further release of TRH and TSH by the hypothalamus and anterior pituitary gland, respectively. **B.** In Graves' disease, a stimulatory autoantibody autonomously activates the TSH receptor in the thyroid gland, resulting in sustained stimulation of the thyroid gland, increased plasma thyroid hormone (*thick lines*), and suppression of TRH and TSH release (*dashed lines*). **C.** In Hashimoto's thyroiditis, a destructive autoantibody attacks the thyroid gland, causing thyroid insufficiency and decreased synthesis and secretion of thyroid hormone (*dashed lines*). Consequently, feedback inhibition on the hypothalamus and anterior pituitary gland does not occur, and plasma TSH levels rise (*thick lines*).

PATHOPHYSIOLOGY

The pathophysiology of thyroid diseases can be understood as a disturbance of the physiologic hypothalamic-pituitary-thyroid axis. For example, a physiologic decrease in thyroid hormones normally activates TSH synthesis and release, which leads to increased release of thyroid hormones by the thyroid gland and to restoration of normal thyroid hormone levels. Thyroid gland pathology can also cause thyroid hormone insufficiency, which also reduces the negative feedback of thyroid hormone on TSH release. Although TSH levels are elevated as a consequence, there is no increase in thyroid hormone release because the diseased thyroid gland cannot respond appropriately.

Most common thyroid diseases are best categorized as conditions that result in increased (hyperthyroid) or decreased (hypothyroid) thyroid hormone secretion. Two common thyroid diseases are **Graves' disease** and **Hashimoto's thyroiditis** (Fig. 28-4). Each is believed to be autoimmune in origin, but Graves' disease causes hyperthyroidism, whereas Hashimoto's thyroiditis ultimately results in hypothyroidism.

Graves' disease demonstrates the importance of plasma thyroid hormone in regulating homeostasis of the hypothalamic-pituitary-thyroid axis. In this syndrome, an IgG autoantibody specific for the TSH receptor is produced. This autoantibody is known as **thyroid-stimulating immunoglobulin (TSIg)**. The antibody acts as an agonist, activating the TSH receptor and thereby stimulating thyroid follicular cells to synthesize and release thyroid hormone. *Unlike TSH, however, TSIg is not subject to negative feedback control; it continues to stimulate thyroid function even when plasma thyroid hormone levels*

rise into the pathologic range. Because the autoantibody in Graves' disease acts independently of the hypothalamic-pituitary-thyroid axis, thyroid hormone homeostasis is disrupted. Clinical symptoms of hyperthyroidism result, and laboratory studies show high plasma thyroid hormone levels, low or undetectable TSH levels, and high TSIg levels. In the introductory case, Ms. L's TSH levels were low because her excess plasma thyroid hormone suppressed release of TSH by her anterior pituitary gland.

Hashimoto's thyroiditis, in contrast, results in selective destruction of the thyroid gland. Antibodies specific for many thyroid gland proteins, including thyroglobulin and thyroid peroxidase, can be found in the plasma of patients with Hashimoto's thyroiditis. As with Graves' disease, the underlying etiology of this disease is thought to be autoimmune. The clinical course of Hashimoto's thyroiditis involves a gradual inflammatory destruction of the thyroid gland with resultant hypothyroidism. Early in the course of the disease, destruction of thyroid follicular cells can release excessive quantities of stored colloid, resulting in transiently increased levels of thyroid hormone. Eventually, the gland is almost completely destroyed, and clinical symptoms of hypothyroidism develop (e.g., lethargy and decreased metabolic rate). Therapy for Hashimoto's thyroiditis involves pharmacologic replacement with oral synthetic thyroid hormone.

Other causes of hypothyroidism and hyperthyroidism include developmental anomalies, subacute (de Quervain's) thyroiditis, and thyroid adenomas and carcinomas. Details of the underlying pathophysiologies differ, but pharmacologic intervention in each case rests on determining whether the patient is hypothyroid, euthyroid, or hyperthyroid.

PHARMACOLOGIC CLASSES AND AGENTS

Pharmacologic treatment of thyroid gland diseases involves either replacement of deficient thyroid hormone or antagonism of excessive thyroid hormone. Replacement is self-evident, while the antagonists work at multiple steps in thyroid hormone synthesis and action (Fig. 28-5). In addition, a number of pharmacologic agents used for nonthyroid disease indications have important effects on peripheral thyroid hormone metabolism. The mechanisms of their action are discussed at the end of this section.

Treatment of Hypothyroidism

Thyroid hormone is a well-established and safe therapy for long-term treatment of hypothyroidism. Therapy aims to replace missing endogenous thyroid hormone with regularly administered exogenous thyroid hormone. The exogenous thyroid hormone is structurally identical to endogenous thyroid hormone (generally T4) and is produced by chemical synthesis.

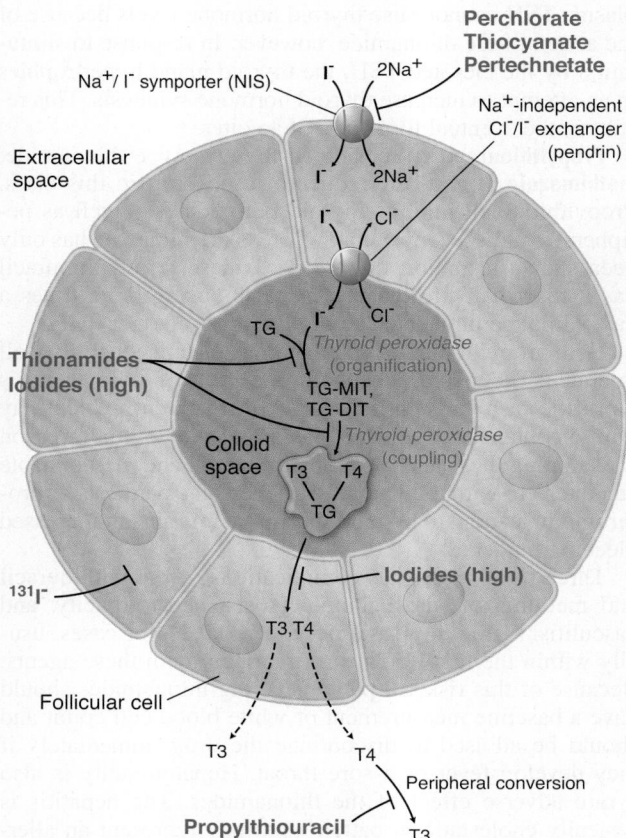

FIGURE 28-5. Pharmacologic interventions affecting thyroid hormone synthesis. Anions with a molecular radius approximately equal to that of the iodide anion (I⁻), such as perchlorate, thiocyanate, and pertechnetate, compete with iodide for uptake by the Na^+/I^- symporter. Radioactive $^{131}I^-$, when concentrated within thyroid cells, causes selective destruction of the thyroid gland. High levels of iodide transiently depress thyroid function by inhibiting organification, coupling, and proteolysis of thyroglobulin. Thionamides, such as propylthiouracil and methimazole, inhibit organification and coupling; propylthiouracil also inhibits peripheral conversion of T4 to T3. TG-MIT, thyroglobulin-monoiodotyrosine; TG-DIT, thyroglobulin-diiodotyrosine.

Many trials with replacement hormone debated whether it would be more efficacious to provide replacement of T3 or T4. T3 is the metabolically more active form of thyroid hormone, and one might have anticipated that replacement of deficient thyroid hormone with T3 would more effectively normalize thyroid homeostasis. However, a number of findings argue against this. First, most thyroid hormone in the blood is in the form of T4, although T4 has lower activity than T3 and is eventually metabolized to T3. Having a large reservoir of thyroid "prodrug" (T4) in the plasma may be important, perhaps as an effective buffer to normalize metabolic rates over a wide range of conditions. Second, the half-life of T4 is 6 days, as compared to the 1-day half-life of T3. The extended half-life of T4 allows a patient to take just one thyroid hormone replacement pill per day. For these reasons, **levothyroxine**, the L-isomer of T4, is still the treatment of choice for hypothyroidism. (One possible exception is myxedema coma, where the faster onset of T3 may provide enhanced recovery from life-threatening hypothyroidism.) The efficacy of thyroid hormone replacement is monitored by assays of plasma TSH and thyroid hormone levels. TSH is an accurate marker of thyroid hormone activity because anterior pituitary gland release of TSH is exquisitely sensitive to feedback control by thyroid hormone in the blood.

Once a patient is taking a stable dose of levothyroxine, monitoring of TSH levels can generally be performed less frequently, such as every 6 months to a year. Sudden alterations in TSH levels despite constant dosing of levothyroxine may be due to drug–drug interactions affecting absorption and metabolism. For example, resins such as **sodium polystyrene sulfonate** (Kayexalate®) and **cholestyramine** may decrease absorption of T4. Adequate gastric acidity is also required for absorption of exogenous levothyroxine; the dose of levothyroxine may therefore need to be increased in patients who become infected with *Helicobacter pylori* or who start taking a proton pump inhibitor. Drugs that increase the activity of certain hepatic P450 enzymes, including **rifampin** and **phenytoin**, increase the hepatic clearance of T4. In such cases, it may be necessary to increase the dose of T4 in order to maintain a euthyroid state.

Treatment of Hyperthyroidism

There are pharmacologic agents that target each step of thyroid hormone synthesis, from initial uptake of iodide, to organification, coupling, and peripheral conversion of T4 to T3. Clinically, both radioactive iodine and thionamides are available for the treatment of hyperthyroidism. β-Adrenergic antagonists are also sometimes used to ameliorate some of the symptoms of hyperthyroidism.

Inhibitors of Iodide Uptake

Iodide is taken up by the thyroid follicular cell via a Na^+/I^- symporter. Certain anions with the approximate atomic radius of iodide, such as **perchlorate**, **thiocyanate**, and **pertechnetate**, compete with iodide for uptake into the thyroid gland follicular cell (Fig. 28-5). This results in a decreased amount of iodide available for thyroid hormone synthesis. The effects of anion uptake inhibitors are usually not immediately apparent because of the large store of preformed thyroid hormone in the colloid.

Anion uptake inhibitors can be used in the treatment of hyperthyroidism; these agents reduce the intrathyroidal supply of iodide available for thyroid hormone synthesis. However, their use is uncommon because of the potential for causing aplastic anemia, and the thionamides (see below) are generally more effective. Because many of these uptake inhibitors are also used as radiopaque contrast materials, it is important to keep this physiologic antagonism in mind whenever a patient has symptoms of hypothyroidism after extensive radiographic studies employing contrast material.

Inhibitors of Organification and Hormone Release
Iodides

Two distinct types of iodide are used in clinical practice. Both take advantage of the thyroid gland's selective uptake and concentration of iodide to levels much higher than that in the blood.

The first agent, $^{131}I^-$, is a radioactive iodine isotope that strongly emits β-particles toxic to cells. The Na^+/I^- symporter expressed on thyroid follicular cell membranes cannot distinguish $^{131}I^-$ from normal stable iodide ($^{127}I^-$). Therefore, $^{131}I^-$ becomes sequestered within the thyroid gland. This makes radioactive $^{131}I^-$ a specific and effective therapy for hyperthyroidism. The concentrated intracellular radioactive iodine continues to emit β-particles, resulting in selective local destruction of the thyroid gland. Radioactive iodine is used to treat thyrotoxicosis, and this agent serves as an alternative to surgery in the treatment of hyperthyroidism. There is a concern that patients may eventually develop hypothyroidism after treatment with radioactive iodine, because it is difficult to ascertain for a given patient the extent to which radioactive $^{131}I^-$ will kill all or most of his or her thyroid follicular cells. *The goal is to administer enough $^{131}I^-$ to result in a euthyroid state, without precipitating hypothyroidism.* This desired result is not always obtained; for example, in the introductory case, Ms. L eventually developed hypothyroidism after treatment with $^{131}I^-$. Regardless, the development of hypothyroidism is easier to manage clinically than hyperthyroidism. Based on epidemiologic studies, it is unlikely that therapeutic doses of radioactive iodine have any effect on the incidence of thyroid cancer.

The second clinically important pharmacologic agent is, paradoxically, stable inorganic iodide. High levels of iodide inhibit thyroid hormone synthesis and release, a phenomenon known as the **Wolff-Chaikoff effect**. This phenomenon is likely mediated by down-regulation of the Na^+/I^- symporter in the thyroid gland. The negative feedback effect of high intrathyroidal iodide concentrations is reversible and transient; thyroid hormone synthesis and release returns to normal a few days after the plasma iodide concentration is increased. Therefore, inorganic iodide is not a useful long-term therapy for hyperthyroidism. This phenomenon does, however, have other important uses. For example, high iodide dosing reduces the size and vascularity of the thyroid gland. Because of this, iodide is often administered before thyroid gland surgery, resulting in technically easier excision of the gland.

Iodide can also have important preventative effects. When the nuclear accident at Chernobyl occurred, there was concern that radioactive iodine released into the air over Poland could cause population-wide thyroid gland destruction. As a preventative measure, millions of Polish children were given large doses of iodide for a number of days to suppress thyroid gland function temporarily and thereby to avoid uptake of environmental radioactive iodine.

Thionamides

The thionamides **propylthiouracil** and **methimazole** are important and useful inhibitors of thyroid hormone production. Thionamides compete with thyroglobulin for oxidized iodide in a process that is catalyzed by the enzyme thyroid peroxidase (Fig. 28-5). *By competing for oxidized iodide, thionamide treatment causes a selective decrease in the organification and coupling of thyroid hormone precursors and thereby inhibits thyroid hormone production.* Iodinated thionamides may also be capable of binding to thyroglobulin, further antagonizing any coupling reactions. Recall that thyroid follicular cells store a large quantity of nascent thyroid hormone in the form of colloid. This colloid can provide a sufficient amount of thyroid hormone for more than a week in the absence of any new synthesis. Because thionamides affect the synthesis but not the secretion of thyroid hormone, the effects of these drugs are not manifested until several weeks after the initiation of treatment (as in the introductory case).

Thionamide treatment often results in goiter formation. For this reason, the drugs are commonly referred to as **goitrogens**. Inhibition of thyroid hormone production by thionamides results in up-regulation of TSH release by the anterior pituitary gland in an attempt to reestablish homeostasis. The increased plasma TSH cannot raise thyroid hormone levels because of the action of the thionamide, however. In response to stimulation by the elevated TSH, the thyroid gland hypertrophies in an attempt to increase thyroid hormone synthesis. This results in the eventual formation of a goiter.

Propylthiouracil is considered the prototype thionamide; **methimazole** is another frequently used drug in this class. Propylthiouracil inhibits thyroid peroxidase as well as peripheral T4 to T3 conversion, whereas methimazole has only been shown to inhibit thyroid peroxidase. Propylthiouracil has a short half-life that necessitates dosing three times a day, while methimazole can be administered once daily.

Both propylthiouracil and methimazole are generally well tolerated. The most frequent adverse effect of these agents is a pruritic rash early in the course of treatment, which may remit spontaneously. Arthralgias are also a common reason for stopping these agents. Propylthiouracil and methimazole can interfere with the vitamin K-dependent synthesis of prothrombin, leading to hypoprothrombinemia and an increased bleeding tendency.

Three rare but serious complications of propylthiouracil and methimazole are agranulocytosis, hepatotoxicity, and vasculitis. Agranulocytosis occurs in <0.1% of cases, usually within the first 90 days of treatment with these agents. Because of this risk, all patients taking thionamides should have a baseline measurement of white blood cell count and should be advised to discontinue the drug immediately if they develop fever or a sore throat. Hepatotoxicity is also a rare adverse effect of the thionamides. The hepatitis is typically cholestatic in pattern and may represent an allergic reaction to the drugs. Severe hepatitis leading to liver failure and death has been associated with propylthiouracil treatment. Vasculitis from these agents can manifest as drug-induced lupus or an antineutrophil cytoplasmic antibody (ANCA)-associated vasculitis.

Because the incidence of serious adverse effects appears to be less frequent with methimazole than with propylthiouracil, methimazole is generally the preferred agent in clinical practice. Two exceptions to this rule are thyroid storm and pregnancy. In the acute management of severe hyperthyroidism (thyroid storm), the additional ability of propylthiouracil to block peripheral conversion of T4 to T3 makes this drug the more attractive agent. In pregnancy, propylthiouracil is the preferred agent because it has a more extensive safety record and because methimazole use during pregnancy has been associated with the development of aplasia cutis.

The thionamides are generally effective at controlling hyperthyroidism. A high percentage of patients taking these agents will go into remission over the course of 6 months to a year and may be able to maintain a euthyroid state after discontinuation of these medications. Some patients, however, will develop persistent hyperthyroidism despite treatment, as in the introductory case. Such patients require more definitive treatment of their hyperthyroidism by either radioactive iodine therapy or surgical removal of the thyroid gland.

Inhibitors of Peripheral Thyroid Hormone Metabolism
Although the majority of thyroid hormone is synthesized in the thyroid gland as T4, thyroid hormone acts at peripheral sites principally as T3. Conversion of T4 to T3 is dependent on a peripheral 5′-deiodinase, and inhibitors of this enzyme are effective adjuncts in treating the symptoms of hyperthyroidism. As mentioned above, propylthiouracil inhibits both organification and coupling in the thyroid gland and peripheral conversion of T4 to T3. Two other agents, β-adrenergic blockers and ipodate, are discussed below.

β-Adrenergic Blockers
β-Adrenergic antagonists are useful therapies for the *symptoms* of hyperthyroidism. Many of the effects of high plasma thyroid hormone levels resemble nonspecific β-adrenergic stimulation (e.g., sweating, tremor, tachycardia), although circulating catecholamine levels are not elevated. It is hypothesized that thyroid hormones may increase the responsiveness of tissues such as the heart to β-adrenergic stimulation, perhaps by up-regulating β-adrenergic receptor expression or altering G protein-mediated signaling. It has also been demonstrated that β-blockers can reduce peripheral conversion of T4 to T3, but this effect is not thought to be clinically relevant. Because of its rapid onset of action and short elimination half-life (9 minutes), **esmolol** is a preferred parenteral β-adrenergic antagonist for the treatment of thyroid storm.

Ipodate
Ipodate is a radiocontrast agent formerly used for visualization of the biliary ducts in endoscopic retrograde cholangiopancreatography (ERCP) procedures. In addition to its usefulness as a radiocontrast agent, ipodate significantly inhibits conversion of T4 to T3 by inhibiting the enzyme 5′-deiodinase. Although ipodate was sometimes used in the past to treat hyperthyroidism, it is no longer commercially available.

Other Drugs Affecting Thyroid Hormone Homeostasis
Lithium
Lithium, a drug used in the treatment of bipolar disorder (see Chapter 15, Pharmacology of Serotonergic and Central Adrenergic Neurotransmission), can cause hypothyroidism. Lithium is actively concentrated in the thyroid gland, and high levels of lithium inhibit thyroid hormone release from thyroid follicular cells. There is some evidence that lithium may inhibit thyroid hormone synthesis as well. The mechanism(s) responsible for these actions is unknown.

Amiodarone
Amiodarone is an antiarrhythmic drug (see Chapter 24, Pharmacology of Cardiac Rhythm) that has both positive and negative effects on thyroid hormone function. Amiodarone structurally resembles thyroid hormone and it contains a high concentration of iodine (each 200-mg tablet of amiodarone contains 75 mg of iodine). Metabolism of amiodarone releases this iodine as iodide, resulting in increased plasma concentrations of iodide. The increased plasma iodide is concentrated in the thyroid gland; this can result in hypothyroidism by the Wolff-Chaikoff effect.

Amiodarone can also cause hyperthyroidism by two mechanisms. In type I thyrotoxicosis, the excess iodide load provided by amiodarone leads to increased thyroid hormone synthesis and release. In type II thyroiditis, an autoimmune thyroiditis is induced that leads to release of excess thyroid hormone from the colloid. Because of its close structural similarity to thyroid hormone, amiodarone may also act as an analogue of thyroid hormone at the level of the receptor.

In addition, amiodarone competitively inhibits type I 5′-deiodinase. This results in decreased peripheral conversion of T4 to T3 and increased plasma concentrations of rT3.

Corticosteroids
Corticosteroids, such as cortisol and glucocorticoid analogues, also inhibit the 5′-deiodinase that converts T4 to T3. Because T4 has less physiologic activity than T3, treatment with corticosteroids reduces net thyroid hormone activity. In addition, corticosteroids suppress TSH levels, likely by inhibiting transcription of TRH in the hypothalamus. Despite these effects on the hypothalamic-pituitary-thyroid axis, chronic use of high-dose corticosteroids does not appear to cause clinically significant hypothyroidism.

Tyrosine Kinase Inhibitors
Tyrosine kinase inhibitors (TKIs) are effective therapeutics for the treatment of many malignancies (see Chapter 40, Pharmacology of Cancer: Signal Transduction). Many of these drugs can also alter thyroid hormone levels. The first TKI found to cause hypothyroidism was **sunitinib**, but subsequently, this same adverse effect was identified in patients treated with other TKIs as well. It has also been recognized that TKIs can induce hyperthyroidism. This apparent paradoxical effect suggests that targeting of receptor tyrosine kinases, such as the vascular endothelial growth factor receptor, may lead to alterations in angiogenesis and/or autoimmunity that affect the hypothalamic-pituitary-thyroid axis. It is likely that the mechanisms of thyroid dysfunction in patients treated with TKIs are multifactorial, and thyroid function must be monitored in such patients.

▌CONCLUSION AND FUTURE DIRECTIONS
Thyroid hormone synthesis consists of a complex set of synthesis and degradation steps. This pathway creates numerous points for pharmacologic intervention, from iodide uptake to peripheral conversion of T4 to T3. Thyroid hormone replacement is a safe and effective long-term therapy for thyroid hormone deficiencies. Several effective therapies exist for the management of thyrotoxicosis. Radioactive iodine and thionamides are commonly used for this purpose, leading to selective destruction of the thyroid gland and antagonism of organification and coupling, respectively.

Future potential therapies for diseases of the thyroid gland may focus on treating the etiology of autoimmune thyroid diseases, such as Graves' disease and Hashimoto's thyroiditis, and better defining the molecular targets of thyroid hormone action.

Acknowledgment

We thank Ehrin J. Armstrong and the late Armen H. Tashjian, Jr. for their valuable contributions to this chapter in the First, Second, and Third Editions of *Principles of Pharmacology: The Pathophysiologic Basis of Drug Therapy.*

Suggested Reading

Biondi B, Wartofsky L. Treatment with thyroid hormone. *Endocr Rev* 2014;35:433–512. (*Extensive discussion of the uses of thyroid hormone as a replacement hormone and a therapeutic agent.*)

Brent GA. Clinical practice. Graves' disease. *N Engl J Med* 2008;358:2594–2605. (*Reviews the clinical approach to Graves' disease and discusses other causes of hyperthyroidism.*)

Cheng SY, Leonard JL, David PJ. Molecular aspects of thyroid hormone actions. *Endocr Rev* 2010;31:139–170. (*A comprehensive treatise on the action of thyroid hormones in the cell.*)

Cooper DS. Antithyroid drugs. *N Engl J Med* 2005;352:905–917. (*An excellent, detailed summary of the clinical uses and adverse effects of methimazole and propylthiouracil.*)

Fekete C, Lechan RM. Central regulation of hypothalamic-pituitary-thyroid axis under physiological and pathophysiological conditions. *Endocr Rev* 2014;35:159–194. (*Review of the regulatory aspects of thyroid physiology.*)

Medical Letter, Inc. Drugs for hypothyroidism and hyperthyroidism. *Treat Guidel Med Lett* 2006;4:17–24. (*Review of therapeutic considerations, including important drug interactions.*)

Portulano C, Paroder-Belenitsky M, Carrasco N. The Na^+/I^- symporter (NIS): mechanism and medical impact. *Endocr Rev* 2014;35:106–149. (*Excellent review of this critical transporter of iodide into the thyroid follicular cell.*)

DRUG SUMMARY TABLE: CHAPTER 28 Pharmacology of the Thyroid Gland

DRUG	CLINICAL APPLICATIONS	*SERIOUS* AND COMMON ADVERSE EFFECTS	CONTRAINDICATIONS	THERAPEUTIC CONSIDERATIONS
THYROID HORMONE REPLACEMENTS **Mechanism—Replace missing endogenous thyroid hormone with exogenous thyroid hormone**				
Levothyroxine (T4) Liothyronine (T3)	Hypothyroidism Myxedema coma	*Hyperthyroidism (shared adverse effect); osteopenia, pseudotumor cerebri, seizure, myocardial infarction (levothyroxine only); thyrotoxicosis (liothyronine only)* Palpitations, excessive sweating (shared adverse effects); weight loss, diarrhea, insomnia, anxiety, fatigue (levothyroxine only); headache (liothyronine only)	Shared contraindications: Uncorrected adrenal cortical insufficiency Untreated thyrotoxicosis Hypersensitivity to thyroid hormones Levothyroxine only: Acute myocardial infarction Liothyronine only: Concomitant use with artificial warming of patients	Cholestyramine and sodium polystyrene sulfonate decrease absorption of synthetic thyroid hormone. Rifampin and phenytoin increase metabolism of synthetic thyroid hormone. Because of its longer elimination half-life, T4 is usually preferred for the treatment of hypothyroidism. T3 may be preferred in myxedema coma due to its faster onset of action.
IODIDE UPTAKE INHIBITORS **Mechanism—Compete with iodide for uptake into the thyroid gland follicular cells via sodium-iodide symporter, thereby decreasing intrathyroidal supply of iodide available for thyroid hormone synthesis**				
Perchlorate Thiocyanate Pertechnetate	Hyperthyroidism Radiocontrast agents	*Aplastic anemia* Gastrointestinal irritation	No major contraindications	Clinical use in hyperthyroidism is limited due to the risk of developing aplastic anemia. Frequently used as radiocontrast agents.
INHIBITORS OF ORGANIFICATION AND THYROID HORMONE RELEASE **Mechanism—Radioactive iodine strongly emits β-particles that are toxic to thyroid follicular cells. High-concentration iodide inhibits iodide uptake and organification via Wolff-Chaikoff effect. Propylthiouracil inhibits thyroid peroxidase and conversion of T4 to T3. Methimazole inhibits thyroid peroxidase.**				
131I⁻ (Radioactive iodine)	Hyperthyroidism	*May worsen ophthalmopathy in Graves' disease, hypothyroidism*	Pregnancy	Alternative to surgery in the treatment of hyperthyroidism. Excess radiation can destroy thyroid, thereby causing hypothyroidism.
Iodide (high concentrations)	Hyperthyroidism	*May worsen toxic goiter symptoms*		Used for temporary suppression of thyroid gland function. Also used before thyroid gland surgery to allow technically easier excision.
Propylthiouracil (PTU) Methimazole	Hyperthyroidism	*Agranulocytosis, hepatotoxicity (shared adverse effects); liver failure (propylthiouracil only); aplastic anemia (methimazole only)* Rash, arthralgias	Hypersensitivity to propylthiouracil or methimazole Pregnancy Breastfeeding (methimazole only)	Methimazole is generally preferred in the treatment of hyperthyroidism due to lower incidence of serious adverse effects. PTU is the preferred agent in thyroid storm due to additional inhibition of peripheral T4 to T3 conversion.
INHIBITORS OF PERIPHERAL THYROID HORMONE METABOLISM **Mechanism—Block 5′-deiodinase, thereby inhibiting T4 to T3 conversion**				
β-Blockers	See Drug Summary Table: Chapter 11 Adrenergic Pharmacology			The sympatholytic effect of β-blockers is more important in treating the symptoms of hyperthyroidism than the minor effect of these drugs on 5′-deiodinase. Esmolol is a preferred β-adrenergic antagonist for treatment of thyroid storm because of its rapid onset of action and short elimination half-life.
Ipodate	Hyperthyroidism	Urticaria, serum sickness, may occasionally exacerbate hyperthyroid symptoms	Hypersensitivity to radiocontrast agents	Formerly used as radiocontrast agent. No longer commercially available.

29

Pharmacology of the Adrenal Cortex

Rajesh Garg and Gail K. Adler

INTRODUCTION

Like the pituitary gland, the adrenal gland consists of two organs fused together during embryologic development. The outer adrenal cortex originates from mesoderm, and the inner adrenal medulla is derived from neural crest cells. The adrenal cortex synthesizes and secretes steroid hormones essential for salt balance, intermediary metabolism, and, in females, androgenic actions. The adrenal medulla synthesizes and secretes the catecholamine epinephrine, which is important, although not essential, for maintaining sympathetic tone. This chapter focuses on the adrenal cortex; because of its importance in neuropharmacology, the adrenal medulla is discussed in Chapter 11, Adrenergic Pharmacology.

The therapeutic utility of adrenocortical hormones spans almost every area of medicine. This is largely because of the usefulness of glucocorticoid analogues as efficacious and potent anti-inflammatory agents. Unfortunately, long-term systemic glucocorticoid therapy also produces a substantial number of predictable but undesirable adverse effects. The physiology of mineralocorticoids has been studied in the etiology of hypertension, cardiovascular disease, and renal disease, and there is considerable interest in the use of mineralocorticoid receptor antagonists as therapies for these disorders. Adrenal androgens, although lacking a definitive therapeutic indication at present, are the focus of investigation for use in female sexual dysfunction. Both deficiency and excess of adrenocortical hormones can cause human disease. Deficiency states are treated by replacing the hormones in the form of therapeutic agents, while inhibitors of adrenocortical biosynthetic enzymes and antagonists at adrenocortical hormone receptors can be used to treat hormone excess.

OVERVIEW OF THE ADRENAL CORTEX

The adrenal cortex synthesizes three classes of hormones: **mineralocorticoids**, **glucocorticoids**, and **androgens**. Histologically, the adrenal cortex is divided into three zones. Moving from the capsule toward the medulla, these regions are the zona glomerulosa, zona fasciculata, and zona reticularis (Fig. 29-1). The glomerulosa is responsible for mineralocorticoid production and is under the control of **angiotensin II**, blood **potassium** concentration, and, to a lesser extent, **adrenocorticotropic hormone (ACTH)**. The fasciculata and reticularis synthesize glucocorticoids and androgens, respectively. Both the fasciculata and reticularis are mainly under the control of ACTH, which, in turn, is regulated by corticotropin-releasing hormone (CRH), vasopressin, and cortisol (see Chapter 27, Pharmacology of the Hypothalamus and Pituitary Gland).

CASE

Eight-year-old Johnny finds that he can barely catch his breath at times, especially while exercising. His asthma comes and goes, but no therapy seems to stop the asthma attacks completely. Although his doctor is concerned that it could stunt Johnny's growth, she eventually prescribes oral prednisone (a glucocorticoid analogue) and tells Johnny's parents to make sure he takes the medication every day. After a few weeks, Johnny's asthma attacks subside, and he is able to have a fairly normal childhood. During this time, the doctor pays close attention to Johnny's linear growth. Two years later, Johnny's doctor decides that a new inhaled glucocorticoid could be a safer medication for him. Johnny switches to the inhaled glucocorticoid and discontinues oral prednisone. Three days later, he develops a respiratory infection and is brought to the emergency department with low blood pressure and a temperature of 103°F. Based on his history of prednisone use, Johnny is immediately given hydrocortisone (cortisol) intravenously, as well as a saline infusion. Johnny recovers and for the next 6 months slowly tapers his oral prednisone dose with continued use of the inhaled glucocorticoid. Eventually, he is able to take the inhaled glucocorticoid alone as an effective therapy for his asthma.

Questions

1. Why are cortisol analogues such as prednisone used for treating asthma?
2. Why did abrupt cessation of oral prednisone precipitate Johnny's clinical presentation in the emergency department?
3. Why are inhaled glucocorticoids safer than oral glucocorticoids for long-term treatment of asthma?
4. Why did the doctor monitor Johnny's linear growth?

Through its mineralocorticoid, glucocorticoid, and adrenal androgen products, the adrenal cortex plays a role in diverse aspects of homeostasis. The following discussion considers the physiology, pathophysiology, and pharmacology of each class of adrenal hormones. The glucocorticoids are discussed first, followed by the mineralocorticoids and the adrenal androgens.

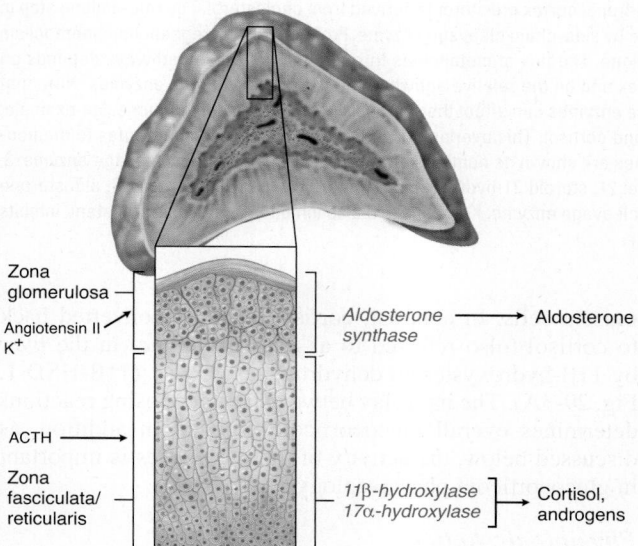

FIGURE 29-1. Regions of the adrenal cortex. The adrenal cortex is divided into three regions. The outermost region, the zona glomerulosa, synthesizes aldosterone and is regulated by circulating levels of angiotensin II, potassium, and, to a lesser extent, adrenocorticotropic hormone (ACTH). The zona fasciculata and zona reticularis synthesize cortisol and adrenal androgens. ACTH released from the anterior pituitary gland stimulates production of both cortisol and adrenal androgens. Tissue-specific expression of enzymes in each zone of the adrenal cortex—aldosterone synthase in the glomerulosa, steroid 11β-hydroxylase and steroid 17α-hydroxylase in the fasciculata/reticularis—determines the specificity of hormone production in that zone.

GLUCOCORTICOIDS

Physiology

Synthesis

Cortisol, the endogenous glucocorticoid, is synthesized from cholesterol. Its synthesis begins with the rate-limiting conversion of cholesterol to pregnenolone, a reaction catalyzed by side-chain cleavage enzyme (Fig. 29-2). This first step converts the 27-carbon cholesterol into a 21-carbon precursor common to all adrenocortical hormones. From this precursor, steroid metabolism can proceed down three different pathways to generate mineralocorticoids, glucocorticoids, or adrenal androgens.

An oxidase enzyme catalyzes each step in the pathway of adrenocortical hormone synthesis. The oxidase enzymes are mitochondrial **cytochromes**, similar to the liver cytochrome P450 oxidase system. Tissue-specific expression of particular oxidase enzymes in each zone of the adrenal cortex provides the biochemical basis for the differences among the hormonal end products of the different zones of the cortex. For example, the zona fasciculata synthesizes cortisol but not aldosterone or androgens (Fig. 29-1). This is because enzymes required uniquely for cortisol synthesis, such as steroid 11β-hydroxylase, are expressed in the zona fasciculata, whereas enzymes required for aldosterone and androgen synthesis are not. The human zona glomerulosa does not express steroid 17α-hydroxylase, which is required for production of cortisol and androgens but is not required for production of aldosterone (Fig. 29-2).

Metabolism

Approximately 90% of circulating cortisol is bound to plasma proteins, the most important of which are **corticosteroid-binding globulin** (**CBG**, also referred to as *transcortin*) and albumin. CBG has high affinity for cortisol but low overall capacity, whereas albumin has low cortisol affinity but high overall capacity. Only molecules of cortisol that are unbound to protein (the so-called free fraction) are bioavailable, that is, available to diffuse through plasma membranes

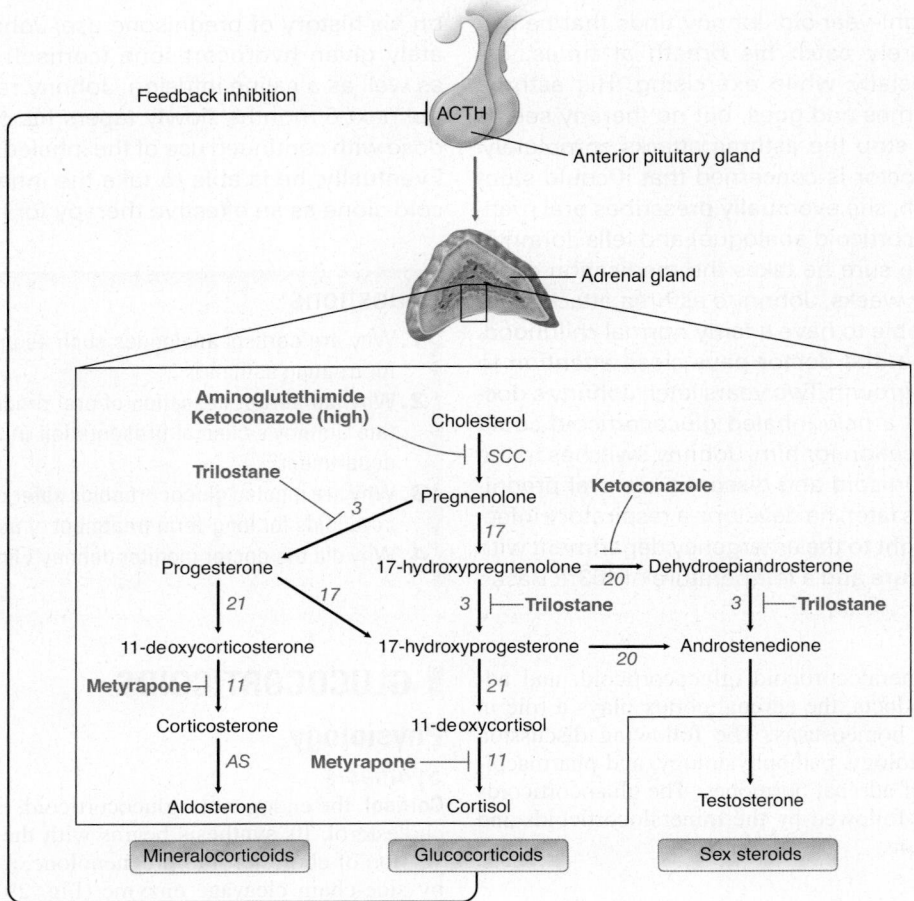

FIGURE 29-2. Hormone synthesis in the adrenal cortex. The hormones of the adrenal cortex are steroids derived from cholesterol. The rate-limiting step in adrenal hormone biosynthesis is the modification of cholesterol to pregnenolone by side-chain cleavage enzyme. From this step, pregnenolone metabolism can be directed toward the formation of aldosterone, cortisol, or androstenedione. The flux of metabolites through each of these pathways depends on the tissue-specific expression of enzymes in the different cell types of the cortex and on the relative activity of the different synthetic enzymes. Note that several enzymes are involved in more than one pathway and that defects in these enzymes can affect the synthesis of more than one hormone. For example, a defect in steroid 21-hydroxylase prevents the synthesis of both aldosterone and cortisol. This overlap of synthetic activities also contributes to the non-selective action of glucocorticoid synthesis inhibitors such as trilostane. Enzymes are shown as numbers or letters—SCC, side-chain cleavage enzyme; 3, 3β-hydroxysteroid dehydrogenase; 17, steroid 17α-hydroxylase; 20, 17, 20-lyase; 21, steroid 21-hydroxylase; 11, steroid 11β-hydroxylase; AS, aldosterone synthase. Aminoglutethimide and high levels of ketoconazole inhibit side-chain cleavage enzyme. Ketoconazole also inhibits 17, 20-lyase. Trilostane inhibits 3β-hydroxysteroid dehydrogenase. Metyrapone inhibits steroid 11β-hydroxylase.

into cells. Thus, the affinity and capacity of plasma binding proteins regulate the availability of active hormone and, consequently, hormone activity.

The liver and kidneys are the primary sites of peripheral cortisol metabolism. Through reduction and subsequent conjugation to glucuronic acid, the liver is responsible for inactivating cortisol in the plasma. The conjugation reaction makes cortisol more water soluble, thus enabling renal excretion. Importantly, the liver and kidneys express different isoforms of the enzyme **11β-hydroxysteroid dehydrogenase**, a regulator of cortisol activity. The two isoforms catalyze opposing reactions. In distal collecting duct cells of the kidney, 11β-hydroxysteroid dehydrogenase type 2 (11β-HSD 2) converts cortisol to the biologically inactive compound **cortisone**, which (unlike cortisol) does not bind to the mineralocorticoid receptor (see below; Fig. 29-3B). Expression of 11β-HSD 2 protects the mineralocorticoid receptor from activation by cortisol in a variety of cell types, including endothelial cells and vascular smooth

muscle cells. In contrast, cortisone can be converted back to cortisol (also referred to as *hydrocortisone*) in the liver by 11β-hydroxysteroid dehydrogenase type 1 (11β-HSD 1, Fig. 29-3A). The interplay between these opposing reactions determines overall glucocorticoid activity. In addition, as discussed below, the activity of these enzymes is important in glucocorticoid pharmacology.

Physiologic Actions

Like other steroid hormones, unbound cortisol diffuses across the plasma membrane into the cytosol of target cells, where the hormone binds to a cytosolic receptor. There are two types of glucocorticoid receptors: the **Type I (mineralocorticoid)** and **Type II glucocorticoid receptors**. The Type I receptor is expressed in the organs of excretion (kidney, colon, salivary glands, sweat glands) and other tissues including the hippocampus, vasculature, heart, adipose tissue, and peripheral blood cells. The Type II receptor has a broader tissue distribution. *The Type I glucocorticoid receptor is synonymous*

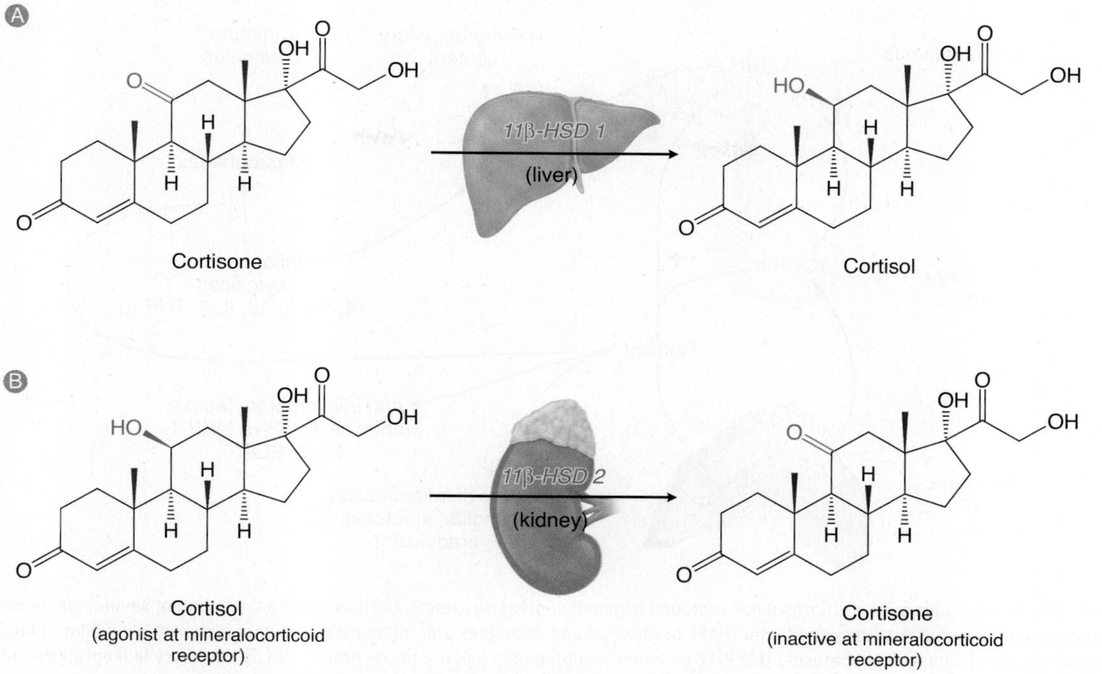

FIGURE 29-3. 11β-Hydroxysteroid dehydrogenase. The enzyme 11β-hydroxysteroid dehydrogenase (11β-HSD) exists in two isoforms, which catalyze opposing reactions. **A.** In the liver, 11β-hydroxysteroid dehydrogenase type 1 (11β-HSD 1) converts 11-keto glucocorticoids such as cortisone to 11-hydroxy glucocorticoids such as cortisol. **B.** In vitro, cortisol is a potent agonist at the mineralocorticoid receptor (MR). In the kidney, however, MRs are "shielded" from cortisol by the action of the enzyme 11β-hydroxysteroid dehydrogenase type 2 (11β-HSD 2), which converts cortisol to inactive cortisone. This mechanism ensures that, at physiologic levels, cortisol does not exert mineralocorticoid effects. At high concentrations, however, cortisol can overwhelm the capacity of 11β-HSD 2, leading to stimulation of renal MRs.

with the mineralocorticoid receptor. The nomenclature is unfortunate, and this chapter hereafter refers to the Type I receptor as the "mineralocorticoid receptor."

Once cortisol binds to its cytosolic receptor and forms a hormone–receptor complex, the complex is transported into the nucleus. In the case of cortisol, a homodimerized hormone–receptor complex binds to gene promoter elements referred to as **glucocorticoid response elements (GREs)** or **negative GREs**, which enhance or inhibit the expression of specific genes, respectively. The glucocorticoid receptor also regulates transcription through direct and indirect interaction with co-activator molecules. Cortisol has profound effects on mRNA expression; about 10% of all human genes are estimated to contain GREs. Because the expression of such a large number of genes is affected by activation of GREs, cortisol has physiologic actions in most tissues. These actions can be divided generally into metabolic effects and anti-inflammatory effects.

Metabolic effects of cortisol increase nutrient availability by raising blood glucose, amino acid, and triglyceride levels. Cortisol increases blood glucose by antagonizing insulin action and by promoting gluconeogenesis in the fasting state. Cortisol also increases muscle protein catabolism, leading to release of amino acids that can be utilized by the liver as fuels for gluconeogenesis. By potentiating growth hormone action on adipocytes, cortisol increases the activity of hormone-sensitive lipase and the subsequent release of free fatty acids (lipolysis). Free fatty acids further increase insulin resistance. Cortisol levels increase as a component of stress responses induced by a wide range of stimuli, such as vigorous exercise, psychological stress, acute trauma, surgery, fear, severe infection, hypoglycemia, and pain. By increasing blood glucose, the physiologic effects of glucocorticoids maintain energy homeostasis during the stress response, thus ensuring that critical organs such as the brain continue to receive nutrients.

Cortisol also has multiple anti-inflammatory actions. Cortisol negatively regulates cytokine release from cells of the immune system by inhibiting nuclear factor κB (NF-κB); this action may be an important mechanism to limit the extent of immune responses and to regulate the inflammatory response. In turn, certain cytokines, including IL-1, IL-2, IL-6, and TNF-α, can stimulate hypothalamic release of CRH, which stimulates ACTH and cortisol release. This series of stimulatory and inhibitory effects creates a feedback loop in which inflammatory cytokines and cortisol are coordinately regulated to control immune and inflammatory responses (Fig. 29-4). Glucocorticoid-mediated suppression of the inflammatory response also has important pharmacologic implications for clinical conditions such as organ transplantation, rheumatoid arthritis, and asthma. Indeed, the introductory case demonstrates that glucocorticoids are an effective therapy for asthma. The exact mechanisms by which glucocorticoids act to ameliorate the symptoms of asthma are unknown but are thought to be related to the ability of glucocorticoids to reduce inflammation in the airways (see below and Chapter 48, Integrative Inflammation Pharmacology: Asthma).

Regulation

The hypothalamic-pituitary unit coordinates the production of cortisol (refer to Chapter 27 for an overview). In response to central circadian rhythms and to stress, neurons in the paraventricular nucleus of the hypothalamus synthesize and

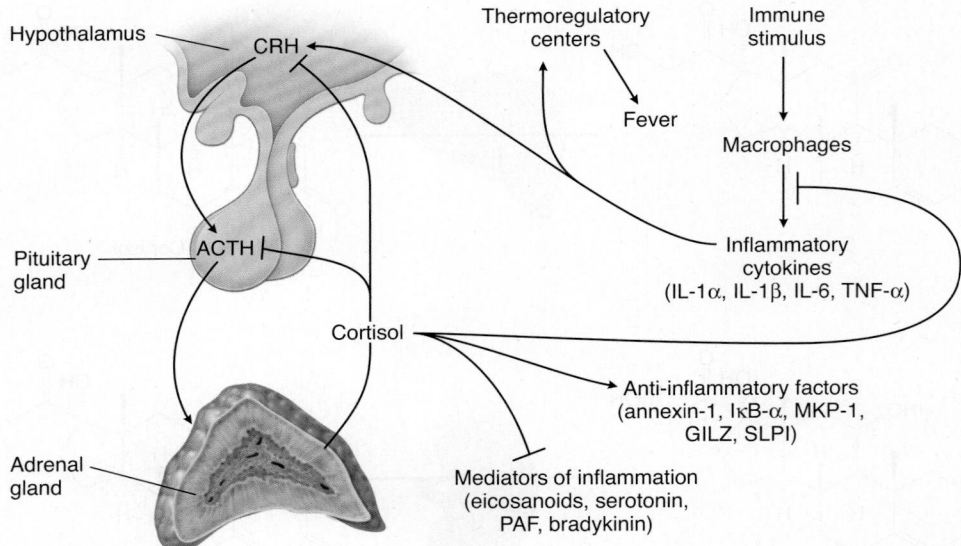

FIGURE 29-4. The immune-adrenal axis. Cortisol has profound immunosuppressive effects. Cortisol inhibits the action of several mediators of inflammation (eicosanoids, serotonin, platelet activating factor [PAF], bradykinin) and stimulates anti-inflammatory factors (annexin-1, inhibitor of nuclear factor κB [IκB-α], mitogen-activated kinase phosphatase-1 [MKP-1], glucocorticoid-induced leucine zipper protein [GILZ], secretory leukoprotease inhibitor [SLPI]). Cortisol also inhibits the release of a number of cytokines from macrophages, including IL-1α, IL-1β, IL-6, and TNF-α. Because these cytokines in turn promote the hypothalamic release of corticotropin-releasing hormone (CRH) and thereby increase serum cortisol levels, it is hypothesized that the stress-induced increase in cortisol limits the extent of the inflammatory response.

secrete **corticotropin-releasing hormone (CRH)**, a peptide hormone. CRH then travels through the hypothalamic-pituitary portal system and binds to G protein-coupled receptors on the surface of corticotroph cells in the anterior pituitary gland. CRH binding stimulates the corticotrophs to synthesize **proopiomelanocortin (POMC)**, a precursor polypeptide that is cleaved into multiple peptide hormones including ACTH. Neurons in the paraventricular nucleus can also respond to stress by synthesizing and secreting arginine vasopressin. This vasopressin is released into the hypothalamic-pituitary portal system together with CRH, and it synergizes with CRH to increase the release of ACTH by the anterior pituitary gland. Interestingly, the stress-responsive parvocellular neurons that secrete CRH and vasopressin into the hypothalamic-pituitary portal system are different from the osmolality-responsive magnocellular neurons that synthesize vasopressin and transport this hormone to the posterior pituitary gland (see Chapter 27), even though both types of neurons are located in the paraventricular nucleus of the hypothalamus.

Proteolytic cleavage of POMC yields not only ACTH but also γ-melanocyte-stimulating hormone (MSH), lipotropin, and β-endorphin. MSH binds to receptors on skin melanocytes, promoting melanogenesis and thereby increasing skin pigmentation. Because of the similarities between the ACTH and MSH peptide sequences, high concentrations of ACTH can also bind to and activate MSH receptors. This action becomes apparent in primary hypoadrenalism (see below), in which increased ACTH levels result in increased skin pigmentation. The role of lipotropin in human physiology is uncertain but is thought to involve control of lipolysis. β-Endorphin is an endogenous opioid that is important for pain modulation and for regulation of reproductive physiology.

Because steroid hormones are able to diffuse freely across cell membranes and because the adrenal gland stores little

cortisol, ACTH regulates cortisol production by promoting synthesis of the hormone. ACTH also has a trophic effect on the zona fasciculata and zona reticularis of the adrenal cortex, and hypertrophy of the cortex can occur in response to chronically elevated levels of ACTH.

As in other endocrine axes, the hormone (cortisol) produced by the target organ (adrenal cortex) exerts negative feedback regulation at the level of both the hypothalamus and the anterior pituitary gland. *High cortisol levels decrease both synthesis and release of CRH and ACTH.* Because ACTH has important trophic effects on the adrenal cortex, the absence of ACTH leads to atrophy of the cortisol-producing zona fasciculata and the androgen-producing zona reticularis. However, the aldosterone-producing zona glomerulosa cells continue to function in the absence of ACTH because angiotensin II and blood potassium continue to stimulate the production of aldosterone.

Pathophysiology

Diseases affecting glucocorticoid physiology can be divided into disorders of hormone deficiency and disorders of hormone excess. Addison's disease is the classic example of adrenocortical insufficiency, while Cushing's syndrome exemplifies cortisol excess.

Adrenal Insufficiency

Addison's disease is an example of a *primary adrenal insufficiency* in which the adrenal cortex is selectively destroyed, most commonly due to a T cell-mediated autoimmune reaction but alternatively due to infection, infiltration, cancer, or hemorrhage. Destruction of the cortex results in decreased synthesis of all classes of adrenocortical hormones. By comparison, *secondary adrenal insufficiency* is caused by hypothalamic or pituitary disorders or by prolonged administration of exogenous glucocorticoids. In secondary adrenal insufficiency, the decrease in ACTH levels causes decreased synthesis of sex hormones and cortisol but does not alter aldosterone synthesis (see earlier discussion).

Regardless of the underlying cause, adrenal insufficiency has serious consequences and can be life threatening if left untreated in the setting of stress. Patients with adrenal insufficiency frequently experience fatigue, loss of appetite, weight loss, dizziness on standing, and nausea. Hyperkalemia is common in primary adrenal insufficiency due to the lack of aldosterone. If adrenal insufficiency is the result of high-dose, prolonged therapy with exogenous glucocorticoids, then the dose of glucocorticoid should be tapered slowly to allow the **hypothalamic-pituitary-adrenal (HPA) axis** time to regain full activity. Importantly, it can take up to 1 year for the HPA axis to recover function after discontinuation of exogenous glucocorticoid treatment.

In the introductory case, Johnny was switched from an oral glucocorticoid to an inhaled glucocorticoid that delivered a much lower systemic concentration of glucocorticoid. His adrenal cortex had atrophied because he had been maintained for 2 years on chronically high doses of prednisone; therefore, he was unable to produce a sufficient amount of cortisol in response to the stress of a respiratory infection. As a result, he arrived in the emergency department with acute adrenal insufficiency and required intravenous therapy with saline and hydrocortisone.

Glucocorticoid Excess

Cushing's syndrome refers to a number of underlying pathophysiologies, all of which increase cortisol production. The term *Cushing's disease* is reserved for ACTH-secreting pituitary adenomas that lead to increased cortisol production (Fig. 27-5C). Other causes of Cushing's syndrome include ectopic secretion of ACTH, most commonly by small cell carcinomas of the lung (Fig. 27-5D), and (rarely) ectopic CRH production. Cushing's syndrome can also result from cortisol-secreting tumors (adenoma or carcinoma) of the adrenal cortex (Fig. 27-5B). However, iatrogenic Cushing's syndrome—secondary to pharmacologic treatment with exogenous glucocorticoids—is by far the most common cause of Cushing's syndrome.

The clinical features of Cushing's syndrome result from chronic overstimulation of target organs by endogenous or exogenous glucocorticoids. These features—which can include centripetal adipose redistribution, hypertension, proximal limb myopathy, osteoporosis, immunosuppression, and diabetes mellitus—reflect amplification of the normal physiologic actions of glucocorticoids in a variety of target tissues. In cases of endogenous Cushing's syndrome, cortisol-mediated activation of mineralocorticoid receptors leads to volume expansion, hypertension, and hypokalemia.

Pharmacologic Classes and Agents

Cortisol and Glucocorticoid Analogues

Drug therapy with glucocorticoids is indicated for two main purposes. First, exogenous glucocorticoids can be used as *replacement* therapy in cases of adrenal insufficiency. The goal of this therapy is to administer physiologic doses of glucocorticoids to ameliorate the effects of the adrenal insufficiency. Second, and more commonly, glucocorticoids are administered at *pharmacologic* doses to suppress inflammation and immune responses associated with disorders such as asthma, rheumatoid arthritis, and organ rejection after transplantation.

Because pharmacologic levels of systemic glucocorticoids invariably result in severe adverse effects, strategies to minimize these untoward responses to glucocorticoids have focused on local delivery of glucocorticoids to the area(s) requiring treatment. By limiting systemic exposure to the drug, HPA axis suppression and other features of iatrogenic Cushing's syndrome can be minimized or avoided. Examples of local glucocorticoid delivery include inhaled glucocorticoids for asthma, topical glucocorticoids for inflammatory skin conditions, and intra-articular glucocorticoids for arthritis.

A large number of glucocorticoid analogues have been synthesized. The following discussion highlights the differences among some commonly used cortisol analogues—including **prednisone**, **prednisolone**, **fludrocortisone**, and **dexamethasone**—by comparing the structures, potencies, and durations of action of these compounds to those of cortisol.

Structure and Potency

Glucocorticoids can be divided into two classes based on the structural moiety present at the 11-carbon position. Compounds with a hydroxyl ($-OH$) group at the 11-carbon position, such as cortisol, possess intrinsic glucocorticoid activity. In contrast, compounds with a carbonyl ($=O$) group at the 11 carbon, such as cortisone, are inactive. The liver enzyme 11β-HSD 1 must reduce the 11-carbonyl compound to its 11-hydroxyl congener in order for the compound to be active (Fig. 29-3). In other words, *cortisone is an inactive prodrug until it is converted by the liver to the active drug cortisol.* The native activity of a glucocorticoid is especially important for topically administered drugs because the skin does not possess appreciable amounts of 11β-HSD 1 (see below). Also, whenever possible, the active drug form is preferred over the inactive prodrug form for patients with liver dysfunction because such patients may not be able to convert the prodrug to its active form.

The basic cortisol "backbone" is essential for glucocorticoid activity, and *all synthetic glucocorticoids are analogues of the endogenous glucocorticoid cortisol* (Fig. 29-5).

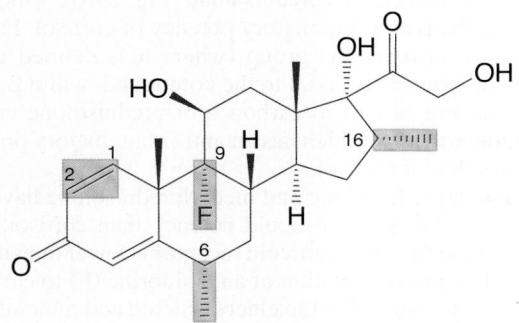

FIGURE 29-5. Synthetic modifications to the cortisol backbone. Four modifications to the cortisol backbone are common in synthetic glucocorticoids. Addition of a 1–2 double bond (*far left box*), a methyl group at carbon 6, or a methyl group at carbon 16 increases the glucocorticoid activity of the compound relative to that of cortisol. Addition of fluorine to carbon 9 increases glucocorticoid activity and markedly increases mineralocorticoid activity; the mineralocorticoid effect is blunted if 9-fluorination is combined with 16-methylation. Simultaneous addition of the 1–2 double bond, methyl at carbon 16, and fluorine at carbon 9 creates dexamethasone, which has very potent glucocorticoid activity and essentially no mineralocorticoid activity.

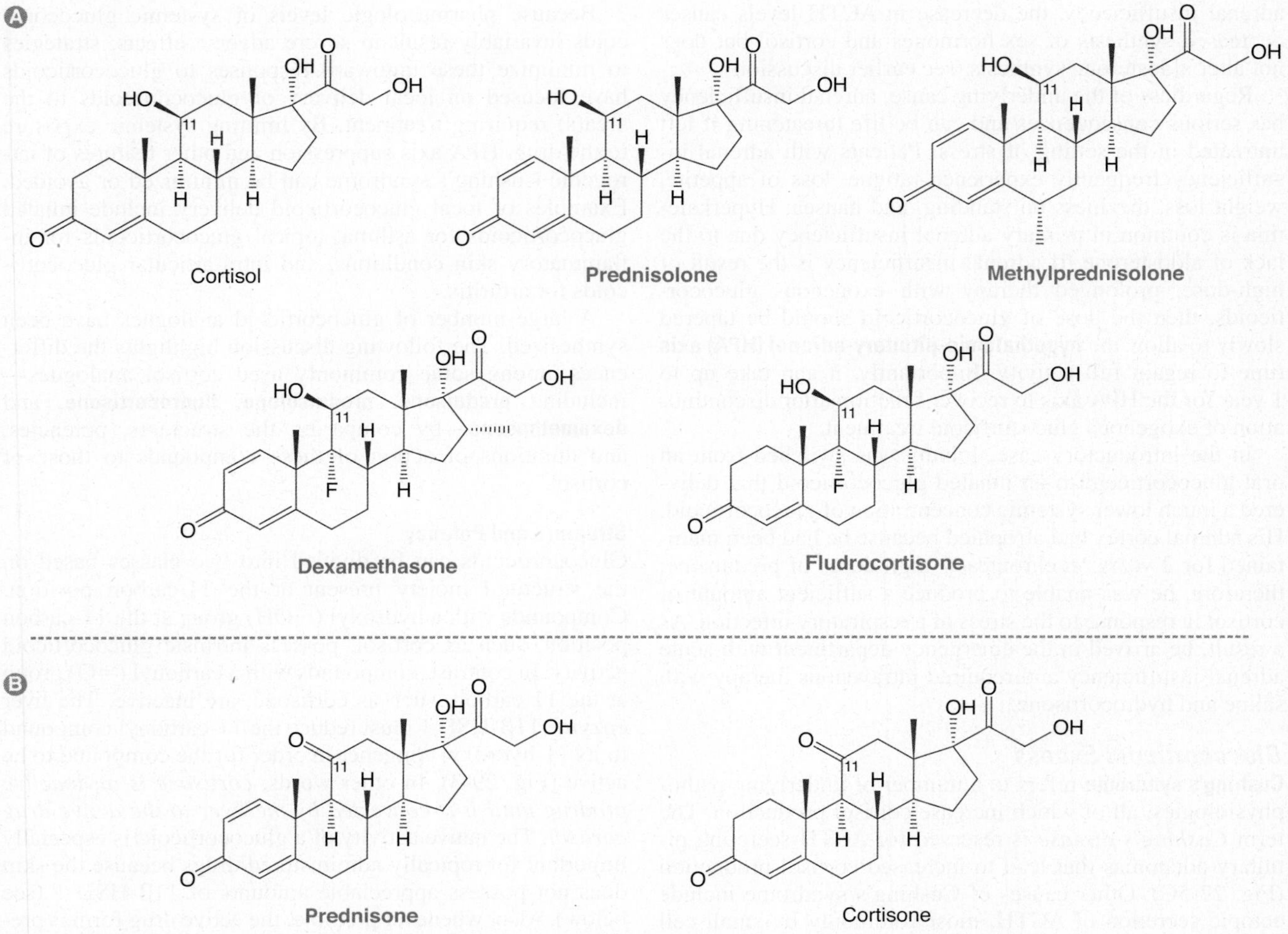

FIGURE 29-6. Glucocorticoid analogues. Panel A shows a number of 11-hydroxy glucocorticoids, while **panel B** shows two 11-keto congeners. Note that the drugs in panel A are physiologically active, while the drugs in panel B are prodrugs that must be activated by 11β-HSD 1 to become active compounds. The structural class to which a glucocorticoid analogue belongs can be an important consideration in therapeutic decision making. For example, because the skin lacks significant 11β-HSD 1 activity, only 11-hydroxy glucocorticoids can be used in topical glucocorticoid creams. HSD, hydroxysteroid dehydrogenase.

For example, addition of a double bond between carbons 1 and 2 of cortisol creates **prednisolone** (Fig. 29-6), which has 4–5 times the anti-inflammatory potency of cortisol. Further addition of an α-methyl group (where α is defined as the side-group orientation axial to the compound, while β is the equatorial orientation) to carbon 6 of prednisolone creates **methylprednisolone**, which has an anti-inflammatory potency 5–6 times that of cortisol.

Although prednisolone and methylprednisolone have significantly higher glucocorticoid potency than cortisol, their potency at the mineralocorticoid receptor is lower than that of cortisol. In contrast, addition of an α-fluorine (F) to carbon 9 of cortisol increases both the glucocorticoid and mineralocorticoid potencies of the resulting compound, known as **fludrocortisone** (Fig. 29-6). Because of its remarkably enhanced mineralocorticoid activity, fludrocortisone is useful in the treatment of mineralocorticoid deficiency states (see below).

Dexamethasone incorporates two of the above changes to the cortisol backbone (1–2 double bond, 9α-fluorine) as well as the addition of an α-methyl group at the 16-carbon position (Fig. 29-6). This compound has more than 18 times the glucocorticoid potency of cortisol but virtually no mineralocorticoid activity.

A number of other permutations have been made to the cortisol backbone in other synthetic glucocorticoids, but the earlier discussion highlights the pertinent structural differences among the most common synthetic glucocorticoids. *Clinically, it is most important to be aware of the potency of each agent relative to cortisol, especially when considering a change from one analogue to another that has different relative glucocorticoid and mineralocorticoid activities.* In general, glucocorticoids used at pharmacologic doses should have minimal mineralocorticoid activity to avoid the consequences of mineralocorticoid excess (i.e., hypokalemia, volume expansion, and hypertension). Table 29-1 summarizes the relative glucocorticoid potencies and mineralocorticoid activities of several common glucocorticoid analogues.

Duration of Action

The duration of glucocorticoid action is a complex pharmacokinetic variable that depends on:

1. Fraction of the drug bound to plasma proteins. More than 90% of circulating cortisol is protein-bound, primarily to CBG and, to a lesser degree, to albumin. In contrast, glucocorticoid analogues generally bind to CBG with low affinity. As a result, approximately

TABLE 29-1 Relative Potencies and Durations of Action of Representative Glucocorticoid Analogues

PHARMACOLOGIC AGENT	RELATIVE GLUCOCORTICOID POTENCY	RELATIVE MINERALOCORTICOID ACTIVITY	DURATION OF ACTION
Hydrocortisone (cortisol)	1	1	Short
Prednisolone	4–5	0.25	Short
Methylprednisolone	5–6	0.25	Short
Dexamethasone	18	<0.01	Long

Short-acting agents have a tissue half-life of < 12 hours, and long-acting agents have a half-life of > 48 hours.

two-thirds of a typical glucocorticoid analogue circulates in the plasma bound to albumin, while the rest is present as free steroid. Because only the free steroid is metabolized, the extent of binding to plasma proteins is a determinant of the drug's duration of action.

2. Affinity of the drug for 11β-HSD 2. Glucocorticoids that have a lower affinity for 11β-HSD 2 have a longer plasma half-life because such drugs are not transformed into inactive metabolites as rapidly.

3. Lipophilicity of the drug. Increased lipophilicity promotes partitioning of the drug into adipose stores; the resulting decrease in the drug's metabolism and excretion extends its plasma half-life.

4. Affinity of the drug for the glucocorticoid receptor. Increased affinity of a glucocorticoid analogue for the glucocorticoid receptor increases the duration of action of the drug, because drug bound to the receptor continues to exert its effect until the drug–receptor complex dissociates.

Together, these four variables result in a characteristic duration of action profile for each glucocorticoid analogue. Table 29-1 summarizes the duration of action of representative analogues as "short" or "long." *In general, glucocorticoid agents with higher anti-inflammatory (glucocorticoid) potency have a longer duration of action.*

Replacement Therapy

Treatment of primary adrenal insufficiency is aimed at physiologically replacing both glucocorticoids and mineralocorticoids. **Oral hydrocortisone** is the glucocorticoid of choice. Because glucocorticoid replacement therapy must continue for life, the therapeutic goal is to administer the smallest possible effective dose of cortisol so as to minimize the adverse effects of chronic glucocorticoid excess. Patients with primary adrenal insufficiency also require mineralocorticoid replacement, as described below. Patients with secondary adrenal insufficiency require only glucocorticoid replacement because mineralocorticoid production is preserved by the renin-angiotensin system (see Chapter 21, Pharmacology of Volume Regulation).

Pharmacologic Dosing

Effects at Pharmacologic Levels. Glucocorticoids are important mediators of the stress response, regulating both glucose homeostasis and the immune system. Glucocorticoids have found wide clinical use as anti-inflammatory agents because of their profound effects on immune and inflammatory processes. Pharmacologic levels of glucocorticoids inhibit **cytokine release** and thereby decrease IL-1, IL-2, IL-6, and TNF-α action (Fig. 29-4). Local regulation of cytokine release is crucial for leukocyte recruitment and activation, and disruption of this signaling process profoundly inhibits immune function. Glucocorticoids also block the synthesis of arachidonic acid metabolites by inhibiting the action of phospholipase A_2. As discussed in Chapter 43, Pharmacology of Eicosanoids, arachidonic acid metabolites such as thromboxanes, prostaglandins, and leukotrienes mediate many of the early steps of inflammation, including vascular permeability, platelet aggregation, and vasoconstriction. By blocking the production of these metabolites, glucocorticoids significantly down-regulate the inflammatory response.

The multiple effects described above make glucocorticoids useful drugs in the treatment of many inflammatory and autoimmune diseases, such as asthma, rheumatoid arthritis, Crohn's disease, polyarteritis nodosa, temporal arteritis, and immune rejection after organ transplantation. It is important to note, however, that *pharmacologic glucocorticoid therapy does not correct the underlying disease etiology but only limits the effects of inflammation.* Thus, discontinuing chronic glucocorticoid therapy often results in the resumption of inflammatory symptoms, unless the disorder has gone into spontaneous remission or been treated by other means.

Endogenous glucocorticoids affect many metabolic processes, and pharmacologic dosing with exogenous glucocorticoids amplifies those actions. Because of this, adverse effects typically accompany prolonged pharmacologic dosing with glucocorticoids. Increased *susceptibility to infection* is a potential adverse effect of long-term immunosuppression by exogenous glucocorticoids. Glucocorticoids raise plasma *glucose levels*, as described above, and pharmacologic doses of glucocorticoids amplify these effects. Insulin resistance and increased plasma glucose concentrations necessitate increased pancreatic β-cell production of insulin to normalize blood glucose levels. As a result, *diabetes mellitus* is a common complication of long-term glucocorticoid administration, especially in patients with decreased pancreatic β-cell reserve.

Pharmacologic dosing of glucocorticoids inhibits the vitamin D-mediated absorption of calcium. This results in *secondary hyperparathyroidism* and, therefore, increases bone resorption. Glucocorticoids also directly suppress osteoblast and osteocyte function. These mechanisms contribute to bone loss, and long-term glucocorticoid therapy often results in *osteoporosis*. Steroid-induced bone resorption can be prevented with bisphosphonates, which inhibit osteoclast function and thus slow the progression of bone loss (see Chapter 32, Pharmacology of Bone Mineral Homeostasis). Chronic administration of glucocorticoids also slows *linear bone growth* in children, and glucocorticoid administration can cause growth retardation. Short stature can be the result in children who take glucocorticoids throughout adolescence. For this reason, Johnny's physician monitored his growth closely while he was treated with oral prednisone.

Pharmacologic doses of glucocorticoids can cause selective atrophy of fast-twitch muscle fibers, resulting in catabolism and weakness of (primarily) the proximal muscles. Glucocorticoids also cause a characteristic redistribution of fat, with peripheral wasting of adipose stores and central obesity. Excessive fat deposition also occurs on the back of the neck (buffalo hump) and face (moon facies).

In considering the potential for adverse effects of glucocorticoids, it is important to understand the concept of a population at risk. Not all individuals treated with glucocorticoids develop the same adverse effects because genetic and environmental variability place different individuals at risk for different sequelae of therapy. For example, a patient with borderline diabetes who is treated with glucocorticoids is likely to develop overt diabetes, whereas a patient with sufficient pancreatic β-cell reserve may not experience this adverse effect. *By carefully defining a patient's risk factors, it is often possible to predict the patient's predisposition for adverse effects of glucocorticoids.*

Withdrawal from Glucocorticoid Treatment. Problems can be associated with the discontinuation of chronic glucocorticoid therapy. During long-term therapy with pharmacologic doses of glucocorticoids, high plasma glucocorticoid levels suppress the release of CRH and ACTH, resulting in atrophy of the adrenal cortex. Abrupt cessation of glucocorticoid therapy can precipitate **acute adrenal insufficiency** because a substantial period of time (months) is required to reactivate the hypothalamic-pituitary-adrenal axis. Even after ACTH secretion recovers, additional months may be required for the adrenal cortex to begin secreting physiologic levels of cortisol. Thus, it is axiomatic that *chronic glucocorticoid treatment should, whenever possible, be tapered slowly with gradually decreasing doses.* This taper allows the hypothalamus, anterior pituitary gland, and adrenal cortex to resume normal function gradually, thus avoiding adrenal insufficiency and, it is hoped, avoiding exacerbation of the underlying inflammatory condition.

Routes of Administration

Several different drug delivery methods allow selective targeting of glucocorticoid to a particular tissue. The relevant concept is that *glucocorticoids can be administered locally at many times the normal plasma concentration while minimizing systemic adverse effects.* Examples of these methods include inhaled, topical, and depot preparations of glucocorticoids. The administration of glucocorticoids during pregnancy is also an example of selective targeting because the placenta can metabolically partition glucocorticoids between mother and fetus.

Inhaled Glucocorticoids. Inhaled glucocorticoids are the formulation of choice in the chronic treatment of asthma. Glucocorticoids reduce asthma symptoms by inhibiting airway inflammatory responses, especially eosinophil-mediated inflammation. The exact mechanism(s) is unknown but is thought to involve inhibition of cytokine release and subsequent inhibition of the inflammatory cascade (see Chapter 48). Because systemic therapy with glucocorticoids can lead to serious adverse effects, efforts have been made to develop inhaled glucocorticoids with low oral bioavailability, thereby allowing high-dose delivery directly to the airway mucosa while minimizing systemic dosing. The goal of inhaled glucocorticoid therapy is to maximize the local-to-systemic ratio of glucocorticoid concentration. Because the inhaled glucocorticoid is delivered directly to the inflamed organ, rather than via the systemic circulation, less inhaled glucocorticoid than oral glucocorticoid is required to control airway inflammation. The inhaled route of administration makes glucocorticoids safer for long-term dosing, especially in children. Microcrystalline powders and metered-dose inhalers of potent glucocorticoids such as **beclomethasone**, **ciclesonide**, **flunisolide**, **fluticasone**, **mometasone**, and **triamcinolone** (Fig. 29-7) are currently available as inhaled formulations.

If a patient treated chronically with systemic glucocorticoids is switched to inhaled glucocorticoids, care must be taken not to stop the systemic dosing abruptly. In the introductory case, acute adrenal insufficiency occurred because Johnny was switched acutely from oral prednisone to an inhaled glucocorticoid. On average, inhaled preparations deliver approximately 20% of the dose to the lung, while the other 80% is swallowed. However, the glucocorticoids available as inhaled formulations (see above) have significant first-pass hepatic metabolism, and the swallowed portion is converted to inactive metabolites by the liver. For example, less than 1% of swallowed fluticasone is systemically bioavailable. Thus, Johnny's abrupt switch from an orally available glucocorticoid to an inhaled formulation caused acute adrenal insufficiency. Acute adrenal insufficiency can be life threatening and should be treated immediately with a large dose of intravenous glucocorticoid; for this reason, Johnny was given an intravenous infusion of hydrocortisone. Eventually, after Johnny was placed back on oral prednisone, he was able to taper the dose slowly and, once his hypothalamic-pituitary-adrenal axis had been reactivated, to use the inhaled glucocorticoid alone.

Oropharyngeal candidiasis is a potential local complication of inhaled glucocorticoid therapy, because some glucocorticoid is delivered directly to the oral and pharyngeal mucosa. This results in local immunosuppression and permits infection with opportunistic organisms. Oropharyngeal candidiasis can be avoided by rinsing the mouth with water after each administration of aerosolized glucocorticoid or by using antifungal mouthwash.

Intranasal administration of a glucocorticoid analogue is an effective therapy for allergic rhinitis. Glucocorticoids profoundly suppress the eosinophilic response and are often superior to antihistamines in the treatment of this disorder.

Cutaneous Glucocorticoids. Topical preparations of glucocorticoids are available for multiple dermatologic disorders, including psoriasis, lichen planus, and atopic dermatitis. Cutaneous administration delivers an extremely low percentage of the glucocorticoid systemically, allowing topical dosing at many-fold higher local concentrations than could be achieved safely with systemic administration. The

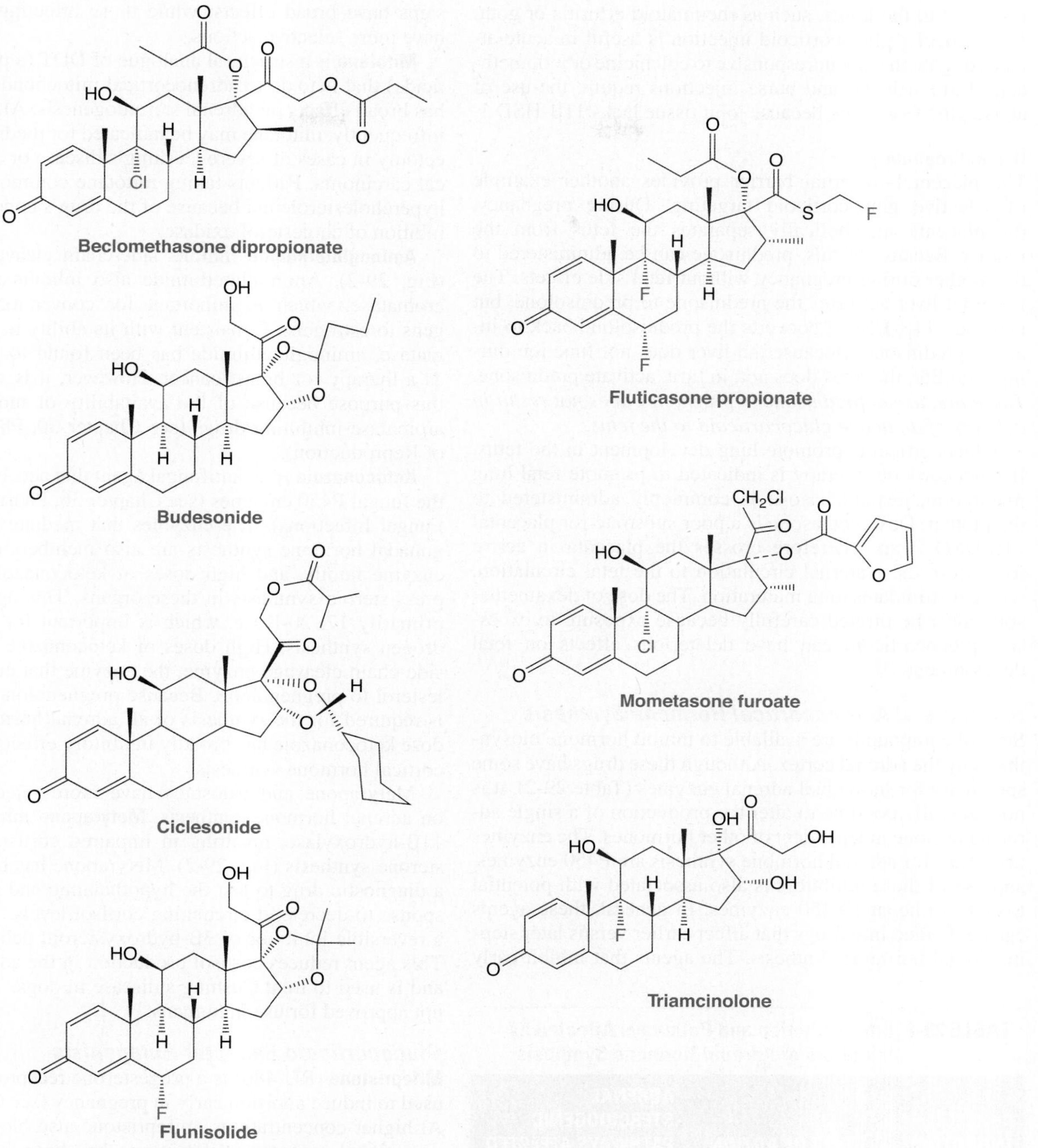

FIGURE 29-7. Structures of common inhaled glucocorticoids. Most of the inhaled glucocorticoids are halogenated analogues of cortisol that are highly potent glucocorticoid agonists with little mineralocorticoid activity (halogen atoms are shown in *blue*). Their high potency allows low doses of the inhaled glucocorticoids to inhibit the local inflammatory response that is a critical component of asthma pathophysiology. In addition, because several of these compounds are subject to almost complete first-pass metabolism in the liver, the fraction of inhaled glucocorticoid that is inadvertently swallowed (80% of the inhaled dose) becomes inactivated so that it is not systemically bioavailable. The fraction of inhaled glucocorticoid delivered to the lung is eventually absorbed into the systemic circulation.

glucocorticoid that is administered must be biologically active because the skin has little, if any, of the 11β-HSD 1 enzyme needed to convert glucocorticoid prodrugs to active compounds. Hydrocortisone, methylprednisolone, and dexamethasone are effective steroids for cutaneous use.

Depot Glucocorticoids. Depot intramuscular preparations of glucocorticoid analogues last for days to weeks and can be an alternative to daily or alternate-day oral glucocorticoids in the treatment of inflammatory diseases. Although depot formulations reduce the necessity for daily oral administration, these preparations are seldom used because the dose cannot be titrated on a frequent basis. Depot preparations of methylprednisolone suspended in polyethylene glycol are commonly used, however, for **intra-articular administration**. This approach can be indicated for inflammatory processes restricted to the joints, such as rheumatoid arthritis or gout. Intra-articular glucocorticoid injection is useful in acute attacks of gout that are unresponsive to colchicine or indomethacin. Intra-articular and bursa injections require the use of active glucocorticoid, because joint tissue lacks 11β-HSD 1.

Use in Pregnancy

The placental–maternal barrier provides another example of selective glucocorticoid targeting. During pregnancy, the placenta metabolically separates the fetus from the mother. Because of this, prednisone can be administered to the mother during pregnancy without fetal side effects. The maternal liver activates the prednisone to prednisolone, but placental 11β-HSD 2 converts the prednisolone back to inactive prednisone. Because the liver does not function during fetal life, the fetus does not, in turn, activate prednisone. *Therefore, use of prednisone in pregnancy does not result in delivery of an active glucocorticoid to the fetus.*

Glucocorticoids promote lung development in the fetus. If glucocorticoid therapy is indicated to promote fetal lung maturation, dexamethasone is commonly administered to the mother. Dexamethasone is a poor substrate for placental 11β-HSD 2 and therefore crosses the placenta in active form from the maternal circulation to the fetal circulation, where it stimulates lung maturation. The dose of dexamethasone must be titrated carefully because exposure to excessive glucocorticoid can have deleterious effects on fetal development.

Inhibitors of Adrenocortical Hormone Synthesis

Several compounds are available to inhibit hormone biosynthesis by the adrenal cortex. Although these drugs have some specificity for individual adrenal enzymes (Table 29-2), it is not generally possible to alter the production of a single adrenal hormone independent of other hormones. The enzymes necessary for adrenal hormone synthesis are P450 enzymes, and use of these inhibitors is also associated with potential toxicity to hepatic P450 enzymes. In general, these agents can be divided into drugs that affect earlier versus later steps in adrenal hormone synthesis. The agents that inhibit early steps have broad effects, while those affecting later steps have more selective actions.

Mitotane is a structural analogue of DDT (a potent insecticide) that is toxic to adrenocortical mitochondria and thus has broad effects on adrenal steroidogenesis. Although used infrequently, mitotane may be indicated for medical adrenalectomy in cases of severe Cushing's disease or adrenocortical carcinoma. Patients taking mitotane commonly develop hypercholesterolemia because of the drug's concomitant inhibition of cholesterol oxidase.

Aminoglutethimide inhibits side-chain cleavage enzyme (Fig. 29-2). Aminoglutethimide also inhibits the enzyme aromatase, which is important for conversion of androgens to estrogens. Consistent with its ability to inhibit aromatase, aminoglutethimide has been found to be effective as a therapy for breast cancer. However, it is not used for this purpose because of the availability of more selective aromatase-inhibiting drugs (see Chapter 30, Pharmacology of Reproduction).

Ketoconazole is an antifungal agent that acts by inhibiting the fungal P450 enzymes (see Chapter 36, Pharmacology of Fungal Infections). The enzymes that mediate adrenal and gonadal hormone synthesis are also members of the P450 enzyme family, and high doses of ketoconazole also suppress steroid synthesis in these organs. This agent inhibits primarily 17, 20-lyase, which is important for adrenal androgen synthesis. High doses of ketoconazole also inhibit side-chain cleavage enzyme, the enzyme that converts cholesterol to pregnenolone. Because pregnenolone generation is required for the synthesis of all adrenal hormones, high-dose ketoconazole has broadly inhibitory effects on adrenocortical hormone synthesis.

Metyrapone and trilostane have more selective effects on adrenal hormone synthesis. **Metyrapone** inhibits steroid 11β-hydroxylase, resulting in impaired cortisol and aldosterone synthesis (Fig. 29-2). Metyrapone has been used as a diagnostic drug to test the hypothalamic and pituitary response to decreased circulating cortisol levels. **Trilostane** is a reversible inhibitor of 3β-hydroxysteroid dehydrogenase. This agent reduces cortisol production in the adrenal cortex and is used to treat Cushing's disease in dogs. Trilostane is not approved for use in humans.

Glucocorticoid Receptor Antagonists

Mifepristone (RU-486) is a progesterone receptor antagonist used to induce abortion early in pregnancy (see Chapter 30). At higher concentrations, mifepristone also blocks the glucocorticoid receptor. Mifepristone has been approved for treatment of hyperglycemia in Cushing's syndrome. Mifepristone potentially could be useful for the treatment of life-threatening elevated glucocorticoid levels, such as in ectopic ACTH syndrome, although its clinical usefulness for this purpose has not been evaluated fully.

■ MINERALOCORTICOIDS

Physiology

Synthesis

Like cortisol, **aldosterone** is a 21-carbon steroid hormone derived from cholesterol. Enzymes unique to aldosterone synthesis are expressed only in the zona glomerulosa. Aldosterone secretion is stimulated by angiotensin II, blood potassium concentration, and ACTH (Fig. 29-1).

TABLE 29-2 Sites of Action and Pathways Affected by Inhibitors of Adrenal Hormone Synthesis

INHIBITOR	SITE OF ACTION	ADRENAL STEROIDOGENIC PATHWAYS AFFECTED
Mitotane	Mitochondria	All
Aminoglutethimide	Side-chain cleavage enzyme	All (aromatase also inhibited in ovary)
Ketoconazole	Primarily 17, 20-lyase	Low concentrations: ↓ Androgen synthesis High concentrations: ↓ Synthesis of all adrenal and gonadal steroid hormones
Metyrapone	Steroid 11β-hydroxylase	Cortisol and aldosterone synthesis
Trilostane	3β-Hydroxysteroid dehydrogenase	All (primarily cortisol and aldosterone synthesis)

Metabolism

Circulating aldosterone binds with low affinity to transcortin, albumin, and a specific aldosterone binding protein. Only 50% to 60% of circulating aldosterone is bound to transport proteins, and aldosterone has a short elimination half-life (20 minutes). Orally administered aldosterone also has high first-pass hepatic metabolism; approximately 75% of the hormone is metabolized to an inactive form during each pass through the liver. As a result, orally administered aldosterone is not an effective replacement therapy for adrenal insufficiency states.

Physiologic Actions

Mineralocorticoids play important roles in regulating sodium reabsorption in the kidney, the colon, and sweat and salivary glands. Circulating aldosterone diffuses across the plasma membrane and binds to a cytosolic **mineralocorticoid receptor** (synonymous with the Type I glucocorticoid receptor). The aldosterone:mineralocorticoid receptor complex is then transported into the nucleus, where it increases or decreases transcription of specific genes through interactions with transcriptional complexes and binding to hormone-responsive-element DNA-binding domains on specific gene promoters. In addition to these transcriptional effects, aldosterone has rapid effects on intracellular signaling pathways. These nongenomic actions appear to be mediated by hormone binding to mineralocorticoid receptors located on the cell surface. The physiologic and pathophysiologic roles of this second signaling mechanism are an active area of investigation.

In the kidney, aldosterone increases transcription of serum and glucocorticoid-induced kinase 1 (SGK1). SGK1 increases $Na^+/K^+ATPase$ activity in the basolateral membrane and induces the apical Na^+ channel of distal nephron cells, resulting in increased sodium reabsorption and potassium secretion across the luminal epithelium of the nephron (see Chapter 21). As a result, sodium retention, potassium excretion, and H^+ excretion are all enhanced by aldosterone. Increased sodium retention is accompanied by increased water retention and, thus, extracellular volume expansion. Excess aldosterone can cause hypokalemic alkalosis and hypertension, while hypoaldosteronism can cause hyperkalemic acidosis and hypotension.

The mineralocorticoid receptor is also expressed in cells not involved in sodium reabsorption, including endothelial cells, vascular smooth muscle cells, cardiomyocytes, adipocytes, neurons, and inflammatory cells. Preclinical studies demonstrate a role for the mineralocorticoid receptor in the pathophysiology of vascular injury, atherosclerosis, heart disease, renal disease, and stroke. Activation of the mineralocorticoid receptor increases oxidative stress, promotes inflammation, regulates adipocyte differentiation, and reduces insulin sensitivity. In humans, antagonists of aldosterone action at the mineralocorticoid receptor, such as spironolactone and eplerenone, reduce morbidity and mortality in heart failure, improve vascular function, reduce cardiac hypertrophy, and reduce albuminuria. These beneficial effects of mineralocorticoid receptor blockade appear to be independent of changes in blood pressure.

Regulation

Three systems regulate aldosterone synthesis: the renin-angiotensin system, blood potassium levels, and ACTH.

The **renin-angiotensin-aldosterone system** is a central regulator of extracellular fluid volume. Decreases in extracellular fluid volume decrease perfusion pressure at the afferent arteriole of the renal glomerulus, which acts as a baroreceptor. This stimulates the juxtaglomerular cells to secrete renin, a protease that cleaves the prohormone angiotensinogen to angiotensin I. Angiotensin I is then converted to angiotensin II by angiotensin converting enzyme, which is expressed at high concentrations by the capillary endothelium of the lungs. Angiotensin II has direct arteriolar pressor effects, and it stimulates aldosterone synthesis by binding to and activating a G protein-coupled receptor in zona glomerulosa cells of the adrenal cortex. In a feedback loop, angiotensin II also inhibits renin secretion.

Potassium loading increases aldosterone synthesis independent of renin activity. Because aldosterone activity at the distal nephron promotes potassium excretion, this control mechanism serves a homeostatic role in regulating potassium balance.

Finally, **ACTH** acutely stimulates aldosterone synthesis in the zona glomerulosa. Changes in ACTH levels contribute to the circadian regulation of aldosterone and to the aldosterone increases associated with acute stress, such as hypoglycemia. Unlike cortisol, aldosterone does not negatively regulate ACTH secretion.

Pathophysiology

Aldosterone Hypofunction

Aldosterone hypofunction (hypoaldosteronism) can result from a primary decrease in aldosterone synthesis or action or from a secondary decrease in aldosterone regulators such as angiotensin II. Most cases of hypoaldosteronism result from decreased aldosterone synthesis. Defects in the gene coding for steroid 21-hydroxylase, an enzyme necessary for both aldosterone and glucocorticoid synthesis, lead to congenital adrenal hyperplasia (discussed below under adrenal androgen pathophysiology) and cause salt wasting as a result of aldosterone deficiency. **Addison's disease**, or primary adrenal insufficiency, results in hypoaldosteronism secondary to destruction of the zona glomerulosa. Most cases of Addison's disease are caused by autoimmune adrenalitis; other causes of adrenal cortex destruction include tuberculosis, metastatic cancer, and hemorrhage. In each case, aldosterone hypofunction can lead to salt wasting, volume depletion, hyperkalemia, and acidosis. Hypoaldosteronism can also result from states of decreased renin production (so-called hyporeninemic hypoaldosteronism, which is common in diabetic renal insufficiency). Both resistance to the action of aldosterone at the level of the mineralocorticoid receptor and inactivating mutations of the aldosterone-regulated epithelial sodium channel in the cortical collecting duct of the nephron result in clinical hypoaldosteronism, despite normal to elevated aldosterone levels in the blood.

Aldosterone Hyperfunction

Primary hyperaldosteronism results from excess aldosterone production by the adrenal cortex. Bilateral zona glomerulosa adrenal hyperplasia and aldosterone-producing adenomas are the two most common causes. Increased aldosterone synthesis leads to positive sodium balance, with consequent extracellular volume expansion, suppression of plasma renin activity, potassium wasting and hypokale-mia, and hypertension. Independent of its effect on blood pressure, primary hyperaldosteronism also has adverse cardiovascular effects, including endothelial dysfunction, increased intima-media thickness, vascular stiffness, and increased left ventricular wall thickness. Primary hyperal-dosteronism is also a cause of insulin resistance. The preva-lence of primary hyperaldosteronism is much higher than initially thought, occurring in 5% to 10% of all patients with hypertension and up to 25% of patients with resistant hypertension.

Pharmacologic Classes and Agents

Mineralocorticoid Receptor Agonists

Pathophysiologic conditions leading to hypoaldosteron-ism necessitate replacement with physiologic doses of a mineralocorticoid. It is not possible to administer al-dosterone itself as a therapeutic agent, because the liver converts more than 75% of oral aldosterone to an inac-tive metabolite during first-pass metabolism. Instead, the cortisol analogue **fludrocortisone**, which has minimal first-pass hepatic metabolism and a high mineralocorticoid-to-glucocorticoid potency ratio, is used. The adverse effects of fludrocortisone therapy are all related to the ability of this agent to mimic a state of mineralocorticoid excess, including hypertension, hypokalemia, and even heart fail-ure. To ensure that an appropriate dose of drug is being administered, it is important to monitor serum potassium and blood pressure levels closely in all patients receiving fludrocortisone.

Mineralocorticoid Receptor Antagonists

Spironolactone (also discussed in Chapters 21 and 30) is a competitive antagonist at the mineralocorticoid receptor, but the drug also binds to and inhibits the androgen and proges-terone receptors to a lesser extent. The latter actions, which result in adverse effects such as gynecomastia in males, limit the usefulness of this agent in some patient subsets. **Eplerenone** is a mineralocorticoid receptor antagonist that binds selectively to the mineralocorticoid receptor, thereby reducing the incidence of gynecomastia relative to spirono-lactone. Both spironolactone and eplerenone can be used as antihypertensive agents, and both are approved for use in pa-tients with heart failure.

Antagonism of the mineralocorticoid receptor can result in significant hyperkalemia. Because many patients with heart failure are prescribed both spironolactone or eplere-none and an angiotensin converting enzyme inhibitor (which also raises blood potassium levels), it is important to monitor potassium levels closely in these patients.

ADRENAL ANDROGENS

Physiology

Sex steroids produced by the adrenal cortex, primarily **dehydroepiandrosterone (DHEA)**, have an uncertain role in human physiology. DHEA seems to be a prohormone that is converted to more potent androgens, primarily testosterone, in the periphery. Adrenocortical androgens are an important source of testosterone in females; these hormones are neces-sary for the development of female axillary and pubic hair at the time of puberty, when adrenal androgen secretion is activated (adrenarche).

Pathophysiology

Congenital adrenal hyperplasia (CAH) and **polycystic ovarian syndrome** are two important diseases related to adrenocorti-cal androgen production. *Congenital adrenal hyperplasia* is a clinical term related to several different inherited enzyme deficiencies in the adrenal cortex. Enzyme defects leading to increased adrenocortical androgen production cause hirsut-ism and virilization in females. Polycystic ovarian syndrome, discussed in Chapter 30, may be caused by congenital adre-nal hyperplasia in a small subset of patients.

The most common form of congenital adrenal hyper-plasia results from a deficiency of **steroid 21-hydroxylase**. Deficiency of 21-hydroxylase results in the inability of adrenocortical cells to synthesize both aldosterone and cortisol (Fig. 29-8). Because cortisol is the main negative feedback regulator of pituitary ACTH release, the decreased cortisol synthesis that results from 21-hydroxylase defi-ciency disinhibits ACTH release. Increased ACTH restores the cortisol level in patients with partial enzyme defects, but it also induces shunting of precursor compounds into the "unblocked" androgen pathway, resulting in greater production of DHEA and androstenedione. The liver sub-sequently converts these compounds into testosterone. In severe 21-hydroxylase deficiency, there may be a virilizing effect on the developing female fetus. As a result, female neonates with severe 21-hydroxylase deficiency typically have masculinized or ambiguous external genitalia. In the male neonate, however, increased adrenal androgens may have little or no noticeable phenotypic effect. Infants with severe 21-hydroxylase deficiency are commonly diagnosed in infancy during an acute salt-wasting crisis, which results from the inability to synthesize aldosterone and cortisol. Mild 21-hydroxylase deficiency may manifest later in life as hirsutism, acne, and oligomenorrhea in young women after menarche.

Treatment of congenital adrenal hyperplasia due to severe enzyme defects requires physiologic replacement doses of glucocorticoids and mineralocorticoids. Treatment of con-genital adrenal hyperplasia in patients with mild enzyme defects may include therapy with exogenous glucocorticoid to suppress excessive hypothalamic and pituitary release of CRH and ACTH, thus decreasing the production of adrenal androgens.

Pharmacologic Classes and Agents

Androgens synthesized by the adrenal gland can be viewed as prohormones. Because no specific receptors for either DHEA or androstenedione have been described, the activity of these hormones depends on their conversion to testoster-one, and subsequently to dihydrotestosterone, in peripheral target tissues. As discussed above, adrenal androgen excess can cause a variety of syndromes in women; the pharma-cologic interruption of excessive androgenic activity is dis-cussed in Chapter 30.

DHEA is not regulated by the US Food and Drug Administration (FDA) and is commonly used as an over-the-counter drug. Population cross-sectional studies have shown a reciprocal relationship between an age-related decline in DHEA levels and the risk of cardiovascular disease and

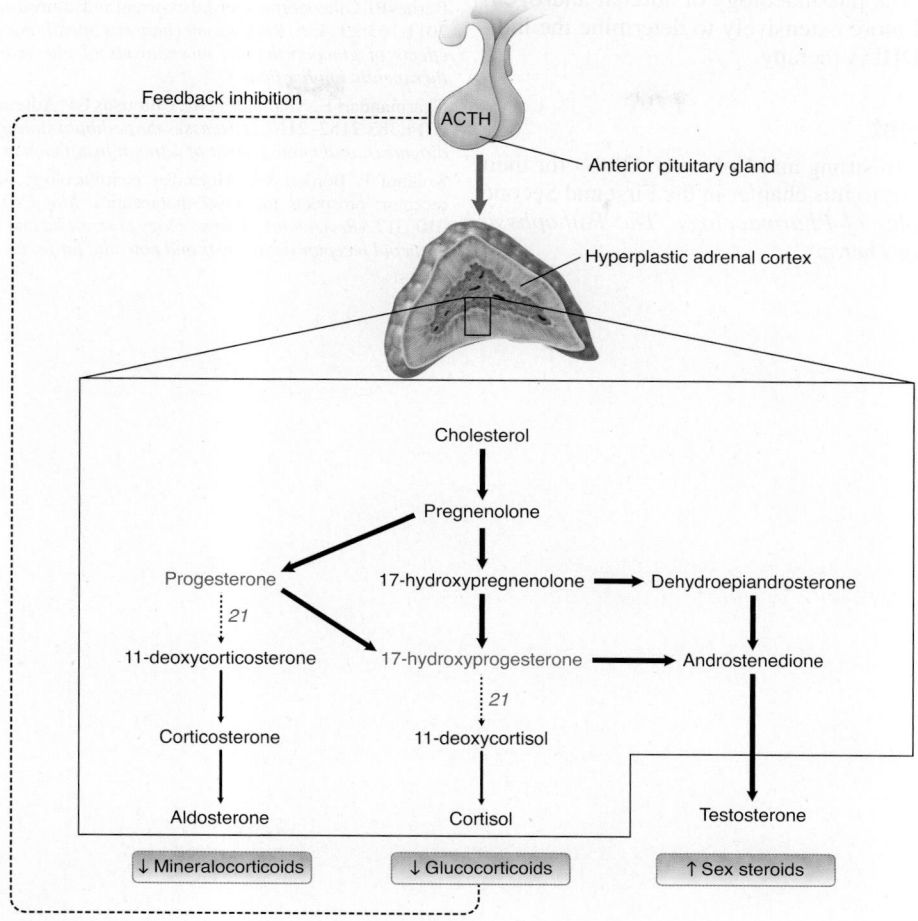

FIGURE 29-8. Congenital adrenal hyperplasia. Steroid 21-hydroxylase deficiency, the most common cause of congenital adrenal hyperplasia, results in impaired biosynthesis of aldosterone and cortisol (*dashed lines*). Therefore, steroid hormone synthesis in the adrenal cortex is shunted toward increased production of sex steroids (*thick lines*). The lack of cortisol production decreases the negative feedback on corticotroph cells of the anterior pituitary gland (*dashed line*), causing increased ACTH release (*thick blue arrow*). Increased levels of ACTH induce adrenal hyperplasia and further stimulate the synthesis of sex steroids. This pathway can be interrupted by administering exogenous cortisol. The deficient enzyme is shown as a number: 21, steroid 21-hydroxylase.

cancer. Replacement therapy with DHEA may be indicated for cases of Addison's disease in which there is bona fide DHEA deficiency. Exogenous DHEA can be converted to testosterone by the liver. As a result, DHEA is commonly abused for its anabolic effects.

CONCLUSION AND FUTURE DIRECTIONS

Aldosterone, cortisol, and adrenal androgens regulate many aspects of basic homeostasis. Aldosterone regulates extracellular fluid volume by promoting sodium reabsorption and fluid retention. Cortisol regulates diverse physiologic processes, including energy homeostasis and inflammatory responses. The physiologic role of adrenal androgens is unknown, but pathophysiologic states causing increased adrenal androgen production have significant masculinizing effects in women. Antagonists of aldosterone are currently used to control high blood pressure and to improve clinical

outcomes in heart failure. Accumulating evidence suggests that antagonists selective for the aldosterone receptor may become important therapies for a range of cardiovascular and renovascular diseases. Efforts are ongoing to develop aldosterone receptor antagonists that are tissue-specific and lack effects on potassium homeostasis. Also, aldosterone synthase inhibitors are being developed and may be used in the future to reduce aldosterone production. Glucocorticoid pharmacology is an immense field, primarily because glucocorticoids are used to suppress inflammation in many different disease states. Chronic glucocorticoid use is associated with a multitude of predictable adverse effects, and future research in this area will attempt to minimize the adverse effects of glucocorticoid therapy while maintaining the anti-inflammatory actions. Such efforts could include the development of tissue-selective glucocorticoid agonists and antagonists (analogous to the selective estrogen receptor modulators), as well as further refinement of drug delivery methods. Attempts are also being made to design sustained-release preparations of hydrocortisone to better mimic the circadian rhythm of cortisol for treatment of Addison's disease. The pharmacology of adrenal androgens needs to be studied more extensively to determine the indications, if any, for DHEA therapy.

Acknowledgment

We thank Ehrin J. Armstrong and Robert G. Dluhy for their valuable contributions to this chapter in the First and Second Editions of *Principles of Pharmacology: The Pathophysiologic Basis of Drug Therapy*.

Suggested Reading

Barnes PJ. Glucocorticosteroids: current and future directions. *Br J Pharmacol* 2011;163:29–43. (*Reviews mechanisms mediating the anti-inflammatory effects of glucocorticoids, mechanisms of glucocorticoid resistance, and therapeutic implications.*)

Charmandari E, Nicolaides NC, Chrousos GP. Adrenal insufficiency. *Lancet* 2014;383:2152–2167. (*Discusses the pathophysiology, clinical presentation, diagnosis, and management of adrenal insufficiency.*)

Kolkhof P, Borden SA. Molecular pharmacology of the mineralocorticoid receptor: prospects for novel therapeutics. *Mol Cell Endocrinol* 2012;350: 310–317. (*Reviews the pharmacology of steroidal and non-steroidal mineralocorticoid receptor antagonists and potential for tissue-specific drugs.*)

DRUG SUMMARY TABLE: CHAPTER 29 Pharmacology of the Adrenal Cortex

DRUG	CLINICAL APPLICATIONS	SERIOUS AND COMMON ADVERSE EFFECTS	CONTRAINDICATIONS	THERAPEUTIC CONSIDERATIONS
GLUCOCORTICOID RECEPTOR AGONISTS Mechanism—Mimic cortisol function by acting as agonists at the glucocorticoid receptor				
Prednisone **Prednisolone** **Methylprednisolone** **Dexamethasone** **Hydrocortisone** **Fluticasone** **Beclomethasone** **Flunisolide** **Triamcinolone** **Budesonide**	Inflammatory conditions in many different organs Autoimmune diseases Replacement therapy for primary and secondary adrenal insufficiency (hydrocortisone only)	*Cushing's syndrome, pulmonary toxicity, increased risk of infection (shared adverse effects); impaired wound healing, psychotic disorder (prednisone, prednisolone, methylprednisolone, dexamethasone, hydrocortisone, and triamcinolone only); cardiotoxicity, seizure, muscle atrophy (prednisone, prednisolone, methylprednisolone, dexamethasone, and hydrocortisone only); decreased body growth (prednisone, methylprednisolone, dexamethasone, flunisolide, and triamcinolone only); electrolyte imbalance (prednisone and methylprednisolone only); hyperglycemia (prednisone, methylprednisolone, dexamethasone, and triamcinolone only); eye toxicity (dexamethasone, fluticasone, beclomethasone, triamcinolone, and budesonide only); thromboembolic disorder, aseptic necrosis of bone (prednisone only)* Hypertension, edema, weight gain, osteoporosis, mood disturbance, headache	Shared contraindications: Hypersensitivity to drug Systemic fungal infection Dexamethasone only: Ocular infection, glaucoma, posterior lens capsule injury Concomitant use with rilpivirine	See Table 29-1 for relative potency and duration of action of individual agents. Pharmacologic glucocorticoid therapy does not correct the underlying disease etiology but rather limits the effects of inflammation. Chronic glucocorticoid treatment should be tapered slowly; abrupt withdrawal of systemic glucocorticoids can lead to acute adrenal insufficiency. Intranasal and inhaled formulations greatly reduce systemic adverse effects; do not switch abruptly from high-dose oral to inhaled glucocorticoids. The intrinsic activity of a glucocorticoid is especially important for topically administered drugs because the skin does not possess appreciable amounts of 11β-HSD 1. Glucocorticoid agents with higher anti-inflammatory potency typically have a longer duration of action. Inhaled glucocorticoids include fluticasone, beclomethasone, flunisolide, triamcinolone, and budesonide.
GLUCOCORTICOID RECEPTOR ANTAGONISTS Mechanism—Competitive antagonist of cortisol action at the glucocorticoid receptor				
Mifepristone (RU-486)	Hyperglycemia in Cushing's syndrome Abortion (through day 70 of pregnancy)	*Prolonged QT interval, prolonged bleeding time, bacterial infection, sepsis* Hypertension, peripheral edema, hypokalemia, nausea, vomiting, diarrhea, cramps, dizziness, abnormal vaginal bleeding, headache, fatigue, glucocorticoid insufficiency despite normal to elevated cortisol levels	Hypersensitivity to mifepristone Chronic adrenal failure Ectopic pregnancy Hemorrhagic disorders Anticoagulation therapy Inherited porphyrias Intrauterine device Undiagnosed adnexal mass Concomitant use with simvastatin, lovastatin, or other CYP3A substrates with a narrow therapeutic range	Mifepristone is a progesterone receptor antagonist used to induce abortion early in pregnancy. At higher concentrations, mifepristone also blocks the glucocorticoid receptor; the latter action makes mifepristone useful for the treatment of select patients with endogenous Cushing's syndrome.

continues

DRUG SUMMARY TABLE: CHAPTER 29 Pharmacology of the Adrenal Cortex continued

DRUG	CLINICAL APPLICATIONS	SERIOUS AND COMMON ADVERSE EFFECTS	CONTRAINDICATIONS	THERAPEUTIC CONSIDERATIONS
INHIBITORS OF GLUCOCORTICOID SYNTHESIS Mechanism—Inhibit various steps in glucocorticoid hormone biosynthesis				
Mitotane	Medical adrenalectomy in cases of severe Cushing's syndrome or adrenocortical carcinoma	*Adrenal insufficiency, prolonged bleeding time, neurological deficit, toxic retinopathy, hemorrhagic cystitis* Rash, gastrointestinal upset, dizziness, lethargy, vertigo	Hypersensitivity to mitotane	Structural analogue of DDT that is toxic to adrenocortical mitochondria. Hypercholesterolemia may result from inhibition of cholesterol oxidase.
Aminoglutethimide	Cushing's syndrome	*Agranulocytosis, aplastic anemia, cortisol insufficiency* Rash, loss of appetite, nausea, dizziness, somnolence	Hypersensitivity to glutethimide or aminoglutethimide	Aminoglutethimide inhibits side-chain cleavage enzyme as well as aromatase, which is important for conversion of androgens to estrogens.
Metyrapone	Diagnostic evaluation of hypothalamic-pituitary-adrenal axis	*Cortisol insufficiency* Hypertension	Hypersensitivity to metyrapone Adrenal cortical insufficiency	Inhibits 11β-hydroxylation, resulting in impaired cortisol synthesis. Treatment with metyrapone results in disinhibition of ACTH secretion; thus, metyrapone can be administered to test ACTH reserve.
Trilostane	Cushing's syndrome in dogs	*Addisonian crisis* Postural hypotension, hypoglycemia, diarrhea, nausea	Adrenal cortical insufficiency Renal or hepatic dysfunction	Trilostane is a reversible inhibitor of 3β-hydroxysteroid dehydrogenase; it decreases aldosterone and cortisol production in the adrenal cortex. Trilostane is not approved for use in humans.
Ketoconazole	See Drug Summary Table: Chapter 36 Pharmacology of Fungal Infections			
MINERALOCORTICOID RECEPTOR AGONISTS Mechanism—Agonist at the mineralocorticoid receptor				
Fludrocortisone	Hypoaldosteronism	*Heart failure, hypertension, hypokalemia, thrombophlebitis, secondary hypocortisolism, decreased body growth, increased intracranial pressure, seizure* Edema, bruising, impaired wound healing, rash, myopathy, hyperglycemia, menstrual irregularities, headache, vertigo	Hypersensitivity to fludrocortisone Systemic fungal infection	The adverse effects of fludrocortisone therapy are related to its ability to mimic a state of mineralocorticoid excess, including hypertension, hypokalemia, and heart failure; serum potassium and blood pressure levels should be monitored closely.
MINERALOCORTICOID RECEPTOR ANTAGONISTS Mechanism—Competitive antagonists of aldosterone action at the mineralocorticoid receptor				
Spironolactone Eplerenone	See Drug Summary Table: Chapter 21 Pharmacology of Volume Regulation			
ADRENAL SEX STEROID Mechanism—DHEA is a prohormone that is converted to testosterone in the periphery				
Dehydroepiandrosterone (DHEA)	Under investigation	Acne, hepatitis, hirsutism, androgenization	Hypersensitivity to dehydroepiandrosterone Breast, ovarian, or prostate cancer Pregnancy	May be used as replacement therapy for cases of Addison's disease with documented DHEA deficiency; DHEA is commonly abused for its anabolic effects.

30

Pharmacology of Reproduction

Ehrin J. Armstrong and Robert L. Barbieri

INTRODUCTION

This chapter presents endocrine pharmacology relevant to both the male and female reproductive tracts. Although men and women differ in their hormonal profiles, androgens and estrogens are both under the control of the anterior pituitary gland gonadotropins, luteinizing hormone (LH) and follicle-stimulating hormone (FSH), and ultimately regulated by hypothalamic release of gonadotropin-releasing hormone (GnRH). Female hormone patterns are temporally more complex and cyclic than male patterns: hormonal control of the menstrual cycle is an illustrative example of how sex hormones are integrated into a complex physiologic system. Understanding the menstrual cycle also provides a basis for understanding the pharmacology of contraception.

A number of diseases are treated pharmacologically via modification of reproductive hormone activity; these range from infertility and endometriosis to breast and prostate cancer. Key concepts in this chapter include (1) the interactions between estrogen and the pituitary gland, (2) the effects of GnRH release frequency on gonadotropin release, (3) the tissue selectivity of estrogen receptor agonists and antagonists, and (4) the various strategies used to antagonize the effects of endogenous sex hormones, from suppression of the hypothalamic-pituitary-reproduction axis to antagonism at the target tissue receptor.

PHYSIOLOGY OF REPRODUCTIVE HORMONES

Synthesis of Progestins, Androgens, and Estrogens

The synthesis of progestins, androgens, and estrogens is closely intertwined. All three groups are steroid hormones derived from the metabolism of cholesterol. The synthesis of these hormones is similar to that of adrenal sex hormones, which is discussed in Chapter 29, Pharmacology of the Adrenal Cortex.

The terminology *progestins*, *androgens*, and *estrogens* denotes a number of related hormones rather than a single molecule in each group (Fig. 30-1). The **progestins** consist of **progesterone**, a common precursor to testosterone and estrogen synthesis (see also Fig. 29-2), and a number of synthetically altered progesterone derivatives used for therapeutic purposes. Progestins generally exert antiproliferative effects on the female endometrium by promoting the endometrial lining to secrete rather than proliferate (see below). Progesterone is also required for the maintenance of pregnancy. **Androgens**, all of which have masculinizing properties, include dehydroepiandrosterone (DHEA), androstenedione, **testosterone**, and **dihydrotestosterone (DHT)**; among the androgens, testosterone is considered the classic circulating androgen and DHT the classic intracellular

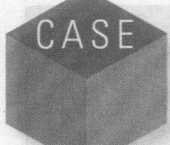

Amy J first notices that her hair is thinning during her teenage years. Even though she loses some hair on her scalp, Ms. J notices excessive hair growth on her face; she sometimes has to shave to remove inappropriate hair growth. At age 24, she goes to her doctor complaining of both her hair problem and the fact that her periods are irregular. On further questioning, the doctor discovers that the longest interval between her menstrual cycles has been 6 months and the shortest 22 days. When Ms. J does have periods, they are heavy and last for more than her previous average of 5 days. The increased hair growth on her face, extremities, abdomen, and breasts had begun around age 15. Ms. J also reports a problem with being overweight since high school, although in middle school, she had been extremely active in soccer, field hockey, and swimming. The doctor orders several tests and finds that Ms. J has mildly elevated free and total testosterone levels and an increased ratio of plasma LH to FSH.

Based on these findings, the doctor tells Ms. J that she probably has a disorder called *polycystic ovarian syndrome* (PCOS). He recommends combination oral contraceptives to regularize her menstrual cycles. He also prescribes spironolactone to ameliorate her problems with hair growth and balding.

Questions

1. What is the pathophysiologic link between excessive hair growth and infertility in polycystic ovarian syndrome?
2. Why was spironolactone prescribed to treat Ms. J's hair problem?
3. How do oral contraceptives act, and how would they help regulate Ms. J's menstrual cycles?

androgen. Androgens are required for conversion to a male phenotype during development and for male sexual maturation. **Estrogens** refer to a number of substances that share a common feminizing activity. **17β-Estradiol** is the most potent naturally occurring estrogen, while estrone and estriol are less potent.

Note that *all estrogens are derived from the aromatization of precursor androgens* (Fig. 30-1). The ovary and placenta most actively synthesize the **aromatase** enzyme that converts androgens to estrogens, but other nonreproductive tissues such as adipose tissue, hypothalamic neurons, and muscle can also aromatize androgens to estrogen. After menopause, the majority of circulating estrogen is derived from adipose tissue. This is also the main source of circulating estrogens in men.

Hormone Action and Metabolism

Progestins, androgens, and estrogens are all hormones that bind to a related superfamily of nuclear hormone receptors; glucocorticoids, mineralocorticoids, vitamin D, and thyroid hormone also bind to the same superfamily of receptors. Once synthesized, these hormones diffuse into the plasma, where they bind tightly to carrier proteins such as sex hormone-binding globulin (SHBG) and albumin. Only the unbound fraction of hormone is able to diffuse into cells and bind to an intracellular receptor. Interestingly, *testosterone is essentially a prohormone*. Testosterone binds to the androgen receptor but with only modest affinity. As a result, testosterone has only modest androgenic activity. Instead, testosterone is converted in target tissues to the more active **dihydrotestosterone** (Fig. 30-2), which binds to the androgen receptor with an affinity tenfold higher than that of testosterone. The formation of dihydrotestosterone from testosterone is catalyzed by the enzyme **5α-reductase**. There are at least two subtypes of 5α-reductase. Differential tissue expression of these enzymes provides some pharmacologic specificity for the 5α-reductase inhibitors. The importance

of dihydrotestosterone as the most active androgen is highlighted in individuals with inherited deficiencies of 5α-reductase. Males lacking this enzyme are phenotypically female because they are unable to convert testosterone to dihydrotestosterone and are thus unable to activate a program of male differentiation during development.

The **estrogen receptor (ER)** is the best studied of the sex hormone receptors and serves as an example for all three receptor types (i.e., estrogen receptor, androgen receptor, and progesterone receptor). Because progestins, androgens, and estrogens are lipophilic steroid hormones, the fraction of hormone that remains unbound to plasma proteins can freely diffuse across the plasma membrane into the cytosol of cells. Once inside the cell, the hormone ligand binds to its specific intracellular receptor, which subsequently dimerizes. For example, association of estrogen with the estrogen receptor causes dimerization of two estrogen–estrogen receptor complexes, and the dimer then binds to **estrogen response elements (EREs)** in promoter regions of DNA. This binding to EREs, together with the recruitment of coactivators or corepressors, enhances or inhibits the transcription of specific genes and thereby causes the physiologic effects of the hormone.

There are two subtypes of estrogen receptors—ERα and ERβ. In addition, it is now recognized that many estrogen receptor actions involve association of the receptor with other transcription cofactors. In other words, dimerization of the estrogen receptor and subsequent binding of the dimer to EREs are insufficient to explain the complex and varied actions of estrogen in different tissues. *The specific transcription factors that are recruited by the estrogen receptor appear to be tissue-dependent and ligand-dependent and probably account for some of the target specificity of estrogen action.* Although the subtypes and molecular associations of the androgen and progesterone receptors have not been studied as thoroughly as those of the estrogen receptor, it is likely that the same complexities exist for these receptors. The recognition that differential binding of modular transcription factors

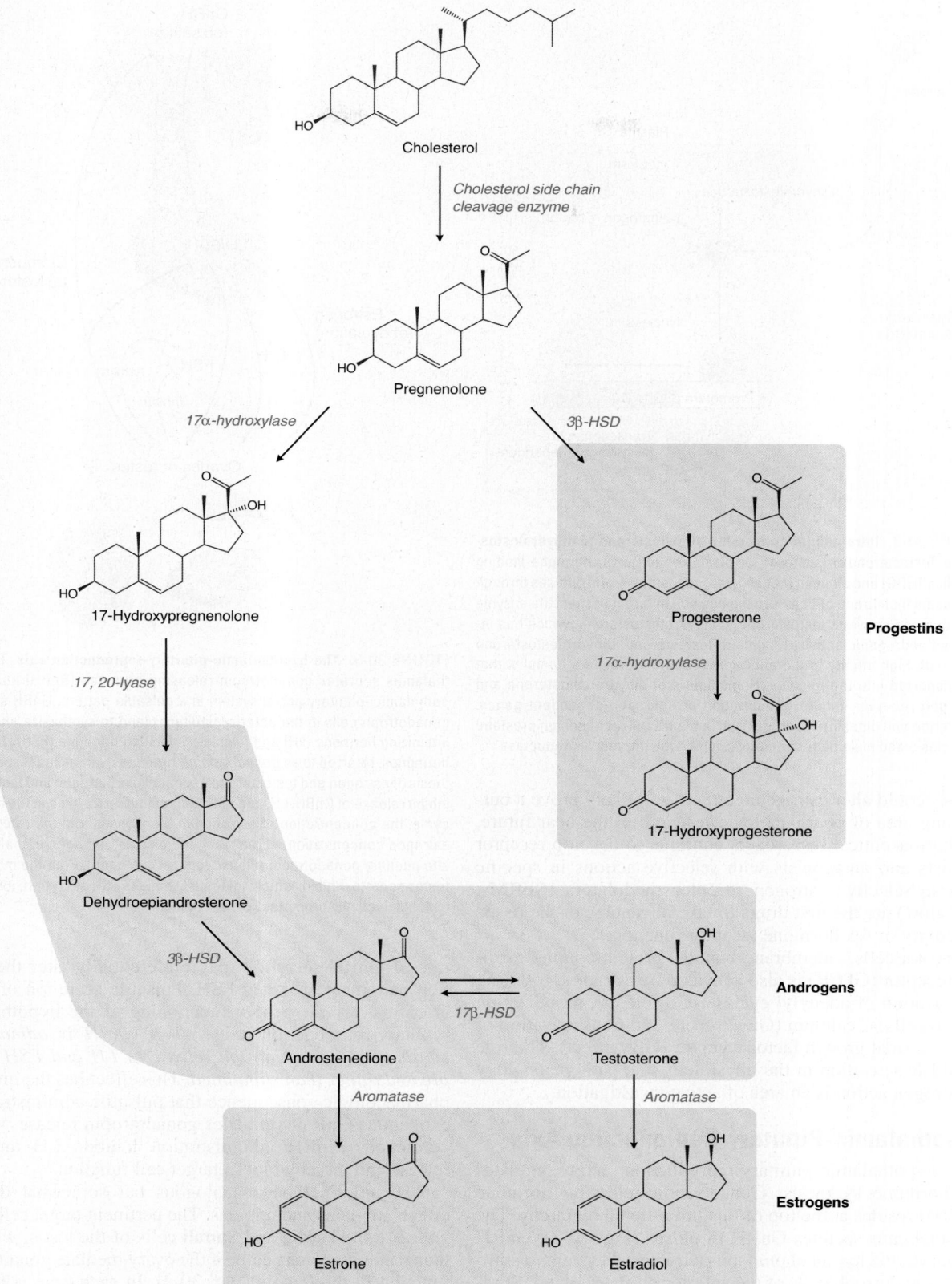

FIGURE 30-1. Synthesis of progestins, androgens, and estrogens. Progestins, androgens, and estrogens are steroid hormones derived from cholesterol. The major progestins include progesterone and 17α-hydroxyprogesterone. The androgens include dehydroepiandrosterone (DHEA), androstenedione, and testosterone. Estrogens include estrone and estradiol. Estrogens are aromatized forms of their conjugate androgens: androstenedione is aromatized to estrone, and testosterone is aromatized to estradiol. Estradiol and estrone are both metabolized to estriol, a weak estrogen (*not shown*). Some of the precursor–product relationships among the hormones are omitted for clarity (see Fig. 29-2). HSD, hydroxysteroid dehydrogenase.

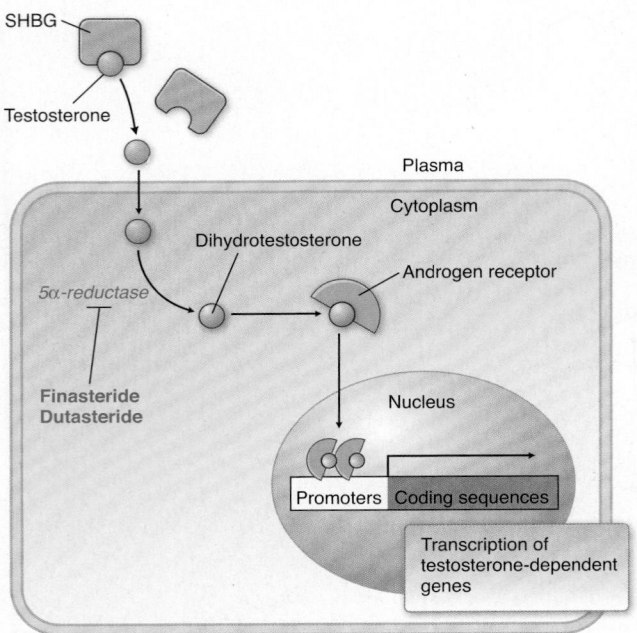

FIGURE 30-2. Intracellular conversion of testosterone to dihydrotestosterone. Testosterone circulates in the plasma bound to sex hormone-binding globulin (SHBG) and albumin (*not shown*). Free testosterone diffuses through the plasma membrane of cells into the cytosol. In target tissues, the enzyme 5α-reductase converts testosterone to dihydrotestosterone, which has increased androgenic activity relative to testosterone. Dihydrotestosterone binds with high affinity to the androgen receptor, forming a complex that is transported into the nucleus. Homodimers of dihydrotestosterone and androgen receptor initiate transcription of androgen-dependent genes. Finasteride and dutasteride, drugs used in the treatment of benign prostatic hyperplasia and male pattern hair loss, inhibit the enzyme 5α-reductase.

to ERs could alter estrogenic effects will likely prove a burgeoning area of pharmacologic research in the near future, as pharmaceutical researchers continue to develop receptor agonists and antagonists with selective actions in specific tissues. Selective estrogen receptor modulators (SERMs, see below) are the first drugs to take advantage of the tissue selectivity of sex hormone receptor function.

In some cells, a membrane-bound G protein-coupled estrogen receptor (GPER) is also activated by estradiol, resulting in activation of adenylyl cyclase ($G\alpha_s$ effect), mobilization of intracellular calcium ($G\beta\gamma$ effect), and transactivation of the epidermal growth factor receptor ($G\beta\gamma$ effect). The role of GPER activation in the physiology and pathophysiology of estrogen action is an area of active investigation.

Hypothalamic-Pituitary-Reproduction Axis

The hypothalamic-pituitary-reproduction axis regulates sex hormone synthesis. Gonadotropin-releasing hormone (GnRH) resides at the top of this three-tiered hierarchy. The hypothalamus secretes GnRH in pulses (Fig. 30-3). GnRH travels via the hypothalamic–pituitary portal system to stimulate gonadotroph cells of the anterior pituitary gland. Stimulation of gonadotroph cells via a G protein-coupled cell surface receptor increases the synthesis and secretion of LH and FSH, which are jointly referred to as the *gonadotropins*.

Although one cell type produces both LH and FSH, the synthesis and release of these two hormones are controlled independently. Current research suggests that the

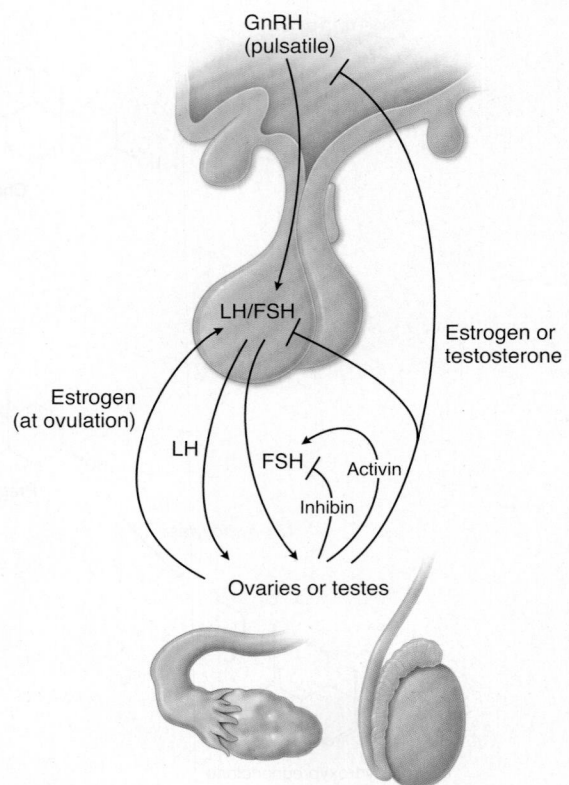

FIGURE 30-3. The hypothalamic-pituitary-reproduction axis. The hypothalamus secretes gonadotropin-releasing hormone (GnRH) into the hypothalamic–pituitary portal system in a pulsatile pattern. GnRH stimulates gonadotroph cells in the anterior pituitary gland to synthesize and release luteinizing hormone (LH) and follicle-stimulating hormone (FSH). These two hormones, referred to as *gonadotropins*, promote ovarian and testicular synthesis of estrogen and testosterone, respectively. Estrogen and testosterone inhibit release of GnRH, LH, and FSH. Depending on the time in the menstrual cycle, the concentration of estrogen in the plasma, and the rate at which estrogen concentration increases in the plasma, estrogen can also stimulate pituitary gonadotropin release (e.g., at ovulation). Both the ovaries and testes secrete inhibin, which selectively inhibits FSH secretion, and activin, which selectively promotes FSH secretion.

rate of GnRH secretion may preferentially alter the secretion patterns of LH and FSH. Pulsatile secretion of GnRH is critical for the proper functioning of the hypothalamic-pituitary-reproduction axis. *When GnRH is administered continuously, gonadotroph release of LH and FSH is suppressed rather than stimulated.* This effect has the important pharmacologic consequence that pulsatile administration of exogenous GnRH stimulates gonadotropin release, whereas continuous GnRH administration inhibits LH and FSH release and thereby blocks target cell function.

LH and FSH have analogous but somewhat different effects in males and females. The pertinent target cells in the male are the **Leydig** and **Sertoli** cells of the testis, while the **thecal** and **granulosa** cells of the ovary mediate gonadotropin function in the female (Fig. 30-4). In each case, a two-cell system is coordinated to mediate sex hormone actions. In the male, LH stimulates testicular Leydig cells to increase the synthesis of testosterone, which then diffuses into neighboring Sertoli cells. In the Sertoli cell, FSH stimulation increases the production of androgen binding protein (ABP), which is important for maintaining the high testicular concentrations

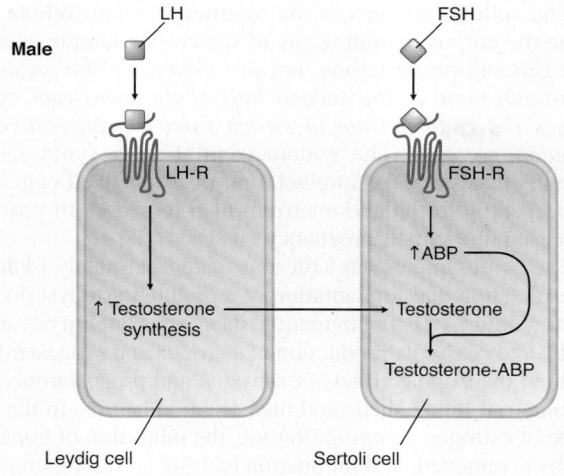

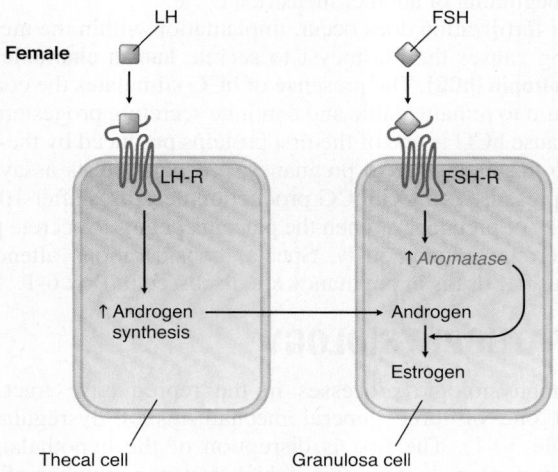

FIGURE 30-4. Two-cell systems for gonadal hormone action. In the **male**, the binding of luteinizing hormone (LH) to the LH receptor (LH-R) activates testosterone synthesis in Leydig cells. Testosterone then diffuses into nearby Sertoli cells, where the binding of follicle-stimulating hormone (FSH) to its receptor (FSH-R) increases levels of androgen binding protein (ABP). ABP stabilizes the high concentrations of testosterone that, together with other FSH-induced proteins synthesized in Sertoli cells, promote spermatogenesis in the nearby germinal epithelium (*not shown*). In the **female**, LH acts in an analogous manner to promote androgen (androstenedione) synthesis in thecal cells. Androgen then diffuses into nearby granulosa cells, where aromatase converts androstenedione to estrone, which is then reduced to the biologically active estrogen, estradiol. FSH increases aromatase activity in granulosa cells, promoting the conversion of androgen to estrogen. Note that dihydrotestosterone is not a substrate for aromatase.

of testosterone necessary for spermatogenesis. In addition, FSH stimulates the Sertoli cell to produce other proteins necessary for sperm maturation. In the female, LH stimulates the thecal cells to synthesize the androgen androstenedione, which is then aromatized to estrone and estradiol in the granulosa cells under the influence of FSH.

Both Sertoli cells and granulosa cells synthesize and secrete the regulatory proteins **inhibin A**, **inhibin B**, and **activin**. Inhibins secreted by the gonad act on the anterior pituitary gland to inhibit the release of FSH, while activin stimulates FSH release. Neither the inhibins nor activin has an effect on anterior pituitary gland LH release (Fig. 30-3). The role of these regulatory proteins in controlling hormone action is still

not completely understood. In the male, testosterone is also an important negative regulator of pituitary gland and hypothalamic hormone release. The role of estrogen in the female is more complex and can involve either positive or negative feedback depending on the prevailing hormonal milieu; this topic is addressed below as part of the menstrual cycle discussion. In the female, the combination of estradiol and progesterone synergistically suppresses GnRH, LH, and FSH secretion by actions at both the hypothalamus and pituitary gland.

Integration of Endocrine Control: The Menstrual Cycle

The female menstrual cycle is governed by the cycling of hormones with an approximate periodicity of 28 days (normal range, 24–35 days). This cycle begins at the onset of puberty and continues uninterrupted (with the exception of pregnancy) until menopause (Fig. 30-5). The start of the cycle, cycle day 1, is arbitrarily defined as the first day of menstruation. Ovulation occurs at the midportion (about day 14) of each cycle. The portion of the menstrual cycle before ovulation is often referred to as the **follicular** or **proliferative** phase; during this time, the developing ovarian *follicle* produces most of the gonadal hormones, which stimulate cellular *proliferation* of the endometrium. Subsequent to ovulation, the **corpus luteum** produces progesterone, and the endometrium becomes *secretory* rather than proliferative. The second half of the menstrual cycle is thus often referred to as the **luteal** or **secretory** phase, depending on whether the ovary or the endometrium is considered as the frame of reference.

At the start of the menstrual cycle, there is low production of estrogen and inhibin A. As a result, the anterior pituitary gland secretes increasing amounts of FSH and LH. These hormones stimulate the maturation of four to six follicles, each of which contains an ovum arrested in the first stage of meiosis. Maturing follicles secrete increasing concentrations of estrogen, inhibin A, and inhibin B. Estrogen causes the follicles to increase the expression of LH and FSH receptors on thecal and granulosa cells, respectively. Receptor up-regulation increases the follicular response to pituitary gland gonadotropins and allows one follicle to secrete increasing quantities of estrogen. The increased plasma estrogen and inhibin levels partially suppress pituitary gland LH and FSH release. In turn, the decreased gonadotropin levels cause other follicles to become atretic, so that usually, only one follicle matures. At the same time, increased estrogen levels stimulate the uterine endometrium to proliferate rapidly.

As the dominant follicle continues to grow, it secretes high, sustained levels of estrogen. Although the mechanism is still not completely understood, the combination of high estrogen levels and the rapid rate of increase of estrogen levels causes a brief positive feedback effect on gonadotroph release of gonadotropins, stimulating rather than inhibiting release of LH and FSH. The resulting midcycle surge of LH and FSH stimulates the dominant follicle to swell and to increase the activity of its proteolytic enzymes. Approximately 40 hours after the onset of the **LH surge**, the follicle ruptures and ovulation occurs. The ovum is released into the peritoneal cavity and is then taken up by a fallopian tube, where it begins its route toward the uterus. If the oocyte becomes fertilized in the fallopian tube, it reaches the uterus approximately 4 days after ovulation and implants into the endometrium approximately 5–6 days after ovulation.

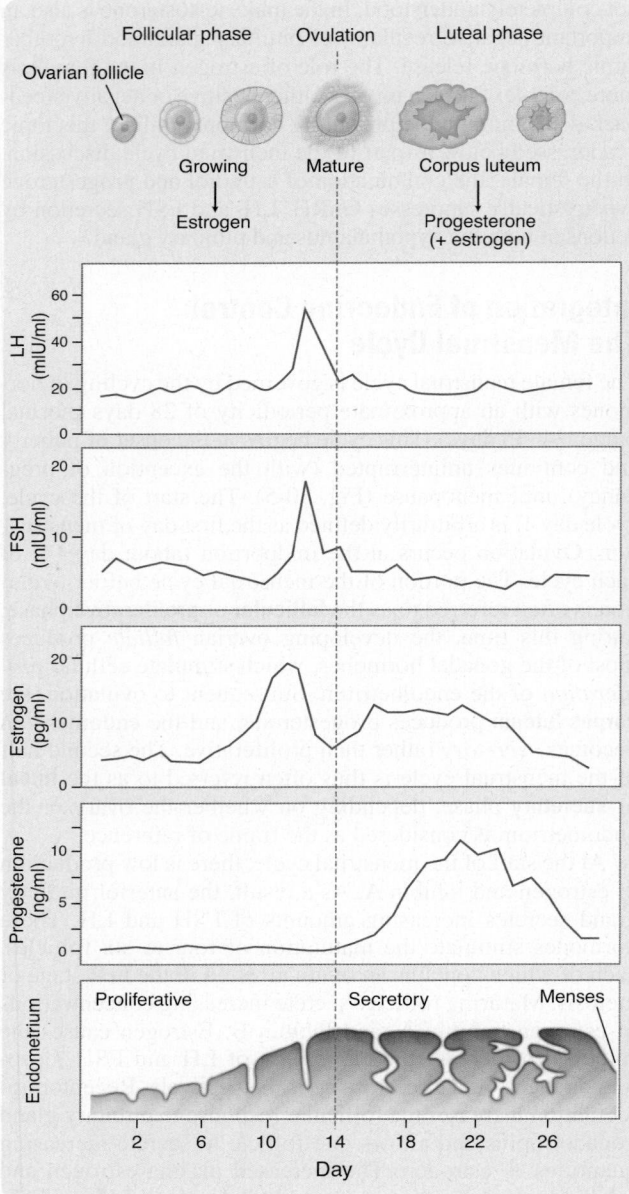

FIGURE 30-5. **The menstrual cycle.** The menstrual cycle is divided into the follicular phase and the luteal phase. Ovulation defines the transition between these two phases. During the follicular phase, gonadotroph cells of the anterior pituitary gland secrete LH and FSH in response to pulsatile GnRH stimulation. Circulating LH and FSH promote growth and maturation of ovarian follicles. Developing follicles secrete increasing amounts of estrogen. At first, the estrogen has an inhibitory effect on gonadotropin release. Just before the midpoint in the menstrual cycle, however, estrogen exerts a brief positive feedback effect on LH and FSH release. This is followed by follicular rupture and release of an egg into the fallopian tube. During the second half of the cycle, the corpus luteum secretes both estrogen and progesterone. Progesterone induces a change in the endometrium from a proliferative to a secretory type. If fertilization and implantation of a blastocyst do not occur within 14 days after ovulation, the corpus luteum involutes, secretion of estrogen and progesterone declines, menses occurs, and a new cycle begins.

The cellular remains of the ruptured ovarian follicle become the corpus luteum. Cells of the corpus luteum secrete estrogen and progesterone, not just estrogen. *The presence of progesterone in the second half of the menstrual cycle causes the endometrium to switch from a proliferative to a secretory state.* The endometrium begins synthesizing proteins necessary for implantation of a fertilized egg. The blood supply to the endometrium also increases to provide increased nutrients if pregnancy ensues.

The corpus luteum has a lifespan of approximately 14 days. If fertilization and implantation of a viable blastocyst do not occur within 14 days of ovulation, the corpus luteum becomes atretic and ceases its production of estrogen and progesterone. Without the trophic effects of estrogen and progesterone, the endometrial lining sheds and menstruation begins. In the absence of estrogen and progesterone, the inhibition of gonadotrophs is removed, and production of FSH and LH increases. This stimulates the development of new ovarian follicles and the beginning of another menstrual cycle.

If fertilization does occur, implantation within the uterine lining causes the blastocyst to secrete **human chorionic gonadotropin (hCG)**. The presence of hCG stimulates the corpus luteum to remain viable and continue secreting progesterone. Because hCG is one of the first proteins produced by the embryo that is unique to pregnancy, pregnancy tests assay for the presence of hCG. hCG production decreases after 10–12 weeks of pregnancy, when the placenta begins to secrete progesterone autonomously. Special considerations attending the use of drugs in pregnancy are discussed in Box 6-1.

▋ PATHOPHYSIOLOGY

Pathophysiologic processes in the reproductive tract reflect one of three general mechanisms of dysregulation (Table 30-1). The first is disruption of the hypothalamic-pituitary-reproduction axis, which causes a number of underlying disorders that can lead to infertility. The second is inappropriate growth of estrogen-dependent or testosterone-dependent tissue. This can lead to breast cancer or prostate cancer, as well as to benign but clinically important conditions such as endometriosis or endometrial hyperplasia. Finally, decreased estrogen secretion, as in menopause, or decreased androgen secretion, as in some aging men, is associated with a number of undesirable health consequences.

TABLE 30-1 General Mechanisms of Reproductive Tract Disorders for Which Pharmacologic Agents Are Currently Used

MECHANISM	EXAMPLES
Disruption of the hypothalamic-pituitary-reproduction axis	Polycystic ovarian syndrome Prolactinoma
Inappropriate growth of hormone-dependent tissue	Breast cancer Prostatic hyperplasia, prostate cancer Endometriosis, endometrial hyperplasia Leiomyomas (uterine fibroids)
Decreased estrogen or androgen secretion	Hypogonadism Menopause

Disruption of the Hypothalamic-Pituitary-Reproduction Axis

The hypothalamic-pituitary-reproduction axis is normally tightly regulated via feedback inhibition or stimulation of hormone activity, with the goal of producing a successful menstrual cycle every month. When this axis is disrupted, infertility can result. Common causes of infertility due to disruption of sex hormone production include polycystic ovarian syndrome and prolactinomas.

Polycystic ovarian syndrome (PCOS) is a complex syndrome characterized by anovulation or oligo-ovulation and by increased levels of plasma androgen. PCOS is a common problem affecting between 3% and 5% of women of reproductive age. The diagnosis is typically clinical, as in the case of Ms. J, and based on the concurrent findings of oligo-ovulation and hirsutism (excessive hair growth). Although multiple etiologies are likely to be responsible for PCOS, all of the etiologies result in increased androgen secretion and suppression of normal ovulatory cycles. The increased androgen secretion results in masculinization; as seen in Ms. J's case, male pattern baldness and inappropriate facial hair growth are common. Many women with PCOS are treated with both an estrogen–progestin contraceptive to suppress ovarian production of testosterone and an antiandrogen, such as spironolactone (see below), to abrogate the masculinizing effects of increased circulating testosterone.

Three primary hypotheses have been advanced to explain the development of PCOS. The first, referred to as the **LH hypothesis**, is based on the observation that many women with PCOS have an increased frequency and amplitude of pituitary LH pulses. In fact, 90% of women with PCOS have increased circulating LH. Increased LH activity stimulates thecal cells of the ovary to synthesize increased amounts of androgens, including androstenedione and testosterone. In addition, the increased LH and androgen levels prevent normal follicle growth, in turn preventing follicle secretion of large amounts of estrogen. The absence of an estrogen "trigger" prevents the LH surge and ovulation. As seen in the introductory case, patients with PCOS menstruate irregularly, and the menstrual periods that they do have tend to have heavy flow.

The second hypothesis, referred to as the **insulin theory**, is based on the observation that many women with PCOS are obese and insulin resistant and secrete increased insulin. Increased insulin decreases the production of sex hormone-binding globulin (SHBG), which results in a higher concentration of free testosterone and therefore greater androgenic effects on peripheral tissues. It has also been observed that insulin can directly synergize with LH to increase androgen production by thecal cells. Interestingly, in women with PCOS, medications that specifically treat insulin resistance, such as metformin, may result in regular ovulatory menses and normalization of testosterone levels.

The third hypothesis is the **ovarian hypothesis**. This explanation posits dysregulation of sex steroid synthesis at the level of the thecal cell. For example, an abnormal increase in the activity of the oxidative enzymes responsible for androgen synthesis could lead to greater thecal cell production of androgens in response to any given stimulus. It is important to note that these hypotheses are not mutually exclusive and that PCOS could result from a combination of two or three mechanisms. When the cellular mechanisms underlying this disease are better elucidated, new pharmacologic therapies can be developed to treat the etiology of the disease rather than its effects.

Prolactinomas are another common cause of infertility among women of reproductive age. These clonal, benign tumors of lactotrophs in the anterior pituitary gland can cause infertility through two parallel pathways. First, increased prolactin levels suppress estrogen synthesis, both by antagonizing the hypothalamic release of GnRH and by decreasing gonadotroph sensitivity to GnRH. This antagonism decreases LH and FSH release and thereby decreases end-organ stimulation by the hypothalamic-pituitary-reproduction axis. The second mechanism, common to all pituitary gland tumors, is a crowding-out or mass effect. Because the pituitary gland is enclosed in the bony sella turcica, lactotroph proliferation in the anterior pituitary gland leads to crowding of other cell types and thereby inhibits the function of nearby gonadotroph cells. Prolactin-secreting tumors typically remain responsive to the inhibitory effect of dopamine agonists. In most cases, chronic administration of dopamine agonists such as **cabergoline** or **bromocriptine** suppresses prolactin secretion and causes the tumor cells to shrink, thereby decreasing the size of the tumor and restoring normal gonadotroph function and ovulation.

Inappropriate Growth of Hormone-Dependent Tissues

The growth of breast tissues is dependent on many hormones, including estrogen, progesterone, androgens, prolactin, and insulin-like growth factors. Many (but not all) breast cancers express the estrogen receptor (ER), and the growth of such cancers is often stimulated by endogenous levels of estrogen and inhibited by antiestrogens. When a **breast carcinoma** is found to express the ER, an estrogen receptor antagonist (either a pure antagonist such as **fulvestrant** or a selective estrogen receptor modulator such as **tamoxifen**; see below) or an estrogen synthesis inhibitor (an aromatase inhibitor such as **anastrozole**, **letrozole**, **exemestane**, or **formestane**) is commonly administered to slow tumor growth. Prostate growth is androgen-dependent and requires the local conversion of testosterone to dihydrotestosterone by type II 5α-reductase in stromal cells of the prostate. Both enzyme inhibition (**finasteride** or **dutasteride**) and receptor antagonist (**flutamide**, **bicalutamide**, **nilutamide**, or **enzalutamide**) strategies are used to treat conditions in which the growth of prostate tissue is dysregulated, such as **benign prostatic hyperplasia** and metastatic **prostate cancer** (see below).

Endometriosis is the growth of endometrial tissue outside the uterus. The fact that endometriosis is usually found in areas surrounding the fallopian tube (ovaries, rectovaginal pouch, and uterine ligaments) has led to the hypothesis that endometriosis could result from retrograde migration of endometrial tissue via the fallopian tubes during menstruation. Other etiologies are possible, however, including metaplastic tissue growth from the peritoneum or spread of endometrial cells to extrauterine sites via lymphatic ducts. There is also evidence of increased aromatase activity in endometrial tissue from such patients. Because foci of endometriosis respond to estrogen stimulation, endometriosis grows and regresses with the menstrual cycle. This can lead to severe pain, abnormal bleeding, and the formation of adhesions in the peritoneal cavity. In turn, adhesion formation can lead to infertility. Because endometriosis is usually estrogen-dependent, treatment with long half-life GnRH agonists often achieves regression of the disease.

Decreased Estrogen or Androgen Secretion

The effects of decreased sex hormone production vary depending on the age of the patient at the onset of symptoms. **Hypogonadism** results if sex hormone production is impaired before adolescence. Patients with hypogonadism do not undergo sexual maturation, but proper hormone replacement can, in many cases, allow the development of secondary sexual characteristics.

Menopause is a normal physiologic response to exhaustion of the ovarian follicles. Throughout a woman's lifetime, follicles are arrested in meiosis. Only a small percentage of follicles mature during the menstrual cycle; the rest eventually become atretic. Menstrual cycles cease when all of the follicles are depleted from the ovaries. Follicle depletion leads to a decrease in estrogen and inhibins (because developing follicles are the main estrogen and inhibin source in premenopausal women) and an increase in LH and FSH (because estrogen and inhibins suppress gonadotropin release). *After menopause, androstenedione continues to be converted to estrone by aromatase in peripheral (mainly adipose) tissues. However, estrone is a less potent estrogen than estradiol.* Because of the relative lack of estrogen after menopause, many women experience hot flashes, vaginal dryness, and decreased libido. Postmenopausal women are also at risk for osteoporosis. The role of estrogen in the maintenance of bone mass is discussed in further detail in Chapter 32, Pharmacology of Bone Mineral Homeostasis.

Men do not experience a sudden decrease in sex hormones in a manner analogous to the female menopause, but androgen secretion does decline gradually with age. Although controversy currently exists over the role of androgen therapy in normal elderly men, androgen replacement is indicated in cases of adult hypogonadism where both low testosterone levels and symptoms of hypogonadism are present.

■ PHARMACOLOGIC CLASSES AND AGENTS

Pharmacologic agents have been developed to target most of the steps in gonadal physiology and pathophysiology. The relevant drug classes include modulators of anterior pituitary gland gonadotroph activity and specific antagonists of peripheral hormone action. In addition, sex hormones are often used as replacement therapy or to modify gonadotropin release (Fig. 30-6).

Inhibitors of Gonadal Hormones

Synthesis Inhibitors

GnRH Agonists and Antagonists

Under physiologic conditions, the hypothalamus releases GnRH in a pulsatile fashion. The frequency of GnRH pulses controls the relative release of LH and FSH by the anterior pituitary gland. In contrast, continuous administration of GnRH

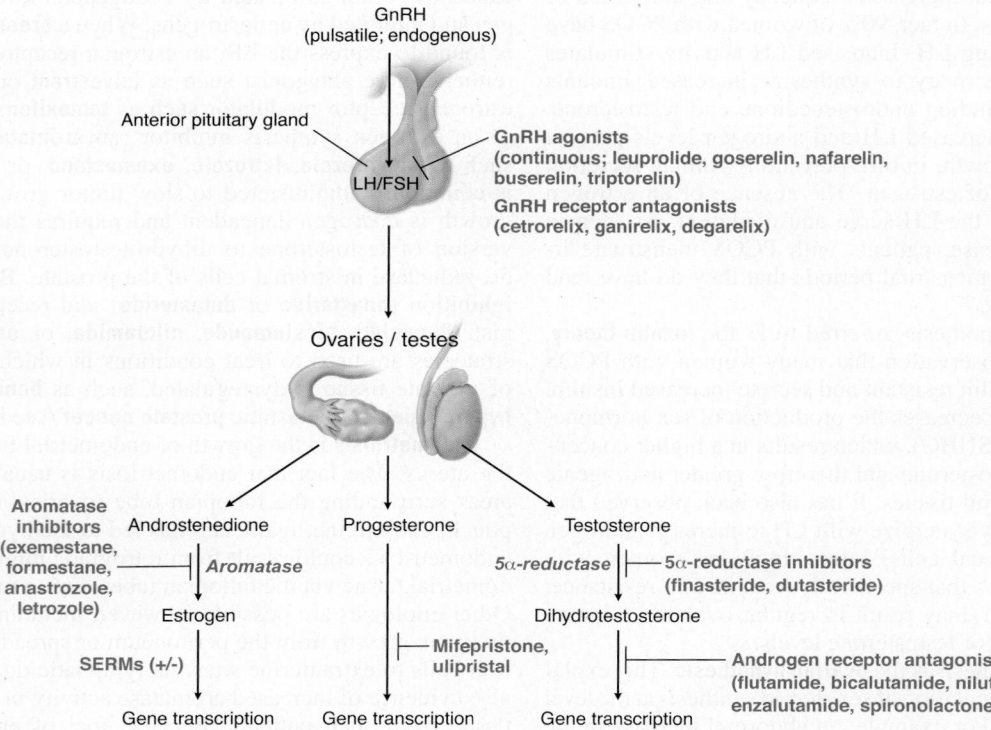

FIGURE 30-6. Pharmacologic modulation of gonadal hormone action. Pharmacologic modulation of gonadal hormone action can be divided into inhibitors of hormone synthesis and hormone receptor antagonists. Continuous administration of GnRH suppresses LH and FSH release from the anterior pituitary gland, thus preventing gonadal hormone synthesis. GnRH receptor antagonists (cetrorelix, ganirelix, degarelix) are also used for this purpose. Finasteride and dutasteride inhibit the enzyme 5α-reductase, thus preventing conversion of testosterone to the more active dihydrotestosterone. Aromatase inhibitors (exemestane, formestane, anastrozole, letrozole) inhibit production of estrogens from androgens. A number of hormone receptor antagonists and modulators prevent the action of endogenous estrogens (some SERMs), androgens (flutamide, bicalutamide, nilutamide, enzalutamide, spironolactone), and progesterone (mifepristone, ulipristal).

suppresses, rather than stimulates, pituitary gonadotroph activity. It is possible to suppress the hypothalamic-pituitary-reproduction axis either by continuous administration of a GnRH agonist (**leuprolide, goserelin, nafarelin, buserelin,** or **triptorelin**) or by administration of a GnRH receptor antagonist (**cetrorelix, ganirelix,** or **degarelix**). Continuous administration of a GnRH agonist is used to treat hormone-dependent tumors such as prostate cancer and, in some cases, breast cancer. Individual agents are discussed in detail in Chapter 27, Pharmacology of the Hypothalamus and Pituitary Gland. Currently available GnRH analogues are peptides and are administered by non-oral routes such as injection or nasal spray. A nonpeptide oral GnRH antagonist, **elagolix,** is in late clinical trials for the treatment of pelvic pain caused by endometriosis.

5α-Reductase Inhibitors

Finasteride and **dutasteride** are inhibitors of 5α-reductase, the enzyme that converts testosterone to dihydrotestosterone. Finasteride is a selective inhibitor of the type II reductase, which is highly expressed in the prostate. Dutasteride is an inhibitor of both type II reductase and type I reductase (which is expressed in skin and prostate). Recall that dihydrotestosterone binds to the androgen receptor with higher affinity than testosterone. *Blocking the local conversion of testosterone to dihydrotestosterone effectively abrogates the local action of testosterone.* Prostate cells are dependent on androgen stimulation for survival, and administration of a reductase inhibitor slows the growth of prostate tissue. Finasteride and dutasteride are approved for treatment of symptoms resulting from benign prostatic hyperplasia, such as decreased urine flow and difficulty initiating urination. These drugs are potential alternatives to transurethral resection of the prostate (TURP), which is a common surgical treatment for symptomatic prostatic hyperplasia. One year of therapy can result in up to 25% reduction in prostate size. These drugs are most effective for patients with larger prostates because the greatest clinical changes are observed in prostates that are already significantly hypertrophied. Adverse effects include decreased libido and erectile dysfunction.

Aromatase Inhibitors

Because estrogens are synthesized from androgen precursors via the action of aromatase, blocking the aromatase enzyme can effectively inhibit estrogen formation. This approach is used to inhibit the growth of estrogen-dependent tumors such as estrogen receptor (ER)-positive breast cancer. A number of highly selective aromatase inhibitors have recently been developed. **Anastrozole** and **letrozole** are competitive inhibitors of aromatase, while **exemestane** and **formestane** bind covalently to aromatase. All of these agents are currently used in the treatment of metastatic breast cancer and in the prevention of recurrences in cancers primarily treated with surgery and radiation. Recent trials suggest that aromatase inhibitors are more effective than estrogen receptor antagonists, such as tamoxifen, for the treatment of breast cancer. However, aromatase inhibitors produce profound suppression of estrogen action, and estrogen is a major regulator of bone density. Therefore, women taking aromatase inhibitors have an increased risk of osteoporotic fractures. Approximately 20% of breast cancer occurs in premenopausal women. In these patients, the combination of a GnRH agonist (to suppress ovarian hormone production) and an aromatase inhibitor (to suppress estrogen formation) has been shown to significantly reduce the risk of distal tumor recurrence.

TABLE 30-2 Tissue-Specific Agonist and Antagonist Activity of Selective Estrogen Receptor Modulators

	BREAST	ENDOMETRIUM	BONE
Estrogen	+++	+++	+++
Tamoxifen	−	+	+
Raloxifene	−	−	++
Bazedoxifene	−	− −	+

Estrogen, the physiologic hormone, has stimulatory effects in breast, endometrium, and bone. Tamoxifen is an antagonist in breast tissue and is therefore used in the treatment of estrogen receptor-positive breast cancer. Raloxifene is an agonist in bone but an antagonist in breast and endometrium. Raloxifene is approved for prevention and treatment of osteoporosis in postmenopausal women and prevention of breast cancer. Bazedoxifene is an antagonist in breast and endometrium but an agonist in bone. Bazedoxifene is approved for treatment of hot flashes and prevention of postmenopausal osteoporosis. Clomiphene (*not shown in the table*) is a SERM that acts as an estrogen receptor antagonist in hypothalamus and anterior pituitary gland; it is used clinically to increase FSH secretion, thereby inducing ovulation.

Receptor Antagonists

Selective Estrogen Receptor Modulators

The term *selective estrogen receptor modulator* (SERM) is based on the observation that certain so-called anti-estrogen drugs are not pure antagonists but rather mixed agonists/antagonists (Table 30-2). These pharmacologic agents inhibit estrogenic effects in some tissues, while promoting estrogenic effects in other tissues. The basis for tissue selectivity may include several mechanisms. First, there are two estrogen receptor subtypes, ERα and ERβ, and the expression of these receptor subtypes is tissue-specific. Second, the ability of the estrogen receptor to interact with other transcription cofactors (coactivators and corepressors) depends on the structure of the ligand that is bound to the receptor.

Figure 30-7 provides an example. Assume that the binding of 17β-estradiol (called *Estrogen* in the figure) to the estrogen receptor causes a conformational change in the receptor, so that two transcriptional cofactors, X and Y, can also bind to the receptor. This complex can then activate three genes: an X-dependent gene, a Y-dependent gene, and a gene that depends on both X and Y. In contrast, the binding of a SERM to the estrogen receptor causes a different conformational change in the receptor, so that transcription factor X is able to bind, but transcription factor Y is not. As a result, the SERM-receptor-X complex can activate the X-dependent gene but not the Y-dependent gene or the (X+Y)-dependent gene.

In addition, assume that transcription factors X and Y are expressed in bone cells but that breast cells express only transcription factor Y. In the breast, this SERM acts as an antagonist because (1) the inability of Y to associate with the SERM-estrogen receptor complex prevents the SERM from activating any estrogen-dependent effects and (2) binding of the SERM to the estrogen receptor competitively inhibits the binding of endogenous estrogen to the receptor. In bone, however, this SERM acts as a partial agonist because it can activate X-dependent but not Y-dependent genes.

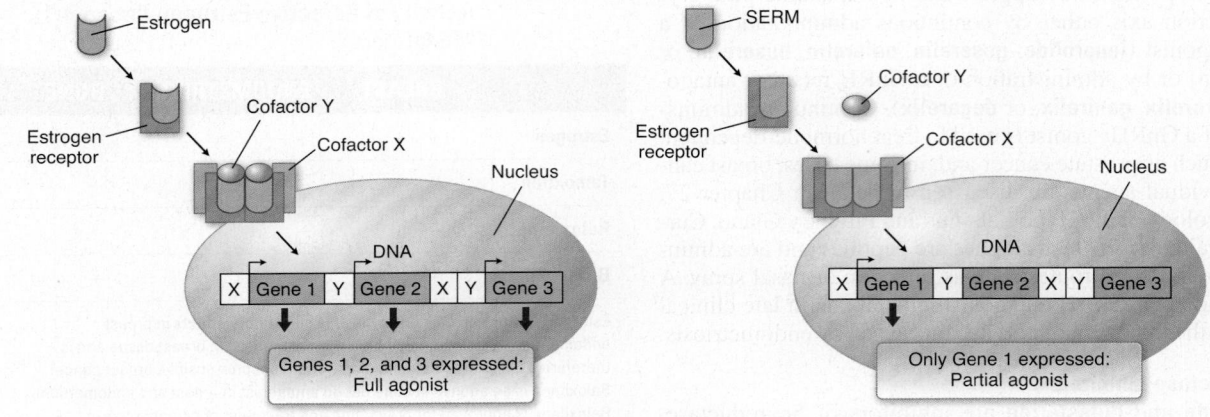

A Bone: both X and Y cofactors expressed

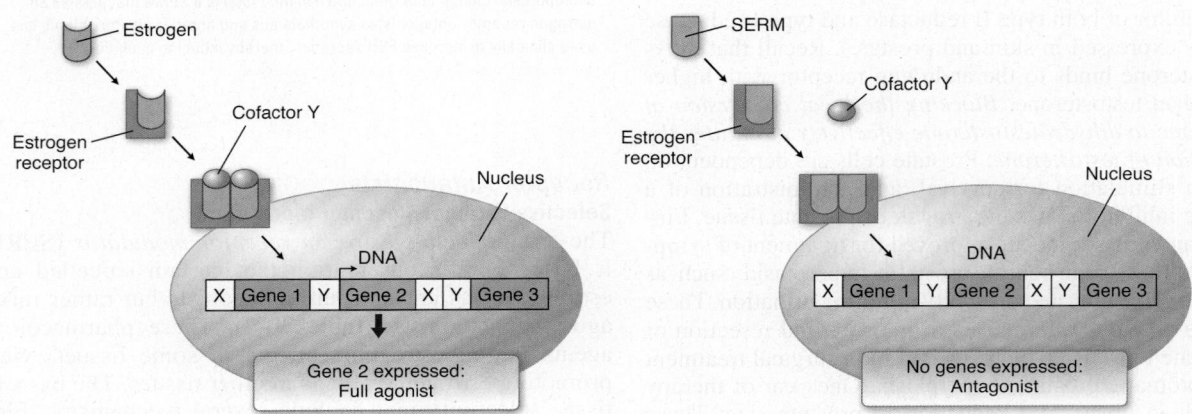

B Breast: only Y cofactor expressed

FIGURE 30-7. A model for the tissue specificity of action of SERMs. Selective estrogen receptor modulators (SERMs) exhibit tissue-specific estrogen receptor antagonist or partial agonist activity. This tissue specificity of action seems to be explained by the following observations: (1) transcriptional coactivators and/or corepressors are expressed in a tissue-specific manner, (2) a SERM–estrogen receptor (ER) complex can associate with some coactivators or corepressors but not others, and (3) genes can be activated or inhibited by different combinations of SERM–ER complexes and coactivators or corepressors. In the example shown, assume that bone cells express coactivators (cofactors) X and Y, whereas breast cells express only coactivator Y. The estrogen–ER complex can associate with X and Y, whereas the SERM–ER complex can associate with only X. **A.** In bone cells, estrogen binding to ER and recruitment of coactivators X and Y induce expression of Genes 1, 2, and 3. The SERM–ER complex cannot bind coactivator Y, and the SERM–ER–cofactor X complex induces expression of only Gene 1. In bone, then, estrogen is a full agonist, whereas the SERM is a partial agonist. **B.** In breast cells, estrogen binding to ER and recruitment of coactivator Y induce expression of Gene 2, but the SERM is unable to promote expression of any gene. In breast, then, the SERM acts as an antagonist. For simplicity, this model shows only coactivators, although corepressors are also involved in SERM action.

These tissue-specific actions of SERMs have important implications for both the desired effects and the adverse effects of pharmacologic agents. If it were possible to design a SERM that inhibits estrogen-dependent growth of breast carcinoma without causing estrogen-induced endometrial hyperplasia, then the undesirable adverse effects of tamoxifen (discussed below) could be reduced. It is likely that SERMs with refined specificity will have important implications for the treatment of osteoporosis, breast cancer, and perhaps even cardiovascular disease. The six SERMs in current clinical use are tamoxifen, raloxifene, toremifene, bazedoxifene, ospemifene, and clomiphene.

Tamoxifen is the only SERM currently approved for use in the treatment and prevention of breast cancer. Tamoxifen has been employed in the palliative treatment of metastatic breast cancer and as adjuvant therapy after lumpectomy. *Tamoxifen is an estrogen receptor antagonist in breast tissue*

but a partial agonist in endometrium and bone. These pharmacodynamic effects result in inhibition of the estrogen-dependent growth of breast cancer but also stimulation of endometrial growth. Because of the latter effect, tamoxifen administration is associated with a fourfold to sixfold increase in the incidence of endometrial cancer. Therefore, in order to minimize the risk of iatrogenic endometrial cancer, tamoxifen is typically administered for no more than 5 years.

Raloxifene is a newer SERM that possesses *estrogen receptor agonist activity in bone but antagonist activity in both breast and endometrial tissue.* Its mechanism of action is illustrated in Figure 30-7 and its molecular structure is shown in Figure 30-8. Consistent with this profile of tissue-specific actions, raloxifene does not appear to increase the incidence of endometrial cancer. The agonist activity of raloxifene in bone decreases bone resorption and thus delays or prevents

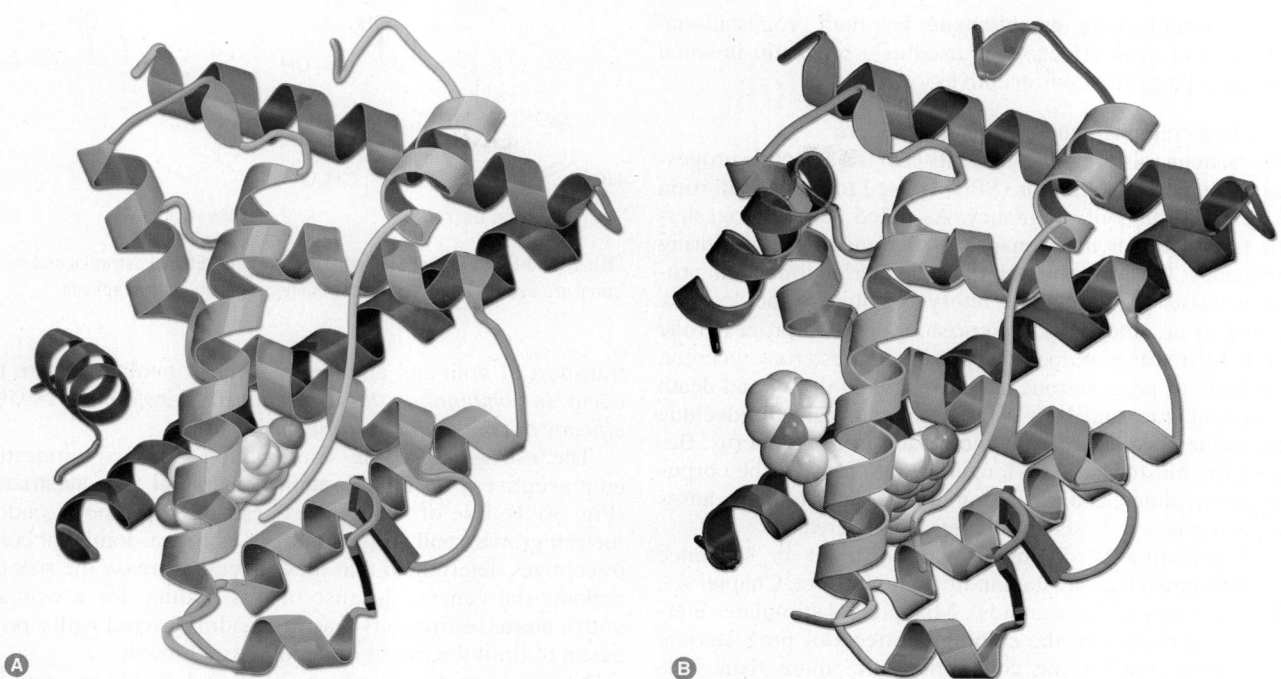

FIGURE 30-8. Structural comparison of estrogen (natural ligand) and raloxifene (SERM) bound to the estrogen receptor. The ligand-binding domain of the human estrogen receptor-alpha is displayed in ribbon format from the yellow-brown N-terminus to the dark blue C-terminus. The natural ligand 17β-estradiol (estrogen) and the selective estrogen receptor modulator (SERM) raloxifene are displayed in space-filling format. **A.** In the estrogen-bound structure, the position of the orange helix (H12) defines the agonist conformation of the receptor that recruits coactivators and thereby regulates transcription of estrogen-regulated genes (see Fig. 30-7). **B.** In the raloxifene-bound structure, the bulky side chain of raloxifene disrupts the agonist conformation of the receptor (note that helix H12 is substantially displaced); in this conformation, the receptor is capable of recruiting some coactivators but not others (see Fig. 30-7).

the progression of osteoporosis in postmenopausal women (discussed in more detail in Chapter 32). Raloxifene is approved for use in prevention of breast cancer and prevention and treatment of osteoporosis. In a large clinical trial comparing raloxifene and tamoxifen for prevention of breast cancer in women at high risk, both agents resulted in a 50% reduction in the development of invasive breast cancer. Tamoxifen treatment was associated with more cases of endometrial hyperplasia, endometrial cancer, cataracts, and deep vein thrombosis than raloxifene. However, tamoxifen also prevented more cases of noninvasive breast cancer than raloxifene.

Toremifene is an estrogen receptor antagonist in breast tissue. It is approved for treatment of metastatic breast cancer in postmenopausal women. **Bazedoxifene** is a unique SERM that blocks estrogen-induced proliferation of the endometrium. In menopausal women with a uterus, the combination of estrogen and bazedoxifene is approved for treatment of hot flashes. Bazedoxifene is also approved for prevention of postmenopausal osteoporosis. **Ospemifene** is an estrogen receptor agonist in vaginal tissue and it improves vulvovaginal atrophy in postmenopausal women. It is approved for treatment of moderate to severe pain with sexual relations in postmenopausal women.

Clomiphene is a SERM used to induce ovulation. *The drug acts as an estrogen receptor antagonist in the hypothalamus and anterior pituitary gland and as a partial agonist in the ovaries.* In women with PCOS, the antagonist activity of clomiphene in the hypothalamus and anterior pituitary gland results in relief of the negative feedback inhibition imposed by endogenous estrogen and, therefore, in the increased release

of GnRH and gonadotropins, respectively. The increased levels of FSH stimulate follicle growth, resulting in an estrogen trigger signal, an LH surge, and ovulation. The main adverse effect is that clomiphene can cause multiple follicles to grow, resulting in increased ovarian size. Unlike the administration of exogenous FSH (see Chapter 27), however, clomiphene use is seldom associated with the ovarian hyperstimulation syndrome. The aromatase inhibitor letrozole can also reduce the negative feedback of estrogen on the hypothalamus and pituitary and induce ovulation in women with PCOS. In obese women with PCOS, letrozole is more effective than clomiphene in inducing ovulation and pregnancy.

Androgen Receptor Antagonists

Androgen receptor antagonists competitively inhibit the binding of endogenous androgens to the androgen receptor. By this mechanism, receptor antagonists block the action of testosterone and dihydrotestosterone on their target tissues. The androgen receptor antagonists include **flutamide**, **bicalutamide**, **nilutamide**, and **enzalutamide**. These agents are approved only for the treatment of metastatic prostate cancer, but flutamide is also used therapeutically in the treatment of benign prostatic hyperplasia. **Spironolactone**, originally approved as an aldosterone receptor antagonist (see Chapter 21, Pharmacology of Volume Regulation), also has significant antagonist activity at the androgen receptor. Like other androgen receptor antagonists, spironolactone can be used as a competitive inhibitor of testosterone action. Ms. J was treated with spironolactone to antagonize the excessive androgen stimulation of her hair follicles and thus to ameliorate her hirsutism. A compound derived from spironolactone, **drospirenone**, has both progestational and antiandrogen effects. It is used as a progestin in some estrogen–progestin contraceptives.

Selective Progesterone Receptor Modulators

Mifepristone (also referred to as **RU-486**) is a selective progesterone receptor modulator (SPRM) used to induce abortion at up to 70 days of pregnancy. As noted above, progesterone is crucial for maintenance of the endometrium during pregnancy; the hormone stabilizes the uterine lining and promotes vessel growth and secretory activities of the decidua. Acting as an antagonist, mifepristone inhibits progesterone action by binding competitively to the progesterone receptor. Blockade of progesterone action results in decay and death of the decidua, and lack of nourishment from the decidua causes the blastocyst to die and detach from the uterus. Because the blastocyst is no longer secreting hCG, the corpus luteum involutes, and involution of the corpus luteum causes progesterone synthesis and secretion to decrease.

Mifepristone is commonly administered in sequence with **misoprostol**, a prostaglandin analogue (see Chapter 43, Pharmacology of Eicosanoids). Misoprostol stimulates uterine contractions, and the combined effects of progesterone antagonism and uterine contractions are more than 95% effective in terminating first-trimester pregnancy. Because mifepristone is administered as a single dose, adverse effects related to progesterone antagonism are rare. Instead, the main potential for complication lies in the subsequent abortion, which can result in excessive vaginal bleeding. In addition, co-administration of misoprostol can cause nausea and vomiting.

Ulipristal, a second SPRM, is approved for use in emergency contraception (see below). **Asoprisnil** is an investigational progesterone receptor modulator that does not cause abortion but inhibits the growth of tissues derived from the endometrium and myometrium. Preliminary studies indicate that ulipristal and asoprisnil may be effective in the treatment of endometriosis and uterine leiomyomata (fibroids). The differences in the tissue specificities of mifepristone, ulipristal, and asoprisnil are probably due to their differences in influencing the binding of transcription cofactors to the progesterone receptor complex.

Hormones and Hormone Analogues: Contraception

The development of safe, efficacious contraceptives for women has revolutionized sexual practices. The two classes of widely used oral contraceptives are **estrogen–progestin combinations** and **progestin-only contraception**. The development of male contraception is an active area of research; current approaches to this therapy are discussed briefly at the end of the section.

Combination Estrogen–Progestin Contraception

Combination estrogen–progestin contraception suppresses GnRH, LH, and FSH secretion and follicular development, thereby inhibiting ovulation. The combination of an estrogen and a progestin is the most potent known method to suppress GnRH, LH, and FSH secretion. Co-administration of estrogen and progestin may also inhibit pregnancy by a number of secondary mechanisms, including alterations in tubal peristalsis, endometrial receptivity, and cervical mucus secretions. The latter actions could together inhibit the proper

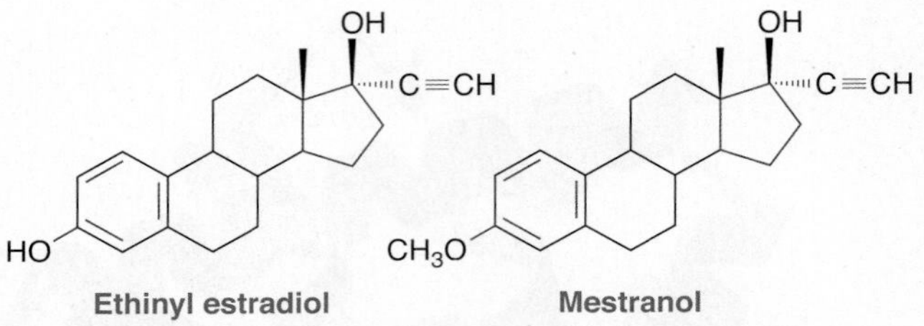

FIGURE 30-9. Structure of synthetic estrogens. Ethinyl estradiol and mestranol are used in combination estrogen–progestin contraceptives.

transport of both egg and sperm, even if ovulation were to occur. *In combination, these mechanisms explain the >95% efficacy of combination oral contraception.*

The estrogen used in combination estrogen–progestin contraceptives is either **ethinyl estradiol** or **mestranol** (Fig. 30-9). Use of "unopposed" estrogens promotes endometrial growth, and early studies of estrogen-dominant contraceptives determined that these agents increase the risk of endometrial cancer. Because of this finding, for a woman with a uterus, estrogen is always co-administered with a progestin to limit the extent of endometrial growth.

Numerous progestins (Figs. 30-10 and 30-11) are used in estrogen–progestin contraceptives, and all are potent progesterone receptor agonists. Ideally, the progestin would possess activity only at progesterone receptors, but almost all currently available progestins also have some androgenic cross-reactivity. Progestins vary in their androgenic activity. On a molar basis, **norgestrel** and **levonorgestrel** have the highest androgenic activity, while **norethindrone** and **norethindrone acetate** (Fig. 30-10) have lower androgenic activity. The so-called

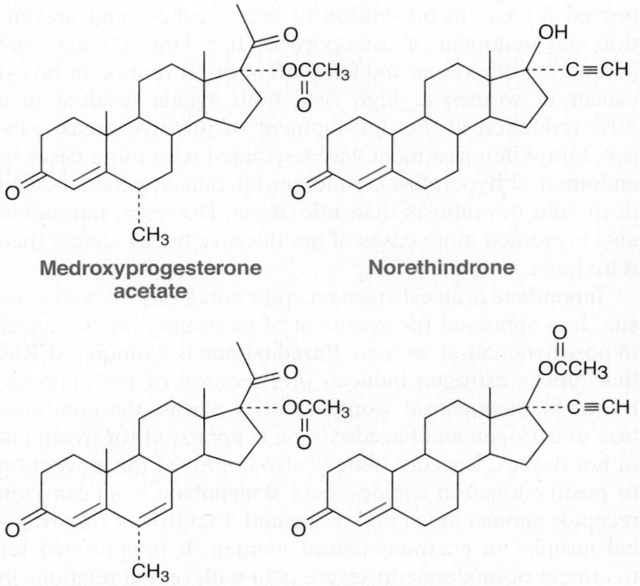

FIGURE 30-10. Structure of synthetic progestins. Medroxyprogesterone acetate is commonly combined with estrogen for hormone therapy in postmenopausal women. Megestrol acetate is often used as therapy for endometrial cancer. Norethindrone was the first progestin to be synthesized in quantities sufficient to mass-produce combination estrogen–progestin contraceptives. Norethindrone acetate is commonly used in contraceptives; it is metabolized to the parent compound, norethindrone.

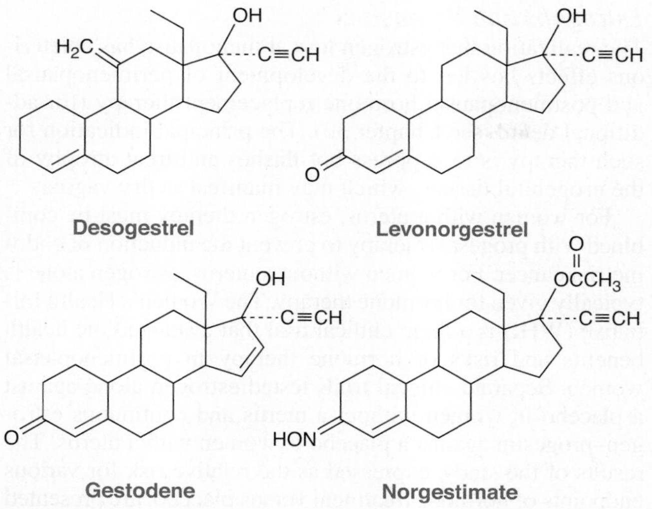

FIGURE 30-11. **Structure of progestins commonly used in oral contraceptives.** Levonorgestrel is the most androgenic of the commonly used progestins. Desogestrel, gestodene, and norgestimate are less androgenic than levonorgestrel.

third-generation progestins—**ethynodiol, norgestimate, gestodene,** and **desogestrel** (Fig. 30-11)—have even lower androgen receptor cross-reactivity. **Drospirenone** is a unique synthetic progestin that also has antiandrogenic activity.

Combination estrogen–progestin contraceptives are available in three delivery systems: a vaginal ring, transdermal patches, and oral tablets. The vaginal ring consists of a silastic cylinder packed with ethinyl estradiol and a progestin, **etonogestrel**. The steroids are released with zero-order kinetics (see Chapter 3, Pharmacokinetics). The ring is placed in the vagina and remains there for 21 days. It is then removed, and 7 days later, a new ring is placed. During the 7 days following removal of the ring, menses may ensue (see below). The contraceptive transdermal patch consists of a matrix that continually releases ethinyl estradiol and a synthetic progestin, **norelgestromin**. The patch is changed weekly for 3 weeks. During the fourth week, no patch is utilized and menses may occur.

Classical regimens of combination oral contraceptive tablets consist of 21 days of drugs followed by 7 days of a placebo pill. The 7-day placebo period removes exogenous hormone stimulation, causing the endometrium to slough and resulting in withdrawal bleeding. Because the administration of progestin throughout the cycle inhibits the proliferative growth of the endometrium, most women experience lighter menstrual periods when taking combination oral contraceptives, and a woman's menstrual cycle often becomes more regular. The 21-7 cycle formulation was meant to simulate a 28-day cycle but is relatively arbitrary. By combining pill packs, "long cycles" of 42 active hormone pills followed by 7 days off hormone pills, or 63 active hormone pills followed by 7 days off hormone pills, can easily be prescribed. "Long cycle" regimens reduce the frequency of menstrual bleeding but may increase the frequency of irregular, unscheduled bleeding—so-called breakthrough bleeding. An even longer cycle formulation of ethinyl estradiol and levonorgestrel is available, in which the drug combination is administered for 84 days followed by 7 days of placebo. This formulation has contraceptive efficacy equal to that of the classical regimen and reduces to four the total number of menstrual cycles

each year. Formulations containing 24 daily hormone pills and 4 days of placebo are also available. An advantage of this formulation is that ovulation is not as likely to occur if a woman forgets to start her new cycle of pills for 3 or 4 days.

Combination oral contraceptive formulations include monophasic and triphasic hormone schedules. The standard formulation, used by the majority of women, is a constant (monophasic) dose of estrogen and progestin for 21 days. Triphasic formulations incorporate a constant dose of estrogen with a dose of progestin that increases each week during the 21 days of the cycle. *The main advantage of triphasic administration is that the total amount of progestin administered over each month is reduced.* Indeed, the general trend in recent years has been to decrease the quantities of administered estrogen and progestin to the smallest amount necessary for inhibition of ovulation. However, there are no clearly established differences in either the adverse effects or the clinical efficacy of monophasic compared to triphasic therapy. In general, the lowest effective dose of ethinyl estradiol is preferred because low-dose estrogen is thought to minimize the risk of deep vein thrombosis (see below).

A number of studies have been performed to assess the adverse effects of long-term contraceptive use. These studies have shown that the incidence of **deep vein thrombosis** and the incidence of **pulmonary embolism** are increased with combination oral contraception. These complications occur infrequently, and the absolute number of adverse events is low. Interestingly, pregnancy is associated with a greater risk of deep vein thrombosis and pulmonary embolism than treatment with estrogen-containing contraceptives. Studies have failed to demonstrate any increase (or decrease) in breast cancer. Use of oral contraceptives is associated with an increase in **gallbladder disease** because estrogens increase the biliary concentration of cholesterol relative to that of bile salts, and the resulting decrease in cholesterol solubility promotes the formation of gallstones. *Oral contraceptives should not be administered to women over 35 who smoke, because the administration of contraceptives to this population is associated with an increase in thrombotic cardiovascular events.*

Recent studies have focused on the benefits rather than the adverse effects of oral contraception. Modern combination oral contraceptives *reduce* the risk of endometrial cancer, probably because constant administration of a progestin inhibits endometrial growth. In addition, exogenous administration of an estrogen–progestin combination reduces the risk of ovarian cancer, probably by lowering circulating levels of gonadotropins. *Overall, the consensus is that oral contraceptives have more beneficial than harmful medical effects.*

Progestin-Only Contraception

In situations where estrogen may be contraindicated, the use of continuous low-dose oral progestins may be warranted. The two progestin-only oral contraceptives available in the United States, commonly referred to as the *mini-pill*, are **norethindrone** and **desogestrel**.

Progestin-only oral contraception prevents ovulation 70–80% of the time, probably because progestins alter the frequency of GnRH pulsing and decrease anterior pituitary gland responsiveness to GnRH. Despite the relatively high frequency of ovulation, this form of contraception is 96–98% effective, suggesting that secondary mechanisms—such as alterations in cervical mucus, endometrial receptivity, and tubal peristalsis—are also at work. Because progesterone inhibits endometrial proliferation and promotes endometrial secretion, it may also be the case that an egg is unable to implant in an endometrium that is continually exposed to progestin. Patients taking these drugs do not typically menstruate, but breakthrough spotting and irregular, light menstrual periods commonly occur during the first year of administration.

Progestin-only contraceptives are also available as injectables and implants. **Medroxyprogesterone acetate** (formulated as 104 mg for subcutaneous injection or 150 mg for intramuscular injection) can be given parenterally every 3 months (Fig. 30-10). This dosage form is especially effective for women who have difficulty remembering to take a daily (pill) or weekly (patch) agent. A silastic implant is also available that releases **etonogestrel** and is effective for 3 years. The implant is typically inserted into the dorsal side of the forearm.

Emergency (Morning-After) Contraception

Emergency contraception refers to the administration of medications to prevent pregnancy after failure of a barrier contraceptive (condom breakage) or recent unprotected intercourse (including sexual assault). Both **levonorgestrel**, a potent progestin, and **ulipristal**, an SPRM, are approved as emergency contraceptives. Emergency hormonal contraception is most effective when administered within 120 hours of the exposure. Both levonorgestrel and ulipristal prevent pregnancy by interfering with ovulation.

Male Contraception

The goal of hormonal male contraception is to suppress endogenous production of sperm reversibly, generating a state of azoospermia (absence of sperm in the ejaculate) without suppressing libido or erectile function. Reliable inhibition of spermatogenesis is a difficult task, because even a 99% reduction in spermatogenesis could result in a sufficient number of viable sperm for fertilization. Initial studies of male contraception centered on the parenteral administration of testosterone esters such as testosterone enanthate or testosterone undecanoate. As an end product of the hypothalamic-pituitary-reproduction axis, testosterone significantly suppresses gonadotropin release. The reduced circulating levels of LH and FSH are unable to stimulate Sertoli cell function, and decreased spermatogenesis results. In a large-scale clinical trial, this approach produced a contraceptive failure rate of 1 per 100 man-years.

Recent clinical trials indicate that the administration of both an androgen and a progestin may be superior to an androgen alone in suppressing spermatogenesis because the combination more completely suppresses GnRH secretion and gonadotropin release. The following combinations have been demonstrated to be effective, reversible male contraceptives: parenteral **testosterone enanthate** plus daily oral levonorgestrel; parenteral **testosterone undecanoate** plus injectable medroxyprogesterone acetate; and transdermal administration of testosterone and a synthetic progestin, **Nestorone®**. The main difficulties with this approach have been the large population variability in the degree of spermatogenesis inhibition (on average, only 60% of men become azoospermic) and the significant adverse effects of acne, weight gain, polycythemia, and a potential increase in prostate size.

Hormones and Hormone Analogues: Replacement

Estrogens, progestins, and androgens are used as replacement therapies in cases of hormone deficiency.

Estrogens and Progestins

The realization that estrogen loss at menopause has deleterious effects has led to the development of perimenopausal and postmenopausal hormone replacement therapy (for additional detail, see Chapter 32). The principal indication for such therapy is to suppress hot flashes and treat atrophy of the urogenital tissues, which may manifest as dry vagina.

For women with a uterus, estrogen therapy must be combined with progestin therapy to prevent the induction of endometrial cancer. For women without a uterus, estrogen alone is typically given for hormone therapy. The Women's Health Initiative (WHI) is a large clinical trial that evaluated the health benefits and risks of hormone therapy in postmenopausal women. Separate clinical trials tested estrogen alone against a placebo in women without a uterus and continuous estrogen–progestin against a placebo in women with a uterus. The results of the study, expressed as the relative risk for various endpoints of hormone treatment versus placebo, are presented in Table 30-3. Estrogen treatment did not increase the risk of coronary heart disease or breast cancer, but it did increase the risk of stroke and it decreased the risk of osteoporotic fracture. Continuous estrogen–progestin treatment increased the risk of stroke, pulmonary embolism, and breast cancer, and it decreased the risk of osteoporotic fracture (see Chapter 32). Given the balance of risks and benefits, the current recommendation for postmenopausal women is to use hormone therapy only to treat bothersome symptoms such as vasomotor symptoms or vaginal dryness and to use the lowest possible dose of hormone therapy for the shortest period of time. After the results of the WHI trial were published in 2002, there was a marked decrease in the number of menopausal women using estrogen–progestin therapy and a parallel reduction in the number of cases of diagnosed breast cancer.

Many synthetic progestins are available for use in hormone therapy for menopausal women. Recent epidemiologic studies

TABLE 30-3 Summary of Findings from the Women's Health Initiative

	ESTROGEN ALONE VS. PLACEBO	CONTINUOUS ESTROGEN–PROGESTIN VS. PLACEBO
Sample size	10,739	16,608
Mean age of subjects	63 years old	63 years old
Mean duration of hormone use	6.8 years	5.2 years
Coronary heart disease	0.91 (0.75–1.12)	1.29 (1.02–1.63)
Breast cancer	0.77 (0.59–1.01)	1.26 (1.00–1.59)
Stroke	1.39 (1.10–1.77)	1.41 (1.07–1.85)
Pulmonary embolism	1.34 (0.87–2.06)	2.13 (1.39–3.25)
Osteoporotic hip fracture	0.61 (0.41–0.91)	0.67 (0.47–0.96)
Osteoporotic vertebral fracture	0.62 (0.42–0.93)	0.65 (0.46–0.92)

Data represent hazard ratios (95% confidence intervals) of various events during treatment with hormone therapy or placebo. Confidence intervals that cross the value of 1.00 are not statistically significant ($p > .05$).

report that micronized progesterone may be associated with a lower risk of breast cancer than other commonly used synthetic progestins such as medroxyprogesterone acetate. Micronization is a process in which the progesterone crystals are synthesized with a diameter in the nanometer range, thus facilitating their absorption when administered orally.

Like contraceptives, hormone therapy is available as oral tablets, transdermal patches, and vaginal rings and tablets. A vaginal ring that elutes estradiol at a controlled dose rate (see Chapter 55, Drug Delivery Modalities) provides local administration of estrogen and minimal systemic absorption of the drug. The vaginal ring is an effective therapy for postmenopausal vaginal dryness and atrophy.

Androgens

Androgen replacement is an effective therapy for hypogonadism. Oral testosterone is ineffective because of its high first-pass metabolism by the liver. Two esters of testosterone, **testosterone enanthate** and **testosterone cypionate**, can be administered intramuscularly. A preparation of either of these agents, injected every 2–4 weeks, increases plasma testosterone to physiologic concentrations in hypogonadal men. Transdermal **testosterone patches** have also been developed; this drug delivery system has the advantages that plasma testosterone levels remain relatively constant and first-pass hepatic metabolism is bypassed. Testosterone is also available in a topical gel formulation; using this preparation on a once-a-day application schedule, plasma testosterone levels gradually increase until they reach physiologic replacement levels after 1 month of application. Testosterone can also be administered as a tablet that adheres to the buccal mucosa, resulting in rapid systemic absorption of the drug.

Aging men sometimes develop symptoms and signs of hypogonadism, such as decreased energy, decreased libido, gynecomastia, decreased muscle mass, and facial hair growth. Recent guidelines recommend that androgen replacement therapy be offered to men only with consistent symptoms and signs of hypogonadism and low plasma testosterone levels (<3.0 ng/mL). Testosterone should not be administered to men with prostate cancer because it may stimulate growth of the tumor. A novel approach is to combine parenteral testosterone replacement with androgen receptor blockade using flutamide. The testosterone replacement stimulates an increase in muscle mass, even in the presence of androgen receptor blockade. However, flutamide does block prostate enlargement caused by testosterone replacement.

Some athletes abuse androgens by self-administration at supratherapeutic levels. Androgens have been demonstrated to increase muscle mass and fat-free mass. In one survey, approximately 5% of high school athletes reported that they had used androgen supplements. Almost every type of androgen has been abused in an attempt to enhance athletic performance, including the adrenal hormone precursors androstenedione and dehydroepiandrosterone. Covert laboratories are continuously inventing new synthetic androgens that have not yet been recognized by standard drug testing programs. These "designer" androgens are meant to enhance athletic performance and to be undetectable by sports regulatory authorities. Pharmacologic doses of androgens suppress the hypothalamic-pituitary-reproduction axis, resulting in suppression of testicular function, decreased sperm production, and impaired fertility. Because many androgens can be converted to estrogens by aromatase, pharmacologic doses of androgens can also cause an increase in plasma estrogen,

resulting in gynecomastia. In addition, high plasma levels of androgens are associated with erythrocytosis, severe acne, and derangements in lipid metabolism (increased low-density lipoprotein [LDL] and decreased high-density lipoprotein [HDL]). Some athletes have recently started to use injections of hCG to stimulate endogenous Leydig cell testosterone production, hoping to avoid detection by sports authorities. SERMs and aromatase inhibitors have also been used by athletes in an attempt to increase endogenous LH secretion and Leydig cell testosterone production.

CONCLUSION AND FUTURE DIRECTIONS

The male and female hormones of reproduction share significant mechanistic overlap with one another. Androgens, estrogens, and progestins are all steroid hormones that exert their physiologic action by binding to intracellular receptors, translocating to the nucleus, and altering gene transcription. Recent evidence suggests that estrogens may also act on membrane receptors to mediate nongenomic effects. Derangements in the physiologic effects of reproductive hormones can involve disruption of the hypothalamic-pituitary-reproduction axis, inappropriate growth of hormone-dependent tissue, or decreased activity of gonadal hormones at target tissues. Currently available pharmacologic agents can modify the endocrine axis (e.g., GnRH agonists), inhibit synthesis of active hormones (e.g., 5α-reductase inhibitors, aromatase inhibitors), or inhibit end-organ effects at the receptor level (e.g., SERMs, SPRMs, antiandrogens). Oral contraceptives, such as estrogen–progestin combinations and progestin-only contraception, disrupt the exquisite cyclicity of the menstrual cycle and thus suppress ovulation. The development of an effective male contraceptive has met a number of obstacles but should represent a major pharmacologic advance in the future. Exciting progress is also being made in the design of new SERMs that possess a variety of tissue-specific activities; such research may result in new agents effective for both prevention of breast cancer and treatment of postmenopausal osteoporosis.

Suggested Reading

Borst SE, Yarrow JG, Conover CF, et al. Musculoskeletal and prostate effects of combined testosterone and finasteride administration in older hypogonadal men: a randomized controlled trial. *Am J Physiol Endocrinol Metab* 2014;306:E433–E442. (*Example of combining testosterone and finasteride.*)

Legro RS, Arslanian SA, Ehrmann DA, et al. Diagnosis and treatment of polycystic ovary syndrome: an Endocrine Society clinical practice guideline. *J Clin Endocrinol Metab* 2013;98:4565–4592. (*Recent clinical recommendations regarding treatment of polycystic ovarian syndrome.*)

Legro RS, Brzyski RG, Diamond MP, et al. Letrozole versus clomiphene for infertility in the polycystic ovary syndrome. *N Engl J Med* 2014;371:119–129. (*Clinical trial that demonstrated improved fertility rates using letrozole among patients with polycystic ovarian syndrome.*)

Manson JE, Chlebowski RT, Stefanick ML, et al. Menopausal hormone therapy and health outcomes during the intervention and extended post-stopping phases of the Women's Health Initiative randomized trials. *JAMA* 2013;310:1353–1368. (*Integrated overview of long-term health benefits and risks with menopausal hormone therapy.*)

Pagani O, Regan MM, Walley BA, et al. Adjuvant exemestane with ovarian suppression in premenopausal breast cancer. *N Engl J Med* 2014;371:107–118. (*Clinical trial that demonstrated reduced rates of recurrent breast cancer with exemestane.*)

Winikoff B, Dzuba IG, Chong E, et al. Extending outpatient medical abortion services through 70 days of gestational age. *Obstet Gynecol* 2012;120:1070–1076. (*Clinical trial of medication pregnancy termination through day 70 of pregnancy.*)

DRUG SUMMARY TABLE: CHAPTER 30 Pharmacology of Reproduction

DRUG	CLINICAL APPLICATIONS	SERIOUS AND COMMON ADVERSE EFFECTS	CONTRAINDICATIONS	THERAPEUTIC CONSIDERATIONS
GONADOTROPIN-RELEASING HORMONE (GnRH) AGONISTS **Mechanism—Continuous: inhibit LH and FSH release; Pulsatile: stimulate LH and FSH release**				
Gonadorelin Goserelin Histrelin Leuprolide Nafarelin Buserelin Triptorelin	See Drug Summary Table: Chapter 27 Pharmacology of the Hypothalamus and Pituitary Gland			
GONADOTROPIN-RELEASING HORMONE (GnRH) ANTAGONISTS **Mechanism—GnRH receptor antagonists**				
Cetrorelix Ganirelix Degarelix	See Drug Summary Table: Chapter 27 Pharmacology of the Hypothalamus and Pituitary Gland			
INHIBITORS OF PERIPHERAL TESTOSTERONE CONVERSION TO DHT **Mechanism—Inhibit 5α-reductase, the enzyme that converts testosterone to dihydrotestosterone in prostate, liver, and skin. Finasteride is a selective inhibitor of type II 5α-reductase, whereas dutasteride inhibits both type I and type II 5α-reductase.**				
Finasteride Dutasteride	Benign prostatic hyperplasia (shared indication) Androgenic alopecia (finasteride only)	*Prostate cancer (shared adverse effect); immune hypersensitivity reaction, angioedema (dutasteride only)* Breast tenderness, decreased libido, erectile dysfunction, ejaculatory disorder	Shared contraindications: Hypersensitivity to drug Known or suspected pregnancy Dutasteride only: Use in women and children	Improve symptoms of decreased urine flow. Potential alternatives to transurethral resection of the prostate (TURP). One year of therapy can result in up to 25% reduction in prostate size. Finasteride is most effective for patients with large prostates. Women should not handle finasteride or dutasteride tablets.
INHIBITORS OF AROMATASE **Mechanism—Anastrozole and letrozole are competitive inhibitors of aromatase, the enzyme that catalyzes the formation of estrogens from androgen precursors. Exemestane and formestane are irreversible (covalent) inhibitors of aromatase.**				
Anastrozole Letrozole Exemestane Formestane	Treatment and prevention of estrogen receptor-positive early-stage, locally advanced, and metastatic breast cancer	*Thrombophlebitis, osteoporotic fractures (shared adverse effects); hepatitis (anastrozole and exemestane only); Stevens-Johnson syndrome, profuse vaginal bleeding, increased risk of neoplasm (anastrozole only); pancytopenia, pleural effusion (letrozole only)* Hypertension, peripheral edema, rash, gastrointestinal upset, arthralgia, bone pain, asthenia, insomnia, headache, depression, dyspnea (shared adverse effects); excessive sweating (letrozole only); alopecia (exemestane only)	Hypersensitivity to drug Pregnancy (anastrozole, letrozole, and exemestane only) Premenopausal women (exemestane only)	Aromatase inhibitors are used to treat estrogen-dependent tumors. Aromatase inhibitors may be more effective than estrogen receptor antagonists or SERMs for the treatment of breast cancer. Due to profound suppression of estrogen action, women taking aromatase inhibitors are at substantial risk for osteoporotic fractures.

SELECTIVE ESTROGEN RECEPTOR MODULATORS (SERMs)

Mechanism—Estrogen antagonist in some tissues and estrogen agonist in other tissues. The basis for tissue selectivity may be related to tissue-specific expression of estrogen receptor subtypes and the differential ability of the ligand–receptor complex to recruit transcriptional coactivators and corepressors.

Drug	Clinical Applications	Serious and Common Adverse Effects	Contraindications	Therapeutic Considerations
Tamoxifen	Prevention of breast cancer Palliative treatment of metastatic breast cancer Adjuvant therapy of breast cancer after primary excision of the tumor (lumpectomy)	*Stevens-Johnson syndrome, contralateral breast cancer, thromboembolic disorder, endometrial cancer, cataract, interstitial pneumonia* Hot flashes, abnormal menstruation, vaginal discharge	Hypersensitivity to tamoxifen History of deep vein thrombosis or pulmonary embolism if used for breast cancer prevention or ductal carcinoma in situ; in patients with invasive breast cancer, benefits of tamoxifen outweigh risks of recurrent thromboembolic disease Pregnancy	An estrogen receptor antagonist in breast tissue and a partial agonist in the endometrium and bone. Because tamoxifen stimulates endometrial growth, tamoxifen administration is associated with a fourfold to sixfold increase in the incidence of endometrial cancer. Usually administered for no more than 5 years in order to minimize the risk of iatrogenic endometrial cancer.
Raloxifene	See Drug Summary Table: Chapter 32 Pharmacology of Bone Mineral Homeostasis			
Bazedoxifene	Menopausal hot flashes Prevention of postmenopausal osteoporosis		None	Available in combination with conjugated equine estrogen. Bazedoxifene can replace progestins in hormone therapy. Bazedoxifene prevents estrogen-induced endometrial hyperplasia.
Ospemifene	Moderate to severe dyspareunia	*Thromboembolic disorder* Flushing, vaginal discharge	Arterial thromboembolic disease Estrogen-dependent neoplasia Genital bleeding Pregnancy	Oral SERM used to improve sexual function and reduce symptoms of vulvovaginal atrophy.
Clomiphene	Female infertility due to ovulatory disorder	*Pancreatitis, vision loss, psychotic disorder, hyperstimulation or hypertrophy of ovaries, ovarian cancer* Vasomotor symptoms, abdominal discomfort, headache, breast pain	Hypersensitivity to clomiphene Pregnancy Uncontrolled thyroid or adrenal dysfunction Liver disease Endometrial carcinoma Ovarian cysts Organic intracranial lesion Abnormal uterine bleeding	An estrogen receptor antagonist in hypothalamus and anterior pituitary gland and a partial agonist in ovaries; disinhibits GnRH release, leading to increased levels of LH and FSH; the increased FSH stimulates follicle growth, resulting in an estrogen trigger signal, an LH surge, and ovulation. Unlike exogenous FSH, clomiphene use is rarely associated with the ovarian hyperstimulation syndrome.

ESTROGEN RECEPTOR ANTAGONIST

Mechanism—Competitively inhibits estrogen binding to receptor, blocking the action of estrogen on target tissues

Drug	Clinical Applications	Serious and Common Adverse Effects	Contraindications	Therapeutic Considerations
Fulvestrant	Treatment of estrogen receptor-positive metastatic breast cancer in postmenopausal women with disease progression following anti-estrogen therapy	*Thromboembolic disorder, liver failure, hypersensitivity reaction, angioedema* Gastrointestinal upset, asthenia, bone pain, vasodilation (hot flashes), headache	Hypersensitivity to fulvestrant Pregnancy	A pure estrogen receptor antagonist with no agonist activity; binds with high affinity to estrogen receptor, preventing receptor dimerization and increasing receptor degradation; sometimes referred to as the first in a new class of selective estrogen receptor down-regulators (SERDs).

continues

DRUG SUMMARY TABLE: CHAPTER 30 Pharmacology of Reproduction *continued*

DRUG	CLINICAL APPLICATIONS	SERIOUS AND COMMON ADVERSE EFFECTS	CONTRAINDICATIONS	THERAPEUTIC CONSIDERATIONS
ANDROGEN RECEPTOR ANTAGONISTS Mechanism—Competitively inhibit dihydrotestosterone and testosterone binding to androgen receptor, blocking the action of testosterone and dihydrotestosterone on target tissues				
Flutamide Bicalutamide Nilutamide Enzalutamide	Metastatic prostate cancer (shared indication) Benign prostatic hyperplasia (finasteride only)	*Hepatotoxicity, disorders of the hematopoietic system, interstitial pneumonitis* Hot flash, diarrhea, nausea, rash (shared adverse effects); seizure (enzalutamide only)	Hypersensitivity to flutamide, bicalutamide, nilutamide, enzalutamide Severe hepatic impairment Use in women Pregnancy	Androgen receptor antagonists compare favorably to leuprolide monotherapy in the treatment of prostate cancer. Most effective when combined with medical or surgical castration.
Spironolactone	Hypertension Edema associated with heart failure, cirrhosis (with or without ascites), or nephrotic syndrome Hypokalemia Primary aldosteronism	*Stevens-Johnson syndrome, toxic epidermal necrolysis, hyperkalemic metabolic acidosis, gastrointestinal hemorrhage, agranulocytosis, systemic lupus erythematosus, breast cancer (not established)* Gynecomastia, gastrointestinal upset, somnolence, abnormal menstruation, impotence	Anuria Hyperkalemia Acute renal insufficiency Concomitant eplerenone use	An aldosterone receptor antagonist that also has significant antagonist activity at the androgen receptor. Used as a competitive inhibitor of testosterone and dihydrotestosterone binding to androgen receptors. Drospirenone (derived from spironolactone) has both progestational and antiandrogen effects; it is used as a progestin in some estrogen–progestin contraceptives.
SELECTIVE PROGESTERONE RECEPTOR MODULATORS Mechanism—Inhibit progesterone binding to receptor; the differences in the tissue specificity of mifepristone, ulipristal, and asoprisnil are likely due to their differences in influencing the binding of transcriptional coactivators and corepressors to the progesterone receptor complex				
Mifepristone (RU-486)	Abortion (through day 70 of pregnancy) Cushing's disease	*Prolonged QT interval, anemia, life-threatening infection* Hypertension, peripheral edema, hypokalemia, gastrointestinal upset, abnormal vaginal bleeding, headache, dizziness, uterine cramping, endometrial hypertrophy, fatigue	Hypersensitivity to mifepristone, misoprostol, or prostaglandins Chronic adrenal failure Ectopic pregnancy Hemorrhagic disorders Anticoagulation therapy Inherited porphyrias Intrauterine device Undiagnosed adnexal mass Corticosteroid therapy Endometrial hyperplasia or endometrial carcinoma	Mifepristone (RU-486) is a progesterone receptor antagonist used to induce abortion. Blockade of progesterone action results in decay and death of the decidua, and lack of nourishment from the decidua causes the blastocyst to die and detach from the uterus. Mifepristone is commonly administered in sequence with misoprostol, a prostaglandin analogue that stimulates uterine contractions; co-administration of misoprostol can cause nausea and vomiting. In 2000, the FDA approved a 49-day gestational limit for mifepristone-misoprostol medication pregnancy termination. Since 2000, evidence has accumulated to support the use of these medications to terminate pregnancy through 70 days of gestational age. At higher concentrations, mifepristone also blocks the glucocorticoid receptor, which makes it potentially useful for treating conditions associated with life-threatening elevated glucocorticoid levels, such as the ectopic ACTH syndrome.
Ulipristal	Emergency contraception	Headache, abdominal pain, nausea, dysmenorrhea, fatigue, dizziness	Known or suspected pregnancy	Prevents pregnancy by interfering with ovulation. Emergency hormonal contraception is most effective when administered within 120 hours of the exposure.

| Asoprisnil | Investigational agent for the treatment of endometriosis and uterine leiomyomata (fibroids) | Under investigation | Under investigation | A progesterone receptor antagonist that inhibits the growth of tissues derived from the endometrium and myometrium; preliminary studies indicate that asoprisnil may be effective in the treatment of endometriosis and uterine leiomyomata (fibroids). |

COMBINATION ESTROGEN–PROGESTIN CONTRACEPTION

Mechanism—Suppress GnRH, LH, and FSH secretion and follicular development, thereby inhibiting ovulation; secondary mechanisms of pregnancy prevention include alterations in tubal peristalsis, endometrial receptivity, and cervical mucus secretions, which together prevent the proper transport of both egg and sperm

Drug	Indication	Adverse effects	Contraindications	Therapeutic considerations
Estrogens: Ethinyl estradiol Mestranol *Progestins:* Norgestrel Levonorgestrel Norethindrone Norethindrone acetate Ethynodiol Norgestimate Gestodene Desogestrel Drospirenone	Contraception (shared indication) Dysfunctional uterine bleeding (levonorgestrel and norethindrone acetate only) Endometriosis (norethindrone acetate only)	*Thromboembolic disorder, gallbladder disease, hypertension, increased risk of neoplasm (shared adverse effects); ectopic pregnancy (levonorgestrel and norethindrone only); pelvic inflammatory disease, uterine perforation (levonorgestrel only); optic neuritis (norethindrone acetate only)* Abnormal menstruation, breakthrough bleeding, breast tenderness, bloating symptoms, migraine, weight change	Shared contraindications: Hypersensitivity to drug Breast cancer Endometrial cancer or other estrogen-dependent neoplasms Cerebral vascular or coronary artery disease Cholestatic jaundice of pregnancy or jaundice with prior hormonal contraceptive use Benign or malignant liver tumors Severe hypertension Prolonged immobilization Pregnancy Female smokers over 35 years of age Thrombotic disorders Levonorgestrel only: Cervicitis, vaginitis, or pelvic inflammatory disease	Because unopposed estrogen increases the risk of endometrial cancer, estrogen is always co-administered with a progestin in women with a uterus. Progestins vary in their androgenic activity. Norgestrel and levonorgestrel have the highest androgenic activity; norethindrone and norethindrone acetate have moderate androgenic activity; ethynodiol, norgestimate, gestodene, and desogestrel have low androgen receptor cross-reactivity; drospirenone is a synthetic progestin that also has antiandrogenic activity. Combination estrogen–progestin contraceptives are available in oral tablets, a vaginal ring, and transdermal patches. Triphasic oral formulations have lower total amounts of progestin each month. The lowest effective dose of ethinyl estradiol is preferred to reduce the risk of deep vein thrombosis. Levonorgestrel is also used for emergency (morning-after) contraception.

PROGESTIN-ONLY CONTRACEPTIVES

Mechanism—Alter frequency of GnRH pulsing and decrease anterior pituitary gland responsiveness to GnRH; secondary mechanisms of pregnancy prevention include alterations in tubal peristalsis, endometrial receptivity, and cervical mucus secretions, which together prevent the proper transport of both egg and sperm

Drug	Indication	Adverse effects	Contraindications	Therapeutic considerations
Desogestrel Norethindrone Medroxyprogesterone acetate (injectable) Etonogestrel (silastic implant)	Contraception (shared indication) Abnormal uterine bleeding (medroxyprogesterone acetate only) Hormone therapy (medroxyprogesterone acetate only)	*Ectopic pregnancy, anaphylaxis, decreased bone mineral density, thromboembolic disorder* Irregular periods, breast tenderness, nausea, dizziness, headache (shared adverse effects); weight gain (medroxyprogesterone acetate only)	Shared contraindications: Hypersensitivity to drug Acute liver disease Benign or malignant liver tumors Known or suspected breast cancer Pregnancy Undiagnosed genital bleeding Medroxyprogesterone acetate and etonogestrel only: Thromboembolic disorders	Breakthrough spotting and irregular, light menstrual periods commonly occur during the first year of administration. Medroxyprogesterone acetate can be given parenterally every 3 months. A silastic implant that releases etonogestrel is effective for 3 years.

continues

DRUG SUMMARY TABLE: CHAPTER 30 Pharmacology of Reproduction *continued*

ANDROGENS USED FOR HORMONE REPLACEMENT

Mechanism—Replacement of testosterone to produce androgenic effects, including growth and maturation of the prostate, seminal vesicles, penis, and scrotum; development of male hair distribution; laryngeal enlargement; vocal cord thickening; and alterations in body musculature and fat distribution

DRUG	CLINICAL APPLICATIONS	SERIOUS AND COMMON ADVERSE EFFECTS	CONTRAINDICATIONS	THERAPEUTIC CONSIDERATIONS
Testosterone enanthate **Testosterone cypionate** **Testosterone transdermal gel or patch**	Hypogonadism Delayed puberty Metastatic breast cancer	*Increased risk of neoplasm, cholestatic jaundice syndrome, benign prostatic hyperplasia, thromboembolic disorder, peliosis hepatis, erythrocytosis* Amenorrhea, virilization, acne, gynecomastia, oral irritation with buccal delivery, skin irritation with transdermal delivery, headache, sense of smell alteration, upper respiratory infection	Hypersensitivity to drug Breast cancer in men Prostate cancer Cardiac, hepatic, or renal disease Use in women Pregnancy	Various delivery routes have been developed for testosterone replacement therapies; testosterone replacement can be administered intramuscularly, transdermally, and via topical gel formulation; the transdermal delivery system has the advantages that plasma testosterone levels remain relatively constant and first-pass hepatic metabolism is bypassed; testosterone can also be administered as a tablet that adheres to the buccal mucosa. Androgen replacement therapy should be offered to men only with consistent symptoms and signs of hypogonadism and low plasma testosterone levels (<3.0 ng/mL); testosterone should not be administered to men with prostate cancer. Some athletes abuse androgens by self-administration at supratherapeutic levels.

Pharmacology of the Endocrine Pancreas and Glucose Homeostasis

31

Giulio R. Romeo and Steven E. Shoelson

INTRODUCTION

This chapter reviews the physiology and pharmacology of insulin, glucagon, and the other major hormones that regulate glucose homeostasis. Diabetes mellitus is clinically the most common disease of these endocrine axes, and the majority of the chapter is devoted to the physiology and pharmacology of insulin. Type 1 diabetes mellitus is caused by an absolute deficiency of insulin secretion, and type 2 diabetes mellitus is caused by insufficient (or dysfunctional) insulin secretion to overcome insulin resistance in target tissues. Medical students may be interested to note that Charles Best, a fourth-year medical student in Canada, had a significant role in the identification of insulin. Along with his mentor, Frederick Banting, Best isolated a pancreatic extract from dogs that could reduce blood glucose in diabetic dogs and humans. Although the 1923 Nobel Prize in Medicine or Physiology was jointly awarded to surgeon Frederick Banting and physiologist J. J. R. MacLeod, Banting shared his award with Best.

BIOCHEMISTRY AND PHYSIOLOGY

Pancreatic Anatomy

The pancreas is a glandular organ that contains both exocrine and endocrine tissue. The exocrine portion—which constitutes 99% of the pancreatic mass—secretes bicarbonate and digestive enzymes into the gastrointestinal (GI) tract. Scattered within the exocrine tissue are nearly one million small islands of endocrine tissue that secrete hormones directly into the blood. These tiny endocrine glands, collectively called **islets of Langerhans**, include several different cell types that secrete different hormones: **α-cells** release **glucagon**; **β-cells** release **insulin** and **amylin**; **δ-cells** release **somatostatin** and gastrin; and PP cells release pancreatic polypeptide.

Energy Homeostasis

The storage and subsequent release of nutrients provides a homeostatic mechanism for sustained cellular nutrition in the absence of continuous feeding. Multiple hormones are

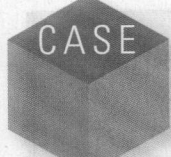

CASE

At her annual check-up, 55-year-old Mrs. S complains of fatigue and frequent urination (polyuria), even at night. She also reports drinking large volumes of fluids (polydipsia) to quench her thirst. These symptoms have worsened during the past 2 years and correlate with a 15-lb weight gain over the same period. Her current body mass index (BMI; the weight in kilograms divided by the square of the height in meters) is 32, thus meeting criteria for class I obesity. She is "frustrated" by her ineffectiveness to curb portion sizes and maintain a routine of physical activity. She denies other urinary symptoms; her kidney function is essentially normal. Her past medical history is remarkable for hyperlipidemia for the past 10 years. Both of her parents died of coronary heart disease in their early 60s.

On physical examination, Mrs. S is moderately obese but otherwise appears normal. Glucose is detected in her urine, but proteins and ketones are not. Her blood tests are significant for elevated glucose (210 mg/dL), total cholesterol (340 mg/dL), and HbA1c (a measure of glucose covalently bound to hemoglobin; 8.2%) levels. The physician explains to Mrs. S that she most likely has type 2 diabetes mellitus. In this disease, the body fails to respond normally to insulin (insulin resistance) and cannot produce a sufficient amount of insulin to overcome this resistance.

The physician discusses that lifestyle interventions (adhering to a balanced diet with controlled total calorie intake as well as increasing her exercise) are the cornerstone of diabetes treatment. The physician also discusses the benefits and risks of antidiabetic medications and prescribes metformin (a biguanide) for her diabetes.

Questions

1. What are the cellular and molecular actions of insulin?
2. What is the etiology of diabetes mellitus, and how is type 1 diabetes mellitus different from type 2 diabetes mellitus?
3. In addition to alleviating her polyuria and polydipsia, why is it important to control Mrs. S's diabetes (i.e., what acute and chronic complications could arise)?
4. What do the blood glucose and HbA1c levels indicate about Mrs. S's diabetes? Are there circumstances under which one parameter could be elevated and the other could be normal?
5. What are the effects of antidiabetic medications on body weight? Why might Mrs. S's physician have chosen metformin to treat her diabetes?

involved in controlling the uptake, utilization, storage, and release of nutrients. Insulin promotes the uptake and storage of glucose and other small, energy-containing molecules. The **"counterregulatory" hormones** oppose the actions of insulin and promote glucose release (Table 31-1). These hormones include (1) glucagon from islet α-cells, (2) the catecholamines norepinephrine and epinephrine from the sympathetic nervous system and adrenal medulla, (3) the glucocorticoid cortisol from the adrenal cortex, and (4) growth hormone from the pituitary gland. **Glucagon-like peptide-1 (GLP-1)** from the GI tract enhances insulin release in response to an ingested meal, while amylin suppresses endogenous production of glucose in the liver.

Blood glucose is easily measured and provides an accurate guide to the current balance of insulin and the counterregulatory hormones. This balance normally keeps blood glucose levels within a narrow range (70–120 mg/dL) regardless of recent food intake. Blood glucose excursions are much greater in patients with diabetes, potentially rising higher than 400 mg/dL in instances of poor control. The drugs used to treat diabetes, particularly insulin and the insulin secretagogues (sulfonylureas and glinides), may reduce blood glucose values below the normal range of 70 mg/dL. Severe hypoglycemia, which is defined by the patient requiring assistance to administer glucose or glucagon to restore normal blood glucose levels, is dangerous because organs—particularly the brain—depend on a constant supply of glucose for proper functioning. Conversely, chronic hyperglycemia is toxic to many cells and tissues.

Energy Repletion and the Fed State

After a meal, complex carbohydrates are broken down to monosaccharides (e.g., glucose, galactose, and fructose) in the lumen of the GI tract and transported into GI epithelial cells by a combination of active and passive apical membrane transporters. Sugars are then transported by basal membrane transporters from the epithelial cell cytosol to intercellular spaces, from which the sugars continue into the bloodstream. Elevated glucose in the blood is the signal for pancreatic β-cells to release insulin, which enters the portal vein. The liver, therefore, receives the highest concentrations of insulin concurrently with the nutrients absorbed from the digestive tract. *The liver and the other energy-storing tissues, such as skeletal muscle and adipose tissue, are the primary target tissues for insulin* (Fig. 31-1). Insulin also acts on pancreatic α-cells to suppress the secretion of glucagon.

The hormone **leptin** is not directly involved in nutrient regulation, but it plays an important role in the neuroendocrine response to energy storage and long-term energy balance. Leptin is secreted by adipocytes and detected by receptors in the hypothalamus. Its concentration in the plasma is proportional to total fat mass. *Thus, leptin signals from the periphery to the central nervous system that energy stores (in the form of adipose tissue) are replete.* Leptin also suppresses appetite, which switches the body from an energy-accumulating state to a state of energy utilization. This allows growth and reproduction to be switched on, whereas the lack of leptin, as occurs in prolonged starvation, results in persistently increased appetite and suppression of energy-utilizing functions.

TABLE 31-1 Effects of Selected Hormones on Energy Homeostasis

HORMONE	SOURCE	TARGET TISSUES	ACTION
Glucagon	α-Cell (pancreas)	Liver (adipose, skeletal muscle)	Promotes glycogenolysis and gluconeogenesis in liver
Insulin	β-Cell (pancreas)	Liver (adipose, skeletal muscle)	Promotes uptake of glucose, amino acids, and fatty acids from blood into cells for storage as glycogen, protein, and triglyceride
Amylin	β-Cell (pancreas)	Central nervous system	Suppresses glucagon release Slows gastric emptying Decreases food intake
Somatostatin	δ-Cell (pancreas) GI tract Hypothalamus	Other islet cells, GI tract, brain, and pituitary gland	Decreases release of insulin and glucagon Decreases GI tract motility and hormone release Decreases growth hormone secretion
Epinephrine	Adrenal medulla	Many	Promotes glycogenolysis in liver Lipolytic via activation of hormone-sensitive lipase
Cortisol	Adrenal cortex	Many	Antagonizes insulin action at target tissues Promotes gluconeogenesis in liver, protein breakdown in muscle
GLP-1	Ileum	Endocrine pancreas, stomach, brain, heart	Increases β-cell mass and insulin secretion Delays gastric emptying Decreases food intake and glucagon secretion
Leptin	Adipocytes	CNS (basomedial hypothalamus)	Signals adequacy of body energy stores Decreases food intake Permits energy-intensive neuroendocrine functions

Physiologically, insulin and glucagon are the two most important hormones controlling glucose homeostasis. Insulin promotes energy storage in target tissues. Glucagon, epinephrine, cortisol, and growth hormone—the "counterregulatory" hormones—act to raise blood glucose and thereby to counteract the effects of insulin. By acting as a "fat sensor," leptin signals total-body energy storage and regulates long-term energy balance. GI, gastrointestinal. GLP-1, glucagon-like peptide-1.

A key intracellular mediator of energy storage is the nuclear receptor **peroxisome proliferator-activated receptor-γ (PPARγ)**. PPARγ is a transcription factor that has roles in both adipose cell differentiation and lipid metabolism. PPARγ activation decreases serum free fatty acid levels and increases lipogenesis in adipose tissue, which increases the storage of fatty acids in adipose tissue. This allows other tissues—such as the liver—to lower their fat content, lower their glucose production, and increase their insulin sensitivity. PPARγ is the target for the thiazolidinedione (TZD) class of diabetes drugs.

Like many small hydrophilic molecules, glucose is freely filtered at the glomerulus but is normally reabsorbed almost completely by the sodium-glucose co-transporter 2 (SGLT-2) in the proximal convoluted tubule. Therefore, the glucose content of the urine is normally negligible. However, the transport maximum (T_{max}) for SGLT-2 is reached at glucose concentrations of 180–200 mg/dL, so, in diabetes, when blood glucose levels are over 200 mg/dL and SGLT-2 is saturated, glucose does appear in the urine. (Urinary glucose "dipsticks" were used by patients with diabetes to monitor glycemic control long before "finger stick" measures of blood glucose came into use.) The principle of losing glucose in the urine has been capitalized on with the development of selective inhibitors of SGLT-2, which cause enough glucose to remain in the urine that blood glucose levels, HbA1c levels, and even body weight are lowered.

Fasting and Starvation
As the blood glucose concentration decreases, pancreatic α-cells release increasing amounts of glucagon and pancreatic

β-cells secrete decreasing amounts of insulin. In contrast to insulin, which promotes the cellular uptake of glucose in the fed state, glucagon mobilizes glucose from the liver by stimulating gluconeogenesis and glycogenolysis. As fasting continues, catecholamine and glucocorticoid levels also increase, promoting the release of fatty acids from adipose tissue and the breakdown of protein to amino acids in muscle.

In low-energy (low adenosine triphosphate [ATP]) states, the enzyme **adenosine 5′-monophosphate-activated protein kinase (AMPK)** also triggers a shift from anabolic to catabolic activities. AMPK is present in tissues throughout the body, and it helps to regulate energy metabolism at both the cellular and organismal levels. Exercise activates AMPK, which increases muscle uptake of glucose. Activated AMPK also decreases glucose production and the synthesis of lipids and proteins by the liver. The pharmacologic effects of metformin and other biguanides are incompletely understood despite intense investigation but are contributed to by both AMPK-dependent and AMPK-independent mechanisms.

Insulin

Biochemistry
Insulin is a 51-amino acid protein composed of two peptide chains that are linked by two disulfide bridges. Its name comes from the Latin *insula* (meaning "island," after the islets of Langerhans). The human pancreas contains approximately 8 mg of insulin, of which 0.5 to 1.0 mg is secreted and replenished daily. Insulin is initially synthesized in pancreatic β-cells as preproinsulin, which is processed first to proinsulin and then insulin and free connecting (C) peptide (Fig. 31-2).

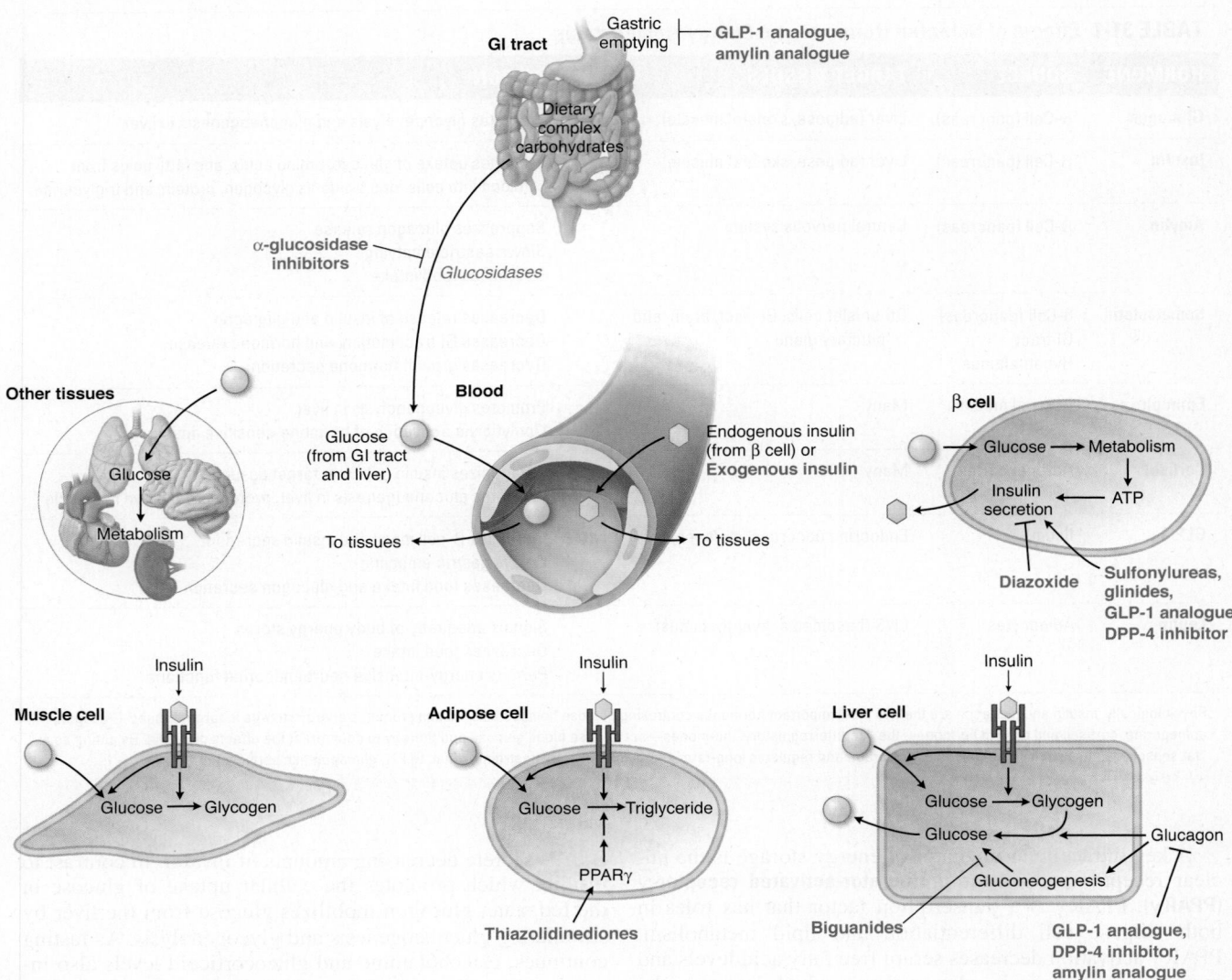

FIGURE 31-1. Physiologic and pharmacologic regulation of glucose homeostasis. Dietary complex carbohydrates are broken down to simple sugars in the GI tract by the action of glucosidases; simple sugars are then absorbed by GI epithelial cells and transported into the blood. Glucose in the blood is taken up by metabolically active tissues throughout the body. Glucose metabolism in pancreatic β-cells increases cytosolic ATP, which stimulates insulin secretion. Released insulin acts on plasma membrane insulin receptors in target tissues (muscle, adipose, liver) to increase glucose uptake and storage as glycogen or triglyceride. Glucose is also taken up by other cells and tissues to fuel metabolism. In muscle and liver, insulin promotes glucose storage as glycogen. In adipose cells, insulin promotes glucose conversion to triglycerides. Peroxisome proliferator-activated receptor γ (PPARγ) also promotes the conversion of glucose to triglycerides in adipocytes. Glucagon promotes both hepatic gluconeogenesis and glycogen breakdown; the newly generated glucose is transported out of the liver cell into the blood. Note that glucose from dietary complex carbohydrates and insulin secreted by pancreatic β-cells both enter the liver in high concentrations through the portal circulation (*not shown*). Pharmacologic interventions that decrease blood glucose levels include delaying gastric emptying with a GLP-1 analogue or an amylin analogue; inhibiting intestinal α-glucosidases with an α-glucosidase inhibitor; administering exogenous insulin; augmenting β-cell insulin secretion with sulfonylureas (SFUs), glinides, or incretins; suppressing glucagon and gluconeogenesis with incretins, an amylin analogue, or biguanides; and enhancing the action of insulin in adipose cells with thiazolidinediones. To treat hyperinsulinemic hypoglycemia, diazoxide inhibits pancreatic β-cell insulin secretion.

Secretion

Resting pancreatic β-cells are poised to secrete insulin, which is preformed and stored in secretory vesicles at the plasma membrane. The low basal rate of insulin secretion is increased dramatically upon exposure of β-cells to glucose.

Glucose enters β-cells via **GLUT2**, a specific plasma membrane transporter. As blood glucose rises (e.g., after feeding), more enters the cell, where it is phosphorylated to glucose-6-phosphate and enters the glycolytic pathway and the citric acid cycle. ATP is produced and ADP consumed by these processes, and the ATP/ADP ratio in the β-cell rises.

This modulates the activity of a membrane-spanning **ATP-sensitive K$^+$ channel (K$^+$/ATP channel)**. *When open, the K$^+$/ATP channel hyperpolarizes the cell by allowing an outward flux of K$^+$, and insulin release is inhibited. When closed, the cell depolarizes and insulin is released.* Because ATP inhibits the channel and ADP activates the channel, a high intracellular ATP/ADP ratio closes the K$^+$/ATP channel. Depolarization of the β-cell activates voltage-gated Ca^{2+} channels to promote the influx of extracellular Ca^{2+} and the fusion of insulin-containing vesicles with the plasma membrane, which increases insulin release into the circulation (Fig. 31-3).

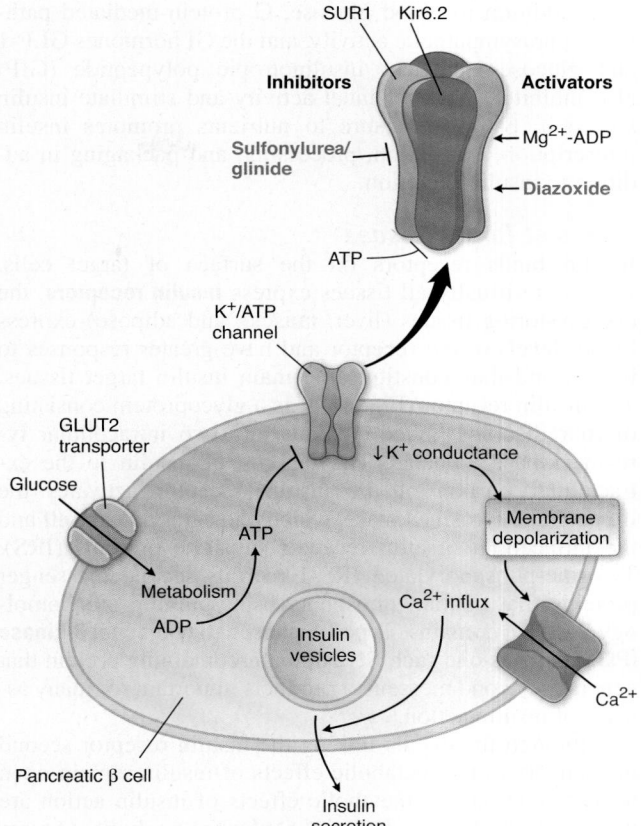

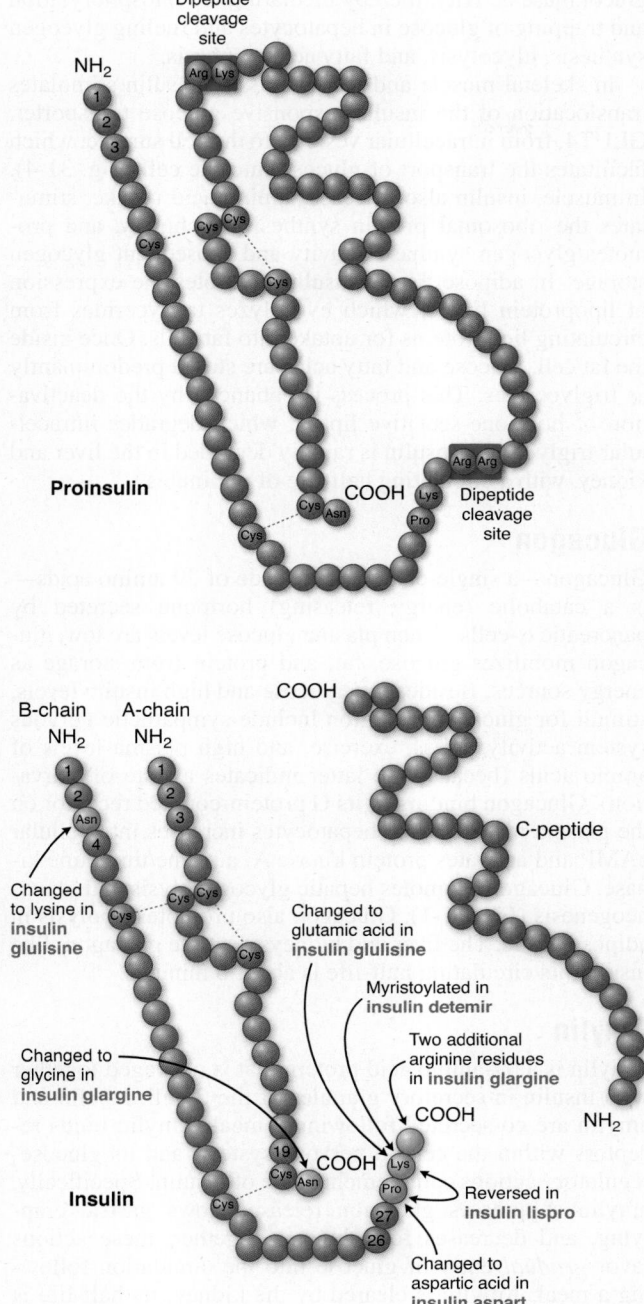

FIGURE 31-2. Processing of human insulin. Preproinsulin is synthesized and exported into the endoplasmic reticulum, where the signal peptide (*not shown*) is cleaved to generate proinsulin **(top panel)**. Intramolecular disulfide bonds (cys–cys) aid in the proper folding of proinsulin. Proinsulin is transported to secretory vesicles, where prohormone convertases act on dipeptide cleavage sites in proinsulin (*boxes*) to generate insulin and connecting (C) peptide. Two disulfide bonds aid in holding the A chain and B chain of insulin together. Insulin and C peptide are secreted together from the pancreatic β-cell **(bottom panel)**. Modifications to insulin's amino acid sequence result in the altered pharmacokinetics of the various insulin analogues; lispro, aspart, and glulisine are rapid-acting insulins, whereas glargine and detemir have slower absorption. The substitutions are: in lispro, the positions of ProB28 and LysB29 are reversed; in aspart, ProB28 is replaced by aspartic acid; in glulisine, AsnB3 and LysB29 are replaced by lysine and glutamic acid, respectively; in glargine, AsnA21 is replaced by glycine, and two additional arginines are added to the carboxyl terminus of the B-chain; and in detemir, a fatty acid (myristic acid) is esterified to the ε-amino group of LysB29.

FIGURE 31-3. Physiologic and pharmacologic regulation of insulin release from pancreatic β-cells. *When the K^+/ATP channel is open in its basal state, less insulin is released; when the K^+/ATP channel is closed, more insulin is released.* In the basal state, the plasma membrane of the β-cell is hyperpolarized, and the rate of insulin secretion from the cell is low. However, when glucose is available, it enters the cell via GLUT2 transporters in the plasma membrane and is metabolized to generate intracellular ATP. ATP binds to and inhibits the plasma membrane K^+/ATP channel. Inhibition of the K^+/ATP channel decreases plasma membrane K^+ conductance; the resulting depolarization of the membrane activates voltage-gated Ca^{2+} channels and thereby stimulates an influx of Ca^{2+}. Ca^{2+} mediates fusion of insulin-containing secretory vesicles with the plasma membrane, leading to insulin secretion. The K^+/ATP channel, an octamer composed of Kir6.2 and SUR1 subunits, is the target of several physiologic and pharmacologic regulators. ATP binds to and inhibits Kir6.2, while sulfonylureas (SFUs) and glinides bind to and inhibit SUR1; all three of these substances promote insulin secretion. The GLP-1 mimetic exenatide, acting as an agonist at G protein-coupled GLP-1 receptors in the plasma membrane of the pancreatic β-cell, also stimulates glucose-dependent insulin secretion. This action of exenatide appears to be mediated by an increase in intracellular cyclic AMP and may involve an indirect effect on the K^+/ATP channel (*not shown*). Mg^{2+}-ADP and diazoxide bind to and activate SUR1, thereby inhibiting insulin secretion. (For clarity, only four of the eight K^+/ATP channel subunits are shown.)

β-cell K^+/ATP channels are octameric structures containing four subunits of Kir6.2 and four subunits of the sulfonylurea receptor, SUR1. The Kir6.2 tetramer forms the pore of the K^+/ATP channel, while the associated SUR1 proteins regulate the channel's sensitivity to ADP and pharmacologic agents, including sulfonylurea and related insulin secretagogue drugs. Mutations in Kir6.2 or SUR1 can result in hyperinsulinemic hypoglycemia because the channel remains closed and the β-cell remains continually depolarized even when the extracellular glucose concentration and the intracellular ATP/ADP ratio are low.

In addition to blood glucose, G protein-mediated pathways, parasympathetic activity, and the GI hormones GLP-1 and glucose-dependent insulinotropic polypeptide (GIP) also inhibit K^+/ATP channel activity and stimulate insulin secretion. β-Cell exposure to nutrients promotes insulin transcription, translation, processing, and packaging in addition to insulin secretion.

Action at Target Tissues

Insulin binds receptors on the surface of target cells. Although virtually all tissues express **insulin receptors**, the energy-storing tissues (liver, muscle, and adipose) express higher levels of the receptor and have greater responses to insulin and thus constitute the main insulin target tissues. The insulin receptor (Fig. 31-4) is a glycoprotein consisting of four disulfide-linked subunits and two intracellular tyrosine kinase domains. The binding of insulin to the extracellular portion of the insulin receptor activates the intracellular tyrosine kinase, which phosphorylates itself and the intracellular insulin receptor substrate proteins (IRS). Tyrosine-phosphorylated IRS-1 recruits second messenger proteins that contain phosphotyrosine-binding src homology 2 (SH2) domains. Type IA **phosphatidylinositol 3-kinase (PI3-kinase)** is one such SH2 domain-containing protein that generates second messenger products important for many aspects of insulin action.

Although the details linking the insulin receptor second messengers to the metabolic effects of insulin remain open to investigation, the metabolic effects of insulin action are well understood: *insulin is the classic anabolic (energy storing) hormone* (Fig. 31-1). In the liver, insulin increases

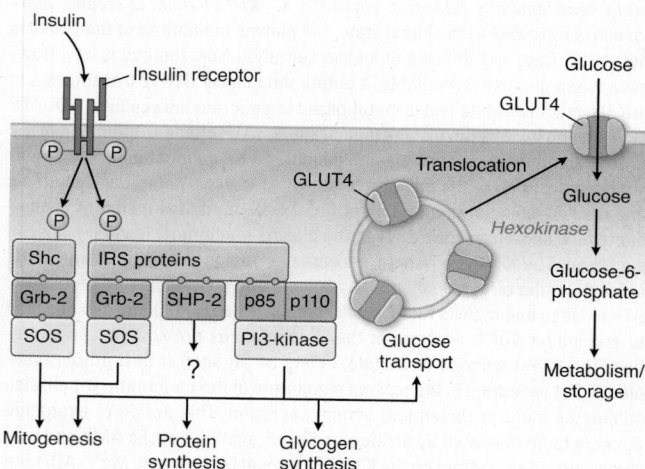

FIGURE 31-4. Downstream effects of insulin receptor activation. Insulin binding to the extracellular portion of the receptor activates tyrosine kinase domains inside the cell, leading to receptor "autophosphorylation" and tyrosine phosphorylation of cytoplasmic substrate proteins including Shc and insulin receptor substrate (IRS) proteins. Phosphorylated Shc promotes mitogenesis. Phosphorylated IRS proteins interact with many other signaling proteins (Grb-2, SHP-2, p85, and p110) to effect changes in cellular function. The IRS interaction with p85 and p110 recruits phosphatidylinositol 3-kinase (PI3-kinase). PI3-kinase activates signaling cascades that control many aspects of cellular insulin action, including glucose transport (via the translocation of GLUT4 glucose transporters to the cell surface), protein synthesis, and glycogen synthesis. Glucose that enters the cell is rapidly phosphorylated by hexokinase and subsequently used for metabolism or stored in the cell as glycogen or triglyceride.

glucokinase activity, thereby mediating the phosphorylation and trapping of glucose in hepatocytes and fueling glycogen synthesis, glycolysis, and fatty acid synthesis.

In skeletal muscle and adipose tissue, insulin stimulates translocation of the insulin-responsive glucose transporter, GLUT4, from intracellular vesicles to the cell surface, which facilitates the transport of glucose into the cell (Fig. 31-4). In muscle, insulin also increases amino acid uptake, stimulates the ribosomal protein synthesis machinery, and promotes glycogen synthase activity and subsequent glycogen storage. In adipose tissue, insulin promotes the expression of lipoprotein lipase, which hydrolyzes triglycerides from circulating lipoproteins for uptake into fat cells. Once inside the fat cell, glucose and fatty acids are stored predominantly as triglycerides. This process is enhanced by the deactivation of hormone-sensitive lipase, which degrades intracellular triglyceride. Insulin is rapidly degraded in the liver and kidney, with a circulating half-life of 6 minutes.

Glucagon

Glucagon—a single-chain polypeptide of 29 amino acids—is a catabolic (energy releasing) hormone secreted by pancreatic α-cells. When plasma glucose levels are low, glucagon mobilizes glucose, fat, and protein from storage as energy sources. Besides low glucose and high insulin levels, stimuli for glucagon secretion include sympathetic nervous system activity, stress, exercise, and high plasma levels of amino acids (because the latter indicates a state of starvation). Glucagon binding to its G protein-coupled receptor on the plasma membrane of hepatocytes increases intracellular cAMP and activates protein kinase A, a serine/threonine kinase. Glucagon promotes hepatic glycogenolysis and gluconeogenesis (Fig. 31-1). Glucagon also promotes lipolysis in adipose tissue. The liver and kidneys degrade glucagon; like insulin, its circulating half-life is about 6 minutes.

Amylin

Amylin is a 37-amino acid protein that is packaged together with insulin in secretory granules of the β-cell. Insulin and amylin are co-secreted following a meal. Amylin binds receptors within the central nervous system, and its glucose-regulatory actions complement those of insulin. Specifically, amylin suppresses glucagon release, slows gastric emptying, and decreases food intake. Together, these actions favor *gradual* entry of glucose into the circulation following a meal. Amylin is cleared by the kidney; its half-life is approximately 10 minutes.

Somatostatin

Somatostatin has 14- and 28-amino acid forms that are selectively produced in pancreatic δ-cells, the gastrointestinal tract, and the hypothalamus. Primary functions of somatostatins are to inhibit (1) the release of pituitary growth hormone and thyroid-stimulating hormone (see Chapter 27, Pharmacology of the Hypothalamus and Pituitary Gland), (2) the secretion of pancreatic insulin and glucagon, and (3) GI motility and the release of various GI hormones. The stimuli for pancreatic somatostatin release are similar to those for insulin (i.e., high plasma levels of glucose, amino acids, and fatty acids). Local somatostatin release allows the hormone to act in a paracrine fashion. The circulating half-life of somatostatin is only 2 minutes.

Incretins

Glucagon-like peptide-1 (GLP-1) and glucagon are both encoded by the glucagon gene, but their sequences are different due to differential mRNA splicing in the enteroendocrine L cells of the distal small intestine and in pancreatic α-cells, respectively. Bioactive forms of GLP-1 are 29 or 30 amino acids in length. Blood levels of GLP-1 are low during fasting and rise after a meal. GLP-1 acts on G protein-coupled receptors located on islet α- and β-cells and in the central and peripheral nervous systems, heart, kidney, lung, and GI tract. *At the pancreatic β-cell, GLP-1 augments insulin secretion in response to an oral glucose load (hence GLP-1's "incretin" effect).* At the pancreatic α-cell, GLP-1 suppresses glucagon secretion. GLP-1 acts in the stomach to delay gastric emptying and at the hypothalamus to decrease appetite. GLP-1 has a short half-life in the circulation (1–2 minutes) due to enzymatic degradation by **dipeptidyl peptidase-4 (DPP-4)**.

PATHOPHYSIOLOGY

Diabetes Mellitus

As early as AD 200, the Greek physician Aretaeus observed patients who had excessive thirst and urination. He named this condition *diabetes*, which is Greek for "to siphon, or pass through." Later, physicians added *mellitus* (Latin for "honeyed, sweet") to the disease name after noticing that diabetic patients produce urine that contains sugar. The designation *diabetes mellitus* also distinguishes this disorder from *diabetes insipidus* (see Chapter 27), in which either the secretion of antidiuretic hormone (ADH) or the response to ADH action in the kidney is dysregulated, such that water

is not reabsorbed in the collecting duct of the nephron and copious amounts of dilute urine are produced.

The syndrome of diabetes mellitus results from a heterogeneous group of metabolic disorders that have hyperglycemia in common (Table 31-2). Hyperglycemia can result from an absolute lack of insulin (**type 1 diabetes mellitus**) or from a relative insufficiency of insulin production in the face of insulin resistance (**type 2 diabetes mellitus**). The pathophysiology of diabetes that occurs during pregnancy or is induced by other causes (e.g., pancreatitis) is beyond the scope of this chapter.

Type 1 Diabetes

Type 1 diabetes mellitus, which accounts for ~5% of cases in the United States, results from the autoimmune destruction of pancreatic β-cells. No insulin is produced in the absence of β-cells, so circulating insulin concentrations are near zero. *The unavailability of insulin to promote nutrient entry into cells, coupled with the unopposed actions of counterregulatory hormones, induces a starvation-like response by the cells and tissues of the body.* Glycogenolysis and gluconeogenesis proceed unchecked in the liver, thereby increasing the concentration of blood glucose even though it is already too high. Skeletal muscle protein breakdown leads to the release of amino acids, which travel to the liver to further fuel gluconeogenesis. In adipose tissue, triglycerides are broken down and glycerol and fatty acids are released into the circulation.

In addition, the liver breaks down fatty acids for use as gluconeogenic fuels and for export as ketone bodies that could be used as fuel by the brain. These ketones equilibrate into β-hydroxybutyrate and acetoacetate. Excessively high concentrations of these "ketoacids" can deplete serum bicarbonate, eventually resulting in a state of high-anion-gap

TABLE 31-2 Type 1 and Type 2 Diabetes Mellitus

	TYPE 1	TYPE 2
Etiology	Autoimmune destruction of pancreatic β-cells	Insulin resistance, with inadequate β-cell function to compensate
Insulin levels	Absent or negligible	Typically higher than normal
Insulin action	Absent or negligible	Decreased
Insulin resistance	Not part of syndrome but may be present (e.g., in obese patients)	Yes
Age of onset	Typically <30 years	Typically >40 years
Acute complications	Ketoacidosis Wasting	Hyperglycemic hyperosmolar syndrome (can lead to seizures and coma)
Chronic complications	Neuropathy Retinopathy Nephropathy Atherosclerotic cardiovascular disease (ASCVD; includes stroke, peripheral arterial disease, and coronary artery disease)	Same as type 1
Pharmacologic interventions	Insulin	Approximately 10 drug classes are available, including insulin if other therapies fail.

Type 1 and type 2 diabetes mellitus are both associated with increased blood glucose levels, but the two diseases result from distinct pathophysiologic pathways. In type 1 diabetes mellitus, autoimmune destruction of pancreatic β-cells leads to an absolute lack of insulin. The etiology of type 2 diabetes is less well understood but seems to involve impaired insulin sensitivity and an inadequate level of compensatory insulin production or an abnormal profile of secretion by pancreatic β-cells. Although type 1 and type 2 diabetes have different acute complications (*see text*), they share similar chronic complications. Insulin is the primary pharmacologic intervention for type 1 diabetes, while type 2 diabetes can be treated with a number of different agents.

metabolic acidosis called **diabetic ketoacidosis (DKA)**. This is a medical emergency that requires immediate, aggressive treatment. DKA is often the initial presentation of type 1 diabetes during childhood or adolescence.

Some patients with residual β-cells can experience a transient "honeymoon" phase, lasting weeks to months, in which adequate endogenous insulin secretion occurs before the eventual complete loss of insulin production. Patients in whom the autoimmune β-cell destruction proceeds in a "smoldering" fashion are often diagnosed in adulthood, a clinical picture referred to as *latent autoimmune diabetes in adults* (LADA).

The genetic predisposition to type 1 diabetes maps strongly to the human leukocyte antigen (HLA) loci, also known as the *major histocompatibility complex* (MHC), which encodes proteins involved in antigen presentation. Other genetic loci weakly contribute to type 1 diabetes. In most patients with type 1 diabetes, autoantibodies to β-cell proteins can be detected. Environmental and nutritional factors influence disease development as well; if one member of an identical twin pair is affected, the incidence of type 1 diabetes in the other twin is about 50%.

Because patients with type 1 diabetes produce little or no endogenous insulin, therapy invariably consists of replacement with exogenous insulin.

Type 2 Diabetes

Type 2 diabetes mellitus, which constitutes >90% of cases in the United States, has historically been thought of as "adult-onset diabetes." The prevalence of type 2 diabetes has dramatically risen over the past three decades and now affects adolescents as well as adults. Obesity is the single most important risk factor, and more than 80% of type 2 diabetic patients are obese. The disorder typically develops gradually, without obvious symptoms at the onset. It is frequently diagnosed either by elevated blood glucose levels in routine screening tests or, as in the introductory case, after the disease has become severe enough to be symptomatic.

The progression to type 2 diabetes often begins with a state of **insulin resistance**. With increasing age and added weight, tissues that were once normally insulin-responsive become relatively refractory to insulin action and require increased insulin levels to respond appropriately. Current investigations are focused on two potential mechanisms for the pathogenesis of insulin resistance: (1) the ectopic accumulation of lipid into liver and muscle and (2) obesity-induced inflammation. Increasing evidence suggests that the immune system plays an important role in insulin resistance, although many of the details remain to be elucidated. In most individuals, the initial insulin resistance is compensated for by increased production of insulin by pancreatic β-cells. Indeed, many individuals with obesity and insulin resistance never progress to frank diabetes because their β-cells continue to compensate by secreting increased amounts of insulin. In some patients like Mrs. S, however, the β-cells eventually fail to keep pace with the increasing demand for insulin.

Although patients with type 2 diabetes generally have higher than normal circulating insulin levels, these levels are insufficient to overcome the insulin resistance in target tissues. The eventual failure of β-cell compensation could result from the loss of β-cells through increased apoptosis (programmed cell death) or from dysfunctional insulin secretion. Type 2 diabetes is a complex, polygenic disorder, meaning that polymorphisms in many genes can contribute to

overall risk, although the degree of risk conferred by each polymorphism is often quite small. A great number of such genes have now been identified. Most of these genes affect pancreatic β-cells, while a relatively small number of the identified type 2 diabetes genes confer risk for either obesity or insulin resistance. Therefore, lean, insulin-sensitive patients with type 2 diabetes have a strong predisposition to β-cell failure. Most of the relatively rare familial, monogenic causes of diabetes are also due to genetic lesions affecting β-cell function. Mild or early type 2 diabetes can be unmasked in predisposed individuals by transient periods of insulin resistance, for example, as occurs during treatment with glucocorticoids (see Chapter 29, Pharmacology of the Adrenal Cortex) or pregnancy (gestational diabetes).

The ability of patients with type 2 diabetes (like Mrs. S) to produce insulin provides the rationale for treating such patients with oral agents that either sensitize target cells to the action of insulin (e.g., metformin, thiazolidinediones) or increase insulin secretion by pancreatic β-cells (e.g., sulfonylureas and other insulin secretagogues). Drugs that control blood glucose levels by slowing the absorption of sugars from the GI tract (e.g., acarbose) are used less frequently. Patients with type 2 diabetes who have lost a great deal of β-cell function or are otherwise difficult to manage with oral agents may benefit from exogenous insulin therapy.

Morbidity and Mortality

Type 1 and type 2 diabetes are associated with both type-specific acute morbidities and common chronic complications. In uncontrolled type 1 diabetes, the lack of insulin and unopposed action of counterregulatory hormones leads to a "metabolic storm" that includes the activation of hormone-sensitive lipase in adipose tissue, the breakdown of triglycerides into glycerol and fatty acids, and the increased flux of fatty acids in the liver mitochondria that fuels ketogenesis. Although ketoacidosis is less common in type 2 diabetes because these patients produce insulin, uncontrolled type 2 diabetes can cause a hyperglycemic hyperosmolar syndrome that leads to mental status changes and can progress to seizures, coma, and death.

Both type 1 and type 2 diabetes are associated with long-term vascular pathology. These **chronic complications** include *accelerated atherosclerotic cardiovascular disease (ASCVD), retinopathy, nephropathy, and neuropathy*. Although the exact mechanisms are unclear, chronic hyperglycemia, chronic hyperlipidemia, and increased inflammatory signaling may all be contributing factors. In treating Mrs. S's diabetes, the goal is not only to correct her hyperglycemia and associated symptoms (e.g., polydipsia) but also to prevent these serious chronic complications. Roughly 80% of diabetic patients die from ASCVD. It is therefore critically important to control concomitant cardiovascular risk factors, such as hypertension and atherogenic dyslipidemia, in addition to lowering blood glucose in these patients.

Two large, multicenter, randomized clinical trials, the Diabetes Control and Complications Trial/Epidemiology of Diabetes Interventions and Complications (DCCT/EDIC) involving type 1 diabetic patients, and the United Kingdom Prospective Diabetes Study involving newly diagnosed type 2 patients, demonstrated that intensive diabetes management dramatically decreases the onset (primary prevention) and delays the progression (secondary prevention) of the microvascular complications of *retinopathy, nephropathy, and neuropathy*. These trials also suggested that intensive blood glucose control initiated early after diagnosis may decrease ASCVD in the long-term. However, causal relationships between glycemic control and risk of ASCVD are less clear in patients with established diabetes.

Self-monitoring of blood glucose is key to confirm "tight" control and to guide changes in diet, exercise activity, and pharmacologic treatment. Blood glucose is measured by finger stick using a monitor that assesses glucose concentration in small samples of capillary blood. In addition, levels of **glycohemoglobin (HbA1c)** provide estimates of the average blood glucose level over the previous 8–12 weeks. HbA1c results from the nonenzymatic glycation of hemoglobin in red blood cells. It is proportional to the average level of glucose in the blood and to the lifespan of the red blood cells (~120 days). HbA1c and blood glucose levels usually rise in parallel, although it is possible for HbA1c to be elevated while blood glucose is normal in a given instance—for example, when the blood glucose level is acutely normal but the glucose levels had been chronically elevated over the previous several months. *HbA1c levels are monitored as a marker of average blood glucose control.* Mrs. S's HbA1c level of 8.2% is concerning because the rate of chronic diabetic complications rises dramatically with HbA1c levels greater than 7.5%. HbA1c levels may be misleadingly low in patients with a shortened red blood cell lifespan (e.g., patients with hemolytic anemia) or in pregnancy.

Hypoglycemia

Hyperinsulinemia is one of several conditions that can result in hypoglycemia, which is a dangerous condition because the brain requires a constant supply of glucose and cannot rely on alternate fuels as readily as peripheral tissues can. Hyperinsulinemia has various causes, the most common of which is iatrogenic (i.e., exogenous insulin or insulin secretagogues used to treat type 1 or type 2 diabetes). A central challenge in the therapy of both type 1 and type 2 diabetes is to normalize glucose levels adequately while avoiding hypoglycemia due to overtreatment. Rarer causes of hypoglycemia include insulinomas (insulin-secreting tumors of pancreatic β-cells) and mutations in the β-cell K^+/ATP channel (e.g., mutations in Kir6.2 or SUR1 that result in constitutive depolarization; see above).

▌ PHARMACOLOGIC CLASSES AND AGENTS

Therapy for Diabetes

Therapeutic agents for treating diabetes target various steps in the regulation of normal glucose homeostasis. Currently available classes of agents include (1) exogenous insulin preparations; (2) metformin, a biguanide; (3) insulin secretagogues (sulfonylureas, D-phenylalanine derivatives, and meglitinides); (4) incretins (GLP-1 receptor agonists and DPP-4 inhibitors); (5) inhibitors of glucose reabsorption in the kidney (SGLT-2 inhibitors); (6) PPAR-γ agonists (thiazolidinediones); (7) analogues of amylin; (8) bile acid sequestrants; (9) inhibitors of intestinal glucose absorption; and (10) dopamine receptor agonists (bromocriptine).

The major goals for the pharmacologic therapy of diabetes are to normalize blood glucose levels and other metabolic parameters in order to reduce the risk of long-term complications. Lifestyle interventions are a cornerstone of the management of both type 1 and type 2 diabetes, and all patients with diabetes should receive personalized diabetes education focused on improved diet and exercise. For patients with type 1 diabetes, the strategy is to provide sufficient exogenous insulin to nearly normalize glycemia without substantially increasing the risk of hypoglycemia. Appropriate treatment of type 1 diabetic patients not only achieves normoglycemia but also reverses the metabolic starvation response mediated by the unopposed action of counterregulatory hormones. For example, insulin treatment reverses amino acid breakdown in muscle and ketogenesis in the liver.

The treatment of type 2 diabetes is multifaceted but nearly always includes recommendations for a balanced diet rich in fiber and low in high-glycemic-index carbohydrates and saturated fats (<7%) and a stepwise program of physical activity with the goal of 150 min/week of aerobic, resistance, and flexibility training. In the clinical vignette, Mrs. S was diagnosed with type 2 diabetes after progressive weight gain, which likely increased her insulin resistance. Exercise and weight loss could dramatically improve her blood glucose control.

If a patient is unable or unwilling to make the necessary changes in lifestyle, which is often the case, then one or more drugs may be used. Currently available drugs offer the potential to individualize diabetes treatment, with decisions about the blood glucose target (i.e., HbA1c level) being guided by age, life expectancy, comorbidities, and the patient's expectations. The choice of pharmacologic regimen should take into account the frequency of administration, efficacy, ease of use, adverse effects, and patient's ability and preference (Table 31-3).

TABLE 31-3 Estimated Frequency of Drug Prescribing for Treatment of Diabetes

DRUG CLASS	PERCENT OF PATIENTS WITH AT LEAST ONE CLAIM	PERCENT OF TOTAL CLAIMS FOR DIABETES MEDICATIONS
Metformin	65	32
Sulfonylureas	41	21
Insulin	29	22
Thiazolidinediones	20	12
DPP-4 inhibitors	12	4
Incretin mimetic	3	2
Meglitinides	2	1
α-Glucosidase inhibitors	0.5	0.2
Amylin analogue	0.4	0.2

Estimates are based on the Medco Health Solutions, Inc., 2009 database of 4.5 million adult patients making at least one claim for a diabetes medication, representing a total of 41 million medication claims. The middle column sums to greater than 100% because some patients were prescribed multiple medications. The right column sums to less than 100% because about 5% of claims were for fixed-dose combination therapies, especially sulfonylurea/metformin and DPP-4 inhibitor/metformin combinations. These results are pooled for all patients with diabetes and do not distinguish between type 1 diabetes and type 2 diabetes. Adapted from Medco Health Solutions Diabetes TRC. Medco Diabetes Drug Usage: 2009. 2010; Medco Health Solutions, Inc.

Tight diabetes control (HbA1c ≤6.5%) might be appropriate in patients with a long life expectancy and low risk of hypoglycemia but may be harmful in elderly patients with a history of severe hypoglycemia and significant CVD. The biguanide metformin is uniformly endorsed as the first option for patients with type 2 diabetes in the absence of contraindications. Currently, ~70% of type 2 diabetic patients in the United States take metformin either alone or in combination with other agents.

Insulin Replacement: Exogenous Insulin

Insulin is not only the foundation for treating patients with type 1 diabetes but also a potentially helpful adjunct for patients with type 2 diabetes when diet and other therapies provide insufficient control of hyperglycemia. The first insulin preparations were derived from pig and cow sources, but current recombinant human preparations are produced in vitro.

The ideal insulin delivery system would mimic normal β-cell insulin delivery into the portal circulation, which causes the liver to be exposed to higher concentrations of insulin than peripheral tissues are. Because insulin is a protein, however, it is rapidly degraded by digestive proteases, and it is not generally effective as an oral agent. Exogenous insulin is therefore administered parenterally, typically by injection with a fine-gauge needle that creates a small depot at the subcutaneous injection site. This route of administration means that the liver and other target tissues are exposed to similar insulin concentrations, which is unnatural because the liver is exposed to too little insulin and peripheral tissues are exposed to too much.

The rate at which the depot of insulin is absorbed depends on a variety of factors, including the solubility of the insulin preparation, the local density of blood and lymphatic vessels, and potential circulatory or subcutaneous factors (e.g., lipoatrophy or lipohypertrophy). All other factors being equal, faster absorption generally translates into faster onset of action, but high interperson and site-to-site variability in rates of absorption alters the action profile of the injected insulin.

Table 31-4 lists the most commonly used insulin preparations according to two categories: **prandial bolus insulins** and **basal insulins**. Patients using insulin usually require both a longer acting basal insulin and a fast-acting prandial bolus insulin for optimal control of hyperglycemia; other therapeutic options are also available (e.g., insulin pumps).

Prandial bolus insulins are used to mimic β-cell release of insulin in response to a nutrient load and thus act rapidly and for relatively short durations. **Regular insulin** is the classic prandial bolus insulin. It is structurally similar to endogenous insulin with the addition of zinc ions to promote stability. Regular insulin tends to aggregate into hexamers, and the dissociation of the hexamers into monomers is the rate-limiting step for absorption. Thirty minutes is required for regular insulin to reach the bloodstream after subcutaneous administration. Thus, regular insulin should be administered 30 minutes prior to a meal.

Several "rapid-acting" engineered insulins are available that enter the circulation more quickly than regular insulin and can be administered just minutes before a meal. The analogues are structurally similar to regular insulin but have been modified slightly to favor dissociation of the hexamer into monomers (Fig. 31-2). The names of these analogues hint at the modifications: in **insulin lispro**, the amino acids *pro*line and *lys*ine at positions B28 and B29 are reversed; in **insulin aspart**, *asp*artic acid replaces proline at B28; in **insulin glulisine**, *lys*ine replaces asparagine at B3 and *glu*tamic acid replaces lysine at B29. In 2014, the US Food and Drug Administration (FDA) approved an *inhaled* human insulin formulation (Afrezza®) with kinetics similar to "rapid-acting" injectable insulin analogues: onsets of action for both are 10–30 minutes, peaks of action are between 30 and 90 minutes, and overall durations of action are 3–5 hours. Inhaled insulin

TABLE 31-4 Commonly Used Insulin Preparations

TYPE AND PREPARATION	CONSTITUENTS	ACTION PROFILE (HOURS)			USAGE
		ONSET	PEAK	DURATION	
Prandial bolus					
Regular	Unmodified insulin	0.5–1	2–3	6–8	Meals or acute hyperglycemia
Lispro	Modified insulin	0.1–0.25	0.5–3	4	Meals or acute hyperglycemia
Aspart	Modified insulin	0.1–0.25	0.5–3	4	Meals or acute hyperglycemia
Glulisine	Modified insulin	0.1–0.25	0.5–3	4	Meals or acute hyperglycemia
Basal					
NPH	Modified insulin, protamine	2–4	4–10	12–18	Basal insulin, insulin of choice in pregnancy
Glargine	Modified insulin	2–4	None	20–24	Basal insulin
Detemir	Modified insulin	2–4	None	20–23	Basal insulin

Modifications to native human insulin consist of either (1) alterations in the amino acid sequence of the molecule or (2) changes in the physical form of the molecule. These changes affect the rate at which insulin is absorbed and the temporal profile of insulin action. Alterations in the amino acid sequence change the tendency for insulin to aggregate. For example, the modification in lispro decreases aggregation, resulting in faster absorption and more rapid action. In contrast, a neutral formulation like glargine increases aggregation and delays the rate of absorption of insulin from its subcutaneous injection site, making this preparation a long-acting dosage form.

should not be used in patients with chronic lung disease, such as asthma or chronic obstructive pulmonary disease (COPD), due to risk of bronchospasm after administration of the drug.

Basal "long-acting" insulins are administered once or twice daily and provide a more constant low-level release of insulin. **NPH (neutral protamine Hagedorn) insulin** is the oldest basal insulin that is still in common use. NPH insulin contains regular insulin suspended with zinc and protamine—an arginine-rich protein isolated from fish sperm. Protamine prolongs the time required for the absorption of insulin because it remains complexed with insulin until proteolytic enzymes cleave the protamine from the insulin. NPH insulin must be gently resuspended prior to administration and can exhibit a wide variability in its action profile. NPH's peak activity occurs between 4 and 10 hours after administration; this variability in peak activity can be associated with an increased risk of hypoglycemia. U-500 insulin is fivefold more concentrated than regular (U-100) insulin in the bottle and initially at the injection site, which promotes hexamerization and retards its absorption. This makes its action profile a "hybrid" between regular U-100 insulin and NPH insulin, since U-500 insulin peaks at 2–5 hours and lasts for up to 12 hours. U-500 insulin is most often used when large daily doses (>200 units) of insulin are needed and is administered 2–3 times a day before meals.

Two engineered long-acting insulin preparations are also available. **Insulin glargine** differs from human insulin by the addition of two arginines after position B30 and the replacement of asparagine A21 with glycine. These modifications raise the pK_a of insulin glargine from acidic to neutral, which renders the insulin less soluble and slows its absorption from the injection site. **Insulin detemir** differs from regular insulin in that myristic acid, a 14-carbon saturated fatty acid, is attached to the side chain of lysine B29. The fatty acid chain promotes binding of the insulin analogue to serum and tissue albumin, which retards the absorption, action, and clearance of the drug. Compared to NPH, the engineered long-acting insulins provide more constant insulin levels that plateau for many hours to provide basal coverage with lower risk of nocturnal hypoglycemia.

A typical basal-bolus regimen consists of a long-acting basal insulin once or twice daily with boluses of fast-acting insulin before meals. Advances in insulin preparations and delivery modalities continue to evolve. Premixed insulin preparations consisting of 25–30% fast-acting and 70–75% long-acting analogues are usually administered twice daily. These may be more convenient for some patients due to the reduced number of injections. Insulin pumps providing a continuous, variable-rate insulin infusion are gaining popularity among patients with type 1 diabetes. Insulin pumps allow programmed delivery at both a continuous rate to mimic basal insulin secretion and peaks to match postprandial glucose excursions. This provides greater flexibility in dosing while avoiding multiple injections but also requires a high degree of patient understanding and involvement.

The major danger with insulin therapy is that administration of insulin in the absence of adequate carbohydrate intake can result in hypoglycemia. While tight glycemic control that aims to maintain near normoglycemia decreases the incidence of diabetic complications, it also increases the frequency of hypoglycemic events, especially after administration of prandial insulin. Appropriate matching of insulin dose and carbohydrate intake is a major goal for diabetes management.

In type 2 diabetic patients such as Mrs. S, insulin resistance is typically more severe in muscle and liver than in fat cells. For this reason, insulin preferentially deposits calories in adipose tissue, and insulin therapy in insulin-resistant patients (especially those who are already obese, like Mrs. S) often leads to weight gain.

Metformin

Hepatic glucose production may be abnormally elevated in type 2 diabetes. **Metformin** acts to decrease glucose production, fatty acid synthesis, and cholesterol synthesis in the liver, potentially through AMPK-dependent and AMPK-independent mechanisms. Metformin also improves glucose uptake in peripheral muscle; the molecular mechanism responsible for this is less well understood. Metformin increases insulin signaling and is especially effective at lowering glucose in type 2 diabetics who are obese and insulin resistant. Metformin is also used for the off-label (not FDA-approved) treatment of other conditions, such as polycystic ovarian syndrome and non-alcoholic fatty liver disease, that are associated with insulin resistance and hyperinsulinemia.

The most common adverse effect of metformin is mild gastrointestinal distress, which is usually transient and can be minimized by slow titration of the dose. A potentially more serious adverse effect is **lactic acidosis**. Because biguanides decrease the flux of metabolic acids through gluconeogenic pathways, lactic acid can accumulate to dangerous levels in biguanide-treated patients. This complication is rarely seen with metformin (as opposed to phenformin, which is not approved for use in the United States). Lactic acidosis may occur more frequently when metformin is taken by patients who have other conditions predisposing to metabolic acidosis, such as hepatic disease, heart failure, sepsis, alcohol abuse, or renal disease (because biguanides are excreted by the kidneys). Current guidelines suggest reducing the metformin dose when the glomerular filtration rate (GFR) is <45 mL/min and discontinuing metformin when GFR is <30 mL/min. Biguanides do not directly affect insulin secretion, and their use is not associated with hypoglycemia. Unlike insulin and insulin secretagogues, biguanides promote a modest decrease in weight or are weight neutral.

Insulin Secretagogues: Sulfonylureas and Glinides

Sulfonylureas (SFUs) have been available in the United States since the 1950s for the treatment of type 2 diabetes. SFUs stimulate insulin release from pancreatic β-cells, thereby increasing circulating insulin to levels sufficient to overcome the insulin resistance. *At the molecular level, SFUs bind the SUR1 subunit of the SFU receptor, which inhibits the β-cell K^+/ATP channel* (Fig. 31-3). The SFUs used to treat type 2 diabetes bind with a higher affinity to SUR1 than to SUR2 isoforms, accounting for their relative β-cell specificity. The inhibition of the K^+/ATP channel by SFUs is functionally similar to the molecular events occurring after a meal, when increased glucose metabolism causes β-cell accumulation of intracellular ATP, membrane depolarization, Ca^{2+} influx, fusion of insulin-containing vesicles with the plasma membrane, and insulin secretion (see above).

SFUs are orally available and metabolized by the liver. Their major adverse effect is hypoglycemia resulting from relative oversecretion of insulin. These medications should be used cautiously in patients who are unable to recognize or respond appropriately to hypoglycemia (e.g., the elderly) and in patients with decreased renal or hepatic function due to impaired clearance. It is controversial whether glyburide bears an especially high risk for hypoglycemia, but the American Geriatric Society recommends that glyburide be avoided in elderly patients. Although SFUs are generally effective, safe, and inexpensive generic drugs that, along with metformin, are mainstays of treatment for type 2 diabetes, their use is waning for two reasons. Unlike some diabetes drugs that maintain efficacy, the SFUs have been shown to lose efficacy over time. In addition, due to their mechanism of action, SFUs and glinides are thought to diminish rather than preserve β-cell function over time. SFUs can cause weight gain secondary to increased insulin activity on adipose tissue. This adverse effect is counterproductive in obese patients such as Mrs. S. Therefore, SFUs are better suited for use in non-obese patients.

Like SFUs, meglitinides and D-phenylalanine derivatives, known collectively as **glinides**, stimulate insulin release by binding SUR1 and inhibiting the β-cell K$^+$/ATP channel. Although they are structurally distinct, SFUs and glinides both bind the SUR1 subunit, albeit at distinct sites on SUR1. The glinides have a rapid onset of action, similar to SFUs, but also a short half-life, making them an attractive option for patients with irregular meal schedules or who are prone to late postprandial hypoglycemia. Similar to SFUs, glinides are associated with weight gain.

GLP-1-Based "Incretin" Therapies: GLP-1 Receptor Agonists (GLP-1Ra's) and DPP-4 Inhibitors

Exenatide, a hormone originally isolated from the salivary glands of the Gila monster, acts as an agonist at human GLP-1 receptors. The drug is injected subcutaneously either twice a day or weekly in its extended-release formulation. **Liraglutide** is a long-acting form of GLP-1 with palmitic acid attached to the side chain of lysine, which causes it to bind serum and tissue albumin much like insulin detemir. This increases its circulating half-life from 1–2 minutes to >12 hours, making it suitable for daily injection. **Albiglutide**, a GLP-1 dimer fused to human albumin, has a half-life of 4–7 days, thereby allowing for weekly injection. These GLP-1 receptor agonists (GLP-1Ra's) can be used in combination with other antidiabetic drugs but not with DPP-4 inhibitors; the latter combination may enhance the risk of pancreatitis.

GLP-1Ra's have several mechanisms of action, including increased glucose-dependent β-cell secretion of insulin, suppressed α-cell secretion of glucagon, slowed gastric emptying (which retards ingested nutrient entry into the circulation), and decreased appetite. The most common adverse effects are nausea and vomiting (20–30%), which often improve with prolonged use but are the most common causes for discontinuation of these therapies (5% of patients).

Medullary thyroid cancer has been observed in rodents treated with GLP-1Ra's but not in humans. GLP-1Ra's carry a "black box" warning for this potential risk. The risk of acute pancreatitis and pancreatic cancer has been debated. The FDA recently issued a press release stating that existing data do not conclusively support a causal link between incretins and pancreatic pathology but also recommending continued monitoring through analysis of ongoing postmarketing clinical trials. Because GLP-1Ra's augment glucose-dependent insulin secretion, they are not associated with hypoglycemia unless used in conjunction with other antidiabetic agents such as SFUs. GLP-1Ra's are associated with weight loss in 10–40% of patients. Indeed, liraglutide at doses higher than those routinely used for treatment of diabetes was approved in late 2014 for treatment of obesity.

Dipeptidyl peptidase-4 (DPP-4) is an endogenous enzyme that cleaves and inactivates GLP-1. The DPP-4 inhibitors thus prolong the half-life of endogenous GLP-1 by inhibiting DPP-4. These drugs increase circulating GLP-1 and insulin concentrations and decrease glucagon concentration. They are used most commonly in combination with metformin (see earlier), although they can also be used alone. Currently approved DPP-4 inhibitors include **sitagliptin**, **saxagliptin**, **linagliptin**, and **alogliptin**. They are taken orally once a day and typically decrease HbA1c levels by 0.5–0.7%. Like metformin, pramlintide, and GLP-1 agonists, DPP-4 inhibitors alone are not associated with hypoglycemia, although an increased risk of hypoglycemia is noted when they are administered with SFUs. They are well tolerated and weight neutral.

Inhibitors of Glucose Reabsorption in the Kidney: SGLT-2 Inhibitors

Glucose excretion in the urine represents the net difference between the amount of glucose filtered at the glomerulus and the amount reabsorbed by low-affinity, high-capacity SGLT-2 transporters in the proximal convoluted tubule. The sodium gradient across the luminal membrane of the proximal tubule cells provides the driving force for glucose reabsorption. Intracellular glucose diffuses into the bloodstream via the transporter GLUT2. SGLT-2 capacity is saturated and the transport maximum for glucose is reached at blood glucose levels of 180–200 mg/dL. Above these levels, as often occurs in diabetes, glucose is excreted in the urine.

Inhibition of SGLT-2 drew interest as a potential therapeutic target when the nonspecific inhibitor phlorizin was found to normalize glucose in experimental models of diabetes. While GI adverse effects and low bioavailability hampered the development of phlorizin for use in humans, the specific SGLT-2 inhibitors **canagliflozin**, **empagliflozin**, and **dapagliflozin** are now approved for treating patients with type 2 diabetes. As an add-on therapy, SGLT-2 inhibitors decrease HbA1c levels by 0.7–1.0% from a baseline of ~8%. Importantly, the mechanism of action of SGLT-2 inhibitors is independent of both insulin secretion and insulin action, which distinguishes this therapeutic class from other antidiabetic therapies. The efficacy of SGLT-2 inhibitors is blunted in patients with reduced GFR (between 30 and 60 mL/min), consistent with their mechanism of action. SGLT-2 inhibitors have a low risk for hypoglycemia, since urine glucose is already negligible at low blood glucose concentrations. The main adverse effects include urinary tract infection, vulvovaginitis, and balanitis, which have been reported more often in female patients and are presumably linked to the presence of glucose in the urine. SGLT-2 inhibitors result in weight loss due to the excretion of glucose in the urine. Of note, SGLT-2 inhibitors are not approved for treatment of patients with type 1 diabetes and have been linked to cases of euglycemic DKA. This risk is especially high in patients who have rapidly decreased their insulin doses after starting SGLT-2 inhibitors, and appears to be the result of increased glucagon secretion.

Thiazolidinediones

The **thiazolidinedione (TZD)** drugs are insulin "sensitizers" that *enhance the action of insulin at target tissues* but do not directly affect insulin secretion. TZDs are synthetic ligands for the transcription factor PPARγ, which affects adipose cell differentiation and lipid metabolism. By activating PPARγ, TZDs promote fatty acid uptake and storage in adipose tissue rather than in skeletal muscle or liver. This decrease in muscle and liver fat content enables tissues to be more sensitive to insulin and suppresses glucose production in the liver.

Rosiglitazone and **pioglitazone** are the currently available TZDs. In addition to redistributing lipid stores among adipose, muscle, and liver, the TZDs have anti-inflammatory properties that may contribute to their efficacy. Adverse effects of TZDs include weight gain of 2–4 kilograms, fluid retention (edema), heart failure, and risk of bone fractures. Rosiglitazone had been associated with an increased risk of myocardial infarction, leading initially to a special warning, but the FDA recently reevaluated the data and suspended that warning.

Amylin Analogue: Pramlintide

Pramlintide was designed as a stable analogue of human amylin, the β-cell hormone that is co-secreted with insulin and may help regulate postprandial glucose levels. Type 1 diabetics lack endogenous amylin, and type 2 diabetics are relatively deficient in amylin. Thus, pramlintide is approved for use in both type 1 diabetics and insulin-requiring type 2 diabetics. Pramlintide's structure is similar to amylin with the exception of three amino acid substitutions that confer improved solubility and stability (three prolines replace an alanine and two serines). Pramlintide slows gastric emptying, reduces postprandial glucagon and glucose release, and promotes satiety. It is administered as a subcutaneous injection before meals. Its most common adverse effect is nausea, which is often limiting but may improve in some patients with continued use. Pramlintide is not associated with hypoglycemia unless it is used in conjunction with other agents that can cause hypoglycemia. Use of pramlintide often results in modest weight loss.

Bile Acid Sequestrants

In addition to its well-characterized cholesterol-lowering effects, **colesevelam** significantly lowers HbA1c levels in patients with type 2 diabetes. Colesevelam binds bile acids in the intestine, leading to an increase in fecal excretion and a decrease in enterohepatic reuptake of these acids. This promotes the conversion of cholesterol to bile acid, leading to hepatic uptake of LDL cholesterol and reduction in serum LDL cholesterol. However, colesevelam also increases triglyceride levels in ~50% of patients.

The glucose-lowering mechanism of colesevelam is likely related to its binding of bile acids. This could alter the activity of the G protein-coupled receptor TGR5 to increase secretion of GLP-1 or other incretins and inhibit hepatic glycogenolysis. As an add-on therapy, colesevelam reduces HbA1c levels by 0.3–0.5%. It is contraindicated in patients with a history of bowel obstruction or severe hypertriglyceridemia. Its main adverse effects are constipation, nausea, and dyspepsia.

Inhibitors of Intestinal Glucose Absorption

α-Glucosidase inhibitors are carbohydrate analogues that delay the absorption of dietary carbohydrates by inhibiting intestinal brush border α-glucosidase enzymes and thus reduce rates of cleavage of complex carbohydrates into glucose. By retarding the absorption of complex carbohydrates, α-glucosidase inhibitors reduce the postprandial peak in blood glucose. α-Glucosidase inhibitors are effective when taken with meals but not at other times.

α-Glucosidase inhibitors may be used as monotherapy or adjunctive therapy. They pose no risk of hypoglycemia and are most useful in postprandial hyperglycemia and for new-onset patients with mild hyperglycemia. Adverse effects that limit the use of α-glucosidase inhibitors include flatulence,

bloating, abdominal discomfort, and diarrhea. These adverse effects are mechanism-based, since delivery of undigested carbohydrate to the distal bowel provides nutrients for colonic bacteria. Thus, α-glucosidase inhibitors are contraindicated in patients with inflammatory bowel disease. A dose-dependent increase in hepatic transaminases is reversible after drug discontinuation. These agents do not promote weight change.

Dopamine Receptor Agonists

Bromocriptine mesylate is a nonselective dopamine agonist that has been used for decades to treat hyperprolactinemia. The antidiabetic mechanism of action is not completely understood. Growing evidence in animals points to suppression of hepatic glucose production by modulating the hepatic–hypothalamic circuitry. Bromocriptine does not augment insulin secretion or insulin sensitivity in peripheral tissues. When administered daily and within 2 hours after awakening, bromocriptine reduces HbA1c levels by ~0.5% in poorly controlled type 2 diabetic patients treated with diet alone or with one other drug. As monotherapy, bromocriptine is either weight neutral or results in modest weight gain (1–2 lb over the first 6 months).

Pharmacologic Management Strategies

As discussed above, patients with type 1 diabetes require insulin therapy. A subset of patients with type 2 diabetes also receive insulin, and both types of patients benefit from individual optimization of therapy using combinations of rapid-acting and long-acting insulin preparations. However, patients with type 2 diabetes rarely receive insulin as an initial therapy. Depending on disease severity, patients with type 2 diabetes may first receive recommendations for altered lifestyle such as diet and exercise. If this is insufficient, an oral medication is initiated, which is invariably metformin providing it is tolerated and not contraindicated. In the case of Mrs. S, in addition to counseling her on lifestyle, most physicians would prescribe metformin because it is safe and effective and does not lead to weight gain; Mrs. S also does not appear to have renal disease or other contraindications. Starting from a HbA1c level of 8.2%, behavioral modification and metformin treatment may result in a reduction of HbA1c level to the target of <7%. Advancement to combination therapy should be considered if monotherapy does not achieve the target HbA1c level. Current evidence does not support a "priority list" among the other oral agents and non-insulin injectables as an add-on(s) to metformin. The decision of which drugs to use in combination with metformin is based on ease of use, cost, adverse effect profile, and patient preference. In general, *combination therapy with drugs that affect different molecular targets, and that have different mechanisms of actions, has the advantage of improving glycemic control while using a lower dose of each drug and thus reducing adverse effects.* See Table 31-5 for a comparison of adverse effects associated with the long-term use of several different therapies for type 2 diabetes.

Therapy for Hyperinsulinemia

Although surgical removal is ultimately the treatment of choice for insulinomas, **diazoxide**, **octreotide**, and, in some cases, **everolimus** may stabilize hypoglycemia preoperatively. Diazoxide binds the SUR1 subunit of K$^+$/ATP channels in pancreatic β-cells and stabilizes the ATP-bound (open) state of the channel so that the β-cells remain hyperpolarized and

TABLE 31-5 Adverse Effects over Ten Years of Use: A Comparison of Several Agents Used as Monotherapy for Type 2 Diabetes Mellitus

AGENT	INCREASE IN WEIGHT (COMPARED TO DIET THERAPY ALONE), KG	SEVERE HYPOGLYCEMIA,* % OF SUBJECTS	SYMPTOMATIC HYPOGLYCEMIA,** % OF SUBJECTS
Insulin	4.0	2.3	36
Sulfonylurea	2.2	0.5	14
Biguanide	0	0	4

Because diabetes is a chronic disease, the long-term implications of therapy are an important consideration. Insulin and sulfonylureas are both capable of lowering blood glucose to dangerous levels, while biguanides lack this adverse effect. In addition, biguanide use is not associated with an increase in body weight, while patients taking insulin or a sulfonylurea tend to gain weight.
*Severe hypoglycemia is defined as hypoglycemia requiring hospitalization or other third-party intervention.
**Symptomatic hypoglycemia is defined as hypoglycemia not requiring hospitalization.
Data from United Kingdom Prospective Diabetes Study (UKPDS), 1998.

less insulin is released. Diazoxide binds channels containing either SUR1 or SUR2 isoforms and is therefore used not only to decrease insulin secretion by pancreatic β-cells but also to hyperpolarize SUR2-expressing cardiac and smooth muscle cells. In a rare form of genetic hyperinsulinemic hypoglycemia, a mutant SUR1 isoform is relatively insensitive to Mg^{2+}-ADP but does respond to diazoxide; in most forms of this disease, however, the mutant channel is not transported to the cell surface, and diazoxide is ineffective.

Octreotide is a somatostatin analogue that is longer acting than endogenous somatostatin. Like somatostatin, this agent blocks hormone release from endocrine-secreting tumors, such as insulinomas, glucagonomas, and thyrotropin-secreting pituitary adenomas. Octreotide has several other clinical indications as well (see Chapter 27).

The mammalian target of rapamycin (mTOR) inhibitor everolimus is FDA-approved for the treatment of neuroendocrine tumors of pancreatic origin. Everolimus has been shown to prolong progression-free survival in patients with nonresectable locally advanced or metastatic neuroendocrine tumors of the pancreas, including insulinoma.

Glucagon as a Therapeutic Agent

Glucagon is used to treat severe hypoglycemia when oral or intravenous glucose administration is not possible. As with insulin, glucagon is administered by subcutaneous injection. The hyperglycemic action of glucagon is transient, and it requires a sufficient hepatic store of glycogen. Glucagon is also used as an intestinal relaxant before radiographic or magnetic resonance imaging (MRI) of the gastrointestinal tract. The mechanism by which glucagon mediates intestinal relaxation remains uncertain.

CONCLUSION AND FUTURE DIRECTIONS

Fuel homeostasis involves the pancreatic hormones insulin, glucagon, amylin, and somatostatin and the GI hormones GLP-1 and GIP. When the levels of these hormones are pathologically altered, an individual can become hyperglycemic (as in diabetes mellitus) or hypoglycemic. Various pharmacologic agents act at several different cellular and molecular sites to normalize blood glucose levels. Exogenous insulin, SFUs, glinides, and incretins increase insulin levels, while diazoxide reduces insulin levels. Metformin and thiazolidinediones increase insulin sensitivity at target tissues. SGLT-2 inhibitors inhibit the reabsorption of glucose in the proximal tubule of the kidney. α-Glucosidase inhibitors slow the intestinal absorption of carbohydrates. Amylin analogues slow gastric emptying. Octreotide, a synthetic form of somatostatin, has wide-ranging inhibitory effects on hormone secretion. Exogenous glucagon can be used to increase plasma glucose levels.

Research on new pharmacologic treatments for early type 1 diabetes include efforts to develop immune modulatory therapies aimed at reversing β-cell dysfunction. For type 2 diabetes, agents may be developed to inhibit the enzymes of glycogen synthesis and glycogenolysis in order to restrain glucose production (e.g., inhibitors of glycogen synthase kinase 3 to promote glycogen synthesis and inhibitors of hepatic glycogen phosphorylase to suppress glycogenolysis), to modulate the microbiome either directly or indirectly, or to target inflammation using small-molecule anti-inflammatory drugs or selected biologics that block the actions of certain cytokines.

Suggested Reading

Drucker DJ. The biology of incretin hormones. *Cell Metab* 2006;3:153–165. (*Reviews basic physiology of GLP-1 and related hormones.*)

Garber AJ, Abrahamson MJ, Barzilay JI, et al. AACE comprehensive diabetes management algorithm 2013. *Endocr Pract* 2013;19:327–336. (*Reviews principles of management of diabetes, including strategies to escalate pharmacologic treatment through combination therapy.*)

Hardie DG, Ross FA, Hawley SA. AMPK: a nutrient and energy sensor that maintains energy homeostasis. *Nat Rev Mol Cell Biol* 2012;13:251–262. (*Reviews function and mechanism of action of potential metformin target.*)

Inzucchi SE, Bergenstal RM, Buse JB, et al. Management of hyperglycemia in type 2 diabetes: a patient-centered approach. *Diabetes Care* 2012;35:1364–1379. (*Clinically oriented approach to treatment of type 2 diabetes, including diet, exercise, insulin and other injectables, oral agents, and combination therapy.*)

Rena G, Pearson ER, Sakamoto K. Molecular mechanism of action of metformin: old or new insights? *Diabetologia* 2013;56:1898–1906. (*Thorough review of mechanism of action of metformin and its relationship with antidiabetic effects.*)

DRUG SUMMARY TABLE: CHAPTER 31 Pharmacology of the Endocrine Pancreas and Glucose Homeostasis

DRUG	CLINICAL APPLICATIONS	SERIOUS AND COMMON ADVERSE EFFECTS	CONTRAINDICATIONS	THERAPEUTIC CONSIDERATIONS
EXOGENOUS INSULIN				
Mechanism—The classic anabolic hormone, insulin promotes carbohydrate metabolism and facilitates glucose, amino acid, and triglyceride uptake and storage in liver, cardiac and skeletal muscle, and adipose tissue				
Prandial bolus insulins: **Regular insulin** **Insulin lispro** **Insulin aspart** **Insulin glulisine** **Inhaled human insulin** ***Basal "long-acting" insulins:*** **NPH insulin** **Insulin glargine** **Insulin detemir**	Type 1 diabetes mellitus Type 2 diabetes mellitus	*Hypoglycemia, hypersensitivity reaction, hypokalemia (shared adverse effects), seizure (insulin glulisine only)* Injection site reaction, lipodystrophy (shared adverse effects); upper respiratory infection (inhaled human insulin only)	Shared contraindications: Hypersensitivity to drug Hypoglycemia Inhaled human insulin only: COPD and asthma	Subcutaneous route is most common; inhaled insulin formulation also available. The "rapid-acting" subcutaneous analogues lispro, aspart, and glulisine offer flexibility and convenience because they can be injected minutes before a meal. Regular insulin is short-acting and must be administered 30 minutes before a meal. Inhaled human insulin is supplied as cartridges containing either 4 or 8 units, which are connected to a whistle-size inhaler; the drug should be administered minutes before or at the time of the meal. NPH is intermediate-acting; it is usually administered twice a day. Insulin glargine and detemir have the advantage of long-acting, steady release without a peak (mimicking "basal" insulin secretion); they are usually injected once a day (detemir can be dosed twice a day in some patients). The major danger with insulin therapy is that hypoglycemia can result from mismatching of insulin administration to carbohydrate intake.
INSULIN SENSITIZERS: BIGUANIDES				
Mechanism—Activate AMP-dependent protein kinase (AMPK) to block synthesis of fatty acids; inhibit hepatic gluconeogenesis and glycogenolysis				
Metformin **Metformin-ER**	Type 2 diabetes mellitus	*Lactic acidosis* Diarrhea, dyspepsia, flatulence, nausea, vomiting, cobalamin deficiency	Hypersensitivity to metformin Iodinated contrast media if acute alteration of renal function is suspected, as this may result in lactic acidosis Metabolic acidosis	Gastrointestinal distress associated with metformin use is usually transient and can be minimized by slow titration of the dose. Incidence of lactic acidosis is low and predictable; lactic acidosis typically occurs with metformin use in patients who have other conditions that predispose to metabolic acidosis. Does not induce hypoglycemia. Lowers serum lipids and is either weight neutral or decreases weight.

continues

DRUG SUMMARY TABLE: CHAPTER 31 Pharmacology of the Endocrine Pancreas and Glucose Homeostasis continued

DRUG	CLINICAL APPLICATIONS	SERIOUS AND COMMON ADVERSE EFFECTS	CONTRAINDICATIONS	THERAPEUTIC CONSIDERATIONS
NON-INCRETIN INSULIN SECRETAGOGUES: SULFONYLUREAS AND GLINIDES (D-PHENYLALANINE DERIVATIVES AND MEGLITINIDES) Mechanism—Sulfonylureas and glinides inhibit the β-cell K+/ATP channel via their binding to the SUR1 subunit, thereby stimulating insulin release from pancreatic β-cells and increasing circulating insulin to levels sufficient to overcome insulin resistance				
First-generation sulfonylureas: Acetohexamide Chlorpropamide Tolazamide Tolbutamide ***Second- and third-generation sulfonylureas:*** Glimepiride Glipizide, Glipizide ER Glyburide (Glibenclamide) Micronized glyburide Gliclazide	Type 2 diabetes mellitus (shared indication) Diagnosis of neoplasm of pancreas (tolbutamide only)	*Hypoglycemia (shared adverse effect); hemolytic anemia (chlorpropamide, glipizide, and glyburide only); Stevens-Johnson syndrome (glimepiride and glipizide only)* Gastrointestinal upset, dizziness, asthenia, headache	Shared contraindications: Hypersensitivity to drug Diabetic ketoacidosis Type 1 diabetes mellitus Glyburide only: Concomitant use of bosentan	Sulfonylureas are still a mainstay of treatment for type 2 diabetes. Metabolism by the liver and/or kidney varies among the different sulfonylureas. The major adverse effect is hypoglycemia; therefore, they should be used cautiously in patients who are unable to recognize or respond to hypoglycemia. Can cause weight gain secondary to increased insulin secretion; therefore, are better suited for non-obese patients.
Meglitinides: Repaglinide ***D-Phenylalanine derivatives:*** Nateglinide	Type 2 diabetes mellitus	*Hypoglycemia (shared adverse effect); cardiac arrhythmia (repaglinide only)* Upper respiratory infection (shared adverse effect); diarrhea, arthralgia, headache (repaglinide only)	Shared contraindications: Hypersensitivity to drug Diabetic ketoacidosis Type 1 diabetes mellitus Repaglinide only: Concomitant therapy with gemfibrozil	Glinides have therapeutic characteristics similar to sulfonylureas.
INCRETINS: GLP-1 RECEPTOR AGONISTS AND DPP-4 INHIBITORS Mechanism—Act via binding to the glucagon-like peptide-1 (GLP-1) receptor (GLP-1R agonists) or by prolonging GLP-1 activity (DPP-4 inhibitors) to enhance glucose-dependent insulin secretion, inhibit glucagon secretion, delay gastric emptying, and decrease appetite				
GLP-1 analogues: Exenatide Exenatide-ER Liraglutide Albiglutide	Type 2 diabetes mellitus	*Pancreatitis, renal failure (shared adverse effects); hypersensitivity reaction (exenatide and albiglutide only); hyperplasia or carcinoma of thyroid (liraglutide and albiglutide only); ALT/SGPT level increased (albiglutide only)* Hypoglycemia, nausea, vomiting, diarrhea (shared adverse effects); injection site reaction (exenatide and albiglutide only); headache (exenatide only); upper respiratory infection (albiglutide only)	Hypersensitivity to drug Personal or family history of medullary thyroid cancer	These agents are delivered by subcutaneous injection. Typically used in combination with any other antidiabetic agent except for DPP-4 inhibitors, since this combination may increase the risk of pancreatitis; the association between incretins and pancreatitis and pancreatic cancer is under scrutiny and is actively monitored by the FDA.

Drug	Clinical Applications	Adverse Effects	Contraindications	Therapeutic Considerations
DPP-4 inhibitors: Sitagliptin Saxagliptin Linagliptin Alogliptin	Type 2 diabetes mellitus	*Pancreatitis (shared adverse effect); anaphylaxis (sitagliptin, linagliptin, and alogliptin only); Stevens-Johnson syndrome (sitagliptin and alogliptin only); rhabdomyolysis, renal failure (sitagliptin only); bone fracture (saxagliptin only)* Hypoglycemia, upper respiratory infection, nasopharyngitis, headache	Hypersensitivity to drug	Dose adjustment is necessary in patients with moderate or severe kidney disease for all DPP-4 inhibitors except linagliptin. May cause hypoglycemia in combination with sulfonylureas and insulin. Digoxin levels should be monitored in patients receiving digoxin and sitagliptin. Interaction with drugs that induce or inhibit CYP3A4.

SODIUM-GLUCOSE CO-TRANSPORTER-2 (SGLT-2) INHIBITORS
Mechanism—Inhibit reabsorption of glucose in the proximal tubule of the kidneys, thereby increasing glucose excretion in the urine

Drug	Clinical Applications	Adverse Effects	Contraindications	Therapeutic Considerations
Canagliflozin Dapagliflozin Empagliflozin	Type 2 diabetes mellitus	*Hypoglycemia (shared adverse effect); hypovolemia, hypersensitivity reaction, renal impairment (canagliflozin and dapagliflozin only); hyperkalemia, pancreatitis (canagliflozin only)* Polyuria, urinary tract infection, vulvovaginitis, balanitis	Hypersensitivity to drug Renal impairment	Modest risk of hypoglycemia. Not indicated in patients with history of urinary tract infections. Can be used as monotherapy or in combination with other drugs. Effects are independent of insulin release or peripheral resistance but require appropriate glomerular filtration. Effects on cardiovascular endpoints not established yet.

INSULIN SENSITIZERS: THIAZOLIDINEDIONES (TZDs)
Mechanism—Bind and stimulate the nuclear hormone receptor peroxisome proliferator-activated receptor-γ (PPARγ), thereby increasing insulin sensitivity in adipose tissue, liver, and muscle

Drug	Clinical Applications	Adverse Effects	Contraindications	Therapeutic Considerations
Pioglitazone Rosiglitazone	Type 2 diabetes mellitus	*Heart failure, hepatotoxicity, diabetic macular edema, pulmonary toxicity (shared adverse effects); malignant bladder tumor, anemia, bone fracture (pioglitazone only)* Edema, weight gain, headache (shared adverse effects); myalgia, upper respiratory infection (pioglitazone only)	Hypersensitivity to drug Heart failure	TZDs do not increase insulin levels and therefore do not induce hypoglycemia. Newer TZDs appear to have less hepatotoxicity. Rosiglitazone use was restricted for several years due to concerns about increased risk of cardiovascular disease; recently, the FDA lifted these restrictions while actively monitoring effects of the drug in individuals at high risk.

AMYLIN ANALOGUE
Mechanism—Co-released with insulin from the β-cell; acts on receptors in the central nervous system to slow gastric emptying, reduce postprandial glucagon and glucose release, and promote satiety

Drug	Clinical Applications	Adverse Effects	Contraindications	Therapeutic Considerations
Pramlintide	Type 1 diabetes mellitus Type 2 diabetes mellitus	*Hypoglycemia* Loss of appetite, nausea	Hypersensitivity to pramlintide Hypoglycemia Gastroparesis	Administered via subcutaneous injection before meals. 30–50% dose reduction in insulin is required when pramlintide is used.

BILE ACID SEQUESTRANT
Mechanism—Binds bile acids and increases GLP-1 release, possibly via activation of the TGR5 receptor; bile acid sequestrant also enhances clearance of LDL cholesterol by up-regulation of the LDL receptor in hepatocytes

Drug	Clinical Applications	Adverse Effects	Contraindications	Therapeutic Considerations
Colesevelam	Type 2 diabetes mellitus Hypercholesterolemia	*Heart disease, pancreatitis* Constipation, indigestion, nausea, nasopharyngitis	History of bowel obstruction Severe hypertriglyceridemia History of hypertriglyceridemia-induced pancreatitis	Very low risk of hypoglycemia. May interact with multiple drugs, including glyburide, levothyroxine, and oral contraceptives.

continues

DRUG SUMMARY TABLE: CHAPTER 31 Pharmacology of the Endocrine Pancreas and Glucose Homeostasis *continued*

DRUG	CLINICAL APPLICATIONS	SERIOUS AND COMMON ADVERSE EFFECTS	CONTRAINDICATIONS	THERAPEUTIC CONSIDERATIONS
α-GLUCOSIDASE INHIBITORS **Mechanism—Carbohydrate analogues that bind avidly to intestinal brush border α-glucosidase enzymes, slowing breakdown and absorption of dietary carbohydrates such as starch, dextrin, and disaccharides**				
Acarbose **Miglitol**	Type 2 diabetes mellitus	*Bowel obstruction* Abdominal pain, diarrhea, flatulence (shared adverse effects); elevated serum aminotransferase levels (miglitol only)	Hypersensitivity to drug Cirrhosis Diabetic ketoacidosis Intestinal disease Inflammatory bowel disease Bowel obstruction	Very low risk of hypoglycemia. Most useful for patients with predominantly postprandial hyperglycemia and for patients with mild hyperglycemia. Gastrointestinal distress usually diminishes with continued use. Serum aminotransferase levels should be monitored during therapy. Modest increases in plasma triglycerides may occur with therapy.
DOPAMINE RECEPTOR AGONISTS **Mechanism— Poorly understood; likely affect hypothalamic–liver circuitry that influences hepatic glucose production; no effects on insulin release**				
Bromocriptine mesylate	Acromegaly Hyperprolactinemia Parkinson's disease Type 2 diabetes mellitus	*Coronary thrombosis, gastrointestinal ulcer, stroke, seizure, psychotic disorder, pleural effusion, pulmonary fibrosis* Constipation, nausea, asthenia, dizziness, headache	Hypersensitivity to bromocriptine mesylate Uncontrolled hypertension Breastfeeding Syncopal migraine Postpartum period in women with a history of severe cardiovascular conditions	Modest risk of hypoglycemia. Should be used as an antidiabetic agent in combination with other drugs. Initial evidence indicates beneficial effects on cardiovascular endpoints through a yet-to-be-established mechanism.
DIAZOXIDE **Mechanism— Binds to SUR1 subunit of K⁺/ATP channels in pancreatic β-cells and stabilizes the ATP-bound (open) state of the channel so that the β-cells remain hyperpolarized; this decreases insulin secretion by the cells**				
Diazoxide	Hypoglycemia due to hyperinsulinism Malignant hypertension	*Cardiac arrest, congestive heart failure, diabetic ketoacidosis, hypoglycemia, bowel obstruction, pancreatitis, thrombocytopenia, optic nerve infarction* Hypotension, hyperglycemia, nausea, vomiting, asthenia, dizziness	Hypersensitivity to diazoxide Functional hypoglycemia	Diazoxide also hyperpolarizes SUR2-containing channels in cardiac and smooth muscle cells and has been used off-label to decrease blood pressure in hypertensive emergencies.
EVEROLIMUS **Mechanism—Inhibits the mammalian target of rapamycin (mTOR) kinase that stimulates cell growth and angiogenesis**				
Everolimus	Hypoglycemia due to insulinoma Advanced kidney cancer Renal angiomyolipomas or subependymal giant cell astrocytoma associated with tuberous sclerosis Renal cell carcinoma Advanced breast cancer, HER2 negative Liver or kidney transplant rejection Pancreatic neuroendocrine tumor	*Anemia, leukopenia, thrombosis, infectious disease, sepsis, seizure, renal failure, interstitial lung disease, pleural effusion* Hypertension, peripheral edema, acne, eczema, dyslipidemia, hypoalbuminemia, hypophosphatemia, hyperglycemia, constipation, diarrhea, nausea, vomiting, increased liver function tests, impaired wound healing, asthenia, amenorrhea, cough, dyspnea, fatigue	Hypersensitivity to everolimus	FDA-approved in patients with unresectable neuroendocrine tumors; improves both progression-free survival and signs/symptoms related to tumor secretion, including hypoglycemia in patients with insulinoma.

SOMATOSTATIN ANALOGUES

Mechanism—Inhibits GHRH release

Octreotide	See Drug Summary Table: Chapter 27 Pharmacology of the Hypothalamus and Pituitary Gland

EXOGENOUS GLUCAGON

Mechanism—A polypeptide hormone, produced by α-cells in the islets of Langerhans in the pancreas, that stimulates gluconeogenesis and glycogenolysis in the liver, resulting in an increase in blood sugar

Glucagon	Hypoglycemia Intestinal relaxant before radiography of gastrointestinal tract	Rash, nausea, vomiting	Hypersensitivity to glucagon Pheochromocytoma Insulinoma	Used to treat severe hypoglycemia when oral or intravenous glucose administration is not possible. The hyperglycemic action of glucagon is transient and depends on a sufficient hepatic store of glycogen.

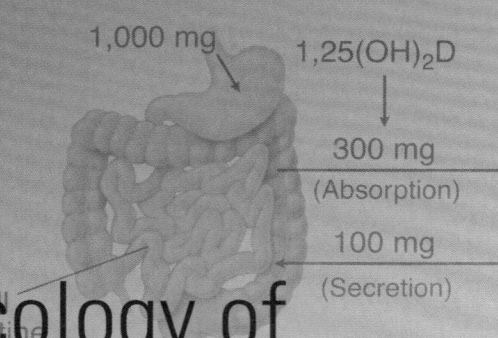

32

Pharmacology of Bone Mineral Homeostasis

David M. Slovik and Ehrin J. Armstrong

INTRODUCTION

The 206 bones of the human skeleton are far from the lifeless structures they are commonly imagined to be. Bones are remodeled continuously and are involved in many functions besides structural support and protection of internal organs, including hematopoiesis and mineral storage. The focus of this chapter is on the critical role of bone in mineral homeostasis, the process and regulation of bone remodeling, the diseases that can result when the delicate balances of mineral homeostasis and bone remodeling are perturbed, and the pharmacologic therapies employed to treat these conditions. A key concept regarding the pharmacologic agents discussed in this chapter is the distinction between bone antiresorptive agents, which slow bone loss, and bone anabolic agents, which have the potential to increase overall bone mass.

PHYSIOLOGY OF BONE MINERAL HOMEOSTASIS

Specialized cells called *osteoblasts* and *osteoclasts* continually remodel the human skeleton in response to mechanical forces and endocrine and paracrine factors. Two of the endocrine factors—parathyroid hormone and vitamin D—control bone metabolism for the purpose of maintaining extracellular calcium homeostasis. Other hormones, such as glucocorticoids, thyroid hormone, gonadal steroids, and fibroblast growth factor 23 (FGF-23), also have important effects on bone integrity. This section reviews the cellular and molecular mechanisms that mediate bone formation and bone resorption and the mechanisms by which hormones (especially parathyroid hormone and vitamin D) maintain plasma calcium levels within a narrow concentration range.

Structure of Bone

Bone consists of 25% organic and 75% inorganic components. The organic component includes the cells (osteoblasts, osteoclasts, osteocytes, bone lining cells, bone stromal cells) and osteoid (a matrix consisting primarily of type I collagen fibers and several low-abundance proteins). The inorganic component consists of crystalline calcium phosphate salts, primarily **hydroxyapatite**. The chemical formula of hydroxyapatite is $(Ca)_5(PO_4)_3OH$. Ninety-nine percent of the calcium in the body is stored in the skeleton, mostly

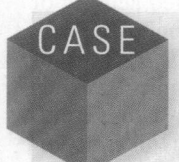

CASE

RS is a 60-year-old Caucasian female living in the northeast who comes to her physician with the recent onset of low back pain that began when she inadvertently stepped into a pothole. She is otherwise healthy and has no history of prior fractures.

Her menstrual periods ceased when she was 54 years old. She had little in the way of postmenopausal symptoms and never took hormone replacement therapy. Menarche was at age 11. She has one child who was born when RS was 38 years old. Her mother died at age 55 with breast cancer, and her sister, age 58, was recently diagnosed with breast cancer. She is lactose intolerant and avoids dairy. Additionally, she does not take calcium or vitamin D supplements and she has very little sunlight exposure with her daily activity. There is no known family history of osteoporosis. Her father and maternal aunt died in their 60s with coronary artery disease.

Her physical examination is unremarkable except for point tenderness over lumbar vertebra L1. Her weight is 135 lb, and she is 64 inches tall but believes she has lost some height over the last year. Laboratory studies are all within normal limits except for a low 25-OH vitamin D level. Lateral x-ray

of the spine shows a compression fracture of L1 and generalized osteopenia. Measurement of bone mineral density (BMD) at the spine and hip reveals values that are 2.6 standard deviations below the healthy peak female value for both sites. Her physician diagnoses postmenopausal osteoporosis and a recent compression fracture of L1. RS asks her physician to discuss with her the available therapeutic options and is particularly interested in the potential risks and benefits of each option.

Questions

1. What medical conditions should be investigated to rule out reversible causes of RS's osteoporosis?
2. Why is RS at particularly high risk for osteoporosis?
3. Given her family history, RS has an increased risk for breast cancer and cardiovascular disease. How does this alter the choice of therapeutic agents that could be prescribed?
4. What are the therapeutic options available for RS? What are the advantages and disadvantages of each option?
5. Should RS take calcium and vitamin D in addition to another therapeutic agent?

as hydroxyapatite. Figure 32-1 illustrates the structure of a long bone.

Mineral Balance

Calcium is absorbed in the small intestine by two mechanisms: facilitated transport, which occurs throughout the small intestine, and calcitriol-dependent active transport, which occurs mainly in the duodenum. In people ingesting 1,000 mg of dietary calcium per day, approximately 300 mg/day is normally absorbed by the intestines (Fig. 32-2). At lower calcium intakes, the efficiency of intestinal calcium absorption is higher, and at higher calcium intakes, the efficiency of absorption is lower. These adjustments contribute importantly to calcium homeostasis, and intestinal calcium absorption can increase to as much as 600 mg/day in the presence of high levels of **calcitriol** (the active form of vitamin D), as discussed below. The absorption of calcium from the intestine is normally balanced by calcium losses through renal excretion (about 200 mg/day) and salivary and biliary secretion (about 100 mg/day; Fig. 32-2). In contrast to calcium absorption, intestinal absorption of inorganic phosphate is not homeostatically regulated and is typically about two-thirds of the ingested phosphate irrespective of dietary intake.

Regulation of Bone Remodeling

Osteoclasts are the cells responsible for bone resorption. **Osteoblasts** are the cells responsible for bone formation. Regulation of these two cell types by mechanical, endocrine,

and paracrine factors determines the balance between bone formation and bone resorption (see below).

The two signaling proteins **RANK ligand (RANKL)** and macrophage colony-stimulating factor (M-CSF) are together both necessary and sufficient for the maturation of osteoclasts. RANKL, a member of the tumor necrosis factor (TNF) superfamily, is synthesized by osteoblasts and by osteoblast precursors, which express RANKL on their cell membranes. RANKL binds to **RANK**, a receptor expressed on osteoclasts and osteoclast precursor cells in the bone marrow. This binding interaction promotes the differentiation of osteoclast precursors into mature osteoclasts (Fig. 32-3). Alternatively, RANKL binds with high affinity to **osteoprotegerin (OPG)**, a soluble extracellular protein synthesized and secreted by osteoblasts. OPG is called a *decoy receptor* because it prevents RANKL from interacting with RANK. Inherited deficiency of RANKL or RANK causes a form of osteopetrosis (defined as defective bone resorption and increased bone mass), while inherited deficiency of OPG causes increased bone resorption and osteoporosis.

To repair its strength over time and to respond adaptively to mechanical stresses, human bone is continually resorbed and reformed. This process is called **remodeling**. Partly because of its large surface area on which remodeling can take place, 25% of trabecular bone is remodeled each year in adults. In contrast, only 3% of cortical bone is remodeled each year. This difference is important because *pathologic conditions that disturb bone remodeling preferentially affect bones with a high content of trabecular bone, such as the vertebral bodies.*

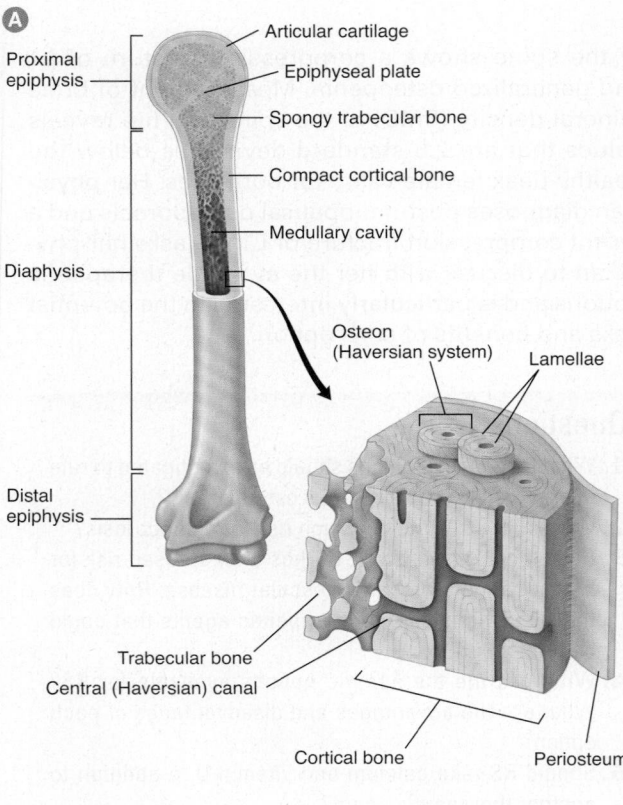

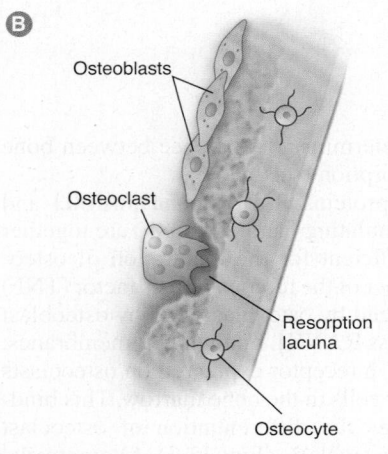

FIGURE 32-1. Structure of bone. A. The upper panel depicts the structure of a long bone (exemplified by the humerus). Note that the diaphysis consists of a thick outer layer or cortex of compact cortical bone surrounding the bone marrow. In the epiphysis, the cortex is thinner and surrounds trabecular bone as well as bone marrow; trabecular bone is also found in the vertebral bodies and much of the pelvis. **B.** The lower panel shows the detailed structure of bone. Bone remodeling is a dynamic balance between the catabolic activity of osteoclasts and the anabolic activity of osteoblasts. Osteoblasts and osteoclasts are found on all inner bone surfaces, including the endosteum that lines cortical bone and the many surfaces in trabecular bone. Bone remodeling is most intense in trabecular bone. Consequently, conditions that disrupt bone remodeling and/or bone mineralization affect trabecular bone preferentially. For example, osteoporotic fractures occur most commonly in vertebral bodies, which are predominantly trabecular bone.

Remodeling is carried out by the coordinated activity of millions of cellular units—**basic multicellular units (BMU)**—consisting of osteoblasts and osteoclasts. The process of resorption begins when physical and/or chemical signals (discussed below) recruit osteoclasts to form a tight ring-like seal with the bone surface and extend villus-like projections toward the surface within this ring. These villi secrete lactic acid, carbonic acid, and citric acid and use carbonic anhydrase to generate protons and a H^+-ATPase to pump the protons onto the bone surface. (Individuals and experimental animals deficient in this carbonic anhydrase have osteopetrosis.) The tight seal creates a closed, ring-shaped microenvironment beneath the osteoclast, within which the secretion of organic acids and protons consumes hydroxide at the bone surface and dissolves hydroxyapatite. The dissolution of hydroxyapatite can be expressed as follows:

$$(Ca)_5(PO_4)_3OH \rightarrow 5Ca^{2+} + 3PO_4^{3-} + OH^- \quad \textbf{Equation 32-1}$$

According to Le Chatelier's principle, OH^- consumption drives this reaction to the right. This is an important mechanism exploited by osteoclasts to resorb the mineral component of bone.

Demineralization of the bone matrix exposes it to proteolysis by cathepsin K, collagenases, and other proteases that are concomitantly secreted by the villi. Although this proteolysis totally degrades much of the exposed bone matrix, some of the type I collagen peptide chains escape into the circulation after partial proteolysis. The blood or urine level of such type I collagen metabolites (e.g., NTX, CTX) is an index of bone turnover, reflecting breakdown of type I collagen and total body bone resorption. Because of its large hydroxyapatite-covered surface area, bone normally adsorbs various nonskeletal proteins and peptides from its environment, including IGF-I and TGF-β. Demineralization exposes these **adsorbed growth factors** to the proteolytic enzymes secreted by osteoclast villi, but some escape proteolysis and affect the cellular activity of neighboring osteoclasts, osteoblasts, and osteocytes.

After about 3 weeks of such bone resorption, cytokines and growth factors liberated from the matrix, together with hormonal and other factors (see below), begin to stimulate local accumulation of osteoblasts via proliferation, differentiation, and reduced apoptosis (programmed cell death). These osteoblasts replace the osteoclasts in the resorption cavity (lacuna) and begin to refill the cavity with concentric layers, or **lamellae**, of unmineralized organic matrix (osteoid) (Fig. 32-3). As osteoblasts fill the cavity with new osteoid, they also secrete **alkaline phosphatase**, which hydrolyzes phosphate esters including pyrophosphate (a potent inhibitor of bone mineralization). The hydrolysis of pyrophosphate also increases the local concentration of inorganic phosphate. Together, the alkaline phosphatase-catalyzed hydrolysis of pyrophosphate and the liberation of inorganic phosphate promote the crystallization of calcium phosphate salts and mineralization of the bone matrix.

As osteoblasts continue to lay down matrix, some eventually become completely surrounded by it and are then called *osteocytes* (Fig. 32-1). Osteocytes are the most numerous bone cell type, comprising 90–95% of the cells in bone. Osteocytes respond to changes in mechanical strain and help control the balance between bone formation and resorption via their secretion of **sclerostin** (a protein that inhibits bone formation) and other factors. Genetic mutations that delete

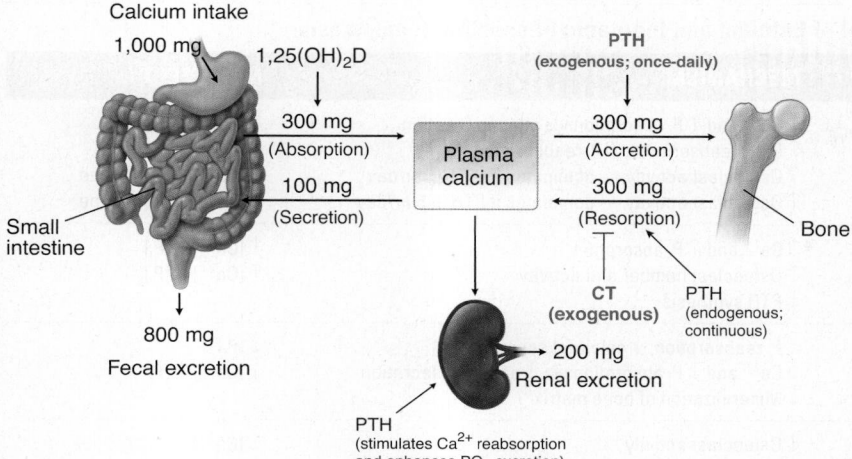

FIGURE 32-2. Daily whole-body calcium balance. In a state of whole-body calcium balance, the fluxes of calcium include net uptake of 200 mg per day from the GI tract and excretion of 200 mg per day by the kidneys. Calcitriol [1,25(OH)$_2$D] enhances absorption of Ca^{2+} from the GI tract. Continuous secretion of parathyroid hormone (PTH) increases bone formation and (even more) bone resorption and stimulates renal tubular reabsorption of calcium; both effects raise plasma Ca^{2+}. Continuous secretion of PTH also enhances renal clearance of inorganic phosphate (PO$_4$). In contrast, once-daily injection of PTH (*in blue*) stimulates new bone formation (accretion) more than it stimulates bone resorption and has only transient (and consequently minor) effects on renal clearance of Ca^{2+} and PO$_4$. Exogenous calcitonin (CT; *also in blue*) inhibits bone resorption.

or inactivate sclerostin increase bone formation without a corresponding increase in bone resorption. Such **uncoupling** leads to a marked increase in bone mass and bone strength in humans and experimental animals. A monoclonal antibody that inactivates sclerostin, and thereby increases bone mass and bone strength throughout the skeleton, is being evaluated

as a potential treatment for osteoporosis. Mature osteocytes normally alter their secretion of sclerostin in bone regions subjected to mechanical loads and thereby play a critical role in skeletal adaptations to gravity and other mechanical loads by localizing bone remodeling responses to such loads.

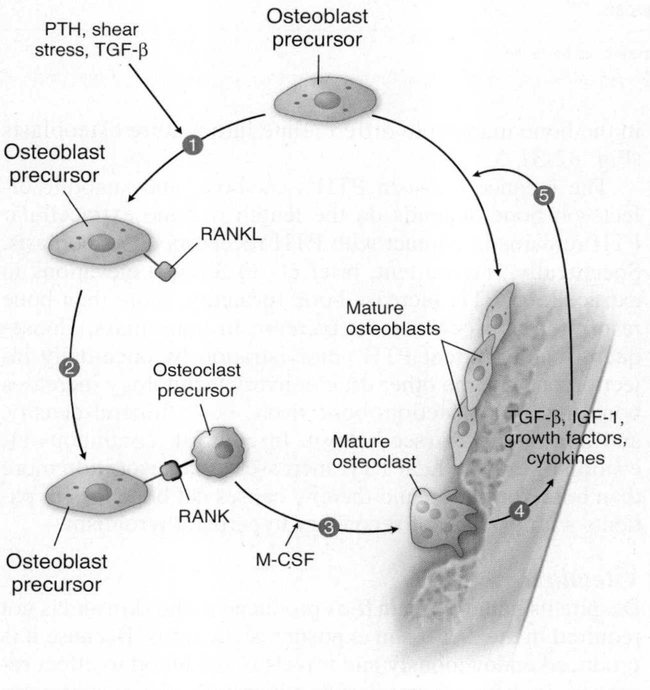

Hormonal Control of Calcium and Phosphate

Calcium is essential for many important physiologic processes, such as neurotransmitter release, muscle contraction, and blood coagulation, and deviations in extracellular calcium levels can have serious consequences. Therefore, the plasma calcium level is tightly regulated. Inorganic phosphate concentrations must also be regulated, in part because changes in plasma inorganic phosphate concentrations affect plasma calcium levels (see below). Three main hormones—parathyroid hormone (PTH), vitamin D, and FGF-23—mediate calcium and phosphate homeostasis. In addition, calcitonin, glucocorticoids, thyroid hormone, and gonadal steroids have lesser effects on calcium and phosphate homeostasis. Table 32-1 summarizes the mechanisms and effects of these hormones on calcium and phosphate homeostasis.

Parathyroid Hormone

The most important endocrine regulator of calcium homeostasis is **parathyroid hormone**, an 84-amino acid peptide hormone secreted by the parathyroid glands. The secretion of PTH is finely regulated in response to plasma calcium levels. Calcium-sensing receptors reside on the plasma membrane of chief cells in the parathyroid gland; when bound by extracellular calcium ions, these G protein-coupled receptors mediate increases in the level of intracellular free calcium, which, in turn, decreases secretion of preformed PTH. By this mechanism, *high plasma calcium levels suppress PTH secretion, while low plasma calcium levels stimulate PTH secretion*. (Note: In many other secretory tissues, an increase in intracellular calcium enhances secretion. Thus, the parathyroid chief cell is unusual in its response to changes in intracellular calcium.)

PTH acts on three organs to raise the plasma calcium concentration: it acts directly on kidney and bone and indirectly on the gastrointestinal (GI) tract (Fig. 32-4). The most rapid physiologic effects of PTH are to increase reabsorption of calcium and decrease reabsorption of inorganic phosphate by the kidney tubules. These actions decrease renal clearance of calcium while increasing renal clearance of inorganic

FIGURE 32-3. Interaction of osteoblasts and osteoclasts in bone remodeling. Bone resorption and bone formation are coupled by the interactions between osteoblasts and osteoclasts. 1. Factors such as parathyroid hormone (PTH), shear stress, and transforming growth factor β (TGF-β) cause osteoblast precursors to express the osteoclast differentiation factor RANK-ligand (RANKL). 2. RANKL binds to RANK, a receptor expressed on osteoclast precursors. 3. The RANKL–RANK binding interaction, together with macrophage colony-stimulating factor (M-CSF), causes osteoclast precursors to differentiate into mature osteoclasts. 4. As mature osteoclasts resorb bone, matrix-bound factors such as TGF-β, insulin-like growth factor 1 (IGF-1), other growth factors, and cytokines are released. 5. These liberated factors stimulate osteoblast precursors to develop into mature osteoblasts, which begin to refill the resorption cavities excavated by the osteoclasts.

TABLE 32-1 Summary of Endocrine Control of Calcium and Inorganic Phosphate Homeostasis

HORMONE	TARGET ORGAN	MECHANISM	NET EFFECT
PTH	GI tract	$\uparrow Ca^{2+}$ and $\uparrow P_i$ absorption via vitamin D action	$\uparrow [Ca^{2+}] \uparrow [P_i]$
	Kidney tubules	$\uparrow Ca^{2+}$ reabsorption; $\downarrow P_i$ reabsorption	$\uparrow [Ca^{2+}] \downarrow [P_i]$
	Bone	$\uparrow$ Osteoclast activity — dominates if PTH 24 hr/day	$\uparrow [Ca^{2+}] \uparrow [P_i] \downarrow$ bone
		$\uparrow$ Osteoblast activity — dominates if PTH 3–5 hr/day	$\downarrow [Ca^{2+}] \downarrow [P_i] \uparrow$ bone
Vitamin D	GI tract	$\uparrow Ca^{2+}$ and $\uparrow P_i$ absorption	$\uparrow [Ca^{2+}] \uparrow [P_i]$
	Bone	$\uparrow$ Osteoclast number and activity	$\uparrow [Ca^{2+}] \uparrow [P_i]$
	Parathyroid glands	$\downarrow$ PTH synthesis	
FGF-23	Kidney tubule	$\downarrow P_i$ reabsorption; $\downarrow$ calcitriol secretion	$\downarrow [P_i]$
	GI tract	$\downarrow Ca^{2+}$ and $\downarrow P_i$ absorption via $\downarrow$ calcitriol secretion	$\downarrow [Ca^{2+}] \downarrow [P_i]$
	Bone	$\downarrow$ Mineralization of bone matrix	
Calcitonin	Bone	$\downarrow$ Osteoclast activity	$\downarrow [Ca^{2+}]$
	Kidney tubule	$\downarrow Ca^{2+}$ reabsorption (pharmacologic doses)	$\downarrow [Ca^{2+}]$
Glucocorticoids	GI tract	$\downarrow Ca^{2+}$ absorption	$\downarrow [Ca^{2+}] \downarrow [P_i]$
	Kidney tubule	$\downarrow Ca^{2+}$ and $\downarrow P_i$ reabsorption (pharmacologic doses)	$\downarrow [Ca^{2+}] \downarrow [P_i]$
	Bone	$\uparrow$ Osteoblast apoptosis, $\downarrow$ osteoblast activity	$\downarrow$ Bone
		$\uparrow$ Osteocyte apoptosis	$\downarrow$ Bone
Thyroid hormone	Bone	$\uparrow$ Resorption $> \uparrow$ formation	$\uparrow [Ca^{2+}] \downarrow$ bone
Gonadal steroids	Bone	$\downarrow$ Osteoclast activity	$\downarrow [Ca^{2+}] \downarrow [P_i]$
		$\uparrow$ Osteoclast apoptosis	$\downarrow$ Bone resorption
		$\downarrow$ Osteoblast apoptosis	

FGF-23, fibroblast growth factor 23; GI, gastrointestinal; P_i, inorganic phosphate; PTH, parathyroid hormone.

phosphate. In this manner, PTH raises plasma calcium levels and decreases plasma inorganic phosphate concentrations.

Another important, although slower, effect of PTH results from its direct actions on bone cells. Physiologic levels of PTH stimulate cell surface PTH receptors on osteoblasts, causing these cells to increase their expression of the osteoclast differentiation factor RANKL (Fig. 32-3) and decrease their expression of its antagonist OPG. The resulting increase in osteoclastic activity increases bone resorption and thereby increases the release of calcium and inorganic phosphate into the circulation. PTH also induces bone marrow stromal cells to secrete cytokines such as IL-6, and these cytokines ultimately stimulate osteoclast proliferation and bone resorption.

Finally, PTH raises plasma calcium levels by an indirect effect on the intestine. PTH stimulates the kidney not only to increase calcium reabsorption and decrease phosphate reabsorption, as described above, but also to increase the enzymatic conversion of 25-hydroxy vitamin D to 1,25-dihydroxy vitamin D (calcitriol). This hydroxylation takes place in cells of the proximal renal tubules. Calcitriol, in turn, increases small intestinal absorption of calcium and (to a lesser extent) inorganic phosphate (discussed below).

Although the release of skeletal calcium and inorganic phosphate could be considered catabolic, PTH simultaneously stimulates new bone formation by promoting differentiation of osteoblast precursors to mature osteoblasts and by enhancing osteoblast survival. Interaction of PTH with its receptor on mature osteoblasts stimulates $G\alpha_s$, which increases adenylyl cyclase activity, which, in turn, increases intracellular cAMP. The PTH-induced increase in cAMP has an anti-apoptotic effect on osteoblasts. In addition, the increase in cAMP promotes osteoblast release of IGF-1, which induces osteoblast precursor cells

in the bone marrow to differentiate into mature osteoblasts (Fig. 32-3).

The balance between PTH's catabolic and anabolic effects on bone depends on the length of time extracellular PTH remains in contact with PTH receptors on osteoblasts. Specifically, intermittent, brief (1- to 3-hour) elevations in extracellular PTH increase bone formation more than bone resorption and cause a net increase in bone mass. Consequently, intermittent PTH administration by once-daily injection or by some other drug delivery technology increases bone matrix production, bone mass, bone mineral density, and bone strength (see below). In contrast, continuous elevation of extracellular PTH increases bone resorption more than bone formation and thereby causes net bone loss in patients with primary or secondary hyperparathyroidism.

Vitamin D

Despite its name, **vitamin D**$_3$ is produced in the skin and is not required in the diet if sun exposure is generous. Because it is produced endogenously and travels in the blood to effect responses in distant target tissues, vitamin D$_3$ is more correctly considered a hormone. The term vitamin D applies to two related compounds, **cholecalciferol** and **ergocalciferol**. Cholecalciferol, or vitamin D$_3$, is generated nonenzymatically in the skin when 7-dehydrocholesterol absorbs a photon of short ultraviolet light (UV-B; Fig. 32-5). Ergocalciferol, or vitamin D$_2$, is produced when ergosterol in plants absorbs such a photon. Vitamins D$_2$ and D$_3$ are each added to dairy products and some other foods; each is available as a dietary supplement; and each is available (in much higher doses) as a prescription drug. Vitamins D$_2$ and D$_3$ have equal biological activities, and "vitamin D" in subsequent paragraphs refers to both the D$_2$ and D$_3$ forms of the hormone.

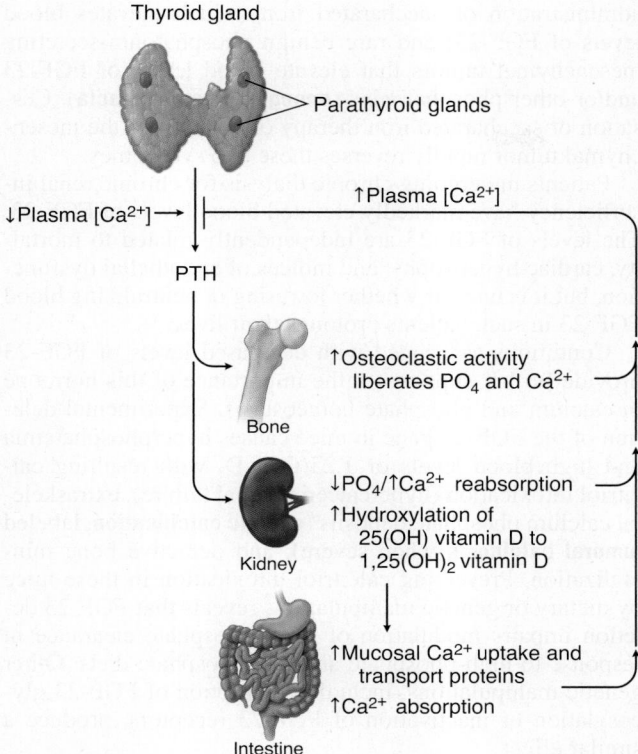

FIGURE 32-4. Summary of the actions of PTH on bone, kidney, and intestine. Decreased plasma $[Ca^{2+}]$ is the primary stimulus for parathyroid hormone (PTH) secretion by the parathyroid glands. PTH raises plasma Ca^{2+} levels via its effects on bone, kidney, and intestine. In bone, PTH promotes increased differentiation of osteoclast precursors into mature osteoclasts. Osteoclasts resorb bone and thereby liberate inorganic phosphate (PO_4) and Ca^{2+} into the plasma. In the kidney, PTH increases tubular reabsorption of Ca^{2+} and decreases proximal and distal tubular reabsorption of PO_4. In addition, PTH stimulates proximal tubule cells to hydroxylate 25(OH) vitamin D, forming 1,25(OH)$_2$ vitamin D. 1,25(OH)$_2$ vitamin D then stimulates intestinal absorption of Ca^{2+} by increasing the expression of mucosal Ca^{2+} uptake and transport proteins. Note that the effect of PTH on the intestine is indirect, via increased renal synthesis of the active form of vitamin D. In a tightly controlled negative feedback loop, increased plasma $[Ca^{2+}]$ inhibits further PTH secretion by the parathyroid glands.

Whether from an endogenous (skin) or an exogenous (dietary) source, vitamin D travels to the liver, where it is either stored or converted to calcifediol [25-hydroxy vitamin D, or 25(OH)D] by the first of two enzymatic hydroxylation steps. The second enzymatic hydroxylation converts calcifediol to the final, active form of vitamin D called *calcitriol* [1α,25-dihydroxy vitamin D, or 1,25(OH)$_2$D]. This second hydroxylation takes place in many tissues, particularly in the proximal tubule of the kidney (where it is PTH-dependent), but does not take place in the intestines because they lack the 1α-hydroxylase enzyme required for the second hydroxylation. *Calcitriol's primary effect on calcium balance is in the small intestine, where it increases the absorption of dietary calcium.* Calcitriol enhances Ca^{2+} absorption by acting on nuclear receptors in the enterocyte to up-regulate the expression of genes coding for multiple brush border proteins. Calcitriol also promotes the transcellular transport of Ca^{2+} through the enterocyte by inducing the expression of (1) a calcium uptake pump on the luminal surface of the enterocyte; (2) calbindin, an intracellular Ca^{2+}-binding

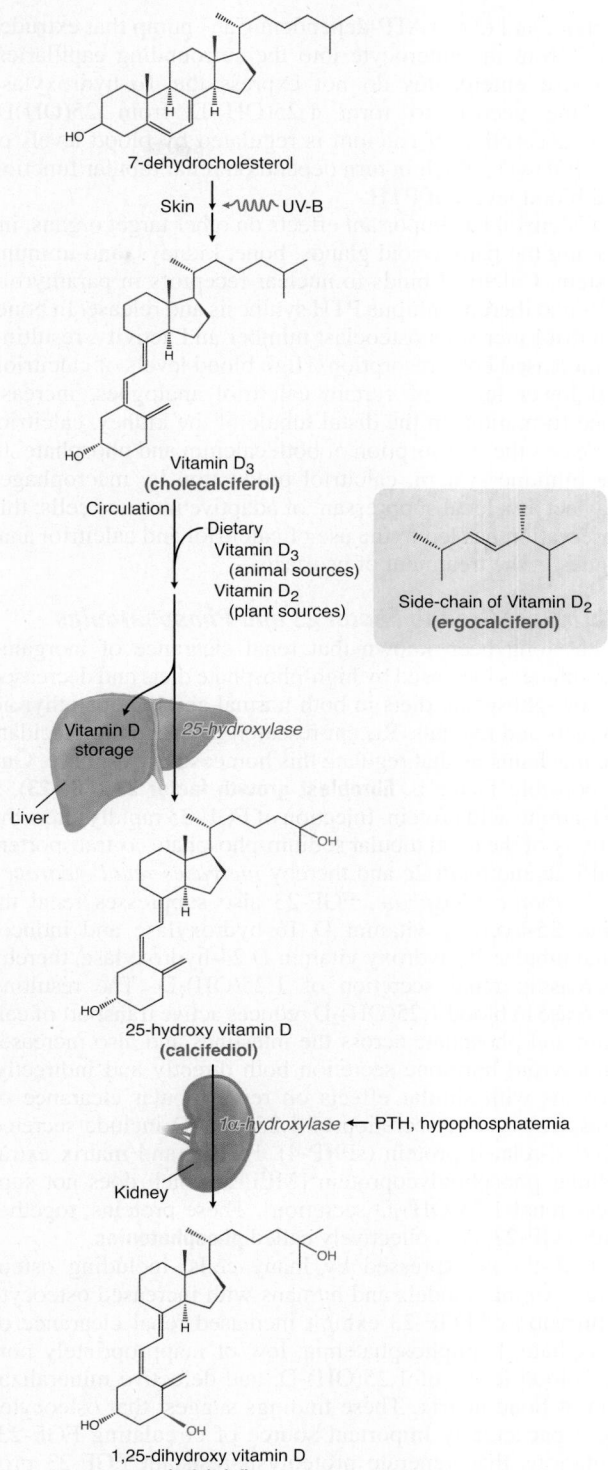

FIGURE 32-5. Photobiosynthesis and activation of vitamin D. Both endogenous and exogenous vitamin D are converted to 25-hydroxy vitamin D in the liver and then to calcitriol in the kidney. Calcitriol is the active metabolite of vitamin D. Endogenous vitamin D$_3$ is synthesized in the skin from 7-dehydrocholesterol in a reaction that is catalyzed by ultraviolet light (UV-B). Exogenous vitamin D can be provided as D$_3$ (from animal sources) or as D$_2$ (from plant sources); D$_3$ and D$_2$ have the same biological activity. Parathyroid hormone (PTH) increases the activity of 1α-hydroxylase in the kidney and thereby stimulates the conversion of 25-hydroxy vitamin D to calcitriol, as does hypophosphatemia.

protein; and (3) an ATP-dependent Ca^{2+} pump that extrudes Ca^{2+} from the enterocyte into the surrounding capillaries. Because enterocytes do not express the 1α-hydroxylase enzyme needed to form $1,25(OH)_2D$ from $25(OH)D$, their absorption of calcium is regulated by blood levels of $1,25(OH)_2D$, which in turn depend on renal tubular function and blood levels of PTH.

Calcitriol has important effects on other target organs, including the parathyroid glands, bone, kidneys, and immune system. Calcitriol binds to nuclear receptors in parathyroid cells and thereby inhibits PTH synthesis and release. In bone, calcitriol increases osteoclast number and activity, resulting in increased bone resorption. High blood levels of calcitriol, and lower levels of certain calcitriol analogues, increase bone formation. In the distal tubule of the kidney, calcitriol increases the reabsorption of both calcium and phosphate. In the immune system, calcitriol production by macrophages may act as a local suppressant of adaptive immune cells; this observation has led to the use of calcitriol and calcitriol analogues in the treatment of psoriasis.

Fibroblast Growth Factor 23 and Phosphatonins

It has long been known that renal clearance of inorganic phosphate is increased by high-phosphate diets and decreased by low-phosphate diets in both normal and hypoparathyroid humans and animals. Recent research has begun to elucidate the mechanisms that regulate this homeostatic response. One responsible factor is **fibroblast growth factor 23** (**FGF-23**), a 251-amino acid protein. Injection of FGF-23 rapidly alters the activity of the renal tubular sodium-phosphate co-transporters NaPi-2a and NaPi-2c and thereby *increases renal clearance of inorganic phosphate*. FGF-23 also suppresses renal tubular 25-hydroxy vitamin D 1α-hydroxylase and induces renal tubular 25-hydroxy vitamin D 24-hydroxylase, thereby decreasing renal secretion of $1,25(OH)_2D$. The resulting decrease in blood $1,25(OH)_2D$ reduces active transport of calcium and phosphate across the intestines and also increases parathyroid hormone secretion both directly and indirectly. Proteins with similar effects on renal tubular clearance of phosphate and/or secretion of $1,25(OH)_2D$ include secreted frizzled-related protein (sFRP-4), FGF-7, and matrix extracellular phosphoglycoprotein [MEPE, which does not suppress renal $1,25(OH)_2D$ secretion]. These proteins, together with FGF-23, are collectively called **phosphatonins**.

FGF-23 is expressed by many cells, including osteocytes. Animal models and humans with increased osteocyte expression of FGF-23 exhibit increased renal clearance of phosphate, hypophosphatemia, low or inappropriately normal blood levels of $1,25(OH)_2D$, and defective mineralization of bone matrix. These findings suggest that osteocytes are a particularly important source of circulating FGF-23. Mutations that generate proteolysis-resistant FGF-23 produce a nearly identical syndrome in mice and humans (e.g., human **autosomal dominant hypophosphatemic rickets, ADHR**). A more common hereditary form of FGF-23/phosphatonin excess in humans is **X-linked hypophosphatemic rickets (XLH)**, caused by mutations in the endopeptidase PHEX. How PHEX mutations elevate blood FGF-23 and/or phosphatonin levels remains controversial.

Nonhereditary causes of hypophosphatemia with increased renal clearance of phosphate, low or inappropriately normal blood levels of $1,25(OH)_2D$, and defective mineralization of bone matrix include repeated intravenous administration of saccharated iron (which elevates blood levels of FGF-23) and rare benign phosphatonin-secreting mesenchymal tumors that elevate blood levels of FGF-23 and/or other phosphatonins (**oncogenic osteomalacia**). Cessation of saccharated iron therapy or ablation of the mesenchymal tumor rapidly reverses these two syndromes.

Patients undergoing chronic dialysis for chronic renal insufficiency have markedly elevated blood levels of FGF-23. The levels of FGF-23 are independently related to mortality, cardiac hypertrophy, and indices of endothelial dysfunction, but it is unclear whether lowering or neutralizing blood FGF-23 in such patients prolongs their lives.

Conditions associated with decreased levels of FGF-23 provide further support for the importance of this hormone in calcium and phosphate homeostasis. Experimental deletion of the FGF-23 gene in mice causes hyperphosphatemia and high blood levels of $1,25(OH)_2D$, with resulting calcitriol intoxication (hypercalcemic renal failure), extraskeletal calcium phosphate deposits (**ectopic calcification**, labeled **tumoral calcinosis** when severe), and defective bone mineralization. Preventing calcitriol intoxication in these mice by dietary or genetic manipulations reveals that FGF-23 deletion impairs modulation of renal phosphate clearance in response to high-phosphate and low-phosphate diets. Other genetic manipulations, including disruption of FGF-23 glycosylation or inactivation of FGF-23 receptors, produce a similar effect.

When humans are fed high-phosphate or low-phosphate diets, their renal clearance of phosphate changes as described above. However, their blood levels of FGF-23 change less than expected, or sometimes not at all. Whether this discordance reflects the importance of other phosphatonins, or other variables, is not yet clear. It is also unclear whether serum inorganic phosphate regulates FGF-23 secretion and/or catabolism, because changes in serum inorganic phosphate are not consistently correlated with changes in serum FGF-23 levels. Although $1,25(OH)_2D$ can increase FGF-23 secretion and blood levels, other mechanisms must be more important regulators of serum FGF-23, because serum FGF-23 is poorly correlated with serum $1,25(OH)_2D$.

Calcitonin, Glucocorticoids, Thyroid Hormone, and Gonadal Steroids

PTH, vitamin D, and FGF-23 are the primary regulators of calcium and phosphate homeostasis, but several other endogenous hormones also have important effects on bone mineral metabolism. These hormones include calcitonin, glucocorticoids, thyroid hormone, estrogens, and androgens.

Calcitonin is important to calcium homeostasis in some animals but less important in humans. This hormone is a 32-amino acid peptide that is synthesized and released by parafollicular C cells of the thyroid gland in response to hypercalcemia. *Calcitonin binds directly to receptors on osteoclasts; this binding inhibits the resorptive activity of the osteoclasts and thereby decreases bone resorption and plasma calcium levels.* In adult humans, endogenous calcitonin has only weak effects on plasma calcium levels, and the elimination of calcitonin secretion after thyroidectomy generally causes no significant changes in plasma calcium levels. Nevertheless, exogenous calcitonin is useful in the emergency treatment of certain forms of hypercalcemia, as discussed below.

Pharmacologic doses of glucocorticoids promote osteocyte and osteoblast apoptosis and inhibit osteoblast maturation and osteoblast activity, thereby decreasing bone formation and, to a lesser extent, bone resorption. Chronic glucocorticoid use is a common cause of iatrogenic bone loss, osteoporosis, and fractures. When taking the history of a patient such as RS, it is important to determine whether she has ever taken glucocorticoids for months at a time, because this would be a significant risk factor for osteoporosis. Pharmacologic doses of glucocorticoids also decrease intestinal absorption of calcium and (at high doses) renal tubular reabsorption of calcium. The latter effects would tend to lower plasma calcium levels; however, glucocorticoid use is not associated with hypocalcemia or changes in blood PTH, presumably because glucocorticoid-induced bone loss releases compensating amounts of skeletal calcium.

Excess thyroid hormone also increases bone turnover. By stimulating bone resorption more than bone formation, prolonged high levels of thyroid hormone can cause bone loss. In fact, low bone mass is a common manifestation of hyperthyroidism. Therefore, the evaluation of RS's osteoporosis should include assessment of her thyroid status and measurement of her serum TSH level to rule out hyperthyroidism (see Chapter 28, Pharmacology of the Thyroid Gland).

Estrogens and androgens inhibit osteoclastic activity and thereby slow the rate of bone turnover and bone loss. Among other effects, these gonadal steroids inhibit the production of RANKL by immune cells and the production by osteoblasts of cytokines such as interleukin-6 that recruit and activate osteoclasts. Estrogen also has a pro-apoptotic effect on osteoclasts and an anti-apoptotic effect on osteoblasts and osteocytes. As described in more detail in Chapter 30, Pharmacology of Reproduction, estrogen exerts its actions principally by binding to the estrogen receptor (ER), which is a nuclear transcription factor. Binding of estrogen facilitates dimerization of the ER, allowing the estrogen–ER complex to recruit coactivator or corepressor molecules and bind to promoter regions of target genes. In this way, estrogen regulates the transcription of target genes encoding, for example, the cytokines that are important in bone turnover.

PATHOPHYSIOLOGY

Bone turnover, including repeated cycles of bone resorption and bone formation, is required to maintain the integrity of the skeleton. **Osteoporosis** and **chronic kidney disease** are two common disorders of bone mineral homeostasis. In osteoporosis, bone turnover is disrupted such that bone resorption exceeds bone formation. In chronic kidney disease, the pathophysiology involves a complex interplay between decreased mineral absorption and **secondary hyperparathyroidism**. A summary of these and related diseases of bone mineral homeostasis—including their mechanisms, clinical features, and treatments—is provided in Table 32-2.

Osteoporosis

Osteoporosis is a common condition in which bone mass is reduced and internal bone architecture is degraded throughout the skeleton due to decreased bone formation, increased bone resorption, or both. The reduced bone mass and architectural deterioration make the bones fragile and predisposes them to fractures after minimal trauma. RS's presentation is typical, with minimal trauma and a sudden twisting motion leading to subsequent back pain from a compression fracture in a lumbar vertebra.

Bone mineral density (BMD) measurements are the principal test used to determine fracture risk. The lower the BMD, the higher the risk of fracture. The mineral content of bones can be measured by their attenuation of x-rays and then adjusted for bone size by dividing the mineral content by the bone's projected two-dimensional area on a simultaneous radiograph. The resulting ratio, termed areal bone mineral density (**aBMD**), differs for different skeletal regions. To eliminate this variability, aBMD measurements are often expressed as standard deviations above or below the mean aBMD of that skeletal region in healthy young adults (T-score) or age-matched people (Z-score). Prospective observational studies have repeatedly shown that fracture incidence in women age 55 or older approximately doubles for every 1.0 standard deviation decrease in T-score. Similarly, aBMD, T-score, and Z-score predict an excised bone's resistance to destructive testing in vitro. Normal aBMD is defined as the mean value measured in healthy young adults $\pm$ 1.0 standard deviation; **osteopenia** is defined as aBMD values between 1.0 and 2.5 standard deviations below the mean for healthy young adults; and **osteoporosis** is defined as aBMD values 2.5 standard deviations or more below the mean for healthy young adults.

Peak bone mass is achieved in young adulthood and is determined by several factors, including dietary calcium, pubertal age, subsequent gonadal hormone status, physical activity, and the interplay of multiple genetic factors that are incompletely defined. *Once peak bone mass is attained, there is a very slow decline in bone mass during mid to late adult life.* This decline probably results from imperfections in the bone remodeling process: osteoblast-mediated bone formation does not fully keep pace with osteoclast-mediated bone resorption. Moreover, with age, osteoblasts have a reduced capacity to proliferate, to synthesize organic bone matrix, and to respond to growth factors. As a result, there is an average loss of 0.7% of bone mass per year, and this rate is accelerated in the years around menopause (Fig. 32-6).

Although the rate of bone remodeling increases in perimenopausal women, annual rates of bone loss do not change until such women are amenorrheic for intervals of 3 months or more (**late perimenopause**). At that time, the lower estrogen levels lead to an increase in osteoclast activity and bone turnover rate, which causes an imbalance between bone formation and bone resorption. The longer lifespan (decreased apoptosis) of osteoclasts in the absence of estrogen allows these cells to excavate deeper cavities in trabecular bone, leading to bone remodeling characterized by widely spaced and thin trabeculae with fewer interconnections. These remodeled trabeculae are structurally weaker in weight-bearing regions than the well-connected, closely spaced, thick trabeculae characteristic of bone in premenopausal women. In cortical bone, deeper cavities coalesce to form porous spaces. The lack of estrogen also leads to increased apoptosis of osteoblasts, rendering these cells unable to keep pace with the osteoclasts, and to increased apoptosis of osteocytes, impairing the mechanosensory network that detects microdamage and stimulates bone repair. Bone loss continues at the same rapid rate for several years after menses cease, after which the rate of annual bone loss decreases by about half. By then, however, the increased

TABLE 32-2 Diseases of Bone Mineral Homeostasis: Mechanisms, Clinical Features, and Treatments

DISEASE	MECHANISM	CLINICAL FEATURES	TREATMENT
Estrogen-deficiency bone loss	Bone resorption > formation	Low bone mass and bone strength	Calcium, vitamin D; selective estrogen receptor modulator (SERM); estrogen; bisphosphonates; RANKL antagonists; calcitonin
Osteoporosis	Bone resorption > formation	Low bone mass and bone strength, fragile bones	Calcium, vitamin D; SERM; estrogen; bisphosphonates; RANKL antagonists; daily subcutaneous parathyroid hormone (PTH); cathepsin K inhibitor (investigational); sclerostin antibodies (investigational)
Chronic kidney disease	↓ Excretion of phosphate ↓ Secretion of 1,25(OH)$_2$D Secondary ↑ PTH	Ectopic calcification, hypocalcemia, osteomalacia, osteitis fibrosa cystica	Phosphate restriction and binders; calcitriol or its analogues; calcimimetics
Hyperphosphatemia-hyperostosis syndrome (HHS), tumoral calcinosis with hyperphosphatemia	Mutant FGF-23 or GALNT3 or Klotho gene; ↓ excretion of phosphate	Ectopic dermal and/or periarticular calcification; hyperostoses	Phosphate restriction and binders
Vitamin D deficiency	Inadequate sunlight or diet	Child: bone deformity, pain, fragility Adult onset: bone pain, fragility	Calcium and vitamin D
D-dependent rickets, type I	Mutant 1-hydroxylase gene	Hypocalcemia, rickets	Calcitriol
D-dependent rickets, type II	Mutant calcitriol receptor	Hypocalcemia, rickets, alopecia	Calcitriol (megadose), intravenous calcium
Oncogenic osteomalacia	Hypersecretion of FGF-23	Elevated blood FGF-23, reduced or inappropriately normal 1,25(OH)$_2$D	Ablate tumor secreting FGF-23
Hypophosphatemia induced by saccharated ferric oxide	Iatrogenic hypersecretion of FGF-23	Elevated blood FGF-23, reduced or inappropriately normal 1,25(OH)$_2$D	Withdraw saccharated ferric oxide
X-linked hypophosphatemia (XLH)	Mutant PHEX protein	Rickets, hypophosphatemia, elevated blood FGF-23, reduced or inappropriately normal 1,25(OH)$_2$D	Neutral potassium phosphate, calcitriol; calcimimetics (investigational)
Autosomal dominant hypophosphatemic rickets (ADHR)	Mutant FGF-23 (degradation-resistant)	Rickets, hypophosphatemia, elevated blood FGF-23, reduced or inappropriately normal 1,25(OH)$_2$D	Neutral potassium phosphate, calcitriol; calcimimetics (investigational)
Autosomal recessive hypophosphatemia (ARHP)	Mutant DMP-1	Rickets, hypophosphatemia, elevated blood FGF-23, reduced or inappropriately normal 1,25(OH)$_2$D, large pulp chambers in teeth	Neutral potassium phosphate, calcitriol; calcimimetics (investigational)
Hypophosphatemic rickets with hypercalciuria (HHRH)	Mutant NaPi2c phosphate transporter or DMP-1	Rickets, hypophosphatemia, hypercalciuria, elevated blood FGF-23 and 1,25(OH)$_2$D, normal or low PTH	Neutral potassium phosphate
Primary hyperparathyroidism	Parathyroid tumor or parathyroid hyperplasia	Hypercalcemia, bone loss, bone pain, bone fragility, renal calculi	Bisphosphonate to stop bone loss; surgical removal; calcimimetics (investigational)
Familial hypocalciuric hypercalcemia (FHH)	Mutant (hypoactive) Ca^{2+}-sensing receptor	Hypercalcemia, hypocalciuria, hypermagnesemia	Observation
Pseudohypoparathyroidism, type 1	Mutant Gα_s; impaired PTH action	Hypocalcemia, seizures, tetany, short metacarpals/tarsals, short height	Calcitriol or megadose vitamin D
Hypoparathyroidism due to CaSR	Mutant (hyperactive) Ca^{2+}-sensing receptor	Low blood PTH, hypocalcemia, seizures, tetany	Calcitriol + chlorthalidone
Hypoparathyroidism	Parathyroid gland absence or decreased activity	Hypocalcemia, seizures, tetany	Calcitriol + chlorthalidone; subcutaneous parathyroid hormone (PTH)
Paget's disease	↑ Local bone turnover	Local bone pain and fragility, hearing loss, high-output heart failure	Bisphosphonates; calcitonin (rarely)

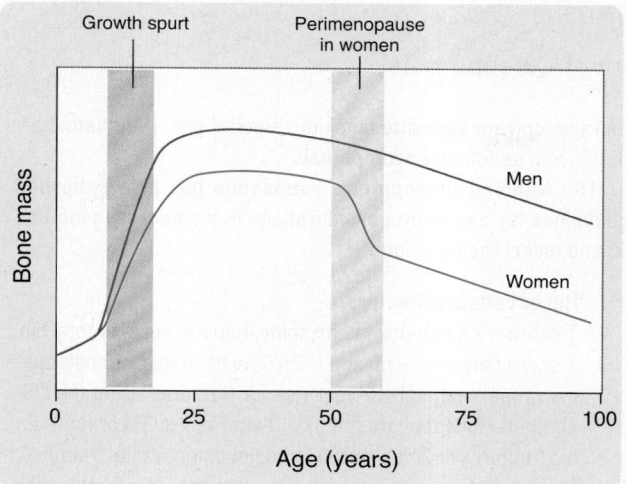

FIGURE 32-6. **Bone mass as a function of age.** In both men and women, bone mass increases with age until a peak is reached in young adulthood; the growth spurt begins earlier and peaks earlier in women compared to men (*not shown*). After the peak, bone mass gradually declines by approximately 0.7% per year. In women, the reduction in the frequency of menses coincides with a sharp decline in bone mass, as the decrease in estrogen production leads to increased bone resorption. As bone mass decreases with age, the skeleton may become sufficiently fragile that minor trauma can cause fractures. The goal of antiresorptive agents is to arrest or slow the loss of bone. In contrast, bone anabolic agents can be used to reverse bone loss that has already occurred and restore bone mass and bone structure.

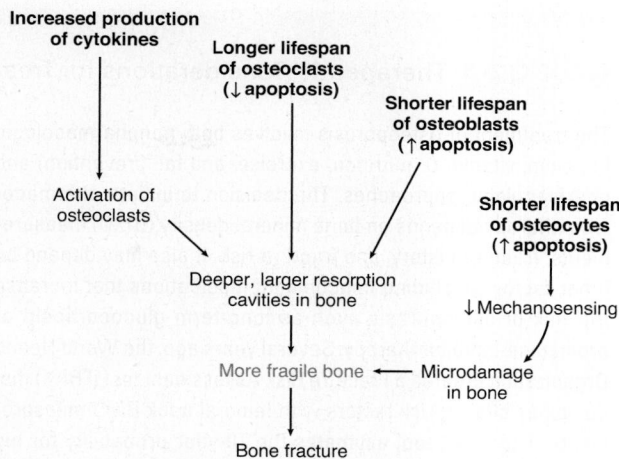

FIGURE 32-7. **Pathophysiologic basis of osteoporosis.** Several interrelated factors contribute to the development of osteoporosis. Many of these factors are activated by the decline in estrogen levels in perimenopausal women. Disinhibited production of cytokines and other regulatory molecules leads to the activation of osteoclasts. Decreased estrogen allows these osteoclasts to have a longer functional lifespan; conversely, the lack of estrogen promotes apoptosis in osteoblasts and osteocytes. The resulting imbalance between osteoclast and osteoblast activity leads to the formation of deep and large resorption cavities, which make the bone fragile and prone to fracture. The relative paucity of osteocytes impairs the mechanosensory network on which repair of microdamage in bone depends. Increased microdamage also predisposes to bone fragility and eventual fracture. Estrogen and raloxifene reverse this pathophysiologic sequence of events by suppressing cytokine production, promoting osteoclast apoptosis, and inhibiting osteoblast and osteocyte apoptosis (*not shown*).

bone resorption and accumulation of microdamage have increased bone fragility. Patient RS, for example, was diagnosed with osteoporosis about 6 years after completing menopause. In summary, the *bone of postmenopausal and late perimenopausal women is characterized by increased osteoclast activity and larger resorption cavities, increased but inadequate osteoblast activity, and impairment of the osteocyte mechanosensory network* (Fig. 32-7).

As discussed above, remodeling takes place to a greater degree in trabecular bone than in compact bone. Because appendicular bones contain trabecular bone only in their metaphyses while axial bones, such as the spine and pelvis, contain trabecular bone throughout, axial bones are more prone than appendicular bones to osteoporotic fractures. Within 25–35 years after menopause, women may lose as much as 35% of their cortical bone mass and as much as 50% of their trabecular bone mass. Therapeutic considerations regarding initiation of treatment for osteoporosis are discussed in Box 32-1.

Certain systemic illnesses and medications induce **secondary osteoporosis**. Common predisposing causes include thyrotoxicosis, hyperparathyroidism, high doses of glucocorticoids, aromatase inhibitor therapy for breast cancer in women, androgen-deprivation therapy for prostate cancer in men, smoking, alcohol abuse, intestinal malabsorption and maldigestion syndromes, cirrhosis, and bone marrow abnormalities. Secondary osteoporosis is best treated by correcting the underlying cause.

Chronic Kidney Disease

Chronic kidney disease causes **secondary hyperparathyroidism** (which enhances the resorption and formation of bone),

osteomalacia (an excess of unmineralized bone matrix), and **osteitis fibrosa cystica** (increased osteoclastic resorption and osteoblastic formation of bone and replacement of hematopoietic cells by bone marrow stromal cells). *Hyperparathyroidism in chronic kidney disease stems from the interplay of several factors, including hyperphosphatemia, increased blood FGF-23 levels, decreased production of $1,25(OH)_2$ vitamin D, and hypocalcemia* (Fig. 32-8). Each of these factors originates as the result of a decrease in renal function, manifested as an impairment in both renal synthetic ability [important for, among other processes, the 1α-hydroxylation step in $1,25(OH)_2$ vitamin D synthesis] and renal tubular function (important for phosphate excretion).

Inadequate levels of $1,25(OH)_2$ vitamin D lead to inadequate intestinal absorption of calcium. The resulting hypocalcemia stimulates synthesis and secretion and suppresses degradation of PTH in parathyroid cells. The low levels of $1,25(OH)_2D$ are also thought to cause a reduction in calcium receptor synthesis in the chief cells of the parathyroid gland. The decrease in calcium receptor number raises the set point for calcium regulation, so that a higher concentration of calcium is required to suppress PTH secretion. By this mechanism, hyperparathyroidism can persist even in the setting of hypercalcemia. In addition, evidence suggests that $1,25(OH)_2D$ normally suppresses both growth of the parathyroid gland and transcription of the PTH gene. Therefore, the deficiency of $1,25(OH)_2D$ in chronic kidney disease causes secondary hyperparathyroidism by several different mechanisms. This understanding has led to the development of several treatments for the metabolic sequelae of chronic kidney disease, including active vitamin D analogues—which bypass the requirement for 1α-hydroxylase activity in the kidney—and the calcimimetic cinacalcet—which adjusts the sensitivity of the calcium-sensing receptor on parathyroid chief cells (see below).

Hyperphosphatemia, resulting from decreased renal excretion of phosphate, further exacerbates the hypocalcemia of chronic kidney disease. Hyperphosphatemia induces hypocalcemia by altering the equilibrium for hydroxyapatite formation and dissolution, as described in Equation 32-1. Hyperphosphatemia also leads to the formation of toxic calcium phosphate precipitates in extraskeletal tissues, as in tumoral calcinosis; in addition, in chronic kidney disease, hyperphosphatemia stimulates increased secretion of FGF-23. Elevated blood FGF-23 suppresses renal secretion of $1,25(OH)_2D$ and has the toxic cardiovascular effects described above. Paradoxically, osteomalacia may coexist with ectopic calcium phosphate deposits because bone matrix does not mineralize normally. Metabolic acidosis due to chronic kidney disease is one factor that inhibits bone mineralization, and other mineralization inhibitors are also involved but are not yet adequately defined.

PHARMACOLOGIC CLASSES AND AGENTS

Significant advances have occurred in recent years in the treatment of osteoporosis and chronic kidney disease. For osteoporosis, the relevant pharmacologic agents can be divided into two main categories: *drugs that inhibit bone resorption (antiresorptive agents)* and *drugs that stimulate bone formation (anabolic agents)*. Antiresorptive agents consist of hormone replacement therapy (HRT), selective estrogen receptor modulators (SERMs), bisphosphonates, RANKL antagonists, calcitonin, and cathepsin K inhibitors (in development). Bone anabolic agents consist of fluoride and parathyroid hormone. For chronic kidney disease, the relevant pharmacologic agents include *drugs that lower plasma phosphate levels* (oral phosphate binders) and *drugs that decrease parathyroid hormone synthesis and secretion* (vitamin D, vitamin D analogues, and calcimimetics).

Oral calcium and vitamin D also have an important role in the prevention and treatment of osteoporosis, rickets, and hypoparathyroidism.

Antiresorptive Agents

Antiresorptive agents prevent or arrest bone loss by suppressing osteoclastic bone resorption. However, because bone resorption and bone formation are closely coupled processes, a decrease in one typically leads to a decrease in the other, via molecular mechanisms that remain to be elucidated. As a result, hormone replacement therapy (HRT), selective estrogen receptor modulators (SERMs), bisphosphonates, RANKL antagonists, and calcitonin induce little increase in bone tissue. The increase in bone mineral density seen during the first 12–18 months of therapy with these drugs represents filling of resorption cavities produced during the previous period of excessive bone resorption, mineralization of this new bone, and completion of mineralization (secondary mineralization) in old bone formed and partially mineralized during the 12–18 months preceding antiresorptive therapy. After the first 12–18 months of therapy with these agents, bone mineral density increases slowly, reflecting the slow formation and mineralization of new bone when resorption is suppressed. Cathepsin K inhibitors are an unusual exception, because they appear to suppress osteoclastic bone resorption without suppressing bone formation.

Hormone Replacement Therapy (HRT)

Estrogens reduce bone resorption by suppressing the transcription of genes coding for RANKL and cytokines such as IL-6 that induce osteoclast proliferation, differentiation, and activation. Estrogen also promotes apoptosis of osteoclasts while inhibiting apoptosis of osteoblasts and osteocytes. Estrogen decreases bone formation, as described above, but less so than more potent antiresorptive agents. Estrogen is usually administered with a progestational agent to reduce the risk of endometrial cancer in women with an intact uterus (see "Estrogens and Progestins" in Chapter 30). Estrogen also relieves postmenopausal hot flashes and vaginal dryness, and the primary indication for estrogen is the treatment of significant menopausal symptoms.

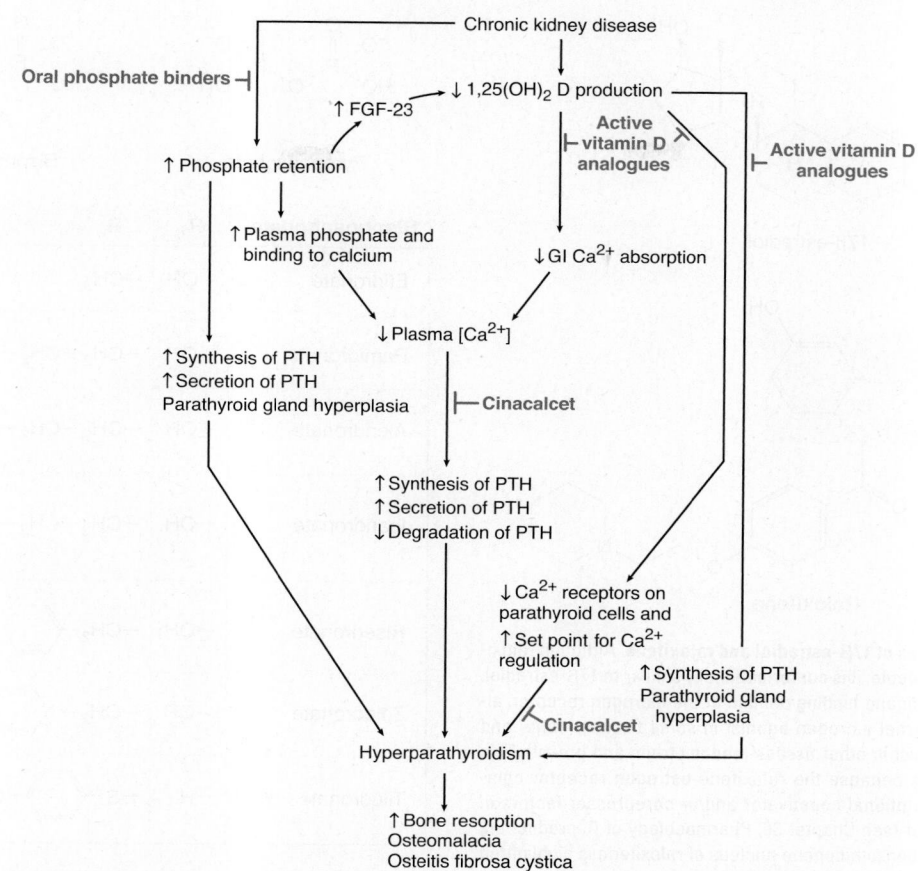

FIGURE 32-8. Pathophysiologic basis for osteomalacia and osteitis fibrosa cystica in chronic kidney disease. In chronic kidney disease, compromised renal function leads to decreased 1,25(OH)$_2$D synthesis and decreased phosphate excretion. The decrease in 1,25(OH)$_2$D causes decreased gastrointestinal (GI) absorption of Ca^{2+}, while the increased phosphate retention causes an increase in the levels of plasma phosphate, which complexes with Ca^{2+}. By these two mechanisms, chronic kidney disease leads to hypocalcemia. Hypocalcemia stimulates secretion of parathyroid hormone (PTH). Decreased levels of 1,25(OH)$_2$D stimulate PTH synthesis and parathyroid gland hyperplasia and lead to a decreased number of Ca^{2+} receptors on parathyroid gland chief cells and an elevated set point for Ca^{2+} regulation. Hyperphosphatemia may stimulate increased synthesis and secretion of PTH directly and also increase levels of FGF-23, leading to decreased levels of 1,25(OH)$_2$D. This combination of complex regulatory events leads to hyperparathyroidism, a syndrome characterized by increased bone resorption, increased amounts of unmineralized osteoid, and osteitis fibrosa cystica. Oral phosphate binders lower plasma phosphate levels by preventing dietary phosphate absorption. Active vitamin D analogues bypass the defect in renal 1α-hydroxylase activity that accompanies chronic kidney disease. Calcimimetics (cinacalcet) modulate the activity of the Ca^{2+}-sensing receptor on chief cells, such that the receptor is activated at lower plasma Ca^{2+} concentrations.

The adverse effects of estrogen can cause patients to discontinue treatment; these include vaginal bleeding and breast tenderness. HRT also increases the risk of venous thromboembolism, in part because oral estrogen promotes the hepatic synthesis of clotting factors. For many women, the greatest concern regarding HRT is the increased long-term risk of breast cancer, which is statistically significant. HRT was once commonly prescribed for postmenopausal osteoporosis, but in 2002, a large US government-sponsored study concluded that the increased risks of breast cancer and stroke outweigh the potential benefits of HRT on bone and other tissues. Because RS has two close relatives with breast cancer, she should strongly consider an alternative to HRT for treatment of her osteoporosis.

Selective Estrogen Receptor Modulators

Selective estrogen receptor modulators (SERMs) are a group of compounds that bind to the estrogen receptor (ER) and have tissue-selective effects on the target organs of estrogen. Depending on the tissue, a SERM is capable of acting as an estrogen agonist or an estrogen antagonist. These tissue-selective effects occur because, in different tissues, SERM–ER complexes bind different tissue-specific hormone response elements and/or different tissue-selective transcriptional corepressors and coactivators (see Chapter 30).

The goal of SERM development is to retain the beneficial effects of estrogen in one or more tissues while eliminating the undesirable effects of estrogen in other tissues. **Raloxifene**, for example, is an estrogen agonist in bone but an estrogen antagonist in the endometrium and breast (Fig. 32-9; see also Fig. 30-7). Raloxifene is approved for prevention and treatment of osteoporosis because it increases vertebral and nonvertebral bone mineral density and decreases vertebral fractures. Raloxifene is also approved for reduction in risk of invasive breast cancer in women with postmenopausal osteoporosis and in postmenopausal women at high risk for invasive breast cancer. Raloxifene lowers low-density lipoprotein (LDL) cholesterol levels slightly but neither increases nor decreases the incidence of heart disease in postmenopausal women. Like estrogen, and to the same extent, raloxifene

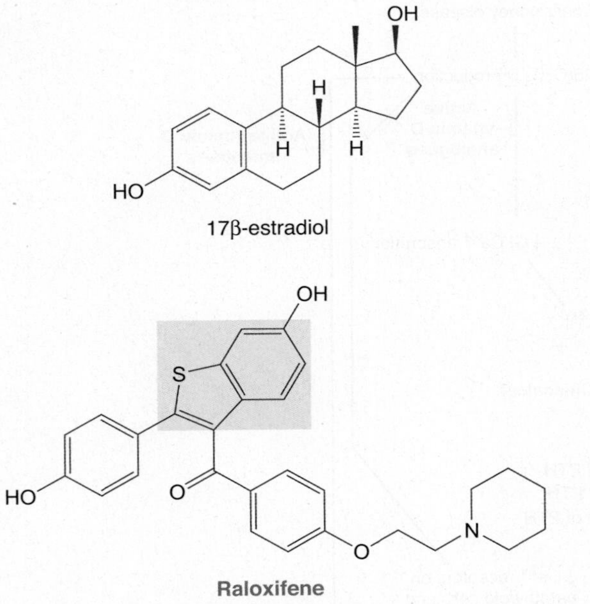

FIGURE 32-9. Structures of 17β-estradiol and raloxifene. Although raloxifene is not a steroid molecule, it is conformationally similar to 17β-estradiol. Raloxifene binds to the ligand binding domain of the estrogen receptor, allowing it to act as a partial estrogen agonist in some tissues (bone) and as an estrogen antagonist in other tissues (endometrium and breast). This selective action occurs because the raloxifene-estrogen receptor complex can recruit transcriptional coactivator and/or corepressor factors in a tissue-specific manner (see Chapter 30, Pharmacology of Reproduction, for further details). The benzothiophene nucleus of raloxifene is highlighted in a *blue box*.

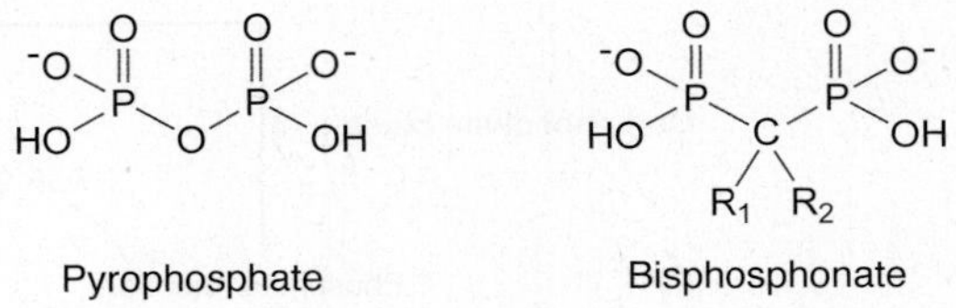

Bisphosphonate	R₁	R₂
Etidronate	—OH	—CH₃
Pamidronate	—OH	—CH₂—CH₂—NH₂
Alendronate	—OH	—CH₂—CH₂—CH₂—NH₂
Ibandronate	—OH	—CH₂—CH₂—N(CH₃)((CH₂)₄—CH₃)
Risedronate	—OH	—CH₂—(pyridine)
Zoledronate	—OH	—CH₂—(imidazole)
Tiludronate	—H	—S—(phenyl)—Cl

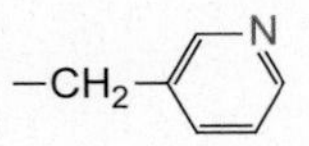

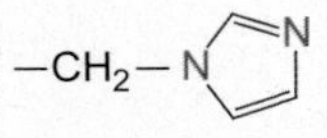

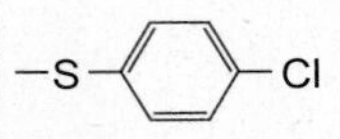

FIGURE 32-10. Structures of pyrophosphate and various bisphosphonates. Note that the P-O-P structure of pyrophosphate is replaced with a P-C-P structure in bisphosphonate. This motif is conserved across the marketed bisphosphonates. The R₁ and R₂ side chains of bisphosphonates differ from one drug to another: side chains containing a nitrogen atom have higher potency, and substitution of a hydroxyl group for a hydrogen atom at R₁ enhances skeletal retention of the drug.

increases the risk of venous thrombosis and pulmonary embolism. *Raloxifene may be the preferred therapy for preventing osteoporosis in women with breast cancer or women with a family history of breast cancer.* Because of her family history of breast cancer, RS could potentially benefit from raloxifene. However, in adequately powered studies raloxifene does not reduce nonvertebral fractures and may therefore not be sufficiently potent to protect RS, who has already had a vertebral fracture and therefore has an increased risk of one or more nonvertebral fractures in the next 3–5 years, including an increased risk of hip fracture.

Bisphosphonates

Bisphosphonates (BPs), currently the most widely used class of antiresorptive drugs, are analogues of pyrophosphate in which the readily hydrolyzable P-O-P bond is replaced by a nonhydrolyzable P-C-P bond. Five widely used bisphosphonates (the so-called amino-bisphosphonates)—**alendronate**, **risedronate**, **ibandronate**, **pamidronate**, and **zoledronate**—have a nitrogen-containing amino, pyridine, or imidazole moiety in the side chain, which greatly enhances their antiresorptive activity (Fig. 32-10).

Because the oxygen atoms in the phosphonate groups coordinate with divalent cations such as calcium, BPs concentrate in mineralized tissues, where they are incorporated into the mineral and remain unmetabolized and biologically active. Once the bone is subsequently resorbed, the acids secreted by osteoclasts dissociate the bone mineral from the BP, which is then excreted or deposited elsewhere in the skeleton or internalized by the osteoclasts. Within osteoclasts,

the amino-bisphosphonates block a step in the **mevalonate pathway**. Disruption of this process decreases prenylation, the covalent attachment of certain lipids (farnesyl and geranylgeranyl moieties) to multiple proteins, including intracellular regulatory proteins such as GTPases. This, in turn, impairs several osteoclastic functions (e.g., H⁺-ATPase activity) and ultimately causes osteoclast apoptosis. BPs appear to inhibit the mevalonate pathway only in osteoclasts, in part because osteoclastic bone resorption greatly increases the concentration of BPs near osteoclasts, and perhaps because the acidic milieu beneath active osteoclasts protonates BPs and thereby facilitates their diffusion across the osteoclast cell membrane.

Intravenous pamidronate and zoledronate rapidly inhibit accelerated bone resorption caused by osteoclast hyperactivity, and these agents are approved for treatment of **hypercalcemia associated with malignancy**. This includes malignancies involving the bone marrow, malignancies metastatic to bone, and malignancies that secrete parathyroid hormone or parathyroid hormone-related peptide (PTHrP). PTHrP is a peptide structurally and functionally similar to PTH, and it causes hypercalcemia by the same mechanisms as PTH. BPs are ineffective in treating hypercalcemia caused by intestinal hyperabsorption of calcium or hypercalcemia caused by impaired renal excretion of calcium (see Box 32-2). Some malignancies (e.g., certain lymphomas and some breast carcinomas) cause hypercalcemia by hypersecreting calcitriol. In such instances, intravenous bisphosphonates are less effective because the malignancy-associated hypercalcemia results from increased absorption of dietary calcium in addition to increased resorption of bone. Similarly, several randomized, double-blind, prospective clinical trials have shown that, although daily or weekly oral alendronate arrests bone loss and increases BMD in patients with mild primary hyperparathyroidism, it does not lower their plasma calcium levels.

Neither oral nor intravenous bisphosphonates are approved for treatment of hypercalcemia due to nonmalignant conditions, but intravenous bisphosphonates are effective therapy if hypercalcemia is caused by increased bone resorption (e.g., resorption associated with prolonged immobilization or paralysis, vitamin A intoxication, hyperthyroidism, or primary hyperparathyroidism with low-calcium diet). Although intravenous ibandronate is not approved for treatment of hypercalcemia, this agent has corrected hypercalcemia caused by increased bone resorption (with or without associated malignancy) in several randomized, double-blind, prospective clinical trials.

Intravenous pamidronate and zoledronate also reduce skeletal complications (bone pain and fractures) in patients with osteolysis caused by bone metastases or multiple myeloma, and both agents are approved for this use. Intravenous bisphosphonates are not approved for this use in patients with other bone marrow malignancies (e.g., leukemia, lymphomas)

BOX 32-2 Treatment of Hypercalcemia and Hypocalcemia

Hypercalcemia and Its Treatment

Hypercalcemia is most commonly treated by one or more of three different approaches: decreasing intestinal calcium absorption, increasing renal calcium excretion, and inhibiting bone resorption.

Emergency treatment of severe hypercalcemia starts with **saline diuresis**. In this treatment, intravenous saline is administered together with a loop diuretic that increases renal calcium excretion, such as furosemide. Calcium reabsorption in the kidney is, in part, passive, driven by the electrochemical gradient associated with sodium reabsorption. By inhibiting sodium reabsorption, loop diuretics decrease calcium reabsorption and, thus, increase renal calcium excretion. Saline diuresis is very effective at rapidly reducing elevated plasma calcium levels. The saline infusion also rehydrates the patient and ensures adequate renal filtration. Hypercalcemia can also be treated rapidly with **calcitonin**. As noted in the text, this agent decreases plasma calcium levels by inhibiting osteoclastic activity. The hypocalcemic effects of calcitonin are rapid but limited in duration because tachyphylaxis develops within several days. The addition of a glucocorticoid can briefly delay tachyphylaxis.

Granulomatous diseases, such as tuberculosis, sarcoidosis, and many others, can cause hypercalcemia because of excessive ectopic calcitriol production by activated mononuclear cells. The resulting increase in calcium absorption by the GI tract can be countered by eliminating dairy products and calcium-fortified orange juice and other calcium-rich foods from the diet and blunted by the administration of **oral phosphate**, which forms insoluble complexes with dietary calcium and thereby decreases calcium absorption. Glucocorticoids (most commonly, prednisone) effectively decrease the ectopic production of calcitriol and accelerate its catabolism. Some malignancies (especially certain lymphomas) cause hypercalcemia because of excessive ectopic calcitriol production, which is treated similarly.

The hypercalcemia of most malignancies (e.g., cancer in the bone marrow or metastatic to bone) is treated by increasing renal calcium excretion and inhibiting bone resorption. Long-term management of such hypercalcemia can be achieved by using intravenous **bisphosphonates (BPs)**. These agents, like calcitonin, lower plasma calcium by inhibiting osteoclastic activity. Unlike calcitonin, BPs do not induce tachyphylaxis. Several BPs are effective for this purpose, but pamidronate and zoledronate are most often used in the United States. Severe or symptomatic acute hypercalcemia (plasma calcium level ≥ 12 mg/dL) is generally treated with a combination of all three of the above approaches: saline diuresis with furosemide, calcitonin, and a bisphosphonate. The first two agents are typically effective within the first 24 hours; bisphosphonates are typically effective by the third day and may also have a prolonged effect.

Hypocalcemia and Its Treatment

Treatment of hypocalcemia depends on the etiology and the severity of the symptoms. Intravenous calcium gluconate should be used for (1) patients with severe symptoms (e.g., carpopedal spasm, tetany, seizures, and/or prolonged QT interval), (2) asymptomatic patients with an acute decrease in plasma calcium levels, and (3) patients with a corrected plasma calcium level of 7.5 mg/dL or lower. Patients with mild symptoms (e.g., tingling or circumoral paresthesias) may be able to be managed with oral calcium and vitamin D. Hypocalcemia can be caused by hypomagnesemia (which is typically due to severe GI or renal loss of magnesium) as a result of target-organ resistance to PTH and a decrease in PTH secretion. In the setting of hypomagnesemia, hypocalcemia is difficult to correct until the plasma magnesium level is normalized. Patients with minimal to no symptoms may be treated with oral magnesium preparations (e.g., sustained-release **magnesium chloride** or oral magnesium oxide), although diarrhea may be a limiting factor. For patients with severe symptoms (e.g., tetany, arrhythmias, and/or seizures) or with very low plasma magnesium concentrations, intravenous magnesium sulfate may be necessary. Ultimately, as the plasma magnesium level increases, an increase in the plasma calcium level follows. When the plasma magnesium concentration is normal (provided that the underlying etiology for hypomagnesemia is resolved), the treatment of hypocalcemia consists principally of oral calcium and vitamin D (either calcitriol or ergocalciferol), supplemented if necessary by chlorthalidone to lower renal clearance of calcium. ■

but are widely used for this purpose despite the lack of proven efficacy in these other illnesses.

Oral alendronate and risedronate and intravenous pamidronate and zoledronate decrease bone turnover and bone pain in patients with Paget's disease and accelerate radiographic healing of the lytic bone lesions and cortical bone fissures characteristic of Paget's disease. All four bisphosphonates are approved for treatment of Paget's disease that is symptomatic, associated with a high risk of complications (fracture, paralysis, and heart failure), or associated with a serum alkaline phosphatase level at least double the upper limit of normal. Paget's disease of bone that is widespread or associated with very severe osteolysis and/or very high serum alkaline phosphatase levels usually requires intravenous zoledronate, but milder Paget's disease can usually be controlled by any of these four bisphosphonates.

Randomized, double-blind, prospective clinical trials have also shown that BPs decrease bone resorption and prevent or arrest bone loss in patients with hyperthyroidism of all types and in skeletal regions immobilized by paraplegia, tetraplegia, hemiplegia, Guillain-Barré syndrome, etc., but no BP is approved for such uses.

In well-controlled clinical trials, oral alendronate, risedronate, and ibandronate and intravenous ibandronate and zoledronate suppress bone resorption, arrest bone loss, and slightly increase spine and hip BMD in postmenopausal women, and all are approved for osteoporosis prevention and treatment in this population. In postmenopausal women, all four of these BPs decrease the risk of new vertebral fractures, and three of the four (all except for ibandronate in the marketed dose) reduce nonvertebral fractures and hip fractures. Therefore, a BP would be a reasonable therapeutic option for RS, but ibandronate is not sufficiently potent because she is at significant risk of nonvertebral fractures. Generic alendronate is the least expensive choice.

BPs also suppress bone resorption, arrest bone loss, and slightly increase spine and hip BMD in women with most other forms of hypogonadism (e.g., iatrogenic estrogen deficiency due to chemotherapy or aromatase inhibitors, or pituitary insufficiency) but are not approved for such uses. Oral alendronate and risedronate and intravenous zoledronate also suppress bone resorption, arrest bone loss, and slightly increase spine and hip BMD in men with idiopathic or hypogonadal low BMD and are approved for such use. Ibandronate is not approved for prevention or arrest of bone loss in men. Oral alendronate and risedronate and intravenous zoledronate are approved for prevention or arrest of bone loss in patients of either sex taking chronic glucocorticoids in doses >7.5 mg prednisone-equivalent per day.

Because of poor intestinal absorption, oral BPs must be swallowed in the morning after an overnight fast, and the patient must swallow nothing but water with the bisphosphonate and for the subsequent 30–60 minutes. Only thereafter can the patient swallow other medications, other liquids, or food. Oral BPs can cause local esophagitis and esophageal erosion; for this reason, patients are advised to swallow bisphosphonates with at least 8 ounces (250 cc) of water and sit upright or stand for the next 30–60 minutes. Oral BPs are contraindicated in patients with delayed esophageal emptying. Intravenous BPs, especially pamidronate or zoledronate, can cause acute renal failure or hepatitis, but this is rare. Renal impairment is less likely if the BP is infused slowly (e.g., zoledronate over 15 minutes or longer and pamidronate

over several hours). All bisphosphonates are excreted by glomerular filtration. When renal function is impaired, the dose of intravenous and oral BP must be reduced or withheld accordingly. No bisphosphonate is approved for use in patients with calculated glomerular filtration rate (GFR) <30–35 mL/min, and all BPs are contraindicated in patients with low plasma ionized calcium levels (measured or estimated by adjustment for the simultaneous plasma albumin level).

Amino-bisphosphonates have been used to treat Paget's disease of bone for more than 20 years and widely used to treat osteoporosis for more than 17 years. Serious adverse effects are rare, but BPs are not metabolizable, and pharmacologically active BP accumulates progressively in the skeleton during chronic therapy. It is unclear whether this is therapeutically desirable (because it prevents bone resorption) or therapeutically undesirable. Prolonged inhibition of bone turnover can prevent repair of the microscopic cracks that normally develop in bone because of repetitive mechanical loads. The accumulation and coalescence of such cracks could, in theory, eventually reduce bone toughness and cause a late increase in fractures among patients treated for many years with potent bisphosphonates. Stopping BPs temporarily or permanently after 5–10 years may be appropriate for certain individuals. In one study in alendronate-treated women, alendronate was randomly withdrawn or continued after their first 5 years of alendronate use. During the next 5 years, symptomatic new spine fractures occurred more frequently in the women randomly allocated to stop alendronate after 5 years. At the end of 10 years, however, there was no difference in morphometric fractures between the two groups.

Occasional patients treated chronically with bisphosphonates develop oversuppression of bone resorption (manifested as subnormal serum and/or urine indices of bone collagenolysis) or complete suppression of new bone formation (as indicated by no new bone formation in bone biopsies taken after in vivo tetracycline labeling). The latter finding is typical of patients who develop a nonhealing stress fracture or an atypical femoral shaft fracture during chronic bisphosphonate therapy, but it is not yet clear whether such findings represent BP overdosage or impaired bone formation intrinsic to these occasional patients. For example, many such patients are taking glucocorticoids chronically for other illnesses.

It is now recognized that some patients taking potent bisphosphonates develop necrotizing osteomyelitis of the alveolar ridge (osteonecrosis of the jaw) after oral surgery. This occurs occasionally in patients taking intravenous bisphosphonates chronically to control hypercalcemia or other skeletal complications of malignancy but occurs rarely in patients taking intravenous or oral bisphosphonates chronically for osteoporosis. The BP doses used to treat patients with cancer are typically 9–10 times higher than those used to treat patients with osteoporosis. In addition, many patients with cancer have increased susceptibility to infection because of chemotherapy, reduced food intake, and other manifestations of widespread malignancy.

RANKL Antagonists

Denosumab is a synthetic, fully humanized monoclonal antibody directed against RANKL that reduces osteoclast numbers and bone resorption in humans and animal models of osteoporosis. Denosumab suppresses bone resorption, arrests bone loss, and slightly increases spine and hip BMD. These results have been observed in multiple patient populations, including women with postmenopausal osteoporosis, women with iatrogenic estrogen deficiency due to aromatase inhibitors, men with idiopathic or hypogonadal osteoporosis, and men with iatrogenic hypogonadism caused by prostate cancer therapy.

Denosumab is approved in a dose of 60 mg subcutaneously every 6 months. With this dosing regimen, it is approved (1) for treatment of women with postmenopausal osteoporosis who are at high risk for fracture, (2) to increase bone mass in men with osteoporosis, (3) to increase bone mass in men with non-metastatic prostate cancer receiving androgen deprivation therapy, and (4) in women receiving adjuvant aromatase inhibitor therapy for breast cancer who are at high risk for fracture.

Denosumab also reduces bone resorption and skeletal complications in patients with malignancies metastatic to bone or involving bone marrow. It is approved in a different dosing regimen, 120 mg every 4 weeks, for prevention of skeletal-related events in patients with bone metastases from solid tumors. Denosumab also reduces bone resorption in patients with rheumatoid arthritis; it is not yet clear whether denosumab increases bone mass or reduces skeletal complications in this disease. The effects of denosumab on hypercalcemia and Paget's disease of bone are not yet clear. Recent studies have reported osteonecrosis of the jaw and atypical femur fractures with denosumab, although these adverse effects are very rare.

Calcitonin

As discussed above, calcitonin binds to and activates a G protein-coupled receptor on osteoclasts, thereby decreasing the resorptive activity of these cells. Because of this action, exogenous calcitonin can be used to treat conditions characterized by high osteoclastic activity, such as certain forms of hypercalcemia, Paget's disease of bone, and postmenopausal osteoporosis.

The synthetic calcitonin marketed in the United States has an amino acid sequence native to salmon because that peptide has a higher affinity for the human calcitonin receptor and a longer half-life than human calcitonin. Salmon calcitonin is a peptide and therefore is administered subcutaneously (for Paget's disease and hypercalcemia) or as a nasal spray (for postmenopausal osteoporosis). Twice-daily subcutaneous injections are useful in the rapid treatment of severe hypercalcemia (see Box 32-2). An important drawback to long-term calcitonin administration is the tachyphylaxis that can result from desensitization of the receptor-signaling pathway. For the treatment of hypercalcemia, short-term administration of glucocorticoids can delay the onset of tachyphylaxis. Clinical trials in patients with Paget's disease show that once-daily subcutaneous salmon calcitonin reduces bone turnover and bone pain and accelerates radiographic healing of osteolytic lesions. However, bisphosphonates have greater therapeutic efficacy than calcitonin for treatment of Paget's disease, particularly when the Paget's disease is severe.

Once-daily intranasal salmon calcitonin slows vertebral bone loss inconsistently in women who are less than 5 years postmenopausal (and therefore losing bone rapidly). In older women with postmenopausal osteoporosis, it reduces spine fractures inconsistently, fails to reduce nonspine fractures, and has inconsistent analgesic properties.

Because of its low efficacy, intranasal salmon calcitonin is not a good therapeutic option for RS. It may be useful in women at least 5 years postmenopausal who are unable or unwilling to take any of the more effective alternatives (e.g., raloxifene, estrogen, bisphosphonates, RANKL inhibitors, or teriparatide). However, there have been recent reports suggesting an increased incidence of cancer with calcitonin use.

Bone Anabolic Agents

Antiresorptive agents slow the rate of bone loss but do not build new bone. For patients who have already lost a large amount of bone mass (BMD more than 3.0 standard deviations below normal) or who have experienced one or more osteoporotic fragility fractures, antiresorptive agents are not optimal therapies. This realization has led to the development of bone anabolic agents, which are drugs that actually increase bone mass and bone strength, not just prevent its loss.

Fluoride

The first bone anabolic agent was fluoride, in doses substantially higher than those ingested in artificially fluoridated water. At such doses, fluoride is a mitogen for osteoblasts and it increases trabecular bone mass while accelerating cortical bone loss. Use of fluoride, however, leads to the conversion of hydroxyapatite to fluoroapatite, which is denser and more brittle. It is unclear whether fluoride prevents vertebral or nonvertebral fractures: studies to date have shown inconsistent results and fluoride is not approved to treat osteoporosis.

Parathyroid Hormone

As noted above, a persistently elevated plasma concentration of PTH, such as occurs in hyperparathyroidism, leads to increased bone remodeling, with more bone resorbed than formed. As a result, bone can become weak and susceptible to fracture and osteitis fibrosa cystica. In contrast, although intermittent exposure of bone cells to PTH also increases bone remodeling, more new bone is formed than old bone resorbed. Thus, *once-daily subcutaneous administration of PTH favors bone anabolism, while continuous exposure to PTH favors bone resorption.*

Native PTH is an 84-amino acid peptide, but N-terminal fragments containing the first 31–34 amino acids of PTH retain essentially all the important functional properties of the native protein. The 1–34 fragment has been shown in clinical trials to act as a powerful anabolic agent that builds new bone. Because **PTH(1–34)** is a peptide, the bioavailability of this agent is close to zero when administered orally. The currently available formulation is a subcutaneous injection that is designed to be self-administered. Alternative dosage forms (e.g., transcutaneous) are in advanced stages of clinical development.

Human PTH(1–34) is approved under the generic name **teriparatide** for the treatment of osteoporosis in postmenopausal women, idiopathic and hypogonadal osteoporosis in men, and glucocorticoid-induced osteoporosis in patients of either sex, and approved for the reduction of spine and nonspine fractures in postmenopausal osteoporotic women at high risk of fracture. Full-length human PTH(1–84) is approved for such uses in some countries but not in the United States (because of hypercalcemia and other adverse effects from the marketed dose). Because prolonged treatment of rodents with either of these peptides causes dramatic bone overgrowth followed by osteosarcomas, teriparatide is used only in patients at high risk of fractures. However, there is no evidence that any parathyroid hormone increases osteosarcomas in humans, and the drug has been approved and available for over 12 years. In humans, the anabolic skeletal effects of teriparatide are attenuated by concomitant alendronate therapy. It is unclear whether concomitant therapy with other bisphosphonates, or prior therapy with any bisphosphonate, does the same.

Treatment of Secondary Hyperparathyroidism in Chronic Kidney Disease

Three pharmacologic approaches are currently available to prevent and modify the metabolic sequelae of chronic kidney disease—oral phosphate binders, calcitriol and its analogues, and calcimimetics.

Oral Phosphate Binders

In patients with chronic kidney disease, or chronic hyperphosphatemia of any cause, the increased plasma phosphate can complex with circulating calcium. The resulting decrease in plasma calcium concentration can lead to hyperparathyroidism, and the precipitation of calcium phosphate in extraskeletal tissues can impair their function. Dietary phosphate restriction and oral phosphate binders can limit both processes.

Aluminum hydroxide was one of the first agents used to treat hyperphosphatemia. Aluminum precipitates phosphate in the gastrointestinal tract, forming nonabsorbable complexes. Although effective at lowering plasma phosphate levels, this approach has been abandoned (except in cases of refractory hyperphosphatemia) because of aluminum toxicity: over the course of years, chronic use of aluminum-based phosphate binders can lead to chronic anemia, osteomalacia, and neurotoxicity.

Oral preparations of **calcium carbonate** and **calcium acetate** can control plasma phosphate. These agents, when administered with meals, bind to dietary phosphate and thereby inhibit its absorption. At the doses required for phosphate binding, however, these agents can also cause iatrogenic hypercalcemia and may increase the risk of vascular calcification.

Sevelamer is a nonabsorbable cationic ion-exchange resin that binds intestinal phosphate, thereby decreasing the absorption of dietary phosphate. Sevelamer also binds bile acids, leading to interruption of the enterohepatic circulation and to decreased cholesterol absorption. Its principal disadvantage is its expense. Sevelamer is used to treat hyperphosphatemia in patients with chronic kidney disease. Sevelamer is also used to correct hyperphosphatemia in patients with the hyperphosphatemia-hyperostosis syndrome (also known as *tumoral calcinosis with hyperphosphatemia*), who are deficient in FGF-23 secretion or action (Table 32-2).

Calcitriol and Its Analogues

Because impaired synthesis of 1α-vitamin D derivatives is one of the main homeostatic disturbances leading to secondary hyperparathyroidism in chronic kidney disease, vitamin D is a logical replacement therapy in this disease. Three active (i.e., 1α-hydroxylated) vitamin D congeners are approved for treatment of secondary hyperparathyroidism. *All of these agents bypass the need for 1α-hydroxylation in the kidney and are therefore useful in the treatment of bone diseases that complicate renal failure.* Active vitamin D increases dietary absorption of calcium, and the resulting increase in plasma calcium level suppresses the secretion of PTH by chief cells of the parathyroid gland. In addition, these agents bind to and activate vitamin D receptors on the chief cells and thereby suppress PTH gene transcription and parathyroid hyperplasia. Care should be taken to avoid hypercalcemia when administering any of the active vitamin D congeners.

Calcitriol [$1,25(OH)_2D_3$] is the dihydroxylated form of vitamin D_3. Calcitriol is available in oral and intravenous forms; some data suggest that the intravenous formulation may be more effective in patients on hemodialysis. Calcitriol should not be administered to patients with chronic kidney disease until hyperphosphatemia has been controlled with diet and/or drugs, because the addition of calcitriol can cause increased plasma levels of both calcium and phosphate.

Paricalcitol [$19\text{-nor-}1,25(OH)_2D_2$] is a synthetic analogue of vitamin D. **Doxercalciferol** [$1\alpha\text{-}(OH)D_2$] is the 1α-hydroxylated form of vitamin D_2; it is 25-hydroxylated to the fully active 1,25-dihydroxy form in the liver. Both paricalcitol and doxercalciferol may lower plasma PTH levels without significantly raising plasma calcium levels.

Calcimimetics

Although vitamin D and its analogues can be effective in the treatment of secondary hyperparathyroidism, these agents can also lead to unwanted hypercalcemia and hyperphosphatemia. The so-called calcimimetics—agents that modulate the activity of the calcium-sensing receptor on chief cells—are effective treatments for hyperparathyroidism that do not cause these unwanted effects. **Cinacalcet**, the first US Food and Drug Administration (FDA)-approved calcimimetic, binds to the transmembrane region of the calcium-sensing receptor and thereby modulates receptor activity by increasing its sensitivity to calcium. Because the cinacalcet-bound receptor is activated at lower calcium concentrations, PTH synthesis and secretion are also suppressed at lower calcium concentrations. As diagrammed in Figure 32-8, these effects interrupt the pathophysiologic sequence of events leading from chronic kidney disease to secondary hyperparathyroidism. Cinacalcet is approved for treatment of secondary hyperparathyroidism in patients with chronic kidney disease on dialysis and for treatment of hypercalcemia associated with parathyroid carcinoma. It is also approved for treatment of severe hypercalcemia in patients with primary hyperparathyroidism who are unable to undergo parathyroid surgery. Unexpectedly, cinacalcet does not arrest or reverse bone loss in patients with either hyperparathyroidism or parathyroid carcinoma, for unclear reasons.

Calcium, Inorganic Phosphate, and Vitamin D

Calcium

Oral calcium has both therapeutic and prophylactic utility. It is administered as a therapy for hypocalcemic states associated with disorders such as vitamin D-dependent rickets and hypoparathyroidism. In severe cases of hypocalcemia, calcium can be administered intravenously. Commonly used intravenous formulations include **calcium gluconate** and **calcium chloride**. Calcium gluconate is preferable because it produces less tissue irritation if extravasated.

To prevent osteoporosis or treat mild hypocalcemia, calcium is typically administered orally as **calcium citrate** or **calcium carbonate**, although some other preparations are sometimes used. Calcium citrate is the more readily absorbed form, but calcium carbonate is the more widely used because of its lower cost, higher ratio of calcium to total weight, wide availability (e.g., Tums®), and antacid properties. Calcium carbonate should be taken with meals. Since calcium carbonate requires gastric acid for absorption, while calcium citrate does not, calcium citrate should be used in patients receiving proton pump inhibitor therapy. Dietary calcium supplementation has been shown in clinical trials to reduce vertebral bone loss modestly in postmenopausal women, although its effects on fracture prevention are less clear. If RS had taken calcium regularly after menopause and during late perimenopause, her vertebral bone loss might have slowed, reducing her risk of a spine fracture. She should now be counseled to take daily calcium (and vitamin D) supplementation as a component of her therapy for osteoporosis. In women over age 50, the total calcium intake (food + supplement) should not exceed 1,100–1,200 mg calcium per day.

Inorganic Phosphate

Inorganic phosphate is administered as a therapy for hypophosphatemia caused by renal phosphate wasting, intestinal phosphate malabsorption, rapid bone remineralization, sepsis, or other disorders. Commonly used preparations are neutral potassium phosphate and neutral sodium phosphate. The potassium salt is usually preferred because sodium can increase renal phosphate clearance by expanding extracellular fluid volume. "Neutral" refers to the pH of the salt when dissolved (acidic salts of inorganic phosphate complicate treatment undesirably). The ratio of phosphate to total weight varies by preparation, so inorganic phosphate should be prescribed by millimoles, not by weight. If hypophosphatemia is severe, potassium phosphate or sodium phosphate can be administered intravenously with careful monitoring of plasma calcium levels. Oral phosphate overdosage causes diarrhea; intravenous phosphate overdosage causes hypocalcemia (see above).

Vitamin D

Vitamin D preparations include **cholecalciferol** (vitamin D_3), **ergocalciferol** (vitamin D_2), **calcifediol** [25(OH)D], and **calcitriol** [1,25(OH)$_2$D$_3$] (Fig. 32-5). Several synthetic vitamin D analogues are also available, as noted above.

Vitamin D is used in the treatment of hypoparathyroidism, rickets, osteomalacia, osteoporosis, and chronic kidney disease. Calcitriol is preferred because of its faster onset and offset (12 hours) and faster approach to steady state (72–96 hours). Because vitamin D increases both plasma calcium and plasma phosphate, the plasma levels of these minerals should be monitored carefully.

In the case of *hypoparathyroidism*, calcitriol is used to increase intestinal absorption of calcium; concomitantly, a thiazide diuretic (preferably chlorthalidone because of its prolonged action) is used to lower renal clearance of calcium. Once the plasma calcium level is normal, renal clearance of phosphate usually increases enough to lower plasma inorganic phosphate levels to normal. If not, oral phosphate binders should be added. Once plasma calcium and inorganic phosphate levels are near normal, urinary calcium excretion must be checked to guard against hypercalciuria.

For type I *vitamin D-dependent rickets* (Table 32-2), calcitriol is used. Type II vitamin D-dependent rickets (Table 32-2) is refractory to conventional doses of calcitriol,

but very high doses have been effective for some patients with this disease.

For *nutritional rickets*, vitamin D is used at low doses as a preventive measure and at higher doses as a treatment. In vitamin D-resistant rickets accompanied by hypophosphatemia, oral neutral potassium phosphate and calcitriol are administered.

Vitamin D and dietary calcium supplements are used in combination to prevent as well as treat *osteoporosis* because many elderly individuals have poor calcium intake and are also vitamin D-deficient, especially if they lack sunlight exposure. Although differences exist in the suggested amount of vitamin D supplements, the range of 800–1,000 international units daily is often accepted; some experts feel that higher doses are necessary. The combination of calcium and vitamin D prevents spine, nonspine, and hip fractures in some studies but not others; this inconsistency may reflect study-to-study differences in the incidence of undiagnosed renal 25-OH vitamin D 1α-hydroxylase deficiency, which would require supplements of calcitriol rather than vitamin D. RS should be counseled to take a daily vitamin D supplement of at least 1,000 international units.

CONCLUSION AND FUTURE DIRECTIONS

Bone is composed of organic and inorganic components. The organic component consists of cells (osteoblasts, osteoclasts, and osteocytes) and an organic matrix called *osteoid* (mainly type I collagen). The inorganic component consists primarily of the calcium phosphate salt hydroxyapatite. The dynamic structure of bone depends on the relative balance between anabolic and resorptive processes and on the physiologic regulators of calcium and phosphate homeostasis.

The most important modulators of bone remodeling and bone mineral homeostasis are parathyroid hormone (PTH), calcitriol, and FGF-23. Through their actions on bone, kidney, and intestine, these hormones preserve bone mineral homeostasis, sometimes at the expense of bone integrity. Bone disorders can result from abnormal levels of these hormones (e.g., high levels of PTH in hyperparathyroidism, low levels of vitamin D in nutritional rickets, and high levels of FGF-23 in hypophosphatemic rickets and oncogenic osteomalacia), increased rates of bone remodeling (e.g., unbalanced bone resorption in osteoporosis and increased formation of disorganized bone in Paget's disease), or failure of organs that are important in maintaining mineral homeostasis (e.g., chronic kidney disease). Bone disorders usually lead to structurally weakened bone because of either (1) a reduction in bone mass because of increased bone resorption or decreased bone formation or (2) the formation of architecturally unsound bone because of excessively rapid bone formation (woven bone) or deficient bone mineralization (rickets and osteomalacia). In turn, structural weakening of bone predisposes to bone fracture or deformity.

Bone disorders can be treated by correcting the underlying hormonal or mineral imbalances (e.g., vitamin D and calcium) or by modulating bone remodeling (e.g., SERMs, bisphosphonates, and RANKL antagonists). Pharmacologic interventions directed at the physiology of bone remodeling can be divided into two main categories: antiresorptive agents and bone anabolic agents. The majority of drugs currently approved for the treatment of osteoporosis are antiresorptive agents. These drugs act by inhibiting osteoclastic bone resorption, thus slowing the loss of bone mass. However, these drugs do not stimulate new bone formation and *do not increase true bone mass (matrix plus mineral)*. Hence, antiresorptive agents do not represent optimal therapy for individuals who have already sustained severe loss of bone mass. The only FDA-approved bone anabolic agent is once-daily PTH, which acts by increasing bone formation and is therefore the most beneficial agent for patients with very low bone mass. The structurally related natural protein, PTH-related protein, has similar effects in animals, and a synthetic analogue of PTHrP increases bone mass in humans and is undergoing additional trials in humans. Most drugs that reduce bone resorption subsequently reduce bone formation. Two important exceptions are currently undergoing clinical trials in humans: a fully-humanized monoclonal antibody that neutralizes sclerostin (an osteocyte-derived glycoprotein that inhibits osteoblast activity) and an oral inhibitor of cathepsin K (a protease expressed in osteoclasts that helps to degrade the bone matrix). The former increases bone formation without increasing bone resorption, and the latter decreases bone resorption without decreasing bone formation. The action of these agents suggests that it may be possible to uncouple bone resorption from bone formation and thereby treat osteoporosis more effectively.

Acknowledgment

We thank Allen S. Liu and Ariel Weissmann for their valuable contributions to this chapter in the First and Second Editions of *Principles of Pharmacology: The Pathophysiologic Basis of Drug Therapy*, Robert M. Neer for his valuable contribution to the Third Edition, and Armen H. Tashjian, Jr. for his valuable contributions to the First, Second, and Third Editions.

Suggested Reading

Andress DL. Vitamin D treatment in chronic kidney disease. *Semin Dial* 2005;18:315–321. (*Reviews progression of chronic kidney disease and indications for vitamin D therapy.*)

Bergwitz C, Juppner H. Disorders of phosphate homeostasis and tissue mineralisation. *Endocr Dev* 2009;16:133–156. (*Current understanding of the pathophysiology, diagnosis, and treatment of abnormal phosphate homeostasis and tissue mineralization.*)

Ebeling PR. Osteoporosis in men. *N Engl J Med* 2008;358:1474–1482. (*Review of an underappreciated public health problem.*)

Lobo RA. Where are we 10 years after the Women's Health Initiative? *J Clin Endocrinol Metab* 2013;98:1771–1780. (*Discussion that updates many of the issues noted in the Women's Health Initiative.*)

Maclean C, Newberry S, Maglione M, et al. Systematic review: comparative effectiveness of treatments to prevent fractures in men and women with low bone density or osteoporosis. *Ann Intern Med* 2008;148:197–213, 423–425, 884–887. (*Excellent overview of the comparative effectiveness of various agents for the treatment of osteoporosis.*)

National Osteoporosis Foundation. *Clinician's guide to prevention and treatment of osteoporosis.* Washington, DC: National Osteoporosis Foundation; 2013. (*An excellent review of evaluating, preventing, and managing osteoporosis.*)

Querfeld U. The therapeutic potential of novel phosphate binders. *Pediatr Nephrol* 2005;20:389–392. (*Review of agents used to lower plasma phosphate levels.*)

Raisz LG. Pathogenesis of osteoporosis: concepts, conflicts, and prospects. *J Clin Invest* 2005;115:3318–3325. (*Current understanding of osteoporosis pathophysiology.*)

Rosen CJ. Postmenopausal osteoporosis. *N Engl J Med* 2005;353:595–603. (*Succinct overview of the clinical management of osteoporosis.*)

Rosen CJ. Vitamin D insufficiency. *N Engl J Med* 2011;364:248–254. (*Discusses current understanding and uncertainties about vitamin D levels and supplementation.*)

Seeman E, Martin TJ. Co-administration of antiresorptive and anabolic agents: a missed opportunity. *J Bone Miner Res* 2015;30:753–764. (*Discussion of potentially combining agents to stimulate bone formation and block bone resorption.*)

Steddon SJ, Cunningham J. Calcimimetics and calcilytics—fooling the calcium receptor. *Lancet* 2005;365:2237–2239. (*New approaches to pharmacologic modulation of the calcium-sensing receptor.*)

Watts NB, Bilezikian JP, Camacho PM, et al. American Association of Clinical Endocrinologists medical guidelines for clinical practice for the diagnosis and treatment of postmenopausal osteoporosis. *Endocr Pract* 2010;16:1–37. (*Detailed and extensive review with a large reference list.*)

DRUG SUMMARY TABLE: CHAPTER 32 Pharmacology of Bone Mineral Homeostasis

DRUG	CLINICAL APPLICATIONS	SERIOUS AND COMMON ADVERSE EFFECTS	CONTRAINDICATIONS	THERAPEUTIC CONSIDERATIONS
HORMONE REPLACEMENT THERAPY **Mechanism—Decreases bone resorption by osteoclasts**				
Estrogen + progestin	See Drug Summary Table: Chapter 30 Pharmacology of Reproduction			
SELECTIVE ESTROGEN RECEPTOR MODULATOR (SERM) **Mechanism—Estrogen receptor agonist in bone, estrogen receptor antagonist in endometrium and breast**				
Raloxifene	Prevention and treatment of osteoporosis Prophylaxis of invasive breast cancer	*Retinal vascular occlusion, venous thromboembolism* Hot flashes, leg cramps	Pregnancy History or presence of venous thromboembolism	Decreases breast cancer incidence.
BISPHOSPHONATES **Mechanism—Decrease bone resorption by osteoclasts**				
Alendronate **Risedronate** **Ibandronate** **Pamidronate** **Zoledronate**	Prevention and treatment of osteoporosis (alendronate, risedronate, ibandronate, and zoledronate only) Paget's disease (alendronate, risedronate, pamidronate, and zoledronate only) Osteolytic lesions of multiple myeloma and breast cancer (pamidronate and zoledronate only) Hypercalcemia associated with malignancy (pamidronate and zoledronate only)	*Arthralgia, myalgia, osteonecrosis of external auditory canal (rare), jaw osteonecrosis primarily in cancer patients (rare), atypical femur fractures (rare) (shared adverse effects); hypersensitivity reaction (alendronate and risedronate only); esophageal ulcer (alendronate, risedronate, and ibandronate only); nephrotoxicity, electrolyte imbalance (risedronate and pamidronate only); heart failure (alendronate only); cardiac arrhythmia, peripheral edema, eye toxicity, benign prostatic hyperplasia (risedronate only)* Gastrointestinal upset (shared adverse effect); backache (risedronate only); upper respiratory infection (ibandronate only); cough, dyspnea, fatigue (pamidronate only)	Shared contradictions: Hypersensitivity to drug Hypocalcemia Alendronate, risedronate, and ibandronate only: Esophageal disease Inability to sit up for 30 minutes after taking drug orally	Extended skeletal effects. Unclear how to define overdosage. Pamidronate and zoledronate are only available IV. IV dosage corrects hypercalcemia in days. Ibandronate is not approved for prevention of bone loss in men.
RANKL ANTAGONIST **Mechanism—Decreases bone resorption by osteoclasts**				
Denosumab	Prevention and treatment of osteoporosis Bone metastases from solid tumors	*Endocarditis, cellulitis, electrolyte imbalance, pancreatitis, hypersensitivity reaction, jaw osteonecrosis in cancer patients (rare), atypical femur fractures (rare)* Gastrointestinal upset, asthenia, upper respiratory infection, dyspnea, fatigue	Hypersensitivity to denosumab Hypocalcemia Pregnancy	Injected subcutaneously every 6 months (osteoporosis) or monthly (malignancy).

continues

DRUG SUMMARY TABLE: CHAPTER 32 Pharmacology of Bone Mineral Homeostasis *continued*

DRUG	CLINICAL APPLICATIONS	*SERIOUS* AND COMMON ADVERSE EFFECTS	CONTRAINDICATIONS	THERAPEUTIC CONSIDERATIONS
CALCITONIN — Mechanism—**Decreases bone resorption by osteoclasts**				
Salmon calcitonin	Hypercalcemia Paget's disease Osteoporosis	*Hypocalcemia, hypersensitivity reaction, seizure, cancer* Flushing, nausea	Hypersensitivity to salmon calcitonin	Nasal spray or subcutaneous. Subcutaneous doses lower plasma calcium levels over hours.
BONE ANABOLIC AGENTS — Mechanism—**Increase bone formation by osteoblasts**				
hPTH 1-34 (teriparatide)	Severe osteoporosis	*Angina* Hypotension, rash, sweating, hyperuricemia, gastrointestinal upset, asthenia, dizziness, cough, rhinitis	Hypersensitivity to teriparatide Paget's disease Open epiphyses Prior radiation therapy Bone malignancy Hypercalcemia	In rodents, long-term use causes osteosclerosis and osteosarcomas.
hPTH 1-84	Hypoparathyroidism	*Hypercalcemia* Paresthesias, nausea, diarrhea	Paget's disease Open epiphyses Prior radiation therapy involving the skeleton Hypercalcemia	In rodents, long-term use causes osteosclerosis and osteosarcomas.
ORAL PHOSPHATE BINDERS — Mechanism—**Decrease gastrointestinal absorption of dietary inorganic phosphate**				
Aluminum hydroxide	Chronic kidney disease Tumoral calcinosis Hyperphosphatemia-hyperostosis syndrome	*Encephalopathy, osteomalacia*	None	Rarely used because of adverse effects due to aluminum accumulation.
Calcium carbonate Calcium acetate	Calcium deficiency (calcium carbonate only) End-stage renal disease (calcium acetate only)	*Myocardial infarction, renal calculi, prostate cancer, milk alkali syndrome (calcium carbonate only)* Constipation, flatulence (calcium carbonate only); hypercalcemia (calcium acetate only)	Hypercalcemia	Acidic gastric pH required for $CaCO_3$ absorption.
Sevelamer	End-stage renal disease Hyperphosphatemia-hyperostosis syndrome	*Bowel obstruction, peritonitis* Gastrointestinal upset	Bowel obstruction	Lowers serum cholesterol by binding bile acids.

VITAMIN D AND ANALOGUES
Mechanism—Increase gastrointestinal absorption of dietary calcium, decrease transcription of PTH gene

Drug	Clinical Applications	Serious and Common Adverse Effects	Contraindications	Therapeutic Considerations
Cholecalciferol (vit D_3) Ergocalciferol (vit D_2) Calcifediol [25(OH)D_3] Calcitriol [1,25(OH)$_2D_3$] Doxercalciferol [1α-(OH)D_2] Paricalcitol [19-nor-1,25(OH)$_2D_2$]	Vitamin D deficiency Hypoparathyroidism Rickets Osteomalacia Osteoporosis Secondary hyperparathyroidism	*Hypervitaminosis D, hypercalcemia, hypophosphatemia, hypercalciuria, gastrointestinal hemorrhage, angioedema* Abnormal lipids, gastrointestinal upset, edema, headache	Hypersensitivity to drug Hypercalcemia Hypervitaminosis D Malabsorption syndrome	Calcitriol is often the preferred agent because of its faster onset and offset (12 hours) and faster approach to steady state (72–96 hours). Calcitriol may cause more hypercalcemia than either paricalcitol or doxercalciferol.

CALCIMIMETIC
Mechanism—Increases sensitivity of calcium-sensing receptor to calcium in parathyroid cells, causing decreased secretion of PTH

Drug	Clinical Applications	Serious and Common Adverse Effects	Contraindications	Therapeutic Considerations
Cinacalcet	Hyperparathyroidism Hypercalcemia associated with parathyroid carcinoma	*Cardiac arrhythmia, heart failure, seizure, electrolyte imbalance, anemia, bone fractures* Paresthesia, gastrointestinal upset, arthralgia, myalgia, asthenia, headache, depression, dehydration, fatigue	Hypocalcemia	Sometimes used off-label to treat other forms of secondary hyperparathyroidism.

CALCIUM
Mechanism—Essential for bone mineralization

Drug	Clinical Applications	Serious and Common Adverse Effects	Contraindications	Therapeutic Considerations
Calcium gluconate (IV) Calcium chloride (IV) Calcium carbonate (oral) Calcium citrate-malate (oral)	Calcium deficiency	*Urolithiasis, prostate cancer* Gastrointestinal upset	Hypercalcemia (shared contraindication) Ventricular fibrillation (calcium gluconate only)	Calcium carbonate must be taken with food unless the patient is known to have normal gastric acid secretion. Calcium citrate is preferred if patient is taking a proton pump inhibitor. Subcutaneous infiltration of IV infusion is less toxic with calcium gluconate than with $CaCl_2$.

INORGANIC PHOSPHATE
Mechanism—Essential for bone mineralization

Drug	Clinical Applications	Serious and Common Adverse Effects	Contraindications	Therapeutic Considerations
Potassium phosphate (pH 7)	Severe hypophosphatemia	*Nephrotoxicity* Diarrhea	Hyperkalemia Hypocalcemia Hyperphosphatemia	Potassium phosphate is usually preferred over sodium phosphate to minimize renal excretion of phosphate and/or to correct coexisting hypokalemia.

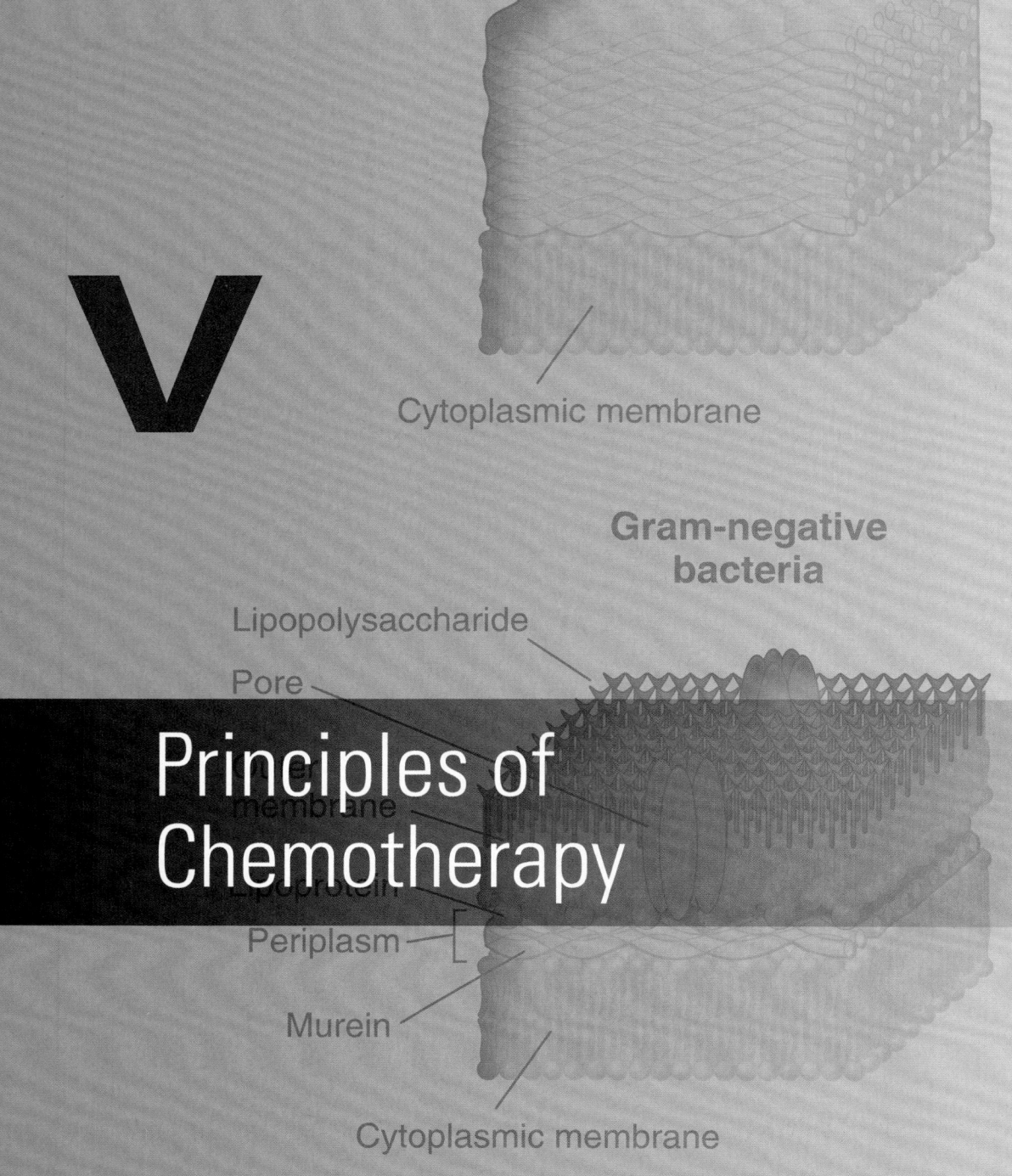

Cytoplasmic membrane

**Gram-negative
bacteria**

Lipopolysaccharide

Pore

membrane

Lipoprotein

Periplasm

Murein

Cytoplasmic membrane

Mycobacteria

Pore

Extractable
phospholipids

Mycolic acids

V

Principles of
Chemotherapy

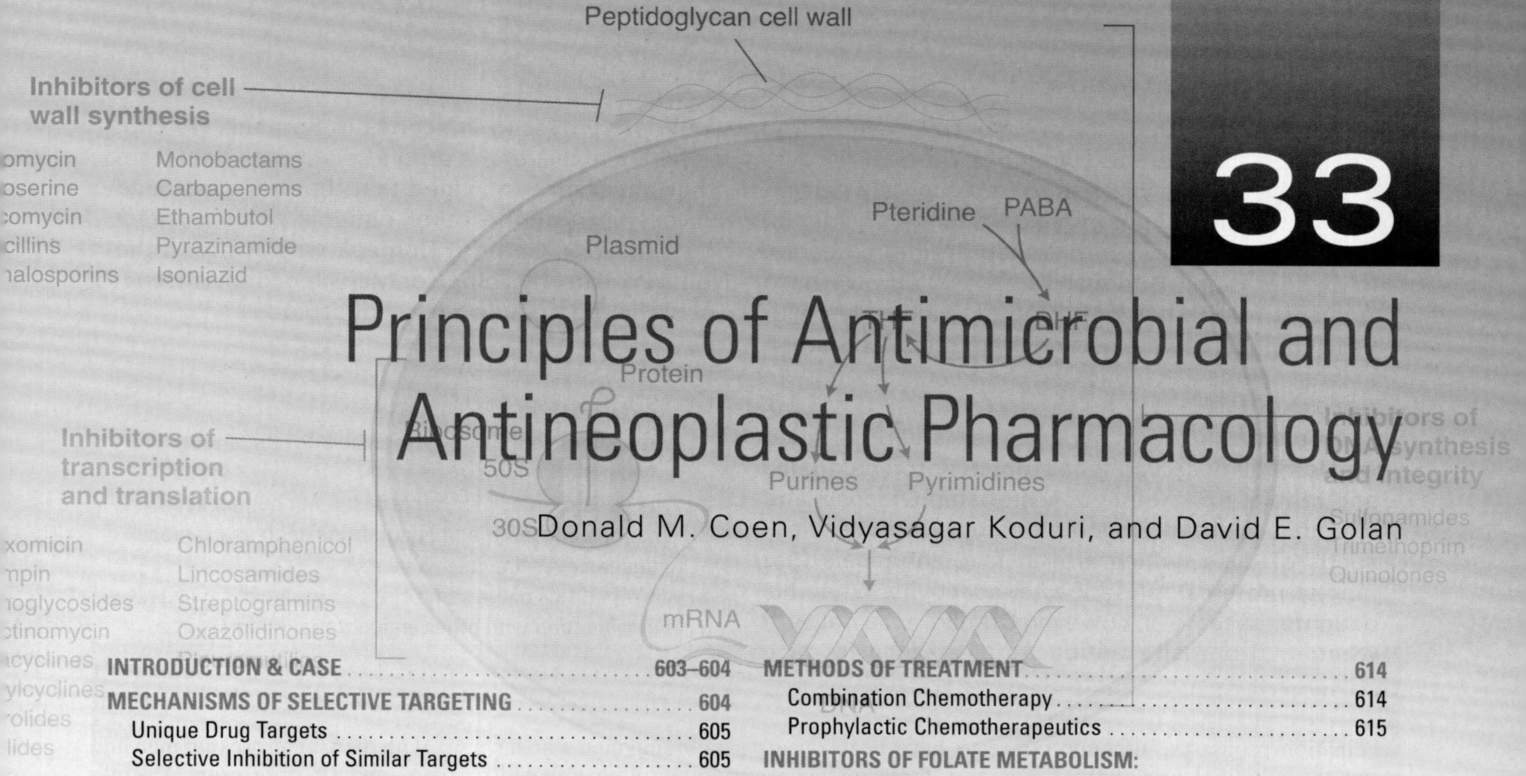

Inhibitors of cell
wall synthesis

...omycin   Monobactams
...oserine   Carbapenems
...comycin   Ethambutol
...cillins   Pyrazinamide
...halosporins Isoniazid

Plasmid

Pteridine   PABA

Principles of Antimicrobial and
Antineoplastic Pharmacology

Protein

Donald M. Coen, Vidyasagar Koduri, and David E. Golan

Inhibitors of
transcription
and translation

...xomicin   Chloramphenicol
...mpin   Lincosamides
...noglycosides Streptogramins
...tinomycin   Oxazolidinones
...cyclines
...ylcyclines
...rolides
...lides

Purines   Pyrimidines

mRNA

INTRODUCTION

While infectious diseases and cancers have different underlying etiologies, from a pharmacologic perspective, the broad principles of treatment are similar. One common thread in these pharmacologic strategies is the *targeting of selective differences between the microbe or cancer cell and the normal host cell*. A second common thread is that *the goal of treatment is complete inhibition of growth of the microbe or cancer cell*. Because both microbes and cancer cells can evolve resistance to drug therapies, the development of new treatments is also a continually evolving process.

Infectious diseases and cancers are among the deadliest afflictions plaguing human societies. The World Health Organization (WHO) has estimated that, in the year 2012, communicable disease accounted for 23% of 56 million deaths worldwide, and malignant neoplasms accounted for a further 14.7%. Among the infectious diseases, the most common causes of mortality worldwide included lower respiratory infections (5.5%), diarrheal diseases (2.7%), HIV/AIDS (2.8%), tuberculosis (1.7%), and malaria (1.2%). In the developed world, cancer (along with heart disease and stroke) is a more significant cause of death than infectious disease. The deadliest cancers in the United States presently include lung cancer (159,260 estimated deaths in 2014), colon cancer (50,310), breast cancer (40,430), pancreatic cancer (39,590), and prostate cancer (29,480). Patterns of both infectious and neoplastic diseases will likely change as increasingly effective treatments and preventive measures are developed and distributed.

This chapter focuses on the principles of antimicrobial and antineoplastic pharmacology, but there are also many important and effective nonpharmacologic strategies to combat microbes and cancer. These strategies include public health measures, vaccinations, and screening. Most public health and vaccination programs aim to prevent infections rather than treat existing infections. Smallpox, for example, was eradicated worldwide in 1977 through aggressive

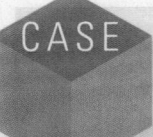

CASE

In 1935, in Wuppertal, Germany, 11-year-old Hildegard Domagk is desperately ill with a streptococcal infection that she contracted after an accidental pinprick with an embroidery needle. In desperation, Hildegard's father, Dr. Gerhard Domagk, injects her with prontosil, a red dye with which he has been experimenting in his laboratory. In what seems like a miracle, she makes a complete recovery.

This story actually began 3 years earlier, when Dr. Domagk observed that prontosil protected mice and rabbits from lethal doses of staphylococci and streptococci. He discovered this by screening thousands of dyes (which are, in fact, chemicals that bind to proteins) for antibacterial activity. When his daughter became ill, however, Domagk was not sure whether prontosil's antibacterial efficacy in mice

would carry over to infections in humans. He kept his personal test of the drug a secret until data from other physicians indicated that the drug had been successful in curing other patients of their infections. In 1939, Gerhard Domagk was awarded the Nobel Prize in Physiology or Medicine for his discovery of the therapeutic benefit of prontosil.

Questions

1. What is the mechanism responsible for the antibacterial action of prontosil?
2. Why does prontosil kill bacteria but not human cells?
3. What has caused the utility of drugs such as prontosil to decline over the past 75 years?
4. Why are drugs of the same class as prontosil now used in combination with other antibacterial agents?

vaccination programs, although concerns have been raised about the potential use of this virus as a bioterror agent. A similar campaign to eradicate polio is ongoing. Reductions in smoking and other environmental carcinogens have had a major impact on cancer mortality. Cancer screening, through regular mammograms, colonoscopy, and other tests, is widely used to detect cancer in its early and more treatable stages. Early detection through the widespread use of Papanicolaou cytologic tests (Pap smears) has caused the mortality of cervical cancer to decrease by more than two-thirds in the United States; cervical cancer has moved from the primary to the 15th leading cause of cancer deaths in women. It is hoped that widespread vaccination against specific types of human papilloma virus, the most common causative agent of cervical cancer, will further reduce the mortality of this cancer.

Effective strategies against disease, including drug therapy, also depend on socioeconomic factors. In affluent countries, the widespread use of antimicrobial drugs and improvements in sanitation and nutrition have markedly reduced mortality from infectious diseases. This progress has only begun to reach the developing world, where otherwise treatable infectious diseases remain major causes of mortality. Since 2012, a growing body of research has supported the use of combination therapy as preexposure prophylaxis (PrEP) in the prevention of HIV infection. In May 2014, the Centers for Disease Control and Prevention (CDC) released new guidelines on the use of tenofovir-emtricitabine to prevent HIV infection in populations at substantial risk,

including men who have sex with men, heterosexual men and women with infected partners, and IV drug users. Despite the importance of public health measures, vaccinations, and screening procedures, drug therapy remains vital to the treatment of microbial disease and cancer. Understanding the general principles and mechanisms of antimicrobial and antineoplastic pharmacology is essential to the safe and effective prescribing of existing drugs and, especially in light of continually evolving mechanisms of resistance, to the discovery of new drugs.

MECHANISMS OF SELECTIVE TARGETING

The goal of antimicrobial and antineoplastic drug therapy is **selective toxicity**: inhibiting pathways or targets that are critical for pathogen or cancer cell survival and replication at concentrations of drug lower than those required to affect critical host pathways. Selectivity can be realized by attacking (1) targets unique to the pathogen or cancer cell that are not present in the host, (2) targets in the pathogen or cancer cell that are similar but not identical to those in the host, and (3) targets in the pathogen or cancer cell that are shared with the host—or are even host rather than pathogen gene products—but that vary in importance between pathogen and host and thus impart selectivity (Table 33-1). These selectively targeted differences range from structures that are unique to individual pathogens, such as the peptidoglycan

TABLE 33-1 Mechanisms of Selective Targeting by Chemotherapeutic Agents

TYPE OF TARGETING	MECHANISM	EXAMPLE
Unique	Drug targets genetic or biochemical pathway that is unique to pathogen	Bacterial cell wall synthesis inhibitor
Selective	Drug targets protein isoform that is unique to pathogen or cancer cell	Dihydrofolate reductase (DHFR) inhibitor
Common	Drug targets a host protein or pathway that is more important to pathogen or cancer cell than to host cell	5-Fluorouracil

cell wall of bacteria, to differences as slight as a single amino acid change in a signaling protein that is otherwise common to cancer cells and normal cells, such as the acquisition of activating mutations in the epidermal growth factor receptor (EGFR) in certain lung cancers. In principle, drugs exhibit the least toxicity to the host when they target unique differences and the most toxicity when they target common pathways. For a given drug, the ratio of the toxic dose to the therapeutic dose is termed the **therapeutic index** (see Chapter 2, Pharmacodynamics) and is an indication of how selective the drug is in producing the desired effects. A highly selective drug such as **penicillin**, which targets the peptidoglycan cell wall unique to bacteria, can be prescribed safely because of the large difference between its therapeutic and toxic concentrations. Drugs such as **erlotinib**, which inhibits mutated EGFRs but cannot fully discriminate between wild-type and mutant receptors, have a much lower therapeutic index and a higher incidence of adverse effects.

As we learn more about the biology of pathogens and cancer cells, more selective drugs are being developed. For example, **imatinib** is a highly selective anticancer agent that targets the kinase domain of a fusion protein that is produced by a novel gene rearrangement. This fusion protein kinase is constitutively active and highly expressed in chronic myelogenous leukemia cells and is important for the growth and survival of these cells. In contrast, the drug has relatively little effect on normal cells, in which the unrearranged protein kinase is less active, less highly expressed, and less critical for cell growth and survival (see Chapter 1, Drug–Receptor Interactions). That being said, it is important to recognize that many potential targets that seem attractive remain unexploited because of issues such as unexpected adverse effects, unfavorable pharmacokinetic properties, or prohibitive costs associated with experimental drugs that have been developed to date against these targets.

In the section below, we discuss examples of targets of antimicrobial and antineoplastic drugs that illustrate the principles of selective toxicity.

Unique Drug Targets

Unique drug targets include metabolic pathways, enzymes, and other gene products that are present in the pathogen or cancer cell but absent in the host. One attractive target for antibacterial drugs is the biochemical pathway that leads to synthesis of the bacterial peptidoglycan cell wall (see Chapter 35, Pharmacology of Bacterial and Mycobacterial Infections: Cell Wall Synthesis). This structure is both biochemically unique and essential for the survival of growing bacteria. Penicillin and other **β-lactam antibiotics** inhibit the transpeptidase enzymes that catalyze the final cross-linking step in peptidoglycan synthesis. Without peptidoglycans, bacterial cell wall synthesis is fatally compromised. Because of their unique specificity for bacterial transpeptidase proteins, the penicillins have minimal host toxicity—in fact, allergic hypersensitivity is the major adverse reaction.

Fungi also present a unique target that is exploited by the currently available antifungal drugs. Like the bacterial cell wall, the fungal cell wall is biochemically unique and essential for survival. The **echinocandins** inhibit the synthesis of β-(1,3)-D-glucan, an essential component of the fungal cell wall. Disruption of cell wall integrity can cause fungal cell lysis. The echinocandins are well tolerated compared to

other antifungal drug classes, with adverse effects unrelated to inhibition of their target, but are limited by their lack of oral bioavailability. Thus, drugs that act on unique targets are often highly selective, with high therapeutic indices.

Selective Inhibition of Similar Targets

Many pathogenic organisms and cancer cells have metabolic pathways similar to those of normal human cells but because of evolutionary divergence or mutation possess enzyme or receptor isoforms that differ in sequence and structure from their normal human counterparts. Drugs can take advantage of these differences, even though they are sometimes subtle. However, the resulting therapeutic indices are usually smaller than with unique targets. Examples of this targeting strategy include an inhibitor of the B-Raf protein kinase and inhibitors of bacterial protein synthesis. B-Raf is part of a signaling pathway downstream of cell surface receptors. A mutant form of B-Raf, with a single amino acid substitution, is frequently expressed in the skin cancer melanoma. Despite this very subtle difference in the protein kinase, the drug **vemurafenib** more potently inhibits the mutant B-Raf than it does the normal enzyme. Because the mutant kinase is required for the growth and survival of many melanomas, vemurafenib treatment can cause dramatic responses in the disease with an acceptable toxicity profile.

In both humans and bacteria, protein synthesis is a multistep process that involves binding of tRNAs and mRNA to the ribosome, decoding of mRNA, synthesis of peptide bonds, translocation of the tRNAs relative to the mRNA, emergence of the polypeptide chain, and release of the polypeptide from the ribosome. The bacterial protein synthesis machinery differs from its human counterpart in the use of a different set of ribosomal RNAs and proteins and, correspondingly, distinct ribosomes. Several drug classes, including the macrolides and aminoglycosides, exploit these differences to selectively inhibit bacterial protein synthesis (see Chapter 34, Pharmacology of Bacterial Infections: DNA Replication, Transcription, and Translation). Macrolide antibiotics such as **erythromycin** bind to the 50S bacterial ribosomal subunit and block translation by preventing emergence of polypeptides from the ribosome. Aminoglycoside antibiotics such as **streptomycin** and **gentamicin** bind to the 30S bacterial ribosomal subunit and disrupt the decoding of mRNA. More generally, the bacterial protein synthesis inhibitors include a wide variety of individual drugs with diverse mechanisms, and the selectivity and dose-limiting toxicities of these drugs are often class- and/or drug-specific. For example, the macrolides rarely cause serious adverse effects, whereas some of the aminoglycosides have dose-limiting ototoxicity and nephrotoxicity. Some adverse effects appear to result from drug binding to human mitochondrial ribosomes in addition to bacterial ribosomes. Thus, selective inhibition of similar targets, as exemplified by mutant B-Raf inhibitors and protein synthesis inhibitors, can result in effects characterized by therapeutic indices that range from low to high, depending on the individual drug or drug class under consideration.

Common Targets

It is often the case that the host and pathogen or cancer share common targets. In these cases, selective toxicity can be achieved when the pathogen or cancer is more affected than the host by inhibition of the target. One striking example is the human chemokine receptor CCR5. This protein is essential for entry of certain strains of HIV into cells but is dispensable for human health as revealed by studies of individuals who, despite frequent exposure to HIV, have remained uninfected due to a deletion in the CCR5 gene. Accordingly, the antiviral drug **maraviroc**, which binds to CCR5 and prevents HIV entry into cells, can help suppress HIV replication with minimal toxicity to patients (see Chapter 38, Pharmacology of Viral Infections).

The paradigm of common targets is most frequently exemplified by antineoplastic drugs. Because tumor cells arise from transformed normal cells, they share nearly all of the cellular machinery needed for growth and replication. However, tumor cells may be more dependent on certain of these pathways than normal cells and therefore can be more sensitive to their inhibition. Also, some of these pathways can be more sensitized in cancer cells than in normal cells to agents that stress the cells, for example, by damaging DNA. These differences can be subtle, and anticancer drugs that attempt to exploit these differences often have narrow therapeutic indices. Therefore, selective inhibition of cancer cell growth remains a major challenge.

Recent discoveries have identified a number of proteins that are mutant or overexpressed in cancer cells, and selective inhibitors of these proteins are entering clinical use with increasing frequency (see Chapter 40, Pharmacology of Cancer: Signal Transduction, and discussion of vemurafenib above). Nonetheless, it is still the case that the selectivity of many currently used antineoplastic drugs is based not on specific mutant protein targets but rather on variations in cancer cell growth behavior and on the increased susceptibility of cancer cells to induction of apoptosis or senescence. Cancer, as a disease of persistent proliferation, requires continued cell division. Therefore, cytotoxic drugs targeting processes involved in DNA synthesis, mitosis, and cell cycle progression may kill rapidly cycling cancer cells preferentially over their normal relatives. (An important correlate to this statement is that many chemotherapeutic strategies are more successful against rapidly growing than slowly growing cancers.) Antimetabolites such as **5-fluorouracil** (**5-FU**) inhibit DNA synthesis in dividing cells (see Chapter 39, Pharmacology of Cancer: Genome Synthesis, Stability, and Maintenance). 5-FU inhibits thymidylate synthase, the enzyme responsible for converting dUMP to dTMP, a pyrimidine building block of DNA. As a pyrimidine analogue, 5-FU is also incorporated into growing RNA and DNA strands, thereby interrupting the synthesis of these strands. By causing DNA damage, 5-FU induces the cell to activate its apoptotic pathway, resulting in programmed cell death. 5-FU is toxic to all human cells undergoing DNA synthesis and, thus, is particularly toxic both for rapidly cycling tumor cells (therapeutic effect) and for high-turnover host tissues such as the bone marrow and gastrointestinal mucosa (adverse effect).

These examples illustrate the importance of studying the cell biology, molecular biology, and biochemistry of microbes and cancer cells to identify specific targets for selective inhibition. Clinically, an awareness of drug mechanisms and the basis of drug selectivity can help to explain the narrow or broad therapeutic indices that have an impact on drug dosing and treatment strategies. Understanding the selectivity of drugs for their targets is also important in combating drug resistance. Thus, the fundamental pharmacologic principles of drug–receptor interactions, therapeutic and adverse effects, and drug resistance form the basis for selective targeting in antimicrobial and antineoplastic drug therapy.

PATHOGENS, CANCER CELL BIOLOGY, AND DRUG CLASSES

Pharmacologic interventions target specific differences between the host and the microbial pathogen or cancer cell. This section examines some of the distinctive characteristics that evolution has bestowed on organisms and the major drug classes that target these molecular differences among host cells, pathogens, and cancer cells.

Bacteria

Bacteria are organisms that often contain unique targets for pharmacologic intervention. Some of these drug targets have been discussed previously and are illustrated in Figure 33-1. Currently available drugs act to interrupt bacterial DNA replication and repair (this chapter and Chapter 34), transcription and translation (Chapter 34), and cell wall synthesis (Chapter 35).

Depending on the role of the drug target in bacterial physiology, antibacterial drugs can produce bacteriostatic or bactericidal effects. Drugs that inhibit the growth of the pathogen without causing cell death are called **bacteriostatic**. These drugs target metabolic pathways that are necessary for bacterial growth but not for bacterial survival. Most protein synthesis inhibitors have a bacteriostatic effect (aminoglycosides are an important exception). The clinical effectiveness of these drugs relies on an intact host immune system to clear the nongrowing (but viable) bacteria. In contrast, **bactericidal** drugs kill bacteria. For example, cell wall synthesis inhibitors such as penicillins and cephalosporins cause bacterial lysis when the bacteria grow in hypertonic or hypotonic environments. Bacterial infections in immunocompetent hosts can often be treated with bacteriostatic drugs, whereas the treatment of bacterial infections in immunocompromised hosts often requires bactericidal drugs.

Bacteriostatic and bactericidal effects must be considered when antibiotics are used in combination (see Chapter 41, Principles of Combination Chemotherapy). *The combination of a bacteriostatic drug with a bactericidal drug can result in* **antagonistic** *effects.* For example, the bacteriostatic drug tetracycline inhibits protein synthesis and thereby retards cell growth and division. The action of this drug antagonizes the effects of a cell wall synthesis inhibitor, such as penicillin, which requires bacterial growth in order to be effective. In contrast, *the combination of two bactericidal drugs can be* **synergistic**; that is, the effect of the combination is greater than the sum of the effects of each drug alone (at the same doses of the two drugs). For example, a penicillin–aminoglycoside combination can have a synergistic effect because inhibition of bacterial cell wall synthesis by the penicillin allows increased entry of the aminoglycoside. The combination of two bacteriostatic drugs can also be synergistic (see "Synergy of DHFR Inhibitors and Sulfonamides" later in this chapter).

Fungi and Parasites

Eukaryotes, which include pathogenic fungi (yeasts and molds) and parasites (protozoa and helminths) as well as all

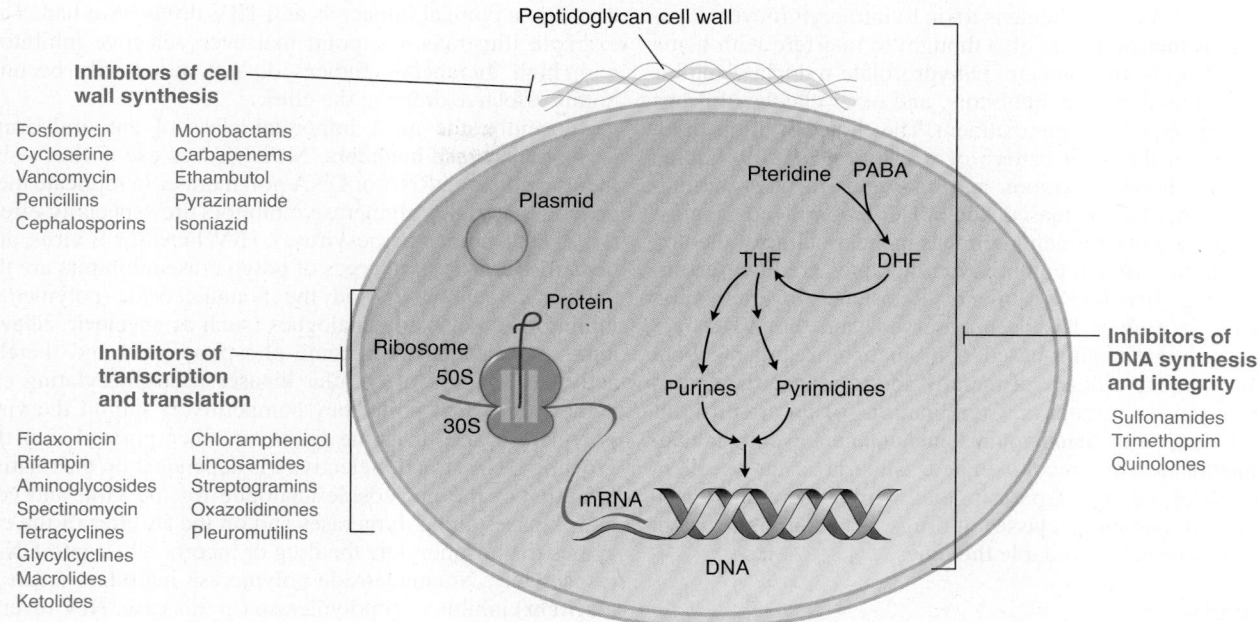

FIGURE 33-1. Sites of action of antibacterial drug classes. Antibacterial drug classes are often divided into three general groups. Drugs in one group inhibit specific enzymes involved in DNA synthesis and integrity: sulfonamides and trimethoprim inhibit the formation or use of folate compounds that are necessary for nucleotide synthesis; quinolones inhibit bacterial type II topoisomerases. Drugs targeting transcription and translation inhibit bacterial processes that mediate RNA and protein synthesis: fidaxomicin inhibits initiation of RNA synthesis by bacterial DNA-dependent RNA polymerase; rifampin inhibits elongation of RNA chains by the same enzyme; aminoglycosides, spectinomycin, tetracyclines, and glycylcyclines inhibit the bacterial 30S ribosomal subunit; macrolides, ketolides, chloramphenicol, lincosamides, streptogramins, oxazolidinones, and pleuromutilins inhibit the bacterial 50S ribosomal subunit. A third group of drugs inhibits specific steps in bacterial cell wall synthesis: fosfomycin and cycloserine inhibit early steps in peptidoglycan monomer synthesis; vancomycin binds to peptidoglycan intermediates, inhibiting their polymerization; penicillins, cephalosporins, monobactams, and carbapenems inhibit peptidoglycan cross-linking; and ethambutol, pyrazinamide, and isoniazid inhibit processes necessary for synthesis of the cell wall and outer membrane of *Mycobacterium tuberculosis*. Several clinically useful antibacterial drugs do not fit into one of these three groups; one recent example is daptomycin. The development of resistance is a problem for all antibacterial agents. Many bacteria carry plasmids (small, circular segments of DNA) with genes that confer resistance to an antibacterial agent or class of agents. PABA, para-aminobenzoic acid; DHF, dihydrofolate; THF, tetrahydrofolate.

multicellular organisms, are more complex than bacteria. Cells in these organisms contain a nucleus and membrane-bound organelles, as well as a plasma membrane. Eukaryotic cells reproduce by mitotic division rather than binary fission. Because of the similarities among human, fungal, and parasitic cells, infections caused by fungi and parasites can be more difficult to target than bacterial infections. However, the burden of disease from these organisms is vast. Parasitic infections caused by protozoa and helminths (worms) affect some 3 billion people worldwide, especially in less developed countries where the consequences of infection can be devastating. In both developed and less developed parts of the world, increasing numbers of patients are immunocompromised from AIDS, cancer chemotherapy, organ transplants, and old age. Such patients are especially susceptible to fungal and parasitic infections, which are becoming more prominent and will require greater attention in the future.

Currently available antifungal drugs can be divided into four main classes. Polyenes (e.g., **amphotericin**, **nystatin**) and azoles (e.g., **miconazole**, **fluconazole**) selectively target ergosterol in the fungal cell membrane, and echinocandins (e.g., **caspofungin**, **micafungin**) inhibit the synthesis of β-(1,3)-D-glucans in the fungal cell wall. Pyrimidines such as **5-fluorocytosine** inhibit DNA synthesis. Another class of miscellaneous antifungals, mostly acids, is used only topically because of unacceptable systemic toxicity. As with antibacterials, antifungals can be fungistatic or fungicidal; this

distinction is usually determined empirically. For example, the azoles interfere with fungal cytochrome P450-mediated ergosterol metabolism. Many azoles (e.g., **itraconazole** and **fluconazole**) are fungistatic. Newer azole agents (e.g., **voriconazole** and **ravuconazole**) may have fungicidal activity against some fungal species. As compared to fungistatic drugs, fungicidal drugs are more efficacious and faster acting and allow more favorable dosing regimens. Antifungal drugs are discussed in further detail in Chapter 36, Pharmacology of Fungal Infections.

Parasites exhibit diverse and complex life cycles and metabolic pathways, and the treatment of parasitic infections utilizes a wide array of drugs (see Chapter 37, Pharmacology of Parasitic Infections). One important protozoal infection is malaria, which is transmitted when the female *Anopheles* mosquito deposits *Plasmodia* sporozoites in the human bloodstream. The parasites leave the circulation and develop into tissue schizonts in the liver. The tissue schizonts rupture, releasing merozoites that enter the circulation to infect red blood cells (erythrocytes). The parasites then mature to trophozoites and, finally, to mature schizonts. Crops of mature schizonts are released into the bloodstream when the erythrocytes rupture, causing the typical cyclic fever associated with malaria. Antimalarial drugs target different stages of the protozoal life cycle. Aminoquinolines (such as the previous first-line drug, **chloroquine**) inhibit the polymerization of heme within the erythrocyte; it is thought that nonpolymerized heme is toxic to intraerythrocytic *Plasmodia*. **Artemisinins** are also thought to interfere with heme metabolism in the parasite. Dihydrofolate reductase inhibitors, protein synthesis inhibitors, and other classes of drugs are also used in malaria treatment. The choice of drugs often depends on the local pattern of resistance. As chloroquine resistance is now common and resistance to most antimalarial agents has increased, the WHO recommends against all single-agent treatment regimens in the first line of therapy for malaria. Instead, combination therapies are now recommended as first-line treatments. Resistance to artemisinin and its derivatives has been observed, and the WHO recommends artemisinin-based combination treatments both to increase the efficacy of therapy and to reduce the spread of drug-resistant malaria. Combinations of an artemisinin-based drug with **amodiaquine**, **mefloquine**, or **sulfadoxine-pyrimethamine** are recommended. Malaria is an excellent example of a complex parasite that, while theoretically susceptible to numerous classes of drugs, is becoming resistant to many currently available therapies.

Viruses

Viruses are noncellular organisms that typically consist of a nucleic acid core of RNA or DNA enclosed in a proteinaceous capsid. Some viruses also possess a host cell-derived lipid envelope containing viral proteins. Viruses lack the capability to synthesize proteins themselves, relying instead on the host cell machinery. Most viruses also encode distinct or even unique proteins not normally produced by human cells, however. Many of these proteins are involved in the viral life cycle, mediating attachment and entry of the virus into the host cell, uncoating of the viral capsid, expression of viral genes, replication of the viral genome, assembly and maturation of the viral particle, and release of viral progeny from the host cell. These virus-specific processes are often targeted by antiviral drugs. A schematic diagram of the general viral life cycle is presented in Figure 33-2 to illustrate the stages of viral replication that can be targeted by antiviral drugs. Because these targets are present only during active viral replication, viruses capable of latency have not been cured by any currently available antiviral drugs.

The HIV protease is an excellent example of a viral protein that has served as a fruitful target for drug development. This enzyme cleaves viral precursor proteins to generate the structural proteins and enzymes necessary for virus maturation. Without HIV protease, only immature and noninfective virions (individual virus particles) are produced. HIV **protease inhibitors** structurally mimic natural substrates of the protease but contain a noncleavable bond. These drugs act as competitive inhibitors at the active site of the enzyme (see Chapter 38). In combination with other classes of anti-HIV drugs, protease inhibitors helped to revolutionize the treatment of patients with HIV/AIDS, converting a nearly invariably fatal disease to a chronic illness.

Influenza viruses offer examples of other classes of proteins that have been successfully targeted. **Zanamivir** and **oseltamivir** target a viral neuraminidase that is vital for virion release from host cells. **Amantadine** and **rimantadine** act on the influenza virus membrane protein M2 (a proton channel) to inhibit viral uncoating. These anti-influenza drugs are effective inhibitors of their targets. However, at least partly because the immune system ordinarily clears influenza infections in less than a week, these agents have not had as dramatic a clinical impact as anti-HIV drugs have had. This example illustrates the point that even selective inhibitors with high therapeutic indices do not necessarily become highly effective drugs in the clinic.

Currently, the most important class of antiviral drugs is the **polymerase inhibitors**. Most viruses use a viral polymerase, either an RNA or DNA polymerase, to replicate their genetic material. Polymerase inhibitors are especially effective against human herpesviruses, HIV, hepatitis B virus, and hepatitis C virus. Two types of polymerase inhibitors are the nucleoside analogues and the nonnucleoside polymerase inhibitors. Nucleoside analogues (such as **acyclovir**, **zidovudine**, and **sofosbuvir**) become phosphorylated and thereby activated by viral or cellular kinases (phosphorylating enzymes), at which point they competitively inhibit the viral polymerase and, in some cases, are incorporated into the growing DNA strand. Selectivity is dependent on the relative affinities of the nucleoside analogue for the viral and cellular kinases and polymerases and on the abilities of the enzymes to phosphorylate the drug or incorporate it into DNA, respectively. Nonnucleoside polymerase inhibitors (such as **efavirenz**) inhibit viral polymerase (in this case, HIV reverse transcriptase), preventing DNA replication, but bind to a different site than the nucleoside analogues do. Mutations in viral polymerase genes are a major mechanism of resistance to polymerase inhibitors. Whether these resistance mutations affect the replicative capacity (fitness) of the virus can play a major role in determining the effectiveness of the therapy.

Chapter 38 provides a detailed discussion of the pharmacology of antiviral drugs.

Cancer Cells

Cancer is a disease of cell proliferation in which normal cells are transformed into cells with dysregulated growth. Neoplastic cells compete with normal cells for energy and nutrition, resulting in deterioration of normal organ function. Cancers also impinge on vital organs by mass effects. Carcinogenesis, chemotherapy, and the log cell kill model of tumor regression are discussed below to provide an overview of cancer pharmacology. Chapters 39 and 40 should be read with these principles in mind, and Chapter 41 provides integrated examples of the clinical applications of combination antineoplastic chemotherapy.

Carcinogenesis and Cell Proliferation

Carcinogenesis occurs in three main steps—transformation, proliferation, and metastasis. **Transformation** denotes a change in phenotype from a cell with normal growth controls to a cell with dysregulated growth. Nonlethal **genetic changes** (mutations) can be inherited in the germ line, can occur spontaneously, or can be caused by environmental agents such as chemicals, radiation, or viruses. If the change is not repaired, the mutated genes (e.g., genes involved in growth regulation and DNA repair) can express altered gene products that allow abnormal cell growth and proliferation. Among other effects, mutations can activate growth-promoting genes, inactivate growth-inhibiting genes, alter apoptosis-regulating genes, confer immortalization, and inactivate DNA repair genes. Additionally, the expression of these genes can be altered by certain heritable changes that do not alter DNA sequence, such as changes in DNA methylation or modifications to histones that package chromosomal DNA. Such **epigenetic changes** can also promote carcinogenesis.

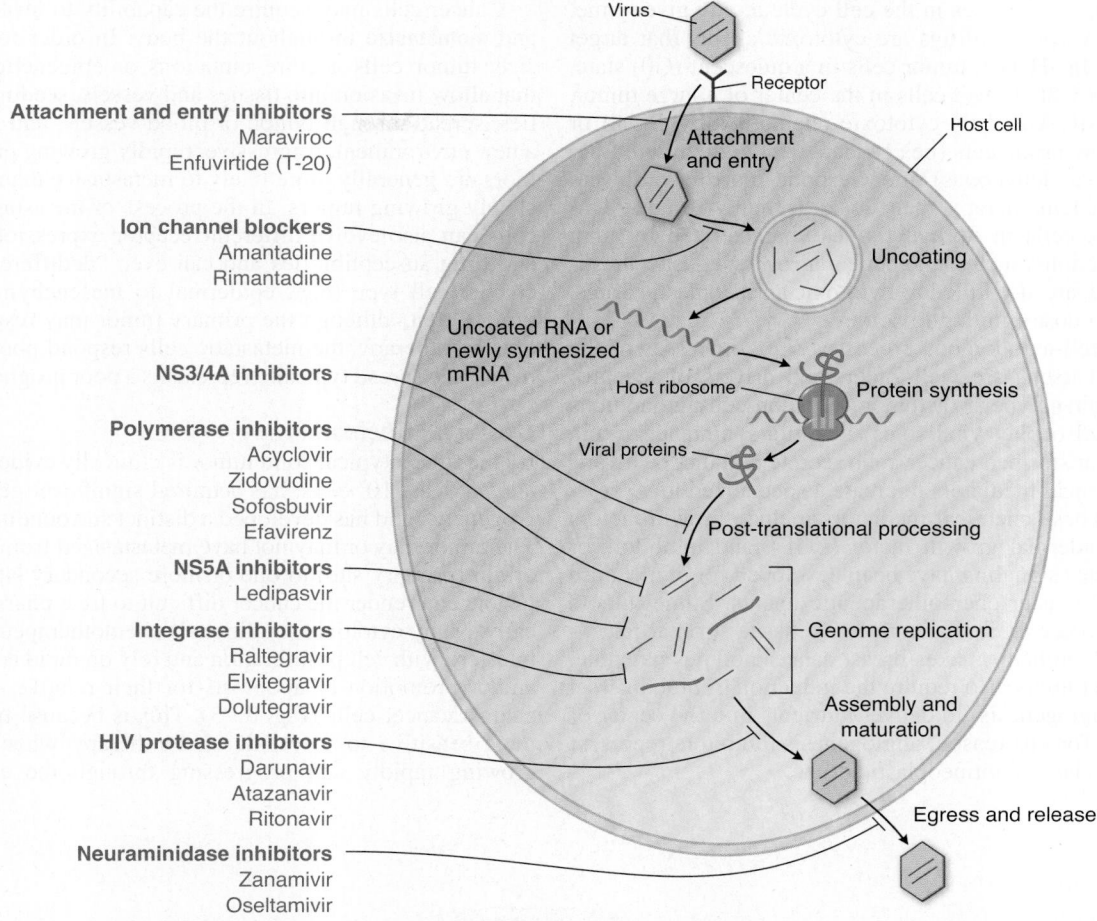

FIGURE 33-2. Stages of the viral life cycle targeted by antiviral drug classes. The viral life cycle begins with attachment of the virus to a host cell receptor and entry of the virus into the cell. The virus then uncoats, sometimes in an endosomal compartment. The uncoated viral nucleic acid is either directly translated into proteins on host ribosomes or undergoes transcription (RNA synthesis) and the newly synthesized mRNAs are translated, the proteins are processed post-translationally, and the viral genome (DNA or RNA) is replicated. The replicated viral genome and viral proteins are assembled into a virion (viral particle), which is then released from the host cell. The process of virion assembly and/or release is often accompanied by maturation of the virus into an infective agent that is able to repeat this life cycle with a new host cell. Depending on the particular virus, the various stages of the viral life cycle may occur in a different order from that shown in this general model. The anti-HIV drugs maraviroc and enfuvirtide (T-20) block the attachment and entry of HIV into host cells. The ion channel blockers amantadine and rimantadine inhibit influenza virus uncoating. The anti-HCV NS3/4A protease inhibitors block viral gene expression by preventing post-translational processing of the viral polyprotein. Polymerase inhibitors are a large class of antiviral agents that include acyclovir, sofosbuvir, and efavirenz; these drugs inhibit viral genome replication by interfering with viral DNA polymerase (acyclovir), viral RNA polymerase (sofosbuvir), and reverse transcriptase (efavirenz). The anti-hepatitis C virus (HCV) drug ledipasvir inhibits viral genome replication by interfering with the viral NS5A protein. The anti-HIV drugs raltegravir, elvitegravir, and dolutegravir inhibit viral genome replication by interfering with the viral integrase. Anti-HIV protease inhibitors, such as darunavir, atazanavir, and ritonavir, inhibit viral maturation. Neuraminidase inhibitors block the release of influenza virus particles from the host cell.

Expression of altered gene products and/or loss of normal gene regulation can cause dysregulated growth. Most cancers are initially clonal (i.e., genetically identical to a single precursor cell) but evolve to heterogeneity as new mutations and epigenetic changes increase the variation among daughter cells. When progeny cells with higher survival capacity are selected, increased cell proliferation ensues, and the tumor progresses to greater and greater heterogeneity. Thus, carcinogenesis, the progression from a normal cell to a malignant tumor, is a multistep process that usually requires an accumulation of multiple alterations. As more is learned about the molecular basis for carcinogenesis, these differences can be targeted for selective drug therapy.

The growth of transformed cells into a tumor requires **proliferation**, or an increase in the number of cells. Dividing human cells progress through a cell cycle (or mitotic cycle) consisting of distinct phases. The two key events in

the cell cycle are the synthesis of DNA during *S phase* and the division of the parent cell into two daughter cells during mitosis or *M phase*. The phase between cell division and DNA synthesis is called *gap 1 (G1)*, and the phase between DNA synthesis and mitosis is called *gap 2 (G2)*. Proteins called *cyclins* and *cyclin-dependent kinases (CDKs)* govern progression through the phases of the cell cycle. Mutations in cyclin and/or CDK genes can result in neoplastic transformation, and loss of normal cell cycle control can result in genetic instability, augmenting the transformed phenotype.

After a cancer cell divides, a daughter cell has four potential fates: it can become quiescent by entering a resting phase called *G0*, enter the cell cycle and proliferate, enter a state of cell-cycle arrest called *senescence*, or die. The ratio of the number of cells that are proliferating to the total number of cells in the tumor is called the **growth fraction**. An average tumor growth fraction is about 20%, because only one in five cells participates in the cell cycle at any given time. Many antineoplastic drugs are cytotoxic agents that target dividing cells. Hence, tumor cells in a quiescent (G0) state, such as nutrient-starved cells in the center of a large tumor, are not easily killed by cytotoxic chemotherapy. Small or rapidly growing cancers (i.e., cancers with high growth fractions, such as leukemias) often respond more favorably to cytotoxic chemotherapy than do large bulky tumors. Unfortunately, cells in normal tissues characterized by high growth fractions, such as the bone marrow and gastrointestinal mucosa, are also killed by cytotoxic antineoplastic drugs, resulting in dose-limiting toxicities.

While cell-autonomous processes (i.e., processes of the cancer cell itself) are well-understood drivers of the proliferative phenotype in a tumor cell, non-cell-autonomous processes also play vital roles in tumor maintenance and growth. Transformed cancer cells secrete and induce a variety of chemical mediators to create a specialized local environment. These chemical mediators include growth factors such as epidermal growth factor (EGF), and inhibitors of growth factor signaling have been developed for clinical use as targeted cancer chemotherapeutic agents. Some tumors create a protective fibrous connective tissue stroma; for example, this property makes breast cancer nodules palpable. Most solid tumors also require the induction of blood vessel growth (angiogenesis) to deliver nutrients into the center of the tumor; for this reason, angiogenesis inhibitors represent a valuable class of antineoplastic drugs.

Cancer cells may acquire the capability to invade tissues and **metastasize** throughout the body. In order to metastasize, tumor cells acquire mutations or epigenetic changes that allow invasion into tissues and vessels, seeding of cavities, spread through lymph or blood vessels, and growth in a new environment. Aggressive, rapidly growing primary tumors are generally more likely to metastasize than indolent, slowly growing tumors. In the process of metastasis, tumor cells can also evolve different receptor expression patterns and drug susceptibilities and can even "dedifferentiate" or change cell type (e.g., epidermal to mesenchymal transition). Often, although the primary tumor may respond well to chemotherapy, the metastatic cells respond poorly. Thus, metastatic spread typically represents a poor prognostic sign.

Cytotoxic Chemotherapy

By the time a typical solid tumor is clinically evident, it contains at least 10^9 cells, has acquired significant genetic heterogeneity, and has developed a distinct surrounding stroma. The tumor may or may not have metastasized from its site of origin (primary site) to one or more secondary sites. These factors can render the cancer difficult to treat pharmacologically. Many cytotoxic (traditional) chemotherapeutic agents interfere with cell proliferation and rely on rapid cell cycling and/or promotion of apoptosis for their relative selectivity against cancer cells (Fig. 33-3). This is because tumors are most sensitive to cytotoxic chemotherapy when they are growing rapidly and progressing through the cell cycle.

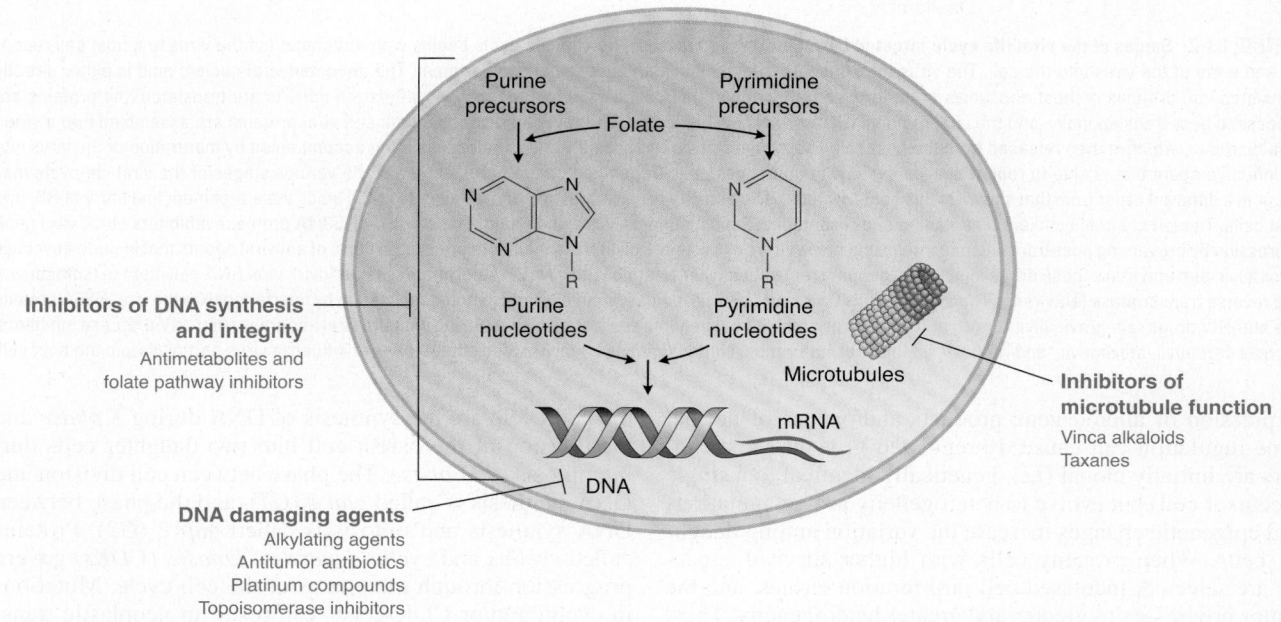

FIGURE 33-3. Cytotoxic antineoplastic drug classes. Many cancer cells divide more frequently than normal cells, and cancer cells can often be killed preferentially by targeting three critical processes in cell growth and division. DNA-damaging agents alter the structure of DNA and thereby promote apoptosis of the cell. These drugs include alkylating agents (which covalently couple alkyl groups to nucleophilic sites on DNA), antitumor antibiotics (which cause free radical damage to DNA), platinum compounds (which cross-link DNA), and topoisomerase inhibitors (which induce damage to DNA by stabilizing topoisomerase-induced strand breaks). Inhibitors of DNA synthesis and integrity block intermediate steps in DNA synthesis; these agents include antimetabolites and folate pathway inhibitors (which inhibit purine and pyrimidine metabolism). Inhibitors of microtubule function interfere with the mitotic spindle that is required for cell division. This group of drugs includes vinca alkaloids, which inhibit microtubule polymerization, and taxanes, which stabilize polymerized microtubules. The classes of targeted antineoplastic agents—such as growth factor receptor and signal transduction antagonists, proteasome inhibitors, angiogenesis inhibitors, tumor-specific monoclonal antibodies, and hormones—are not shown (see Chapter 40).

These metabolically active cells are susceptible to drugs that interfere with cell growth and division (the **mitotoxicity hypothesis**). Many cytotoxic antineoplastic drugs interfere with the cell cycle at a particular phase; such drugs are called **cell-cycle specific**. Other cytotoxic antineoplastic drugs act independently of the cell cycle and are called **cell-cycle nonspecific** (Fig. 33-4). Inhibitors of DNA synthesis, such as antimetabolites, are S-phase specific. Microtubule poisons, such as taxanes and vinca alkaloids, interfere with spindle formation during M phase. Alkylating agents that damage DNA and other cellular macromolecules act during all phases of the cell cycle. These various classes of drugs can be administered in combination, using cell-cycle specific drugs to target mitotically active cells and cell-cycle nonspecific agents to kill both cycling and noncycling tumor cells (see Chapter 41).

The mitotoxicity hypothesis of cytotoxic cancer therapy leaves some puzzles unresolved, however. Although cytotoxic chemotherapy is often toxic to the bone marrow, gastrointestinal mucosa, and hair follicles, these tissues usually

recover, while (in successful treatment) cancers with similar growth kinetics are eradicated. *It has now been established that almost all chemotherapeutic drugs also cause apoptosis of cancer cells.* DNA damage is normally sensed by molecules, such as p53, that arrest the cell cycle in order to allow time for the damage to be repaired. If the damage is not repaired, a cascade of biochemical events is triggered, which can result in **apoptosis** (programmed cell death). Therefore, a cancer cell that is defective in its capability for DNA repair may undergo apoptosis, whereas a normal cell can repair its DNA and recover. Cancers that express wild-type p53, such as most leukemias, lymphomas, and testicular cancers, are often highly responsive to chemotherapy. In contrast, cancers that acquire a mutation in p53, including many pancreatic, lung, and colon cancers, are often minimally responsive or even resistant to DNA-damaging drugs, because DNA damage does not trigger apoptosis in these cells.

Advances in cancer cell biology over the past several decades have led to the development of classes of therapeutic agents that more selectively target the molecular pathways responsible for the dysregulated growth of cancer cells. Because specific cancers may become "addicted" to a particular growth factor or signal transduction pathway for their survival (independent of their proliferation rate), selective targeting of these pathways can provide a basis for selective killing of cancer cells. This concept and the many classes of targeted antineoplastic agents that have been developed—including growth factor receptor and signal transduction antagonists, proteasome inhibitors, angiogenesis inhibitors, and tumor-specific monoclonal antibodies—are discussed in Chapter 40.

Log Cell Kill Model

The **log cell kill model** is based on experimentally observed rates of tumor growth and tumor regression in response to cytotoxic chemotherapy. Tumor growth is typically exponential, with a doubling time (i.e., time required for the total number of cancer cells to double) that depends on the type of cancer. For example, testicular cancer often has a doubling time of less than 1 month, whereas colon cancer tends to double every 3 months. In solid tumors, the cancer may grow exponentially until a clinically observable tumor size is achieved. *The log cell kill model states that the cell destruction caused by cytotoxic cancer chemotherapy is first-order;* that is, each dose of chemotherapy kills a constant fraction of cells. If the tumor starts with 10^{12} cells and 99.99% are killed, then 10^8 malignant cells will remain. The next dose of chemotherapy will then kill 99.99% of the remaining cells, and so on. Unlike antibacterial drugs, which can often be used in a constant high dose until the bacteria are eradicated, most cytotoxic antineoplastic drugs must be used intermittently to reduce toxic side effects. Intermittent dosing allows partial recovery of normal cells but also provides time for cancer cell regrowth and for evolution of drug resistance in the cancer cells. As shown in Figure 33-5, intermittent "cycles" of cytotoxic chemotherapy are administered until all the cancer cells are killed or the tumor develops resistance. Drug-resistant cells continue to grow exponentially despite treatment, eventually resulting in death of the host. Improvements in the rates of eradication of malignant cell populations by cytotoxic drugs are likely to require either higher doses of these agents (which are limited by toxicity) or initiation of therapy at a time when the tumor contains

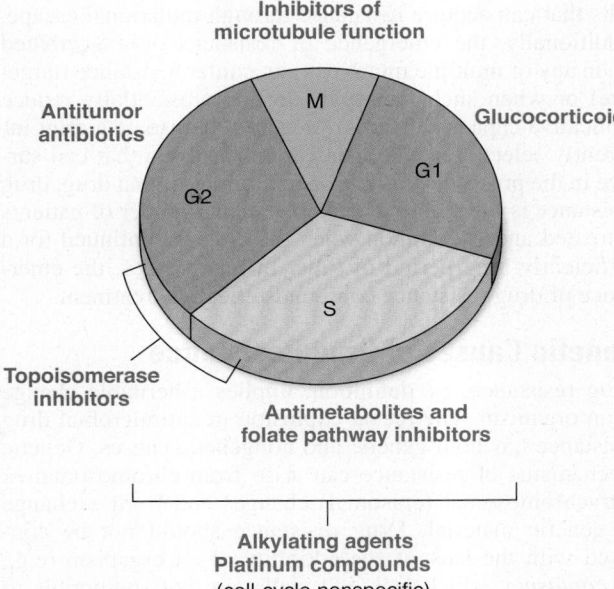

FIGURE 33-4. Cell-cycle specificity of some cytotoxic antineoplastic drug classes. The cell cycle is divided into four phases. Cell division into two identical daughter cells occurs during mitosis (M phase). Cells then enter the gap 1 (G1) phase, which is characterized by active metabolism in the absence of DNA synthesis. Cells replicate their DNA during the synthesis (S) phase. After completion of S phase, the cell prepares for mitosis during the gap 2 (G2) phase. Some cytotoxic antineoplastic drugs exhibit specificity for different phases of the cell cycle, depending on their mechanism of action. Inhibitors of microtubule function affect cells in M phase; glucocorticoids affect cells in G1; antimetabolites and folate pathway inhibitors affect cells in S phase; antitumor antibiotics affect cells in G2; topoisomerase inhibitors affect cells in S phase and G2. Alkylating agents and platinum compounds affect cell function in all phases and are therefore cell-cycle nonspecific. The differential cell-cycle specificity of the various drug classes allows them to be used in combination to target different populations of cells. For example, cell-cycle specific drugs can be administered to target actively replicating neoplastic cells, whereas cell-cycle nonspecific agents can be used to target quiescent (nonreplicating) neoplastic cells. The classes of targeted antineoplastic agents—such as growth factor receptor and signal transduction antagonists, proteasome inhibitors, angiogenesis inhibitors, tumor-specific monoclonal antibodies, and hormones—are not shown (see Chapter 40).

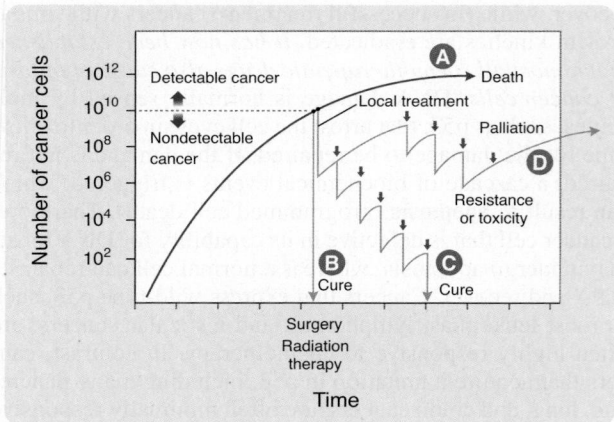

FIGURE 33-5. Log cell kill model of tumor growth and regression. The log cell kill model predicts that the effects of cytotoxic antineoplastic chemotherapy can be modeled as a first-order process. That is, a given dose of drug kills a constant *fraction* of tumor cells, and the number of cells killed depends on the total number of cells remaining. The four curves (*A–D*) represent four possible outcomes of antineoplastic therapy. **Curve A** is the growth curve of untreated cancer. The cancer continues to grow over time, eventually resulting in the death of the patient. **Curve B** represents curative local treatment (surgery and/or radiation therapy) before metastatic spread of the malignancy. **Curve C** represents local treatment of the primary tumor, followed immediately by systemic cytotoxic chemotherapy administered in cycles (*down arrows*) to eradicate the remaining metastatic cancer cells. Note that each cycle of chemotherapy reduces the number of cancer cells by a constant fraction (here, by about two "logs," or about 99%) and that some cancer growth occurs as the normal tissues are given time to recover between cycles of cytotoxic chemotherapy. **Curve D** represents local treatment followed by systemic chemotherapy that fails when the tumor becomes resistant to the drugs or when toxic drug effects occur that are intolerable to the patient. Note that 10^9 to 10^{10} cancer cells must typically be present for a tumor to be detectable; for this reason, multiple cycles of chemotherapy are required to eradicate the cancer, even when there is no detectable tumor remaining.

fewer cells (which often implies earlier detection). (In contrast, it seems that, for certain targeted antineoplastic agents, higher doses do not contribute further to efficacy once a sufficiently high dose is achieved to inhibit the target.) Adjuvant therapies, such as surgery and radiation, are other important modalities used to reduce the number of tumor cells before chemotherapy is initiated.

■ MECHANISMS OF DRUG RESISTANCE

Drug resistance is a major problem in all of antimicrobial and antineoplastic pharmacology. Although resistance to current drug therapies is emerging relatively rapidly, the rate of introduction of new drugs (especially antimicrobial drugs) is relatively slow. Formerly curable acute diseases such as gonorrhea and typhoid fever are becoming more difficult to treat due to drug resistance, and chronic or endemic infections such as tuberculosis or malaria are growing increasingly resistant worldwide. In some parts of China, up to 99% of gonorrhea isolates are multidrug resistant. In the United States, 60% of hospital-acquired (nosocomial) infections due to Gram-positive bacteria are caused by drug-resistant microbes. Tuberculosis, the fourth leading cause of infectious disease deaths worldwide, currently has an estimated 5% overall multidrug resistance (MDR) rate, although the rate of MDR in new cases of tuberculosis is as

high as 20–30% in some Asian countries (e.g., Azerbaijan, Belarus, Estonia, Kazakhstan, Kyrgyzstan, Russian Federation, and Uzbekistan). The appearance of MDR tuberculosis in the United States is of special concern because of the airborne spread of this organism. Despite these ominous trends, only several new classes of antibiotics—exemplified by new transcription inhibitors (e.g., **fidaxomicin**), glycylcyclines (**tigecycline**), streptogramins (**quinupristin/dalfopristin**), oxazolidinones (**linezolid**), pleuromutilins (**retapamulin**), and lipopeptides (**daptomycin**)—have entered clinical use in the past four decades, and some of these have only limited clinical utility. The numerous examples of rapidly emerging drug-resistant organisms suggest that this problem must be addressed promptly.

Because pathogens and cancer cells are primed to evolve rapidly in response to adaptive pressure, resistance can eventually appear with the use of any antimicrobial or antineoplastic drug. In a population of microbes or transformed cells, cells that contain genetic changes promoting replication in the presence of the drug will survive. Thus, high cell number, rapid growth rate, and high mutation rate all promote the development of a heterogeneous population of cells that can acquire resistance through mutational escape. Additionally, the emergence of resistance is exacerbated when any of multiple mutations can confer resistance (target size) or when such mutations do not substantially reduce replicative capacity (fitness). Because the use of a drug inherently selects for pathogens or cancer cells that can survive in the presence of high concentrations of that drug, drug resistance is inevitable when a sufficient number of patients is treated and is common when the drug is continued for a sufficiently long period of time. In many cases, the emergence of drug resistance confounds effective treatment.

Genetic Causes of Drug Resistance

Drug resistance, by definition, implies a heritable change in an organism. The recent explosion in antimicrobial drug resistance has both genetic and nongenetic causes. Genetic mechanisms of resistance can arise from chromosomal or extrachromosomal (episomal) changes and from exchange of genetic material. Drug resistance should not be confused with the lack of susceptibility of an organism (e.g., *Mycoplasma*, which lack cell walls, are not susceptible to penicillins) or with other mechanisms by which organisms can become less susceptible to drugs (e.g., by adaptation in the absence of genetic change such as the formation of biofilms). Table 33-2 lists the major mechanisms of drug resistance that can be caused by either chromosomal mutation or genetic exchange.

Chromosomal mutations typically occur in genes that code for drug targets or in genes that code for drug transport or metabolism systems. These mutations can then be transferred to daughter cells (**vertical transmission**) to create drug-resistant pathogens or cancer cells. Alternatively, bacteria can acquire resistance by gaining genetic material from other bacteria (**horizontal transmission**). For example, methicillin-resistant *Staphylococcus aureus* (MRSA) and vancomycin-resistant enterococcus (VRE) are able to cause highly feared nosocomial infections because these bacteria have acquired resistance genes. Bacteria acquire genetic material by three main mechanisms: conjugation, transduction, and transformation. In **conjugation**, chromosomal or plasmid DNA is transferred directly between bacteria. DNA can

TABLE 33-2 Mechanisms of Genetic Drug Resistance

MECHANISM	EXAMPLE: ANTIMICROBIAL	EXAMPLE: ANTINEOPLASTIC
Reduced Intracellular Drug Concentration		
Inactivate drug	Inactivation of β-lactam antibiotics by β-lactamase	Inactivation of antimetabolites by deaminase
Prevent uptake of drug	Prevention of aminoglycoside entry by altered porins	Decreased methotrexate entry by decreased expression of reduced folate carrier
Promote efflux of drug	Efflux of multiple drugs by multidrug resistance (MDR) membrane efflux pump	Efflux of multiple drugs by p170 membrane efflux pump (MDR1)
Target-Based Mechanisms		
Alter drug target	Expression of altered peptidoglycan that no longer binds vancomycin	Expression of mutant DHFR that no longer binds methotrexate
Overexpress drug target	Overexpression of dihydropteroate synthase or dihydrofolate reductase (DHFR)	Overexpression of DHFR, thymidylate synthase, or topoisomerase
Overproduce endogenous ligand or substrate	Overproduction of substrate para-aminobenzoic acid (PABA) causes resistance to sulfonamides	Overproduction of substrate asparagine and/or glutamine causes resistance to L-asparaginase (under investigation)
Bypass metabolic requirement for target	Loss of inhibition of host kinase bypasses requirement for viral kinase, causing resistance to the investigational antiviral drug maribavir	Activation of alternative signaling pathway confers vemurafenib resistance in melanoma
Insensitivity to Apoptosis	Not applicable	p53 mutation or loss

also be transferred from one cell to another by a bacterial virus, or bacteriophage, in a process called **transduction**. In **transformation**, naked DNA in the environment is taken up by the bacteria.

Drug resistance in bacteria is most often caused by the transfer of plasmids, which are extrachromosomal strands of DNA that contain drug resistance genes. Transfer of a DNA plasmid is especially important for drug resistance because this mechanism occurs at high rates both within and between bacterial species and because multiple drug resistance genes can be transferred simultaneously.

Reduced Intracellular Drug Concentration

Drugs must reach their targets in order to be effective. Both microbes and cancer cells have evolved mechanisms to reduce drug concentrations before the drugs reach their targets. One major mechanism entails the *inactivation of drugs*. Many bacteria acquire resistance to β-lactam antibiotics, such as penicillins, cephalosporins, and carbapenems, through expression of a hydrolytic enzyme, **β-lactamase**, which cleaves the β-lactam ring and thereby inactivates the drug. A single β-lactamase enzyme can hydrolyze 10^3 penicillin molecules per second, significantly reducing the intracellular concentration of active drug. As another example, cancer cells that overexpress a deaminase enzyme can rapidly inactivate purine or pyrimidine analogues such as 5-FU and make the drugs less effective.

Pathogens and cancer cells can also acquire mutations that *prevent uptake of the drug* into the cell or otherwise prevent access of the drug to the target molecule. For example, cancer cells with mutated folate-transport systems become resistant to folate analogues, such as **methotrexate**, that require active transport into cells in order to inhibit dihydrofolate reductase (DHFR).

Finally, both bacteria and cancer cells can acquire the ability to cause active *drug efflux* from the cell. Bacteria typically possess membrane pumps to transport lipophilic or amphipathic molecules (such as antibiotics) in and out of the cells. Overproduction of these membrane proteins or their variants can mediate active pumping of an antibiotic out of the cell faster than the drug can enter the cell. Despite the achievement of therapeutic blood levels of the antibiotic, this active efflux mechanism can cause intrabacterial drug concentrations to be ineffectively low. Similarly, the emergence of multidrug resistant cancers is often associated with cancer cell overexpression of membrane proteins, such as the **P-glycoprotein** (p170 or **MDR1**), which actively pump antineoplastic drugs out of the cell. These efflux pumps are especially important because they are capable of pumping out more than one type of drug, thus allowing pathogens or cancer cells to become resistant to multiple drugs of different classes.

It is worth noting that heritable changes are not the only class of mechanisms leading to reduced intracellular drug concentration. For example, the brain is protected by a *blood–brain barrier* that acts to exclude pathogens and toxins, but it also excludes many antibiotics and chemotherapeutic agents. This makes treatment of central nervous system infections and brain cancers more difficult. Certain infections are characterized by the formation of abscesses, and the hard wall of the abscess can similarly act to exclude antibiotics.

Target-Based Mechanisms

Pathogens and cancer cells can also evolve to alter or overexpress drug targets or evolve other changes related to the drug target that result in drug resistance. One common mechanism for development of drug resistance is *alteration of the target of a drug*. In vancomycin-resistant enterococcus, the *vanHAX* genes encode a novel enzymatic pathway that alters surface peptidoglycan synthesis such that the sequence terminates in D-Ala-D-lactate instead of the normal D-Ala-D-Ala. This substitution does not affect peptidoglycan cross-linking in the synthesis of the bacterial cell wall and thus does not alter the integrity of the cell wall, but it does lower by 1,000-fold the binding affinity of **vancomycin** for the dipeptide.

Almost all examples of antiviral drug resistance are due to alteration of targets through mutation of the genes encoding the targets. For example, resistance to the anti-herpesvirus drug **acyclovir** occurs through mutations in the viral thymidine kinase gene, which encodes the enzyme that activates the drug, or the viral DNA polymerase gene, which encodes the enzyme inhibited by the triphosphate form of the drug (see Fig. 38-7). In bacteria and cancer cells, both alteration and *overexpression* of the enzyme targets of cytotoxic antineoplastic drugs—such as DHFR, thymidylate synthase, and topoisomerase—can reduce the fraction of the targets that bind drug, thus reducing potency and conferring drug resistance.

Variations on this mechanism are to *overproduce an endogenous ligand or substrate* that competes with the drug for the drug target, as occurs with resistance of bacteria to sulfonamides (see under "Inhibitors of Folate Metabolism"), or to alter the target, ligand, or substrate so that the target binds the ligand more tightly, processes the substrate more efficiently, or is less necessary for microbial or cancer cell growth and survival. For example, mutations that alter sites of cleavage by HIV protease so that they are processed more readily can contribute to resistance to protease inhibitors. Yet another target-based mechanism, which is becoming increasingly important in resistance to targeted anticancer drugs, is to *bypass the metabolic requirement for the target*. For example, as mentioned above, melanomas often depend on inappropriate signaling by a mutant B-Raf protein kinase for their growth and survival, and targeting of this mutant kinase by inhibitors such as vemurafenib can result in dramatic regressions of the tumors. However, resistance arises frequently. One resistance mechanism involves activation of an entirely different signaling pathway to drive proliferation of the melanoma cells.

Insensitivity to Apoptosis

Drug resistance in cancer cells can occur through chromosomal or extrachromosomal mutations or epigenetic changes that are then passed to daughter cells to create a resistant tumor. Although anticancer drugs act at a variety of molecular targets, most, if not all, ultimately cause cell death by inducing apoptosis. In general, drug-induced **molecular lesions** can lead to cell-cycle arrest, activation of repair processes, senescence, or apoptosis. Mutations in key proteins associated with the control of apoptosis, such as p53 and Bcl-2, can result in failure to induce the apoptotic response to DNA damage and can thereby reduce the sensitivity of tumor cells to many anticancer drugs. As noted above, tumors with wild-type p53, such as many leukemias, lymphomas, and testicular cancers, are often highly responsive to chemotherapy. In contrast, many pancreatic, lung, and colon cancers have a high incidence of p53 mutations and are minimally responsive to chemotherapy.

Thus, the causes of drug resistance include changes in chromosomal DNA or episomal DNA, epigenetic changes, and external acquisition of genetic material. Resistance can be caused by drug inactivation, decreased drug uptake, increased drug efflux, alteration or overexpression of the target structure or pathway, bypass of the requirement for the target, repair of drug-induced lesions, and insensitivity to apoptosis. *Resistance is probably the major limiting factor in the effective treatment of both infections and cancer.* Drug therapy is a dynamic balance, an "evolutionary arms race," between the design of new drugs and the evolution of changes leading to drug resistance.

Practices That Promote Drug Resistance

One of the most important causes of drug resistance is the overprescription of antimicrobial drugs that are not indicated for the clinical situation. Overprescription is a problem not only in humans but also in the treatment and prophylaxis of animal infections. Such widespread use promotes drug resistance, which can then be transferred from one microorganism to another by the mechanisms described above. Because low drug concentrations in vivo can permit multiple cycles of replication and selection for resistant variants, low patient adherence can also promote resistance, as can the erratic drug availability found in parts of the developing world (and even in some communities in the developed world). International travel promotes a global disease community, ensuring that the multidrug-resistant tuberculosis found in Russia or Peru will eventually emerge in hospitals in the United States. Finally, demographic shifts and other trends have led to the formation of large populations that are susceptible to infections, such as immunocompromised cancer patients, AIDS patients, and the elderly population.

METHODS OF TREATMENT

Combination Chemotherapy

The development of drug resistance depends on such factors as the number of microorganisms or cancer cells in the pretreatment population, the rate of replication or "generation time" of the organism or cell, the intrinsic rate of mutation in the population, the target size for resistance mutations, and the replicative capacity (fitness) of the resistant organism or cell. Compared to treatment with a single agent, treatment with a combination of drugs can significantly decrease the probability that resistance will develop. Combination chemotherapy is the standard-of-care in tuberculosis and HIV therapy and most antineoplastic drug regimens. Despite potential or real drawbacks of increased toxicities and cost, there can be several major reasons to administer multiple drugs simultaneously in a combination chemotherapy regimen; the rationales are discussed in further detail in Chapter 41. First, the use of multiple drugs with different mechanisms of action targets multiple steps in microbial or cancer cell growth, leading to the maximum achievable effect. Second, provided that resistance to one drug does not also confer resistance to others in the combination, the use of combinations of drugs makes it more difficult for resistance to develop because, while the likelihood of development of a resistance mutation to one drug is relatively high, the concurrent emergence of separate mutations against several different drugs is less likely. The probability of resistance to multiple drugs is the product of the probabilities of resistance to the individual drugs in the combination; for example, if resistance to each drug has a probability of 10^{-3} (which would be high), then the probability of resistance to three drugs would be 10^{-9}. Third, the use of lower doses of synergistically acting drugs in the combination can reduce drug-associated adverse effects. This is especially important in antimicrobial chemotherapy, where synergistic activity of drug combinations has been clearly demonstrated. Fourth, because many cytotoxic antineoplastic drugs have distinct dose-limiting adverse effects (toxicities), it is often possible to give each drug to its maximally tolerated dose while achieving increased overall cell killing.

Finally, the concept of combination chemotherapy is being redefined as new treatments become available. In the future, immunotherapies, hormone therapies, and biotherapies will become increasingly integrated into combination chemotherapy regimens (see Chapter 54, Protein Therapeutics).

Prophylactic Chemotherapeutics

In most instances, antimicrobial and antineoplastic drugs are used to treat overt disease. These classes of drugs can also be used to prevent diseases from occurring (chemoprophylaxis), both before a potential exposure and after a known exposure. The potential benefit of chemoprophylaxis must always be weighed against the risk of evolving drug-resistant pathogens or cancer cells and the potential for toxicity attributable to the chemoprophylactic agent. Antimicrobial chemoprophylaxis is frequently used in high-risk patients to prevent infection. Travelers to malaria-infested areas, for example, often take prophylactic antimalarial drugs such as **mefloquine** (see Chapter 37). Chemoprophylaxis is also used in some types of surgery to prevent wound infections. Antibiotics are commonly administered prophylactically during surgical procedures that could release bacteria into the wound site, such as colon resection. In certain situations, immunocompromised patients are given antibacterial, antifungal, antiviral, and/or antiparasitic drugs prophylactically to prevent opportunistic infections. For example, **acyclovir** can protect previously infected immunocompromised patients against disease caused by reactivation of latent herpes simplex virus.

Chemoprophylaxis or preemptive therapy can also be used in healthy persons after exposures to certain pathogens. Prophylactic therapy after known or suspected exposure to gonorrhea, syphilis, bacterial meningitis, HIV, and other infections can often prevent disease. The risk of seroconversion after a single needle stick exposure to HIV-infected blood is approximately 0.3% (95% confidence interval [CI] = 0.2–0.5%). Although limited data are available regarding the reduction of risk achievable with prophylaxis, the CDC currently recommends postexposure treatment with a three-drug antiretroviral therapy regimen (e.g., **raltegravir, tenofovir [TDF]**, and **emtricitabine [FTC]**) for 4 weeks. Several antiretroviral drug combinations, such as **zidovudine + lamivudine** and TDF + FTC, have been shown to reduce maternal transmission of HIV, representing chemoprophylaxis for the fetus (see Chapter 38).

■ INHIBITORS OF FOLATE METABOLISM: EXAMPLES OF SELECTIVE TARGETING AND SYNERGISTIC DRUG INTERACTIONS

Folic acid is a vitamin that participates in multiple enzymatic reactions involving the transfer of one-carbon units. These reactions are essential for the biosynthesis of DNA and RNA precursors; the amino acids glycine, methionine, and glutamic acid; the formyl-methionine initiator tRNA; and other essential metabolites. Given the importance of folate metabolism in the biochemistry of the cell, it is not surprising that agents inhibiting folate biosynthesis and interfering with the folate cycle have been used widely in the treatment of bacterial infections, parasitic infections, and cancer. These drug classes also provide excellent examples of the principles of chemotherapy.

Folate Metabolism

The structure of folic acid contains three chemical moieties (Fig. 33-6A): a pteridine ring system, **para-aminobenzoic acid (PABA)**, and the amino acid glutamate. (Because of its ability to absorb ultraviolet light, PABA is the active ingredient in many topical sunscreens.) For humans, folate is an essential vitamin that must be provided intact in the diet. In bacteria and certain protozoans, however, folate is synthesized from precursors, as shown in Figure 33-7.

Both dietary folate and folate synthesized from precursors enter the folate cycle (Fig. 33-7). In this cycle, dihydrofolate is reduced to tetrahydrofolate by dihydrofolate reductase (DHFR). Tetrahydrofolate then participates in many metabolic interconversions that involve one-carbon transfers. For example, tetrahydrofolate is an essential donor of carbon atoms in the synthesis of inosine monophosphate (IMP) (leading to adenosine monophosphate [AMP] and guanosine monophosphate [GMP]) and in the conversion of deoxyuridine monophosphate (dUMP) to deoxythymidine monophosphate (dTMP) (see Fig. 39-2). In all of these reactions, tetrahydrofolate donates a carbon atom and, in the process, is oxidized to dihydrofolate. For further rounds of one-carbon transfers to occur, the dihydrofolate must be reduced to tetrahydrofolate by DHFR.

Inhibitors of Folate Metabolism

Antimetabolites are agents that inhibit nucleotide and DNA synthesis (see Chapter 39). This chapter uses one class of antimetabolites, the **inhibitors of folate metabolism**, to exemplify the basis for selective targeting of antimicrobial and antineoplastic drugs according to the distinctiveness of the drug target. As described above, selectivity can take the form of (1) a protein or a biochemical pathway that is unique to the pathogen or cancer cell, (2) a structure (isoform) of a protein that is specific to the pathogen or cancer cell, or (3) a requirement for a host protein or pathway that is specific to the pathogen or cancer cell. Where relevant, the following discussion emphasizes the basis for selectivity of each therapeutic agent.

Inhibitors of folate metabolism include inhibitors of dihydropteroate synthase and inhibitors of dihydrofolate reductase. In each case, drugs that structurally resemble the physiologic substrate of the enzyme act as enzyme inhibitors.

Unique Drug Targets: Antimicrobial Dihydropteroate Synthase Inhibitors

Bacteria and certain protozoans are unable to take up folic acid from the environment and therefore must synthesize the vitamin de novo from PABA, pteridine, and glutamate using the enzyme dihydropteroate synthase (Fig. 33-7). Mammalian cells, in contrast, use folate receptors and folate carriers in the plasma membrane of the gastrointestinal lining to scavenge the intact vitamin. This fundamental metabolic difference between pathogen and host cells helps make dihydropteroate synthase an excellent target for antimicrobial therapy. The **sulfa** drugs, such as **sulfamethoxazole** and **sulfadiazine**, are PABA analogues that competitively inhibit dihydropteroate synthase and thereby prevent the synthesis of folic acid in the pathogens. The lack of folic acid, in turn, prevents synthesis of purines, pyrimidines, and some amino acids and eventually results in cessation of pathogen growth. Sulfa drugs are usually bacteriostatic (i.e., they usually prevent bacterial growth

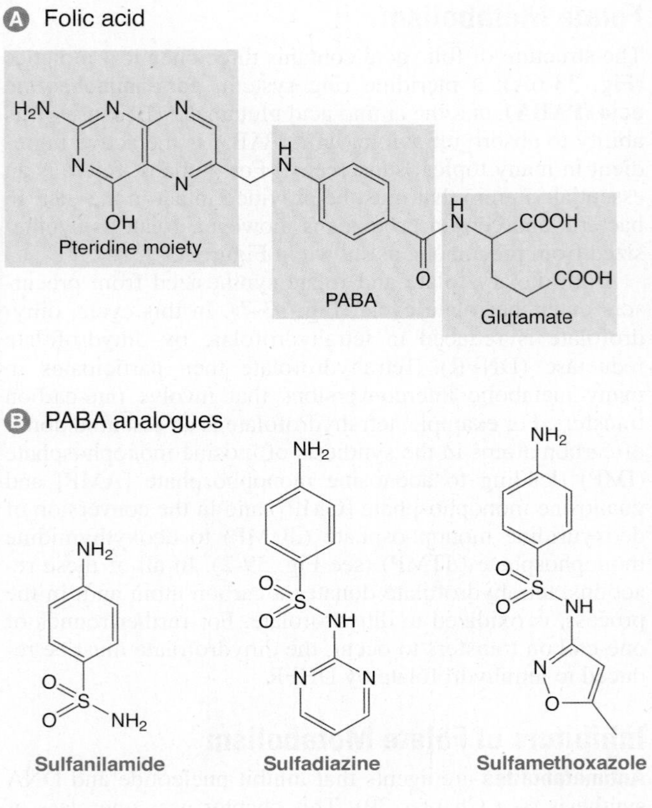

A Folic acid

B PABA analogues

Sulfanilamide   Sulfadiazine   Sulfamethoxazole

C Folate analogues

Methotrexate

Trimethoprim   Pyrimethamine

FIGURE 33-6. Structures of folic acid, PABA analogues (sulfonamides), and folate analogues (dihydrofolate reductase inhibitors). A. Folic acid is formed by the condensation of pteridine, para-aminobenzoic acid (PABA), and glutamate (see Fig. 33-7). Folate is the deprotonated form of folic acid. **B.** PABA analogues (sulfonamides) structurally resemble PABA. These drugs inhibit dihydropteroate synthase, the enzyme that catalyzes the formation of dihydropteroic acid from PABA and pteridine (see Fig. 33-7). **C.** Folate analogues (dihydrofolate reductase inhibitors) structurally resemble folic acid. These drugs inhibit dihydrofolate reductase, the enzyme that converts dihydrofolate to tetrahydrofolate.

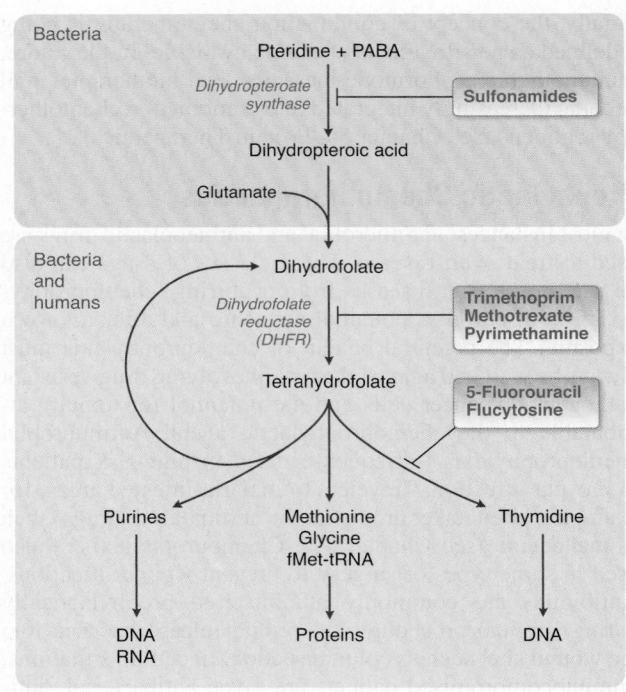

FIGURE 33-7. Folate synthesis and functions. Folate synthesis begins with the formation of dihydropteroic acid from pteridine and para-aminobenzoic acid (PABA); this reaction is catalyzed by dihydropteroate synthase. Glutamate and dihydropteroic acid condense to form dihydrofolate (DHF). DHF is reduced to tetrahydrofolate (THF) by dihydrofolate reductase (DHFR). THF and its congeners (*not shown*) serve as one-carbon donors in numerous reactions necessary for the biosynthesis of DNA, RNA, and proteins. In each such reaction, the reduced folate (THF) becomes oxidized to DHF, and the THF must then be regenerated via reduction by DHFR. Inhibitors of folate metabolism target three steps in the folate pathway. Sulfonamides inhibit dihydropteroate synthase; trimethoprim, methotrexate, and pyrimethamine inhibit DHFR; and 5-fluorouracil (5-FU) and flucytosine inhibit thymidylate synthase (see Fig. 39-4). Note that bacteria and certain parasites synthesize folate de novo from pteridine and PABA, whereas humans require dietary folate.

but do not kill the bacteria). However, in some settings in which thymine is unavailable, such as in urine, they can be bactericidal (thymine-less death). There are two structural classes of sulfa drugs: sulfonamides and sulfones.

Sulfonamides and Sulfones

As demonstrated in the case of Hildegard Domagk, **sulfonamides** were the first modern agents to be employed in the treatment of bacterial infections (prontosil is a sulfonamide precursor). Figure 33-6 shows the similarity in structure between PABA and the sulfonamide analogues **sulfanilamide**, **sulfadiazine**, and **sulfamethoxazole**. Sulfonamides are highly selective for dihydropteroate synthase. Because microbial growth requires activity of this enzyme, and the enzyme is not expressed in mammalian cells, this drug class has very few adverse effects (except in the special case of neonates, noted below).

Despite the exquisite selectivity of the sulfonamides, the development of resistance to these drugs has resulted in their diminished use. Resistance to sulfonamides most frequently develops because of (1) overproduction of the endogenous substrate, PABA, or (2) a mutation in the PABA binding site on dihydropteroate synthase, resulting in reduced affinity of the enzyme for sulfonamides. Some resistant streptococci produce levels of PABA that are 70-fold higher than the normal value.

Because of the high incidence of sulfonamide resistance in the bacterial and parasite populations, these drugs are rarely administered as single agents. Instead, they are commonly administered in combination with a synergistic drug such as **trimethoprim** or **pyrimethamine**, as discussed below.

Sulfonamides compete with bilirubin for binding sites on serum albumin and can cause kernicterus in newborns. **Kernicterus**, a condition characterized by markedly elevated concentrations of unconjugated (free) bilirubin in the blood of neonates, can lead to severe brain damage. For this reason, newborns should not be treated with sulfonamides.

Dapsone, a member of the **sulfone** class of dihydropteroate synthase inhibitors, is used in the treatment of leprosy and as a second-line agent in the prevention of *Pneumocystis jiroveci* pneumonia (PCP). The mechanism of action of dapsone is the same as that of the sulfonamides, and dapsone and trimethoprim or pyrimethamine can also be used as a synergistic drug combination (see discussion below). Because dapsone is an oxidizing agent, approximately 5% of patients can develop **methemoglobinemia** after administration of the drug. Susceptible patients are typically deficient in the erythrocyte enzyme glucose-6-phosphate dehydrogenase, which is involved in the detoxification of endogenous and exogenous oxidizing agents.

Selective Inhibition of Similar Targets: Antimicrobial Dihydrofolate Reductase Inhibitors

Dihydrofolate reductase (DHFR) is the enzyme that is used by all organisms to reduce dihydrofolate (DHF) to tetrahydrofolate (THF). Several drugs, including **trimethoprim**, **pyrimethamine**, and **methotrexate**, are folate analogues that competitively inhibit DHFR and prevent the regeneration of THF from DHF (Figs. 33-6 and 33-7). By doing so, these drugs prevent the synthesis of purine nucleotides as well as the methylation of dUMP to dTMP (see above). Pharmacologic inhibition of DHFR is used both in the treatment of infection and in cancer chemotherapy.

Many inhibitors of DHFR have been developed. As shown in Table 33-3, **methotrexate** is a potent (sub-nanomolar) inhibitor of DHFR, although it exhibits little selectivity amongst the mammalian, bacterial, and protozoal isoforms of the enzyme. In contrast, inhibitors with structures that are more divergent from that of folate, such as **trimethoprim** and **pyrimethamine** (see Fig. 33-6), show considerable selectivity of DHFR inhibition among the various isoforms of the enzyme. Trimethoprim is a potent and selective antibacterial agent; pyrimethamine is a potent and selective antiprotozoal drug; and methotrexate is an antineoplastic agent used to treat many different malignancies.

Why are trimethoprim and pyrimethamine each selective for specific isoforms of DHFR, while methotrexate is not? For example, a 50% reduction in the activity of bacterial DHFR can be achieved at a trimethoprim concentration of $0.007 \, \mu M$, while comparable inhibition of human DHFR requires a trimethoprim concentration of $350 \, \mu M$ (Table 33-3). In part, this may be because methotrexate closely resembles dihydrofolate, which is the normal substrate for DHFR. While the amino acid sequences of DHFRs amongst bacteria, protozoans, and humans vary substantially, these isoforms have been evolutionarily constrained to maintain their

TABLE 33-3 IC$_{50}$ Values for Three Dihydrofolate Reductase Inhibitors

DHFR Inhibitor	DHFR Isoform		
	E. coli DHFR	Malarial DHFR	Mammalian DHFR
Trimethoprim	**7**	1,800	350,000
Pyrimethamine	2,500	**0.5**	1,800
Methotrexate	0.1	0.7	**0.2**

IC$_{50}$ is the concentration of drug required for 50% enzyme inhibition. All values are reported in nM (10^{-9} M) units. Boldface indicates the DHFR isoform targeted for therapy. Trimethoprim and pyrimethamine are selective inhibitors of the *E. coli* and malarial isoforms of DHFR, respectively. In contrast, methotrexate is a nonselective inhibitor of all three DHFR isoforms. DHFR, dihydrofolate reductase.

enzymatic activity in the conversion of DHF to THF and therefore remain sensitive to drugs such as MTX that closely mimic the enzymatic substrate. In contrast, drugs such as trimethoprim and pyrimethamine, which are poorer mimics of the enzymatic substrate, are able to take advantage of these sequence differences, which translate to structural differences, and more selectively target individual isoforms. The basis for selectivity thus resides in differences in enzyme structure that are largely irrelevant for binding of the natural substrate but that have an important role in analogue (drug) binding. Increased understanding of the structural basis for DHFR inhibition may lead to the development of still more selective agents.

Trimethoprim

Trimethoprim is a folate analogue that selectively inhibits bacterial DHFR (Fig. 33-6C; Table 33-3) and thereby prevents the conversion of DHF to THF. As with the sulfonamides, trimethoprim is usually bacteriostatic, although it, too, can lead to thymine-less death in certain settings. Because trimethoprim is excreted unchanged in the urine, it can be used as a single agent to treat uncomplicated urinary tract infections. For most infections, however, trimethoprim is used in combination with sulfamethoxazole. The rationale for this combination antibacterial chemotherapy is described below.

Pyrimethamine

Pyrimethamine is a folate analogue that selectively inhibits parasitic DHFR (Fig. 33-6C; Table 33-3). Pyrimethamine is currently the only effective chemotherapeutic agent against toxoplasmosis; for this indication, it is typically administered in combination with sulfadiazine. Pyrimethamine has also been used to treat malaria, although widespread resistance has limited its effectiveness in recent years. Further discussion of the therapeutic applications of pyrimethamine and sulfadiazine can be found in Chapter 37.

Common Targets: Antineoplastic Dihydrofolate Reductase Inhibitors

Methotrexate

As described above, **methotrexate (MTX)** is a folate analogue that reversibly inhibits DHFR. In mammalian cells, DHFR inhibition causes a critical shortage of intracellular supplies of tetrahydrofolate, resulting in inhibition of de novo purine and thymidylate synthesis and, therefore, cessation of DNA and RNA synthesis. Because the synthesis of DNA is halted, mammalian cells treated with methotrexate are arrested in the S phase of the cell cycle.

The basis for the relative selectivity of methotrexate for cancer cells compared to normal cells is thought to be that rapidly growing cancer cells have an increased requirement for metabolites, such as purines and thymidylate, that are critical to DNA synthesis and that are generated by folate-dependent enzymes. In addition, malignant cells may be more susceptible than normal cells to the apoptosis-inducing effects of MTX (see discussion below). Of note, the usefulness of high-dose MTX in cancer chemotherapy has been greatly improved by the application of **folinic acid rescue**. In this technique, folinic acid (N-5 formyltetrahydrofolate, also called **leucovorin**) is administered to the patient several hours after an otherwise lethal dose of methotrexate. The rationale for this technique is that the malignant cells are killed selectively, while the normal cells are "rescued" by the folinic acid. The molecular mechanism underlying folinic acid rescue is unclear. One hypothesis suggests that normal (nonmalignant) cells are able to concentrate the folinic acid (and, thus, to protect themselves from the effects of MTX), whereas malignant cells have a reduced rate of folinic acid transport (and, therefore, are preferentially harmed by high doses of MTX). Another hypothesis suggests that high-dose MTX induces apoptosis in malignant cells but cell-cycle arrest in normal cells; the normal cells are then able to use the folinic acid to resume cell growth and division, while the malignant cells are already committed to programmed cell death.

MTX is used to treat many tumor types, including carcinomas of the breast, lung, and head and neck, acute lymphoblastic leukemia, and choriocarcinoma. MTX is also used to treat psoriasis and certain autoimmune diseases such as rheumatoid arthritis. Methotrexate toxicity is manifested primarily in rapidly dividing host cells, causing damage to the gastrointestinal mucosa and the bone marrow. These effects are generally reversible after therapy is discontinued. MTX is extremely toxic to the fetus because folic acid is essential for the proper differentiation of fetal cells and for closure of the neural tube. MTX has undergone clinical trials as an abortion-inducing agent, either alone or in combination with the prostaglandin analogue **misoprostol**, and is sometimes used off-label to terminate early-stage ectopic pregnancy.

Synergy of DHFR Inhibitors and Sulfonamides

Both trimethoprim and pyrimethamine can be used in combination with sulfonamides to block sequential steps in the biosynthetic pathway leading to tetrahydrofolate (Fig. 33-7). This type of combination chemotherapy, called **sequential blockade**, has been effective in the treatment of certain parasitic infections (pyrimethamine and sulfadiazine) and bacterial infections (trimethoprim and sulfamethoxazole). One rationale for the use of a DHFR inhibitor and a sulfa drug in combination is the marked synergistic interaction between these two classes of drugs (see Chapter 41). The sulfonamide decreases the intracellular concentration of dihydrofolate; this increases the effectiveness of the DHFR inhibitor, which competes with dihydrofolate for binding to the enzyme. The sulfa/DHFR inhibitor combination can also be effective in treating strains of bacteria and parasites that exhibit resistance to monotherapy with a DHFR inhibitor. Typically, this

drug resistance phenotype is caused by the expression of a structurally altered DHFR that has a lower affinity for the inhibitor. The trade-off for the bacteria or parasite is often that the altered DHFR also has a lower affinity for the natural ligand dihydrofolate. In such strains, sulfonamide treatment can decrease the intracellular concentration of dihydrofolate to the point that the altered DHFR cannot meet the metabolic requirements of the cell.

Another important rationale for the use of a combination such as trimethoprim/sulfamethoxazole is that resistance to trimethoprim alone or sulfamethoxazole alone develops rather quickly, whereas resistance to the drug combination develops much more slowly. As discussed earlier in the chapter, because the two drugs act on different enzymes, two different mutations would need to occur simultaneously for the bacteria to develop resistance to the drug combination, and the likelihood that two mutations will occur simultaneously is much lower than the likelihood that one mutation will occur (see Chapter 41).

CONCLUSION AND FUTURE DIRECTIONS

Many of the principles underlying the pharmacologic treatment of microbial diseases and cancer are similar. Pharmacologic treatments of both infection and cancer rely on selective inhibition of the pathogen or cancer cell to prevent its growth or survival, with a minimum of adverse effects that could interfere with host function. Selective inhibition of a unique target, such as the bacterial cell wall, is, in principle, ideal. Often, less selective therapies must be employed, targeting a molecule or pathway that is similar or even identical between the pathogen or cancer cell and the host. Even highly selective drugs aimed at an entirely unique target can be rendered ineffective if the microbe or cancer cell mutates to become resistant. Both microbes and cancer cells grow rapidly, with the potential for evolving or acquiring mutations that confer resistance. Physicians attempt to circumvent the development of resistance by initiating treatment early, using maximally tolerated doses of drugs, and administering multiple drugs in combination. Despite these strategies, however, resistance has become a major impediment to successful therapy. As more is learned about the biology of microbes and cancer cells and more unique targets are discovered, it is hoped that treatments will become more selective, less toxic, and less prone to the development of drug resistance.

Antimetabolite-based therapies, such as the inhibition of folate metabolism, have a long and storied history and have taught us a great deal about the principles of selective toxicity in the treatment of infections and cancer. Despite the advent of novel anticancer therapies directed at newly identified driver mutations, transcription factors, or immune regulators, antimetabolite therapies remain both a cornerstone of current cancer treatment and the subject of active investigation. For example, a recent analysis of expression patterns of metabolic enzymes in matched tumor and normal tissue samples showed that tumors overexpress TSTA3, PYCR1, and MTHFD2. These enzymes play critical roles in fucosylation, proline synthesis, and mitochondrial one-carbon metabolism, respectively—metabolic processes that are currently less appreciated in cancer pathophysiology. Methylenetetrahydrofolate dehydrogenase ($NADP^+$ dependent) 2

(MTHFD2) is the mitochondrial paralog of an enzyme that plays a vital role in one-carbon transfers. In the mitochondria, MTHFD2 acts to generate formate (likely through glycine catabolism) that is exported to the cytosol, conjugated to THF by the cytosolic paralog MTHFD1, and then used for nucleotide synthesis. This finding adds to our appreciation of the complexity of folate metabolism and, in particular, the role of mitochondria and mitochondrial paralogs of folate-dependent enzymes in nucleotide synthesis. Although much more work needs to be done, TSTA3, PYCR1, and MTHFD2 may together represent novel metabolic targets in the treatment of cancer and, in the case of MTHFD2, deepen our understanding of folate metabolism and open the door to the development of novel drugs. The work that Gerhard Domagk began 80 years ago continues to yield new knowledge and the promise of new therapies.

Acknowledgment

We thank Heidi Harbison, Harris S. Rose, and Quentin J. Baca for their valuable contributions to this chapter in the First, Second, and Third Editions of *Principles of Pharmacology: The Pathophysiologic Basis of Drug Therapy*.

Suggested Reading

American Cancer Society Statistics. http://www.cancer.org/docroot/STT/stt_0.asp. (*Source of cancer statistics provided in this chapter.*)

Antimicrobial Resistance Prevention Initiative: proceedings of an expert panel on resistance. *Am J Med* 2006;119(6 Suppl 1):S1–S76. (*Series of seven articles and discussion on mechanisms of antimicrobial drug resistance.*)

Bennett JE, Dolin R, Blaser MJ, eds. *Mandell, Douglas, and Bennett's principles and practice of infectious diseases*. 8th ed. Philadelphia: Churchill Livingstone; 2014. (*Authoritative textbook on clinical management of infectious diseases.*)

Coen DM, Richman DD. Antiviral agents. In: Knipe DM, Howley PM, Cohen JI, et al., eds. *Fields virology*. 6th ed. Philadelphia: Lippincott Williams & Wilkins; 2013:338–373. (*Detailed review of the mechanisms and uses of antiviral drugs.*)

Fischbach MA, Walsh CT. Antibiotics for emerging pathogens. *Science* 2009;325:1089–1093. (*Overview of the need for new antibiotics to treat infections with multidrug-resistant organisms and discussion of approaches to identifying novel classes of antibiotics.*)

Kuhar DT, Henderson DK, Struble KA, et al. Updated US Public Health Service guidelines for the management of occupational exposures to human immunodeficiency virus and recommendations for postexposure prophylaxis. *Infect Control Hosp Epidemiol* 2013;34:875–892. (*Comprehensive guidelines for postexposure prophylaxis for the prevention of HIV infection, including an extensive reference list.*)

LaFemina R, ed. *Antiviral research: strategies in antiviral drug discovery*. Washington, DC: ASM Press; 2009. (*Review of strategies used to discover antiviral drugs.*)

Moscow JA, Schneider E, Sikic BI, et al. Drug resistance and its clinical circumvention. In: Hong WK, Bast RC Jr, Hait W, et al., eds. *Holland-Frei cancer medicine*. 8th ed. Hamilton, Ontario, Canada: BC Decker and American Association for Cancer Research; 2009:597–610. (*Discusses mechanisms of resistance to antineoplastic agents.*)

Nilsson R, Jain M, Madhusudhan N, et al. Metabolic enzyme expression highlights a key role for MTHFD2 and the mitochondrial folate pathway in cancer. *Nat Commun* 2014;5:3128–3133. (*Demonstrates role of MTHFD2 in cancer.*)

US Public Health Service. Preexposure prophylaxis for the prevention of HIV infection in the United States – 2014: a clinical practice guideline. www.cdc.gov/hiv/pdf/PrEPguidelines2014.pdf. (*Comprehensive guidelines for preexposure prophylaxis for the prevention of HIV infection, including an extensive reference list.*)

Vousden KH, Prives C. Blinded by the light: the growing complexity of p53. *Cell* 2009;137:413–431. (*Review of p53 mechanisms, functions, and pharmacology.*)

Walsh CT. *Antibiotics: actions, origins, resistance*. Washington, DC: ASM Press; 2003. (*Reviews structural and chemical basis of antibiotic action and resistance.*)

WHO Statistical Information System. http://www.who.int/whosis/. (*Source of world health statistics provided in this chapter.*)

DRUG SUMMARY TABLE: CHAPTER 33 Principles of Antimicrobial and Antineoplastic Pharmacology

DRUG	CLINICAL APPLICATIONS	*SERIOUS* AND COMMON ADVERSE EFFECTS	CONTRAINDICATIONS	THERAPEUTIC CONSIDERATIONS
ANTIMICROBIAL DIHYDROPTEROATE SYNTHASE INHIBITORS Mechanism—PABA analogues that competitively inhibit microbial dihydropteroate synthase and thereby prevent the synthesis of folic acid				
Sulfonamides: **Sulfanilamide** **Sulfadiazine** **Sulfamethoxazole** **Sulfadoxine (See Chapter 36)** **Sulfalene (See Chapter 36)**	Susceptible vaginal infections (sulfanilamide) Toxoplasmosis, *Haemophilus influenzae*, chancroid, inclusion conjunctivitis, meningococcal meningitis, nocardiosis, recurrent rheumatic fever, trachoma (sulfadiazine) Atypical mycobacterial infection, chancroid (sulfamethoxazole) *Pneumocystis jiroveci* pneumonia, shigellosis, traveler's diarrhea, urinary tract infection, granuloma inguinale, acute otitis media (sulfamethoxazole/trimethoprim)	*Kernicterus in newborns, crystalluria, Stevens-Johnson syndrome, agranulocytosis, aplastic anemia, hepatic failure* Gastrointestinal disturbance, rash	Hypersensitivity to sulfonamides Infants less than 2 months old Pregnant women at term Breastfeeding Megaloblastic anemia due to folate deficiency	Because of the high incidence of sulfonamide resistance, sulfonamides are commonly administered in combination with a synergistic drug such as trimethoprim or pyrimethamine. Sulfonamides compete with bilirubin for binding sites on serum albumin and can cause kernicterus in newborns. Avoid co-administration with PABA, which is the natural substrate for dihydropteroate synthase.
Sulfones: **Dapsone**	Acne vulgaris Leprosy Dermatitis herpetiformis	*Hemolytic anemia, methemoglobinemia, aplastic anemia, agranulocytosis, toxic epidermal necrolysis, pancreatitis, toxic hepatitis, suicidal ideation*	Hypersensitivity to dapsone Glucose-6-phosphate dehydrogenase (G6PD) deficiency	Dapsone and trimethoprim or pyrimethamine can be used as a synergistic drug combination. Patients susceptible to hemolytic anemia and methemoglobinemia are typically deficient in the erythrocyte enzyme G6PD.
ANTIMICROBIAL DIHYDROFOLATE REDUCTASE INHIBITORS Mechanism—Folate analogues that competitively inhibit microbial dihydrofolate reductase (DHFR) and thereby prevent the regeneration of tetrahydrofolate from dihydrofolate				
Trimethoprim	Urinary tract infection See above for applications of sulfamethoxazole/trimethoprim combination therapy	*Stevens-Johnson syndrome, erythema multiforme, anaphylaxis, megaloblastic anemia* Rash, pruritus	Hypersensitivity to trimethoprim Megaloblastic anemia due to folate deficiency	Selectively inhibits bacterial DHFR. Trimethoprim is bacteriostatic and can be used as a single agent to treat uncomplicated urinary tract infection. Typically used in combination with sulfamethoxazole.
Pyrimethamine (See Chapter 36)	Toxoplasmosis Malaria	*Stevens-Johnson syndrome, leukopenia, megaloblastic anemia, anaphylaxis* Rash	Hypersensitivity to pyrimethamine Megaloblastic anemia due to folate deficiency	Selectively inhibits parasitic DHFR. Typically used in combination with sulfadiazine for treatment of toxoplasmosis. Folic acid may interfere with the efficacy of pyrimethamine.

ANTINEOPLASTIC DIHYDROFOLATE REDUCTASE INHIBITOR
Mechanism—Folate analogue that competitively inhibits mammalian DHFR and thereby prevents the regeneration of tetrahydrofolate from dihydrofolate

| Methotrexate | Many tumor types, including carcinomas of the breast, lung, head and neck; acute lymphoblastic leukemia; choriocarcinoma

Autoimmune diseases including psoriasis, rheumatoid arthritis | *Thromboembolic disorder, erythema multiforme, Stevens-Johnson syndrome, myelosuppression, hepatotoxicity, kidney disease, interstitial pulmonary disease, leukoencephalopathy, seizure, malignant lymphoma, opportunistic infection*

Gastrointestinal disturbance, stomatitis, alopecia, photosensitivity, rash, headache, bronchitis, nasopharyngitis | Hypersensitivity to methotrexate

Pregnancy

Breastfeeding

Patients with psoriasis or rheumatoid arthritis who also have alcoholism, alcoholic liver disease, chronic liver disease, preexisting blood dyscrasia, or laboratory evidence of immunodeficiency syndrome | The use of high-dose methotrexate in cancer chemotherapy has been broadened by the application of folinic acid rescue.

Methotrexate toxicity to the gastrointestinal mucosa and bone marrow is generally reversible after therapy is discontinued.

Extremely toxic to the fetus because folic acid is essential for differentiation of fetal cells and for neural tube closure.

Avoid co-administration of polio vaccine in immunosuppressed patients receiving methotrexate as a component of chemotherapy.

Avoid concurrent alcohol intake.

Use extreme caution with co-administration of naproxen and phenylbutazone due to sporadic case reports of deaths.

Co-administration with trimethoprim may result in severe methotrexate toxicity.

Oral absorption of methotrexate can be decreased by up to 50% in patients receiving oral antibiotic mixtures containing paromomycin, neomycin, nystatin, and vancomycin. |

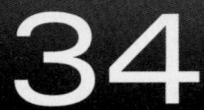

34

Pharmacology of Bacterial Infections: DNA Replication, Transcription, and Translation

Alexander J. McAdam and Donald M. Coen

■ INTRODUCTION

The central dogma processes—DNA replication, transcription, and translation—are generally similar in bacteria and humans. DNA is replicated and transcribed into RNA, and messenger RNA is translated into protein. However, there are important differences in the biochemistry of bacterial and human central dogma processes, and these differences can be exploited for the development and clinical use of antibiotics. Three such differences are targeted by the currently available antibacterial chemotherapeutic drugs: (1) *topoisomerases*, which regulate supercoiling of DNA and mediate segregation of replicated strands of DNA; (2) *RNA polymerases*, which transcribe DNA into RNA; and (3) *ribosomes*, which translate messenger RNA (mRNA) into protein. This chapter briefly reviews the biochemistry of central dogma processes in bacteria and discusses certain relevant differences between these processes in bacteria and humans. With this background, the chapter discusses the mechanisms by which pharmacologic agents interrupt bacterial DNA replication, transcription, and translation.

■ BIOCHEMISTRY OF BACTERIAL DNA REPLICATION, TRANSCRIPTION, AND TRANSLATION

The central dogma of molecular biology begins with the structure of DNA, which is the macromolecule that carries

genetic information. To transmit all of the genetic information in a cell to two progeny cells, the parental DNA must be copied in its entirety (replicated), and the two resulting copies must be segregated—one copy going to each progeny cell. In order to express the genes that are present in the DNA, these specific portions of the DNA are copied (transcribed) into RNA. Some RNAs (mRNAs) are then read (translated) by the protein synthesis machinery in order to produce proteins. Certain other RNAs, such as transfer RNAs (tRNAs) and ribosomal RNAs (rRNAs), perform complex functions essential to protein synthesis. It is important to note that the following discussion of these bacterial processes is vastly simplified in order to emphasize the steps that are inhibited by antibiotics.

DNA Structure

DNA is composed of two strands of polymerized deoxyribonucleotides that wind around one another in a "double helix" conformation. The 3′-hydroxyl group of each nucleotide's deoxyribose ring is joined by a phosphate group to the 5′-hydroxyl group of the next nucleotide, thereby forming the phosphodiester backbone of each side of the double helical "ladder" (Figs. 34-1 and 34-2). The purines **adenine** *(A)* and **guanine** *(G)* and the pyrimidines **thymine** *(T)* and **cytosine** *(C)*, which are covalently linked to the deoxyribose ring, associate with one another (*A* with *T*, *G* with *C*) via hydrogen bonds to form the "rungs" of the ladder (Fig. 34-2). *It is the*

CASE

It is the summer of 1976. Participants returning from an American Legion convention in Philadelphia are falling severely ill with a mysterious type of pneumonia. The outbreak centers on the Bellevue Stratford Hotel, where 150 hotel occupants and 32 passersby contract "Legionnaires' disease." Twenty-nine victims ultimately die. Conventional sputum stains, cultures, and even autopsy material show no consistent pathogens. The terror of an unknown epidemic disease sparks rumors and news reports of poison gases, tainted water supplies, terrorists, and deadly viruses.

Several months later, laboratory and field investigation teams from the Centers for Disease Control and Prevention (CDC) identify the causative aerobic Gram-negative bacterium and name it *Legionella pneumophila*. It is observed that patients treated with erythromycin, a macrolide antibiotic, and tetracycline have better outcomes than those treated with other agents. Today, newer macrolides, such as azithromycin, and fluoroquinolones are often used for treating Legionnaires' disease—as well as many chlamydial, streptococcal, and staphylococcal infections.

Questions

1. Why are some antibiotics such as quinolones and aminoglycosides bactericidal, while other antibiotics such as tetracyclines and macrolides are bacteriostatic?

2. Which step in translation is blocked by tetracyclines and which by macrolides?

3. How do bacteria develop resistance to macrolide and fluoroquinolone antibiotics? Do they need to acquire exogenous DNA in order to become resistant to these antibiotics?

linear sequence of bases that encodes the genetic information of a cell. How the nucleotide precursors to these bases are synthesized is reviewed in Chapter 39, Pharmacology of Cancer: Genome Synthesis, Stability, and Maintenance. DNA structure is essentially the same between bacteria and eukaryotes. However, bacterial chromosomes are usually circular DNAs, while eukaryotic chromosomes, including our own, are linear molecules.

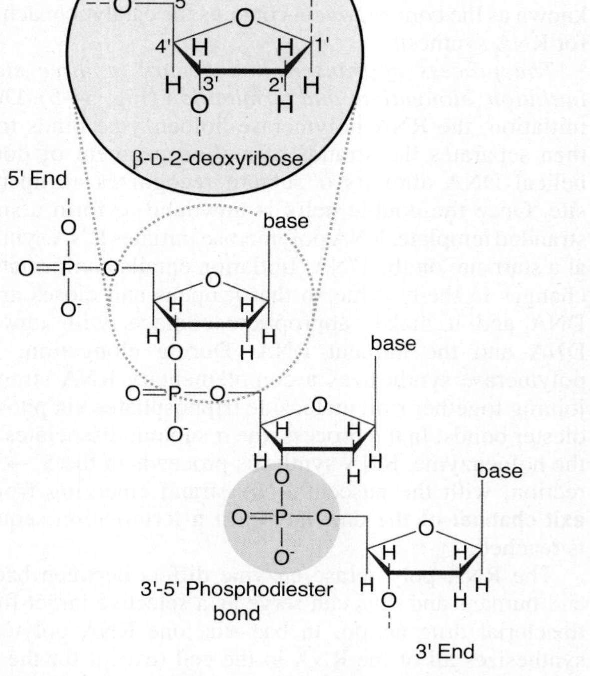

DNA Replication, Segregation, and Topoisomerases

The faithful replication and segregation of bacterial DNA to progeny cells involve numerous steps, many of which could make good targets for antibacterial drugs. To date, the enzymes in this process that have been most successfully targeted are **topoisomerases**. These enzymes perform several functions during DNA replication and segregation.

During DNA replication in both bacterial and eukaryotic cells, complementary strands of DNA are synthesized bidirectionally, forming two so-called replication forks. To initiate this process, the two DNA strands that compose the double helix must unwind and separate. In so doing, the DNA strands form excess **"supercoils"** in which the helical polymer overtwists as it rotates in the same direction as the turn of the helix. Supercoils increase tension in DNA strands and thereby interfere with further unwinding. In the absence of a process to relieve the stress created by the supercoils, the entire chromosome would have to rotate; this process would be complex and energy-consuming and could entangle the entire molecule.

Moreover, when DNA replication is completed, the two progeny DNA copies are wrapped around each other. In bacteria, because the chromosomes are circular, the intertwined progeny copies form interlocking rings (catenanes). These intertwined rings must be separated (resolved) before they can be segregated to the progeny cells.

Topoisomerases perform both of these functions—removing excess DNA supercoils during DNA replication and separating intertwined progeny DNA. *Topoisomerases catalyze these activities by breaking, rotating, and resealing DNA strands.* There are two types of topoisomerases. **Type I topoisomerases** form and reseal single-stranded breaks in DNA to decrease positive supercoiling (Fig. 34-3). **Type II topoisomerases** form and reseal double-stranded

FIGURE 34-1. Backbone structure of DNA. DNA is a polymer of nucleotides in which a phosphodiester bond connects the 2′-deoxyribose sugars of each neighboring nucleotide. The phosphodiester bond links the 3′-OH of one deoxyribose to the 5′-OH of the next deoxyribose, thus forming the backbone of the DNA strand.

β-D-2-deoxyribose

5′ End

3′-5′ Phosphodiester bond

3′ End

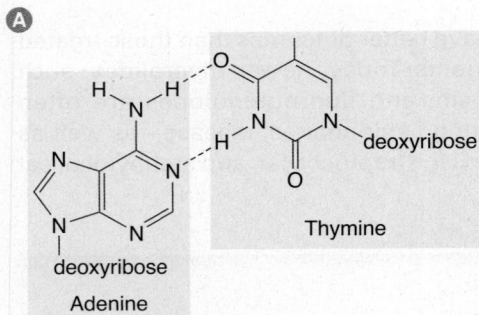

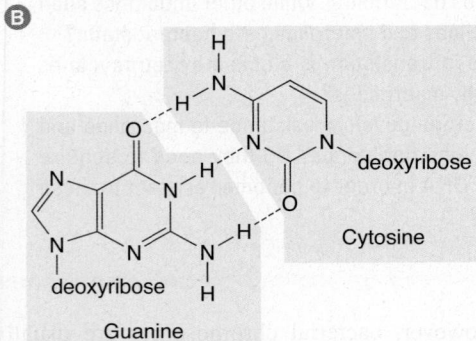

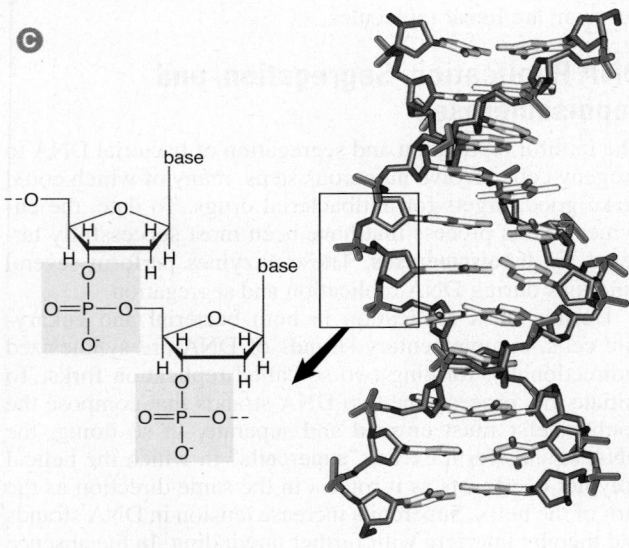

FIGURE 34-2. Hydrogen bonding between DNA strands. A and **B**. The *dashed lines* indicate hydrogen bonds between complementary bases on opposite DNA strands. Adenine *(A)* and thymine *(T)* form two hydrogen bonds, while guanine *(G)* and cytosine *(C)* form three hydrogen bonds. **C.** These *A-T* and *G-C* base pairs form the "rungs" of the DNA double helical "ladder." Note that the deoxyribose moieties and phosphodiester bonds are located on the outside of the DNA double helix, while the purine and pyrimidine bases stack in the center of the DNA molecule.

breaks (Fig. 34-4). Both types of topoisomerases can remove excess DNA supercoils during DNA replication. However, only type II topoisomerases can resolve intertwined copies of double-stranded DNA to permit segregation of the DNA to daughter cells. Type II enzymes are both more complex and more versatile than type I topoisomerases, and the type II enzyme is a more common molecular target for chemotherapeutic agents.

The mechanism of action of a type II topoisomerase proceeds in two steps. First, the enzyme binds a segment of DNA and forms covalent bonds with phosphates from each strand, thereby nicking both strands. Second, the enzyme causes a second stretch of DNA from the same molecule to pass through the break, relieving supercoiling (Fig. 34-4). This passage of double-stranded DNA through a double-stranded break permits separation of intertwined copies of DNA following replication and, thereby, segregation of DNA into progeny cells.

Two main type II topoisomerases are present in bacteria. The first to be identified, **DNA gyrase**, is a type II topoisomerase that is unusual in that it can introduce negative supercoils before the DNA strands separate and thereby neutralize positive supercoils that form during DNA unwinding. The second is **topoisomerase IV**. DNA gyrase is particularly crucial for segregation in some bacteria, while topoisomerase IV is the critical enzyme in other bacteria.

Because supercoiling is important for transcription as well as segregation, topoisomerases influence this central dogma process as well. Given their multiple functions, topoisomerases are usually engaged with DNA, and this is important for their roles as drug targets. These enzymes are important not only as antibacterial drug targets but also as targets for cancer chemotherapy (see Chapter 39).

Bacterial Transcription

Gene expression begins with transcription, which involves the synthesis of single-stranded RNA transcripts from a DNA template. Transcription is catalyzed by the enzyme **RNA polymerase**. In bacteria, five subunits (2 α, 1 β, 1 β', and 1 σ) associate to form the holoenzyme. As discussed below, the σ subunit is instrumental for initiating transcription, while the rest of the RNA polymerase enzyme—also known as the *core enzyme*—contains the catalytic machinery for RNA synthesis.

The process of transcription occurs in three stages: initiation, elongation, and termination (Fig. 34-5). During initiation, the RNA polymerase holoenzyme binds to and then separates the strands of a short segment of double-helical DNA after its σ subunit recognizes an upstream site. Once the double helix is unwound to form a single-stranded template, RNA polymerase initiates RNA synthesis at a start site on the DNA. Initiation entails conformational changes in the enzyme so that it opens and closes around DNA and it makes appropriate contacts with unwound DNA and the nascent RNA. During elongation, RNA polymerase synthesizes a complementary RNA strand by joining together ribonucleoside triphosphates via phosphodiester bonds. In the process, the σ subunit dissociates from the holoenzyme. RNA synthesis proceeds in the 5'→3' direction, with the nascent RNA strand emerging from an **exit channel** of the enzyme, until a termination sequence is reached.

The RNA polymerase enzyme differs between bacteria and humans and thus can serve as a selective target for antibacterial drug action. In bacteria, one RNA polymerase synthesizes all of the RNA in the cell (except for the short RNA primers needed for DNA replication, which are made by **primase**). In contrast, eukaryotes express three different nuclear RNA polymerases, and each enzyme is considerably more complex in its subunit structure than the bacterial counterpart.

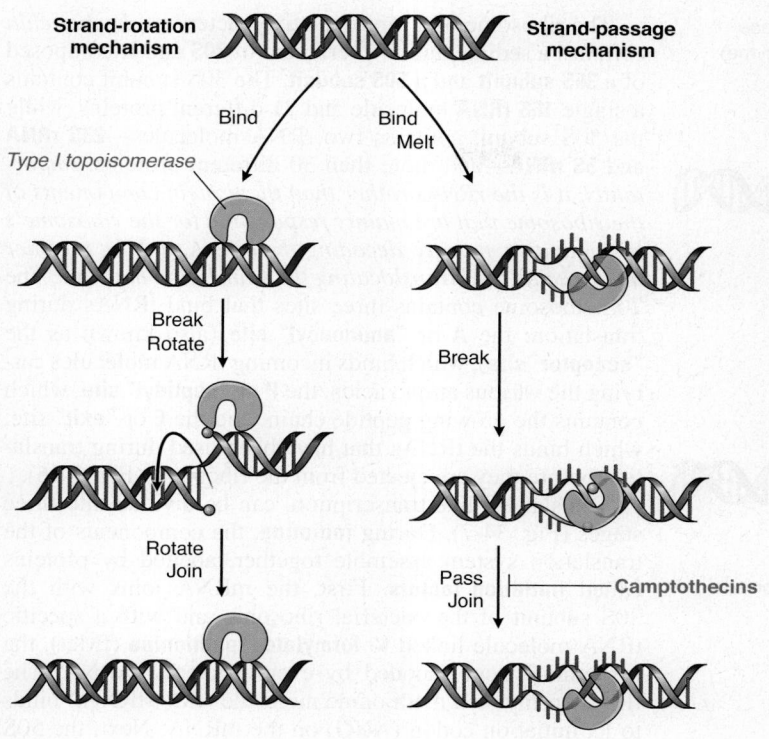

Strand-rotation mechanism

Strand-passage mechanism

Bind

Bind
Melt

Type I topoisomerase

Break
Rotate

Break

Rotate
Join

Pass
Join — **Camptothecins**

FIGURE 34-3. Regulation of DNA supercoiling by type I topoisomerases. Two mechanisms have been proposed for the action of type I topoisomerases. In the strand-rotation model, type I topoisomerase binds to opposite strands of the DNA double helix. The topoisomerase then nicks one strand and remains bound to one of the nicked ends (*filled green circle*). The unbound end of the nicked strand is able to unwind by one or more turns and is then joined (religated) to its parent strand. In the strand-passage model, type I topoisomerase binding to the DNA double helix results in melting (separation) of the two DNA strands. The DNA-bound topoisomerase then introduces a nick into one strand, while remaining bound to each end of the broken DNA strand (*filled green circles*). The broken strand is then passed through the helix and joined (religated), resulting in a net unwinding of the DNA. Camptothecins, which are used in cancer chemotherapy (see Chapter 39), inhibit the joining of the broken strand of DNA after strand passage.

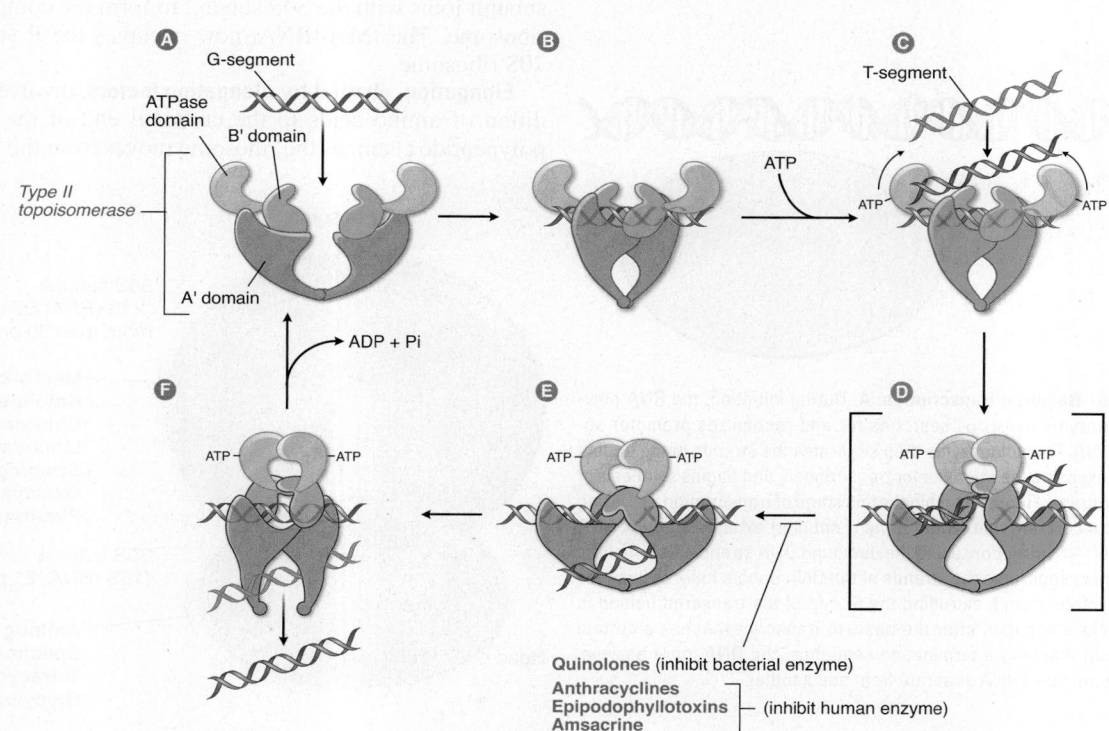

(A) G-segment

ATPase domain

B' domain

Type II topoisomerase

A' domain

ADP + Pi

(B)

(C) T-segment

ATP

ATP — — ATP

(D) ATP — — ATP

(E) ATP — — ATP

(F) ATP — — ATP

Quinolones (inhibit bacterial enzyme)

Anthracyclines
Epipodophyllotoxins ⎤ (inhibit human enzyme)
Amsacrine ⎦

FIGURE 34-4. Regulation of DNA supercoiling by type II topoisomerases. A. The type II topoisomerase enzymes contain A', B', and ATPase domains. The A' and B' domains engage a segment of the DNA double helix (G-segment). **B.** Interaction with the G-segment induces a conformational change in the type II isomerase, causing it to "lock" around the DNA G-segment. **C.** ATP binds to the ATPase domains of the topoisomerase, and a second segment of the DNA double helix (T-segment) enters and is "locked" into the B' domains. **D.** Once the enzyme is engaged with both DNA segments, the topoisomerase cuts both strands of the G-segment DNA. **E.** This double-stranded break in the G-segment allows the T-segment to pass through the G-segment to the opposite side of the topoisomerase. **F.** The T-segment is released from the topoisomerase, and the G-segment break is resealed. ATP is hydrolyzed to ADP, ADP dissociates from the topoisomerase, and the cycle begins anew. The result of each cycle is to change the coiling of DNA or, when two separate circular DNA molecules are involved, to resolve catenanes. Quinolone antibiotics inhibit passage of the T-segment and resealing of the G-segment by bacterial type II topoisomerases. At therapeutic concentrations, quinolones also promote topoisomerase subunit dissociation, resulting in double-stranded breaks in the DNA and killing of the bacteria. Several classes of cancer chemotherapeutic agents, including the anthracyclines, epipodophyllotoxins, and amsacrine, inhibit passage of the T-segment and resealing of the G-segment by human type II topoisomerases, thereby causing double-stranded DNA breaks and inducing apoptosis of the cancer cells (see Chapter 39).

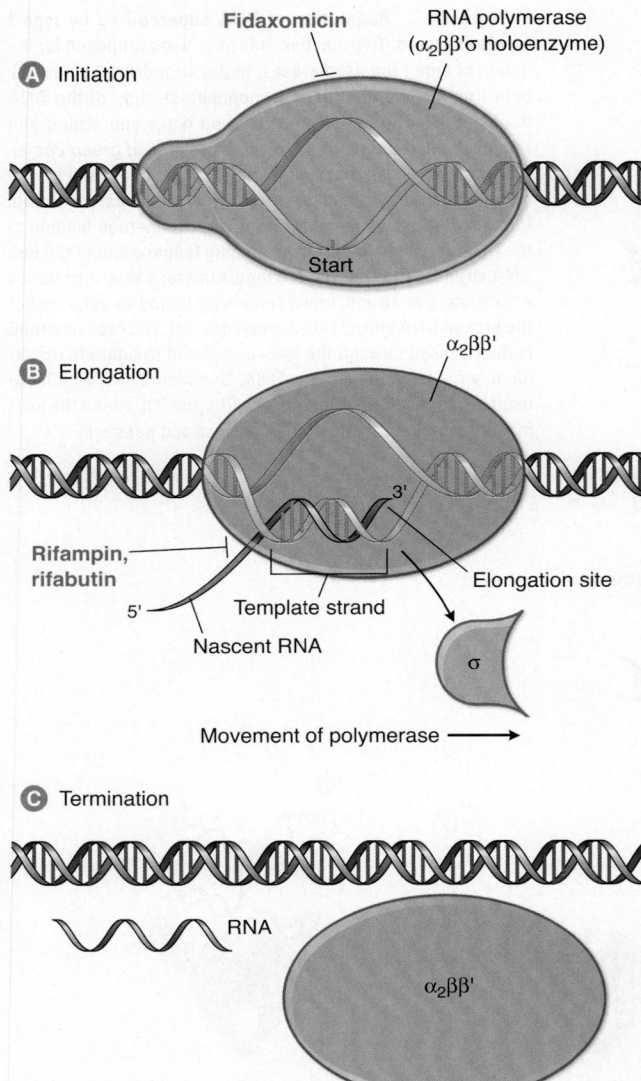

FIGURE 34-5. Bacterial transcription. A. During initiation, the RNA polymerase holoenzyme ($\alpha_2\beta\beta'\sigma$) searches for and recognizes promoter sequences on DNA. The holoenzyme then separates the strands of the double helical DNA, exposing the start site for transcription, and begins synthesis of the new RNA strand. Fidaxomicin blocks this stage of transcription. **B.** During elongation, the core enzyme (without the σ subunit) extends the new RNA strand in the $5' \rightarrow 3'$ direction, using the unwound DNA strand as a template. RNA polymerase separates the strands of the DNA double helix as it moves along the template strand, extruding the 5' end of the transcript behind it. Rifampin blocks elongation after the nascent transcript reaches a certain length. **C.** Upon reaching a termination sequence, the DNA, core enzyme, and newly synthesized RNA separate from one another.

Bacterial Protein Synthesis

Once the mRNA transcripts are synthesized from a DNA template, these transcripts are translated by the bacterial translational machinery. Although the overall process of translation is similar between bacteria and higher organisms, there are a number of pharmacologically exploitable differences in the details of the mechanisms. In particular, the composition of the rRNA molecules differs between bacterial and human ribosomes. Thus, bacterial ribosomes can also serve as selective targets for antibiotics.

The ribosome of a representative bacterium, *Escherichia coli*, has a sedimentation coefficient of **70S** and is composed of a **30S subunit** and a **50S subunit**. The 30S subunit contains a single **16S rRNA** molecule and 21 different proteins, while the 50S subunit contains two rRNA molecules—**23S rRNA** and **5S rRNA**—and more than 30 different proteins. *Importantly, it is the rRNAs rather than the protein components of the ribosome that are mainly responsible for the ribosome's key activities, namely, decoding the mRNA, linking together amino acids, and translocating the translation machine.* The 70S ribosome contains three sites that bind tRNAs during translation: the **A** or **"aminoacyl" site** (also known as the **"acceptor" site**), which binds incoming tRNA molecules carrying the various amino acids; the **P** or **"peptidyl" site**, which contains the growing peptide chain; and the **E** or **"exit"** site, which binds the tRNAs that have been used during translation before they are ejected from the ribosome (Fig. 34-6).

Translation, like transcription, can be divided into three stages (Fig. 34-7). During **initiation**, the components of the translation system assemble together, abetted by proteins called **initiation factors**. First, the mRNA joins with the 30S subunit of the bacterial ribosome and with a specific tRNA molecule linked to **formylated methionine** (fMet), the first amino acid encoded by every bacterial mRNA. The tRNA-formylated methionine molecule (fMet-tRNA$_f$) binds to its initiation codon (AUG) on the mRNA. Next, the 50S subunit joins with the 30S subunit to form the complete 70S ribosome. The fMet-tRNA$_f$ now occupies the P site of the 70S ribosome.

Elongation, abetted by **elongation factors**, involves the addition of amino acids to the carboxyl end of the growing polypeptide chain, as the ribosome moves from the 5'-end to

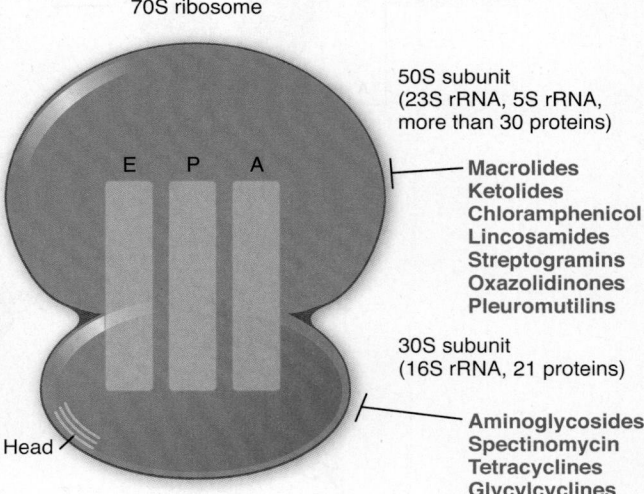

FIGURE 34-6. The bacterial 70S ribosome. The bacterial 70S ribosome consists of a 30S subunit, which has a structural feature known as the *head*, and a 50S subunit. Each subunit is composed of ribosomal RNA (rRNA) and numerous proteins. The rRNAs are mainly responsible for most of the important activities of the ribosome and are the targets of antibiotic drugs that inhibit translation. Aminoglycosides, spectinomycin, tetracyclines, and glycylcyclines bind to 16S rRNA in the 30S subunit. Macrolides, ketolides, chloramphenicol, lincosamides, streptogramins, oxazolidinones, and pleuromutilins bind to 23S rRNA in the 50S subunit. *A,* aminoacyl site (site of binding of aminoacyl tRNA); *P,* peptidyl site (site of binding of tRNA that is covalently joined to the elongating peptide chain); *E,* exit site (site of binding of tRNA that has been ejected from the P site during translocation).

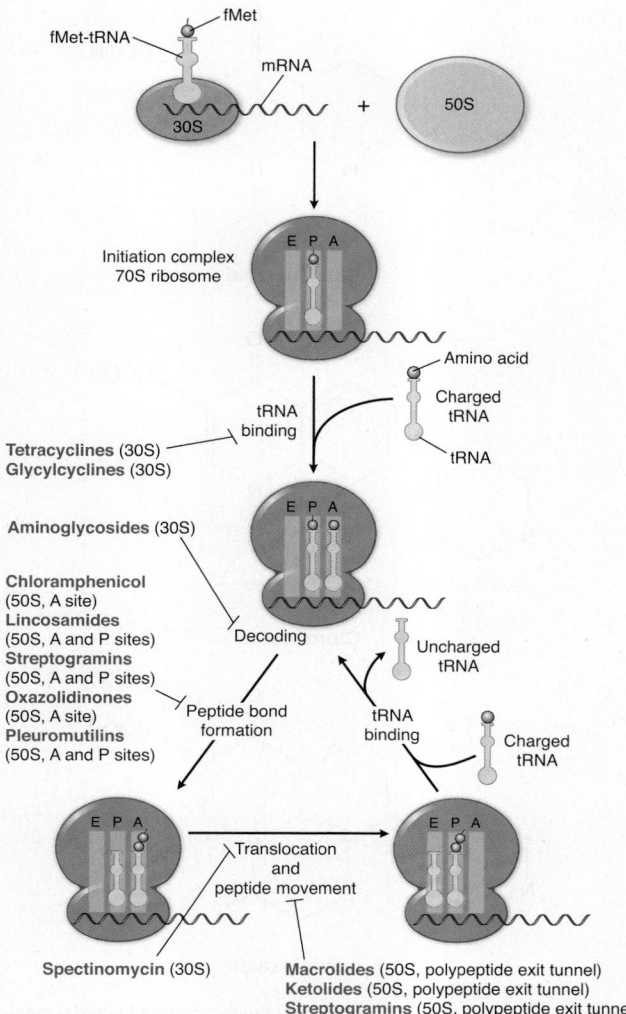

FIGURE 34-7. Bacterial translation. Bacterial translation begins with the assembly of an initiation complex containing a 30S ribosomal subunit, mRNA, formyl-methionine-linked tRNA, and a 50S ribosomal subunit. This assembly step is dependent on the binding of fMet-tRNAf to an initiator codon in the mRNA. The assembled 70S ribosome contains the aminoacyl (A), peptidyl (P), and exit (E) sites. The A site contains a triplet codon of mRNA and allows the anticodon of an incoming amino acid-linked tRNA (i.e., charged tRNA) to bind to its corresponding codon. The decoding function of 16S rRNA helps ensure that binding of the mRNA codon to the correct tRNA, but not an incorrect tRNA, leads to conformational changes that position the amino acid on the charged A site tRNA near the amino acid on the charged P site tRNA within the peptidyl transfer center of the 23S rRNA in the 50S subunit. There, formation of a peptide bond occurs between the amino acid occupying the A site and the carboxy terminus of the nascent peptide residing in the P site. Once the peptide bond has formed, the tRNA–mRNA complex translocates from the A site to the P site, the tRNA molecule that had occupied the P site translocates to the E site, from which it dissociates, and the elongating polypeptide chain moves out through the exit tunnel. The A site is now empty, and introduction of the next charged tRNA molecule into the A site completes the cycle. Translation continues until a stop codon is encountered in the mRNA, at which point the newly synthesized protein is released from the ribosome.

Pharmacologic agents that inhibit translation interfere with the activities of the bacterial ribosome. Aminoglycosides bind to 16S rRNA in the 30S subunit and interfere with decoding, thus resulting in the synthesis of proteins containing incorrect amino acids; tetracyclines and glycylcyclines block aminoacyl tRNA binding to the A site; chloramphenicol, lincosamides, streptogramins, oxazolidinones, and pleuromutilins inhibit the peptide bond formation activity of the 50S subunit. Spectinomycin inhibits translocation, and macrolides, ketolides, and streptogramins inhibit peptide movement through the exit tunnel of the ribosome.

the 3′-end of the mRNA that is being translated. tRNA molecules carrying specific amino acids (aminoacyl tRNAs) enter the ribosomal A site, and their three base anticodons base-pair to their complementary codons on the mRNA. Utilization of the correct tRNA requires not only anticodon–codon recognition between tRNA and mRNA, respectively, but also **decoding** functions provided largely by the 16S rRNA in the **decoding center** of the 30S ribosomal subunit. Binding of the correct tRNA to its codon in the A site leads to several conformational changes—in 16S rRNA within the decoding center, in a region of 23S rRNA of the 50S subunit that protrudes into the decoding center, in the A site tRNA, and in protein elongation factors. These movements culminate in the positioning of the tRNA-bound amino acid in the A site so that it is close to the fMet (on the P site tRNA) in a region of the 50S subunit known as the **peptidyl transferase center**. This center, which is formed largely by the 23S rRNA, catalyzes the formation of a peptide bond between fMet and the next amino acid. Once the peptide bond is formed linking fMet to the next amino acid, which, in turn, is linked to the tRNA in the A site, the tRNA in the A site is said to have "accepted" the fMet.

After the peptide bond has been formed, the ribosome undergoes more conformational changes, including rotation ("ratcheting") of the 30S subunit relative to the 50S subunit and a swiveling motion of the "head" of the 30S subunit, so that both subunits advance three nucleotides toward the 3′-end of the mRNA. In this multistep process, the tRNAf that was originally linked to the fMet is ejected from the P site and binds to the E site, the tRNA that is now linked to two amino acids shifts from the A site to the unoccupied P site, and the A site becomes available. This process is known as **translocation**. As these translocation events occur, the nascent polypeptide starts to move through the **exit tunnel** of the ribosome. In this manner, polypeptide chain elongation results from multiple cycles of aminoacyl tRNA binding to the A site, peptide bond formation, and translocation.

During **termination**, proteins called **release factors** recognize the termination codon in the A site and activate discharge of the newly synthesized protein and dissociation of the ribosome–mRNA complex, with the 70S ribosome separating into its 50S and 30S subunits.

Three general points are worth noting about bacterial translation. First, *the two ribosomal subunits demonstrate segregated functions*: the 30S subunit is largely responsible for faithful decoding of the mRNA message, while the 50S subunit catalyzes peptide bond formation. Translocation, however, involves both subunits. Second, *these functions are performed mainly by the RNA components of the ribosome*. Third, *inhibitors of protein synthesis affect the process of translation at different steps and, indeed, have greatly helped dissect these steps.*

■ PHARMACOLOGIC CLASSES AND AGENTS

Three general categories of drugs target bacterial DNA replication, transcription, and translation: (1) drugs that target type II topoisomerases, (2) drugs that target RNA polymerase, and (3) drugs that target ribosomes. Quinolone antibiotics are broad-spectrum agents that not only inhibit certain topoisomerases but also convert these enzymes into DNA-damaging agents. Fidaxomicin and rifamycin derivatives bind to and inhibit bacterial RNA polymerase. Fidaxomicin is used to treat colitis caused by *Clostridium difficile*, and one rifamycin derivative, rifampin, is a mainstay in the therapy of tuberculosis. Multiple classes of drugs bind bacterial ribosomes to inhibit protein synthesis. Specifically, aminoglycosides, spectinomycin, tetracyclines, and glycylcyclines bind the 30S ribosomal subunit, while macrolides, ketolides, chloramphenicol, lincosamides, streptogramins, oxazolidinones, and pleuromutilins target the 50S ribosomal subunit. These inhibitors of protein synthesis generally act on both Gram-positive and Gram-negative organisms and are therefore in wide clinical use (see Chapter 35, Pharmacology of Bacterial and Mycobacterial Infections: Cell Wall Synthesis, for a discussion of Gram-positive and Gram-negative bacteria).

Elucidation of the mechanisms of action of the agents described below has depended crucially on the field of bacterial genetics. In particular, the molecular targets of antibiotics have been identified by (1) isolating bacteria that are resistant to the particular antibiotic (e.g., rifampin), (2) showing that the target molecule (e.g., RNA polymerase) exhibits biochemical resistance to the antibiotic, and (3) demonstrating that the drug-resistance mutation lies within the gene encoding the target (e.g., the gene encoding the β subunit of RNA polymerase). More recent work, using nuclear magnetic resonance spectroscopy and x-ray crystallography, has further elucidated the structures of the targets as well as the molecular nature of the various drug–target interactions. Indeed, the 2009 Nobel Prize in Chemistry was awarded for crystallographic analyses of ribosomes and their binding to certain antibiotics.

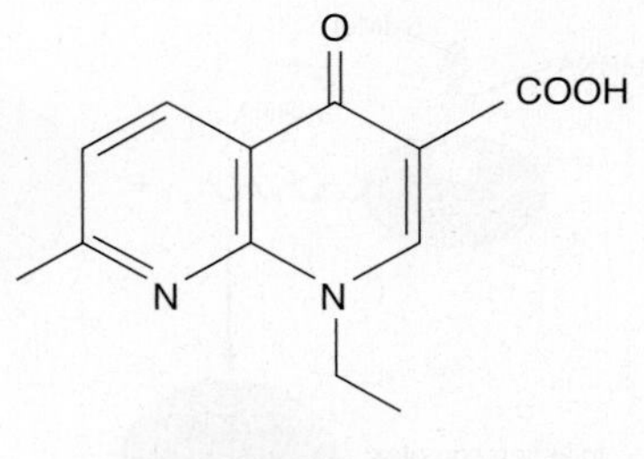

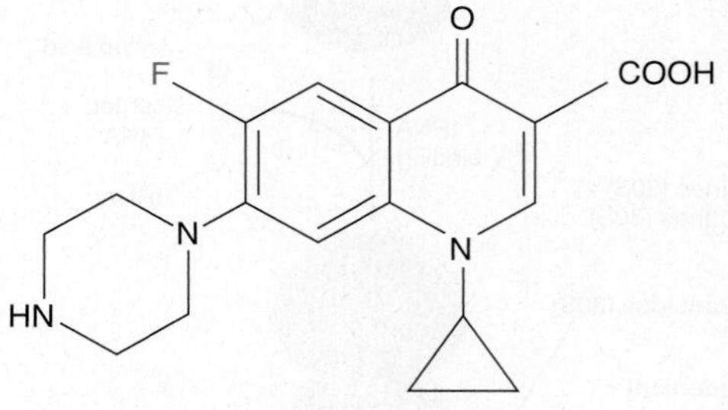

Inhibitors of Topoisomerases: Quinolones

Quinolones are a major class of bactericidal antibiotics that act by inhibiting bacterial type II topoisomerases. One of the earliest quinolones to enter clinical use was **nalidixic acid** (Fig. 34-8), and the mechanism of action of the quinolones was elucidated largely by studying this drug. **Fluoroquinolones** (all ending in "-floxacin") have a fluorine atom at position 6 (Fig. 34-8), which increases the potency and spectrum of bacteria killed by these agents compared to nalidixic acid. The older fluoroquinolones, **ciprofloxacin**, **norfloxacin**, and **ofloxacin**, are used to treat urinary tract infections and gastrointestinal infections caused by Gram-negative bacteria, including *E. coli*, *Klebsiella pneumoniae*, *Campylobacter jejuni*, and *Enterobacter*, *Salmonella*, and *Shigella* species. Newer fluoroquinolones, including **gemifloxacin**, **moxifloxacin**, and **levofloxacin**, retain activity against Gram-negative bacteria and also have activity against *Streptococcus pneumoniae* and bacteria that cause atypical pneumonia (*Mycoplasma pneumoniae*, *Chlamydophila pneumoniae*, and *Legionella pneumophila*), so these drugs are commonly used to treat bacterial pneumonia. Levofloxacin and moxifloxacin have activity against *Mycobacterium tuberculosis* and are sometimes used in combination with other antimycobacterial drugs to treat tuberculosis. Fluoroquinolone resistance is common in staphylococci, so other antibiotics are usually used to treat infections with these organisms. Bacteria typically evolve resistance to the quinolones through chromosomal mutations in the genes that encode type II topoisomerases or through alterations in

FIGURE 34-8. Structures of antimicrobial drugs targeting bacterial topoisomerases. Nalidixic acid, ciprofloxacin, and levofloxacin are quinolone antibiotics that inhibit bacterial type II topoisomerases.

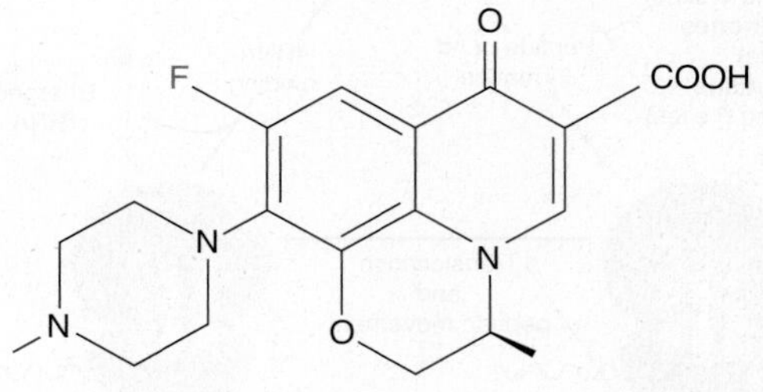

the expression of membrane porins and efflux pumps that determine the concentration of drug inside the bacteria. Adverse effects are infrequent but can include nausea, vomiting, and diarrhea and, rarely, tendinitis, tendon rupture, and peripheral neuropathy.

Quinolones act by inhibiting one or both of the two type II topoisomerases in sensitive bacteria: **DNA gyrase** (topoisomerase II) and **topoisomerase IV**. Selectivity of action results from differences in structure between the bacterial and eukaryotic forms of these enzymes. Quinolones primarily inhibit DNA gyrase in Gram-negative organisms, and they inhibit topoisomerase IV in Gram-positive organisms such as *Streptococcus pneumoniae*. The mechanism of action of the quinolones involves subverting the function of bacterial type II topoisomerases. Ordinarily, type II topoisomerases bind to and break both strands of a DNA molecule, allowing another stretch of the same molecule to pass through the double-stranded DNA break (Fig. 34-4). Quinolones inhibit these enzymes before the second segment of DNA can pass through, thereby stabilizing the form of the complex in which the DNA polymer is broken. At low concentrations, quinolones inhibit type II topoisomerases reversibly, and their action is bacteriostatic. At higher concentrations, however—which are readily achieved in patients—quinolones convert the topoisomerases into DNA-damaging agents by stimulating dissociation of the enzyme subunits from the broken DNA. DNA with double-stranded breaks cannot be replicated (unless the breaks are repaired), and transcription cannot proceed through such breaks. The double-stranded breaks themselves and/or the bacterial response to the double-stranded breaks lead ultimately to cell death. Thus, at therapeutic doses, the quinolone antibiotics are bactericidal.

Inhibitors of Transcription: Fidaxomicin and Rifamycin Derivatives

Fidaxomicin is a macrocyclic antibiotic with an 18-membered macrolactone ring (Fig. 34-9). The use of fidaxomicin is limited to treatment of *C. difficile* colitis. Fidaxomicin is as effective as standard therapy with oral vancomycin for initial clinical cure of *C. difficile* colitis, and patients treated with fidaxomicin are less likely to have recurrence of disease

within 4 weeks of initial cure. The selectivity of fidaxomicin stems from its high potency and bactericidal action against *C. difficile*; it is much less potent against the Gram-negative bacteria that compose the desirable intestinal flora.

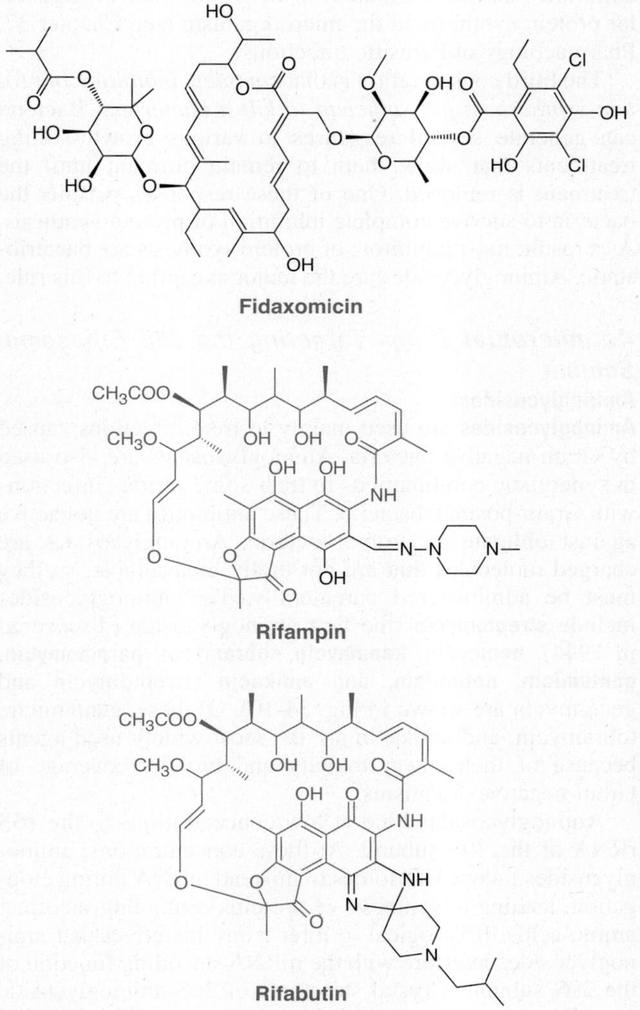

The mechanism by which fidaxomicin inhibits transcription is not well understood, but it differs from the mechanism by which rifamycin derivatives act (see below). Fidaxomicin acts at the initiation stage of RNA synthesis, after binding of RNA polymerase to DNA and before separation of the strands of the DNA double helix (Fig. 34-5). Fidaxomicin resistance mutations encode amino acid substitutions in a region of the enzyme that is involved in the conformational changes that occur during initiation; this region also makes contact with unwound DNA and nascent RNA. Fidaxomicin-resistant bacteria remain susceptible to rifampin, which is consistent with the conclusion that the two drugs act through different mechanisms.

Because very little fidaxomicin is absorbed from the gastrointestinal tract, it can be administered orally to achieve concentrations in the colon that greatly exceed those needed to kill *C. difficile*. Fidaxomicin is generally well tolerated, but adverse effects can include nausea, vomiting, abdominal pain, gastrointestinal hemorrhage, neutropenia, and anemia. Acute hypersensitivity reactions to fidaxomicin have occasionally been reported.

Rifampin (also known as **rifampicin**) and its structural relative, **rifabutin**, are two semisynthetic derivatives of the naturally occurring antibiotic rifamycin B (Fig. 34-9). Although rifampin can be used for prophylaxis of meningococcal disease and for treatment of some other bacterial infections, its major use is in the treatment of tuberculosis and other mycobacterial infections. Rifampin is particularly effective against phagosome-dwelling mycobacteria because it is bactericidal for intracellular as well as extracellular bacteria. Furthermore, rifampin increases the in vitro activity of **isoniazid**, another first-line drug used in the combination therapy of tuberculosis (see Chapter 35 and Chapter 41, Principles of Combination Chemotherapy).

Rifamycin derivatives exert their bactericidal activity against mycobacteria by forming a highly stable complex with the DNA-dependent RNA polymerase, thereby inhibiting RNA synthesis. The drugs target the β subunit of bacterial RNA polymerase. Rifampin permits the initiation of transcription but then blocks elongation once the length of the nascent RNA reaches two to three nucleotides. Exactly how this occurs for all rifamycin derivatives and all bacterial RNA polymerases has not been completely resolved; however, for one bacterial RNA polymerase, there is crystallographic evidence that rifampin occludes the exit channel by which the nascent RNA emerges from the enzyme. Rifampin displays high selectivity for bacteria, as mammalian polymerases (even those of mitochondria, which are considered bacteria-like) are inhibited by rifampin only at far higher concentrations. Hence, rifampin is generally well tolerated, and the incidence of adverse effects (typically, rash, fever, nausea, vomiting, and jaundice) is low.

Because the rapid emergence of resistance makes single-drug therapy of tuberculosis not only ineffective but also counterproductive, rifampin is administered in combination with other antituberculosis drugs. In vitro experiments show that 1 out of every 10^6 to 10^8 tubercle bacilli can develop resistance to rifampin via a one-step mutational process that

FIGURE 34-9. Structures of antimicrobial drugs targeting bacterial RNA polymerases. Fidaxomicin inhibits bacterial DNA-dependent RNA polymerase at the initiation stage, while rifampin and rifabutin, which are derivatives of rifamycin B, inhibit at the elongation stage. The rifamycin B backbone of rifampin and rifabutin is shown in *blue*.

appears to affect the binding site of the drug on the polymerase. However, as a component of a multidrug therapeutic regimen, rifampin can markedly reduce the lifetime rate of reactivation of latent tuberculosis (see Chapter 41).

Inhibitors of Translation

Three general considerations apply to inhibitors of bacterial translation. First, *translation inhibitors target either the 30S or 50S subunit of the bacterial ribosome.* The following discussion of translation inhibitors is presented in terms of 30S versus 50S inhibition (Table 34-1).

The second consideration concerns selectivity. *In addition to their inhibitory effects on bacterial ribosomes, protein synthesis inhibitors can affect mammalian mitochondrial ribosomes, cytosolic ribosomes, or both.* Inhibition of host ribosomes is one common mechanism by which these drugs cause adverse effects. For some antibiotics, such as chloramphenicol, inhibition of mammalian ribosomes represents a major drawback and can lead to serious, even lethal, adverse effects. Tetracyclines can also inhibit mammalian ribosomes in vitro; fortunately, however, this class of drugs is concentrated selectively in bacterial cells. Certain other translation inhibitors exhibit little or no inhibition of mammalian ribosomes at clinically relevant concentrations; for these agents, the dose-limiting toxicities appear to be attributable to other mechanisms. As with most orally available, broad-spectrum antibiotics, gastrointestinal adverse events appear to be due to elimination of normal gut flora.

An interesting twist on the issue of selectivity emerged in the 1990s. It was discovered that certain aminoglycoside, macrolide, and lincosamide antibiotics demonstrate some efficacy against eukaryotic microorganisms (e.g., protozoan parasites) that cause opportunistic infections in patients with AIDS and in other immunocompromised individuals. In these microorganisms, it appears that the activity of the antibiotics can be attributed to their inhibition of organellar protein synthesis in the microorganism (see Chapter 37, Pharmacology of Parasitic Infections).

The third consideration is that *complete inhibition of protein synthesis is not sufficient to kill a bacterium.* Bacteria can generate several responses to various growth-stifling treatments that allow them to remain dormant until the treatment is removed. One of these responses permits the bacteria to survive complete inhibition of protein synthesis. As a result, most inhibitors of protein synthesis are bacteriostatic. Aminoglycosides are the major exception to this rule.

Antimicrobial Drugs Targeting the 30S Ribosomal Subunit

Aminoglycosides

Aminoglycosides are used mainly to treat infections caused by Gram-negative bacteria. Aminoglycosides are also used in synergistic combinations to treat some serious infections with Gram-positive bacteria. These antibiotics are not active against obligate anaerobic bacteria. Aminoglycosides are charged molecules that are not orally bioavailable, so they must be administered parenterally. The aminoglycosides include **streptomycin** (the first aminoglycoside, discovered in 1944), **neomycin**, **kanamycin**, **tobramycin**, **paromomycin**, **gentamicin**, **netilmicin**, and **amikacin** (streptomycin and gentamycin are shown in Fig. 34-10). Of these, gentamicin, tobramycin, and amikacin are the most widely used agents because of their lower toxicity and broader coverage of Gram-negative organisms.

Aminoglycosides bind at low concentrations to the 16S rRNA of the 30S subunit. At these concentrations, aminoglycosides induce ribosomes to misread mRNA during elongation, leading to synthesis of proteins containing incorrect amino acids. It is logical to infer from this effect that aminoglycosides interfere with the mRNA-decoding function of the 30S subunit. Crystal structures of 30S-aminoglycoside complexes have greatly aided our understanding of the decoding process. How aminoglycosides affect decoding has been studied structurally mainly for paromomycin. There are two current models for the induction of misreading by paromomycin binding to the 30S subunit. In one model, paromomycin binding causes conformational changes in

TABLE 34-1 Sites and Mechanisms of Action of Antibacterial Translation Inhibitors

DRUG OR DRUG CLASS	SITE OF ACTION	MECHANISM OF ACTION
Drugs targeting the 30S ribosomal subunit		
Aminoglycosides	16S rRNA	Induce misreading; halt protein synthesis at higher concentrations
Spectinomycin	16S rRNA	Inhibits translocation by blocking swiveling of the head of the 30S subunit
Tetracyclines and glycylcyclines	16S rRNA	Block aminoacyl tRNA binding to A site
Drugs targeting the 50S ribosomal subunit		
Macrolides and ketolides	23S rRNA	Inhibit translocation by blocking the exit tunnel from which the growing polypeptide chain emerges
Chloramphenicol	23S rRNA	Inhibits peptide bond formation by interfering with positioning of the aminoacyl moiety in the A site of the peptidyl transferase center
Lincosamides	23S rRNA	Inhibit peptide bond formation by binding to the A site and, possibly, the P site in the peptidyl transferase center
Streptogramins	23S rRNA	Inhibit peptide bond formation by binding to the A site and P site in the peptidyl transferase center and block the polypeptide exit tunnel
Oxazolidinones	23S rRNA	Inhibit peptide bond formation by blocking productive binding of the aminoacyl moiety in the A site of the peptidyl transferase center
Pleuromutilins	23S rRNA	Inhibit peptide bond formation by binding to the A site and P site in the peptidyl transferase center

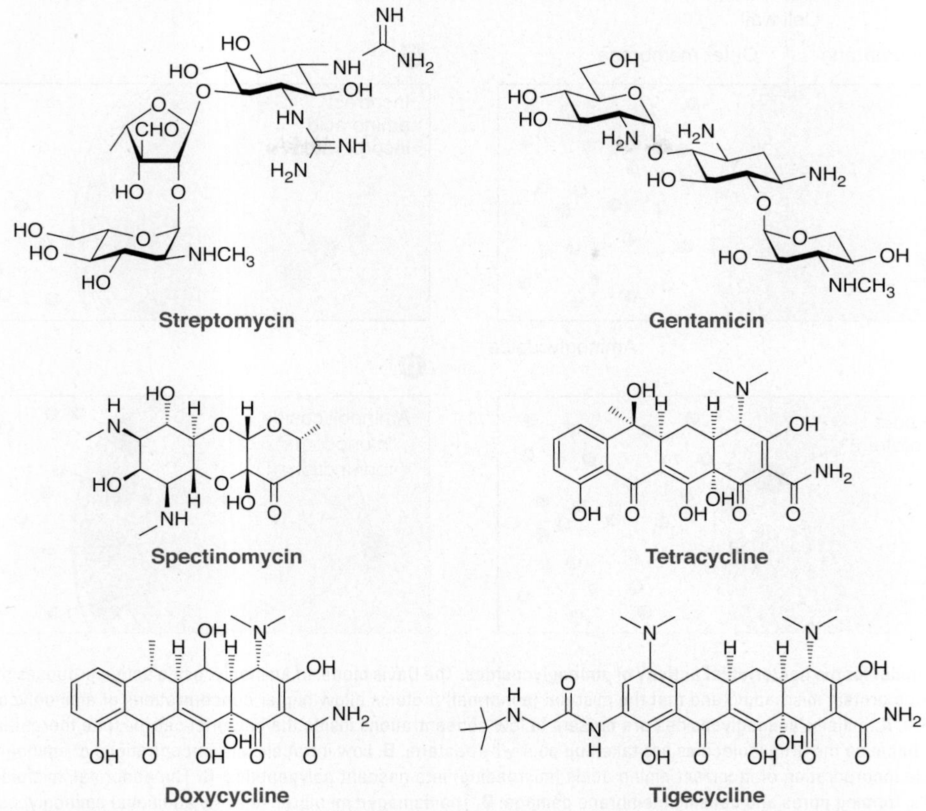

FIGURE 34-10. Structures of antimicrobial drugs targeting the 30S ribosomal subunit. Streptomycin and gentamicin are aminoglycosides. Spectinomycin is a structural relative of the aminoglycosides. Tetracycline and doxycycline are tetracyclines. Tigecycline is a glycylcycline.

particular nucleotides of the 16S rRNA that monitor codon–anticodon interactions, thereby mimicking changes caused by binding of the correct (cognate) tRNA anticodon to an mRNA codon in the A site. It is thought that these conformational changes induce the subsequent conformational changes that result in peptide bond formation, even when the incorrect tRNA is present in the A site. (Consistent with this model, streptomycin also induces misreading, and it binds at a different, but nearby, site to stabilize the 30S subunit in a state similar to that induced by binding the correct tRNA.) A second model stems from the observation that crystal structures of 70S ribosomes containing either incorrect or correct tRNAs exhibit the same conformational changes thought to lead to peptide bond formation. When added to these ribosomes, paromomycin induces a conformational change in a 16S nucleotide that promotes movement of a region of 23S rRNA that protrudes into the decoding center. This model posits that the conformational change in 23S rRNA allows retention of the incorrect tRNA in the A site, so that peptide bond formation and thus misreading can occur.

At higher concentrations, aminoglycosides completely inhibit protein synthesis. Exactly how this occurs is not understood, although in vitro, there is evidence that at least some aminoglycosides inhibit translocation and, in fact, stimulate tRNA movement in the opposite direction (reverse translocation). Certain aminoglycosides can bind at high concentrations to the 23S rRNA of the 50S subunit and prevent the dissociation of 70S ribosomes into individual subunits following termination of translation. In treated bacteria, not only does misreading occur, but ribosomes also become trapped at the AUG initiation codons of mRNA. Eventually, translation halts, despite the presence of ribosomes that are not bound to drug.

In contrast to other protein synthesis inhibitors, aminoglycosides are **bactericidal**. This is an important feature in the treatment of serious infections. Although the precise mechanism for bactericidal activity is not known, one appealing model, developed by the late Bernard Davis, has gained some acceptance (Fig. 34-11). The **Davis model** frames bacterial cell death in terms of the concentration-dependent effects of aminoglycosides. When drug first enters the cell, it is poorly transported across bacterial membranes. At these initial low concentrations, misreading occurs, leading to synthesis of misfolded proteins. Some of these proteins insert into membranes and cause the formation of membrane pores, which allow aminoglycosides to flood the cell and halt protein synthesis completely. As a result, the damage to the membrane cannot be repaired, and leakage of ions and, later, larger molecules leads to cell death. An alternative model also invokes misreading and protein misfolding as key steps in bactericidal action but posits that the misfolded proteins activate a stress-response sensor that contributes to membrane damage and DNA damage, and thus to cell death.

Another important aspect of aminoglycoside activity is that these drugs act **synergistically** with agents that inhibit peptidoglycan synthesis, such as β-lactams and glycopeptide antibiotics. Therefore, aminoglycosides and β-lactams are commonly used in combination (see Chapter 41). The explanation most commonly suggested for this synergy is that inhibition of cell wall synthesis increases the entry of

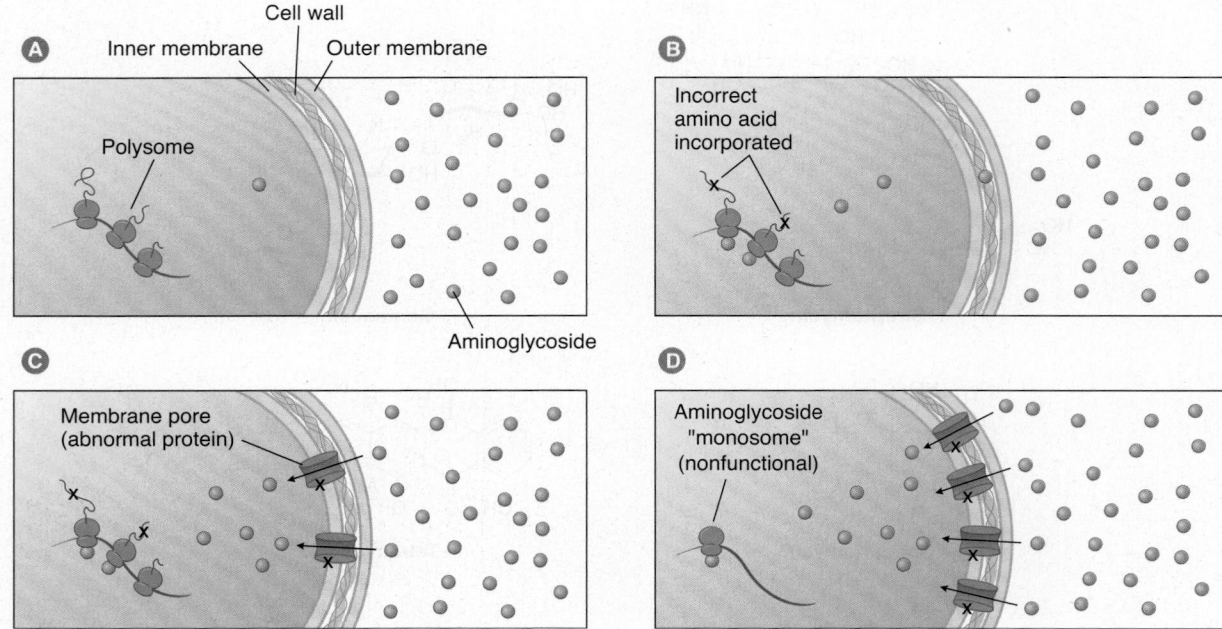

FIGURE 34-11. Davis model for the bactericidal activity of aminoglycosides. The Davis model of aminoglycoside action proposes that low concentrations of aminoglycosides induce protein misreading and that the misread (abnormal) proteins allow higher concentrations of aminoglycosides to enter the cell and halt protein synthesis. **A.** Initially, aminoglycosides are present at low concentrations inside the bacterial cell, despite therapeutic (high) extracellular concentrations of drug, because the drug molecules are taken up poorly by bacteria. **B.** Low intracellular concentrations of aminoglycoside bind to bacterial ribosomes and cause incorporation of incorrect amino acids (misreading) into nascent polypeptides. **C.** The abnormal, misfolded proteins insert into the bacterial membranes, forming pores and causing membrane damage. **D.** The damaged membranes allow additional aminoglycoside molecules to flood into the cell, causing complete inhibition of ribosome activity. The effect is irreversible, perhaps because of trapping of drug inside the cell ("caging"). The membrane damage cannot be repaired because new proteins cannot be synthesized, and cell death ensues.

aminoglycosides into the bacteria. The synergy between β-lactams and the aminoglycosides contrasts sharply with the antagonism between β-lactams and the bacteriostatic inhibitors of protein synthesis discussed below.

Three general mechanisms have been established for resistance to aminoglycosides. First, and clinically most common, is the plasmid-encoded production of a transferase enzyme or enzymes that inactivate aminoglycosides by adenylation, acetylation, or phosphorylation. Second, drug entry into the cell can be impaired, perhaps by alteration or elimination of porins or other proteins involved in drug transport. Third, the drug target on the 30S ribosomal subunit can become resistant to drug binding by virtue of mutation or the activity of a plasmid-encoded enzyme.

In addition to several general types of toxicity, such as hypersensitivity reactions and drug-induced fever, aminoglycosides can cause three specific adverse effects: ototoxicity, nephrotoxicity, and neuromuscular blockade. Of these, **ototoxicity** (manifesting as either auditory or vestibular damage that is usually irreversible) is the most important factor restricting aminoglycoside use. The aminoglycosides accumulate and persist in the perilymph and endolymph of the inner ear and, at high concentrations, they damage hair cells. There is excellent evidence from human genetic studies that ototoxicity is caused, at least in part, by aminoglycoside inhibition of host mitochondrial ribosomes. An alternative view is based on the finding that aminoglycosides bind to phospholipids in the cell membrane and to iron. Drug binding to iron can generate free radicals, which may be agents of damage in the inner ear.

Aminoglycosides also cause **acute renal failure** that is usually reversible. Aminoglycoside concentrations can reach high levels in renal proximal tubular cells due to receptor-mediated endocytosis via a specific receptor called megalin in clathrin-coated pits. The biochemical mechanism responsible for the subsequent toxicity is poorly understood, although both mitochondrial poisoning and perturbation of the plasma membrane are suspected. At very high concentrations, aminoglycosides can produce reversible nondepolarizing **neuromuscular blockade**, potentially causing respiratory paralysis. This effect is thought to result from drug competition with calcium at presynaptic sites, leading to reduction in acetylcholine release, failure of the postsynaptic end-plate to depolarize, and muscle paralysis.

Spectinomycin

Spectinomycin (Fig. 34-10) also binds to the 16S rRNA of the 30S ribosomal subunit but at a location different from those bound by aminoglycosides. Spectinomycin permits formation of the 70S ribosome but inhibits translocation. This appears to be due to inhibition of swiveling of the head of the 30S subunit during translocation. Unlike the aminoglycosides, spectinomycin does not induce codon misreading and is not bactericidal. Spectinomycin is administered parenterally and is used clinically only as an alternative therapy for gonorrheal infections.

Tetracyclines and Glycylcyclines

Tetracyclines have been used clinically for many years. Four **tetracyclines** are available for use in humans in the United States: **tetracycline**, **demeclocycline**, **doxycycline**, and **minocycline**. All are close structural relatives and can be considered as a group (tetracycline and doxycycline are shown in Fig. 34-10). Although differences in clinical efficacy are minor, doxycycline and minocycline are most often used because they can be administered at less frequent dosing intervals than tetracycline and because, unlike tetracycline, their absorption is not significantly reduced when taken orally with food. Tetracyclines are bacteriostatic broad-spectrum antibiotics that are used widely.

Tetracyclines bind reversibly to the 16S rRNA of the 30S subunit and inhibit protein synthesis by blocking the binding of aminoacyl tRNA to the A site on the mRNA–ribosome complex. This action prevents the addition of further amino acids to the nascent peptide. However, inhibition of protein synthesis does not account entirely for the high bacterial selectivity of tetracyclines, because these drugs can also halt eukaryotic protein synthesis *in vitro* at concentrations not much higher than those required to inhibit bacterial protein synthesis. *Rather, the high selectivity of tetracyclines derives from the active accumulation of these drugs in bacteria but not in mammalian cells.* Tetracyclines enter Gram-negative bacteria by passive diffusion through porin proteins in the outer membrane, followed by active (energy-dependent) transport across the inner cytoplasmic membrane. Uptake into Gram-positive bacteria occurs similarly via an energy-dependent transport system. In contrast, mammalian cells lack the active transport system found in susceptible bacteria.

Since the bacterial selectivity of tetracyclines results from drug-concentrating mechanisms, it follows that resistance can occur through increased drug efflux or decreased drug influx. In fact, plasmid-encoded **efflux pumps** represent the most widespread mechanism employed by tetracycline-resistant microbes. A second form of resistance arises through the production of proteins that bind the ribosome and interfere with the binding of tetracyclines. A third mechanism of resistance involves the enzymatic inactivation of tetracyclines.

An important pharmacokinetic feature of the tetracyclines is the interaction of these drugs with foods and oral drugs containing divalent and trivalent cations. Absorption of oral tetracycline is inhibited by about half if taken with food (particularly calcium-rich dairy products), so tetracycline should be taken when the stomach is empty. In contrast, doxycycline and minocycline may be taken with food. Intestinal absorption of all tetracyclines is inhibited by medicines containing divalent and trivalent cations, such as antacids. The same interaction with cations—specifically calcium—causes sequestration of the drug in developing bones and teeth, potentially leading to reduced skeletal growth and permanent brown discoloration of the teeth in children. Gastrointestinal distress and renal toxicity are the two most problematic adverse effects of the tetracyclines. Nausea, vomiting, and diarrhea occur with all tetracyclines but are more common with tetracycline (which is taken on an empty stomach) than with doxycycline and minocycline. All tetracyclines are excreted in both urine and bile. Urine is the primary route of excretion for tetracycline, and this drug is associated with renal toxicity in people with preexisting renal failure. Lower fractions of doxycycline and minocycline are eliminated via the kidney, making these drugs safer for use in patients with kidney disease. Finally, a red rash occurs on sun-exposed skin (photosensitivity) in some patients taking tetracyclines.

Tigecycline is the first member of a newer class of antibiotics—**glycylcyclines**. The four-ring structure of tigecycline resembles that of the tetracyclines (Fig. 34-10), as does its mechanism of action. Tigecycline has a broader spectrum of activity than tetracyclines and has been approved for intravenous administration in the treatment of serious skin and abdominal infections and of community-acquired pneumonia caused by susceptible organisms. The US Food and Drug Administration (FDA) warns that tigecycline should be reserved for use only when alternative treatments are not suitable, because of a higher rate of mortality in patients treated with tigecycline than with other antibiotics.

Antimicrobial Drugs Targeting the 50S Ribosomal Subunit

The clinically available antibiotics that target the 50S subunit —macrolides, ketolides, chloramphenicol, lincosamides, streptogramins, oxazolidinones, and pleuromutilins—bind to a small region of 23S rRNA near the peptidyl transferase active center. Small differences in their binding sites and differences in their chemical structures are responsible for differences in their detailed mechanisms of action.

Macrolides and Ketolides

Macrolides are named for their large lactone rings. Attached to these rings are one or more deoxy sugars. **Erythromycin** (Fig. 34-12) is the best-known member of this group. Two semisynthetic derivatives of erythromycin, **azithromycin** and **clarithromycin**, are broader in spectrum and better tolerated than erythromycin and are therefore growing in use. As illustrated in the introductory case, macrolides have proven to be especially important in the treatment of pulmonary infections, including Legionnaires' disease. These agents display excellent lung tissue penetration, and just as important, they have intracellular activity against *Legionella*.

Macrolides are bacteriostatic antibiotics that bind to a specific segment of 23S rRNA. They act during the elongation stage of protein synthesis by blocking the exit tunnel from which nascent peptides emerge, as clearly illustrated by a crystal structure of erythromycin bound to the 50S subunit (Fig. 34-13A). As a result, short nascent peptides are synthesized (akin to the short nascent transcripts synthesized by bacterial RNA polymerase in the presence of rifamycin derivatives), and then translation stops. Interestingly, however, certain proteins can be synthesized even in the presence of macrolides. Evidently, the drugs do not completely block the exit tunnel, and some polypeptides can "slither" past the block.

Macrolide use is complicated by the problem of resistance, which is usually plasmid encoded. One mechanism employed by some resistant *Enterobacteriaceae* is the production of esterases or phosphotransferases that modify macrolides. Modification of the ribosomal binding site by chromosomal mutation represents a second mechanism of resistance. Some bacteria reduce the permeability of their membrane to macrolides or (more commonly) increase active drug efflux. Production of a methylase that modifies the 23S rRNA target site of the macrolides, leading to decreased drug binding, accounts for the vast majority of resistance to macrolides in Gram-positive organisms. Constitutive production of methylase also confers resistance to the structurally unrelated compounds **clindamycin** and **streptogramin B**, which bind 23S rRNA close to the macrolide target site (see discussion below).

Adverse reactions to erythromycin typically involve the gastrointestinal tract or the liver. Gastrointestinal intolerance represents the most frequent reason for discontinuing erythromycin, as the drug can directly stimulate gut motility and

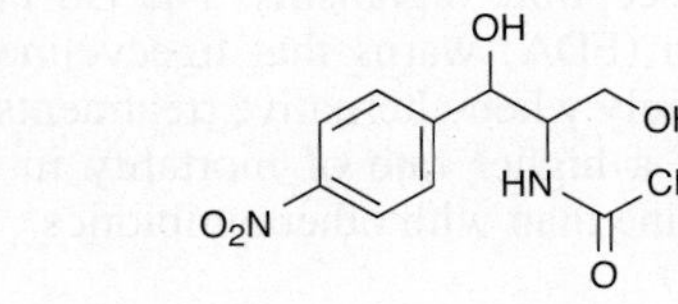

FIGURE 34-12. Structures of antimicrobial drugs targeting the 50S ribosomal subunit. Chloramphenicol, erythromycin (a macrolide), clindamycin (a lincosamide), quinupristin (a streptogramin), dalfopristin (a streptogramin), linezolid (an oxazolidinone), and retapamulin (a pleuromutilin) each inhibit bacterial translation by targeting the 50S ribosomal subunit.

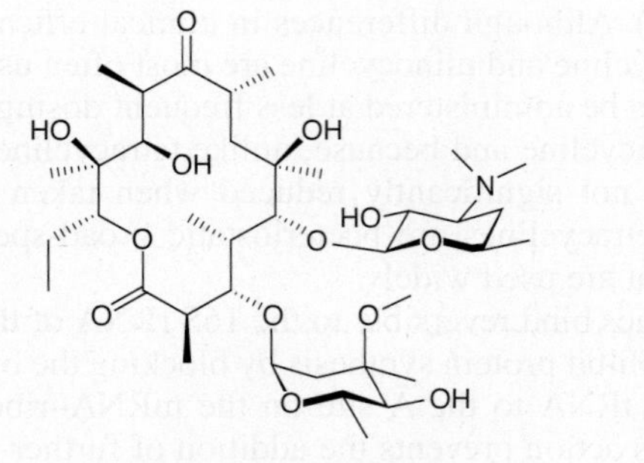

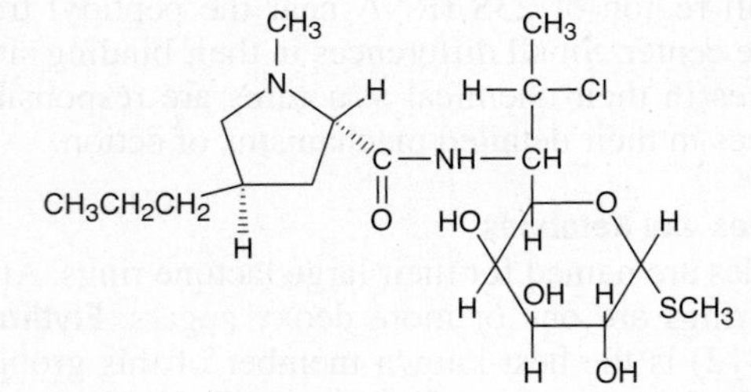

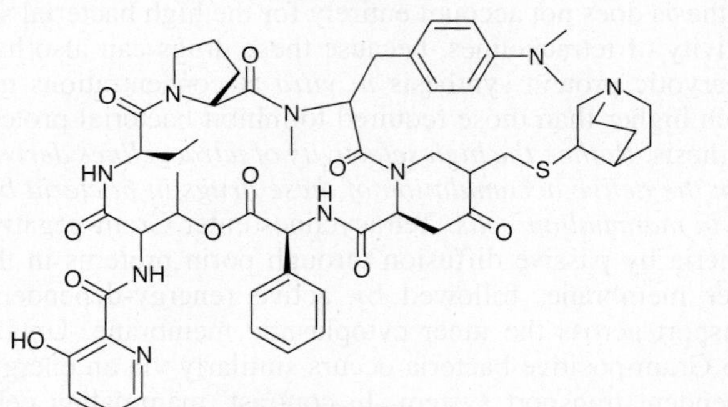

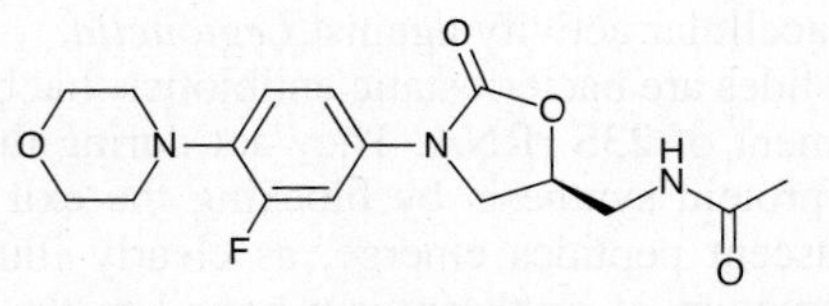

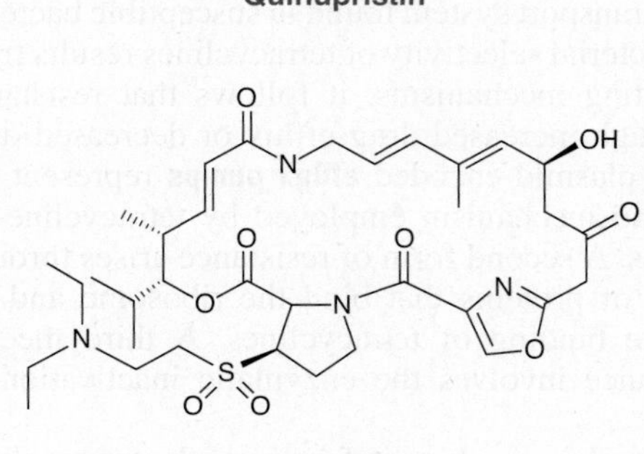

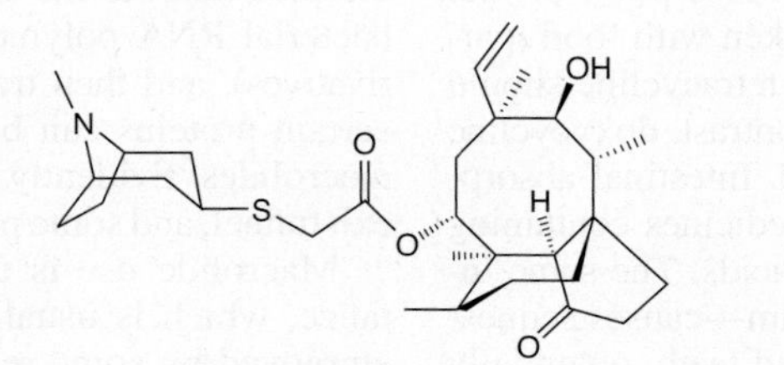

cause nausea, vomiting, diarrhea, and sometimes anorexia. Erythromycin can also produce acute cholestatic hepatitis (with fever, jaundice, and impaired liver function), probably as a hypersensitivity reaction. Metabolites of erythromycin can inhibit certain cytochrome P450 isozymes in the liver and thus increase the plasma concentration of numerous drugs that are also metabolized by these liver enzymes. Azithromycin and clarithromycin are generally well tolerated, although these drugs can also cause liver impairment.

Telithromycin, a third semisynthetic derivative of erythromycin, was approved by the FDA in 2004. Formally known

as a **ketolide** rather than a macrolide, telithromycin has a mechanism of action similar to that of the macrolides, but with a higher affinity for the 50S ribosomal subunit due to its ability to bind an additional site on 23S rRNA. Its higher affinity for the 50S subunit and its lack of induction of expression of some genes mediating resistance allows telithromycin to be used in treating infections due to some Gram-positive cocci that are resistant to macrolides. Telithromycin is also bactericidal against certain Gram-positive bacteria, but it is not clear why. Telithromycin can be involved in numerous drug–drug interactions and in rare cases of fulminant hepatic

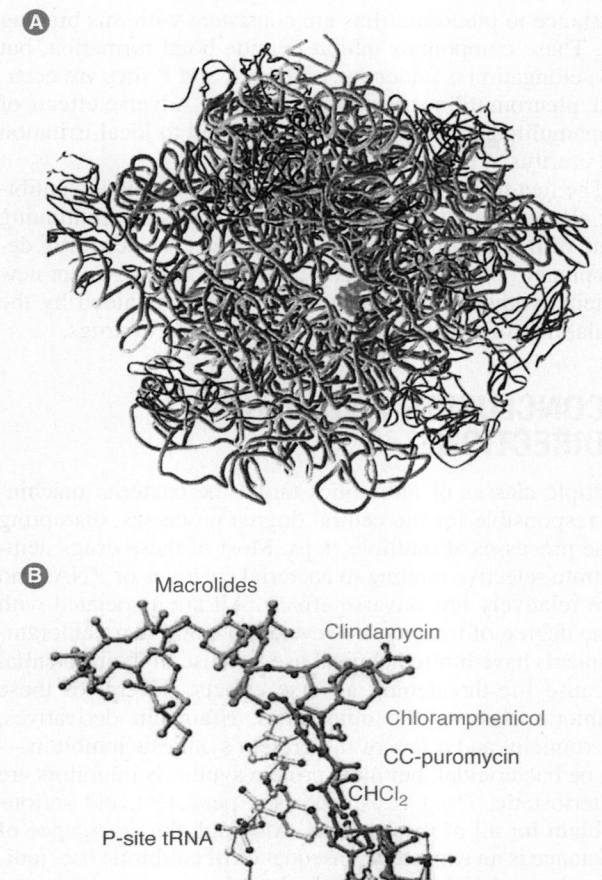

FIGURE 34-13. **Mechanism of action of erythromycin, clindamycin, and chloramphenicol revealed by crystallographic analysis of drug binding to the 50S ribosomal subunit. A.** Erythromycin *(red)* binds to a specific segment of 23S rRNA and blocks the exit tunnel from which nascent peptides emerge. **B.** Clindamycin and macrolides have partially overlapping binding sites on the 50S ribosomal subunit, as do clindamycin and chloramphenicol. The positions of the A-site tRNA and P-site tRNA are also shown. The exact binding locations and conformations of the drugs vary in crystal structures of drug-bound ribosomes from different species.

necrosis. Telithromycin is contraindicated in patients with myasthenia gravis since it exacerbates weakness and can lead to respiratory compromise in patients with this disease.

Chloramphenicol
Chloramphenicol (Fig. 34-12) is a bacteriostatic broad-spectrum antibiotic that is active against both aerobic and anaerobic Gram-positive and Gram-negative organisms. The most highly susceptible organisms include *Haemophilus influenzae*, *Neisseria meningitidis*, and some strains of *Bacteroides*. However, the potential for serious toxicity has limited the systemic use of chloramphenicol. The drug is still used occasionally in the treatment of typhoid fever, bacterial meningitis, and rickettsial diseases but only when safer alternatives cannot be used, as in the case of resistance or serious drug allergy.

Chloramphenicol binds to 23S rRNA and inhibits peptide bond formation, apparently by occupying a site that interferes with proper positioning of the aminoacyl moiety of tRNA in the A site in the peptidyl transferase center (Fig. 34-13B).

Microbes have developed resistance to chloramphenicol by two major mechanisms. Low-level resistance has emerged in large chloramphenicol-susceptible populations by the selection of mutants with decreased permeability to the drug. The more clinically significant type of chloramphenicol resistance has arisen from the spread of specific plasmid-encoded **acetyltransferases** (at least three types of which have been characterized) that inactivate the drug.

The fundamental mechanism underlying the toxicity of chloramphenicol appears to involve inhibition of mitochondrial protein synthesis. One manifestation of this toxicity is the **gray baby syndrome**, which can occur when chloramphenicol is administered at high doses to newborn infants. Because newborns lack an effective glucuronic acid conjugation mechanism for the degradation and detoxification of chloramphenicol, the drug can accumulate to toxic levels and cause vomiting, flaccidity, hypothermia, gray color, respiratory distress, and metabolic acidosis. More frequently, chloramphenicol causes dose-related, reversible depression of erythropoiesis and gastrointestinal distress (nausea, vomiting, and diarrhea). **Aplastic anemia**, a rare but potentially fatal toxicity, occurs via an idiopathic mechanism that is unrelated to dose.

Of special interest are the adverse effects that chloramphenicol can cause in tandem with other drugs. Like the macrolides, chloramphenicol increases the half-life of certain drugs, such as phenytoin and warfarin, by inhibiting the cytochrome P450 enzymes that metabolize these drugs. Chloramphenicol also antagonizes the bactericidal effects of penicillins and aminoglycosides, as do other bacteriostatic inhibitors of microbial protein synthesis.

Lincosamides
The major **lincosamide** in clinical use is **clindamycin** (Fig. 34-12). Clindamycin blocks peptide bond formation, apparently through interactions with the A site (like chloramphenicol) (Fig. 34-13B), and, possibly, also through interactions with the P site.

The most important indication for clindamycin is the treatment of serious intra-abdominal or gynecological infections that are likely to include penicillin-resistant *Bacteroides fragilis* and other intestinal anaerobes. Clindamycin is a cause of **pseudomembranous colitis** caused by *Clostridium difficile* overgrowth. An infrequent member of the normal fecal flora, *C. difficile* is selected for during the administration of clindamycin or other broad-spectrum oral antibiotics to which it is not susceptible. *C. difficile* elaborates a cytotoxin that can cause colitis characterized by mucosal ulcerations, severe diarrhea, and fever. This serious adverse effect is a major concern with the use of oral clindamycin.

Streptogramins
In 1999, the FDA approved the first drug in the **streptogramin** class of protein synthesis inhibitors. The drug is a mixture of two distinct chemicals: **dalfopristin**, a group A streptogramin, and **quinupristin**, a group B streptogramin (Fig. 34-12). Dalfopristin/quinupristin was approved for the treatment of serious or life-threatening infections caused by vancomycin-resistant *Enterococcus faecium* or *Streptococcus pyogenes*. Common adverse effects of dalfopristin/quinupristin include elevated bilirubin, pain with administration, and joint and muscle pain.

Streptogramins inhibit protein synthesis by binding to the peptidyl transferase center of bacterial 23S rRNA. Mutations and modifications affecting this region can confer resistance. The A component binds to a location overlapping both the A site and the P site in the peptidyl transferase center, and it can inhibit peptidyl transferase in vitro. The binding site for the B component overlaps with that of the macrolides, and it is thought that, like the macrolides, quinupristin blocks the emergence of nascent peptides from the ribosome. When dalfopristin binds the ribosome, the ribosome changes conformation such that it binds quinupristin with higher affinity, leading to synergy between the two streptogramin components.

Streptogramins are unusual among the 50S antibiotics in that they are bactericidal against many, but not all, susceptible bacterial species. A clear explanation for this phenomenon remains elusive; the current hypothesis is that, unlike the other 50S antibiotics, the streptogramins induce a conformational change in the ribosome that is reversible only after subunit dissociation.

Oxazolidinones

In 2000, the FDA approved **linezolid** (Fig. 34-12), the first drug in the **oxazolidinone** class of antibacterial agents. In 2014, **tedizolid phosphate**, a prodrug of tedizolid, became the second oxazolidinone to be approved. Both drugs are orally available and demonstrate excellent activity against drug-resistant Gram-positive bacteria, including methicillin-resistant *S. aureus* (MRSA), penicillin-resistant streptococcus, and vancomycin-resistant enterococcus (VRE), but have very little activity against Gram-negative bacteria. Although there was initially controversy regarding the precise mechanism of action of oxazolidinones, crystallographic analyses have located the binding site of linezolid in a pocket of the A site where the amino acid moiety in aminoacyl tRNA normally binds. Moreover, mutations in 23S rRNA can confer drug resistance. These results and those of biochemical studies suggest that oxazolidinones block productive interactions of aminoacyl tRNAs with the A site in the peptidyl transferase center. Linezolid has occasionally been associated with serious adverse effects, including myelosuppression and neuropathy, but tedizolid appears to be associated with lower rates of these adverse effects.

Pleuromutilins

In 2007, the FDA approved **retapamulin** (Fig. 34-12), the first drug in the **pleuromutilin** class of antibiotics. This drug is used as a topical treatment for minor bacterial skin infections (impetigo), and its mechanism of action is relatively well understood. Like linezolid, pleuromutilins bind to a pocket in the A site of the peptidyl transferase center where aminoacyl tRNA normally binds. Distinct from linezolid, pleuromutilin binding also extends into the P site. Thus, the binding site of pleuromutilins is similar to that of group A streptogramins. The locations of mutations conferring resistance to pleuromutilins are consistent with this binding site. These compounds inhibit peptide bond formation, but once elongation is underway and the A and P sites are occupied, pleuromutilins are no longer active. Adverse effects of retapamulin are minor and largely limited to local irritation and pruritus at the site of use.

The fact that three of the most recently developed antibiotic classes inhibit the ribosome emphasizes the continuing value of this complex structure as a target for new drug development. There is much continuing effort to discover new protein synthesis inhibitors, and this work is aided by the availability of structures of ribosomes bound to drugs.

▌CONCLUSION AND FUTURE DIRECTIONS

Multiple classes of antibiotics target the bacterial machinery responsible for the central dogma processes, disrupting these processes at multiple steps. Most of these drugs demonstrate selective binding to bacterial enzymes or RNAs and have relatively few adverse effects. All are associated with some degree of toxicity, however, and some (e.g., chloramphenicol) have limited clinical use because of their potential to cause life-threatening adverse effects. Several of these antibiotic classes—the quinolones, rifamycin derivatives, fidaxomicin, and a few of the protein synthesis inhibitors—can be bactericidal, but most protein synthesis inhibitors are bacteriostatic. Drug resistance is a persistent and serious problem for all of these agents. Although the emergence of resistance is an expected consequence of antibiotic use, judicious drug administration, multidrug therapies, and the continued development of new antibacterial agents can combat the emergence of resistance. The development of fidaxomicin and the newer classes of bacterial ribosome inhibitors represents an important advance in the search for drugs that are effective against resistant bacteria. Further elucidation of the mechanism of action of these drugs will both inform basic biology and define new biochemical targets for pharmacologic intervention.

Suggested Reading

Kannan K, Vazquez-Laslop N, Mankin AS. Selective protein synthesis by ribosomes with a drug-obstructed exit tunnel. *Cell* 2012;151:508–520. (*This report changed thinking about the mechanisms of macrolide and ketolide antibiotics by showing that they permit the synthesis of subsets of bacterial proteins despite blocking the polypeptide exit tunnel.*)

Louie TJ, Miller MA, Mullane KM, et al. Fidaxomicin versus vancomycin for *Clostridium difficile* infection. *New Engl J Med* 2011;364:422–431. (*Clinical trial evaluating use of fidaxomicin for C. difficile infection.*)

Walsh CT. *Antibiotics: actions, origins, resistance.* Washington, DC: ASM Press; 2003. (*Reviews antibiotic synthesis, action, and mechanisms of resistance.*)

Wilson DN. Ribosome-targeting antibiotics and mechanisms of bacterial resistance. *Nat Rev Microbiol* 2014;12:35–48. (*Reviews molecular mechanisms of action of and resistance to these antibiotics.*)

DRUG SUMMARY TABLE: CHAPTER 34 Pharmacology of Bacterial Infections: DNA Replication, Transcription, and Translation

DRUG	CLINICAL APPLICATIONS	SERIOUS AND COMMON ADVERSE EFFECTS	CONTRAINDICATIONS	THERAPEUTIC CONSIDERATIONS
INHIBITORS OF TOPOISOMERASES: QUINOLONES **Mechanism**—Inhibit bacterial type II topoisomerases. At therapeutic concentrations, quinolones have a bactericidal effect by causing dissociation of the topoisomerase from cleaved DNA, leading to double-stranded DNA breaks and cell death.				
Ciprofloxacin **Gemifloxacin** **Levofloxacin** **Moxifloxacin** **Norfloxacin** **Ofloxacin**	Respiratory tract infection (ciprofloxacin, gemifloxacin, levofloxacin, moxifloxacin, and ofloxacin only) Gastrointestinal tract infection (ciprofloxacin, levofloxacin, and moxifloxacin only) Infection of skin/subcutaneous tissue (ciprofloxacin, levofloxacin, moxifloxacin, and ofloxacin only) Urinary tract infection (ciprofloxacin, levofloxacin, norfloxacin, and ofloxacin only) Eye infection (levofloxacin, moxifloxacin, norfloxacin, and ofloxacin only) Bone infection (ciprofloxacin only) Ear infection (ofloxacin only)	*Prolonged QT interval, myasthenia gravis exacerbation, cartilage damage, tendon rupture, peripheral neuropathy (shared adverse effects); severe hypersensitivity reaction, bone marrow depression, hepatotoxicity, nephrotoxicity, retinal detachment (ciprofloxacin, levofloxacin, moxifloxacin, norfloxacin, and ofloxacin only); Clostridium difficile diarrhea (ciprofloxacin, norfloxacin, and ofloxacin only); seizure (ciprofloxacin and ofloxacin only); increased intracranial pressure, pancreatitis, psychotic disorder (ciprofloxacin only); extrapyramidal disease (ofloxacin only)* Rash, gastrointestinal disturbance (shared adverse effects); burning sensation in eye (ofloxacin only)	Shared contraindication: Hypersensitivity to quinolones Ciprofloxacin only: Concomitant tizanidine administration	Bacteria evolve resistance through chromosomal mutations in the genes that encode type II topoisomerases or through alterations in the expression of membrane porins and efflux pumps that determine drug levels inside the bacteria. Avoid co-administration with drugs that prolong QT interval due to increased risk of cardiotoxicity. Limited use in children under 18 years of age due to arthropathy in juvenile animals and increased adverse events involving joints and surrounding tissues (e.g., tendons) in pediatric patients.
Nalidixic Acid	Urinary tract infection	*Prolonged QT interval, porphyria, metabolic acidosis, paralytic ileus, hemolytic anemia, thrombocytopenia, hypersensitivity reaction, cartilage damage, tendon rupture, increased intracranial pressure, peripheral neuropathy, seizure, psychotic disorder*	Hypersensitivity to nalidixic acid Concomitant use with chemotherapeutic alkylating agents History of seizure disorder Infants under 3 months of age Mothers who are breastfeeding Porphyria	One of the earliest quinolones to enter clinical use. Nalidixic acid is no longer marketed in the United States.
INHIBITORS OF TRANSCRIPTION: FIDAXOMICIN AND RIFAMYCIN DERIVATIVES **Mechanism**—Form a stable complex with bacterial DNA-dependent RNA polymerase, thereby inhibiting RNA synthesis				
Fidaxomicin	Treatment of *Clostridium difficile*-associated diarrhea	*Bowel obstruction, gastrointestinal hemorrhage, neutropenia, anemia* Gastrointestinal upset	Hypersensitivity to fidaxomicin	Efficacy is similar to standard therapy for initial cure, with lower rate of relapse with fidaxomicin.

continues

DRUG SUMMARY TABLE: CHAPTER 34 Pharmacology of Bacterial Infections: DNA Replication, Transcription, and Translation *continued*

DRUG	CLINICAL APPLICATIONS	SERIOUS AND COMMON ADVERSE EFFECTS	CONTRAINDICATIONS	THERAPEUTIC CONSIDERATIONS
Rifabutin **Rifampin**	Mycobacterial infections, including tuberculosis (shared indication) Prophylaxis of meningococcal disease (rifampin only)	*Agranulocytosis, hypersensitivity reaction (shared adverse effects); hepatotoxicity, nephrotoxicity (rifampin only)* Rash, gastrointestinal upset, elevated liver function tests, discoloration of saliva, tears, sweat, and urine (rifabutin only)	Shared contraindications: Hypersensitivity to drug Concomitant use with rilpivirine Rifampin only: Concomitant use with atazanavir, darunavir, fosamprenavir, saquinavir, or tipranavir	Rifampin is not used as a single agent because of rapid development of resistance. Rifampin may reduce cyclosporine concentration and efficacy. Avoid concurrent administration of clarithromycin with rifabutin because clarithromycin increases plasma concentration of rifabutin and rifabutin reduces plasma concentration of clarithromycin.

ANTIMICROBIAL DRUGS TARGETING THE 30S RIBOSOMAL SUBUNIT
Mechanism—Bind to 16S rRNA of the 30S ribosomal subunit and elicit concentration-dependent effects on protein synthesis. Aminoglycosides are bactericidal, evidently due to induction of mRNA misreading; misread mRNA causes synthesis of aberrant proteins that may activate oxidative stress pathways and/or insert into the cell membrane, forming pores that eventually lead to cell death. Other drugs are bacteriostatic.

DRUG	CLINICAL APPLICATIONS	SERIOUS AND COMMON ADVERSE EFFECTS	CONTRAINDICATIONS	THERAPEUTIC CONSIDERATIONS
Aminoglycosides: **Amikacin** **Gentamicin** **Kanamycin** **Neomycin** **Netilmicin** **Paromomycin** **Streptomycin** **Tobramycin**	Serious Gram-negative infections	*Respiratory paralysis (shared adverse effect); nephrotoxicity (shared adverse effect excepting tobramycin); ototoxicity (amikacin, gentamicin, kanamycin, neomycin, netilmicin, and tobramycin only); neuromuscular blockade (amikacin, gentamicin, kanamycin, neomycin, and netilmicin only); facial paresthesia (streptomycin only)* Gastrointestinal upset, rash	Shared contraindication: Hypersensitivity to aminoglycosides Neomycin and paromomycin only: Gastrointestinal disease	Act synergistically with β-lactam antibiotics. Resistance can occur by three mechanisms: 1. Plasmid-encoded production of a transferase enzyme or enzymes that inactivate aminoglycosides 2. Impaired drug entry, possibly by alteration or elimination of porins or other proteins involved in drug transport 3. Mutation of the drug target on the 30S ribosomal subunit
Spectinomycin	Gonorrhea (alternative therapy)	Injection site pain, nausea, dizziness, insomnia	Hypersensitivity to spectinomycin	Permits formation of the 70S ribosome but inhibits translocation.
Tetracyclines: **Demeclocycline** **Doxycycline** **Minocycline** **Tetracycline**	Used to treat a variety of infections, notably those due to *Propionibacterium acnes, Vibrio cholerae, Borrelia burgdorferi, Helicobacter pylori, Mycoplasma pneumoniae, Chlamydia* species, and rickettsial species (shared indications) Malaria prophylaxis (doxycycline only)	*Nephrotoxicity (demeclocycline and tetracycline only); hypersensitivity reaction, Clostridium difficile diarrhea, hepatotoxicity, pseudotumor cerebri (doxycycline, minocycline, and tetracycline only)* Photosensitivity, gastrointestinal upset, tooth discoloration, headache (shared adverse effects)	Shared contraindication: Hypersensitivity to drug Tetracycline only: Last half of pregnancy, infancy, childhood up to 8 years of age	Tetracyclines antagonize the bactericidal effects of penicillins, and this antagonism likely occurs with any combination of a bacteriostatic inhibitor of protein synthesis and a β-lactam drug or an aminoglycoside. Tetracyclines are actively transported into bacterial cells. Resistance occurs by plasmid-encoded efflux pumps, production of proteins that interfere with binding of tetracyclines to the ribosome, or enzymatic inactivation of tetracyclines. Tetracycline should be taken on an empty stomach because calcium products interfere with absorption. Avoid co-administration with acitretin due to increased risk of elevated intracranial pressure.

Drug	Clinical Applications	Serious and Common Adverse Effects	Contraindications	Therapeutic Considerations
Glycylcyclines: Tigecycline	Complicated skin or subcutaneous infection; Complicated abdominal infection; Community-acquired bacterial pneumonia	*Septic shock, Clostridium difficile diarrhea, pancreatitis, hepatotoxicity, hypersensitivity reaction, pseudotumor cerebri*; Gastrointestinal upset	Hypersensitivity to tigecycline	Structure is similar to tetracyclines.

ANTIMICROBIAL DRUGS TARGETING THE 50S RIBOSOMAL SUBUNIT
Mechanism—Bind to a small region of 23S rRNA of the 50S ribosomal subunit near the peptidyl transferase active center. All drugs are bacteriostatic except for streptogramins, which can be bactericidal.

Drug	Clinical Applications	Serious and Common Adverse Effects	Contraindications	Therapeutic Considerations
Macrolides and Ketolides: Azithromycin, Clarithromycin, Erythromycin, Telithromycin	Erythromycin is used to treat a variety of infections, notably those due to *Propionibacterium acnes, Legionella pneumophila, Mycoplasma pneumoniae,* and *Chlamydia* species. Clarithromycin has increased activity against *H. influenzae.* Azithromycin has increased activity against *H. influenzae* and *Moraxella catarrhalis*	*Prolonged QT interval, hepatotoxicity, hypersensitivity reaction (shared adverse effects); exacerbation of myasthenia gravis (azithromycin and telithromycin only); Eaton-Lambert syndrome, corneal erosion (azithromycin only); Clostridium difficile diarrhea (clarithromycin and erythromycin only); pancreatitis, seizure, ototoxicity, interstitial nephritis (erythromycin only); respiratory failure (telithromycin only)*; Gastrointestinal disturbance	Shared contraindications: Hypersensitivity to drug; Hepatic dysfunction; Clarithromycin and telithromycin only: QT prolongation or ventricular arrhythmias; Concomitant use with pimozide; Clarithromycin only: Concomitant use with HMG-CoA reductase inhibitors metabolized by CYP3A4; Telithromycin only: Myasthenia gravis	Resistance can be conferred by chromosomal mutations leading to alteration of the 50S ribosomal binding site, production of methylases that alter the 50S binding site, or production of esterases that degrade macrolides. Macrolides and ketolides inhibit hepatic metabolism of cyclosporine, carbamazepine, warfarin, and theophylline and can lead to toxic levels of these drugs. Macrolides eliminate certain species of intestinal flora that inactivate digoxin, thereby leading to greater oral absorption of digoxin in some patients.
Chloramphenicol	Broad-spectrum antibiotic active against bacteria (especially anaerobes) and rickettsiae	*Aplastic or hypoplastic anemia, leukemia, thrombocytopenia, hepatotoxicity, hypersensitivity reaction, optic atrophy, paroxysmal nocturnal hemoglobinuria, gray baby syndrome*	Hypersensitivity to chloramphenicol	Most adverse effects are due to inhibition of mitochondrial function. Inhibits hepatic metabolism of warfarin, phenytoin, tolbutamide, and chlorpropamide and thereby potentiates their effects.
Lincosamides: Clindamycin	Bacterial infections due to anaerobic organisms	*Erythema multiforme, Clostridium difficile diarrhea, agranulocytosis, increased liver function tests, jaundice*; Gastrointestinal upset, rash	Hypersensitivity to clindamycin	Clindamycin is associated with overgrowth of *C. difficile*, which can result in pseudomembranous colitis.

continues

DRUG SUMMARY TABLE: CHAPTER 34 Pharmacology of Bacterial Infections: DNA Replication, Transcription, and Translation *continued*

DRUG	CLINICAL APPLICATIONS	SERIOUS AND COMMON ADVERSE EFFECTS	CONTRAINDICATIONS	THERAPEUTIC CONSIDERATIONS
Streptogramins: **Dalfopristin/** **Quinupristin**	Vancomycin-resistant *Enterococcus faecium* (VREF) Skin infections caused by *Staphylococcus aureus* or *Streptococcus pyogenes*	Injection site inflammation, gastrointestinal disturbance, hyperbilirubinemia, arthralgia, myalgia, headache	Hypersensitivity to dalfopristin/quinupristin	Should not be co-administered with SSRIs due to risk of serotonin syndrome. Co-administration with pimozide should be avoided due to increased risk of cardiotoxicity (QT prolongation, torsades de pointes, cardiac arrest).

Oxazolidinones: **Linezolid** **Tedizolid** **phosphate**	Linezolid only:
	  Gram-positive bacterial infections, especially vancomycin-resistant enterococcus, methicillin-resistant *S. aureus* (MRSA), *S. agalactiae, S. pneumoniae* (including drug-resistant strains), and *S. pyogenes*
	  Nosocomial pneumonia
	  Complicated diabetic foot infections
	Tedizolid phosphate only:
	  Acute bacterial skin and subcutaneous tissue infections caused by Gram-positive cocci
		Clostridium difficile diarrhea, peripheral neuropathy, disorder of optic nerve (shared adverse effects); lactic acidosis, myelosuppression, hepatotoxicity, serotonin syndrome (linezolid only); neutropenia (tedizolid phosphate only)
		Gastrointestinal upset, headache
			Shared contraindication: Hypersensitivity to drug
			Linezolid only:
			  Concomitant use of monoamine oxidase inhibitors (MAOIs)
				Available in both oral and IV formulations.
				Tedizolid phosphate approved in 2014.

Pleuromutilins: **Retapamulin**	Impetigo due to MSSA or *Streptococcus pyogenes*	*Hypersensitivity reaction* Application site irritation	No specific contraindications	Topical application for bacterial skin infections.

Pharmacology of Bacterial and Mycobacterial Infections: Cell Wall Synthesis

David W. Kubiak, Ramy A. Arnaout, and Sarah P. Hammond

INTRODUCTION

In 1928, Alexander Fleming made a chance discovery that would revolutionize the treatment of bacterial infections. He observed that certain molds produce a compound that inhibits the growth of bacteria. The compound he isolated was **penicillin**, the first in a long line of antibiotics that act by inhibiting the biosynthesis of **peptidoglycan**, the major component of the bacterial cell wall. The unique chemical and structural properties of peptidoglycan make it an attractive and prominent target for antibacterial chemotherapy. The emergence and spread of antibiotic resistance increasingly complicate the clinical use of cell wall synthesis inhibitors, however. This chapter reviews the biochemistry of peptidoglycan synthesis and describes the mechanisms of action, uses, and limitations of the antibiotics that interfere with this pathway. These limitations include resistance, toxicity, and drug–drug interactions. Antibiotics that target other essential components of the bacterial cell wall are also discussed.

BIOCHEMISTRY OF BACTERIAL CELL WALL SYNTHESIS

Cell Wall Structure and Function

Peptidoglycan, named for its peptide and sugar composition, is a three-dimensional meshwork of peptide-cross-linked sugar polymers that surrounds the bacterial cell just outside its cytoplasmic membrane (Fig. 35-1). Peptidoglycan is also known as *murein,* after the Latin *murus* (wall). Nearly all clinically important bacteria produce peptidoglycan. The major exceptions are *Mycoplasma pneumoniae*, which can cause atypical pneumonia, and the intracellular form (or "reticulate body") of *Chlamydia trachomatis*, which can cause a sexually transmitted infection. Peptidoglycan is critically important for the survival of bacteria, which experience large fluctuations in osmotic pressure depending on their environment. The peptidoglycan meshwork wrapped around the cell provides the tensile strength required to withstand high turgor pressures that would otherwise cause the plasma

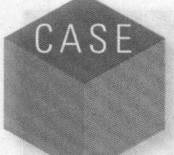

CASE

Samantha T is a 50-year-old woman who presents to an urgent care center with a sore area on her left medial thigh. She reports that she scratched her thigh on some exercise equipment at her local gym, where she works out 6 days a week. The area slowly became red, warm, and tender over the next 4 days. Over the past 24 hours, she has felt that the sore spot is "ready to burst." On examination, Ms. T has a 2- × 2-cm, round, fluctuant area on the left thigh, with a surrounding patch of erythema that covers a 6- × 7-cm area of the thigh. She undergoes incision and drainage of the abscess in the urgent care office and the purulent material is sent for culture, which later grows methicillin-sensitive *Staphylococcus aureus* (MSSA). She is treated with dicloxacillin.

Ms. T returns to the urgent care clinic 10 days later and reports that the left thigh wound is nearly completely healed but that she now has profuse diarrhea and fever. She feels light-headed when standing. She reports that she has been living with her elderly father, who has several chronic medical ailments and was recently treated for *Clostridium difficile* infection. Ms. T is referred to her local emergency room for treatment of dehydration, and she is treated with intravenous fluids. A stool sample tests positive for *Clostridium difficile* toxin. Ms. T is treated with oral vancomycin and her diarrhea resolves over the course of the next week.

Questions

1. Which test can help determine the cause of Ms. T's skin and soft tissue infection before the culture result is available?
2. What type of antibiotic is dicloxacillin and what is its mechanism of action?
3. Is dicloxacillin an appropriate drug for treatment of an MSSA skin infection?
4. What is the mechanism of action of vancomycin?
5. Why is vancomycin administered orally instead of intravenously to treat *C. difficile* infection?

membrane to rupture. Since peptidoglycan is essential for bacterial survival, its biosynthesis is a major target for antibiotics. The largest and most widely used class of bacterial cell wall synthesis inhibitors, the beta-lactam (β-lactam) antibiotics, inhibit the transpeptidase enzymes that mediate peptide cross-linking of the sugar polymers.

Bacteria are conventionally divided into two groups, **Gram-positive** and **Gram-negative**, based on the relative ability of the bacteria to retain the purple color of the gentian violet component of the Gram stain after being washed with an organic solvent such as acetone. Gram-positive bacteria retain the stain and appear purple, whereas Gram-negative bacteria lose the stain and appear pink from the subsequently applied safranin counterstain. Gram staining is frequently used to help identify the bacteria present in a specimen of body fluid such as urine, sputum, or pus. The Gram stain is one test that the urgent care clinician used to determine what type of organism was causing Ms. T's skin abscess and cellulitis in the introductory case. The ability to retain Gram stain results from two distinguishing characteristics of cell wall architecture (Fig. 35-1). First, Gram-negative bacteria possess an outer membrane, an asymmetric bilayer in

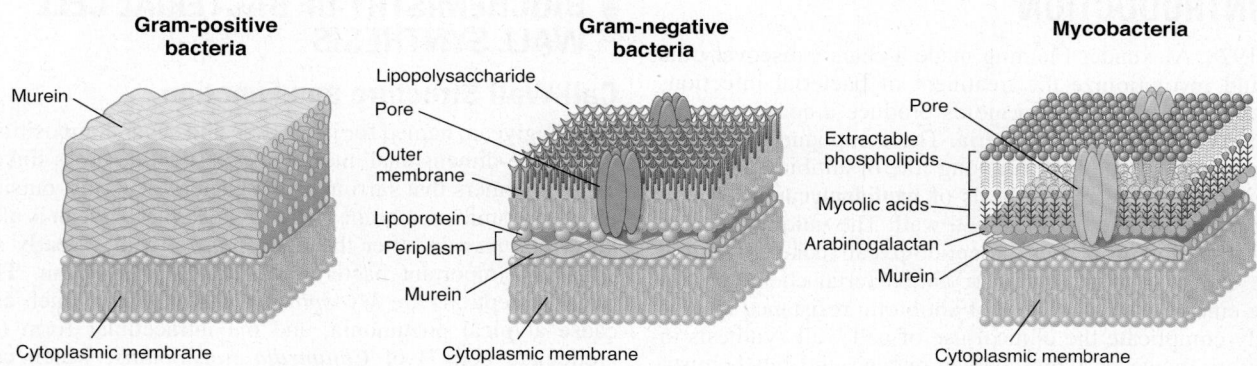

FIGURE 35-1. Bacterial cell wall architecture. In Gram-positive bacteria **(left)**, the cell wall is composed of a thick layer of murein, through which nutrients, waste products, and antibiotics can diffuse. Lipoteichoic acids in the outer leaflet of the cytoplasmic membrane intercalate through the cell wall to the outer surface of Gram-positive bacteria (*not shown*); the hydrophilic side chains of these molecules are involved in bacterial adherence, feeding, and evasion of the host immune system. In Gram-negative bacteria **(center)**, the murein layer is thinner and is surrounded by a second, outer lipid bilayer membrane. Hydrophilic molecules cross this outer membrane through channels, which are formed by a cylindrical arrangement of pore proteins (porins). Gram-negative bacteria have lipopolysaccharide (LPS) in the outer membrane; LPS is a major antigen for the immune response to Gram-negative organisms. The cell wall of mycobacteria **(right)**, which include the causative agents of tuberculosis (*M. tuberculosis*) and leprosy (*M. leprae*), is analogous to that of Gram-negative bacteria. The main difference between the surface architecture of mycobacteria and that of Gram-negative bacteria is in the lipid structures outside the murein layer. In mycobacteria, the outer membrane contains arabinogalactan-linked mycolic acids, extractable phospholipids, and other lipid components. One simplified model for the organization of the mycobacterial outer membrane is shown.

which the outer leaflet is composed of lipopolysaccharide. This structurally unusual membrane forms a permeability barrier that excludes a wide variety of molecules and limits the penetration of Gram stain into the periplasm, the space between the inner and outer membranes where the peptidoglycan layer is located. Second, Gram-positive bacteria have a very thick murein layer, whereas Gram-negative bacteria have only a thin layer. Since Gram stain binds to peptidoglycan, and the binding capacity and accessibility of the thick murein layer are much greater in Gram-positive than Gram-negative organisms, the Gram-positive bacteria stain purple.

The outer membrane of Gram-negative bacteria not only limits the penetration of Gram stain into the periplasm, but it also prevents the penetration of many other molecules, including antibiotics that target peptidoglycan synthesis—such as vancomycin and bacitracin. Hence, although Gram-negative organisms express the molecular targets for these antibiotics, they are not susceptible. To enable uptake of hydrophilic nutrients and excretion of hydrophilic waste products, Gram-negative bacteria have outer membrane **porins**—beta-barrel proteins that traverse the outer membrane and allow certain molecules to pass in and out (see Fig. 35-1). Porins are important pharmacologically because it is through these pores that most hydrophilic antibiotics with activity against Gram-negative organisms gain access to the murein layer and to the structures beneath this layer. Also important pharmacologically are the **lipopolysaccharides (LPS)** that compose the outer leaflet of the outer membrane of Gram-negative bacteria. Lipopolysaccharides are amphipathic molecules that protect bacteria from toxic hydrophilic host molecules such as bile salts. Lipopolysaccharides are also important for bacterial adherence to host cells and for evasion of the host immune response. Polymyxin is a topically used antibiotic that facilitates its own entry into the periplasm by binding to LPS and disrupting the integrity of the outer membrane. Once in the periplasm, polymyxin permeabilizes the inner membrane, discharging the membrane potential so that bacterial cells no longer generate the energy required for survival. Although polymyxin is too toxic for systemic use in people, its mechanism of action suggests that it may be possible to develop less toxic molecules that breach the outer membrane and allow the passage of antibiotics to their molecular targets in Gram-negative bacteria.

Gram-positive bacteria do not have an outer membrane; the extracellular enzymes involved in cell wall synthesis are therefore accessible to a wider range of antibiotics than those that can penetrate Gram-negative organisms. However, the cell wall of Gram-positive organisms is not composed simply of peptidoglycan; there is also a set of other cell wall polymers that play important roles in adherence to host tissue and other aspects of pathogenicity. These include **lipoteichoic acids** and **wall teichoic acids**, anionic polymers that are typically composed of acyclic sugar-phosphate repeats functionalized with D-alanine and cyclic sugars such as glucose. Lipoteichoic acids are anchored in the bacterial membrane and extend into the peptidoglycan layers. Wall teichoic acids are covalently attached to peptidoglycan and extend through and beyond its outermost layer. These polymers are important for bacterial infection of the host, and the pathways of teichoic acid biosynthesis are possible targets for antibiotics. In some Gram-positive organisms, including *Staphylococcus aureus*, the peptidoglycan layers are also functionalized with proteins that are required for pathogenesis. These proteins

are covalently attached to uncross-linked peptides in peptidoglycan by enzymes called **sortases**. Sortases have also been suggested as possible targets for antibiotics.

These important structural differences between the cell envelopes of Gram-negative and Gram-positive bacteria lead to differential access of antibiotics to cellular targets and also present different opportunities for the development of new antibiotics. Despite this, peptidoglycan biosynthesis, which is conserved among Gram-negative and Gram-positive organisms, remains the most important antibacterial cell envelope target. In fact, the peptidoglycan biosynthetic pathway is one of a very small number of broad-spectrum antibacterial targets that exist in bacterial pathogens. The other broad-spectrum targets include DNA synthesis, RNA synthesis, and protein synthesis (see Chapter 34, Pharmacology of Bacterial Infections: DNA Replication, Transcription, and Translation). Of these processes, only peptidoglycan biosynthesis is unique to bacteria.

Peptidoglycan Biosynthesis

Peptidoglycan biosynthesis occurs in three major stages. The first stage is intracellular and involves the synthesis of murein monomers from amino-acid and sugar building blocks; the second and third stages involve the export of these murein monomers to the surface of the inner membrane, followed by their polymerization into linear peptidoglycan polymers and their cross-linking into two-dimensional lattices and three-dimensional mats (Fig. 35-2). Because the details of bacterial cell wall synthesis can be daunting, it is helpful to keep in mind the three major stages—*monomer synthesis, glycan polymerization,* and *polymer cross-linking*—in the discussion that follows. In principle, any of the biochemical steps in peptidoglycan biosynthesis could be a target for antibiotics; in practice, clinically used antibiotics target only a few of the steps in these stages. A vast number of secondary metabolites produced by soil and marine microorganisms also block peptidoglycan biosynthesis, providing a reservoir of structurally and functionally novel compounds for possible clinical development as our existing antibiotics fail due to the spread of resistance.

Synthesis of Murein Monomers

The **murein monomer** is a disaccharide comprising N-acetylglucosamine connected via a beta linkage to the C4 hydroxyl of N-acetyl muramic acid, which is functionalized on the C3 lactate moiety with a peptide (Fig. 35-2). The first phase of peptidoglycan synthesis takes place in the cytoplasm and involves the conversion of UDP-N-acetylglucosamine (UDP-NAG), a nucleotide-sugar used as a building block in many cell wall polymers, to UDP-N-acetyl muramic acid pentapeptide (UDP-NAM-peptide; also known as the *Park nucleotide*). The first two enzymes in this process, MurA and MurB, convert the C3 hydroxyl of NAG to lactate. **MurA**, also known as *enolpyruvate transferase,* transfers enolpyruvate from **phosphoenolpyruvate (PEP)** to UDP-NAG to form UDP-NAG pyruvate enol ether (Box 35-1). The flavoenzyme **MurB** (also known as *UDP-NAG-enolpyruvate reductase*) then reduces the double bond to produce UDP-NAM, which has a free carboxylate to serve as the handle for the peptide chain. UDP-NAM is a sugar unique to bacteria, and its biosynthesis thus provides opportunities for selective antibiotics. One clinically used antibiotic that blocks the biosynthesis of UDP-NAM is **fosfomycin**, a PEP analogue that inhibits MurA.

A Murein monomer synthesis (cytoplasmic phase)

B Completion of murein monomer synthesis, and murein monomer export, polymerization, and cross-linking

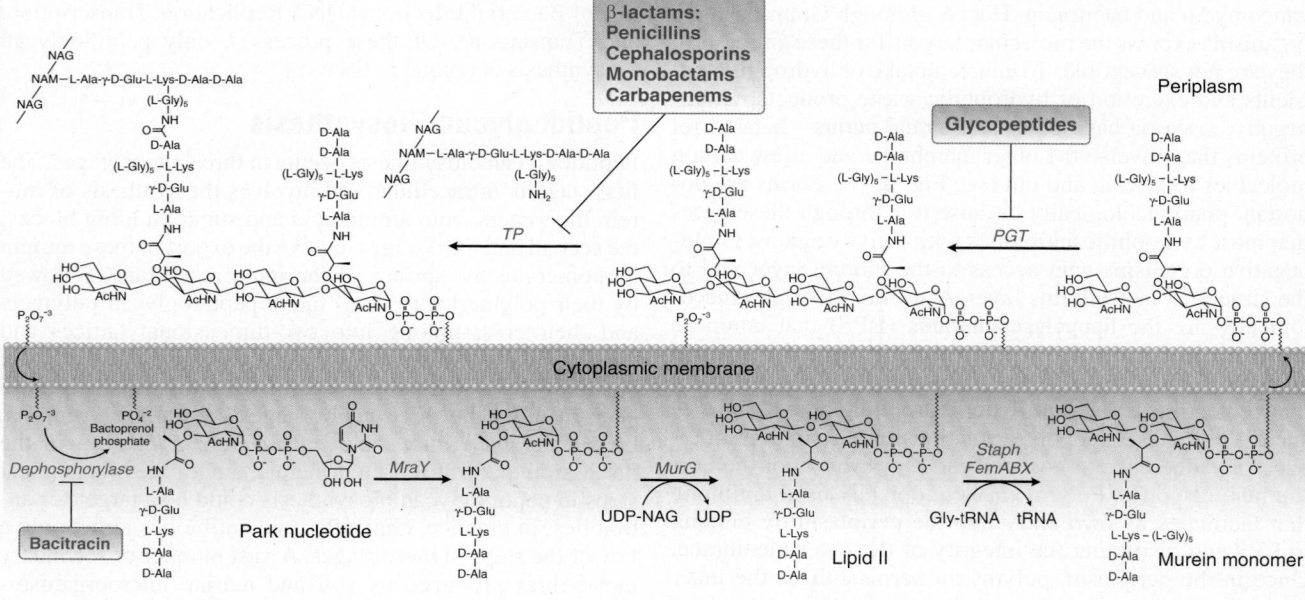

FIGURE 35-2. Bacterial cell wall biosynthesis and its inhibition by pharmacologic agents. Bacterial cell wall biosynthesis can be divided into three major stages. **A.** In the cytoplasmic phase of murein monomer synthesis, glucose is amidated and phosphorylated to glucosamine-1-phosphate (*not shown*), which is acetylated and conjugated to a uridine diphosphate (UDP) nucleotide by the enzyme GlmU (*not shown*) to form UDP-N-acetylglucosamine (UDP-NAG). Addition of phosphoenolpyruvate (PEP) by enolpyruvate transferase (MurA) and reduction of the resulting product by MurB form UDP-N-acetyl muramic acid (UDP-NAM). NAG and NAM are the two sugar building blocks for subsequent cell wall synthesis. MurC, MurD, and MurE sequentially add the amino acids L-alanine, D-glutamate, and L-lysine to UDP-NAM. In some bacteria, diaminopimelic acid (DAP) is added instead of L-lysine. Alanine racemase converts L-alanine to D-alanine, and D-Ala-D-Ala ligase B (DdlB) forms the dipeptide D-Ala-D-Ala. This dipeptide is then added to the L-Ala-D-Glu-L-Lys (or L-Ala-D-Glu-DAP) tripeptide by MurF, resulting in a UDP-NAM molecule linked to five amino acids (Park nucleotide). Fosfomycin is a selective inhibitor of MurA. Cycloserine inhibits both alanine racemase and D-Ala-D-Ala ligase B, thereby preventing the addition of alanine residues to the growing peptide chain. **B.** The NAM–pentapeptide complex is transferred from UDP to the lipid carrier bactoprenol by the enzyme MraY, and NAG is added from UDP-NAG by MurG. In some bacteria, one to five amino acids can then be added to L-lysine or DAP to form a branched peptidoglycan; the amino acids are added from amino acyl tRNA. (Here, as an example, five glycine residues are added from glycyl-tRNA.) This completes the synthesis of the murein monomer.

In the murein monomer export and polymerization stage, the bactoprenol–peptidoglycan complex is transported from the bacterial inner membrane to the periplasmic space, where peptidoglycan glycosyltransferases (PGTs) join the murein monomer to the growing peptidoglycan chain. Simultaneously, the bactoprenol is liberated to facilitate another round of murein monomer translocation. Bactoprenol diphosphate is dephosphorylated to bactoprenol phosphate by dephosphorylase, regenerating the form of the lipid carrier that can react with the Park nucleotide.

In the final stage of cell wall biosynthesis, adjacent glycopeptide polymers are cross-linked in a reaction catalyzed by bacterial transpeptidases (TPs). In the example shown, a transpeptidase cross-links a glycine pentapeptide on one peptidoglycan chain to a D-Ala residue on an adjacent peptidoglycan chain; as shown in detail in Figure 35-3, the terminal D-Ala residue is displaced in this reaction.

Bacitracin inhibits bactoprenol dephosphorylation and thereby interrupts murein monomer synthesis and export. The glycopeptides vancomycin, telavancin, dalbavancin, and oritavancin bind the D-Ala-D-Ala terminus of the bactoprenol-conjugated murein monomer unit and thereby prevent the PGT-mediated addition of murein monomer to the growing peptidoglycan chain. The β-lactam antibiotics (penicillins, cephalosporins, monobactams, and carbapenems) inhibit the transpeptidase enzymes that cross-link adjacent peptidoglycan polymers.

BOX 35-1 Enzymes of Cell Wall Biosynthesis

Like most enzymes, the enzymes of cell wall biosynthesis are known by multiple names. The Mur naming convention used here is the emerging standard, but the enzymes are also still known by the following descriptive names (among others):

GlmU   Diamine N-acetyltransferase
MurA   Enolpyruvate transferase
MurB   UDP–NAG-enolpyruvate reductase
MurC   UDP–NAM-L-Ala synthetase
MurD   UDP–NAM-L-Ala-D-Glu synthetase

MurE   UDP–NAM-L-Ala-D-Glu-2,6-diaminopimelate synthetase
MurF   UDP–NAM-tripeptide-D-Ala-D-Ala synthetase
MraY   UDP–NAM-pentapeptide:undecaprenol-phosphate transferase
MurG   Undecaprenoldiphospho-NAM-pentapeptide: NAG transferase

Note: Undecaprenol is another name for bactoprenol. ∎

The peptide component of UDP-NAM-peptide is assembled on the C3 lactate from amino acids and dipeptides by a series of ATP-dependent ligases. **MurC, MurD**, and **MurE** sequentially add the amino acids L-alanine, D-glutamate, and a diamino acid—either L-lysine or **diaminopimelic acid (DAP)**—to UDP-NAM. DAP differs from lysine in having a carboxyl group as well as an amine on the side chain. Most Gram-positive bacteria use L-lysine, whereas a minority of Gram-positive and all known Gram-negative bacteria use DAP. This is noteworthy because m-DAP is not found in humans, and therefore, it offers a unique target for future drug development.

Peptide formation continues with the addition of a D-alanyl-D-alanine dipeptide (D-Ala-D-Ala) to the growing chain. The dipeptide is synthesized from two molecules of L-alanine in two reactions. Because amino acids are usually available in the environment in the L-conformation—which is the conformation found in most mammalian proteins—the first reaction requires the transformation of two molecules of L-alanine into D-alanine. This reaction is catalyzed by the enzyme **alanine racemase**. (Similarly, a glutamate racemase converts L-glutamate to D-glutamate to provide the building block for the second amino acid in the peptide chain.) In the second reaction, an ATP-dependent enzyme called *D-Ala-D-Ala synthetase* (or **D-Ala-D-Ala ligase B [DdlB]**) joins the two D-alanines together after first activating one as the AMP-ester. The resulting D-Ala-D-Ala dipeptide is added to the UDP-NAM-tripeptide by **MurF** to form UDP-NAM-L-Ala-D-Glu-L-Lys (or m-DAP-)-D-Ala-D-Ala, a molecule referred to as the **Park nucleotide** (Fig. 35-2A).

The second phase of peptidoglycan synthesis takes place on the inner surface of the cytoplasmic membrane and begins with the transfer of UDP-NAM-peptide to a phospholipid carrier embedded in the membrane (Fig. 35-2B). This carrier is called *bactoprenol phosphate* or, alternatively, *undecaprenol phosphate* in recognition of the fact that it is assembled from 11 five-carbon isoprene units. **Bactoprenol phosphate (BP)** is called a *carrier* because murein monomers as well as many other cell wall precursors are assembled on it, delivered by it to the surface of the plasma membrane, and then released in a process that regenerates the carrier for further cycles of reaction and precursor transport. The reaction by which UDP-NAM-peptide is anchored to the carrier lipid is mediated by an integral membrane protein called **MraY**. This enzyme catalyzes a diphosphate exchange reaction, so called

because the uridine diphosphate linkage to the NAM-peptide is replaced with an undecaprenol diphosphate linkage, in a chemical exchange reaction illustrated in Figure 35-2B. This reaction is thermodynamically neutral since the products contain the same types of bonds as the starting materials, and indeed, MraY is a readily reversible enzyme. Once the NAM-peptide is anchored to the carrier lipid on the cytoplasmic surface of the membrane, a membrane-associated enzyme called **MurG** catalyzes the transfer of N-acetyl glucosamine to the C4 hydroxyl of the NAM sugar to produce a lipid-anchored NAM-NAG disaccharide commonly known as **Lipid II**. Finally, in some Gram-positive bacteria, including *S. aureus*, a linker peptide, typically composed of five glycine residues, is usually added to the lysine (or DAP) side chain amine. The additional amino acids in the branching peptide are not added in the same fashion as those in the main peptide chain. Rather than being activated as AMP-esters for attack by nucleophilic amines, these amino acids are activated by ester bonds to tRNA molecules.

In *S. aureus*, three different enzymes (**FemA, FemB**, and **FemX**) assemble the glycine pentapeptide branch from the appropriately charged tRNAs. FemX, which attaches the first glycine, is essential for survival. FemA and FemB (which add the next four glycines) are not essential for survival, but their deletion compromises the viability of the organism by affecting cross-linking and integrity of the cell wall. Thus, these enzymes are potential targets for antibiotic development. In Gram-negative bacteria, the murein monomers are usually cross-linked to one another directly, without the use of a branching peptide.

These steps complete the synthesis of a **murein monomer**. Before the final stages of cell wall synthesis can take place, the murine monomer must be transferred from the inner surface of the cytoplasmic membrane to the outer surface. How this is accomplished is an active area of investigation and may be a potential target for new antimicrobial agents.

Glycan Polymerization

Murein monomers on the external surface of the cytoplasmic membrane undergo **polymerization** to make long glycan chains through several rounds of glycosylation. Polymerization is catalyzed by enzymes called **peptidoglycan glycosyltransferases** (**PGTs**, or formerly, transglycosylases). These enzymes catalyze several rounds of elongation by addition of disaccharide subunits to the reducing end of the growing polymer without releasing it. With each glycosylation reaction, bactoprenol diphosphate is released and returns to the inner surface of the cytoplasmic membrane, where it loses a phosphate group to form bactoprenol phosphate; this step is catalyzed by a **dephosphorylase**. Bactoprenol phosphate is now ready to accept another Park nucleotide (Fig. 35-2B).

The PGTs are often found as N-terminal catalytic domains in bifunctional proteins that also have a C-terminal transpeptidation domain; however, they can also be found as monofunctional PGTs (known as *MGTs*). Most bacteria have a number of structurally related PGTs, some bifunctional and some monofunctional. Their enzymatic activities are similar in vitro, but they are presumed to play different roles in cells. For example, in rod-shaped organisms, some PGTs are dedicated to the synthesis of side wall peptidoglycan, whereas others are dedicated to the synthesis of septal peptidoglycan. Nevertheless, these enzymes can partially substitute for one another, complicating a detailed understanding of their specific roles. One possible way of understanding this biological complexity is that bacteria have evolved to have multiple overlapping systems to ensure survival should specific problems arise in an individual machine. This partial redundancy can be a disadvantage from the standpoint of antibiotic treatment.

Polymer Cross-Linking

In the final stage of cell wall synthesis, murein chains are cross-linked to one another by enzymes called **transpeptidases (TPs)**. Because transpeptidases were first identified as the molecular targets of penicillin, they are also called **penicillin-binding proteins (PBPs)**. The PGT domain couples murein monomers to produce glycan strands. These oligosaccharide chains must then be cross-linked through their stem peptides to produce the murein found in bacterial cell walls. The transpeptidation reaction takes place in two steps: activation and coupling. In the **activation step**, a serine hydroxyl in the active site of a TP enzyme attacks the D-Ala-D-Ala amide bond of one of the stem peptides on the glycan polymer, forming a covalent enzyme–peptidoglycan intermediate and releasing alanine. In the **coupling step**, a free amino group on the terminal amino acid of the interbridge peptide (glycine for many Gram-positive bacteria) or on DAP (Gram-negative bacteria) then attacks this intermediate, producing a new amide bond cross-link between the two stem peptides and regenerating the active enzyme (Figs. 35-2B and 35-3). **Penicillin**, a β-lactam, apparently mimics the terminal D-Ala-D-Ala substrate: it binds in the TP active site, where it then reacts with the serine nucleophile to form a covalent enzyme–penicillin complex (Fig. 35-3). This modification inactivates the enzyme, thereby resulting in lower degrees of cell wall cross-linking; in turn, this compromises the integrity of the cell wall and eventually causes cell lysis (see discussion below).

Bacteria typically contain several TPs with different but overlapping specificities. As described above for PGTs, these different enzyme isoforms are used to build different parts of the wall. *Escherichia coli*, for example, has six transpeptidases, some of which build the cylindrical middle of this rod-shaped bacteria, and others of which build its hemispherical ends. It is believed that differences in the number and type of cross-links and glycan chain length give each bacterial species its characteristic shape and size and the cell

wall of each species its characteristic thickness. Consistent with this hypothesis, it has been found that the complement of transpeptidases differs from species to species and especially between rods such as *E. coli* and *C. perfringens* and spherical cocci such as streptococci and staphylococci.

It is thought that, in some cases, bacteria exploit the presence of multiple TPs to develop antibiotic resistance in the clinic. A major form of resistance develops in *S. aureus* when strains acquire a resistant TP that is capable of cross-linking peptidoglycan even when exposed to the β-lactam methicillin, which typically inactivates TPs in a manner similar to penicillin (see discussion below). The cell wall produced by methicillin-resistant *S. aureus* (MRSA) in the presence of drug has lower levels of cross-linking than in the absence of drug, which is presumed to be due to the inefficiency of the resistant TP. One possible strategy for overcoming MRSA is to further weaken the cross-linking ability of this resistant TP.

Mycobacterial Cell Wall Synthesis

The cell wall structures described above are found in the vast majority of clinically relevant bacteria, including Gram-positive cocci such as streptococci and staphylococci, Gram-negative rods such as *E. coli* and *Pseudomonas aeruginosa*, and Gram-positive rods such as *C. perfringens*. However, a discussion of cell wall structure would not be complete without mentioning the unusual cell envelopes of the Corynebacteriae, a group of bacteria that includes the important pathogens *Mycobacterium tuberculosis* and *Mycobacterium leprae*. These bacteria are classified as high G+C (i.e., a high percentage of guanine and cytosine in their DNA) Gram-positives, but their cell envelopes have characteristics of both Gram-positive and Gram-negative bacteria.

Unlike other Gram-positives, the Corynebacteriae have an outer membrane. The NAM sugars in the peptidoglycan layer that surrounds the cytoplasmic (inner) membrane have covalently attached NAG-arabinogalactan polymers to which are attached mycolic acids. The mycolic acids have long alkyl chains containing as many as 90 carbons, and these alkyl chains form a waxy layer that make the bacteria resistant to acid decolorization (acid-fast). The mycolic acids are essential for the assembly of the outer membrane, but the organizational details are unclear. In addition to mycolic acids, the outer membrane of mycobacteria contains secreted phospholipids called **extractable lipids** (see Fig. 35-1). Mycobacteria have outer membrane porins, but their structures are different from the structures of the porins found in Gram-negative bacteria.

The synthesis of **NAG-arabinogalactan** begins with the transfer of a molecule of NAG phosphate from UDP-NAG to mycobacterial bactoprenol phosphate. Next, a molecule of the sugar rhamnose is added, followed by the addition of the several galactose and arabinose units that make up arabinogalactan. **Arabinosyl transferase** catalyzes the addition of the arabinose units. **Mycolic acid** is a long, complex, branched fatty acid. The starting materials for its synthesis include long, saturated hydrocarbon chains that are synthesized from two-carbon units carried by acetyl CoA. The enzyme **fatty acid synthetase 1 (FAS1)** catalyzes the formation of these saturated hydrocarbon chains, and the enzyme **fatty acid synthetase 2 (FAS2)** catalyzes the linkage of these chains. The linked product then undergoes several enzymatic transformations

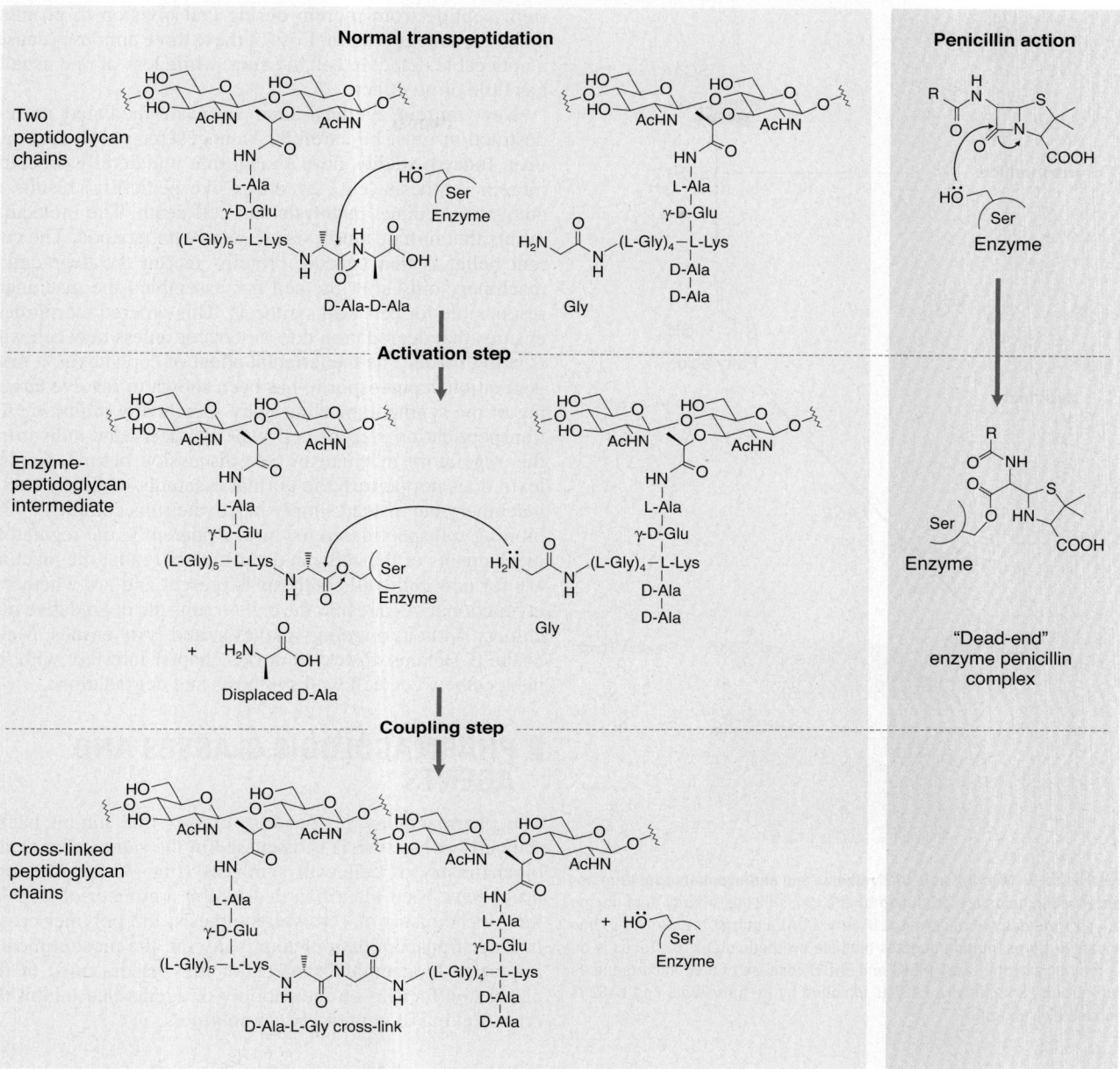

FIGURE 35-3. Transpeptidase action and its inhibition by penicillin. The left side of the figure shows the mechanism by which transpeptidases catalyze transpeptidation, a reaction that occurs in bacteria but not in mammalian cells. **Top panel:** A nucleophilic hydroxyl group in the active site of the transpeptidase (Enzyme) attacks the peptide bond between the two D-Ala residues at the terminus of a pentapeptide moiety on one peptidoglycan chain. **Middle panel:** The terminal D-alanine residue is displaced from the peptidoglycan chain, and an enzyme-D-alanine-peptidoglycan intermediate is formed. This intermediate is then attacked by the amino terminus of a polyglycine pentapeptide linked at its carboxy terminus to L-lysine or diaminopimelic acid on an adjacent peptidoglycan chain (see Fig. 35-2). **Bottom panel:** As the enzyme is liberated from the intermediate, a new peptide bond (cross-link) is formed between the terminal glycine residue on one peptidoglycan chain and the enzyme-activated D-alanine residue on the adjacent peptidoglycan chain. The free enzyme can then catalyze another transpeptidation reaction. The right side of the figure shows the mechanism by which penicillin interferes with transpeptidation, leading to the formation of a penicilloyl-enzyme "dead-end" complex. In this form, the enzyme is incapable of catalyzing further transpeptidation (cross-linking) reactions.

to become mycolic acid. Mycolic acid is eventually added to NAG-arabinogalactan, which, in turn, is attached to NAM to organize and form a major component of the mycobacterial outer membrane (Figs. 35-1 and 35-4). In principle, any step in this process is susceptible to pharmacologic intervention. As discussed below, standard antimycobacterial treatment regimens include antibiotics that target both the synthesis of NAG-arabinogalactan and the early reactions of mycolic acid synthesis.

The mycobacterial cell envelope is thick, asymmetric, and highly impermeable to both hydrophilic and hydrophobic substances. *M. tuberculosis* is among the most challenging pathogens to eradicate because (1) its cell envelope resists entry of many antibiotics and (2) the organism grows very slowly; note that cell-wall-active antibiotics are typically most effective against bacteria that are actively growing and making new cell wall rapidly. Special treatment regimens, involving long-term therapy with combinations of antibiotics, are required to cure tuberculosis.

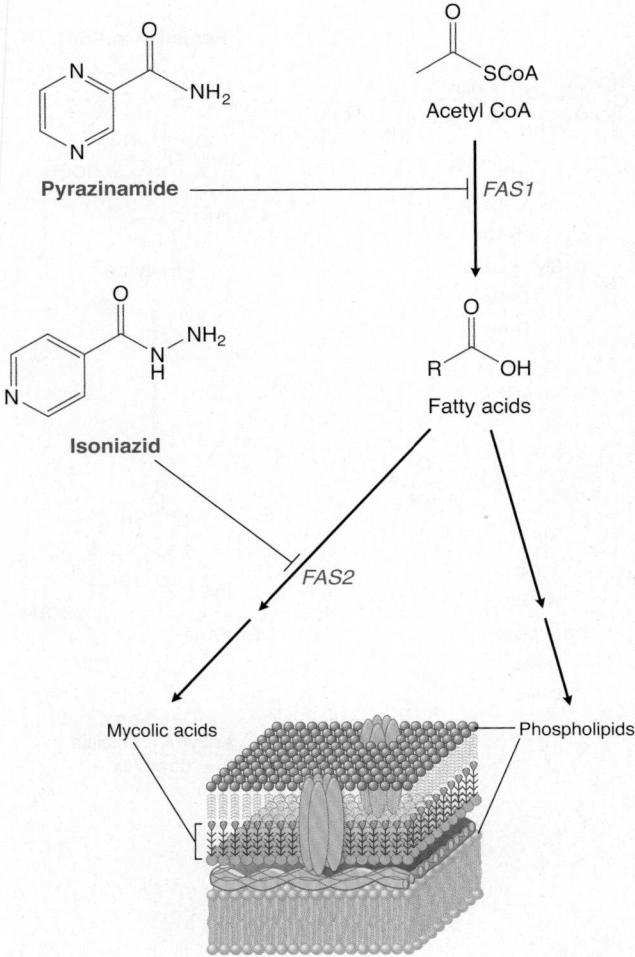

FIGURE 35-4. Mycolic acid biosynthesis and antimycobacterial drug action. Mycolic acids are produced by the cross-linking of fatty acid chains derived from acetyl coenzyme A (Acetyl CoA). Each of the arrows in this simplified representation denotes multiple synthetic steps; the focus is on the fatty acid synthetases (FAS1 and FAS2) because of their importance as drug targets. Specifically, FAS1 is inhibited by pyrazinamide, and FAS2 is inhibited by isoniazid.

Autolysins and Cell Wall Degradation

Although the cell wall provides stability, it is a dynamic structure; it is continuously modified by synthetic and degradative enzymes that are finely tuned to allow the sacculus to grow and divide without lysing. For bacteria to grow, bacterial cell walls must expand; for expansion to occur, new murein units must be incorporated into the existing cell wall. This is difficult to accomplish in a "finished" cell wall, which is composed of specific lengths of glycan polymers with particular degrees of cross-linked stem peptides. In addition, for a bacterium to divide, its cell wall must at some point be broken to allow two daughter cells to separate. Bacteria address these issues by using highly regulated **autolysins**. These enzymes punch small holes in the cell wall that allow for remodeling and expansion. Different autolysins exhibit preferences for different bonds in murein. Similar to the synthetic enzymes, many are functionally redundant but play necessary roles in the cell. For example, in *E. coli*, three autolysins called *NAM-L-alanine amidases* cleave the

stem peptide from murein during cell division to promote daughter cell separation. Loss of these three amidases causes a noticeable defect in cell division, while loss of one usually has little or no effect.

New murein synthesis and autolysin-mediated murein destruction must be carefully balanced for bacteria to survive. Indeed, studies have shown that unilaterally blocking murein synthesis (e.g., by drugs like penicillin) results in autolysin-mediated **autolysis** and cell death. The molecular events that initiate autolysis are poorly understood. The current belief is that specific proteins recruit the degradative machinery only after the cell has assembled the machinery responsible for cell wall synthesis. This ordered recruitment ensures that degradation does not occur unless new cell wall is being made. The **bactericidal effect** of cephalexin, a first-generation cephalosporin, has been shown to involve targeting of the synthetic machinery by specifically inhibiting the transpeptidation step of cell wall synthesis and subverting this regulatory mechanism (see discussion below). Cephalexin does not perturb the normal assembly of the synthetic machinery but instead simply inactivates this complex by inhibiting transpeptidase enzymes. Apparently, the regulatory mechanisms of the cell can determine only that the machinery for new cell wall synthesis is present and not whether it is functional. As a result, the cell recruits the degradative machinery without ongoing synthesis, and lysis ensues. Many of the β-lactams discussed in this chapter interfere with the balance between cell wall synthesis and degradation.

PHARMACOLOGIC CLASSES AND AGENTS

The pharmacology of the drug classes that inhibit bacterial cell wall synthesis is discussed in the same order as the biochemistry of cell wall synthesis (Fig. 35-2). Although drugs have been identified that inhibit a number of steps in the biochemistry of cell wall synthesis, the polymer cross-linking (transpeptidation) step is, by far, the most clinically important biochemical target. For this reason, most of the discussion focuses on the panoply of agents that inhibit the cross-linking of peptidoglycan polymers.

Inhibitors of Murein Monomer Synthesis

Fosfomycin

Fosfomycin (also written **phosphomycin**) is a phosphoenolpyruvate (PEP) analogue that inhibits bacterial enolpyruvate transferase (also known as *MurA*) by covalent modification of the enzyme's active site. Given that PEP is a key intermediate in (mammalian) glycolysis, it may come as a surprise that this agent does not interfere with carbohydrate metabolism in human cells; this selectivity of antibacterial action likely results from structural differences between the mammalian and bacterial enzymes that act on PEP. Thus, fosfomycin has no appreciable effect on human enolase, pyruvate kinase, or carboxykinase, and the drug is relatively nontoxic.

Fosfomycin enters the cell via transporters for glycerophosphate or glucose-6-phosphate that are normally used by bacteria to take up these nutrients from the environment. Fosfomycin is especially effective against Gram-negative bacteria that infect the urinary tract, including *E. coli*, because it is excreted unchanged in the urine. A single 3-g dose of oral fosfomycin tromethamine has been shown to be as effective as multiple doses of other agents in the treatment of uncomplicated urinary tract infections. As a rule, fosfomycin is less effective against Gram-positive bacteria because these bacteria generally lack selective glycerophosphate and glucose-6-phosphate transporters, although it is often active against *Enterococcus faecalis*. Resistance to fosfomycin is typically caused by mutations in these transporters; in addition, a temperature-sensitive *E. coli* strain has been found in which a mutation in enolpyruvate transferase results in reduced affinity of the enzyme for both PEP and fosfomycin. Adverse effects of fosfomycin are uncommon; between 1% and 10% of patients develop headache, diarrhea, or nausea. Significant drug interactions are also rare. The absorption of oral fosfomycin can be decreased by co-administration with promotility agents such as metoclopramide, and probenecid can reduce renal clearance of the drug. Intravenous disodium fosfomycin (which has not been approved by the US Food and Drug Administration [FDA] for use in the United States) has been shown to have antibacterial synergy in vitro with β-lactams, aminoglycosides, and fluoroquinolones.

Cycloserine

Cycloserine, a structural analogue of D-Ala, is a second-line agent used to treat multidrug-resistant *M. tuberculosis* infection (Fig. 35-5). Cycloserine inhibits both the alanine racemase that converts L-Ala to D-Ala and the D-Ala-D-Ala ligase that joins together two D-Ala molecules (Fig. 35-2A). Cycloserine is an irreversible inhibitor of these enzymes and, in fact, binds these enzymes more tightly than does their natural substrate, D-Ala. Resistance to cycloserine occurs by multiple mechanisms, some of which are still unknown; known mechanisms include overexpression of alanine racemase and mutations in the alanine uptake system. As with many small molecules, including fosfomycin, cycloserine is excreted in the urine. Adverse effects include seizures, psychosis, and neurological syndromes such as peripheral neuropathy. Patients with neuropsychiatric disease, alcoholism, and chronic kidney disease should avoid the drug. Alcohol, isoniazid, and ethionamide potentiate its toxicity; pyridoxine may mitigate cycloserine-induced peripheral neuropathy. Cycloserine inhibits the hepatic metabolism of phenytoin.

Bacitracin

So named because it was first identified in a species of *Bacillus*, **bacitracin** is a peptide antibiotic that interferes with the dephosphorylation of bactoprenol diphosphate, rendering the bactoprenol lipid carrier useless for further rounds of murein monomer synthesis and export (Fig. 35-2B). Bacitracin is

therefore notable among the cell wall synthesis inhibitors for having a lipid, rather than a protein or peptide, as its target. Bacitracin inhibits dephosphorylation by forming a complex with bactoprenol diphosphate that involves the drug's imidazole and thiazoline rings. This interaction requires a divalent metal ion, usually Zn^{2+} or Mg^{2+}; hence, drugs that act as metal chelators could interfere with the activity of bacitracin. Due to its significant kidney, neurological, and bone marrow toxicity, bacitracin is not used systemically. It is most commonly used topically for superficial dermal or ophthalmologic infections. Because bacitracin is not absorbed when administered orally, the antibiotic remains within the gut lumen and is thus used occasionally for gut decontamination prior to colorectal surgery.

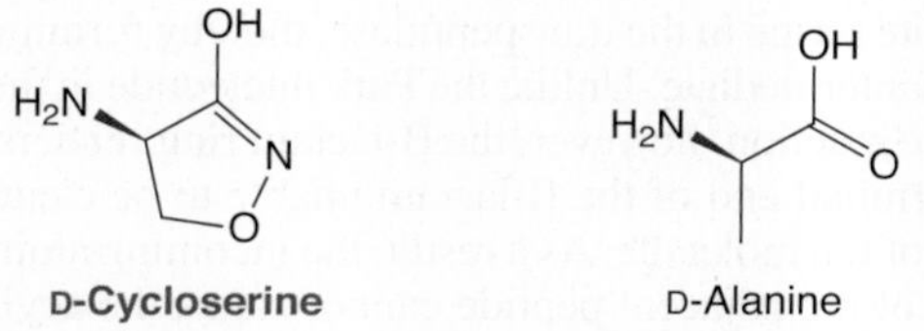

Inhibitors of Murein Polymerization

Vancomycin, Telavancin, Dalbavancin, and Oritavancin

Vancomycin, the agent used to treat *C. difficile* infection in the introductory case, is a glycopeptide with bactericidal activity against Gram-positive rods (such as *Clostridia*) and Gram-positive cocci. **Telavancin**, **dalbavancin**, and **oritavancin** are related lipoglycopeptides with a similar spectrum of action. Gram-negative rods are resistant to the action of these drugs. These agents interrupt cell wall synthesis by binding tightly to the D-Ala-D-Ala terminus of the murein monomer unit, inhibiting **peptidoglycan polymerization** and thereby blocking the addition of murein units to the growing polymer chain. Telavancin and oritavancin have, in addition to the D-Ala-D-Ala-binding moiety, a lipid side chain that interacts with the bacterial cell membrane; this lipid anchor both enhances drug binding to the D-Ala-D-Ala terminus and effects depolarization of the bacterial membrane, resulting in higher antibacterial potency than vancomycin.

Dalbavancin is synthesized from a natural glycopeptide. The amidation of the carboxyl group of the peptide provides enhanced activity against staphylococci, including coagulase-negative staphylococci (CoNS). In addition, the lack of an acetylglucosamine group in dalbavancin allows for increased activity against resistant enterococci. Oritavancin is also derived from a naturally occurring glycopeptide. The addition of an N-alkyl-*p*-chlorophenylbenzyl substituent on the disaccharide sugar results in increased activity against enterococci, including vancomycin-resistant strains. Dalbavancin and oritavancin have prolonged elimination half-lives, allowing for once-weekly dosing.

Intravenous vancomycin is most commonly used to treat serious infections such as pneumonia, bacteremia, and endocarditis caused by methicillin-resistant *Staphylococcus aureus* (MRSA) (see discussion below). Intravenous telavancin is used to treat serious skin infections and pneumonias caused by susceptible strains of staphylococci (including MRSA) and streptococci. Dalbavancin and oritavancin are used to treat serious skin and soft tissue infections caused by susceptible stains of staphylococci (including MRSA) and streptococci; both drugs also have utility in treating enterococcal infections. Oral vancomycin is commonly used to treat gastrointestinal infections caused by *C. difficile*; when administered orally, it is poorly absorbed and therefore remains within the gastrointestinal tract.

The adverse effects of vancomycin include skin flushing or rash—the so-called **red man syndrome**—which is due to release of histamine and can be avoided by decreasing the rate of intravenous infusion or preadministering antihistamines.

FIGURE 35-5. Structure of cycloserine. Cycloserine is a structural analogue of D-alanine that inhibits the racemic interconversion of L-alanine to D-alanine by alanine racemase. Cycloserine also inhibits the activity of D-Ala-D-Ala ligase B, the enzyme that catalyzes the formation of the D-Ala-D-Ala dipeptide that is subsequently utilized in the synthesis of murein monomers (see Fig. 35-2A).

Vancomycin has also been associated with nephrotoxicity and rarely ototoxicity, particularly when other nephrotoxic or ototoxic medications such as gentamicin are co-administered. Patients with underlying renal dysfunction need adjusted dosing and measurement of drug levels in order to mitigate nephrotoxicity. Drug fever, hypersensitivity rash, and drug-induced neutropenia can also occur. Telavancin appears to have a toxicity profile similar to that of vancomycin, with a slightly lower risk of infusion-related reactions but a higher incidence of nephrotoxicity. Dalbavancin does not appear to cause infusion-related reactions or nephrotoxicity; the most common adverse event in clinical trials was mild gastrointestinal upset. Oritavancin has similar toxicities to vancomycin except for a much lower risk of renal toxicity. Telavancin and oritavancin can bind to artificial phospholipid surfaces in some commercially available anticoagulation assays, resulting in falsely prolonged prothrombin, activated partial thromboplastin, and activated clotting times (PT, aPTT, and ACT, respectively). This also results in a falsely elevated international normalized ratio (INR). In order to minimize this interference, blood drawn for these assays should be taken near the time of the trough plasma concentration of telavancin or oritavancin.

Resistance to vancomycin, telavancin, dalbavancin, and oritavancin most commonly arises through the acquisition of DNA encoding enzymes that catalyze the formation of D-Ala-D-lactate instead of D-Ala-D-Ala. As with D-Ala-D-Ala, D-Ala-D-lactate is incorporated into the murein monomer unit and participates readily in the transpeptidase reaction, but the D-Ala-D-lactate dipeptide is not bound by vancomycin and related glycopeptides. Two enzymes mediate the synthesis of D-Ala-D-lactate: VanH, a dehydrogenase that generates D-lactate from pyruvate, and VanA, a ligase that links D-Ala to D-lactate. VanH and VanA are encoded on a transposable element that can be found on either the bacterial chromosome or an extrachromosomal plasmid. This element also encodes enzymes that degrade D-Ala-D-Ala, thereby removing any residual targets of vancomycin. In clinical practice, bacteria resistant to vancomycin (such as vancomycin-resistant enterococci [VRE]) are often resistant to most other antibacterials; plasmid-mediated spread of vancomycin resistance is therefore a serious medical problem. A few cases of vancomycin-resistant *S. aureus* (VRSA) due to acquisition of enterococcal resistance genes have been reported. Vancomycin-intermediate *S. aureus* (VISA) has also been described; these organisms have a thicker murein layer in which increased amounts of free D-Ala-D-Ala act as a decoy target for vancomycin. Dalbavancin and oritavancin are more stable than vancomycin and telavancin against the development of resistance to *Staphylococcus* and *Streptococcus* species. Oritavancin may be active against *Enterococcus* strains that exhibit resistance to the other glycopeptides.

Inhibitors of Polymer Cross-Linking

β-Lactam Antibiotics: General Considerations

With more than 30 different agents currently in use, including the original **penicillin** and the **dicloxacillin** used in the introductory case, the β-lactams are the largest and most widely prescribed class of antibiotics that inhibit bacterial cell wall synthesis. The various agents in this class differ in chemical structure (Fig. 35-6) and consequently in spectrum of action, but all β-lactams share the same antibiotic mechanism of action: *inhibition of murein polymer cross-linking*.

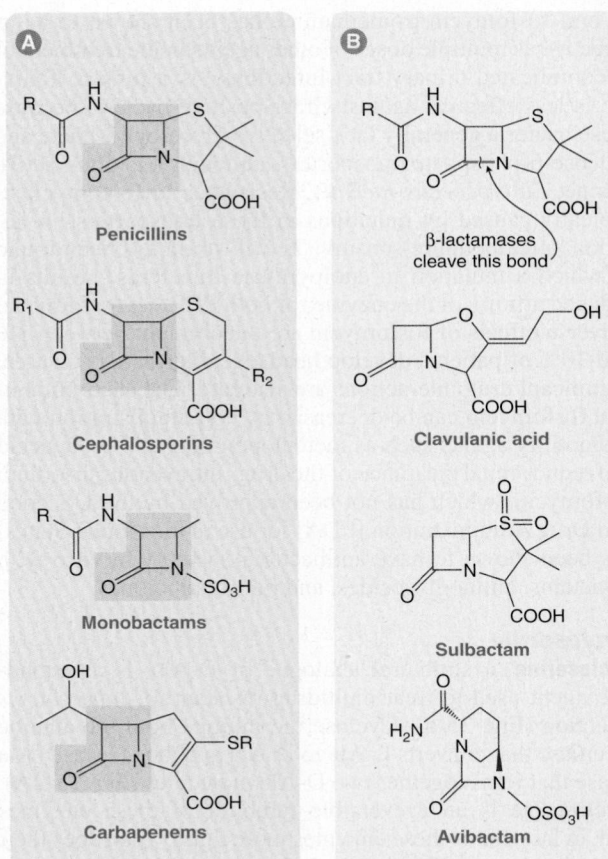

FIGURE 35-6. Structural features of β-lactam antibiotics and β-lactamase inhibitors. A. The β-lactam family members (penicillins, cephalosporins, monobactams, and carbapenems) differ from one another in their backbone structures; individual drugs within these subclasses also differ in their R groups. Note the four-membered β-lactam ring that is common to all four families (*blue boxes*); it is this ring that gives the agents their ability to block the transpeptidation reaction (and also their name). **B.** Bacteria expressing β-lactamases are able to cleave the β-lactam bond (*blue line*) that is required for antibiotic action. The β-lactamase inhibitors clavulanic acid, sulbactam, and avibactam act as decoys by binding to (and thereby inhibiting) β-lactamase enzymes. Note the structural similarity between the β-lactamase inhibitors and the β-lactam antibiotics.

Chemically, the key to this mechanism of action is the presence of a four-membered β-**lactam ring** (Fig. 35-6). This ring makes every β-lactam a structural analogue of the terminal D-Ala-D-Ala dipeptide of the Park nucleotide and hence a substrate for one or more bacterial transpeptidases. As with the Park nucleotide, the β-lactam reacts covalently with the active-site serine in the transpeptidase, thereby forming an acyl enzyme intermediate. Unlike the Park nucleotide in the normal substrate reaction, however, the β-lactam ring renders the carboxy terminal end of the β-lactam unable to be cleaved from the rest of the molecule. As a result, the incoming amino terminal end of the adjacent peptide cannot attack the acyl enzyme intermediate, and the transpeptidase reaches a *"dead-end"* **complex** (Fig. 35-3). (This mode of irreversible enzyme inhibition is sometimes called **suicide substrate inhibition**.) Provided that the cells are growing, transpeptidase inhibition results in autolysin-mediated autolysis and cell death. Hence, as a rule, β-lactams are **bactericidal** for actively dividing bacteria.

The various subclasses of β-lactam agents fall into four families—the **penicillins**, the **cephalosporins** (which are further subdivided into five "generations"), the **monobactams**, and the **carbapenems**. Each of these subclasses differs structurally in the chemical substituents that are attached to the β-lactam ring (see Fig. 35-6). In general, the development of these families resulted from pharmacologists' efforts in the laboratory to improve on penicillin's antibiotic **spectrum of action** and to stay ahead of the spread of **antibiotic resistance**. Recall that spectrum of action refers to the number and variety of bacterial species against which an antibiotic shows bactericidal or bacteriostatic activity. Hence, broad-spectrum β-lactams are typically active against Gram-negative as well as Gram-positive bacteria, whereas narrow-spectrum β-lactams are typically effective only against Gram-positive organisms.

Bacterial transpeptidases are located in the periplasmic space between the cytoplasmic membrane and the cell wall. Hence, to exert their effects, β-lactams must traverse the cell wall and, in the case of Gram-negative bacteria, the outer membrane as well. A β-lactam's spectrum of action is determined by two factors: its ability to penetrate the outer membrane and cell wall and, once in the periplasmic space, its ability to inhibit specific transpeptidases. Both hydrophilic and (to a lesser extent) hydrophobic agents diffuse through the thick murein layer of Gram-positive bacteria, but hydrophilic agents pass through the outer membrane pores of Gram-negative bacteria much more readily than do hydrophobic agents. As a result, hydrophilic agents such as **ampicillin**, **amoxicillin**, and, especially, **piperacillin** and **ticarcillin** tend to have broad spectra of action, whereas hydrophobic agents such as **oxacillin**, **cloxacillin**, **dicloxacillin**, **nafcillin**, **methicillin**, and **penicillin G** tend to have narrow spectra of action (see discussion below for details). This means that some Gram-negative bacteria are inherently resistant to narrow-spectrum β-lactams simply by virtue of the permeability barrier presented by their outer membrane. (Similarly, **intracellular bacteria**, that is, bacteria that live within human cells, such as *Chlamydia*, are, in general, also inherently resistant to β-lactams, both because mammalian cells tend to lack β-lactam uptake mechanisms and because these bacteria tend either to have unique cell wall architectures or to lack cell walls altogether.)

The second factor that determines a β-lactam's spectrum of action is the extent to which the drug, after accessing the periplasmic space, inhibits a particular transpeptidase. In large part, this is determined by the β-lactam's affinity for the transpeptidase. As noted above, bacteria typically have several transpeptidase enzymes that differ subtly in their substrate specificity and cross-linking activity; these differences are especially prominent between rods and cocci. Most β-lactams have selectivity for several different transpeptidases; others, such as the penicillin analogue methicillin that was previously used against *S. aureus*, are specific for just one.

Antibiotic resistance can be encoded by either **chromosomal (intrinsic)** or **acquired (extrinsic)** genes. For β-lactams, chromosomal resistance in Gram-positive bacteria is most commonly conferred by a chromosomally encoded mutation in a transpeptidase-encoding gene that abolishes the transpeptidase's ability to bind a particular β-lactam or by acquisition of a gene encoding a transpeptidase with low affinity for the β-lactam. This mechanism is the cause of resistance to methicillin in *S. aureus*, as mentioned above, and

the mechanism by which pneumococci acquire resistance to penicillin. However, resistance to β-lactams by genetically altered transpeptidases is the exception, not the rule, because most β-lactams are active against multiple transpeptidases that would all need to be mutated in order to abolish the drugs' effectiveness.

Most resistance to β-lactams is conferred by proteins called **β-lactamases** that are encoded on the chromosome or on extrachromosomal DNA **plasmids**. As their name implies, β-lactamases are enzymes that inactivate β-lactams via (hydrolytic) cleavage of the β-lactam ring. More than 100 different β-lactamases have been identified, each with activity against a particular β-lactam or set of β-lactams. β-Lactamases are secreted in Gram-positive bacteria; in Gram-negative bacteria, these enzymes are retained in the periplasmic space between the cell wall and outer membrane. Gram-negative bacteria produce much less β-lactamase than Gram-positive bacteria do, but because the Gram-negatives concentrate the β-lactamase where it is needed in the periplasmic space, the β-lactamase is more effective at conferring resistance. This concentration effect, coupled with the strong permeability barrier to penicillins afforded by the bacterial outer membrane, makes Gram-negative bacteria largely refractory to penicillin therapy.

That many β-lactamases are encoded on plasmids is of special clinical importance. Because plasmids are easily transferred by conjugation from one bacterium to another, the resistance conferred by the plasmid can sweep rapidly through a bacterial population. Moreover, plasmids can "jump strains," spreading resistance from one strain to another. Organisms such as *Klebsiella pneumoniae* and *E. coli* may also produce **extended-spectrum β-lactamases (ESBLs)** and **carbapenemases** that render them resistant to most β-lactam antibiotics, including penicillins, cephalosporins, the monobactam **aztreonam**, and the carbapenems. Other bacteria, such as *Enterobacter* species, may overexpress a chromosomally encoded β-lactamase that produces similarly broad resistance to β-lactams.

Pharmacologists have responded to the challenge of β-lactamases in two ways. First, as noted above, new families of β-lactams have been developed with structures that make them less susceptible to cleavage by existing β-lactamases. Second, **β-lactamase inhibitors** have been developed that can be co-administered with β-lactam antibiotics. β-Lactamase inhibitors are β-lactam-like molecules that bind to the active site of β-lactamases and thereby prevent the β-lactamases from destroying the β-lactam antibiotics with which the lactamase inhibitors are co-administered. Four examples of β-lactamase inhibitors are **clavulanic acid (clavulanate)**, **sulbactam**, **tazobactam**, and **avibactam** (Fig. 35-6). Avibactam is a novel β-lactamase inhibitor recently developed for use in combination with ceftazidime to provide enhanced activity against resistant Gram-negative bacteria.

β-Lactams act synergistically with **aminoglycosides**, the bactericidal inhibitors of protein synthesis discussed in Chapter 34. (For more on synergy, see Chapter 41, Principles of Combination Chemotherapy.) Aminoglycosides inhibit protein synthesis by binding to the 30S ribosomal subunit in the cytoplasm of the cell. To access the cytoplasm, aminoglycosides must diffuse passively across the cell wall before being transported actively across the cytoplasmic membrane. It is thought that the cell walls of some bacteria, such as enterococci, are poorly permeable to aminoglycosides when these drugs are

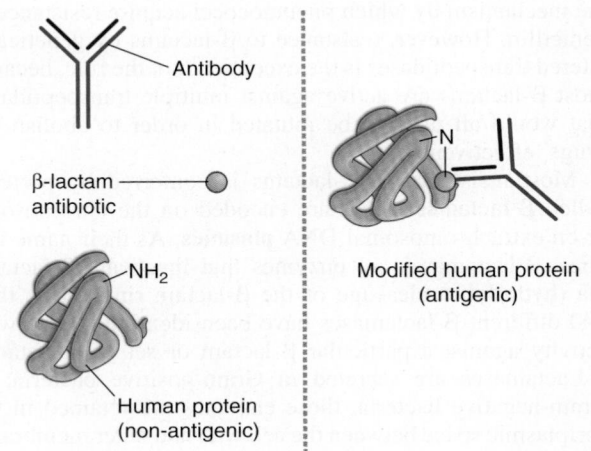

FIGURE 35-7. β-Lactam toxicity. In the absence of modification, human proteins are generally nonantigenic. β-Lactams can modify amino groups on human proteins, creating an immunogenic β-lactam hapten. This new antigenic determinant can be recognized as "nonself" by antibodies of the host immune system.

administered as single agents. Because β-lactams increase cell wall permeability, co-administration of a β-lactam facilitates the uptake of an aminoglycoside and thus enhances its effect.

Hypersensitivity reactions are the most common adverse effects of β-lactams. As small molecules, β-lactams would not be expected to stimulate immune responses by themselves, and indeed they do not. However, β-lactam rings can react with amino groups on human proteins to create a hapten–carrier complex (Fig. 35-7). The β-lactam–protein conjugate can then provoke a hypersensitivity response. The most serious of these reactions is **anaphylaxis**, which typically occurs within an hour of drug administration and leads to bronchospasm, angioedema, and/or cardiovascular collapse. Urticaria, morbilliform drug rash, serum sickness, and drug fever may also occur. Proteins on the surface of red blood cells can also be modified by penicillin, leading to drug-induced autoimmune hemolytic anemia. Rarely, β-lactam antibiotics cause drug-induced lupus. For most individuals, this process is strongly dose dependent: the likelihood of a hypersensitivity reaction increases with each administration of a β-lactam. β-Lactams of a given class often cross-react with each other, but β-lactams of one class are less often cross-reactive with β-lactams of another class. Patients with a penicillin allergy should not receive ampicillin or other penicillins due to the high risk of cross-reactivity. Patients with a penicillin allergy other than serum sickness or anaphylaxis generally may receive a cephalosporin or a carbapenem. **Aztreonam** (a monobactam) is unique in that it has no cross-reactivity with either penicillins or carbapenems; however, cross-reactivity between aztreonam and ceftazidime (a cephalosporin), presumably due to a shared side chain, has been reported. Although allergic reactions to carbapenems can occur in patients with penicillin allergy, they are rare.

β-Lactam Antibiotics: Specific Agents
Penicillins
As noted above, there are four structurally distinct subclasses of β-lactam antibiotics (see Fig. 35-6A). The first of these subclasses, the penicillins, can be further divided into five groups according to their spectra of action.

The first group of penicillins includes **penicillin G**, which is intravenously administered, and **penicillin V**, its gastric acid-stable oral counterpart. Penicillin V is used to treat dental infections and to prevent recurrent rheumatic fever in patients with a prior episode and recurrent streptococcal cellulitis in patients with lymphedema. Penicillin G is used to treat serious infections with Gram-positive bacteria such as pneumococcus and *S. pyogenes* (some strains of each), Gram-negative diplococci such as *Neisseria* species (except penicillinase-producing *N. gonorrhoeae*), Gram-positive rods of the genera *Clostridium* and *Actinomyces*, and spirochetes such as syphilis and *Leptospira*. High-dose penicillin G may cause seizures, in addition to the already mentioned hypersensitivity reactions and rash. All penicillins can cause acute interstitial nephritis. Drug–drug interactions are rare, but the anticoagulant effects of warfarin may be potentiated by concomitant penicillin administration.

The second group consists of the **antistaphylococcal penicillins**, including **oxacillin**, **cloxacillin**, **dicloxacillin**, **nafcillin**, and **methicillin**. These drugs are structurally resistant to staphylococcal β-lactamase, which is encoded by plasmid genes in most clinical isolates. Because of their relative hydrophobicity, however, antistaphylococcal penicillins lack activity against Gram-negative bacteria. (Recall also that methicillin binds to only a single transpeptidase.) Thus, oral antistaphylococcal penicillins are used mostly for skin and soft tissue infections. Intravenous antistaphylococcal penicillins are predominantly used for more serious methicillin-sensitive *S. aureus* skin and soft tissue infections or other serious infections, such as bacteremia, endocarditis, or osteomyelitis. Use of the oral antistaphylococcal penicillins (cloxacillin and dicloxacillin) is somewhat limited by their gastrointestinal adverse effects (nausea and antibiotic-associated diarrhea) and occasionally by secondary development of *C. difficile* infection. Adverse effects of intravenous nafcillin include phlebitis at the injection site; agranulocytosis and acute interstitial nephritis occur at a higher rate than with the other penicillins. Nafcillin is an inducer of hepatic isoenzyme CYP3A4 and can decrease the plasma levels of drugs that are substrates for CYP3A4. Oxacillin can cause hepatotoxicity, which is reversible with discontinuation of the drug. The utility of antistaphylococcal penicillins in treating *S. aureus* has been compromised by the emergence of MRSA strains. Patients with MRSA infection are typically treated with vancomycin or with non-cell wall-active agents such as trimethoprim-sulfamethoxazole, doxycycline, linezolid, or tedizolid.

Ampicillin and **amoxicillin** are members of the third group of penicillins, the **amino penicillins**, which have a positively charged amino group on the R side chain (see Fig. 35-6A). This positive charge enhances diffusion through porin channels but does not confer resistance to β-lactamases. These agents are effective against a variety of Gram-positive cocci, Gram-negative cocci such as *Neisseria gonorrhoeae* and *N. meningitidis*, and Gram-negative rods such as *E. coli* and *Haemophilus influenzae*, but their spectrum is limited by sensitivity to most β-lactamases. Intravenous ampicillin is used most commonly to treat invasive enterococcal infections and *Listeria* meningitis; oral amoxicillin is used to treat uncomplicated ear, nose, and throat infections, to prevent endocarditis in high-risk patients undergoing dental work, and as a component of combination therapy for *Helicobacter pylori* infection. Rash is the most common adverse effect.

The spectrum of both agents is broadened when they are co-administered with β-lactamase inhibitors such as clavulanic acid (with amoxicillin) or sulbactam (with ampicillin) to treat β-lactamase-producing organisms such as *S. aureus*, *H. influenzae*, *E. coli*, *Klebsiella*, and anaerobes. Sulbactam itself has activity against *Acinetobacter*.

Agents in the fourth group of penicillins, the **carboxy penicillins**, are also broad in spectrum. The carboxyl group on the R side chain provides a negative charge that confers resistance to some β-lactamases but is less effective than a positively charged amino group in facilitating diffusion through porin channels. To overcome this limitation in diffusion, high doses are used. Resistance to the chromosomally encoded β-lactamases of *Enterobacter* and *Pseudomonas* adds these organisms to the spectrum of the carboxy penicillins. This group includes **ticarcillin**.

A fifth group, the **ureido penicillins**, is represented by **piperacillin**. This drug has both positive and negative charges on the R side chain and is generally more potent than the carboxy penicillins. Its spectrum of action is similar to that of the carboxy penicillins; in addition, ureido penicillins have activity against *Klebsiella* and enterococci. Piperacillin is currently available only in combination with the β-lactamase inhibitor tazobactam.

Cephalosporins

Cephalosporins differ structurally from penicillins by having a six-membered rather than a five-membered accessory ring attached to the β-lactam ring (Fig. 35-6A).

First-generation cephalosporins (**cefazolin**, **cephalexin**, and **cefadroxil**) are active against Gram-positive species as well as the Gram-negative rods *Proteus mirabilis* and *E. coli*, both of which cause urinary tract infections, and *Klebsiella pneumoniae*, which causes pneumonia in addition to urinary tract infections. These agents are sensitive to many β-lactamases but are not degraded by the chromosomally encoded β-lactamase of *K. pneumoniae* and the common staphylococcal β-lactamase. Cephalexin and cefadroxil are both administered orally and are used to treat skin and soft tissue infections and streptococcal pharyngitis. The intravenous agent cefazolin is also used to treat serious skin and soft tissue infections and is used for surgical prophylaxis and treatment of serious infections due to MSSA in individuals unable to take an antistaphylococcal penicillin.

Second-generation cephalosporins can be divided into two groups. **Cefuroxime**, which represents the first group, has increased activity against *H. influenzae* compared to the first-generation cephalosporins; **cefotetan** and **cefoxitin**, which represent the second group, demonstrate increased activity against *Bacteroides*. In general, second-generation cephalosporins are resistant to more β-lactamases than are first-generation cephalosporins. Thus, cefuroxime can be used to treat community-acquired pneumonia, and cefotetan is used to treat intra-abdominal and pelvic infections, including pelvic inflammatory disease. Adverse effects of these agents include diarrhea, mild liver enzyme elevation, and hypersensitivity reactions; rarely, agranulocytosis or interstitial nephritis can occur.

Third-generation cephalosporins (**ceftriaxone**, **cefotaxime**, and **cefpodoxime**) are resistant to many β-lactamases and are thus highly active against Enterobacteriaceae (*E. coli*, indole-positive *Proteus*, *Klebsiella*, *Enterobacter*, *Serratia*, and *Citrobacter*) as well as *Neisseria* and *H. influenzae*.

The third-generation cephalosporins are less active against Gram-positive organisms than are the first-generation drugs; despite that, they have good activity against penicillin-intermediate *S. pneumoniae* (although cephalosporin resistance can occur). Common uses include treatment of pneumonia, community-acquired meningitis due to *S. pneumoniae*, uncomplicated gonococcal infection, culture-negative endocarditis, and Lyme disease involving the central nervous system or joints. In addition to the adverse effects already mentioned, ceftriaxone can cause cholestatic hepatitis, albeit uncommonly. **Ceftazidime** is another commonly used third-generation cephalosporin; its spectrum differs from the other agents in that it has significant activity against *Pseudomonas aeruginosa* and minimal activity against Gram-positive organisms. It is used predominantly to treat hospital-acquired Gram-negative bacterial infections and documented infections with *P. aeruginosa* and as empiric therapy for neutropenic patients with fever. Gram-negative bacteria that have acquired extended-spectrum β-lactamase activity are resistant to third-generation cephalosporins.

Cefepime is the only currently available fourth-generation cephalosporin. Like ceftriaxone, it is highly active against Enterobacteriaceae, *Neisseria*, *H. influenzae*, and Gram-positive organisms; additionally, it is as active as ceftazidime against *P. aeruginosa*. Cefepime is also more resistant to the chromosomally encoded β-lactamases of *Enterobacter* than are third-generation cephalosporins. Unlike ceftazidime, however, cefepime is not approved for treatment of meningitis. An uncommon adverse effect is the development of autoantibodies against red blood cell antigens, typically without significant hemolysis. In addition, cefepime can infrequently cause neurotoxicity including myoclonus and encephalopathy, particularly in the elderly and in patients with impaired renal function; for the latter patients, the antibiotic requires dose adjustment.

Ceftaroline is a fifth-generation cephalosporin. This drug is distinct in having antimicrobial activity against multidrug-resistant *S. aureus*—including methicillin-resistant, vancomycin-intermediate *S. aureus* and vancomycin-resistant strains—as well as *S. pneumoniae* and respiratory Gram-negative pathogens such as *Moraxella catarrhalis* and *H. influenzae*, including β-lactamase-expressing strains. Ceftaroline is only available intravenously and is approved for treatment of community-acquired pneumonia and skin infections.

Ceftolozane is a novel intravenous cephalosporin currently available in combination with the β-lactamase inhibitor tazobactam. It is FDA approved for the treatment of complicated urinary tract infections and complicated intra-abdominal infections. Ceftolozane is structurally similar to ceftazidime but has a more heavily substituted pyrazole at the 3-position side chain that confers greater stability against β-lactamase-producing *Pseudomonas aeruginosa* compared to ceftazidime. It has antimicrobial activity against many Gram-negative aerobes, β-lactamase-producing Enterobacteriaceae, and *Pseudomonas aeruginosa*. It lacks activity against carbapenemase-producing *Klebsiella pneumoniae*. While it is active against most streptococci, it has limited activity against staphylococci. The addition of tazobactam broadens ceftolozane's activity against various anaerobes, such as *Bacteroides* species and *Prevotella* species, but not *Clostridium* species.

As noted above, cephalosporins can generally be used in patients with non-life-threatening allergic reactions to penicillins. Nevertheless, cephalosporins can cause hypersensitivity reactions themselves and should be used with caution in patients with known cephalosporin hypersensitivity. Interestingly, **cefotetan** and **cefoperazone** (another third-generation cephalosporin) contain an N-methylthiotetrazole (NMTT) side chain that causes two unique adverse effects. The first is an alcohol intolerance syndrome known as the **disulfiram-like reaction** (disulfiram is a drug that inhibits alcohol metabolism; see Chapter 19, Pharmacology of Drugs of Abuse). The second involves an effect on vitamin K metabolism that results in decreased synthesis of vitamin K-dependent coagulation factors; thus, cefotetan and cefoperazone should be used with caution in patients taking warfarin and in patients with underlying coagulation abnormalities (see Chapter 23, Pharmacology of Hemostasis and Thrombosis). Cefotetan, like most of the cephalosporins, can also cause antibody-mediated hemolysis.

Monobactams and Carbapenems

The only available monobactam, **aztreonam**, is active against most Gram-negative bacteria, including *P. aeruginosa*, but it has no activity against Gram-positive organisms. Aztreonam is particularly useful in patients with serious penicillin allergy who have infections due to resistant Gram-negative organisms because of its lack of cross-allergenicity with penicillins; however, Gram-negative bacteria with extended-spectrum β-lactamases are resistant to the drug. It is available intravenously for treatment of systemic infections and in an inhaled form for prevention of pulmonary exacerbations in patients with cystic fibrosis, who are commonly colonized with *P. aeruginosa*.

Four carbapenems are currently used in clinical practice: **imipenem**, **meropenem**, **doripenem**, and **ertapenem**. All four are broadly active against most Gram-positive, Gram-negative, and anaerobic organisms. None is active against MRSA, VRE, or *Legionella*; and Gram-negative bacteria with carbapenemases (especially *K. pneumoniae*) exhibit resistance to these drugs. Importantly, ertapenem is much less active against *P. aeruginosa* and *Acinetobacter* than the other three agents; the benefit of ertapenem is its once-daily dosing. Because imipenem is inactivated by the human renal enzyme dehydropeptidase I, this drug is co-administered with the dehydropeptidase inhibitor **cilastatin**. Neither meropenem, doripenem, nor ertapenem is inactivated by the renal enzyme. All four agents are typically administered intravenously, but ertapenem and imipenem can also be administered intramuscularly. No oral carbapenems are currently available. All carbapenems can cause hypersensitivity reactions and IV site phlebitis; at high plasma drug levels, imipenem and meropenem can cause seizures. Probenecid can increase meropenem levels, and all carbapenems can decrease valproate levels.

Inhibitors of Cell Membrane Stability

Daptomycin is a cyclic lipopeptide antibiotic. Its exact mechanism of action is unclear, but the drug appears to integrate into the membranes of Gram-positive bacteria. Oligomerization of daptomycin may then result in the formation of pores, leading to potassium efflux, membrane depolarization, and cell death. Daptomycin is administered intravenously and is approved for the treatment of complicated skin infections and bacteremia (including bacteremia from right-sided endocarditis) caused by *Staphylococcus aureus*.

Daptomycin also has therapeutic efficacy in the treatment of Gram-positive bacterial infections and specifically may be active in the treatment of methicillin-resistant *Staphylococcus aureus* and vancomycin-resistant enterococcal infections. Adverse effects include myopathy and eosinophilic pneumonia. Because of the association with myopathy, caution should be exercised when co-administering statins with daptomycin. Daptomycin can bind to artificial phospholipid surfaces in some commercially available anticoagulation assays, resulting in falsely prolonged PT and aPTT. In order to minimize this interference, blood drawn for these assays should be taken near the time of the trough plasma concentration of daptomycin.

Antimycobacterial Agents

Ethambutol, Pyrazinamide, and Isoniazid

Ethambutol, **pyrazinamide**, and **isoniazid (INH)** are three of the five first-line agents used to treat tuberculosis (rifampin and streptomycin, discussed in Chapter 34, are the other two). Patients with active tuberculosis and without a history of prior therapy are started on a four-drug regimen if the local prevalence of isoniazid resistance is higher than 4%. If isoniazid resistance is rare, a three-drug regimen without ethambutol can be used (see Chapter 41).

Ethambutol, a bacteriostatic agent, decreases arabinogalactan synthesis by inhibiting the arabinosyl transferase that adds arabinose units to the growing arabinogalactan chain. Pyrazinamide and INH inhibit mycolic acid synthesis. Pyrazinamide is a prodrug; it must be converted to its active form, pyrazinoic acid, by the enzyme pyrazinamidase. Pyrazinoic acid inhibits FAS1, the enzyme that synthesizes the fatty acid precursors of mycolic acid. Isoniazid and the related second-line agent **ethionamide** target the FAS2 complex and are bactericidal, although the exact mechanism of bacterial killing is unknown. The targets of pyrazinamide and isoniazid are summarized in Figure 35-4.

Treatment of active tuberculosis requires multidrug therapy. Since resistance to antimycobacterial agents usually occurs by mutation, a powerful argument in favor of this strategy is based on the frequency of resistance mutations and the number of bacteria present in a clinical infection. Each tuberculous lesion in an infected lung can contain 10^8 bacteria. The frequency of mutants resistant to any single antimycobacterial drug is about 1 in 10^6 bacteria. This frequency means that, in each tuberculous lesion, an average of about 100 bacteria will already be resistant to an antimycobacterial drug, even before that drug is administered. Combination therapy with just two drugs reduces the likelihood of encountering preexisting resistance to just 1 bacterium in 10^{12}; treatment with four drugs lowers this probability to 1 in 10^{24} (see Chapter 41).

Antimycobacterial agents can cause serious adverse effects. Ethambutol is associated with optic neuritis; patients report impaired visual acuity, loss of color discrimination, constricted visual fields, and/or central and peripheral scotomata. Symptoms usually occur after more than a month of therapy and are reversible; however, sudden-onset irreversible blindness has been reported. Therefore, patients taking ethambutol must be seen regularly for eye examination by an ophthalmologist to assess both visual acuity and color discrimination. Pyrazinamide is associated with arthralgias and (usually asymptomatic) hyperuricemia; more importantly, it commonly causes hepatotoxicity that can be severe and irreversible. Whereas patients who experience mild hepatotoxicity due to INH may be rechallenged with the drug, patients who experience pyrazinamide-induced hepatotoxicity should not be rechallenged. Isoniazid is associated with hepatitis as well as peripheral neuropathy. INH-induced hepatotoxicity can be mild, manifesting only as minor liver enzyme elevation not requiring cessation of the drug (occurs in 10–20% of patients), or it can be severe, leading to symptomatic hepatitis (occurs in 0.1% of patients overall, with increased risk in older patients with underlying liver disease who are also taking rifampin). Neurological manifestations of INH toxicity include paresthesias, peripheral neuropathy, and ataxia; this toxicity is due to INH's competitive inhibition of pyridoxine in neurotransmitter synthesis and can be prevented by pyridoxine supplementation. Isoniazid can also inhibit or induce cytochrome P450 enzymes and thereby interact with multiple other drugs, including rifampin, the antiseizure medications carbamazepine and phenytoin, azole-type antifungals, and alcohol. Isoniazid is a weak monoamine oxidase inhibitor; administered with serotonergic agents such as meperidine or fluoxetine, it may cause serotonin syndrome.

Resistance to these drugs, and to antimycobacterial agents in general, results from chromosomal mutations. Ethambutol resistance most often results from mutations in the arabinosyl transferase gene, some of which cause overexpression of the target enzyme. Resistance to isoniazid usually results from an inactivating mutation in the mycobacterial enzyme **catalase-peroxidase**, which converts isoniazid into its antimycobacterial form. Mutations in the *inhA* gene, which is required for mycolic acid synthesis, also confer resistance to INH. Resistance to pyrazinamide is generally due to mutations in the pyrazinamidase gene, which result in the inability to convert the prodrug into its active form.

▌CONCLUSION AND FUTURE DIRECTIONS

The bacterial cell wall presents unique antibacterial targets. This structure consists of a three-dimensional mat of cross-linked peptide-sugar polymers called *murein* and is synthesized in three stages: (1) synthesis of murein monomers, (2) polymerization of monomers into murein polymers, and (3) cross-linking of polymers to complete the wall.

Antibacterial agents act in all three stages of cell wall synthesis: fosfomycin and cycloserine act in the first stage; vancomycin, telavancin, dalbavancin, oritavancin, and bacitracin act in the second stage; and the β-lactams, the largest and most important group, act in the third stage. β-Lactams—which include the penicillins, cephalosporins, monobactams, and carbapenems—are bactericidal; autolytic cell death most likely results from the unopposed action of wall remodeling proteins called *autolysins*. Structural and chemical differences among the β-lactams determine their spectra of activity against bacteria with different cell wall architectures.

Resistance to β-lactam antibiotics is generally conferred by plasmid-encoded β-lactamases. Pharmacologists have addressed this mechanism of resistance by (1) developing new β-lactam agents, for example, the second- and third-generation cephalosporins that are resistant to degradation by many β-lactamases, and (2) co-administering β-lactam "decoys," such as clavulanic acid and sulbactam, that serve as β-lactamase inhibitors. Because β-lactamases can be encoded on plasmids, they can spread through bacterial (and human) populations with great speed, making antibiotic development an ongoing "arms race."

Antimycobacterial agents act by blocking various steps in the synthesis of molecules, such as mycolic acid and arabinogalactan, that are unique to the mycobacterial cell wall. Resistance to these agents is typically due to chromosomal mutation, but combination therapy is critically important to avoid the development of mutational resistance. Future innovations will likely include the development of new agents directed against the additional unique molecular targets that are presented by the biochemistry of the bacterial cell wall.

Acknowledgment

We thank Robert R. Rando, Anne G. Kasmar, Tania Lupoli, David C. Hooper, Daniel Kahne, and Suzanne Walker for their valuable contributions to this chapter in the First, Second, and Third Editions of *Principles of Pharmacology: The Pathophysiologic Basis of Drug Therapy*.

Suggested Reading

Bush K. Alarming β-lactamase-mediated resistance in multidrug-resistant Enterobacteriaceae. *Curr Opin Microbiol* 2010;13:558–564. (*Reviews β-lactam resistance in Gram-negative bacteria, focusing on recent reports of ESBL- and carbapenemase-mediated resistance.*)

Drawz SM, Papp-Wallace KM, Bonomo RA. New β-lactamase inhibitors: a therapeutic renaissance in an MDR world. *Antimicrob Agents Chemother* 2014;58:1835–1846. (*Reviews approved and investigational drugs for the treatment of extended-spectrum β-lactamase-producing organisms.*)

El Zoeiby A, Sanschagrin F, Levesque RC. Structure and function of the Mur enzymes: development of novel inhibitors. *Mol Microbiol* 2003;47:1–12. (*Reviews the structure, catalytic action, and inhibition of MurA–MurF.*)

Favrot L, Ronning DR. Targeting the mycobacterial envelope for tuberculosis drug development. *Expert Rev Anti Infect Ther* 2012;10:1023–1036. (*Reviews the structure of the mycobacterial cell wall and its potential targets for drug development.*)

Gale EF, Cundliffe E, Reynolds PE, Richmond MH, Waring MJ. *The molecular basis of antibiotic action.* 2nd ed. London: John Wiley; 1981. (*Classic treatise on antibiotics that describes the experiments leading to the determination of many of the mechanisms of action discussed in this chapter.*)

Guskey MT, Tsuji BT. A comparative review of the lipoglycopeptides: oritavancin, dalbavancin, and telavancin. *Pharmacotherapy* 2010;30:80–94. (*Discusses glycopeptide agents recently approved for use in the United States*)

Howden BP, Davies JK, Johnson PD, Stinear TP, Grayson ML. Reduced vancomycin susceptibility in *Staphylococcus aureus*: resistance mechanisms, laboratory detection, and clinical implications. *Clin Microbiol Rev* 2010;23: 99–139. (*Reviews VISA and VRSA, including definitions, risk factors, and mechanisms of resistance.*)

Jacoby GA, Munoz-Price LS. The new beta-lactamases. *N Engl J Med* 2005; 352:380–391. (*Reviews the pharmacology of β-lactamases.*)

Mdluli K, Kaneko T, Upton A. The tuberculosis drug discovery and development pipeline and emerging drug targets. *Cold Spring Harb Perspect Med* 2015;5:a021154. (*Reviews approved and investigational drugs for the treatment of tuberculosis.*)

Rattan A, Kalia A, Ahmad N. Multidrug-resistant *Mycobacterium tuberculosis*: molecular perspectives. *Emerg Infect Dis* 1998;4:195–209. (*Discusses the problem of resistance in tuberculosis.*)

Shahid M, Sobia F, Singh A, et al. Beta-lactams and beta-lactamase-inhibitors in current- or potential-clinical practice: a comprehensive update. *Crit Rev Microbiol* 2009;35:81–108. (*Discusses novel beta-lactamase inhibitors and their combinations with beta-lactams.*)

Terico AT, Gallagher JC. Beta-lactam hypersensitivity and cross-reactivity. *J Pharm Pract* 2014;27:530–544. (*Reviews hypersensitivity and cross-reactivity of β-lactams.*)

DRUG SUMMARY TABLE: CHAPTER 35 Pharmacology of Bacterial and Mycobacterial Infections: Cell Wall Synthesis

DRUG	CLINICAL APPLICATIONS	SERIOUS AND COMMON ADVERSE EFFECTS	CONTRAINDICATIONS	THERAPEUTIC CONSIDERATIONS
INHIBITORS OF MUREIN MONOMER SYNTHESIS Mechanism—See specific drug				
Fosfomycin (PO)	Urinary tract infections caused by E. coli, Enterococcus faecalis	Headache, diarrhea, nausea	Hypersensitivity to fosfomycin	Phosphoenolpyruvate (PEP) analogue that inhibits bacterial enolpyruvate transferase (MurA) by covalent modification of the enzyme's active site, thereby inhibiting the synthesis of UDP-NAM from UDP-NAG. An intravenous formulation (available only outside United States) has exhibited synergism with β-lactams, aminoglycosides, and fluoroquinolones. Decreased absorption when co-administered with drugs that increase gastrointestinal motility (e.g., metoclopramide).
Cycloserine (PO)	M. tuberculosis	*Seizures* Confusion, dizziness, headache, somnolence	Hypersensitivity to cycloserine Epilepsy Depression, anxiety, psychosis Severe renal insufficiency Alcohol abuse	Inhibits both alanine racemase and D-Ala-D-Ala ligase. Alcohol, isoniazid, and ethionamide potentiate cycloserine toxicity. Pyridoxine may prevent cycloserine-induced peripheral neuropathy. Cycloserine inhibits hepatic metabolism of phenytoin.
Bacitracin (PO and topical use only)	Cutaneous and eye infections (topical only) Superficial bacterial infection of skin	*Nephrotoxicity if systemic absorption occurs* Contact dermatitis (topical use only)	Hypersensitivity to bacitracin	Inhibits dephosphorylation of bactoprenol diphosphate.
INHIBITORS OF MUREIN POLYMER SYNTHESIS Mechanism—Bind to the D-Ala-D-Ala terminus of the murein monomer unit and inhibit peptidoglycan glycosyltransferase (PGT), thereby preventing addition of murein units to the growing polymer chain				
Vancomycin (IV; PO for C. difficile infection only) **Telavancin (IV)** **Dalbavancin (IV)** **Oritavancin (IV)**	Shared indications: Methicillin-resistant S. aureus infections (IV) Serious skin infections involving staphylococci and streptococci (IV) Vancomycin and telavancin only: Nosocomial pneumonia including ventilator-associated pneumonia Vancomycin only: C. difficile enterocolitis Infective endocarditis and bacteremia	*Anaphylaxis (shared adverse effect); nephrotoxicity (vancomycin and telavancin only); Clostridium difficile diarrhea (vancomycin, dalbavancin, and oritavancin only); cardiac arrest, hypotension, bone marrow suppression, ototoxicity (vancomycin only); prolonged QT interval, bleeding risk, osteomyelitis (oritavancin only)* Gastrointestinal upset	Shared contraindication: Hypersensitivity to drug Oritavancin only: Unfractionated heparin sodium use within 48 hours	Increased nephrotoxicity when administered with aminoglycosides. Red man syndrome can be avoided by slowing infusion rate or preadministering antihistamines. Resistance to vancomycin most commonly arises through acquisition of DNA encoding enzymes that catalyze formation of D-Ala-D-lactate. Telavancin has slightly greater nephrotoxicity than vancomycin. Telavancin and oritavancin may result in false increases in coagulation tests.

INHIBITORS OF POLYMER CROSS-LINKING: PENICILLINS

Mechanism—β-Lactams inhibit transpeptidase by forming a covalent ("dead-end") acyl enzyme intermediate. Penicillins have a five-membered accessory ring attached to the β-lactam ring.

Drug	Clinical Applications	Serious and Common Adverse Effects	Contraindications	Therapeutic Considerations
Penicillin G (IV) **Penicillin benzathine (IM)** **Penicillin V (PO)**	Penicillin-sensitive *S. aureus* and *S. pyogenes*, oral anaerobes, *N. meningitidis, Clostridia* species Syphilis Yaws Leptospirosis Prophylaxis of rheumatic fever Dental infections	*Anaphylaxis (shared adverse effect); congestive heart failure, electrolyte imbalance, coma, seizure (penicillin G only); Clostridium difficile infection (penicillin V only)* Rash, fever, injection site reaction, gastrointestinal upset, Jarisch-Herxheimer reaction when used to treat syphilis	Hypersensitivity to penicillins	Anticoagulant effects of warfarin may be potentiated by concomitant penicillin administration. β-Lactamase sensitive.
Oxacillin (IV) **Cloxacillin (PO)** **Dicloxacillin (PO)** **Nafcillin (IV)**	Skin and soft tissue infections or systemic infection with β-lactamase-producing, methicillin-sensitive *S. aureus*	*Anaphylaxis, Clostridium difficile infection (cloxacillin, nafcillin, and dicloxacillin only); nephrotoxicity (dicloxacillin and nafcillin only); hepatotoxicity (dicloxacillin only); hypokalemia, bone marrow depression (nafcillin only)* Gastrointestinal upset (shared adverse effect); rash (oxacillin only)	Hypersensitivity to penicillins	β-Lactamase resistant. Narrow-spectrum antibacterial activity; used mainly to treat skin and soft tissue infections or documented methicillin-sensitive *S. aureus* infections. Nafcillin is a hepatic CYP3A4 enzyme inducer and can decrease plasma concentrations of CYP3A4 substrates.
Ampicillin (IV/PO) **Amoxicillin (PO)** **Amoxicillin/clavulanic acid (PO)** **Ampicillin/sulbactam (IV)**	Ampicillin: Invasive enterococcal infections Infectious disease of the genitourinary system Respiratory tract infection Amoxicillin: Uncomplicated ear, nose, and throat infections Component of combination therapy for *Helicobacter pylori* infection Infectious disease of the genitourinary system Infection of the skin and subcutaneous tissue Lower respiratory tract infection Amoxicillin/clavulanic acid and ampicillin/sulbactam: β-Lactamase-producing organisms such as *S. aureus, H. influenzae, E. coli, Klebsiella, Acinetobacter, Enterobacter*, anaerobes	*Erythema multiforme, Stevens-Johnson syndrome, toxic epidermal necrolysis, anaphylaxis, Clostridium difficile infection (shared adverse effects); agranulocytosis, thrombocytopenia (ampicillin only)* Rash, diarrhea	Hypersensitivity to penicillins	Broad-spectrum antibacterial activity. Ampicillin and amoxicillin are β-lactamase sensitive as single agents; clavulanic acid and sulbactam are β-lactamase inhibitors. Positively charged amino group on side chain enhances diffusion through porin channels of Gram-negative bacteria.

continues

DRUG SUMMARY TABLE: CHAPTER 35 Pharmacology of Bacterial and Mycobacterial Infections: Cell Wall Synthesis *continued*

DRUG	CLINICAL APPLICATIONS	*SERIOUS* AND COMMON ADVERSE EFFECTS	CONTRAINDICATIONS	THERAPEUTIC CONSIDERATIONS
Piperacillin/Tazobactam (IV)	Primarily used to treat *P. aeruginosa* infection, peritonitis, and hospital-acquired pneumonia due to resistant Gram-negative organisms	*Erythema multiforme, Stevens-Johnson syndrome, toxic epidermal necrolysis, Clostridium difficile infection, anaphylaxis* Rash, gastrointestinal upset	Hypersensitivity to penicillins	Broad-spectrum antibacterial activity but primarily used against *P. aeruginosa.* Generally β-lactamase sensitive.

INHIBITORS OF POLYMER CROSS-LINKING: CEPHALOSPORINS
Mechanism—β-Lactams inhibit transpeptidase by forming a covalent ("dead-end") acyl enzyme intermediate. Cephalosporins have a six-membered accessory ring attached to the β-lactam ring.

DRUG	CLINICAL APPLICATIONS	*SERIOUS* AND COMMON ADVERSE EFFECTS	CONTRAINDICATIONS	THERAPEUTIC CONSIDERATIONS
Cefazolin (IV) **Cephalexin (PO)** **Cefadroxil (PO)**	*Proteus mirabilis, E. coli, Klebsiella pneumoniae* Skin and soft tissue infections Surgical prophylaxis	*Stevens-Johnson syndrome, Clostridium difficile infection, anaphylaxis (shared adverse effects); hepatotoxicity (cefazolin and cefadroxil only); renal toxicity (cephalexin only); leukopenia, encephalopathy, seizure (cefazolin only); thrombocytopenia (cefadroxil only)* Gastrointestinal upset (shared adverse effect); rash (cefazolin only)	Hypersensitivity to cephalosporins	First-generation cephalosporins. Relatively good Gram-positive coverage (*Staphylococcus* species and *Streptococcus* species). Sensitive to many β-lactamases.
Cefuroxime (IV) **Cefotetan (IV)** **Cefoxitin (IV)**	Shared indication: *H. influenzae* Cefotetan and cefoxitin only: *Enterobacter* species, *Neisseria* species, *P. mirabilis, E. coli, K. pneumoniae*	*Stevens-Johnson syndrome, toxic epidermal necrolysis, anaphylaxis, Clostridium difficile infection (shared adverse effects); seizure (cefotetan and cefoxitin only); hemolytic anemia (cefotetan only)*	Hypersensitivity to cephalosporins	Second-generation cephalosporins. Relatively broader Gram-negative coverage than first-generation cephalosporins. More β-lactamase resistant than first-generation cephalosporins. Cefuroxime is primarily used in community-acquired pneumonia. Cefotetan and cefoxitin are primarily used in intra-abdominal and pelvic infections and for surgical prophylaxis.

Drug	Clinical Applications	Adverse Effects	Contraindications	Therapeutic Considerations
Cefotaxime (IV) **Cefpodoxime (PO)** **Ceftriaxone (IV/IM)** **Cefoperazone (IV/IM)** **Ceftazidime (IV)**	Cefotaxime only: *H. influenzae* Ceftriaxone only: *N. gonorrhoeae, Borrelia burgdorferi, H. influenzae,* most *Enterobacteriaceae* Ceftazidime only: *P. aeruginosa*	*Cardiac arrhythmia, erythema multiforme, Stevens-Johnson syndrome, toxic epidermal necrolysis, anaphylaxis, Clostridium difficile infection (shared adverse effects); granulocytopenic disorder (cefotaxime only); hemolytic anemia, kernicterus of newborn, renal failure, lung toxicity (ceftriaxone only); gastrointestinal hemorrhage (cefoperazone only); asterixis, coma, encephalopathy, myoclonus, seizure (ceftazidime only)* Injection site pain (IV formulations only); rash, gastrointestinal upset	Shared contraindication: Hypersensitivity to cephalosporins Ceftriaxone only: Concurrent administration of calcium-containing IV solutions in neonates, due to risk of fatal salt precipitation in lung and kidneys Hyperbilirubinemic neonates, due to increased risk of kernicterus	Third-generation cephalosporins. Highest CNS penetration of the cephalosporins. Resistant to many β-lactamases. Highly active against *Enterobacteriaceae* but less active against Gram-positive organisms than are first-generation cephalosporins.
Cefepime (IV)	*Enterobacteriaceae, Neisseria, H. influenzae, P. aeruginosa,* Gram-positive organisms	*Stevens-Johnson syndrome, toxic epidermal necrolysis, Clostridium difficile infection, anaphylaxis, encephalopathy, myoclonus, seizure*	Hypersensitivity to cephalosporins	Fourth-generation cephalosporin. Resistant to many β-lactamases.
Ceftaroline (IV)	Methicillin-resistant *S. aureus* infections, vancomycin-resistant *S. aureus* infections, *S. pneumoniae, Moraxella catarrhalis, Haemophilus influenzae*	Same as cefazolin, except ceftaroline may cause drug-induced hemolytic anemia and may cause significant leukopenia or neutropenia	Hypersensitivity to cephalosporins (rarely cross-react with penicillins)	Fifth-generation cephalosporin. Ceftobiprole is a fifth-generation cephalosporin in late-stage clinical trials with a similar spectrum of action.

INHIBITORS OF POLYMER CROSS-LINKING: MONOBACTAMS/CARBAPENEMS
Mechanism—β-Lactams inhibit transpeptidase by forming a covalent ("dead-end") acyl enzyme intermediate.

Drug	Clinical Applications	Adverse Effects	Contraindications	Therapeutic Considerations
Aztreonam (IV)	Gram-negative bacteria Used in penicillin-allergic patients	*Clostridium difficile infection, gastrointestinal hemorrhage, neutropenia, ototoxicity, nephrotoxicity*	Hypersensitivity to aztreonam	A monobactam. No Gram-positive activity.
Imipenem/cilastatin (IV/IM) **Meropenem (IV)** **Doripenem (IV)** **Ertapenem (IV/IM)**	Gram-positive and Gram-negative bacteria except MRSA, VRE, and *Legionella* (ertapenem is not active against *Pseudomonas* or *Acinetobacter*)	*Anaphylaxis (imipenem/cilastatin, meropenem, and doripenem only); Clostridium difficile infection, jaundice (meropenem only); Stevens-Johnson syndrome, toxic epidermal necrolysis, seizure, interstitial pneumonia (doripenem only)* Injection site pain (shared adverse effect); headache (doripenem only)	Shared contraindication: Hypersensitivity to drug Imipenem/cilastatin and ertapenem only: Hypersensitivity to amide local anesthetics Imipenem/cilastatin only: Severe shock or heart block Meropenem and doripenem only: Hypersensitivity to β-lactam antibiotics	Cilastatin inhibits renal dehydropeptidase I, which would otherwise inactivate imipenem. Probenecid may increase meropenem levels. All four agents decrease valproate levels.

continues

DRUG SUMMARY TABLE: CHAPTER 35 Pharmacology of Bacterial and Mycobacterial Infections: Cell Wall Synthesis *continued*

DRUG	CLINICAL APPLICATIONS	*SERIOUS* AND COMMON ADVERSE EFFECTS	CONTRAINDICATIONS	THERAPEUTIC CONSIDERATIONS
INHIBITORS OF CELL MEMBRANE STABILITY **Mechanism**—Daptomycin integrates into membranes of Gram-positive bacteria, leading to formation of pores that cause potassium efflux, membrane depolarization, and cell death.				
Daptomycin (IV)	Complicated skin infections Bacteremia or right-sided endocarditis from *S. aureus*	*Rhabdomyolysis, eosinophilic pneumonia* Diarrhea, vomiting	Hypersensitivity to daptomycin	Daptomycin should be co-administered with a statin with caution due to risk of myopathy.
ANTIMYCOBACTERIAL AGENTS **Mechanism**—See specific drug				
Ethambutol (PO)	*Mycobacterium* species	*Optic neuritis, blindness, peripheral neuropathy, neutropenia, thrombocytopenia* Hyperuricemia, mania, nausea, vomiting	Known optic neuritis Patients unable to report visual changes, such as young children Optic neuritis	Decreases arabinogalactan synthesis by inhibiting the arabinosyl transferase that adds arabinose units to the growing arabinogalactan chain. Mycobacteriostatic and used in combination with other antimycobacterials, including rifampin and streptomycin.
Pyrazinamide (PO)	*Mycobacterium* species	*Anemia, hepatotoxicity* Nausea, vomiting, hyperuricemia, arthralgia	Hypersensitivity to pyrazinamide Acute gout Severe hepatic dysfunction	Pyrazinamide is a prodrug that must be converted to its active form pyrazinoic acid, which inhibits fatty acid synthetase 1 (FAS1). Used in combination with other antimycobacterials, including rifampin and streptomycin.
Isoniazid (IV/IM/PO) **Ethionamide (PO)**	*Mycobacterium* species	*Hepatotoxicity (shared adverse effect); neurotoxicity (paresthesias, peripheral neuropathy, ataxia), systemic lupus erythematosus, seizure, hematologic abnormalities, rhabdomyolysis (isoniazid only); encephalopathy (ethionamide only)* Gastrointestinal upset (ethionamide only)	Shared contraindications: Hypersensitivity to drug Active liver disease Isoniazid only: Concomitant use with serotonergic agents	Inhibit mycolic acid synthesis by targeting fatty acid synthetase 2 (FAS2). Can inhibit or induce cytochrome P450 enzymes and thus interact with other drugs, such as rifampin, antiseizure medications (carbamazepine and phenytoin), azole antifungals, and alcohol. Mycobactericidal and used in combination with other antimycobacterials, including rifampin and streptomycin. Isoniazid neurotoxicity can be prevented by pyridoxine supplementation.

IV, intravenous administration
IM, intramuscular administration
PO, oral administration

36

Pharmacology of Fungal Infections

Chelsea Ma and April W. Armstrong

INTRODUCTION

Fungi are free-living microorganisms that exist as **yeasts** (single-cell, round fungi), **molds** (multicellular filamentous fungi), or a combination of the two (so-called dimorphic fungi). All fungi are eukaryotic organisms. Because of their phylogenetic similarity, fungi and humans have homologous metabolic pathways for energy production, protein synthesis, and cell division. Consequently, *there is greater difficulty in developing selective antifungal agents than in developing selective antibacterial agents*. The success of many antibacterial agents has resulted from the identification of unique molecular targets in bacteria, emphasizing the necessity for identifying unique fungal targets that can be exploited.

Certain patient populations are particularly susceptible to fungal infections (mycoses). These populations include surgical and intensive care unit (ICU) patients, patients with prostheses, and patients with compromised immune defenses. In the past three to four decades, the extensive use of broad-spectrum antibiotics, the wider use of long-term intravenous catheters, and infection with human immunodeficiency virus (HIV) have correlated with an increasing incidence of opportunistic and systemic mycoses. Additionally, the successes of organ transplantation, immunosuppressive therapy, and cancer chemotherapy have contributed to an increasing number of chronically immunosuppressed patients, who are particularly susceptible to fungal infections.

Traditionally, the diagnosis of fungal infections has relied on culture-based methods and direct examination of specimens under light microscopy. However, the indolent growth of fungi makes culturing inefficient, while direct microscopic examination may not be reliable or provide definitive speciation. These disadvantages have important clinical implications because prognosis often correlates inversely with the duration of time from clinical presentation to accurate diagnosis. Consequently, one major focus of modern mycology is the development of rapid, nonculture-based methods of early diagnosis. New diagnostic techniques rely on the polymerase chain reaction (PCR), western blot, antigen detection, and identification of fungal metabolites. Because many of these techniques are still investigational, they must be performed in parallel with traditional culture-based methods.

The treatment options for opportunistic and systemic fungal infections were once thought to be limited. These options are now expanding, however. Fungal processes that have been exploited in the development of antifungal agents include nucleic acid synthesis, mitosis, and membrane synthesis and stability. Traditional antifungal agents, such as azoles and polyenes, are directed against molecular targets involved in the synthesis and stability of the fungal membrane. The echinocandins, a relatively newer class of antifungal agents, target an enzyme complex involved in the synthesis of the fungal cell wall. As the emergence of resistant fungi increases, it will become increasingly important to identify and exploit new molecular targets for antifungal therapy.

BIOCHEMISTRY OF THE FUNGAL MEMBRANE AND CELL WALL

Although fungi have a cellular ultrastructure similar to that of animal cells, there are a number of unique biochemical differences that have been exploited in the development of antifungal drugs. To date, the most important biochemical difference lies in the principal sterol used to maintain plasma membrane structure and function. Mammalian cells use cholesterol for this purpose, whereas fungal cells use

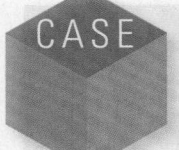

CASE

James F, a 31-year-old HIV-positive man, presents to his physician with a 3-week history of fever, cough, and chest pain after touring Southern California. His history is notable for past intravenous drug use. Clinical evaluation and chest x-ray reveal a left lower lobe infiltrate and left paratracheal adenopathy. Sputum cultures are positive for *Coccidioides immitis*, and blood tests are notable for an elevated titer of antibodies directed against this fungal pathogen. The physician makes a preliminary diagnosis of pulmonary coccidioidomycosis and prescribes a course of amphotericin B.

Over the next several days, however, Mr. F does not improve. He goes to the emergency department with fever, chills, sweats, cough, fatigue, and headaches. His temperature is 100°F, but he shows no evidence of meningitis or peripheral adenopathy. Lung examination reveals diffuse wheezing over the left lung fields, noted on both inspiration and expiration.

Bronchoscopy shows narrowing of the tracheal lumen by numerous mucosal granulomas from the left mainstem bronchus to the level of the midtrachea. Fungal culture grows *Coccidioides immitis*, a definitive diagnosis of chronic pulmonary coccidioidomycosis is made, the granulomas are bronchoscopically removed, and amphotericin B is continued. A week later, Mr. F's symptoms begin to subside, amphotericin B is discontinued, and a course of fluconazole is initiated.

Questions

1. What factors predisposed Mr. F to fungal infection?
2. What are the mechanisms of action of amphotericin B and fluconazole?
3. What adverse effects could Mr. F experience as a consequence of treatment with amphotericin B and fluconazole?

the structurally distinct sterol **ergosterol**. The biosynthesis of ergosterol involves a series of steps, two of which are targeted by currently available antifungal drugs (Fig. 36-1). The enzymes that catalyze ergosterol synthesis are localized in fungal microsomes, which contain an electron transport system nearly identical to that found in mammalian liver microsomes. The first targeted step, the conversion of **squalene** to **lanosterol**, is catalyzed by the enzyme **squalene epoxidase**. This enzyme is the molecular target of the **allylamine** and **benzylamine** antifungal agents. The fungus-specific cytochrome P450 enzyme **14α-sterol demethylase** mediates the key reaction in the second targeted step, the conversion of lanosterol to ergosterol. **Imidazole** and **triazole** antifungal agents inhibit 14α-sterol demethylase. Therefore, allylamine, benzylamine, imidazole, and triazole antifungal agents all inhibit the biosynthesis of ergosterol. Because ergosterol is necessary for the maintenance of plasma membrane structure and function, these agents compromise fungal membrane integrity. Ergosterol synthesis inhibitors suppress fungal cell growth under most circumstances (**fungistatic** effect), although they can sometimes cause fungal cell death (**fungicidal** effect).

Fungal cells are surrounded by a cell wall, a rigid structure that has been studied intensively as a new and important target for antifungal therapy. The major components of the fungal cell wall are **chitin**, **β-(1,3)-D-glucan**, **β-(1,6)-D-glucan**, and cell wall glycoproteins (especially proteins containing complex mannose chains, or **mannoproteins**). Chitin is a linear polysaccharide consisting of more than 2,000 N-acetylglucosamine units joined by β-(1,4) linkages; these chains are bundled into microfibrils that form the fundamental scaffold of the cell wall. β-(1,3)-D-glucan and β-(1,6)-D-glucan, which are polymers of glucose units joined by β-(1,3) and β-(1,6) glycosidic linkages, respectively, are the most abundant components of the cell wall. These glucan polymers are covalently linked to the chitin scaffold. The cell wall glycoproteins comprise a diverse group of proteins that are noncovalently associated with other cell wall components or are covalently linked to chitin, glucan, or other cell wall proteins. Because mammalian cells do not have cell walls, drugs directed against the fungal cell wall would be expected to have a high therapeutic index. **Echinocandin** antifungal agents target **β-(1,3)-D-glucan synthase**, the enzyme that adds glucose residues from the donor molecule UDP-glucose to the growing polysaccharide chain. By inhibiting cell wall biosynthesis, echinocandins disrupt fungal cell wall integrity. Echinocandins often have fungicidal activity, although these agents are fungistatic under some circumstances (see "Suggested Reading").

Fungal adhesion represents a third potential target for antifungal drugs. Adhesion to host cells is mediated by the binding of fungal **adhesins** to host cell receptors. In yeasts, for example, aspartyl proteases and phospholipases mediate adhesion. Compounds that block adhesive interactions between fungal cells and mammalian cells are currently under development.

PATHOPHYSIOLOGY OF FUNGAL INFECTIONS

Mycoses (fungal infections) can be divided into superficial, cutaneous, subcutaneous, systemic or primary, and opportunistic infections. Few fungi possess sufficient virulence to be considered primary pathogens capable of initiating serious infections in immunocompetent hosts. However, immunocompromised hosts can develop serious systemic infections with fungi that are not pathogenic in normal individuals. In the introductory case, Mr. F's HIV infection likely increased his risk of infection with *Coccidioides immitis*. Thus, the pathogenesis of fungal infections is based on the interplay between a host's immune system and the pathogenicity of the particular fungal organism. Polymorphonuclear leukocytes, cell-mediated immunity, and humoral immunity are all important components of the host immune defense against fungal pathogens.

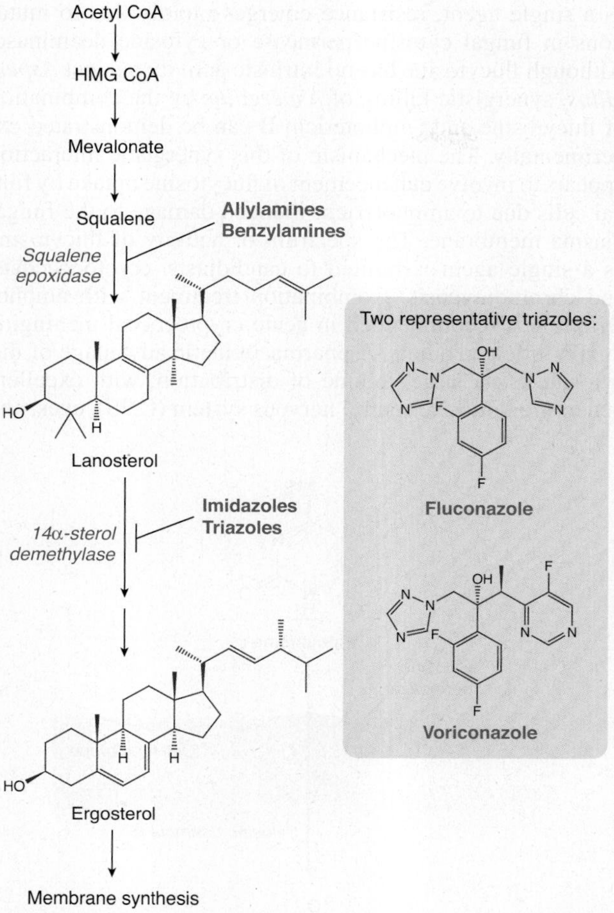

FIGURE 36-1. Ergosterol synthesis pathway. Ergosterol is synthesized in fungal cells from acetyl CoA building blocks. One of the intermediates, squalene, is converted to lanosterol by the action of squalene epoxidase. Allylamines and benzylamines inhibit squalene epoxidase. 14α-Sterol demethylase, a cytochrome P450 enzyme not expressed in mammalian cells, catalyzes the first step in the conversion of lanosterol to the unique fungal sterol ergosterol. Imidazoles and triazoles inhibit 14α-sterol demethylase and thereby prevent the synthesis of ergosterol, which is the principal sterol in fungal membranes. Fluconazole and voriconazole are two representative triazoles.

The pathogenesis of fungal infections is only partly understood, and different fungi possess distinct virulence factors that are unique to the pathogen. Adhesion is an initial step in the early stages of infection. Adhesion and localization can occur on skin, mucosal, and prosthetic device surfaces. For example, *Candida* species adhere to a variety of surfaces via a combination of specific ligand–receptor interactions as well as nonspecific forces such as van der Waals and electrostatic interactions. Virulent pathogens are subsequently able to invade the colonized surface and proliferate in deep tissue, sometimes reaching the systemic circulation. Systemic dissemination can be accelerated by local tissue injury, such as that caused by cancer chemotherapy, ischemia, or the presence of a prosthetic device. In addition, some pathogens secrete lytic enzymes to enable invasive growth and systemic dissemination. *C. immitis* breaches the respiratory mucosa by producing an alkaline proteinase capable of digesting structural proteins in lung tissue. *C. immitis* also produces a 36-kDa extracellular proteinase capable of degrading human elastin, collagen, immunoglobulins, and hemoglobin.

Fungal cell wall composition plays an important role in the pathogenesis of fungal infections. Pathogens such as *Blastomyces dermatitidis*, *Histoplasma capsulatum*, and *Paracoccidioides brasiliensis* modulate the complement of glycoproteins in their cell walls in response to host immune system interactions. For example, the cell wall of *B. dermatitidis* contains a 120-kDa glycoprotein, BAD-1 (formerly WI-1), which elicits a potent humoral and cellular immune response. Avirulent strains of *B. dermatitidis* have increased expression of BAD-1, which is recognized by the host immune system and leads to elimination of the pathogen through phagocytosis. In contrast, the cell wall of virulent strains of *B. dermatitidis* contains high levels of α-(1,3)-glucan, which is inversely correlated with the amount of BAD-1 detectable on the cell surface. It is speculated that the increased amount of α-(1,3)-glucan in the cell wall effectively masks the BAD-1 surface glycoprotein, thereby allowing the virulent strains to evade host immune detection and destruction.

The ability of a fungal pathogen to change from one morphotype to another is termed **phenotype switching**. By responding to changes in the microenvironment, *Candida* species are capable of undergoing yeast-to-hyphae transformation. The hyphal forms of *Candida* species possess a "sense of touch" that allows them to grow in crevices and pores, thereby increasing their infiltrative potential. Similarly, *B. dermatitidis* undergoes transformation from conidia (small, asexual reproductive structures) to the larger yeast forms. The larger forms offer an important survival advantage because they are capable of resisting the phagocytic action of neutrophils and macrophages.

PHARMACOLOGIC CLASSES AND AGENTS

The ideal antifungal agent would possess four characteristics: broad spectrum of action against a variety of fungal pathogens, low drug toxicity, multiple routes of administration, and excellent penetration into the cerebrospinal fluid (CSF), urine, and bone. With the recent expansion in identifying novel targets of antifungal therapy, treatment options for superficial and deep fungal infections are improving. Some antifungal agents can be used to treat both superficial and deep mycoses (in some cases, using different formulations), while others are restricted to narrower indications. In this section, the currently available antifungal drugs are categorized according to their molecular targets and mechanisms of action. The primary molecular targets for antifungal therapy are enzymes and other molecules involved in fungal DNA synthesis, mitosis, plasma membrane synthesis, and cell wall synthesis (Fig. 36-2). Because the clinical trials used to support regulatory approval of new drugs often exclude children and women of childbearing potential (see Chapter 52, Clinical Drug Evaluation and Regulatory Approval), the safety of some of the newer antifungal agents is not precisely determined in these patient populations. The treating physician must therefore weigh the risks of treatment against the expected benefits.

Inhibitor of Fungal Nucleic Acid Synthesis: Flucytosine

Flucytosine is the name of the fluorinated pyrimidine 5-fluorocytosine. Flucytosine is selectively taken up by fungal

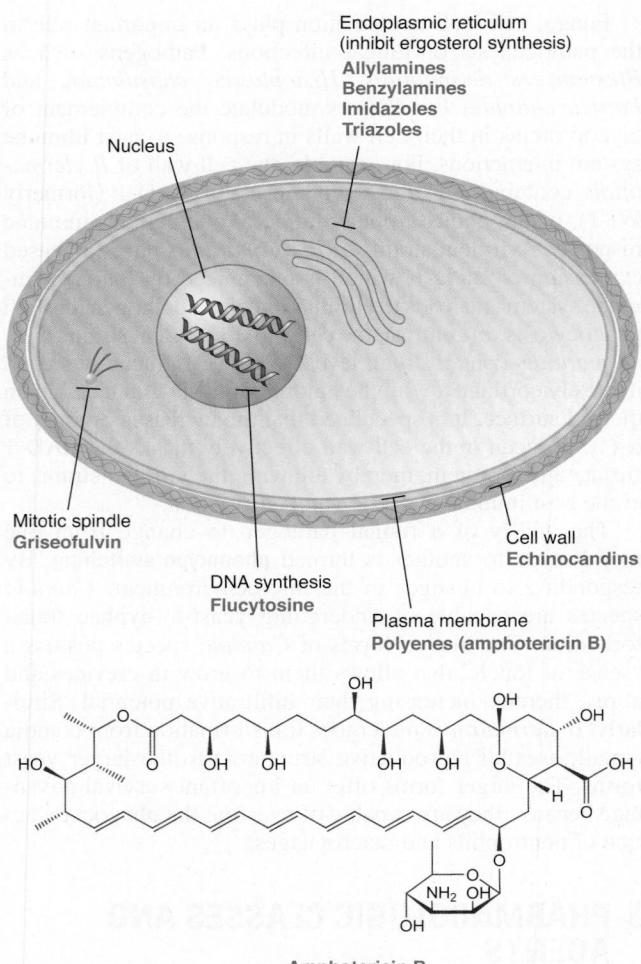

FIGURE 36-2. Cellular targets of antifungal drugs. The currently available antifungal agents act on distinct molecular targets. Flucytosine inhibits fungal DNA synthesis. Griseofulvin inhibits fungal mitosis by disrupting mitotic spindles. Allylamines, benzylamines, imidazoles, and triazoles inhibit the ergosterol synthesis pathway in the endoplasmic reticulum. Polyenes bind to ergosterol in the fungal membrane and thereby disrupt plasma membrane integrity. Amphotericin B is a representative polyene. Echinocandins inhibit fungal cell wall synthesis.

cells via cytosine-specific permeases that are expressed only in fungal membranes. Lacking these transporters, mammalian cells are protected. Inside the fungal cell, the enzyme cytosine deaminase converts flucytosine to 5-fluorouracil (5-FU). (5-FU is itself an antimetabolite that is used in cancer chemotherapy; see Chapter 39, Pharmacology of Cancer: Genome Synthesis, Stability, and Maintenance.) Subsequent reactions convert 5-FU to 5-fluorodeoxyuridylic acid monophosphate (5-FdUMP), which is a potent inhibitor of **thymidylate synthase**. Inhibition of thymidylate synthase results in inhibition of DNA synthesis and cell division (Fig. 36-3). Flucytosine appears to be fungistatic under most circumstances. Although mammalian cells lack cytosine-specific permeases and cytosine deaminase, fungi and bacteria in the intestine can convert flucytosine to 5-fluorouracil, which can cause adverse effects in host cells.

Flucytosine is typically used in combination with amphotericin B to treat systemic mycoses; when the drug is used

as a single agent, resistance emerges rapidly due to mutations in fungal cytosine permease or cytosine deaminase. Although flucytosine has no intrinsic activity against *Aspergillus*, synergistic killing of *Aspergillus* by the combination of flucytosine and amphotericin B can be demonstrated experimentally. The mechanism of this synergistic interaction appears to involve enhancement of flucytosine uptake by fungal cells due to amphotericin-induced damage to the fungal plasma membrane. The spectrum of activity of flucytosine as a single agent is limited to candidiasis, cryptococcosis, and chromomycosis. Combination treatment with amphotericin B is recommended in acute cryptococcal meningitis in HIV-infected adults. A pharmacokinetic advantage of flucytosine is its large volume of distribution, with excellent penetration into the central nervous system (CNS), eyes, and

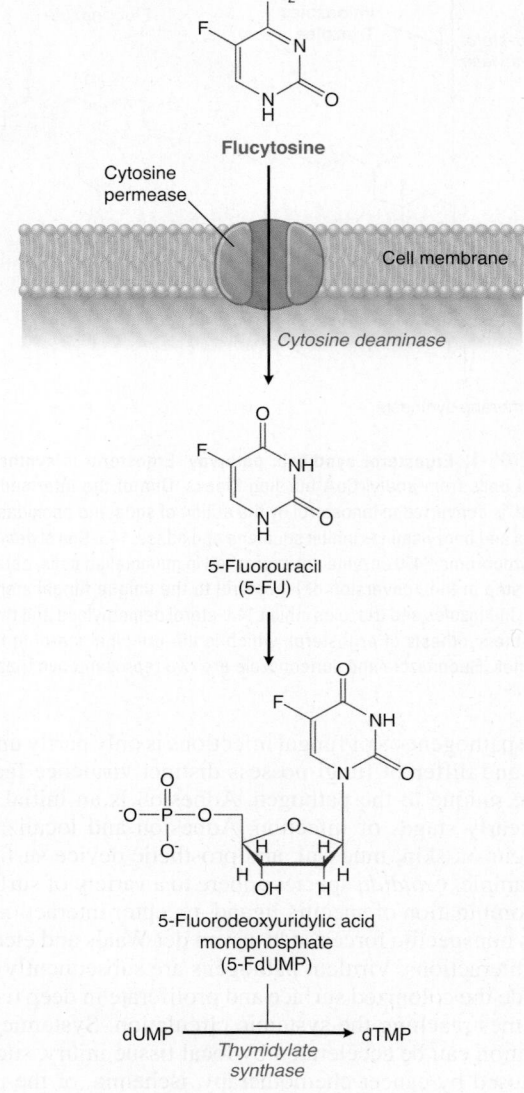

FIGURE 36-3. Mechanism of action of flucytosine. Flucytosine enters the fungal cell via a transmembrane cytosine permease. Inside the cell, cytosine deaminase converts flucytosine to 5-fluorouracil (5-FU), which is subsequently converted to 5-fluorodeoxyuridylic acid monophosphate (5-FdUMP). 5-FdUMP inhibits thymidylate synthase and thereby blocks the conversion of deoxyuridylate (dUMP) to deoxythymidylate (dTMP). In the absence of dTMP, DNA synthesis is inhibited.

urinary tract. Dose-dependent adverse effects include bone marrow suppression leading to leukopenia and thrombocytopenia, nausea, vomiting, diarrhea, and hepatic dysfunction. Flucytosine is contraindicated during pregnancy.

Inhibitor of Fungal Mitosis: Griseofulvin

Derived from *Penicillium griseofulvum* in the 1950s, **griseofulvin** inhibits fungal mitosis by binding to tubulin and a microtubule-associated protein and thereby disrupting assembly of the mitotic spindle. The drug is also reported to inhibit fungal RNA and DNA synthesis. Griseofulvin accumulates in keratin precursor cells and binds tightly to keratin in differentiated cells. The prolonged and tight association of griseofulvin with keratin allows new growth of skin, hair, or nail to be free of dermatophyte infection. Griseofulvin appears to be fungistatic under most circumstances.

The therapeutic use of oral griseofulvin is currently limited, due to the availability of topical antifungal medications as well as other oral antifungal agents with fewer adverse effects. Griseofulvin can be used to treat fungal infection of the skin, hair, and nail due to *Trichophyton*, *Microsporum*, and *Epidermophyton*. The drug is not effective against yeast (such as *Pityrosporum*) and dimorphic fungi. Doses should be taken at 6-hour intervals because blood levels of griseofulvin can be variable; absorption is enhanced if the drug is taken with a fatty meal. It is important to continue treatment until the infected skin, hair, or nail is completely replaced by normal tissue.

Griseofulvin use is not associated with a high incidence of serious adverse effects. A relatively common (up to 15%) adverse effect is headache, which tends to disappear as therapy continues. Other nervous system effects include lethargy, vertigo, and blurred vision; these adverse effects can be exacerbated by the consumption of alcohol. Occasionally, hepatotoxicity or albuminuria without renal insufficiency can be observed. Hematologic adverse effects—including leukopenia, neutropenia, and monocytosis—can occur during the first month of therapy. Serum sickness, angioedema, exfoliative dermatitis, and toxic epidermal necrolysis are extremely rare but potentially life-threatening adverse effects. Chronic use can sometimes result in increased fecal protoporphyrin levels. Concurrent administration with barbiturates decreases the gastrointestinal absorption of griseofulvin. Because griseofulvin induces hepatic cytochrome P450 enzymes, it can increase the metabolism of warfarin and potentially reduce the efficacy of low-estrogen oral contraceptive medications. Griseofulvin should be avoided during pregnancy, since fetal abnormalities have been reported.

Inhibitors of the Ergosterol Synthesis Pathway

Inhibitors of Squalene Epoxidase: Allylamines and Benzylamines

In the ergosterol synthesis pathway (Fig. 36-1), squalene is converted to lanosterol by the action of **squalene epoxidase**. Inhibitors of squalene epoxidase prevent the formation of lanosterol, which is a precursor for ergosterol. These drugs also promote accumulation of the toxic metabolite squalene in the fungal cell, making them fungicidal under most circumstances. The antifungal agents that inhibit squalene epoxidase can be divided into **allylamines** and **benzylamines** based on their chemical structures: **terbinafine** and **naftifine** are allylamines, whereas **butenafine** is a benzylamine.

Terbinafine is available in both oral and topical formulations. When taken orally, the drug is 99% protein-bound in the plasma, and it undergoes first-pass metabolism in the liver. Because of this first-pass metabolism, the oral bioavailability of terbinafine is 40%. The drug's elimination half-life is extremely long, approximately 300 hours, because terbinafine accumulates extensively in the skin, nails, and fat. The oral form of terbinafine is used in the treatment of onychomycosis, tinea corporis, tinea cruris, tinea pedis, and tinea capitis. Terbinafine is not recommended in patients with renal or hepatic failure or in pregnant women. Very rarely, the oral form of terbinafine can lead to hepatotoxicity, Stevens-Johnson syndrome, neutropenia, and exacerbation of psoriasis or subacute cutaneous lupus erythematosus. Liver function enzymes should be monitored during the treatment course. Plasma levels of terbinafine are increased by co-administration with cimetidine (a cytochrome P450 inhibitor) and decreased by co-administration with rifampin (a cytochrome P450 inducer). Topical terbinafine is available in cream or spray form and is indicated for tinea pedis, tinea cruris, and tinea corporis.

Similar to terbinafine, **naftifine** is a squalene epoxidase inhibitor that has broad-spectrum antifungal activity. Naftifine is only available topically as a cream or gel; it is effective in tinea corporis, tinea cruris, and tinea pedis.

Butenafine, a benzylamine, is a topical antifungal agent with a mechanism of action and spectrum of antifungal activity similar to that of the allylamines. Topical allylamines and benzylamines are more effective than topical azole agents against common dermatophytes, especially those causing tinea pedis. However, topical terbinafine and butenafine are less effective than topical azoles against *Candida* skin infections (see below).

Inhibitors of 14α-Sterol Demethylase: Imidazoles and Triazoles

Another important molecular target in the ergosterol synthesis pathway is **14α-sterol demethylase**, a microsomal cytochrome P450 enzyme that catalyzes the first step in the conversion of lanosterol to ergosterol. The **azoles** are antifungal agents that inhibit fungal 14α-sterol demethylase. The resulting decrease in ergosterol synthesis and accumulation of 14α-methyl sterols disrupt the tightly packed acyl chains of the phospholipids in fungal membranes. Destabilization of the fungal membrane leads to dysfunction of membrane-associated enzymes, including those in the electron transport chain, and may ultimately lead to cell death. Azoles are not completely selective for the fungal P450 enzyme, however, and they can also inhibit hepatic P450 enzymes. While the extent of hepatic P450 enzyme inhibition varies among the azoles, *drug–drug interactions are an important consideration whenever an azole antifungal agent is prescribed*. For example, cyclosporine is an immunosuppressive drug used to prevent graft rejection in recipients of allogeneic kidney, liver, and heart transplants. It is metabolized by hepatic P450 enzymes and excreted in the bile. To minimize the risk of cyclosporine-associated nephrotoxicity and hepatotoxicity, patients concomitantly receiving an azole antifungal agent should be treated with lower doses of cyclosporine.

As a group, the azoles have a wide range of antifungal activity and are clinically useful against *B. dermatitidis*, *Cryptococcus neoformans*, *H. capsulatum*, *Coccidioides* species, *P. brasiliensis*, dermatophytes, and most *Candida* species. Azoles have intermediate clinical activity against *Fusarium*, *Sporothrix schenckii*, *Scedosporium apiospermum*, and *Aspergillus* species. Pathogens mediating zygomycosis (invasive fungal infections caused by *Zygomycetes* species) and *Candida krusei* are resistant to azoles. The azoles are generally fungistatic rather than fungicidal against susceptible organisms.

The azole antifungal agents can be categorized into two broad classes, **imidazoles** and **triazoles**, which share the same mechanism of action and similar antifungal spectrum. Because systemically administered triazoles tend to have less effect than systemically administered imidazoles on human sterol synthesis, recent drug development has focused primarily on triazoles.

The imidazole antifungal class includes **ketoconazole**, **clotrimazole**, **luliconazole**, **miconazole**, **econazole**, **butoconazole**, **oxiconazole**, **sertaconazole**, **sulconazole**, and **tioconazole**. **Ketoconazole** was introduced in 1977 as the prototypic drug in this class. Ketoconazole is available in both oral and topical formulations. Its broad spectrum of action includes *C. immitis*, *C. neoformans*, *Candida* species, *H. capsulatum*, *B. dermatitidis*, and a variety of dermatophytes. The pharmacokinetic and adverse effect profiles of ketoconazole limit its clinical utility. (In fact, oral ketoconazole has been replaced by itraconazole for the treatment of many mycoses; see discussion below.) Gastrointestinal absorption of oral ketoconazole depends on conversion of the drug to a salt in the acidic environment of the stomach. Thus, ketoconazole cannot be used if the patient has achlorhydria or is receiving bicarbonate, antacids, H_2-blockers, or proton pump inhibitors. Ketoconazole has little penetration into the CSF and urine, which limits its efficacy in CNS and urinary tract infections. In approximately 20% of patients, the drug causes nausea, vomiting, or anorexia; hepatic dysfunction occurs in 1–2% of patients.

Ketoconazole potently inhibits hepatic P450 enzymes and therefore affects the metabolism of many other drugs. At therapeutic doses, it also inhibits the P450 enzymes 17, 20-lyase and side-chain cleavage enzyme in the adrenal gland and gonads, thereby decreasing steroid hormone synthesis. Persistent adrenal insufficiency has been reported in association with ketoconazole therapy; at high doses of the drug, significant inhibition of androgen synthesis can result in gynecomastia and impotence. This dose-dependent adverse effect has been exploited therapeutically by some clinicians, who prescribe ketoconazole to inhibit androgen production in patients with advanced prostate cancer and to inhibit corticosteroid synthesis in patients with advanced adrenal cancer.

Topical ketoconazole is widely used to treat common dermatophyte infections and seborrheic dermatitis. Topical ketoconazole has been shown to have anti-inflammatory activity comparable to that of hydrocortisone. The cream formulation contains sulfites and therefore should be avoided in patients with sulfite hypersensitivity.

Clotrimazole, **luliconazole**, **miconazole**, **econazole**, **butoconazole**, **oxiconazole**, **sertaconazole**, **sulconazole**, and **tioconazole** are topical imidazole antifungal agents used to treat superficial fungal infections of the stratum corneum, squamous mucosa, and cornea. All of these agents are comparable to one another in efficacy. In addition to inhibiting 14α-sterol demethylase, miconazole affects fatty acid synthesis and inhibits fungal oxidative and peroxidase enzymes. The currently available topical azoles are generally not effective against hair or nail fungal infections, and topical azoles should not be used to treat subcutaneous or systemic mycoses. Topical azole agents are available for cutaneous and vaginal application, and selection of a particular agent should be based on cost and availability. Rare adverse effects of these agents include itching, burning, and sensitization.

The triazole class of antifungal agents includes **itraconazole**, **fluconazole**, **voriconazole**, **terconazole**, **posaconazole**, and **isavuconazole**; one additional member of this class, **ravuconazole**, is currently in clinical trials. **Itraconazole** is available in both oral and intravenous formulations. Given its broad spectrum of activity, itraconazole has largely replaced oral ketoconazole for the treatment of many mycoses. The absorption of oral itraconazole is maximized in an acidic gastric environment. However, because the oral bioavailability of itraconazole is unpredictable, intravenous administration is sometimes preferred. Itraconazole is oxidized in the liver to the active metabolite hydroxyitraconazole, which is more than 90% bound to plasma protein. Hydroxyitraconazole inhibits fungal 14α-sterol demethylase. Compared to ketoconazole and fluconazole, itraconazole shows increased activity in aspergillosis, blastomycosis, and histoplasmosis. Itraconazole is not efficiently transported into the CSF, urine, or saliva; however, itraconazole can be used in certain meningeal fungal infections due to the high drug levels achieved in the meninges. Hepatotoxicity is the major adverse effect associated with itraconazole therapy. Other adverse effects include nausea, vomiting, abdominal pain, diarrhea, hypokalemia, pedal edema, and hair loss.

Posaconazole is an oral triazole developed from itraconazole. Posaconazole is fungistatic against most species of *Candida*, *Cryptococcus*, *Trichosporon*, and some species of *Fusarium*. It is also active against multidrug-resistant *Candida*, *Aspergillus*, and *Zygomycetes* isolates. Posaconazole is used primarily in the prophylaxis and treatment of invasive fungal infections. The most common adverse effects are nausea, vomiting, diarrhea, rash, hypokalemia, thrombocytopenia, and abnormal liver function tests. Interactions may occur with co-administration of cimetidine, rifabutin, and phenytoin, and these drugs should be avoided in patients on posaconazole. Moreover, cyclosporine, tacrolimus, and midazolam dosages should be reduced in patients taking posaconazole.

Fluconazole is currently the most widely used antifungal drug. Fluconazole is a hydrophilic triazole that is available in both oral and intravenous formulations. The bioavailability of oral fluconazole is nearly 100%, and, unlike ketoconazole and itraconazole, its absorption is not influenced by gastric pH. Once absorbed, fluconazole diffuses freely into CSF, sputum, urine, and saliva. Fluconazole is excreted primarily by the kidneys.

Its relatively low adverse effect profile (see below) and excellent CSF penetration make fluconazole the drug of choice for systemic candidiasis and cryptococcal meningitis. Due to the morbidity associated with intrathecal amphotericin B administration, fluconazole is also the drug of choice for coccidioidal meningitis. While fluconazole is active against blastomycosis, histoplasmosis, and sporotrichosis, it is less effective than itraconazole against these infections. Fluconazole is not effective against aspergillosis.

Fungal resistance to fluconazole develops readily, and *Candida* species are the most notable pathogens to develop resistance (e.g., *C. glabrata*). Mechanisms of drug resistance include mutation of fungal P450 enzymes and overexpression of multidrug efflux transporter proteins.

Numerous drug interactions have been noted with fluconazole. As examples, fluconazole can increase the levels of amitriptyline, cyclosporine, phenytoin, and warfarin, and the levels and effects of fluconazole can be decreased by carbamazepine, isoniazid, and phenobarbital. Adverse effects of fluconazole include nausea, vomiting, abdominal pain, and diarrhea in about 10% of patients, as well as reversible alopecia with prolonged oral therapy. Rare cases of Stevens-Johnson syndrome and hepatic failure have been reported.

Ravuconazole, a fluconazole derivative that is currently in clinical trials, demonstrates an expanded spectrum of antifungal activity in vitro against multiple fungal species, including *Aspergillus* and the relatively resistant *Candida* species *C. krusei* and *C. glabrata*.

Voriconazole is a triazole antifungal agent that is available in both oral and parenteral forms. It is the drug of choice in the treatment of invasive aspergillosis and other molds such as *Fusarium* and *Scedosporium*. Voriconazole is fungicidal against essentially all species of *Aspergillus*, and its spectrum of activity also includes *Candida* species (including *C. krusei* and *C. glabrata*) and a number of newly emerging fungi. It is ineffective in the treatment of zygomycosis. Compared to amphotericin, voriconazole is associated with significantly better outcomes, particularly in difficult-to-treat cases such as allogeneic bone marrow transplant recipients, patients with CNS infections, and patients with disseminated infections. Voriconazole inhibits hepatic P450 enzymes to a significant extent, and lower doses of cyclosporine or tacrolimus are used when these drugs are combined with voriconazole. Due to accelerated voriconazole metabolism, co-administration with ritonavir, rifampin, and rifabutin is contraindicated. The intravenous formulation of voriconazole should not be used in patients with renal failure because the cyclodextrin excipient accumulates and can cause CNS toxicity. Hepatic toxicity is common but can usually be managed by decreasing the dose. Unusual visual symptoms (photophobia and colored lights) can occur at peak plasma concentrations of voriconazole; typically, these symptoms last for 30–60 minutes.

Isavuconazole is a triazole antifungal agent approved by the US Food and Drug Administration (FDA) in March 2015 for the treatment of invasive aspergillosis and invasive mucormycosis. It is available in oral and parenteral formulations with equivalent bioavailability.

Terconazole is a topical triazole used to treat vaginal candidiasis. Its mechanism of action and spectrum of antifungal activity are similar to those of the other topical azoles. Terconazole is available as a vaginal suppository that is inserted at bedtime.

Inhibitors of Fungal Membrane Stability: Polyenes

Amphotericin B, **nystatin**, and **natamycin** are **polyene** macrolide antifungal agents. These drugs act by binding to ergosterol and disrupting fungal membrane stability. The three agents are natural products derived from *Streptomyces* species. For decades, amphotericin B provided the only effective treatment for systemic mycoses, including candidiasis, cryptococcal meningitis, invasive aspergillosis, zygomycosis, coccidioidomycosis, blastomycosis, and histoplasmosis. Both its therapeutic effect and its toxicity are related to its affinity for plasma membrane sterols. Fortunately, *the affinity of amphotericin B for ergosterol is 500 times greater than its affinity for cholesterol*. The binding of amphotericin B to ergosterol produces channels or pores that alter fungal membrane permeability and allow for leakage of essential cellular contents, leading ultimately to cell death. The concentration of membrane-associated ergosterol in a given fungal species determines whether amphotericin B is fungicidal or fungistatic for that species. Resistance to amphotericin B, although less frequent than with other antifungal agents, is attributable to a decrease in the ergosterol content of the fungal membrane. In addition to its pore-forming activity, amphotericin B appears to destabilize fungal membranes by generating toxic free radicals upon oxidation of the drug.

Because amphotericin B is highly insoluble, it is supplied as a buffered deoxycholate colloidal suspension. This suspension is poorly absorbed from the gastrointestinal tract and must be administered intravenously. Once in the bloodstream, more than 90% of the drug binds rapidly to tissue sites, while the remainder binds to plasma proteins. Penetration of amphotericin B into the CSF is extremely low (2–4%). Hence, intrathecal therapy may be necessary for treatment of serious meningeal disease. The drug also diffuses poorly into vitreous humor and amniotic fluid.

The toxicity of amphotericin B limits its clinical use. Adverse effects are divided into three groups: immediate systemic reactions, renal effects, and hematologic effects. Systemic reactions can include cytokine storm, in which amphotericin B elicits release of tumor necrosis factor-alpha (TNF-α) and interleukin-1 (IL-1) from cells of the host immune system. In turn, TNF-α and IL-1 cause fever, chills, rigors, and hypotension within the first several hours after drug administration. These responses can usually be minimized by decreasing the rate of drug administration or by pretreatment with antipyretic agents (e.g., acetaminophen, nonsteroidal anti-inflammatory drugs [NSAIDs], or hydrocortisone).

Renal toxicity of amphotericin B is a serious adverse effect. The mechanism of renal toxicity is unknown but may be related to amphotericin-mediated vasoconstriction of afferent arterioles, leading to renal ischemia. Renal toxicity is often the limiting factor in determining the extent of the therapeutic response to amphotericin B. It may be necessary to discontinue therapy temporarily if the blood urea nitrogen (BUN) exceeds 50 mg/dL or the serum creatinine exceeds 3 mg/dL. (BUN and creatinine are surrogate measures of renal function.) Renal tubular acidosis, cylindruria (the presence of renal cell casts in the urine), and hypokalemia can occur to such a degree that electrolyte replacement is required. In the introductory case, treatment with amphotericin B was discontinued as soon as Mr. F's acute symptoms resolved in order to prevent renal toxicity.

Hematologic toxicity of amphotericin B is also common; anemia is probably secondary to decreased production of erythropoietin. The renal and hematologic toxicities of amphotericin B are cumulative and dose-related. Therapeutic measures that can minimize these toxicities include avoidance of other nephrotoxic drugs, such as aminoglycosides and cyclosporine, and maintenance of euvolemia to provide adequate renal perfusion.

Attempts to reduce nephrotoxicity have also led to the development of lipid formulations of amphotericin B. The strategy is to package amphotericin B in liposomes or other lipid carriers, with the goal of preventing high drug exposure to the proximal tubule of the nephron. **Amphotec**®, **Abelcet**®, and **AmBisome**® are all FDA-approved lipid-containing preparations of amphotericin B. They are equal in efficacy to each other and to native amphotericin deoxycholate.

These formulations are less toxic than the native compound but more expensive.

Nystatin, a structural relative of amphotericin B, is a polyene antifungal agent that also acts by binding ergosterol and causing pore formation in fungal cell membranes. The drug is used topically to treat candidiasis involving the skin, vaginal mucosa, and oral mucosa. Nystatin is not absorbed systemically from the skin, vagina, or gastrointestinal tract.

Natamycin, another polyene antifungal agent that binds ergosterol in the fungal cell membrane, is primarily used to treat *Aspergillus* or *Fusarium* corneal infections. It is also indicated in the treatment of blepharitis and conjunctivitis. Natamycin accumulates in the corneal stroma but not in intraocular fluid and is effective at low concentrations.

Inhibitors of Fungal Wall Synthesis: Echinocandins

The key components of the fungal cell wall are chitin, β-(1,3)-D-glucan, β-(1,6)-D-glucan, and cell wall glycoproteins. Because human cells do not have a cell wall, fungal cell wall components represent unique targets for antifungal therapy, and antifungal agents directed at these targets are likely to be relatively nontoxic. **Echinocandins** are a class of antifungal agents that target fungal cell wall synthesis by noncompetitively inhibiting the synthesis of β-(1,3)-D-glucans. Disruption of cell wall integrity results in osmotic stress, lysis of the fungal cell, and ultimately fungal cell death. The three antifungal agents in the echinocandin class are **caspofungin**, **micafungin**, and **anidulafungin**; all are semisynthetic lipopeptides derived from natural products. The echinocandins have in vitro and in vivo antifungal activity against *Candida* and *Aspergillus* species. All three echinocandins are fungicidal against *Candida* species, including *C. krusei* and *C. glabrata*, and fungistatic against *Aspergillus* species. They have poor activity against zygomycetes. All three agents are available only in parenteral form because they are insufficiently bioavailable for oral use.

Caspofungin was the first echinocandin to be approved. The drug is used as primary therapy for esophageal candidiasis and candidemia, as salvage therapy for *Aspergillus* infections, and as empiric therapy for febrile neutropenia. Like the other echinocandins, caspofungin is highly protein-bound (97%) in the plasma; it is metabolized in the liver via peptide bond hydrolysis and N-acetylation; and it penetrates poorly into the CSF (although animal data indicate that the echinocandins do have some activity in the CNS). Caspofungin does not require dose adjustment for renal insufficiency, but dose adjustment is required for patients with moderate hepatic dysfunction. Because co-administration with cyclosporine significantly increases plasma concentrations of caspofungin and elevates liver function enzymes, this drug combination is generally not recommended unless the expected benefits outweigh the risks. Similarly, co-administration with tacrolimus significantly increases plasma concentrations of tacrolimus. To achieve therapeutic plasma concentrations, caspofungin dosing may need to be increased in patients receiving nelfinavir, efavirenz, phenytoin, rifampin, carbamazepine, or dexamethasone.

Micafungin is approved for the treatment of esophageal candidiasis and as antifungal prophylaxis for recipients of hematopoietic stem cell transplants. It is also effective against candidemia and pulmonary aspergillosis. **Anidulafungin** is approved for the treatment of esophageal candidiasis and candidemia. Several small case series have reported the use of echinocandins in combination with amphotericin B, flucytosine, itraconazole, or voriconazole in patients with refractory fungal infections. **Aminocandin** is an investigational echinocandin with a spectrum of activity similar to that of the other echinocandins. It has a half-life threefold to fourfold greater than that of the other echinocandins, thus permitting less frequent administration.

Echinocandins are generally well tolerated; their adverse-effect profile is comparable to that of fluconazole. Because echinocandins contain a peptide backbone, symptoms related to histamine release can be observed (see "Suggested Reading"). Other adverse effects include headache, fever (more common with caspofungin), rash, abnormal liver function tests, and, rarely, hemolysis.

Chelator of Polyvalent Cations: Ciclopirox

Ciclopirox is a synthetic hydroxypyridone antifungal agent whose mechanism of action is poorly understood. In experimental studies, the drug chelates the polyvalent cations Fe^{+3} and Al^{+3}. Chelation of these ions inhibits numerous metal-dependent enzymes responsible for electron transport, DNA and RNA synthesis, energy production, catalase activity, and peroxide degradation within fungal cells. Ciclopirox also demonstrates mild anti-inflammatory properties that may be due to inhibition of 5-lipoxygenase and cyclooxygenase.

Ciclopirox is approved for the treatment of seborrheic dermatitis, tinea versicolor, tinea corporis, tinea pedis, cutaneous candidiasis, and onychomycosis. It is administered as a topical cream, gel, lotion, shampoo, or lacquer. No serious adverse effects have been associated with topical use of ciclopirox. Common adverse effects include a burning sensation with application, pruritus, and contact dermatitis.

▌ CONCLUSION AND FUTURE DIRECTIONS

The development of antifungal agents has progressed significantly since the introduction of amphotericin B. As the population of immunocompromised patients increases, opportunistic fungal infections that are resistant to conventional antifungal therapy pose new challenges to researchers and clinicians. For example, new antifungal therapy is greatly needed in the treatment of zygomycosis. Effective *topical* antifungal agents are eagerly sought for the treatment of nail and hair dermatophytosis, because oral therapies for these superficial fungal infections carry risks such as hepatotoxicity. The development of protease inhibitors and phospholipase inhibitors represent new frontiers in the treatment of *Candida* and *Cryptococcal* species, respectively. As novel and unique molecular targets are identified in fungal pathogens, newer antifungal agents will be developed with the goal of minimizing mechanism-based ("on-target") toxicity while expanding antifungal spectrum of action.

Acknowledgment

We thank Lorne W. Murray, Robert H. Rubin, Charles R. Taylor, and Ali Alikhan for their valuable contributions to this chapter in the First, Second, and Third Editions of *Principles of Pharmacology: The Pathophysiologic Basis of Drug Therapy.*

Suggested Reading

Gauwerky K, Borelli C, Korting HC. Targeting virulence: a new paradigm for antifungals. *Drug Discov Today* 2009;14:214–222. (*Discusses virulence factors of fungi and their inhibitors, with an emphasis on new options for antifungal development, including inhibitors of the secreted aspartyl protease of C. albicans.*)

Miceli MH, Kauffman CA. Isavuconazole: a new broad-spectrum triazole antifungal agent. *Clin Infect Dis* 2015;61:1558–1565. (*Discusses the use of this recently approved agent.*)

Naeger-Murphy N, Pile JC. Clinical indications for newer antifungal agents. *J Hosp Med* 2008;4:102–111. (*Discusses the use of echinocandins and triazoles in several common and/or important clinical situations.*)

Ostrosky-Zeichner L, Casadevall A, Galgiani JN, Odds FC, Rex JH. An insight into the antifungal pipeline: selected new molecules and beyond. *Nat Rev Drug Discov* 2010;9:719–727. (*Discusses development of polyenes, azoles, echinocandins, and investigational antifungal drugs, including vaccines and antibody-based immunotherapy.*)

Patterson TF. Advances and challenges in management of invasive mycosis. *Lancet* 2005;366:1013–1025. (*Focused discussion of fungal pathogens that occur in immunocompromised hosts and management strategies for these opportunistic pathogens.*)

Ruiz-Herrera J, Elorza MV, Valentin E, Sentandreu R. Molecular organization of the cell wall of *Candida albicans* and its relation to pathogenicity. *FEMS Yeast Res* 2006;6:14–29. (*Comprehensive review of the fungal cell wall.*)

Scher RK, Nakamura N, Tavakkol A. Luliconazole: a review of a new antifungal agent for the topical treatment of onychomycosis. *Mycoses* 2014;57:389–393. (*Discusses the development and therapeutic potential of luliconazole, the latest FDA-approved antifungal agent.*)

DRUG SUMMARY TABLE: CHAPTER 36 Pharmacology of Fungal Infections

DRUG	CLINICAL APPLICATIONS	SERIOUS AND COMMON ADVERSE EFFECTS	CONTRAINDICATIONS	THERAPEUTIC CONSIDERATIONS
INHIBITOR OF FUNGAL NUCLEIC ACID SYNTHESIS: FLUCYTOSINE Mechanism—Flucytosine is converted in several steps to 5-FdUMP, which inhibits thymidylate synthase and thereby interferes with DNA synthesis.				
Flucytosine	Candidiasis Cryptococcosis	*Cardiotoxicity, bone marrow suppression (leukopenia, thrombocytopenia), renal failure* Gastrointestinal disturbance, psychosis, headache	Hypersensitivity to flucytosine	Mutations in cytosine permease or cytosine deaminase account for the development of resistance. The combination of flucytosine and amphotericin B exhibits synergistic killing of *Aspergillus*. Use with caution in patients with renal impairment.
INHIBITOR OF FUNGAL MITOSIS: GRISEOFULVIN Mechanism—Binds to tubulin and a microtubule-associated protein, thereby disrupting assembly of the mitotic spindle				
Griseofulvin	Fungal infection of the skin, hair, or nail due to *Trichophyton, Microsporum,* or *Epidermophyton*	*Hepatotoxicity, albuminuria, leukopenia, neutropenia, monocytosis, serum sickness, angioedema, toxic epidermal necrolysis* Headache, lethargy, vertigo, blurred vision, increased fecal protoporphyrin levels, erythema multiforme, photosensitivity, lupus erythematosus exacerbation	Pregnancy Porphyria and hepatic failure Hypersensitivity to griseofulvin	Continue treatment until the infected skin, hair, or nail is completely replaced by normal tissue. Concurrent administration with barbiturates decreases gastrointestinal absorption of griseofulvin. Griseofulvin induces hepatic P450 enzymes, which may result in increased metabolism of warfarin and reduced efficacy of low-estrogen oral contraceptives.
INHIBITORS OF SQUALENE EPOXIDASE: ALLYLAMINES AND BENZYLAMINES Mechanism—Inhibit conversion of squalene to lanosterol by inhibiting squalene epoxidase				
Terbinafine **Naftifine** **Butenafine**	Onychomycosis tinea corporis, tinea cruris (shared indications) Tinea capitis, dermal mycosis (terbinafine only) Tinea pedis (naftifine and butenafine only) Pityriasis versicolor (butenafine only)	*Hepatotoxicity, hearing loss, exanthematous pustulosis, Stevens-Johnson syndrome, toxic epidermal necrolysis, neutropenia (shared adverse effects); exacerbation of psoriasis or subacute cutaneous lupus erythematosus (oral terbinafine only); agranulocytosis (naftifine only)* Headache, nasopharyngitis, gastrointestinal disturbance (shared adverse effects); change or loss of taste and smell, depression (terbinafine only); burning sensation and local irritation of the skin (topical applications only)	Hypersensitivity to terbinafine, naftifine, or butenafine	Terbinafine and naftifine are allylamines, whereas butenafine is a benzylamine. Plasma levels of terbinafine are increased by co-administration with cimetidine and decreased by co-administration with rifampin. Naftifine is only available topically as a cream or gel. Topical allylamine and benzylamine agents are more effective than topical azole agents against common dermatophytes, especially those causing tinea pedis.

INHIBITORS OF 14α-STEROL DEMETHYLASE: IMIDAZOLES AND TRIAZOLES

Mechanism—Inhibit first enzymatic step in conversion of lanosterol to ergosterol by inhibiting 14α-sterol demethylase; the resulting decrease in ergosterol synthesis and accumulation of 14α-methyl sterols disrupt the tightly packed acyl chains of the phospholipids in the fungal membrane.

Drug	Clinical Applications	Serious and Common Adverse Effects	Contraindications	Therapeutic Considerations
Imidazole antifungals: **Ketoconazole** **Butoconazole** **Clotrimazole** **Econazole** **Luliconazole** **Miconazole** **Oxiconazole** **Sertaconazole** **Sulconazole** **Tioconazole**	Coccidioides immitis, Cryptococcus neoformans, Candida species, Histoplasma capsulatum, Blastomyces dermatitidis, and a variety of dermatophytes (ketoconazole only) Superficial fungal infections of the stratum corneum, squamous mucosa, and cornea (butoconazole, clotrimazole, econazole, luliconazole, miconazole, oxiconazole, sertaconazole, sulconazole, and tioconazole only)	*QT prolongation, ventricular tachycardia, ventricular fibrillation, torsades de pointes, hepatotoxicity (ketoconazole only)* Gastrointestinal disturbance (ketoconazole only); pruritus and burning (butoconazole, clotrimazole, econazole, luliconazole, miconazole, oxiconazole, sertaconazole, sulconazole, and tioconazole only)	Hypersensitivity to ketoconazole, butoconazole, clotrimazole, econazole, luliconazole, miconazole, oxiconazole, sertaconazole, sulconazole, or tioconazole Concomitant use with alprazolam, colchicine, eplerenone, ergot alkaloids, felodipine, irinotecan, lurasidone, oral midazolam, nisoldipine, tolvaptan, or oral triazolam (ketoconazole only) Concomitant use with CYP3A4-metabolized HMG-CoA reductase inhibitors (e.g., lovastatin, simvastatin) (ketoconazole only) Concomitant use with disopyramide, dofetilide, dronedarone, methadone, pimozide, quinidine, or ranolazine (ketoconazole only) Liver disease (ketoconazole only) Hypersensitivity to milk protein (miconazole only)	Ketoconazole is available both orally and topically. Ketoconazole inhibits CYP3A4 and increases levels of many drugs, including warfarin, tolbutamide, phenytoin, cyclosporine, H1-antihistamines, and others. Agents that decrease gastric acidity interfere with ketoconazole absorption. Butoconazole, clotrimazole, econazole, luliconazole, miconazole, oxiconazole, sertaconazole, sulconazole, and tioconazole are topical imidazole antifungal agents. Topical azoles should be applied to the skin twice a day for 3–6 weeks, whereas vaginal preparations should be used once a day for 1–7 days at bedtime.
Triazole antifungals: **Fluconazole** **Itraconazole** **Posaconazole** **Terconazole** **Voriconazole** **Isavuconazole**	Aspergillosis, blastomycosis, candidiasis, histoplasmosis, onychomycosis (itraconazole only) Candidiasis, cryptococcal meningitis (fluconazole only) Aspergillosis, candidiasis, Fusarium, Monosporium apiospermum (voriconazole only) Vulvovaginal candidiasis (terconazole only) Aspergillosis prophylaxis, candidiasis prophylaxis and treatment (posaconazole and voriconazole only) Invasive aspergillosis, invasive mucormycosis (isavuconazole only)	*Hepatic toxicity, Stevens-Johnson syndrome, toxic epidermal necrolysis, agranulocytosis, seizure (shared adverse effects)* *QT prolongation, torsades de pointes (fluconazole and posaconazole only)* *Heart failure, pancreatitis, pulmonary edema (itraconazole only)* *Toxic encephalopathy, optic disc edema, optic neuritis, renal failure, malignant melanoma, squamous cell carcinoma (voriconazole only)* Gastrointestinal disturbance (itraconazole, fluconazole, posaconazole, and isavuconazole only) Edema, rhinitis (itraconazole only) Headache (itraconazole, posaconazole, and terconazole only) Hypokalemia, refractory candidiasis, fever (posaconazole only) Visual disturbance (voriconazole only) Hypokalemia, dyspnea, cough, edema, back pain (isavuconazole only)	Pregnancy (shared contraindication) Hypersensitivity to drug Co-administration with dofetilide, oral midazolam, pimozide, levacetylmethadol, quinidine, lovastatin, simvastatin, or triazolam (itraconazole and fluconazole only) Co-administration with ergot alkaloids metabolized by CYP3A4, such as dihydroergotamine, ergotamine, ergonovine, and methylergonovine (posaconazole, voriconazole, and isavuconazole only) History of heart failure (itraconazole only) Concomitant use with drugs utilizing P-glycoprotein-mediated gastrointestinal absorption (itraconazole only) Concomitant use with efavirenz at standard doses of 400 mg/day or higher (voriconazole only) Familial short QT syndrome (isavuconazole only)	Fluconazole and itraconazole inhibit CYP3A4. The 0.4% terconazole cream is used for 7 days, whereas the 0.8% cream is used for 3 days for vulvovaginal candidiasis. Ravuconazole is in clinical trials.

continues

DRUG SUMMARY TABLE: CHAPTER 36 Pharmacology of Fungal Infections *continued*

INHIBITORS OF FUNGAL MEMBRANE STABILITY: POLYENES
Mechanism—Bind to ergosterol and form pores that after fungal membrane permeability and stability

DRUG	CLINICAL APPLICATIONS	*SERIOUS* AND COMMON ADVERSE EFFECTS	CONTRAINDICATIONS	THERAPEUTIC CONSIDERATIONS
Amphotericin B	Potentially life-threatening aspergillosis, cryptococcosis, North American blastomycosis, systemic candidiasis, coccidioidomycosis, histoplasmosis, systemic candidiasis, zygomycosis, American mucocutaneous leishmaniasis, *Basidiobolus, Conidiobolus*, mucormycosis, sporotrichosis	*Renal toxicity (renal tubular acidosis, cylindruria, hypokalemia), cytokine storm (fever, chills, hypotension), anemia, asystole, cardiac arrest, cardiac arrhythmia, ventricular fibrillation, Stevens-Johnson syndrome, toxic epidermal necrolysis, agranulocytosis, encephalopathy, seizure* Weight loss, gastrointestinal disturbance, arthralgia, myalgia, headache, malaise	Hypersensitivity to amphotericin B	Amphotericin B is supplied as a buffered deoxycholate colloidal suspension, which must be administered intravenously; intrathecal therapy may be necessary for serious meningeal disease. Lipid formulations of amphotericin B are designed to reduce drug exposure to the proximal tubule of the nephron and thereby minimize nephrotoxicity. Amphotec®, Abelcet®, and AmBisome® are all FDA-approved lipid-containing preparations of amphotericin B. Combination treatment with flucytosine is recommended in acute cryptococcal meningitis in HIV-infected adults.
Nystatin	Mucocutaneous candidiasis	*Stevens-Johnson syndrome* Rare contact dermatitis	Hypersensitivity to nystatin	Nystatin is not absorbed systemically from the skin, vagina, or gastrointestinal tract. Nystatin is used clinically for topical treatment of candidiasis involving the skin, vaginal mucosa, or oral mucosa.
Natamycin	Keratitis, conjunctivitis, blepharitis caused by *Aspergillus, Candida, Cephalosporium, Fusarium*, and *Penicillium*	Eye irritation	Hypersensitivity to natamycin	For ophthalmic use only.

INHIBITORS OF FUNGAL WALL SYNTHESIS: ECHINOCANDINS

Mechanism—Noncompetitively inhibit synthesis of β-(1,3)-D-glucans, which leads to disruption of cell wall integrity

Caspofungin Micafungin Anidulafungin	Esophageal candidiasis, candidemia, salvage therapy of *Aspergillus* infections, empiric therapy of febrile neutropenia (caspofungin only) Esophageal candidiasis, antifungal prophylaxis for recipients of hematopoietic stem cell transplants, candidemia (micafungin only) Esophageal candidiasis, candidemia (anidulafungin only)	*Stevens-Johnson syndrome, pancreatitis, hepatic necrosis, liver failure, sepsis, nephrotoxicity, pleural effusion, respiratory failure, angioedema (caspofungin only)* *Atrial fibrillation, cardiac arrest, myocardial infarction, pericardial effusion, hemolytic anemia, liver failure, encephalopathy, intracranial hemorrhage, seizure, renal failure (micafungin only)* *Deep vein thrombosis, hepatic necrosis, hypokalemia, seizure (anidulafungin only)* Pruritus, rash, gastrointestinal disturbance, hypotension, increased liver enzymes, thrombophlebitis, headache, fever	Hypersensitivity to caspofungin, micafungin, or anidulafungin	All three echinocandins are fungicidal against *Candida* species, including *C. krusei* and *C. glabrata*, and fungistatic against *Aspergillus* species. Co-administration of cyclosporine with caspofungin significantly increases plasma concentration of caspofungin and elevates liver function enzymes. Co-administration with tacrolimus significantly increases plasma concentration of tacrolimus. Caspofungin dose should be adjusted for patients with moderate liver dysfunction.

CHELATOR OF POLYVALENT CATIONS: CICLOPIROX

Mechanism—Chelates polyvalent cations, thereby inhibiting enzymes responsible for electron transport, DNA repair, energy production, and peroxide degradation within fungal cells

Ciclopirox	Tinea versicolor Tinea corporis Tinea pedis Onychomycosis Cutaneous candidiasis Seborrheic dermatitis	Contact dermatitis, pruritus, burning sensation	Hypersensitivity to ciclopirox	Ciclopirox is not for ophthalmic, intravaginal, or oral use. Use with caution in women who are nursing, since it is unknown whether ciclopirox is secreted in human milk.

37

Pharmacology of Parasitic Infections

Louise C. Ivers and Edward T. Ryan

INTRODUCTION

More than one billion people worldwide are infected with parasites. Parasites of medical importance include protozoa (such as the organisms that cause malaria, toxoplasmosis, giardiasis, amebiasis, leishmaniasis, and trypanosomiasis) and helminths ("worms"). Worms that infect humans include cestodes ("flatworms" or "tapeworms," such as the worm that causes taeniasis), nematodes ("roundworms," which cause filariasis, strongyloidiasis, and ascariasis), and trematodes ("flukes," such as the worms that cause schistosomiasis).

Ideally, antiparasitic drugs should be targeted to structures or biochemical pathways present or accessible only in parasites. Many antiparasitic drugs act by unknown or poorly defined mechanisms of action, however. This chapter focuses on a number of the better defined agents, including those active against *Plasmodia* species (which cause malaria), *Entamoeba histolytica* (which causes amebiasis), and *Onchocerca volvulus* (which causes onchocerciasis, a filarial infection referred to as *river blindness*). In each of these cases, antiparasitic agents interfere with metabolic requirements of the parasite: the dependence of malarial plasmodia on heme metabolism, the dependence of luminal parasites on specific fermentation pathways, and the dependence of helminths on neuromuscular activity. These three examples

are not all-inclusive but rather emphasize opportunities to use or design pharmacologic agents to interrupt metabolic requirements specific to parasites.

MALARIAL PLASMODIA

Each year, approximately 200 million individuals in more than 90 countries develop malaria, and over a half million individuals die of malaria. Malaria is the most important parasitic disease of humans and one of the most important infections of humans. Human malaria is caused by one of five species of plasmodial parasites: ***Plasmodium falciparum***, ***P. vivax***, ***P. ovale***, ***P. malariae***, and ***P. knowlesi***. The most serious type of malaria is that caused by *P. falciparum*.

Physiology of Malarial Plasmodia

Life Cycle

The life cycle of malaria involves a parasite, a mosquito vector, and a human host (Fig. 37-1). An ***Anopheles*** spp. mosquito can ingest sexual forms of malarial parasites (gametocytes) when taking a blood meal from an infected human. After fusion of the male and female gametocytes and maturation of the zygote within the mosquito, **sporozoites** are released from an oocyst. The sporozoites, which migrate to the mosquito's salivary glands, can be inoculated into the blood of another human host

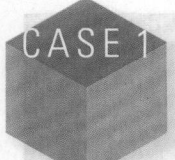

CASE 1

Binata, a 3-year-old girl living in a remote area of a central African country, is in good health when, one day, she begins to feel hot, has sweats and shaking chills, stops eating, and becomes intermittently listless and lethargic. Several days later, these symptoms climax in a seizure and coma, prompting Binata's parents to rush her to the local health care clinic. In the clinic, the unconscious child's neck is supple, but she is febrile to 103°F. Her lungs are clear to auscultation, and there is no rash. A smear of Binata's peripheral blood discloses *P. falciparum* ring trophozoites in approximately 10% of her erythrocytes. Binata is given the only antimalarial medicines available at the clinic, chloroquine and pyrimethamine/sulfadoxine; however, the child does not improve, and she dies within 24 hours.

Questions

1. Why did Binata die?
2. Why did Binata not improve after receiving antimalarial drugs?
3. How often does a child die of malaria?

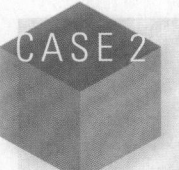

CASE 2

Mr. G is a 36-year-old married software engineer who was born and raised in India. He comes to the United States and is completely well for 6 months. He then begins to experience episodes of fever, headache, and body aches. One week later, he goes to his physician, who examines a smear of Mr. G's blood, diagnoses malaria, and prescribes chloroquine for treatment. Therapy with chloroquine resolves his symptoms completely. However, Mr. G notes recurrence of fevers and the other symptoms 3 months later and returns to his doctor's office.

Questions

4. What is a likely explanation for the return of Mr. G's fever?
5. How can Mr. G's treatment be modified so that his illness will not return?

during a subsequent blood meal. In the human, sporozoites leave the blood and multiply in the liver, forming **tissue schizonts**. This *exoerythrocytic hepatic stage* is asymptomatic. In a typical *P. falciparum* infection, 1–12 weeks after the infective bite, the liver cells release parasites into the bloodstream as **merozoites**. A single sporozoite can produce more than 30,000 merozoites. Merozoites invade erythrocytes, multiply asexually, and form **blood schizonts**. This is the *erythrocytic stage*. Infected erythrocytes eventually rupture, releasing another generation of merozoites that continue the erythrocytic cycle. Rare merozoites also mature into gametocytes. Ingestion of these circulating gametocytes by an appropriate mosquito completes the life cycle. The clinical symptoms of malaria, most distinctively fever, are caused by the intravascular lysis of erythrocytes and subsequent release of merozoites into the blood. The fevers that Binata and Mr. G experienced were associated with these hemolytic episodes. Binata, unfortunately, developed cerebral malaria due to *P. falciparum*.

P. falciparum-infected erythrocytes express "knobs" on their surface that are composed of both host and parasite proteins. Parasite proteins include PfEMP-1, a protein family composed of approximately 100–150 gene products that mediate attachment of infected erythrocytes to cellular receptors—including CD36, ICAM-1, ELAM-1, and chondroitin sulfate—on endothelial surfaces in the human host. This intravascular binding during a malarial episode occurs only during *P. falciparum* infection and contributes to intravascular "sludging" of erythrocytes. Endothelial attachment lessens the amount of time during which infected erythrocytes circulate systemically, thereby decreasing the likelihood that infected erythrocytes will be cleared via splenic

sequestration. Sludging also accounts, in large part, for the pathophysiology of malaria caused by *P. falciparum*. Sludging can affect any organ, including the brain, lungs, and kidneys; damage to these organs leads to tissue hypoxia, focal necrosis, and hemorrhage. In Binata's case, the brain was involved (so-called cerebral malaria).

Untreated, cerebral malaria is almost uniformly fatal, and, even with optimal treatment, cerebral malaria has a case fatality rate exceeding 20%. Binata was treated with two drugs that have historically been quite important in treating individuals with malaria but which, unfortunately, are now ineffective in most places in the world because of widespread drug-resistant *P. falciparum*. Largely because of their low cost and availability, these drugs (chloroquine and a fixed combination of pyrimethamine and sulfadoxine) were widely used in many developing areas of the world to treat older children and adults with partial immunity to malaria, but these agents have little clinical use in treating nonimmune individuals such as Binata. Due to the increasing ineffectiveness of these older agents, it is now recommended that individuals in sub-Saharan Africa with malaria be treated with an artemisinin derivative in combination with a second agent (see below).

Unfortunately, Binata's story has been all too common. On average, worldwide, a child dies of malaria every 75 seconds; of these deaths, more than 90% occur in sub-Saharan Africa, more than 90% occur in children under 5 years of age, and more than 95% are caused by *P. falciparum* infection. No pharmacologic agent has yet been developed that interferes with the recently elucidated role of PfEMP-1 in the endothelial attachment of malarially infected erythrocytes.

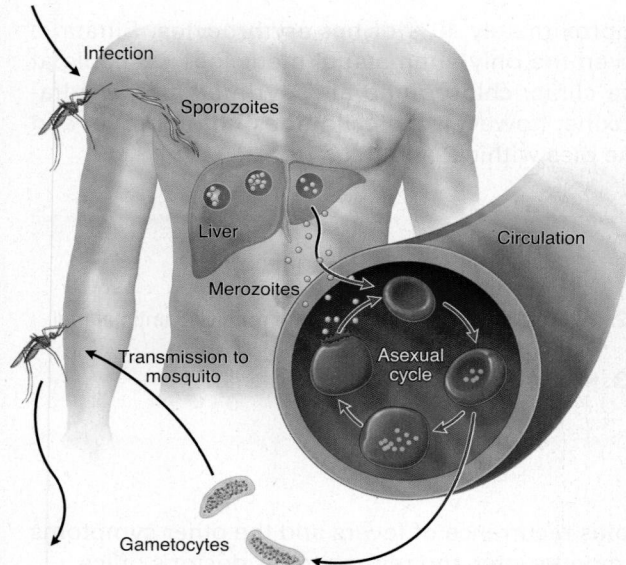

FIGURE 37-1. Life cycle of malaria. Malarial plasmodia have a complex life cycle that relies on both humans and *Anopheles* spp. mosquitoes. Gametocytes from an infected human are transferred to a mosquito during a blood meal. In the mosquito stomach, a zygote forms and matures to become an oocyst on the outside wall of the stomach (*not shown*). Sporozoites released from the oocyst migrate to the salivary glands. During its next blood meal, the mosquito transfers *Plasmodium* spp. sporozoites from its saliva to another human. Sporozoites enter the host's bloodstream and travel to the liver. Sporozoites replicate in the liver and then lyse infected hepatocytes, releasing merozoites into the circulation. Merozoites infect erythrocytes, undergoing asexual cycles of erythrocytic infection and lysis. Some merozoites differentiate into gametocytes, which can be ingested by another mosquito and thereby continue the cycle of infection. *P. vivax* and *P. ovale* can also form dormant hypnozoites, which can remain in infected hepatocytes for months to years before release into the circulation (*not shown*).

In Mr. G's case, a peripheral blood smear showed *P. vivax* parasites inside his erythrocytes. Because *P. falciparum* and *P. malariae* infections involve only one cycle of hepatic cell invasion, drugs that eliminate these species from erythrocytes are usually sufficient to clear the infection. Unfortunately, *P. vivax* and *P. ovale* also have dormant hepatic forms (**hypnozoites**) that release merozoites over months to 1–2 years. Therefore, individuals infected with *P. vivax* or *P. ovale* should be treated with agents that are effective against not only blood-stage plasmodia but also liver-stage parasites (see below). Because chloroquine does not eliminate hepatic forms of *P. vivax* and *P. ovale*, Mr. G's *P. vivax* infection recurred.

Heme Metabolism

Plasmodia have a limited capacity for de novo amino acid synthesis; instead, they rely on amino acids released from ingested host **hemoglobin** molecules. Within red blood cells, plasmodia degrade hemoglobin in a digestive vacuole, which is an elaborate lysosome with an acidic pH (Fig. 37-2). Hemoglobin is sequentially degraded to its constituent amino acids by plasmodial aspartic proteases (plasmepsins), a cysteine protease (falcipain), and a metalloprotease (falcilysin). Degradation of hemoglobin releases protonated basic amino acids and a toxic heme metabolite, ferriprotoporphyrin IX. Ferriprotoporphyrin IX is detoxified by polymerization to crystalline hemozoin. If ferriprotoporphyrin IX does not

polymerize, it causes lysosomal membrane damage and toxicity to the malarial parasite. Quinoline antimalarials (see below) are believed to act by inhibiting heme polymerization, thereby creating an environment that is toxic to intraerythrocytic plasmodia.

Electron Transport Chain

Malarial plasmodia also possess mitochondria with a tiny genome (approximately 6 kb) that encodes only three **cytochromes** (large protein complexes involved in electron transport and oxidative phosphorylation). These cytochromes, together with a number of mitochondrial-targeted proteins

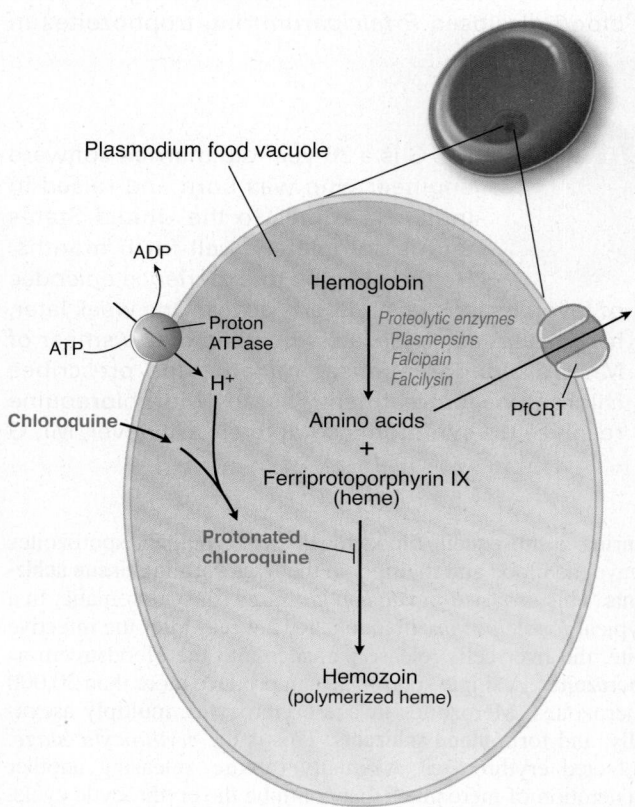

FIGURE 37-2. Proposed mechanisms of heme metabolism in the plasmodial food vacuole. Malarial plasmodia possess a specialized food vacuole that maintains an acidic intravacuolar environment by the action of a proton ATPase in the vacuolar membrane. Within the vacuole, human hemoglobin is used as a food source. Hemoglobin is proteolyzed to amino acids by several plasmodial-derived proteolytic enzymes, including plasmepsins, falcipain, and falcilysin. Protonated amino acids are then removed from the food vacuole through the PfCRT transporter. Degradation of hemoglobin also releases heme (ferriprotoporphyrin IX). Free ferriprotoporphyrin IX can react with oxygen to produce superoxide (O_2^-); oxidant defense enzymes, which may include plasmodial-derived superoxide dismutase and catalase, convert the potentially cytotoxic superoxide to H_2O (*not shown*). Plasmodia polymerize ferriprotoporphyrin IX into the nontoxic derivative hemozoin; evidence suggests that polymerization requires the activity of positively charged histidine-rich proteins (*not shown*). The iron moiety in ferriprotoporphyrin IX can also be oxidized from the ferrous (Fe^{2+}) to the ferric (Fe^{3+}) state, with concomitant production of hydrogen peroxide (H_2O_2). Many antimalarial agents are thought to disrupt the process of malarial heme metabolism; proposed mechanisms of drug action include inhibition of heme polymerization, enhancement of oxidant production, and reaction with heme to form cytotoxic metabolites. The inhibition of ferriprotoporphyrin IX polymerization by protonated chloroquine is shown.

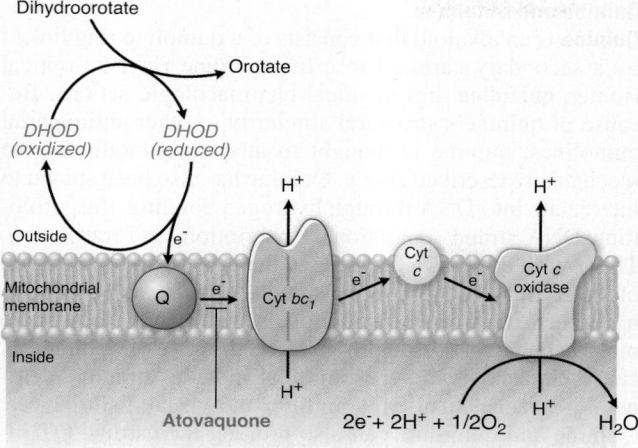

FIGURE 37-3. The mitochondrial electron transport chain in plasmodia. The electron transport chain consists of a series of oxidation/reduction steps that culminate in the donation of electrons to oxygen, forming water. In plasmodia, the electron transport chain acts as an electron acceptor for reduced dihydroorotate dehydrogenase (DHOD), an enzyme that is essential for plasmodial pyrimidine synthesis. In this cascade, reduced ubiquinone (Q) transfers electrons to the cytochrome bc_1 complex ($Cyt\ bc_1$), which then passes electrons to cytochrome c ($Cyt\ c$) and, finally, to cytochrome c oxidase ($Cyt\ c\ oxidase$). In a 4-electron reduction of molecular oxygen (*shown here as the half-reaction*), cytochrome c oxidase donates electrons to oxygen to form water. This chain of electron transfers also involves the pumping of protons across the mitochondrial membrane by Cyt bc_1 and Cyt c oxidase; the resulting electrochemical gradient of protons is used to generate ATP (*not shown*). Atovaquone antagonizes the interaction between ubiquinone and the plasmodial cytochrome bc_1 complex, thereby disrupting pyrimidine synthesis by preventing the regeneration of oxidized DHOD.

derived from the plasmodial nuclear genome, make up a rudimentary electron transport chain similar in organization to that found in mammals (Fig. 37-3). In this electron transport chain, integral proteins of the mitochondrial inner membrane are reduced and then oxidized as they transport electrons from one intermediate protein to another. The energy liberated by electron transport is used to drive proton pumping across the mitochondrial membrane, and the energy stored in the proton gradient drives ATP synthesis. In this electron transport chain, oxygen is the final electron acceptor, resulting in the reduction of oxygen to water.

Plasmodia derive most of their ATP directly from glycolysis and probably do not use mitochondrial electron transport as a significant source of energy. However, plasmodia do rely on electron transport for the oxidation of key enzymes involved in nucleotide synthesis. For example, **dihydroorotate dehydrogenase** (**DHOD**), the enzyme that mediates an early step in pyrimidine synthesis (see Chapter 39, Pharmacology of Cancer: Genome Synthesis, Stability, and Maintenance), catalyzes the oxidation of dihydroorotate to orotate. As part of this reaction, DHOD is reduced, and the enzyme must be reoxidized before it can continue with another cycle of catalysis. **Ubiquinone**, an integral membrane protein located near the beginning of the electron transport chain, accepts electrons from reduced DHOD, thus regenerating the oxidized form of DHOD necessary for pyrimidine synthesis. Because plasmodia depend on de novo pyrimidine synthesis for DNA replication, interrupting the ability of ubiquinone to oxidize DHOD can disrupt plasmodial DNA replication (see below).

Pharmacology of Antimalarial Agents

The currently available antimalarial agents target four physiologic pathways in plasmodia: heme metabolism (**chloroquine, quinine, mefloquine,** and **artemisinin**), electron transport (**primaquine** and **atovaquone**), protein translation (**doxycycline, tetracycline,** and **clindamycin**), and folate metabolism (**sulfadoxine-pyrimethamine** and **proguanil**). The following section discusses the pharmacologic agents that target these pathways.

Clinically, antimalarials can be classified into agents used for prophylaxis (to prevent malaria in individuals residing in or traveling through a malaria zone), agents used for treating individuals with acute blood-stage malaria, and agents used to eliminate hypnozoite liver-stage malarial infections. Generally, agents used for prophylaxis must be well tolerated and easy to administer.

Inhibitors of Heme Metabolism

For many centuries, agents that disrupt intraerythrocytic malarial parasites have been the foundation of antimalarial treatment regimens. Most of these compounds are congeners of quinoline and, as a result, are all believed to possess similar mechanisms of action. Artemisinin, discussed at the end of this section, is also thought to act by inhibiting heme metabolism, although its structure is different from that of the quinolines.

Chloroquine

For the past 2,000 years, humans have used the roots of *Dichroa febrifuga* or the leaves of hydrangea in the treatment of individuals with malaria. More recently, the bark of the **cinchona** tree was found to be a more effective remedy. In all these plants, a **quinoline** compound is the pharmacologically active antiplasmodial agent. **Chloroquine**, a 4-aminoquinoline, was introduced in 1935 for use in the treatment of malaria. Chloroquine is a weak base that, in its neutral form, freely diffuses across the membrane of the parasite's food vacuole. Once inside the acidic environment of the vacuole, chloroquine is rapidly protonated, making it unable to diffuse out of the vacuole. As a result, protonated chloroquine accumulates to high concentrations inside the parasite's food vacuole, where it binds to ferriprotoporphyrin IX and inhibits the polymerization of this heme metabolite. Accumulation of unpolymerized ferriprotoporphyrin IX leads to oxidative membrane damage and is toxic to the parasite. *Chloroquine thus poisons the parasite by preventing the detoxification of a toxic product of hemoglobin catabolism* (Fig. 37-2).

Chloroquine is concentrated by as much as 100-fold in parasitized erythrocytes compared to uninfected erythrocytes. In addition, the concentration of chloroquine required to alkalinize lysosomes of mammalian cells is much higher than that needed to raise the pH in malarial food vacuoles. Therefore, chloroquine is relatively nontoxic to humans, although the drug commonly causes pruritus in darkly pigmented individuals, and it can exacerbate psoriasis and porphyria. Taken in supratherapeutic doses, however, chloroquine can cause vomiting, retinopathy, hypotension, confusion, and death. In fact, chloroquine is used globally in suicides each year (largely because it is inexpensive, available, and toxic at high doses), and accidental ingestion by children can be fatal.

When initially introduced, chloroquine was a first-line drug used against all types of malaria; however, it is now ineffective against most strains of *P. falciparum* in Africa, Asia, and South America (Fig. 37-4). Hypotheses regarding the mechanisms responsible for chloroquine resistance are based on the finding that chloroquine-resistant plasmodia accumulate less chloroquine inside food vacuoles than chloroquine-sensitive plasmodia do. In the food vacuole, protonated amino acids are generated by the parasite as it degrades hemoglobin. These protonated amino acids exit the lysosome by means of a transmembrane protein called *PfCRT*, encoded by *pfcrt* on *P. falciparum* chromosome 7. A number of mutations in PfCRT have been associated with chloroquine resistance; for example, a substitution of threonine for lysine at position 76 (K76T) is highly correlated with chloroquine resistance. This mutated PfCRT probably pumps protonated chloroquine out of the food vacuole. This altered pump action could also be detrimental to the parasite, perhaps because of altered amino acid export and/or changes in vacuole pH. Many *P. falciparum* strains with mutations in *pfcrt* carry a second mutation in the gene *pfmdr1* encoding Pgh1, a food vacuole membrane protein involved in pH regulation. It is speculated that this second mutation provides a "corrective" action that allows chloroquine-resistant *P. falciparum* to continue growth in the presence of a *pfcrt* mutation.

Strains of *P. vivax* with decreased susceptibility to chloroquine are now reported with increasing frequency in areas of Papua New Guinea, Indonesia, and other focal areas of Oceania and Latin America, although the exact mechanism of decreased susceptibility to chloroquine in these strains has not been fully established. Despite concerns regarding increasing resistance, chloroquine remains a drug of choice for treating most individuals with malaria caused by *P. vivax*, *P. ovale*, *P. malariae*, and *P. knowlesi* and by chloroquine-sensitive strains of *P. falciparum*. It can also be used prophylactically to prevent malaria caused by sensitive strains of plasmodia.

Quinine and Quinidine

Quinine is an alkaloid that consists of a quinoline ring linked by a secondary carbinol to a quinuclidine ring. Its optical isomer, **quinidine**, has identical pharmacologic actions. Because of quinine's structural similarity to other antimalarial quinolines, quinine is thought to attack plasmodia by the mechanism described above. Quinine has also been shown to intercalate into DNA through hydrogen bonding, thus inhibiting DNA strand separation, transcription, and translation. The overall effect is a decrease in the growth and replication of the erythrocytic form of plasmodia. Quinine and quinidine have been used to treat individuals with acute blood-stage malaria but are not used prophylactically. Use of quinine can cause **cinchonism**, a syndrome that includes tinnitus, deafness, headaches, nausea, vomiting, and visual disturbances. Quinine and quinidine can also prolong the cardiac QT interval (see Chapter 24, Pharmacology of Cardiac Rhythm).

Mefloquine

Mefloquine is a quinoline compound that is structurally related to other antimalarial agents. Unlike quinine, mefloquine does not bind to DNA. Its exact mechanism of action is unknown, although mefloquine appears to disrupt polymerization of heme in intraerythrocytic malarial parasites. Mefloquine has a number of adverse effects, including nausea, cardiac conduction abnormalities (including bradycardia, prolongation of the QT interval, and arrhythmia), and neuropsychiatric effects, including vivid dreams/nightmares, insomnia, anxiety, depression, hallucinations, seizures, and, rarely, psychosis. The mechanism(s) responsible for these adverse effects is unknown. In 2013, the US Food and Drug Administration (FDA) issued a black box warning related to these neurologic and psychiatric adverse effects. Mefloquine can be used both therapeutically and prophylactically. Strains of *P. falciparum* resistant to both chloroquine and mefloquine have been reported in areas of Southeast Asia.

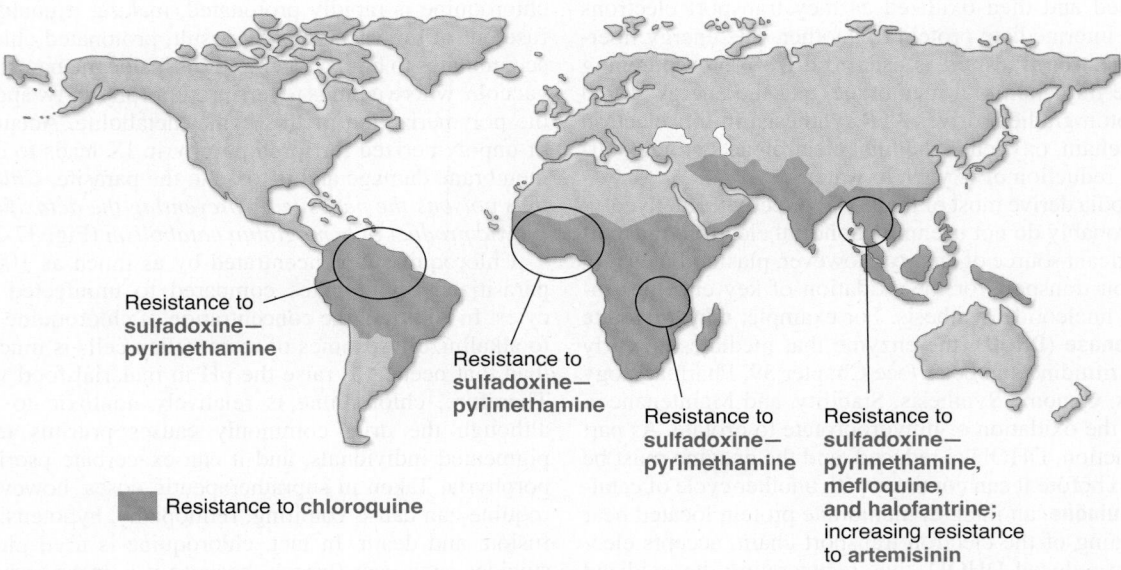

FIGURE 37-4. Geographic distribution of drug-resistant *Plasmodium falciparum*. Historically, chloroquine was the drug of choice for prophylaxis and treatment of individuals with *P. falciparum* malaria. Unfortunately, *P. falciparum* is now resistant to chloroquine in most areas of the world (*blue shading*). In many areas, *P. falciparum* is also resistant to other antimalarial agents, including sulfadoxine–pyrimethamine, mefloquine, and halofantrine. (Halofantrine is associated with potentially lethal cardiac toxicity and is therefore seldom used.)

Artemisinin

Artemisinin, from the wormwood plant *Artemisia annua*, has been used in China (where it is known as *qinghao*) for centuries in the treatment of individuals with fever. Artemisinin derivatives have now become the first-line drug for treating individuals with falciparum malaria. The compound is both a sesquiterpene lactone and a cyclic endoperoxide. When activated by free or heme-bound iron, it forms a carbon-centered free-radical compound (Fig. 37-5). This free radical has the ability to alkylate many proteins as well as heme. The mechanism of specificity of the drug for plasmodia-infected erythrocytes is unknown—potential sources of specificity include artemisinin's requirement for heme for free radical formation and artemisinin's preferential accumulation in plasmodia. Drug action may relate to free radical production in the food vacuole of the parasite and subsequent inhibition of PfATP6, the parasite Ca^{2+} ATPase that is the ortholog of the mammalian SERCA calcium pump (see Chapter 25, Pharmacology of Cardiac Contractility). Administration of artemisinin and its derivatives (**artesunate**, **artemether**, **dihydroartemisinin**) is associated with a rapid decrease in the level of malaria parasites in the blood of an infected individual and rapid resolution of symptoms in patients with blood-stage malaria. Unlike many of the other antimalarials, artemisinins affect blood-stage gametocytes and thus can decrease transmission of malaria from an infected human. Artemisinin is not effective as a prophylactic agent against malaria.

Due to the short half-life of artemisinins and the subsequent risk of recrudescence of malaria, and to decrease the likelihood of drug resistance, the World Health Organization (WHO) strongly recommends against use of artemisinins as monotherapy. Artemisinins should be used as fixed combinations, usually including a rapidly acting artemisinin

and a second agent with a longer half-life (referred to as *artemisinin combination therapy [ACT]*). Combinations include artemether–lumefantrine, artesunate–mefloquine, artesunate–amodiaquine, and dihydroartemisinin–piperazine. Oral, parenteral, and rectal suppository formulations are available. The WHO now recommends that ACT should be used as the first-line treatment for chloroquine-resistant *P. falciparum* malaria. In comparison to quinine, artesunate is superior and is associated with a decreased risk of death, more rapid parasite clearance, and lower incidence of adverse events. In vitro resistance to artemisinin has been associated with mutations in the parasite calcium pump PfATP6 (see above). Unfortunately, increasing resistance to artemisinin has now been reported in a number of countries in Southeast Asia, although clinical response to ACT remains acceptable.

Overall, artemisinin and its derivatives are better tolerated than most other antimalarial agents. In laboratory animals, intramuscular injection of oil-based formulations of artemisinin has been shown to cause brainstem neuropathy; this potentially lethal effect has not been observed in humans, but some studies have found evidence suggesting that artemisinins may be associated with auditory impairment and other neurotoxic effects in humans. Hypoglycemia occurs less often than with quinine-based therapy. Safety data in pregnancy are lacking.

Inhibitors of Electron Transport

Although the electron transport chain is a ubiquitous feature of eukaryotic cells, two agents have been developed that appear to selectively interrupt the plasmodial electron transport chain. This selectivity is due to different molecular structures of the same biochemical target rather than the presence of a unique enzymatic pathway in plasmodia

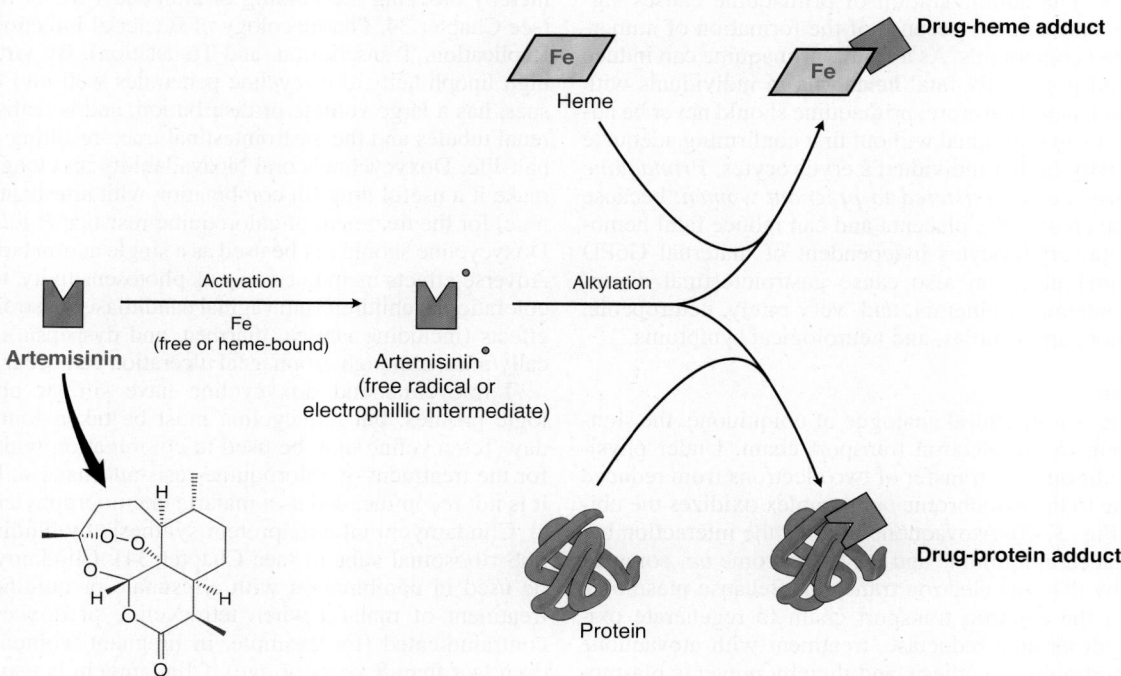

FIGURE 37-5. Proposed mechanism of action of artemisinin. Artemisinin is a cyclic endoperoxide that forms a free radical after activation by iron (Fe). The mechanism of action of artemisinin is not known with certainty but may involve alkylation of macromolecules such as heme and proteins, resulting in the formation of artemisinin–heme adducts and artemisinin–protein adducts that are toxic to plasmodia. One such adduct may involve PfATP6, a parasite Ca^{2+}ATPase (*not shown*).

(see Chapter 33, Principles of Antimicrobial and Antineoplastic Pharmacology).

Primaquine

Primaquine was approved in 1952 for the treatment of malaria. Because primaquine attacks the hepatic stage of malaria caused by *P. vivax* and *P. ovale*, it is used to prevent recrudescence of these infections and is the only standard drug currently available for this use. In Mr. G's case, primaquine can be prescribed to clear the hepatic stage of his malaria and prevent recurrence of his symptoms. Primaquine severely disrupts the metabolic processes of plasmodial mitochondria. The antimalarial activity is probably attributable to **quinone**, a primaquine metabolite that interferes with the function of **ubiquinone** as an electron carrier in the respiratory chain. Another potential mechanism of action involves the ability of certain primaquine metabolites to cause nonspecific oxidative damage to plasmodial mitochondria.

Primaquine is predominantly used to clear hepatic hypnozoites from individuals with malaria caused by *P. vivax* or *P. ovale*. Strains of *P. vivax* have intrinsic variability in their susceptibility to primaquine. For example, the Chesson strain, first isolated from an American soldier in Papua New Guinea in the 1940s, is less susceptible than other strains to primaquine. Because of this variability, an increased dose of primaquine (compared to the most common dose administered historically) is now recommended as standard treatment. Primaquine may also be used as a prophylactic agent.

Individuals with **glucose-6-phosphate dehydrogenase (G6PD) deficiency** have a limited ability to protect their erythrocytes against oxidative damage. G6PD is needed to reduce $NADP^+$ to NADPH, which converts oxidized **glutathione** to reduced glutathione. Reduced glutathione protects erythrocytes by catalyzing the breakdown of toxic oxidant compounds. The administration of primaquine causes significant oxidative stress because of the formation of numerous oxidized compounds. As a result, primaquine can induce massive and potentially fatal **hemolysis** in individuals with G6PD deficiency. Therefore, primaquine should never be administered to an individual without first confirming adequate G6PD activity in that individual's erythrocytes. *Primaquine should never be administered to pregnant women*, because primaquine crosses the placenta and can induce fatal hemolysis in fetal erythrocytes independent of maternal G6PD status. Primaquine can also cause gastrointestinal disturbances, methemoglobinemia, and, very rarely, neutropenia, hypertension, arrhythmias, and neurological symptoms.

Atovaquone

Atovaquone is a structural analogue of ubiquinone, the shuttling protein in the electron transport chain. Under physiologic conditions, the transfer of two electrons from reduced ubiquinone to the cytochrome bc_1 complex oxidizes the ubiquinone (Fig. 37-3). Atovaquone inhibits the interaction between reduced ubiquinone and the cytochrome bc_1 complex and thereby disrupts electron transport. Because plasmodia depend on the electron transport chain to regenerate oxidized dihydroorotate reductase, treatment with atovaquone disrupts pyrimidine synthesis and thereby prevents plasmodia from replicating their DNA. It is likely that inhibition of the electron transport chain also disrupts other steps in the intermediary metabolism of the parasite that depend on oxidation/reduction cycling of proteins.

The cytochrome bc_1 complex is a ubiquitous feature of eukaryotic organisms. The selectivity of atovaquone for plasmodia likely relies on differences in the sequences of amino acids between human and plasmodial ubiquinone–cytochrome bc_1 binding regions. Atovaquone inhibits the activity of plasmodial cytochrome bc_1 with approximately 100-fold selectivity compared to the human form of the protein. However, this selectivity is easily disrupted; a single point mutation in the cytochrome bc_1 complex can render plasmodia resistant to atovaquone. For this reason, atovaquone is not used as a single agent. Atovaquone can be co-administered with **doxycycline**, a protein synthesis inhibitor, or as a fixed combination with **proguanil**, a dihydrofolate reductase inhibitor (see discussion below). Proguanil and atovaquone are synergistic in their antimalarial activity. Interestingly, this synergy may not be related to proguanil's action as an antifolate, because other inhibitors of dihydrofolate reductase do not have synergistic effects with atovaquone. Instead, when administered with atovaquone, proguanil may act as an uncoupling agent in mitochondrial membranes, thereby enhancing atovaquone-mediated mitochondrial depolarization.

Atovaquone is generally well tolerated; its use is associated with a low incidence of adverse gastrointestinal effects and an occasional rash. In combination with a second antimalarial drug, atovaquone can be used both therapeutically and prophylactically.

Inhibitors of Translation
Doxycycline, Tetracycline, and Clindamycin

Agents that disrupt parasite protein synthesis include **doxycycline**, **tetracycline**, and **clindamycin**. Doxycycline is a structural isomer of tetracycline and is produced semisynthetically from oxytetracycline or methacycline. Doxycycline inhibits parasite protein synthesis by binding to the 30S ribosomal subunit, thereby blocking the binding of aminoacyl tRNA to mRNA (see Chapter 34, Pharmacology of Bacterial Infections: DNA Replication, Transcription, and Translation). By virtue of its high lipophilicity, doxycycline penetrates well into body tissues, has a large volume of distribution, and is reabsorbed in renal tubules and the gastrointestinal tract, resulting in a long half-life. Doxycycline's oral bioavailability and long half-life make it a useful drug (in combination with artesunate or quinine) for the treatment of chloroquine-resistant *P. falciparum*. Doxycycline should not be used as a single antimalarial agent. Adverse effects include cutaneous photosensitivity, tooth discoloration in children, and vaginal candidiasis; gastrointestinal effects (including nausea, diarrhea, and dyspepsia) are typically mild, although esophageal ulceration can occur rarely.

Tetracycline and doxycycline have similar pharmacologic profiles, but tetracycline must be taken four times a day. Tetracycline may be used in combination with quinine for the treatment of chloroquine-resistant malaria; however, it is not recommended as a malaria chemoprophylactic.

Clindamycin inhibits protein synthesis by binding to the 50S ribosomal subunit (see Chapter 34). Clindamycin may be used in combination with artesunate or quinine for the treatment of malaria when tetracycline or doxycycline is contraindicated (for example, in pregnant women or children less than 8 years of age). Clindamycin is usually well tolerated, especially in children; its major adverse effect is an increased risk of antibiotic-associated diarrhea caused by *Clostridium difficile*. Clindamycin is not used as a malaria chemoprophylactic.

Inhibitors of Folate Metabolism

Folic acid is a vitamin involved in the transfer of one-carbon units in a variety of biosynthetic pathways, including those of DNA and RNA precursors and certain amino acids (see Chapter 33). In humans, folate is an essential vitamin and must be ingested in the diet. In parasites and bacteria, folate is synthesized de novo, providing a useful target for selective drug action. Inhibition of folate metabolism can result in successful treatment of parasitic infections. In the context of malaria, antifolate drugs act against parasite-specific isoforms of dihydropteroate synthetase and dihydrofolate reductase. Combination therapies that include a sulfonamide and pyrimethamine were historically used. Two antimalarial formulations are available, **sulfadoxine–pyrimethamine** and the less frequently used **sulfalene–pyrimethamine**.

Sulfadoxine–Pyrimethamine

Sulfadoxine is a para-aminobenzoic acid (PABA) analogue that competitively inhibits parasite dihydropteroate synthetase, an essential enzyme in the folic acid synthesis pathway. **Pyrimethamine** is a folate analogue that competitively inhibits parasite dihydrofolate reductase, the enzyme that converts dihydrofolate to tetrahydrofolate (see Figs. 33-6 and 33-7). In combination, sulfadoxine and pyrimethamine act synergistically to inhibit growth of the malarial parasite.

Sulfonamide–pyrimethamine combinations were initially highly effective against blood schizont stages of *P. falciparum* malaria, but not against gametocytes, and were less effective against other species of malaria. Both drugs are highly protein-bound, resulting in long elimination half-lives. The long half-life of the combination provided selective pressure for the development of drug resistance in areas with high-level malaria transmission, and increasing resistance to this combination made it ineffective for treatment and prophylaxis in many parts of the world (Fig. 37-4).

Individuals infected with sensitive strains of malaria may be treated with sulfadoxine–pyrimethamine as a convenient single dose. The most serious drug reactions involve hypersensitivity to the sulfonamide component of the combination. Severe skin reactions such as Stevens-Johnson syndrome or erythema multiforme have been reported, but the incidence of these adverse effects is rare after single-dose therapy for malaria. Adverse hematologic effects include megaloblastic anemia, leukopenia, and thrombocytopenia. Sulfonamide–pyrimethamine is not used as a chemoprophylactic agent against malaria.

Proguanil

Proguanil is a derivative of pyrimidine and, like pyrimethamine, is an inhibitor of dihydrofolate reductase. Proguanil acts against the hepatic, pre-erythrocytic forms of *P. falciparum* and *P. vivax*. Proguanil has been used for prophylaxis in combination with chloroquine in areas of the world where chloroquine resistance is not widespread. However, other prophylactic agents are significantly more effective, and this combination is not recommended. Proguanil may be used in a synergistic combination with atovaquone for both treatment and prevention of malaria (discussed above). Proguanil is usually well tolerated, but it has been associated with oral ulcerations, pancytopenia, thrombocytopenia, and granulocytopenia.

Antimalarial Drug Resistance

Antimalarial drug resistance is a major public health problem and a significant barrier to the effective treatment of individuals with malaria. In association with the collapse of effective prevention efforts, lack of political will, and socioeconomic factors, the waning efficacy of antimalarial drugs contributed significantly to the increased burden of malaria morbidity and mortality observed worldwide from the 1980s to the early 2000s.

Chloroquine was the standard therapy for treating individuals with malaria for many years after its introduction in 1946. Resistance was first reported in the 1950s and steadily increased since then; at present, resistance has been reported everywhere in the world except on the island of Hispaniola and in focal parts of Central America, South America, and Asia. The chloroquine-resistance *P. falciparum* haplotype has recently been detected in Haiti, but clinical resistance has not yet been reported. Childhood mortality doubled in eastern and southern Africa in the 1980s and 1990s as chloroquine and sulfadoxine–pyrimethamine resistance increased; chloroquine resistance was associated with an overall doubling of childhood mortality from malaria during this period, with increases as high as 11-fold in certain areas. Similarly, *P. vivax* resistance to chloroquine was unknown until 1989 but is now endemic in Indonesia and Papua New Guinea. Reports of chloroquine-resistant *P. vivax* have also emerged in South America, Brazil, Myanmar, and India.

Resistance to sulfadoxine–pyrimethamine was reported after the combination was introduced in 1971 as a second-line therapy for treating individuals with chloroquine-resistant *P. falciparum*. Resistance to sulfadoxine–pyrimethamine was initially reported in Southeast Asia but is now relatively widespread in South America and prevalent in Africa as well.

Strains of *P. falciparum* resistant to mefloquine were noted in Southeast Asia following the widespread introduction of this agent in the 1980s. Mefloquine resistance has not spread more widely as yet, in large measure due to the fact that the drug is not now routinely used to treat individuals with malaria.

Strains of *P. falciparum* with increasing resistance to artemisinin were first reported in Cambodia and have also been reported in Vietnam, Myanmar, and Thailand.

Many factors contribute to the development of drug resistance by malaria parasites, including inappropriate and/or unsupervised drug use, inconsistent drug availability, poor adherence to treatment regimens due to adverse effects and other factors, inconsistent quality of drug manufacturing, presence of counterfeit drugs, and prohibitive drug costs. Combining therapies to reduce the development of resistance is a strategy that has long been employed in the treatment of individuals with tuberculosis, leprosy, and HIV infection, and this approach is strongly recommended in the treatment of individuals with malaria. The WHO has demanded cessation of production of all stand-alone artemisinin products and has requested that only two-drug, fixed-combination, artemisinin-containing products be manufactured. Although rapidly acting artemisinins reduce parasite burden by a factor of 10^4 with every treatment cycle, resulting in rapid clearance of parasites from the bloodstream, the short half-life of artemisinins favors the possibility of recrudescence of infection and the risk of selective pressure for drug resistance. To counter these risks, the WHO recommends combining an artemisinin with a slowly eliminated blood schizonticidal agent.

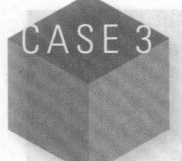

CASE 3   Mr. S, a 29-year-old American journalist, returns from a trip to Southeast Asia. He feels fine for 5 weeks but then begins to experience mild diarrhea, abdominal pain, and malaise. He does not attribute his symptoms to the trip, because they developed well after he returned home. Furthermore, Mr. S's wife shared the same food and water during the trip, and she remains well. As a result, Mr. S ignores the symptoms for a week, but he eventually goes to his physician when the symptoms do not abate spontaneously. Physical examination reveals tenderness in the right upper quadrant of the abdomen. Blood tests are notable for elevated liver enzymes, and a computed tomography (CT) scan reveals a liver abscess. Stool examination is positive for heme and for *E. histolytica* cysts. He is prescribed metronidazole for 10 days, after which he takes paromomycin for an additional week. Follow-up imaging confirms regression of Mr. S's liver abscess.

Questions

6. Why is Mr. S's wife asymptomatic?

7. What are the potential adverse effects of metronidazole?

8. Why was Mr. S prescribed paromomycin after a course of metronidazole?

OTHER PROTOZOA

In addition to plasmodium, other medically important protozoa include *Entamoeba histolytica*, the organism that causes amebiasis; *Giardia lamblia*, the organism that causes giardiasis; *Cryptosporidium hominis/parvum*, the organism that causes cryptosporidiosis; *Trypanosoma brucei rhodesiense* and *T. b. gambiense*, the causative agents of African sleeping sickness; *Trypanosoma cruzi*, the causative agent of Chagas' disease; and *Leishmania* spp., the causative agents of leishmaniasis. Because more is known about *E. histolytica*, the following physiology section focuses on this parasite; however, the pharmacology section includes not only agents effective against amebiasis but also agents effective against African sleeping sickness, Chagas' disease, and leishmaniasis.

Physiology of Luminal Protozoa

The enteric protozoa *Entamoeba dispar* and *E. histolytica* are morphologically indistinguishable, although these two species can be differentiated using specific monoclonal antibodies. *E. dispar* does not cause invasive disease (i.e., it does not compromise the gut epithelium), but *E. histolytica* can cause an asymptomatic carrier state, invasive colitis, or so-called metastatic infections (usually hepatic abscesses).

Five percent to 10% of individuals who live in poverty in the developing world have serologic evidence of previous *E. histolytica* infection. It is estimated that 50 million cases of dysentery are caused by *E. histolytica* each year, resulting in tens of thousands of deaths. Because Mr. S's wife shared the same food and water with her husband, she was also likely infected with *E. histolytica*. For unclear reasons, she excreted *E. histolytica* asymptomatically, while her husband developed invasive disease.

Life Cycle of *Entamoeba histolytica*

Colonic infection with *E. histolytica* occurs as a result of ingestion of cysts through the fecal–oral route, for example, drinking contaminated water. Whether intestinal invasion occurs may be a function of the number of cysts ingested, the strain of the parasite, the motility of the host gastrointestinal tract, and the presence of appropriate enteric bacteria to serve as nourishment for the ameba. Disease results when active trophozoites invade the intestinal epithelium, and secondary spread to the liver can occur via the portal circulation (Fig. 37-6). As its name implies, *E. histolytica* lyses and destroys human tissue. Trophozoites typically multiply superficial to the muscularis mucosae of the intestines and spread laterally. They may also penetrate more deeply, occasionally perforating the intestinal wall and spreading locally. Seeding of the liver is also common. In Mr. S's case, a CT scan revealed involvement of the liver with formation of an abscess.

E. histolytica exists in two forms: the inactive but infective **cyst** and the active **trophozoite**. Cysts are ingested in contaminated food or water. Excystation occurs in the small intestine, where the trophozoites mature. The trophozoite form is capable of invading host tissue. Inside the human body, the trophozoites move using pseudopods and ingest bacteria, other protozoa, and host red blood cells. A trophozoite can convert to a binucleated cyst form, which matures into a tetranucleated cyst that travels through the colon but is not capable of mucosal invasion (Fig. 37-6).

Symptoms due to amebiasis vary from diarrhea and abdominal cramps to fulminant dysentery and hepatic abscess formation. Fewer than 40% of individuals with amebic dysentery develop fever, and microscopic evaluation of the stool typically discloses few neutrophils. The onset of symptoms can range from a few days to a year after exposure, or symptoms may never occur. Mr. S's symptoms did not develop until at least a month after exposure, giving him reason not to attribute his symptoms to his travels.

Fermentation Pathways

E. histolytica and other luminal parasites are a diverse group of eukaryotes with novel adaptations to their anaerobic niche. For example, *E. histolytica* lacks **fermentation enzymes** (lactate dehydrogenase and pyruvate decarboxylase) that are present in yeast and other eukaryotes. Ameba also lack enzymes of oxidative phosphorylation, the Krebs cycle, and pyruvate dehydrogenase. Instead, ameba (and many anaerobic organisms) utilize novel enzymes to provide a source for the electron transfers that drive metabolism.

Ameba are obligate fermenters of glucose to ethanol (Fig. 37-7). Many of these fermentation enzymes, which are missing in humans, yeast, and most eubacteria, contain a set of

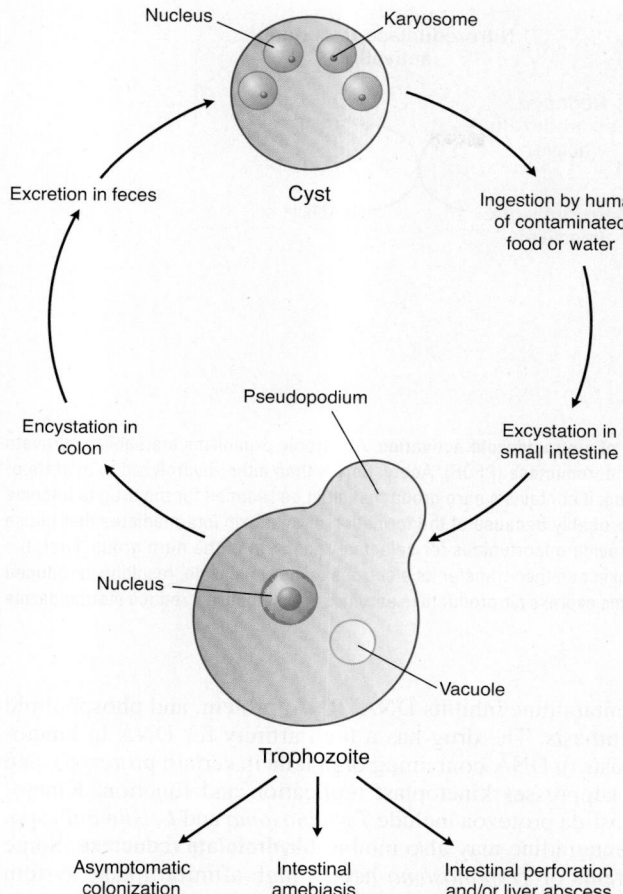

Cyst

Nucleus   Karyosome

Excretion in feces

Ingestion by human of contaminated food or water

Encystation in colon

Excystation in small intestine

Pseudopodium

Nucleus

Vacuole

Trophozoite

Asymptomatic colonization

Intestinal amebiasis

Intestinal perforation and/or liver abscess

FIGURE 37-6. Manifestations of amebiasis. Ingestion of *Entamoeba histolytica* cysts can result in several different clinical outcomes, ranging from asymptomatic excretion of the cysts to invasive disease. Asymptomatic infection occurs when the ingested cysts excyst (mature) in the small intestine but do not invade the intestinal mucosa. These trophozoites then encyst in the colon, and excretion occurs in the feces. Invasive disease results when active trophozoites invade the intestinal epithelium. This invasion can result in asymptomatic colonization, intestinal amebiasis (amebic dysentery)—which is characterized by diarrhea and abdominal cramps—or intestinal perforation. Spread of infection via the portal vein can cause liver abscesses.

iron–sulfur centers called **ferredoxins** that transfer electrons under strongly reducing (anaerobic) conditions. This activity is in contrast to that of heme and cytochromes, which use iron centers to transfer electrons under oxidizing (aerobic) conditions. **Pyruvate-ferredoxin oxidoreductase** (**PFOR**), which contains a single ferredoxin domain, catalyzes the decarboxylation of pyruvate to acetyl CoA, with the production of CO_2. PFOR activity also produces reduced ferredoxin, which can reduce protons to form hydrogen gas or reduce $NADP^+$ to NADPH. Acetyl CoA is reduced to ethanol via alcohol dehydrogenase E (ADHE), with the recovery of two NAD^+ cofactors. Anaerobic bacteria (e.g., *Helicobacter* spp. and *Clostridia* spp.) express PFORs, ferredoxins, and ADHEs similar to those of luminal protozoa. Indeed, phylogenetic analyses suggest that most of the genes encoding parasite fermentation enzymes, and many of the genes encoding parasite enzymes involved in core energy metabolism, have been laterally transferred from anaerobic bacteria. Although lateral gene transfer is extraordinarily frequent between bacteria, it

is extremely rare between bacteria and higher eukaryotes, which (except for parasites such as *E. histolytica* that share environmental niches with bacteria) maintain their gametes in a sterile environment.

Pharmacology of Antiprotozoal Agents

Metronidazole

Metronidazole is inactive until it is reduced within host or microbial cells that possess a large negative redox potential; such redox potentials are present in many anaerobic or microaerophilic luminal parasites. Activation can occur by interaction with reduced ferredoxin or with specific nitroreductases (Fig. 37-7). Activated metronidazole forms reduced cytotoxic compounds that bind to proteins, membranes, and DNA in target cells, causing severe damage.

Metronidazole sensitivity is directly related to the presence of PFOR activity. Most eukaryotes and eubacteria lack PFOR and therefore fail to activate metronidazole. However, in poorly oxygenated tissues such as abscesses, metronidazole can be activated. Because PFOR is expressed in protozoa but has no counterpart in mammalian systems, the drug is selectively toxic for ameba and anaerobic organisms.

The widespread use of metronidazole has led to drug resistance in *Helicobacter pylori*, a common bacterial cause of gastritis and peptic ulcers (see Chapter 47, Integrative Inflammation Pharmacology: Peptic Ulcer Disease). This resistance is due to a null mutation in the *rdxA* gene, which encodes an oxygen-insensitive NADPH nitroreductase. Low-level resistance to metronidazole has also been observed in a number of anaerobic protozoa, including trichomonads (caused by decreased expression of ferredoxin), *Giardia* (caused by decreased PFOR activity and decreased drug permeability), and ameba (caused by increased expression of **superoxide dismutase**). Metronidazole resistance among luminal parasites has not yet become clinically important, however.

There are three explanations for the slow development of resistance to metronidazole among luminal parasites. First, luminal parasites are generally diploid, so a single mutation will not typically confer resistance. This contrasts with the case of haploid bacteria and certain haploid stages of *P. falciparum*, in which resistance develops more quickly. Second, luminal parasites have few metabolic alternatives to PFOR activity. Third, metronidazole is hydrophilic, so overexpression or modification of P-glycoprotein, which confers resistance to hydrophobic drugs, does not increase metronidazole efflux.

Adverse effects of metronidazole include gastrointestinal discomfort, headaches, occasional neuropathy, a metallic taste, and nausea. Metronidazole also causes nausea and flushing when taken concomitantly with alcohol (a so-called disulfiram-like effect, caused by inhibition of ethanol metabolism). Metronidazole is active against *E. histolytica* trophozoites in tissues, but it has much less activity against intraluminal ameba (probably, in large part, because of the drug's extensive absorption in the upper gastrointestinal tract, leading to its low drug concentration in the lumen of the colon, where the ameba live). Therefore, individuals with invasive amebiasis are typically treated first with metronidazole (to eradicate trophozoites that are actively invading human tissue) and then with a second agent that has more intraluminal activity, such as **iodoquinol** or **paromomycin**. The latter two agents kill ameba by unknown mechanisms but are poorly absorbed from the gastrointestinal tract and therefore reach high concentrations in the lumen of the colon.

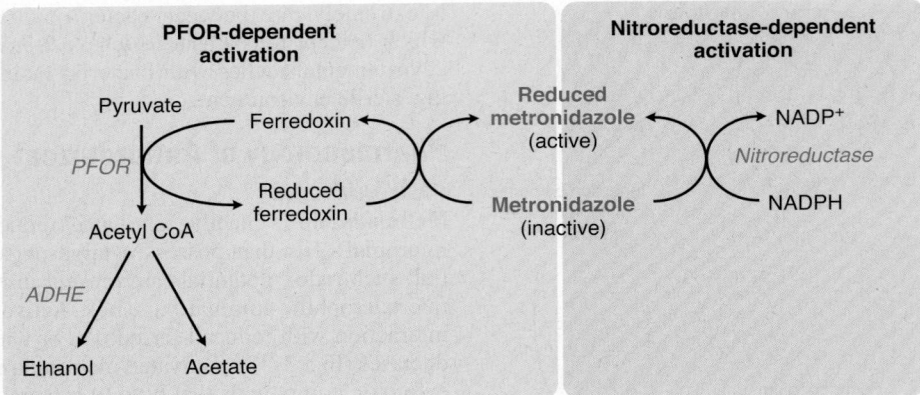

FIGURE 37-7. Fermentation enzymes of anaerobic organisms and mechanisms of metronidazole activation. Anaerobic organisms metabolize pyruvate to acetyl CoA; this conversion is catalyzed by the enzyme pyruvate-ferredoxin oxidoreductase (PFOR). Acetyl CoA is then either hydrolyzed to acetate or oxidized to ethanol by alcohol dehydrogenase E (ADHE). Metronidazole is a prodrug; it contains a nitro group that must be reduced for the drug to become active. Reduced metronidazole is highly effective against anaerobic organisms, probably because of the formation of cytotoxic intermediates that cause DNA, protein, and membrane damage. Two aspects of anaerobic metabolism provide opportunities for selective reduction of the nitro group. First, the reaction catalyzed by PFOR results in the reduction of ferredoxin; reduced ferredoxin can then transfer its electrons to metronidazole, resulting in reduced (active) metronidazole and reoxidized ferredoxin. Second, many anaerobic organisms express nitroreductase enzymes that selectively reduce metronidazole and, in the process, oxidize NADPH to $NADP^+$.

Tinidazole

Tinidazole, a second-generation nitroimidazole related to metronidazole, is also effective against a number of protozoa and is licensed for the treatment of giardiasis, amebiasis, and vaginal trichomoniasis. Its mechanism of action is unclear but is believed to be similar to that of metronidazole and related to the generation of cytotoxic free radicals. A particular benefit of tinidazole is that the duration of a therapeutic course of the drug is shorter than that of metronidazole. Tinidazole is also better tolerated than metronidazole, but it is similarly ineffective as a luminicidal agent for the treatment of ameba infections. Adverse effects are rare and mild, including gastrointestinal discomfort and the occasional development of a metallic taste. Tinidazole is not recommended for use during the first trimester of pregnancy, during breastfeeding, and in children less than 3 years of age.

Nitazoxanide

Nitazoxanide is a nitrothiazolyl-salicylamide derivative structurally related to metronidazole. Nitazoxanide has a broad spectrum of action, including activity against protozoa, anaerobic bacteria, and helminths. It is approved in the United States for use in children with giardiasis and in adults and children with cryptosporidiosis. As a structural analogue of thiamine pyrophosphate, nitazoxanide inhibits the PFOR that converts pyruvate to acetyl CoA in protozoa and anaerobic bacteria (Fig. 37-7). Its mechanism of action against helminths is unclear. After oral administration, nitazoxanide is rapidly hydrolyzed to the active metabolite tizoxanide. The active metabolite is excreted in urine, bile, and feces. Nitazoxanide is usually well tolerated with few reported adverse effects.

Other Antiprotozoal Agents

Pentamidine can be used to treat early-stage African trypanosomiasis (African sleeping sickness), which is caused by *Trypanosoma brucei gambiense* and certain strains of *T. b. rhodesiense*. Early-stage trypanosomiasis is defined as disease that does not involve the central nervous system (CNS).

Pentamidine inhibits DNA, RNA, protein, and phospholipid synthesis. The drug has a high affinity for DNA in kinetoplasts (a DNA-containing organelle in certain protozoa), and it suppresses kinetoplast replication and function. Kinetoplastida protozoa include *Trypanosoma* and *Leishmania* spp. Pentamidine may also inhibit **dihydrofolate reductase**. Some strains of *Trypanosoma* have a high-affinity uptake system for the drug, contributing to its selectivity. Pentamidine can cause fatigue, dizziness, hypotension, pancreatitis, and kidney damage. Pentamidine is now used most commonly as a third- or fourth-line treatment for individuals with ***Pneumocystis jiroveci (P. carinii)*** pneumonia (PCP), a common infection in patients with AIDS.

Suramin is another drug used to treat early-stage African trypanosomiasis. Suramin interacts with many macromolecules and inhibits numerous enzymes, including those involved in energy metabolism (e.g., glycerol phosphate dehydrogenase). It also inhibits RNA polymerase and thus interferes with parasite replication. Suramin can cause pruritus, paresthesias, vomiting, and nausea. The biochemical basis for suramin's relative selectivity for African trypanosomiasis is not well understood.

Melarsoprol is used as a first-line drug in the treatment of late-stage African trypanosomiasis (i.e., disease that involves the CNS). Melarsoprol was developed by conjugating the heavy metal chelator dimercaptopropanol to the trivalent arsenic of melarsen oxide. The drug is insoluble in water and is instead dissolved in propylene glycol. Blood trypanosomes lack a functional tricarboxylic acid cycle and are entirely dependent on glycolysis for ATP production. Melarsoprol inhibits trypanosomal pyruvate kinase, thereby inhibiting glycolysis and decreasing ATP production. Affected trypanosomes quickly lose motility and lyse. Melarsoprol also inhibits the uptake of adenine and adenosine by trypanosomal transporters. Mammalian cells are less permeable to the drug than are trypanosomes, and the drug has some selectivity on this basis. Unfortunately, melarsoprol is still quite toxic to humans (4–6% death rate). Melarsoprol is administered intravenously and can cause severe phlebitis.

It is also corrosive to plastics, limiting storage and administration options. In addition, 5–10% of individuals with late-stage African trypanosomiasis develop intense inflammation of the brain after administration of melarsoprol (*reactive encephalopathy*); this complication is associated with a mortality rate of greater than 50%. Concomitant administration of corticosteroids lessens the likelihood of reactive encephalopathy. Polyneuropathy after melarsoprol administration is also common (10%) and can be lessened by concomitant administration of thiamine.

Eflornithine (α-difluoromethylornithine) is a much less toxic alternative to melarsoprol in the treatment of African trypanosomiasis caused by *T. b. gambiense* (West Africa sleeping sickness). Eflornithine is highly effective against both early- and late-stage West African sleeping sickness but not against East African trypanosomiasis (caused by *T. b. rhodesiense*). Eflornithine is a selective and irreversible inhibitor of **ornithine decarboxylase** and thus of polyamine synthesis. Ornithine decarboxylase converts ornithine to putrescine; this is a rate-limiting step in the synthesis of putrescine and the polyamines spermine and spermidine. Polyamines are involved in nucleic acid synthesis and the regulation of protein synthesis. *T. b. gambiense* organisms are susceptible to eflornithine, possibly because of the slow turnover of ornithine decarboxylase in these parasites; *T. b. rhodesiense* organisms have a higher rate of turnover (as do human cells) and are less sensitive.

Nifurtimox is used in the treatment of New World trypanosomiasis (Chagas' disease), which is caused by *Trypanosoma cruzi*. The drug undergoes reduction and generates toxic intracellular oxygen radicals in the parasite. It first forms reduced intermediates such as nitro anion radicals. These radicals can then be reoxidized and, in the process, generate **superoxide** anions, which react with water to produce cytotoxic hydrogen peroxide. Some parasites, such as trypanosomes, lack **catalase** and other enzymes capable of degrading hydrogen peroxide. Such parasites are thus sensitive to the toxicity of nitro aromatic drugs. Mammalian cells are protected because of their complement of antioxidant enzymes such as catalase, glutathione peroxidase, and superoxide dismutase. Nifurtimox can cause anorexia, vomiting, memory loss, sleep disorders, and seizures.

Sodium stibogluconate and **meglumine antimonate** are used to treat leishmaniasis, which is caused by parasites of the genus *Leishmania*. These agents contain pentavalent antimony and act by an unknown mechanism. It is postulated that these drugs inhibit the glycolytic pathway and fatty acid oxidation, processes that are crucial for intermediary metabolism. Pentavalent antimony can also have many non-specific effects, such as modification of sulfhydryl groups. These drugs can cause bone marrow suppression, a prolonged QT interval, pancreatitis, and rash.

Resistance of *Leishmania* to antimonial agents is being recognized with increasing frequency, especially in South Asia. Alternative agents include **amphotericin** and **miltefosine**. The mechanism of action of miltefosine is unknown. It is a synthetic ether phospholipid analogue that is chemically similar to natural phospholipids present in cell membranes. Miltefosine has been shown to have antineoplastic, immunomodulatory, and antiprotozoal activity. It is presumed that the cytostatic and cytotoxic effects of miltefosine are caused by inhibition of enzyme systems associated with plasma membranes (such as protein kinase C) and inhibition of phosphatidylcholine biosynthesis. Miltefosine may also inhibit platelet activating factor-induced responses and inositol phosphate formation. The immunomodulatory effects of miltefosine include T-cell activation, interferon-gamma production in peripheral mononuclear cells, and increased interleukin-2 receptor and HLA-DR expression. The drug received FDA approval in 2014 and can be administered orally to treat patients with leishmaniasis. Use of miltefosine may be associated with late clinical relapse of leishmaniasis.

HELMINTHS

Helminths are multicellular worms with digestive, excretory, nervous, and reproductive systems. Parasitic helminths can infect the liver, blood, intestines, and other tissues in human hosts. Clinically significant worms can be divided phylogenetically into three classes: **nematodes** (roundworms), **trematodes** (flukes), and **cestodes** (tapeworms). The presence of a rudimentary nervous system provides a number of possible targets for antihelminthic agents. The physiology of *Onchocerca volvulus*, which causes onchocerciasis ("river blindness"), provides an example of potential targets for antihelminthic drugs. Although the majority of the following discussion focuses on the physiology and pharmacology of onchocerciasis, several other antihelminthic agents are also presented.

Physiology of Helminths

Humans can become infected with helminths when they ingest food or water contaminated with eggs or larvae. In addition, larvae in soil can penetrate human skin, and insects can transmit still other larvae through bites. If humans are the definitive host, the eggs or larvae develop into adult worms

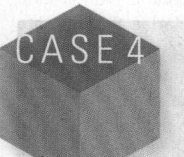

CASE 4   Thumbi is a boy who enjoys fishing in a river near his village in the Democratic Republic of Congo. At the age of 13, he emigrates with his family to the United States. Shortly thereafter, he begins to scratch his arms and legs vigorously. Six months later, his mother brings him to a dermatologist. Physical examination reveals a macular and papular rash with excoriations on the arms and legs, as well as a few subcutaneous nodules. Examination of peripheral blood discloses high-level eosinophilia.

A nodule is excised and examined by a pathologist, leading to a diagnosis. Thumbi begins treatment with ivermectin but returns the next day feverish and feeling more itchy than before.

Questions

9. What did the pathologist see in the subcutaneous nodule?

10. Why did Thumbi feel worse immediately after treatment with ivermectin?

that can migrate through tissues and enter the sexual stage. During the sexual stage, adult worms release additional eggs or larvae, which can then pass out of the host through the gastrointestinal or urinary tracts. Larvae in humans can also be ingested by insects during a blood meal. In the environment or within vector hosts, eggs or larvae then become infective for humans, and the cycles start over.

Life Cycle of Onchocerca volvulus

Onchocerciasis is one of eight human filarial infections (a specific type of nematodal worm infection). In Thumbi's case, an infected *Simulium* spp. blackfly bit and inoculated *O. volvulus* larvae into his skin in Africa. Adult worms then developed in Thumbi's subcutaneous tissues. These adult male and female filarial worms came to rest in subcutaneous nodules, in which they mated (Fig. 37-8). Adult worms are large (3–80 cm in length), look like angel-hair pasta, and can live for 10–15 years. The nodules have a characteristic appearance that was recognized by the pathologist. From these nodules (onchocercomata), gravid females release millions of microfilariae, which migrate freely through the skin and cornea. If ingested by a *Simulium* fly, additional maturation can occur, and the cycle can continue. The diagnosis of onchocerciasis is usually based on microscopic detection of microfilariae in skin snips, not on pathological examination of excised onchocercomata. Microfilariae are small (200–400 μm); as they degenerate and die, they cause local inflammatory reactions, provoking itching, dermatitis, and, eventually, scarring. When microfilariae die in the cornea, they induce a punctate keratitis that, over years, leads to scarring and blindness. Such ocular involvement made onchocerciasis a leading cause of infectious blindness in the world (along with trachoma) and is the reason onchocerciasis is also referred to as "river blindness" (also reflecting the fact that the blackflies carrying the larvae inhabit areas with flowing streams, such as the one in which Thumbi enjoyed fishing). Without treatment, Thumbi could well become one of the thousands of individuals in the world who are currently blind or visually impaired from onchocerciasis.

Neuromuscular Activity

The subcuticular layer of longitudinal muscle in nematodes is inhibited by **glutamate** and **gamma-aminobutyric acid (GABA)** and excited by **acetylcholine**. The motor neurons of invertebrates are unmyelinated, making them more vulnerable to neurotoxins than the myelinated somatic motor neurons of humans. (See Chapter 9, Principles of Nervous System Physiology and Pharmacology, for more information on the human nervous system.) Many antihelminthic agents modulate parasite neuromuscular activity by enhancing inhibitory signaling, antagonizing excitatory signaling (nondepolarizing block), or tonically stimulating excitatory signaling (depolarizing block).

Pharmacology of Antihelminthic Agents

Agents That Interrupt Neuromuscular Activity
Ivermectin

Ivermectin is a semisynthetic macrocyclic lactone that acts against a broad range of helminths and arthropods and that has been used most extensively to treat and control onchocerciasis. Ivermectin's exact mechanism of action is unclear, but studies in *Caenorhabditis elegans* (a soil helminth that is studied extensively in eukaryotic biology as a simple model organism) suggest that the mechanism of action

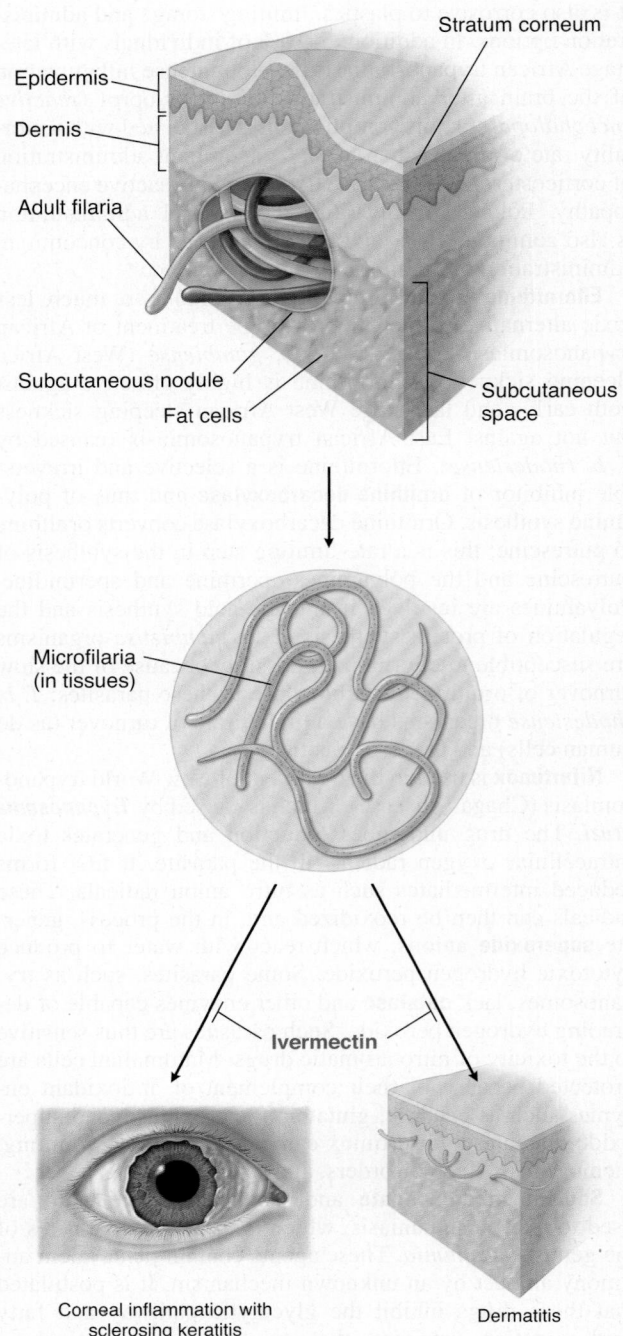

FIGURE 37-8. Life cycle of *Onchocerca volvulus*. Adult filarial worms mate in subcutaneous nodules in humans, releasing microfilariae that migrate through the skin and subcutaneous tissues and cause dermatitis and pruritus as they die. Microfilariae that die in the cornea induce ocular inflammation, which can lead to corneal scarring and blindness ("river blindness"). Ivermectin, the agent of choice for treating individuals with onchocerciasis, is effective only against microfilariae; the drug does not kill adult filarial worms.

involves potentiation and/or direct activation of **glutamate-gated chloride channels** in nematode plasma membranes. This results in hyperpolarization of neuromuscular cells and causes pharyngeal paralysis. (Note that the glutamate-gated chloride channels in nematodes mediate *inhibitory* neurotransmission, unlike the *excitatory* glutamate-gated cation channels in humans.) Ivermectin is also thought to affect **GABA** inhibitory transmission by potentiating the release of GABA from presynaptic terminals, directly activating GABA receptors, and/or potentiating the binding of GABA to its receptor. All of these effects increase GABA-mediated transmission of signals in peripheral nerves, resulting in hyperpolarization. The net effect is variable, depending on the nematode model system under study, but *the ultimate result is blockade of neuromuscular transmission and paralysis of the worm.*

Pharyngeal paralysis of *O. volvulus* inhibits nutrient uptake and kills developing larvae (microfilariae). Unfortunately, ivermectin does not kill adult filarial worms. It does, however, destroy microfilariae in utero, thereby preventing production and release of new microfilariae from adult female worms for at least 6 months. Thus, ivermectin is used to prevent microfilaria-mediated ocular damage and to decrease human-to-vector transmission (because microfilariae are infectious to *Simulium* flies), but it cannot cure human hosts of *O. volvulus* infection. Because the drug is noncurative, it is typically administered to infected humans every 6–12 months for the life expectancy of the adult worms (5–10 years).

Ivermectin does interact with GABA receptors in vertebrates, but its affinity for invertebrate GABA receptors is about 100-fold greater. Cestodes and trematodes lack high-affinity ivermectin receptors, which may explain the resistance of these organisms to the drug. GABA receptors in humans are present mainly in the CNS, but because ivermectin does not cross the blood–brain barrier, the drug is generally well tolerated. When the blood–brain barrier is hyperpermeable, as in patients with meningitis, ivermectin can be more toxic and can result in headaches, ataxia, and coma. Adverse effects of ivermectin are usually attributable to inflammatory or allergic responses to dying microfilariae (i.e., Mazzotti reaction) and include headaches, dizziness, weakness, rash, pruritus, edema, abdominal pain, hypotension, and fever. This is why Thumbi felt worse the day after initiation of treatment.

Ivermectin is widely used to treat animals with nematode infections, and resistance to ivermectin is already recognized in livestock parasites. Although the exact mechanism of resistance is unknown, the P-glycoprotein may be involved. In studies of mice, hypersensitivity to ivermectin results from disruption of the *mdr1a* gene, which encodes a P-glycoprotein membrane transporter. Furthermore, analysis of P-glycoprotein cDNA from *Haemonchus contortus* (a nematode of veterinary importance) shows 65% homology to P-glycoprotein/multidrug resistance (MDR) protein sequences in mice and humans. P-glycoprotein mRNA expression is higher in ivermectin-selected strains of *H. contortus* than in unselected strains, and verapamil, which reverses multidrug resistance by blocking P-glycoprotein channels, increases the efficacy of ivermectin. Fortunately, clinically important resistance in humans has not yet been documented.

In addition to its use in the treatment of onchocerciasis, ivermectin is used to treat strongyloidiasis and cutaneous larva migrans (both are nematodal infections) and scabies (an ectoparasitic infestation).

Piperazine and Pyrantel Pamoate

Piperazine and **pyrantel pamoate** are antihelminthic agents of primarily historical interest. They are discussed briefly in the Drug Summary Table.

Other Antihelminthic Agents

Albendazole, **mebendazole**, and **thiabendazole** inhibit tubulin polymerization by binding to β-tubulin. Evidence suggests that these agents are selective for the nematodal isoform of β-tubulin, thus decreasing host toxicity. Inhibition of tubulin polymerization disrupts nematodal motility and DNA replication (see Chapter 39), leading to degenerative changes in integumental and intestinal cells of helminths and, eventually, causing immobilization and death of the worms. The effects of the drugs against immotile tissue forms of cestodal larval parasites (e.g., cysticercosis and echinococcosis) are less well understood but may also involve β-tubulin binding. In this case, the drugs disrupt the integumental integrity of the protoscolex, a larval structure that eventually becomes the "head" of the adult cestode. Thiabendazole causes significant nausea, vomiting, and anorexia at therapeutic doses and is rarely used. Mebendazole and albendazole are better tolerated, and albendazole has the highest oral bioavailability of the three drugs.

Praziquantel is the drug of choice for treating adult cestode (tapeworm) and trematode (fluke) infections. Most importantly, praziquantel is the drug of choice for treating individuals with schistosomiasis, a trematodal infection that causes considerable morbidity and mortality worldwide. Although the exact mechanism of praziquantel's action is unknown, it appears to increase parasite membrane permeability to calcium, resulting in contraction and paralysis of the worms. The main adverse effects of praziquantel include nausea, headache, and abdominal discomfort.

Diethylcarbamazine (**DEC**), a piperazine derivative, is the drug of choice for treating certain filarial infections, including lymphatic filariasis. Its use in the treatment of filarial onchocerciasis has been largely supplanted by the use of ivermectin (predominantly because of ivermectin's tolerability and ease of administration). Unlike ivermectin, however, DEC kills adult filarial worms and is thus a curative agent. DEC's mechanism of action is unknown; current hypotheses include stimulation of innate immune mechanisms, inhibition of microtubule polymerization, and inhibition of arachidonic acid metabolism. DEC is reasonably well tolerated at low doses; its major adverse effects include anorexia, headache, and nausea. Administration of DEC can, however, precipitate Mazzotti reactions in individuals with heavy microfilarial burdens, and such reactions can be fatal. Administration of gradually increasing doses of DEC minimizes this possibility. DEC is excreted by the kidneys, and dosing may need to be adjusted in individuals with decreased kidney function.

Antibacterial agents may also have a role in treating certain helminthic infections. For example, *O. volvulus* has been found to contain an obligate symbiont (*Wolbachia* endobacteria) important in helminth fertility, and the use of doxycycline to treat individuals with onchocerciasis leads to decreased fertility, embryogenesis, and viability of *O. volvulus*.

■ CONCLUSION AND FUTURE DIRECTIONS

The development of new antiparasitic agents will rely on continued exploitation of molecular and metabolic differences between parasites and hosts. Recent advances in the application of molecular biological and genetic techniques to study parasitic eukaryotes, and detailed knowledge of parasite, vector, and host genomes, transcriptomes, and proteomes, should facilitate the development of more selective agents effective against many parasitic infections. The development of resistance to antiparasitic agents is of increasing concern, most notably among malarial and leishmanial parasites, and will necessitate both the judicious use of currently available agents and the development of new agents, including antiparasitic vaccines.

Despite long-standing efforts to develop effective treatments for malaria, the disease remains a major global cause of morbidity and mortality, although progress is being made. Development of an effective malaria vaccine could have a major impact on this global burden. However, the development of an effective vaccine has been hampered by a number of difficult scientific challenges, including the diversity of parasite species and strains, the diversity of parasite life forms, the intracellular location of the parasites, and the ability of *P. falciparum* to undergo antigenic variation. The situation has been worsened by the lack of meaningful economic incentives for vaccine development. Unfortunately, the complexity of the parasites and of their intimate relationship with infected hosts suggests that the development of effective antiparasite vaccines (especially against malaria) will be difficult.

Suggested Reading

Babokhov P, Sanyaolu AO, Oyibo WA, Fagbenro-Beyioku AF, Iriemenam NC. A current analysis of chemotherapy strategies for the treatment of human African trypanosomiasis. *Pathog Glob Health* 2013;107:242–252. (*Reviews treatment options and strategies for treating human African trypanosomiasis ["sleeping sickness"].*)

Dorlo TP, Balasegaram M, Beijnen JH, de Vries PJ. Miltefosine: a review of its pharmacology and therapeutic efficacy in the treatment of leishmaniasis. *J Antimicrob Chemother* 2012;67:2576–2597. (*Reviews use of miltefosine in patients with leishmaniasis.*)

Fairhurst RM, Nayyar GM, Breman JG, et al. Artemisinin-resistant malaria: research challenges, opportunities, and public health implications. *Am J Trop Med Hyg* 2012;87:231–241. (*Discusses implications of increasing artemisinin resistance among malaria-causing Plasmodium falciparum.*)

González P, González FA, Ueno K. Ivermectin in human medicine, an overview of the current status of its clinical applications. *Curr Pharm Biotechnol* 2012;13:1103–1109. (*Reviews current uses of this important antiparasitic agent.*)

Martin C, Gavotte L. The bacteria Wolbachia in filariae, a biological Russian dolls' system: new trends in antifilarial treatments. *Parasite* 2010;17:79–89. (*Discusses the potential of using drugs that target bacteria [Wolbachia] within parasites to treat patients with parasitic infections.*)

DRUG SUMMARY TABLE: CHAPTER 37 Pharmacology of Parasitic Infections

ANTIMALARIAL AGENTS: INHIBITORS OF HEME METABOLISM
Mechanism—Decrease the metabolism and/or removal of toxic heme products, resulting in increased toxicity to the plasmodia

DRUG	CLINICAL APPLICATIONS	SERIOUS AND COMMON ADVERSE EFFECTS	CONTRAINDICATIONS	THERAPEUTIC CONSIDERATIONS
Chloroquine	Malaria, all species	AV block, heart failure, prolonged QT interval, Stevens-Johnson syndrome, neutropenia, extrapyramidal disease, seizure, retinopathy	Visual field changes Hypersensitivity to 4-aminoquinoline compounds	Protonated chloroquine accumulates inside the parasite's food vacuole, where it binds to ferriprotoporphyrin IX (heme) and inhibits its polymerization; accumulation of unpolymerized ferriprotoporphyrin IX leads to oxidative membrane damage. Most strains of *P. falciparum* in Africa, Asia, and South America have developed resistance to chloroquine. Kills only erythrocytic stage of plasmodial infections. Used therapeutically and prophylactically.
Quinine Quinidine (See Chapter 24)	Malaria, especially *P. falciparum*	Prolonged PR interval, prolonged QT interval, torsades de pointes, wide QRS complex, agranulocytosis, thrombocytopenia, disseminated intravascular coagulation, hemolysis, thrombocytopenic purpura, hepatotoxicity, ototoxicity, renal failure Cinchonism	Glucose-6-phosphate dehydrogenase (G6PD) deficiency Myasthenia gravis Hypersensitivity to mefloquine, quinidine, or quinine Optic neuritis Prolonged QT interval	Mechanism similar to chloroquine; additionally, quinine intercalates into DNA. Used to treat acute blood-stage malaria but not used prophylactically.
Mefloquine	Chloroquine-resistant malaria	Prolonged QT interval, seizure, suicidal ideation, pneumonitis Gastrointestinal disturbance, dizziness, dream disorder, headache, insomnia, somnolence, anxiety	Depression Generalized anxiety disorder Psychosis Schizophrenia Seizure disorder Hypersensitivity to mefloquine	Appears to inhibit polymerization of heme to hemozoin inside intraerythrocytic malarial parasites. Used therapeutically and prophylactically.
Artemisinin Artesunate Artemether Dihydroartemisinin	Malaria, all species	Hemolytic anemia, bradycardia, potential neurotoxic effects	Hypersensitivity to artemisinin and its derivatives	Form carbon-centered free radicals that alkylate heme. First-line therapy for uncomplicated and complicated malaria in combination with a second antimalarial agent. Not used prophylactically. Oral artemether–lumefantrine is commercially available in the United States for treatment of uncomplicated malaria. Intravenous artesunate is available through the Centers for Disease Control and Prevention Investigational New Drug program for treatment of complicated *P. falciparum* malaria.

continues

DRUG SUMMARY TABLE: CHAPTER 37 Pharmacology of Parasitic Infections continued

DRUG	CLINICAL APPLICATIONS	SERIOUS AND COMMON ADVERSE EFFECTS	CONTRAINDICATIONS	THERAPEUTIC CONSIDERATIONS
ANTIMALARIAL AGENTS: INHIBITORS OF ELECTRON TRANSPORT Mechanism—Inhibit the plasmodial electron transport chain				
Primaquine	*P. vivax* *P. ovale*	*Hemolytic anemia, methemoglobinemia, leukopenia* Gastrointestinal distress	Glucose-6-phosphate dehydrogenase (G6PD) deficiency Pregnancy Concomitant medications that cause bone marrow suppression Rheumatoid arthritis Systemic lupus erythematosus	Disrupts metabolism in plasmodial mitochondria, likely by inhibiting ubiquinone and by nonspecific oxidative damage. Used to eradicate hypnozoites of *P. vivax* and *P. ovale*; sometimes used as primary prophylaxis against all malarial plasmodia. Kills both liver and erythrocyte-stage malarial parasites.
Atovaquone	*Pneumocystis carinii (jiroveci)* pneumonia	*Stevens-Johnson syndrome, methemoglobinemia, liver failure* Rash, gastrointestinal distress, headache, asthenia, headache, insomnia, cough, dyspnea, rhinitis, fever	Hypersensitivity to atovaquone	Inhibits the interaction between reduced ubiquinone and the cytochrome bc_1 complex. Often used in combination with proguanil or doxycycline.
ANTIMALARIAL AGENTS: INHIBITORS OF TRANSLATION Mechanism—Inhibit protein synthesis by binding to 30S ribosomal subunit (doxycycline and tetracycline) or 50S ribosomal subunit (clindamycin)				
Doxycycline Tetracycline Clindamycin	Malaria, all species (See Chapter 34 for other indications.)	*Stevens-Johnson syndrome, toxic epidermal necrolysis, Clostridium difficile diarrhea, hepatotoxicity (shared adverse effects); pseudotumor cerebri (doxycycline and tetracycline only); phototoxicity, acidosis, azotemia, serum blood urea nitrogen elevated, bulging fontanelle, raised intracranial pressure (tetracycline only)* Photosensitivity, gastrointestinal disturbance, nasopharyngitis, tooth discoloration	Hypersensitivity to doxycycline, tetracycline, or clindamycin Last half of pregnancy and childhood up to 8 years of age	In combination with quinine, doxycycline or tetracycline is used for the treatment of chloroquine-resistant *P. falciparum.* Clindamycin is used in combination with quinine when the use of doxycycline or tetracycline is contraindicated (for example, in pregnant women and children less than 8 years old).
ANTIMALARIAL AGENTS: INHIBITORS OF FOLATE METABOLISM Mechanism—See specific drug				
Sulfadoxine–pyrimethamine Sulfalene–pyrimethamine	*P. falciparum*	*Stevens-Johnson syndrome, toxic epidermal necrolysis, megaloblastic anemia, thrombocytopenia, hepatitis, nephrotoxicity* Gastrointestinal distress, urticaria, headache	Blood dyscrasias Infants less than 2 months old Pregnancy or breastfeeding Severe liver or renal disease Hypersensitivity to pyrimethamine or sulfonamides	Sulfadoxine and sulfalene are PABA analogues that competitively inhibit plasmodial dihydropteroate synthetase. Pyrimethamine is a folate analogue that competitively inhibits plasmodial dihydrofolate reductase. Effective against blood schizont stages of *P. falciparum* but not against gametocytes Sulfadoxine–pyrimethamine can be administered as a single dose, but worldwide resistance to this combination has markedly restricted its utility.

Drug	Indications	Contraindications	Adverse Effects	Mechanism/Notes
Proguanil	Malaria, all species	Prophylaxis of *P. falciparum* malaria in patients with severe renal impairment	*Pancytopenia, thrombocytopenia, granulocytopenia* Oral ulcerations, gastrointestinal distress, pruritus, headache	Pyrimidine derivative that inhibits plasmodial dihydrofolate reductase. Primarily active against the hepatic, pre-erythrocytic forms of *P. falciparum* and *P. vivax*. In combination with chloroquine, used for prophylaxis in areas where chloroquine resistance is not widespread. Also used in combination with atovaquone for treatment and prevention of malaria.

ANTIPROTOZOAL AGENTS
Mechanism—See specific drug

Drug	Indications	Contraindications	Adverse Effects	Mechanism/Notes
Metronidazole Tinidazole	Anaerobic bacteria Amebiasis Giardiasis Trichomoniasis Rosacea	Shared contraindications: Hypersensitivity to metronidazole or other nitroimidazole agents Hypersensitivity to parabens (gel formulation) First trimester of pregnancy Concomitant alcohol administration leads to disulfiram-like reaction Tinidazole only: Lactation	*Stevens-Johnson syndrome, toxic epidermal necrolysis, leukopenia, aseptic meningitis, encephalopathy, peripheral neuropathy, seizure, disorder of optic nerve, ototoxicity, hemolytic uremic syndrome* Gastrointestinal disturbance, headache, metallic taste, vaginitis	Metronidazole is activated by enzymes in parasites and anaerobic bacteria to form reduced cytotoxic compounds that damage microbial proteins, membranes, and DNA. Active against *E. histolytica* trophozoites in tissues but much less active against intraluminal ameba. Individuals with invasive amebiasis are typically treated first with metronidazole and then with a second agent such as iodoquinol or paromomycin. Tinidazole is a second-generation nitroimidazole related to metronidazole; compared to metronidazole, it is better tolerated and requires a shorter duration of treatment.
Nitazoxanide	Giardiasis Cryptosporidiosis	Hypersensitivity to nitazoxanide	Gastrointestinal upset, headache	Structurally related to metronidazole. Inhibits the pyruvate-ferredoxin oxidoreductase (PFOR) enzyme that converts pyruvate to acetyl CoA in protozoa and anaerobic bacteria. Mechanism of action against helminths unclear.
Pentamidine	*Pneumocystis carinii (jiroveci)* pneumonia Early-stage African trypanosomiasis	Hypersensitivity to pentamidine	*Pancreatitis, cardiac arrhythmia, hypotension, hypoglycemia, leukopenia, thrombocytopenia, nephrotoxicity, bronchospasm* Rash, gastrointestinal upset, liver enzyme abnormalities	Inhibits DNA, RNA, protein, and phospholipid synthesis and may inhibit dihydrofolate reductase activity. Has a high affinity for DNA in kinetoplasts and suppresses kinetoplast replication and function. Used as a third- or fourth-line treatment for individuals with *Pneumocystis carinii (jiroveci)* pneumonia.
Suramin	Early-stage African trypanosomiasis	Hypersensitivity to suramin	Pruritus, paresthesias, vomiting, nausea	Inhibits RNA polymerase and glycerol phosphate dehydrogenase.

continues

DRUG SUMMARY TABLE: CHAPTER 37 Pharmacology of Parasitic Infections *continued*

DRUG	CLINICAL APPLICATIONS	SERIOUS AND COMMON ADVERSE EFFECTS	CONTRAINDICATIONS	THERAPEUTIC CONSIDERATIONS
ANTIPROTOZOAL AGENTS *(continued)* Mechanism—See specific drug				
Melarsoprol	Late-stage African trypanosomiasis	*Reactive encephalopathy, death* Fever, phlebitis, neuropathy	Hypersensitivity to melarsoprol	First-line drug for late-stage African trypanosomiasis, in which the disease involves the central nervous system. Melarsoprol inhibits trypanosomal pyruvate kinase, thereby inhibiting glycolysis and decreasing ATP production; melarsoprol also inhibits adenine and adenosine uptake by trypanosomal transporters. Treatment can be associated with 4–6% death rate. Concomitant administration of corticosteroids lessens the likelihood of reactive encephalopathy. Concomitant administration of thiamine lessens the likelihood of polyneuropathy.
Eflornithine	West African trypanosomiasis (intravenous) Hair removal (topical)	*Myelosuppression, thrombocytopenia, seizure, ototoxicity* Acne, stinging of the skin	Hypersensitivity to eflornithine	Active against early- and late-stage West African trypanosomiasis (caused by *T. b. gambiense*) but not effective against East African trypanosomiasis (caused by *T. b. rhodesiense*). Eflornithine is a selective and irreversible inhibitor of ornithine decarboxylase; *T. b. gambiense* organisms may be susceptible to eflornithine because of their slow turnover of ornithine decarboxylase. In the United States, topical formulation of eflornithine is used for hair removal.
Nifurtimox	New World trypanosomiasis (Chagas' disease)	*Pancytopenia, neuropathy, seizures* Vomiting, anorexia, memory loss, sleep disorders	Hypersensitivity to nifurtimox	Generates toxic intracellular oxygen radicals in the parasite; mammalian cells are protected by the activity of antioxidant enzymes such as catalase, glutathione peroxidase, and superoxide dismutase.
Sodium stibogluconate Meglumine antimonate	Leishmaniasis	*Myelosuppression, chemical pancreatitis, prolonged QT interval, kidney dysfunction* Rash	Hypersensitivity to sodium stibogluconate or meglumine antimonate	Contain pentavalent antimony and act by an unknown mechanism; postulated to inhibit the glycolytic pathway and fatty acid oxidation.
Miltefosine	Visceral leishmaniasis (oral) Cutaneous leishmaniasis	*Stevens-Johnson syndrome, leukocytosis, thrombocytosis* Gastrointestinal upset, dizziness, headache, pruritus, rash	Sjögren-Larson syndrome Breastfeeding Pregnancy Hypersensitivity to miltefosine	A synthetic ether phospholipid analogue similar to natural phospholipids in cell membranes. Has antineoplastic, immunomodulatory, and antiprotozoal activity. May inhibit enzyme systems associated with plasma membranes (such as protein kinase C) and phosphatidylcholine biosynthesis. May also inhibit platelet activating factor–induced responses and inositol phosphate formation. Immunomodulatory effects include T-cell activation, interferon-gamma production, and increased interleukin-2 receptor and HLA-DR expression. FDA approved in 2014.

ANTHELMINTHIC AGENTS

Mechanism—All mechanisms lead to paralysis and death of worms; see specific drug for individual mechanisms.

Drug	Therapeutic Uses	Serious and Common Adverse Effects	Contraindications	Notes
Ivermectin	Onchocerciasis Intestinal strongyloidiasis Pediculosis capitis	*Seizure* Inflammatory or allergic responses to dying microfilariae (Mazzotti reaction), including itching, fever, dizziness, headache	Hypersensitivity to ivermectin	Potentiates both glutamate-gated chloride channels in nematode cell membranes and release of GABA from presynaptic terminals → hyperpolarization of neuromuscular cells and pharyngeal paralysis. Does not kill adult filarial worms and therefore cannot cure human hosts of *O. volvulus* infection. Ivermectin does not cross the blood–brain barrier; however, the drug has increased CNS toxicity (headaches, ataxia, coma) when the blood–brain barrier is hyperpermeable (as in meningitis). Ivermectin resistance has been found in livestock parasites but not (to date) in humans; in livestock parasites, the P-glycoprotein may be involved in ivermectin resistance.
Albendazole Mebendazole Thiabendazole	Cysticercosis (shared indication) Echinococcosis (albendazole only) Ancylostomiasis, ascariasis, enterobiasis, trichuriasis (mebendazole only)	*Stevens-Johnson syndrome, agranulocytosis, leukopenia, pancytopenia, thrombocytopenia, hepatotoxicity, acute renal failure (shared adverse effects); seizures (mebendazole only)* Gastrointestinal disturbance, headache	Hypersensitivity to albendazole, mebendazole, thiabendazole	Inhibit tubulin polymerization by binding to β-tubulin → degenerative changes in integumental and intestinal cells of helminths. Thiabendazole causes significant nausea, vomiting, and anorexia at therapeutic doses and is rarely used. Mebendazole and albendazole are better tolerated; albendazole has the highest oral bioavailability of the three drugs. Dose reduction is required for patients with renal insufficiency.
Praziquantel	Schistosomiasis Liver fluke infections	*Cardiac arrhythmia, seizure* Headache, gastrointestinal disturbance	Hypersensitivity to praziquantel Concomitant use with CYP inducers, such as rifampin Ocular cysticercosis	Increases parasite membrane permeability to calcium → contraction and paralysis of worms.
Diethylcarbamazine	Filariasis	*Mazzotti reactions in individuals with heavy microfilarial burdens* Anorexia, headache, nausea	Hypersensitivity to diethylcarbamazine	Mechanism of action unknown; postulated to stimulate innate immune system, inhibit microtubule polymerization, and inhibit arachidonic acid metabolism. Kills adult filarial worms and is considered a curative agent. Excreted by the kidneys; consider dose adjustment in individuals with decreased kidney function.
Pyrantel pamoate	Pinworm infections	Gastrointestinal disturbance, dizziness, headache, somnolence	Hypersensitivity to pyrantel pamoate	Causes constant release of acetylcholine → persistent activation of parasite nicotinic acetylcholine receptors → tonic paralysis. Largely replaced by more effective and better tolerated agents.
Piperazine	Roundworm infection	*Seizures* Gastrointestinal disturbance, pruritus	Hypersensitivity to piperazine History of seizures	GABA agonist → flaccid paralysis. Rarely used.

38

Pharmacology of Viral Infections

Jonathan Z. Li and Donald M. Coen

INTRODUCTION

Viral infections are among the leading causes of morbidity and mortality worldwide. Although much progress has been made on antiviral drug development, public health measures and prophylactic vaccines remain the primary means by which society controls the spread of viral infections. The persistence of the acquired immunodeficiency syndrome (AIDS) epidemic makes this painfully clear. Despite advances in anti-human immunodeficiency virus (HIV) drug therapies, AIDS continues to be a common cause of death, particularly in some African nations, where as many as one adult in four is infected with HIV. This enormous prevalence is largely attributable to failures in public health measures and the lack of an effective vaccine against HIV in a setting where anti-HIV drugs are too expensive and the healthcare delivery system is too fragmented.

Despite this bleak statistic, the array of drugs available to combat viruses has been instrumental in saving millions of lives each year and in improving the quality of life for countless others with viral illnesses. This chapter describes the physiology of viral replication and the steps in the viral life cycle that are targeted by current antiviral medications. Key concepts for the chapter include: (1) viruses replicate intracellularly and utilize host cell machinery; (2) despite this mode of replication, multiple targets have been exploited

for antiviral drug therapy; and (3) most current antiviral drugs exploit differences between the structures and functions of viral and human proteins to achieve selectivity of antiviral action.

PHYSIOLOGY OF VIRAL REPLICATION

Viruses replicate by co-opting the host cell's metabolic machinery. Based on this fact, one might think that there would be fewer differences between viruses and their human hosts to exploit for drug development than between bacteria and humans. However, all viruses encode proteins that are substantially different from their human counterparts. Additionally, certain host proteins are more important for viral replication than they are for human health. In principle, antiviral drugs could target many of these proteins. In practice, however, relatively few viral proteins and even fewer host proteins have thus far served as useful targets for therapy. Nevertheless, it is a testament to the remarkable progress in antiviral drug development that the number of viral proteins that have been exploited for antiviral therapy is greater than the number of bacterial proteins that have been exploited for antibacterial therapy. However, most antiviral drugs are active against only one or a few viruses while most antibacterial drugs target multiple bacterial species. This difficulty arises because viruses are a heterogeneous group of

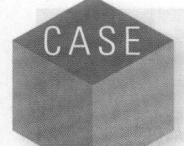

CASE

The year is 1993. Mr. M, a 26-year-old man, complains to Dr. Rose, his primary care physician, of a sore throat, fever, and fatigue for the past several weeks. On physical examination, Dr. Rose notes bilateral cervical lymphadenopathy, consistent with the patient's "flu-like symptoms." Dr. Rose thinks it likely that Mr. M has an infection, possibly a simple "cold," the "flu," or strep throat. Because of Mr. M's mononucleosis-like symptoms, Dr. Rose also includes human cytomegalovirus (HCMV), Epstein-Barr virus (EBV), toxoplasmosis, and HIV in her differential diagnosis. Laboratory antibody tests for *Streptococcus*, HCMV, EBV, toxoplasmosis, and HIV infection are negative. Mr. M is concerned about the possibility of HIV infection and the lack of truly effective therapies for AIDS, although he denies any unprotected sexual activity, intravenous (IV) drug use, or other potential exposure risks. Dr. Rose tells Mr. M that his symptoms will likely resolve with rest but that he should return for follow-up within 6 months. She explains to Mr. M that, if he has recently been infected with HIV, his body would not yet have produced sufficient antibodies to become evident on an anti-HIV antibody test.

Five years later, Mr. M returns to Dr. Rose's office. He has not seen any physician in the interim and now presents with new symptoms. There are multiple open lesions on his lips and in his mouth, and he confides that he has similar lesions in his genital area. An ELISA test is positive for anti-HIV antibodies,

and a viral load measurement shows high levels of HIV RNA in his blood. Mr. M's CD4 count is 100 per mm^3 (normal range, 800–1,200 per mm^3). Dr. Rose immediately prescribes a drug regimen of zidovudine (AZT), lamivudine (3TC), and ritonavir, explaining to Mr. M that a combination of anti-HIV drugs is his best option for reducing the viral load and forestalling more serious disease. In addition, Dr. Rose prescribes oral valacyclovir, a prodrug of acyclovir, to treat Mr. M's oral and genital herpes.

Over the next 3 years, Mr. M's HIV viral load falls to undetectable levels and his condition improves. The herpes infections are also kept in check. Today, Mr. M appears in good health and he takes his medications diligently, which is easier now with a once-a-day pill containing efavirenz, emtricitabine, and tenofovir.

Questions

1. What is acyclovir's mechanism of action?
2. Why does acyclovir not ordinarily cause significant toxicity in humans, while AZT does?
3. What are the mechanisms of action of the three anti-HIV drugs prescribed by Dr. Rose in 1998? In the once-a-day pill Mr. M is taking today?
4. Why is combination antiretroviral therapy required to effectively treat HIV infections?
5. What potential adverse effects could Mr. M experience from long-term treatment with ritonavir?

infectious agents, whereas most bacteria share a common cell wall structure and distinct DNA replication, transcription, and translation machineries.

Viral Life Cycle

Viruses exist as small particles called **virions**. Virions consist of a nucleic acid genome packaged into a virus-encoded protein shell called a **capsid**. In some viruses, the capsid is surrounded by an **envelope**, a lipid bilayer membrane that contains virus-encoded envelope proteins. Viral genomes can consist of DNA or RNA and can be single- or double-stranded.

Almost all viruses have the same general life cycle for replication (Fig. 38-1) with some variations. Figure 38-2 illustrates the specific life cycle for HIV, which, as a retrovirus, contains RNA that is copied into DNA. At the start of infection, the virus attaches to the host cell. This **attachment** is mediated by proteins on the viral surface that bind specifically to a particular host membrane component. For example, the HIV viral envelope contains the glycoprotein gp120, a transmembrane protein that mediates binding and attachment of the virus to host cells expressing CD4 and chemokine receptors such as CCR5 or CXCR4 (Fig. 38-2). Next, the virion undergoes **entry** by crossing a host cell membrane

into the cytoplasm. In the case of HIV, the process of entry depends on gp41, a viral envelope protein that fuses together the membranes of HIV and the target cell.

The virion then loses enough of its capsid proteins—the stage of **uncoating**—that its nucleic acid becomes available for **gene expression**. (For retroviruses, uncoating does not lead directly to gene expression; instead, it allows reverse transcription of the viral RNA genome into DNA to occur—as described below, this is a step in genome replication.) Viral gene expression entails **transcription** of the viral genome into mRNA, **translation** of mRNA into protein on cellular ribosomes, and a variety of processing events including splicing of mRNA precursors and **proteolytic cleavage** of viral **polyproteins** into their individual protein units. For many viruses, gene expression begins with transcription. For certain RNA viruses, such as hepatitis C virus (HCV), the first step in gene expression is translation of the viral RNA. Many viruses encode proteins that execute or abet certain of these steps in gene expression, and these proteins can serve as drug targets.

Genome replication is the next stage of the cycle. This stage requires a supply of ribonucleoside triphosphates for RNA viruses and deoxyribonucleoside triphosphates for DNA viruses. For DNA viruses, the generation of these deoxyribonucleoside triphosphates occurs via two

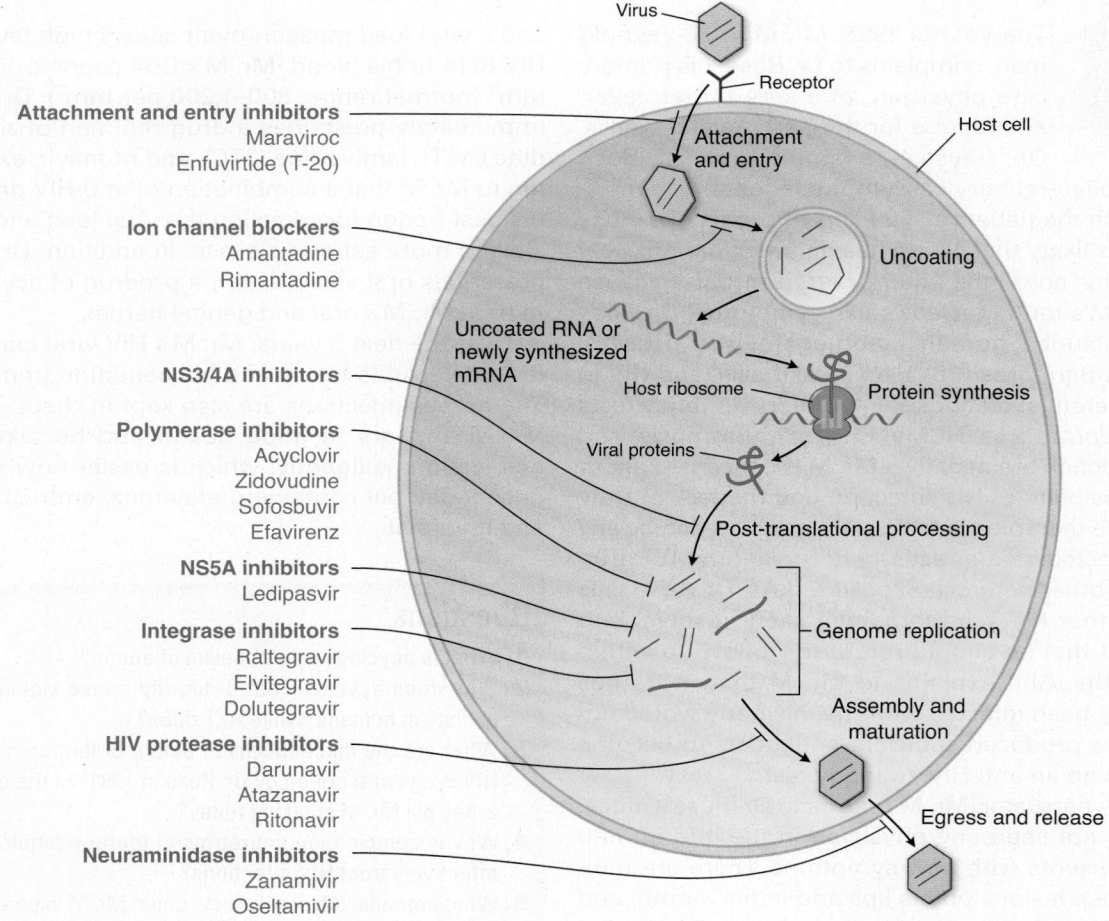

FIGURE 38-1. Viral life cycle and pharmacologic intervention. The viral life cycle can be divided into a sequence of stages, each of which is a potential site for pharmacologic intervention. Shown is a generic replication cycle of viruses in cells, alongside which are listed the names of drug classes and examples of individual agents that block each stage. Many of the currently approved antiviral agents are nucleoside analogues or nonnucleoside compounds that target genome replication, typically by inhibiting viral DNA polymerase or reverse transcriptase. Several other drug classes target other stages in the viral life cycle, including attachment and entry, uncoating, gene expression, assembly and maturation, and egress and release. It should be noted that the individual features of viral replication differ for each type of virus, often presenting unique targets for pharmacologic intervention and drug development. See the legend to Figure 33-2 for additional details.

pathways: the salvage pathway, which employs the pharmacologically relevant enzyme thymidine kinase, and the de novo pathway, which includes the enzyme thymidylate kinase. Nucleoside triphosphates are incorporated into new viral genomes by a viral or cellular polymerase (see Chapter 39, Pharmacology of Cancer: Genome Synthesis, Stability, and Maintenance, for more detail on nucleotide metabolism). In the case of herpes simplex viruses 1 and 2 (which will be collectively referred to as *HSV*), the generation of deoxyribonucleoside triphosphates includes phosphorylation of nucleosides via the salvage pathway by a viral thymidine kinase; a viral DNA polymerase then adds deoxyribonucleoside triphosphates to the growing DNA genome. Exploitation of this two-step process has led to the development of some of the most effective and safe antivirals currently available, because *differences between human and viral kinases and polymerases allow drugs to take advantage of two different steps in a single pathway*. For many viruses, genome replication requires other kinds of proteins. One example is the HCV NS5A protein.

Viral proteins that are synthesized intracellularly assemble with viral genomes within the host cell in a process known as **assembly**. For a number of viruses, assembly is followed by a process known as viral **maturation**, which is essential for newly formed virions to become infectious. This process typically involves cleavage of viral polyproteins by proteases. For some viruses, maturation occurs within the host cell; for others, such as HIV, it occurs outside the host cell. Viruses **egress** from the cell either by cell lysis or by budding through the cell membrane. For influenza viruses, the newly formed virions require an additional step of **release** from the extracellular surface of the host cell membrane.

In summary, nearly all viruses replicate via the following stages: attachment, entry, uncoating, gene expression, genome replication, assembly, and egress. Some viruses have additional stages such as maturation and release. The stages of retrovirus infection occur in a different order from those of most other viruses, and retroviruses have additional steps and stages in their life cycle. For example, genome replication of HIV includes the additional step of **integration**, in which the viral genome is incorporated into the host

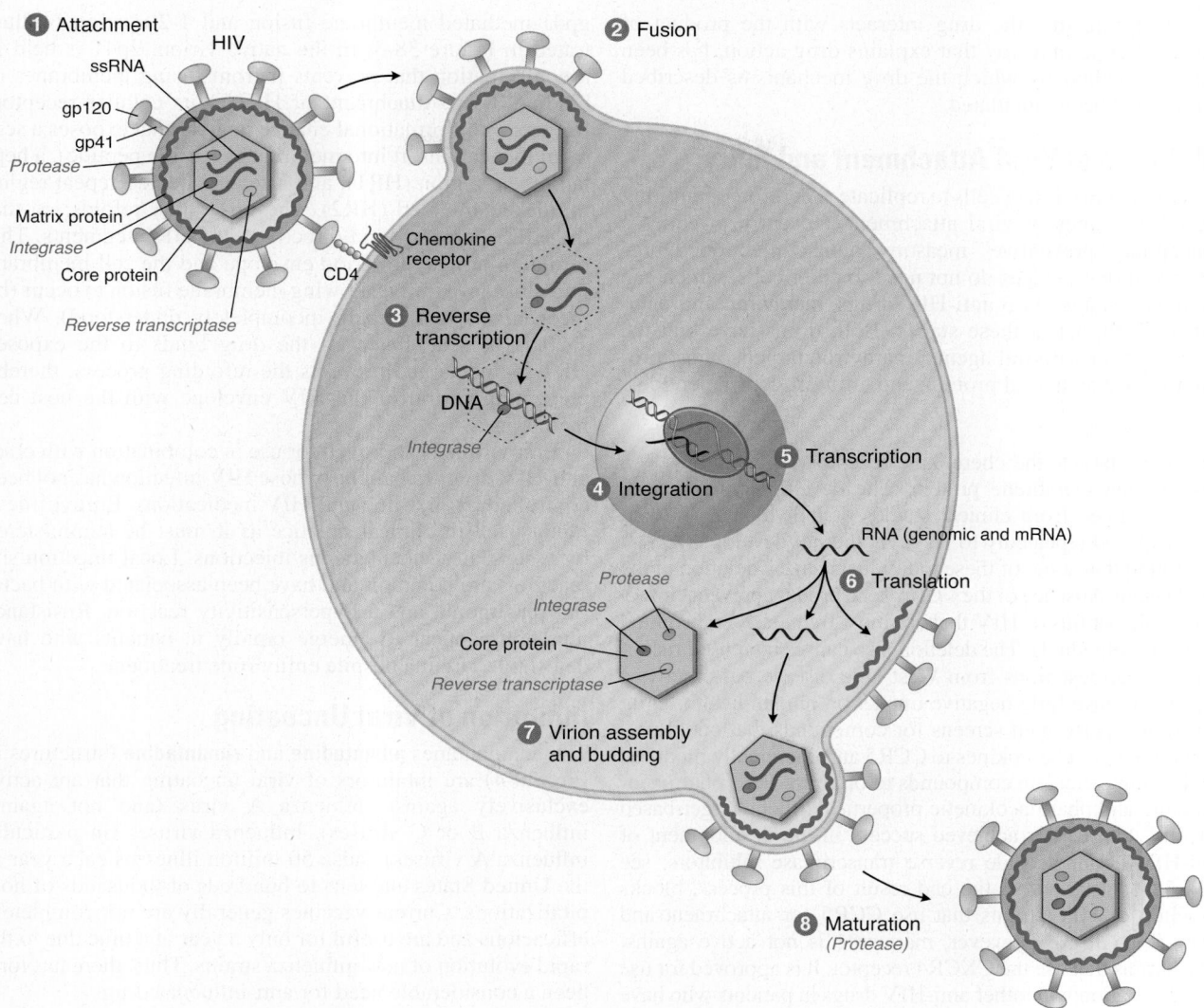

FIGURE 38-2. Life cycle of HIV. HIV is a retrovirus that infects CD4 cells. **1.** Virus attachment is dependent on binding interactions between viral gp41 and gp120 proteins and host cell CD4 and certain chemokine receptors. **2.** Fusion of the viral membrane (envelope) with the host cell plasma membrane allows the HIV genome complexed with certain virion proteins to enter the host cell. **3.** Uncoating permits the single-stranded RNA (ssRNA) HIV genome to be copied by reverse transcriptase into double-stranded DNA. **4.** The HIV DNA is integrated into the host cell genome in a reaction that depends on HIV-encoded integrase. **5.** Gene transcription and post-transcriptional processing by host cell enzymes produce genomic HIV RNA and viral mRNA. **6.** The viral mRNA is translated into proteins on host cell ribosomes. **7.** The proteins assemble into immature virions that bud from the host cell membrane. **8.** The virions undergo proteolytic cleavage, maturing into fully infective virions. Currently approved anti-HIV drugs target viral attachment and fusion, reverse transcription, integration, and maturation. The development of drug resistance can be significantly retarded by using combinations of drugs that target a single stage (e.g., two or more inhibitors of reverse transcription) or more than one stage in the HIV life cycle (e.g., reverse transcriptase inhibitors and protease inhibitors).

genome (Fig. 38-2). Specific host and/or viral proteins are involved in each of these stages. Differences between viral and host proteins at any of these stages can be targeted for antiviral therapy.

Different viruses have vastly different arrays of genes. Some, such as hepatitis B virus (HBV), have compact genomes that encode only coat proteins and a few proteins used mainly in gene expression and genome replication. Others, such as herpesviruses, encode scores of proteins that perform many different functions. The viral proteins that most frequently have served as targets for antiviral drugs are enzymes involved in genome replication, although multiple other proteins acting at different stages in the viral life cycle serve as targets, too.

PHARMACOLOGIC CLASSES AND AGENTS

This section of the chapter reviews the mechanisms of antiviral drugs that target different stages of the viral life cycle. Understanding the mechanisms of antiviral drugs has relied strongly on studies of viruses that are resistant to these drugs. Resistance to an antiviral drug usually implies that the drug acts, at least in part, by interfering directly with a virus-specific process rather than by incapacitating a host cell process. In most cases, then, mutations that confer resistance to an antiviral drug affect the target(s) of that drug and suggest that the drug acts selectively against that target. Thus, mapping drug-resistance mutations to viral genes, along with demonstrating that the drug interacts with the product of that viral gene in a way that explains drug action, has been a major method by which the drug mechanisms described below have been elucidated.

Inhibition of Viral Attachment and Entry

All viruses must infect cells to replicate. Therefore, inhibiting the initial stages of viral attachment and entry provides a conceptual "preventive" measure against infection. Drugs that act at these stages do not need to enter cells, which can be an advantage. Two anti-HIV drugs, **maraviroc** and **enfuvirtide (T-20)**, act at these stages. Both drugs have unusual properties for antiviral agents: maraviroc targets a host protein rather than a viral protein, and enfuvirtide is a peptide.

Maraviroc

Maraviroc targets the chemokine receptor CCR5, which is a host plasma membrane protein. The development of maraviroc stemmed from clinical studies of individuals who had been exposed repeatedly to HIV, yet did not develop AIDS. It was found that some of these individuals have a deletion in the *CCR5* gene. Absence of the CCR5 gene product prevents infection by the strains of HIV that are most frequently transmitted between individuals. The deletion also causes increased risk of clinical manifestations from West Nile disease but otherwise appears to have little negative impact on human health. Drug companies performed screens for compounds that could prevent binding of chemokines to CCR5 and chemically modified the leading candidate compounds to optimize their pharmacodynamic and pharmacokinetic properties. (Such "target-based screens" had earlier achieved success in the development of anti-HIV nonnucleoside reverse transcriptase inhibitors; see Box 38-1.) Maraviroc, the end result of this process, blocks infection of HIV strains that use CCR5 for attachment and entry (Fig. 38-3). However, maraviroc is not active against HIV strains that use the CXCR4 receptor. It is approved for use in combination with other anti-HIV drugs in patients who have undetectable levels of CXCR4-using virus (which requires a genotypic or phenotypic diagnostic test of viral tropism).

Enfuvirtide (T-20)

Enfuvirtide, also known as *T-20*, is a peptide that is structurally similar to a segment of gp41, the HIV protein that mediates membrane fusion. The proposed mechanism for gp41-mediated membrane fusion and T-20 action is illustrated in Figure 38-3. In the native virion, gp41 is held in a conformation that prevents it from fusing membranes or binding T-20. Attachment of HIV to its cellular receptors triggers a conformational change in gp41 that exposes a segment that can insert into membranes (fusion peptide), a heptad repeat region (HR1), and a second heptad repeat region mimicked by T-20 (HR2). The gp41 then refolds, so that the HR2 segments bind directly to the HR1 segments. This refolding brings the virion envelope and the cell membrane into close proximity, allowing membrane fusion to occur (by mechanisms that remain incompletely understood). When T-20 is present, however, the drug binds to the exposed HR1 segments and prevents the refolding process, thereby preventing fusion of the HIV envelope with the host cell membrane.

Enfuvirtide is approved for use in combination with other anti-HIV drugs in patients whose HIV infection has not been controlled by first-line anti-HIV medications. Enfuvirtide is rarely used in clinical practice as it must be administered by twice-daily subcutaneous injections. Local injection site reactions are common and have been associated with bacterial pneumonia and a hypersensitivity reaction. Resistance mutations appear to emerge rapidly in patients who have detectable viremia despite enfuvirtide treatment.

Inhibition of Viral Uncoating

The adamantanes **amantadine** and **rimantadine** (structures in Fig. 38-4) are inhibitors of viral uncoating that are active exclusively against influenza A virus (and not against influenza B or C viruses). Influenza viruses (in particular influenza A viruses) cause 50 million illnesses each year in the United States and tens to hundreds of thousands of hospitalizations. Current vaccines generally are not completely efficacious and are useful for only a year at a time due to the rapid evolution of new influenza strains. Thus, there has long been a considerable need for anti-influenza drugs.

A well-supported model for the mechanism of action of the adamantanes is diagrammed in Figure 38-4. Influenza virions enter cells via receptor-mediated endocytosis and are internalized into endosomes (see Chapter 1, Drug–Receptor Interactions). As endosomes acidify because of the action of an endosomal proton pump, two events occur. First, the conformation of the viral envelope protein **hemagglutinin** changes

---

BOX 38-1 Development of Nonnucleoside Reverse Transcriptase Inhibitors and CCR5 Antagonist

The nonnucleoside reverse transcriptase inhibitors (NNRTIs) were discovered by using target-based, high-throughput screening methods. The gene encoding HIV RT was overexpressed in *E. coli*, and large amounts of RT were purified and used in an RT assay that could be easily automated. Using this assay, many thousands of compounds were screened for the ability to inhibit RT. Candidate compounds were then tested for specificity in a counter-screen by checking their ability to inhibit an unrelated polymerase. The compounds that emerged were chemically modified to improve their stability, pharmacokinetics, and toxicity profile. This process eventually yielded NNRTIs that are highly specific, inhibiting HIV-1 RT at low concentrations while not inhibiting even the RT of the closely related virus HIV-2.

The CCR5 antagonist maraviroc was also developed using a target-based, high-throughput screen. In this case, the assay was designed to discover lead compounds that prevented the binding of endogenous ligands (chemokines) to CCR5. As with the development of the NNRTIs, the lead compounds were then tested for specificity against CCR5 and chemically modified to optimize their potency, antiviral activity, pharmacokinetics, and toxicity profile. The end result was maraviroc, a selective CCR5 antagonist that is used in combination antiretroviral treatment of adults infected with CCR5-tropic HIV-1. ∎

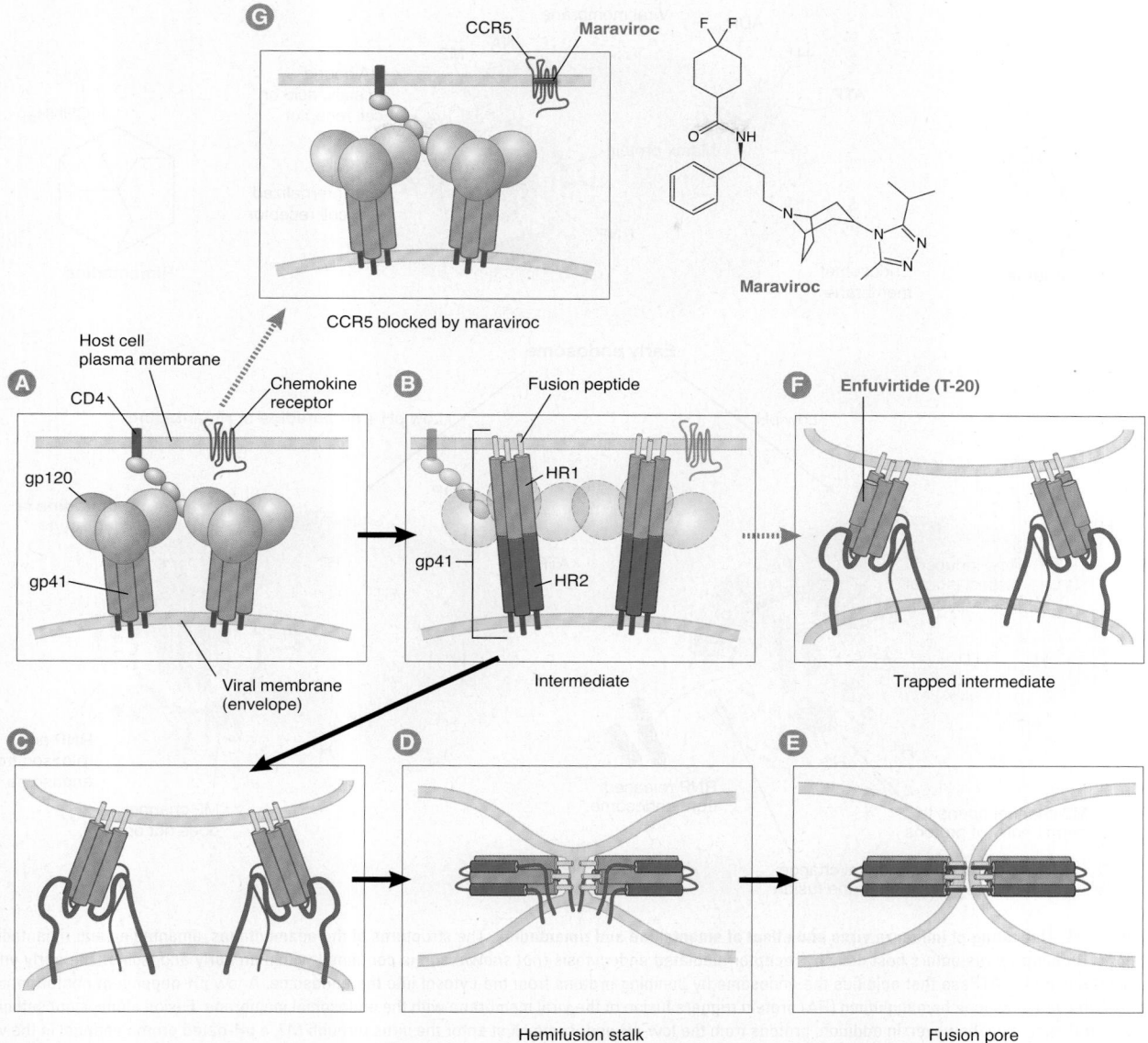

FIGURE 38-3. Model for HIV gp41-mediated fusion and maraviroc and enfuvirtide (T-20) action. A. HIV glycoproteins exist in trimeric form in the viral membrane (envelope). Each gp120 molecule is depicted as a ball attached noncovalently to gp41. **B.** The binding of gp120 to CD4 and certain chemokine receptors in the host cell plasma membrane causes a conformational change in gp41 that exposes the fusion peptide, heptad-repeat region 1 (HR1) and heptad-repeat region 2 (HR2). The fusion peptide inserts into the host cell plasma membrane. **C.** gp41 undergoes further conformational changes, characterized mainly by unfolding and refolding of the HR2 repeats. **D.** Completed refolding of the HR regions creates a hemifusion stalk, in which the outer leaflets of the viral and host cell membranes are fused. **E.** Formation of a complete fusion pore allows viral entry into the host cell. **F.** Enfuvirtide (T-20) is a synthetic peptide drug that mimics HR2, binds to HR1, and prevents the HR2–HR1 interaction (*dashed arrow*). Therefore, the drug traps the virus–host cell interaction at the attachment stage, preventing membrane fusion and viral entry. **G.** Maraviroc is a small-molecule antagonist of the CCR5 chemokine receptor; the drug blocks cellular infection of HIV strains that use CCR5 for attachment and entry (*dashed arrow*). The structure of maraviroc is shown.

drastically. This conformational change permits fusion of the influenza virus envelope with the endosome membrane (see the above discussion of HIV-mediated membrane fusion). By itself, this action could liberate viral ribonucleoprotein (including the virion's RNA genome), but that would not be sufficient to permit its transcription: a second pH-dependent event within the virion is also required. This entails the influx of protons through a proton channel called **M2** in the viral envelope, which causes dissociation of the virion **matrix protein** from the rest of the ribonucleoprotein. Amantadine and rimantadine inhibit the influx of protons through M2.

As hydrophobic molecules with a positive charge at one end, these drugs resemble blockers of cellular ion channels (see Chapters 12, Local Anesthetic Pharmacology, and 24, Pharmacology of Cardiac Rhythm), and indeed the adamantanes appear to simply "plug" (physically occlude) the channel.

Amantadine can cause light-headedness and difficulty concentrating; these adverse effects are likely due to its effects on host ion channels. Indeed, the unintended effects of amantadine on host channels likely account for this drug's other therapeutic use—the treatment of Parkinson's disease (see Chapter 14, Pharmacology of Dopaminergic

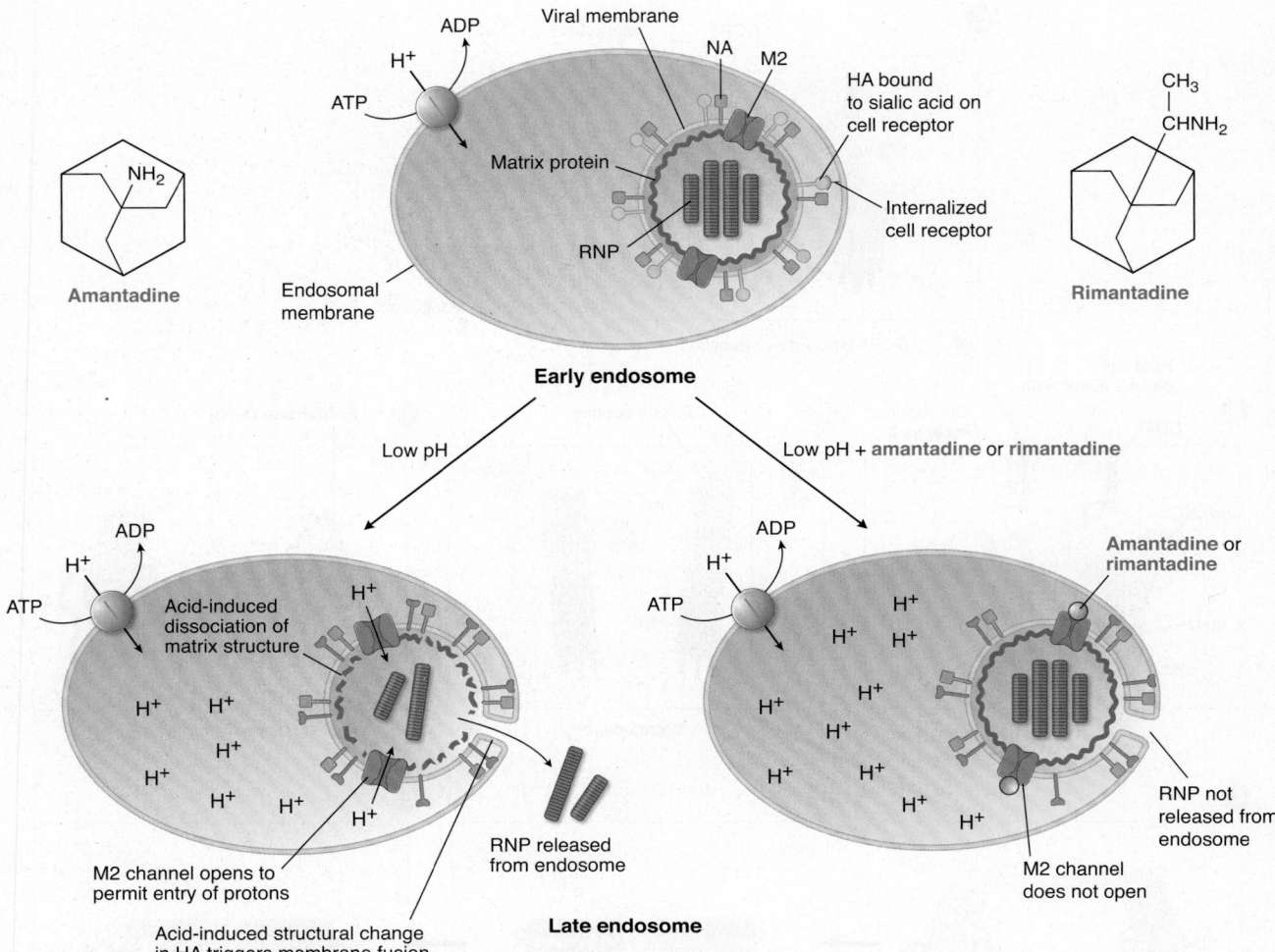

FIGURE 38-4. Uncoating of influenza virus and effect of amantadine and rimantadine. The structures of the adamantanes, amantadine and rimantadine, are shown. Influenza virus enters host cells by receptor-mediated endocytosis (*not shown*) and is contained within an early endosome. The early endosome contains an H^+-ATPase that acidifies the endosome by pumping protons from the cytosol into the endosome. A low pH-dependent conformational change in the viral envelope hemagglutinin (HA) protein triggers fusion of the viral membrane with the endosomal membrane. Fusion alone is not sufficient to cause viral uncoating, however. In addition, protons from the low-pH endosome must enter the virus through M2, a pH-gated proton channel in the viral envelope that opens in response to acidification. The entry of protons through the viral envelope causes dissociation of matrix protein from the influenza virus ribonucleoprotein (RNP), releasing RNP and thus the genetic material of the virus into the host cell cytosol. Amantadine and rimantadine block M2 ion channel function and thereby inhibit acidification of the interior of the virion, dissociation of matrix protein, and uncoating. Note that the drug is shown as "plugging" the channel. NA, neuraminidase.

Neurotransmission). **Rimantadine** is an analogue of amantadine that has a similar antiviral mechanism and fewer adverse effects compared to amantadine, especially the neurological effects that can be problematic in the elderly. However, resistance to adamantanes develops rapidly, and resistant viruses retain nearly complete replication capacity (fitness) and pathogenicity. Indeed, adamantanes are no longer recommended for use in the United States due to the high rates of drug resistance, and they have been supplanted by neuraminidase inhibitors (see "Inhibition of Viral Release").

Inhibition of Viral Gene Expression

HCV causes serious liver disease and more deaths in the United States than does HIV. After entry of HCV into the cell and uncoating in endosomes, the first step in HCV gene expression is translation of the viral genome. The translation product is a so-called polyprotein that encompasses proteins from multiple viral genes, and the next, crucial step in HCV gene expression is cleavage of the polyprotein into individual proteins (Fig. 38-5A). Certain of these individual proteins then replicate HCV RNA, producing new genomes to be translated and cleaved. Other viral proteins assemble RNA-containing viral particles that are then released from the cell. HCV encodes a protease, called *NS3/4A*, which is essential for several of the cleavages of the polyprotein. Additionally, this enzyme may play a role in counteracting host innate immune responses, particularly those elicited by interferon alpha.

Given the success of drugs targeting the HIV protease, which is required for the maturation step in its virus' life cycle (see "Inhibition of Viral Maturation"), there was considerable interest in developing drugs that target the HCV

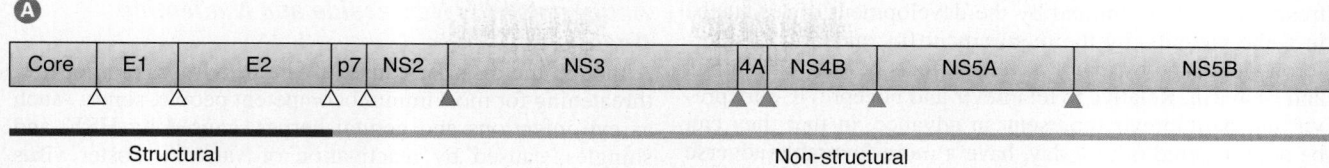

FIGURE 38-5. The HCV polyprotein and anti-HCV protease inhibitors. A. The HCV RNA genome is translated into a polyprotein, which is shown as a long rectangle, with the segments corresponding to the indicated individual viral proteins. The polyprotein is then cleaved into the individual proteins by host peptidases (sites of cleavage are indicated by *open triangles*), the viral NS2 protease (*green triangle*), and the viral NS3/4A protease (*blue triangles*). (Modified from Ray SC, Bailey JR, Thomas DL. Hepatitis C virus. In: Knipe DM, Howley PM, Cohen JI, et al, eds. *Fields virology.* 6th ed. Philadelphia: Lippincott Williams & Wilkins; 2013:795–824.) **B.** The structures of telaprevir, boceprevir, simeprevir, and paritaprevir are shown. Telaprevir and boceprevir covalently react with their target via ketoamide groups, while simeprevir and paritaprevir are noncovalent inhibitors with macrocyclic structures. These drugs are approved for use only in combination with other anti-HCV therapies.

NS3/4A protease. In 2011, two such drugs, **telaprevir** (which is no longer marketed) and **boceprevir** (Fig. 38-5B), were the first agents that act directly against HCV (direct-acting antivirals, DAAs) to be approved by the US Food and Drug Administration (FDA). In 2013 and 2014, respectively, the NS3/4A inhibitors **simeprevir** and **paritaprevir** (Fig. 38-5B), which can be administered once a day, were approved. All four drugs were developed by an iterative approach similar to that used to discover inhibitors of the HIV protease (see discussion below and Fig. 38-11), although, among other differences, telaprevir and boceprevir covalently react with their target via ketoamide groups rather than binding tightly via noncovalent interactions like the anti-HIV drugs. Simeprevir and paritaprevir are noncovalent inhibitors with

macrocyclic structures that increase the affinity of binding by decreasing entropic effects. All four drugs inhibit HCV NS3/4A protease with higher potency than they do human proteases.

None of the NS3/4A inhibitors are approved for use as monotherapies. Telaprevir, boceprevir, and simeprevir are approved for use in combination with interferon alpha (modified by pegylation to permit less frequent dosing) and ribavirin (see below for further information on these two agents), which was the previous standard of care for HCV therapy. The addition of the protease inhibitors results in a substantially higher rate of "sustained virological response," which is tantamount to cure of HCV infection. However, these interferon-based combinations entail 6 months or more of treatment and are limited by the development of resistance in some patients, by the requirement for injection of interferon alpha, and by major adverse effects of interferon alpha and ribavirin. Relative to telaprevir and boceprevir, simeprevir and paritaprevir represent an advance, in that they can be administered once a day, have a more favorable adverse effect profile, and are also approved for use in combination with particular DAAs that inhibit HCV genome replication (see below)—simeprevir with sofosbuvir; paritaprevir with ombitasvir and dasabuvir—in a regimen that requires no interferon alpha and, in many cases, only 3 months of treatment. However, each of the protease inhibitors is approved for only certain genotypes of HCV, and resistance can arise. Indeed, it is strongly recommended that testing for resistance occur prior to use of simeprevir. Paritaprevir is formulated together with the anti-HIV protease inhibitor ritonavir (see below), which increases paritaprevir serum levels by blocking its hepatic metabolism and is not recommended for use in patients with decompensated liver disease. Depending on the HCV subtype, the DAA combination containing paritaprevir may be co-administered with ribavirin, which has its own toxicities. Newer NS3/4A protease inhibitors are under development.

Inhibition of Viral Genome Replication— Polymerase Inhibitors

The vast majority of drugs that inhibit viral genome replication inhibit a polymerase. Most viruses encode their own polymerases. These enzymes are required to replicate the viral genomes and differ in various ways from human polymerases, making them excellent targets for antiviral drugs. Viruses expressing polymerases that have been successfully targeted to yield drugs approved by the FDA include certain human herpesviruses, HIV, HBV, and HCV. Most of these drugs are so-called **nucleoside analogues** (Fig. 38-6). Several, as discussed below, are **nonnucleoside inhibitors** of a polymerase. The latter do not structurally resemble physiologic nucleosides.

All nucleoside analogues must be activated by phosphorylation, usually to the triphosphate form, in order to exert their effect. In their phosphorylated form, these agents mimic nucleoside triphosphates, which are the natural substrates of polymerases. *Nucleoside analogues inhibit polymerases by competing with the natural triphosphate substrate; these analogues are also typically incorporated into the growing DNA or RNA chain, where they often terminate elongation.* Either or both of these features—enzyme inhibition and incorporation into DNA or RNA—can be important for antiviral activity.

The more efficiently cellular enzymes phosphorylate the nucleoside analogue, and the more potently the phosphorylated forms inhibit cellular enzymes, the more toxic the nucleoside analogue will be. Therefore, selectivity depends on how much more efficiently viral enzymes phosphorylate the drug than cellular enzymes do, as well as how much more potently and effectively viral DNA synthesis is inhibited than analogous cellular functions are. The challenge in designing nucleoside analogues is to make the drug appear enough like a natural nucleoside that it can be activated and its triphosphate can inhibit a viral polymerase, but not so much like a natural nucleoside that it inhibits cellular processes. All nucleoside analogues employ variations on this theme to achieve their respective degrees of selectivity.

Antiherpesvirus Nucleoside and Nucleotide Analogues

Although the diseases caused by herpesviruses are not life-threatening for most immunocompetent people, some—such as eye infections and genital herpes, caused by HSV, and shingles, caused by reactivation of varicella zoster virus (VZV)—can be serious nonetheless. For immunocompromised patients such as Mr. M, herpesvirus diseases such as HSV esophagitis and HCMV retinitis or neurologic disease can be devastating or even fatal. Herpesviruses also have the property of **latency**, in which viral genomes reside inside a cell and abundantly express a few genes (at most), thus avoiding immune surveillance. The viruses can then reactivate long after the primary infection and cause disease. No currently available antiviral drug attacks viruses during latency; rather, all available drugs act only on actively replicating virus.

Herpesvirus replication corresponds roughly to the schematic in Figure 38-1. All herpesviruses contain double-stranded DNA encoding a variety of proteins involved in DNA replication. These proteins are categorized in two groups. The first group, which includes the viral **DNA polymerase**, participates directly in DNA replication and is essential for virus replication. The second group participates indirectly, for example, by helping to synthesize the deoxyribonucleoside triphosphates necessary for DNA replication. For some herpesviruses, including HSV and VZV, one of these proteins is a viral **thymidine kinase (TK)**. Some other viruses, including HCMV, do not encode a TK but instead encode a protein kinase that induces the expression of cellular enzymes that synthesize deoxyribonucleoside triphosphates. Proteins in the second group are not essential for virus replication in cell culture or in certain cells in mammalian hosts because cellular enzymes can substitute for their activities. Herpesvirus DNA polymerases and kinases are sufficiently different from their cellular counterparts to enable development of selective antiviral nucleoside analogues.

Acyclovir

Acyclovir (ACV) is a drug used against HSV and VZV. Acyclovir illustrates the fundamental mechanisms of nucleoside analogues, and it is the drug that convinced the medical community that antivirals could be safe and effective. Acyclovir was discovered in a screen of compounds for activity against HSV replication. It exhibits a high therapeutic index (toxic dose/effective dose) because of its high selectivity. Accordingly, acyclovir toxicity is generally a clinical problem only when the drug is administered intravenously at high doses for very serious infections or in the setting of renal insufficiency.

The structure of acyclovir consists of a guanine base attached to a broken (acyclic) and incomplete sugar ring (Fig. 38-6). Despite the lack of a complete sugar ring, HSV and VZV TK can phosphorylate acyclovir much more efficiently than any mammalian enzyme can. Therefore, HSV- and VZV-infected cells contain much more phosphorylated acyclovir than do uninfected cells; this finding accounts for much of acyclovir's antiviral selectivity.

Phosphorylation of ACV produces the compound ACV monophosphate. This compound is then converted to ACV diphosphate and ACV triphosphate by cellular enzymes (Fig. 38-7A). ACV triphosphate inhibits the herpesvirus DNA polymerase; moreover, it inhibits viral DNA polymerase more potently than cellular DNA polymerases. In vitro, inhibition of HSV DNA polymerase is a three-step process.

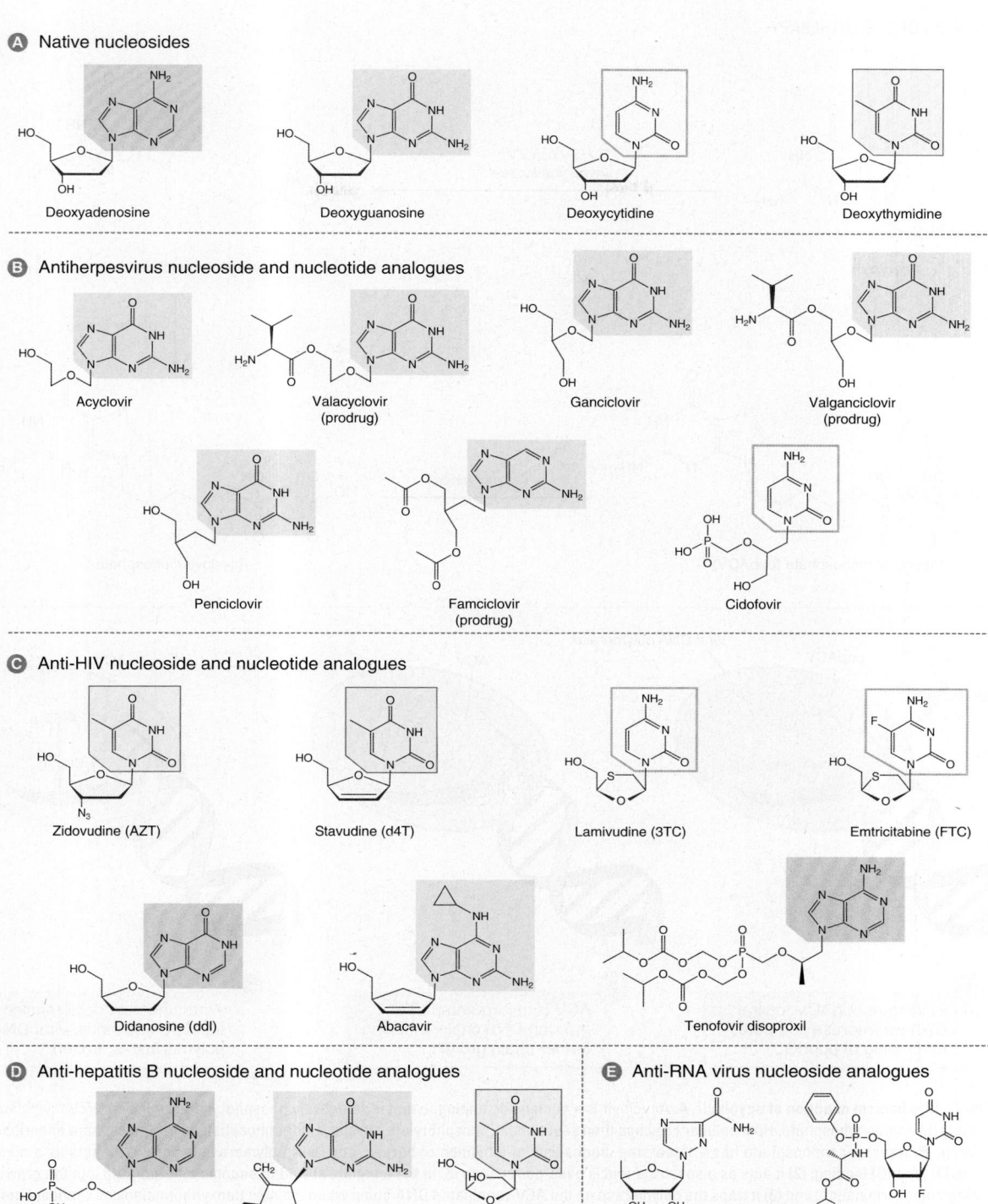

FIGURE 38-6. Antiviral nucleoside and nucleotide analogues. A. The nucleosides used as precursors for DNA synthesis are depicted in their *anti* conformations. Each nucleoside consists of a purine (adenine and guanine) or pyrimidine (cytosine and thymidine) base attached to a deoxyribose sugar. These deoxyribonucleosides are phosphorylated in stepwise fashion to the triphosphate forms (*not shown*) for use in nucleic acid synthesis. **B.** Except for cidofovir, the antiherpesvirus nucleoside and nucleotide analogues are structural mimics of deoxyguanosine. For example, acyclovir consists of a guanine base attached to an acyclic sugar. Cidofovir, which mimics the deoxyribonucleotide deoxycytidine monophosphate, uses a phosphonate (C–P) bond to mimic the physiologic P–O bond of the native nucleotide. Valacyclovir, famciclovir, and valganciclovir are more orally bioavailable prodrugs of acyclovir, penciclovir, and ganciclovir, respectively.
C. Anti-HIV nucleoside and nucleotide analogues mimic a variety of endogenous nucleosides and nucleotides and contain variations not only in the sugar but also in base moieties. For example, AZT is a deoxythymidine mimic that has a 3'-azido group in place of the native 3'-OH. Stavudine and lamivudine also contain modified sugar moieties linked to natural base moieties. Tenofovir, which is shown as its prodrug tenofovir disoproxil, is a phosphonate analogue of deoxyadenosine monophosphate. Of the analogues that contain modified base moieties, didanosine mimics deoxyinosine and is converted to dideoxyadenosine, while emtricitabine contains a fluoro-modified cytosine and abacavir contains a cyclopropyl-modified guanine. **D.** Telbivudine is an L-stereoisomer of thymidine, adefovir is a phosphonate analogue of the endogenous nucleotide deoxyadenosine monophosphate, and entecavir is a deoxyguanosine analogue with an unusual moiety substituting for deoxyribose. These three compounds, together with lamivudine and tenofovir (see **panel C**), are approved for use in the treatment of HBV infection.
E. Sofosbuvir, which contains uracil linked to a modified sugar linked to a phosphoramidite that is modified to increase uptake by liver cells, is approved for use against the RNA virus HCV. Ribavirin, which contains a purine mimic attached to ribose, is approved for use against the RNA viruses HCV and RSV.

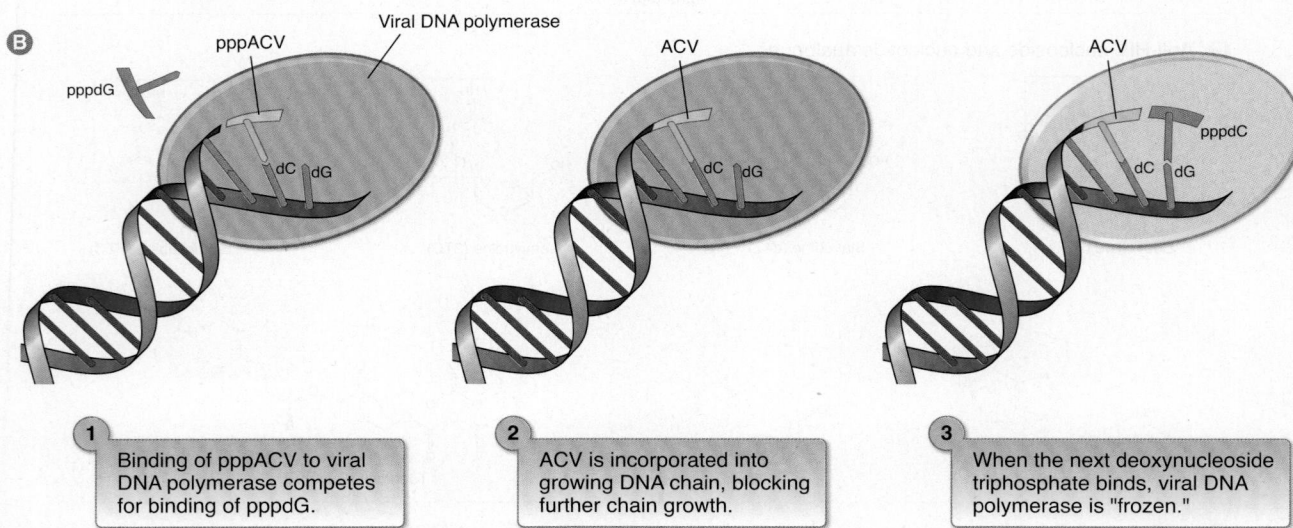

FIGURE 38-7. **Mechanism of action of acyclovir. A.** Acyclovir is a nucleoside analogue that is selectively phosphorylated by HSV or VZV thymidine kinase to generate acyclovir monophosphate. Host cellular enzymes then sequentially phosphorylate acyclovir monophosphate to its diphosphate and triphosphate (pppACV) forms. **B.** Acyclovir triphosphate has a three-step mechanism of inhibition of herpesvirus DNA polymerase in vitro: **(1)** it acts as a competitive inhibitor of dGTP (pppdG) binding; **(2)** it acts as a substrate and is base-paired with dC in the template strand to become incorporated into the growing DNA chain, causing chain termination; and **(3)** it traps the polymerase on the ACV-terminated DNA chain when the next deoxyribonucleoside triphosphate (*shown here as dCTP, or pppdC*) binds.

In the first step, ACV triphosphate competitively inhibits deoxyguanosine triphosphate (dGTP) incorporation (note that high concentrations of dGTP can reverse inhibition at this early step). Next, ACV triphosphate acts as a substrate and is incorporated into the growing DNA chain opposite a C residue. The polymerase translocates to the next position on the template but cannot add a new deoxyribonucleoside triphosphate because there is no 3′-hydroxyl on ACV triphosphate; hence, ACV triphosphate is an obligate chain terminator. Finally, provided that the next deoxyribonucleoside triphosphate is present, the viral polymerase freezes in a "dead-end complex," leading to apparent inactivation of the enzyme (Fig. 38-7B). (The mechanism of polymerase "freezing" is incompletely understood.) Interestingly, cellular DNA polymerase α does not undergo inactivation to the dead-end complex. It is not yet known whether the inactivating step is important in vivo or whether ACV incorporation and chain termination alone are sufficient to inhibit viral replication.

Acyclovir resistance occurs infrequently during treatment of immunocompetent patients with cold sores or genital herpes. It occurs relatively often (5–10% of patients), however, during treatment of immunocompetent patients with HSV eye infections and immunocompromised hosts with various herpetic diseases.

Valacyclovir is a prodrug form of acyclovir that has approximately fivefold higher oral bioavailability than acyclovir (Fig. 38-6). This compound, which contains an acyclovir structure covalently attached to a valine moiety, is rapidly converted to acyclovir after oral administration.

Famciclovir and Penciclovir

Famciclovir (Fig. 38-6) is the diacetyl 6-deoxy analogue of **penciclovir**, the active form of the drug. Famciclovir is well absorbed orally and subsequently modified by an esterase and an oxidase to yield penciclovir. In humans, this results in approximately 70% oral bioavailability. Like acyclovir, penciclovir consists of a guanine linked to an acyclic sugar-like molecule that lacks a 2′ position but retains the 3′ position and has a CH_2 group in place of the ether oxygen.

Penciclovir's mechanism of action is similar to that of acyclovir (Fig. 38-7), with some quantitative differences. Famciclovir is used in the treatment of HSV infections and shingles, and penciclovir ointment is used to treat cold sores caused by HSV.

Ganciclovir

HCMV is much less sensitive to acyclovir than HSV and VZV are, primarily because much less phosphorylated acyclovir accumulates in HCMV-infected cells than in HSV- or VZV-infected cells. **Ganciclovir** is a nucleoside analogue that was originally synthesized as a derivative of acyclovir with the intention of developing another anti-HSV drug, but it proved too toxic for that indication. It turned out, however, that ganciclovir is much more potent than acyclovir against HCMV, and ganciclovir was the first antiviral drug approved for use against HCMV.

Like penciclovir, ganciclovir contains a guanine linked to an acyclic sugar-like molecule that lacks a 2′ position and retains the 3′ CHOH group that is missing in acyclovir (Fig. 38-6), but unlike penciclovir, ganciclovir retains the ether oxygen. Thus, ganciclovir more closely resembles the natural compound, deoxyguanosine, and this resemblance may account for its greater toxicity. (In fact, ganciclovir is so toxic that it should be used only for serious infections.)

As mentioned above, HCMV does not encode a homolog of HSV TK (which phosphorylates ganciclovir very efficiently) but rather encodes a viral protein kinase that induces expression of host cell enzymes. Remarkably, this viral protein kinase, called **UL97**, directly phosphorylates ganciclovir, leading to a 30-fold increase in the amount of phosphorylated ganciclovir in infected cells compared to uninfected cells. Ganciclovir triphosphate inhibits HCMV DNA polymerase more potently than it does cellular DNA polymerases. Although ganciclovir is not an obligate chain terminator, its incorporation does result in chain termination after the next nucleotide is incorporated. The mechanism of chain termination involves an exonuclease activity of the viral DNA polymerase, which rapidly excises any nucleotides that are incorporated thereafter.

Thus, as with acyclovir and HSV, *ganciclovir is selective against HCMV at two steps: phosphorylation and DNA polymerization.* However, the selectivity against HCMV at each step is not as great as the selectivity of acyclovir against HSV; accordingly, ganciclovir is more toxic than acyclovir. Toxicity is most commonly manifested as bone marrow suppression, especially neutropenia. Ganciclovir resistance due to mutations in either or both the UL97 and DNA polymerase genes is a clinical problem in a substantial fraction of patients.

Valganciclovir is a prodrug form of ganciclovir that has higher oral bioavailability than ganciclovir. Valganciclovir is a valine ester of ganciclovir, making the relationship between valganciclovir and ganciclovir similar to that between valacyclovir and acyclovir (Fig. 38-6).

Cidofovir

This phosphonate-containing acyclic cytosine analogue represents a twist on the mechanism of action of antiherpesvirus nucleoside analogues. Indeed, cidofovir can be considered a nucleo*tide* rather than a nucleo*side* analogue. With its phosphonate group, **cidofovir** mimics deoxycytidine monophosphate (dCMP); thus, in effect, it is already phosphorylated (Fig. 38-6). Therefore, cidofovir does not require viral kinases for its phosphorylation, and, accordingly, it is active against UL97-mutant viruses that are resistant to ganciclovir. As predicted by its structural resemblance to a phosphorylated compound, cidofovir is not orally available and is therefore administered intravenously. Nevertheless, this drug enters cells with reasonable efficiency. It is further phosphorylated (twice) by cellular enzymes to yield an analogue of dCTP, which inhibits herpesvirus DNA polymerases more potently than cellular DNA polymerases. Like ganciclovir, cidofovir is not an obligate chain terminator, but it can induce chain termination. Cidofovir is approved for use in the treatment of HCMV retinitis in patients with HIV/AIDS. Cidofovir diphosphate has a long intracellular half-life; therefore, its use requires relatively infrequent dosing (only once each week or less). Because of its mechanism of renal clearance, cidofovir must be co-administered with probenecid. (Probenecid inhibits a proximal tubule anion transporter and thereby decreases cidofovir excretion.) Nephrotoxicity is a major problem, and great care must be taken in administering this drug.

Other Antiherpesvirus Nucleoside Analogues

Several nucleoside analogues with antiherpesvirus activity were developed and approved before the development of acyclovir. These agents are more toxic than acyclovir and so are not widely used, but are listed in the Drug Summary Table.

Anti-HIV Nucleoside and Nucleotide Analogues

HIV is a retrovirus. All retroviruses contain an RNA genome within a capsid surrounded by a lipid envelope studded with glycoproteins. The capsid also contains three enzymes that are especially important from a pharmacologic perspective: reverse transcriptase, integrase, and protease. All three enzymes are essential for HIV replication (Fig. 38-2). **Reverse transcriptase (RT)** is a DNA polymerase that can copy both DNA and RNA. RT copies the RNA retrovirus genome into double-stranded DNA after the virus enters a cell. The viral DNA is then integrated into the host genome through the action of the viral enzyme **integrase** (see below). Subsequently, cellular RNA polymerase copies the integrated viral DNA back into RNA to make both full-length genomic viral RNA and the mRNAs that encode the various viral proteins. The structural proteins assemble onto the full-length genomic RNA, and soon thereafter, the virus buds through the cell membrane and matures into a form capable of infecting new cells. The **protease** cleaves viral proteins during assembly and maturation (see discussion below). Without these cleavages, the viral particles that are formed remain functionally immature and noninfectious.

Similar to herpesviruses, HIV forms latent infections in humans, and no available antiviral drug attacks HIV during latency. Rather, the available drugs act only on replicating virus.

Zidovudine

Zidovudine (azidothymidine [AZT]) was the first FDA-approved anti-HIV drug. Although it has largely been supplanted by newer nucleoside analogues with higher efficacy, lower toxicity, and improved pharmacokinetic properties, AZT illustrates many of the important principles of anti-HIV nucleoside analogues. Like the antiherpesvirus nucleoside analogues described above, AZT has an altered sugar moiety. Specifically, AZT contains a thymine base attached to a sugar in which the normal 3′ hydroxyl has been converted to an azido group (Fig. 38-6). Thus, like acyclovir, AZT is an obligate chain terminator.

AZT is a substrate for cellular thymidine kinase, which phosphorylates AZT to AZT monophosphate. (Unlike herpesviruses, HIV does *not* encode its own kinase.) AZT monophosphate is then converted to the diphosphate form by cellular thymidylate kinase and to the triphosphate form by cellular nucleoside diphosphate kinase. Thus, unlike acyclovir and ganciclovir, there is no selectivity at the activation step, and *phosphorylated AZT accumulates in almost all dividing cells in the body, not just infected cells*. The accumulation of phosphorylated AZT in almost all dividing cells largely accounts for the increased toxicity of AZT compared to a drug such as acyclovir.

AZT triphosphate targets HIV reverse transcriptase and is a substantially more potent inhibitor of HIV RT than of the human DNA polymerases that have been tested. The mechanism by which AZT inhibits RT is not entirely resolved, but incorporation of AZT triphosphate into the growing DNA chain is clearly important for antiviral activity.

Resistance to AZT inexorably appeared in patients when it was used as a monotherapy. High-level resistance was typically associated with the accumulation of several mutations in the gene encoding HIV RT. Like all polymerases, HIV RT catalyzes not only a forward reaction but also a back-reaction in which the two linked phosphates (pyrophosphate), which are cleaved from the nucleoside triphosphate or drug triphosphate during incorporation, can combine with the newly extended primer template to regenerate the triphosphate and the original primer template. With HIV RT, this "excision" reaction can be supported by ATP as well as by pyrophosphate. Many mutations that cause resistance to AZT and some other nucleoside analogues favor this ATP-dependent excision reaction.

Thus, AZT can be compared with acyclovir and ganciclovir (Table 38-1). Acyclovir is the most selective of these drugs because it is highly selective at both the activation (kinase) and inhibition (polymerase) steps. AZT is probably the least selective of the three drugs because it is nonselective at the activation step. Although AZT is relatively selective at the inhibition step, phosphorylated forms of AZT inhibit important cellular enzymes. For example, AZT monophosphate is both a substrate and an inhibitor of cellular thymidylate kinase, which is essential for cellular replication. Ganciclovir is intermediate in selectivity, with modest selectivity at both the activation and inhibition steps.

AZT toxicity is a serious clinical problem and led to its being administered in doses lower than those that achieve maximum efficacy. In particular, AZT causes bone marrow suppression, which is manifested most commonly as neutropenia and anemia. AZT toxicity appears to be caused not only by the effects of AZT triphosphate on cellular polymerases but also by the effects of AZT monophosphate on cellular thymidylate kinase (see above). The limited clinical effectiveness of AZT and problems with its toxicity and resistance led to the development of other anti-HIV drugs and to the use of combination chemotherapy for HIV (Box 38-2).

Other Anti-HIV Nucleoside Analogues with Mechanisms of Resistance Similar to That of AZT

Most anti-HIV nucleoside analogues—other than lamivudine and emtricitabine (see below)—have mechanisms of action and mechanisms of resistance similar to those of AZT (Fig. 38-6 and Drug Summary Table). Most exhibit toxicities that are thought to be due, at least in part, to inhibition of mitochondrial DNA polymerase by drug triphosphates, but these vary from drug to drug. Several of these drugs can be used at efficacious doses with much less toxicity than AZT. **Tenofovir**, which contains a phosphonate like the anti-HCMV drug cidofovir, is formulated as an orally available prodrug, tenofovir disoproxil (Fig. 38-6); the prodrug can be administered just once a day. Tenofovir has been combined with other drugs that have different resistance mechanisms, which also can be administered once a day, to provide a much simpler treatment regimen than the original anti-HIV combinations.

Lamivudine and Emtricitabine

Two nucleoside analogues—**lamivudine (3TC)** and **emtricitabine (FTC)**—differ from the other anti-HIV nucleoside analogues in their structure and mechanism of resistance. These drugs are L-stereoisomers, not the standard D-stereoisomer of biological nucleosides and the other anti-HIV nucleoside analogues, and they contain a sulfur atom in their five-membered ring (Fig. 38-6). Like AZT and the other anti-HIV nucleoside analogues, 3TC and FTC are

TABLE 38-1 Selectivity of Action of Antiviral Nucleoside Analogues Is Determined by Specificity of Viral and Cellular Kinases and Polymerases

DRUG	KINASE SPECIFICITY	POLYMERASE SPECIFICITY
Acyclovir	Viral TK >> Cellular kinases	Viral DNA polymerase >> Cellular DNA polymerase
Ganciclovir	Viral UL97 > Cellular kinases	Viral DNA polymerase > Cellular DNA polymerase
Zidovudine (AZT)	Cellular TK	Viral RT >> Cellular DNA polymerase

Drugs are presented in order of selectivity of action: >>, large difference in specificity; >, modest difference in specificity. TK, thymidine kinase; RT, reverse transcriptase.

obligate chain terminators. However, resistance to these compounds is not usually conferred by the same mutations that confer resistance to the other anti-HIV nucleoside analogues. Rather, alteration of a single residue drastically reduces incorporation of these compounds into the growing primer template. As a result, 3TC or FTC have frequently been combined with one of the other anti-HIV nucleoside analogues, since resistance to one compound does not usually result in resistance to the other (Box 38-2). Additionally, 3TC and FTC are biotransformed to relatively weak inhibitors of mitochondrial DNA polymerase. FTC can be administered just once a day and is often used in combination with other once-a-day anti-HIV drugs.

Anti-HBV Nucleoside and Nucleotide Analogues

In addition to their use in treating HIV infections, 3TC/FTC and tenofovir are used in patients with chronic HBV infections and evidence of active virus replication. (FTC is not FDA-approved for treatment of HBV but is often used in patients who are co-infected with HIV and HBV.) Three other nucleoside analogues are also approved for use against HBV: these include **adefovir**, which, like cidofovir and tenofovir, is a nucleoside phosphonate; **telbivudine**, which is simply L-thymidine; and **entecavir**, which is an unusual deoxyguanosine analogue (Fig. 38-6).

HBV is an unusual DNA virus. Within the HBV virion is a partially double-stranded DNA genome and a viral DNA

BOX 38-2 Combination Antiviral Therapy in the Treatment of HIV

When AZT was first introduced, monotherapy with this drug delayed disease progression in HIV-infected individuals and prolonged the survival of patients with advanced AIDS. In the late 1980s and early 1990s, this was a major advance in treatment. Since then, however, the drawbacks of AZT as monotherapy have become well recognized. AZT causes considerable toxicity—including anemia, nausea, headache, insomnia, arthralgia, and, rarely, lactic acidosis—and it effects only a modest (threefold to tenfold) and transient decrease in the viral load of HIV in plasma. Most patients treated with AZT as monotherapy inexorably progressed to AIDS. AZT-resistant virus could be detected in most of these patients, and it is generally accepted that these AZT-resistant variants contributed to the low long-term efficacy of AZT monotherapy.

Similar problems have been encountered with the use of most other anti-HIV drugs as monotherapy. When 3TC, the NNRTIs, or protease inhibitors were used as single agents, although the initial antiviral efficacy was greater than that of AZT (>30-fold reduction in the concentration of HIV in plasma), it was still incomplete, and resistance developed even more quickly than it did with AZT. Toxicities, unfavorable pharmacokinetic properties, and drug–drug interactions are also significant problems with many of the available agents.

Because of these drawbacks, combination chemotherapy (i.e., the use of "drug cocktails"; see Chapter 41, Principles of Combination Chemotherapy) has become the standard of care for HIV-infected individuals. The cocktails are more efficacious than single agents, inducing larger decreases in the viral load of HIV. Combination chemotherapy also decreases the emergence of resistance, both because virus replication is more efficaciously inhibited and, therefore, the chances for mutations to arise during replication are reduced, and because multiple mutations are required to confer resistance to all the drugs in the cocktail. In theory, combination chemotherapy can permit each drug to be used at lower doses, thereby reducing toxicity. It is now widely accepted that patients diagnosed with HIV infection should start therapy immediately with combination chemotherapy rather than with a single drug. Indeed, all new anti-HIV drugs are now approved by the FDA for combination use only, and certain combinations of drugs are combined into single pills. In 2006, the first single pill co-formulated regimen of tenofovir, emtricitabine, and efavirenz was approved for use on a once-a-day basis. Several other one-pill once-daily co-formulated regimens have been approved since then, and the reduced pill burden has been shown to improve both adherence and clinical outcome.

In antibacterial and antineoplastic combination chemotherapy, it is typical that only agents affecting different targets are combined (see Chapter 41). However, in anti-HIV combination chemotherapy, two or even three RT inhibitors (e.g., tenofovir, emtricitabine, and efavirenz) have been combined with evident benefit. One factor accounting for this success could be the incomplete efficacy of each drug alone; combining these drugs could allow for greater efficacy. (Because some of these drugs have toxicity profiles that differ from one another, it is possible to combine these agents without a significant increase in overall toxicity.) A second factor is that mutations conferring resistance to one drug do not ordinarily confer resistance to the other drugs. For example, mutants resistant to AZT and most other nucleoside analogues remain sensitive to 3TC or FTC and to NNRTIs. A third possible factor is that mutations conferring resistance to one drug can suppress the effects of mutations conferring resistance to another drug, although the clinical significance of this finding is controversial. A fourth possible factor—perhaps the most important—is that many resistance mutations decrease the "fitness" of the virus; that is, its ability to replicate in the patient. Thus, under some circumstances, it may even be beneficial to include in a combination therapy regimen a drug to which the virus is resistant in order to maintain selective pressure in favor of that less-fit, drug-resistant virus.

In many patients undergoing combination anti-HIV therapy (often called **highly active antiretroviral therapy** or **HAART**), the concentration of virus in the blood drops below the limit of detection (fewer than 20-50 copies of HIV RNA/mL in a standard test). However, anti-HIV drugs, like antiherpesvirus drugs, attack only replicating virus and not latent virus, and the best evidence is that HAART will need to be maintained life-long. Despite this limitation, HAART has been a tremendous success story, saving millions of lives worldwide and preventing countless additional infections. ∎

polymerase that also functions as an RT. Upon entry into the cell nucleus, this polymerase completes the synthesis of the viral DNA. The resulting DNA does not ordinarily integrate; rather, it serves as an episomal template for transcription by cellular RNA polymerase, which copies it into RNA to make both full-length genomic RNA and the mRNAs that encode the various viral proteins. Structural proteins, including the viral polymerase, then assemble onto the full-length genomic RNA. Within the resulting particles, which are still inside the infected cell, the polymerase copies the RNA into partially double-stranded DNA. Finally, the virus particle buds out of the cell, acquiring a lipid envelope. The triphosphate forms of the five different nucleoside analogues are potent inhibitors of the HBV polymerase; they become incorporated into the growing DNA chain and cause chain termination (although some are not obligate chain terminators).

Drug resistance is an important consideration in the treatment of HBV with these drugs. Resistance to 3TC/FTC and telbivudine occurs relatively rapidly due to mutations similar to those that confer resistance of HIV to 3TC and FTC. Multiple mutations are required for resistance to entecavir, which may contribute to the relatively slow development of resistance to this drug in patients. Interestingly, some of these mutations do not confer resistance per se but rather seem to increase fitness in the presence of the other mutations. Adefovir, telbivudine, and entecavir are all relatively well tolerated. Mitochondrial toxicity is a risk for all of these drugs. Cases of myopathy and peripheral neuropathy have been reported with telbivudine, and lactic acidosis has been reported with all of the anti-HBV nucleoside analogues.

Anti-HCV Nucleoside and Nucleotide Analogues

The RNA virus HCV encodes an RNA-dependent RNA polymerase. Based on the success of nucleoside analogue inhibitors of viral DNA polymerase, much effort has gone into developing such inhibitors of HCV RNA polymerase. The first of these to be approved is **sofosbuvir** (Fig. 38-6), which contains uracil. Recall that uracil is the base in uridine, a normal nucleoside precursor of RNA. Despite its activity as an RNA polymerase inhibitor, sofosbuvir does not contain a hydroxyl group at the 2′ position of the sugar moiety. Instead, that position is modified with fluorine and a methyl group. Like cidofovir, tenofovir, and adefovir, sofosbuvir contains a phosphate mimic—but in this case, a phosphoramidite rather than a phosphonate—that can be further phosphorylated by cellular enzymes to a triphosphate mimic that has a long cellular half-life. The phosphoramidite is further modified with additional groups that are cleaved off in hepatocytes; i.e., sofosbuvir is a prodrug. At concentrations that show little or no cytotoxicity, including mitochondrial toxicity, sofosbuvir is highly efficacious at inhibiting HCV RNA polymerase and genome replication.

Although certain mutations in the gene coding for the viral RNA polymerase can confer resistance to sofosbuvir, such mutations do not readily arise during treatment with the drug, evidently because they decrease viral fitness. Presumably, the enzyme would need to change its active site for resistance to occur, and such changes would be expected to impair enzyme efficiency. As the first DAA approved for use in an all-oral regimen without interferon alpha (but with ribavirin) against certain genotypes of HCV, sofosbuvir transformed HCV treatment. It has subsequently been approved for use without ribavirin in combination with the protease inhibitor

simeprevir (see above) or the NS5A inhibitor ledipasvir (see below) against certain HCV genotypes. In many cases, only a 2- to 3-month course of combination antiviral treatment is needed to cure the disease. Sofosbuvir is generally well tolerated, and serious adverse reactions have been limited.

Nonnucleoside DNA Polymerase Inhibitors

Nucleoside analogues can inhibit cellular as well as viral enzymes. As a result, efforts have been made to discover compounds with different structures that can more selectively target viral enzymes. The first such compound to be used clinically was **foscarnet (phosphonoformic acid [PFA]**; Fig. 38-8). Foscarnet has a relatively broad spectrum of activity *in vitro* (including against HIV), but clinically, it is used to treat certain serious HSV and HCMV infections in which therapy with acyclovir or ganciclovir has not succeeded (e.g., because of resistance). Mechanistically, foscarnet differs from nucleoside analogues in that it does not require activation by cellular or viral enzymes; rather, foscarnet inhibits viral DNA polymerase directly by mimicking the pyrophosphate product of DNA polymerization. Moreover, a crystal structure suggests that foscarnet occupies the position of two of the phosphates on the *incoming* deoxyribonucleoside triphosphate, thus stalling the polymerase. Selectivity results from the increased sensitivity of viral DNA polymerase to foscarnet relative to cellular enzymes. As might be expected of a compound that so closely mimics a natural compound (pyrophosphate), foscarnet's selectivity is not as high as acyclovir's; it inhibits cell division at concentrations not much higher than its effective antiherpesvirus concentration. Major drawbacks to foscarnet use include its lack of oral bioavailability and its poor solubility; renal impairment is its major dose-limiting toxicity. Resistance can also arise.

Nonnucleoside Reverse Transcriptase Inhibitors

The nonnucleoside reverse transcriptase inhibitors (NNRTIs) **efavirenz**, **nevirapine**, **delavirdine**, **etravirine**, and **rilpivirine** were developed using the rational approach of target-based, high-throughput screening (Box 38-1 and Fig. 38-8). Indeed, the NNRTIs were among the first successes of this now widely used approach. Unlike the nucleoside analogues, these drugs inhibit their target directly, without the need for chemical modification. X-ray crystallographic studies have shown that NNRTIs bind near the catalytic site of RT. NNRTIs permit RT to bind a nucleoside triphosphate and primer template but inhibit the joining of the two. The NNRTIs are orally bioavailable, and their adverse effects (most commonly, rash) are typically less serious than those of foscarnet and most nucleoside analogues. The main limitation of NNRTI use is that resistance develops rapidly; just a single mutation that prevents drug binding is sufficient for high-level resistance with little fitness cost. This limitation requires that these drugs must be used in combination with other anti-HIV drugs (Box 38-2).

One NNRTI, **efavirenz**, was the first anti-HIV drug to be taken once a day. In 2006, a single pill combining efavirenz, tenofovir, and FTC was approved by the FDA for once-a-day administration. Since then, a co-formulated single pill containing rilpivirine, tenofovir, and FTC has also become available. While efavirenz-containing treatments are frequently associated with neuropsychiatric adverse effects, the rilpivirine-based regimen is recommended as first-line treatment only for HIV-1-infected individuals with viral RNA load <100,000 copies/mL and CD4 count >200 cells/mm^3.

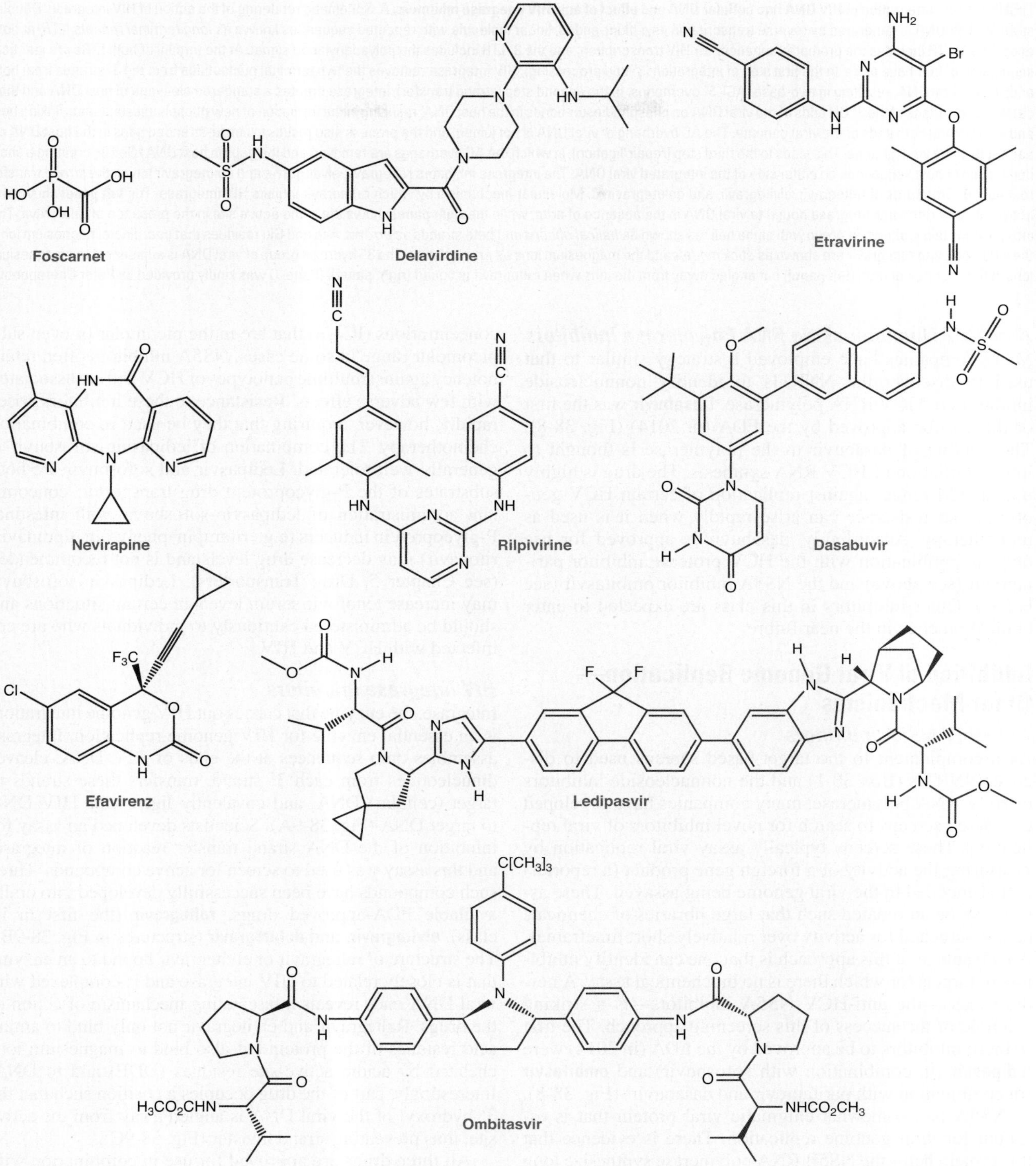

FIGURE 38-8. Nonnucleoside DNA polymerase and reverse transcriptase inhibitors and NS5A inhibitors. Foscarnet is a pyrophosphate analogue that inhibits viral DNA and RNA polymerases. Foscarnet is approved for the treatment of HSV and HCMV infections that are resistant to antiherpesvirus nucleoside analogues. The nonnucleoside reverse transcriptase inhibitors (NNRTIs) delavirdine, etravirine, nevirapine, rilpivirine, and efavirenz inhibit HIV-1 reverse transcriptase. The NNRTIs are approved in combination with other antiretroviral drugs for the treatment of HIV-1 infection. Note that the structures of the NNRTIs are significantly different from those of the anti-HIV nucleoside and nucleotide analogues (compare with Fig. 38-6). Dasabuvir inhibits HCV RNA polymerase. The anti-HCV NS5A inhibitors, ledipasvir and ombitasvir, have twofold symmetric elements, which permit very tight binding to the dimeric NS5A protein. These compounds are approved for treatment of HCV disease in combination with other anti-HCV drugs.

FIGURE 38-9. **Integration of HIV DNA into cellular DNA and effect of anti-HIV integrase inhibitors. A.** Schematic rendering of the action of HIV integrase. Double-stranded HIV DNA is generated by reverse transcription as a blunt-ended, linear molecule with repeated sequences known as *long terminal repeats (LTR)* at both ends. The 5′ LTR includes the promoter/enhancer for HIV transcription, and the 3′ LTR includes the polyadenylation signal. At the termini of both LTRs are identical sequences of four base pairs. In the first step of integration (3′ end processing), HIV integrase removes the two terminal nucleotides from the 3′ strands from both ends of the viral DNA, resulting in two-base (AC), 5′ overhangs. In the second step (strand transfer), integrase creates a staggered cleavage of host DNA and then catalyzes the attack of the 3′ OH ends of the viral DNA on phosphodiester bonds in the host DNA, resulting in the formation of new phosphodiester bonds linking host and viral DNA at both ends of the viral genome. The AC overhang of viral DNA is not joined, and the process also results in single-stranded gaps in the host DNA on each side of the viral genome. This leads to the third step (repair/ligation), in which the AC overhangs are removed and the gaps in host DNA filled in, creating a short duplication of host sequences on either side of the integrated viral DNA. The integrase inhibitors raltegravir, elvitegravir, and dolutegravir inhibit the strand transfer reaction. **B.** Structures of raltegravir, elvitegravir, and dolutegravir. **C.** Molecular mechanism by which raltegravir inhibits HIV integrase. The **left panel** shows the active site of a retroviral integrase bound to viral DNA in the absence of drug, while the **right panel** shows the same active site in the presence of raltegravir. The integrase protein is shown in *green* with alpha helices shown as *helical ribbons* and beta strands as *arrows*. Asp and Glu residues that coordinate magnesium ions, the viral DNA, and raltegravir are shown as *stick models* and the magnesium ions as *gray spheres*. The 3′-hydroxyl group of viral DNA is adjacent to the magnesium ions in the absence of drug (**left panel**) but angled away from the ions when raltegravir is bound (**right panel**). (Panel C was kindly provided by Peter Cherepanov.)

Anti-HCV Nonnucleoside RNA Polymerase Inhibitors

Many companies have employed a strategy similar to that used to discover the NNRTIs to identify nonnucleoside inhibitors of HCV RNA polymerase. **Dasabuvir** was the first of these to be approved by the FDA (in 2014) (Fig. 38-8). The binding of dasabuvir to the polymerase is thought to inhibit initiation of HCV RNA synthesis. The drug is highly potent (nM range) against replication of certain HCV genotypes, but resistance can arise rapidly when it is used as monotherapy. Accordingly, dasabuvir is approved for use only in combination with the HCV protease inhibitor paritaprevir (see above) and the NS5A inhibitor ombitasvir (see below). Other inhibitors in this class are expected to enter clinical practice in the near future.

Inhibition of Viral Genome Replication—Other Mechanisms

Anti-HCV NS5A Inhibitors

As a complement to the target-based screens used to discover NNRTIs (Box 38-1) and the nonnucleoside inhibitors of HCV RNA polymerase, many companies have developed cell-based screens to search for novel inhibitors of viral replication. These screens typically assay viral replication by measuring the activity of a foreign gene product (a reporter) that is encoded in the viral genome being assayed. These assays can be automated such that large libraries of chemicals can be screened for activity over relatively short timeframes. An advantage of this approach is that one can identify inhibitors of targets for which there is no biochemical assay. A new drug class—the anti-HCV NS5A inhibitors—is a striking example of the success of this screening approach. The first of these inhibitors to be approved by the FDA (in 2014) were **ledipasvir** (in combination with sofosbuvir) and **ombitasvir** (in combination with paritaprevir and dasabuvir) (Fig. 38-8).

NS5A is a somewhat enigmatic viral protein that is essential for viral genome replication. There is evidence that this protein helps the NS5B RNA polymerase synthesize long chains of RNA. NS5A is also thought to alter the host cell environment in order to abet viral RNA synthesis and to have roles at later stages of infection. The protein is a dimer, and NS5A inhibitors similarly display either rough (ledipasvir) or complete (ombitasvir) twofold symmetry. This structure promotes tight binding of the drugs, with each half of the molecule engaging an NS5A monomer. Additionally, it appears that drug binding to a small fraction of NS5A molecules in the infected cell is sufficient to inhibit HCV replication. These features collectively lead to remarkably potent inhibition of HCV genome replication, with 50% inhibitory concentrations (IC_{50}'s) that are in the picomolar or even sub-picomolar range in some cases. NS5A inhibitors often retain potency against multiple genotypes of HCV and are associated with few adverse effects. Resistance to these inhibitors arises rapidly, however, requiring that they be used in combination chemotherapy. The combination of ledipasvir–sofosbuvir is generally well tolerated. Ledipasvir and sofosbuvir are both substrates of the P-glycoprotein drug transporter; concomitant administration of ledipasvir–sofosbuvir with intestinal P-glycoprotein inducers (e.g., rifampin, phenytoin, tipranavir/ritonavir) may decrease drug levels and is not recommended (see Chapter 5, Drug Transporters). Ledipasvir–sofosbuvir may increase tenofovir serum levels in certain situations and should be administered cautiously to individuals who are co-infected with HCV and HIV.

HIV Integrase Inhibitors

Integrase, the enzyme that carries out HIV genome integration, is an essential enzyme for HIV genome replication. Integrase assembles onto sequences at the ends of HIV DNA, cleaves dinucleotides from each 3′ strand, transfers these strands to target (cellular) DNA, and covalently ligates the HIV DNA to target DNA (Fig. 38-9A). Scientists developed an assay for inhibition of the DNA strand transfer reaction of integrase, and this assay was used to screen for active compounds. Three such compounds have been successfully developed into orally available FDA-approved drugs, **raltegravir** (the first in its class), **elvitegravir**, and **dolutegravir** (structures in Fig. 38-9B). The structure of raltegravir or elvitegravir bound to an enzyme that is closely related to HIV integrase and is complexed with viral DNA ends reveals a fascinating mechanism of action of the drugs. Raltegravir and elvitegravir not only bind to amino acid residues of the protein but also bind to magnesium ions chelated by acidic active-site residues (DDE) and to DNA. Interestingly, part of the drug occupies a position such that the 3′-hydroxyl of the viral DNA is angled away from the active site, thus preventing strand transfer (Fig. 38-9C).

All three drugs are approved for use in combination with other anti-HIV drugs in HIV-infected individuals, including those who have not previously been treated with antiretroviral drugs (treatment-naïve). Of note, raltegravir is approved for use in pediatric cases, and elvitegravir is formulated as a once-a-day pill with FTC, tenofovir, and an inhibitor of the cytochrome P450 enzyme that metabolizes elvitegravir (cobicistat). Dolutegravir has a higher barrier to genetic resistance than raltegravir and elvitegravir do, and dolutegravir remains active against many viruses that are resistant to the other two integrase inhibitors. Dolutegravir is available as a single co-formulated tablet with abacavir and lamivudine.

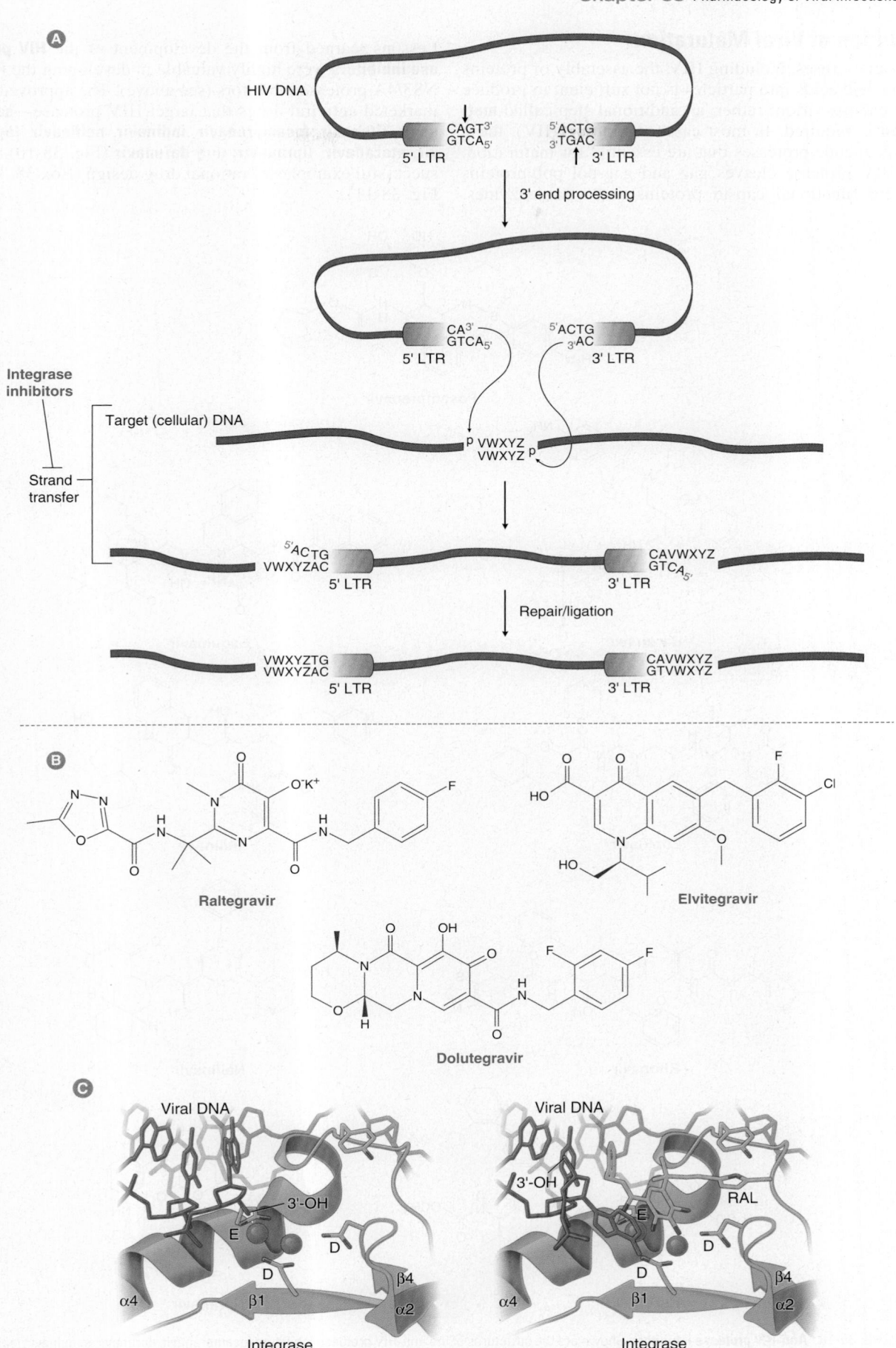

Raltegravir

Elvitegravir

Dolutegravir

Inhibition of Viral Maturation

For many viruses, including HIV, the assembly of proteins and nucleic acids into particles is not sufficient to produce an infectious virion; rather, an additional step called **maturation** is required. In most cases (including HIV), these viruses encode proteases that are essential for maturation. The HIV protease cleaves gag and gag-pol polyproteins to yield functional capsid proteins and viral enzymes.

Lessons learned from the development of the **HIV protease inhibitors** were highly valuable in developing the HCV NS3/4A protease inhibitors (see above). The approved and marketed antiviral drugs that target HIV protease—**saquinavir**, **ritonavir**, **fosamprenavir**, **indinavir**, **nelfinavir**, **lopinavir**, **atazanavir**, **tipranavir**, and **darunavir** (Fig. 38-10)—are successful examples of rational drug design (Box 38-3 and Fig. 38-11).

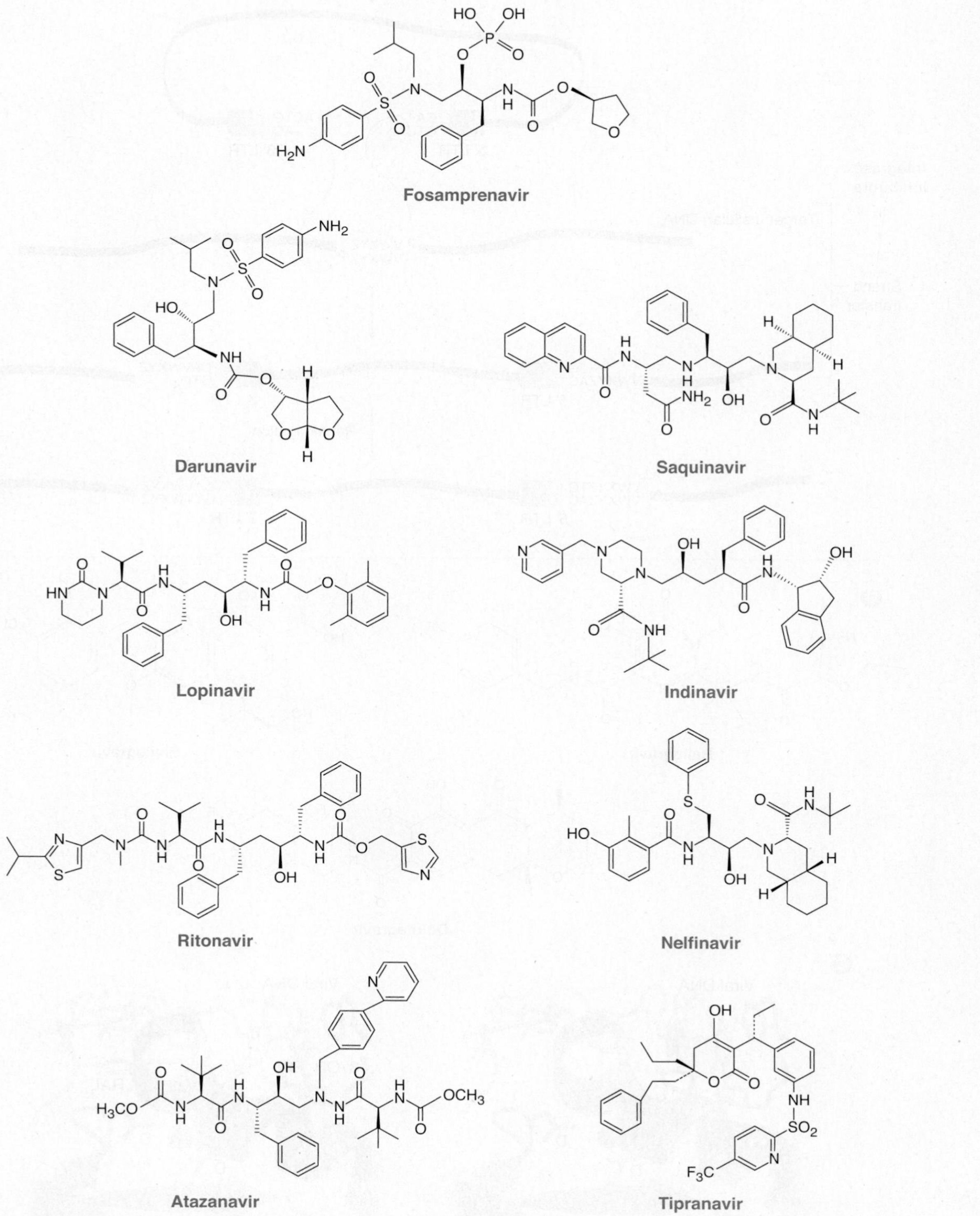

FIGURE 38-10. Anti-HIV protease inhibitors. Shown are the structures of the anti-HIV protease inhibitors fosamprenavir, darunavir, saquinavir, lopinavir, indinavir, ritonavir, nelfinavir, atazanavir, and tipranavir. These compounds mimic peptides (peptidomimetics), and all but tipranavir contain peptide bonds.

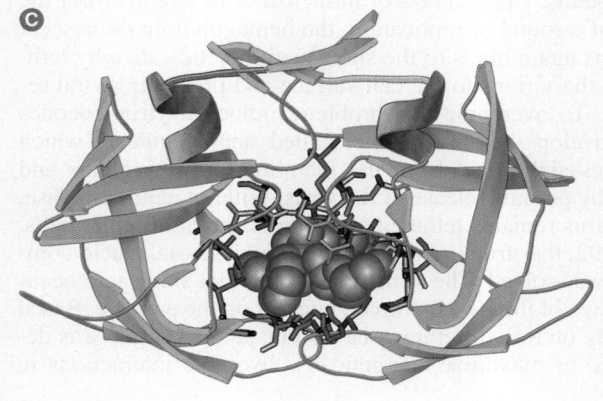

A *pol* Substrate sequence — Protease attack — Model of transition state on substrate sequence; Rotational axis of symmetry

P_{-3} P_{-2} P_{-1} (Phe) P_1 (Pro) P_2

B

A-74702
Protease IC_{50} > 200 μM

A-74704
Protease IC_{50} = 5 nM
Antiviral activity < 1 μM

A-75925
Protease IC_{50} < 1 nM
Antiviral activity < 1 μM
Poor aqueous solubility

A-77003
Protease IC_{50} < 1 nM
Antiviral activity = 0.1 μM
Good solubility
Poor oral bioavailability

Ritonavir
Protease IC_{50} < 1 nM
Antiviral activity = 25 nM
Fair solubility
Good oral bioavailability

FIGURE 38-11. Steps in the evolution of ritonavir. A. The HIV *pol* gene product has a phenylalanine (Phe)–proline (Pro) sequence that is unusual as a cleavage site for human proteases. HIV protease cleaves this Phe–Pro bond. The transition state of the protease reaction includes a rotational axis of symmetry. **B.** Structure-based development of a selective HIV protease inhibitor began with a compound (A-74702) that contained two phenylalanine analogues and a CHOH moiety between them. This compound, which had weak inhibitory activity, was then modified to maximize antiprotease activity while also maximizing antiviral activity, aqueous solubility, and oral bioavailability. The maximization of antiprotease activity was measured as a progressive reduction in IC_{50}, the drug concentration required to cause 50% inhibition of the enzyme. See Box 38-3 for details. **C.** Structure of ritonavir (space-filling structure) bound to HIV protease, with beta strands shown as green arrows, alpha helices in purple, and the amino acids that bind ritonavir depicted in stick form.

BOX 38-3 Development of Ritonavir

The development of ritonavir is an example of structure-based ("rational") drug design. Scientists began with a model of the transition state that forms during the cleavage of a substrate by HIV protease (Fig. 38-11). An analogue of the transition state was designed using just one residue on each side of the cleavage site. Knowing that HIV protease is a symmetric dimer, the scientists chose to use the same residue—phenylalanine—on both sides of the cleavage site, with a CHOH group that mimics the transition state as the center of symmetry. This molecule, A-74702, was a very weak inhibitor of HIV protease, but adding symmetric groups at both ends to form A-74704 (Fig. 38-11, where Val is valine and Cbz is carbobenzyloxy) resulted in a >40,000-fold increase in potency (IC_{50} = 5 nM). All attempts to modify A-74704 to improve aqueous solubility also reduced potency, however, so a related potent inhibitor, A-75925, in which the center of symmetry was a C-C bond between two CHOH groups, became the scaffold for further modifications. Symmetric changes to both ends of the molecule resulted in a soluble, highly potent inhibitor, A-77003. This compound was not orally bioavailable, however. Further modifications, which removed a central OH group and altered other moieties at each end of the molecule, resulted in a compound—ritonavir—that was less soluble but had improved antiviral activity and good oral bioavailability. Therapeutically achievable plasma concentrations of ritonavir greatly exceed the concentration required for antiviral activity. In the process of structure-based drug design, successive modifications to these molecules took advantage of x-ray structures of HIV protease complexed to each inhibitor. By examining these structures, scientists were able to make informed guesses about which specific chemical groups to add or subtract. The result was the therapeutically useful HIV protease inhibitor ritonavir. ∎

For several reasons, HIV protease was (and remains) an attractive target for pharmacologic intervention. First, it is essential for HIV replication. Second, a point mutation is sufficient to inactivate the enzyme, suggesting that a small molecule might successfully inhibit activity. Third, the sequences cleaved by HIV protease are conserved and somewhat unusual, suggesting both specificity and a starting point for drug design. Fourth, HIV protease—unlike the human proteases most closely related to it—is a symmetric dimer of two identical subunits, each of which contributes to the active site, again suggesting both specificity and a starting point for drug design. Fifth, the enzyme can be easily overexpressed and assayed, and its crystal structure has been solved. All of these factors increased the likelihood that a drug discovery effort would be successful.

The HIV protease inhibitor ritonavir provides an example of rational drug design. Ritonavir is a peptidomimetic (i.e., it mimics the structure of a peptide; see Box 38-3 and Fig. 38-11). Its design began with the identification of one of the natural substrates of HIV protease, a site for cleaving a longer protein into reverse transcriptase. This site is unusual in that it contains a phenylalanine–proline (Phe–Pro) bond (Fig. 38-11A); mammalian enzymes rarely, if ever, cleave at such a site. To take advantage of the symmetric dimer feature of the HIV protease structure, correspondingly symmetric inhibitors were designed in which the Pro was replaced with a Phe. Moreover, CHOH was used in place of the native C=O of the peptide bond in order to mimic the transition state of protease catalysis, which is the catalytic intermediate that binds the enzyme most tightly (Fig. 38-11). The designed inhibitors, unlike the original peptide and the native transition state, cannot be cleaved by the enzyme. How these symmetric inhibitors evolved into ritonavir is discussed in Box 38-3 (also see Fig. 38-11).

Although clever design is no guarantee that a drug will be active against a virus by the expected mechanism, the protease inhibitors do act as expected. (Interestingly, darunavir inhibits not only the activity of the protease but also its dimerization.) The compounds are potent in cell culture, albeit often less potent against virus replication than against enzyme activity in vitro. As expected, HIV-infected cells exposed to protease inhibitors continue to make viral proteins, but these proteins are not processed efficiently. Viral particles bud from the infected cells, but these particles are immature and noninfectious.

Used in combination with other anti-HIV drugs, protease inhibitors have had a major impact on AIDS therapy (Box 38-2). Currently, ritonavir-boosted atazanavir and darunavir are the two protease inhibitors recommended as components of first-line therapy. The main adverse effects of atazanavir are indirect hyperbilirubinemia and jaundice. Darunavir has a sulfonamide moiety and its main adverse effect is a rash. All protease inhibitors also alter fat distribution and cause metabolic abnormalities, which has limited their use. The mechanisms of these adverse effects remain poorly understood.

Inhibition of Viral Release

Rational design has also led to the development of inhibitors of influenza virus neuraminidases. The rationale for these inhibitors, which block viral release from the host cell, follows from the mechanism of viral attachment and release. Influenza virus attaches to cells via interactions between hemagglutinin, a protein on the viral envelope, and sialic acid moieties, which are present on many cell surface glycoproteins. Upon egress of influenza virus from cells at the end of a round of replication, the hemagglutinin on nascent virions again binds to the sialic acid moieties, thereby tethering the virions to the cell surface and preventing viral release. To overcome this problem, influenza virus encodes an envelope-bound enzyme, called **neuraminidase**, which cleaves sialic acid from the membrane glycoproteins and thereby permits release of the virus. Without neuraminidase, the virus remains tethered and cannot spread to other cells. In 1992, the structure of the neuraminidase–sialic acid complex was solved. The structure showed that sialic acid occupies two of three well-formed pockets on the enzyme. Based largely on this structure, a new sialic acid analogue was designed to maximize energetically favorable interactions in

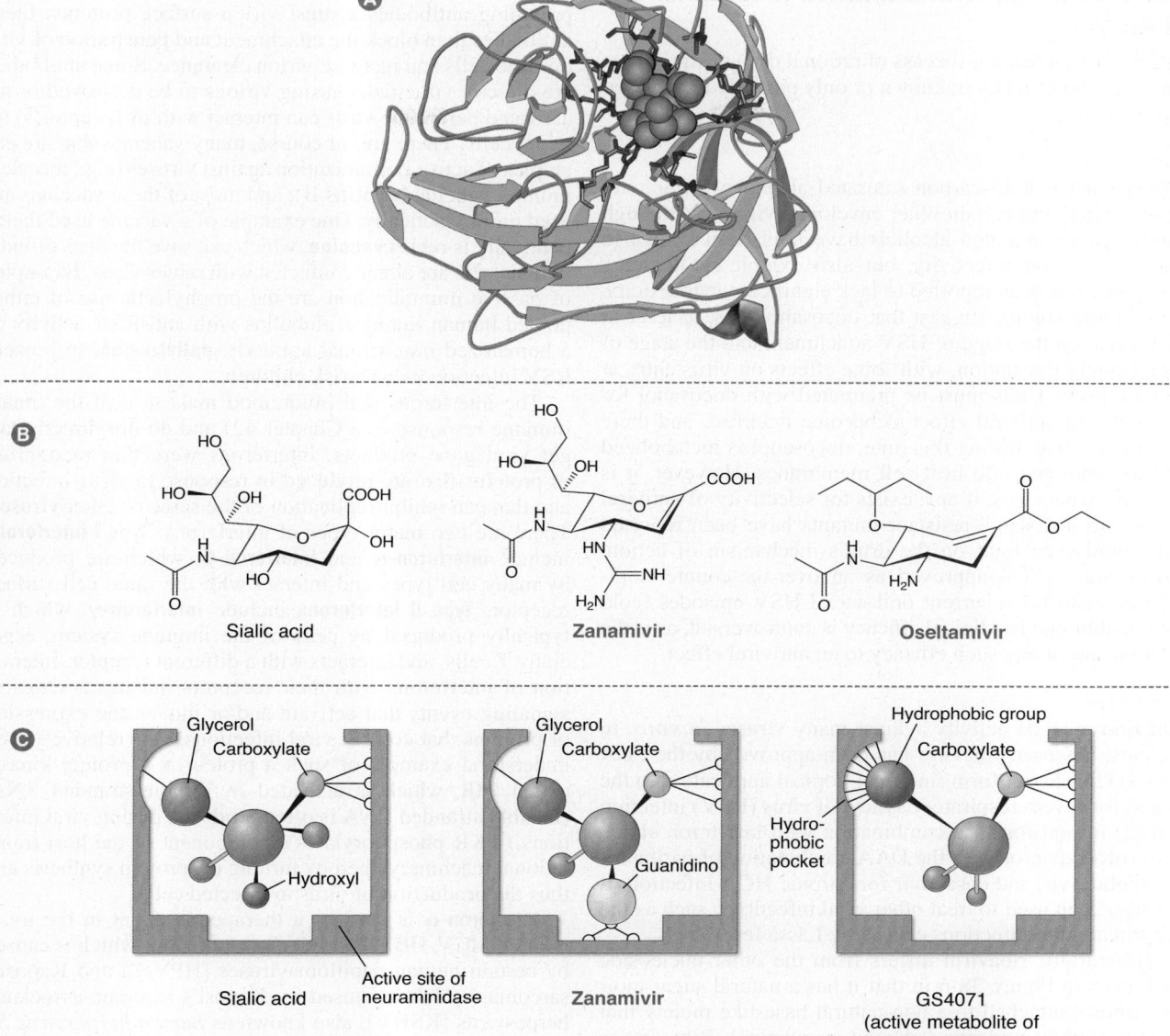

FIGURE 38-12. Structure-based design of neuraminidase inhibitors. A. Shown is a model of sialic acid (*space-filling structure*) bound to the influenza A virus neuraminidase, with the amino acids that bind sialic acid depicted in *stick form*. This structure was used to design transition state analogues that bind more tightly to neuraminidase than sialic acid does, resulting in potent inhibitors of the enzyme. **B.** Structures of sialic acid and the neuraminidase inhibitors zanamivir and oseltamivir. **C.** Schematic diagram of the active site of influenza virus neuraminidase, depicting the binding of sialic acid, zanamivir, and GS4071 to several different features of the active site. (Oseltamivir is the ethyl ester prodrug of GS4071.)

all three of the potential binding pockets (Fig. 38-12). This compound, now known as **zanamivir**, inhibits neuraminidase with a K_i of about 0.1 nM. Zanamivir is active against both influenza A and influenza B, with potencies of about 30 nM. However, zanamivir has low oral bioavailability and must be administered by inhaler.

Efforts to improve on zanamivir's pharmacokinetics resulted in a new drug, **oseltamivir** (Fig. 38-12), whose oral availability is approximately 75%. Oseltamivir binds well to two of the three binding pockets of the neuraminidase. When taken prophylactically, oseltamivir reduces the number of flu cases in susceptible populations (e.g., nursing home residents). Both oseltamivir and zanamivir reduce the duration of flu symptoms in most patients who are already infected with the virus. However, this reduction is only

1 day on average, and even this modest effect (although it can be quite meaningful to the "flu" sufferer) requires that the drugs be taken within 2 days of the onset of symptoms. Oseltamivir is also used to treat patients who are at high risk for severe infection (e.g., immunocompromised individuals) or those who already have severe infection. Concerns about H5N1 avian influenza ("bird flu") or the 2009 H1N1 ("swine flu") pandemic strain have led to stockpiling of oseltamivir. Although mutations that cause resistance to neuraminidase inhibitors reduce viral fitness and were not detected in treated patients for a number of years, influenza strains have since evolved with additional mutations that compensate for the loss of fitness. Regardless, the neuraminidase inhibitors represent a triumph of rational drug design.

Antiviral Drugs with Unknown Mechanisms of Action

Despite the increasing success of rational drug design, some antiviral agents act by unknown or only partially understood mechanisms.

Docosanol

n-**Docosanol** is a 22-carbon saturated alcohol with activity against HSV and certain other enveloped viruses. Although shorter chain saturated alcohols have long been known to inactivate virion infectivity, but also exhibit cytotoxicity, docosanol has been reported to lack significant cytotoxicity. Cell culture studies suggest that docosanol acts, at least in part, between the stage of HSV attachment and the stage of viral protein translation, with some effects on virus entry at certain doses. Cells must be pretreated with docosanol for hours for an antiviral effect to become manifest, and there is evidence that, during this time, docosanol is metabolized and incorporated into host cell membranes. However, it is not clear what basis, if any, exists for selectivity of antiviral action; no docosanol-resistant mutants have been reported that could shed light on the drug's mechanism of action. Docosanol is FDA-approved as an over-the-counter topical treatment for recurrent oral–facial HSV episodes (cold sores), although its clinical efficacy is controversial, as is the relationship of any such efficacy to an antiviral effect.

Ribavirin

Ribavirin exhibits activity against many viruses in vitro. In patients, however, ribavirin has been approved by the FDA only (1) in aerosol form (in effect, topical application to the lungs) for severe respiratory syncytial virus (RSV) infection and (2) in oral form, in combination with interferon alpha, with sofosbuvir, or with the DAA combination of paritaprevir, ombitasvir, and dasabuvir for chronic HCV infection. It has also been used to treat other viral infections, such as the life-threatening infections caused by Lassa fever virus.

Structurally, ribavirin differs from the other nucleoside analogues in Figure 38-6 in that it has a natural sugar moiety (ribose) attached to a non-natural base-like moiety that most resembles a purine (adenine or guanine). Ribavirin is converted to monophosphate, diphosphate, and triphosphate forms by cellular enzymes. The phosphorylated forms can inhibit various host and viral enzymes, and the triphosphate derivative can also be incorporated into RNA by viral RNA polymerases and induce deleterious mutations. There is also evidence that ribavirin can enhance immune responses. Which of these proposed mechanisms of ribavirin action are relevant for the therapeutic effect of the drug on viral infections in humans is not firmly established. Indeed, for HCV, ribavirin by itself has little if any effect on the levels of virus in treated patients. Moreover, ribavirin has important toxicities, including anemia. Regardless, learning more about the mechanisms of ribavirin action may lead to improved antiviral therapies.

Drugs That Modulate the Immune System

Three classes of drugs that make explicit use of host immune processes are used to treat viral infections. These classes include immunization, interferons, and imiquimod. For background on the immune system, see Chapter 42, Principles of Inflammation and the Immune System.

Active and **passive immunization** inhibit viral infection by providing antibodies against virion surface proteins; these antibodies then block the attachment and penetration of virions into cells and increase virion clearance. Some antibodies are directly virucidal, causing virions to be destroyed or inactivated before the virus can interact with its receptor(s) on target cells. There are, of course, many vaccines that are examples of active immunization against viruses (e.g., measles, mumps, rubella, hepatitis B), and most of these vaccines are used prophylactically. One example of a vaccine used therapeutically is **rabies vaccine**, which can save the lives of individuals who are already infected with rabies virus. Examples of passive immunization are the prophylactic use of either pooled human immune globulins with anti-RSV activity or a humanized monoclonal antibody, **palivizumab**, to prevent RSV infection in high-risk children.

The interferons and imiquimod make use of the innate immune response (see Chapter 42) and do not directly target viral gene products. Interferons were first recognized as proteins that are produced in response to virus infection and that can inhibit replication of the same or other viruses. There are two major types of interferons. **Type I interferons** include **interferon-α** and **interferon-β**, which are produced by many cell types and interact with the same cell surface receptor. **Type II interferons** include **interferon-γ**, which is typically produced by cells of the immune system, especially T cells, and interacts with a different receptor. Interaction of interferons with their receptors induces a series of signaling events that activate and/or induce the expression of proteins that combat viral infections. One relatively well understood example of such a protein is a protein kinase, called **PKR**, which is activated by double-stranded RNA. (Double-stranded RNA is often produced during viral infections.) PKR phosphorylates a component of the host translational machinery, thereby turning off protein synthesis and thus the production of virus in infected cells.

Interferon-α is used as a therapeutic agent in the treatment of HCV, HBV, condyloma acuminata (which is caused by certain human papillomaviruses [HPVs]), and Kaposi's sarcoma (which is caused by Kaposi's sarcoma-associated herpesvirus [KSHV], also known as *human herpesvirus 8*). Interferon-α is usually administered in a form that has been modified with polyethylene glycol (pegylated) to improve its pharmacokinetic profile after injection. Although the mechanism by which interferons inhibit the replication of certain viruses is reasonably well understood (e.g., by inducing PKR), the mechanisms by which interferons act against HCV, HBV, HPVs, and KSHV remain poorly understood. Interestingly, all of these viruses encode proteins that inhibit interferon action. Understanding the mechanism of this inhibition may aid understanding of the action of interferons in inhibiting viral replication. This is an active area of investigation.

Interferon-α is also used to treat certain relatively rare malignancies, and **interferon-β** is used to treat multiple sclerosis. Again, the mechanisms by which interferons exert their therapeutic effects in these clinical settings are poorly understood. For multiple sclerosis, there is evidence that, while boosting innate immune responses, type I interferons also suppress certain inflammatory responses.

Imiquimod is approved for the treatment of certain diseases caused by HPVs. Imiquimod interacts with the Toll-like receptors TLR7 and TLR8 to boost innate immunity, including the secretion of interferons. Toll-like receptors are membrane proteins that recognize pathogen-associated molecular patterns. Activation of Toll-like receptors induces intracellular signaling events that are important for defense against pathogens. In the case of imiquimod, it is not clear exactly how this stimulation results in effective treatment of disease caused by HPV.

CONCLUSION AND FUTURE DIRECTIONS

The various stages in the viral life cycle provide a basis for understanding the mechanisms of action of currently available antiviral drugs and for developing new antiviral therapies. The vast majority of antiviral drugs available today inhibit viruses at the genome replication stage by taking advantage of structural and functional differences between viral and host polymerases. In addition, maraviroc and enfuvirtide (T-20) inhibit HIV attachment and entry, adamantanes inhibit influenza A uncoating, protease inhibitors inhibit viral gene expression (HCV) and viral maturation (HIV), and neuraminidase inhibitors inhibit influenza release. It is important to bear in mind, however, that many of these drugs inhibit only one virus (e.g., HIV), and, in some cases, only one species of that virus (e.g., HIV-1 but not HIV-2). Only a tiny fraction of viruses known to cause human disease can be treated effectively with the antiviral therapies that are currently available. Nevertheless, great strides have been made. At this writing, new antiviral small-molecule drugs are under review at the FDA, and many other small molecules, antibodies, and other modalities, such as oligonucleotides that block viral gene expression by RNA interference, are under investigation. (An antisense DNA-based oligonucleotide that blocks HCMV replication has been FDA-approved [fomivirsen], but it is no longer marketed and whether it actually acts by blocking viral gene expression has not been established.) In the case of Mr. M, the treatment of HIV with a combination of drugs could reduce viral loads to undetectable levels and delay the progression of AIDS for many years. Although antiviral therapies do not yet represent either prevention or cure for this disease, such therapies have already decreased the morbidity and mortality of HIV/AIDS in millions of individuals, essentially converting HIV infection from a death sentence to a manageable chronic disease.

Acknowledgment

We thank Robert W. Yeh for his valuable contributions to this chapter in earlier editions of *Principles of Pharmacology: The Pathophysiologic Basis of Drug Therapy* and Peter Cherepanov for Figure 38-9C, illustrating the mechanism of integrase inhibitors.

Suggested Reading

Coen DM, Richman DD. Antiviral agents. In: Knipe DM, Howley PM, Cohen JI, et al., eds. *Fields virology*. 6th ed. Philadelphia: Lippincott Williams & Wilkins; 2013. (*Detailed review of the general and specific aspects of the mechanisms and uses of antiviral drugs.*)

Dorr P, Westby M, Dobbs S, et al. Maraviroc (UK-427,857), a potent, orally available, and selective small-molecule inhibitor of chemokine receptor CCR5 with broad-spectrum anti-human immunodeficiency virus type 1 activity. *Antimicrob Agents Chemother* 2005;49:4721–4732. (*Describes the development of an antiviral drug, maraviroc, that acts by blocking a host target.*)

Hare S, Gupta SS, Valkov E, Engelman A, Cherepanov P. Retroviral intasome assembly and inhibition of strand transfer. *Nature* 2010;464:232–236. (*Presents the crystal structure of a retroviral integrase bound to viral DNA and integrase inhibitors, thereby elucidating mechanisms of integrase action and drug inhibition.*)

Hay AJ, Wolstenholme AJ, Skehel JJ, Smith MH. The molecular basis of the specific anti-influenza inhibition of amantadine. *EMBO J* 1985;4: 3021–3024. (*This classic paper illustrates how viral genetics can be used to identify a drug target.*)

Sofia MJ, Bao D, Chang W, et al. Discovery of a β-D-2′-deoxy-2′-α-fluoro-2′-β-*C*-methyluridine nucleotide prodrug (PSI-7977) for the treatment of hepatitis C virus. *J Med Chem* 2010;53:7202–7218. (*Describes the iterative process undertaken to discover sofosbuvir.*)

von Itzstein M, Wu WY, Kok GB, et al. Rational design of potent sialidase-based inhibitors of influenza virus replication. *Nature* 1993;363:418–423. (*Describes the structure-based design of zanamivir.*)

DRUG SUMMARY TABLE: CHAPTER 38 Pharmacology of Viral Infections

DRUG	CLINICAL APPLICATIONS	SERIOUS AND COMMON ADVERSE EFFECTS	CONTRAINDICATIONS	THERAPEUTIC CONSIDERATIONS
INHIBITORS OF VIRAL ATTACHMENT AND ENTRY Mechanism—Maraviroc blocks the chemokine receptor CCR5. Enfuvirtide blocks HIV attachment and entry by inhibiting gp41-mediated fusion of the HIV envelope with the host plasma membrane.				
Maraviroc	Human immunodeficiency virus (HIV)	*Hepatotoxicity, myocardial infarction/ischemia, immune reconstitution syndrome, risk of infection, severe hypersensitivity reaction* Rash, dizziness, upper respiratory infection, fever, gastroparesis	Hypersensitivity to maraviroc Renal impairment Simultaneous treatment with potent CYP3A inhibitor or inducer	Maraviroc blocks infection of HIV strains that use CCR5 for attachment and entry, but it is not active against HIV strains that use the CXCR4 receptor. Used in combination with other anti-HIV drugs in patients who have undetectable levels of CXCR4-tropic virus.
Enfuvirtide (T-20)	HIV	*Guillain–Barré syndrome, renal insufficiency, thrombocytopenia, neutropenia, eosinophilia, bacterial pneumonia* Peripheral neuropathy, sixth nerve palsy, conjunctivitis, injection site reaction	Hypersensitivity to enfuvirtide	Enfuvirtide is a peptide that must be administered parenterally, with twice-daily injections. Used in combination with other anti-HIV drugs in patients whose HIV has not been controlled on other anti-HIV medications.
INHIBITORS OF VIRAL UNCOATING Mechanism—Inhibit influenza A uncoating by blocking M2, a proton channel that acidifies the interior of the virus; acidification is necessary for dissociation of viral matrix protein from the viral ribonucleoprotein.				
Amantadine Rimantadine	Shared indication: Influenza A Amantadine only: Parkinsonism	*Neuroleptic malignant syndrome, exacerbation of mental disorder, hypersensitivity reaction* Orthostatic hypotension, peripheral edema, gastrointestinal disturbance, confusion, dizziness, insomnia, irritability, hallucination	Hypersensitivity to amantadine or rimantadine	Rimantadine causes fewer neurological effects than amantadine. The use of these drugs has been largely supplanted by neuraminidase inhibitors.
INHIBITORS OF VIRAL GENE EXPRESSION Mechanism—Inhibit hepatitis C virus (HCV) gene expression by inhibition of the viral NS3/4A protease. This protease cleaves the polyprotein that is the primary translation product of HCV RNA, thereby permitting the expression of functional viral proteins.				
Telaprevir Boceprevir Simeprevir Paritaprevir	Chronic hepatitis C, genotype 1	Photosensitivity, rash, nausea, hyperbilirubinemia, headache, fatigue	Specific contraindications have not been determined.	Used in combination with other anti-HCV drugs. Telaprevir was voluntarily discontinued by the manufacturer in 2014 and boceprevir will be voluntarily discontinued by the manufacturer in 2015.
ANTIHERPESVIRUS NUCLEOSIDE AND NUCLEOTIDE ANALOGUES Mechanism—Phosphorylation of drug by viral kinases leads to inhibition of DNA synthesis in virus-infected cells. Acyclovir, valacyclovir, penciclovir, famciclovir, ganciclovir, and valganciclovir are phosphorylated by viral kinases and then inhibit viral DNA polymerase. Cidofovir is phosphorylated by cellular enzymes and then inhibits HCMV DNA polymerase.				
Acyclovir Valacyclovir	Herpes simplex virus (HSV) Varicella-zoster virus (VZV)	*Renal failure (intravenous administration), thrombotic thrombocytopenic purpura in immunocompromised patients, hemolytic uremic syndrome (shared adverse effects); aseptic meningitis, encephalopathy, seizure (valacyclovir only)* Gastrointestinal disturbance, rash, headache, fatigue	Hypersensitivity to acyclovir or valacyclovir	Valacyclovir is a prodrug of acyclovir with higher oral bioavailability.

Drug	Clinical Uses	Adverse Effects	Contraindications	Notes
Penciclovir Famciclovir	HSV	*Erythema multiforme (famciclovir only)* Headache (shared adverse effect); gastrointestinal disturbance, dysmenorrhea (famciclovir only)	Hypersensitivity to penciclovir or famciclovir	Famciclovir is a diacetyl 6-deoxy prodrug analogue of penciclovir, the active form of the drug.
Ganciclovir Valganciclovir	Human cytomegalovirus (HCMV) Ganciclovir only: Herpes simplex keratitis	*Cardiac arrest, Stevens-Johnson syndrome, gastrointestinal perforation, pancreatitis, hepatotoxicity, anaphylaxis, rhabdomyolysis, retinal detachment, nephrotoxicity (ganciclovir only)* Gastrointestinal disturbance, neutropenia, thrombocytopenia, fever, ocular infection (shared adverse effects); rash (ganciclovir only); anemia, tremor, upper respiratory infection (valganciclovir only)	Shared contraindication: Hypersensitivity to drug Ganciclovir only: Severe neutropenia Severe thrombocytopenia	Valganciclovir is a prodrug of ganciclovir with higher oral bioavailability.
Cidofovir	HCMV retinitis	*Nephrotoxicity, anemia, neutropenia, metabolic acidosis, decreased intraocular pressure, serious infection* Headache, rash, alopecia, oral candidiasis, asthenia, headache, ocular infection	Hypersensitivity to drug Renal insufficiency Concomitant nephrotoxic agents	Must be co-administered with probenecid. Long half-life, requiring only once-weekly dosing.
Vidarabine Idoxuridine Trifluridine	HSV keratitis	Eye irritation, lacrimation, light intolerance	Hypersensitivity to vidarabine, idoxuridine, or trifluridine	Early anti-HSV drugs with increased toxicity relative to other agents. Used as ophthalmic preparations. Vidarabine has been voluntarily discontinued in the United States.

ANTI-HIV NUCLEOSIDE AND NUCLEOTIDE ANALOGUES
Mechanism—Anti-HIV nucleoside and nucleotide analogues are phosphorylated by cellular kinases and then inhibit viral reverse transcriptase.

Drug	Clinical Uses	Adverse Effects	Contraindications	Notes
Zidovudine (AZT) Stavudine (d4T) Lamivudine (3TC) Emtricitabine (FTC) Didanosine (ddI) Abacavir	HIV (3TC and FTC also used for HBV; see below)	*Neutropenia, anemia, pancreatitis, lactic acidosis, hepatomegaly with steatosis, peripheral neuropathy (shared adverse effects); myocardial infarction, fatal hypersensitivity (didanosine and abacavir only); rhabdomyolysis, optic neuritis, nephrotoxicity (didanosine only)* Gastrointestinal disturbance, headache, rash, malaise	Shared contraindication: Hypersensitivity to zidovudine, stavudine, lamivudine, emtricitabine, didanosine, or abacavir Didanosine only: Concomitant use of allopurinol or ribavirin Abacavir only: Hepatic impairment	All drugs in this class are used in combination with other anti-HIV drugs. Most toxicity is due to inhibition of mitochondrial DNA polymerase by drug triphosphates. Lamivudine is less toxic, possibly due to L-stereoisomer structure. Emtricitabine is administered once daily.
Tenofovir	HIV	*Lactic acidosis, hepatotoxicity, renal toxicity*	Hypersensitivity to tenofovir	Administered as a once-daily dose.

ANTI-HBV NUCLEOSIDE AND NUCLEOTIDE ANALOGUES
Mechanism—Anti-HBV nucleoside and nucleotide analogues are phosphorylated by cellular enzymes and then inhibit HBV DNA polymerase.

Drug	Clinical Uses	Adverse Effects	Contraindications	Notes
Lamivudine (3TC) Emtricitabine (FTC) Telbivudine Adefovir Entecavir	HBV (3TC and FTC also used for HIV; see above); FTC is not FDA approved for HBV but is often used in HIV–HBV co-infected patients	*Lactic acidosis, hepatotoxicity (shared adverse effects); rhabdomyolysis (telbivudine only); renal toxicity (adefovir only)* Rash, gastrointestinal disturbance, fatigue, cough	Shared contraindication: Hypersensitivity to drug Telbivudine only: Concomitant use with pegylated interferon alfa-2a	Differences in rates of resistance development in patients can have therapeutic consequences. Entecavir dose should be adjusted for patients with moderate renal insufficiency.

continues

DRUG SUMMARY TABLE: CHAPTER 38 Pharmacology of Viral Infections continued

DRUG	CLINICAL APPLICATIONS	SERIOUS AND COMMON ADVERSE EFFECTS	CONTRAINDICATIONS	THERAPEUTIC CONSIDERATIONS
ANTI-HCV NUCLEOSIDE AND NUCLEOTIDE ANALOGUES Mechanism—Anti-HCV nucleoside and nucleotide analogues are phosphorylated by cellular enzymes and then inhibit HCV RNA polymerase.				
Sofosbuvir	Chronic hepatitis C	*Pancytopenia, suicidal ideation* Diarrhea, anemia, headache, insomnia, fatigue	Concomitant ribavirin or peginterferon alfa in women who are or may become pregnant and in men with pregnant female partners	Used in combination with other anti-HCV drugs.
NONNUCLEOSIDE DNA POLYMERASE INHIBITORS Mechanism—Inhibit viral DNA polymerase directly by mimicking the pyrophosphate product of the DNA polymerization reaction				
Foscarnet	HSV HCMV	*Renal impairment, electrolyte imbalance, seizures, pancreatitis* Anemia, fever, gastrointestinal disturbance, headache	Hypersensitivity to foscarnet Concurrent administration of arsenic trioxide, bepridil, levomethadyl, mesoridazine, pimozide, probucol, thioridazine, ziprasidone, intravenous pentamidine	Renal impairment is the major dose-limiting toxicity.
NONNUCLEOSIDE REVERSE TRANSCRIPTASE INHIBITORS (NNRTIs) Mechanism—Bind near the catalytic site of reverse transcriptase and thereby impair the enzyme's joining of deoxyribonucleotides with the primer template strand				
Efavirenz Nevirapine Delavirdine Etravirine Rilpivirine	HIV	*Hypersensitivity reaction (shared adverse effects); hepatotoxicity (efavirenz, nevirapine, and etravirine only); prolonged QT (efavirenz only); psychotic disorder, suicidal ideation (efavirenz and rilpivirine only); rhabdomyolysis (nevirapine and etravirine only); nephrotoxicity (rilpivirine only)* Rash, dizziness, insomnia, gastrointestinal upset (shared adverse effects); dyslipidemia (efavirenz, nevirapine, and rilpivirine only)	Shared contraindications: Hypersensitivity to drug Concurrent administration of drugs metabolized by CYP3A4 is contraindicated for all of the NNRTIs—must verify metabolism of concurrent medications before prescribing NNRTIs. Nevirapine only: Hepatic impairment	Resistance develops rapidly, requiring the use of these drugs in combination with other anti-HIV drugs.
ANTI-HCV NONNUCLEOSIDE RNA POLYMERASE INHIBITORS Mechanism—Directly inhibit HCV RNA polymerase				
Dasabuvir	Hepatitis C	*Hepatotoxicity* Rash, gastrointestinal disturbance, anemia, asthenia, insomnia, fatigue	Hypersensitivity to dasabuvir Concomitant use of ethinyl estradiol-containing products Concomitant use of potent CYP2C8 inhibitors	Used in combination with other anti-HCV drugs.
ANTI-HCV NS5A INHIBITORS Mechanism—Inhibit NS5A, a viral protein required for HCV genome replication and certain later stages in the viral life cycle				
Ledipasvir Ombitasvir	Hepatitis C (chronic, genotype 1)	Diarrhea, nausea, elevated serum lipase and bilirubin, headache, insomnia, fatigue	Specific contraindications have not been determined.	Used in combination with other anti-HCV drugs. NS5A inhibitors have a low barrier to resistance.

INHIBITORS OF VIRAL INTEGRATION
Mechanism—Inhibit integrase, the viral enzyme that facilitates the integration of HIV into the cellular genome

| Raltegravir Elvitegravir Dolutegravir | HIV | *Hypersensitivity reaction, renal failure (shared adverse effects); suicidal ideation, rhabdomyolysis (raltegravir and elvitegravir only); hepatotoxicity (dolutegravir only)* Insomnia, nausea, headache, fatigue, gastrointestinal disturbance, dyslipidemia | Shared contraindication: Hypersensitivity to drug Dolutegravir only: Concomitant use with dofetilide | Approved for use only in combination with other anti-HIV drugs. Elvitegravir is formulated with tenofovir and FTC in a once-a-day pill. Dolutegravir is active against certain HIV mutants that are resistant to the other two inhibitors. |

INHIBITORS OF VIRAL MATURATION
Mechanism—Inhibit HIV protease, which is required for viral maturation; HIV virions replicate and bud from the cell, but these particles are noninfectious.

| Saquinavir Ritonavir Fosamprenavir Indinavir Nelfinavir Lopinavir Atazanavir Tipranavir Darunavir | HIV | *Heart block, Stevens-Johnson syndrome, hemolytic anemia, pancytopenia, pancreatitis, psychosis, suicidal ideation, nephrotoxicity (shared adverse effects); hepatotoxicity, intracranial hemorrhage (tipranavir only)* Dyslipidemia (↑ cholesterol, ↑ triglycerides), lipodystrophy, hyperglycemia, gastrointestinal disturbance | Hypersensitivity to drug Severe hepatic impairment Concurrent administration of CYP3A4 substrates with narrow therapeutic indices, including ergot derivatives, pimozide, midazolam, triazolam QT prolongation Refractory hypokalemia or hypomagnesemia Concomitant use with flecainide or propafenone, when fosamprenavir is combined with ritonavir | Used in combination with other anti-HIV drugs. Lopinavir is administered in combination with ritonavir; ritonavir inhibits CYP3A4, thus increasing plasma levels of lopinavir. Many protease inhibitors are inducers and/or inhibitors of P450 enzymes, especially CYP3A4, with numerous pharmacokinetic drug–drug interactions. Fosamprenavir is a prodrug form of amprenavir. |

INHIBITORS OF VIRAL RELEASE
Mechanism—Inhibit influenza virus neuraminidase, causing newly synthesized virions to remain attached to host cell

| Zanamivir Oseltamivir | Influenza A and B | *Cardiac arrhythmias, bronchospasm, respiratory depression, seizure, delirium (shared adverse effects); erythema multiforme, gastrointestinal hemorrhage, hepatitis (oseltamivir only)* Cough, headache, nasal symptoms (zanamivir only); gastrointestinal disturbance (oseltamivir only) | Hypersensitivity to zanamivir or oseltamivir | Inhibit both influenza A and influenza B. Zanamivir is administered by inhaler. Oseltamivir is approved for both prophylaxis and treatment; zanamivir is indicated only for treatment. Oseltamivir is used to treat serious human disease due to H5N1 (avian flu) and H1N1 (swine flu). |

continues

DRUG SUMMARY TABLE: CHAPTER 38 Pharmacology of Viral Infections *continued*

DRUG	CLINICAL APPLICATIONS	*SERIOUS* AND COMMON ADVERSE EFFECTS	CONTRAINDICATIONS	THERAPEUTIC CONSIDERATIONS
ANTIVIRAL DRUGS WITH UNKNOWN MECHANISMS OF ACTION Mechanism—See specific drug				
Fomivirsen	CMV retinitis (second-line)	Inflammatory disorders of the eye, transiently elevated intraocular pressure	Hypersensitivity to fomivirsen IV or intravitreal cidofovir therapy within 2–4 weeks due to risk for exaggerated ocular inflammation	Fomivirsen was designed as an intravitreally administered antisense nucleotide, but the actual mechanism of action is uncertain. Fomivirsen has been voluntarily discontinued by the manufacturer.
Ribavirin	Respiratory syncytial virus (RSV) Hepatitis C virus (in combination with other anti-HCV therapies)	*Bradyarrhythmia, hypotension, pancreatitis, hemolytic anemia, thrombotic thrombocytopenic purpura, hepatotoxicity, bacterial infection, suicide* Rash, gastrointestinal disturbance, headache, conjunctivitis, fatigue	Co-administration with didanosine Pregnancy or women of childbearing potential Creatinine clearance <50 mL/min Significant cardiac disease Hemoglobinopathies Autoimmune hepatitis (in combination with peginterferon alfa-2a) Severe hepatic decompensation	Ribavirin may inhibit host and/or viral enzymes, may be incorporated into viral RNA to induce deleterious mutations, and/or may enhance host immune responses. Administered in aerosol form for treatment of RSV
Docosanol	Herpes simplex virus (HSV)	Application site reaction	Hypersensitivity to docosanol	Docosanol lacks significant cytotoxicity. Administered topically.
ANTIVIRAL DRUGS THAT MODULATE THE IMMUNE SYSTEM Mechanism—Interferons activate signaling cascades that lead to production of antiviral proteins, including protein kinase R, which turn off host translational machinery in virus-infected cells. Imiquimod interacts with toll-like receptors to boost innate immunity, including the secretion of interferons.				
Interferon-α	Hepatitis C virus (HCV) Hepatitis B virus (HBV) Kaposi's sarcoma	*Gastric hemorrhage, aplastic anemia, neutropenia, thrombocytopenia, increased liver enzymes, autoimmune diseases, psychotic disorder* Depression, altered mental status, influenza-like symptoms	Hypersensitivity to interferon-α	Used as an antiviral drug in combination with ribavirin and/or with oral antiviral agents. Modified with polyethylene glycol (pegylated) to improve pharmacokinetic profile. Also used to treat chronic myelogenous leukemia, hairy cell leukemia, malignant melanoma, and renal cell carcinoma.
Imiquimod	Human papilloma virus (HPV)	*Cardiac arrhythmia, Henoch-Schönlein purpura, erythema multiforme, idiopathic thrombocytopenic purpura, stroke, angioedema* Skin irritation including erythema, superficial erosion and crusting, and burning sensation	Hypersensitivity to imiquimod	Wash hands before and after application. Also used to treat basal cell carcinoma and actinic keratosis.

Pharmacology of Cancer: Genome Synthesis, Stability, and Maintenance

David A. Barbie and David A. Frank

INTRODUCTION

Cancer therapy has traditionally been based on the principle that tumor cells are traversing the cell cycle frequently and are thus more sensitive than normal cells to interference with DNA synthesis and mitosis. Indeed, the **antimetabolites**, a class of agents that are analogues of endogenous folates, purines, and pyrimidines, and that function as inhibitors of the enzymes of nucleotide synthesis, were some of the first drugs to be tested as chemotherapeutic agents. In the late 1940s, Sidney Farber and colleagues administered the antifolate compound **aminopterin** to patients with acute leukemia and observed temporary remissions in more than half of the patients.

Because of their rapid growth and division, cancer cells are also thought to be more sensitive than normal cells to the effect of DNA-damaging agents. Also in the late 1940s, **nitrogen mustards**—derivatives of agents that had been found to cause bone marrow suppression through wartime exposures—were tested in patients with lymphoma and leukemia and shown to induce remissions.

These and other findings have since led to the development of multiple classes of antineoplastic drugs designed to interfere with the building blocks of DNA synthesis and mitosis, or to produce DNA damage and chromosomal instability, and thereby to promote cytotoxicity and programmed cell death (**apoptosis**). Unfortunately, the therapeutic window of these drugs is narrow because they also affect normal cells that routinely undergo cell division in tissues such as the gastrointestinal tract and bone marrow. That being said, cancer cells can often be induced to undergo apoptosis more readily than normal cells, providing some degree of selectivity. Use of combination chemotherapy with agents from different classes has helped to enhance efficacy while minimizing overlapping dose-limiting toxicities, but the ability to cure patients with most types of advanced cancer remains limited. In part, this limited efficacy is due

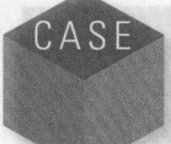

CASE

One day, JL, a 23-year-old graduate student who has heretofore been in good health, notices while showering that he has developed a hard lump in his left testis. Concerned by the finding, JL's physician orders an ultrasound examination, which shows a solid mass suggestive of cancer. The testis is removed surgically; pathologic review confirms the diagnosis of testicular cancer. A chest x-ray reveals several lung nodules, which are thought to represent metastatic spread of the cancer. JL is treated with several cycles of combination chemotherapy, including bleomycin, etoposide, and cisplatin. The lung nodules disappear completely. One year later, JL is able to resume his studies, and there are no signs of recurrence of the cancer. Nonetheless, at every subsequent follow-up visit, JL's physician asks him whether he is developing shortness of breath.

Questions

1. How did serendipity lead to the discovery of cisplatin, the most efficacious drug against testicular cancer?
2. What is the molecular target of each of the drugs in JL's combination chemotherapy regimen?
3. Why does JL's physician inquire about shortness of breath at each follow-up visit?
4. By what mechanisms could bleomycin, etoposide, and cisplatin act synergistically against JL's testicular cancer?

to the development of multiple **resistance** mechanisms, including the failure of tumor cells to undergo apoptosis in response to DNA damage or stress. In addition, it is increasingly apparent that populations of **cancer stem cells** may have low proliferation rates and other properties that render them resistant to cytotoxic chemotherapy.

BIOCHEMISTRY OF GENOME SYNTHESIS, STABILITY, AND MAINTENANCE

The central dogma of molecular biology states that DNA contains all the information necessary to encode cellular macromolecules—specifically, that DNA is transcribed into RNA, and RNA is then translated into proteins. Antimetabolites inhibit the synthesis of nucleotides, which are the building blocks of both DNA and RNA. Figure 39-1A provides an overview of nucleotide synthesis, and Figure 39-1B shows the steps at which some of the drugs discussed in this chapter inhibit nucleotide metabolism.

Nucleotide Synthesis

Nucleotides, the precursors of DNA and RNA, include the **purine** nucleotides and the **pyrimidine** nucleotides. Purines and pyrimidines are the bases that are used to determine the chemical code within DNA and RNA. Adenine and guanine are purines; cytosine, thymine, and uracil are pyrimidines. **Nucleosides** are derivatives of purines and pyrimidines that are conjugated to ribose or deoxyribose. **Nucleotides** are monophosphate, diphosphate, and triphosphate esters of the corresponding nucleosides. For example, an adenine base covalently linked to a ribose sugar and a diphosphate ester is called **adenosine diphosphate** (**ADP**). The various purine and pyrimidine bases, nucleosides, and nucleotides are shown in Table 39-1.

Nucleotide synthesis involves three general sets of sequential reactions: (1) synthesis of ribonucleotides, (2) reduction of ribonucleotides to deoxyribonucleotides, and (3) conversion of deoxyuridylate (dUMP) to deoxythymidylate (dTMP) (Fig. 39-2). Ribonucleotide synthesis differs for purines and pyrimidines; therefore, the synthesis of each class of molecules is discussed individually. All ribonucleotides are reduced to deoxyribonucleotides by a single enzyme, **ribonucleotide reductase**. Deoxyribonucleotides generated from ribonucleotides and from dUMP are used for DNA synthesis. Because folate is an essential cofactor for the synthesis of purine ribonucleotides and dTMP, folate metabolism is discussed separately (see Chapter 33, Principles of Antimicrobial and Antineoplastic Pharmacology).

Purine Ribonucleotide Synthesis

Adenine and **guanine**, the purine bases shown in Table 39-1, are synthesized as components of ribonucleotides (for RNA synthesis) and deoxyribonucleotides (for DNA synthesis). Derivatives of adenine and guanine, which include ATP, GTP, cAMP, and cGMP, are also used for energy storage and cell signaling. Purine synthesis begins with the assembly of **inosinate** (**IMP**) from a ribose phosphate, moieties derived from the amino acids glycine, aspartate, and glutamine, and one-carbon transfers catalyzed by **tetrahydrofolate** (**THF**), as shown in Figure 39-2. Because of the central role of THF in purine synthesis, one important chemotherapeutic strategy is to reduce the amount of THF available to the cell and thereby to inhibit purine synthesis.

Figure 39-3 shows the central role of IMP in purine synthesis. IMP can be aminated to AMP or oxidized to GMP. In turn, AMP and GMP can be converted to ATP and GTP, respectively, and then incorporated into RNA, or reduced to dAMP and dGMP, respectively, as described below.

Purine bases, nucleosides, and nucleotides are readily interconverted by multiple enzymes within the cell. In one such reaction, the enzyme **adenosine deaminase** (**ADA**) catalyzes the irreversible conversion of adenosine or 2′-deoxyadenosine to inosine or 2′-deoxyinosine, respectively. Inhibition of ADA causes the intracellular stores of adenosine and 2′-deoxyadenosine to exceed those of the other purines, ultimately resulting in metabolic effects that are toxic to the cell (see discussion of pentostatin below).

Pyrimidine Ribonucleotide Synthesis

Pyrimidine ribonucleotides are synthesized according to the metabolic pathway shown in Figure 39-4. The basic pyrimidine ring, orotate, is assembled from carbamoyl phosphate and aspartate. Orotate then reacts with a ribose phosphate; the decarboxylation product of this reaction yields

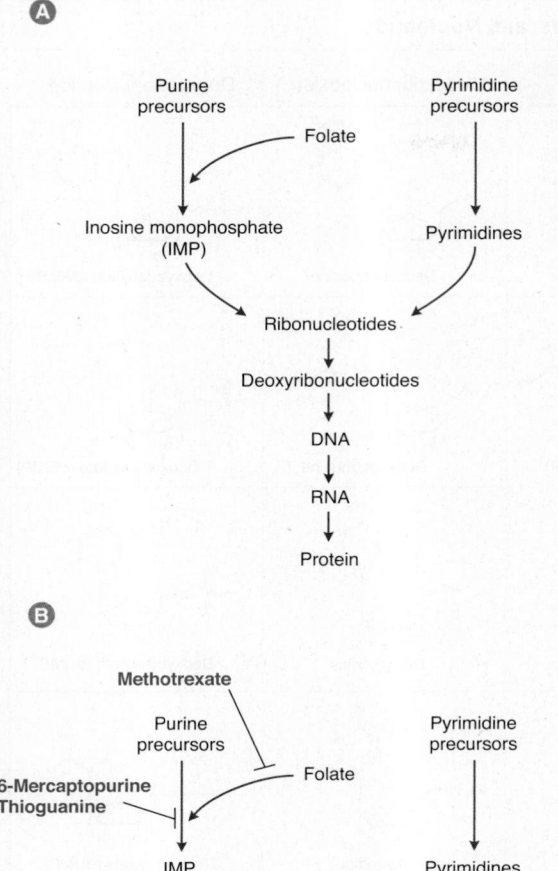

FIGURE 39-1. Overview of de novo nucleotide biosynthesis. A. Folate is an essential cofactor in the synthesis of inosine monophosphate (IMP), from which all purine nucleotides are derived. Pyrimidine synthesis does not require folate, although folate is required for the methylation of deoxyuridylate (dUMP) to deoxythymidylate (dTMP) (see Fig. 39-2). Ribonucleotides contain one of the purine or pyrimidine bases linked to ribose phosphate. Subsequent reduction of the ribose at the 2′ position produces deoxyribonucleotides. Deoxyribonucleotides are polymerized into DNA, while ribonucleotides are used to form RNA (*not shown*). The central dogma of molecular biology states that the DNA code determines the sequence of RNA (transcription) and that RNA is then translated into protein. **B.** Methotrexate inhibits dihydrofolate reductase (DHFR) and thereby prevents the utilization of folate in purine nucleotide and dTMP synthesis. 6-Mercaptopurine and thioguanine inhibit the formation of purine nucleotides. Hydroxyurea inhibits the enzyme that converts ribonucleotides to deoxyribonucleotides. Fludarabine, cytarabine, and cladribine are purine and pyrimidine analogues that inhibit DNA synthesis. 5-Fluorouracil inhibits the enzyme that converts dUMP to dTMP (*not shown*). Sulfonamides are discussed in Chapter 33.

uridylate (**UMP**). As with IMP in purine synthesis, UMP has a central role in pyrimidine synthesis. UMP is itself a nucleotide component of RNA, as well as the common precursor of the RNA and DNA components cytidylate (CMP), deoxycytidylate (dCMP), and deoxythymidylate (dTMP). CTP is formed by the amination of UTP.

Ribonucleotide Reduction and Thymidylate Synthesis

The ribonucleotides ATP, GTP, UTP, and CTP, which are required for RNA synthesis, are assembled on a DNA template and linked to form RNA. Alternatively, ribonucleotides can be reduced at the 2′ position on ribose to form the deoxyribonucleotides dATP, dGTP, dUTP, and dCTP. The conversion of ribonucleotides to deoxyribonucleotides is catalyzed by the enzyme **ribonucleotide reductase**. (In actuality, ribonucleotide reductase uses as substrates the diphosphate forms of the four ribonucleotides to produce dADP, dGDP, dUDP, and dCDP; nucleotides can, however, be readily interconverted among their monophosphate, diphosphate, and triphosphate forms.)

Note, in Figures 39-2 through 39-4, that ribonucleotide reductase catalyzes the formation of the DNA precursors dATP, dGTP, and dCTP. The DNA precursor dTTP is not synthesized directly by ribonucleotide reductase, however. Rather, dUMP must be modified to form dTMP. As demonstrated in Table 39-1, dTMP is the product of dUMP methylation. The methylation of dUMP to dTMP is catalyzed by **thymidylate synthase**, with methylenetetrahydrofolate (MTHF) serving as the donor of the methyl group (Fig. 39-4). As MTHF donates its methyl group, it is oxidized to dihydrofolate (DHF). DHF must be reduced to THF by **dihydrofolate reductase** (**DHFR**) and then converted to MTHF in order to serve as the cofactor for another cycle of dTMP synthesis. Inhibition of DHFR prevents the regeneration of tetrahydrofolate and thereby inhibits the conversion of dUMP to dTMP, eventually resulting in an insufficient cellular level of dTMP for DNA replication.

Nucleic Acid Synthesis

Provided that sufficient levels of nucleotides are available, DNA and RNA can be synthesized, and protein synthesis, cell growth, and cell division can occur. Many drugs, including the antimetabolites discussed in this chapter, inhibit both DNA and RNA synthesis. To avoid repetition, a detailed discussion of DNA and RNA synthesis is provided in Chapter 34, Pharmacology of Bacterial Infections: DNA Replication, Transcription, and Translation. For the purposes of this chapter, the reader should be aware that *RNA and DNA are formed by polymerization of ribonucleotides and deoxyribonucleotides, respectively.* RNA polymers are elongated by the enzyme **RNA polymerase**, and DNA is elongated by **DNA polymerase**. Although antimetabolites primarily inhibit the enzymes that mediate nucleotide synthesis, some antimetabolites also inhibit DNA and RNA polymerases (see below).

DNA Repair and Chromosome Maintenance

Mutations and other DNA lesions can arise spontaneously or as a result of exposure to DNA-damaging chemical agents or radiation. Several general pathways exist for repair of these lesions, including **mismatch repair** (**MMR**) for DNA replication errors, **base excision repair** (**BER**) for small base modifications and single-strand breaks, **nucleotide excision repair** (**NER**) for removal of bulky adducts, and

TABLE 39-1 Purine and Pyrimidine Derivatives: Bases, Nucleosides, and Nucleotides

		Base	Ribonucleoside	Ribonucleotide	Deoxyribonucleoside	Deoxyribonucleotide
Purines		Adenine (A)	Adenosine	Adenylate (AMP)	Deoxyadenosine	Deoxyadenylate (dAMP)
		Guanine (G)	Guanosine	Guanylate (GMP)	Deoxyguanosine	Deoxyguanylate (dGMP)
Pyrimidines		Cytosine (C)	Cytidine	Cytidylate (CMP)	Deoxcytidine	Deoxycytidylate (dCMP)
		Uracil (U)	Uridine	Uridylate (UMP)	Deoxyuridine	Deoxyuridylate (dUMP)
		Thymine (T)	NONE	NONE	Deoxythymidine	Deoxythymidylate (dTMP)

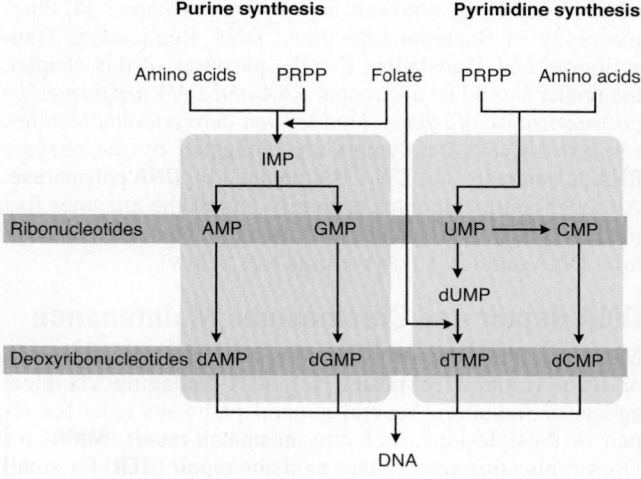

Purine synthesis / **Pyrimidine synthesis**

FIGURE 39-2. Nucleotide synthesis. Purine synthesis **(left)** begins with the formation of inosine monophosphate (IMP) from amino acids, phosphoribosylpyrophosphate (PRPP), and folate. IMP is aminated to adenylate (AMP) or oxidized to guanylate (GMP). The ribonucleotides AMP and GMP are reduced to form the deoxyribonucleotides deoxyadenosine monophosphate (dAMP) and deoxyguanosine monophosphate (dGMP), respectively. (The conversion of ribonucleotides to deoxyribonucleotides actually takes place at the level of the corresponding diphosphates and triphosphates, e.g., ADP → dADP and ATP → dATP.) Pyrimidine synthesis **(right)** begins with the formation of orotate from aspartate and carbamoyl phosphate (see Fig. 39-4). Orotate is ribosylated and decarboxylated to uridylate (UMP); amination of UMP yields cytidylate (CMP). (The conversion of UMP to CMP actually takes place at the level of the corresponding triphosphates, i.e., UTP → CTP.) The ribonucleotides UMP and CMP are reduced to form the deoxyribonucleotides deoxyuridine monophosphate (dUMP) and deoxycytidine monophosphate (dCMP). dUMP is converted to deoxythymidine monophosphate (dTMP) in a reaction that depends on folate. At the level of the corresponding triphosphates (*not shown*), deoxyribonucleotides are incorporated into DNA, and ribonucleotides are incorporated into RNA (*not shown*). Note the central role of folate as an essential cofactor in the synthesis of purine nucleotides and dTMP.

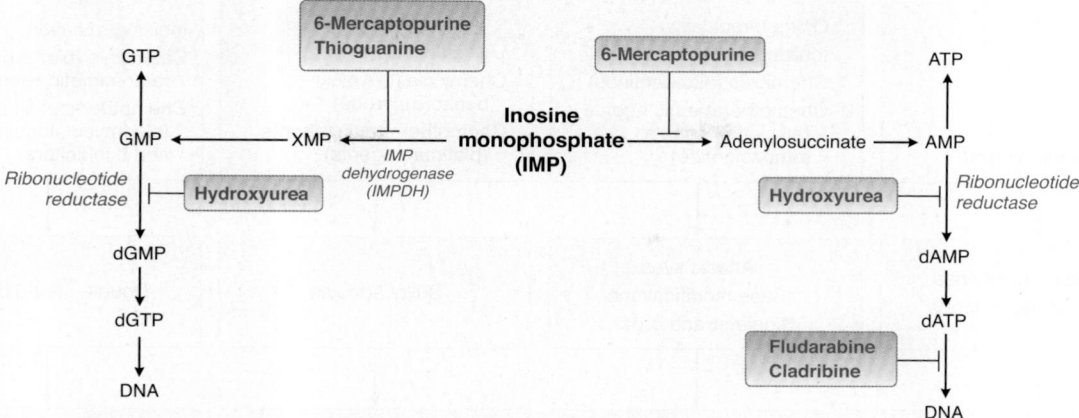

FIGURE 39-3. Details of purine synthesis. Inosine monophosphate, or IMP, occupies a central position in the synthesis of purine nucleotides. IMP is oxidized by IMP dehydrogenase (IMPDH) to xanthylate (XMP), which is converted to guanosine monophosphate (GMP). GMP can be incorporated into DNA or RNA as deoxyguanosine triphosphate (dGTP) or guanosine triphosphate (GTP), respectively. Alternatively, IMP can be aminated to adenosine monophosphate (AMP) through an adenylosuccinate intermediate. AMP can be incorporated into DNA or RNA as deoxyadenosine triphosphate (dATP) or adenosine triphosphate (ATP), respectively. 6-Mercaptopurine and thioguanine inhibit IMPDH and thus interrupt GMP synthesis. 6-Mercaptopurine also inhibits the conversion of IMP to adenylosuccinate and thus interrupts AMP synthesis. Hydroxyurea inhibits ribonucleotide reductase and thus inhibits formation of the deoxyribonucleotides required for DNA synthesis. Fludarabine and cladribine are halogenated adenosine analogues that inhibit DNA synthesis.

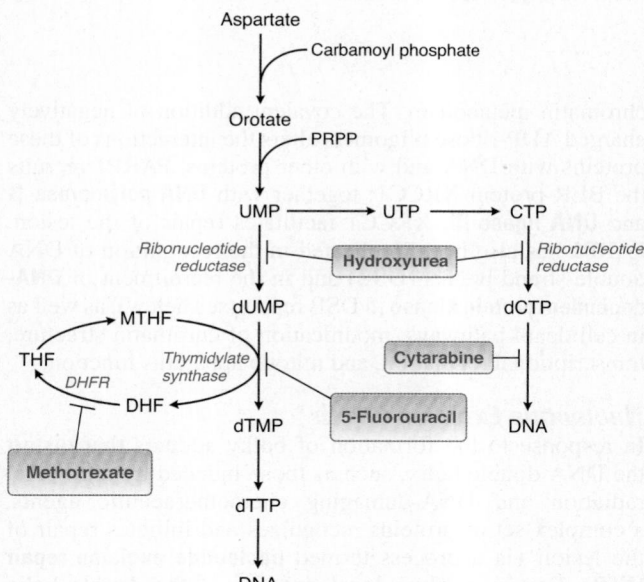

FIGURE 39-4. Details of pyrimidine synthesis. Aspartate (an amino acid) and carbamoyl phosphate combine to form orotate, which then combines with phosphoribosylpyrophosphate (PRPP) to form uridylate (UMP). UMP occupies a central position in the synthesis of pyrimidine nucleotides. UMP can be sequentially phosphorylated to uridine triphosphate (UTP). UTP is incorporated into RNA (*not shown*) or aminated to form cytidine triphosphate (CTP). CTP is incorporated into RNA (*not shown*) or reduced by ribonucleotide reductase to deoxycytidine triphosphate (dCTP), which is incorporated into DNA. Alternatively, UMP can be reduced to deoxyuridylate (dUMP). Thymidylate synthase converts dUMP to deoxythymidylate (dTMP) in a reaction that depends on folate. dTMP is phosphorylated to deoxythymidine triphosphate (dTTP), which is incorporated into DNA. Hydroxyurea inhibits the formation of deoxyribonucleotides and thereby inhibits DNA synthesis. Cytarabine, a cytidine analogue, inhibits the incorporation of dCTP into DNA. 5-Fluorouracil inhibits dTMP synthesis by inhibiting thymidylate synthase. Methotrexate inhibits dihydrofolate reductase (DHFR), the enzyme responsible for regenerating tetrahydrofolate (THF) from DHF. By inhibiting DHF reductase, this drug inhibits the formation of methylenetetrahydrofolate (MTHF), which is the folate compound required for dTMP synthesis.

homologous recombination or **nonhomologous end-joining** for double-strand breaks (Fig. 39-5). DNA repair pathways are important not only because they can alter the efficacy of chemotherapy but also because loss of these pathways frequently contributes to tumor development via impairment of genomic integrity and facilitation of mutations in oncogenes and tumor suppressor genes. **Telomeres**, the repeat sequences that cap the ends of chromosomes, also play an important role in genome stability and prevention of chromosome fusions. The enzyme **telomerase**, which prevents telomere shortening in cancer cells, represents a key component in the process of immortalization and oncogenic transformation.

Mismatch Repair

During DNA replication, errors such as single-base mismatches and insertions or deletions of microsatellite repeat sequences (microsatellite instability) are recognized and repaired by proteins of the mismatch repair (MMR) system. For single-base mismatches, recognition involves a heterodimer between the MSH2 protein and MSH6, while for insertion/deletion loops, MSH2 can also partner with MSH3 (Fig. 39-6). These complexes recruit the proteins MLH1 and PMS2 (as well as MLH3 for insertion/deletion loops), which, in turn, recruit exonucleases and components of the DNA replication machinery for excision and repair of the lesion. Germline mutations in MLH1, PMS2, MSH2, or MSH6 are associated with 70–80% of cases of **hereditary nonpolyposis colon cancer**. In addition, **microsatellite instability**, a hallmark of defective MMR, is observed in 15–25% of sporadic colorectal cancers.

Base Excision Repair

DNA single-strand breaks (SSB), which may be formed directly by ionizing radiation or indirectly due to enzymatic excision of a modified base by a DNA glycosylase, activate the enzyme **poly(ADP-ribose) polymerase 1 (PARP1)** (Fig. 39-7). At the site of the break, PARP1 transfers ADP-ribose moieties from nicotinamide adenine dinucleotide (NAD) to itself and to a number of other proteins involved in DNA and

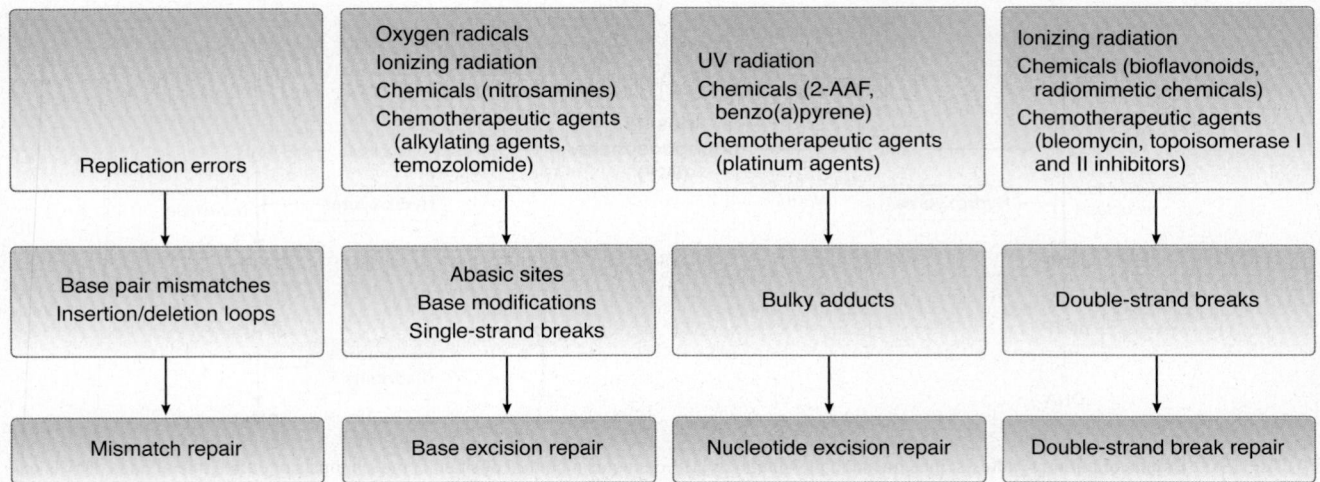

FIGURE 39-5. Mechanisms of DNA damage and repair. Several general pathways mediate repair of DNA lesions in response to DNA damage. Replication errors typically result in base pair mismatches or insertion/deletion loops in regions of microsatellite DNA repeats; these lesions are repaired by the mismatch repair (MMR) pathway. Oxygen radicals, ionizing radiation, and various chemicals and chemotherapeutic agents can cause abasic site formation, base modifications, and single-strand breaks, which are repaired by the base excision repair (BER) pathway. Ultraviolet (UV) irradiation and certain DNA-modifying chemicals and chemotherapeutic agents can cause the formation of bulky adducts that are excised and repaired by the nucleotide excision repair (NER) pathway. Ionizing radiation, radiomimetic chemicals, bleomycin, and natural (bioflavonoids) and chemotherapeutic (camptothecins, anthracyclines, epipodophyllotoxins) topoisomerase inhibitors can induce double-strand DNA breaks that trigger repair by the double-strand break (DSB) repair pathway. 2-AAF, 2-acetylaminofluorene.

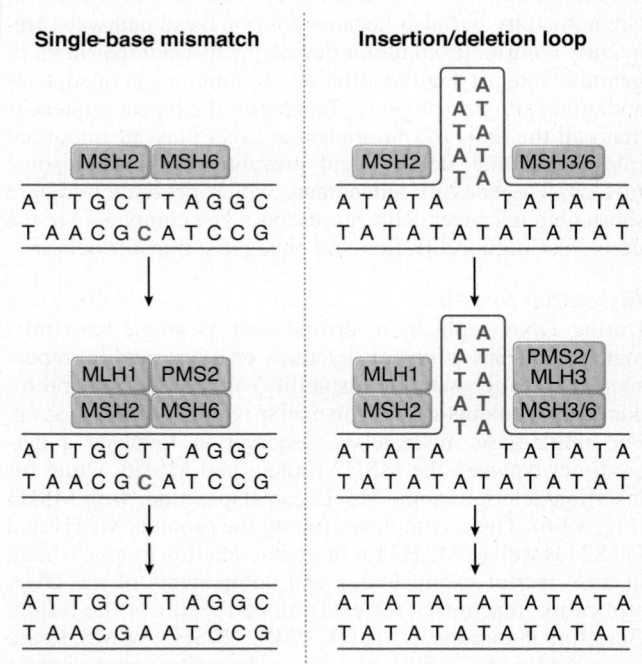

FIGURE 39-6. Mismatch repair pathway. Replication errors can result in single-base mismatches or insertion/deletion loops in microsatellite repeat regions, the latter as a result of intrastrand complementary base-pairing. Single-base mismatches are recognized by an MSH2/MSH6 heterodimer, and insertion/deletion loops are recognized by an MSH2/MSH3 or MSH2/MSH6 heterodimer. Additional components of the mismatch repair machinery are then recruited, including MLH1/PMS2 for single-base mismatches or MLH1/PMS2 or MLH1/MLH3 for insertion/deletion loops. Exonucleases and components of the DNA replication machinery are subsequently recruited for excision and repair of the lesions.

chromatin metabolism. The covalent addition of negatively charged ADP-ribose oligomers alters the interactions of these proteins with DNA and with other proteins. PARP1 recruits the BER protein XRCC1; together with **DNA polymerase β** and **DNA ligase III**, XRCC1 facilitates repair of the lesion. PARP1 has also been implicated in the recognition of DNA double-strand breaks (DSB) and in the recruitment of **DNA-dependent protein kinase** in DSB repair (see below), as well as in cell death pathways, modification of chromatin structure, transcriptional regulation, and mitotic apparatus function.

Nucleotide Excision Repair

In response to the formation of bulky adducts that distort the DNA double helix, such as those induced by ultraviolet radiation and DNA-damaging chemotherapeutic agents, a complex set of proteins recognizes and initiates repair of the lesion via a process termed **nucleotide excision repair (NER)**. Repair involves local opening of the double helix around the site of the damage, incision of the damaged strand on both sides of the lesion, excision of the oligonucleotide containing the lesion, and, finally, DNA repair synthesis and ligation. The endonuclease **ERCC1** plays an important role in targeted excision of the DNA lesion. The genes involved in nucleotide excision repair were in part identified from study of the clinical syndromes **xeroderma pigmentosa** and **Cockayne syndrome**, which are rare photosensitivity disorders that exhibit defects in NER.

Double-Strand Break Repair

In response to a double-strand break, activation of the ataxia telangiectasia mutated (ATM) kinase results in generation of the phosphorylated histone gamma-H2AX at the site of the break. Together with the protein MDC1, gamma-H2AX recruits to the locus of DNA damage a complex (MRN) containing the proteins Mre11, Rad50, and Nijmegen breakage syndrome gene 1 (NBS1) (Fig. 39-8). The breast and ovarian

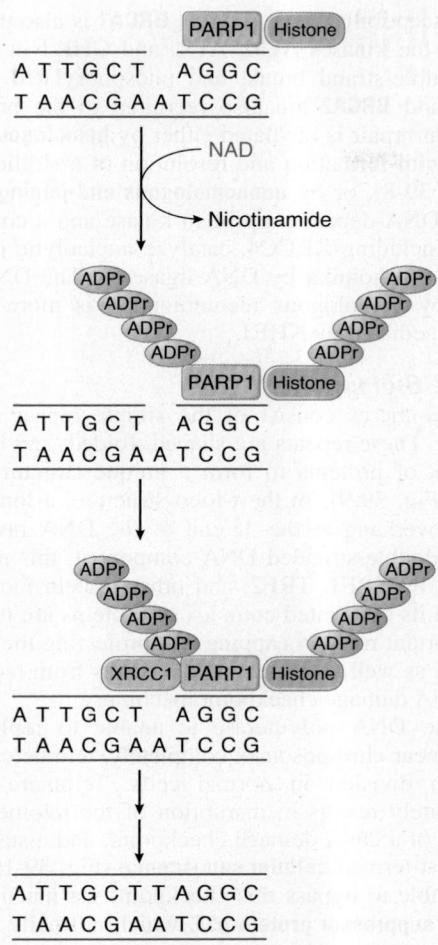

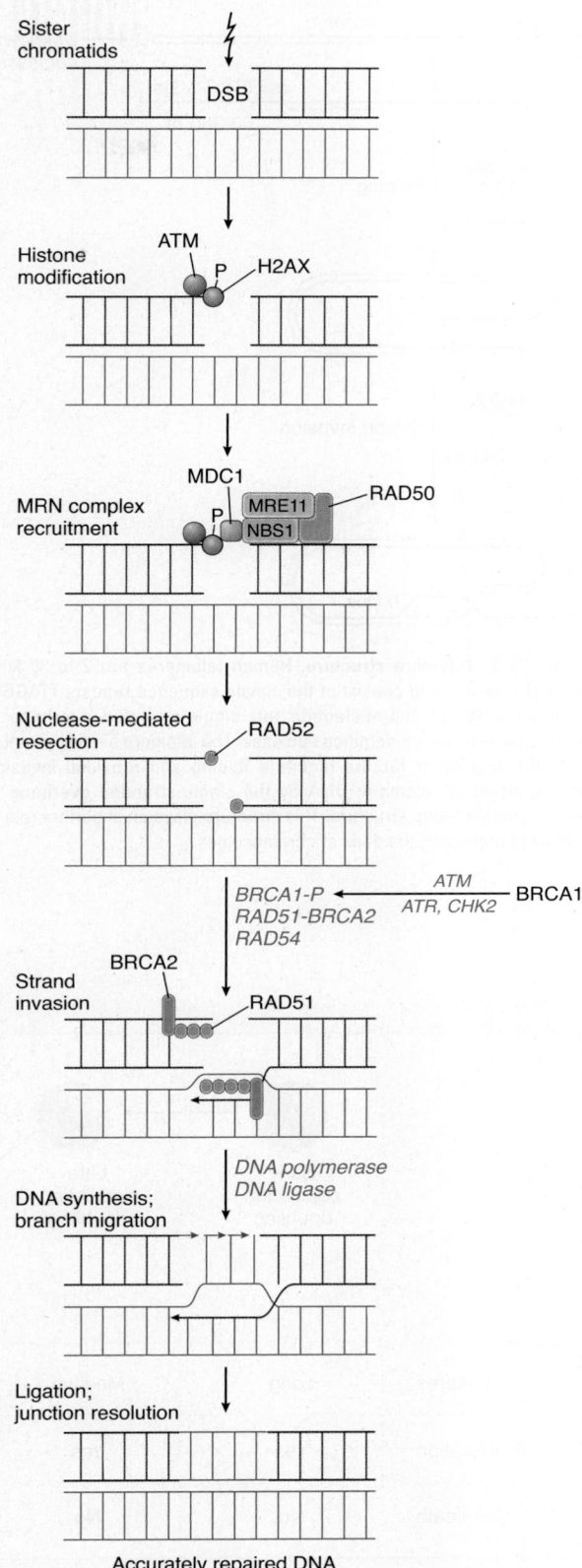

FIGURE 39-7.   Base excision repair pathway. The enzyme poly(ADP-ribose) polymerase 1 (PARP1) is recruited to single-strand break sites resulting from ionizing radiation or base lesion excision. PARP1 poly-ADP ribosylates a variety of targets at the site of injury, including itself and histones. The proteins modified with ADP-ribose (ADPr) oligomers then recruit additional proteins, such as XRCC1, which, in turn, recruit DNA polymerase β and DNA ligase III to repair the lesion.

FIGURE 39-8.   Double-strand break repair pathway. The ataxia telangiectasia mutated (ATM) kinase recognizes and binds to double-strand DNA break sites. Upon activation, the ATM kinase marks the site by generating the phosphorylated histone gamma-H2AX. Gamma-H2AX and the protein MDC1 recruit the Mre11/Rad50/Nijmegen breakage syndrome gene 1 (NBS1) complex (MRN) to the site of injury. After RAD52 is recruited and nucleases mediate DNA resection, BRCA1 is recruited to the site and phosphorylated by ATM, ATR, and CHK2 kinases. Together with RAD51 and BRCA2, phosphorylated BRCA1 facilitates repair of the double-strand break by homologous recombination (*depicted in the figure*) or nonhomologous end-joining (NHEJ; *not shown*).

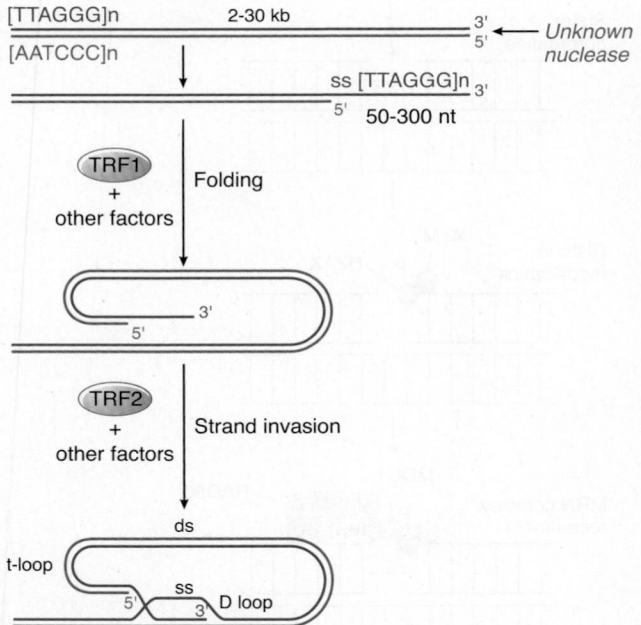

FIGURE 39-9. Telomere structure. Human telomeres are 2 to 30 kilobases (kb) in length and consist of the simple sequence repeats TTAGGG. A 3′-terminal 50- to 300-nucleotide (nt) single-stranded overhang is generated by an as yet unidentified nuclease. The telomere binding proteins TRF1, TRF2, and other factors facilitate folding and proximal invasion of double-stranded telomeric DNA by the single-stranded overhang to generate a stable t-loop structure. This structure plays an important role in capping and protecting the ends of chromosomes.

cancer susceptibility gene product **BRCA1** is also phosphorylated by the kinases ATM, ATR, and CHK2 in response to the double-strand break, and phosphorylated BRCA1, RAD51, and **BRCA2** are also recruited to the break site. Subsequent repair is mediated either by **homologous recombination**, with formation and resolution of a Holliday junction (Fig. 39-8), or by **nonhomologous end-joining** (**NHEJ**), in which DNA-dependent protein kinase and a complex of proteins, including XRCC4, catalyze nucleolytic processes that allow end-joining by DNA ligase IV. The DNA repair effected by homologous recombination is more accurate than that mediated by NHEJ.

Telomere Biology

Human telomeres consist of the simple repeat sequence TTAGGG. These repeats are shaped, folded, and bound by a complex of proteins to form a unique structure termed a *t-loop* (Fig. 39-9). In the t-loop structure, a long single-stranded overhang at the 3′ end of the DNA invades the proximal double-stranded DNA component; this process is facilitated by TRF1, TRF2, and other protein factors. The t-loop and its associated complex of proteins are thought to play important roles in capping and protecting the chromosome end, as well as protecting telomeres from recognition by the DNA damage checkpoint machinery.

Because DNA polymerase is unable to replicate the ends of linear chromosomes completely, telomeres shorten with each division in normal cells. Telomere shortening ultimately results in disruption of the telomeric caps, activation of a DNA damage checkpoint, and a state of cell cycle arrest termed **cellular senescence** (Fig. 39-10). When cells are able to bypass this checkpoint via inactivation of the **tumor suppressor protein p53**, which normally regulates

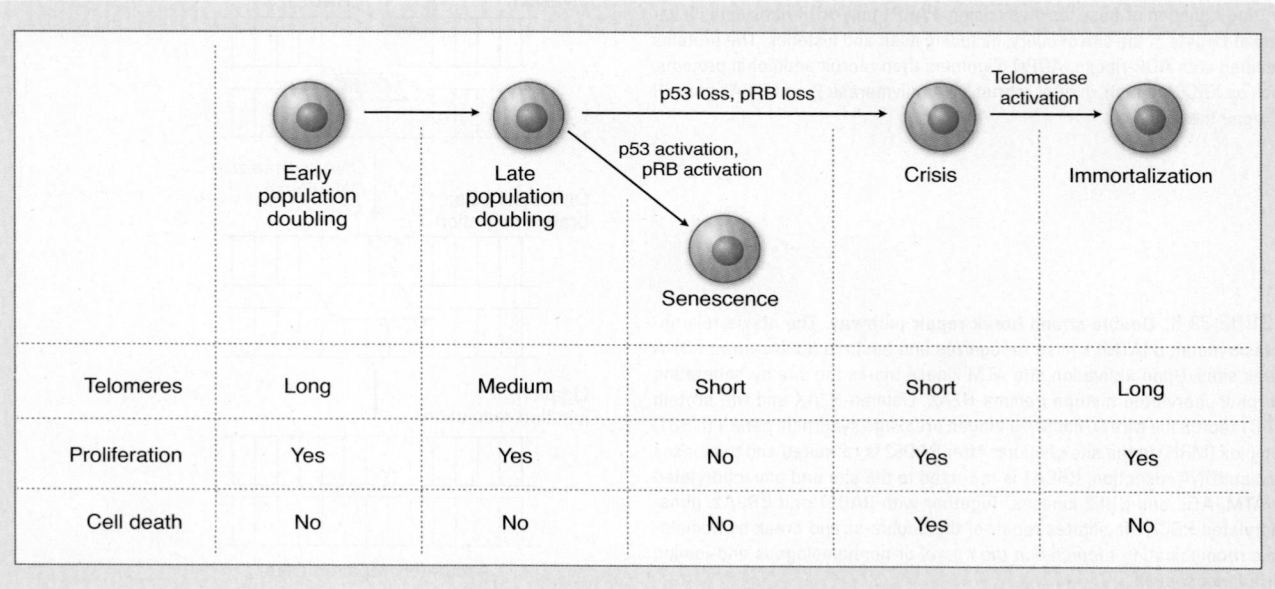

	Early population doubling	Late population doubling	Senescence	Crisis	Immortalization
Telomeres	Long	Medium	Short	Short	Long
Proliferation	Yes	Yes	No	Yes	Yes
Cell death	No	No	No	Yes	No

FIGURE 39-10. Chromosome maintenance and its relationship to immortalization. As primary cells undergo successive population doublings, telomeres progressively shorten due to the inability of DNA polymerase to replicate the ends of linear chromosomes. Ultimately, a checkpoint is triggered, mediated by the proteins p53 and pRB, which results in a state of growth arrest termed *cellular senescence*. Senescence can be bypassed by inactivation of p53 and pRB; ultimately, however, the critically short telomeres cause the cells to enter a state termed *crisis* and to die. Activation of telomerase allows cells to maintain adequate telomere length and divide indefinitely, resulting in immortalization. Notably, exogenous expression of telomerase alone in primary cells is sufficient for these cells to bypass senescence and become immortalized.

cell cycle arrest or apoptosis in response to DNA damage, chromosome fusions are observed. It is thought that the progressive shortening of telomeres with age promotes genomic instability and contributes to oncogenesis. However, cells also continue to die under these conditions. Activation of the enzyme **telomerase**, which is a reverse transcriptase that uses an RNA template to synthesize TTAGGG repeats, allows cells to restore telomere length and divide indefinitely. Telomerase activation is observed in normal germline cells and some stem cell populations and has been shown to maintain the presence of the 3′ overhang in normal cells. The immortalization process associated with telomerase activation is also essential for tumor formation and maintenance. In a minority of tumors, an alternative lengthening of telomeres (ALT) pathway is activated.

Microtubules and Mitosis

Once a cell has replicated its DNA, it is prepared to undergo mitosis. In this process, chromosomes condense and are segregated into two identical daughter cells. The cell cycle transitions from DNA replication (S phase) to G2 phase and then to mitosis (M phase) are complex and depend on the coordinated action of a number of so-called **cyclin-dependent kinases** (**CDKs**; see Chapter 33). Progression through mitosis is also facilitated by enzymes that include aurora kinases and polo-like kinases. Many cancer cells exhibit dysregulation of cell cycle timing and abnormalities in mitosis. Thus, pharmacologic inhibition of these regulatory kinases is an active area of cancer research. Currently, however, the microtubule machinery represents the primary target of agents that act in mitosis.

Microtubules are cylindrical, hollow fibers composed of polymers of tubulin, which is a heterodimeric protein consisting of **α-tubulin** and **β-tubulin** subunits (Fig. 39-11). α-Tubulin and β-tubulin are encoded by separate genes, but they have similar three-dimensional structures. Both α- and β-tubulin bind GTP; in addition, β-tubulin (but not α-tubulin) can hydrolyze GTP to GDP. Microtubules originate from a central microtubule organizing center (the centrosome, which includes two centrioles and associated proteins), where **γ-tubulin** (a protein with homology to α-tubulin and β-tubulin) nucleates tubulin polymerization. Nascent microtubules assemble into protofilaments, which are longitudinal polymers of tubulin subunits. Each protofilament interacts laterally with two other protofilaments to form a hollow-core tube, 24 nm in diameter, which consists of 13 protofilaments arranged concentrically. *Because tubulin is a heterodimer, this tube has inherent asymmetry*; the end of a microtubule nearest the centrosome is bordered by α-tubulin and is called the (−) (*minus*) end, while the end of a microtubule extending from the centrosome is bordered by β-tubulin and is called the (+) (*plus*) end (Fig. 39-11). Tubulin units are added at different rates to the (−) and (+) ends; the (+) end grows (adds tubulin) twice as fast as the (−) end.

Microtubules are not static structures. Rather, they possess an inherent property known as **dynamic instability** (Fig. 39-12). Tubulin heterodimers add to the end of the microtubule with GTP bound to both α-tubulin and β-tubulin subunits. As the microtubule grows, the β-tubulin of each tubulin heterodimer hydrolyzes its GTP to GDP. The hydrolysis of GTP to GDP introduces a conformational change in tubulin that destabilizes the microtubule. The exact mechanism of this destabilization is unknown, but it may be related to a

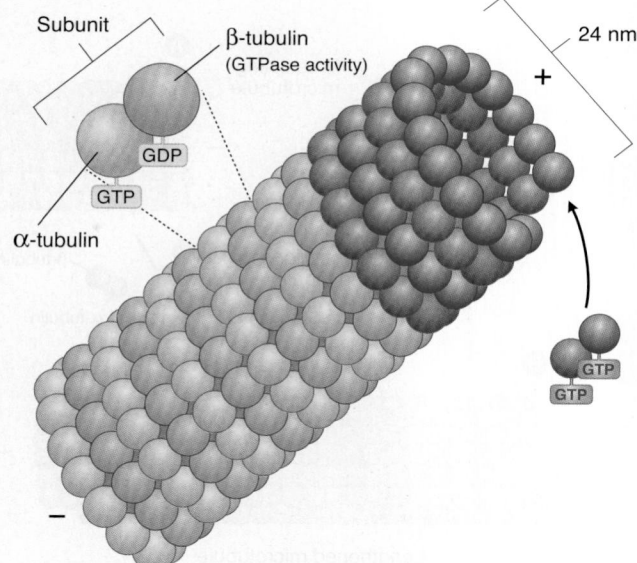

FIGURE 39-11. Microtubule structure. Microtubules are hollow cylindrical tubes that polymerize from tubulin subunits. Each tubulin subunit is a heterodimer composed of α-tubulin (*shades of purple*) and β-tubulin (*shades of blue*). Both α-tubulin and β-tubulin bind GTP (*dark shades of purple and blue*); β-tubulin hydrolyzes GTP to GDP after the tubulin subunit is added to the end of a microtubule (*lighter shades of purple and blue*). Microtubules are dynamic structures that grow and shrink lengthwise; the cylindrical tubes are composed of 13 subunits arranged concentrically, resulting in a diameter of 24 nm. Note that microtubules have an inherent structural asymmetry. One end of a microtubule is limited by α-tubulin and is referred to as the (−) (*minus*) end; the opposite end is limited by β-tubulin and is referred to as the (+) (*plus*) end.

decrease in the strength of lateral protofilament interactions or an increase in the tendency for protofilaments to "curve" away from the straight microtubule.

Therefore, microtubule stability is determined by the rate of microtubule polymerization relative to the rate of GTP hydrolysis by β-tubulin. If a microtubule polymerizes tubulin faster than β-tubulin hydrolyzes GTP to GDP, then, in the steady state, there is a cap of GTP-bound β-tubulin at the (+) end of the microtubule. This GTP cap provides stability to the microtubule structure, allowing further polymerization of the microtubule. Conversely, if tubulin polymerization proceeds more slowly than the hydrolysis of GTP to GDP by β-tubulin, then, in the steady state, the (+) end of the microtubule is enriched with GDP-bound β-tubulin. This GDP-bound tubulin conformation is unstable and causes rapid depolymerization of the microtubule. The ability of microtubules to assemble and disassemble rapidly is important for their many physiologic roles. Pharmacologic agents can disrupt microtubule function either by preventing the assembly of tubulin into microtubules or by stabilizing existing microtubules (and thereby preventing microtubule disassembly).

Microtubules have important physiologic roles in mitosis, intracellular protein trafficking, vesicular movement, and cell structure and shape. Mitosis is the physiologic role that is targeted pharmacologically; the other physiologic roles, however, predict many of the adverse effects of drugs that interrupt microtubule function.

Recall that microtubules nucleate from centrosomes, which consist of centrioles and other associated proteins. In mitosis,

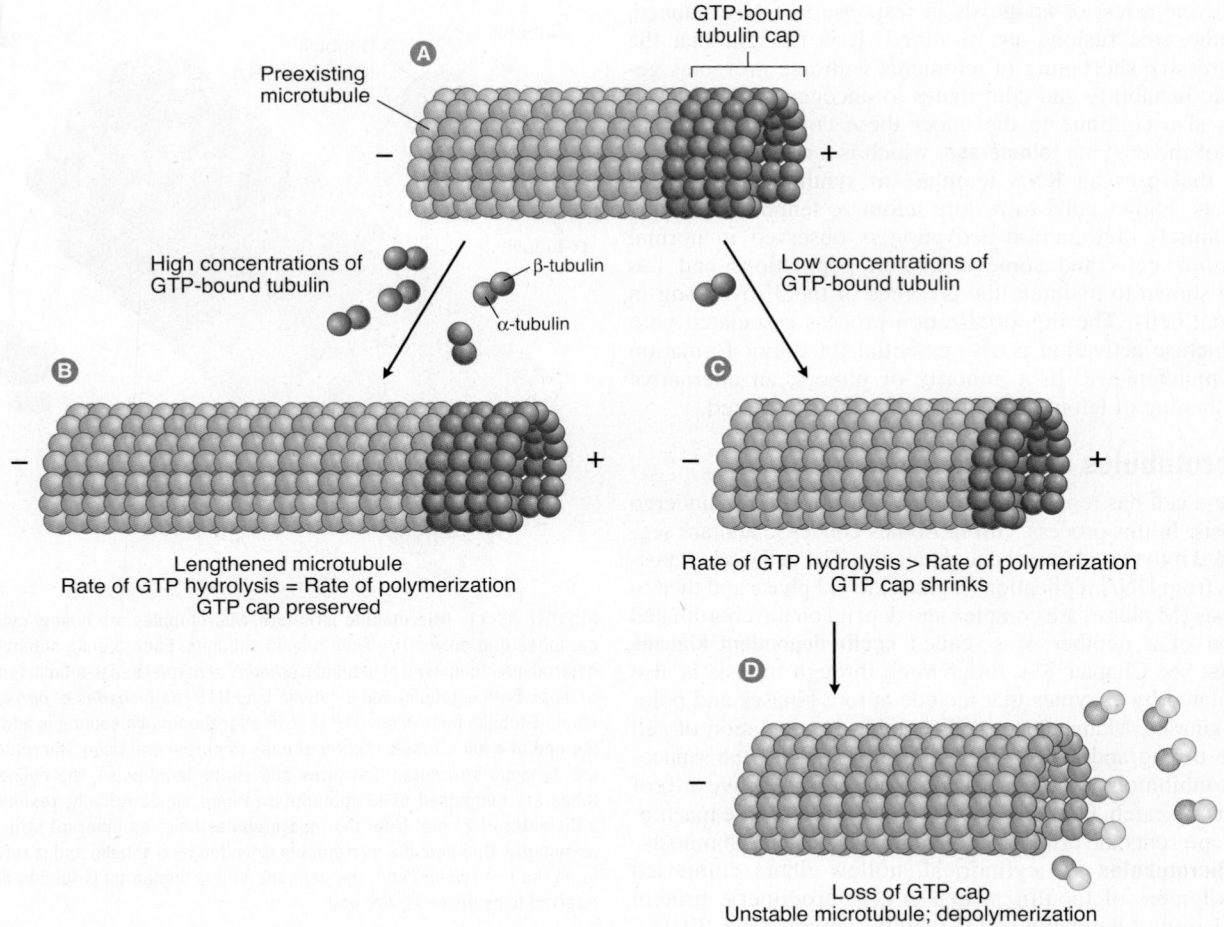

FIGURE 39-12. Dynamic instability of microtubules. A. A preexisting microtubule is characterized by tubulin subunits that have predominantly hydrolyzed the GTP on β-tubulin to GDP (*light purple and light blue*). However, β-tubulin subunits that have recently been added to the microtubule have not yet hydrolyzed GTP (*dark purple and dark blue*). The GTP-bound tubulin subunits form a GTP-bound tubulin cap at the (+) end of the microtubule. **B.** In the presence of a high concentration of GTP-bound free tubulin subunits, new GTP-bound tubulin is added to the (+) end of the microtubule at a rate that equals or exceeds the rate of GTP hydrolysis by β-tubulin. Maintenance of a GTP-bound tubulin cap results in a stable microtubule. **C.** In the presence of a low concentration of GTP-bound free tubulin subunits, new GTP-bound tubulin is added to the (+) end of the microtubule at a rate less than the rate of GTP hydrolysis by β-tubulin. This results in shrinkage of the GTP-bound tubulin cap. **D.** A microtubule that lacks a GTP-bound tubulin cap is unstable and undergoes depolymerization.

the two centrosomes align at opposite ends of the cell. Microtubules are extremely dynamic during M phase; they grow and shrink during M phase at rates much greater than during other phases of the cell cycle. This increased dynamic instability during M phase allows microtubules to locate and attach to the chromosomes. The microtubules emanating from each centrosome bind to kinetochores, which are proteins that attach to the centromere of a chromosome. Once the kinetochore of each chromosome is attached to a microtubule, microtubule-associated proteins act as motors to align the kinetochore-bound chromosomes at the equator of the cell (defined by the midpoint between the two centrosomes). When every chromosome has aligned at the equator, the microtubules shorten, separating a diploid pair of chromosomes into each half of the cell. Finally, cytokinesis (division of the cytoplasm) occurs, and two daughter cells are formed. Although many other proteins are involved in the regulation of mitosis, microtubules have a critical role in the process. Disruption of microtubule function freezes cells in M phase, leading eventually to the activation of programmed cell death (apoptosis).

PHARMACOLOGIC CLASSES AND AGENTS

Traditional antineoplastic chemotherapy can be subdivided into several classes of agents. The antimetabolite drugs are compounds that either inhibit the enzymes involved in nucleotide synthesis and metabolism or are incorporated as analogues into DNA and result in chain termination or strand breaks. These drugs act primarily during the S phase of the cell cycle, when cells are undergoing DNA replication. Another broad class of agents, which induce cytotoxicity by modification of DNA structure and generation of DNA damage, includes alkylating agents, platinum compounds, bleomycin, and topoisomerase inhibitors. These drugs exert their effects during multiple phases of the cell cycle. The final category of agents inhibits microtubule assembly or depolymerization, disrupting the mitotic spindle and interfering with mitosis. For a summary of the major classes of chemotherapeutic agents, their cell cycle specificity, and major toxicities, see Table 41-2 (Chapter 41, Principles of Combination Chemotherapy).

Inhibitors of Thymidylate Synthase

Thymidylate (dTMP) is synthesized by the methylation of 2′-deoxyuridylate (dUMP). This reaction, which is catalyzed by thymidylate synthase, requires MTHF as a cofactor (Fig. 39-4). **5-Fluorouracil** (**5-FU**; Fig. 39-13) inhibits DNA synthesis, primarily by interfering with the biosynthesis of thymidylate. 5-FU is first converted to 5-fluoro-2′-deoxyuridylate (FdUMP) by the same pathways that convert uracil to dUMP. FdUMP then inhibits **thymidylate synthase** by forming, together with MTHF, a stable, covalent ternary enzyme–substrate–cofactor complex. Cells deprived of dTMP for a sufficient period of time undergo so-called thymineless death. 5-FU can also be metabolized to floxuridine triphosphate (FUTP), which can be incorporated into mRNA in place of uridylate and can thereby interfere with RNA processing. Either inhibition of thymidylate synthase by FdUMP or interference with RNA processing by FUTP, or a combination of the two mechanisms, could explain the toxic effect of 5-FU on cells. However, certain 5-FU congeners that inhibit thymidylate synthase but are not incorporated into RNA show antitumor efficacy similar to that of 5-FU. This finding points to thymidylate synthase inhibition as the dominant mechanism of 5-FU action.

5-FU is used as an antineoplastic agent, especially in the treatment of carcinomas of the breast and gastrointestinal tract. 5-FU has also been used in the topical treatment of premalignant keratoses of the skin and of multiple superficial basal cell carcinomas. Because 5-FU depletes thymidylate from normal cells as well as cancer cells, this agent is highly toxic and must be used with care.

Capecitabine is an orally bioavailable prodrug of 5-FU. It is absorbed across the gastrointestinal mucosa and converted by a series of three enzymatic reactions to 5-FU. Capecitabine is approved for the treatment of metastatic colorectal cancer and as second-line therapy in metastatic breast cancer. Clinical trials have demonstrated that the efficacy of oral capecitabine is similar to that of intravenous 5-FU.

Elucidation of the mechanism of action of 5-FU has led to the use of a **5-FU/folinic acid** (leucovorin) combination as first-line chemotherapy for colorectal cancer. Because 5-FU inhibits thymidylate synthase by forming a ternary complex involving the enzyme (thymidylate synthase), substrate (5-FdUMP), and cofactor MTHF, it was hypothesized that increasing the levels of MTHF would potentiate the activity of 5-FU. Clinical trials proved this hypothesis to be correct by showing that the efficacy of the combined regimen is greater than that of 5-FU alone. This is an important example of the use of mechanistic knowledge to improve the clinical effectiveness of a drug.

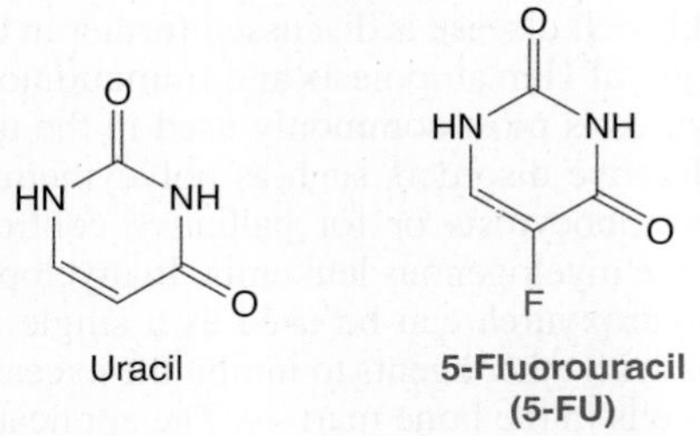

Pemetrexed is a folate analogue that, similar to endogenous folate and the dihydrofolate reductase (DHFR) inhibitor methotrexate (see Chapter 33), is transported into cells by the reduced folate carrier and polyglutamated by the intracellular enzyme folylpolyglutamate synthase. Polyglutamated pemetrexed is a potent inhibitor of thymidylate synthase and a much weaker inhibitor of DHFR; similar to 5-FU, its cytotoxic effect is likely due to the induction of "thymineless" cell death. (Note that the 5-FU derivative 5-FdUMP inhibits thymidylate synthase by binding to the dUMP [substrate] site on the enzyme, whereas pemetrexed inhibits thymidylate synthase by binding to the MTHF [cofactor] site on the enzyme.) Pemetrexed is approved for the treatment of all subtypes of non-small cell lung cancer except for the squamous subtype, due to lack of efficacy of the drug in this subtype. Pemetrexed is also used in combination with cisplatin (see below) in the treatment of malignant pleural mesothelioma. To reduce toxicity to normal cells, patients treated with pemetrexed are also given folic acid and vitamin B_{12} supplementation.

Inhibitors of Purine Metabolism

6-Mercaptopurine (**6-MP**) and **azathioprine** (**AZA**), a prodrug that is nonenzymatically converted to 6-MP in tissues, are inosine analogues that inhibit interconversions among purine nucleotides (Fig. 39-14). 6-Mercaptopurine contains a sulfur atom in place of the keto group at C-6 of the purine ring. After its entry into cells, mercaptopurine is converted by the enzyme

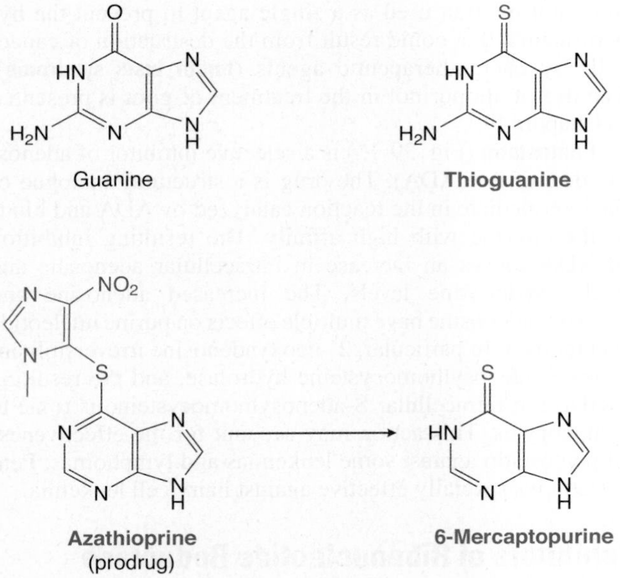

FIGURE 39-14. Structures of guanine, thioguanine, azathioprine, and 6-mercaptopurine. Thioguanine, azathioprine, and 6-mercaptopurine are structural analogues of purines. Thioguanine resembles guanine and can be ribosylated and phosphorylated in parallel with endogenous nucleotides. The nucleotide forms of thioguanine irreversibly inhibit IMPDH (see Fig. 39-3) and, upon incorporation into DNA, inhibit DNA replication. Azathioprine is a prodrug form of 6-mercaptopurine; azathioprine reacts with sulfhydryl compounds in the liver (e.g., glutathione) to release 6-mercaptopurine. The nucleotide form of 6-mercaptopurine, 6-thioinosine-5′-monophosphate (T-IMP), inhibits the enzymes that convert IMP to AMP and GMP (see Fig. 39-3). T-IMP also inhibits the first committed step in purine nucleotide synthesis.

FIGURE 39-13. Structures of uracil and 5-fluorouracil. Note the structural similarity between uracil and 5-fluorouracil (5-FU). Uracil is the base in dUMP, the endogenous substrate for thymidylate synthase (see Fig. 39-4), and 5-FU is metabolized to FdUMP, an irreversible inhibitor of thymidylate synthase.

hypoxanthine-guanine phosphoribosyltransferase (HGPRT; see Chapter 49, Integrative Inflammation Pharmacology: Gout) to the nucleotide form, 6-thioinosine-5'-monophosphate (T-IMP). T-IMP is thought to inhibit purine nucleotide synthesis by several mechanisms. First, T-IMP inhibits the enzymes that convert IMP to AMP and GMP, including inosine monophosphate dehydrogenase (IMPDH) (Fig. 39-3). Second, T-IMP (as with AMP and GMP) is a "feedback" inhibitor of the enzyme that synthesizes phosphoribosylamine, which is the first step in purine nucleotide synthesis. Both of these mechanisms lead to marked decreases in the cellular levels of AMP and GMP, which are essential metabolites for DNA synthesis, RNA synthesis, energy storage, cell signaling, and other functions. 6-MP may also inhibit DNA and RNA synthesis by less well-characterized mechanisms.

The major clinical application of 6-MP is in acute lymphoblastic leukemia (ALL), especially in the maintenance phase of a prolonged combination chemotherapy regimen. 6-MP is also active against normal lymphocytes and can be used as an immunosuppressive agent. For unknown reasons, the prodrug AZA is a superior immunosuppressant compared to 6-MP and is typically the drug of choice for this application. AZA is discussed in detail in Chapter 46, Pharmacology of Immunosuppression.

Both the effectiveness and the toxicity of 6-MP are potentiated by **allopurinol**. Allopurinol inhibits xanthine oxidase, thereby preventing the oxidation of 6-MP to its inactive metabolite 6-thiouric acid. (In fact, allopurinol was discovered in an effort to inhibit the metabolism of 6-MP by xanthine oxidase.) Co-administration of allopurinol and 6-MP allows the dose of 6-MP to be reduced by two-thirds (although toxicity is proportionally increased as well). Allopurinol is often used as a single agent to prevent the hyperuricemia that could result from the destruction of cancer cells by chemotherapeutic agents (**tumor lysis syndrome**). The use of allopurinol in the treatment of gout is presented in Chapter 49.

Pentostatin (Fig. 39-15) is a selective inhibitor of adenosine deaminase (ADA). The drug is a structural analogue of the intermediate in the reaction catalyzed by ADA and binds to the enzyme with high affinity. The resulting inhibition of ADA causes an increase in intracellular adenosine and 2'-deoxyadenosine levels. The increased adenosine and 2'-deoxyadenosine have multiple effects on purine nucleotide metabolism. In particular, 2'-deoxyadenosine irreversibly inhibits S-adenosylhomocysteine hydrolase, and the resulting increase in intracellular S-adenosylhomocysteine is toxic to lymphocytes. This action may account for the effectiveness of pentostatin against some leukemias and lymphomas. Pentostatin is especially effective against hairy cell leukemia.

Inhibitors of Ribonucleotide Reductase

Hydroxyurea inhibits ribonucleotide reductase by scavenging a tyrosyl radical at the active site of the enzyme. In the absence of this free radical, ribonucleotide reductase is unable to convert nucleotides to deoxynucleotides, and DNA synthesis is thereby inhibited.

Hydroxyurea is approved for use in the treatment of adult sickle cell disease and certain neoplastic diseases. The mechanism of action of hydroxyurea in the treatment of sickle cell disease may or may not be related to inhibition of ribonucleotide reductase. As an alternative to this mechanism,

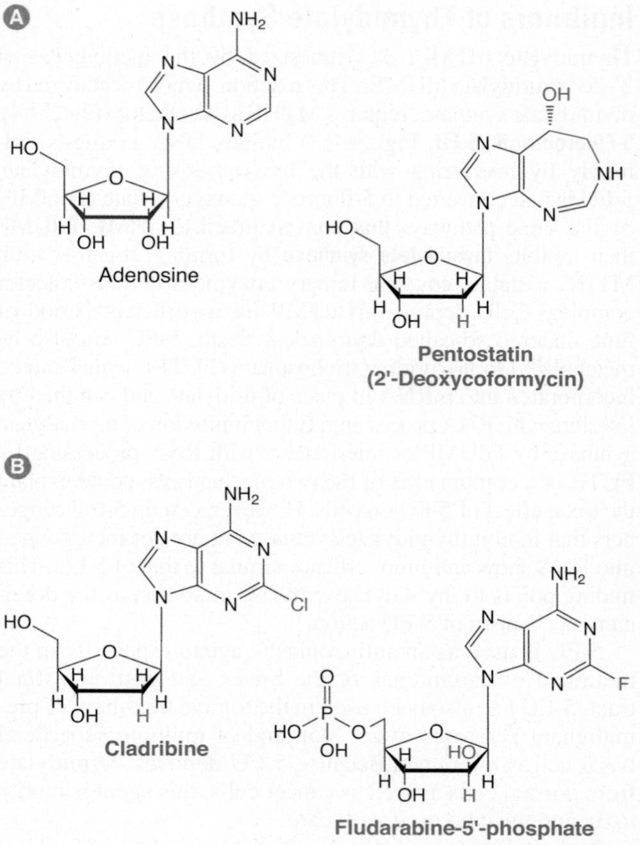

FIGURE 39-15. Structures of adenosine, pentostatin, cladribine, and fludarabine. A. Pentostatin inhibits adenosine deaminase (ADA), the enzyme that converts adenosine and 2'-deoxyadenosine to inosine and 2'-deoxyinosine, respectively. Pentostatin binds to ADA with very high affinity ($K_d = 2.5 \times 10^{-12}$ M) because it structurally resembles the intermediate (transition state) in this enzymatic reaction. **B.** Cladribine and fludarabine-5'-phosphate are also adenosine analogues. Cladribine is a chlorinated purine analogue that is incorporated into DNA and causes DNA strand breaks. Fludarabine phosphate is a fluorinated purine analogue that is incorporated into DNA and RNA; this drug also inhibits DNA polymerase and ribonucleotide reductase.

hydroxyurea has been shown to increase the expression of the fetal isoform of hemoglobin (HbF), which inhibits the polymerization of sickle hemoglobin (HbS) and thereby decreases red blood cell sickling under conditions of hypoxia. Hydroxyurea significantly decreases the incidence of painful (vaso-occlusive) crisis in patients with sickle cell disease. The mechanism by which hydroxyurea increases HbF production is unknown. The role of hydroxyurea in the treatment of sickle cell disease is discussed further in Chapter 45, Pharmacology of Hematopoiesis and Immunomodulation.

Hydroxyurea is most commonly used in the treatment of myeloproliferative disorders such as polycythemia vera and essential thrombocytosis or for palliative control of blood counts in acute myelogenous leukemia. In myeloproliferative disorders, hydroxyurea can be used as a single agent or in combination with other agents to inhibit the excessive growth of myeloid cells in the bone marrow. The applications of hydroxyurea for these indications have been limited somewhat by concerns that long-term hydroxyurea use may be leukemogenic; therefore, this may be an example of the phenomenon that certain antitumor agents can also cause cancer.

Purine and Pyrimidine Analogues That Are Incorporated into DNA

A number of antimetabolites exert their major therapeutic effect by acting as "rogue" nucleotides. These drugs are substrates for the various pathways of nucleotide metabolism, including ribosylation, ribonucleotide reduction, and nucleoside and nucleotide phosphorylation. The sugar triphosphate forms of these drugs can then be incorporated into DNA. Once incorporated into DNA, these compounds disrupt the structure of DNA, resulting in DNA chain termination, DNA strand breakage, and inhibition of cell growth. **Thioguanine** is a guanine analogue in which a sulfur atom replaces the oxygen atom at C-6 of the purine ring (Fig. 39-14). As with 6-mercaptopurine, thioguanine is converted by HGPRT to its nucleotide form, 6-thioguanosine-5'-monophosphate (6-thioGMP). Unlike T-IMP, the nucleotide form of 6-mercaptopurine, 6-thioGMP is a good substrate for guanylyl kinase, the enzyme that catalyzes the conversion of GMP to GTP. By this mechanism, 6-thioGMP is converted to 6-thioGTP, which is incorporated into DNA. Within the structure of DNA, 6-thioGTP interferes with RNA transcription and DNA replication, resulting in cell death. 6-ThioGMP also irreversibly inhibits IMPDH and thereby depletes cellular pools of GMP (Fig. 39-3). Thioguanine is used in the treatment of acute myelogenous leukemia. Major adverse effects of thioguanine include bone marrow suppression and gastrointestinal injury.

Fludarabine-5'-phosphate (Fig. 39-15) is a fluorinated purine nucleotide analogue that is structurally related to the antiviral agent vidarabine (see Chapter 38, Pharmacology of Viral Infections). The triphosphate form of fludarabine is incorporated into DNA and RNA, causing DNA chain termination. Fludarabine triphosphate also inhibits DNA polymerase and ribonucleotide reductase and thereby decreases nucleotide and nucleic acid synthesis in cells. The relative importance of these actions in mediating the cellular toxicity of the drug remains to be elucidated. Fludarabine-5'-phosphate is used in the treatment of lymphoproliferative disorders, especially chronic lymphocytic leukemia (CLL) and low-grade B-cell lymphomas.

Cladribine is a chlorinated purine analogue that is structurally related to fludarabine-5'-phosphate (Fig. 39-15). Cladribine triphosphate is incorporated into DNA, causing strand breaks. Cladribine also depletes intracellular pools of the essential purine metabolites NAD and ATP. Cladribine is approved for use in the treatment of hairy cell leukemia and has been used experimentally in the treatment of other types of leukemia and lymphoma.

Cytarabine (araC) is a cytidine analogue that is metabolized to araCTP (Fig. 39-16). AraCTP competes with CTP for DNA polymerase, and incorporation of araCTP into DNA results in chain termination and cell death (Fig. 39-4). Synergism between cytarabine and cyclophosphamide has been noted, presumably because of the reduced DNA repair caused by cytarabine's inhibition of DNA polymerase. Cytarabine is used to induce and maintain remission in acute myelogenous leukemia; it is especially effective for this indication when combined with an anthracycline (see below).

5-Azacytidine is a cytidine analogue. The triphosphate metabolite of 5-azacytidine is incorporated into DNA and RNA (Fig. 39-16). Once incorporated into DNA, azacytidine interferes with cytosine methylation, altering gene expression and promoting cell differentiation. Azacytidine and its 2'-deoxy

FIGURE 39-16. Structures of cytidine, cytarabine, and 5-azacytidine. Cytarabine and 5-azacytidine are both analogues of the nucleoside cytidine. Cytarabine has an arabinose sugar in place of ribose (note the chirality of the hydroxyl group *highlighted in blue*). The incorporation of cytarabine triphosphate (araCTP) into DNA inhibits further nucleic acid synthesis, because the replacement of 2'-deoxyribose by arabinose interrupts strand elongation. 5-Azacytidine has an azide group (*highlighted in blue*) within the pyrimidine ring; this drug is incorporated into nucleic acids and interferes with the methylation of cytosine bases.

derivative **decitabine** (5-aza-2'-deoxycytidine) are approved for the treatment of myelodysplastic disease.

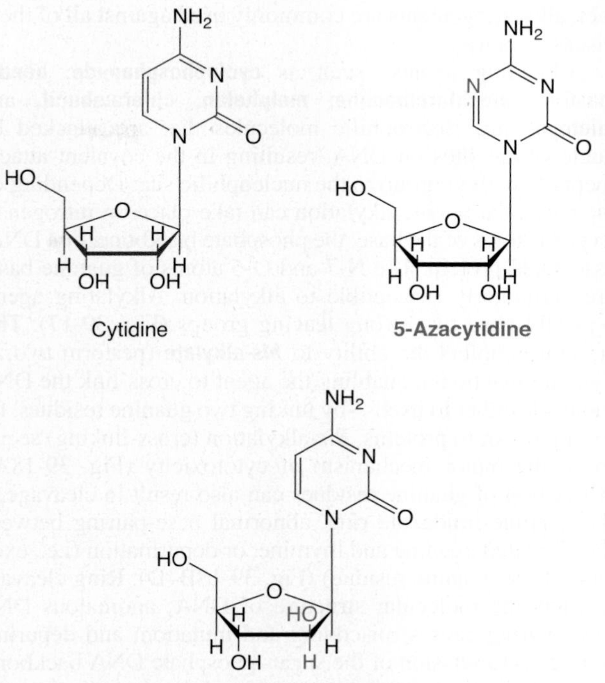

Gemcitabine is a fluorinated cytidine analogue in which the hydrogen atoms on the 2' carbon of deoxycytidine are replaced by fluorine atoms. The diphosphate form of gemcitabine inhibits ribonucleotide reductase; the triphosphate form of gemcitabine is incorporated into DNA, interfering with DNA replication and resulting in cell death. Gemcitabine is active in several solid tumors, including pancreatic, breast, bladder, and non-small cell lung cancer, and is also used in regimens for hematologic malignancies such as Hodgkin's disease.

Agents That Directly Modify DNA Structure

Alkylating Agents

The advent of modern chemotherapy dates to the 1940s, when highly reactive alkylating agents were first noted to induce remissions in otherwise untreatable malignancies. The clinical use of these agents was sparked by observations that nitrogen mustards, derivatives of wartime agents that caused dramatic suppression of hematopoietic cells, could have therapeutic utility in blood-derived malignancies such as leukemias and lymphomas. Soon thereafter, it was suggested that alkylating agents could also be useful in treating epithelial tumors, mesenchymal tumors, carcinomas, and sarcomas; in fact, alkylating agents are commonly used against all of these diseases today.

Alkylating agents—such as **cyclophosphamide**, **bendamustine**, **mechlorethamine**, **melphalan**, **chlorambucil**, and **thiotepa**—are electrophilic molecules that are attacked by nucleophilic sites on DNA, resulting in the covalent attachment of an alkyl group to the nucleophilic site. Depending on the particular agent, alkylation can take place on nitrogen or oxygen atoms of the base, the phosphate backbone, or a DNA-associated protein. The N-7 and O-6 atoms of guanine bases are particularly susceptible to alkylation. Alkylating agents typically have two strong leaving groups (Fig. 39-17). This structure confers the ability to *bis*-alkylate (perform two alkylating reactions), enabling the agent to cross-link the DNA molecule either to itself—by linking two guanine residues, for example—or to proteins. *Bis*-alkylation (cross-linking) seems to be the major mechanism of cytotoxicity (Fig. 39-18A). Alkylation of guanine residues can also result in cleavage of the guanine imidazole ring, abnormal base-pairing between the alkylated guanine and thymine, or depurination (i.e., excision of the guanine residue) (Fig. 39-18B–D). Ring cleavage disrupts the molecular structure of DNA; anomalous DNA base-pairing causes miscoding and mutation; and depurination leads to scission of the sugar–phosphate DNA backbone. Importantly, the mutations caused by these processes can increase the risk of developing new cancers.

Although all nitrogen mustards are relatively reactive, the individual agents vary in the speed with which they react with nucleophiles; this fact has significant impact on their clinical use. Highly unstable compounds, such as mechlorethamine, cannot be administered orally because such agents alkylate target molecules within seconds to minutes. Because of this high reactivity, these molecules are powerful vesicants (causing blisters) and can severely damage skin and soft tissue if they leak out of blood vessels. The rapid reactivity of alkylating agents can be exploited by infusing the drug directly into the site of a tumor. For example, thiotepa can be instilled into the bladder to treat superficial bladder cancers. In contrast to mechlorethamine and thiotepa, chlorambucil and melphalan are much less reactive and can be administered orally. Cyclophosphamide is particularly useful because it is a nonreactive prodrug that requires activation by the hepatic cytochrome P450 system; this agent can be administered either orally or intravenously (Fig. 39-19).

Nitrosoureas, such as **bendamustine** and BCNU (**carmustine**; Fig. 39-17), target DNA in much the same way as do cyclophosphamide and other alkylating agents. Like cyclophosphamide, these compounds require bioactivation. Unlike most alkylating agents, however, nitrosoureas also attach carbamoyl groups to their DNA-associated targets. It is not clear whether carbamoylation contributes significantly to the activity of nitrosoureas. Regardless of the mechanism, however, bendamustine treatment results in significantly greater survival compared with traditional cyclophosphamide-based regimens when combined with **rituximab** (see Chapter 46) for indolent B-cell non-Hodgkin's lymphomas (NHL).

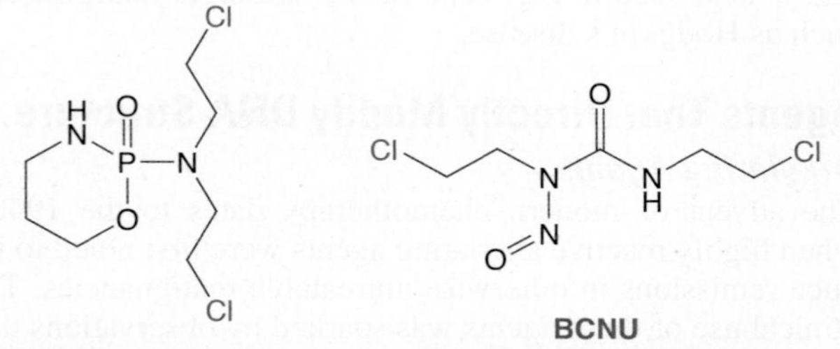

Some alkylating agents are better than others at targeting specific tumors. For example, nitrosoureas are useful in the treatment of brain tumors, because their high lipid solubility enables them to cross the blood–brain barrier. Similarly, the alkylating antibiotic **mitomycin** targets hypoxic tumor cells, such as those at the center of a solid tumor, because it requires bioreductive activation, which occurs more readily in low-oxygen environments.

Several nonclassical alkylating agents also deserve mention as clinically useful drugs. The first is **dacarbazine**, a synthetic molecule that is a component of a potentially curative combination chemotherapy regimen for Hodgkin's disease. Dacarbazine also has some activity in treating melanoma and sarcomas. **Procarbazine** is an orally active drug that is used against Hodgkin's disease. A metabolite of procarbazine functions as a monoamine oxidase inhibitor, and toxicity related to this activity—such as tyramine sensitivity, hypotension, and dry mouth—can occur. **Temozolomide**, an oral alkylating agent, is an imidazotetrazine derivative of dacarbazine. Temozolomide is widely used in the treatment of gliomas and of glioblastoma multiforme in particular. Its action is synergistic with radiation, and it enhances survival in glioblastoma when used in combination with radiotherapy for this disease. Finally, **altretamine** is useful for treating refractory ovarian cancer. Although it is structurally related to alkylating agents of the triethylenemelamine class (such as thiotepa), whether the mechanism of action of this drug involves DNA alkylation remains controversial.

Through natural selection, tumor cells can develop resistance to a single alkylating agent as well as cross-resistance to other drugs in the same class. Several mechanisms for resistance have been reported. Highly reactive drugs can be deactivated by intracellular nucleophiles such as **glutathione**. Alternatively, cells can become resistant by reducing uptake of the drug or accelerating DNA repair. One enzyme, **O^6-methylguanine-DNA methyltransferase (MGMT)**, prevents permanent DNA damage by removing alkyl adducts to the O^6 position of guanine before DNA cross-links are formed. Increased expression of this enzyme in neoplastic cells is associated with resistance to alkylating agents. Conversely, *MGMT* gene silencing predicts clinical benefit from temozolomide in glioblastoma.

Alkylating agent toxicity is dose-dependent and can be severe. As a rule, adverse effects result from damage to DNA in normal cells. Three cell types are preferentially affected by alkylating agents. First, toxicity typically manifests in rapidly proliferating tissues, such as bone marrow, gastrointestinal and genitourinary tract epithelium, and hair follicles. This results in myelosuppression, gastrointestinal distress, and alopecia (hair loss). Second, organ-specific toxicity can result from low activity of a DNA damage repair pathway in that tissue. Third, a tissue can be preferentially affected because the toxic compound accumulates in that tissue; for example, **acrolein** (a byproduct of the activation of cyclophosphamide

FIGURE 39-17. Structures of cyclophosphamide and BCNU. Cyclophosphamide and BCNU (carmustine) each have two chloride leaving groups (*blue*). The presence of two leaving groups allows these alkylating agents to *bis*-alkylate and thereby cross-link macromolecules such as DNA. The ability to cross-link DNA is crucial to the DNA damage caused by these agents.

Cyclophosphamide

BCNU (Carmustine, a nitrosourea)

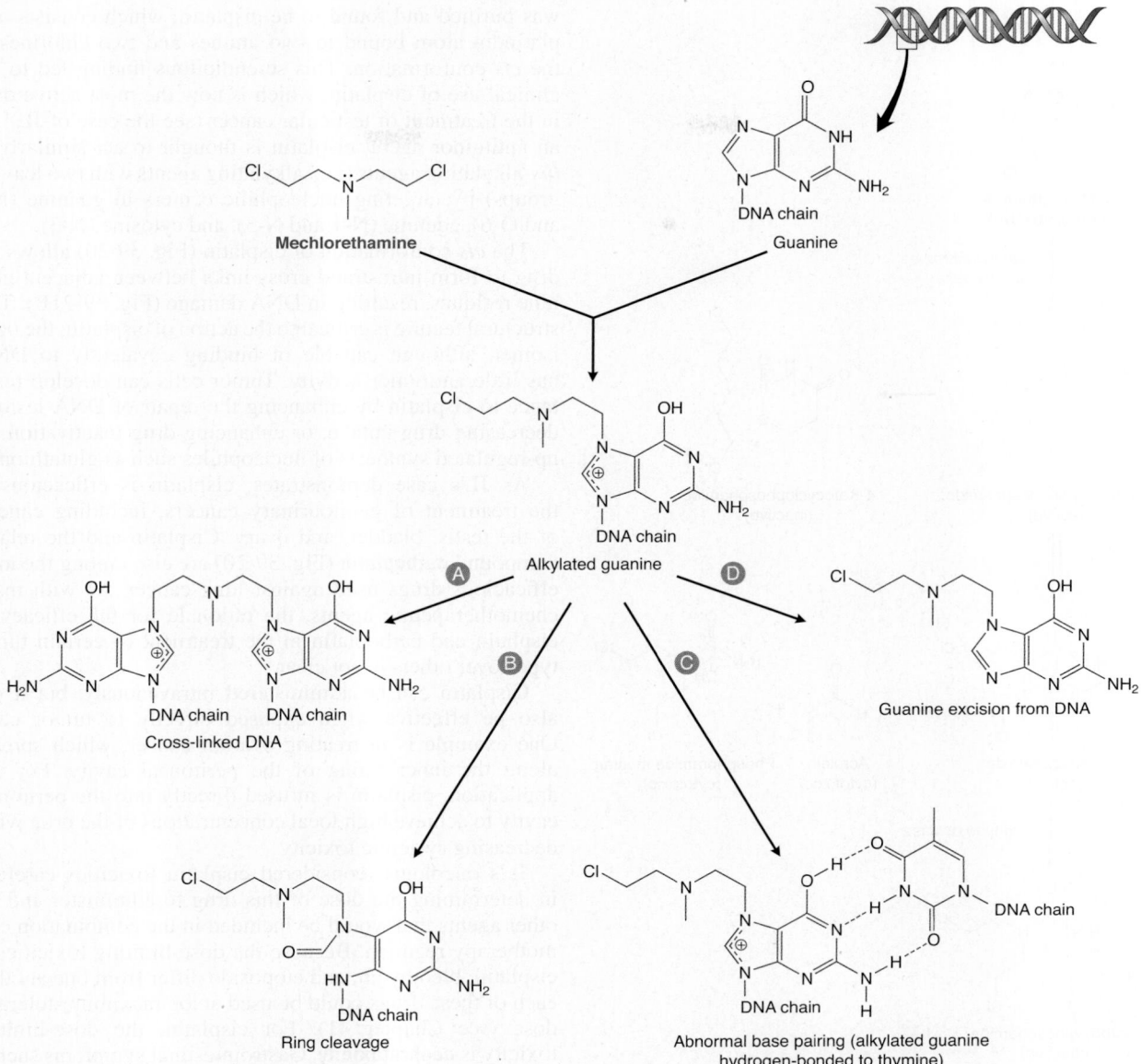

FIGURE 39-18. Biochemical outcomes of guanine alkylation. In reactions such as those exemplified here with mechlorethamine, guanine alkylation can cause several types of DNA damage. The nitrogen of mechlorethamine performs a nucleophilic attack on one of its own β-carbons, resulting in an unstable intermediate that is highly electrophilic (*not shown*). The nucleophilic N-7 of guanine reacts with this unstable intermediate, resulting in an alkylated guanine. Four potential outcomes can result from this initial alkylation, all of which cause structural damage to DNA. **A.** The process of alkylation can be repeated, with a second guanine acting as a nucleophile. The resulting cross-linking of DNA appears to be a major mechanism by which alkylating agents damage DNA. **B.** Cleavage of the imidazole ring disrupts the structure of the guanine base. **C.** The alkylated guanine can hydrogen-bond to thymine rather than cytosine, leading to a mutation in the DNA. **D.** Excision of the alkylated guanine residue results in a depurinated DNA strand.

or its analogue **ifosfamide**) can produce hemorrhagic cystitis because of accumulation and concentration in the bladder (Fig. 39-19). This toxicity can be treated by using the sulfhydryl-containing molecule **mesna**, which is also concentrated in the urine and rapidly inactivates the acrolein.

The immune response requires rapid proliferation of lymphocytes; this makes lymphocytes especially vulnerable to damage by alkylating agents. Thus, in addition to their anticancer activity, alkylating agents such as cyclophosphamide are also effective at immunosuppression. This "toxicity" has been put to clinical use: administered at doses lower than those used for antineoplastic therapy, alkylating agents are used to treat autoimmune diseases and organ rejection (see Chapter 46).

One approach to limiting toxicity has been to develop alkylating agents that accumulate preferentially inside tumor cells. An example of one such agent is melphalan, or phenylalanine mustard; this agent was designed to target melanoma cells, which accumulate phenylalanine for the biosynthesis of melanin. Another example is **estramustine**, in which the mustard component is conjugated to estrogen; this agent was designed to target breast cancer cells that express the estrogen receptor. Interestingly, neither melphalan nor estramustine works as intended, although they both have clinical utility; through mechanisms that are still poorly understood, melphalan is active against multiple myeloma, and estramustine is used to treat prostate cancer.

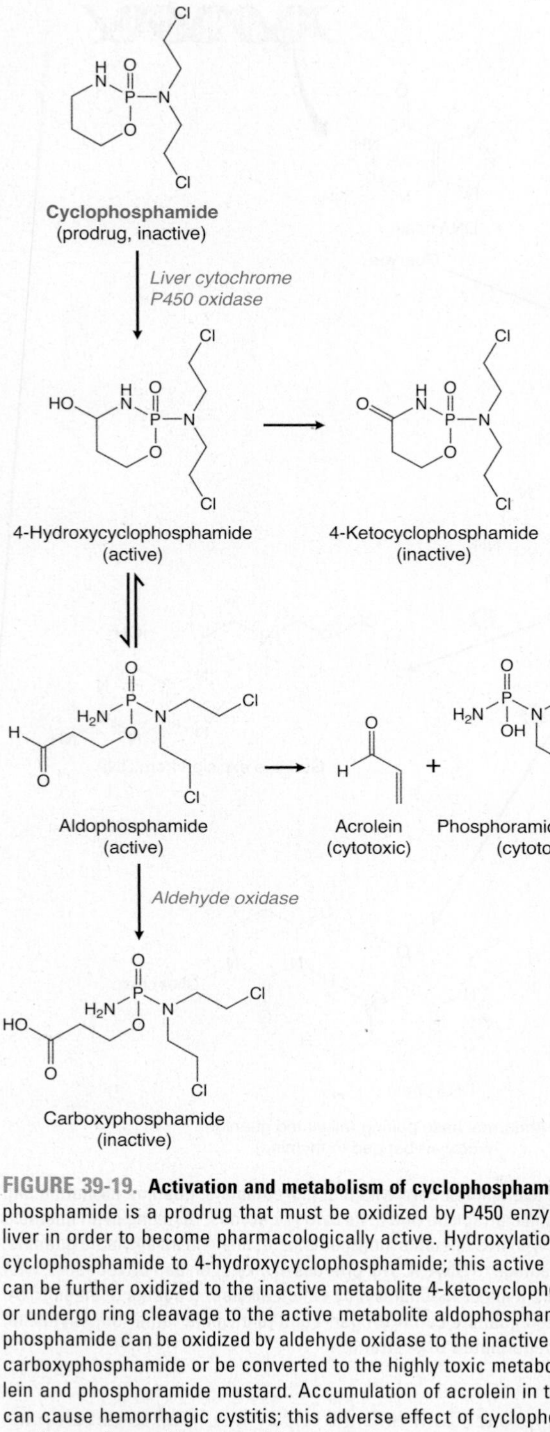

Cyclophosphamide
(prodrug, inactive)

*Liver cytochrome
P450 oxidase*

4-Hydroxycyclophosphamide
(active)

4-Ketocyclophosphamide
(inactive)

Aldophosphamide
(active)

Acrolein
(cytotoxic)

Phosphoramide mustard
(cytotoxic)

Aldehyde oxidase

Carboxyphosphamide
(inactive)

FIGURE 39-19. Activation and metabolism of cyclophosphamide. Cyclophosphamide is a prodrug that must be oxidized by P450 enzymes in the liver in order to become pharmacologically active. Hydroxylation converts cyclophosphamide to 4-hydroxycyclophosphamide; this active metabolite can be further oxidized to the inactive metabolite 4-ketocyclophosphamide or undergo ring cleavage to the active metabolite aldophosphamide. Aldophosphamide can be oxidized by aldehyde oxidase to the inactive metabolite carboxyphosphamide or be converted to the highly toxic metabolites acrolein and phosphoramide mustard. Accumulation of acrolein in the bladder can cause hemorrhagic cystitis; this adverse effect of cyclophosphamide can be ameliorated by co-administration of mesna, a sulfhydryl compound that inactivates the acrolein (*not shown*).

Platinum Compounds

The introduction of **cisplatin** (*cis*-diamminedichloroplatinum [II]) into clinical use in the 1970s transformed previously intractable tumors, such as testicular cancer, into curable ones. As with the alkylating agents, the anticancer properties of cisplatin were discovered by a chance observation. While studying the effects of electricity on bacteria, investigators found that a product of the platinum electrode was inhibiting DNA synthesis in the microbes. The compound

was purified and found to be cisplatin, which consists of a platinum atom bound to two amines and two chlorines in the *cis* conformation. This serendipitous finding led to the clinical use of cisplatin, which is now the most active drug in the treatment of testicular cancer (see the case of JL). As an antitumor agent, cisplatin is thought to act similarly to *bis*-alkylating agents (i.e., alkylating agents with two leaving groups) by targeting nucleophilic centers in guanine (N-7 and O-6), adenine (N-1 and N-3), and cytosine (N-3).

The *cis* conformation of cisplatin (Fig. 39-20) allows the drug to form intrastrand cross-links between adjacent guanine residues, resulting in DNA damage (Fig. 39-21B). This structural feature is critical to the action of cisplatin; the *trans* isomer, although capable of binding covalently to DNA, has little antitumor activity. Tumor cells can develop resistance to cisplatin by enhancing the repair of DNA lesions, decreasing drug uptake, or enhancing drug inactivation via up-regulated synthesis of nucleophiles such as glutathione.

As JL's case demonstrates, cisplatin is efficacious in the treatment of genitourinary cancers, including cancers of the testis, bladder, and ovary. Cisplatin and the related compound **carboplatin** (Fig. 39-20) are also among the most efficacious drugs used against lung cancer. As with many chemotherapeutic agents, the rationale for the efficacy of cisplatin and carboplatin in the treatment of certain tumor types over others is not clear.

Cisplatin can be administered intravenously, but it can also be effective when exposed directly to tumor cells. One example is in treating ovarian cancer, which spreads along the inner lining of the peritoneal cavity. For this application, cisplatin is infused directly into the peritoneal cavity to achieve high local concentrations of the drug while decreasing systemic toxicity.

JL's oncologist considered cisplatin toxicities carefully in determining the dose of this drug to administer and the other agents that would be included in the combination chemotherapy regimen. Because the dose-limiting toxicities of cisplatin, bleomycin, and etoposide differ from one another, each of these drugs could be used at the maximum-tolerated dose (see Chapter 41). For cisplatin, the dose-limiting toxicity is **nephrotoxicity**. Gastrointestinal symptoms such as nausea and vomiting are also common; this is of concern because dehydration due to protracted vomiting can exacerbate cisplatin-induced kidney damage and lead to irreversible renal failure. Neurotoxicity, primarily manifested as paresthesias of the hands and feet and hearing loss, also occurs

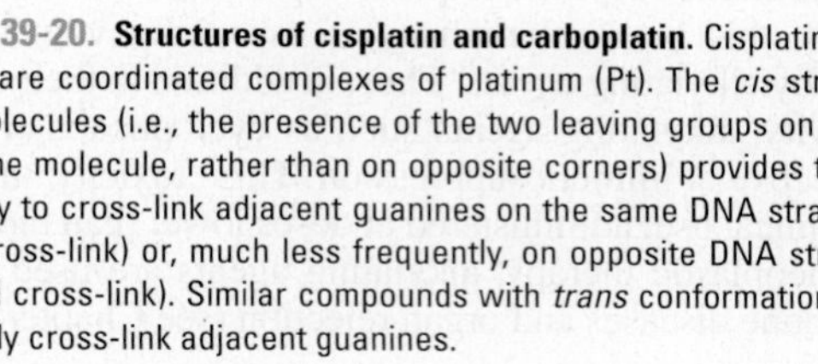

Cisplatin

Carboplatin

FIGURE 39-20. Structures of cisplatin and carboplatin. Cisplatin and carboplatin are coordinated complexes of platinum (Pt). The *cis* structure of these molecules (i.e., the presence of the two leaving groups on the same side of the molecule, rather than on opposite corners) provides them with the ability to cross-link adjacent guanines on the same DNA strand (intrastrand cross-link) or, much less frequently, on opposite DNA strands (interstrand cross-link). Similar compounds with *trans* conformations cannot effectively cross-link adjacent guanines.

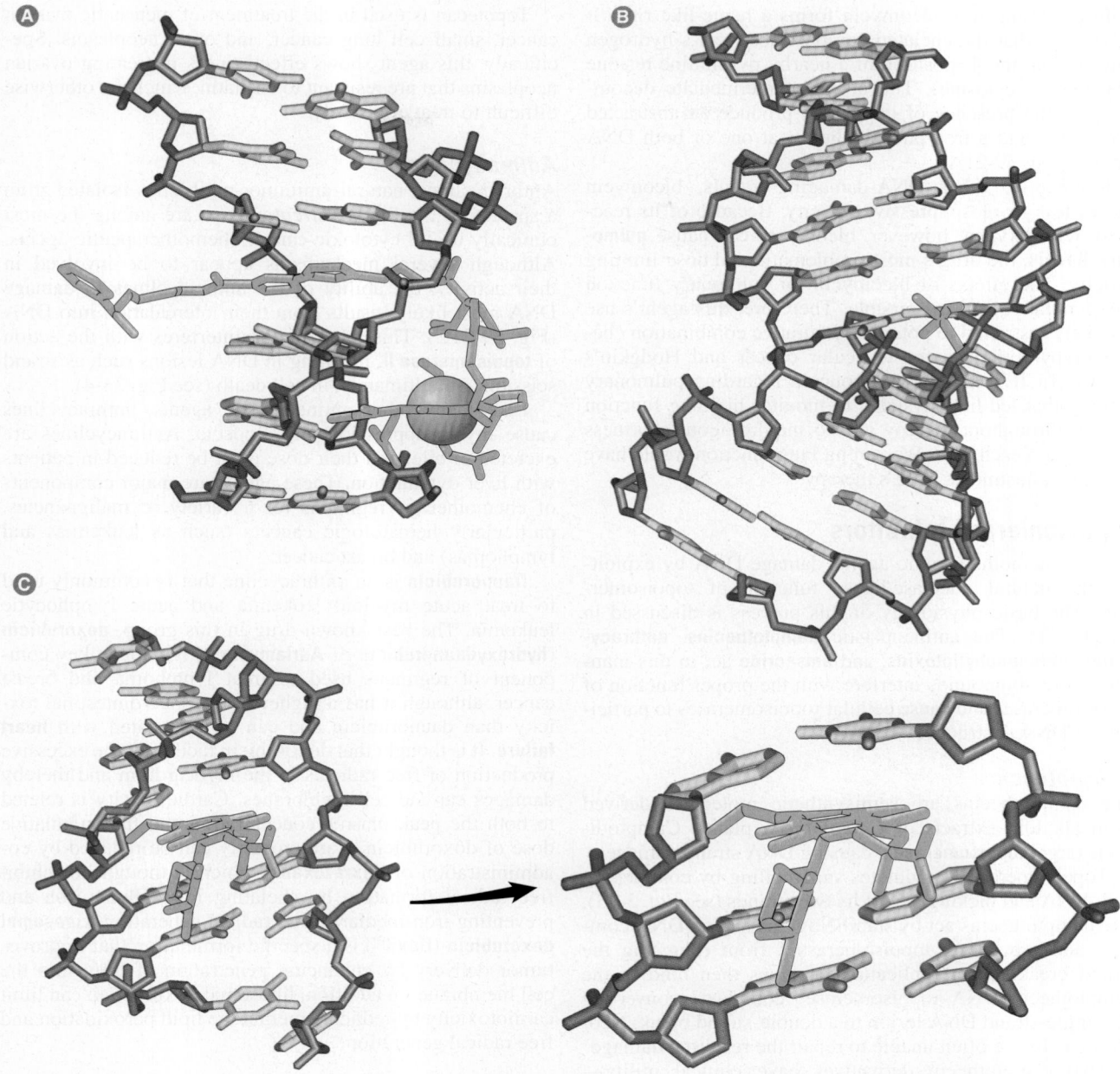

FIGURE 39-21. Interactions of bleomycin, platinum compounds, and anthracyclines with DNA. A. Bleomycin (*highlighted in orange*) binds to the DNA double helix and thereby exposes nucleotides in DNA to the iron (II) atom (*large red ball*) that is complexed to bleomycin. In the presence of molecular oxygen, the iron–bleomycin complex causes single-strand and double-strand breaks in DNA by a free radical mechanism. **B.** Platinum complexes (*highlighted in orange*) cross-link N-7 atoms on adjacent guanine residues, forming intrastrand DNA cross-links. **C.** Daunorubicin, an anthracycline (*highlighted in orange*), intercalates into DNA structure (*see expanded view on right*) and thereby prevents the strand passage and religation steps that are part of the catalytic cycle of type II topoisomerase (see Fig. 34-4). Anthracyclines may also damage DNA by a free radical mechanism.

frequently. Thiol-containing compounds, such as **amifostine**, can ameliorate cisplatin nephrotoxicity without diminishing its antitumor effects. **Carboplatin**, a cisplatin analogue that is less nephrotoxic, has replaced cisplatin in many chemotherapy regimens. **Oxaliplatin**, a third platinum compound, has activity in the treatment of colorectal cancer and other gastrointestinal malignancies. Like cisplatin, oxaliplatin causes cumulative neurotoxicity; oxaliplatin also induces a unique acute neurotoxicity that is exacerbated by exposure to cold temperatures.

Bleomycin

The **bleomycins**, a family of natural glycopeptides synthesized by a species of *Streptomyces*, have prominent cytotoxic activity. A mixture of several of these glycopeptides, differing only in side chains, is used clinically (Fig. 39-21A). Bleomycin binds DNA and chelates iron (II), leading to the formation of free radicals that cause single- and double-strand DNA breaks. As with many chemotherapeutic agents, multidrug-resistance mechanisms, such as increased drug efflux from tumor cells, can reduce tumor susceptibility to bleomycin.

In chelating iron, bleomycin forms a heme-like ring. It is believed that the chelated complex abstracts a hydrogen radical from the 4′ position of a nearby pyrimidine residue (thymine or cytosine). The unstable intermediate decomposes in the presence of oxygen to produce an abstracted pyrimidine and a free phosphodiester at one or both DNA strands (Fig. 39-21A).

Relative to other DNA-damaging agents, bleomycin causes less myelosuppressive toxicity. Because of its reactivity with oxygen, however, bleomycin can cause **pulmonary fibrosis**, the drug's most problematic and dose-limiting toxicity. The effects of bleomycin on pulmonary function are cumulative and irreversible. Therefore, this agent's use is largely restricted to potentially curative combination chemotherapy regimens for testicular cancer and Hodgkin's disease. In JL's case, it was concern regarding pulmonary toxicity that led his physician to monitor his lung function closely throughout therapy and to inquire about shortness of breath on each visit. Worsening lung function would have required adjustments in JL's therapy.

Topoisomerase Inhibitors

Several chemotherapeutic agents damage DNA by exploiting the natural nuclease/ligase function of topoisomerases. The basic physiology of this process is discussed in Chapter 34. The antineoplastic **camptothecins**, **anthracyclines**, **epipodophyllotoxins**, and **amsacrine** act in this manner. These compounds interfere with the proper function of topoisomerases and cause cellular topoisomerases to participate in DNA destruction.

Camptothecins

The camptothecins are semisynthetic molecules derived from alkaloid extracts of *Camptotheca* plants. Camptothecins target **topoisomerase I**, causing DNA strand damage.

Topoisomerase I modulates supercoiling by complexing with DNA and nicking one of its two strands (see Fig. 34-3). The camptothecins act by stabilizing this nicked DNA complex and preventing topoisomerase I from religating the strand break. Other replication enzymes then bind to the camptothecin–DNA–topoisomerase complex, converting the single-strand DNA lesion to a double-strand break. Neoplastic cells are often unable to repair the resulting damage.

Two camptothecin derivatives have clinical utility—**irinotecan** and **topotecan**. Irinotecan was initially introduced for the treatment of advanced colon cancer, although it may also be effective in treating other tumor types. It is a water-soluble prodrug that is cleaved by the enzyme carboxylesterase to release the lipophilic metabolite **SN-38**. Although SN-38 is approximately 1,000-fold more active than irinotecan in inhibiting topoisomerase I, it is more highly protein-bound than irinotecan and has a much shorter half-life in vivo. Thus, the relative contribution of SN-38 to the anticancer effects of irinotecan is unclear. Irinotecan use is limited by severe gastrointestinal toxicity, leading to potentially life-threatening diarrhea. As with many other chemotherapeutic agents, irinotecan also causes dose-dependent bone marrow suppression. SN-38 is metabolized by UDP-glucuronosyltransferase (UGT) A1, and patients with abnormalities in this enzyme (Gilbert's syndrome) are highly susceptible to irinotecan toxicity. This finding supports the hypothesis that SN-38 is an important contributor to the effects of irinotecan.

Topotecan is used in the treatment of metastatic ovarian cancer, small cell lung cancer, and other neoplasms. Specifically, this agent shows effectiveness in treating ovarian neoplasms that are resistant to cisplatin, which are otherwise difficult to treat effectively.

Anthracyclines

Anthracyclines, natural antitumor antibiotics isolated from a species of the fungus *Streptomyces*, are among the most clinically useful cytotoxic cancer chemotherapeutic agents. Although several mechanisms appear to be involved in their activity, the ability of the anthracyclines to damage DNA most likely results from their intercalation into DNA (Fig. 39-21C). This intercalation interferes with the action of **topoisomerase II**, resulting in DNA lesions such as strand scission and, ultimately, in cell death (see Fig. 34-4).

Like many other antineoplastic agents, anthracyclines cause myelosuppression and alopecia. Anthracyclines are excreted in bile, and their dose must be reduced in patients with liver dysfunction. These agents are major components of chemotherapy regimens for a variety of malignancies, particularly hematologic cancers (such as leukemias and lymphomas) and breast cancer.

Daunorubicin is an anthracycline that is commonly used to treat acute myeloid leukemia and acute lymphocytic leukemia. The best known drug in this group, **doxorubicin** (**hydroxydaunorubicin** or **Adriamycin®**), remains a key component of regimens used to treat lymphoma and breast cancer, although it has a higher risk of gastrointestinal toxicity than daunorubicin and can be associated with **heart failure**. It is thought that doxorubicin facilitates the excessive production of free radicals in the myocardium and thereby damages cardiac cell membranes. Cardiotoxicity is related to both the peak plasma concentration and the cumulative dose of doxorubicin. Cardiotoxicity can be reduced by co-administration of **dexrazoxane**, which is thought to inhibit free radical formation by chelating intracellular iron and preventing iron-mediated free radical generation. **Liposomal doxorubicin** (**Doxil®**) is a specific formulation that improves tumor delivery by enhancing penetration of drug into the cell membrane. In addition, liposomal doxorubicin can limit cardiotoxicity by reducing membrane lipid peroxidation and free radical generation.

Epipodophyllotoxins

Like anthracyclines, **epipodophyllotoxins** appear to act primarily by inhibiting topoisomerase II-mediated religation of double-strand DNA breaks (see Fig. 34-4). The antineoplastic agents **etoposide (VP-16)** and **teniposide (VM-26)** are semisynthetic derivatives of a compound isolated from the plant *Podophyllum*. These drugs bind topoisomerase II and DNA, trapping the complex in its cleavable state. Tumor cells often develop resistance to etoposide by increasing their expression of **P-glycoprotein**. This protein normally serves as an efflux pump to rid the cell of toxic molecules such as natural metabolic side-products, but it can also remove chemotherapeutic agents derived from natural products before those agents have exerted their cytotoxic effect. Etoposide is useful for treating testicular cancer, lung cancer, and leukemia, while both etoposide and teniposide are used to treat various lymphomas. Bone marrow suppression is the chief toxicity of the two epipodophyllotoxins in clinical use.

Combining drugs that damage DNA directly, such as cisplatin and bleomycin, with drugs that inhibit topoisomerase II, such as etoposide, can have powerful synergistic anticancer effects. This synergy may relate to the role of topoisomerases in repairing DNA damage or to the combined ability of these drug classes to induce sufficient DNA damage to trigger apoptosis. In practice, drugs of these classes are co-administered in many successful antineoplastic regimens. As JL's case demonstrates, the combination of etoposide, bleomycin, and cisplatin can cure most cases of metastatic testicular cancer.

Amsacrine

Amsacrine is another example of a chemotherapeutic agent that acts primarily by inhibiting topoisomerase II-mediated religation of double-strand DNA breaks. This compound targets DNA by intercalating between base pairs, distorting the double helix, producing DNA–protein cross-links, and creating both single- and double-strand DNA lesions. Its clinical use is generally restricted to the treatment of recurrent leukemia and ovarian cancer.

Microtubule Inhibitors

Microtubules depend on dynamic instability for physiologic functioning. Without the ability to change length quickly, microtubules can do little other than lend structural support to a quiescent cell. Although microtubules play important roles in many aspects of cellular physiology, drugs that inhibit microtubule function are preferentially toxic to M-phase cells. Vinca alkaloids inhibit microtubule polymerization, while taxanes inhibit microtubule depolymerization. Two other inhibitors of microtubule polymerization, griseofulvin and colchicine, are discussed in Chapter 36, Pharmacology of Fungal Infections and Chapter 49, respectively.

Inhibitors of Microtubule Polymerization: Vinca Alkaloids

The vinca alkaloids **vinblastine** and **vincristine** are natural products originally isolated from the periwinkle plant, *Vinca rosea*. Vinca alkaloids bind to β-tubulin on a portion of the molecule that overlaps with the GTP-binding domain (Fig. 39-22). The binding of vinca alkaloids to β-tubulin at the (+) end of microtubules inhibits tubulin polymerization and thereby prevents microtubule extension. Because microtubules must constantly add tubulin to maintain stability (i.e., they must retain a GTP-bound tubulin cap), inhibition of tubulin addition eventually leads to the depolymerization of existing microtubules (Fig. 39-12).

Vinblastine is used to treat certain lymphomas and, as part of a multidrug regimen (with cisplatin and bleomycin), to treat metastatic testicular cancer. Pharmacologic doses of the drug cause nausea and vomiting. **Myelosuppression** is the dose-limiting adverse effect of vinblastine.

Vincristine plays an important role in the chemotherapy of pediatric leukemias. It is also a component of chemotherapy regimens used to treat Hodgkin's disease and some non-Hodgkin's lymphomas. Pharmacologic doses of vincristine cause nausea and vomiting. Vincristine causes some myelosuppression, but not to the same degree as vinblastine. **Peripheral neuropathy** is usually the dose-limiting adverse effect of vincristine; this toxicity may result from inhibition of the microtubule trafficking function in long peripheral nerves that extend from the spinal cord to the extremities.

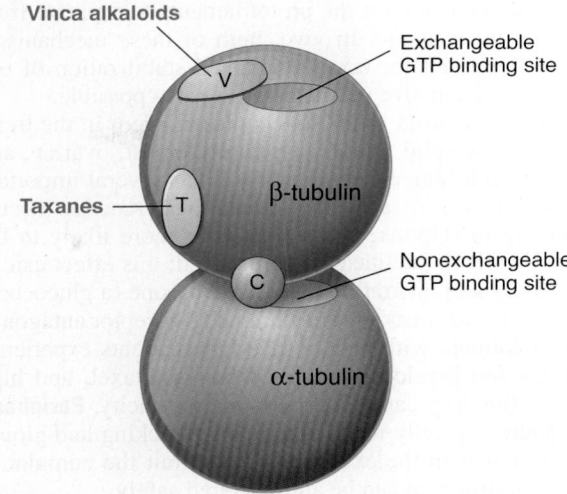

FIGURE 39-22. Tubulin binding sites of microtubule-inhibiting drugs. The tubulin heterodimer is composed of α-tubulin (*purple*) and β-tubulin (*blue*). α-Tubulin and β-tubulin both bind GTP. The GTP on α-tubulin is not hydrolyzed; for this reason, the GTP binding site on α-tubulin is referred to as the *nonexchangeable GTP binding site*. β-Tubulin hydrolyzes GTP to GDP; for this reason, the GTP binding site on β-tubulin is referred to as the *exchangeable GTP binding site*. The two major classes of antineoplastic microtubule inhibitors bind to distinct sites on the tubulin heterodimer. Vinca alkaloids, which inhibit microtubule polymerization, bind to a site on β-tubulin located near the exchangeable GTP binding site (*V*). Vinca alkaloids bind preferentially at the (+) end of microtubules and thereby inhibit the addition of new tubulin subunits to the microtubule. Taxanes, which stabilize polymerized microtubules, bind to a different site on β-tubulin (*T*). Taxanes may stabilize either the interactions between tubulin subunits or the shape of microtubule protofilaments. Colchicine binds to a site located at the interface between α-tubulin and β-tubulin (*C*). Colchicine is not used in cancer chemotherapy but is used in the treatment of gout (see Chapter 49).

Eribulin is an analogue of a natural product from the *Halichondria* genus of marine sponges. It binds to the (+) end of microtubules and inhibits microtubule dynamics. Eribulin was approved in 2010 for use in the treatment of metastatic breast cancer.

Inhibitors of Microtubule Depolymerization: Taxanes

The taxanes, which include **paclitaxel**, **docetaxel**, and **cabazitaxel**, are natural products originally derived from the bark of the western yew tree. Taxanes bind to the β-tubulin subunit of microtubules at a site distinct from the vinca alkaloid binding site (Fig. 39-22). Paclitaxel has been shown to bind to the *inside* of microtubules. Unlike the vinca alkaloids, taxanes promote microtubule polymerization and inhibit depolymerization. Stabilization of the microtubules in a polymerized state arrests cells in mitosis and eventually leads to programmed cell death (apoptosis).

Two leading hypotheses have been proposed for the apparent microtubule-stabilizing properties of taxanes. First, taxanes could strengthen the lateral interactions between microtubule protofilaments. Increased lateral interactions would decrease the tendency for protofilaments to "peel away" from the microtubule cylinder. Second, taxanes could straighten individual protofilaments. Once β-tubulin hydrolyzes GTP to GDP, protofilaments have a tendency to "curl," which produces a strain on the integrity of the microtubule cylinder. By straightening protofilaments, taxanes could reduce the tendency for the protofilaments to separate from the intact microtubule. In vivo, both of these mechanisms may be important for taxane-mediated stabilization of microtubules; alternative mechanisms are also possible.

Paclitaxel is used as an antineoplastic agent in the treatment of many solid tumors, especially breast, ovarian, and non-small cell lung cancer. Paclitaxel has several important adverse effects. An acute hypersensitivity reaction occurs commonly in response to paclitaxel, or more likely to the vehicle in which paclitaxel is solubilized; this effect can be obviated by administration of dexamethasone (a glucocorticoid receptor agonist) and a histamine H_1 receptor antagonist before treatment with paclitaxel. Many patients experience myalgias and myelosuppression from paclitaxel, and high doses of the drug can cause pulmonary toxicity. **Peripheral neuropathy**, typically manifesting as a "stocking and glove" sensory deficit in the extremities, can limit the cumulative amount of drug that can be administered safely.

Abraxane® is an albumin-bound form of paclitaxel with a mean particle size of 130 nanometers. The albumin-bound paclitaxel nanoparticles do not cause a hypersensitivity reaction, do not require premedication, and cause less myelosuppression than traditional, solvent-based paclitaxel. Abraxane® is approved for the treatment of metastatic breast cancer and, in combination with gemcitabine, for the first-line treatment of pancreatic cancer.

Docetaxel is most commonly used in the treatment of breast cancer, non-small cell lung cancer, and prostate cancer. As with paclitaxel, docetaxel causes an acute hypersensitivity reaction that can be obviated by preadministration of glucocorticoids. Docetaxel occasionally exhibits the drug-specific adverse effect of fluid retention, which likely arises from increased capillary permeability. Docetaxel does not cause neuropathy as frequently as paclitaxel does. The myelosuppression associated with docetaxel is profound, however, and is usually dose-limiting.

Cabazitaxel is a third taxane that has recently been approved for the treatment of hormone-refractory prostate cancer after failure of docetaxel-based treatment. Treatment with cabazitaxel is also associated with significant neutropenia.

■ CONCLUSION AND FUTURE DIRECTIONS

The antineoplastic agents described in this chapter exert their effects on the genome by preventing efficient DNA replication, inducing DNA damage, and interfering with mitosis. Because many normal cells as well as cancer cells are transiting through the cell cycle, these agents are associated with multiple dose-limiting toxicities. In addition, although cancer cells are susceptible to DNA damage, in some instances, mutations in key checkpoint proteins such as p53 prevent the apoptosis that would otherwise be induced by these agents.

Novel approaches are being developed to target DNA damage more specifically. For example, it has been shown that mice deficient in PARP1 are able to overcome the defect in single-strand break repair by converting single-strand breaks to double-strand breaks and then repairing the DNA by the DSB repair pathway. Furthermore, normal human cells treated in culture with PARP1 inhibitors are capable of undergoing normal cell division, although these cells do manifest increased susceptibility to DNA damage as a consequence of defective single-strand break repair. In contrast, cells deficient in BRCA1 or BRCA2, which are involved in DSB repair, are killed in response to treatment with PARP1 inhibitors; compared to normal cells, BRCA1⁻ or BRCA2⁻ cells are up to 1,000-fold more sensitive to the action of PARP1 inhibitors. Presumably, the BRCA1⁻ and BRCA2⁻ cells are more sensitive due to impairment of both single-strand break and DSB repair pathways, resulting in lethal accumulation of DNA damage. Based on these findings, **PARP1 inhibitors** are currently in clinical trials for the treatment of BRCA-deficient breast cancer and ovarian cancer, and may be effective in other tumors in which the DNA damage response is compromised. The investigational PARP1 inhibitor **olaparib** has had mixed results in general but may show particular activity in tumors with BRCA mutations.

The observation that telomerase is expressed in most cancer cells and is key to the process of immortalization highlights this enzyme as an important target in future cancer therapy. Although telomerase is expressed to some degree in stem cells and normally cycling cells, most normal cells lack telomerase expression. Therefore, the dependency of tumor cells on the immortalized state could provide **telomerase inhibitors** with a favorable therapeutic index. However, effective agents have yet to be discovered, and one concern is that multiple cell divisions may be required for telomere length to shorten to a level that is critical for cell survival. Combinations of telomerase inhibitors with traditional cytotoxic agents or newer molecularly targeted therapies could yield synergistic effects. Such strategies, as well as those described in Chapter 40, Pharmacology of Cancer: Signal Transduction, will help to advance cancer therapy by moving beyond general cytotoxic approaches and focusing treatment instead on the molecular abnormalities responsible for driving oncogenesis.

Suggested Reading

Bishr M, Saad F. Overview of the latest treatments for castration-resistant prostate cancer. *Nat Rev Urol* 2013;10:522–528. (*Discusses recent advances in the treatment of prostate cancer, including a review of cabazitaxel.*)

Brody LC. Treating cancer by targeting a weakness. *N Engl J Med* 2005;353:949–950. (*Discusses advances in targeted cancer therapy.*)

Gazdar A. DNA repair and survival in lung cancer. *N Engl J Med* 2007;356:771–773. (*Discusses DNA repair pathway status in relationship to survival and chemotherapy responsiveness.*)

O'Sullivan Coyne G, Chen A, Kummar S. Delivering on the promise: poly ADP ribose polymerase inhibition as targeted anticancer therapy. *Curr Opin Oncol* 2015;27:475–481. (*Reviews the development and clinical activity of PARP inhibitors as anticancer drugs.*)

Peltomaki P. Role of DNA mismatch repair defects in the pathogenesis of human cancer. *J Clin Oncol* 2003;21:1174–1179. (*Reviews the pathophysiology of DNA repair mechanisms.*)

Van der Jagt R. Bendamustine for indolent non-Hodgkin lymphoma in the front-line or relapsed setting: a review of pharmacokinetics and clinical trial outcomes. *Exp Rev Hematol* 2013;6:525–537. (*Reviews the pharmacology of bendamustine.*)

DRUG SUMMARY TABLE: CHAPTER 39 Pharmacology of Cancer: Genome Synthesis, Stability, and Maintenance

DRUG	CLINICAL APPLICATIONS	SERIOUS AND COMMON ADVERSE EFFECTS	CONTRAINDICATIONS	THERAPEUTIC CONSIDERATIONS
INHIBITORS OF THYMIDYLATE SYNTHASE Mechanism—Inhibit thymidylate synthase, thereby decreasing cellular availability of dTMP and causing "thymineless" cell death				
Fluorouracil (5-FU)	Breast cancer Gastrointestinal cancers Skin cancer (topical application) Actinic keratosis	*Cardiotoxicity, coronary atherosclerosis, thrombophlebitis, gastrointestinal ulcer, myelosuppression, immune hypersensitivity reaction, cerebellar syndrome, visual changes, stenosis of lacrimal system* Alopecia, rash, photosensitivity, gastrointestinal upset, stomatitis, headache	Hypersensitivity to fluorouracil or capecitabine Severe bone marrow depression Poor nutritional state Serious infection Dihydropyrimidine dehydrogenase deficiency Pregnancy	5-FU is a uracil analogue that, after intracellular modification, inhibits thymidylate synthase by binding to the deoxyuridylate (substrate) site on the enzyme. In addition to inhibiting thymidylate synthase, 5-FU interferes with protein synthesis after the drug metabolite FUTP is incorporated into mRNA. Folinic acid can be used to potentiate the action of 5-FU.
Capecitabine	Metastatic colorectal cancer Breast cancer	Same as fluorouracil Additionally: *Stevens-Johnson syndrome, toxic epidermal necrolysis, hyperbilirubinemia* Edema	Hypersensitivity to capecitabine or fluorouracil Dihydropyrimidine dehydrogenase deficiency Severe renal impairment	Orally available prodrug form of 5-FU.
Pemetrexed	Non-small cell lung cancer Malignant pleural mesothelioma (in combination with cisplatin)	*Stevens-Johnson syndrome, toxic epidermal necrolysis, gastrointestinal obstruction, myelosuppression, neuropathy, renal failure, interstitial pneumonitis, pulmonary embolism* Peeling of skin, fatigue, gastrointestinal upset, stomatitis	Hypersensitivity to pemetrexed Severe renal impairment	Pemetrexed is a folate analogue that, after intracellular modification, inhibits thymidylate synthase by binding to the methylenetetrahydrofolate (cofactor) site on the enzyme. Co-administered with folic acid and vitamin B_{12} to reduce hematologic and gastrointestinal toxicity.
INHIBITORS OF PURINE METABOLISM Mechanism—Drug metabolites inhibit IMPDH and other synthetic enzymes, thereby interfering with AMP and GMP synthesis				
6-Mercaptopurine (6-MP) **Azathioprine**	6-Mercaptopurine only: Acute lymphoid leukemia Azathioprine only: Immunosuppression in renal transplantation Rheumatoid arthritis	*Pancreatitis, myelosuppression, hepatotoxicity, increased risk of infection or malignancy (shared adverse effects); hyperuricemia (6-mercaptopurine only); pericarditis, leukoencephalopathy (azathioprine only)* Gastrointestinal upset (shared adverse effect); rash (6-mercaptopurine only)	Shared contraindications: Pregnancy Hypersensitivity to azathioprine or 6-mercaptopurine Azathioprine only: Rheumatoid arthritis with prior treatment with alkylating agents	Effectiveness and toxicity increased by allopurinol. Azathioprine is a less toxic prodrug of 6-mercaptopurine. Azathioprine is used for immunosuppression of autoimmune diseases.

continues

DRUG SUMMARY TABLE: CHAPTER 39 Pharmacology of Cancer: Genome Synthesis, Stability, and Maintenance *continued*

DRUG	CLINICAL APPLICATIONS	SERIOUS AND COMMON ADVERSE EFFECTS	CONTRAINDICATIONS	THERAPEUTIC CONSIDERATIONS
Pentostatin	Hairy cell leukemia	*Hyponatremia, myelosuppression, renal failure, neurotoxicity, immune hypersensitivity reaction* Rash, shaking chills, gastrointestinal upset, myalgia, asthenia, upper respiratory infection, headache, fever, fatigue	Hypersensitivity to pentostatin	Selective inhibitor of adenosine deaminase (ADA).

INHIBITORS OF RIBONUCLEOTIDE REDUCTASE
Mechanism—Inhibit ribonucleotide reductase, the enzyme that converts ribonucleotides to deoxyribonucleotides

DRUG	CLINICAL APPLICATIONS	SERIOUS AND COMMON ADVERSE EFFECTS	CONTRAINDICATIONS	THERAPEUTIC CONSIDERATIONS
Hydroxyurea	Hematologic malignancies Head and neck cancers Ovarian carcinoma Cervical carcinoma Non-Hodgkin's lymphoma Sickle cell disease	*Gangrenous disorder, skin cancer, myelosuppression, secondary leukemia with long-term use*	Hypersensitivity to hydroxyurea Severe bone marrow depression	Inhibits ribonucleotide reductase by scavenging an essential tyrosyl radical at the active site of the enzyme. In sickle cell disease, hydroxyurea is thought to act by increasing hemoglobin F.

PURINE AND PYRIMIDINE ANALOGUES THAT ARE INCORPORATED INTO DNA
Mechanism—Incorporation into DNA and RNA results in inhibition of DNA polymerase, thereby causing cell death

DRUG	CLINICAL APPLICATIONS	SERIOUS AND COMMON ADVERSE EFFECTS	CONTRAINDICATIONS	THERAPEUTIC CONSIDERATIONS
Thioguanine	Acute myelogenous leukemia	*Myelosuppression, hyperuricemia, intestinal perforation, hepatotoxicity, infection* Gastrointestinal upset, stomatitis	Prior resistance to thioguanine or 6-mercaptopurine	Guanine analogue.
Fludarabine-5′-phosphate	B-cell chronic lymphocytic leukemia	*Autoimmune hemolytic anemia, myelosuppression, neurotoxicity, leukoencephalopathy, pulmonary toxicity, graft versus host disease, tumor lysis syndrome* Gastrointestinal upset, asthenia, paresthesia, fatigue, cough, infection, shivering	Hypersensitivity to fludarabine	Purine nucleotide analogue.
Cladribine	Hairy cell leukemia	*Stevens-Johnson syndrome, toxic epidermal necrolysis, febrile neutropenia, myelosuppression, nephrotoxicity, neurotoxicity, infection* Rash, injection site reaction, nausea, headache, fatigue	Hypersensitivity to cladribine	Adenosine analogue.

Drug	Clinical Applications	Serious and Common Adverse Effects	Contraindications	Therapeutic Considerations
Cytarabine (araC)	Acute lymphoblastic leukemia Acute myelogenous leukemia Chronic myelogenous leukemia Meningeal leukemia	*Myelosuppression, neuropathy, kidney disease, infection* Thrombophlebitis, rash, hyperuricemia, gastrointestinal disturbance, ulcers of mouth or anus	Hypersensitivity to cytarabine	Cytidine analogue.
5-Azacytidine Decitabine	Myelodysplastic syndrome	*Myelosuppression (shared adverse effect); renal failure (5-azacytidine only); atrial fibrillation, heart failure, Sweet's syndrome, infection, intracranial hemorrhage, pleural effusion, pulmonary edema (decitabine only)* Peripheral edema, rash, gastrointestinal upset, electrolyte disturbance, arthralgia, asthenia, dizziness, headache, insomnia, shivering, lethargy, cough, infection	Hypersensitivity to 5-azacytidine or decitabine	Cytidine analogues.
Gemcitabine	Pancreatic cancer Non-small cell lung cancer Breast cancer Ovarian cancer	*Capillary leak syndrome, bullous eruption, myelosuppression, febrile neutropenia, pulmonary toxicity, hepatotoxicity, leukoencephalopathy, hemolytic uremic syndrome, renal failure, infection* Edema, rash, alopecia, gastrointestinal upset, stomatitis, hyperglycemia, hypomagnesemia, paresthesia, fever	Hypersensitivity to gemcitabine Pregnancy	Cytidine analogue.

AGENTS THAT DIRECTLY MODIFY DNA STRUCTURE: ALKYLATING AGENTS
Mechanism—Covalently bind DNA, often cross-link to DNA or associated proteins

Drug	Clinical Applications	Serious and Common Adverse Effects	Contraindications	Therapeutic Considerations
Cyclophosphamide	Autoimmune diseases Leukemias and lymphomas Advanced mycosis fungoides Neuroblastoma Ovarian cancer Retinoblastoma Breast cancer Malignant histiocytosis Multiple myeloma	*Cardiotoxicity, epidermal necrolysis, Stevens–Johnson syndrome, myelosuppression, hemorrhagic cystitis, pyelitis, azoospermia, oligozoospermia, interstitial pneumonitis, increased risk of infection or malignancy* Alopecia, rash, gastrointestinal upset, leukopenia, amenorrhea	Hypersensitivity to cyclophosphamide Urinary outflow obstruction	Acrolein, a metabolite of cyclophosphamide, causes hemorrhagic cystitis; this adverse effect can be prevented by co-administration with mesna.

continues

DRUG SUMMARY TABLE: CHAPTER 39 Pharmacology of Cancer: Genome Synthesis, Stability, and Maintenance *continued*

DRUG	CLINICAL APPLICATIONS	*SERIOUS* AND COMMON ADVERSE EFFECTS	CONTRAINDICATIONS	THERAPEUTIC CONSIDERATIONS
Bendamustine **Mechlorethamine** **Melphalan** **Estramustine** **Chlorambucil** **Mitomycin** **Thiotepa** **Carmustine** **Dacarbazine** **Procarbazine** **Temozolomide** **Altretamine** **Ifosfamide**	Bendamustine: Indolent lymphoma, chronic lymphoid leukemia Mechlorethamine: Leukemia and Hodgkin's disease, lymphosarcoma, mycosis fungoides, polycythemia vera, squamous cell carcinoma of bronchus Melphalan: Multiple myeloma, ovarian tumor Estramustine: Prostate cancer Chlorambucil: Leukemia, lymphoma, mycosis fungoides Mitomycin: Gastric cancer, pancreatic cancer Thiotepa: Bladder cancer, breast cancer, Hodgkin's disease, ovarian cancer Carmustine: Brain cancer, lymphoma, multiple myeloma Dacarbazine: Hodgkin's disease, melanoma Procarbazine: Hodgkin's disease Temozolomide: Anaplastic astrocytoma and glioblastoma multiforme Altretamine: Ovarian cancer Ifosfamide: Germ cell testicular cancer	*Same as cyclophosphamide*	Shared contraindication: Hypersensitivity to drug Mechlorethamine only: Presence of known infectious disease Estramustine only: Active thrombophlebitis or thromboembolic disorder Mitomycin only: Coagulation disorder, pregnancy, or thrombocytopenia Thiotepa only: Hepatic, renal, or bone marrow dysfunction Procarbazine and altretamine only: Severe bone marrow depression Altretamine only: Severe neurologic toxicity Ifosfamide only: Urinary outflow obstruction	Bendamustine treatment shows significantly greater survival compared with traditional cyclophosphamide-based regimens when combined with rituximab for indolent B-cell non-Hodgkin's lymphoma. Thiotepa is instilled directly in the bladder. Carmustine is a nitrosourea that attaches a carbamoyl group to target proteins. Ifosfamide is ordinarily co-administered with mesna.

AGENTS THAT DIRECTLY MODIFY DNA STRUCTURE: PLATINUM COMPOUNDS
Mechanism—Cross-link intrastrand guanine bases

DRUG	CLINICAL APPLICATIONS	*SERIOUS* AND COMMON ADVERSE EFFECTS	CONTRAINDICATIONS	THERAPEUTIC CONSIDERATIONS
Cisplatin **Carboplatin**	Genitourinary cancers	*Myelosuppression (shared adverse effect); neurotoxicity, leukoencephalopathy, peripheral neuropathy, ototoxicity, nephrotoxicity (cisplatin only); visual disturbances (carboplatin only)* Alopecia, electrolyte imbalance, gastrointestinal upset, abnormal liver function tests (carboplatin only)	Shared contraindications: Hypersensitivity to cisplatin or carboplatin Severe bone marrow depression Cisplatin only: Renal or hearing impairment Carboplatin only: Significant bleeding	Cisplatin can be injected intraperitoneally for treatment of ovarian cancer. Co-administration of amifostine and cisplatin can limit nephrotoxicity.

Drug	Clinical Applications	Serious and Common Adverse Effects	Contraindications	Therapeutic Considerations
Oxaliplatin	Colorectal cancer	*Metabolic acidosis, neurotoxicity, pharyngolaryngeal dysesthesia, myelosuppression, colitis, bowel obstruction, pancreatitis, hepatic dysfunction, transient visual loss, hearing loss, hemolytic uremic syndrome, interstitial nephritis, pulmonary fibrosis, angioedema* Gastrointestinal disturbance, abnormal liver function tests, back pain, paresthesia, cough, fever, fatigue	Hypersensitivity to oxaliplatin	Acute neurotoxicity is exacerbated by exposure to cold temperatures.

AGENTS THAT DIRECTLY MODIFY DNA STRUCTURE: BLEOMYCIN
Mechanism—Binds oxygen and chelates Fe(II); binds DNA and leads to strand breaks via a free radical mechanism

Drug	Clinical Applications	Serious and Common Adverse Effects	Contraindications	Therapeutic Considerations
Bleomycin	Testicular cancer Hodgkin's disease Non-Hodgkin's lymphoma Squamous cell carcinoma	*Pulmonary fibrosis, vascular disease, myocardial infarction, Raynaud's disease, gangrenous disorder, cerebral edema, hepatotoxicity, nephrotoxicity, pulmonary fibrosis* Hyperkeratosis, hyperpigmentation, stomatitis, fever	Hypersensitivity to bleomycin	Effects on pulmonary function are dose-limiting and irreversible.

TOPOISOMERASE INHIBITORS
Mechanism—Inhibit topoisomerase I or topoisomerase II, leading to DNA strand breakage

Drug	Clinical Applications	Serious and Common Adverse Effects	Contraindications	Therapeutic Considerations
Irinotecan **Topotecan**	Irinotecan only: Colorectal cancer Topotecan only: Small cell lung cancer Cervical carcinoma Ovarian cancer	*Life-threatening diarrhea, gastrointestinal perforation, myelosuppression, febrile neutropenia, interstitial lung disease* Alopecia, weight loss, gastrointestinal upset, eosinophilia, increased bilirubin, asthenia, headache, dizziness, cough, infection	Shared contraindication: Hypersensitivity to irinotecan or topotecan Topotecan only: Severe bone marrow depression	Irinotecan and topotecan are camptothecins that inhibit topoisomerase I. Action is specific to S phase of cell cycle.
Doxorubicin **Daunorubicin** **Epirubicin**	Doxorubicin and daunorubicin only: Leukemia Lymphoma Doxorubicin and epirubicin only: Breast cancer Doxorubicin only: AIDS-related Kaposi's sarcoma Ovarian cancer Bladder cancer Thyroid cancer Gastrointestinal cancer Nephroblastoma Osteosarcoma Non-small cell and small cell lung cancer	*Heart failure (especially doxorubicin), myelosuppression, severe neutropenia (shared adverse effects); hepatic dysfunction, septic shock, radiation pneumonitis, tumor lysis syndrome (doxorubicin only); hyperuricemia (daunorubicin only); pulmonary embolism (epirubicin only)* Alopecia, gastrointestinal upset (shared adverse effects); rash, lethargy, conjunctivitis, keratitis, amenorrhea, infection (epirubicin only)	Shared contraindications: Hypersensitivity to doxorubicin, daunorubicin, or epirubicin Preexisting heart failure Doxorubicin and epirubicin only: Severe bone marrow depression Doxorubicin only: Severe liver dysfunction Epirubicin only: Prior cumulative maximum dose of anthracyclines	Doxorubicin, daunorubicin, and epirubicin are anthracyclines that inhibit topoisomerase II. Excreted in bile (reduce dose in patients with liver dysfunction). Action is specific to G2 phase of cell cycle. Liposomal doxorubicin improves tumor delivery and lessens cardiotoxicity.

continues

DRUG SUMMARY TABLE: CHAPTER 39 Pharmacology of Cancer: Genome Synthesis, Stability, and Maintenance *continued*

DRUG	CLINICAL APPLICATIONS	*SERIOUS* AND COMMON ADVERSE EFFECTS	CONTRAINDICATIONS	THERAPEUTIC CONSIDERATIONS
Etoposide **Teniposide**	Etoposide only: Testicular cancer, small cell carcinoma of lung Teniposide only: Acute lymphoblastic leukemia	Same as doxorubicin	Hypersensitivity to etoposide or teniposide	Etoposide and teniposide are epipodophyllotoxins that inhibit topoisomerase II. Action is specific to late S and G2 phases of cell cycle.
Amsacrine	Recurrent leukemia Ovarian cancer	ECG changes including QT prolongation, paralytic ileus, myelosuppression, convulsion, azoospermia, hepatotoxicity Alopecia, gastrointestinal disturbance	Hypersensitivity to amsacrine	Inhibits topoisomerase II.

AGENTS THAT INHIBIT MICROTUBULE POLYMERIZATION
Mechanism—Bind tubulin subunits and prevent microtubule polymerization

DRUG	CLINICAL APPLICATIONS	*SERIOUS* AND COMMON ADVERSE EFFECTS	CONTRAINDICATIONS	THERAPEUTIC CONSIDERATIONS
Vinblastine	Metastatic testicular cancer Lymphoma AIDS-related Kaposi's sarcoma Breast cancer Choriocarcinoma Malignant histiocytosis Mycosis fungoides	*Myelosuppression, stroke, neurotoxicity, acute respiratory distress syndrome* Hypertension, alopecia, bone pain, gastrointestinal upset	Bacterial infection Significant granulocytopenia	Bone marrow suppression is dose-limiting.
Vincristine	Leukemias Hodgkin's disease Non-Hodgkin's lymphoma Mantle cell lymphoma Rhabdomyosarcoma Nephroblastoma Mycosis fungoides	*Syndrome of inappropriate antidiuretic hormone secretion (SIADH), neurotoxicity, paralysis, vocal cord palsy, vision loss, ototoxicity* Alopecia, gastrointestinal disturbance	Hypersensitivity to vincristine Charcot-Marie-Tooth syndrome Intrathecal use	Peripheral neuropathy is dose-limiting.
Eribulin	Metastatic breast cancer in patients who have received at least two previous chemotherapy regimens, including both an anthracycline and a taxane	*Myelosuppression, peripheral neuropathy, QT prolongation* Alopecia, gastrointestinal disturbance, abnormal liver function tests, arthralgia, myalgia, asthenia, headache, fatigue, fever	Congenital long QT syndrome	Peripheral neuropathy and myelosuppression are dose-limiting.

AGENTS THAT INHIBIT MICROTUBULE DEPOLYMERIZATION
Mechanism—Bind polymerized tubulin and inhibit microtubule depolymerization

Paclitaxel Abraxane®	Shared indications: Breast cancer Non-small cell lung cancer Paclitaxel only: AIDS-related Kaposi's sarcoma Abraxane® only: Pancreatic cancer	Cardiac arrest, stroke, myelosuppression, pulmonary toxicity, pneumothorax, pulmonary embolism, severe hypersensitivity reaction, neutropenic sepsis, peripheral neuropathy, vocal cord palsy Edema, alopecia, rash, gastrointestinal upset, abnormal liver function tests, arthralgia, myalgia, visual disturbance, fatigue, infection	Hypersensitivity to paclitaxel or Abraxane® Severe neutropenia	Peripheral neuropathy is dose-limiting.
Docetaxel Cabazitaxel	Shared indication: Prostate cancer Docetaxel only: Breast cancer Gastric cancer Head and neck cancer Non-small cell lung cancer	Myelosuppression, renal failure, colitis (shared adverse effects); Stevens-Johnson syndrome, toxic epidermal necrolysis, interstitial pneumonitis, pulmonary embolism (docetaxel only); bowel obstruction (cabazitaxel only) Alopecia, gastrointestinal upset, asthenia, peripheral neuropathy, infection (shared adverse effects); edema, rash, stomatitis, abnormal liver function tests, amenorrhea (docetaxel only); hematuria, cough, fatigue (cabazitaxel only)	Hypersensitivity to docetaxel or cabazitaxel Severe neutropenia	Myelosuppression is dose-limiting.

40

Pharmacology of Cancer: Signal Transduction

David A. Barbie and David A. Frank

INTRODUCTION

Traditional antineoplastic therapy has consisted of agents directed against DNA replication and cell division. These drugs exhibit some degree of selectivity against cancer cells, which tend to have a higher growth fraction and, in some cases, an increased susceptibility to DNA damage compared to normal cells. However, the therapeutic window of these drugs is narrow, resulting in toxicity to normal stem cells and in hematologic and gastrointestinal adverse effects. With the impressive advances in basic tumor cell biology over the last several decades and the identification of numerous oncogenes and tumor suppressor genes, the potential exists for development of agents that are targeted more specifically at the molecular circuitry responsible for the dysregulated proliferation of cancer cells. An early example of such a drug was the selective estrogen receptor modulator **tamoxifen** (see Chapter 30, Pharmacology of Reproduction). Tamoxifen is still one of the most active agents in the treatment of hormone receptor-positive breast cancer, with a relatively modest adverse effect profile. Subsequently, the remarkable success of **imatinib mesylate** in the treatment of chronic myelogenous leukemia has suggested that, in some cases, tumor cells are dependent on oncogenes such as BCR-Abl for their survival. Like tamoxifen, imatinib remains in wide use today. This chapter highlights the basic principles and agents of targeted cancer therapy, detailing recent advances and directions for the future.

BIOCHEMISTRY OF INTERCELLULAR AND INTRACELLULAR SIGNAL TRANSDUCTION

Growth Factors and Growth Factor Receptors

External signals stimulate cell growth and proliferation via the interaction of growth factors with specific cell surface receptors. Growth factor receptors typically contain an extracellular ligand-binding domain, a hydrophobic transmembrane domain, and a cytoplasmic domain that has either intrinsic tyrosine kinase activity or an associated protein tyrosine kinase (Fig. 40-1). In general, binding of the growth factor ligand results in receptor oligomerization, a conformational change in the cytoplasmic domain of the receptor, and tyrosine kinase activation. Intracellular targets are subsequently phosphorylated, propagating a signal that culminates in progression through the cell cycle and cellular proliferation.

One example of a receptor tyrosine kinase is the **epidermal growth factor receptor (EGFR)**, which possesses intrinsic tyrosine kinase activity and is a member of the broader ErbB family of proteins, including EGFR (ErbB1), HER2/*neu* (ErbB2), ErbB3, and ErbB4. Binding of epidermal growth factor (EGF) or transforming growth factor-α (TGF-α) to EGFR results in receptor homodimerization and propagation of a growth signal. In addition, heterodimerization between

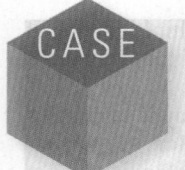

MW is a 65-year-old woman with metastatic non-small cell lung cancer. She has never smoked, and her primary tumor is an adenocarcinoma with bronchioalveolar features. Her oncologist considers treatment with carboplatin and pemetrexed but also sends genetic testing of her tumor for mutations in the epidermal growth factor receptor (EGFR) and for genetic rearrangements of anaplastic lymphoma kinase (ALK), ROS1, and RET. Her tumor is found to harbor an activating mutation in the EGFR kinase domain at codon 858, resulting in a substitution of arginine for leucine (L858R). MW is therefore treated with the oral EGFR tyrosine kinase inhibitor (TKI) erlotinib. She develops a skin rash and diarrhea but otherwise tolerates this medication well. Restaging computed tomography scans are performed 2 months after starting treatment with erlotinib. These scans reveal a dramatic reduction in MW's tumor burden, and after 6 months, there is no residual evidence of cancer. Unfortunately, MW subsequently develops recurrence of her disease. A repeat biopsy reveals that the tumor now also shows amplification of the MET receptor tyrosine kinase. She decides to participate in a clinical trial of a MET inhibitor for treatment of her recurrent non-small cell lung cancer.

Questions

1. How does signaling through EGFR promote cell growth and survival?

2. By what mechanism does erlotinib inhibit EGFR and inhibit cancer cell growth?

3. How does amplification of MET expression lead to tumor recurrence despite treatment with erlotinib?

4. What is the most common mechanism of EGFR TKI resistance, and how might this be overcome?

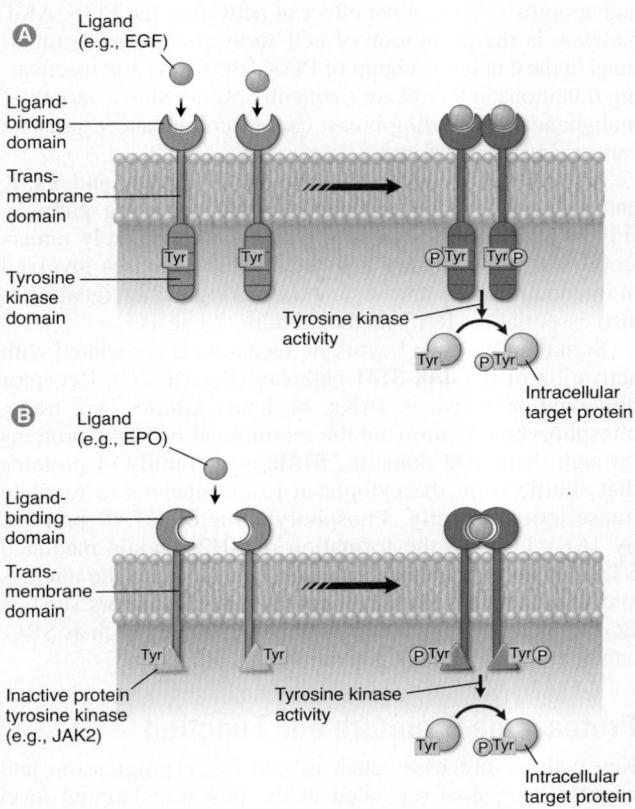

FIGURE 40-1. Structure and function of growth factor receptors. A. Growth factor receptors exemplified by the epidermal growth factor (EGF) receptor contain an extracellular ligand-binding domain, a hydrophobic transmembrane domain, and a cytoplasmic domain with intrinsic tyrosine kinase activity. Binding of ligand results in receptor homodimerization (or heterodimerization with other family members), triggering activation of the tyrosine kinase, autophosphorylation of the receptor on tyrosine (*Tyr*) residues, and phosphorylation of intracellular target proteins. **B.** Growth factor receptors exemplified by the type I cytokine receptors (such as the erythropoietin [EPO] receptor) lack intrinsic tyrosine kinase activity. Instead, the receptors are associated with intracellular protein tyrosine kinases such as JAK2. Upon ligand-induced receptor dimerization, the associated kinase is activated and autophosphorylated on tyrosine residues, resulting in recruitment and phosphorylation of intracellular target proteins.

family members can occur, yielding further diversity in the signal that is transduced. ErbB receptors are expressed on epithelial cells and are often activated or overexpressed in a variety of carcinomas (e.g., EGFR in non-small cell lung cancer and HER2/*neu* in breast cancer).

Other examples of receptor tyrosine kinases include the insulin-like growth factor receptor 1 (IGF1R), platelet-derived growth factor receptor (PDGFR), fibroblast growth factor receptor (FGFR), C-KIT, Bruton's tyrosine kinase (BTK), FMS-like tyrosine kinase (FLT3), anaplastic lymphoma kinase (ALK), ROS1, RET, and MET. Signaling through these receptors activates the growth of certain hematopoietic and mesenchymal tissues, and dysregulation of these receptors is frequently observed in specific myeloproliferative disorders, leukemias, sarcomas, and epithelial cancers (Table 40-1).

Other hematopoietic receptors rely on interaction with an associated cytoplasmic tyrosine kinase for transduction of a growth signal. For example, type I cytokine receptors such as the erythropoietin receptor (EpoR), thrombopoietin receptor (TpoR), and G-CSF receptor (GCSFR) form specifically oriented homodimers upon binding of ligand, resulting in activation of the associated tyrosine kinase JAK2, which leads to further signaling and ultimately to cell growth. Activating mutations of the receptors themselves (e.g., EpoR) have been implicated in conditions such as congenital polycythemia. A common activating mutation in JAK2, resulting in the conversion of valine to phenylalanine at position 617 (V617F), has been found in a majority of patients with the myeloproliferative disorder polycythemia vera and in a significant fraction of patients with essential thrombocythemia and myeloid metaplasia with myelofibrosis.

Intracellular Signal Transduction Pathways

Activation of a growth factor receptor initiates the transduction of a series of intracellular signals, culminating in events such as cell cycle entry, promotion of protein translation and cell growth, and enhanced cell survival. Two broad categories of pathways activated by receptor tyrosine kinases are the **RAS-MAP kinase** pathway and the **phosphatidylinositol-3-kinase (PI3K)**-AKT pathway (Fig. 40-2).

TABLE 40-1 Receptor Tyrosine Kinases Associated with Cancer

RECEPTOR TYROSINE KINASE	MALIGNANCY OR MYELOPROLIFERATIVE DISORDER
EGFR (ErbB1)	Non-small cell lung cancer Head and neck cancer Colon cancer Pancreatic cancer Glioblastoma
HER2/*neu* (ErbB2)	Breast cancer Ovarian cancer Head and neck cancer
PDGFR	Hypereosinophilic syndrome Mast cell disease Dermatofibrosarcoma protuberans Gastrointestinal stromal tumor (GIST)
FGFR3	Multiple myeloma Bladder cancer
C-KIT	Gastrointestinal stromal tumor (GIST) Systemic mastocytosis
FLT3	Acute myelogenous leukemia
RET	Multiple endocrine neoplasia type 2 Familial medullary thyroid carcinoma
MET	Hepatocellular carcinoma Melanoma Glioblastoma Epithelial malignancies

The Kirsten *ras* gene was initially identified as a retroviral oncogene in rats and subsequently found to have several human homologues, including K-*ras*, H-*ras*, and N-*ras*. The protein (RAS) encoded by *ras* is targeted to the plasma membrane by the farnesyltransferase-mediated addition of a hydrophobic farnesyl group to its COOH-terminus; this targeting brings RAS into close proximity to activated receptor tyrosine kinases. Intracellular nonreceptor tyrosine kinases such as ABL and SRC, also originally identified as oncogene products, can activate signaling through RAS as well (Fig. 40-2A).

Upon activation by binding to GTP, RAS triggers a series of phosphorylation events mediated by the kinases RAF, MEK, and ERK (MAP kinase), the targets of which include transcription factors that promote activation of genes involved in proliferation. For example, activation of cyclin D transcription results in cyclin D expression and binding to its catalytic partners, cyclin-dependent kinases 4 and 6 (CDK4 and CDK6) (Fig. 40-3). These complexes initiate phosphorylation of the **retinoblastoma protein (pRB)**, thereby lifting pRB's repression of the transcription factor E2F. E2F mediates the expression of components of the DNA replication machinery and enzymes involved in nucleotide synthesis. Thus, phosphorylation of pRB by cyclin D–CDK4/6 and subsequent activation of other cyclin–CDK complexes (such as cyclin E–CDK2) result in the transition from G1 to S phase and progression through the cell cycle. While such signaling cascades might seem unnecessarily complicated, they allow for the integration of diverse extracellular and intracellular signals, the opportunity for multiple points of feedback control, and the tight regulation of critical events such as cellular proliferation.

A second key intracellular signaling pathway is controlled by the lipid kinase **PI3K**. Stimulation of receptors for growth factors such as insulin or insulin-like growth factors (IGFs) commonly leads to activation of PI3K via an associated insulin receptor substrate protein (IRS). ErbB family members can also activate this pathway via phospholipase C-γ (PLC-γ), and RAS can also promote signaling through this pathway (Fig. 40-2B). Activation of PI3K results in generation of phosphatidylinositol-3,4,5-trisphosphate (PIP3) from plasma membrane phospholipids, activation of phosphoinositide dependent kinase-1 (PDK-1) via translocation to the cell membrane, and phosphorylation of AKT by PDK-1. This pathway is negatively regulated by the lipid phosphatase PTEN, which degrades PIP3. Downstream effects of AKT activation include promotion of translation and cell growth by the mammalian target of rapamycin (mTOR). In addition, phosphorylation of the forkhead family of transcription factors (FOXO) by AKT results in their exclusion from the nucleus, preventing expression of genes involved in cell cycle arrest, stress resistance, and apoptosis. Thus, a net effect of activating the PI3K-AKT pathway is the promotion of cell survival. Activating mutations in the catalytic subunit of PI3K (PI3KCA) and inactivating mutations in PTEN are frequently observed in a variety of malignancies, including breast cancer, colon cancer, prostate cancer, and glioblastoma.

In addition to activating the MAP kinase and PI3K pathways, RAS also activates the **RAL** signaling pathway (Fig. 40-2B). RAL signaling remains incompletely understood, but this pathway activates specific kinases involved in innate immunity and vesicle trafficking. RAL signaling is also essential for RAS-mediated tumorigenesis.

Signaling via type I cytokine receptors is associated with activation of the **JAK-STAT** pathway (Fig. 40-2C). Receptor dimerization activates JAKs, or Janus kinases, via transphosphorylation, allowing the recruitment of STAT proteins through their SH2 domains. **STATs** are a family of proteins that shuttle from the cytoplasm to the nucleus to regulate transcription directly. Phosphorylation of STAT proteins by JAKs leads to the formation of SH2 domain-mediated STAT homo- or heterodimers that translocate to the nucleus and regulate transcription. Growth factor receptors such as EGFR, as well as intracellular tyrosine kinases such as SRC, can also signal through activation of STATs.

Proteasome Structure and Function

Key cellular processes such as cell cycle progression and apoptosis are also regulated at the post-translational level by protein degradation. One of the major systems involved in this control is the **ubiquitin–proteasome pathway**, which comprises three enzymes that target specific proteins for ubiquitin conjugation and degradation by the proteasome (Fig. 40-4A). **Ubiquitin** is a 9-kDa protein that derives its name from its widespread distribution in tissues and its conservation across eukaryotes. The first enzyme involved in the process, E1, uses ATP to activate ubiquitin. The second enzyme in the cascade, E2, is a ubiquitin-conjugating enzyme that transiently carries ubiquitin and acts in conjunction with the third enzyme, the ubiquitin ligase E3, to form a polyubiquitin chain that is transferred to the target protein on an internal lysine residue.

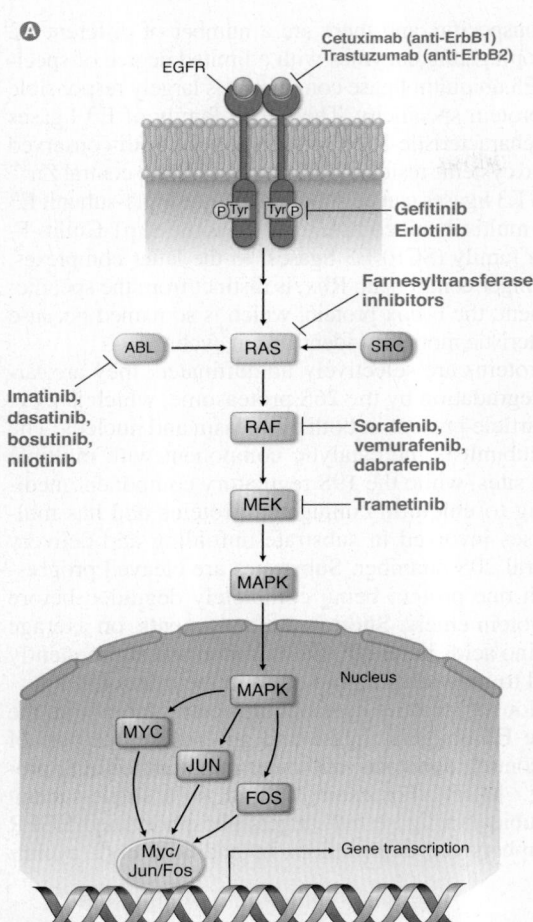

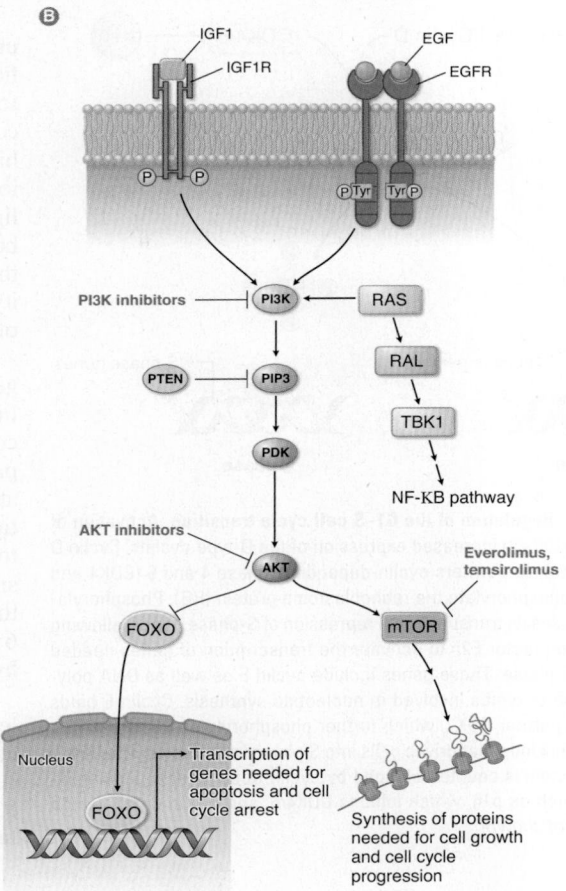

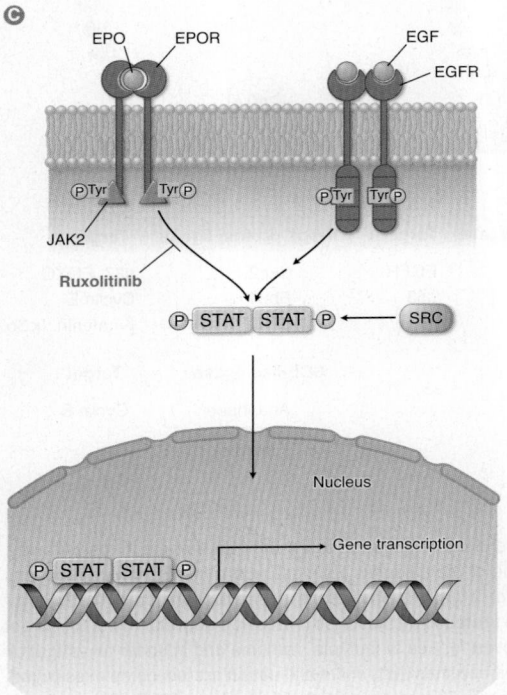

FIGURE 40-2. Intracellular signaling pathways. A. The RAS-MAP kinase pathway is activated by multiple growth factor receptors (here exemplified by the EGF receptor, EGFR) as well as several intracellular tyrosine kinases such as SRC and ABL. RAS is recruited to the plasma membrane by farnesylation and activated by binding to GTP. Activated RAS stimulates a sequence of phosphorylation events mediated by RAF, MEK, and ERK (MAP) kinases. Activated MAP kinase (MAPK) translocates to the nucleus and activates proteins such as MYC, JUN, and FOS that promote the transcription of genes involved in cell cycle progression. Cetuximab and trastuzumab act as antagonists at the EGF receptor (ErbB1) and HER2 receptor (ErbB2), respectively. Gefitinib and erlotinib inhibit the receptor tyrosine kinase. Farnesyltransferase inhibitors prevent RAS activation. Imatinib, dasatinib, bosutinib, and nilotinib inhibit ABL kinase; sorafenib, vemurafenib, and dabrafenib inhibit RAF kinase; and trametinib inhibits MEK kinase. **B.** The PI3 kinase (PI3K) pathway is activated by a number of growth factor receptors (here exemplified by the insulin-like growth factor receptor 1 [IGF1R] and the epidermal growth factor receptor [EGFR]). Activated PI3K generates phosphatidylinositol-3,4,5-trisphosphate (PIP3), which activates phosphoinositide dependent kinase-1 (PDK). In turn, PDK phosphorylates AKT. PTEN is an endogenous inhibitor of AKT activation. Phosphorylated AKT transduces multiple downstream signals, including activation of the mammalian target of rapamycin (mTOR) and inhibition of the FOXO family of transcription factors. mTOR activation promotes the synthesis of proteins required for cell growth and cell cycle progression. Because the FOXO family of transcription factors activates the expression of genes involved in cell cycle arrest, stress resistance, and apoptosis, inhibition of FOXO promotes cell proliferation and resistance to apoptosis. RAS activates not only the MAP kinase pathway diagrammed in panel **A** but also the PI3K pathway diagrammed in panel **B** and the NF-κB pathway diagrammed in Figure 40-5B. Activation of the NF-κB pathway by RAS involves direct activation of RAL, which activates the serine/threonine kinase TBK1. Everolimus and temsirolimus inhibit mTOR, and inhibitors of PI3K and AKT are in development. **C.** The STAT pathway is activated by SRC and by a number of growth factor receptors (here exemplified by the erythropoietin receptor [EPOR], which signals to STAT proteins through JAK2 kinase, and by the EGF receptor [EGFR], which signals to STAT proteins indirectly). Phosphorylation of STAT induces SH2 domain-mediated homodimerization, and phosphorylated STAT homodimers translocate to the nucleus and activate transcription. Ruxolitinib inhibits JAK2; this agent is used to treat myelofibrosis. Ruxolitinib and other JAK2 inhibitors are under evaluation for the treatment of polycythemia vera and essential thrombocythemia, which often share a common activating mutation in JAK2 (V617F).

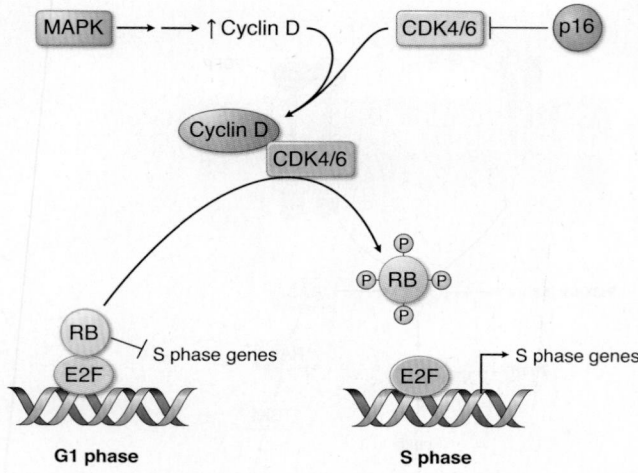

FIGURE 40-3. Regulation of the G1–S cell cycle transition. Activation of MAP kinase results in increased expression of the D-type cyclins. Cyclin D binds to its catalytic partners cyclin-dependent kinase 4 and 6 (CDK4 and CDK6), which phosphorylate the retinoblastoma protein (RB). Phosphorylation of RB releases its transcriptional repression of S-phase genes, allowing the transcription factor E2F to activate the transcription of genes needed for entry into S phase. These genes include cyclin E as well as DNA polymerase and the enzymes involved in nucleotide synthesis. Cyclin E binds to its catalytic partner CDK2, which further phosphorylates RB, creating a positive feedback loop that drives cells into S phase (*not shown*). The CDK2/CDK4/CDK6 system is counterbalanced by cyclin-dependent kinase inhibitors (CDKIs) such as p16, which inhibits CDK4/6, and p21 and p27, which inhibit CDK2 (*not shown*).

E1 is nonspecific, and there are a number of different E2 ubiquitin-conjugating enzymes with a limited degree of specificity. The E3 ubiquitin ligase component is largely responsible for target protein specificity. The RING family of E3 ligases contains a characteristic RING finger domain with conserved histidine and cysteine residues complexed with two central Zn^{2+} ions. RING E3 ligases can be subdivided into single-subunit E3 ligases and multisubunit complexes such as the Skp1-Cullin-F-box protein family (SCF) E3 ligases. In the latter complexes, the RING finger component, Rbx, is distinct from the specificity component, the F-box protein, which is so named because of a characteristic motif first identified in cyclin F.

Once proteins are selectively ubiquitinated, they are targeted for degradation by the 26S proteasome, which is a cylindrical particle present in both cytoplasm and nucleus. The core 20S subunit is the catalytic component with multiple proteolytic sites, while the 19S regulatory component mediates binding to ubiquitin-conjugated proteins and has multiple ATPases involved in substrate unfolding and delivery to the central 20S chamber. Substrates are cleaved progressively, with one protein being completely degraded before the next protein enters. Short peptide segments, on average 6 to 10 amino acids in length, are extruded and subsequently hydrolyzed to individual amino acids in the cytosol.

Regulation of protein degradation occurs largely at the level of the E3 ubiquitin ligase and governs key aspects of cell cycle control, apoptosis, and other important cellular processes (Fig. 40-4B). For example, CBL is a single-subunit RING E3 ubiquitin ligase that targets phosphorylated EGFR family members for degradation. In addition, both cyclins

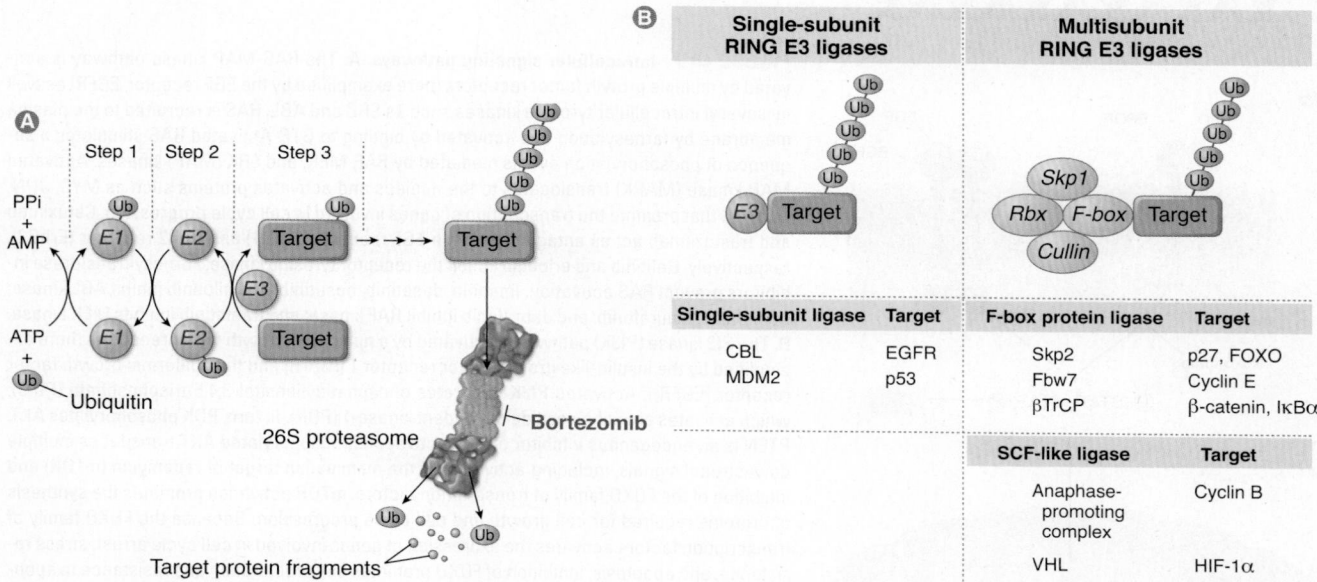

FIGURE 40-4. The ubiquitin–proteasome pathway. A. Ubiquitin (Ub) is activated by ATP-dependent conjugation to E1, the first enzyme in the pathway. Activated ubiquitin is then passed from the active-site cysteine of E1 to the active-site cysteine of the ubiquitin-conjugating enzyme E2, which functions coordinately with the ubiquitin ligase E3 to attach ubiquitin to protein targets. Polyubiquitination of target proteins results in their recognition by the 26S proteasome, which consists of a 19S outer regulatory subunit and a 20S internal core chamber. The proteasome mediates proteolytic degradation of the target protein into short peptide fragments. Bortezomib is a proteasome inhibitor that has been approved for use in multiple myeloma and is under investigation for use in other malignancies. **B.** The RING family of E3 ubiquitin ligases consists of single-subunit enzymes **(left)** and multisubunit protein complexes **(right)**. Single-subunit ligases include CBL, which targets EGFR for degradation, and MDM2, which targets p53 for degradation. Multisubunit RING E3 ligase complexes include SCF and SCF-like family members, which are named for their Skp1, Cullin, and F-box protein subunits. The F-box protein component mediates target protein specificity; for example, Skp2 targets p27 and FOXO for degradation, Fbw7 targets cyclin E for degradation, and βTrCP targets β-catenin and IκBα for degradation. SCF-like ligase complexes include the anaphase-promoting complex, which targets cyclin B for degradation, and VHL, which targets hypoxia-inducible factor-1α (HIF-1α) for degradation.

and cyclin-dependent kinase inhibitors are major targets for ubiquitin-mediated proteasomal degradation. The anaphase-promoting complex is a multisubunit RING-containing E3 ligase that is activated by phosphorylation late in mitosis, triggering degradation of cyclin B and progression through mitosis. Regulation of the G1–S cell cycle transition is in part mediated by the cyclin-dependent kinase inhibitor p27, which inhibits cyclin E–CDK2 and cyclin A–CDK2 complexes. Degradation of p27 is regulated by another SCF E3 ligase, which binds p27 via its F-box specificity component Skp2. Thus, overexpression of Skp2, which is found in a number of tumor types, can promote cell cycle progression by degrading p27. Degradation of FOXO by Skp2 is a second mechanism by which overexpression of Skp2 may promote tumorigenesis. Yet another SCF E3 ligase complex regulates cyclin E activity by targeting it for degradation via the F-box protein Fbw7. Loss of Fbw7 has been implicated in tumor progression due to high levels of cyclin E.

Another example of an E3 ligase with a critical role in the regulation of apoptosis and cell cycle regulation is MDM2, a single-subunit RING E3 ligase that targets p53 for degradation. Activation of MDM2 is linked to impairment of apoptosis and promotion of tumorigenesis via loss of p53. MDM2 is inhibited by the p14ARF protein, which shares the same genomic locus as the CDK4/6 inhibitor p16. Disruption of this locus, which is one of the most common events in cancer, leads ultimately to both p53 and pRB inactivation.

Other key cellular pathways regulated by ubiquitin-mediated proteasomal degradation include the Wnt signaling pathway and the nuclear factor-kappa B (NFκB) pathway. Both pathways are targeted by the common F-box protein βTrCP, which recognizes phosphorylated substrates (Fig. 40-5). Activation of Wnt signaling prevents phosphorylation of β-catenin, which allows it to escape recognition by βTrCP and ubiquitin ligation by SCF E3 ligase. Unphosphorylated β-catenin then translocates to the nucleus with its partners TCF/LEF and activates transcription of genes such as myc and cyclin D1. This pathway is also regulated by the *adenomatous polyposis coli* (APC) gene, which forms

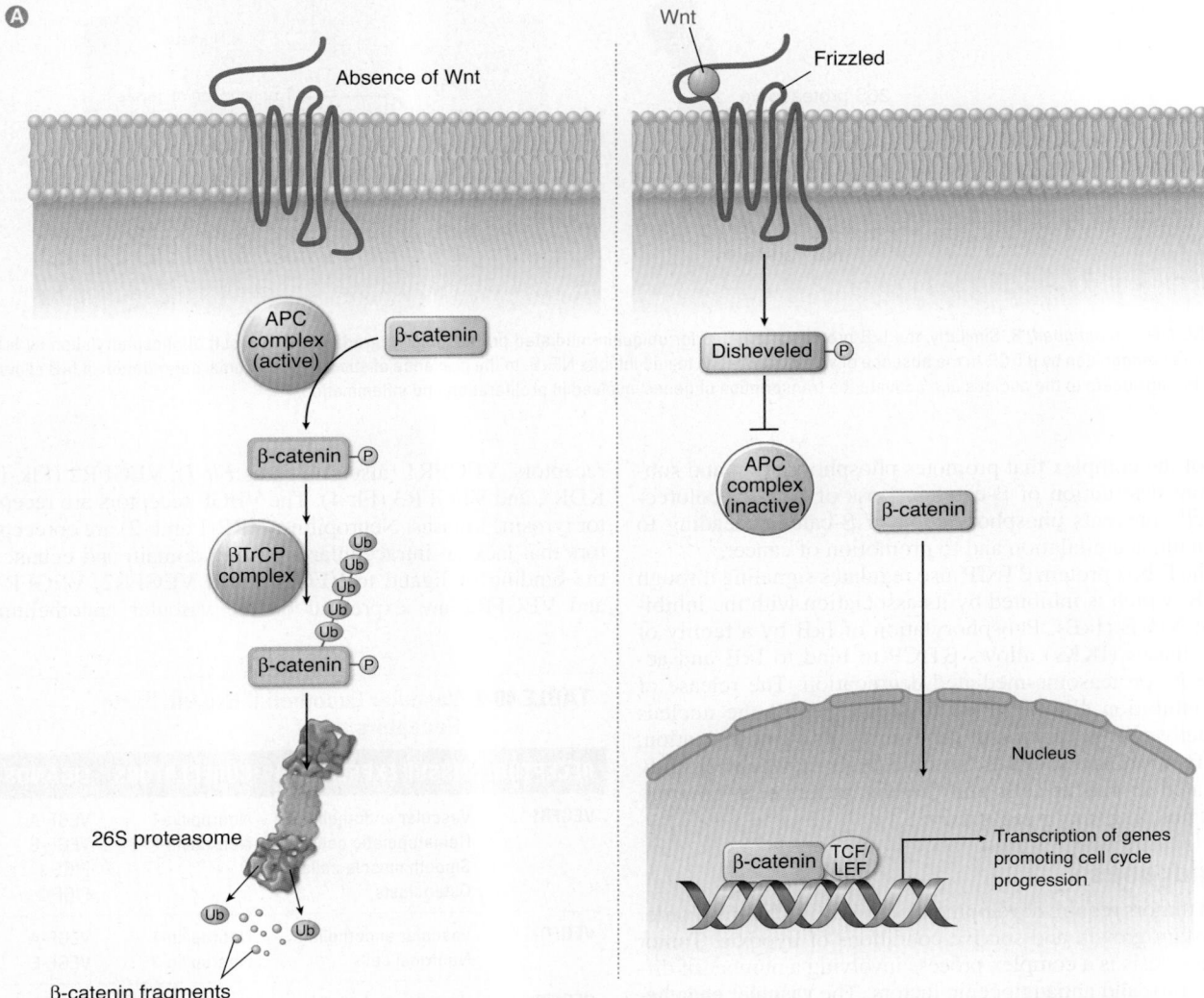

FIGURE 40-5. Wnt signaling and NFκB pathways. A. In the absence of Wnt signaling, β-catenin is phosphorylated by the adenomatous polyposis coli (APC) protein complex. Phosphorylated β-catenin is recognized by βTrCP and thereby targeted for ubiquitin-mediated proteasomal degradation. Activation of Wnt signaling inhibits APC function, allowing β-catenin to accumulate and translocate to the nucleus. In the nucleus, β-catenin complexes with its partners TCF/LEF and activates the transcription of genes promoting cell cycle progression. Hereditary or acquired loss of APC allows accumulation of β-catenin, contributing to oncogenesis in colon cancer. *(continued)*

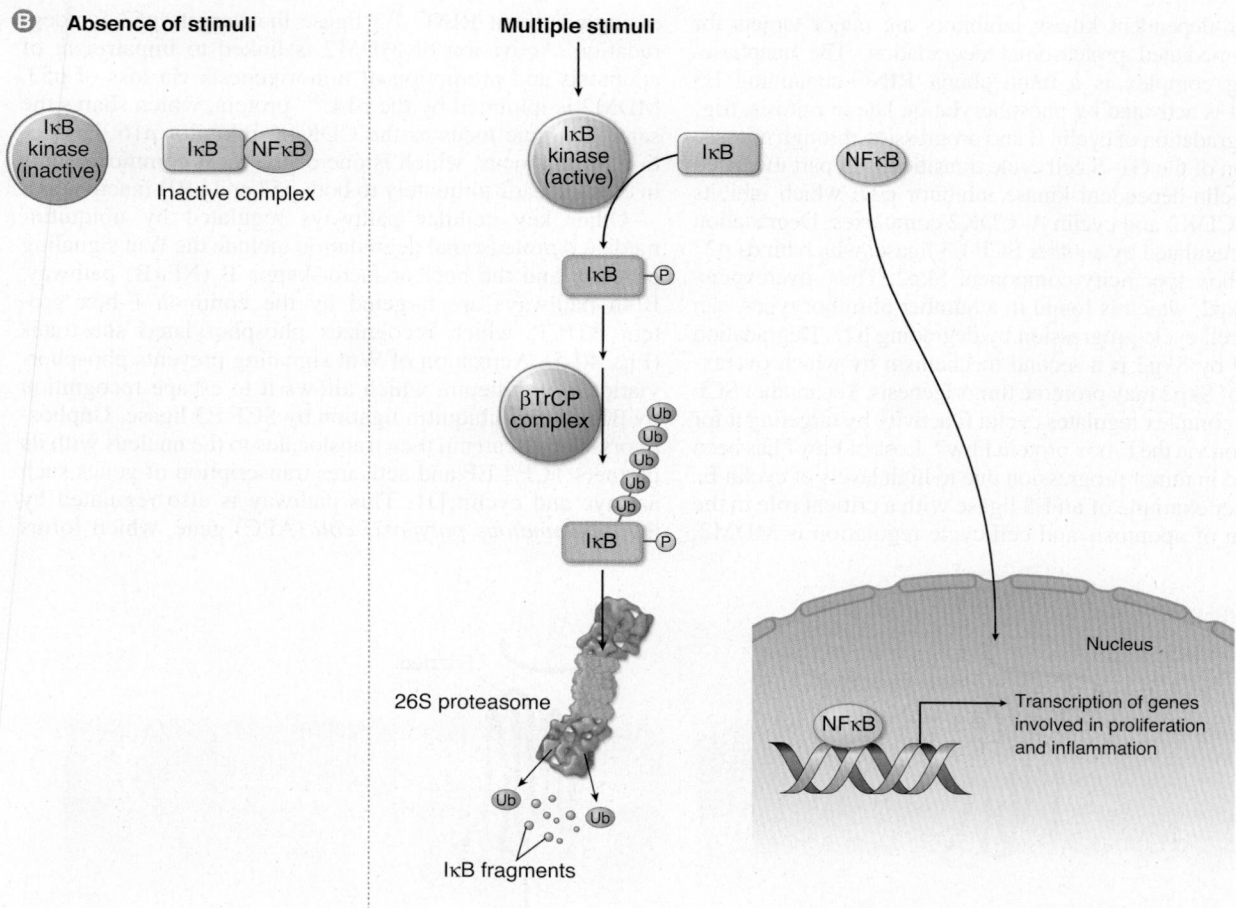

B **Absence of stimuli**   **Multiple stimuli**

IκB kinase (inactive)   IκB   NFκB
                             Inactive complex

IκB kinase (active)   IκB   NFκB

IκB —(P)

βTrCP complex   Ub Ub Ub Ub Ub

IκB —(P)

26S proteasome

Ub   Ub

IκB fragments

Nucleus

NFκB → Transcription of genes involved in proliferation and inflammation

FIGURE 40-5. *(continued)* **B.** Similarly, the IκB protein is targeted for ubiquitin-mediated proteasomal degradation as a result of phosphorylation by IκB kinase and recognition by βTrCP. In the absence of stimuli, IκB binds to and inhibits NFκB. In the presence of stimuli, proteasomal degradation of IκB allows NFκB to translocate to the nucleus and activate the transcription of genes involved in proliferation and inflammation.

part of the complex that promotes phosphorylation and subsequent destruction of β-catenin. Loss of APC in colorectal cells prevents phosphorylation of β-catenin, leading to β-catenin accumulation and to promotion of cancer.

The F-box protein βTrCP also regulates signaling through NFκB, which is inhibited by its association with the inhibitor of NFκB (IκB). Phosphorylation of IκB by a family of IκB kinases (IKKs) allows βTrCP to bind to IκB and activate its proteasome-mediated degradation. The release of IκB inhibition allows NFκB to translocate to the nucleus and activate transcription of genes involved in inflammation, proliferation, and survival. Specific IKKs may be aberrantly activated in cancer cells and thereby generate an environment favoring tumor cell survival.

Angiogenesis

Solid tumors require development of a neovasculature in order to sustain growth and survive conditions of hypoxia. Tumor angiogenesis is a complex process involving a number of different pro- and antiangiogenic factors. The **vascular endothelial growth factor (VEGF)** family of proteins and receptors has emerged as a key regulator of this process. The VEGF family consists of seven ligands, including VEGF-A, -B, -C, -D, and -E and placenta growth factor (PlGF)-1 and -2 (Table 40-2). These ligands have varying affinities for the major VEGF

receptors, VEGFR1 (also known as *Flt-1*), VEGFR2 (Flk-1/KDR), and VEGFR3 (Flt-4). The VEGF receptors are receptor tyrosine kinases. Neuropilins (NRP-1 and -2) are coreceptors that lack an intracellular signaling domain and enhance the binding of ligand to VEGFR1 and VEGFR2. VEGFR1 and VEGFR2 are expressed on the vascular endothelium

TABLE 40-2 Vascular Endothelial Growth Factor Receptors

RECEPTOR	TISSUE EXPRESSION	CORECEPTORS	LIGANDS
VEGFR1	Vascular endothelium Hematopoietic cells Smooth muscle cells Osteoclasts	Neuropilin-1 Neuropilin-2	VEGF-A VEGF-B PlGF-1 PlGF-2
VEGFR2	Vascular endothelium Neuronal cells	Neuropilin-1 Neuropilin-2	VEGF-A VEGF-E
VEGFR3	Vascular endothelium Lymphatic endothelium Monocytes and macrophages	None	VEGF-C VEGF-D

VEGFR, vascular endothelial growth factor receptor; PlGF, placenta growth factor.

and play key roles in angiogenic signaling, while signaling through VEGFR3 appears to play a major role in lymphangiogenesis (i.e., development of new lymphatic vessels). VEGFR2, which appears to be the major proangiogenic receptor targeted by VEGF-A, signals via both a RAF/MAP kinase pathway to promote proliferation of endothelial cells and a PI3K/AKT pathway to promote endothelial cell survival. VEGF also potently induces vascular permeability, utilizing similar signaling pathways both to promote the formation of transendothelial vesicular organelles and to open interendothelial junctions. Invasion and migration of endothelial cells is promoted by activation of matrix metalloproteinases and serine proteases and by reorganization of intracellular actin.

Activation of VEGF is mediated by stimuli such as hypoxia, by cytokines and growth factors, and by a variety of oncogenes and tumor suppressor genes. Regulation of the response to hypoxia is mediated by **von Hippel-Lindau** protein (**VHL**), a component of an SCF-like RING E3 ubiquitin ligase complex that targets **hypoxia-inducible factor-1α (HIF-1α)** for degradation (Fig. 40-6). Loss of VHL is the defining event in the inherited VHL syndrome and is a frequent finding in sporadic clear cell renal carcinoma.

Under normoxic conditions, HIF-1α undergoes oxygen-dependent hydroxylation, which allows VHL binding and subsequent ubiquitin-mediated degradation. Under hypoxic conditions, HIF-1α is not hydroxylated and VHL is unable to bind it. Native HIF-1α is thus allowed to translocate to the nucleus and pair with its binding partner HIF-1β to activate transcription of hypoxia-inducible genes such as VEGF, PDGF-β, and TGF-α. In this manner, angiogenesis is stimulated by hypoxic conditions or by inappropriate activation of HIF-1 due to loss of VHL expression in tumors.

Cytokines such as IL-1 and IL-6, as well as prostaglandin products of COX-2 activation, can also stimulate VEGF production. Signaling via EGFR family members, PDGFR, and the insulin-like growth factor-1 receptor (IGF-1R) have also been shown to induce VEGF expression. Finally, activation of oncogenes such as RAS, SRC, and BCR-Abl and inactivation of tumor suppressor genes such as p53 and PTEN can result in VEGF production and thus promote angiogenesis and tumor maintenance.

PHARMACOLOGIC CLASSES AND AGENTS

Growth Factor Receptor and Signal Transduction Antagonists

The identification of specific pathways that are dysregulated in certain tumors affords the potential to target key components of these pathways in a more selective manner.

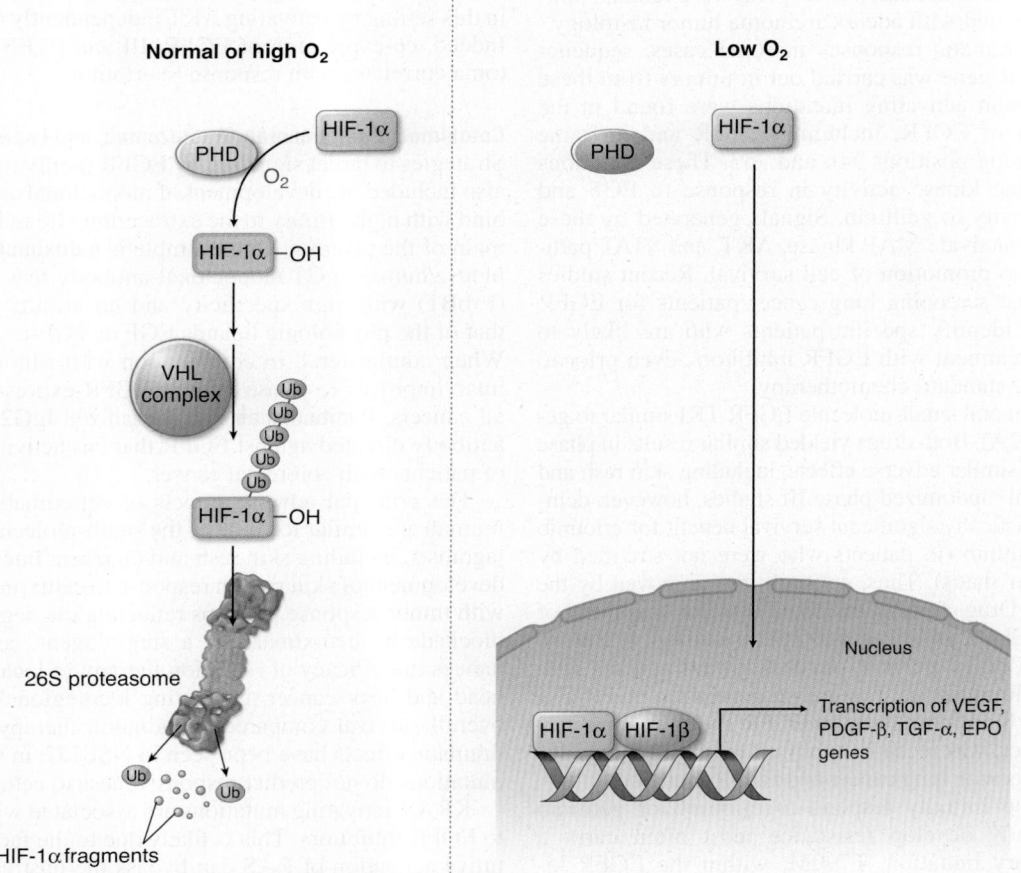

FIGURE 40-6. Regulation of the response to hypoxia. Left panel: Under normal or high oxygen conditions, hypoxia-inducible factor-1α (HIF-1α) is hydroxylated (in an oxygen-dependent reaction) by the prolyl hydroxylase PHD. Hydroxylated HIF-1α is recognized by VHL and thereby targeted for ubiquitin-mediated proteasomal degradation. **Right panel:** PHD is inactive under low oxygen conditions, allowing HIF-1α to accumulate and translocate to the nucleus. In the nucleus, HIF-1α complexes with HIF-1β and activates the transcription of hypoxia-inducible genes such as VEGF, PDGF-β, TGF-α, and erythropoietin (EPO).

While the growth factor and signal transduction pathways described above are active during normal cell physiology, some tumors may become dependent on one pathway in particular for their growth and survival. Conversely, in normal cells, the redundancy of signaling pathways allows for compensation, as exemplified by the observation that inactivation of the EGFR gene in the mouse causes minimal defects. Thus, the therapeutic window of the newer targeted agents tends to be wider than that of traditional cytotoxic chemotherapy, with a different spectrum of adverse effects.

EGF Receptor Antagonists
Gefitinib, Erlotinib, and Afatinib

The expression of EGFR on epithelial cells and its amplification and/or activation in a significant fraction of non-small cell lung cancers (NSCLCs) led to the development and testing of small-molecule EGFR tyrosine kinase inhibitors (TKIs) in patients with advanced NSCLC. The first of these agents to be tested was **gefitinib**. Gefitinib is an orally bioavailable drug that competes with ATP for binding to the cytoplasmic tyrosine kinase domain of EGFR and thereby acts as a reversible inhibitor of EGFR tyrosine kinase activity (Fig. 40-2A). In patients with metastatic NSCLC who had received multiple prior chemotherapy regimens, response rates to gefitinib were on the order of 10% in studies conducted in the United States and 20% in trials conducted in Japan and Europe. During the course of these studies, it was noted that patients who tended to respond were female, nonsmokers, Asian, and with adenocarcinoma tumor histology.

Given the dramatic responses in some cases, sequencing of the EGFR gene was carried out in tumors from these patients. Common activating mutations were found in the kinase domain of EGFR, including L858R and in-frame deletions spanning positions 746 and 753. These mutations enhance tyrosine kinase activity in response to EGF and increase sensitivity to gefitinib. Signals generated by these mutant EGFRs activate MAP kinase, AKT, and STAT pathways, leading to promotion of cell survival. Recent studies have shown that screening lung cancer patients for EGFR mutations can identify specific patients who are likely to benefit from treatment with EGFR inhibitors, even prior to the initiation of standard chemotherapy.

Erlotinib is an oral small-molecule EGFR TKI similar to gefitinib (Fig. 40-2A). Both drugs yielded similar results in phase II studies, with similar adverse effects, including skin rash and diarrhea. Pivotal randomized phase III studies, however, demonstrated a statistically significant survival benefit for erlotinib but not for gefitinib (in patients who were not stratified by EGFR mutation status). Thus, erlotinib was approved by the US Food and Drug Administration (FDA) for treatment of metastatic NSCLC, while gefitinib is still utilized in Europe and Asia; both drugs are now directed toward patients with activating EGFR mutations. The second-generation EGFR TKI **afatinib**, which binds covalently to EGFR and is thus an irreversible inhibitor, was recently approved by the FDA specifically for patients with lung cancer and EGFR mutations.

Patients who initially respond to erlotinib or gefitinib but subsequently develop resistance most often carry a single secondary mutation, T790M, within the EGFR kinase domain. EGF receptors carrying both activating mutations and the T790M secondary mutation exhibit reduced sensitivity to inhibition by erlotinib and gefitinib. Despite their covalent cross-linking to EGFR, second-generation irreversible inhibitors such as afatinib have failed to overcome resistance generated by the T790M mutation, in part due to toxicity associated with inhibition of the wild-type kinase. Novel third-generation EGFR TKIs that are also irreversible yet bind selectively to the T790M mutant protein are entering the clinic and showing promising activity for the large group of patients who develop acquired resistance to erlotinib or gefitinib. Amplification of MET is another mechanism of acquired resistance to EGFR inhibition. MET is a receptor tyrosine kinase that is normally under the control of the ligand hepatocyte growth factor (HGF). MET amplification allows cancer cells to re-activate downstream survival pathways that are blocked by EGFR inhibition. **MET inhibitors** are currently in clinical development; these agents could potentially be used in combination with EGFR antagonists to combat acquired drug resistance.

Erlotinib has shown less impressive activity in a wide variety of other epithelial malignancies in which EGFR is overexpressed, including colon cancer, pancreatic cancer, and head and neck cancer. EGFR is frequently amplified, mutated, or overexpressed in patients with glioblastoma, but response rates of only 10–20% are seen with EGFR antagonists, similar to the response rates in patients with advanced NSCLC. A constitutively active EGFR genomic deletion variant, EGFRvIII, has been identified in a significant fraction of patients with glioblastoma. Because this mutant receptor relies on PI3K/AKT signaling, it was hypothesized that loss of PTEN might impair response to EGFR inhibitors in this setting by activating AKT independently (Fig. 40-2B). Indeed, co-expression of EGFRvIII and PTEN in glioblastoma correlates with response to erlotinib.

Cetuximab, Panitumumab, Trastuzumab, and Lapatinib

Strategies to target signaling by EGFR family members have also included the development of monoclonal antibodies that bind with high affinity to the extracellular ligand-binding domain of the receptor. One example is **cetuximab**, a chimeric mouse/human IgG1 monoclonal antibody that binds EGFR (ErbB1) with high specificity and an affinity greater than that of the physiologic ligands EGF or TGF-α (Fig. 40-2A). When administered in combination with irinotecan, cetuximab improves response rates in EGFR-expressing colorectal cancers. **Panitumumab** is a humanized IgG2 monoclonal antibody directed against EGFR that has activity in a subset of patients with colorectal cancer.

The principal adverse effects of cetuximab and panitumumab are similar to those of the small-molecule EGFR antagonists, including skin rash and diarrhea. Interestingly, the development of skin rash in response to cetuximab correlates with tumor response, perhaps reflecting the degree of EGFR blockade by cetuximab. As a single agent, cetuximab enhances the efficacy of radiation therapy in locally advanced head and neck cancer, improving locoregional control and overall survival compared to radiation therapy alone. Less dramatic effects have been seen in NSCLC, in which EGFR mutations do not predict responsiveness to cetuximab.

KRAS activating mutations are associated with resistance to EGFR inhibitors. This is likely due to the fact that constitutive activation of RAS can bypass the upstream blockade in EGFR signaling (Fig. 40-2A). To help predict responsiveness to EGFR inhibitor therapy, routine testing of KRAS mutational status is now performed in tumors such as lung cancer and colon cancer.

Trastuzumab, another chimeric mouse/human IgG monoclonal antibody, is directed against ErbB2 (HER2) (Fig. 40-2A). Approximately 25–30% of breast cancers are associated with amplification and overexpression of *HER2/neu*; these cancers also display more aggressive behavior. HER2 amplifies the signal generated by other ErbB family members via the formation of heterodimers. Trastuzumab down-regulates HER2 and thereby disrupts this signaling. In vivo, trastuzumab also appears to induce antibody-dependent cellular cytotoxicity and inhibit angiogenesis.

Trastuzumab has significant activity in breast cancers with high levels of HER2 amplification. In addition to the intrinsic activity of trastuzumab in the advanced and metastatic breast cancer settings, treatment of HER2-amplified breast cancers with trastuzumab in the adjuvant setting (i.e., after surgical resection of the tumor) enhances the efficacy of chemotherapy and reduces rates of cancer recurrence by 50%. The principal adverse effect of trastuzumab is cardiotoxicity, particularly when used in combination with anthracyclines. Trastuzumab does not cross the blood–brain barrier, and thus CNS relapse of breast cancer may occur.

Lapatinib, a small-molecule dual EGFR/HER2 inhibitor, has also been approved for the treatment of metastatic breast cancer with HER2 overexpression. Lapatinib crosses the blood–brain barrier and shows activity against brain metastases. **Trastuzumab emtansine (T-DM1)** is an antibody–drug conjugate that links trastuzumab to the cytotoxic agent mertansine and specifically delivers this toxin to HER2-expressing cells. T-DM1 has shown significant activity in trastuzumab-refractory breast cancer.

ALK/ROS1 Inhibitors
Crizotinib and Ceritinib
The success of erlotinib in treating EGFR-mutant lung cancers encouraged investigators to study mutations in other growth factor receptors in patients with cancer. It was discovered that a subset of smokers with adenocarcinoma harbor rearrangements in the ALK receptor tyrosine kinase. Based on this finding, **crizotinib**, initially identified as a MET and ALK TKI, was repurposed for this population of lung cancer patients and found to exhibit remarkable activity, leading to its approval by the FDA. As with EGFR TKIs, however, treatment with crizotinib leads to acquired resistance through a variety of mechanisms.

Recently, the second-generation ALK TKI **ceritinib** was approved by the FDA based on its ability to overcome crizotinib resistance, and additional inhibitors and drug combination strategies are being developed. Lung adenocarcinomas in light smokers continue to be subdivided further into oncogene-dependent genotypes, such as those characterized by ROS1 and RET rearrangements. Crizotinib also inhibits ROS1 and has activity in the subgroup of lung cancers with ROS1 rearrangements. Several multitargeted kinase inhibitors such as **sunitinib** and **cabozantinib** are being evaluated for RET-rearranged lung cancers.

BCR-Abl/C-KIT/PDGFR Inhibition
Imatinib
Imatinib is a small-molecule tyrosine kinase inhibitor that was initially developed as a 2-phenylaminopyrimidine derivative specific for PDGFR. Imatinib was subsequently found to be a potent inhibitor of ABL kinases, including the BCR-Abl fusion protein generated as a result of the t(9;22)

chromosomal translocation (Philadelphia chromosome) found in **chronic myelogenous leukemia** (**CML**) (Fig. 40-2A). Imatinib was also found to inhibit the receptor tyrosine kinase C-KIT. *Imatinib is the canonical example of a targeted therapeutic agent, because BCR-Abl is uniquely expressed by leukemic cells and is essential for their survival.*

Initial in vitro studies demonstrated that imatinib potently and specifically inhibits the growth of cells expressing BCR-Abl. Subsequent evaluation of an oral formulation in mice demonstrated suppression of growth of human BCR-Abl-positive tumors with minimal adverse effects. Early studies of imatinib in patients with chronic-phase CML yielded impressive results, with normalization of blood counts (a hematologic response) in 95% of patients and significant reduction in cells expressing the Philadelphia chromosome (a cytogenetic response) in 41% of patients. In a phase III study, imatinib was superior to standard treatment with interferon and cytarabine in patients with chronic-phase CML, with a hematologic response rate of 95% and a complete cytogenetic response in 76% of patients. Treatment of accelerated or blast-phase CML with imatinib is less effective but is associated with some responses. Imatinib is relatively well tolerated; its principal adverse effects are myelosuppression, superficial edema, nausea, muscle cramps, skin rash, and diarrhea.

Mutation of C-KIT, the receptor for stem cell factor (SCF), is found frequently in **gastrointestinal stromal tumor** (**GIST**) and in the myeloproliferative disorder **systemic mastocytosis**. In GIST, mutations and in-frame deletions of C-KIT are typically found in the juxtamembrane domain, resulting in constitutive activation of the tyrosine kinase in the absence of ligand. In contrast, in systemic mastocytosis, the characteristic C-KIT-activating mutation D816V is within the tyrosine kinase domain itself. Imatinib has shown significant activity in advanced gastrointestinal stromal tumor, but it has proven largely ineffective in the treatment of systemic mastocytosis. Indeed, biochemical studies show that the drug is not effective at targeting C-KIT kinases with the D816V mutation.

Both **idiopathic hypereosinophilic syndrome** and a variant of systemic mastocytosis with eosinophilia are characterized by expression of the FIPL1-PDGFRA fusion protein. This protein, which is generated by an interstitial chromosomal deletion, causes constitutive signaling through PDGFRA. Inhibition of PDGFRA by imatinib has been a successful therapeutic approach in both conditions.

Dasatinib, Bosutinib, and Nilotinib
Most patients with CML experience durable remissions with imatinib treatment. However, a fraction of patients show evidence of the BCR-Abl transcript when sensitive tests such as reverse transcriptase polymerase chain reaction (RT-PCR) are used for detection, even in cases in which a complete cytogenetic response is observed. Moreover, some patients with CML develop acquired resistance to imatinib, occasionally due to amplification of BCR-Abl but more commonly due to acquisition of resistance mutations. Crystallographic studies show that imatinib targets the ATP-binding site of ABL when the activation loop of the kinase is closed, thereby stabilizing the protein in an inactive conformation (see Fig. 1-2). A minority of resistance mutations interfere directly with imatinib binding, while most resistance mutations affect the ability of ABL to adopt the closed conformation to which imatinib binds.

A second class of tyrosine kinase inhibitors, the SRC–ABL inhibitors, bind to the ATP-binding site in ABL irrespective of the conformational status of the activation loop. One of these drugs, **dasatinib**, is more potent than imatinib and has significantly greater efficacy than imatinib against wild-type BCR-Abl. Dasatinib also inhibits the activity of most clinically relevant imatinib-resistant BCR-Abl isoforms, with the exception of the T315I mutation (Fig. 40-2A). **Bosutinib** is another SRC–ABL inhibitor that inhibits most BCR-Abl resistance alleles, with the exception of T315I and V299L.

Investigators have used a structure-based approach to improve the efficacy of imatinib, substituting alternative binding groups for the N-methylpiperazine group. This approach has resulted in the development of **nilotinib**. The affinity of nilotinib for wild-type BCR-Abl is significantly higher than that of imatinib, and nilotinib inhibits most imatinib-resistant mutants with the exception of T315I (Fig. 40-2A). Dasatinib, bosutinib, and nilotinib have shown significant activity in patients with CML who have developed resistance to imatinib and are approved by the FDA for this setting. Another potent and broad-spectrum inhibitor, **ponatinib**, which inhibits VEGFR and FGFR family members in addition to ABL, SRC, and other kinases, has shown activity even in the resistant T315I population but is associated with increased vascular toxicity.

BTK Inhibitors

Ibrutinib is a covalent and relatively selective inhibitor of BTK, which is expressed in B cells and promotes B-cell receptor signaling and lymphocyte survival. Ibrutinib has shown remarkable activity in refractory B-cell malignancies such as mantle cell lymphoma and was also recently approved by the FDA for the treatment of chronic lymphocytic leukemia (CLL). Ibrutinib is currently under evaluation for the treatment of a variety of other B-cell malignancies, including diffuse large B-cell lymphoma and plasma cell dyscrasias such as multiple myeloma and Waldenstrom's macroglobulinemia.

FLT3 Inhibitors

One of the most common mutations in **acute myelogenous leukemia (AML)**, occurring in approximately 25–30% of patients, involves internal tandem duplication within the juxtamembrane domain of the FLT3 receptor tyrosine kinase. This mutation results in ligand-independent dimerization and activation of signaling via the RAS/MAPK and STAT pathways. Several FLT3 inhibitors have been developed and demonstrate anti-leukemia cell activity in vitro. **Sorafenib**, a multitargeted kinase inhibitor developed against RAF but also with activity against VEGFR (see below) and FLT3, has shown significant activity in patients with relapsed/refractory AML carrying FLT3 mutations.

JAK2 Inhibitors

Although BCR-Abl was discovered decades ago to be the pathophysiologically important lesion in CML, the genetic basis of the other major **myeloproliferative disorders** (polycythemia vera, essential thrombocythemia, and myeloid metaplasia with myelofibrosis) remained obscure. It is now apparent that a common activating mutation in JAK2 (V617F) underlies the aberrant signaling and proliferation in most cases, although how one mutation leads to this spectrum of disorders remains unclear (see Fig. 40-2C). The V617F mutation is located in the pseudokinase domain of JAK2, and disruption of this autoinhibitory region leads to unchecked activity of the kinase. In vitro, selective JAK2 inhibitors cause cells containing the JAK2 V617F mutation to be growth inhibited and undergo apoptosis; in animal models, JAK2 inhibitors demonstrate therapeutic efficacy against JAK2(V617F)-induced hematologic disease. **Ruxolitinib** is the first JAK2 inhibitor to be approved by the FDA, based on its activity in myelofibrosis. Ruxolitinib is also under evaluation for the treatment of polycythemia vera and essential thrombocythemia, as are several other JAK2 inhibitors, such as **momelotinib**, that have entered late-stage clinical trials. These and other JAK inhibitors are also being evaluated for use in the treatment of a variety of solid tumors that aberrantly activate cytokine signaling pathways.

RAS/MAP Kinase Pathway Inhibition

Oncogenic mutation of *ras* is one of the most common events in malignancy, occurring in approximately 30% of human cancers. K-*ras* mutations are frequently observed in non-small cell lung cancer, colorectal cancer, and pancreatic carcinoma, while H-*ras* mutations are found in kidney, bladder, and thyroid cancers, and N-*ras* mutations occur in melanoma, hepatocellular carcinoma, and hematologic malignancies. However, despite the frequency of these mutations, inhibition of RAS has thus far been difficult to achieve and has yielded minimal clinical success. Most efforts have focused on targeting farnesylation of RAS and inhibiting downstream effectors.

Farnesylation of RAS is essential for its association with the plasma membrane and its subsequent activation. Several farnesyltransferase inhibitors (FTIs) have been developed that inhibit RAS farnesylation (Fig. 40-2A). While these inhibitors demonstrate activity against RAS in vitro, some RAS mutants exhibit resistance. Moreover, there are many other targets of farnesylation that could be inhibited by FTIs, and such inhibition is likely responsible for the cytotoxic effects of these drugs. FTIs that have been tested clinically include **tipifarnib** and **lonafarnib**. Tipifarnib has demonstrated activity in relapsed/refractory AML, although responses appear to be independent of *ras* mutations. Clinical testing of FTIs in solid tumors has not yet met with success.

Immediately downstream of RAS is the serine/threonine kinase RAF, which phosphorylates MEK, which in turn phosphorylates MAP kinase, leading to transcription factor activation (Fig. 40-2A). There are three RAF family members—A-RAF, B-RAF, and C-RAF. Activating mutations in B-RAF have been found in a significant fraction of malignant melanomas and are also observed at a lower frequency in lung, colorectal, ovarian, and thyroid cancers. **Sorafenib** was initially designed as a C-RAF inhibitor, but it also inhibits B-RAF, among other kinases. Sorafenib has shown significant activity against melanoma cell lines that contain activating B-RAF mutations but has been less impressive clinically. **Vemurafenib** is a more potent and selective inhibitor of B-RAF that was designed to target the common B-RAF V600E mutation observed in melanoma. Vemurafenib treatment of patients with B-RAF(V600E)-mutant melanoma has been associated with significant responses and has led to approval of the drug by the FDA, although resistance invariably develops. **Dabrafenib** is another potent B-RAF inhibitor with activity in this population of melanoma patients.

There are two MEK homologues directly downstream of RAF: MEK1 and MEK2. Both of these homologues have dual serine/threonine kinase activity, phosphorylating and activating ERK1 and ERK2. **Trametinib** is a highly potent inhibitor of both MEK1 and MEK2 (Fig. 40-2A). Based on its activity in B-RAF-mutant melanoma, trametinib has been approved by the FDA for this indication. "Vertical inhibition" (or sequential inhibition) of the RAF-MEK-ERK pathway by combining dabrafenib and trametinib results in further response and delayed resistance in patients with B-RAF-mutant melanoma. These inhibitors are also being explored for use in the subset of lung cancers that harbor B-RAF mutations.

MEK inhibitors are also being explored as a downstream method of targeted therapy for KRAS-driven cancers. However, clinical-stage MEK inhibitors such as trametinib and **selumetinib** have shown limited single-agent activity in KRAS-mutated lung and pancreatic cancers, likely due to the fact that KRAS engages multiple other pathways in parallel. MEK inhibitors are currently being combined with traditional chemotherapy as one strategy to enhance activity. Another approach involves combining MEK inhibitors with targeted inhibitors against downstream signaling components of the RAS/PI3K/AKT/mTOR or RAS/RAL/cytokine pathways. Clinical trials evaluating these combination therapy strategies for KRAS-driven lung and gastrointestinal cancers are underway.

PI3K/AKT/mTOR Inhibitors

Signaling via the PI3K/AKT pathway leads to downstream activation of the mammalian target of rapamycin (mTOR) (Fig. 40-2B). mTOR is a serine/threonine kinase that regulates multiple cellular functions, including cell growth and proliferation, via activation of protein synthesis. mTOR regulation is accomplished in part by activation of the 40S ribosomal protein S6 kinase (p70^{S6k}) and inactivation of the 4E-binding protein (4E-BP1), which regulates translation of certain mRNAs. Dysregulated mTOR activity is seen in a wide variety of malignancies in which the PI3K pathway is activated or PTEN is lost. In addition, hamartoma syndromes such as tuberous sclerosis result in activation of mTOR. The tuberous sclerosis protein complex (TSC1/2) acts as an intermediary between AKT and mTOR: native TSC1/2 inhibits mTOR, and activation of AKT results in phosphorylation of TSC1/2 and subsequent de-repression of mTOR.

TOR was originally identified in a screen for mutations in yeast that conferred resistance to rapamycin, and mTOR was subsequently discovered as its mammalian homologue. **Rapamycin** (also known as **sirolimus**) binds to FKBP12, a member of the FK506-binding protein family, and the rapamycin–FKBP12 complex binds to mTOR and inhibits its activity. In addition to its immunosuppressive properties, rapamycin promotes cell cycle inhibition, apoptosis, and angiogenesis inhibition by blocking translation of downstream targets of mTOR such as cyclin D1, c-MYC, the antiapoptotic protein BAD, and HIF-1α.

A number of rapamycin derivatives are currently undergoing clinical testing in a wide variety of malignancies, including **temsirolimus** and **everolimus**. Both are soluble ester analogues of rapamycin that demonstrate dose-dependent inhibition of tumor cell growth in vitro. Temsirolimus is approved for treatment of renal cell carcinoma and has shown activity in breast cancer and mantle cell non-Hodgkin's lymphoma.

Everolimus is approved for treatment of renal cell carcinoma, breast cancer, and pancreatic cancer. Toxicities include skin rash, mucositis, thrombocytopenia, and leukopenia.

It is likely that particular subsets of patients will benefit from mTOR inhibitors, and future clinical trials will be designed accordingly. For example, in renal cell carcinoma, activation of HIF-1α due to loss of VHL expression has been shown to sensitize cells to mTOR inhibition and may explain the clinical activity of temsirolimus in a subset of patients. Studies of patients with bladder cancer who show a dramatic response to temsirolimus therapy have led to the identification of activating mutations in mTOR, which may, in future studies, identify a population of patients predicted to benefit from this drug. Everolimus treatment is effective in patients with subependymal giant cell astrocytomas due to TSC loss, leading to approval of the drug for this indication. Furthermore, because particular pathways such as estrogen receptor or EGFR signaling are dependent on PI3K/AKT/mTOR signaling (Fig. 40-2B), combination therapies using estrogen receptor or EGFR antagonists and mTOR inhibitors are being explored.

A variety of PI3K and AKT inhibitors are in clinical development. In addition, because rapamycin derivatives inhibit only a portion of mTOR function, and result in feedback activation of AKT signaling, second-generation mTOR inhibitors have been developed and are in clinical trials. These agents are competitive inhibitors of mTOR that bind to the active site of the enzyme. Moreover, since feedback activation of PI3K/AKT signaling typically involves engagement of IGF1R, strategies to target this receptor directly are also undergoing clinical testing.

Proteasome Inhibitors

In light of the importance of ubiquitin-mediated proteasomal degradation in regulating the cell cycle, apoptosis, and other processes involved in neoplastic transformation, proteasome inhibitors have been tested in vitro and in vivo for antitumor effects. The small molecule **bortezomib**, a dipeptide with a linked boronate moiety, targets with high affinity and specificity an active-site N-terminal threonine residue within the 20S catalytic subunit of the proteasome (Fig. 40-4A). Bortezomib induces growth inhibition and apoptosis of tumor cells with relatively few toxic effects on normal cells. Clinically, the effects of bortezomib are reversible, requiring intravenous dosing on a twice-weekly schedule.

Bortezomib has demonstrated considerable efficacy in clinical trials involving patients with multiple myeloma. Principal adverse effects include neuropathy, thrombocytopenia, and neutropenia. Given its relatively modest adverse effect profile, bortezomib has also been incorporated into combination regimens for primary therapy of multiple myeloma, with some of the highest response rates seen to date in this disease. In addition, bortezomib is being tested alone and in combination with standard chemotherapy in a wide variety of other malignancies.

Several mechanisms have been proposed to explain the efficacy of bortezomib in multiple myeloma. One mechanism involves inhibition of NFκB through stabilization of IκB (Fig. 40-5B). Since NFκB activates the transcription of genes promoting cell proliferation and blocking apoptosis in response to inflammation and other stimuli, antagonism of these actions by bortezomib would be expected to lead to growth inhibition and apoptosis. A second proposed mechanism involves accumulation of misfolded proteins, leading to cell death. Like the plasma cells from which they arise, multiple myeloma cells synthesize large amounts of immunoglobulin. The proteasome may play an important role in degrading misfolded proteins in these cells, and inhibition of proteasome function by bortezomib could be lethal in this setting. It has also been proposed that bortezomib can cause stabilization of CDK inhibitors and of p53. Indeed, mutation of p53 is associated with resistance to bortezomib. A second mechanism of bortezomib resistance involves increased expression of heat shock protein-27 (HSP-27), and studies designed at inhibiting heat shock proteins are underway both to overcome bortezomib resistance and to enhance its efficacy.

Carfilzomib is a second-generation proteasome inhibitor that exhibits stronger and irreversible binding to the proteasome and can overcome bortezomib resistance. This drug and other second-generation proteasome inhibitors in development may further advance the treatment of multiple myeloma and other cancers.

Angiogenesis Inhibitors

Recognition of the primary role of VEGF and its receptors in the regulation of angiogenesis has led to strategies to block VEGF function as a means of disrupting tumor vasculature. The most successful approaches to date have included the development of neutralizing antibodies against VEGF or VEGFR and small-molecule inhibitors of the VEGFR tyrosine kinase domain.

Anti-VEGF and Anti-VEGFR Antibodies

Bevacizumab is a recombinant humanized mouse IgG1 monoclonal antibody directed against VEGF-A, one of the major proangiogenic VEGF family members (Table 40-2). In mouse models, blocking VEGF with a monoclonal antibody inhibits angiogenesis and growth of human tumor xenografts. Early clinical studies were designed to test the efficacy of bevacizumab in metastatic renal cell carcinoma, because most of these cancers overexpress VEGF as a result of loss of VHL expression and consequent HIF-1 activation.

Incorporation of bevacizumab into standard chemotherapy regimens has yielded success in several tumor types. Addition of bevacizumab to chemotherapy for metastatic colon cancer has shown significant improvements in response rates and in survival. Improvement in survival has also resulted from the addition of bevacizumab to carboplatin and paclitaxel for the treatment of metastatic NSCLC, although patients with cerebral metastasis, squamous cell tumor histology, and central tumors were excluded from these studies because intratumoral bleeding could lead to potentially fatal cerebral hemorrhage or severe hemoptysis. Significant activity has also been seen in metastatic renal cell carcinoma and glioblastoma, and bevacizumab is also approved for use in these settings.

The potentiation of cytotoxic chemotherapy by bevacizumab and its modest activity as a single agent suggest that its mechanism of action may not be as simple as induction of tumor hypoxia and starvation of nutrients. Activation of VEGFR signaling increases vascular permeability, resulting in high interstitial fluid pressures in tumors. This high interstitial fluid pressure is postulated to prevent optimal delivery of chemotherapy to the tumor. Indeed, inhibition of VEGF with bevacizumab has been shown to decrease vascular permeability, reduce interstitial fluid pressure, and improve drug delivery to tumors.

Adverse effects of bevacizumab include proteinuria, hypertension, risk of thrombosis or bleeding, risk of gastrointestinal perforation, and impairment of wound healing. **Ramucirumab**, a recombinant IgG1 monoclonal antibody that binds VEGFR-2, shares a similar adverse effect profile, consistent with on-target toxicity related to inhibition of this signaling axis. Ramucirumab has recently been approved by the FDA for the treatment of metastatic gastric cancer and gastroesophageal junction adenocarcinoma.

VEGFR Inhibitors

Other strategies to inhibit VEGF signaling have included the development of small-molecule inhibitors of VEGFR tyrosine kinase activity. The small-molecule inhibitors of VEGFR are of special interest because these agents inhibit multiple receptor tyrosine kinases (Table 40-3). For example, **vandetanib** inhibits VEGFR-1, VEGFR-2, VEGFR-3, RET, and EGFR. RET is the oncogene that predisposes to multiple endocrine neoplasia (MEN) type 2 disease and medullary thyroid cancer, and vandetanib has been approved by the FDA for the latter indication. **Cabozantinib**, an inhibitor of VEGFR, C-KIT, RET, FLT3, and MET, among other kinases, is also effective in the treatment of metastatic medullary thyroid cancer.

The treatment of clear cell renal cell carcinoma provides another example of how the broad activity of these agents could be utilized. Loss of VHL expression and activation of HIF-1 result in expression of VEGF, PDGF-β, and TGF-α in a substantial fraction of these tumors, and inhibition of VEGF alone with bevacizumab has yielded only modest benefit in patients with metastatic renal carcinoma. More significant activity has been seen with the receptor tyrosine kinase inhibitors **sunitinib**, which inhibits VEGFRs, PDGFR, C-KIT, RET, and FLT3, and **sorafenib**, which inhibits not only B-RAF but also VEGFRs, PDGFR, C-KIT, RET, and FLT3. **Pazopanib** and **axitinib** are two other multitargeted VEGFR TKIs that have activity in this setting. Given the

TABLE 40-3 Examples of Vascular Endothelial Growth Factor Receptor Inhibitors

VEGFR TYROSINE KINASE INHIBITORS	TARGETS
Sunitinib	VEGFR-1, VEGFR-2, VEGFR-3, PDGFR, C-KIT, RET, FLT3, CSF-1R
Sorafenib	VEGFR-1, VEGFR-2, VEGFR-3, PDGFR, C-KIT, RET, FLT3, B-RAF
Pazopanib	VEGFR-1, VEGFR-2, VEGFR-3, PDGFR, C-KIT, FGFR-1, FGFR-3, Itk, Lck, c-Fms
Axitinib	VEGFR-1, VEGFR-2, VEGFR-3, PDGFR, C-KIT
Cabozantinib	VEGFR-1, VEGFR-2, VEGFR-3, C-KIT, RET, FLT3, MET
Vandetanib	VEGFR-1, VEGFR-2, VEGFR-3, RET, EGFR

VEGFR, vascular endothelial growth factor receptor; PDGFR, platelet-derived growth factor receptor; FLT3, FMS-like tyrosine kinase; FGFR, fibroblast growth factor receptor; Itk, interleukin-2 receptor inducible T-cell kinase; EGFR, epidermal growth factor receptor.

refractory nature of renal cell carcinoma to traditional chemotherapy, the development and use of these new agents, based on a deeper understanding of the tumor cell biology, represents a major advance in the treatment of this tumor.

Sunitinib, sorafenib, and other multitargeted VEGFR inhibitors also have activity in a variety of other solid tumors. For example, sunitinib is effective in the treatment of GISTs that are refractory to imatinib, and sorafenib is utilized for therapy of hepatocellular carcinoma. **Regorafenib**, another broad-spectrum inhibitor of VEGFR and other receptor tyrosine kinases, is approved for use in metastatic colorectal cancer.

Thalidomide and Lenalidomide

Thalidomide is a synthetic glutamic acid derivative that was found to have sedative and antiemetic properties and was marketed outside the United States during the mid-1950s as a treatment for morning sickness in pregnant women. Tragically, thalidomide was discovered to be teratogenic, causing severe developmental deformities including stunted limb development (phocomelia). Thalidomide was subsequently shown to have immunomodulatory properties, inhibiting the synthesis of TNF-α and demonstrating efficacy in the treatment of erythema nodosum leprosum (ENL). In addition, it was hypothesized that the abnormal limb development caused by thalidomide was due to antiangiogenic properties, and indeed, it has since been shown that thalidomide inhibits basic fibroblast growth factor (bFGF)-induced angiogenesis. Thalidomide has also been shown to costimulate T cells. Given its combination of properties, thalidomide is now termed an **immunomodulatory drug (IMiD)**.

Because increased microvascular density in the bone marrow is associated with poor outcomes in multiple myeloma, thalidomide was initially tested in patients with advanced disease and found to have significant clinical activity. Currently, the combination of thalidomide and dexamethasone is a standard first-line regimen for patients with multiple myeloma. Principal adverse effects include risk of thrombosis, neuropathy, constipation, and somnolence. Although thalidomide was initially evaluated for the treatment of multiple myeloma due to its immunomodulatory and antiangiogenic properties, the precise mechanism of its anticancer activity has remained unclear.

Lenalidomide is a synthetic second-generation IMiD analogue of thalidomide. While maintaining the antiangiogenic activity of thalidomide, lenalidomide also exhibits enhanced inhibition of TNF-α and costimulation of T cells as well as direct antitumor activity with induction of apoptosis. Lenalidomide shows activity even in thalidomide-refractory multiple myeloma and, when combined with bortezomib and dexamethasone, yields very high response rates in the primary treatment of multiple myeloma. The incidence of thrombosis with lenalidomide is markedly reduced compared to that with thalidomide, and lenalidomide causes less neuropathy, constipation, and somnolence as well. Lenalidomide also shows significant activity in the treatment of myelodysplastic syndromes, principally in patients with a deletion of the long arm of chromosome 5 (del 5q) or with normal cytogenetics. The main adverse effects of lenalidomide are myelosuppression and thrombocytopenia.

The molecular mechanism of lenalidomide action was recently identified. Lenalidomide binds to cereblon, a multisubunit E3 ubiquitin ligase (Fig. 40-4). The binding of lenalidomide to cereblon directs its activity to the B-cell transcription factors Ikaros family zinc finger proteins 1 and 3 (IKZF1 and IKZF3), resulting in their proteasomal degradation. This discovery not only illuminates the particular efficacy of this class of drugs in multiple myeloma but may also lead to the development of third-generation inhibitors with even more specific activity and therapeutic benefit in myeloma or other diseases.

Tumor-Specific Monoclonal Antibodies

Most hematologic malignancies express specific cell surface markers that have been used to subclassify the malignancies by immunohistochemistry and flow cytometry. The development of chimeric monoclonal antibodies against several of these antigens has provided the opportunity for targeted antibody therapy in a number of these disorders (Table 54-1).

Although the mechanism of action of monoclonal antibodies is incompletely understood, it is likely related to the induction of antibody-dependent cell-mediated cytotoxicity and apoptosis. For example, B-cell lymphomas characteristically express the CD20 cell surface antigen, which is normally found almost exclusively on mature B cells. The anti-CD20 IgG1 monoclonal antibody **rituximab** has demonstrated significant single-agent activity and enhancement of the effects of chemotherapy in B-cell non-Hodgkin's lymphoma (NHL) and is now routinely used in the therapy of this disorder. Principal adverse effects include immunosuppression due to the targeting of normal mature B cells and hypersensitivity reactions related to the chimeric nature of the antibody. **Ofatumumab** is another humanized anti-CD20 antibody that binds CD20 with higher affinity than rituximab and with a slower dissociation rate; this agent has shown efficacy in refractory CLL.

Alemtuzumab is a humanized monoclonal antibody directed against the pan-leukocyte antigen CD52. This agent has been used in the treatment of CLL and as a component of conditioning regimens for stem cell transplantation. Because alemtuzumab induces lysis of both T-cell and B-cell populations, its principal adverse effect is significant immunosuppression, including increased risk for *Pneumocystis jiroveci* pneumonia and for fungal, cytomegalovirus, and herpesvirus infections. Therefore, prophylaxis for opportunistic infections is required.

Conjugation of radioactive isotopes to anti-CD20 antibodies, such as iodine-131 (^{131}I) **tositumomab** and yttrium-90 (^{90}Y) **ibritumomab tiuxetan**, has allowed targeted radioimmunotherapy of B-cell NHL. Ibritumomab in particular has been incorporated into treatment regimens for patients with refractory disease.

In addition to the aforementioned trastuzumab emtansine, two further examples of antibody–toxin conjugates are denileukin diftitox and gemtuzumab ozogamicin. **Denileukin diftitox**, a recombinant fusion protein composed of fragments of diphtheria toxin and human IL-2, targets the CD25 component of the IL-2 receptor and has demonstrated activity in T-cell NHL. **Gemtuzumab ozogamicin** is a conjugate between the antitumor antibiotic calicheamicin and a monoclonal antibody directed against CD33, which is expressed on the surface of leukemic blasts in more than 80% of patients with AML.

■ CONCLUSION AND FUTURE DIRECTIONS

Elucidation of the molecular and biochemical circuitry that regulates normal cell proliferation and identification of the key mutations that promote oncogenesis have provided the ability to target specific pathways that are dysregulated in tumors. The success of imatinib in the treatment of CML demonstrates that cancers can become dependent on oncogenes such as BCR-Abl, requiring oncoprotein signaling for continued proliferation and survival. Although inhibitors of receptor tyrosine kinases and intracellular kinases have a higher therapeutic index than traditional antineoplastic therapies and have had some success in certain tumors, responses are neither durable nor complete in many cases. The identification of subsets of tumors in which specific pathways are activated, such as the EFGR mutation in NSCLC, will guide therapy and improve response rates. Oncogenic microarray signatures and correlations between specific mutations and sensitivity to targeted agents will facilitate the design of clinical trials focusing on subsets of patients with the highest likelihood of response. Efficacy will also be improved with second- and third-generation drugs that have higher selectivity for targets and the ability to overcome resistance mutations.

It is clear, however, that multiple factors contribute to tumor development, including downstream mutations in pathways regulating cell cycle progression, apoptosis, proteasomal degradation, and angiogenesis. The biology of these processes and of tumor cell invasion and acquisition of metastatic potential will likely provide novel targets for directed therapy. As with combination chemotherapy, the successful targeted therapies of the future will likely involve inhibition of multiple pathways using a combination of agents directed at the defects found in individual tumors. Furthermore, systematic approaches involving RNA interference and other genetic or chemical screens may identify previously unanticipated vulnerabilities associated with specific cancer genotypes, a concept derived from "synthetic lethal" screening in yeast. The improved selectivity inherent in such strategies will likely give them a superior therapeutic index compared to traditional combination antineoplastic chemotherapy and will hopefully be met with greater clinical success.

Suggested Reading

Bartlett JB, Dredge K, Dalgleish AG. The evolution of thalidomide and its IMiD derivatives as anticancer agents. *Nat Rev Cancer* 2004;4:314–322. (*Historic and scientific overview of thalidomide and its derivatives.*)

Hanahan D, Weinberg RA. Hallmarks of cancer: the next generation. *Cell* 2011;144:646–674. (*Seminal overview of the characteristic genetic changes leading to oncogenesis.*)

Kaelin WG Jr. The concept of synthetic lethality in the context of anticancer therapy. *Nat Rev Cancer* 2005;5:689–698. (*Novel approaches to cancer genotype-guided drug development.*)

Krause DS, van Etten RA. Tyrosine kinases as targets for cancer therapy. *N Engl J Med* 2005;353:172–187. (*Overview of tyrosine kinase inhibition in cancer therapy.*)

Laplante M, Sabatini DM. mTOR signaling in growth control and disease. *Cell* 2012;149:274–293. (*Reviews the role of the mTOR pathway in health, disease, and aging, with a focus on treatments targeting this pathway.*)

Lu G, Middleton RE, Sun H, et al. The myeloma drug lenalidomide promotes the cereblon-dependent destruction of Ikaros proteins. *Science* 2014;343:305–309. (*Demonstrates the molecular mechanism of action of lenalidomide.*)

Mani A, Gelmann EP. The ubiquitin-proteasome pathway and its role in cancer. *J Clin Oncol* 2005;23:4776–4789. (*Biochemical details of ubiquitin pathways.*)

Shaw AT, Hsu PP, Awad MM, Engelman JA. Tyrosine kinase gene rearrangements in epithelial malignancies. *Nat Rev Cancer* 2013;13:772–787. (*Reviews the etiology, pathogenesis, clinical features, and targeted treatments for epithelial cancers with ALK, ROS1, and RET mutations.*)

Tan CS, Gilligan D, Pacey S. Treatment approaches for EGFR-inhibitor-resistant patients with non-small-cell lung cancer. *Lancet Oncol* 2015;16:e447–459. (*Overview of EGFR pathways and treatments in non-small cell lung cancer.*)

DRUG SUMMARY TABLE: CHAPTER 40 Pharmacology of Cancer: Signal Transduction

INHIBITORS OF EGFR (ErbB1) AND HER2/neu (ErbB2)
Mechanism—Small-molecule and monoclonal antibody inhibitors of EGFR and HER2/neu; see specific drug

DRUG	CLINICAL APPLICATIONS	SERIOUS AND COMMON ADVERSE EFFECTS	CONTRAINDICATIONS	THERAPEUTIC CONSIDERATIONS
Gefitinib	Non-small cell lung cancer	*Interstitial lung disease, liver toxicity* Rash, diarrhea	Hypersensitivity to gefitinib	Reversible inhibitor of the EGFR (ErbB1) cytoplasmic tyrosine kinase domain; competes with ATP binding to the kinase domain.
Erlotinib	Non-small cell lung cancer Pancreatic cancer	*Cardiac arrhythmia, Stevens-Johnson syndrome, toxic epidermal necrolysis, gastrointestinal perforation, pancreatitis, deep vein thrombosis, anemia, stroke, perforation of cornea, interstitial lung disease, liver toxicity, renal failure* Edema, alopecia, rash, gastrointestinal upset, infection, myalgia, headache, conjunctivitis, anxiety, depression, cough, fatigue	Hypersensitivity to erlotinib	Erlotinib is a reversible inhibitor of the EGFR (ErbB1) cytoplasmic tyrosine kinase domain; it competes with ATP binding to the kinase domain.
Afatinib	Non-small cell lung cancer	*Impaired left ventricular function, bullous eruption, hand-foot syndrome, severe diarrhea, hepatotoxicity, interstitial lung disease* Rash, decreased appetite, stomatitis	None	Second-generation EGFR tyrosine kinase inhibitor. Binds to EGFR covalently and is thus an irreversible inhibitor.
Cetuximab Panitumumab	Colorectal cancer Head and neck cancer	*Hypomagnesemia, interstitial lung disease, renal failure (shared adverse effects); cardiac arrest, leukopenia, neutropenia, pulmonary embolism (cetuximab only); keratitis (panitumumab only)* Rash, weight loss, gastrointestinal disturbance, asthenia, headache, neuropathy, infection, fatigue	Hypersensitivity to cetuximab or panitumumab	Monoclonal antibodies that bind to extracellular domain of EGFR (ErbB1). Cetuximab shows improved response rates in EGFR-expressing colorectal cancer when combined with irinotecan. Development of rash in response to cetuximab is predictive of tumor response.
Trastuzumab	Breast cancer or metastatic gastric cancer with HER2 overexpression	*Cardiotoxicity, neutropenia, thrombocytopenia, anemia, thrombosis, hepatotoxicity, nephrotic syndrome, interstitial lung disease* Edema, rash, gastrointestinal upset, stomatitis, infection, arthralgia, myalgia, asthenia, dizziness, fatigue, shivering	Hypersensitivity to trastuzumab	Monoclonal antibody directed against ErbB2 (HER2). Treatment with trastuzumab in the adjuvant setting enhances the efficacy of chemotherapy and reduces rates of recurrence.
Trastuzumab emtansine	Breast cancer with HER2 overexpression	*Left ventricular dysfunction, anemia, neutropenia, thrombocytopenia, hepatotoxicity, interstitial lung disease* Gastrointestinal upset, musculoskeletal pain, headache, fatigue	None	Effective in HER2-positive breast cancer previously treated with trastuzumab and taxol.
Lapatinib	Breast cancer with HER2 overexpression	*Left ventricular dysfunction, prolonged QT interval, anemia, thrombocytopenia, hepatotoxicity, interstitial lung disease* Rash, gastrointestinal upset, abnormal liver function, headache, insomnia, fatigue	Hypersensitivity to lapatinib	Lapatinib is a reversible inhibitor of both EGFR and ErbB2. Lapatinib can prolong the QT interval.

continues

DRUG SUMMARY TABLE: CHAPTER 40 Pharmacology of Cancer: Signal Transduction *continued*

DRUG	CLINICAL APPLICATIONS	*SERIOUS* AND COMMON ADVERSE EFFECTS	CONTRAINDICATIONS	THERAPEUTIC CONSIDERATIONS
INHIBITORS OF ALK, ROS1, AND MET Mechanism—Small-molecule inhibitors of tyrosine kinases, including anaplastic lymphoma kinase (ALK), ROS1, and MET				
Crizotinib **Ceritinib**	Non-small cell lung cancer	*Prolonged QT interval, hepatotoxicity, interstitial lung disease (shared adverse effects); neutropenia, pulmonary embolism (crizotinib only); hyperglycemia, seizure, pneumothorax, tuberculosis, cachexia, sepsis (ceritinib only)* Gastrointestinal upset (shared adverse effects); edema, visual disturbance (crizotinib only); anemia, fatigue (ceritinib only)	None	Inhibit oncogenic fusion proteins that promote gene expression, cell proliferation, and cell survival in cancer. Targeted for a subset of lung cancers with rearrangements in the ALK tyrosine kinase. Ceritinib overcomes acquired resistance to crizotinib. Crizotinib also inhibits ROS1 and has activity in a subgroup of lung cancers with ROS1 rearrangements.
INHIBITORS OF BCR-ABL, C-KIT, AND PDGFR Mechanism—Small-molecule tyrosine kinase inhibitors active against ABL kinases (including BCR-Abl fusion protein), C-KIT, and PDGFR				
Imatinib	Chronic myelogenous leukemia (CML) and acute lymphoblastic leukemia (ALL) expressing the Philadelphia chromosome Gastrointestinal stromal tumor (GIST) expressing C-Kit (CD117) Idiopathic hypereosinophilic syndrome Dermatofibrosarcoma protuberans Myelodysplastic syndrome Myeloproliferative disorder Systemic mast cell disease	*Cardiac tamponade, heart failure, Stevens-Johnson syndrome, toxic epidermal necrolysis, gastrointestinal perforation, pancreatitis, myelosuppression, hepatotoxicity, cerebral edema, optic disc edema, sensorineural hearing loss, renal failure, pleural effusion, tumor lysis syndrome, secondary malignant neoplastic disease* Edema, night sweats, rash, weight gain, gastrointestinal upset, arthralgia, myalgia, asthenia, dizziness, headache, insomnia, infection, fatigue	Hypersensitivity to imatinib	Hematologic and cytogenetic response (disappearance of Philadelphia chromosome) is observed in a large fraction of patients with chronic-phase CML; molecular response (disappearance of BCR-Abl) is observed in a smaller fraction.
Dasatinib **Nilotinib** **Bosutinib** **Ponatinib**	Shared indication: Chronic myelogenous leukemia Dasatinib and ponatinib only: Acute lymphoblastic leukemia expressing the Philadelphia chromosome	*Prolonged QT interval, gastrointestinal hemorrhage, myelosuppression, hepatotoxicity (shared adverse effects); pericardial effusion, pleural effusion, pulmonary edema (dasatinib and bosutinib only); cerebral hemorrhage (dasatinib and nilotinib only); tumor lysis syndrome (nilotinib only); pancreatitis, renal failure (bosutinib only); arterial thrombosis, glaucoma, keratitis (ponatinib only)* Edema, rash, alopecia, night sweats, gastrointestinal upset, electrolyte imbalance, musculoskeletal pain, headache, fatigue, dyspnea, infection	Shared contraindication: Hypersensitivity to drug Nilotinib only: Hypokalemia, hypomagnesemia, long QT syndrome	Dasatinib and nilotinib have greater efficacy than imatinib against wild-type BCR-Abl in vitro, and they inhibit imatinib-resistant BCR-Abl isoforms with the exception of the T315I mutation. Ponatinib is associated with serious vascular toxicity (8% of ponatinib-treated patients in clinical trials manifested cardiovascular, cerebrovascular, or peripheral vascular thrombosis).
INHIBITORS OF BTK Mechanism—Small-molecule inhibitor of Bruton's tyrosine kinase (BTK)				
Ibrutinib	Chronic lymphoid leukemia Mantle cell lymphoma	*Atrial fibrillation, gastrointestinal hemorrhage, anemia, thrombocytopenia, neutropenia, subdural hematoma, renal failure, increased susceptibility to infection and malignancy* Peripheral edema, rash, gastrointestinal upset, arthralgia, myalgia, dizziness, fatigue	None	Interrupts B-cell receptor signaling. Under evaluation for treatment of other B-cell malignancies, including diffuse large B-cell lymphoma and plasma cell dyscrasias.

INHIBITORS OF JAK2

Mechanism—Small-molecule inhibitor of Janus kinase (JAK) 1 and 2, including JAK2 (V617F) mutant kinase

Ruxolitinib	Myelofibrosis	*Anemia, neutropenia, thrombocytopenia, leukoencephalopathy* Dizziness, headache	Under evaluation for treatment of polycythemia vera and essential thrombocythemia.

INHIBITORS OF RAS/MAP KINASE PATHWAYS

Mechanism—Small-molecule inhibitors of wild-type and mutant B-RAF (sorafenib, vemurafenib, dabrafenib); small-molecule inhibitor of MEK 1 and 2 (trametinib)

Sorafenib Vemurafenib Dabrafenib Trametinib	Sorafenib only: Renal cell carcinoma Hepatocellular carcinoma Thyroid cancer Vemurafenib, dabrafenib, and trametinib only: Malignant melanoma	*Cardiovascular disease, susceptibility to malignancy and infection (shared adverse effects); Stevens-Johnson syndrome, toxic epidermal necrolysis, gastrointestinal hemorrhage, hepatitis, cerebral hemorrhage, leukoencephalopathy (sorafenib and vemurafenib only); interstitial lung disease (sorafenib, vemurafenib, and trametinib only); anemia (trametinib and dabrafenib only); pancreatitis, iritis, uveitis, renal failure, pulmonary embolism (dabrafenib only)* Alopecia, rash, gastrointestinal upset, fatigue (shared adverse effects); electrolyte imbalance (sorafenib and dabrafenib only); hypertension, elevated amylase and lipase levels, depressed blood cell counts (sorafenib only); peripheral edema, night sweats, arthralgia, myalgia, headache (dabrafenib only)	Shared contraindications: Hypersensitivity to drug Sorafenib only: Combination with carboplatin and paclitaxel in patients with squamous cell lung cancer	Vemurafenib, dabrafenib, and trametinib have significant activity against melanomas with activating B-RAF mutations. Sorafenib also inhibits VEGFRs, PDGFR, and other receptor tyrosine kinases. Dabrafenib and trametinib combination results in stronger response and delayed resistance in patients with B-RAF-mutant melanoma.

mTOR INHIBITORS

Mechanism—mTOR is a serine-threonine kinase that regulates cell growth and proliferation via activation of translation; rapamycin and analogues bind to FKBP12, and the drug–FKBP12 complex binds to mTOR and inhibits its activity

Rapamycin (sirolimus)	Prophylaxis for renal transplant rejection	*Susceptibility to infection or malignancy, thrombosis, pancytopenia, lymphocele, kidney disease, leukoencephalopathy, interstitial lung disease, pulmonary embolism, pulmonary hemorrhage, angioedema* Edema, rash, hyperlipidemia, gastrointestinal upset, arthralgia, headache, infection	Hypersensitivity to rapamycin	In addition to inhibiting mTOR, rapamycin also blocks downstream targets of mTOR such as cyclin D1, c-MYC, the antiapoptotic protein BAD, and HIF-1. Avoid co-administration with drugs that induce or inhibit CYP3A4.
Temsirolimus Everolimus	Shared indication: Renal cell carcinoma Everolimus only: Angiomyolipoma of kidney Subependymal giant cell astrocytoma Breast cancer Liver or renal transplant rejection Pancreatic cancer	*Renal failure, pneumonia, interstitial lung disease, myelosuppression (shared adverse effects); Stevens-Johnson syndrome, gastrointestinal perforation (temsirolimus only); thrombosis, seizure (everolimus only)* Edema, rash, asthenia, mucositis, electrolyte imbalance, fatigue, infection (shared adverse effects); hyperlipidemia, amenorrhea, menorrhagia (everolimus only)	Shared contraindication: Hypersensitivity to temsirolimus or everolimus Temsirolimus only: Elevated bilirubin	Temsirolimus and everolimus are ester analogues of rapamycin.

continues

DRUG SUMMARY TABLE: CHAPTER 40 Pharmacology of Cancer: Signal Transduction *continued*

DRUG	CLINICAL APPLICATIONS	*SERIOUS* AND COMMON ADVERSE EFFECTS	CONTRAINDICATIONS	THERAPEUTIC CONSIDERATIONS
PROTEASOME INHIBITORS				
Mechanism—Inhibit an active-site N-terminal threonine residue within the 20S catalytic subunit of the proteasome				
Bortezomib **Carfilzomib**	Shared indication: Multiple myeloma Bortezomib only: Mantle cell lymphoma	*Heart failure, neutropenia, thrombocytopenia, liver failure, neuropathy, tumor lysis syndrome (shared adverse effects); leukoencephalopathy, pneumonia, angioedema, toxic epidermal necrolysis (bortezomib only); renal failure, anemia (carfilzomib only)* Gastrointestinal upset, infection, headache (shared adverse effects); hypotension, rash, arthralgia, myalgia, asthenia, dizziness, insomnia (bortezomib only); peripheral edema, fatigue (carfilzomib)	Hypersensitivity to bortezomib, carfilzomib, boron, or mannitol	Because of its relatively modest adverse effects, bortezomib is used in combination regimens for primary therapy of multiple myeloma, with good response rates. Carfilzomib exhibits strong and irreversible binding to proteasome and can overcome bortezomib resistance.
ANGIOGENESIS INHIBITORS				
Mechanism—Neutralizing antibodies against VEGF or VEGFR and small-molecule inhibitors of the VEGFR tyrosine kinase domain; see specific drug				
Bevacizumab **Ramucirumab**	Bevacizumab only: Metastatic colorectal cancer Non-small cell lung cancer Glioblastoma multiforme Renal cell carcinoma Ramucirumab only: Metastatic gastric cancer Gastroesophageal junction adenocarcinoma	*Arterial thromboembolism, hypertensive crisis, impaired wound healing, gastrointestinal perforation, leukoencephalopathy (shared adverse effects); bladder, vaginal, bronchopleural, or bile duct fistula, heart failure, nephrotic syndrome, angioedema, necrotizing fasciitis (bevacizumab only); hemorrhage (ramucirumab only)* Hypertension, headache (shared adverse effects); alopecia, hand-foot syndrome, gastrointestinal upset, asthenia, dizziness, infection (bevacizumab only); hyponatremia, diarrhea (ramucirumab only)	Hypersensitivity to bevacizumab or ramucirumab	Bevacizumab is an IgG1 monoclonal antibody directed against VEGF-A. Ramucirumab is an IgG1 monoclonal antibody directed against VEGFR-2.
Sunitinib	Renal cell carcinoma Gastrointestinal stromal tumor Pancreatic cancer	*Left ventricular dysfunction, prolonged QT interval, tissue necrosis, gastrointestinal perforation, pancreatitis, hemorrhage, thrombocytopenia, aseptic necrosis of jaw bone, leukoencephalopathy, pulmonary embolism, pulmonary hemorrhage, tumor lysis syndrome* Rash, gastrointestinal upset, thyroid dysfunction, asthenia, fatigue	Hypersensitivity to sunitinib	Sunitinib inhibits VEGFR-1, VEGFR-2, PDGFR, and other receptor tyrosine kinases.
Pazopanib **Vandetanib** **Cabozantinib**	Pazopanib only: Renal cell carcinoma Soft tissue sarcoma Vandetanib and cabozantinib only: Medullary thyroid carcinoma	*Leukoencephalopathy, cardiotoxicity (shared adverse effects); hemorrhage, pancreatitis (pazopanib and vandetanib only); myelosuppression (pazopanib and cabozantinib only); hepatotoxicity, arterial thrombosis, pneumothorax, pulmonary embolism (pazopanib only); Stevens-Johnson syndrome, sepsis, interstitial lung disease (vandetanib only); gastrointestinal perforation, gastrointestinal or tracheoesophageal fistula, aseptic necrosis of jaw bone (cabozantinib only)* Gastrointestinal upset, headache, fatigue (shared adverse effects); electrolyte imbalance (pazopanib and cabozantinib only); hypothyroidism, myalgia, (pazopanib only); rash (vandetanib and cabozantinib only)	Shared contraindication: Hypersensitivity to pazopanib, vandetanib, or cabozantinib Vandetanib only: Congenital long QT syndrome	Pazopanib inhibits VEGFR-2, PDGFR-β, KIT, and other receptor tyrosine kinases. Vandetanib and cabozantinib inhibit RET, the oncogene that predisposes to medullary thyroid carcinoma. Pazopanib can prolong the QT interval.

Thalidomide	Multiple myeloma Erythema nodosum leprosum	*Cardiac arrhythmia, Stevens-Johnson syndrome, toxic epidermal necrolysis, gastrointestinal perforation, thrombotic disorder, neutropenia, seizure, angioedema, tumor lysis syndrome* Edema, rash, weight changes, hypocalcemia, gastrointestinal upset, somnolence, tremor, asthenia, fatigue, infection	Hypersensitivity to thalidomide Pregnancy Women capable of becoming pregnant Males not using latex condom	An immunomodulatory drug that inhibits basic fibroblast growth factor (bFGF)-induced angiogenesis; also, costimulates T cells. Combination of thalidomide with dexamethasone is a standard first-line regimen for multiple myeloma.
Lenalidomide	Multiple myeloma Myelodysplastic syndrome Mantle cell lymphoma	*Same as thalidomide, except for lower incidence of thrombosis, gastrointestinal upset, and somnolence*	Pregnancy Women capable of becoming pregnant Males not using latex condom	Analogue of thalidomide with enhanced inhibition of TNF-α and improved T-cell costimulatory properties, while maintaining antiangiogenic activity. Combination of lenalidomide with bortezomib and dexamethasone has very high response rates in multiple myeloma.

TUMOR-SPECIFIC MONOCLONAL ANTIBODIES AND OTHER RECOMBINANT PROTEINS
Mechanism—See specific drug; also, see Chapter 54, Protein Therapeutics

Rituximab **Tositumomab** **Ibritumomab** **Alemtuzumab** **Denileukin diftitox** **Gemtuzumab ozogamicin** **Ofatumumab**	Rituximab, tositumomab, ibritumomab, and denileukin diftitox only: Lymphoma Rituximab, alemtuzumab, ofatumumab, and gemtuzumab ozogamicin only: Leukemia Rituximab only: Hemolytic anemia Evans syndrome Graft-versus-host disease Thrombocytopenic purpura Minimal change disease Pemphigus vulgaris Sjögren's syndrome Post-transplant lymphoproliferative disorder Rheumatoid arthritis Systemic lupus erythematosus Waldenström's macroglobulinemia	*Cardiac arrhythmias, myelodysplastic syndrome, significant immunosuppression (including increased risk of developing opportunistic bacterial, fungal, and viral infections), hypersensitivity, anaphylactoid reaction related to chimeric antibody (shared adverse effects); leukoencephalopathy (rituximab, alemtuzumab, and ofatumumab only); nephrotoxicity (rituximab and alemtuzumab only); bowel obstruction, tumor lysis syndrome (ofatumumab and rituximab only); Stevens-Johnson syndrome, toxic epidermal necrolysis, liver failure, keratitis, angioedema (rituximab only); pleural effusion (tositumomab only)* Rash, gastrointestinal upset, infection, fatigue (shared adverse effects); hypotension, edema, neuropathy, musculoskeletal pain, headache, shivering (rituximab, tositumomab, ibritumomab, alemtuzumab, denileukin diftitox, and gemtuzumab ozogamicin only)	Hypersensitivity to drug	Rituximab: anti-CD20 antibody. Tositumomab: anti-CD20 antibody. Ibritumomab: anti-CD20 antibody. Alemtuzumab: anti-CD52 antibody. Denileukin diftitox: fusion protein of diphtheria toxin and IL-2. Gemtuzumab ozogamicin: conjugate of anti-CD33 antibody and calicheamicin (antitumor antibiotic). Voluntarily withdrawn from the US market in 2010 due to high rate of fatal toxicity seen in post-approval study. Ofatumumab: anti-CD20 antibody that binds with higher affinity than rituximab and with a slower dissociation rate.

41

Principles of Combination Chemotherapy

Quentin J. Baca, Donald M. Coen, and David E. Golan

INTRODUCTION

Many infections and some cancers can be success-fully treated with single-drug therapies. Such regimens often fail, however, when pathogens or tumors develop resistance to chemotherapeutic agents, when multiple pathogens with different drug susceptibilities are simulta-neously present, or when the dose of the therapeutic agent is limited by toxicity. Under these circumstances, combi-nation chemotherapy may offer decisive advantages. The drugs in a multidrug regimen can interact synergistically to enhance the antimicrobial or antineoplastic effective-ness of the combination and can decrease the likelihood that resistance will emerge. Combinations are frequently used when treatment must be initiated before the defini-tive identification of the pathogen, and synergistic combi-nations can be used to reduce toxicity when the individual drugs in the combination have low therapeutic indices. Although combination chemotherapy opens new avenues for the expedient elimination of a pathogen or tumor, it also introduces the potential for multiple adverse effects and drug interactions. The goal of any combination drug regimen should be to efficiently remove the offending pathogen or tumor without incurring unacceptable host toxicity.

ANTIMICROBIAL COMBINATION THERAPY

In the treatment of microbial infections, drug combinations are used (1) to prevent the emergence of drug resistance, (2) to enhance the activity (efficacy) of the drug therapy against a specific infection (synergy), (3) to reduce toxic-ity to the host, (4) to treat multiple simultaneous infections (sometimes called *polymicrobial infections*), and (5) to treat a life-threatening infection empirically before the microor-ganism causing the infection has been identified. Because microbes are genetically distant from humans, antimicrobial drug combinations can target several different molecules that are specific to the microbe(s), potentially without a concomitant increase in adverse effects. In contrast, anti-neoplastic drug combinations are often limited by adverse effects (see below). The following section provides a con-ceptual framework for the different types of antimicrobial drug interactions and discusses specific examples of antimi-crobial combination therapy.

Minimum Inhibitory Concentration and Minimum Bactericidal Concentration

Antimicrobial agents with activity against a pathogenic bacterial, protozoal, or fungal microorganism can be

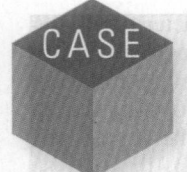

CASE

Mr. M is a 27-year-old man from rural Haiti who presents to a clinic with a chronic cough. He cannot afford treatment at a private clinic, so he goes to a drugstore and asks the pharmacist for appropriate medication. The pharmacist thinks that Mr. M could have tuberculosis, and he sells Mr. M a 2-week supply of isoniazid and rifampin. Mr. M takes both drugs for a couple of days, but they make him nauseated, and he decides to take just the isoniazid for 2 weeks. His symptoms resolve.

Three months later, Mr. M's cough returns. This time, he notices blood in his sputum and he has night sweats. He takes the remainder of the 2-week supply of rifampin and experiences a brief lull in his symptoms. Within a few days, however, his cough, bloody sputum, and night sweats return. Because he does not have enough money to buy additional drugs, he travels to the nearest government hospital to seek free care and medications. The government doctor takes three sputum samples, all of which are positive for acid-fast bacilli. The doctor also sends sputum to the laboratory for culture, but since *Mycobacterium tuberculosis* (the causative agent of

tuberculosis) is slow-growing, she also starts Mr. M on a multidrug regimen consisting of isoniazid, rifampin, pyrazinamide, and ethambutol for 2 months, followed by isoniazid and rifampin for 4 months.

Several weeks later, the culture reveals that Mr. M's tuberculosis is not susceptible to either isoniazid or rifampin. Mr. M's doctor is now seeking a new recommendation for treatment.

Questions

1. Why did the government doctor prescribe four different drugs for Mr. M?
2. How is resistance transferred from one generation of tubercle bacilli to the next? How does this resistance-transfer mechanism compare to the mechanism by which penicillin resistance is transferred?
3. Why were Mr. M's initial efforts at treatment unsuccessful? What treatment strategy could have been employed to avoid Mr. M's treatment failure?
4. Does Mr. M have multidrug-resistant tuberculosis (MDR-TB)? Should he stay on the four-drug regimen that includes isoniazid and rifampin? If not, how should his treatment be modified?

characterized by the **minimum inhibitory concentration (MIC)** and the **minimum bactericidal concentration (MBC)** for the drug–pathogen pair. The MIC is defined as the lowest concentration of drug that inhibits growth of a culture of the microorganism after 18–24 hours of incubation in vitro. The MBC is defined as the lowest concentration of drug that kills 99.9% of a culture of the microorganism after 18–24 hours of incubation in vitro. In general, the MBC is higher than the MIC. Comparisons between the MICs or MBCs and the clinically achievable concentrations of antimicrobial drugs allow these drugs to be grouped broadly into two categories: *cidal* and *static* (Table 41-1; also see Chapter 33, Principles of Antimicrobial and Antineoplastic Pharmacology). An antimicrobial agent is *static* (e.g., bacterio*static*, fungi*static*) if its MIC is within the therapeutic range of the drug but

its MBC is not. The agent is *cidal* (e.g., bacteri*cidal*, fungi*cidal*) if its MBC is within the therapeutic range of the drug. Note that the MIC and MBC refer to a specific drug–microbe pair under a specific set of conditions. Many drugs with activity against an organism are static in one growth medium but cidal in another or are cidal at sufficiently high concentrations in vitro. Furthermore, for any particular drug, the MIC and MBC may differ from one microbe to the next. Indeed, a drug may be static against one organism and cidal against another. As an operational definition, we can state that, *at therapeutic concentrations, cidal drugs kill the microorganism, while static drugs merely arrest microbial growth.* In this definition, the therapeutic concentration refers to plasma drug levels that are sufficient for pharmacologic activity (here, killing or arresting the growth of the microorganism) without unacceptable toxicity to the patient. For example, most inhibitors of bacterial cell wall synthesis are bactericidal, whereas most inhibitors of bacterial protein synthesis are bacteriostatic (see Chapter 34, Pharmacology of Bacterial Infections: DNA Replication, Transcription, and Translation, and Chapter 35, Pharmacology of Bacterial and Mycobacterial Infections: Cell Wall Synthesis).

As noted in Chapter 33, an important distinction between static and cidal drugs lies in their clinical applications. *In general, the successful use of static drugs to treat infections requires an intact host immune system.* This is because static drugs do not kill microorganisms but only prevent them from multiplying. Accordingly, such drugs rely on the host's immune and inflammatory mechanisms to effect clearance of organisms from the body. These drugs are more efficacious when initiated early in the course of an infection (i.e., when the infectious burden is lower). Furthermore, removal of a

TABLE 41-1 Examples of Bactericidal and Bacteriostatic Antibiotics

BACTERIOSTATIC ANTIBIOTICS	BACTERICIDAL ANTIBIOTICS	
	CONCENTRATION-DEPENDENT	TIME-DEPENDENT
Chloramphenicol	Aminoglycosides	β-Lactams
Clindamycin	Bacitracin	Isoniazid
Ethambutol	Quinolones	Metronidazole
Macrolides		Pyrazinamide
Sulfonamides		Rifampin
Tetracyclines		Vancomycin
Trimethoprim		

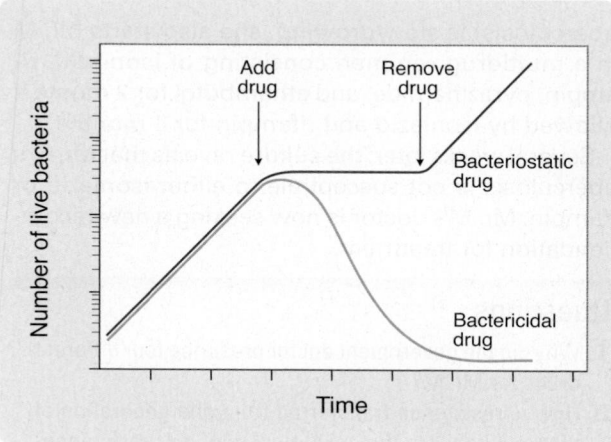

FIGURE 41-1. **Comparison of the effects of bacteriostatic and bactericidal drugs on bacterial growth kinetics in vitro.** In the absence of drug, bacteria grow with exponential (first-order) kinetics. A bactericidal drug kills the target organism, as demonstrated by the time-dependent decrease in the number of live bacteria. A bacteriostatic drug prevents microbial growth without killing the bacteria. Removal of a bacteriostatic drug is followed by an exponential increase in bacterial number as the previously inhibited bacteria resume growth. Bacteriostatic drugs eradicate infections by limiting the growth of the infecting organism for a long enough period of time to allow the host immune system to kill the bacteria.

static drug before the immune system has completely cleared the infection can result in resumption of microbial growth and reappearance of infection (Fig. 41-1).

According to their mechanism of cell killing, bactericidal agents can be further characterized as **time-dependent** or **concentration-dependent** (Fig. 41-2). Time-dependent bactericidal agents exhibit a constant rate of killing that is independent of drug concentration, provided that the drug

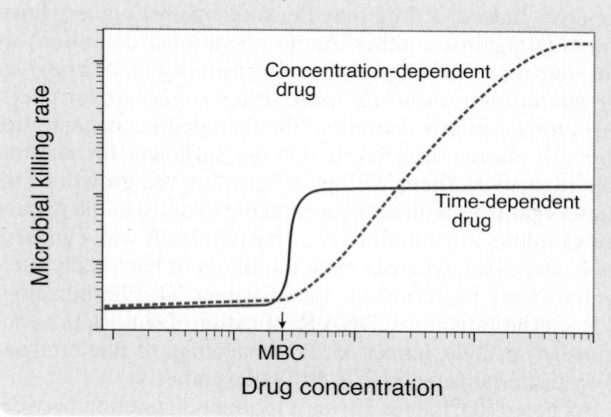

FIGURE 41-2. **Relationship between rate of microbial killing and drug concentration for time-dependent and concentration-dependent bactericidal drugs.** Time-dependent bactericidal agents exhibit a constant rate of microbial killing at concentrations of drug greater than the minimum bactericidal concentration (MBC) (*solid line*). In contrast, concentration-dependent bactericidal agents exhibit increased killing with increasing drug concentration (*dashed line*). Note that the efficacy of concentration-dependent bactericidal agents eventually plateaus because the effective concentration of the drug becomes limited by the rate of drug diffusion to its molecular target.

concentration is higher than the minimum bactericidal concentration (MBC). Thus, the overriding consideration for the clinical use of such agents is not the absolute drug concentration that is achieved, but the duration of time during which the drug concentration remains in the therapeutic range (which is defined as [drug] > MBC). In contrast, concentration-dependent bactericidal agents exhibit a rate of killing that increases with drug concentration for [drug] > MBC. For such agents, a single very large dose may be sufficient to eliminate the infection.

Types of Drug Interactions—Synergy, Additivity, and Antagonism

The discussion has thus far considered the general properties of drugs used as single agents to treat a microbial infection. When such drugs are used in combination with other agents, these effects can be modified (either enhanced or diminished). In fact, some drugs that have little or no activity against an organism when used as single agents can show high activity when used in combination with another agent. One example of this concept involves the treatment of *Enterococcus faecalis*, a Gram-positive organism that exhibits little susceptibility to **aminoglycosides**. Recall that aminoglycosides are thought to kill bacteria by inducing misreading of the genetic code and translation of defective proteins, which cause further cellular damage (see Chapter 34). In the case of *E. faecalis*, aminoglycosides are unable to penetrate the organism's thick cell wall to reach their target, the 30S ribosomal subunit. However, when used in combination with a cell wall synthesis inhibitor such as **vancomycin** or a **β-lactam** antibiotic, aminoglycosides are able to reach the bacterial ribosomes and effectively kill the bacteria (see Chapter 35). The potentiating effect of the cell wall synthesis inhibitor on the activity of the aminoglycoside is an example of the important pharmacologic concept of **synergy**.

From this example, one could ask whether combining two drugs with individual activity against a particular microbe always results in a more efficacious drug combination. Surprisingly, for many combinations, this turns out not to be the case. In fact, when two drugs with activity against the same pathogen are combined, the drugs can interact to diminish the efficacy of the combination relative to each alone (**antagonism**). Alternatively, the drugs may not interact, and the effect of the combination is simply the sum of the effects of each drug used individually (**additivity**). The interaction between two antimicrobial drugs is often quantified by selecting a particular endpoint (e.g., inhibition of bacterial growth) and then measuring the effect of various combinations of the two drugs that reach this endpoint. When such data are plotted, additional information can be obtained (Fig. 41-3). The x- and y-intercepts correspond to the MICs of each of the two drugs, and the concavity of the curve indicates the nature of the interaction between the two drugs—concave-up is synergistic; concave-down is antagonistic; linear is additive. The following discussion provides a mathematical rationale for these relationships.

Suppose that Drugs A and B inhibit a particular enzyme required for bacterial growth. In this case, the ratio $[A]/MIC_A$ would represent the fraction of bacterial growth inhibition that can be attributed to the presence of Drug A. This is known as the *fractional inhibitory concentration of A (FIC$_A$)*. Similarly, $FIC_B = [B]/MIC_B$ is the fraction

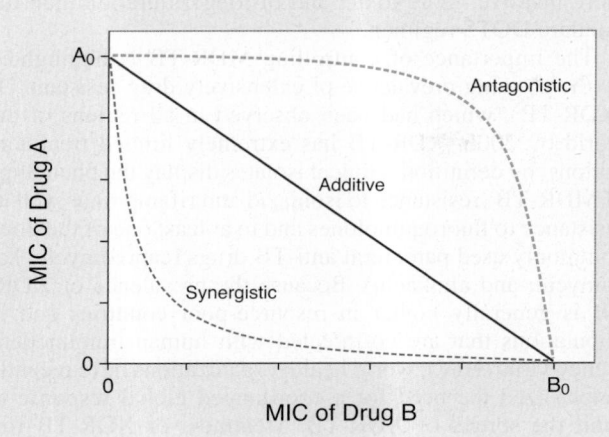

FIGURE 41-3. Quantification of additive, synergistic, and antagonistic drug interactions. Drug combinations can exhibit additive, synergistic, or antagonistic effects. The nature of this interaction can be depicted graphically by observing the effect of each drug on the other's minimum inhibitory concentration (MIC). If two drugs have an additive interaction, then the addition of increasing amounts of Drug B to Drug A results in a linear decrease in the MIC of Drug A; in this case, each of the two drugs can be thought of as interchangeable. If two drugs have a synergistic interaction, then the addition of Drug B to Drug A results in a significantly lower MIC for Drug A (i.e., there is an increase in the potency of Drug A). If two drugs have an antagonistic interaction, then the addition of Drug B to Drug A does not significantly lower the MIC of Drug A; in some cases (*not shown*), higher doses of each drug must be administered to achieve the same effect as that of each drug used alone. A_0 and B_0 are the MICs of Drugs A and B, respectively, when used as single agents.

of growth inhibition that can be attributed to Drug B. Now, suppose that the concentration of A is decreased by a small amount, $-d[A]$. To compensate for this loss of growth inhibition ($dFIC_A = -d[A]/MIC_A$), the concentration of B must be increased by an amount $+d[B]$.

For additive drugs, the ratio $-d[A]/d[B]$ (which is the same as the slope of the curve in Fig. 41-3) is a constant because one unit of A has exactly the same activity as (MIC_A/MIC_B) units of B. For example, A and B could bind to independent sites on the enzyme (i.e., each drug has no effect on the binding of the other drug).

In contrast, if A and B are synergistic, then the amount of B ($d[B]$) required to compensate for a decrease in A ($-d[A]$) depends on the amount of A that is already present. Because of the potentiating effect of Drug A on Drug B, $d[B]$ is smaller for higher $[A]$ (i.e., $d^2[A]/d[B]^2 > 0$, which corresponds to the concave-up curve in Fig. 41-3). For example, the binding of A could induce a conformational change in the enzyme that enhances the binding of B.

By extension, A and B are antagonistic if the amount of B required to compensate for a small decrease in the concentration of A is larger for higher $[A]$ (i.e., $d^2[A]/d[B]^2 < 0$, which corresponds to the concave-down curve in Fig. 41-3). For example, the binding of A could induce a conformational change in the enzyme that reduces the binding of B.

Because of its intuitiveness and simplicity, the mathematical model described above is often used to define synergy, additivity, and antagonism. However, the experimental determination and quantitative analysis of the effects of

multiple drugs are complex topics that are beyond the scope of this text. The interested reader is referred to the work of TC Chou (1984, 2006) for an extensive treatment of this subject.

Several generalizations can be made concerning the nature of drug interactions between different classes of antimicrobial agents. First, many bacteriostatic drugs (e.g., **tetracycline**, **erythromycin**, **chloramphenicol**) antagonize the action of bactericidal drugs (e.g., **vancomycin**, **penicillin**) by inhibiting cell growth and/or preventing the cellular processes that are required for cidal drugs to act (described below in more detail). Second, two bactericidal drugs usually act synergistically in combination. One notable exception to the latter generalization is that **rifampin**, a bactericidal inhibitor of RNA polymerase, antagonizes other bactericidal drugs by inhibiting cell growth. Finally, the interactions between two bacteriostatic drugs are often additive but cannot be predicted in all cases.

Examples of Antimicrobial Combination Therapy

Tuberculosis

The treatment of tuberculosis illustrates one of the principal reasons that combinations of drugs are used—to suppress the emergence of resistance. In the course of this illness, tuberculous bacilli (also called *mycobacteria*) are inhaled and phagocytosed by alveolar macrophages, in which the bacilli multiply within intracellular vacuoles. A predominantly T-cell–mediated lymphocytic response is elicited, and the macrophages and helper T cells form large granulomas that wall off the infected sites. Activated macrophages are usually able to keep the infection under control by killing the multiplying bacilli but are unfortunately unable to eradicate the infection completely. Tissue damage is caused by the release of neutral proteases and reactive oxygen intermediates from activated macrophages, with the end result that central necrosis occurs in the tuberculous cavities in the lungs. Inside each of these cavities, as many as 10^8 to 10^9 living bacilli may be held in check by macrophages and helper T cells.

Successful cure of tuberculosis infections typically requires the use of combinations of drugs with antimycobacterial activity. Commonly used drugs include **isoniazid**, **rifampin**, **pyrazinamide**, and **ethambutol** (see Chapter 35). As illustrated in the case of Mr. M, a standard regimen could consist of 2 months of isoniazid, rifampin, pyrazinamide, and ethambutol, followed by 4 months of isoniazid and rifampin. **Kanamycin** and other second-line drugs are sometimes substituted for one or two drugs in this regimen if resistance develops. Isoniazid and rifampin are often the preferred drugs in such regimens because of their ability to kill intracellular as well as extracellular mycobacteria.

As noted in Chapter 35, resistance to antimycobacterial drugs develops primarily through chromosomal mutations, and the frequency of resistance to any one of the drugs is about 1 in 10^6 bacteria. These mutations are passed on to daughter cells when the bacteria replicate, leading to establishment of a drug-resistant population. Chapter 35 discusses the implications of the fact that a tuberculous cavity contains 10^8 to 10^9 bacteria, while the frequency of mutants resistant to a single drug is about 1 in 10^6. On average, then, 100 bacteria will already be resistant to each drug in any single lesion, even before that drug is administered. Moreover, treatment with only one drug would result in selection for bacilli that are resistant to that drug. In the case of Mr. M, his initial 2 weeks of isoniazid treatment likely killed all the isoniazid-susceptible bacilli in his cavity. This accounts for the cessation in his symptoms after 2 weeks of treatment. However, the 100 or so isoniazid-resistant bacilli that were selected for by Mr. M's use of monotherapy remained alive and multiplied. If he had taken rifampin as well as isoniazid, only 1 in 10^{12} bacilli would likely have been resistant to both drugs, and he might have eradicated the infection.

Over the 3 months during which Mr. M stopped taking isoniazid, the isoniazid-resistant bacilli remaining in his lungs multiplied, leading to a relapse in his symptoms. He then began taking rifampin. Of the 10^8 to 10^9 isoniazid-resistant bacilli in each lesion, again there was a 1 in 10^6 probability that a bacillus had mutated to acquire rifampin resistance. By taking rifampin for 2 weeks, he killed all the rifampin-susceptible bacilli but selected for rifampin-resistant organisms. He was therefore left with bacilli that were both isoniazid-resistant and rifampin-resistant—the phenotype of **multidrug-resistant tuberculosis (MDR-TB)**.

Mr. M will require a new drug regimen for treatment of MDR-TB. Ideally, the regimen should be constructed using drugs that have been shown to be effective in susceptibility tests. Also, at least initially, drugs that are part of his current treatment plan should be avoided (i.e., pyrazinamide and ethambutol), because his bacilli may have developed resistance to these agents. Isoniazid and rifampin should certainly be avoided. Treatment for MDR-TB should begin with at least four new drugs to which Mr. M's TB isolate has proven susceptibility. Such regimens usually include daily dosing of a parenteral aminoglycoside (**kanamycin** or **amikacin**) or peptide antibiotic (**capreomycin**), together with a fluoroquinolone (**levofloxacin** or **moxifloxacin**), for at least 4–6 months. Three to five oral drugs should be co-administered with the aminoglycoside and fluoroquinolone for 18–24 months after the sputum culture converts to negative. **Ethionamide** and **clofazimine** are second-line drugs that could be included in the regimen. Newer drugs that could be included are **linezolid**, **bedaquiline**, and **delamanid**. Note that, as a whole, the second-line regimen will be significantly more toxic than the first-line regimen. If bacilli isolated from Mr. M's sputum prove to be susceptible to pyrazinamide and/or ethambutol, these agents could replace some of the more toxic drugs.

Considering all the issues discussed above, MDR-TB is to be avoided at all costs. Patients with drug-susceptible tuberculosis require access to combination therapy as well as help in adhering to the combination therapy to avoid the emergence of drug-resistant bacilli. This rationale is the basis for **DOTS (Directly Observed Therapy Short Course)**, the World Health Organization (WHO)-recommended strategy for tuberculosis treatment. DOTS is a public health program that has five components: (1) political commitment and resources for TB control, (2) the use of sputum-smear microscopy for accurate diagnosis of TB infection, (3) a standardized 6- to 8-month treatment that is directly observed by a community health worker for at least the first 2 months, (4) a regular and uninterrupted supply of medicines, and (5) standardized recording and reporting of each patient's treatment and progress to central authorities. When used in cases of drug-susceptible TB, DOTS has a remarkable cure rate and can prevent the development of resistance. As noted above, treatment of MDR-TB requires therapy that is more intensive, more invasive, more toxic, and of longer duration than the standard DOTS regimen.

The importance of controlling MDR-TB is highlighted by the growing prevalence of extensively drug-resistant TB (XDR-TB), which had been observed in all regions of the world by 2006. XDR-TB has extremely limited treatment options; by definition, clinical isolates display the phenotype of MDR-TB (resistance to isoniazid and rifampin) as well as resistance to fluoroquinolones and to at least one of the three commonly used parenteral anti-TB drugs (capreomycin, kanamycin, and amikacin). Because the prevalence of XDR-TB is generally higher in resource-poor countries and in populations that are co-infected with human immunodeficiency virus (HIV), world health organizations have recently emphasized the need for a coordinated global response to limit the spread of XDR-TB. Treatment of XDR-TB frequently involves the use of up to five drugs, guided by drug susceptibility testing.

Synergistic Combinations

A second reason for using a combination drug regimen is to take advantage of the synergy between the actions of the two drugs. This consideration is especially important in the setting of infections that are not readily handled by the immune defenses of immunocompromised patients. In the immunocompetent patient, bacteriostatic and bactericidal drugs are often equally efficacious in eliminating an infection. Bactericidal drugs are strongly preferred, however, in the setting of immunocompromised patients (e.g., HIV/AIDS patients, immunosuppressed transplant patients, and neutropenic cancer patients), endovascular infection (e.g., bacterial endocarditis), or meningitis. The reason for using bactericidal combinations in the immunocompromised patient should be obvious—the host does not have sufficient numbers of functioning lymphocytes and/or neutrophils to eliminate even a nondividing bacterial population. In the case of endocarditis, the reason is not so straightforward. In this case, although there is not a deficiency in the absolute number of leukocytes, the phagocytes are unable to efficiently penetrate the thick "vegetation"—composed of a meshwork of fibrin, platelets, and bacterial products—that surrounds the bacteria. Bactericidal drug combinations are sometimes indicated for meningitis to maximize the probability of overcoming the poor opsonization of bacteria by antibody and complement in the immunologically privileged site of the meninges, especially if the responsible organism is not known (see Chapter 9, Principles of Nervous System Physiology and Pharmacology).

One example of antibacterial synergy involves the use of a **penicillin** and an **aminoglycoside** to treat a common cause of subacute bacterial endocarditis, *Streptococcus viridans*. As described above, the mechanism of synergy relies on the penicillin inhibiting cell wall biosynthesis, which allows the aminoglycoside to penetrate the thick peptidoglycan layer of this Gram-positive organism.

Two other commonly used synergistic combinations include (1) the antifungal combination of **amphotericin B** and **flucytosine** and (2) the antibacterial and antiprotozoal combination of a **sulfonamide** and **trimethoprim** or **pyrimethamine**. These classic examples illustrate two basic mechanisms whereby one drug can potentiate the activity of another. It is thought that, analogous to the action of penicillins, which enhance the uptake of aminoglycosides by Gram-positive bacteria, amphotericin B enhances flucytosine uptake by fungal cells by damaging ergosterol-rich fungal cell membranes (see Chapter 36, Pharmacology of Fungal Infections). Only after penetrating the fungal membrane can flucytosine be converted into its active form (5-fluorouracil, which is converted to 5-FdUMP, an irreversible inhibitor of thymidylate synthase) by a fungal-specific deaminase. Amphotericin B has a low therapeutic index when used as a single agent (primarily as a consequence of its nephrotoxicity), but its synergistic effect in combination with flucytosine allows a reduction in the dose of amphotericin B required to treat a systemic fungal infection such as cryptococcal meningitis (with a corresponding reduction in toxicity).

Sulfamethoxazole and **trimethoprim** are commonly used in combination in the treatment of *Pneumocystis jiroveci* pneumonia, an opportunistic infection frequently encountered in patients with AIDS, as well as many urinary tract infections caused by Gram-negative enteric organisms. An analogous combination, **sulfadoxine** and **pyrimethamine**, is used in the treatment of malaria, toxoplasmosis, and other protozoal infections. These combinations illustrate a second mechanism whereby drugs can exert a synergistic effect. The mechanism of synergy is based on the sulfa drug's inhibition of production of dihydrofolate, which ordinarily competes with the second drug for binding to its target, dihydrofolate reductase (see Chapter 33). The product of this enzyme, tetrahydrofolate, is a required substrate for purine biosynthesis and for many one-carbon transfer reactions and is thus necessary for microbial DNA replication and cell division (see Fig. 33-7).

Co-administration of Penicillins with β-Lactamase Inhibitors

The combination of a β-lactam antibiotic and a β-lactamase inhibitor (e.g., **clavulanic acid**, **sulbactam**, **tazobactam**) illustrates a mechanism of drug interaction that is not technically synergistic (because the β-lactamase inhibitor has no antibacterial activity on its own) but that shares a functional similarity with the drug combinations discussed above. Clavulanic acid is an inhibitor of β-lactamase, an enzyme used by many β-lactam-resistant Gram-positive and Gram-negative bacteria to inactivate penicillins (see Chapter 35). By preventing the hydrolysis and inactivation of penicillins, clavulanic acid (and other β-lactamase inhibitors) greatly increases the potency of penicillins (and other β-lactams) against bacteria that express β-lactamase. This combination has been effective in the treatment of infections due to penicillin-resistant *Streptococcus pneumoniae*, which is a common cause of otitis media in infants. Such organisms have typically acquired resistance to penicillins through a plasmid-encoded β-lactamase.

Polymicrobial and Life-Threatening Infections

Combinations of antimicrobial drugs are used not only to prevent the emergence of resistance and to act synergistically against a specific, known pathogen but also to treat polymicrobial infections and infections in which treatment must be initiated before the microbe causing the infection is identified. Consider, for example, the case of a ruptured appendix or colonic diverticulum that has leaked bacteria into the peritoneal cavity and formed an intra-abdominal abscess. Such an abscess is likely to contain a wide spectrum of microorganisms—much too broad to be targeted effectively by a single antibiotic. After draining the abscess, treatment with a combination of antibacterial agents such as a **fluoroquinolone** or **β-lactam**—to kill aerobic Gram-negative Enterobacteriaceae (e.g., *Escherichia coli*)—and **clindamycin** or **metronidazole**—to kill anaerobes (e.g., *Bacteroides fragilis*; see Chapter 37, Pharmacology of Parasitic Infections)—often results in clearance of the infection. (Note that it may sometimes be necessary to treat with antagonistic drug combinations in order to cover the spectrum of microorganisms that are likely to be present.) In cases where presumptive treatment is indicated before the causative microorganism is identified, body fluids such as blood, sputum, urine, and cerebrospinal fluid (CSF) should be submitted for culture before initiating therapy. A combination of drugs with activity against the microbes that are most likely to be involved in the infection (or that could result in the most serious outcome) is then administered until a positive bacteriologic identification is made and drug susceptibility results are obtained. At that point, it may be possible to discontinue unnecessary drugs and implement specific monotherapy.

Unfavorable Drug Combinations

As mentioned above, antagonistic drug combinations can sometimes be used in combination chemotherapy regimens, although this situation is to be avoided if possible. Antagonism is most commonly observed when static drugs are used in combination with cidal drugs. For example, **tetracyclines** are bacteriostatic antimicrobials that antagonize the bactericidal activity of **penicillins** (see Chapter 34). Recall that the bactericidal activity of penicillins depends on cell growth. By inhibiting the transpeptidation reaction involved in bacterial cell wall cross-linking, the penicillins create an imbalance between cell wall synthesis and autolysin-mediated cell wall degradation. If the bacterial cell continues to grow, this leads to spheroplast formation and eventually to osmotic lysis. A protein synthesis inhibitor such as tetracycline, which arrests cell growth, would therefore antagonize the effect of a β-lactam. Similarly, **imidazoles** and **triazoles** are fungistatic agents that antagonize the fungicidal activity of **amphotericin B** (see Chapter 36). The mechanism of antagonism can be appreciated by noting that amphotericin B acts by binding ergosterol and forming pores in the fungal membrane, whereas imidazoles and triazoles inhibit a microsomal cytochrome P450-dependent enzyme, 14α-sterol demethylase, which is involved in ergosterol biosynthesis. Thus, the imidazoles and triazoles oppose the action of amphotericin B by decreasing the concentration of the target for the latter drug. Despite these considerations, static and cidal antimicrobial drugs are sometimes used clinically in combination when no good alternatives exist. In such cases, it may be necessary to increase the dose of one or both drugs to compensate for the antagonistic drug–drug interaction. The resulting increase in the therapeutic drug concentration(s) can increase the likelihood of adverse effects.

▌ ANTIVIRAL COMBINATION THERAPY

For certain viruses, no drug provides long-term suppressive benefit when used as a single agent. This phenomenon, which is due largely to the development of drug resistance, has been most studied with HIV.

The viral life cycle is central to understanding the reason that monotherapy for HIV fails to suppress long-term viral replication (see Chapter 38, Pharmacology of Viral

Infections; Fig. 38-2). After virus attachment, entry, and uncoating, the viral enzyme reverse transcriptase (RT) synthesizes double-stranded DNA from the single-stranded viral RNA genome. The DNA is then integrated into the host cell genome and transcribed over and over using the host cell's transcription machinery. These complete genomic transcripts are eventually packaged into virions that infect new cells. However, HIV RT is relatively unfaithful, so replication error rates are quite high. In addition, transcription of the integrated DNA into RNA is also error prone. As a result, on average, every new HIV particle contains one mutation relative to its parental virus. The resulting error rate is not so high as to be intolerable to the virus, but it is sufficiently high that, after repeated cycles of infection, reverse transcription, and transcription, a substantial number of viruses encode altered targets of anti-HIV therapy and thereby acquire resistance, even prior to treatment.

In the setting of high mutation rates, combination antiviral therapy is beneficial. Combinations of RT inhibitors (as first shown for zidovudine and lamivudine) are more effective than one RT inhibitor alone, in part because resistance to one nucleoside analogue does not necessarily confer resistance to another. The current standard of care for treatment of HIV infection is "triple therapy." Triple therapy can use many combinations—for example, two nucleoside analogue RT inhibitors and a nonnucleoside reverse transcriptase inhibitor (NNRTI), two nucleoside analogues and a protease inhibitor, or two nucleoside analogues and an integrase inhibitor. Clinical trials have shown that such combinations are able to reduce viral RNA plasma levels below the limit of detection (typically, 50 copies/mL). At such low levels of viral replication, the probability of resistance emerging to any one of the drugs is greatly reduced. Thus, for example, it has been shown that combinations remain effective for much longer periods of time than does any single agent.

Although combination formulations of common anti-HIV therapies have reduced "pill burden," simplified treatment, and increased adherence, the adverse effects of some combinations can result in reduced adherence. Despite these concerns, data from randomized clinical trials now provide conclusive evidence for the use of combination antiretroviral therapy regardless of the stage of disease. Therefore, treatment guidelines in the United States as well as those developed by WHO now recommend universal treatment of all patients with HIV infection, regardless of CD4 T-cell counts.

Combination chemotherapy has also become common for treatment of other viruses that require prolonged therapy and have high mutation rates, such as hepatitis B virus (HBV) and hepatitis C virus (HCV). For HIV, HBV, and HCV, an important strategy in designing combination regimens is to include drugs that are less likely to select for resistant mutants because the mutants that are selected are also less fit.

ANTINEOPLASTIC COMBINATION CHEMOTHERAPY

Several intrinsic difficulties are faced in the administration of antineoplastic chemotherapy. *Cancer cells can be thought of as "altered self" cells that maintain similarities to normal, noncancerous cells, often making it difficult to target the cancer cells selectively.* Also, many cancer chemotherapeutic agents have serious adverse effects that limit their dose and frequency of administration. Despite these hurdles, combination chemotherapy has led to remarkable advances in the treatment of cancer, including the examples of Hodgkin's disease and testicular cancer discussed at the end of this section. Table 41-2 provides an overview of the major antineoplastic drug classes that are currently available, including their mechanisms of action, cell cycle specificities, major resistance mechanisms, and dose-limiting toxicities. Note that all these drug classes have been discussed in previous chapters; the following discussion integrates relevant information about the individual drugs in a clinical context.

General Considerations

To appreciate the challenges that must be faced in treating cancer with drug therapies, it is useful to examine the current model for oncogenic transformation. Normal somatic cells undergo differentiation as they mature from a small regenerating stem cell population. Because cells lose the ability to divide as they progress along their differentiation pathway, malignancies tend to arise in populations of immature or undifferentiated cells. At the molecular level, the process of malignant transformation involves multiple steps, including the loss of tumor suppressor gene products (e.g., p53 and Rb) and the activation of proto-oncogenes (e.g., RAS and c-MYC) through processes such as somatic mutation, DNA translocation, and gene amplification. Acquired alterations in genes that regulate the progression of cells through the cell cycle confer a growth advantage on malignant cells, which proliferate in the absence of normal growth regulatory signals. Some of the most aggressive transformed cells multiply at a rate of about two divisions a day. At this rate, a single such cell could give rise to a clinically detectable mass of 1 g (10^9 cells) in just 15 days, and a tumor burden of 1 kg (10^{12} cells), which is often incompatible with life, could be achieved in 20 days.

Fortunately, oncogenesis usually occurs much more slowly than this—a fact that supports the concept of screening for many types of cancer (e.g., cervical, prostate, and colon). A malignant cell can give rise to a small colony of cells (10^6 cells) rather quickly, but further growth is held in check by the limited availability of oxygen and nutrients. Because oxygen can diffuse passively in tissues over a distance of only 2–3 mm, cells in the center of the growing tumor mass become hypoxic and enter the G0 (resting) phase. Accordingly, the percentage of cells that are actively dividing (i.e., the growth fraction of the tumor) decreases as tumor size increases. Moreover, the continued proliferation of cells at the tumor margins causes a further decrease in the pO_2 in the center of the tumor, and hypoxic tumor cells begin to die (central necrosis). The tumor continues to grow, albeit at a slower rate, because the rate of cell division at the margins exceeds the rate of central necrosis. At some point, hypoxic tumor cells can express or induce the stromal expression of angiogenic factors (e.g., vascular endothelial growth factor [VEGF]) that induce vascularization and thus oxygenation of the tumor. Vascularization can be accompanied by a sudden increase in the growth fraction as cells are pulled out of G0 phase and into the cell cycle.

Because a single malignant cell can expand clonally to give rise to a tumor, it is thought that every malignant cell must be destroyed to effect a cure of the cancer. This hypothesis, together with the "log-kill" hypothesis for tumor cell killing

TABLE 41-2 Classes of Cancer Chemotherapeutic Agents with Selected Examples

DRUG CLASS	MECHANISM OF ACTION	MAJOR RESISTANCE MECHANISM	DOSE-LIMITING TOXICITY
Alkylating agents Cyclophosphamide	Cross-link DNA, RNA, protein (Cell cycle nonspecific)	↑ DNA repair, ↓ drug uptake, ↑ drug inactivation	Bone marrow
Platinum complexes Cisplatin	DNA intrastrand cross-links (G-G) (Cell cycle nonspecific)	↑ DNA repair, ↓ drug uptake, ↑ drug inactivation	Kidney
Antimetabolites **Folic acid metabolism** Methotrexate **Purine analogues** Mercaptopurine **Pyrimidine analogues** Fluorouracil	Disrupt nucleotide synthesis, utilization, incorporation (Cell cycle S-phase specific)	↓ drug uptake, ↓ drug activation, ↑ drug inactivation, ↑ or altered target enzyme, salvage pathway	Bone marrow
Substituted urea Hydroxyurea	Inhibits ribonucleotide reductase (Cell cycle S-phase specific)	↑ DNA repair, ↓ drug uptake, ↑ drug inactivation	Bone marrow
Natural products **Bleomycin**	DNA strand scission (Cell cycle G2-phase specific)	↑ DNA repair?, ↓ drug uptake?, ↑ drug inactivation?, ↑ drug efflux?	Pulmonary fibrosis
Camptothecins Camptothecin	Inhibit topoisomerase I (Cell cycle S-phase specific)	↑ drug efflux?	Bone marrow
Anthracyclines Doxorubicin	DNA intercalation, inhibit topoisomerase II, lipid peroxidation (Cell cycle G2-phase specific)	↑ drug efflux	Bone marrow, cardiotoxicity
Epipodophyllotoxins Etoposide	Inhibit topoisomerase II (Cell cycle S/G2-phase specific)	↑ drug efflux	Bone marrow, GI toxicity (diarrhea)
Vinca alkaloids Vincristine	Disrupt microtubule assembly (Cell cycle M-phase specific)	↑ drug efflux	Bone marrow, neuropathy
Taxanes Paclitaxel	Disrupt microtubule disassembly (Cell cycle M-phase specific)	↑ drug efflux	Bone marrow (mild)
Differentiating agents Tretinoin	Retinoic acid receptor α agonist (Induce differentiation of cancer cells)	PML-RAR-α fusion gene mutation	Retinoic acid syndrome
Endogenous pathway modifiers **Hormone modulators** Prednisone	Glucocorticoid receptor agonist	Loss of hormone sensitivity (↑ or altered target receptor)	Cushingoid syndrome
Tamoxifen	Estrogen receptor antagonist/ modulator	Loss of estrogen-dependent growth	Endometrial cancer, thrombosis
Anastrozole	Aromatase inhibitor	Loss of estrogen-dependent growth	Osteoporosis
Flutamide	Androgen receptor antagonist	Loss of androgen-dependent growth	Hepatotoxicity
Leuprolide	GnRH receptor agonist	Loss of androgen-dependent growth	Osteoporosis
Immunomodulatory drugs Interferon-α	Interferon receptor agonist, specific mechanism unknown		Bone marrow, neurotoxicity, cardiotoxicity
Interleukin-2	IL-2 receptor agonist (stimulates T- and B-cell proliferation and differentiation)		Hypotension, pulmonary edema
(See Table 54-2 for more examples)			
Targeted delivery of compounds or proteins **Toxin conjugates** Denileukin diftitox	Delivers diphtheria toxin to cells expressing IL-2 receptor	Reduction in receptor expression	Severe edema, flu-like systemic symptoms
Small-molecule conjugates Gemtuzumab ozogamicin	Delivers calicheamicin to myeloid leukemia cells expressing CD33	Reduction in receptor expression	Hepatotoxicity, infusion reactions
Radiotherapy conjugates Iodine-131 tositumomab	Delivers radioactive iodine to cells expressing CD20	Reduction in receptor expression	Hypersensitivity reactions, bone marrow
(See Table 54-5 for more examples)			

continues

TABLE 41-2 Classes of Cancer Chemotherapeutic Agents with Selected Examples *continued*

DRUG CLASS	MECHANISM OF ACTION	MAJOR RESISTANCE MECHANISM	DOSE-LIMITING TOXICITY
Growth factor receptor and signal transduction antagonists			
Cetuximab	Binds to and inhibits epidermal growth factor receptor (EGFR)	EGFR mutation	Skin, GI toxicity (diarrhea)
Trastuzumab	Binds to ErbB2 (HER2/*neu*) cell surface receptor and controls cancer cell growth	Signaling pathway modulation, binding site disruption	Cardiotoxicity
BCR-Abl/C-KIT/PDGFR inhibitors	Inhibit protein tyrosine kinase domain	Mutation in target enzyme (e.g., BCR-Abl mutation)	Skin, GI (diarrhea), fluid retention
(See Chapter 40 and Table 54-4 for more examples)			
Proteasome inhibitors			
Bortezomib	Inhibits protein degradation by proteasome	p53 mutation, ↑ HSP-27 expression	Neurotoxicity, bone marrow
Angiogenesis inhibitors			
Bevacizumab	Binds to and neutralizes vascular endothelial growth factor (VEGF)	Multiple adaptive and/or intrinsic mechanisms to evade VEGF dependence of tumor angiogenesis	Kidney (proteinuria), hypertension

(see Chapter 33), suggests that *multiple cycles of chemotherapy must be administered at the highest tolerable doses and the most frequent tolerable intervals to achieve a cure.* Antineoplastic chemotherapy usually follows first-order kinetics (i.e., a constant *fraction* of tumor cells is killed with each cycle of chemotherapy). These kinetics of tumor cell killing are unlike the time-dependent killing characteristic of many antimicrobial drugs, which follows zero-order kinetics (i.e., a fixed *number* of microbes is killed per unit time).

Adding to the difficulty of curative cancer treatment is the phenomenon of tumor progression, in which a clonally derived population of malignant cells becomes heterogeneous through the accumulation of multiple genetic and epigenetic alterations. When subjected to immune surveillance or the administration of an antineoplastic agent, subclones of the tumor with relatively nonantigenic or drug-resistant phenotypes are selected. Mutations that confer drug resistance are of particular concern, because many transformed cells, having lost the ability to repair DNA damage, are characterized by genomic instability. Thus, deletions, gene amplifications, translocations, and point mutations are not infrequent events and can result in antineoplastic drug resistance through any of the mechanisms shown in Table 41-3.

With the possible exception of some recently developed classes of antineoplastic therapies directed against molecular targets that are selectively expressed by a malignant clone of cells (e.g., a monoclonal antibody directed against a tumor cell antigen or an enzyme inhibitor directed against a mutated signal transduction molecule; see Chapter 1, Drug–Receptor Interactions; Chapter 40, Pharmacology of Cancer: Signal Transduction; and Chapter 54, Protein Therapeutics), antineoplastic chemotherapy has focused on differences in the cell cycle between rapidly dividing and normal cells. Some of these agents act by inducing DNA damage and subsequent apoptosis in all phases of the cell cycle, whereas others act selectively in one phase of the cell cycle (see Chapter 33, especially Fig. 33-4). Unfortunately, such drugs are also associated with significant

TABLE 41-3 Mechanisms of Tumor Resistance to Cytotoxic Chemotherapeutic Agents

MECHANISM OF TUMOR RESISTANCE	EXAMPLES
Pharmacokinetic Mechanisms	
Insufficient accumulation of drug	
Insufficient uptake of drug	Methotrexate
Efflux of drug from tumor cell (MDR phenotype)	Vinca alkaloids, etoposides, doxorubicin
Unfavorable metabolism of drug or prodrug	
Insufficient activation of prodrug	5-FU, 6-MP, Ara-C, 6-TG
Increased inactivation of drug	Ara-C
Cytidine deaminase overexpression	6-TG, 6-MP
Alkaline phosphatase overexpression	
Pharmacodynamic Mechanisms	
Overexpression, alteration, or loss of target molecule*	
Dihydrofolate reductase	Methotrexate
Decreased concentration of cofactor	5-FU
Increased concentration of competing molecule	Ara-C metabolite (dCTP)
Increased repair of drug-induced lesions in DNA, proteins, or lipids (membranes)	Alkylating agents
Increased utilization of alternate pathways	Antimetabolites
Loss of drug-induced apoptosis	Most antineoplastics

*Due to DNA mutation, amplification, deletion, or epigenetic change; altered transcription or post-transcriptional processing; altered translation or post-translational modification; or altered target stability.

toxicity, especially in tissues that normally have a high rate of cell turnover (e.g., bone marrow, hair follicles, intestinal epithelia). Accordingly, neutropenia, thrombocytopenia, anemia, alopecia, nausea, and oral and intestinal ulcerations are common adverse effects of many cytotoxic antineoplastic agents.

Although many rapidly growing lymphomas and leukemias seem to melt away with antineoplastic chemotherapy, more indolent solid tumors must often be treated with adjuvant (i.e., chemotherapy-enhancing) radiation therapy and/or surgery. By the time these tumors come to clinical attention, they may be large and may have metastasized. In such cases, surgical removal of the primary tumor is often followed by radiation therapy and/or systemic chemotherapy, using agents that penetrate the various tissues that could be sites of metastatic disease (e.g., brain, liver).

In summary, cancer therapy must eliminate every malignant cell from the body, making high doses of chemotherapeutic agents desirable. (In practice, immune mechanisms may be able to clear small numbers of remaining cancer cells if these cells are sufficiently immunogenic. Monoclonal antibody therapies that enhance the immunogenicity of cancer cells have recently been approved; these "immune checkpoint inhibitors" block immune co-regulatory pathways such as B7/CTLA-4 and PD-1/PD-L1.) However, the toxicity of these relatively nonselective agents limits their achievable doses. Moreover, resistance to these drugs can develop. Finally, because these agents target mainly rapidly dividing cells, antineoplastic drugs are less effective against large solid tumors with low growth fractions. Each of these considerations points to the need for combination drug regimens to treat cancer. The basic pharmacologic principles for such regimens are discussed below.

Rationale for Combination Chemotherapy

Combination antineoplastic drug regimens typically include agents that act on different molecular targets, at different phases of the cell cycle, and with different dose-limiting toxicities (Table 41-2). This strategy targets asynchronously dividing tumor cells, reduces the emergence of drug resistance, and allows each drug to be given at its highest tolerable dose, thereby maximizing efficacy without excessive toxicity. Recent advances in supportive therapy have also increased the maximum tolerated doses for many cytotoxic antineoplastic agents. For example, the routine use of antiemetics, autologous bone marrow transplantation, hematopoietic growth factors (e.g., **GM-CSF**, **G-CSF**, **erythropoietin**), and prophylactic broad-spectrum antibiotics has reduced the complications of myelosuppressive chemotherapy regimens. Similarly, **allopurinol** treatment to prevent the hyperuricemia that could result from widespread release and metabolism of purines from necrotic tumor cells (i.e., **tumor lysis syndrome**) has reduced the morbidity associated with high doses of systemic chemotherapy (see Chapter 49, Integrative Inflammation Pharmacology: Gout). Finally, so-called **leucovorin rescue** after high-dose **methotrexate** administration selectively spares nonmalignant cells from death associated with tetrahydrofolate depletion (see Chapter 33).

Unlike the treatment of bacterial and viral infections, cytotoxic chemotherapy for cancer often employs an intermittent dosing strategy. The main rationale for this strategy is to avoid unacceptable toxicity to normal cells and tissues, for example, by allowing time for bone marrow recovery. Intermittent dosing may also have the advantage of "pulling" some nondividing cells out of the G0 phase of the cell cycle and making them more susceptible to subsequent cycles of chemotherapy. The latter rationale has prompted the use of adjuvant radiation therapy and the inclusion of cell cycle nonspecific drugs in certain combination chemotherapy regimens; both of these strategies have been noted to increase the growth fractions of tumors in some studies. Despite these considerations, continuous delivery of cytotoxic chemotherapeutic agents is occasionally beneficial in treating slowly cycling tumors (e.g., multiple myeloma) or in cases where bolus infusion of drug is associated with significantly higher toxicity (e.g., **anthracyclines**). Many of the growth factor receptor and signal transduction antagonists used in cancer chemotherapy are less toxic than the older cytotoxic antineoplastic agents. The reduced toxicity of these antagonists permits their use in daily dosing regimens, both as single agents and in combination with cytotoxic chemotherapy. One example of such a combination is **lapatinib** (an inhibitor of EGFR and HER2) and **capecitabine** (a prodrug form of fluorouracil) in the treatment of HER2-positive metastatic breast cancer (see Chapter 40).

Finally, some antineoplastic drug combinations take advantage of known synergies. A clinically important example is the interaction between **5-fluorouracil (5-FU)** and **methotrexate**. These drugs are used in combination in the treatment of many adenocarcinomas, including breast, colon, and prostate cancers. Both drugs are S-phase specific and have common dose-limiting toxicities (bone marrow and intestinal mucosal damage), so their use in combination may seem surprising (see Chapter 33 and Chapter 39, Pharmacology of Cancer: Genome Synthesis, Stability, and Maintenance). The mechanism of synergy appears to involve the ability of methotrexate to enhance activation of 5-FU. Recall that methotrexate inhibits purine biosynthesis and that 5-FU is metabolized by cellular salvage pathways that ultimately convert the drug into the active form 5-FdUMP. The first step in the activation of 5-FU requires 5-phosphoribosyl 1-pyrophosphate (PRPP) and is catalyzed by the enzyme phosphoribosyl transferase: 5-FU + PRPP → 5-FUMP + PP$_i$. Methotrexate increases cellular levels of PRPP, likely due to decreased PRPP utilization in purine synthesis pathways. The elevated PRPP levels favor the conversion of 5-FU to 5-FUMP, which is ultimately converted to 5-FdUMP by the action of ribonucleotide reductase and other enzymes.

Examples of Antineoplastic Combination Chemotherapy

Hodgkin's Disease

The treatment of Hodgkin's disease (HD) illustrates the rational use of cytotoxic antineoplastic drug combinations. In this disease, there is clonal proliferation of Reed-Sternberg (RS) cells within a dense, reactive inflammatory cell background. HD originates in a single lymph node and progresses in a contiguous fashion involving adjacent lymphoid tissues. The RS cell is the neoplastic cell; this cell seems to be of B-cell origin, making the disease a true lymphoma. Pathologic subtypes of classical HD, defined on the basis of RS cell morphology and the pattern of surrounding reactive inflammatory changes, include nodular sclerosing, mixed cellularity, lymphocyte-rich, and lymphocyte-depleted HD.

Patients typically present with lymphadenopathy (cervical, supraclavicular, axillary, or inguinal) and/or systemic

TABLE 41-4 The Cotswold/Ann Arbor Staging System for Hodgkin's Disease (HD)*

STAGE	DESCRIPTION	SUBCLASSIFICATION
I	Involvement of a single lymph node region or lymphatic organ (e.g., thymus)	IA: No systemic symptoms IB: Systemic symptoms (e.g., fever, night sweats, weight loss) IE: Involvement of one area of a single organ outside the lymph system
II	Involvement of two or more lymph node regions on the same side of the diaphragm	IIA: No systemic symptoms IIB: Systemic symptoms IIE: Extranodal contiguous extension from one lymph node region into a nearby organ
III	Involvement of nodal regions on both sides of the diaphragm	IIIA: No systemic symptoms IIIB: Systemic symptoms IIIS: Splenic involvement IIIE: Extranodal contiguous extension
IV	Diffuse or disseminated disease involving one or more extralymphatic organs (e.g., liver, bone marrow, lungs, cerebrospinal fluid)	IVA: No systemic symptoms IVB: Systemic symptoms

*Note: Bulky disease or massive disease (denoted by adding the letter X to the stage) is sometimes used to describe HD tumor masses that measure at least one-third of the diameter of the chest or that are at least 10 cm in diameter in non-chest sites.

symptoms including fever, malaise, pruritus, night sweats, and weight loss. The stage of the disease determines treatment; patients with early-stage disease (stages I and II) receive radiation therapy with or without chemotherapy, and patients with advanced-stage disease (stages III and IV) require combination chemotherapy (Table 41-4).

Before the introduction of alkylating agents in the mid-1960s, single-agent chemotherapy for advanced HD resulted in a median survival of 1 year. With the development of **MOPP** (**mechlorethamine**, **vincristine** [**oncovin**], **procarbazine**, and **prednisone**), the first successful antineoplastic drug combination for HD, half of these patients were cured of their disease. Treatment remained limited by significant toxicity, however, including early gastrointestinal and neurological complications as well as late sterility and secondary malignancies (myelodysplastic syndrome, acute nonlymphocytic leukemia, and non-Hodgkin's lymphoma). Further investigation led to the development of the **ABVD** (**doxorubicin** [**adriamycin**], **bleomycin**, **vinblastine**, and **dacarbazine**) combination, which is less toxic and more effective than MOPP. ABVD is the current standard of care for early-stage HD and a preferred treatment option for advanced-stage HD; trials of novel combination therapies are also underway.

The rationale for the ABVD drug combination comes from the knowledge that it combines both cell cycle selective and nonselective agents as well as drugs with different dose-limiting toxicities. Compared to MOPP, ABVD is associated with significantly fewer hematological and gonadal complications and secondary malignancies.

Testicular Cancer

Principles of antineoplastic combination chemotherapy are also exemplified in the treatment of testicular cancer. This tumor arises from the spermatogenic epithelium of the testis and is usually detected as a testicular mass on physical examination. The tumor metastasizes through lymphatic channels to pelvic and periaortic lymph nodes before disseminating widely through hematogenous routes. Treatment of local disease (without evidence of metastasis) involves surgical removal of the affected testis with or without pelvic radiation. Advanced disease requires systemic treatment with combination chemotherapy. One standard-of-care regimen is **BEP** (Fig. 41-4). Of the three drugs commonly used in this regimen (**bleomycin**, **etoposide**, and **cisplatin**), cisplatin is a cell cycle nonspecific drug that may draw nondividing tumor cells into the actively cycling pool, where they are susceptible to the synergistic action of the cell cycle specific agents bleomycin and etoposide. The drugs in this combination have different molecular targets, act on different phases of the cell cycle, and have different dose-limiting toxicities. Intermittent dosing allows each affected organ (lung, bone marrow, and kidney, respectively) time to recover between cycles. Administered after surgical removal of the primary tumor, such a regimen usually results in a cure.

Treatment of Refractory or Recurrent Disease

Despite the fact that combination chemotherapy has resulted in vastly improved survival for some cancers, many cancers become refractory to standard combination chemotherapy. If a standard chemotherapy regimen fails, options include experimental drug therapies, palliative care, or novel drugs approved for use after treatment failure. Many patients choose to enroll in experimental clinical trials. This decision may be

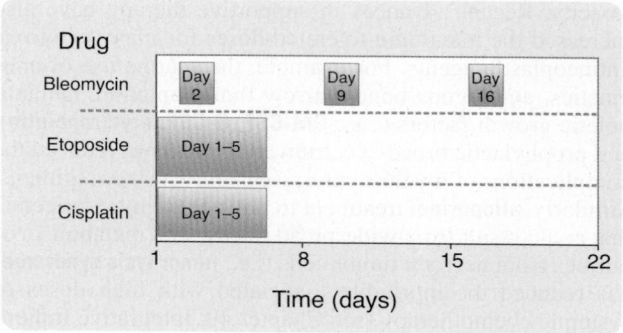

FIGURE 41-4. **The bleomycin-etoposide-platinum (BEP) combination chemotherapy regimen for testicular cancer.** The BEP regimen used to treat testicular cancer consists of a combination of bleomycin, etoposide, and a platinum compound. Cisplatin, a platinum compound often used in this regimen, is a cell cycle nonspecific agent; this drug may draw nondividing cells into the cell cycle, where they can be killed by the G2-phase-specific agent bleomycin and the S/G2-phase-specific agent etoposide. The intermittent dosing schedule limits drug toxicity and allows time for the bone marrow to recover from drug-induced myelosuppression. The 3-week cycle shown is typically administered four times in succession (12 weeks total).

based on the hope that an investigational agent could prove efficacious but with the understanding that the true benefit may be realized only by future patients. Palliative and hospice care are alternatives to continued drug treatment in cases of advanced metastatic disease. An increasing number of agents with novel mechanisms of action are becoming available for disease that is otherwise refractory to treatment. Many of these agents selectively target tumor-specific antigens and signal transduction pathways, as discussed in Chapters 40 and 54. Other agents are being designed and tested to target recently discovered pathways that allow tumors to alter cellular energetics and evade immune destruction (see above). Optimizing combinations of these and other antineoplastic agents for efficacy and safety will be an important challenge for the future.

CONCLUSION AND FUTURE DIRECTIONS

The principles of combination chemotherapy highlight the importance of combination drug treatment in a variety of clinical situations. The use of drug combinations has greatly enhanced the effectiveness of treatment of both infectious and neoplastic diseases. The advantages offered by multidrug regimens over individual drug therapy (monotherapy) include increased antimicrobial, antiviral, and antineoplastic efficacy; decreased overall drug resistance; decreased host toxicity; and broader coverage of suspected pathogenic organisms. These advantages are illustrated in the rational use of drug combinations to treat infections with *Mycobacterium tuberculosis* and HIV, as well as neoplastic disorders such as Hodgkin's disease and testicular cancer. Treatment of multidrug-resistant microorganisms such as MDR-TB and MDR-HIV remains a special challenge, as does treatment of genetically heterogeneous cancers with low growth fractions such as lung, colon, breast, and prostate cancers. Continued refinement of combination chemotherapy regimens will rely on increased understanding of molecular targets and metabolic pathways used by microorganisms and cancer cells.

Acknowledgment

We thank Shreya Kangovi and Gia Landry for initial drafts of the case of Mr. M and the discussion in the chapter related to his case. We thank Ryan L. Albritton for his valuable contributions to this chapter in the First and Second Editions of *Principles of Pharmacology: The Pathophysiologic Basis of Drug Therapy* and Daniel Kuritzkes for helpful comments.

Suggested Reading

Canellos GP, Anderson JR, Propert KJ, et al. Chemotherapy of advanced Hodgkin's disease with MOPP, ABVD, or MOPP alternating with ABVD. *N Engl J Med* 1992;327:1478–1484. (*ABVD remains a standard of care for advanced Hodgkin's disease.*)

Chou TC. Theoretical basis, experimental design, and computerized simulation of synergism and antagonism in drug combination studies. *Pharmacol Rev* 2006;58:621–681. (*Detailed analysis of models for synergistic, antagonistic, and additive drug combinations.*)

Chou TC, Talalay P. Quantitative analysis of dose-effect relationships: the combined effects of multiple drugs or enzyme inhibitors. *Adv Enzyme Regul* 1984;22:27–55. (*Detailed analysis of models for synergistic, antagonistic, and additive drug combinations.*)

Dancey JE, Chen HX. Strategies for optimizing combinations of molecular targeted anticancer agents. *Nat Rev Drug Discov* 2006;5:649–659. (*Discusses principles for determining combinations of antineoplastic agents that could be most promising to test in preclinical and clinical trials.*)

Edge SB, Byrd DR, Compton CC, Fritz AG, Greene FL, Trottie A III, eds. *AJCC cancer staging manual.* 7th ed. New York: Springer; 2010:607–611. (*Lists staging criteria for human cancers.*)

Gunthard HF, Aberg JA, Eron JJ, et al. Antiretroviral treatment of adult HIV infection: 2014 recommendations of the International Antiviral Society—USA Panel. *JAMA* 2014;312:410–425. (*Reviews combination therapies recommended for treatment of HIV.*)

Hanahan D, Weinberg RA. Hallmarks of cancer: the next generation. *Cell* 2011;144:646–674. (*Reviews hallmarks of cancer and discusses therapeutic targeting of pathways required for tumor growth and progression.*)

Harvey RJ. Synergism in the folate pathway. *Rev Infect Dis* 1982;4:255–260. (*Describes kinetics of synergism between trimethoprim and the sulfonamides.*)

Luo J, Solimini NL, Elledge SJ. Principles of cancer therapy: oncogene and non-oncogene addiction. *Cell* 2009;136:823–837. (*Reviews antineoplastic therapies targeting the hallmarks of cancer and proposes principles for developing new antineoplastic therapies and combinations.*)

Momtaz P, Postow MA. Immunologic checkpoints in cancer therapy: focus on the programmed death-1 (PD-1) receptor pathway. *Pharmgenomics Pers Med* 2014;7:357–365. (*Reviews pathways of immune evasion in cancer and therapeutic rationale for development of immune checkpoint inhibitors that block CTLA-4 and PD-1 pathways.*)

Paltiel AD, Walensky RP, Schackman BR, et al. Expanded HIV screening in the United States: effect on clinical outcomes, HIV transmission, and costs. *Ann Intern Med* 2006;145:797–806. (*Compares benefits, risks, and costs of screening for HIV.*)

Panel on Antiretroviral Guidelines for Adults and Adolescents. Guidelines for the use of antiretroviral agents in HIV-1-infected adults and adolescents. http://aidsinfo.nih.gov/contentfiles/lvguidelines/adultandadolescentgl.pdf. (*Reviews combination therapies recommended for treatment of HIV.*)

World Health Organization. *Guidelines for the programmatic management of drug-resistant tuberculosis: 2011 update.* Geneva, Switzerland: World Health Organization; 2011. http://www.ncbi.nlm.nih.gov/books/NBK148644/. (*Evaluates evidence and recommends treatment regimens for multidrug-resistant tuberculosis and extensively drug-resistant tuberculosis.*)

Zumla A, Raviglione M, Hafner R, von Reyn CF. Tuberculosis. *N Engl J Med* 2013;368:745–755. (*Reviews current recommendations for treatment and status of selected trials of treatment for latent tuberculosis infection, drug-sensitive active tuberculosis, and drug-resistant active tuberculosis.*)

VI

Pluripotent hematopoietic
stem cell

Trilineage
~~myeloid stem cell~~

Principles of Inflammation and
Immune Pharmacology

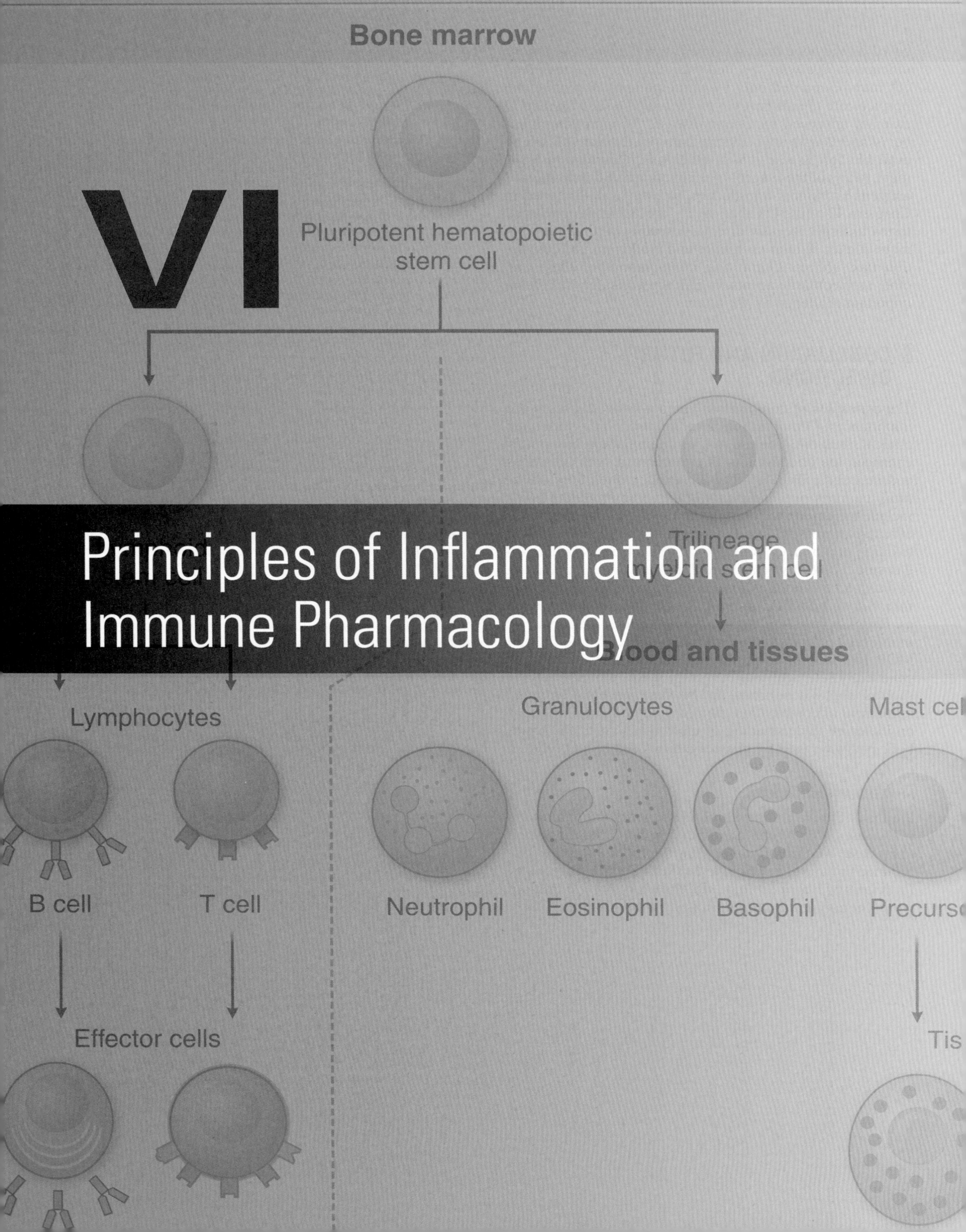

Blood and tissues

Lymphocytes

Granulocytes

Mast cell

B cell

T cell

Neutrophil

Eosinophil

Basophil

Precursor

Effector cells

Tis

Principles of Inflammation and the Immune System

Eryn L. Royer and April W. Armstrong

INTRODUCTION

Inflammation and the immune system are closely intertwined. Inflammation is composed of a complex web of responses to tissue injury and infection, characterized by the classic signs of *rubor* (redness), *calor* (heat), *tumor* (swelling), *dolor* (pain), and *functio laesa* (loss of function). The immune system includes the cells and soluble factors, such as antibodies and complement proteins, which mediate the inflammatory response; these cells and factors both eliminate the inciting inflammatory stimulus and initiate immunologic memory.

A normal inflammatory response is an acute process that resolves after removal of the inciting stimulus. Diseases of inflammation and immunity can occur due to inappropriate inflammation or when the normal inflammatory response progresses to chronic inflammation, either because of a long-term inappropriate response to a stimulus (e.g., allergies) or because the offending agent is not removed (e.g., chronic infection, transplantation, and autoimmunity).

Two pharmacologic strategies are used to target the pathophysiology of immune diseases. The first involves modification of the signaling mediators of the inflammatory process or suppression of components of the immune system. This is the rationale for drugs that modulate eicosanoid pathways (Chapter 43, Pharmacology of Eicosanoids), histamine (Chapter 44, Histamine Pharmacology), and cells of the immune system (Chapter 45, Pharmacology of Hematopoiesis

and Immunomodulation, and Chapter 46, Pharmacology of Immunosuppression). This approach is still in its infancy, because it depends on understanding the molecular events in the relevant pathway, but it promises to yield multiple new drugs in the foreseeable future.

The second pharmacologic approach, used in diseases such as peptic ulcer disease (Chapter 47, Integrative Inflammation Pharmacology: Peptic Ulcer Disease), asthma (Chapter 48, Integrative Inflammation Pharmacology: Asthma), and gout (Chapter 49, Integrative Inflammation Pharmacology: Gout), involves modification of the underlying pathophysiologic stimulus, thus removing the impetus for inflammation. The difference between these two approaches is, at times, indistinct and will continue to overlap as the pathophysiology of chronic inflammatory disease is better understood at the molecular level.

This chapter provides sufficient background on the physiology of inflammation and the immune system to understand the subsequent chapters in this section of the textbook. The treatment is necessarily brief, with an emphasis on pharmacologically relevant targets of the inflammatory response. The chapter is organized in four parts. First, a general overview of the immune system is presented. Second, the molecular signals that mediate cellular communication and inflammation are introduced. Third, the immune and inflammatory cells and signaling molecules are discussed in the context of an integrated inflammatory response. Fourth, chronic

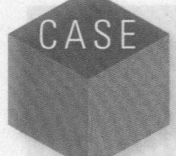

Mark is stressed—he has to take the US Medical Licensing Examination (USMLE) in 2 weeks, and he has barely begun to study. Throwing aside any pretense of a balanced lifestyle, Mark travels to the microbiology lab late one night to review techniques for performing a Gram stain. While applying the gentian violet component of the Gram stain, Mark cuts his thumb on the edge of the microscope slide. Thinking he lacks the time to clean his thumb properly, Mark continues to study furiously. Over the next 5 hours, Mark's thumb becomes progressively swollen, warm, red, and tender. Mark retains focus and continues to study through the evening. By that night, however, he develops a fever and increased swelling in the thumb. By the third day, pus builds up at the site. By the fourth day, however, Mark's body seems to have gotten the better of the offending agent. The swelling decreases, the site loses its distinctive angry red appearance, and his fever abruptly subsides. Relieved that he has not become a casualty of his own procrastination, Mark continues studying and performs well on his exam, not least because his wound has provided him with fundamental insights into immunology.

Questions

1. Which substance likely caused Mark's immune system to activate in response to bacteria in his wound?
2. Which mediators accounted for Mark's fever?
3. What changes in the vasculature accounted for the immediate swelling of Mark's thumb?
4. Which chemical signals mediated the inflammatory response in Mark's thumb?

inflammation, a pathologic state that is often associated with autoimmunity, is presented. For a more comprehensive presentation of this rapidly changing subject, see "Suggested Reading" at the end of this chapter.

OVERVIEW OF THE IMMUNE SYSTEM

The fundamental role of the immune system is to distinguish self from nonself. "Nonself" can be an infectious organism, a transplanted organ, or an endogenous tissue that is mistaken for something foreign. Because protection against infection is the classic role of the immune system, the terms *infection* and *infectious agent* are generally used to denote the inciting stimulus for an immune response. The immune system can be stimulated to react against any nonself agent.

Skin and other barrier tissues form the first line of defense against any infection. (In the introductory case, Mark's infection occurred only after he cut his skin.) Once an offending agent penetrates these barriers, the immune system mounts a response. The immune response consists of innate and adaptive responses. **Innate** responses are stereotyped reactions to a stimulus (e.g., release of histamine, phagocytosis of a bacterium). In some cases, innate responses are sufficient to neutralize the offending agent. Cells of the innate immune system, especially antigen-presenting cells, can also process the offending agent into small fragments; this processing is necessary for activation of the adaptive immune system. **Adaptive** responses are neutralizing reactions that are specific to the offending agent (e.g., antibodies, cytotoxic T cells). In general, then, *the innate immune system recognizes nonself and activates the response to an offending nonself agent; the adaptive immune system generates a response that specifically neutralizes or kills that agent.*

Many different cell types are involved in the immune system, and these cell types interact in a complex web of signaling and communication to create the overall response. The cells of the immune system derive from two types of pluripotent cells in the bone marrow: **myeloid** stem cells and **lymphoid** stem cells. The lymphoid stem cell is sometimes called the **common lymphoid stem cell** because it gives rise to both B cells and T cells. In general, myeloid stem cells give rise to precursor cells of the innate immune system, whereas lymphoid stem cells generate precursor cells of the adaptive immune system; there are some exceptions. Figure 42-1 depicts the myeloid and lymphoid stem cells and the mature cell types into which the precursor cells differentiate. The derivation of these cell types is also discussed in Chapter 45. A helpful conceptual framework is to envision the innate immune system as the immunologic memory of a *species*, which is invariant over the lifetime of an individual and generally the same among individuals of the species. In contrast, the adaptive immune system establishes the immunologic memory of an *individual* over his or her lifetime, depending on that individual's exposure to pathogens, vaccines, or other immunologic stimuli. Adaptive immunity, therefore, is relatively unique to each individual.

Innate Immunity

Cells of the innate immune system are the first responders to an offending agent that has penetrated the skin or another barrier (Table 42-1). Innate immune cells perform three important tasks. First, these cells defend against bacterial and parasitic infections, either by neutralizing the infectious agent with secreted cytotoxic proteins or by phagocytosis (engulfing) of the bacterium or parasite. Second, phagocytosis of the offending agent initiates proteolytic digestion of microbial macromolecules to fragments (antigens) that are then displayed, together with major histocompatibility complex (MHC) class II proteins, on the surface of antigen-presenting cells. In turn, these antigen-presenting cells, which include macrophages and dendritic cells, activate cells of the adaptive immune system. Third, innate immune cells secrete numerous cytokines (see below) that further amplify the immune response. The major cell types of the innate immune system include **granulocytes** (neutrophils, eosinophils, and basophils), **mast cells**, and **antigen-presenting cells** (macrophages and dendritic cells). Some immunologists consider natural killer (NK) cells, NK T cells, and γδ T cells to have innate immune roles; the biology of these cell types is beyond the scope of this text.

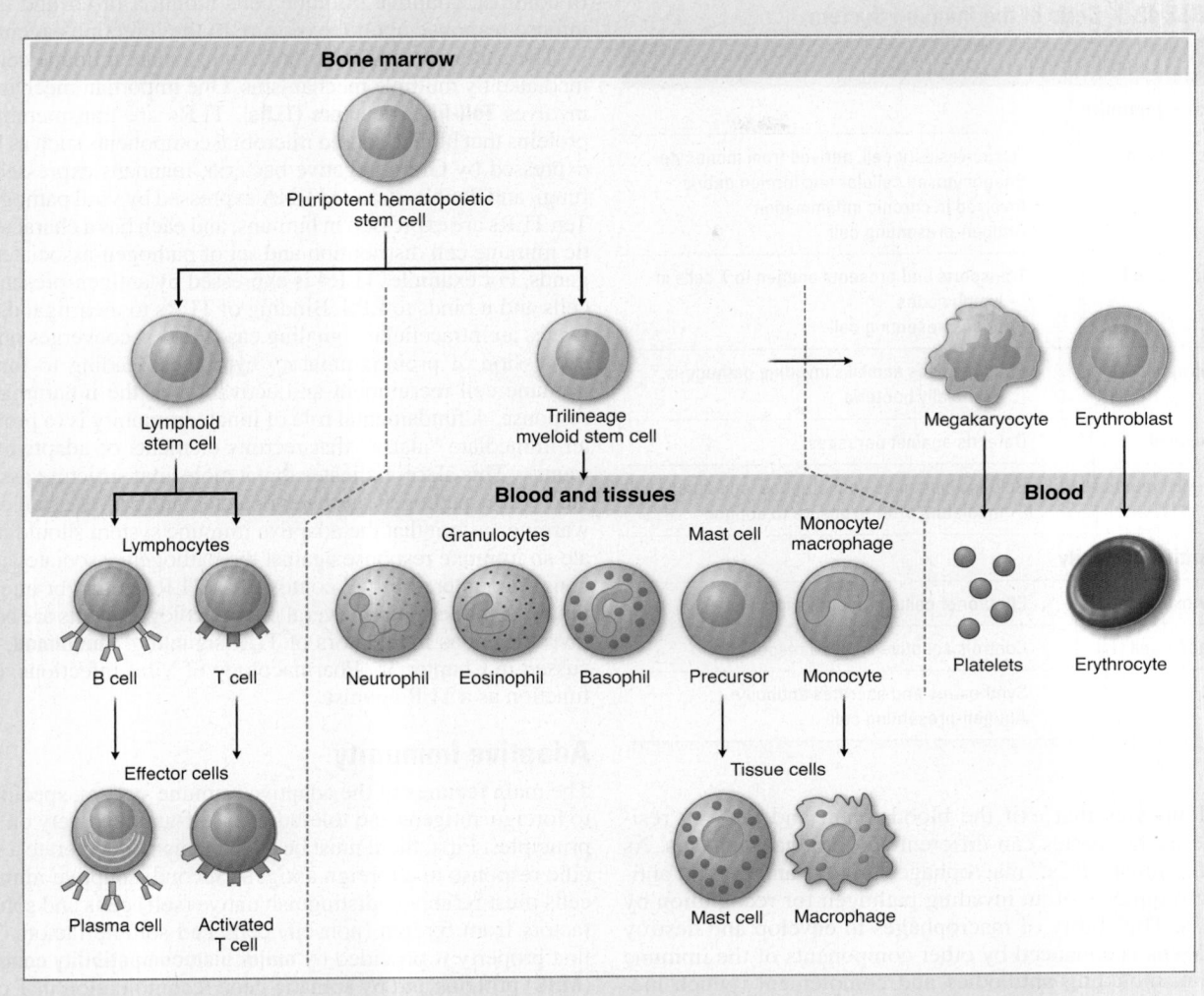

Bone marrow

Pluripotent hematopoietic stem cell

Lymphoid stem cell

Trilineage myeloid stem cell

Megakaryocyte   Erythroblast

Blood and tissues

Lymphocytes

Granulocytes

Mast cell

Monocyte/ macrophage

Blood

B cell   T cell

Neutrophil   Eosinophil   Basophil

Precursor   Monocyte

Platelets

Erythrocyte

Effector cells

Tissue cells

Plasma cell   Activated T cell

Mast cell   Macrophage

FIGURE 42-1. Development of cells of the immune system. All hematopoietic cells develop from the pluripotent hematopoietic stem cell. This cell gives rise to the lymphoid stem cell and the trilineage myeloid stem cell. The lymphoid stem cell and its progenitor cells (*not shown*) give rise to mature lymphocytes (B cells and T cells), the cells that mediate adaptive immune responses. When exposed to specific antigens, B cells differentiate into antibody-producing plasma cells, and T cells adopt an activated phenotype. The myeloid stem cell and its progenitor cells, including megakaryocytes, erythroblasts, and myeloid precursors (*not shown*), proliferate and differentiate into mature neutrophils, eosinophils, basophils, mast cells, monocytes, platelets, and erythrocytes. In the tissues, monocytes differentiate into macrophages or dendritic cells, and mast cell precursors differentiate into mast cells. (See Fig. 45-1 for more details about the differentiation of cell lineages in the bone marrow.)

Granulocyte is a descriptive term based on the appearance of the cytoplasmic granules within these cells. **Neutrophils**, the most abundant cell type of the innate immune system and the "first responders" in inflammation, are phagocytic cells primarily responsible for defense against bacterial infection. These cells envelop invading bacteria in phagocytic vesicles and destroy the bacteria within these vesicles using enzymes such as myeloperoxidase. **Eosinophils** are circulating granulocytes primarily involved in defense against parasitic infections. Because parasites are often too large to engulf, eosinophils attach to a parasite's exterior and secrete cytotoxic substances directly on the parasite. Both **basophils** (circulating) and **mast cells** (tissue-resident) bind IgE antibody, display this IgE on the cell surface, and maintain histamine-containing granules that are released when exogenous antigen binds to and cross-links the IgE. Basophils and mast cells are important in allergic responses. Eosinophils and

basophils are so named because they exhibit eosinophilic and basophilic patterns, respectively, when stained with Wright-Giemsa stain.

Antigen-Presenting Cells

Antigen-presenting cells (APCs) process the macromolecules (especially proteins) of an invading agent to display the processed fragments on the surface of the APC. In this form, the fragments serve as molecular fingerprints used by cells of the adaptive immune system to recognize the invading agent. APCs are important initiators of immune responses because, in addition to displaying nonself antigens to T cells (see below), they provide the costimulatory signals that are necessary for T-cell activation. The concept of **costimulation**, in which two separate signals are required to initiate an immune response to a stimulus, is discussed below.

TABLE 42-1 Cells of the Immune System

CELL TYPE	FUNCTION
Innate Immunity	
Macrophage	Tissue-resident cell, derived from monocyte Phagocytoses cellular and foreign debris Involved in chronic inflammation Antigen-presenting cell
Dendritic cell	Transports and presents antigen to T cells in lymph nodes Antigen-presenting cell
Neutrophil	Phagocytoses and kills invading pathogens, especially bacteria
Eosinophil	Defends against parasites
Basophil/mast cell	Release histamine, leukotrienes, and other mediators after exposure to antigen
Adaptive Immunity	
Cytotoxic T cell (T_C)	Effector of cellular adaptive immunity
Helper T cell (T_H)	Controls adaptive immune responses
B cell	Synthesizes and secretes antibody Antigen-presenting cell

Monocytes that exit the bloodstream and take up residence in the tissues can differentiate into **macrophages**. As "professional APCs," macrophages process and present antigenic fragments of an invading pathogen for recognition by T cells. The ability of macrophages to envelop and destroy pathogens is enhanced by other components of the immune system, including antibodies and complement (which mediate opsonization) and cytokines (which enhance killing ability). In addition, macrophages produce cytokines such as TNF-α that modify immune responses. **Dendritic cells** are the most important APCs for the initiation of adaptive immune responses. In the nonlymphoid tissues, dendritic cells engulf and process foreign antigens. Dendritic cells then migrate to lymphoid tissues, where they present these cognate antigens to T cells via specific molecular interactions.

Activation of the Innate Immune Response

Innate immune cells respond to common determinants that are present on many invading agents (for example, lipopolysaccharide [LPS] in the outer membrane of Gram-negative bacteria). In this role, innate immune cells use **pattern recognition** to phagocytose a class of infectious agents rather than a specific infectious agent. In contrast, adaptive immune cells, as discussed below, mount a specific response to the three-dimensional conformation of a particular antigen, referred to as an **epitope**. From a teleological perspective, innate immunity provides a broad gating function, attempting to counteract harmful effects of foreign invaders in a rapid manner and to determine whether an infectious agent should be further attacked by adaptive immunity, while adaptive immunity provides a specialized response that is specific to the particular invading infectious agent. In an individual, innate immune cells respond in the same way and to the same extent to repeated infections with the same agent.

In contrast, adaptive immune cells mount a faster and more intense response upon reexposure to the infectious agent.

The pattern recognition function of innate immune cells is mediated by multiple mechanisms. One important mechanism involves **Toll-like receptors (TLRs)**. TLRs are transmembrane proteins that bind to shared microbial components such as LPS expressed by Gram-negative bacteria, mannans expressed by fungi, and double-stranded RNA expressed by viral pathogens. Ten TLRs are expressed in humans, and each has a characteristic immune cell distribution and set of pathogen-associated ligands. For example, TLR4 is expressed by antigen-presenting cells and it binds to LPS. Binding of TLRs to their ligands activates an intracellular signaling cascade that converges on the expression of proinflammatory cytokines, leading to further immune cell recruitment and activation of the inflammatory response. A fundamental role of innate immunity is to provide an immediate "alarm" that recruits elements of adaptive immunity. This alarm indicates that a molecular structure associated with a pathogen has been detected and serves as an early warning system that the adaptive immune system should initiate an immune response against the pathogen-associated antigens encountered in the context of a TLR agonist or another innate immune signal. Several pharmacologic agents are being investigated as modulators of TLR signaling. **Imiquimod**, discussed in Chapter 38, Pharmacology of Viral Infections, may function as a TLR agonist.

Adaptive Immunity

The main features of the adaptive immune system, specificity to foreign antigens and tolerance to self-antigens, rely on two principles. First, there must be a mechanism to generate a specific response to a foreign antigen. Second, adaptive immune cells must be able to distinguish native (self) cells and soluble factors from foreign (nonself) cells and soluble factors. The first property is provided by **major histocompatibility complex (MHC)** proteins and by somatic gene recombination in T cells and B cells, whereas the second property is provided by signals from the innate immune system, by regulated immune cell development, and by costimulation.

Major Histocompatibility Complex

MHC proteins are transmembrane proteins that bind and display on their surface proteolytically degraded protein fragments and, in some cases, glycolipid antigens. There are two classes of MHC proteins: MHC class I and MHC class II. MHC class I proteins primarily display fragments of cytosolic proteins (Fig. 42-2). All nucleated cells express MHC class I proteins; the repertoire of protein fragments displayed by MHC class I proteins on a cell provides a fingerprint for all the proteins expressed within that cell. If a cell is expressing a recognizable pattern of proteins, then it will not be attacked by the immune system. However, if foreign (e.g., viral) proteins are being generated within the cell, then proteolytic fragments of those viral proteins will be displayed on MHC class I proteins at the surface of the cell, and the immune system will recognize that cell as virally infected. Antigens presented by MHC class I proteins are recognized by T cells bearing the cell surface protein CD8. (The designation "CD" stands for *cluster of differentiation* or *cluster designation* and is a system for naming an ever-growing list of cell-associated antigens. Each antigen must be defined by at least two different monoclonal antibodies in order to earn the CD designation. CD antigens now number in the hundreds and are present on leukocytes and other cell types.)

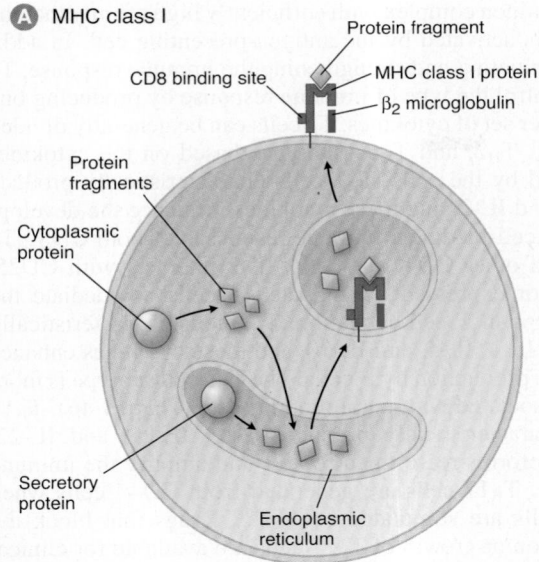

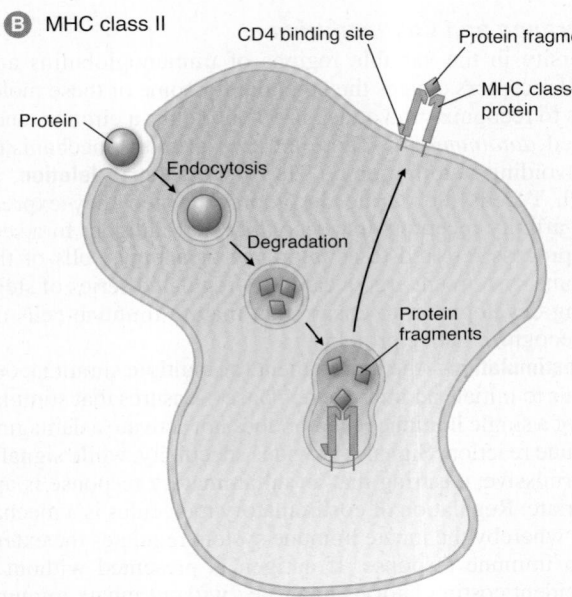

FIGURE 42-2. Class I and class II major histocompatibility complex proteins. **A.** A representative fraction of cytoplasmic proteins are proteolytically degraded in the cytosol, and the protein fragments are transported to the endoplasmic reticulum (ER). A fraction of secretory proteins are degraded directly in the ER. MHC class I protein, in association with β_2 microglobulin, binds a fragment of the degraded cytoplasmic or secretory protein in the ER. The MHC class I:protein fragment complex is transported to the cell surface, where it serves as a fingerprint for the diversity of proteins expressed by that cell. The CD8 binding site on MHC class I ensures that the class I protein:antigen complex interacts only with cytotoxic T cells, which express CD8. All nucleated human cells express MHC class I proteins. **B.** Antigen-presenting cells phagocytose and degrade bacteria and other foreign agents, generating protein fragments that bind to MHC class II protein in the ER. The MHC class II:protein fragment complex is transported to the cell surface, where it serves to display all the potentially nonself antigens that have been ingested by that cell. The CD4 binding site on MHC class II ensures that the class II protein:antigen complex interacts only with helper T cells, which express CD4. Professional antigen-presenting cells (B cells, macrophages, and dendritic cells) are usually the only cell types that express MHC class II proteins, but other cells can be induced to express class II proteins and present antigens under some circumstances.

MHC class II proteins display protein fragments derived from endocytic vesicles. In contrast to class I proteins, which are expressed on all nucleated cells, MHC class II proteins are expressed mostly on antigen-presenting cells (e.g., macrophages and dendritic cells), although some other cell types can be induced to express MHC class II proteins. Endocytic vesicles contain antigenic protein fragments derived from infectious agents after phagocytosis and proteolytic processing of those agents. Therefore, the protein fragments expressed on MHC class II proteins generally identify extracellular foreign agents (e.g., bacteria). As discussed below, T cells bearing the cell surface protein CD4 recognize antigens presented by MHC class II proteins. In the process, these T cells stimulate the antigen-presenting cells to produce soluble factors called *cytokines* and *chemokines*, which, in turn, aid the T cells in responding to the antigen. In general, then, *protein fragments bound to MHC class I identify infected cells, whereas fragments bound to MHC class II identify infectious agents.* However, because of the phenomenon of cross-presentation, some proteins generated in the cytosol can be presented by MHC class II to CD4$^+$ T cells, and some phagocytosed antigens can be presented by MHC class I to CD8$^+$ T cells.

Immune Diversity

While MHC proteins provide a mechanism for distinguishing infected cells and infectious agents from uninfected cells, **somatic gene recombination** and other processes for generating diversity provide a mechanism for generating a specific response to an infection. By recombination, **immunoglobulin** and **T-cell receptor** genes semi-randomly create millions of modular three-dimensional protein structures, referred to as *variable regions*. Recombined variable regions may undergo somatic hypermutation to create additional diversity that, in the aggregate, can recognize almost any structure. This is the primary mechanism by which the immune system generates an astounding diversity of immune responses.

Humoral and Cellular Immunity

Adaptive immunity is generally divided into **humoral immunity** and **cellular immunity**. In the basic (simplified) model of the immune system, the primary cells mediating humoral immunity are B cells, and those mediating cellular immunity are T cells (Table 42-1). The humoral response involves the production of **antibodies** specific for an antigen. Mature B cells are characterized by CD19 and CD20 expression, and they can differentiate into plasma cells. Upon antigen stimulation, plasma cells secrete antibodies against *extracellular* infectious agents such as bacteria. In contrast, the cellular response involves activation and clonal expansion of **T cells** that recognize a specific antigen. Some T cells recognize infected cells and then lyse those cells using cytotoxic proteins called **perforins** and **granzymes**. Cellular immune responses are therefore effective against many *intracellular* infectious agents such as viruses.

In addition to their role in cellular immunity, T cells control the extent of immune responses. Each T cell evolves so that it is activated by only one specific MHC:antigen complex. All T cells express an MHC:antigen-specific T-cell receptor (TCR). T cells are divided into cytotoxic T cells (T$_C$) and helper T cells (T$_H$) based on the type of coreceptor expressed and the function imparted by that coreceptor (Fig. 42-3).

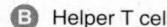

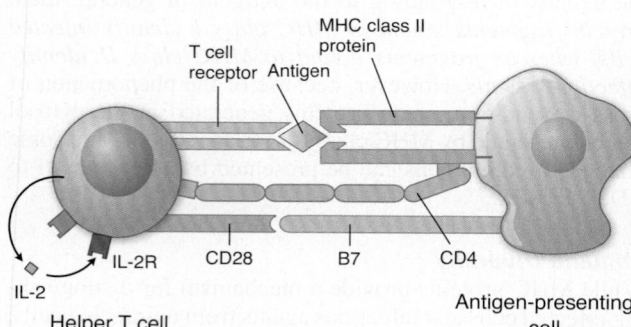

FIGURE 42-3. Activation of cytotoxic and helper T cells. T cells mediate and regulate the cellular immune response. **A.** Cytotoxic T cells (T$_C$) are the primary *mediators* of cellular immunity. These cells express T-cell receptors (TCR) and CD8. The TCR identifies nonself antigens bound to MHC proteins, and CD8 ensures that T$_C$ cells interact only with cells expressing MHC class I proteins. In the example shown, the interaction of a T$_C$ cell with the MHC class I protein of a virus-infected cell leads to activation of the T$_C$ cell and subsequent killing of the virus-infected cell. **B.** Helper T cells (T$_H$) are the primary *regulators* of cellular immunity. These cells express TCR and CD4. CD4 binds to MHC class II proteins on antigen-presenting cells (APCs); this interaction ensures that T$_H$ cells interact only with cells expressing MHC class II proteins. An additional degree of specificity is provided by the interaction of CD28 on T$_H$ cells with proteins of the B7 family on APCs; this "costimulatory signal" is required for T$_H$ cell activation. In the example shown, the interaction of a T$_H$ cell with the MHC class II and B7 proteins of an antigen-presenting cell leads to activation of the T$_H$ cell. The activated T$_H$ cell secretes IL-2 and expresses the IL-2 receptor (IL-2R); this autocrine pathway stimulates further T$_H$ cell proliferation and activation. IL-2 and other cytokines secreted by the T$_H$ cell activate not only T$_H$ cells but also T$_C$ cells and B cells.

T$_C$ cells are the *mediators* of cellular adaptive immunity. These cells express the CD8 coreceptor, which recognizes a constant (i.e., antigen-independent) domain on MHC class I proteins. This coreceptor function allows the antigen-specific TCR on T$_C$ cells to bind a specific class I MHC:antigen complex with sufficiently high affinity that the T$_C$ cell is activated by the cell expressing the class I MHC:antigen complex. Specific activation of the T$_C$ cell initiates a chain of events, including the secretion of membrane-penetrating perforins and apoptosis-inducing granzymes, which result in the death of the cell displaying the foreign antigen.

T$_H$ cells are primarily the *regulators* of adaptive immunity. T$_H$ cells are identified by their expression of the CD4 coreceptor, which recognizes an antigen-independent domain on MHC class II proteins. This coreceptor function allows the antigen-specific TCR on T$_H$ cells to bind a specific class II

MHC:antigen complex with sufficiently high affinity that the T$_H$ cell is activated by the antigen-presenting cell. In addition to initiating and strengthening the immune response, T$_H$ cells control the type of immune response by producing one or another set of cytokines. T$_H$ cells can be generally divided into T$_H$1, T$_H$2, and T$_H$17 subtypes based on the cytokines produced by the cells. T$_H$1 cells characteristically produce IFN-γ and IL-2, and these cytokines influence the development of cell-mediated immune responses of both CD8$^+$ T$_C$ cells and other CD4$^+$ T$_H$ cells. IL-2 interacts with CD25, a receptor expressed on activated T cells, to mediate the early steps in T cell activation. T$_H$2 cells characteristically produce IL-4, IL-5, and IL-10, and these cytokines enhance antibody production by B cells. The T$_H$2 cell subtype is more often associated with autoimmunity (see Chapter 46). T$_H$17 cells characteristically produce IL-17, IL-21, and IL-22. IL-17 isoforms recruit neutrophils and amplify the immune response. T$_H$17 cells are generated from CD4$^+$ cells when these cells are stimulated by IL-23. Drugs that block the maturation or growth of T$_H$17 cells are available for clinical use in the treatment of certain autoimmune diseases.

Tolerance and Costimulation

Diversity in the variable regions of immunoglobulins and T-cell receptors creates the potential for some of these molecules to recognize and attack native proteins, a circumstance termed *autoimmunity*. There are two primary mechanisms for avoiding autoimmunity. The first is **clonal deletion**, in which T cells die during development when they express high-affinity receptors that recognize self-antigen. In a second process referred to as **tolerance** or **anergy**, cells of the immune system undergo a carefully regulated series of steps during development to ensure that mature immune cells do not recognize native proteins.

Costimulation—the requirement for multiple simultaneous signals to initiate an immune response—ensures that stimulation of a single immune receptor does not activate a damaging immune reaction. Signal 1 provides specificity, while signal 2 is permissive, ensuring that an inflammatory response is appropriate. Regulation of costimulatory molecules is a mechanism whereby the innate immune system regulates the extent of an immune response. If antigen is presented without a coincident costimulatory signal (i.e., without innate immune activation), then anergy may result, whereby a cell becomes unreactive and will not respond to further antigenic stimuli. Drugs that induce anergy could be therapeutically attractive because such agents could allow long-term acceptance of an organ graft or limit the extent of an autoimmune disease.

For T cells, signal 1 is mediated by the MHC:antigen:TCR interaction. Signal 2 is mediated predominantly by the interaction of **CD28** on T cells with B7-1 (also called CD80) or B7-2 (CD86) on activated antigen-presenting cells (Fig. 42-4). Resting T cells present CD28, which can bind either B7-1 or B7-2. B7-1 and B7-2 are not normally present on antigen-presenting cells, but their expression is increased by the innate immune system during an immune response to a pathogen. The lack of expression of B7 molecules in the absence of an innate immune response may help to limit inappropriate adaptive immune responses. When a T cell receives both signal 1 and signal 2, the T cell is activated, IL-2 is expressed, and clonal expansion of T$_H$ cells specific for that foreign epitope occurs. Activated T cells eventually down-regulate CD28 expression and up-regulate

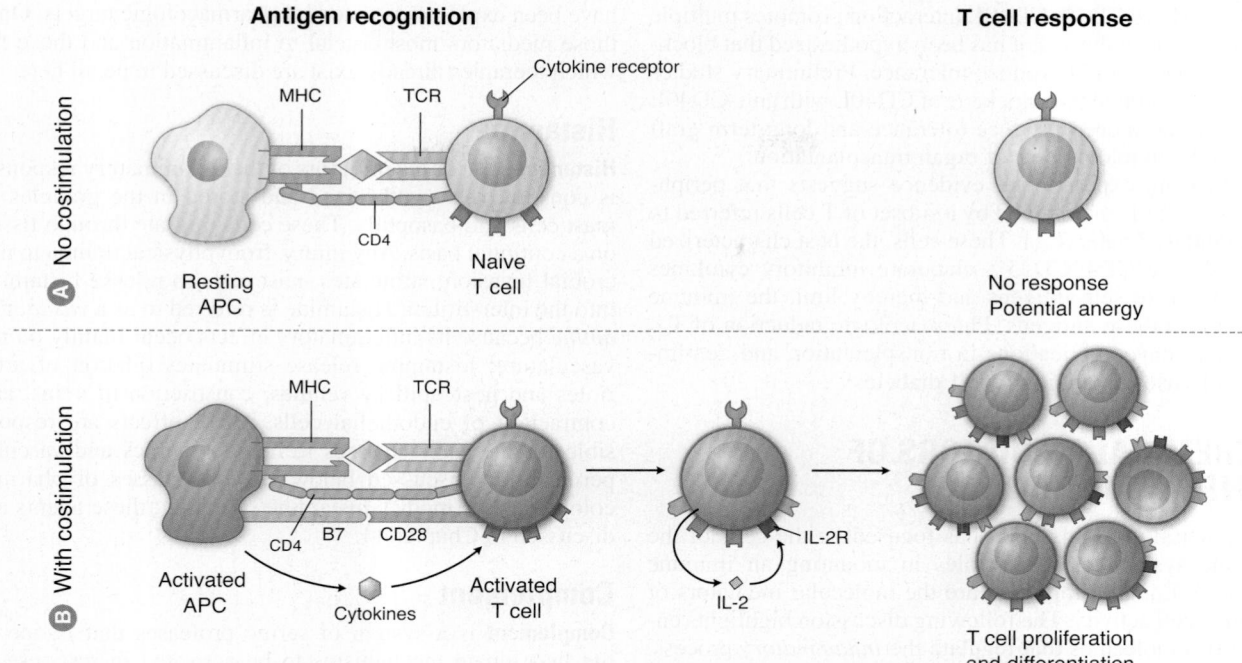

FIGURE 42-4. Costimulation in the T-cell activation pathway. Two signals are required for activation of a T-cell response to antigen. **A.** If an antigen-presenting cell (APC) presents an antigen to a T cell in the absence of an appropriate costimulatory signal, the T cell does not respond and may become anergic. **B.** If an APC presents both the antigen and a costimulatory molecule such as B7, the T cell proliferates and differentiates in response to the antigenic stimulus. Cytokines secreted by the activated APC augment T cell activation.

CTLA-4 expression. **CTLA-4**, like CD28, binds B7-1 and B7-2 but with much higher affinity than CD28. In contrast to the activating CD28 signal, interaction of CTLA-4 with B7-1 or B7-2 inhibits T cell proliferation. This appears to be a physiologic mechanism for self-limitation of the immune response. Other inhibitory **immune checkpoint** signals are discussed in Chapter 46.

CD40 ligand (CD40L) is another mediator of costimulation. Activated T cells express CD40L (CD154). CD40 is expressed on antigen-presenting cells, including B cells and macrophages

(Fig. 42-5). Interaction of T_H cell CD40L with B cell CD40 promotes B cell activation, isotype switching, clonal expansion, and affinity maturation. Interaction of T_H cell CD40L with macrophage CD40 promotes macrophage expression of B7-1 and B7-2. These molecules, as mentioned above, are crucial for costimulation of T cells. This pathway thus provides a positive feedback mechanism whereby activated T cells can promote further expansion of activated T cells. In addition, the increased expression of B7-1 and B7-2 on macrophages is important for promoting CD8$^+$ T_C cell activation.

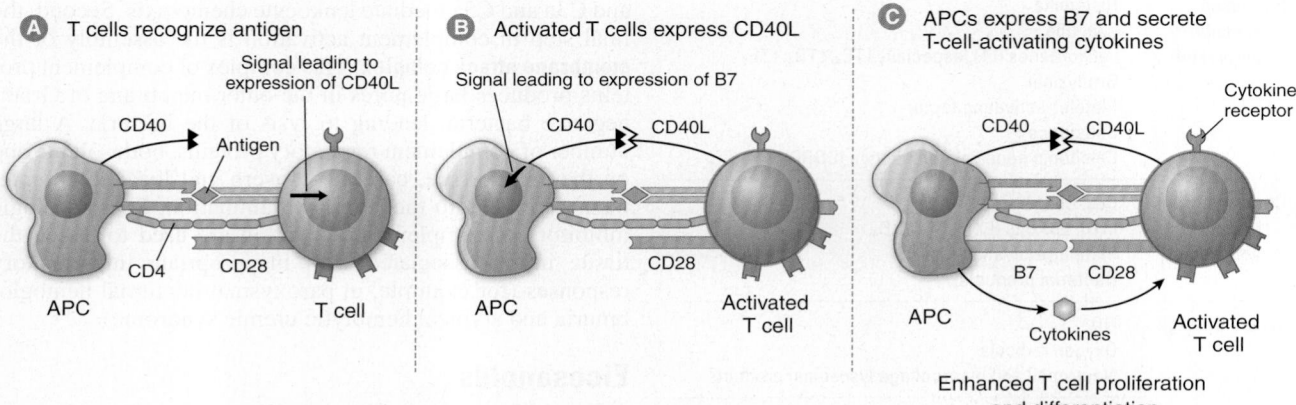

FIGURE 42-5. Costimulation and the CD40–CD40L interaction. A. An antigen-presenting cell (APC) presents MHC class II-bound antigen to a CD4$^+$ T cell. T-cell recognition of antigen initiates an intracellular signaling cascade that leads to expression of CD40 ligand (CD40L) at the T-cell surface. **B.** CD40L on the activated T cell binds to CD40 on the surface of the APC. Activation of CD40 generates an intracellular signaling cascade that leads to expression of B7 on the APC surface. **C.** Enhanced T-cell proliferation and differentiation are promoted by costimulation of the T cell by the MHC class II:antigen complex (which binds to the T-cell receptor), CD40 (which binds to T-cell CD40L), and B7 (which binds to T-cell CD28). Cytokines secreted by the activated APC augment T-cell proliferation and differentiation.

Because the CD40–CD40L interaction promotes multiple costimulation pathways, it has been hypothesized that blockade of CD40L could produce tolerance. Preliminary studies have demonstrated that blockade of CD40L with anti-CD40L antibody can indeed produce tolerance and long-term graft survival in animal models of organ transplantation.

Increasing experimental evidence suggests that peripheral tolerance is maintained by a subset of T cells referred to as **regulatory T cells (T_{reg})**. These cells, the best characterized of which are $CD4^+CD25^+$, elaborate inhibitory cytokines in response to self-antigens and thereby limit the immune response to these antigens. Pharmacologic induction of T_{reg} cells may have applications in transplantation and autoimmune diseases, including type 1 diabetes.

CHEMICAL MEDIATORS OF INFLAMMATION

The discussion to this point has focused on the cells of the immune system and their roles in mounting an immune response. Equally important are the molecular mediators of immune cell activity. The following discussion highlights endogenous molecules that regulate the *inflammatory* process. (Note that signaling pathways for *immune* cells are discussed mainly in Chapter 46, although there is some overlap among the endogenous mediators of inflammation and immunity, especially among the cytokines.) The list of mediators is long (Table 42-2), and essentially all of these signaling systems

TABLE 42-2 Chemical Mediators of the Inflammatory Response

RESPONSE	MEDIATORS
Vasodilation	Histamine C3a, C5a (complement components) Prostaglandins (PG) PGI_2, PGE_1, PGE_2, PGD_2 Nitric oxide (NO) Bradykinin Plasmin
Increased vascular permeability	Histamine C3a, C5a Leukotrienes (LT), especially LTC_4, LTD_4, LTE_4 Bradykinin Platelet-activating factor Substance P Calcitonin gene-related peptide (CGRP)
Chemotaxis and leukocyte activation	C3a, C5a LTB_4, lipoxins (LX) LXA_4, LXB_4 Platelet-activating factor Bacterial products
Tissue damage	NO Oxygen radicals Neutrophil and macrophage lysosomal products
Fever	PGE_2, PGI_2, LTB_4, LXA_4, LXB_4 Interleukin-1 (IL-1), IL-6, tumor necrosis factor (TNF)
Pain	PGE_2, PGI_2, LTB_4 Bradykinin Substance P CGRP

have been explored as potential pharmacologic targets. Only those mediators most crucial to inflammation and those for which therapies already exist are discussed in detail here.

Histamine

Histamine, one of the initiators of the inflammatory response, is constitutively synthesized and stored in the granules of mast cells and basophils. These cells migrate through tissue on a continual basis. Any injury, from physical trauma to microbial invasion, stimulates mast cells to release histamine into the interstitium. Histamine is referred to as a *vasoactive amine* because its inflammatory effects occur mainly on the vasculature: histamine release stimulates dilation of arterioles and postcapillary venules, constriction of veins, and contraction of endothelial cells. These effects are responsible for the early changes in hemodynamics and vascular permeability discussed below. Several classes of pharmacologic agents modify histamine signaling; these agents are discussed in Chapter 44.

Complement

Complement is a system of serine proteases that is one of the first innate mechanisms to be activated in response to injury. The complement system can be activated by antigen–antibody interactions (the classical pathway), by direct interactions with foreign surfaces (the alternative pathway), or by interactions with certain complex carbohydrates (the lectin pathway). In each pathway, a series of proteolytic reactions converts a complement precursor protein, referred to by the letter "C" followed by a number (for example, C3), into its active form(s), indicated by the letter "a" or "b" (for example, C3a and C3b; in this case, both forms are active). The general scheme of this pathway is analogous to that of the coagulation cascade (see Chapter 23, Pharmacology of Hemostasis and Thrombosis), in which precursor proteins are proteolytically cleaved to active products that contribute to the actions of the cascade.

After activation, complement triggers inflammatory responses by two mechanisms. First, several cleavage products of the complement cascade are potent stimulators of inflammation. For example, C3b is an important opsonin, and C3a and C5a mediate leukocyte chemotaxis. Second, the final step in complement activation is the assembly of the **membrane attack complex**. This complex of complement proteins produces large pores in the outer membrane of Gram-negative bacteria, leading to lysis of the bacteria. A large number of complement regulatory proteins, both soluble and on the cell surface, carefully govern and localize complement activation to the site of inflammation. Pharmacologic inhibitors of complement activation are used to lessen the tissue injury associated with inappropriate inflammatory responses (for example, in paroxysmal nocturnal hemoglobinuria and atypical hemolytic uremic syndrome).

Eicosanoids

Eicosanoids are metabolites of arachidonic acid, a fatty acid component of phospholipids in the inner leaflet of the plasma membrane of many cell types. Inflammatory mediators such as cytokines and complement stimulate the enzymatic release of arachidonic acid from the plasma membrane. Multiple biochemical reactions ensue, resulting in the formation of prostaglandins, leukotrienes, and other eicosanoids.

Notably, certain arachidonic acid derivatives are proinflammatory, whereas others serve to limit inflammation. This underscores the fact that acute inflammation is a self-limited process and that the process of pathogen destruction is intimately tied to the process of tissue repair. Chapter 43 is devoted to an in-depth discussion of eicosanoid physiology, pathophysiology, and pharmacology.

Cytokines

Cytokines are proteins that act in a paracrine manner to regulate leukocyte activity. **Interleukins** and **tumor necrosis factor (TNF)** family members are cytokines secreted primarily by cells of the hematopoietic lineage. Interleukin-1 (IL-1) and tumor necrosis factor-α (TNF-α) are among the key cytokines elaborated in the acute inflammatory response; these cytokines were two of the mediators responsible for Mark's fever. Another member of the TNF family is the B lymphocyte stimulator (BLyS), which promotes B cell survival and differentiation. Located on T cells and B cells, TNF receptors contain membrane glycoprotein CD30, which is important in cellular proliferation and survival and serves as a pharmacologic target (see Chapter 46). **Chemokines** are a subset of cytokines that promote immune cell trafficking, transmigration, and localization to sites of inflammation. For example, macrophage chemoattractant protein-1 (MCP-1) promotes monocyte transmigration and activation. Other notable cytokines include the hematopoietic growth factors granulocyte-monocyte colony-stimulating factor (GM-CSF) and granulocyte colony-stimulating factor (G-CSF) (see Chapter 45).

Because cytokines affect the proliferation and function of cells that mediate innate and adaptive immune responses, selective inhibition or stimulation of cytokine action has the potential to modulate immune and inflammatory responses. Pharmacologic uses for cytokine and anticytokine therapies are discussed in Chapter 45 and Chapter 46, respectively.

Other Agents

As noted in Table 42-2, other signaling molecules also coordinate the inflammatory response. These include kinins, platelet-activating factor, nitric oxide, oxygen radicals, and other leukocyte and bacterial products released during phagocytosis. Although pharmacologic agents have been developed to modulate each of these pathways, there are, as yet, no approved anti-inflammatory drugs that specifically interrupt the action of these mediators.

▌ THE INFLAMMATORY RESPONSE

The cells and soluble mediators of the immune system interact with one another to generate the **inflammatory response**, which typically occurs in four phases. First, the vasculature around a site of injury reacts to recruit cells of the immune system. Second, circulating immune cells migrate from these vessels into the injured tissues, and the mechanisms of innate and adaptive immunity (see above) serve to neutralize and remove the inciting stimulus. Next, the process of repair and tissue healing ensues and the acute inflammatory process is terminated. If the process of acute inflammation is not halted but continues to smolder, chronic inflammation can occur.

Dilation of Vessels

Within hours of being cut, Mark's thumb begins to exhibit the five classic signs of inflammation presented in the introduction. Initially, these signs and symptoms result from alterations in vascular hemodynamics at the site of injury. Injury to a tissue causes the release of inflammatory mediators (discussed earlier) that dilate arterioles and postcapillary venules; in turn, vasodilation leads to increased blood flow to the site of injury, causing the clinical signs of redness and warmth. Inflammatory mediators also cause contraction of vascular endothelial cells, leading to increased capillary permeability and the development of an exudate (i.e., interstitial fluid with a high protein content); in turn, the exudate causes the clinical manifestation of swelling. Pain develops due to both increased tissue pressure and the action of various inflammatory mediators.

Recruitment of Cells

Increased vascular permeability also allows cells in the blood to enter the interstitium. Cellular migration out of the blood is not random; rather, leukocyte recruitment is orchestrated to optimize clearing of the infection and local repair of the injured tissue (Fig. 42-6). At the onset of an inflammatory response, the endothelial cells at the site of injury are activated to express adhesion molecules that bind specific receptors expressed by leukocytes. For example, **intercellular adhesion molecules** (**ICAMs**) and **vascular cell adhesion molecules** (**VCAMs**) expressed by the vascular endothelium bind integrins expressed on the cell surface of leukocytes. This interaction causes the leukocytes, which normally roll along the surface of the endothelium by means of loose, transient binding interactions, to adhere tightly to the activated endothelium at the site of injury. The adherent leukocytes then bind other endothelial cell receptors that promote **transmigration** (diapedesis) of the leukocytes from the vasculature into the interstitium. Specificity of the immune response is achieved according to the pattern of adhesion molecules expressed by the activated endothelium and by the various types of leukocytes; for example, neutrophils dominate the early inflammatory response, while monocytes predominate after 24 hours.

Chemotaxis

Once the cells of the immune system cross the endothelial barrier, they migrate through the interstitium to the specific site of injury or infection. Immune cell targeting is accomplished by the process of **chemotaxis**, or chemical signaling. Inflammatory mediators released at the site of injury, such as N-formyl peptides derived from bacterial proteins or endogenous mediators such as C5a and leukotriene B$_4$ (LTB$_4$), create a chemical gradient to which the leukocytes respond, allowing them to crawl preferentially toward the site of the inflammatory reaction.

Phagocytosis

Upon their arrival at the site of injury or infection, neutrophils, macrophages, and other cells of the immune system are ready to perform their duties. However, these cells require one further stimulus to activate their killing machinery. Foreign substances must be coated by an opsonin before they can be ingested (phagocytosed) by leukocytes. **Opsonins** are

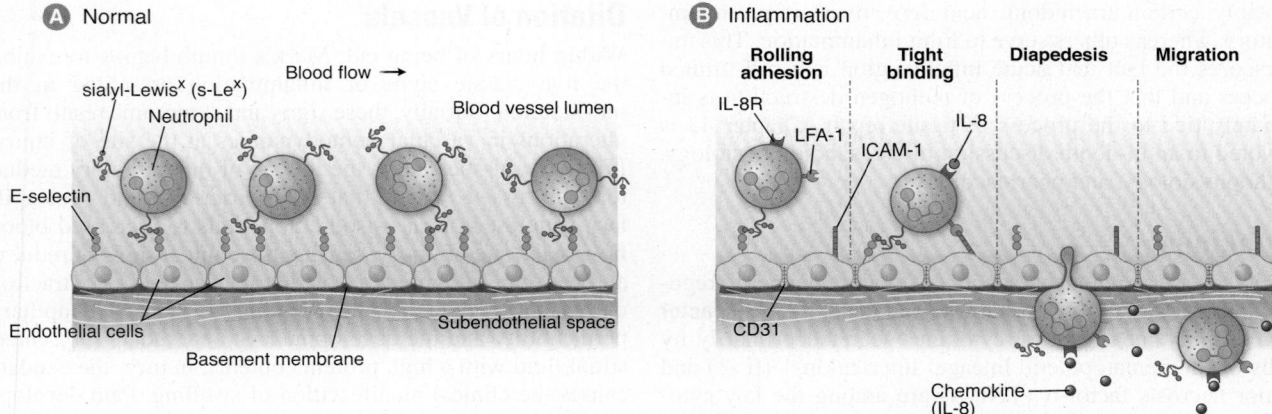

FIGURE 42-6. Overview of the inflammatory response. A. Leukocytes circulating in the blood interact with selectins expressed on the surface of vascular endothelial cells. In the absence of inflammation, the interaction between leukocytes and endothelial cells is weak, and leukocytes either flow past or roll along the endothelium. Neutrophil rolling is mediated by the interaction between endothelial cell E-selectin and neutrophil sialyl-Lewis^x (s-Le^x). **B.** During the inflammatory response, endothelial cells up-regulate their expression of intercellular adhesion molecules (ICAMs). ICAM expression increases the potential for strong binding interactions between leukocytes and the activated endothelial cells. For example, ICAM-1 on endothelial cells binds tightly to LFA-1 on neutrophils. The enhanced cell–cell interaction leads to tethering (rolling, activation, and firm adhesion) of leukocytes to endothelial cell surfaces and initiates the process of leukocyte diapedesis and transmigration from the vascular space into extravascular tissues. Leukocytes migrate through injured tissue in response to chemokines such as IL-8, which are inflammatory mediators released by injured cells and by other immune cells that have already reached the site of injury.

molecular adaptors that coat foreign surfaces and signal leukocytes that a particle should be attacked. The major opsonins consist of complement, immunoglobulins (antibodies), and **collectins** (plasma proteins that bind to certain microbial carbohydrates). The interaction of a phagocytic cell with an opsonized particle initiates engulfment and destruction of the offending agent. This step is also a crucial point of interaction between innate and adaptive immunity. Antigen-presenting cells process engulfed particles and present their antigens to B cells and T cells, which then react to the antigens. In the introductory case, Mark's cut presumably allowed bacteria to penetrate his skin barrier, leading to infection. The presence of these bacteria initiated an inflammatory response that included phagocytosis of bacteria by APCs, presentation of bacterial antigens to T_H cells, activation and expansion of T_H cells, T_H cell activation of further APC-mediated phagocytosis, and synthesis and secretion of antibodies specific for the bacteria.

Resolution

Tissue repair and reestablishment of homeostasis are the final events in the acute inflammatory response. The same mediators that activate inflammation also initiate a cascade of tissue repair; this process is mediated by the release of growth factors and cytokines, including epidermal growth factor (EGF), platelet-derived growth factor (PDGF), basic fibroblast growth factor-2 (bFGF-2), transforming growth factor-$\beta1$ (TGF-$\beta1$), IL-1, and TNF-α. These factors act as mitogens for endothelial cells and fibroblasts and ultimately stimulate healing and scar formation through angiogenesis (formation of new blood vessels) and the formation of granulation tissue. In the introductory case, the granulation tissue and eventual scar will be the only record of Mark's acute inflammatory event. Of note, angiogenesis can be a pathologic state when it is associated with abnormal blood vessel growth or tumor growth, and pharmacologic inhibitors of angiogenesis are currently being used to treat

age-related macular degeneration (where abnormal blood vessels obscure vision) and as antineoplastic agents (see Chapter 40, Pharmacology of Cancer: Signal Transduction).

CHRONIC INFLAMMATION

Chronic inflammation is a pathologic state characterized by the continued and inappropriate response of the immune system to an inflammatory stimulus. Chronic inflammation accounts for the symptoms of many autoimmune diseases and may be an important cause of organ transplant rejection. In contrast to the acute inflammatory response, which is dominated by neutrophils, one of the hallmarks of chronic inflammation is the predominance of macrophages. Activated macrophages secrete collagenases and growth factors in addition to inflammatory mediators such as proteases and eicosanoids. These secreted products initiate and maintain a cycle of tissue injury and repair, leading to tissue remodeling. Over time, chronic inflammation can cause relentless tissue destruction. Promising treatments for chronic inflammation could include cytokine inhibitors that neutralize mediators of the signaling cascades that perpetuate chronic inflammation. These agents are discussed in Chapter 46.

CONCLUSION AND FUTURE DIRECTIONS

The immune system intricately regulates the response to tissue injury and infection. A complete review of immunology is beyond the scope of this text; instead, the discussion in this chapter presents a broad overview and highlights elements of immunity that may be addressed pharmacologically. Innate immune mechanisms respond to patterned elements shared among a class of infectious agents, such as bacterial lipopolysaccharide or viral RNA. The innate immune system also processes these agents and presents them to lymphocytes, thereby activating the adaptive immune system.

The adaptive immune system develops a response specific to an infectious agent or inflammatory stimulus. As part of the inflammatory response, the adaptive immune response also includes mechanisms that mediate tolerance to distinguish self from nonself; dysregulation of these mechanisms may lead to chronic inflammation and autoimmune disease. Many anti-inflammatory drugs act to deplete populations of innate or adaptive immune cells; this concept is discussed in more detail in Chapter 46.

The chemical mediators of the inflammatory response—including histamine, complement, eicosanoids, and cytokines—are also major targets of current pharmacologic therapies. Macromolecular drugs are playing an increasingly important role in modulation of these chemical mediators; for example, anticytokine antibodies that inhibit tumor necrosis factor-α have been developed for the treatment of rheumatoid arthritis, psoriatic arthritis, and inflammatory bowel disease. A second approach to the modulation of inflammatory responses is to target the intracellular signaling cascades responsible for the initiation of immune responses. Cyclosporine, discussed in Chapter 46, is an example of such a drug. As the number of agents available for treatment of immune disorders grows, it will also be important to determine whether macromolecular agents and small-molecule signaling inhibitors can be used in combination to target multiple steps in inflammation.

Suggested Reading

Dinarello CA. Anti-inflammatory agents: present and future. *Cell* 2010; 140:935–950. (*A signaling-oriented overview of targets for development of new anti-inflammatory agents.*)

Ibelgaufts H. COPE: cytokines & cells online pathfinder encyclopedia. http://www.copewithcytokines.de/cope.cgi. (*Website that describes all known actions of cytokines.*)

Iwasaki A, Medzhitov R. Control of adaptive immunity by the innate immune system. *Nat Immunol* 2015;16:343–353. (*Advances in understanding interactions between the innate and adaptive immune systems.*)

Littman DR, Rudensky AY. Th17 and regulatory T cells in mediating and restraining inflammation. *Cell* 2010;140:845–858. (*Discusses advances in T cell subsets and regulatory T cell biology.*)

Matesanz-Isabel J, Sintes J, Llinas L, de Salort J, Lázaro A, Engel P. New B-cell CD molecules. *Immunol Lett* 2011;134:104–112. (*An updated classification of molecules with the CD designation.*)

Murphy KM, Travers P, Walport M. *Janeway's immunobiology.* 8th ed. New York: Garland Publishing; 2011. (*A general immunology textbook.*)

Pier GB, Lyczak JB, Wetzler L. *Immunology, infection and immunity.* Washington, DC: ASM Press; 2004. (*A detailed text with a focus on immunologic mechanisms.*)

43

Pharmacology of Eicosanoids

David M. Dudzinski and Charles N. Serhan

▌ INTRODUCTION

Autacoids are substances that are rapidly synthesized in response to specific stimuli, act quickly in the local environment, and remain active for only a short time before degradation. **Eicosanoids** represent a chemically diverse family of autacoids that are mostly derived from arachidonic acid. Research on eicosanoids has defined their vital roles in inflammatory, neoplastic, and cardiovascular physiology and pathophysiology. Numerous pharmacologic interventions in eicosanoid pathways—including the nonsteroidal anti-inflammatory drugs (NSAIDs), cyclooxygenase-2 (COX-2) inhibitors, leukotriene inhibitors, and others—are useful in the clinical management of inflammation, pain, and fever. Given the diverse bioactivities of eicosanoids, future research in eicosanoid physiology and pharmacology may lead to the development of new therapeutics for the inflammatory and autoimmune bases of asthma, glomerulonephritis, cancer, wound healing, cardiovascular diseases, and other clinical conditions.

▌ PHYSIOLOGY OF EICOSANOID METABOLISM

Eicosanoids are centrally involved in a number of metabolic pathways that exhibit diverse roles in inflammation and cellular signaling. The vast majority of these pathways center on reactions involving the metabolism of arachidonic acid (Fig. 43-1). The following section considers the biochemical steps leading to arachidonic acid generation and then discusses the cyclooxygenase, lipoxygenase, epoxygenase, and isoprostane pathways of arachidonic acid metabolism. The word *eicosanoid* arises from the Greek root meaning twenty, and the term classically refers to unbranched 20-carbon molecules derived from arachidonic acid oxygenation. The term eicosanoid also applies broadly to various other molecules—such as resolvins, protectins, and maresins—that are derived from docosahexaenoic acid, a 22-carbon precursor. The term *docosanoids* is sometimes also used to describe these 22-carbon structures.

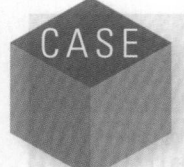

CASE

Ms. G, a 44-year-old Native American female, visits her physician because of joint pain and progressive fatigue. Her history reveals general joint stiffness and pain for the past 3 weeks. The pain is worst in the metacarpophalangeal and proximal interphalangeal joints and is especially prominent in the early morning. Ms. G is advised to take ibuprofen as needed, and this medication provides relief of her pain for some time.

Six months later, Ms. G has continued to take ibuprofen daily and she notes indigestion and new vomiting of "coffee grounds"-like material. Her physician recommends cessation of ibuprofen and an upper gastrointestinal endoscopic examination, which reveals gastric mucosal erosion and hemorrhage. Her physician is also concerned about interval progression in Ms. G's joint stiffness and pain and refers her to a rheumatology clinic. She reports to the rheumatologist that her pain has progressed to include both feet, both hands and wrists, both elbows, some cervical vertebrae, and the left shoulder. Over the past few months, she has hours of morning pain, has noted difficulty with basic household tasks, and has avoided physical activity. On examination, the metacarpophalangeal and proximal interphalangeal joints of both hands are found to be swollen, tender, and warm; Ms. G also has characteristic ulnar deviation of her fingers and "swan-neck" deformities.

Skin nodules are apparent on the extensor surface of both forearms. Laboratory tests show an elevated erythrocyte sedimentation rate (ESR), low hemoglobin, and positive rheumatoid factor. Synovial fluid aspirate is notable for leukocytosis. Hand radiographs show erosion and osteopenia.

Because the symptoms, examination, laboratory studies, and radiographs are consistent with a diagnosis of moderately to severely active rheumatoid arthritis, Ms. G is initially started on a course of celecoxib (a COX-2 selective inhibitor), etanercept (a TNF-α antagonist), and prednisone (a glucocorticoid). Over the subsequent months, the joint pain, swelling, and tenderness decrease noticeably. Joint function in the hands is restored, and Ms. G is able to resume some physical activity.

Questions

1. Which eicosanoid mediators may be causing Ms. G's joint pains?

2. By what mechanism do glucocorticoids such as prednisone affect eicosanoid levels and/or bioactivity?

3. By what mechanism did ibuprofen cause Ms. G's gastric erosion and hemorrhage?

4. What are the potential concerns regarding long-term use of celecoxib?

5. By what mechanism does etanercept affect eicosanoid levels and/or bioactivity?

Generation of Arachidonic Acid and Omega-3 Fatty Acids

Arachidonic acid (all-cis-5,8,11,14-eicosatetraenoic acid) is the common precursor to the vast majority of eicosanoids (Fig. 43-1). Arachidonic acid must be biosynthesized from the essential fatty acid precursor **linoleic acid** (all-cis-9,12-octadecadienoic acid), which humans can obtain only from dietary sources. **Eicosapentaenoic acid** (all-cis-5,8,11,14,17-eicosapentaenoic acid; **EPA**) and **docosahexaenoic acid** (all-cis-4,7,10,13,16,19-docosahexaenoic acid; **DHA**) are the precursors to resolvins, protectins, and maresins. Humans can obtain EPA and DHA either from dietary sources or from biotransformation of the essential fatty acid precursor α-**linolenic acid** (all-cis-9,12,15-octadecatrienoic acid). α-Linolenic acid, EPA, and DHA are also called **omega-3 fatty acids** because they contain a double bond between the third and fourth carbons from the terminal (ω) end of the molecule.

Within cells, arachidonic acid does not exist as a free fatty acid but rather is esterified to the sn_2 position of membrane phospholipids, predominantly phosphatidylcholine and phosphatidylethanolamine. Arachidonic acid is released from cellular phospholipids by the enzyme **phospholipase A$_2$** (Fig. 43-1), which hydrolyzes the acyl ester bond. *This important reaction, which represents the first step in the arachidonic acid cascade, is the overall rate-determining step in the generation of eicosanoids.*

There are membrane-bound and soluble isoforms of phospholipase A$_2$, classified as secretory (sPLA$_2$) and cytoplasmic (cPLA$_2$), respectively. The numerous phospholipase A$_2$ isoforms are differentiated based on molecular weight, pH sensitivity, regulation and inhibition characteristics, calcium requirements, and substrate specificity. The existence of multiple isoforms allows for calibrated regulation of the enzyme in different tissues to achieve selective biological responses. Phospholipase A$_2$ isoforms relevant to inflammation are stimulated by cytokines (such as TNF-α, GM-CSF, and IFN-γ) and growth factors (such as epidermal growth factor [EGF] and the MAP kinase–protein kinase C [MAPK–PKC] cascade). Although glucocorticoids were once thought to inhibit phospholipase A$_2$ directly, it has now been shown that this action is mediated by inducing the synthesis of **lipocortins,** a family of phospholipase A$_2$-regulatory proteins. One of the lipocortins, annexin 1, mediates some of the antiinflammatory actions of glucocorticoids (see below).

Cyclooxygenase Pathway

Unesterified intracellular arachidonic acid is converted by **cyclooxygenase**, **lipoxygenase**, or the cytochrome-containing **epoxygenase** enzymes; the specific enzyme dictates the particular class of local eicosanoids that are generated. *The cyclooxygenase pathway leads to the formation of* **prostaglandins**, **prostacyclin**, *and* **thromboxanes**; *the lipoxygenase pathways lead to* **leukotrienes** *and* **lipoxins**; *and the*

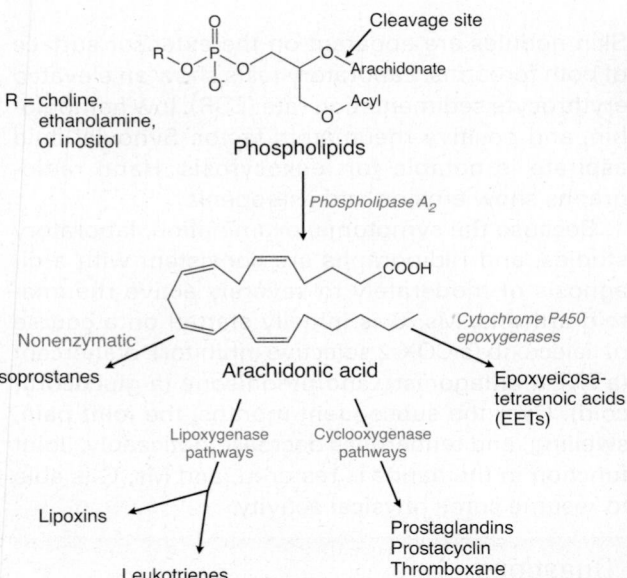

FIGURE 43-1. Overview of the role of arachidonic acid in eicosanoid pathways. Phospholipase A_2 acts on phosphatidylcholine (PC), phosphatidylethanolamine (PE), and phosphatidylinositol (PI) to release arachidonic acid. Phospholipase A_2 cleaves the ester bond *(marked by the arrow at "cleavage site")* to release arachidonic acid. Unesterified arachidonic acid is then used as substrate for the cyclooxygenase, lipoxygenase, and epoxygenase pathways. The cyclooxygenase pathways produce prostaglandins, prostacyclin, and thromboxane. The lipoxygenase pathways produce leukotrienes and lipoxins. The epoxygenase pathway produces epoxyeicosatetraenoic acids (EETs). Nonenzymatic peroxidation of arachidonic acid generates isoprostanes.

TABLE 43-1 Comparison of COX-1 and COX-2

PROPERTY	COX-1	COX-2
Expression	Constitutive	Inducible; not normally present in most tissues Constitutive in parts of nervous system
Tissue location	Ubiquitous expression	Inflamed and activated tissues
Cellular localization	Endoplasmic reticulum (ER)	ER and nuclear membrane
Substrate selectivity	Arachidonic acid, eicosapentaenoic acids	Arachidonic acid, γ-linolenate, α-linolenate, linoleate, eicosapentaenoic acids
Role	Protection and maintenance functions	Proinflammatory and mitogenic functions
Induction	Generally no induction hCG can up-regulate COX-1 in amnion	Induced by LPS, TNF-α, IL-1, IL-2, EGF, IFN-γ mRNA rises 20- to 80-fold upon induction Regulated over 1–3 hours
Inhibition	Pharmacologic: NSAIDs (low-dose aspirin)	In vivo: Anti-inflammatory glucocorticoids, IL-1β, IL-4, IL-10, IL-13 Pharmacologic: NSAIDs, COX-2 selective inhibitors

COX, cyclooxygenase; EGF, epidermal growth factor; hCG, human chorionic gonadotropin; IFN, interferon; IL, interleukin; LPS, lipopolysaccharide; NSAID, nonsteroidal anti-inflammatory drug; TNF, tumor necrosis factor.

epoxygenase pathways lead to epoxyeicosatetraenoic acids (Fig. 43-1).

Cyclooxygenases (also known as *prostaglandin H synthases*) are glycosylated, homodimeric, membrane-bound, heme-containing enzymes that are ubiquitous in animal cells from invertebrates to humans. *Two cyclooxygenase isoforms, denoted* **COX-1** *and* **COX-2***, are found in humans.* Although COX-1 and COX-2 share ~60% sequence homology and near-superimposable three-dimensional structures, the genes are located on different chromosomes, and the enzymes differ in cellular, genetic, physiologic, pathologic, and pharmacologic profiles (Tables 43-1 and 43-2). Each cyclooxygenase enzyme catalyzes two sequential reactions. The first reaction, the cyclooxygenase step, is the oxygen-dependent cyclization of arachidonic acid to prostaglandin G_2 (PGG_2); the second reaction, the peroxidase step, is the reduction of PGG_2 to PGH_2 (Fig. 43-2).

As a result of differences in cellular localization, regulatory profile, tissue expression, and substrate requirements, COX-1 and COX-2 ultimately produce different sets of eicosanoid products that are involved in different pathways and functions. Constitutively expressed COX-1 is believed to function in physiologic, or "housekeeping," activities such as vascular homeostasis, maintenance of renal and gastrointestinal blood flow, renal function, intestinal mucosal proliferation, platelet function, and antithrombogenesis. A number of "as-needed," or specialized, functions are attributed to the products of the inducible COX-2 enzyme, including roles in inflammation, fever, pain, transduction of painful stimuli in the spinal cord, mitogenesis (particularly in the gastrointestinal epithelium),

renal adaptation to stresses, deposition of trabecular bone, ovulation, placentation, and uterine contractions of labor. The role of constitutive COX-2 expression in areas of the nervous system, such as the hippocampus, hypothalamus, and amygdala, remains to be elucidated.

TABLE 43-2 Major Adverse Effects of Nonselective COX Inhibitors and COX-2 Selective Inhibitors

ADVERSE EFFECT	NONSELECTIVE COX INHIBITORS (NSAIDs)	COX-2 SELECTIVE INHIBITORS
Gastric ulceration	+	+/−*
Inhibit platelet function	+	−
Inhibit labor induction	+	+
Impair renal function	+	+
Hypersensitivity reaction	+	?

*The gastrointestinal toxicity of COX-2 selective inhibitors may be less than that of nonselective COX inhibitors, but there is still some incidence of toxicity.

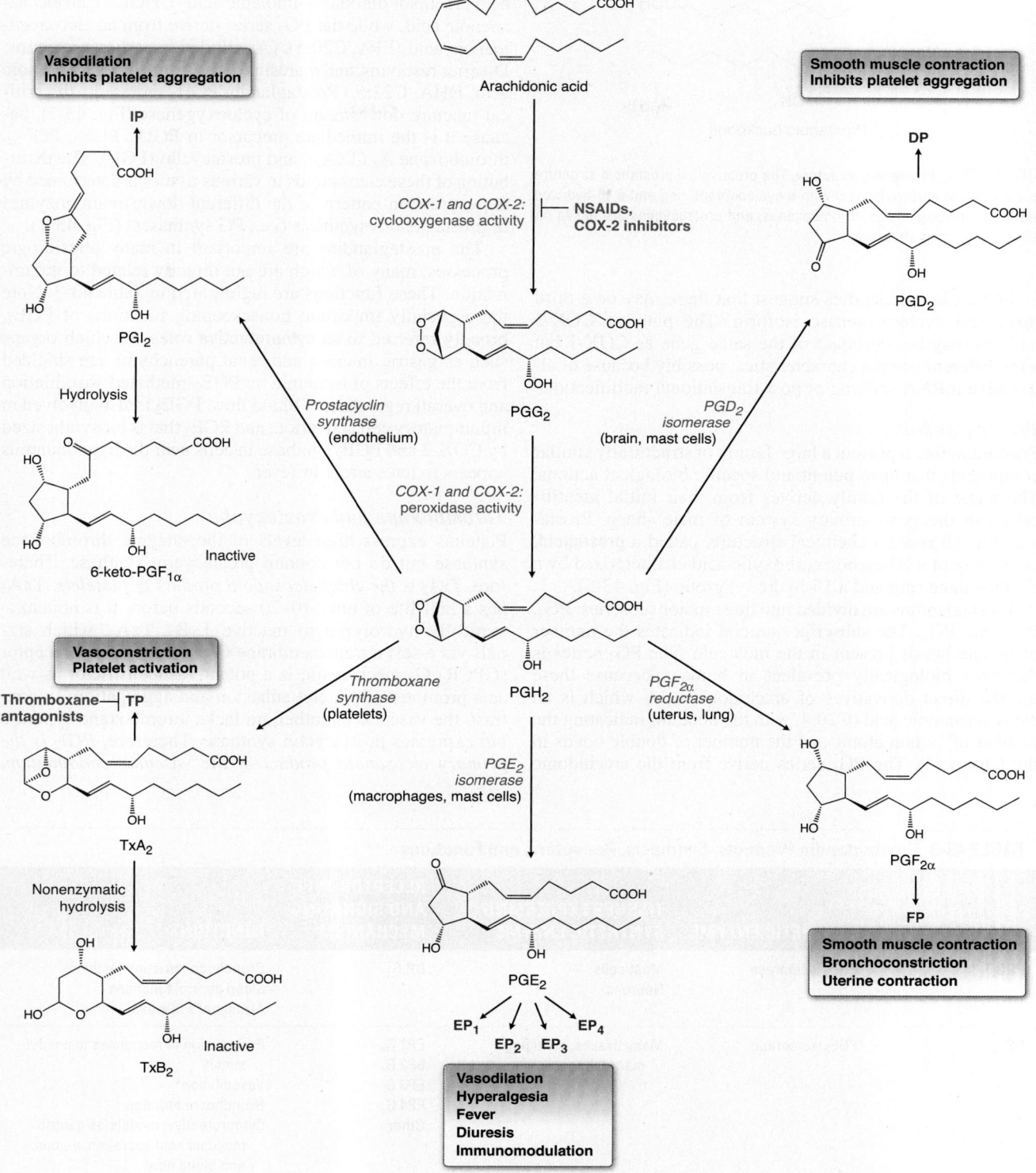

FIGURE 43-2. Prostaglandin biosynthesis, function, and pharmacologic inhibition. The biosynthetic pathways from arachidonic acid to prostaglandins, prostacyclin, and thromboxane are depicted. Tissue-specific enzyme expression determines the tissues in which the various PGH_2-derived products are biosynthesized. NSAIDs and COX-2 inhibitors are the most important classes of drugs that modulate prostaglandin production. COX, cyclooxygenase; PG, prostaglandin; Tx, thromboxane; DP, PGD_2 receptor; EP, PGE_2 receptor; FP, $PGF_{2\alpha}$ receptor; IP, PGI_2 receptor; TP, TxA_2 receptor; NSAID, nonsteroidal anti-inflammatory drug. Note that DP, EP, FP, IP, and TP are all G protein-coupled receptors.

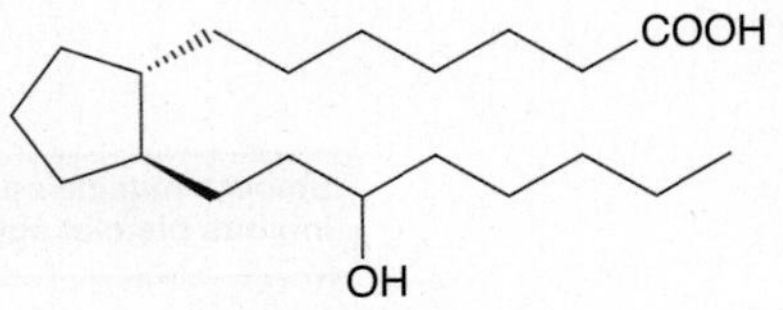

FIGURE 43-3. Prostanoid structure. The prototypical prostanoid structure is a 20-carbon carboxylic acid with a cyclopentane ring and a 15-hydroxyl group. All prostaglandins, thromboxanes, and prostacyclins are based on this common core structure.

Protein kinetic studies suggest that there may be a third functional cyclooxygenase isoform. The putative COX-3 isoform may be a product of the same gene as COX-1 but with different protein characteristics, possibly because of alternative mRNA splicing or post-translational modification.

Prostaglandins

Prostaglandins represent a large family of structurally similar compounds that have potent and specific biological actions. The name of the family derives from their initial identification in the genitourinary system of male sheep. Prostaglandins all share a chemical structure, called a **prostanoid**, consisting of a 20-carbon carboxylic acid characterized by a cyclopentane ring and a 15-hydroxyl group (Fig. 43-3).

Prostaglandins are divided into three major subseries: PG_1, PG_2, and PG_3. The subscript numeral indicates the number of double bonds present in the molecule. The PG_2 series is the most biologically prevalent in humans because these are the direct derivatives of arachidonic acid, which is an eicosatetraenoic acid (C20:4, with the notation indicating the number of carbon atoms and the number of double bonds in the fatty acid). The PG_1 series derive from the arachidonic acid precursor dihomo-γ-linolenic acid (DHGLA), an eicosatrienoic acid, while the PG_3 series derive from an eicosapentaenoic acid (EPA, C20:5). (As alluded to earlier, protectins, D-series resolvins, and maresins derive from docosahexaenoic acid, DHA, C22:6.) Prostaglandin PGH_2 represents the critical juncture downstream of cyclooxygenase (Fig. 43-2), because it is the immediate precursor to PGD_2, PGE_2, $PGF_{2\alpha}$, thromboxane A_2 (TxA_2), and prostacyclin (PGI_2). The distribution of these eicosanoids in various tissues is determined by the expression pattern of the different downstream enzymes of prostaglandin synthesis (i.e., PG synthases) (Fig. 43-2).

The prostaglandins are important in many physiologic processes, many of which are not directly related to inflammation. These functions are highlighted in Table 43-3. Note the especially important housekeeping functions of PGE_2, broadly referred to as **cytoprotective** roles, in which organs such as gastric mucosa and renal parenchyma are shielded from the effects of ischemia by PGE_2-mediated vasodilation and overall regulation of blood flow. PGE_2 is also involved in inflammatory cell activation, and PGE_2 that is biosynthesized by COX-2 and PGE_2 synthase in cells near the hypothalamus appears to have a role in fever.

Thromboxane and Prostacyclin

Platelets express high levels of the enzyme thromboxane synthase but do not contain prostacyclin synthase. Therefore, *TxA_2 is the chief eicosanoid product of platelets.* TxA_2 has a half-life of only 10–20 seconds before it is nonenzymatically hydrolyzed to inactive TxB_2. TxA_2, which signals via a seven transmembrane G protein-coupled receptor (GPCR) G_q mechanism, is a potent vasoconstrictor as well as a promoter of platelet adhesion and aggregation. In contrast, the vascular endothelium lacks thromboxane synthase but expresses prostacyclin synthase. Therefore, *PGI_2 is the primary eicosanoid product of the vascular endothelium.*

TABLE 43-3 Prostaglandin Products, Synthesis, Receptors, and Functions

PROSTAGLANDIN	SYNTHETIC ENZYME	TISSUES EXPRESSING SYNTHETIC ENZYME	RECEPTOR TYPE AND SIGNALING MECHANISM	FUNCTIONS
PGD_2	PGD_2 isomerase	Mast cells Neurons	DP G_s	Bronchoconstriction (asthma) Sleep control functions Alzheimer's disease
PGE_2	PGE_2 isomerase	Many tissues, including macrophages and mast cells	EP1 G_q EP2 G_s EP3 G_i EP4 G_s Other	Potentiation of responses to painful stimuli Vasodilation Bronchoconstriction Cytoprotective: modulates gastric mucosal acid secretion, mucus, and blood flow Inflammatory cell activation Fever Mucus production Possibly erectile function
$PGF_{2\alpha}$	$PGF_{2\alpha}$ reductase	Vascular smooth muscle Uterine smooth muscle Bronchial smooth muscle	FP G_q	Vascular tone Reproductive physiology (abortifacient) Bronchoconstriction

The prostanoid receptors are all G protein-coupled receptors. DP, prostaglandin (PG) D_2 receptor; EP, PGE_2 receptor; FP, $PGF_{2\alpha}$ receptor

PGI_2, which signals via G_s, functions as a vasodilator, venodilator, and inhibitor of platelet aggregation. In other words, PGI_2 is the physiologic antagonist of TxA_2. The vasodilatory actions of PGI_2, like those of PGE_2, also confer cytoprotective properties.

The local balance between TxA_2 and PGI_2 levels contributes to regulation of arterial resistance (and thus blood pressure) and to thrombogenesis. Imbalances can lead to hypertension, ischemia, thrombosis, coagulopathy, myocardial infarction, and stroke. In certain populations of the northern latitudes (including Inuit, Greenland, Irish, and Danish populations), the incidence of heart disease, stroke, and thromboembolic disorders is less than in other populations. The diet of these northern peoples is richer in fish oils and, as a result, contains relatively larger amounts of marine oils (including EPA and DHA). Analogous to the conversion of arachidonic acid into TxA_2 and PGI_2, EPA is converted into TxA_3 and PGI_3. Importantly, the vasoconstricting and platelet aggregating effects of TxA_3 are relatively weak. As a result, the thromboxane–prostacyclin balance could be tipped toward vasodilation, platelet inhibition, and antithrombogenesis. This is one possible contributor to the observation that these northern populations have a lower incidence of heart disease and is cited as one rationale for increasing dietary fish consumption. Novel marine oil-derived mediators that possess potent anti-inflammatory and pro-resolving actions have also recently been discovered (see "Lipoxins, Resolvins, Protectins, and Maresins" section).

Lipoxygenase Pathway

Besides the cyclooxygenase pathway, the other major metabolic fate of arachidonic acid is the lipoxygenase pathway, which leads to the formation of leukotrienes and lipoxins. Lipoxygenases are enzymes that catalyze the insertion of molecular oxygen into arachidonic acid, using non-heme iron to generate specific hydroperoxides. Three lipoxygenases, 5-lipoxygenase, 12-lipoxygenase, and 15-lipoxygenase (5-LOX, etc.), are the major LOX isoforms found in humans (Table 43-4). The lipoxygenases are numbered based on the carbon position in arachidonic acid on which they catalyze the insertion of molecular oxygen. The immediate products of lipoxygenase reactions are **hydroperoxyeicosatetraenoic acids** (**HPETEs**). HPETEs can be reduced to the corresponding **hydroxyeicosatetraenoic acids** (**HETEs**) by glutathione peroxidase-dependent enzymes. 5-HPETE formed by 5-LOX is the direct precursor to leukotriene A_4 (LTA_4), which itself is the precursor to all bioactive leukotrienes (Fig. 43-4). Lipoxygenases are also involved in converting 15-HETE and LTA_4 to lipoxins (Fig. 43-5).

5-LOX requires translocation to the nuclear membrane for enzymatic activity. The protein **5-lipoxygenase-activating protein** (**FLAP**) helps 5-LOX translocate to the nuclear membrane, form an active enzyme complex, and accept the arachidonic acid substrate from phospholipase A_2.

Leukotrienes

Leukotriene biosynthesis begins with the 5-LOX-mediated conversion of 5-HPETE to leukotriene A_4 (LTA_4). Therefore, *5-LOX catalyzes the first two steps in leukotriene biosynthesis* (Fig. 43-4). It is not known whether 5-HPETE diffuses out of the 5-LOX catalytic site between these steps or remains bound to the same 5-LOX enzyme for both reactions.

LTA_4 is next converted to either LTB_4 or LTC_4. The enzyme LTA_4 hydrolase converts LTA_4 to LTB_4 in neutrophils and erythrocytes. The conversion of LTA_4 to LTC_4 occurs in mast cells, basophils, eosinophils, and macrophages by the addition of a γ-glutamylcysteinylglycine tripeptide (glutathione). LTC_4, LTD_4, LTE_4, and LTF_4, which represent the **cysteinyl leukotrienes**, are interconverted by removal of amino acid portions of the γ-glutamylcysteinylglycine tripeptide (Fig. 43-4).

LTB_4 acts via two G protein-coupled receptors, BLT_1 and BLT_2. Binding of LTB_4 to BLT_1, which is expressed mainly in tissues involved in host defense and inflammation (leukocytes, thymus, spleen), leads to proinflammatory sequelae such as neutrophil chemotaxis, aggregation, and transmigration across epithelium and endothelium. LTB_4 up-regulates neutrophil lysosomal function and generates reactive oxygen

TABLE 43-4 Tissue Expression of Lipoxygenases and Products of Lipoxygenase Action

LIPOXYGENASE	TISSUE EXPRESSION	PRODUCTS	PATHWAYS	NOTES
5-LOX	Neutrophils Macrophages Mast cells Eosinophils	5-HPETE/5-HETE LTA_4 Epoxytetraene "	Leukotrienes/lipoxins Lipoxins Lipoxins/aspirin-triggered lipoxins	Requires FLAP for activity

12-LOX
  Platelet type
 	
  Epidermal type
  Leukocyte type
	Platelets
	Megakaryocytes (tumors)
	Skin
	Macrophages
	GI system
	Brain
		12-HPETE/12-HETE
		Epoxytetraene
		"
		"
		"
		"
			Lipoxins
			"
			"
			"
			"
			"	

15-LOX	Macrophages Monocytes Airway epithelium	15-HPETE/15-HETE Epoxytetraene "	Lipoxins " "	

FLAP, 5-lipoxygenase activating protein; GI, gastrointestinal; HETE, hydroxyeicosatetraenoic acid; HPETE, hydroperoxyeicosatetraenoic acid; LOX, lipoxygenase; LT, leukotriene.

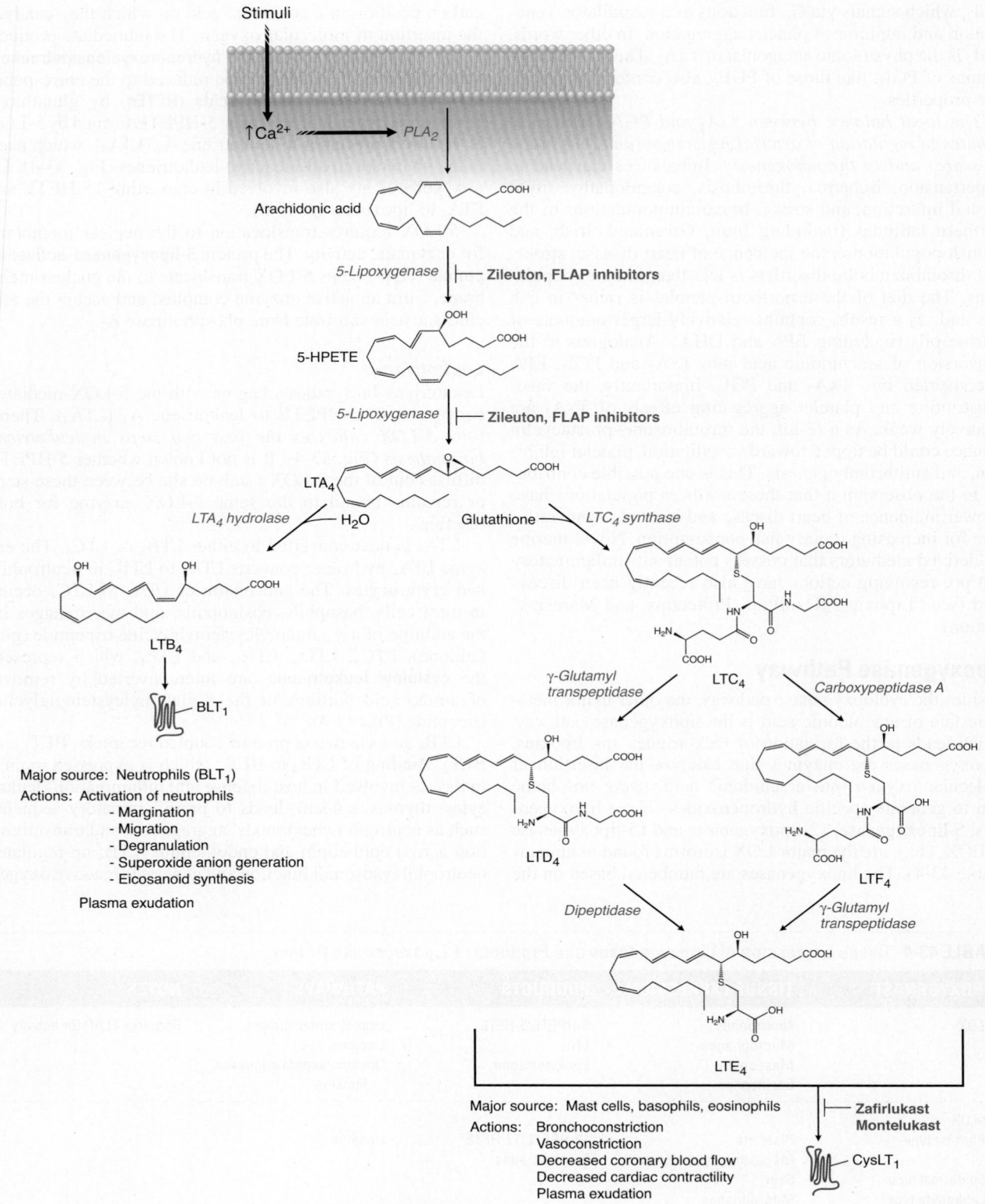

Stimuli

$\uparrow Ca^{2+}$ ⟶ PLA_2

Arachidonic acid

COOH

5-Lipoxygenase ⊣ **Zileuton, FLAP inhibitors**

5-HPETE

COOH

5-Lipoxygenase ⊣ **Zileuton, FLAP inhibitors**

LTA_4

COOH

LTA₄ hydrolase — H_2O Glutathione — *LTC₄ synthase*

LTB_4

COOH

LTC_4

⟶ BLT₁

γ-Glutamyl transpeptidase   *Carboxypeptidase A*

Major source: Neutrophils (BLT₁)

Actions: Activation of neutrophils
- Margination
- Migration
- Degranulation
- Superoxide anion generation
- Eicosanoid synthesis

Plasma exudation

LTD_4

LTF_4

Dipeptidase   *γ-Glutamyl transpeptidase*

LTE_4

Major source: Mast cells, basophils, eosinophils

Actions: Bronchoconstriction
Vasoconstriction
Decreased coronary blood flow
Decreased cardiac contractility
Plasma exudation

⊣ **Zafirlukast Montelukast**

⟶ CysLT₁

FIGURE 43-4. Leukotriene biosynthesis, function, and pharmacologic inhibition. The biosynthetic pathways from arachidonic acid to the leukotrienes are shown. Zileuton and 5-lipoxygenase activating protein (FLAP) inhibitors prevent the conversion of arachidonic acid to 5-HPETE and LTA₄; zileuton has been used in the chronic management of asthma. Zafirlukast and montelukast are antagonists at CysLT₁, the receptor for all cysteinyl leukotrienes (mainly LTC₄ and LTD₄); these drugs are used in the chronic management of asthma. The cysteinyl leukotrienes also interact with CysLT₂ (*not shown*). BLT₁ and BLT₂ are LTB₄-related G protein-coupled receptors; BLT₁ is the major LTB₄ receptor. BLT₂ (*not shown*) is the G protein-coupled receptor for 12-HHT, a cyclooxygenase product (see text for details).

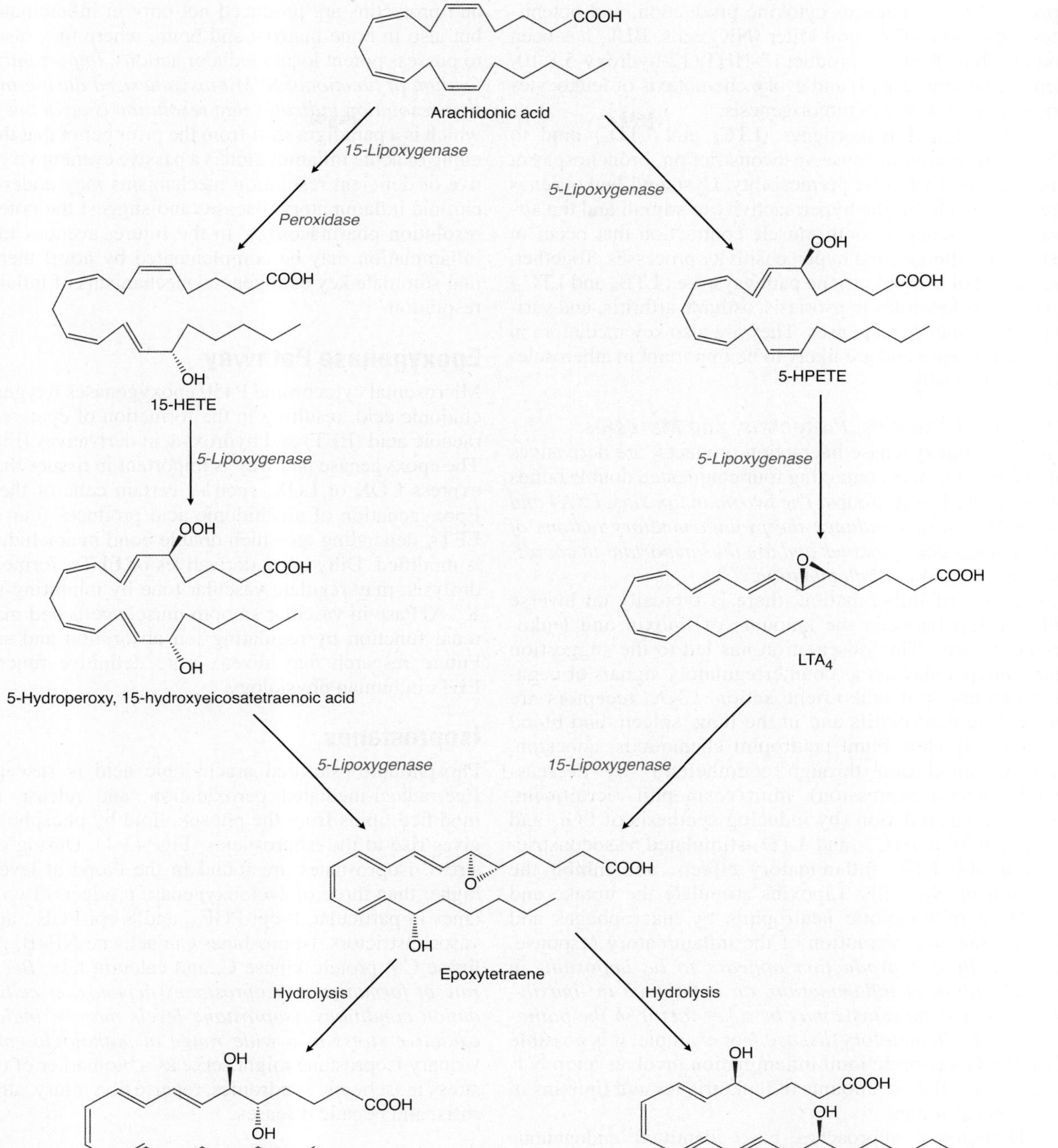

FIGURE 43-5. **Lipoxin biosynthesis.** Two main routes lead to biosynthesis of the lipoxins. In each pathway, sequential lipoxygenase reactions are required to generate epoxytetraene, which then undergoes hydrolysis to yield the lipoxins. **Left pathway:** Arachidonic acid is converted to 15-HETE by sequential activity of 15-lipoxygenase and peroxidase. 15-HETE is converted by 5-lipoxygenase to the chemical intermediate 5-hydroperoxy, 15-hydroxyeicosatetraenoic acid, and 5-lipoxygenase acts on this intermediate to form an epoxytetraene. **Right pathway:** Arachidonic acid is converted to 5-HPETE by 5-lipoxygenase, and 5-HPETE is converted to LTA$_4$ by further action of 5-lipoxygenase. LTA$_4$ is converted to epoxytetraene by 15-lipoxygenase. **Common pathway:** Epoxytetraene is hydrolyzed to the active lipoxins LXA$_4$ and LXB$_4$. The lipoxins have both anti-inflammatory and pro-resolving roles, are counterregulators of leukotriene action, and regulate many cytokines and growth factors. LXA$_4$ is a selective agonist at the G protein-coupled receptor FPR2/ALX.

species (ROS), enhances cytokine production, and potentiates the actions of natural killer (NK) cells. BLT_2 has been found to bind the COX product 12-HHT (12-hydroxy-5,8,10-heptadecatrienoic acid) and evoke chemotaxis of leukocytes and may play a role in tumorigenesis.

The cysteinyl leukotrienes (LTC_4 and LTD_4) bind to $CysLT_1$ receptors to cause vasoconstriction, bronchospasm, and increased vascular permeability. Cysteinyl leukotrienes are responsible for the hyperreactivity to stimuli and the airway and vascular smooth muscle contraction that occur in asthmatic, allergic, and hypersensitivity processes. Together, both arms of the leukotriene pathways (i.e., LTB_4 and LTC_4/LTD_4) play key roles in psoriasis, asthma, arthritis, and various inflammatory responses. They are also key mediators in vascular disease and are likely to be important in atherosclerosis and obesity.

Lipoxins, Resolvins, Protectins, and Maresins

Lipoxins (**lipox**ygenase **in**teraction products) are derivatives of arachidonic acid containing four conjugated double bonds and three hydroxyl groups. *The two main lipoxins, LXA4 and LXB4 (Fig. 43-5), balance the proinflammatory actions of leukotrienes and cytokines and are thus important in coordinating resolution of inflammation.*

At sites of inflammation, there is typically an inverse relationship between the amounts of lipoxin and leukotriene present. This observation has led to the suggestion that lipoxins may act as counterregulatory signals or negative regulators of leukotriene action. LXA_4 receptors are present on neutrophils and in the lung, spleen, and blood vessels. Lipoxins blunt neutrophil chemotaxis, adhesion, and transmigration through endothelium (by decreasing P-selectin expression), limit eosinophil recruitment, stimulate vasodilation (by inducing synthesis of PGI_2 and PGE_2), inhibit LTC_4- and LTD_4-stimulated vasoconstriction, inhibit LTB_4 inflammatory effects, and inhibit the function of NK cells. Lipoxins stimulate the uptake and clearance of apoptotic neutrophils by macrophages and thereby mediate resolution of the inflammatory response. *Because lipoxin production appears to be important in the resolution of inflammation, an imbalance in lipoxin–leukotriene homeostasis may be a key factor in the pathogenesis of inflammatory disease.* For example, it is possible that Ms. G's chronic joint inflammation involves an imbalance in the relative amounts of leukotrienes and lipoxins in her affected joints.

Metabolomic approaches have identified endogenous families of omega-3-derived mediators, called *resolvins, protectins*, and *maresins*, that control both the magnitude and duration of inflammation (Fig. 43-6). Together with lipoxins, they constitute a chemical genus of specialized pro-resolving mediators (SPM). Resolvins, protectins, and maresins are biosynthesized from essential omega-3 fatty acid precursors, especially EPA and DHA.

The mapping of these endogenous inflammation-resolution circuits provides new avenues to probe the molecular bases of many widely occurring inflammatory diseases. Each of the resolvins, protectins, and maresins possesses multiple potent and stereoselective actions in human cells and in animal disease models. In general, these specialized local mediators limit neutrophil recruitment to sites of inflammation and stimulate macrophages to take up and remove apoptotic cells from the inflammatory site. Resolvins and protectins are produced not only in inflammatory sites but also in bone marrow and brain, where they also appear to possess potent local mediator actions. *Importantly, identification of functional SPM biosynthesized during inflammation-resolution indicates that resolution is an active process, which is a paradigm shift from the prior belief that the dampening of acute inflammation is a passive event in vivo.* Defective or deficient resolution mechanisms may underlie some chronic inflammatory diseases and suggest the potential for resolution pharmacology. In the future, avenues to control inflammation may be complemented by novel therapeutics that stimulate key endogenous mechanisms of inflammation resolution.

Epoxygenase Pathway

Microsomal cytochrome P450 epoxygenases oxygenate arachidonic acid, resulting in the formation of epoxyeicosatetraenoic acid (EET) and hydroxyacid derivatives (Fig. 43-1). The epoxygenase pathway is important in tissues that do not express COX or LOX, such as certain cells of the kidney. Epoxygenation of arachidonic acid produces four different EETs, depending on which double bond in arachidonic acid is modified. Dihydroxy derivatives of EETs, formed by hydrolysis, may regulate vascular tone by inhibiting the Na^+/K^+ ATPase in vascular smooth muscle cells and may affect renal function by regulating ion absorption and secretion. Future research may reveal more definitive functions for EETs in human physiology.

Isoprostanes

Phospholipid-esterified arachidonic acid is susceptible to free-radical-mediated peroxidation, and release of these modified lipids from the phospholipid by phospholipase A_2 gives rise to the isoprostanes (Fig. 43-1). During oxidative stress, isoprostanes are found in the blood at levels much higher than those of cyclooxygenase products. Two isoprostanes in particular, 8-epi-$PGF_{2\alpha}$ and 8-epi-PGE_2, are potent vasoconstrictors. Isoprostanes can activate NFκB, phospholipase Cγ, protein kinase C, and calcium flux. *Because the rate of formation of isoprostanes depends on cellular oxidation conditions, isoprostane levels may be indicative of oxidative stress in a wide range of pathologic conditions.* Urinary isoprostane might serve as a biomarker of oxidative stress in ischemic syndromes, reperfusion injury, atherosclerosis, and hepatic diseases.

Metabolic Inactivation of Local Eicosanoids

Prostaglandins, leukotrienes, thromboxanes, and lipoxins are inactivated by hydroxylation, β-oxidation (resulting in a loss of two carbons), or ω-oxidation (to dicarboxylic acid derivatives). These degradation processes render the molecules more hydrophilic and excretable in the urine.

Integrated Inflammation Schema

As described above, eicosanoids are generated locally in numerous complex reactions. It is not necessary to remember each mediator but rather to understand the general scheme of these biosynthetic pathways. This section, along with Table 43-5, provides a concise overview of the physiologic functions of eicosanoids relevant to inflammation and host defense.

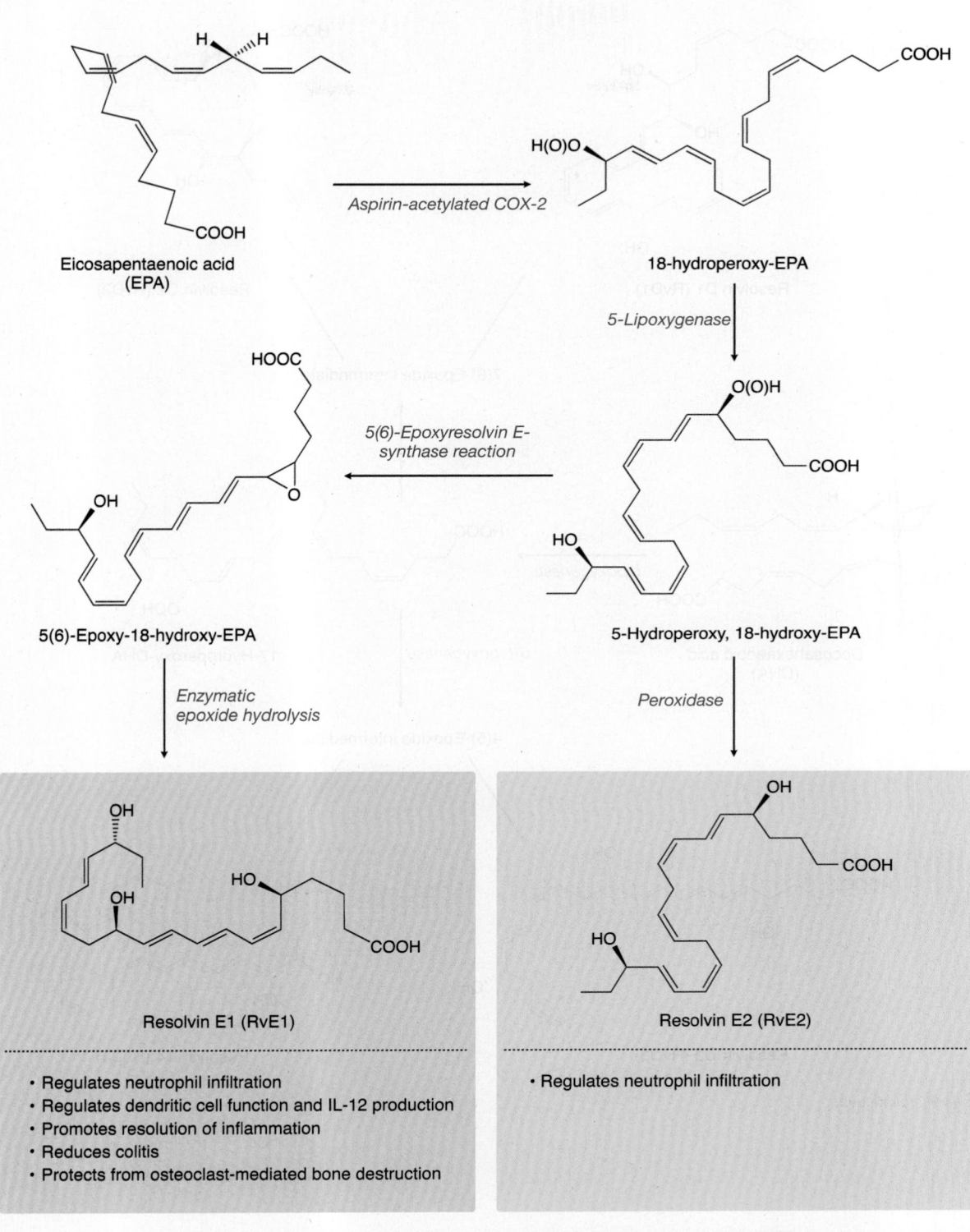

FIGURE 43-6. Resolvins, protectins, and maresins: biosynthesis and actions of novel families of omega-3-derived mediators. A. EPA is the precursor to E-series resolvins. **B and C.** DHA is the precursor to D-series resolvins, protectins, and maresins. Some of the major endogenous anti-inflammatory and pro-resolving functions are listed below some of the mediators. In addition, resolvin D1 regulates neutrophil infiltration and resolvin D2 enhances microbial phagocytosis and clearance. *(continued)*

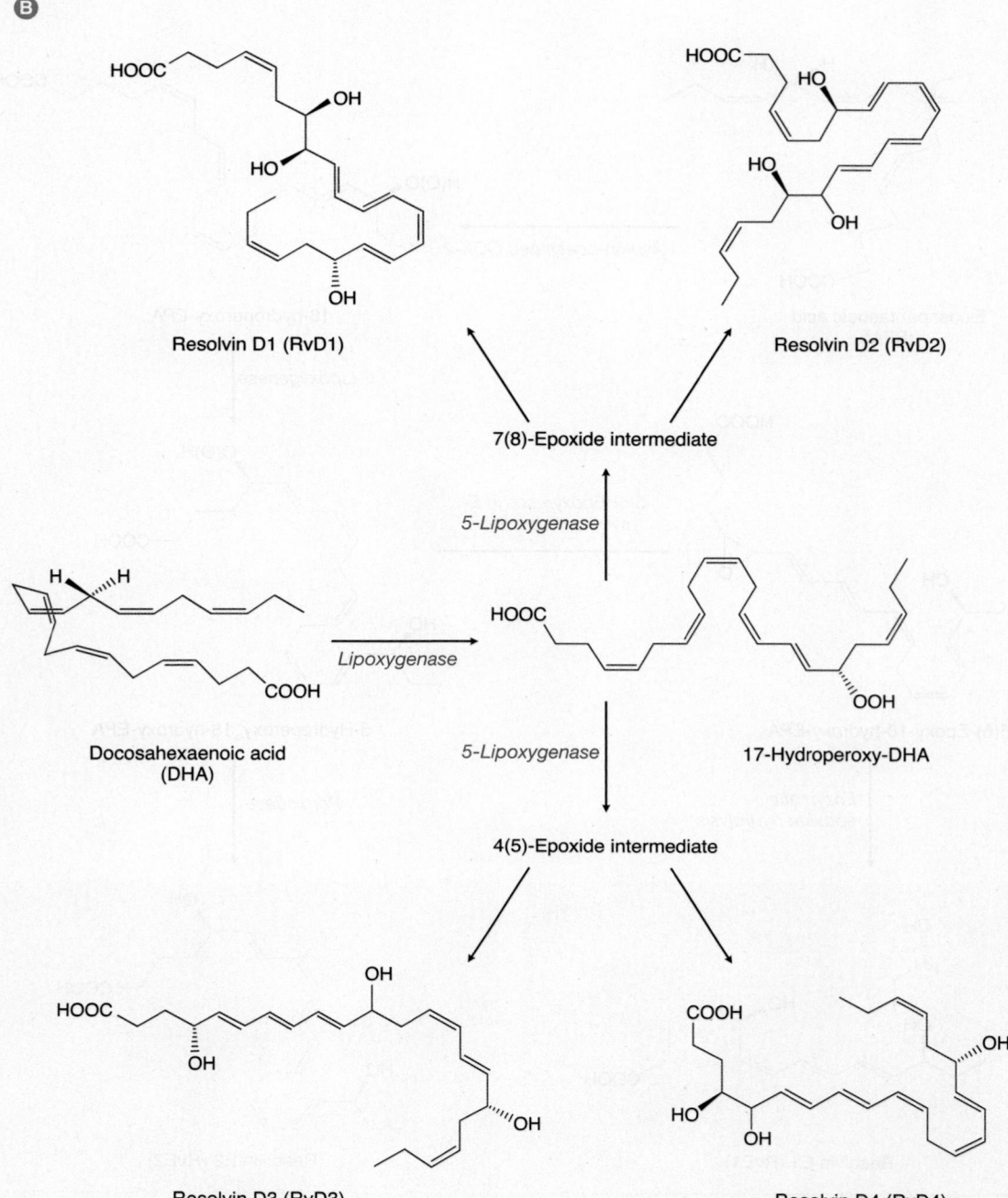

FIGURE 43-6. *(continued)*

C
H
H
COOH
Docosahexaenoic acid (DHA)
Lipoxygenase
HOOC
OOH
17-Hydroperoxy-DHA
Enzymatic epoxidation and hydrolysis
OH
COOH
OH
Protectin D1 (PD1)
• Regulates neutrophil and T-cell infiltration
• Regulates TNF and interferon production
• Promotes resolution of inflammation
• Reduces peritonitis and airway inflammation
• Protects brain from ischemia/reperfusion injury
• Mitigates kidney ischemia injury
H
H
COOH
Docosahexaenoic acid (DHA)
12/15-Lipoxygenases
O(O)H
COOH
14-hydroperoxy-DHA
Enzymatic epoxidation and conversion
COOH
OH
OH
Maresin 1 (MaR1)
• Regulates neutrophil infiltration
• Promotes resolution of inflammation

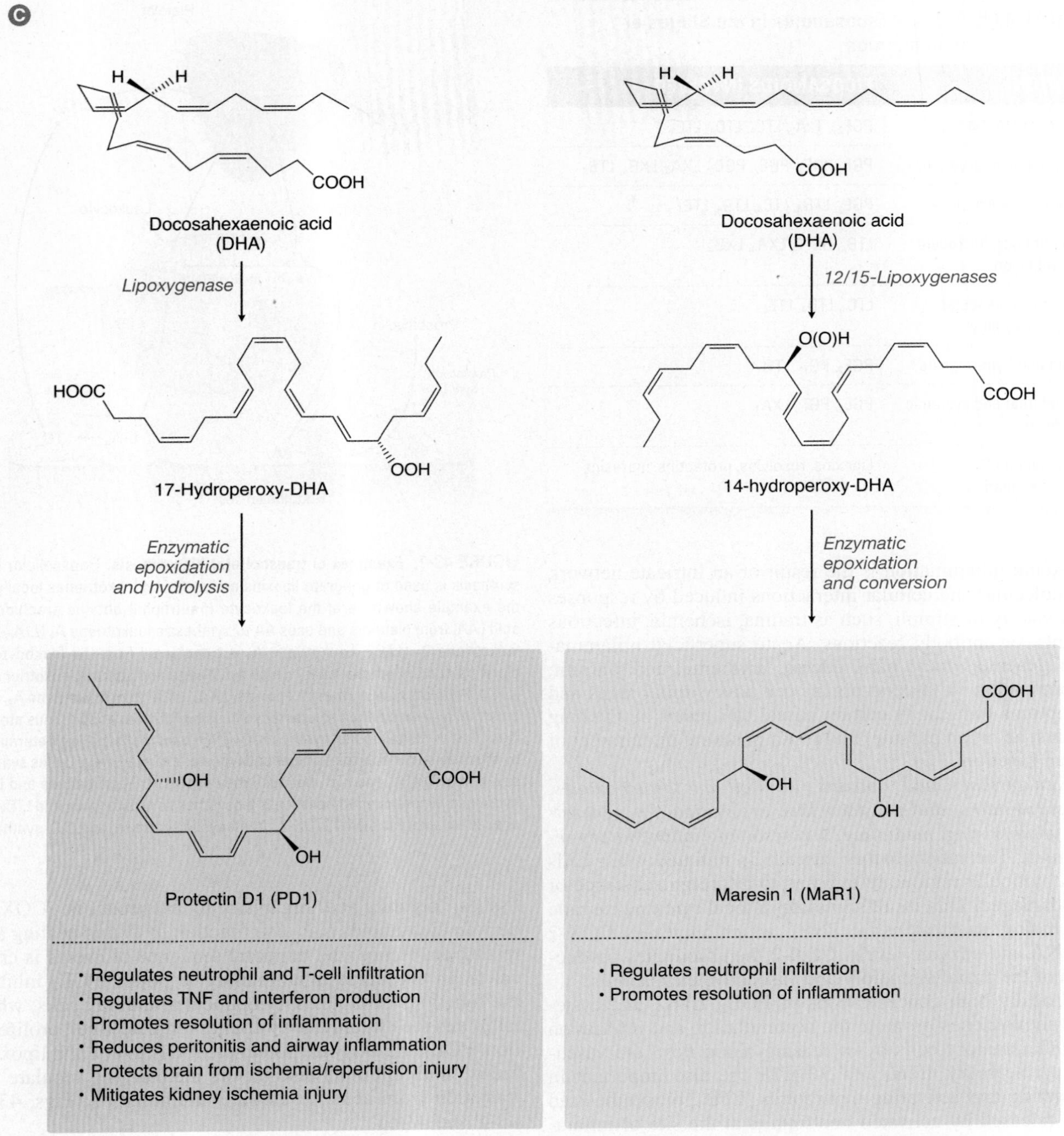

FIGURE 43-6. *(continued)*

TABLE 43-5 Roles of Eicosanoids in the Stages of Inflammation

ACTION	EICOSANOIDS INVOLVED
Vasoconstriction	$PGF_{2\alpha}$, TxA_2, LTC_4, LTD_4, LTE_4
Vasodilation (erythema)	PGI_2, PGE_1, PGE_2, PGD_2, LXA_4, LXB_4, LTB_4
Edema (swelling)	PGE_2, LTB_4, LTC_4, LTD_4, LTE_4
Chemotaxis, leukocyte adhesion	LTB_4, HETE, LXA_4, LXB_4
Increased vascular permeability	LTC_4, LTD_4, LTE_4
Pain and hyperalgesia	PGE_2, PGI_2, LTB_4
Local heat and systemic fever	PGE_2, PGI_2, LXA_4
Resolution of inflammation	Lipoxins, resolvins, protectins, maresins

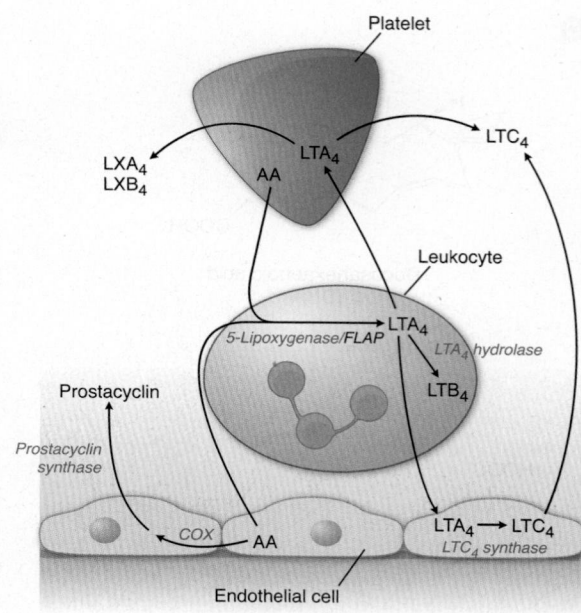

FIGURE 43-7. Examples of transcellular biosynthesis. Transcellular biosynthesis is used to generate lipoxins and cysteinyl leukotrienes locally. In the example shown here, the leukocyte (neutrophil) obtains arachidonic acid (*AA*) from platelets and uses AA to synthesize leukotriene A_4 (*LTA$_4$*) and leukotriene B_4 (*LTB$_4$*). Leukotriene A_4 is transferred from the leukocyte to platelets and endothelial cells, which synthesize and secrete leukotriene C_4 (*LTC$_4$*). Platelets also synthesize lipoxins (*LXA$_4$, LXB$_4$*) from leukotriene A_4, and endothelial cells synthesize prostacyclin using AA from endogenous stores. Note that the eicosanoids synthesized within each cell type are determined by the enzymatic repertoire of that cell type: for example, neutrophils synthesize primarily LTA_4 and LTB_4 because they express 5-lipoxygenase and LTA_4 hydrolase, whereas endothelial cells biosynthesize prostacyclin and LTC_4 because they express COX-1, COX-2, prostacyclin synthase, and LTC_4 synthase.

Acute inflammation is the result of an intricate network of molecular and cellular interactions induced by responses to a variety of stimuli, such as trauma, ischemia, infectious agents, or antibody reactions. Acute superficial inflammation generates local pain, edema, erythema, and warmth; inflammation in visceral organs can have similar signs and symptoms (which, in certain cases, can result in swelling against an organ capsule) and result in severe impairment of organ function.

Leukotrienes and lipoxins, as well as thromboxanes, prostaglandins, and prostacyclins, are critical for generating, maintaining, mediating, and resolving inflammatory responses. The inflammatory cascade is initiated when cells in a particular region are exposed to a foreign substance or are damaged. That insult stimulates a local cytokine cascade (including interleukins or TNF), which increases COX-2 mRNA and enzyme levels. COX-2 then facilitates production of the proinflammatory and vasoactive eicosanoids.

Locally high concentrations of PGE_2, LTB_4, and cysteinyl leukotrienes promote the accumulation and infiltration of inflammatory cells by increasing blood flow and vascular permeability. LTB_4 and 5-HETE are also important in attracting and activating neutrophils. LTB_4, biosynthesized and released by activated neutrophils at the site of inflammation, recruits and activates additional neutrophils and lymphocytes so that these cells adhere to endothelial surfaces and transmigrate into the interstitial spaces. Increased vascular permeability also results in fluid leak and cellular infiltration, causing edema.

With the aggregation of a multitude of inflammatory cells, **transcellular biosynthetic routes** are exploited to generate eicosanoids (Fig. 43-7). *In transcellular biosynthesis, eicosanoid intermediates are donated from one cell type to another to generate a greater diversity of local chemical mediators.* This demonstrates the importance of cellular adhesion and cell–cell interaction in inflammatory and immune responses.

Feedback mechanisms are designed to ensure that the inflammatory response cannot proceed unchecked. Lipoxins help resolve inflammation and promote the return of the tissues, organs, and organism to homeostasis. COX-2-derived eicosanoids may also function in wound healing and resolution. Hence, the temporal sequence of events is critical to an organized inflammatory response. PGE_2 inhibits the functions of B and T lymphocytes and NK cells, while LTB_4 and the cysteinyl leukotrienes regulate T-cell proliferation. PGE_2 and PGI_2 are potent pain sensitizers, and lipoxins reduce nociception. These factors mediate and regulate the transition from acute to chronic inflammation (Figs. 43-2, 43-4, and 43-6).

PATHOPHYSIOLOGY OF EICOSANOIDS

Inflammation and the immune response are the body's mechanisms for combating foreign invaders and trauma. The overall scheme is designed to remove the inciting stimulus and resolve tissue damage. In some cases, the response mechanism itself causes local tissue damage, such as when activated neutrophils inadvertently release proteases and reactive oxygen species into the local milieu. In other settings, if the inflammatory reactions persist for too long or if the immune system misidentifies a component of self as foreign, misdirected responses can cause significant and chronic tissue injury.

Profiled briefly in the following discussion are selected inflammatory diseases in which eicosanoids are implicated, including asthma, inflammatory bowel disease, rheumatoid arthritis, glomerulonephritis, cancer, and cardiovascular disease. Other diseases not discussed here, but having a possible eicosanoid-related inflammatory basis, include certain skin disorders, reperfusion injuries, Alzheimer's disease, and adult respiratory distress syndrome.

Asthma

Asthma is an airway inflammatory disorder typified by intermittent attacks of dyspnea, coughing, and wheezing. Symptoms result from chronic airway inflammation, hyperreactivity, constriction, and obstruction. In asthma, antigens in the lungs stimulate cytokine cascades leading to the generation of both prostaglandins (e.g., PGD_2) and leukotrienes. LTB_4 attracts inflammatory cells and promotes cellular aggregation. LTB_4 acts particularly on B lymphocytes to cause cell activation, proliferation, and differentiation. LTB_4 also promotes expression of $Fc\epsilon RII$ receptors (i.e., receptors for the Fc portion of IgE antibodies) on mast cells and basophils; these receptors bind IgE that is released by antigen-stimulated B lymphocytes. LTC_4 and LTD_4 are extremely potent bronchoconstrictive compounds, more than 1,000 times as potent as histamine. These cysteinyl leukotrienes also cause the airway epithelium to secrete mucus, while impairing the clearance of mucus by inhibiting the beating of cilia on airway epithelium. Mucus secretion is exacerbated by neutrophils and eosinophils, which become part of the inflammatory exudate clogging the airways. LTD_4 and LTE_4 also recruit eosinophils to asthmatic airways; eosinophils integrate signals from T lymphocytes and, when activated, release factors that damage the airway epithelium and enhance local airway inflammation.

In mouse models of asthma in which either the 5-LOX or $CysLT_1$ gene is knocked out, reduced airway hyperresponsiveness and leukocyte infiltration are observed. These results underscore the important role of leukotrienes in the pathogenesis of asthma. The role of leukotriene inhibitors in asthma treatment is discussed below; for additional information, refer to Chapter 48, Integrative Inflammation Pharmacology: Asthma.

Inflammatory Bowel Disease

Crohn's disease and ulcerative colitis are idiopathic, chronic, relapsing, ulcerative, and inflammatory diseases of the gastrointestinal tract. Although the diseases are pathologically distinct, elevated LTB_4 production in the affected mucosa results in abnormal leukocyte infiltration into the parenchyma in both conditions. Chronic inflammation and leukocyte infiltration lead to progressive mucosal damage, with overt histologic changes. Crohn's disease is characterized by focal damage, fissuring ulcers, and granulomas, while mucosal inflammation and colonic dilatation are found in ulcerative colitis. Both diseases increase the risk of adenocarcinoma of the colon in the affected areas. Stable analogues of lipoxin A_4 are effective treatments in mouse models of Crohn's disease and bowel inflammation and may represent a promising new pharmacologic approach to the treatment of inflammatory bowel disease.

Rheumatoid Arthritis

Rheumatoid arthritis is a chronic, systemic, autoimmune, and inflammatory disease that primarily attacks the joints but also affects the skin, cardiovascular system, lungs, and muscles. Rheumatoid arthritis affects up to 1.5% of North Americans and is three times more prevalent in females than in males. Autoimmune targeting of normal joint proteins results in inflammation, with resultant local release of cytokines, TNF, growth factors, and interleukins, all of which induce COX-2 expression. *Levels of COX-2 enzyme and PGE_2 are markedly elevated in the synovial fluid of affected joints.* PGE_2 stimulates pain pathways, and other COX-2-derived eicosanoids and 5-LOX-derived leukotrienes activate the surrounding endothelium to recruit inflammatory cells. Macrophages release collagenase and proteases, while lymphocyte activity leads to immune complex formation; both processes further damage joint tissue and provide substrates that accelerate chronic inflammation. Common findings include synovitis, leukocytosis, rheumatoid nodules, and the presence of rheumatoid factor (a circulating antibody directed against IgG).

As a Native American woman in her fifth decade, Ms. G is in a higher risk group for rheumatoid arthritis. Autoimmune destruction of her joints resulted in the findings of a high erythrocyte sedimentation rate (consistent with a state of chronic inflammation), synovial leukocytosis, radiographic findings of bone loss, and the progressive loss of joint mobility and function. For additional information on rheumatoid arthritis, refer to Chapter 46, Pharmacology of Immunosuppression.

Glomerulonephritis

Glomerulonephritis delineates a large group of inflammatory renal conditions that may ultimately lead to renal failure through deterioration of renal hemodynamics and glomerular filtration. Local complement activation promotes neutrophil and macrophage infiltration. Infiltration of the glomerulus is a characteristic early pathologic finding that correlates with abnormal levels of LTB_4, which is biosynthesized by LTA_4 hydrolase in the kidney mesangium, and which facilitates neutrophil adhesion to the glomerular mesangium and epithelium. LTA_4 is also a substrate for the biosynthesis of LTC_4 and LTD_4. All of the cysteinyl leukotrienes (LTC_4, LTD_4, LTE_4, and LTF_4) promote endothelial and mesangial proliferation. Cysteinyl leukotrienes also directly affect glomerular function; specifically, LTC_4 and LTD_4 decrease renal blood flow and glomerular filtration rate (GFR) by vasoconstricting arterioles and contracting mesangial spaces. Studies with inhibitors have confirmed the roles of leukotrienes in glomerulonephritis: LOX inhibitors administered at early stages of glomerulonephritis prevent glomerular inflammation and evidence of structural damage, and both LOX inhibitors and LTD_4 receptor antagonists increase GFR and decrease proteinuria.

Interestingly, the kidney mesangium expresses both LTA_4 hydrolase and 12-LOX, conferring the ability to synthesize either LTB_4 or LXA_4 from leukocyte-derived LTA_4. At low concentrations, LTA_4 is used primarily for LTB_4 formation; this condition corresponds to the initiation of inflammation. Conversely, when LTA_4 concentrations are relatively high, as in long-standing inflammation, LTA_4 is converted mostly into LXA_4, which provides an autoinhibitory, counter-regulatory impact on the inflammatory response. In the glomerulus, LXA_4 counteracts the deleterious proinflammatory consequences of leukotrienes as well as the effect of leukotrienes on GFR, in part by raising afferent arteriolar flow via vasodilation.

Cancer

Long-term epidemiologic studies have suggested a correlation between chronic NSAID therapy and decreased incidence of colorectal cancer. Human colorectal adenomas and carcinomas express abundant COX-2; similar results have been found with gastric adenocarcinomas and breast tumors. In these tissues, COX-2 is believed to generate PGE_2 and other eicosanoids that promote tumor growth. The perinuclear localization of the COX-2 enzyme (Table 43-1) suggests the potential for an intracellular function of eicosanoid products in oncogenesis. Some eicosanoid derivatives can bind to homologues of the retinoic acid receptor (RXR) family of transcription factors, which are involved in many functions including the regulation of cell growth and differentiation. Overexpression of COX-2 would generate eicosanoids that could flood RXR signaling pathways and provide excessive growth stimuli. A COX-2 inhibitor is being sought as a prophylactic therapy for patients with familial adenomatous polyposis, who are at increased risk for colorectal cancer (see "COX-2 Inhibitors" section). There is also evidence that aspirin may be a chemoprotective agent in colorectal cancer.

Cardiovascular Disease

Platelet-derived thromboxane A_2 is an important mediator of thrombosis in acute coronary syndromes and other cardiovascular diseases; the COX inhibitor aspirin is an effective antiplatelet agent in the prophylaxis and treatment of these diseases (see below and Chapter 23, Pharmacology of Hemostasis and Thrombosis). Intravascular leukotriene production during the rupture of atheromatous plaques is also thought to contribute to the pathophysiology of acute coronary syndromes. Genetic polymorphisms in 5-lipoxygenase, FLAP, and LTA_4 hydrolase may be linked to myocardial infarction.

▍ PHARMACOLOGIC CLASSES AND AGENTS

Pharmacologic intervention in eicosanoid biosynthesis and action is particularly useful for controlling inflammation and restoring homeostasis. Pharmacologic interventions can be directed at any of the number of steps outlined above to achieve the desired effects with tissue, spatial, and temporal selectivity. Strategies include altering the expression of key enzymes, competitively and noncompetitively inhibiting the activity of specific enzymes (e.g., PGE_2 synthase), activating receptors with exogenous receptor agonists, and preventing receptor activation with exogenous receptor antagonists. As with all aspects of medicine, therapeutic benefits must be weighed against the possible adverse effects.

Phospholipase Inhibitors

Inhibition of phospholipase A_2 prevents the release of arachidonic acid from cellular phospholipids, the rate-limiting step in eicosanoid biosynthesis. In the absence of proinflammatory mediators derived from arachidonic acid, inflammation is limited.

Glucocorticoids (also known as *corticosteroids*, including **prednisone**, **prednisolone**, and **dexamethasone**) are a mainstay of therapy in a multitude of autoimmune and inflammatory

diseases. Glucocorticoids induce a family of secreted calcium- and phospholipid-dependent proteins called **lipocortins**. Lipocortins interfere with the action of phospholipase A_2 and thereby limit the availability of arachidonic acid. Annexins, such as annexin 1 and annexin 1-derived peptides, are also induced by glucocorticoids. In turn, annexins act at G protein-coupled receptors on leukocytes to block proinflammatory responses and enhance endogenous anti-inflammatory mechanisms; one anti-inflammatory mechanism involves activation of the lipoxin A_4 receptor. Glucocorticoids also inhibit the action of COX-2 and the formation of prostaglandins by several mechanisms: (1) repressing COX-2 gene and enzyme expression; (2) repressing the expression of cytokines that activate COX-2; and (3) as noted above, limiting the available pool of COX-2 substrate (arachidonic acid) by indirectly blocking phospholipase A_2. Because of this profound and global suppression of immune and inflammatory responses, glucocorticoids are used to treat a number of autoimmune conditions (see Chapter 46).

Small-molecule inhibitors of specific phospholipases are under investigation; these compounds may offer the potential for decreased adverse effects compared to those associated with glucocorticoid use. See Chapter 29, Pharmacology of the Adrenal Cortex, for a more extensive discussion of the effects of glucocorticoids.

Cyclooxygenase Inhibitors

Cyclooxygenase pathway inhibitors are some of the most frequently prescribed drugs in medicine. The nonsteroidal anti-inflammatory drugs (NSAIDs) and acetaminophen are the most commonly used agents in this class.

Traditional Nonselective Inhibitors: NSAIDs

NSAIDs are clinically important because of their combined anti-inflammatory, antipyretic, and analgesic properties. The ultimate goal of most NSAID therapies is to inhibit the COX-mediated generation of proinflammatory eicosanoids and to limit the extent of inflammation, fever, and pain. The antipyretic activity of NSAIDs is likely related to their ability to decrease the levels of PGE_2, particularly in the region of the brain surrounding the hypothalamus. *Despite the benefits of current NSAIDs, these drugs only suppress the signs of the underlying inflammatory response but may not necessarily reverse or resolve the inflammatory process.*

A multitude of NSAIDs have been developed over the last century; most are polycyclic carboxylic acid derivatives. Except for aspirin, all NSAIDs act as reversible, competitive inhibitors of cyclooxygenase (Fig. 43-2). These drugs block the hydrophobic channel of the cyclooxygenase protein where the substrate arachidonic acid binds, thereby preventing conversion of arachidonic acid to PGG_2. Traditional NSAIDs inhibit both COX-1 and COX-2 to different degrees. Because of inhibition of COX-1, long-term NSAID therapy has many deleterious effects. The cytoprotective roles of the COX-1 eicosanoid products are eliminated, leading to a spectrum of **NSAID-induced gastropathy** including dyspepsia, gastrotoxicity, subepithelial damage and hemorrhage, gastric mucosal erosion, frank ulceration, and gastric mucosal necrosis. As in Ms. G's case, patients with gastric ulceration can have bleeding into the stomach, where reaction of hemoglobin with stomach acid results in hematemesis, or vomiting of material that has the color and consistency of "coffee grounds." Regulation of blood flow to the kidney is similarly perturbed, decreasing GFR and potentially causing renal ischemia, papillary necrosis, interstitial nephritis, and renal failure. The results of studies on the effects of COX-2 inhibitors (see below) have prompted reinvestigation of the effects of COX-1 inhibitors and traditional NSAIDs, with the finding that these classes of drugs may also be associated with cardiac risks. The US Food and Drug Administration (FDA) asked nonprescription NSAID manufacturers to update labeling with specific information about cardiovascular risks and to "remind patients of the limited dose and duration of treatment of these products." Epidemiologic studies suggest that up to 20–30% of hospitalizations of patients over the age of 60 may be due to complications of NSAID use.

The organic acid functionality of NSAIDs confers important pharmacokinetic properties on these drugs, including near-complete absorption from the gut, binding to plasma albumin, accumulation in cells at the site of inflammation, and efficient renal excretion. NSAIDs can be divided into short (<6 hours) and long (>10 hours) half-life classes. NSAIDs with long elimination half-lives include **naproxen**, **salicylate**, **piroxicam**, and **phenylbutazone**.

Chemical classification of the NSAIDs is based on the structure of a key moiety in each subclass (Fig. 43-8). The following discussion groups the NSAIDs by chemical class; a discussion of the choice of a particular NSAID for a given clinical situation follows the descriptions of the individual agents.

Salicylates
Salicylates include **aspirin** (acetylsalicylic acid) and its derivatives. Aspirin is the oldest of the NSAIDs and is widely used to treat mild to moderate pain, headache, myalgia, and arthralgia. *In contrast to other NSAIDs, aspirin acts in an* **irreversible** *manner by acetylating the active-site serine residue in both COX-1 and COX-2.* Acetylation of COX-1 destroys the enzyme's cyclooxygenase activity, preventing the formation of COX-1-derived prostaglandins, thromboxanes, and prostacyclin. Salicylates (along with indomethacin, piroxicam, and ibuprofen) may also inhibit the neutrophil oxidative burst by reducing NADPH oxidase activity.

Daily low-dose aspirin is used as an antithrombogenic agent for management of acute coronary syndromes, chronic atherosclerotic disease, and ischemic stroke. Recall that aspirin is antithrombogenic because of its irreversible inhibition of COX, which prevents platelets from biosynthesizing TxA_2. Within an hour of oral aspirin administration, the COX-1 activity in existing platelets is irreversibly destroyed. Platelets, lacking nuclei, cannot synthesize new protein. Therefore, the irreversibly acetylated COX-1 enzymes cannot be replaced by freshly synthesized proteins, and the platelets' cyclooxygenase activity is irreversibly inhibited for their circulating lifetime (about 10 days). Although aspirin also irreversibly inhibits vascular endothelial cell COX-1 and COX-2, the endothelial cells can synthesize new COX protein and thus can rapidly resume synthesis of PGI_2. *A single administration of aspirin thus decreases for several days the amount of thromboxane that can be generated, shifting the vascular TxA_2-PGI_2 balance toward PGI_2-mediated vasodilation, platelet inhibition, and antithrombogenesis.*

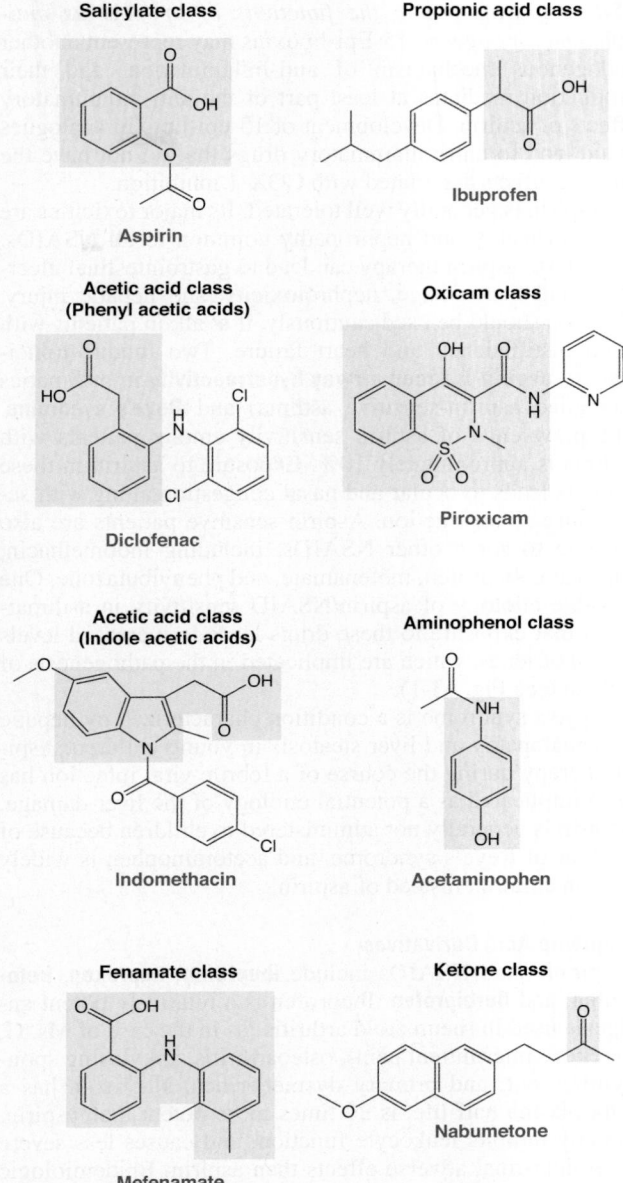

FIGURE 43-8. Structural classes of NSAIDs. NSAIDs are generally hydrophobic molecules, most of which have a carboxylic acid group. NSAIDs are categorized by class depending on one or more of the key moieties in the structure. The moiety that is common to members of each class is highlighted by a box. The structure helps to determine the pharmacokinetic properties of each particular NSAID. Note that acetaminophen is not actually an NSAID, because it has only weak anti-inflammatory properties; this drug is included here because, like NSAIDs, acetaminophen is commonly used for its analgesic and antipyretic effects.

Aspirin-mediated inhibition of COX-2 prevents the generation of prostaglandins. Unlike COX-1, which is totally inactivated by aspirin, the aspirin-modified COX-2 enzyme retains a distinct part of its catalytic activity and can form a new product, 15-(R)-HETE, from arachidonic acid. By analogy to lipoxin biosynthesis (Fig. 43-5), 5-LOX then converts 15-(R)-HETE to 15-epi-lipoxins, which are relatively stable stereoisomers (carbon 15-position epimers) of lipoxins that are collectively called **aspirin-triggered lipoxins (ATLs)**.

15-Epi-lipoxins mimic the functions of lipoxins as anti-inflammatory agents. 15-Epi-lipoxins may represent another endogenous mechanism of anti-inflammation, and their production mediates at least part of the anti-inflammatory effects of aspirin. Development of 15-epi-lipoxin analogues could lead to anti-inflammatory drugs that do not have the adverse effects associated with COX-1 inhibition.

Aspirin is generally well tolerated. Its major toxicities are the gastropathy and nephropathy common to all NSAIDs. Long-term aspirin therapy can lead to gastrointestinal ulceration and hemorrhage, nephrotoxicity, and hepatic injury. NSAIDs should be used cautiously, if at all, in patients with renal insufficiency and heart failure. Two unique toxicities are **aspirin-induced airway hyperreactivity** in asthmatics (so-called aspirin-sensitive asthma) and **Reye's syndrome**. The prevalence of aspirin sensitivity among patients with asthma is approximately 10%. Exposure to aspirin in these patients leads to ocular and nasal congestion along with severe airway obstruction. Aspirin-sensitive patients are also reactive to some other NSAIDs, including indomethacin, naproxen, ibuprofen, mefenamate, and phenylbutazone. One possible etiology of aspirin/NSAID sensitivity in asthmatics is that exposure to these drugs leads to increased levels of leukotrienes, which are implicated in the pathogenesis of asthma (see Fig. 43-1).

Reye's syndrome is a condition characterized by hepatic encephalopathy and liver steatosis in young children. Aspirin therapy during the course of a febrile viral infection has been implicated as a potential etiology of the liver damage. Aspirin is generally not administered to children because of the fear of Reye's syndrome, and acetaminophen is widely used in children instead of aspirin.

Propionic Acid Derivatives

Propionic acid NSAIDs include **ibuprofen**, **naproxen**, **ketoprofen**, and **flurbiprofen**. Ibuprofen is a relatively potent analgesic used in rheumatoid arthritis (as in the case of Ms. G, to relieve intermittent pain), osteoarthritis, ankylosing spondylitis, gout, and primary dysmenorrhea. Naproxen has a long plasma half-life, is 20 times more potent than aspirin, directly inhibits leukocyte function, and causes less severe gastrointestinal adverse effects than aspirin. Epidemiologic studies have suggested that naproxen may be the least cardiotoxic NSAID, but the current evidence for this finding is insufficient to support a separate clinical indication.

Acetic Acid Derivatives

Acetic acid NSAIDs include the indoleacetic acids—**indomethacin**, **sulindac**, and **etodolac**—and the phenylacetic acids **diclofenac** and **ketorolac** (a substituted phenylacetic acid derivative). Besides inhibiting cyclooxygenase, many of the acetic acid NSAIDs promote the incorporation of unesterified arachidonic acid into triglyceride, thus reducing the availability of the substrate for cyclooxygenase and lipoxygenase. Indomethacin is a direct inhibitor of neutrophil motility, but it is not tolerated by patients as well as ibuprofen. Diclofenac also reduces intracellular arachidonic acid concentrations by altering cellular fatty acid transport. Diclofenac is a more potent anti-inflammatory than indomethacin and naproxen and is used widely in the treatment of pain associated with renal stones. Ketorolac is a strong analgesic that is available in both intravenous and intramuscular preparations. It is used particularly in

postsurgical patients; however, in part due to its potency and adverse effects, ketorolac is used for no more than 3–5 days.

The acetic acid NSAIDs are mostly used to relieve symptoms in the long-term treatment of rheumatoid arthritis, osteoarthritis, ankylosing spondylitis, and other musculoskeletal disorders. Indomethacin also has specific uses in the treatment of gout and pericarditis and in promoting the closure of a patent ductus arteriosus in newborns by inhibiting the vasodilatory eicosanoids PGE_2 and PGI_2. Use of acetic acid NSAIDs causes gastrointestinal ulceration and, rarely, hepatitis and jaundice.

Oxicam Derivatives

Piroxicam is as efficacious as aspirin, naproxen, and ibuprofen in the treatment of rheumatoid arthritis and osteoarthritis and may be better tolerated. Piroxicam has additional effects in the modulation of neutrophil function by inhibiting collagenase, proteoglycanase, and the oxidative burst. Because of its extremely long half-life, piroxicam can be administered once daily. As with other NSAIDs, piroxicam displays gastrointestinal adverse effects such as gastric ulceration, and it prolongs the bleeding time because of its antiplatelet effect.

Fenamate Derivatives

The two fenamate NSAIDs are **mefenamate** and **meclofenamate**. Both inhibit cyclooxygenases but also antagonize prostanoid receptors to various degrees. Because fenamates have less anti-inflammatory activity and are more toxic than aspirin, there is little advantage to their use. Mefenamate is used only for primary dysmenorrhea, and meclofenamate is used in the treatment of rheumatoid arthritis and osteoarthritis.

Ketone NSAIDs

Nabumetone is a ketone prodrug that is oxidized in vivo to the active acid form. Compared to other nonselective NSAIDs, nabumetone has preferential activity against COX-2. The incidence of gastrointestinal adverse effects is relatively low, although headache and dizziness are frequently reported.

Acetaminophen

Acetaminophen is sometimes classified with the NSAIDs, but it is technically not an NSAID: *although acetaminophen has analgesic and antipyretic effects similar to aspirin, the anti-inflammatory effect of acetaminophen is insignificant because of its weak inhibition of cyclooxygenases.* Nonetheless, acetaminophen therapy is widely used, especially in patients (such as children) who are at risk for the adverse effects of aspirin. The most important adverse effect of acetaminophen is hepatotoxicity, and clinicians are advised both to monitor and reduce the dose of acetaminophen in combination with other analgesics and to reduce the total daily dose of acetaminophen. Modification of acetaminophen by hepatic cytochrome P450 enzymes produces a reactive metabolite, which is normally detoxified by conjugation with glutathione. An overdose of acetaminophen can overwhelm glutathione stores, leading to cellular and oxidative damage and, in severe cases, to acute hepatic necrosis (see Chapter 6, Drug Toxicity).

Selection of the Appropriate NSAID

The anti-inflammatory, analgesic, and antipyretic effects of the NSAIDs vary among the many agents. However, despite differences in chemistry, tissue selectivity, enzyme selectivity, pharmacokinetics, and pharmacodynamics, the differences in efficacy may not be clinically significant. Overall, the rationale and choice of NSAID do not generally make a substantial difference in treating rheumatoid arthritis or osteoarthritis. However, successful NSAID therapy is still considered more of an art than a science, and therapy for each patient should be directed at achieving the desired anti-inflammatory, analgesic, and antipyretic effects while minimizing adverse effects. The adverse gastric effects of long-term NSAID therapy can be reduced by co-administration of histamine H_2 receptor antagonists or proton pump inhibitors (refer to Chapter 47, Integrative Inflammation Pharmacology: Peptic Ulcer Disease).

COX-2 Inhibitors

As noted earlier, long-term NSAID therapy can be associated with severe gastrointestinal adverse effects that are thought to be caused by inhibition of gastrointestinal COX-1. It was hypothesized that selective inhibition of COX-2 could have the theoretical advantage of inhibiting the chemical mediators responsible for inflammation while maintaining the cytoprotective effects of the products of COX-1 activity.

COX-2 Selective Inhibitors

Although COX-2 was identified only in the 1990s, intense research swiftly led to the development of COX-2 selective inhibitors for clinical use. *Compared with COX-1, COX-2 has a larger hydrophobic channel through which substrate (arachidonic acid) enters the active site.* Subtle structural differences between COX-2 and COX-1 allowed the development of drugs that act preferentially on COX-2.

The COX-2 selective inhibitors—**celecoxib**, **rofecoxib**, **valdecoxib**, and **meloxicam** (Fig. 43-9)—are sulfonic acid derivatives that exhibit 100-fold greater selectivity for COX-2 than for COX-1. The relative inhibition of the two cyclooxygenase isozymes in any given tissue is also a function of drug metabolism, pharmacokinetics, and possibly enzyme polymorphisms. The COX-2 selective inhibitors have anti-inflammatory, antipyretic, and analgesic properties similar to the traditional NSAIDs, but they do not share the antiplatelet actions of the COX-1 inhibitors. Various coxibs had been approved for treatment of osteoarthritis, rheumatoid arthritis, acute pain in adults, and primary dysmenorrhea. However, relative to other NSAIDs, the safety profile of the COX-2 selective inhibitors is uncertain. At the present time, only celecoxib is an approved drug in the United States. Rofecoxib was withdrawn by the manufacturer from the worldwide market in 2004 because of an increase in myocardial infarction and stroke with prolonged use; valdecoxib was then withdrawn in 2005.

The increased thrombogenicity of COX-2 inhibitors, uncovered in clinical use, may be due to prolonged inhibition of vascular COX-2 within endothelial cells, leading to reduced PGI_2 formation. In addition, inhibition of COX-2 may generate problems in wound healing, angiogenesis, and the resolution of inflammation. COX-2 selective inhibitors are much more expensive than equivalent doses of many NSAIDs, especially aspirin and indomethacin. Note that Ms. G's physician attempted to take advantage of the relative gastrointestinal safety of COX-2 selective inhibitors when she was switched from ibuprofen to a COX-2 inhibitor, in part because of symptomatic and endoscopic evidence

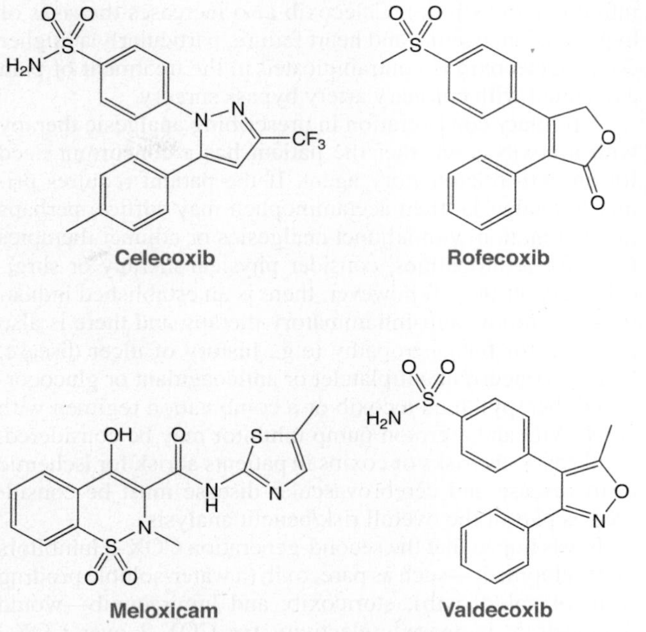

FIGURE 43-9. **COX-2 selective inhibitors.** COX-2 selective inhibitors are hydrophobic sulfonic acid derivatives. Like traditional NSAIDs, these molecules block the hydrophobic channel leading to the active site of cyclooxygenase and thus inhibit the enzyme. Note that COX-2 selective inhibitors are generally larger molecules than NSAIDs. These drugs preferentially inhibit COX-2 compared to COX-1 because the hydrophobic channel of COX-2 is larger than that of COX-1. (That is, COX-2 selective inhibitors are too bulky to access the smaller hydrophobic channel of the COX-1 enzyme.) The COX-2 selective inhibitors display approximately 100-fold greater selectivity for COX-2 compared to COX-1.

of NSAID-induced gastropathy. It is being increasingly recognized, however, that the COX-2 inhibitors may not have as significant an advantage over traditional NSAIDs as previously thought in reducing gastropathy and gastrointestinal bleeding. For example, one study with rofecoxib demonstrated a fivefold increase in significant upper gastrointestinal bleed compared to placebo. One possible mechanism for this toxicity could be the adverse effect of COX-2 inhibitors on the healing of gastric ulcerations.

Celecoxib remains the only FDA-approved COX-2 selective inhibitor. Currently approved indications include osteoarthritis, rheumatoid arthritis, juvenile rheumatoid arthritis (>2 years of age), ankylosing spondylitis, acute pain in adults, and primary dysmenorrhea. Celecoxib is also considered as an adjunct to usual care (e.g., surgery, endoscopic surveillance) to reduce the number of adenomatous colorectal polyps in individuals with **familial adenomatous polyposis**. Celecoxib decreases the activity of peroxisome proliferator-activated receptor δ (PPARδ), a transcription factor that heterodimerizes with the RXR transcription factors involved in growth regulation. It is not yet clear whether COX-2 inhibitors bind directly to PPARδ or whether their action leads to the production of other molecules that inhibit PPARδ. In either case, inhibition of PPARδ prevents signaling through the PPARδ pathway and thus removes a potent mitogenic stimulus that could promote the development of colon cancer.

Like other coxibs, celecoxib carries a label warning of increased, possibly fatal, and possibly dose- and duration-dependent cardiovascular thrombotic events (myocardial infarction and stroke). Celecoxib also increases the risks of hypertension, edema, and heart failure, particularly at higher doses. Celecoxib is contraindicated in the treatment of pain associated with coronary artery bypass surgery.

A primary consideration in prescribing analgesic therapy with a coxib is whether the patient has a concurrent need for an anti-inflammatory agent. If the patient requires primarily analgesia, then acetaminophen may suffice, perhaps in combination with adjunct analgesics or adjunct therapies (e.g., for arthropathies, consider physical therapy or surgical intervention). If, however, there is an established indication for chronic anti-inflammatory therapy and there is also a risk factor for gastropathy (e.g., history of ulcer disease, elderly, concurrent antiplatelet or anticoagulant or glucocorticoid therapy), then a coxib or a combination regimen with an NSAID and a proton pump inhibitor may be considered. In all cases, the risks of coxibs in patients at risk for ischemic heart disease and cerebrovascular disease must be considered as part of the overall risk/benefit analysis.

It was hoped that the second-generation COX-2 inhibitors in development—such as parecoxib (a water-soluble prodrug form of valdecoxib), etoricoxib, and lumiracoxib—would demonstrate increased selectivity for COX-2 over COX-1 and would not have the adverse cardiovascular effects of the existing COX-2 inhibitors. However, none of these agents has achieved FDA approval, and further clinical development in this class of drugs remains in question.

Cytokine Inhibitors
The proinflammatory cytokines TNF-α and IL-1 enhance prostaglandin production and up-regulate COX-2. Novel molecular technologies have provided the ability to inhibit the action of these cytokines and thus to inhibit the process whereby an injurious stimulus activates COX-2 and initiates the inflammatory response. Five antibody-based TNF-α antagonists are currently available: **etanercept**, **infliximab**, **adalimumab**, **golimumab**, and **certolizumab pegol**. Etanercept consists of the extracellular domain of the TNF-α receptor coupled to human IgG1; infliximab is a humanized mouse monoclonal antibody directed against TNF-α; and adalimumab, golimumab, and certolizumab pegol are humanized monoclonal IgG1 antibodies or Fab antibody fragments directed against TNF-α.

TNF-α antagonists were first approved for treatment of rheumatoid arthritis. With few adverse effects, these drugs halt joint destruction and bone erosion, decrease pain, calm swollen and tender joints, and limit overall disease progression in rheumatoid arthritis. Anti-TNF antibody drugs have also been approved for use in a variety of other autoimmune diseases (see Chapter 46), such as ankylosing spondylitis, psoriatic arthritis, plaque psoriasis, juvenile idiopathic arthritis (>4 years of age for adalimumab and >2 years of age for etanercept), Crohn's disease (adalimumab, certolizumab pegol, and infliximab), and ulcerative colitis (infliximab). Years of experience with this class of drugs has shown an increased risk of serious infections, including disseminated or extrapulmonary tuberculosis, invasive fungal infections (*Aspergillus* and endemic fungi such as *Histoplasma*), hepatitis B virus reactivation, and opportunistic infections. Patients are routinely tested for latent tuberculosis prior to initiation of therapy and must be monitored for active tuberculosis during treatment. Other adverse effects include a small but possibly increased risk of lymphoma, demyelinating disease, heart failure, and pancytopenia.

Lipoxins, ATLs, and lipoxin-stable analogues also block the actions of TNF-α, providing a potential new treatment approach (see below).

Anakinra is a recombinant form of the human IL-1 receptor produced in *Escherichia coli*; this drug is approved for use in patients with rheumatoid arthritis who have failed one or more disease-modifying antirheumatic agents. **Canakinumab** is a recombinant monoclonal IgG1 antibody directed against human IL-1 beta. Additional IL-1 antagonists are being developed for use in inflammatory and autoimmune diseases. For more information on these agents, refer to Chapter 46.

Prostanoid Receptor Mimetics
Several applications for prostanoid receptor agonists are listed in the Drug Summary Table at the end of this chapter.

Thromboxane Antagonists
Both TxA$_2$ receptor antagonists and thromboxane synthase inhibitors could theoretically represent powerful and selective agents capable of inhibiting platelet activity and protecting against thrombosis and vascular disease. Thromboxane antagonists could serve as "super" platelet inhibitors in the management of patients with cardiovascular disease. TxA$_2$ receptor antagonists, unlike aspirin, would also be expected to block the vasoconstrictive action of the isoprostanes. Compounds such as **dazoxiben** and **pirmagrel** inhibit thromboxane synthase, and **ridogrel** is a TxA$_2$ receptor antagonist. These thromboxane antagonists have not yet found clinical utility, however, because the clinical benefit of these drugs is not significantly greater than that of aspirin, which is far less expensive; in addition, other inhibitors of platelet aggregation, which antagonize the P2Y$_{12}$ subtype of platelet ADP receptor, are in widespread clinical use already (see Chapter 23).

Leukotriene Inhibition
Lipoxygenase Inhibition
Inhibition of 5-lipoxygenase has the potential to represent a major therapeutic modality in diseases involving leukotriene-mediated pathophysiology, including asthma, inflammatory bowel disease, and rheumatoid arthritis. Lipoxygenase inhibition is an attractive therapeutic approach in these diseases because leukotrienes are potent, locally acting mediators.

Several strategies are possible for the design of lipoxygenase inhibitors, based on the structure, function, and mechanism of the lipoxygenase enzymes. Suicide inhibitors of lipoxygenase (e.g., derivatives of arachidonic acid with triple bonds instead of double bonds), which become covalently bound to the active site and render it inactive, have been developed but are not available for clinical use. Radical scavengers such as catechols, butylated hydroxytoluene (BHT), and α-tocopherol trap the radical intermediates in the lipoxygenase reaction and thereby prevent the functioning of the enzyme, but these nonspecific compounds cannot be used clinically for lipoxygenase inhibition.

Drugs that impair or alter the ability of lipoxygenase to utilize its nonheme iron would be expected to inhibit the activity of the enzyme. The only lipoxygenase inhibitor available for clinical use is **zileuton** (Fig. 43-10A), a benzothiophene derivative of N-hydroxyurea that inhibits 5-LOX by chelating its nonheme iron. In asthma, zileuton induces bronchodilation, improves symptoms, and generates long-lasting improvement in pulmonary function tests. Zileuton is

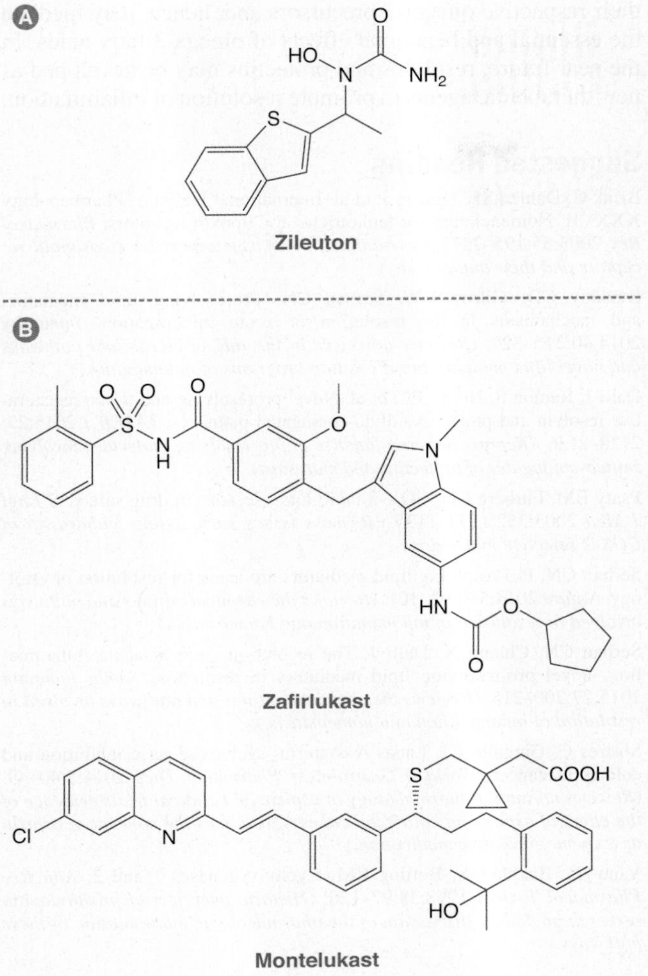

FIGURE 43-10. Leukotriene pathway inhibitors. A. Zileuton is a 5-lipoxygenase inhibitor that blocks the biosynthesis of leukotrienes from arachidonic acid. **B.** Zafirlukast and montelukast are CysLT$_1$ receptor antagonists. All three drugs are approved for the prophylaxis and chronic treatment of asthma. None of these drugs is effective in the treatment of acute asthma attacks.

effective in the treatment of asthma induced by cold, drugs, and allergens. However, because of its low bioavailability, low potency, and significant adverse effects such as liver toxicity, zileuton is not as widely used as the other antileukotriene asthma drugs (see below).

5-Lipoxygenase Activating Protein (FLAP) Inhibition

Interfering with the role of FLAP could represent an alternative approach to the selective inhibition of 5-LOX activity and leukotriene function. Recall that 5-LOX is activated after the enzyme translocates to the nuclear membrane and docks with FLAP, and that FLAP binds arachidonic acid released by phospholipase A$_2$ and shuttles it to the 5-LOX active site. FLAP inhibitors have been developed that both prevent and reverse LOX binding to FLAP and block the arachidonic acid binding site, but no FLAP inhibitors are currently available for clinical use.

Leukotriene Synthesis Inhibitors

Other than zileuton, no specific inhibitors of the enzymes involved in leukotriene synthesis are available for clinical use. Specific LTA$_4$ hydrolase inhibitors, which block LTB$_4$

biosynthesis, are currently in development. **Adenosine**, acting via its receptors on neutrophils, inhibits LTB$_4$ biosynthesis by regulating arachidonic acid release and, possibly, by interfering with the influx of calcium. Furthermore, adenosine is thought to have a role in limiting cell and tissue injury during inflammation. High cell turnover at inflammatory sites generates high local concentrations of adenosine, which may decrease LTB$_4$ biosynthesis and reduce leukocyte recruitment and activation. Selective adenosine receptor agonists could be considered for development as pharmacologic agents in the control of inflammation.

Leukotriene Receptor Antagonists

Leukotriene receptor antagonism represents a receptor-based mechanism for inhibiting leukotriene-mediated bronchoconstriction and other effects (Fig. 43-4). Cysteinyl leukotriene receptor (CysLT1) antagonists are effective against asthma induced by antigen, exercise, cold, or aspirin. These agents significantly improve bronchial tone, pulmonary function tests, and asthma symptoms. **Montelukast** and **zafirlukast** (Fig. 43-10B) are the currently available cysteinyl leukotriene receptor antagonists; the main clinical application for these antagonists is in the treatment of asthma.

More potent CysLT1 antagonists are in development, including pobilukast, tomelukast, and verlukast. Further research will likely elucidate cysteinyl leukotriene receptor subtypes and their respective tissue distributions, which could offer the possibility of tissue-targeted antagonism and the application of these tissue-selective antagonists to other conditions such as rheumatoid arthritis, inflammatory bowel disease, and various allergic disorders.

Lipoxins, Aspirin-Triggered Lipoxins, Resolvins/Protectins/Maresins, and Lipoxin-Stable Analogues

Lipoxins, ATLs, and the omega-3-derived resolvins, protectins, and maresins all offer the potential to antagonize the inflammatory actions of leukotrienes and other inflammatory mediators and to promote resolution of inflammation. Stable oral and parenteral analogues of these compounds could represent a novel approach to treatment of inflammation, since they are agonists of endogenous anti-inflammation and pro-resolution pathways rather than direct enzyme inhibitors or receptor antagonists. Because lipoxins are endogenous regulators, they would be expected to have selective actions with few adverse effects. Stable analogues of lipoxins and ATLs are currently being developed, and second-generation lipoxin-stable analogues have shown efficacy in enhancing the resolution of recurring bouts of acute inflammation in skin inflammation and gastrointestinal inflammation models. Peptido-conjugates of the proresolving mediators have recently been identified that stimulate tissue regeneration and enhance clearance and killing of microbes. This approach to the treatment of inflammation remains to be established in human trials.

▌ CONCLUSION AND FUTURE DIRECTIONS

Eicosanoids are critical mediators of homeostasis and of many pathophysiologic processes, especially those involving host defense and inflammation. Arachidonic acid is the important substrate and is converted into prostaglandins, thromboxanes, prostacyclin, leukotrienes, lipoxins, isoprostanes, and epoxyeicosatetraenoic acids. Prostaglandins have diverse roles in vascular tone regulation, gastrointestinal regulation, uterine physiology, analgesia, and inflammation. Prostacyclin and thromboxane coordinately control vascular tone, platelet activation, and thrombogenesis. Leukotrienes (LTC_4, LTD_4) are the chief mediators of bronchoconstriction and airway hyperactivity; LTB_4 is a major activator of leukocyte chemotaxis and infiltration. Lipoxins antagonize the effects of leukotrienes, reduce the extent of inflammation, and activate resolution pathways.

Pharmacologic interventions at many critical points in these pathways are useful in limiting inflammatory sequelae. Glucocorticoids inhibit several steps in eicosanoid generation, including the rate-determining step involving phospholipase A_2. However, chronic glucocorticoid use is associated with many serious adverse effects, including osteoporosis, muscle wasting, and abnormal carbohydrate metabolism. Cyclooxygenase inhibitors block the first step of prostanoid synthesis and prevent the generation of prostanoid mediators of inflammation. Lipoxygenase inhibitors, FLAP inhibitors, leukotriene synthesis inhibitors, and leukotriene receptor antagonists prevent leukotriene signaling, thereby limiting inflammation and its deleterious effects. Future drug development efforts will allow selective targeting of eicosanoid pathways involved in many clinical conditions.

Systems biology has revealed mechanisms underlying inflammatory disease and has created a new discipline of resolution pharmacology. Essential omega-3 fatty acids, in particular EPA and DHA, are precursors to pro-resolving and anti-inflammatory SPM that serve a physiologic role leading to programmed resolution of inflammation (Fig. 43-6). These new bioactive mediators are many times more potent than their respective omega-3 precursors and, hence, may mediate the essential and beneficial effects of omega-3 fatty acids. In the near future, resolvins and protectins may be developed as new therapeutic agents to promote resolution of inflammation.

Suggested Reading

Brink C, Dahlen SE, Drazen J, et al. International Union of Pharmacology XXXVII. Nomenclature for leukotriene and lipoxin receptors. *Pharmacol Rev* 2003;55:195–227. (*International consensus report on eicosanoid receptors and their antagonists.*)

Buckley CD, Gilroy DW, Serhan CN. Proresolving lipid mediators and mechanisms in the resolution of acute inflammation. *Immunity* 2014;40:315–327. (*Reviews advances in the role of eicosanoid pathways and novel lipid mediators in resolution programs of inflammation.*)

Dalli J, Ramon S, Norris PC, et al. Novel proresolving and tissue regenerative resolvin and protectin sulfido-conjugated pathways. *FASEB J* 2015;29: 2120–2136. (*Reports two new families of pro-resolving molecules involving sulfido-conjugates of protectins and maresins.*)

Psaty BM, Furberg CD. COX-2 inhibitors—lessons in drug safety. *N Engl J Med* 2005;352:1133–1135. (*Reviews issues surrounding withdrawal of COX-2 selective inhibitors.*)

Serhan CN. Pro-resolving lipid mediators are leads for resolution physiology. *Nature* 2014;510:92–101. (*Reviews the chemical entities and pathways involved in resolution of inflammation and homeostasis.*)

Serhan CN, Chiang N, Dalli J. The resolution code of acute inflammation: novel pro-resolving lipid mediators in resolution. *Semin Immunol* 2015;27:200–215. (*Reviews the chemical entities and pathways involved in resolution of inflammation and homeostasis.*)

Sostres C, Gargallo CJ, Lanas A. Aspirin, cyclooxygenase inhibition and colorectal cancer. *World J Gastrointest Pharmacol Ther* 2014;5:40–49. (*Reviews antitumor pharmacology of aspirin and clinical trials evidence of the effect of aspirin on colorectal cancer; discusses the concept of aspirin as a chemopreventive medication.*)

Vane JR, Bakhle YS, Botting RM. Cyclooxygenases 1 and 2. *Ann Rev Pharmacol Toxicol* 1998;38:97–120. (*Historic overview of prostaglandin research, including discussion of the pharmacologic manipulation of these pathways.*)

DRUG SUMMARY TABLE: CHAPTER 43 Pharmacology of Eicosanoids

NONSTEROIDAL ANTI-INFLAMMATORY DRUGS (NSAIDs)
Mechanism—Inhibit cyclooxygenase-1 (COX-1) and cyclooxygenase-2 (COX-2), decreasing the biosynthesis of downstream eicosanoids and thereby limiting the inflammatory response

DRUG	CLINICAL APPLICATIONS	SERIOUS AND COMMON ADVERSE EFFECTS	CONTRAINDICATIONS	THERAPEUTIC CONSIDERATIONS
Aspirin	Mild to moderate pain Headache, myalgia, arthralgia Prophylaxis of stroke and myocardial infarction (antiplatelet effect) Carotid endarterectomy Coronary artery bypass graft Percutaneous coronary intervention Angina Fever Pericarditis	*Gastrointestinal ulcer, bleeding, Reye's syndrome, age-related macular degeneration, bronchospasm, angioedema* Tinnitus, ecchymosis, gastrointestinal disturbance	Aspirin hypersensitivity Syndrome of asthma, rhinitis, and nasal polyps Children and teenagers with chickenpox or flu symptoms, due to risk of Reye's syndrome	The oldest of the NSAIDs. Widely used to treat mild to moderate pain, headache, myalgia, and arthralgia. In contrast to other NSAIDs, aspirin acts in an irreversible manner by acetylating the active site serine residue in both COX-1 and COX-2. Aspirin increases plasma concentration of acetazolamide, which leads to CNS toxicity. Ibuprofen may inhibit the antiplatelet effect of aspirin. Limited reports suggest that salicylates may enhance methotrexate toxicity. Aspirin increases the risk of bleeding in anticoagulated patients.
Propionic acids: Ibuprofen Naproxen Ketoprofen Flurbiprofen **Acetic acids:** Indomethacin Sulindac Etodolac Diclofenac Ketorolac **Oxicams:** Piroxicam **Fenamates:** Mefenamate Meclofenamate **Ketones:** Nabumetone	Shared indications: Mild to moderate pain Fever Arthritis Dysmenorrhea Naproxen only: Tendinitis	*Congestive heart failure, myocardial infarction, aseptic meningitis, stroke, amblyopia, hearing loss, gastrointestinal hemorrhage, ulceration, perforation, nephrotoxicity, liver failure, vanishing bile duct syndrome, agranulocytosis, anemia, neutropenia, thrombocytopenia, Stevens-Johnson syndrome, toxic epidermal necrolysis (shared adverse effects); pseudoporphyria (naproxen only)* Gastrointestinal disturbance, tinnitus	Gastrointestinal or intracranial bleeding Coagulation defects Asthma, urticaria, or allergic-type reactions after taking NSAIDs, due to risk of severe, even fatal, anaphylactic reactions Significant renal insufficiency Significant heart failure	Naproxen has a longer half-life, is 20 times more potent, and causes fewer gastrointestinal adverse effects than aspirin. Naproxen may also have the lowest cardiovascular adverse effect rate of the non-aspirin NSAIDs. Ketorolac is available for intravenous and intramuscular use and is used for analgesia in postsurgical patients; it is used for no more than 3–5 days. Piroxicam has a long half-life; once-daily dosing. Nabumetone has the greatest selectivity of these agents for COX-2. Fenamates have limited use; compared to aspirin, fenamates have less anti-inflammatory activity and higher toxicity.

continues

DRUG SUMMARY TABLE: CHAPTER 43 Pharmacology of Eicosanoids *continued*

DRUG	CLINICAL APPLICATIONS	SERIOUS AND COMMON ADVERSE EFFECTS	CONTRAINDICATIONS	THERAPEUTIC CONSIDERATIONS
ACETAMINOPHEN Mechanism—Weak inhibitor of peripheral cyclooxygenases				
Acetaminophen	Fever Mild to moderate pain	*Acute generalized exanthematous pustulosis, Stevens-Johnson syndrome, toxic epidermal necrolysis, liver failure, pneumonitis* Headache, gastrointestinal disturbance	Hypersensitivity to acetaminophen Significant liver dysfunction	Although acetaminophen has analgesic and antipyretic effects similar to aspirin, the anti-inflammatory effect of acetaminophen is insignificant because of its weak inhibition of peripheral cyclooxygenases. Generally safe for use in patients undergoing surgery and dental procedures. Acetaminophen overdose is a leading cause of hepatic failure. Antidote for acetaminophen overdose is N-acetylcysteine.
COX-2 SELECTIVE INHIBITORS Mechanism—Selective inhibition of COX-2				
Celecoxib	Arthritis (osteoarthritis, rheumatoid arthritis) Primary dysmenorrhea Acute pain in adults	*Myocardial infarction, torsades de pointes, heart failure, stroke, gastrointestinal bleeding, ulceration, perforation, thrombosis, nephrotoxicity, bronchospasm, angioedema, Stevens-Johnson syndrome, toxic epidermal necrolysis* Hypertension, gastrointestinal disturbance, headache	Hypersensitivity to sulfonamides Hypersensitivity to celecoxib Asthma, urticaria, or allergic-type reactions after taking NSAIDs, due to risk of severe, even fatal, anaphylactic reactions Coronary artery bypass graft surgery	Decreases efficacy of ACE inhibitors. Incidence of gastropathy and nephropathy may be less than that associated with NSAIDs but may still be significant. Valdecoxib and rofecoxib withdrawn from US and European markets due to possible increase in cardiovascular mortality.
GLUCOCORTICOIDS Mechanism—Inhibit COX-2 action and prostaglandin biosynthesis by inducing lipocortins, activating endogenous anti-inflammatory pathways, and other mechanisms				
Prednisone Prednisolone Methylprednisolone Dexamethasone	See Drug Summary Table: Chapter 29 Pharmacology of the Adrenal Cortex			
CYTOKINE ANTAGONISTS Mechanism—Etanercept, infliximab, adalimumab, golimumab, and certolizumab pegol inhibit TNF-α; anakinra inhibits IL-1; canakinumab inhibits IL-1β				
Etanercept Infliximab Adalimumab Golimumab Certolizumab pegol	See Drug Summary Table: Chapter 46 Pharmacology of Immunosuppression			
Anakinra Canakinumab	See Drug Summary Table: Chapter 46 Pharmacology of Immunosuppression			

PROSTANOID MIMETICS
Mechanism—Prostanoid receptor agonists; see specific drug

Drug	Indication	Contraindications	Adverse effects	Notes
Alprostadil	Maintenance of patent ductus arteriosus; Cyanotic congenital heart disease; Erectile dysfunction	Sickle cell anemia or trait; Leukemia, myeloma; Neonatal respiratory distress syndrome; Anatomical deformation of the penis, penile implant, Peyronie's disease; Hypersensitivity to alprostadil	*Cardiac arrest, gastrointestinal obstruction, disseminated intravascular coagulation (DIC), infantile cortical hyperostosis, priapism*; Hypotension, tachycardia, bradycardia, flushing, fever, penile fibrosis, penile discomfort	PGE_1 analogue with vasodilator properties. Used primarily for maintaining patent ductus arteriosus in tetralogy of Fallot, Eisenmenger pulmonary hypertension, and aortic valve atresia.
Misoprostol	Cytoprotective and antisecretory effects against gastric ulcers in long-term NSAID therapy	Pregnancy; Hypersensitivity to prostaglandins	*Rare anemia, rare cardiac arrhythmia, gastrointestinal hemorrhage, rupture of uterus, toxic shock syndrome, abortion-related clostridial infection*; Gastrointestinal disturbance	PGE_1 analogue with vasodilator properties. Also used in peptic ulcer disease (see Chapter 47). Cytoprotective effects likely mediated by increasing gastric mucus and bicarbonate production; antisecretory effects mediated via inhibition of basal and nocturnal gastric acid secretion by parietal cells.
Carboprost	Abortion in second trimester; Postpartum hemorrhage	Acute pelvic inflammatory disease; Cardiac, pulmonary, renal, or hepatic disease; Hypersensitivity to carboprost	*Pulmonary edema, excessive uterine bleeding*; Gastrointestinal disturbance with prevalent diarrhea, flushing, leukocytosis	$PGF_{2\alpha}$ analogue that stimulates uterine contraction for abortifacient activity; luteolytic activity controls fertility.
Latanoprost Bimatoprost Travoprost	Shared indication: Ocular hypertension; Latanoprost and bimatoprost only: Open-angle glaucoma; Bimatoprost only: Hypotrichosis of the eyelashes	Hypersensitivity to latanoprost, bimatoprost, or travoprost	*Macular retinal edema (shared adverse effects); bacterial keratitis and uveitis (travoprost only)*; Blurred vision, eye discomfort, conjunctival hyperemia, hyperpigmentation of eyelid, iris pigmentation (shared adverse effects); abnormal hair growth, eyelid erythema, upper respiratory infection (bimatoprost only)	$PGF_{2\alpha}$ analogues with vasodilator properties; ocular hypotensive agents.
Epoprostenol Iloprost Treprostinil	Pulmonary hypertension	Shared contraindications: Hypersensitivity to epoprostenol, iloprost, or treprostinil; Heart failure with severe left ventricular dysfunction; Use in patients developing pulmonary edema; Treprostinil only: Severe liver dysfunction	*Hemorrhage, splenomegaly, sepsis (epoprostenol only); bronchospasm (iloprost only); gastrointestinal hemorrhage, hemoptysis, sepsis, pneumonia (treprostinil only)*; Tachycardia, hypotension, chest pain, flushing, gastrointestinal disturbance, musculoskeletal pain, jaw pain, arthralgia, dizziness, headache, anxiety, influenza-like illness (shared adverse effects); vasodilation, cough (iloprost and treprostinil only)	Prostacyclin analogues that stimulate vasodilation of pulmonary and systemic arterial vasculature; also inhibit platelet aggregation. Available in intravenous and inhaled/nebulizer forms.

continues

DRUG SUMMARY TABLE: CHAPTER 43 Pharmacology of Eicosanoids *continued*

DRUG	CLINICAL APPLICATIONS	SERIOUS AND COMMON ADVERSE EFFECTS	CONTRAINDICATIONS	THERAPEUTIC CONSIDERATIONS
LIPOXYGENASE INHIBITOR Mechanism—Inhibits 5-lipoxygenase, which catalyzes the formation of leukotrienes from arachidonic acid				
Zileuton	Asthma	*Hepatotoxicity, altered behavior, hallucinations, suicidal ideation* Urticaria, abdominal discomfort, dizziness, headache, insomnia	Active liver disease Elevated liver enzymes Hypersensitivity to zileuton	Avoid concurrent use of dihydroergotamine, ergoloid mesylates, ergonovine, and methylergonovine due to an increased risk of ergotism (nausea, vomiting, vasospastic ischemia).
LEUKOTRIENE RECEPTOR ANTAGONISTS Mechanism—Selective antagonists of the cysteinyl leukotriene (CysLT) type-1 receptor				
Montelukast Zafirlukast	Shared indication: Chronic asthma Montelukast only: Perennial allergic rhinitis Seasonal allergic rhinitis Exercise-induced asthma	*Allergic granulomatosis angiitis, Stevens-Johnson syndrome, toxic epidermal necrolysis, altered behavior, suicidal ideation (shared adverse effects); hepatitis, liver failure, hallucinations (zafirlukast only)* Headache	Hypersensitivity to montelukast or zafirlukast	Montelukast and zafirlukast are not indicated for acute asthma attacks and are generally not appropriate as monotherapy for asthma. Both drugs are excreted in breast milk.

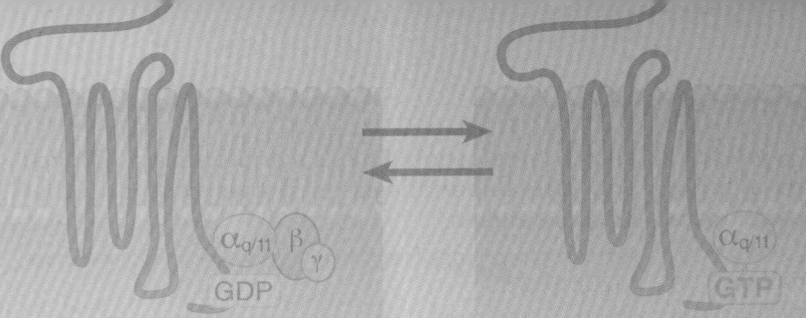

44

Histamine Pharmacology

Elizabeth A. Brezinski and April W. Armstrong

■ INTRODUCTION

Histamine is a biogenic amine found in many tissues, including mast cells, basophils, lymphocytes, neurons, and gastric enterochromaffin-like cells. It is an autacoid—that is, a molecule secreted locally to increase or decrease the activity of nearby cells. *Histamine is a major mediator of allergic and inflammatory processes: it also has significant roles in the regulation of gastric acid secretion, neurotransmission, and immune modulation.* Knowledge of the diverse actions of histamine has led to the development of a number of widely used pharmacologic agents that regulate the effects of histamine in pathologic states. This chapter focuses on the pharmacologic actions of H$_1$-antihistamines; H$_2$-antihistamines are discussed in Chapter 47, Integrative Inflammation Pharmacology: Peptic Ulcer Disease.

■ PHYSIOLOGY OF HISTAMINE

Histamine Synthesis, Storage, and Release

Histamine is synthesized from the amino acid L-histidine. The enzyme **histidine decarboxylase** catalyzes the decarboxylation of histidine to 2-(4-imidazolyl)ethylamine, commonly known as **histamine** (Fig. 44-1). The synthesis of histamine occurs in mast cells and basophils of the immune system, enterochromaffin-like (ECL) cells in the gastric mucosa, and certain neurons in the central nervous system (CNS) that use histamine as a neurotransmitter. Oxidative pathways in the liver rapidly degrade circulating histamine to inert metabolites. One major metabolite of histamine, imidazole acetic acid, can be measured in the urine to determine the amount of histamine that has been released systemically.

Histamine synthesis and storage can be divided into two "pools": a slowly turning over pool and a rapidly turning over pool. The **slowly turning over pool** is located in mast cells and basophils. Histamine is stored in large granules in these inflammatory cells, and the release of histamine involves complete degranulation of the cells. Degranulation can be triggered by allergic processes, anaphylaxis, or cellular destruction from trauma, cold, or other insults. This pool is termed *slowly turning over* because several weeks are required to replenish the stores of histamine after degranulation has occurred. The **rapidly turning over pool** is located in gastric ECL cells and in histaminergic CNS neurons. These cells synthesize and release histamine as required for gastric acid secretion and neurotransmission, respectively. Unlike mast cells and basophils, ECL cells and histaminergic neurons do not store histamine. Instead, the production and release of histamine in these cells depend on physiologic stimuli. In the gut, for example, histidine decarboxylase is activated after the ingestion of food.

Actions of Histamine

Histamine has a broad spectrum of actions involving many organs and organ systems. To understand the roles of histamine, it is useful to consider the physiologic effects of histamine in each tissue (Table 44-1). These effects include actions on bronchial smooth muscle, vascular smooth muscle, vascular endothelium, afferent nerve terminals, heart, gastrointestinal tract, and CNS.

On smooth muscle, histamine causes some muscle fibers to contract and others to relax. In the human respiratory system, histamine causes **bronchoconstriction** (the effect varies in other species). However, the sensitivity of bronchial

CASE

Ellen, a generally healthy 76-year-old grandmother, suffers from allergic rhinitis. Every spring, she develops a runny nose, itchy eyes, and sneezing. To relieve her symptoms, she takes an over-the-counter antihistamine, diphenhydramine. She is annoyed by the unpleasant effects that accompany her allergy medication. Every time she takes her antihistamine, Ellen feels drowsy and her mouth feels dry. She makes an appointment with her doctor, who subsequently advises Ellen to take loratadine. Upon taking her new allergy medication, Ellen's symptoms are relieved and she experiences no drowsiness or other adverse effects.

Questions

1. Why does Ellen develop seasonal allergic rhinitis?
2. What is the mechanism of action of diphenhydramine and loratadine?
3. Why does diphenhydramine cause drowsiness and dry mouth, and why doesn't loratadine cause drowsiness or dry mouth?

smooth muscle to histamine varies among individuals; those with asthma may be up to 1,000 times more sensitive to histamine-mediated bronchoconstriction than nonasthmatic individuals. Other smooth muscles—such as those in the bowel, bladder, iris, and uterus—also contract on exposure to histamine, but these effects are not thought to play a large role physiologically or clinically.

In vascular smooth muscle, histamine dilates postcapillary venules and terminal arterioles. Veins, however, constrict on exposure to histamine. *The vasodilatory effect on the postcapillary venule bed is the most prominent effect of histamine on the vasculature.* During infection or injury, histamine-induced venule dilation engorges the local microvasculature with blood, enhancing the access of immune cells that initiate repair processes to the damaged area. This engorgement explains the **erythema** observed in inflamed tissues.

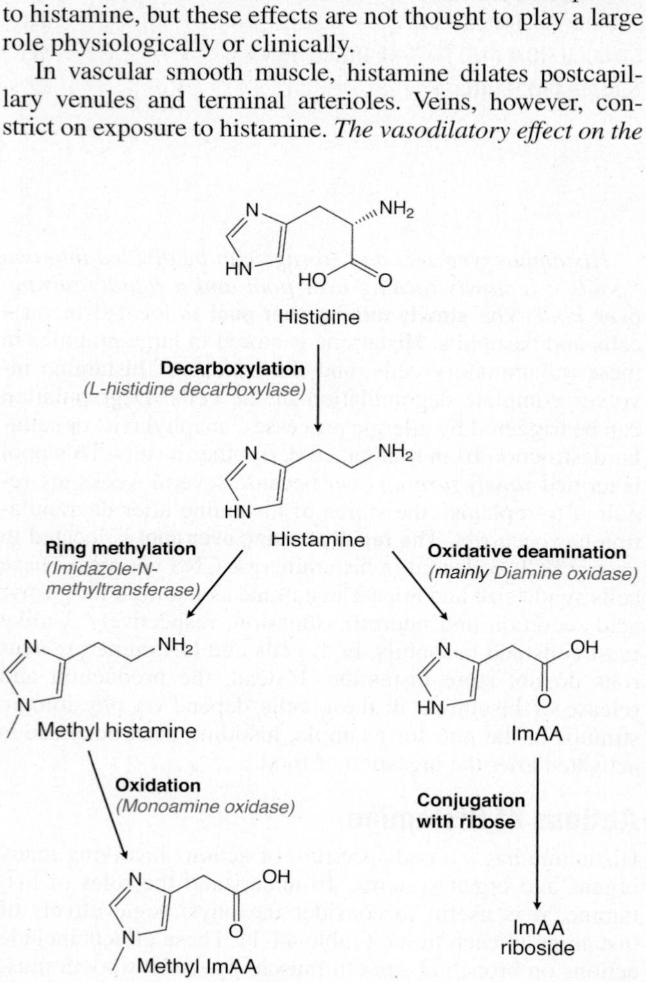

Histamine also causes contraction of vascular endothelial cells. *Histamine-induced endothelial cell contraction causes these cells to separate from one another, allowing release of plasma proteins and fluid from postcapillary venules and thereby causing* **edema**. Thus, histamine is a key mediator of local responses at sites of injury.

Peripheral sensory nerve terminals also respond to histamine. The sensations of **itch** and **pain** result from a *direct depolarizing action of histamine on afferent nerve terminals*. This effect is responsible for the pain and itch experienced after an insect bite, for example.

The combined actions of histamine on vascular smooth muscle, vascular endothelial cells, and peripheral nerve terminals are responsible for the **wheal-and-flare** response noted after histamine release in the skin. **Endothelial cell contraction** causes the edematous wheal response, while the red, painful flare results from **vasodilation** and **sensory nerve stimulation**. Histamine also causes a similar process to occur in the nasal mucosa. Endothelial cell contraction, increased vascular permeability, glandular hypersecretion, and stimulation of irritant receptors contribute to mucosal edema and rhinorrhea, as well as the itching and sneezing typical of allergic rhinitis.

The cardiac effects of histamine consist of minor increases in the force and rate of cardiac contraction. Histamine enhances Ca^{2+} influx into cardiac myocytes, leading to increased inotropy. The increase in heart rate is caused by an increase in the rate of phase 4 depolarization in sinoatrial nodal cells.

The primary role of histamine in the gastric mucosa is to potentiate gastrin-induced acid secretion. *Histamine is one of three molecules that stimulate acid secretion in the stomach, the others being gastrin and acetylcholine.* Activation of histamine receptors in the stomach leads to an increase in intracellular Ca^{2+} in parietal cells and results in increased secretion of hydrochloric acid by the gastric mucosa.

Finally, histamine functions as a neurotransmitter in the CNS. Histaminergic neurons originate in the tuberomammillary nucleus of the hypothalamus and project diffusely throughout the brain and spinal cord. Although the functions of histamine in the CNS are not well understood, histamine

FIGURE 44-1. Histamine synthesis and degradation. Histamine is synthesized from histidine in a decarboxylation reaction catalyzed by L-histidine decarboxylase. The liver metabolizes histamine into inert by-products. Histamine can be methylated on the imidazole ring or oxidatively deaminated. These degradation products can then undergo further oxidation or conjugation with ribose. Diamine oxidase is also known as *histaminase*. ImAA, imidazole acetic acid.

TABLE 44-1 Major Physiologic Actions of Histamine

TISSUE	EFFECT OF HISTAMINE	CLINICAL MANIFESTATIONS	RECEPTOR SUBTYPE
Lungs	Bronchoconstriction	Asthma-like symptoms	H_1
Vascular smooth muscle	Postcapillary venule dilation Terminal arteriole dilation Venoconstriction	Erythema	H_1
Vascular endothelium	Contraction and separation of endothelial cells	Edema, wheal response	H_1
Peripheral nerves	Sensitization of afferent nerve terminals	Itch, pain	H_1
Heart	Minor increase in contractility and heart rate	Minor	H_2
Stomach	Increased gastric acid secretion	Peptic ulcer disease, heartburn	H_2
CNS	Neurotransmitter	Circadian rhythms, wakefulness	H_3

CNS, central nervous system.

is believed to be important in the maintenance of sleep–wake cycles (circadian rhythms), cognitive processes (attention, memory, and learning), and feeding behaviors (appetite suppression).

Histamine Receptors

Histamine actions are mediated by the binding of histamine to one of four receptor subtypes: H_1, H_2, H_3, and H_4. All four subtypes are seven-transmembrane, G protein-coupled receptors, and all demonstrate constitutive activity independent of agonist binding. The receptor isoforms differ in their expression levels, second messenger pathways, and tissue distributions (Table 44-2).

The **H_1 receptor** activates G protein-mediated hydrolysis of phosphatidylinositol-4,5-bisphosphate (PIP_2), leading to increased intracellular concentrations of inositol trisphosphate (IP_3) and diacylglycerol (DAG). IP_3 triggers the release of Ca^{2+} from intracellular stores, increasing cytosolic Ca^{2+} concentration and activating downstream pathways. DAG activates protein kinase C, leading to phosphorylation of numerous cytosolic target proteins. In some tissues, such as bronchial smooth muscle, the increase in cytosolic Ca^{2+} causes smooth muscle contraction by Ca^{2+}/calmodulin-mediated activation of myosin light chain kinase, which phosphorylates myosin light chain. In other tissues, especially precapillary arteriolar sphincters and postcapillary venules, the increase in cytosolic Ca^{2+} causes smooth muscle relaxation by inducing the synthesis of nitric oxide (see Chapter 22, Pharmacology of Vascular Tone). H_1 receptor stimulation also leads to the activation of NFκB, an important and ubiquitous transcription factor that promotes the expression of adhesion molecules and proinflammatory cytokines.

H_1 receptors are expressed primarily on vascular endothelial cells and smooth muscle cells. These receptors mediate **inflammatory** and **allergic reactions**. Tissue-specific responses to H_1 receptor stimulation include (1) edema, (2) erythema, (3) bronchoconstriction, and (4) sensitization of primary afferent nerve terminals. H_1 receptors are also expressed on postsynaptic neurons in the tuberomammillary nucleus of the hypothalamus, cerebral cortex, and limbic system. These neurons appear to be involved in the control of circadian rhythms, wakefulness, and energy metabolism.

*The major function of the **H_2 receptor** is to mediate gastric acid secretion in the stomach.* This receptor subtype is expressed on parietal cells in the gastric mucosa, where histamine acts synergistically with gastrin and acetylcholine to regulate acid secretion (see Chapter 47). H_2 receptors are also expressed on cardiac muscle cells, on some immune cells, and on certain postsynaptic neurons in the CNS. H_2 receptors on parietal cells activate a G protein-dependent cyclic AMP cascade, leading to enhanced proton pump-mediated delivery of protons into the gastric fluid.

Whereas H_1 and H_2 receptor subtypes have been well characterized, H_3 and H_4 receptor subtypes and their downstream actions are areas of active investigation. **H_3 receptors** are predominantly located on presynaptic neurons in distinct regions of the CNS, including the cerebral cortex, basal ganglia, and tuberomammillary nucleus of the hypothalamus. H_3 receptors appear to function as both autoreceptors and heteroreceptors, thereby limiting the synthesis and release of histamine as well as other neurotransmitters, including dopamine, acetylcholine, norepinephrine, GABA, and serotonin. This complex interaction between histamine and various neurotransmitter systems contributes to histamine's wide-

TABLE 44-2 Histamine Receptor Subtypes

RECEPTOR SUBTYPE	POSTRECEPTOR SIGNALING MECHANISM	TISSUE DISTRIBUTION
H_1	$G_{q/11} \rightarrow$ Increased IP_3, DAG, and intracellular Ca^{2+}, activated NFκB	Smooth muscle, vascular endothelium, brain
H_2	$G_s \rightarrow$ Increased cAMP	Gastric parietal cells, cardiac muscle, mast cells, brain
H_3	$G_{i/o} \rightarrow$ Decreased cAMP	CNS, gastric mucosa
H_4	$G_{i/o} \rightarrow$ Decreased cAMP, increased intracellular Ca^{2+}	Hematopoietic cells

G, G protein; cAMP, cyclic adenosine monophosphate; IP_3, inositol trisphosphate; DAG, diacylglycerol; NFκB, nuclear factor kappa B; CNS, central nervous system.

spread effects on CNS functions, including wakefulness, appetite, and memory. The downstream effects of H_3 receptor activation are mediated via a decrease in cAMP.

H_4 receptors are primarily localized to cells of hematopoietic origin, primarily mast cells, eosinophils, dendritic cells, and basophils. H_4 receptors share 40% homology with H_3 receptors and bind many H_3 receptor agonists, although with lower affinity. Coupling of the H_4 receptor to $G_{i/o}$ leads to decreased cAMP and activation of phospholipase $C\beta$, and downstream events result in increased intracellular Ca^{2+}. H_4 receptors are of particular interest because they are thought to play an important role in inflammation; activation of H_4 receptors mediates histamine-induced leukotriene B_4 production, adhesion molecule up-regulation, and chemotaxis of mast cells, eosinophils, and dendritic cells. H_4 receptors also appear to play a role in modulating itch and pain.

PATHOPHYSIOLOGY

Histamine is an essential mediator of immune and inflammatory responses. Histamine plays a prominent role in the **IgE-mediated type I hypersensitivity reaction**, also known as the **allergic reaction**. In a localized allergic reaction, an allergen (antigen) first penetrates an epithelial surface (e.g., skin, nasal mucosa). The allergen can also be delivered systemically, as in the case of an allergic response to penicillin.

With the aid of T-helper (T_H) cells, the allergen stimulates B lymphocytes to produce IgE antibodies that are specific for that allergen. The IgE then binds to Fc receptors on mast cells and basophils, in a process known as *sensitization*. Once these immune cells are "sensitized" with IgE antibodies, they are able to detect and respond rapidly to a subsequent exposure to the allergen. Upon such an exposure, the allergen binds to and cross-links the IgE/Fc receptor complexes, triggering cell degranulation (Fig. 44-2).

Histamine released by mast cells and basophils binds to H_1 receptors on vascular smooth muscle cells and vascular endothelial cells. Activation of these receptors increases local blood flow and vascular permeability. This completes the initial stage of the inflammatory response. Prolonged inflammation requires the activity of other immune cells. The histamine-induced local vasodilation allows such immune cells greater access to the injured area, while the increased vascular permeability facilitates movement of the immune cells into the tissue.

Mast cell degranulation can also occur as a response to local tissue damage in the absence of a humoral immune response. For example, trauma or chemical damage can physically disrupt the mast cell membrane and thereby initiate the degranulation process. Histamine release allows for enhanced access of macrophages and other immune cells, which can begin to repair the damaged area.

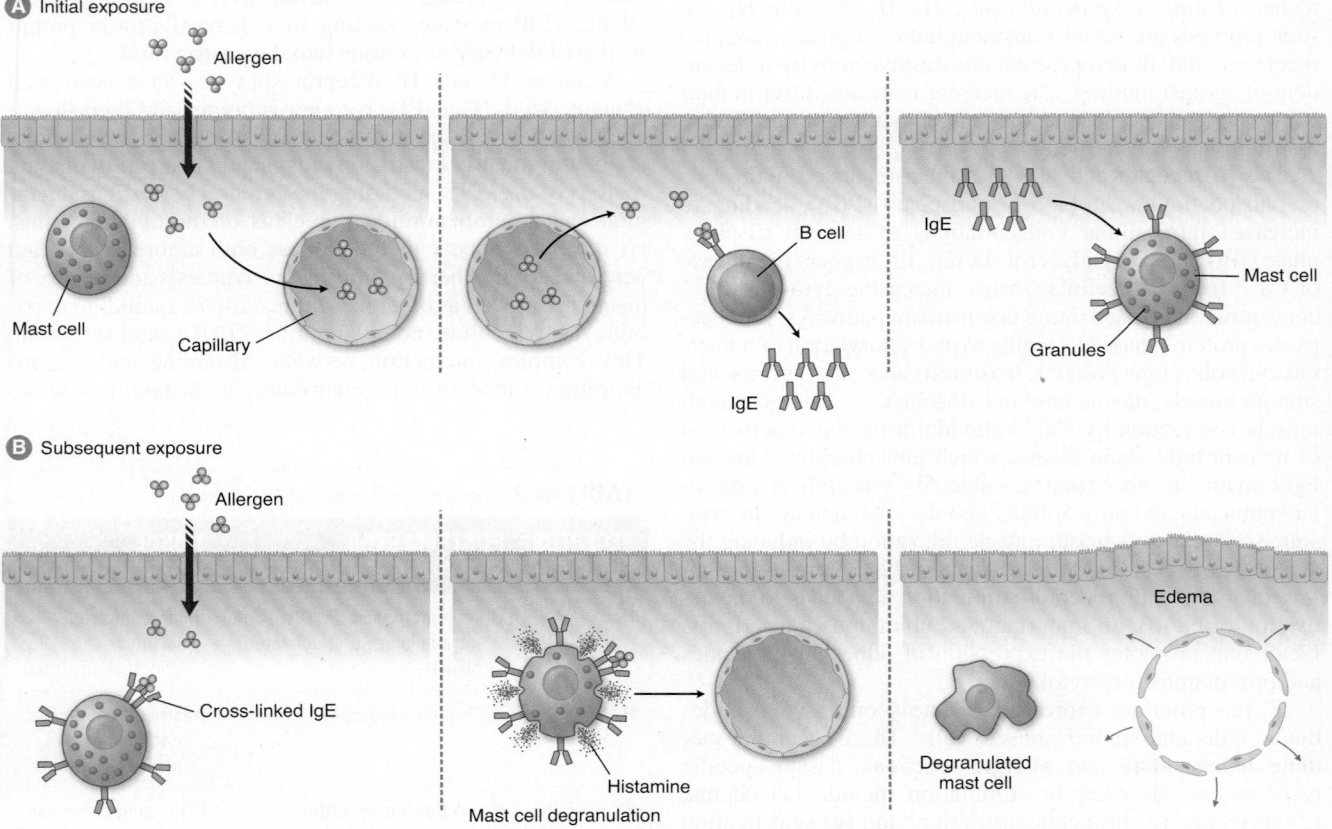

FIGURE 44-2. Pathophysiology of the IgE-mediated hypersensitivity reaction. Allergen-induced mast cell degranulation requires two separate exposures to the allergen. **A.** On initial exposure, the allergen must penetrate epithelial surfaces so that it can encounter cells of the immune system. Activation of the immune response causes B lymphocytes to secrete allergen-specific IgE antibodies. These IgE molecules bind to Fc receptors on mast cells, leading to sensitization of the mast cells. **B.** On subsequent exposure, the multivalent allergen cross-links two IgE/Fc receptor complexes on the mast cell surface. Receptor cross-linking causes the mast cell to degranulate. Local histamine release results in an inflammatory response, shown here as edema.

Clinical Manifestations of Histamine Pathophysiology

The IgE-mediated hypersensitivity reaction is responsible for initiation of certain inflammatory disorders, including **allergic rhinitis** and **acute urticaria** (hives). In the introductory case, Ellen suffered from allergic rhinitis, with a runny nose, itchy eyes, and sneezing. In allergic rhinitis, an environmental allergen, such as pollen, crosses the nasal epithelium and enters the underlying tissue. There, the allergen encounters previously sensitized mast cells and cross-links IgE/Fc receptor complexes on the mast cell surface. Consequently, the mast cell degranulates and releases histamine, which binds to H_1 receptors in the nasal mucosa and local tissues. Stimulation of the H_1 receptors causes blood vessel dilation and increases vascular permeability, leading to edema. This swelling in the nasal mucosa is responsible for the nasal congestion that is experienced in allergic rhinitis. The accompanying itching, sneezing, runny nose, and tearing result from the combined action of histamine and other inflammatory mediators, including kinins, prostaglandins, and leukotrienes. These molecules initiate the hypersecretion and irritation characteristic of allergic rhinitis.

Mast cell activation also occurs in acute urticaria. Here, an allergen, such as penicillin, enters the body, either through ingestion or parenterally, and reaches the skin through the circulation. Histamine release results in a disseminated wheal-and-flare response, creating pruritic, erythematous, and edematous plaques on the skin.

Histamine and Anaphylaxis

Systemic mast cell degranulation can cause the life-threatening condition known as **anaphylaxis**. Typically, anaphylactic shock is initiated in a previously sensitized individual by a hypersensitivity reaction to an insect bite, an antibiotic such as penicillin, or ingestion of certain highly allergenic foods such as peanuts. An allergen that is distributed systemically, either by intravenous injection or by absorption into the circulation, can stimulate mast cells and basophils to release massive amounts of histamine throughout the body. The resulting systemic vasodilation and extravasation of plasma into the interstitium cause severe hypotension. Systemic histamine release also causes bronchoconstriction and epiglottal swelling, which can be lethal within minutes if not treated rapidly by the administration of epinephrine, as described below.

▌ PHARMACOLOGIC CLASSES AND AGENTS

Histamine pharmacology employs three approaches, each of which leads to blockade of histamine action (Table 44-3). The first, and the most frequently used, approach is to administer **antihistamines**, which typically are inverse agonists or competitive antagonists selective for the H_1, H_2, H_3, or H_4 receptor. H_1-antihistamines are discussed below in detail: their mechanism of action involves stabilization of the inactive conformation of the H_1 receptor to decrease signaling events that would lead to the inflammatory response. A second strategy is to prevent mast cell degranulation induced by binding of an antigen to the IgE/Fc receptor complex on mast cells. **Cromolyn** and **nedocromil** use this strategy

TABLE 44-3 Strategies of Histamine Pharmacology

STRATEGY	EXAMPLE OF PHARMACOLOGIC AGENT	EXAMPLE OF DISEASE TREATED
Administer inverse agonist of histamine receptor	Diphenhydramine, loratadine	Allergies
Prevent mast cell degranulation	Cromolyn, nedocromil	Asthma
Administer physiologic antagonist to counter the pathological effects of histamine	Epinephrine	Anaphylaxis

to prevent asthma attacks (see Chapter 48, Integrative Inflammation Pharmacology: Asthma); these compounds disrupt the chloride current through mast cell membranes, which is a key step in the degranulation process. The third strategy is to administer a drug that functionally counteracts the effects of histamine. An example of this approach is the use of **epinephrine** to treat anaphylaxis. Epinephrine is an adrenergic agonist that induces bronchodilation and vasoconstriction (see Chapter 11, Adrenergic Pharmacology); these actions counter the bronchoconstriction, vasodilation, and hypotension caused by histamine in anaphylactic shock.

H_1-Antihistamines

Mechanism of Action

Historically, H_1-antihistamines were referred to as *H_1 receptor antagonists*, based on experiments in tracheal smooth muscle that showed a drug-induced parallel shift in the histamine concentration–response relationship (see Chapter 2, Pharmacodynamics). Recently, however, advances in histamine pharmacology have shown that *H_1-antihistamines are inverse agonists rather than receptor antagonists*.

H_1 receptors appear to coexist in two conformational states—the inactive and active conformations—that are in equilibrium with one another in the absence of histamine or antihistamine (Fig. 44-3). In the basal state, the receptor tends toward constitutive activation. Histamine acts as an agonist for the active conformation of the H_1 receptor, and histamine binding shifts the equilibrium further toward the active receptor state. In comparison, antihistamines are **inverse agonists**. Inverse agonists bind preferentially to the inactive conformation of the H_1 receptor and shift the equilibrium toward the inactive state. Thus, even in the absence of endogenous histamine, inverse agonists reduce constitutive receptor activity (see Chapter 2).

Classification of First- and Second-Generation H_1-Antihistamines

The finding that histamine is a major mediator of the allergic hypersensitivity reaction led to the discovery of the first **H_1-antihistamines** by Bovet and Staub in 1937. Clinically useful drugs that inhibit the actions of histamine began to appear in the 1940s. *Currently, H_1-antihistamines parse into two categories: first-generation and second-generation H_1-antihistamines* (see the Drug Summary Table for details of H_1-antihistamine classification).

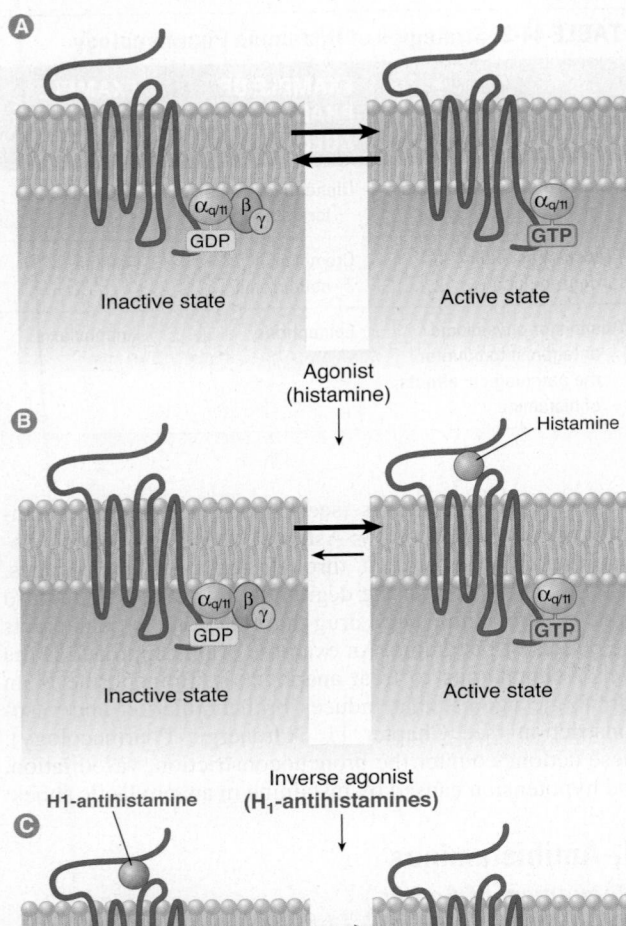

FIGURE 44-3. Simplified two-state model of H₁ receptor. A. H₁ receptors coexist in two conformational states—the inactive and active states—which are in conformational equilibrium with one another. **B.** Histamine acts as an agonist for the active conformation of the H₁ receptor and histamine binding shifts the equilibrium toward the active conformation. **C.** Antihistamines act as inverse agonists that bind and stabilize the inactive conformation of the H₁ receptor, thereby shifting the equilibrium toward the inactive receptor state.

H₁-antihistamines are less selective for the H₁ receptor and may additionally bind cholinergic, α-adrenergic, and serotonergic receptors at therapeutic doses.

The **second-generation H1-antihistamines** can be structurally categorized into four main subclasses—alkylamines, piperazines, phthalazinones, and piperidines. Widely used second-generation H₁-antihistamines include **loratadine**, **cetirizine**,

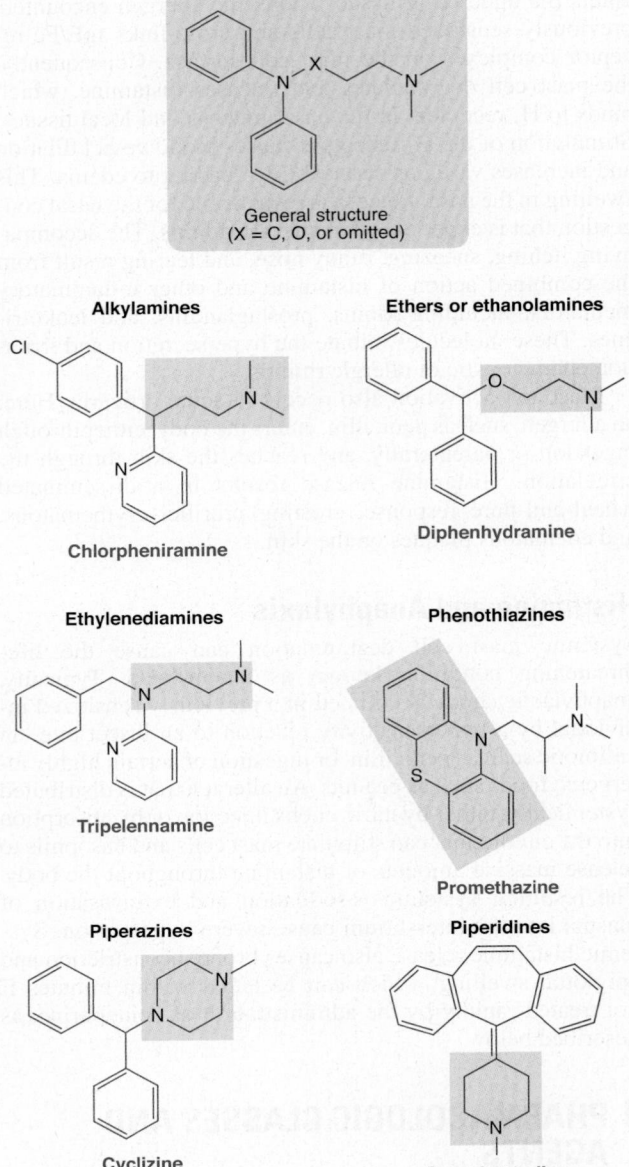

FIGURE 44-4. Structure of first-generation H₁-antihistamines. The general structure of the first-generation H₁-antihistamines consists of a substituted ethylamine backbone with two terminal aromatic rings. (Note the similarity between the ethylamine moiety in these drugs and the ethylamine side chain of histamine shown in Fig. 44-1.) Each of the six subclasses (*denoted by blue boxes*) is a variation on this general structure. First-generation H₁-antihistamines are neutral compounds at physiologic pH and readily cross the blood–brain barrier. In contrast, second-generation H₁-antihistamines (e.g., loratadine, cetirizine, fexofenadine) are ionized at physiologic pH and do not appreciably cross the blood–brain barrier (*not shown*). This difference in blood–brain barrier penetration underlies the differential extent of sedation associated with use of the first- and second-generation H₁-antihistamines.

The basic structure of the **first-generation H₁-antihistamines** consists of two aromatic rings linked to a substituted ethylamine backbone. These drugs are divided into six main subgroups based on their substituted side chains—ethanolamines, ethylenediamines, alkylamines, piperazines, phenothiazines, and piperidines (Fig. 44-4). **Diphenhydramine**, **hydroxyzine**, **chlorpheniramine**, and **promethazine** are among the most frequently used first-generation H₁-antihistamines. First-generation H₁-antihistamines are neutral at physiologic pH and readily cross the blood–brain barrier, where they block the actions of histaminergic neurons in the CNS. Compared to the second-generation H₁-antihistamines, first-generation and **fexofenadine**. Newer second-generation H$_1$-antihistamines include **levocetirizine**, the active enantiomer of cetirizine, and **desloratadine**, an active metabolite of loratadine. Second-generation H$_1$-antihistamines are ionized at physiologic pH and do not appreciably cross the blood–brain barrier. The differences in lipophilicity and selectivity between the first- and second-generation H$_1$-antihistamines account for their differential adverse effect profiles, notably, the tendency to cause CNS depression (drowsiness) and dry mouth (anticholinergic effect).

Pharmacologic Effects and Clinical Uses

Antihistamines are used in a broad spectrum of clinical conditions, including allergy, itching, nausea, vomiting, motion sickness, and insomnia. Despite the known contributions of histamine to bronchoconstriction and anaphylaxis, the currently available antihistamines have a limited role in the treatment of asthma or anaphylactic reactions.

Allergy Disorders

H$_1$-antihistamines are most useful in the treatment of allergic disorders to relieve symptoms of rhinitis, conjunctivitis, urticaria, and pruritus. H$_1$-antihistamines strongly block the increased capillary permeability necessary for the formation of edema and are therefore more effective when used prophylactically than after an allergic reaction has begun. The anti-inflammatory properties of H$_1$-antihistamines are attributable to suppression of the NFκB pathway and subsequent reduction in proinflammatory cytokine transcription, chemotaxis, and adhesion molecule expression.

The first- and second-generation H$_1$-antihistamines are equally efficacious in the treatment of chronic urticaria and allergic rhinitis. However, due to their favorable adverse effect profiles, second-generation antihistamines are generally preferred for long-term clinical use. Although most oral H$_1$-antihistamines do not appreciably relieve symptoms of nasal congestion, topical nasal antihistamines, such as **olopatadine** and **azelastine**, have been shown to be beneficial, particularly when they are combined with intranasal corticosteroids. The most recently approved topical H$_1$ antihistamine for allergy disorders is **bepotastine besilate** ophthalmic solution, which alleviates both ocular and non-ocular symptoms of allergic conjunctivitis.

Generalized Itching

Hydroxyzine and **doxepin** are potent antipruritic agents, and their clinical effectiveness is likely related to their pronounced CNS effects. Doxepin, a tricyclic antidepressant, is best used in patients with depression, since even small doses can cause confusion and disorientation in nondepressed patients. Compared to oral H$_1$-antihistamines, topical H$_1$-antihistamines (including nasal and ophthalmic preparations) have a more rapid onset of action, but they require multiple administrations each day. Cutaneous preparations of antihistamines, administered for pruritic dermatoses, may paradoxically cause allergic dermatitis.

Nausea and Motion Sickness

First-generation H$_1$-antihistamines can be used to counter motion sickness as well as chemotherapy- and migraine-related nausea and vomiting. By inhibiting histaminergic signals from the vestibular nucleus to the vomiting center in the medulla, H$_1$-antihistamines such as **dimenhydrinate**, **diphenhydramine**, **meclizine**, and **promethazine** are useful as antiemetic agents.

Insomnia

Due to their prominent CNS depressive effects, first-generation H$_1$-antihistamines such as **diphenhydramine**, **doxylamine**, and **pyrilamine** are also used to treat insomnia. While effective in promoting sleep, the increased incidence of adverse effects, including the tendency to cause next-day sedation, limits their usefulness in clinical practice. Standard doses of first-generation antihistamines have been shown to cause a reduction in alertness and psychomotor performance similar in magnitude to social alcohol consumption. For this reason, first-generation antihistamines are contraindicated in individuals who are required to maintain alertness or precision.

Several commonly prescribed psychiatric medications, including trazodone (antidepressant) and quetiapine (antipsychotic), are also frequently utilized in the treatment of insomnia due to their antihistaminergic properties in the CNS.

Limited Use: Asthma and Anaphylaxis

H$_1$-antihistamines have limited efficacy in bronchial asthma and should not be used as monotherapy for asthma. While H$_1$-antihistamines appear to inhibit constriction of bronchial smooth muscle in guinea pigs, this effect is much less pronounced in humans because of contributions from other mediators such as leukotrienes and serotonin.

H$_1$-antihistamines alone are also ineffective for systemic anaphylaxis or severe angioedema with laryngeal swelling. In these conditions, the contributions from other local mediators are unaffected by H$_1$-antihistamine treatment, and epinephrine remains the treatment of choice.

Pharmacokinetics

Oral H$_1$-antihistamines are well absorbed from the gastrointestinal tract, and they reach peak plasma concentrations in 2–3 hours. The duration of effect varies depending on the particular H$_1$-antihistamine agent. Most H$_1$-antihistamines are metabolized by the liver, and dose adjustments should be considered in patients with severe liver disease. As inhibitors of hepatic cytochrome P450 enzymes, H$_1$-antihistamines may affect the metabolism of other drugs utilizing the cytochrome P450 system. Co-administration of agents competing for the same enzymes can reduce the metabolism of an H$_1$-antihistamine and increase its serum level.

Adverse Effects

The major adverse effects of H$_1$-antihistamines are CNS toxicity, cardiac toxicity, and anticholinergic effects. Adverse effect profiles of second-generation H$_1$-antihistamines have been thoroughly investigated, but long-term safety studies of first-generation H$_1$-antihistamines are lacking despite their use for over six decades.

Because of their high lipophilicity, first-generation H$_1$-antihistamines readily penetrate the blood–brain barrier. These drugs antagonize the neurotransmitter effects of histamine on H$_1$ receptors in the CNS (especially the hypothalamus) and the periphery. As noted above, the high CNS penetration accounts for the sedating action of these drugs. In the introductory case, Ellen experienced sedation when she took diphenhydramine for her allergic rhinitis. Factors that increase the risk of CNS toxicity include low body mass, severe hepatic or renal dysfunction, and concomitant use of drugs, such as alcohol, that impair CNS function.

The low CNS penetration of second-generation H_1-antihistamines is attributable to several features of the molecules. First, as noted earlier, these compounds are ionized at physiologic pH and so do not diffuse readily across membranes. Second, they exhibit high binding affinity to albumin as well as to the P-glycoprotein efflux pump on the luminal surface of the vascular endothelium, thereby limiting their distribution into the CNS. Second-generation H_1-antihistamines are often preferred for extended use because of their limited sedative effects. For example, the second-generation H_1-antihistamines loratadine, desloratadine, and fexofenadine are the only oral H_1-antihistamines permitted for use by airline pilots.

H_1-antihistamines that prolong the QT interval can cause cardiac toxicity, especially in patients with preexisting cardiac dysfunction. Some earlier second-generation H_1-antihistamines had serious cardiotoxic effects at high plasma concentrations. Two of these drugs, terfenadine and astemizole, were withdrawn by the US Food and Drug Administration (FDA) because they caused prolonged QT intervals that sometimes led to ventricular arrhythmias. The mechanism by which H_1-antihistamines prolong the QT interval is thought to involve inhibition of the I_{Kr} current and not blockade of the H_1 receptor. The human ether-a-go-go-related gene (*hERG*) encodes the α subunit of the potassium channel mediating the I_{Kr} current, and in vitro testing using variants of hERG is now available for assessing whether a medication has the potential to inhibit the I_{Kr} current.

Anticholinergic adverse effects, which are more prominent with first-generation than with second-generation H_1-antihistamines, include pupillary dilation, dry eyes, dry mouth, and urinary retention and hesitancy. Elderly individuals may demonstrate increased sensitivity to the anticholinergic and sedative effects of first-generation H_1-antihistamines and may also experience more drug–drug interactions due to a greater number of concomitant medications. The α-adrenergic blockade and subsequent hypotension associated with some first-generation antihistamines further predispose older individuals to falls.

Young children also appear to be more susceptible to adverse effects related to antihistamine use. Because of the unfavorable adverse effect profile and limited evidence for the efficacy of antihistamines in young children, the FDA advises against the use of cough and cold preparations containing antihistamines in children less than 2 years of age.

Overdose of first-generation H_1-antihistamines can cause severe CNS depression presenting as somnolence, ataxia, and coma. In young children and the elderly, where paradoxical stimulation is more common, acute poisoning may cause hallucinations, irritability, and convulsions before progressing to respiratory failure and cardiovascular collapse. The CNS effects are also generally accompanied by marked anticholinergic symptoms, such as dehydration, pupillary dilation, and fever.

Other Antihistamines

Competitive antagonists and inverse agonists have also been developed against the H_2, H_3, and H_4 receptors. Considerable interest was generated by the development of selective **H_2 receptor antagonists** that inhibit histamine-induced gastric acid secretion. H_2 receptor antagonists, which are discussed in detail in Chapter 47, differ in structure from H_1-antihistamines in that they contain an intact five-membered ring (instead of two or more bulky aromatic rings) and an uncharged, bulky side chain (Fig. 44-5; see also Fig. 47-5). These agents act

FIGURE 44-5. Structure of H_2 receptor antagonists. H_2 receptor antagonists have a thioethanolamine backbone (*highlighted in blue box*) that is N-substituted with a bulky side chain and that terminates in a single five-membered ring. (Compare the bulky N-substituted side chain of the H_2 antagonists with the simple tertiary amine of the H_1-antihistamines in Fig. 44-4, and compare the small five-membered imidazole or furan ring of the H_2 antagonists with the pair of bulky aromatic rings of the H_1-antihistamines.) These structural differences enable cimetidine, ranitidine, and other H_2 antagonists to bind selectively to H_2 receptors in the gastric mucosa, thereby decreasing the production of gastric acid.

as reversible, competitive antagonists of histamine binding to H_2 receptors on gastric parietal cells and thereby reduce gastric acid secretion. Clinical indications include acid reflux disease (heartburn) and peptic ulcer disease. Many of these agents are also available over the counter for the symptomatic treatment of heartburn. **Cimetidine** and **ranitidine** are two of the most commonly used H_2 receptor antagonists. A significant adverse effect of cimetidine involves inhibition of cytochrome P450-mediated drug metabolism, which can result in undesirable elevations in the serum levels of certain concomitantly administered drugs. H_2 receptors are also expressed in the CNS and in cardiac muscle, but the therapeutic doses of H_2 receptor antagonists are sufficiently low that CNS and cardiovascular adverse effects are negligible.

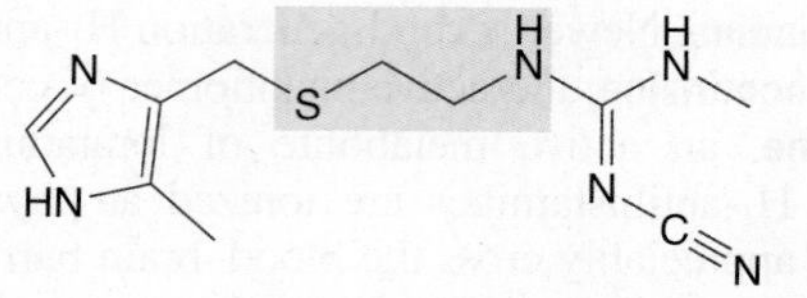

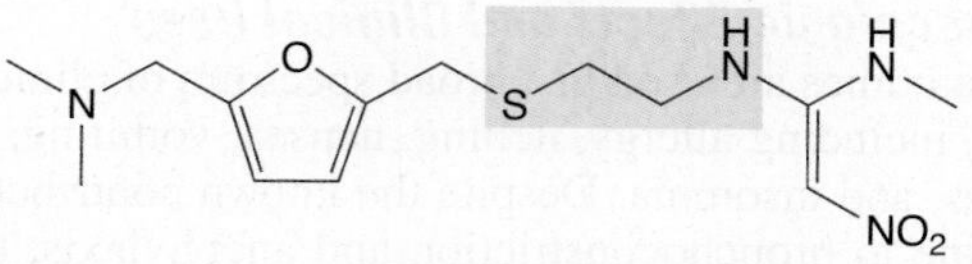

The pharmacology of H_3 and H_4 receptors is an active area of investigation. To date, no drugs selectively directed against H_3 and H_4 receptors have been approved for clinical use. **H_3 receptors** are thought to provide *feedback inhibition* of certain effects of histamine in the CNS and in ECL cells. In animal studies, H_3 receptor antagonists induce wakefulness and improve attention, effects that are thought to be mediated by overstimulation of cortical H_1 receptors. H_3 receptor antagonists that have been developed for experimental use include **thioperamide**, **clobenpropit**, **ciproxifan**, and **proxyfan**. **Pitolisant**, formerly known as *tripolisant*, is an H_3 receptor-selective inverse agonist in late-phase clinical development for the treatment of narcolepsy.

Similar to H_3 receptors, **H_4 receptors** couple with $G_{i/o}$ to decrease intracellular cAMP concentrations. Because H_4 receptors are selectively expressed on cells of hematopoietic origin, especially mast cells, basophils, and eosinophils, there is considerable interest in elucidating the role of the H_4 receptor in the inflammatory process. H_4 receptor antagonists represent a promising area of drug development to treat inflammatory conditions that involve mast cells and eosinophils.

CONCLUSION AND FUTURE DIRECTIONS

Histamine plays a key role in diverse physiologic processes including allergy, inflammation, neurotransmission, and gastric acid secretion. Drugs targeting H_1 and H_2 receptors have substantially increased the pharmacologic options for treatment of allergy and peptic ulcer disease. While most H_1-antihistamines demonstrate similar efficacy in the treatment of allergic rhinitis and urticaria, significant differences exist in the adverse effect profiles of first- and second-generation H_1-antihistamines.

The more recent elucidation of the H_3 and H_4 receptor subtypes has renewed interest in the role of histamine in CNS-related disorders. H_3-specific receptor targeting may provide new therapies for a number of cognitive, neuroendocrine, and neuropsychiatric conditions. Clinical and preclinical research is currently underway evaluating prototypic H_3 antagonists in pathological processes such as sleep–wake disorders (narcolepsy and insomnia), neuropsychiatric diseases (Alzheimer's disease, ADHD, dementia, depression, and schizophrenia), neurologic disorders (epilepsy), nociceptive processes (neuropathic pain), and feeding and energy homeostasis (obesity and diabetes). The H_4 receptor is also an emerging molecular target for drug development, as it is thought to play an important role in inflammatory conditions involving mast cells and eosinophils. Agents directed against H_4 receptors might one day be employed to treat a variety of inflammatory conditions, such as asthma, allergic rhinitis, inflammatory bowel disease, and rheumatoid arthritis.

Acknowledgment

We thank Joseph C. Kvedar, Cindy Chambers, Ashish Sahasrabudhe, and Robert R. Rando for their valuable contributions to the First, Second, and Third Editions of *Principles of Pharmacology: The Pathophysiologic Basis of Drug Therapy*.

Suggested Reading

Bhowmik M, Khanam R, Vohora D. Histamine H3 receptor antagonists in relation to epilepsy and neurodegeneration: a systemic consideration of recent progress and perspectives. *Br J Pharmacol* 2012;167:1398–1414. (*Comprehensively reviews the current state of H_3 receptor antagonist research with a focus on epilepsy and neurodegenerative disorders.*)

Leurs R, Church MK, Taglialatela M. H_1-antihistamines: inverse agonism, anti-inflammatory actions and cardiac effects. *Clin Exp Allergy* 2002;32:489–498. (*Mechanism-based discussion of H_1-antihistamines as inverse agonists.*)

Nicolas JM. The metabolic profile of second-generation antihistamine. *Allergy* 2000;55:46–52. (*Discussion of differences among second-generation drugs.*)

Simons FE. Advances in H1-antihistamines. *N Engl J Med* 2004;351:2203–2217. (*Comprehensively summarizes the mechanism of action and clinical uses of H_1-antihistamines.*)

Thurmond RL, Gelfand EW, Dunford PJ. The role of histamine H1 and H4 receptors in allergic inflammation: the search for new antihistamines. *Nat Rev Drug Discov* 2008;7:41–53. (*Reviews the role of histamine in inflammation and immune modulation, with emphasis on the role of the H_4 receptor.*)

Zampeli E, Tiligada E. The role of histamine H4 receptor in immune and inflammatory disorders. *Br J Pharmacol* 2009;157:24–33. (*Reviews H_4 receptor biology and pharmacology.*)

DRUG SUMMARY TABLE: CHAPTER 44 Histamine Pharmacology

FIRST-GENERATION H$_1$-ANTIHISTAMINES
Mechanism—Inverse agonists that bind preferentially to the inactive conformation of the H$_1$ receptor and shift the equilibrium toward the inactive receptor state

DRUG	CLINICAL APPLICATIONS	SERIOUS AND COMMON ADVERSE EFFECTS	CONTRAINDICATIONS	THERAPEUTIC CONSIDERATIONS
Ethanolamines: **Diphenhydramine** **Carbinoxamine** **Clemastine** **Dimenhydrinate**	Allergic rhinitis Anaphylaxis (*adjunctive* to epinephrine) Insomnia Motion sickness Parkinsonism Urticaria	Xerostomia, sedation, dizziness, dyskinesia, dry eyes, dry nasal mucosa	Shared contraindications: Hypersensitivity to drug Children younger than 2 years of age Nursing mother Carbinoxamine and clemastine only: Lower respiratory tract symptoms including asthma MAOI therapy	In general, first-generation H$_1$-antihistamines have greater CNS and anticholinergic adverse effects than second-generation H$_1$-antihistamines. Diphenhydramine (trade name Benadryl®) is available in oral solid, oral liquid, intramuscular, intravenous, and topical preparations. Diphenhydramine may raise thioridazine plasma levels, thereby increasing the risk of arrhythmia.
Ethylenediamines: **Pyrilamine** **Tripelennamine**	Same as diphenhydramine	Same as diphenhydramine	Hypersensitivity to pyrilamine or tripelennamine Narrow-angle glaucoma Stenosing peptic ulcer Symptomatic prostatic hypertrophy Bladder neck obstruction Pyloroduodenal obstruction Lower respiratory tract symptoms, including asthma Premature infants, neonates, nursing mothers MAOI therapy	Same as diphenhydramine.
Alkylamines: **Chlorpheniramine** **Brompheniramine**	Shared indication: Allergic rhinitis Brompheniramine only: Anaphylaxis Urticaria	Xerostomia, gastrointestinal upset, somnolence	Shared contraindications: Hypersensitivity to chlorpheniramine or brompheniramine MAOI therapy Brompheniramine only: Focal central nervous system lesions	Same as diphenhydramine.
Piperidines: **Cyproheptadine**	Same as diphenhydramine	Same as diphenhydramine	Hypersensitivity to cyproheptadine Newborn or premature infants Nursing mothers MAOI therapy Angle-closure glaucoma Stenosing peptic ulcer Pyloroduodenal obstruction Bladder neck obstruction	Same as diphenhydramine. Cyproheptadine is available as an oral tablet.
Phenothiazines: **Promethazine**	Allergy Motion sickness Nausea and vomiting Postoperative pain Sedation	*Prolonged QT interval, agranulocytosis, leukopenia, thrombocytopenia, jaundice, neuroleptic malignant syndrome, respiratory depression* Rash, gastrointestinal upset, xerostomia, dizziness, extrapyramidal disease, sedation	Hypersensitivity to promethazine Children younger than 2 years of age Comatose states Lower respiratory tract symptoms, including asthma	Promethazine is used primarily to relieve preoperative anxiety and reduce postoperative nausea and vomiting. Tablets, subcutaneous or intra-arterial injection, suppositories.

Drug	Clinical Applications	Serious and Common Adverse Effects	Contraindications	Therapeutic Considerations
Piperazines: **Hydroxyzine** **Cyclizine** **Meclizine**	Hydroxyzine only: Pruritus Anxiety Vomiting Cyclizine and meclizine only: Motion sickness Vertigo	Same as diphenhydramine	Hypersensitivity to hydroxyzine, cyclizine, or meclizine Hydroxyzine only: Early pregnancy	Hydroxyzine is a potent antipruritic agent.
Tricyclic dibenzoxepins: **Doxepin**	Anxiety Depression Pruritus Insomnia	*Ventricular arrhythmia, agranulocytosis, leukopenia, thrombocytopenia, suicidal ideation, nephrotoxicity* Hypotension, gastrointestinal upset, somnolence, dizziness, urinary retention, infection	Hypersensitivity to doxepin MAOI therapy Glaucoma Urinary retention	Doxepin is a tricyclic antidepressant; it is best used in patients with depression, as even small doses can cause confusion and disorientation in nondepressed patients.

SECOND-GENERATION H₁-ANTIHISTAMINES

Mechanism—Inverse agonists that bind preferentially to the inactive conformation of the H₁ receptor and shift the equilibrium toward the inactive receptor state

Drug	Clinical Applications	Serious and Common Adverse Effects	Contraindications	Therapeutic Considerations
Piperazines: **Cetirizine** **Levocetirizine**	Allergic rhinitis Urticaria	*Oculogyric crisis* Xerostomia, asthenia, headache, fatigue	Hypersensitivity to cetirizine or levocetirizine Levocetirizine only: End-stage renal disease, hemodialysis	In general, second-generation H₁-antihistamines have less severe anticholinergic effects and are less sedating than first-generation H₁-antihistamines because of reduced penetration into the CNS.
Alkylamines: **Acrivastine**	Allergic rhinitis	Same as cetirizine	Hypersensitivity to acrivastine Severe hypertension Severe coronary artery disease MAOI therapy	Same as cetirizine. Acrivastine is only available in combination with pseudoephedrine.
Piperidines: **Loratadine** **Desloratadine** **Ebastine** **Mizolastine** **Fexofenadine** **Levocabastine** **Bepotastine besilate**	Shared indications: Allergic rhinitis Urticaria Levocabastine and bepotastine besilate only: Allergic conjunctivitis	Xerostomia, headache, somnolence, fatigue (shared adverse effects); pharyngitis (desloratadine and bepotastine besilate only); myalgia, dysmenorrhea (desloratadine only); gastrointestinal upset (fexofenadine only); taste disorder, eye irritation (bepotastine besilate only)	Hypersensitivity to drug Levocabastine only: Soft contact lens	Same as cetirizine. Levocabastine and bepotastine besilate are administered as ophthalmic solutions.
Phthalazinones: **Azelastine**	Allergic rhinitis Vasomotor rhinitis Allergic conjunctivitis	Bitter taste, headache, somnolence, eye and nasal irritation, sneezing, fatigue	Hypersensitivity to azelastine	Same as cetirizine. Administered as a nasal spray or ophthalmic solution.
Tricyclic dibenzoxepins: **Olopatadine**	Allergic rhinitis Allergic conjunctivitis	*Epistaxis, ulcer of nose* Taste alteration, headache, eye irritation, pharyngitis	Hypersensitivity to olopatadine	Administered as a nasal spray or ophthalmic solution.

H₂ RECEPTOR ANTAGONISTS

Drug				
Cimetidine **Famotidine** **Nizatidine** **Ranitidine**	See Drug Summary Table: Chapter 47 Integrative Inflammation Pharmacology: Peptic Ulcer Disease			

45

Pharmacology of Hematopoiesis and Immunomodulation

Andrew J. Wagner, Ramy A. Arnaout, and George D. Demetri

INTRODUCTION

Many clinical situations are characterized by deficiencies of red blood cells, white blood cells, and/or platelets—cells of the hematopoietic system. This chapter describes the pharmacologic agents that can be used to stimulate production of hematopoietic cells; it is also important to note the nonpharmacologic alternatives, which could include transfusion and bone marrow transplantation. Blood cell production is controlled physiologically by hematopoietic growth factors, a diverse but functionally overlapping group of glycoproteins produced by the body in response to certain signals. For example, hypoxia stimulates the synthesis and release of the erythroid lineage growth factor erythropoietin, which in turn stimulates the production of erythrocytes in an attempt to relieve the hypoxia. The main pharmacologic strategy used to stimulate the production of blood cells is to administer exogenous growth factors or synthetic growth factor analogues. This chapter provides an introduction to the cells of the hematopoietic system, the growth factors that stimulate their production, and the pharmacologic agents used to increase blood cell production. An outline of the immunomodulatory agents used in anticancer therapy is also presented.

PHYSIOLOGY OF HEMATOPOIESIS

The cells of the hematopoietic system are functionally diverse (Table 45-1). Red blood cells, or **erythrocytes**, carry oxygen; many types of white blood cells, from **granulocytes** and **macrophages** to **lymphocytes**, fight infection and help protect against cancer; and **platelets** help control bleeding. Nonetheless, these cells have one feature in common: they all develop from a common cell in the bone marrow called the **pluripotent hematopoietic stem cell** (Fig. 45-1). Hematopoietic stem cells are induced to differentiate along committed lineages into red blood cells, white blood cells, or platelets through interactions with glycoproteins called **hematopoietic growth factors**.

Central Role of Hematopoietic Growth Factors

Hematopoietic growth factors and cytokines constitute a heterogeneous group of molecules that regulate blood cell production, maturation, and function. Nearly 36 such factors have been identified, ranging in size from 9 to 90 kDa. The membrane-associated receptors for these factors

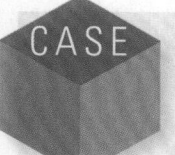CASE

Fifty-two-year-old Mrs. M presents with a lump in her left breast. Subsequent mammogram, core biopsy, and lumpectomy lead to the diagnosis of infiltrating ductal carcinoma that is localized but lymph node–positive. She begins adjuvant chemotherapy with doxorubicin and cyclophosphamide. Ten days after the first cycle of chemotherapy, her white blood cell count (WBC) drops, as expected; over the next 9 days, her WBC recovers to its normal value. By the third cycle of chemotherapy, Mrs. M is moderately anemic, with a hematocrit of 28% (normal, 37–48%), and she feels quite fatigued. Seven days after the fourth cycle of chemotherapy, her WBC plummets to 800 cells per microliter (µL) of blood (normal, 4,300–10,800 cells/µL), and her absolute neutrophil count (ANC) is 300 cells/µL. In this setting, she develops shaking chills and a fever to 102°F. She is admitted to the hospital, where she receives parenteral antibiotics, and she remains there for 5 days until her ANC rises to an acceptable level. Mrs. M completes her cycles of doxorubicin and cyclophosphamide chemotherapy, continues chemotherapy with paclitaxel, and receives local radiation therapy.

Mrs. M is well for 2 years but then presents with pain in the left leg. Workup reveals that the cancer has metastasized to her left femur and liver. She begins chemotherapy with doxorubicin and docetaxel but again develops severe neutropenia and fever. She becomes short of breath while climbing stairs, and her hematocrit is 27%. Her iron stores are normal. Thereafter, her chemotherapy is supplemented with pegylated recombinant human G-CSF (PEG-filgrastim) and an analogue of human erythropoietin (darbepoetin). Neutropenia and fever do not recur, and by 4 weeks after the initiation of erythropoietin therapy, her hematocrit rises to 34.5% and she has normal exercise tolerance. The chemotherapy yields excellent palliative results. One year later, she is still in remission and leading an active life.

Questions

1. Are G-CSF and erythropoietin multilineage growth factors or lineage-specific growth factors?
2. How does erythropoietin increase the number of erythrocytes in the blood?
3. How do analogues of hematopoietic growth factors such as darbepoetin and PEG-filgrastim differ from endogenous, "natural" hematopoietic growth factors?
4. What are the important adverse effects of erythropoietin?

TABLE 45-1 Hematopoietic Cells, Growth Factors, and Growth Factor Analogues

CELL TYPE	MAJOR FUNCTION(S)	LINEAGE-SPECIFIC GROWTH FACTOR	DEFICIENCY STATE	THERAPEUTIC AGENTS
Red blood cell (erythrocyte)	Oxygen transport	Erythropoietin (EPO)	Anemia	Epoetin alfa, PEG-epoetin beta, darbepoetin alfa
Platelet (thrombocyte)	Hemostasis	Thrombopoietin (TPO)	Thrombocytopenia	Eltrombopag, romiplostim, IL-11
Monocyte/macrophage	Phagocytosis of bacteria and cellular and chemical debris, stimulation of T lymphocytes	M-CSF	—	—
Neutrophil	Phagocytosis of bacteria, immune stimulation	G-CSF	Neutropenia	Filgrastim, PEG-filgrastim, sargramostim
Eosinophil	Control of parasites	IL-5	—	—
B lymphocyte	Production of antibody, stimulation of T lymphocytes	Specific interleukins	Various immunodeficiency syndromes	—
T lymphocyte	Killing of virus- and bacteria-infected cells, control of immune responses	Specific interleukins	Various immunodeficiency syndromes	rhIL-2
NK cell	Killing of cancer cells	—	—	—

NK, natural killer; M-CSF, monocyte colony-stimulating factor; G-CSF, granulocyte colony-stimulating factor; IL-5, interleukin-5; PEG, polyethylene glycol; IL-11, interleukin-11; rhIL-2, recombinant human interleukin-2.

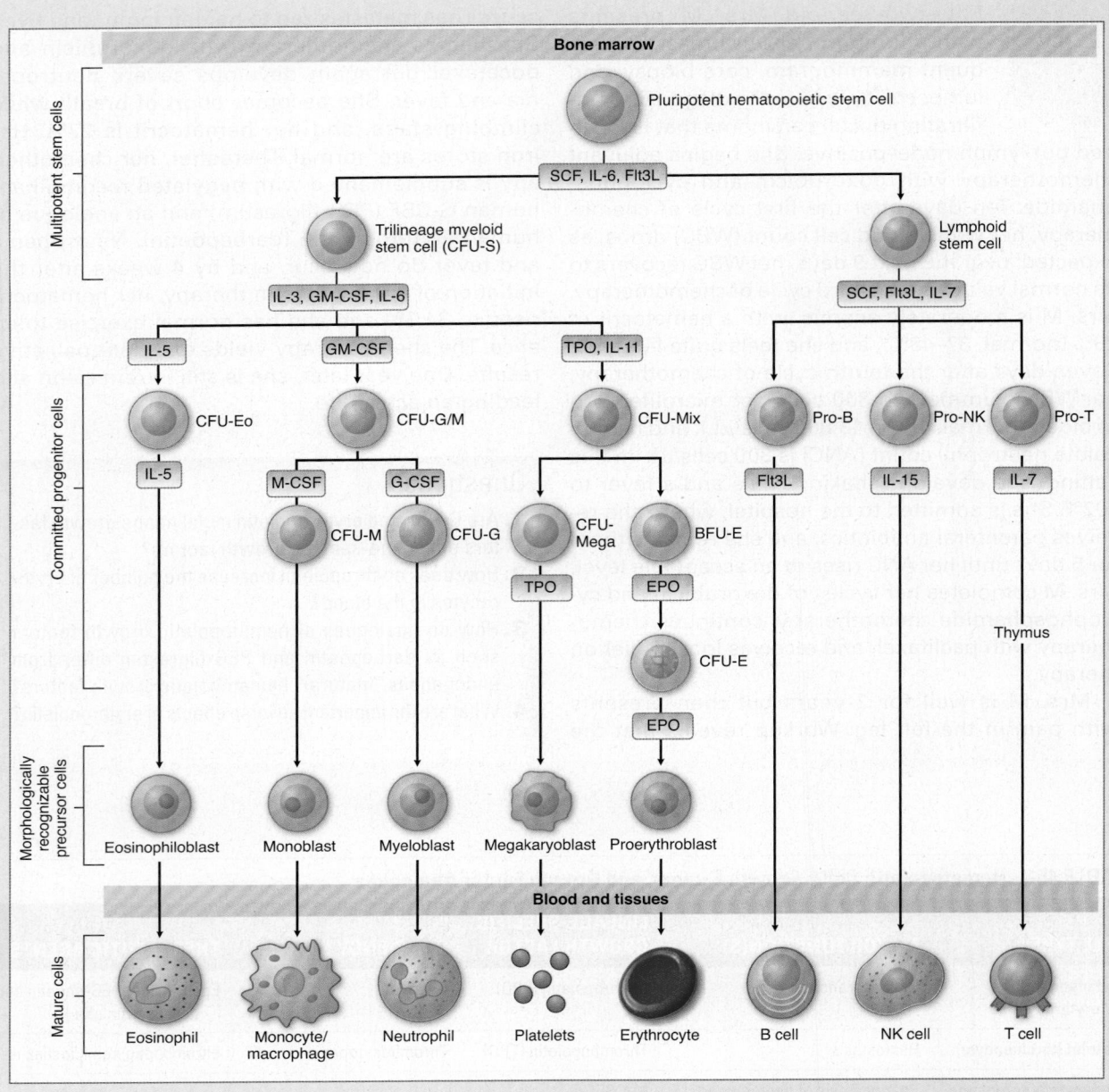

FIGURE 45-1. Development of cells of the hematopoietic system. Mature cells of the hematopoietic system all develop from pluripotent stem cells that reside in the bone marrow. The type of mature cell that develops is dependent on the extracellular milieu and the exposure of stem cells and progenitor cells to specific growth factors. The pluripotent hematopoietic stem cell differentiates into a trilineage myeloid stem cell (CFU-S) or a lymphoid stem cell. Depending on the growth factors that are present, CFU-S cells differentiate into granulocytes (eosinophils, neutrophils), monocyte/macrophages, platelets, or erythrocytes. Lymphoid stem cells differentiate into B cells, natural killer (NK) cells, or T cells. Except for the terminal differentiation of pro-T cells to mature T cells, which takes place in the thymus, the differentiation of all hematopoietic stem cells, progenitor cells, and precursor cells occurs in the bone marrow. Of the growth factors illustrated here, G-CSF, GM-CSF, erythropoietin (EPO), and IL-11 are currently used as therapeutic agents. BFU, burst-forming unit; CFU, colony-forming unit; CSF, colony-stimulating factor; IL, interleukin; SCF, stem cell factor; TPO, thrombopoietin.

belong to at least six receptor superfamilies, and genes encoding the factors are found on 11 different chromosomes. Conceptually, growth factors can be divided into two groups: **multilineage** (also called **general**, **early-acting**, or **pleiotropic**) growth factors, which stimulate multiple lineages, and **lineage-specific** (also called **lineage-dominant** or **late-acting**) growth factors, which stimulate differentiation and survival of a single lineage. Many growth factors and

cytokines act synergistically with one another, sometimes with overlapping effects.

Multilineage Growth Factors

Multilineage growth factors include **stem cell factor** (also called **steel factor** or **KIT ligand**), **interleukin-3 (IL-3)**, **granulocyte-monocyte colony-stimulating factor (GM-CSF)**, insulin-like growth factor 1, IL-9, IL-11, and others. Many of these growth factors are discussed below with respect to the development of individual hematopoietic cell types. The relevant pharmacologic principle is that multilineage growth factors might be appropriate for treating conditions such as **pancytopenia** in which multiple hematopoietic lineages are affected.

The ability of multilineage growth factors to stimulate multiple lineages results from two features of their molecular and cellular physiology. First, the receptors for these growth factors are both structurally related and modular; this commonality makes them somewhat interchangeable. Second, the signal transduction cascades activated by binding of these growth factors to their receptors involve a common family of signaling proteins, the JAK-STAT proteins. In the myeloproliferative diseases polycythemia vera, essential thrombocytosis, and myeloid metaplasia with myelofibrosis, the JAK2 kinase is constitutively activated by a point mutation that leads to a single amino acid substitution (V617F) in the protein product of the gene. These diseases are characterized by clonal proliferation of all lineages, highlighting the general role of the JAK-STAT pathway in hematopoiesis. Pharmacologists have exploited the commonalities of multilineage growth factor signaling to design synthetic growth factors with novel properties (see below).

Lineage-Specific Growth Factors

For a growth factor to be lineage-specific, at least one of two conditions must be met: (1) the expression of the growth factor's receptor(s) must be limited to progenitor and/or precursor cells within a single lineage and/or (2) the growth factor must induce inhibitory or apoptotic signals in cells of other lineages. **Erythropoietin** is one example of a lineage-specific growth factor; **thrombopoietin**, whose actions are essentially limited to the platelet lineage, is another. Other so-called lineage-specific growth factors are more properly considered lineage-selective, because they have secondary effects on lineage(s) other than the lineage of their primary action. Such factors include **G-CSF**, which primarily promotes the differentiation of neutrophils, and a number of **interleukins**, which have selective actions on certain myeloid and lymphoid lineages (see below). From a pharmacologic perspective, lineage-specific growth factors represent selective therapeutics that can be used to treat a deficiency of a single hematopoietic cell type. Some growth factors may also have unique effects against certain cancers, perhaps due to their prodifferentiation and promaturation properties.

Erythrocyte Production (Erythropoiesis)

Erythrocytes are uniquely suited to their role of transporting oxygen from the lungs to the tissues of the body. These cells contain high concentrations of **hemoglobin**, a protein that binds and releases oxygen molecules in response to the partial pressure of oxygen in the blood and tissues. Each hemoglobin molecule consists of four similar polypeptide chains, and each chain contains a binding site for molecular oxygen. The major form of adult hemoglobin, which has two alpha and two beta chains ($\alpha_2\beta_2$), is called **hemoglobin A (HbA)**. Fetal hemoglobin, or **hemoglobin F (HbF)**, contains gamma (γ) chains instead of β chains ($\alpha_2\gamma_2$). HbF predominates during the latter 6 months of fetal life and has a higher affinity for oxygen than HbA does, which helps facilitate the transfer of oxygen from mother to fetus. After birth, DNA methylation inactivates the γ globin gene, and expression of the β globin gene rises. It is important to note that expression of the α, β, and γ globin chains is regulated independently, making possible a multitude of **hemoglobinopathies** in which the α or β chains are abnormal or underexpressed because of an inherited mutation. In **sickle cell anemia**, a point mutation in the β globin gene results in the production of an abnormal hemoglobin—**hemoglobin S (HbS)**—that polymerizes upon deoxygenation, causing morphologic "sickling" of erythrocytes and leading to hemolytic anemia, painful vaso-occlusive crises, and profound end-organ damage. This autosomal recessive disease is the most common inherited blood disorder in the United States, affecting more than 70,000 individuals. Another common hemoglobinopathy is β **thalassemia**, in which the β chain is structurally and functionally normal but underexpressed.

Upon their release from the bone marrow, normal erythrocytes circulate in the blood with a lifespan of approximately 120 days. The number of erythrocytes in the blood is determined by the balance between new erythrocyte production in the bone marrow and erythrocyte loss due to cell destruction (hemolysis) and bleeding. This number is measured clinically as either the hemoglobin level (the concentration of hemoglobin per unit volume of blood) or the **hematocrit** (the percentage of blood volume that is composed of erythrocytes). The normal hemoglobin level ranges from 14 g/dL to 17 g/dL in men and 12 g/dL to 15 g/dL in women, and the normal hematocrit ranges from 42% to 50% in men and 37% to 46% in women. These gender differences are often attributed to increased blood loss through physiologic—that is, menstrual—bleeding in women and enhanced erythropoiesis induced by androgens (through unclear mechanisms) in men. A hemoglobin level or hematocrit below the normal range is defined as **anemia**.

Erythropoietin

Erythrocyte production, or **erythropoiesis**, proceeds under the control of several growth factors. The major growth factor controlling erythropoiesis is erythropoietin, a heavily glycosylated protein that is produced mainly by the liver in the fetus and by the kidney after birth. A lineage-specific growth factor, erythropoietin has received great clinical attention because it stimulates all but the earliest intermediates in the erythroid lineage but does not significantly affect other lineages. Its physiologic importance is attested to by experiments in mice and pathologic conditions in humans, both of which show that the absence of erythropoietin results in severe anemia. Furthermore, rare activating mutations of the erythropoietin receptor have been described in patients with primary familial and congenital polycythemia, a disorder manifested by isolated erythrocytosis and increased responsiveness to erythropoietin. Such was the case for Eero Mantyranta, a Finnish cross-country skier who won several gold medals in the 1964 Olympics but was accused of blood "doping" (receiving erythrocyte transfusions to artificially increase oxygen-carrying capacity) because of an abnormally high hematocrit. He was exonerated 30 years later when researchers identified an activating mutation of the erythropoietin receptor in samples from him and his family.

Given the role of erythrocytes in transporting oxygen, it is not surprising that erythropoietin production is triggered

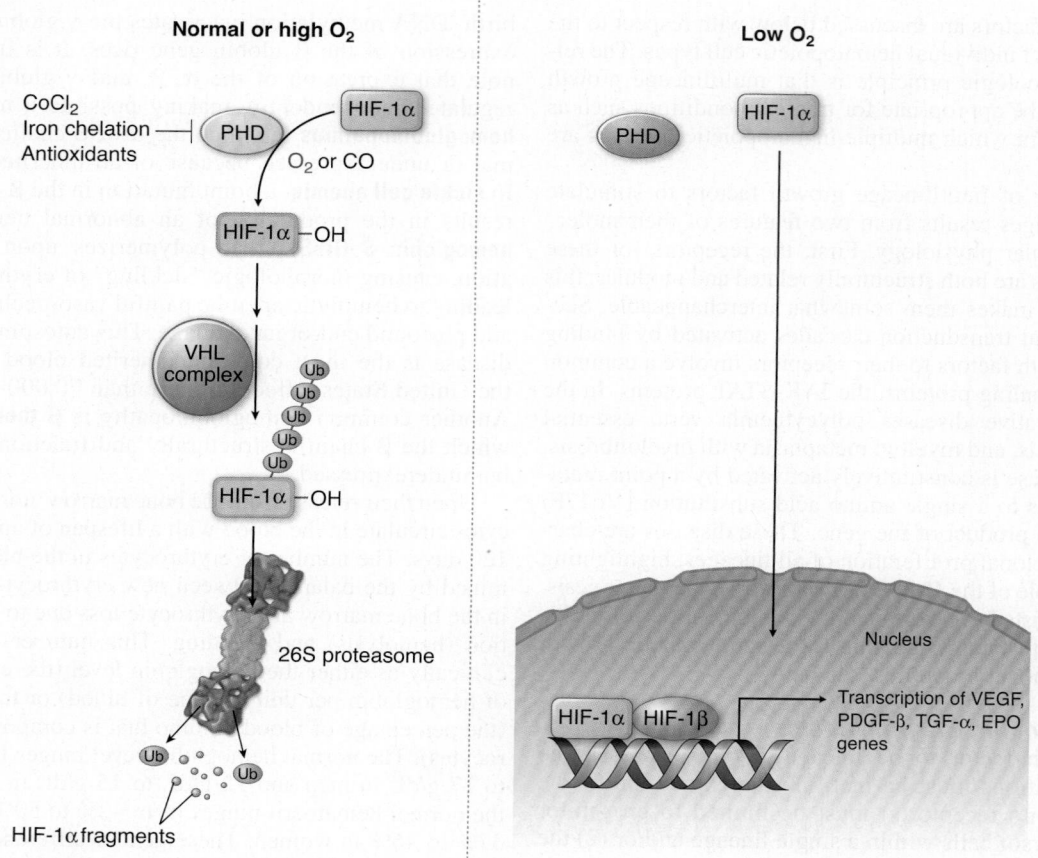

FIGURE 45-2. **Regulation of erythropoietin synthesis.** Synthesis of erythropoietin by the kidney is increased when the oxygen content of the blood is low and decreased when the oxygen content of the blood is normal or high. The physiologic O_2 sensor is an iron-containing dioxygenase, prolyl hydroxylase (PHD). (In vitro experiments using $CoCl_2$, iron chelation, antioxidants, and CO demonstrated the identity of the O_2 sensor as an iron-containing protein.) Under conditions of normal or high O_2 (**left panel**), activated PHD hydroxylates proline residues on hypoxia-inducible factor 1α (HIF-1α). This post-translational modification enhances HIF-1α binding to the ubiquitin ligase pVHL (VHL complex), leading to ubiquitination (Ub) and proteolytic degradation of HIF-1α by the 26S proteasome. Under low oxygen conditions (**right panel**) the prolyl hydroxylase is inactivated, allowing HIF-1α to accumulate, translocate to the nucleus, and induce the expression of a number of genes, including the gene encoding erythropoietin (EPO). In pathologic conditions, such as chronic kidney disease, the cells of the kidney that normally synthesize EPO are injured. These injured cells cannot synthesize adequate amounts of EPO, even under conditions of hypoxia, and anemia ensues. Recombinant human EPO can be administered exogenously to supply the missing growth factor and thereby treat the anemia. See text for discussion of the risks and benefits of EPO treatment in patients with anemia and chronic kidney disease.

by hypoxia. Erythropoietin expression is strongly induced by **hypoxia-inducible factor 1 alpha (HIF-1α)**, which binds to an enhancer element in the erythropoietin gene and activates gene transcription (Fig. 45-2). The level of HIF-1α within a cell is heavily influenced by the local oxygen tension. Under normal or high oxygen conditions, HIF-1α is hydroxylated by prolyl hydroxylase (PHD) via its Fe (II)-dependent dioxygenase activity. Prolyl hydroxylation of HIF-1α facilitates its binding to the von Hippel-Lindau (pVHL) E3 ubiquitin ligase complex, thus targeting HIF-1α for proteasomal degradation. Under hypoxic conditions, prolyl hydroxylation of HIF-1α does not occur, HIF-1α does not associate with pVHL, and HIF-1α instead translocates to the nucleus, where it enhances transcription of the hypoxia-inducible genes, including erythropoietin. In the rare autosomal recessive disease familial erythrocytosis 2 (also called *Chuvash polycythemia*, after the ethnic population of the mid-Volga River region in which it was first described), both germline copies of pVHL are mutated so as to prevent association with HIF-1α, reducing the degradation of HIF-1α and leading to elevated levels of erythropoietin and other target genes.

After transcription and translation, the 166-amino acid, 18-kDa erythropoietin protein is glycosylated to 34–39 kDa, its terminal arginine is cleaved, and the protein is secreted and transported in the circulation to the bone marrow. There, it binds to erythropoietin receptors expressed on the surface of BFU-E and all subsequent progenitor and precursor cells in the erythroid lineage, including the erythrocyte's immediate precursor cell, the **reticulocyte**. Then, through a complex intracellular signaling cascade mediated by JAK-STAT, erythropoietin receptor activation enhances the proliferation and differentiation of erythroid-lineage cells, including the terminal differentiation of reticulocytes to erythrocytes. Erythropoiesis completes a negative feedback loop on erythropoietin production, because the more erythrocytes in the blood (i.e., the higher the hemoglobin level and hematocrit) the higher the oxygen-carrying capacity of the blood. In the absence of cardiopulmonary disease, the higher oxygen-carrying capacity resolves the hypoxia and thereby removes the stimulus for increased erythropoietin production.

Table 45-2 lists the mechanisms of several prominent pathologic conditions that stimulate or inhibit erythropoiesis.

TABLE 45-2 Pathologic Conditions That Stimulate or Inhibit Erythropoiesis

CONDITION	MECHANISM
Stimulate Erythropoiesis	
Bleeding Hemolysis High altitude Pulmonary disease	Induce tissue hypoxia
JAK2-activating mutations in myeloproliferative disorders	Increase intracellular JAK-STAT signaling
Inhibit Erythropoiesis	
Chronic kidney disease	Decreases erythropoietin synthesis in kidney
Iron, folate, or vitamin B_{12} deficiency Chronic inflammatory conditions Sideroblastic anemia Thalassemia Malignant infiltration of bone marrow Aplastic anemia, pure red cell aplasia Drug-induced bone marrow toxicity	Decrease erythroblast differentiation and erythrocyte production

Leukocyte Production (Myelopoiesis and Lymphopoiesis)

White blood cells, or **leukocytes**, are essential cells of the immune system. There are two main categories of leukocytes, corresponding to the two main branches of the immune system. Cells of the **innate branch** of the immune system include granulocytes (**neutrophils**, **eosinophils**, and **basophils**), **monocyte/macrophages**, and variants of the macrophage lineage. Neutrophils target bacteria, eosinophils target parasites, and basophils participate in hypersensitivity responses. Macrophages also target bacteria, but these cells and their variants—**dendritic cells**, **Langerhans cells**, and **osteoclasts**, among others—have important additional functions. Macrophages play key roles in stimulating and regulating both the innate and adaptive branches of the immune system during infection and in clearing biological debris. Dendritic cells and Langerhans cells are important for initiating and targeting the immune response. These cells transport antigen from the site of inoculation to lymph nodes, where lymphocyte responses are coordinated. Osteoclasts are essential for bone resorption. Cells of the **adaptive branch** of the immune system are called **lymphocytes**. The two types of lymphocytes are B cells, which make antibodies, and T cells, and which target virus-infected and neoplastic cells (among other functions). "Adaptive" refers to the ability of these cells to recognize and respond to specific infectious agents and other targets (see Chapter 42, Principles of Inflammation and the Immune System).

All white blood cells develop from pluripotent hematopoietic stem cells (Fig. 45-1). Under the influence of growth factors, these stem cells differentiate into either **myeloid stem cells** or **lymphoid stem cells**. Myeloid stem cells further differentiate into the various cells of the innate branch of the immune system (as well as erythrocytes and platelets), while lymphoid stem cells differentiate into cells of the adaptive branch of the immune system. The growth factors that regulate these differentiation pathways are discussed in the following sections.

Granulocyte-Stimulating Factors

The differentiation of pluripotent stem cells into myeloid stem cells is fostered by certain multilineage growth factors such as stem cell factor and IL-3. Further differentiation of myeloid stem cells into neutrophils and monocyte/macrophages is controlled by the multilineage growth factor **granulocyte-monocyte colony-stimulating factor (GM-CSF)** and the lineage-specific growth factors **granulocyte colony-stimulating factor (G-CSF)** and **monocyte colony-stimulating factor (M-CSF)**. The differentiation of myeloid stem cells into eosinophils is controlled by **interleukin-5 (IL-5)**.

GM-CSF has relatively broad effects on cells of the myeloid lineage. Produced mainly by macrophages and T cells, this 18- to 28-kDa glycoprotein stimulates the differentiation of myeloid stem cells and progenitor cells into morphologically recognizable precursors of eosinophils, monocyte/macrophages, and neutrophils. GM-CSF also enhances the activity of these mature leukocytes and promotes the differentiation of macrophages into Langerhans cells. Some of the effects of GM-CSF are indirect. For example, the effects of GM-CSF on neutrophil production and function may result not only from direct GM-CSF stimulation of neutrophil precursors but also from GM-CSF-stimulated secretion of other cytokines (such as TNF and IL-1) by other cells. Like other hematopoietic growth factors, GM-CSF signals through the JAK-STAT signaling pathway.

G-CSF has effects that are more lineage-selective than those of GM-CSF. G-CSF is an 18-kDa glycoprotein that, like GM-CSF, signals through the JAK-STAT signaling cascade. G-CSF is released into the circulation by monocytes, macrophages, epithelial cells, and fibroblasts at sites of infection. In the bone marrow, G-CSF stimulates the production of neutrophils, which in turn enhance the ability of the immune system to fight infection. Locally released G-CSF stimulates neutrophil-mediated phagocytosis.

The effects of M-CSF (also known as CSF1) are restricted to the differentiation and activation of monocyte/macrophages and their various related cells (including a subset of osteoclasts). In a positive feedback loop, these are also the cells that produce M-CSF. M-CSF exists in alternatively spliced 70–80 kDa and 40–50 kDa isoforms. A rare benign tumor called *pigmented villonodular synovitis* has recently been shown to contain a genetic translocation involving CSF1. This translocation leads to dysregulated expression of CSF1 and the formation of an inflammatory mass composed predominantly of proliferating macrophages and histiocytes.

IL-5 is produced by a subset of helper T cells. This growth factor selectively promotes the differentiation, adhesion, degranulation, and survival of eosinophils. As such, IL-5 is believed to play an important role in the pathophysiology of allergic reactions and asthma.

Lymphocyte-Stimulating Factors

Regulatory proteins called **interleukins** control lymphocyte development and activation. To date, more than 30 members of this family have been defined. Family members are numbered IL-1, IL-2, and so forth. Interleukins regulate not only lymphocyte differentiation but also multiple and overlapping aspects of innate and adaptive immune responses, including stimulation of T cells and macrophages. Several interleukins are described above as granulocyte-stimulating factors; others are discussed below in the context of platelet production.

IL-2 and **IL-7** are two interleukins critical to white blood cell differentiation. IL-2 is a 45-kDa protein produced by

T cells. Because it drives proliferation of T cells and B cells, IL-2 once received much attention as a potential immunostimulant. Investigations of this hypothesis showed, however, that mice lacking IL-2 exhibit *lymphoproliferative* rather than *lymphopenic* diseases. This unexpected finding underscores the principle that growth factors and immune cells have diverse functions in vivo, including, as in this case, regulatory or suppressive (tolerogenic) effects as well as stimulatory effects. This finding also points out that uncontrolled proliferation can ensue if differentiation is not regulated normally, a process that may underlie some types of cancer. IL-7, produced by cells in the spleen, thymus, and bone marrow stroma, is a multilineage lymphostimulatory growth factor that enhances the growth and differentiation of B cells and T cells.

The **interferons** constitute a second family of regulatory proteins that modulate lymphocyte growth and activity. Like the interleukins, these proteins can stimulate the activity of T cells and macrophages. Interferons have prominent antiviral actions and are sometimes used in the treatment of infections such as hepatitis B and C (see Chapter 38, Pharmacology of Viral Infections). Other effects of interferons include promoting the terminal differentiation of lymphocytes, suppressing cell division (in some situations), and exerting direct cytotoxic effects on cells under stress. The three types of interferons—called *IFN-α, IFN-β,* and *IFN-γ*—have different biological actions. The cellular effects of interferons, like those of hematopoietic growth factors, are mediated by specific cell surface receptors and JAK-STAT signal transduction cascades.

Platelet Production (Thrombopoiesis)

Platelets—sometimes called **thrombocytes**—are essential for clot formation. These small cells, which lack a nucleus and do not synthesize new proteins, have a half-life of about 10 days in the circulation. The production of platelets, like that of all formed elements of the hematopoietic system, is controlled by both multilineage and lineage-specific growth factors (Fig. 45-3). The most important multilineage growth factors that stimulate platelet production are IL-11, IL-3, GM-CSF, stem cell factor, and IL-6. Not surprisingly, these factors also stimulate the production of erythrocytes because platelets and erythrocytes share a common progenitor, the CFU-Mix cell. Whether CFU-Mix cells become erythrocytes or platelets depends on their subsequent exposure to lineage-specific growth factors. Differentiation into BFU-E and other cells of the erythroid lineage is promoted by erythropoietin, while differentiation into CFU-Mega cells and then into megakaryocytes (which then form platelets) is promoted by the lineage-specific growth factor thrombopoietin (Fig. 45-1).

Thrombopoietin

Thrombopoietin (TPO) is produced in the liver and, to a lesser extent, in the proximal convoluted tubule of the kidney. Like erythropoietin, thrombopoietin is a heavily glycosylated protein (35 kDa) that has its major effect on a single cell lineage; also like erythropoietin, thrombopoietin signals through a JAK-STAT transduction cascade. However, unlike erythropoietin, thrombopoietin is not regulated in its activity at the level of gene expression, because thrombopoietin is expressed constitutively. Instead, by an interesting functional mechanism, circulating levels of thrombopoietin are regulated by the thrombopoietin receptor (also known as *Mpl*), which is the protein product of the gene *c-mpl*.

Structurally and functionally, the thrombopoietin receptor resembles the receptors for IL-3, erythropoietin, and GM-CSF. It is found both on platelet progenitors—CFU-S, CFU-Mix, CFU-Mega, and megakaryocytes—and on platelets themselves. Thrombopoietin has different effects on these cell types, however. On platelet progenitors, the binding of thrombopoietin to its receptor promotes cell growth and differentiation. In contrast, thrombopoietin receptors on platelets act as molecular sponges to bind excess thrombopoietin and thereby prevent platelet overproduction if platelets are in adequate supply. Thrombopoietin also enhances platelet function by sensitizing these cells to the proaggregatory effects of thrombin and collagen (see Chapter 23, Pharmacology of Hemostasis and Thrombosis).

■ PHARMACOLOGIC CLASSES AND AGENTS

The hematopoietic growth factors used clinically can be divided into two groups. First, recombinant or synthetic growth factor analogues are used to treat deficiencies of the various hematopoietic cell populations. This group includes the G-CSF and erythropoietin analogues administered to Mrs. M. Second, some growth factors have therapeutic use in the treatment of various malignancies.

Agents That Stimulate Erythrocyte Production

The erythroid lineage-specific actions of erythropoietin make this growth factor an obvious candidate for use in the treatment of some forms of anemia. Anemia can result from any of a large number of underlying conditions that either interrupt the normal process of erythropoiesis or result in the premature loss or destruction of mature erythrocytes (Table 45-2). One common indication for erythropoietin therapy is chronic kidney disease, in which loss of functional kidney tissue results in elimination of the cells that, in normal physiology, are responsible for erythropoietin production. Another potential indication for erythropoietin is anemia induced by anticancer therapies, which can

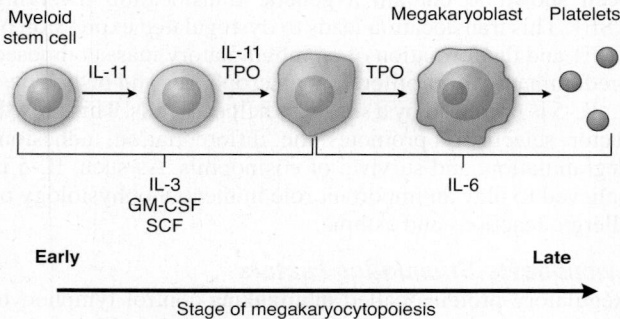

FIGURE 45-3. Growth factors involved in platelet production. Several growth factors are involved in platelet production (megakaryocytopoiesis). IL-11 acts primarily in the early stages; this growth factor stimulates production of GM-CSF and acts synergistically with IL-3 and stem cell factor (SCF) to increase the proliferation and differentiation of megakaryocyte progenitors. IL-6 and thrombopoietin (TPO) act primarily in the late stages of megakaryocytopoiesis. Both recombinant human IL-11 (oprelvekin) and TPO receptor agonists (eltrombopag and romiplostim) can be used therapeutically to increase platelet production.

be directly toxic to bone marrow or kidney or can induce a state of relative resistance to endogenous erythropoietin by mechanisms that may involve proinflammatory cytokines, oxidative stress, and antierythropoietin antibodies. (Cancer can also cause anemia through bleeding, poor nutrition, and infiltration of the bone marrow by tumor cells; these causes can often be diagnosed and treated directly.) Chemotherapy-induced anemia and its associated symptoms, such as those experienced by Mrs. M, can therefore be treated with erythropoietin under some circumstances.

Erythropoiesis-Stimulating Agents (ESAs)

There are currently three erythropoiesis-stimulating agents (ESAs) in clinical use in North America: **recombinant human erythropoietin (rhEPO)** (also known as **epoetin alfa**), **methoxy polyethylene glycol (PEG)-epoetin beta**, and **darbepoetin alfa** (formerly known as *novel erythropoiesis stimulating protein* or **NESP**). Like endogenous erythropoietin, epoetin alfa, PEG-epoetin beta, and darbepoetin alfa act by stimulating the erythropoietin receptor and inducing erythropoiesis. rhEPO increases the hematocrit level by at least 6% in half to three-quarters of patients receiving the drug, depending on the etiology of the anemia and the dose of rhEPO administered.

rhEPO and darbepoetin are very similar in structure; in fact, the two agents differ only in the number of sialic acid (carbohydrate) groups that are attached to the protein. The development of darbepoetin began with the observation that more sialic acid groups confer higher potency on erythropoietin. Darbepoetin's two extra sialic acid groups also give this drug a threefold longer half-life than erythropoietin, enabling less frequent administration. PEG-epoetin beta's polyethylene glycol coating gives this drug a longer half-life than either erythropoietin or darbepoetin. All three agents are proteins and must therefore be administered parenterally.

In addition to its well-characterized role in stimulating erythropoiesis, erythropoietin may also play a role in glial and neuronal cell survival following noxious stimuli or ischemic injury. Clinical studies of the neuroprotective effects of erythropoietin are ongoing.

Administration of erythropoietin to nonanemic or mildly anemic patients can lead to polycythemia, blood hyperviscosity, and stroke or myocardial infarction. Eighteen young cyclists died unexpectedly after the illegal introduction of erythropoietin into the world of professional cycling in the 1980s, possibly as a consequence of these adverse effects. Another serious adverse effect of certain preparations of recombinant erythropoietin became evident between 1998 and 2003. More than 200 patients who received one formulation of recombinant erythropoietin developed pure red cell aplasia and were found to have developed neutralizing antibodies against erythropoietin. The exact cause of the immune response is not well understood; one hypothesis involves the exposure of erythropoietin neoantigens as a result of partial denaturation of the therapeutic protein preparation. Erythropoietin and darbepoetin may also induce hypertension, and the use of these drugs is contraindicated in patients with uncontrolled hypertension. The mechanism responsible for erythropoietin-induced hypertension remains to be elucidated.

Clinical studies have found that patients with anemia and chronic kidney disease are at higher risk for death, serious cardiovascular events, and stroke when they are treated with erythropoiesis-stimulating agents to target a hemoglobin level of greater than 11 g/dL. The mechanisms responsible for these effects are an area of active investigation. Current US Food and Drug Administration (FDA) guidelines recommend that the use of erythropoiesis-stimulating agents should be considered when the hemoglobin level of patients with chronic kidney disease is less than 10 g/dL, and that the dosing should be individualized to use the lowest dose of ESA sufficient to reduce the need for erythrocyte transfusions.

Studies have suggested that erythropoietin may also decrease survival and increase the risk of tumor progression or recurrence in patients with breast, non-small cell lung, head and neck, lymphoid, and cervical cancers, despite an improvement in the patients' chemotherapy-induced anemia. The mechanisms and implications of these findings remain controversial. Potential explanations could include expression of the erythropoietin receptor on some cancer cells, synergistic toxicity due to combining erythropoietin therapy with chemotherapy and radiation therapy, and increased thrombogenicity associated with the elevated hemoglobin levels induced by erythropoietin therapy. These observations have led the FDA to alter the label of erythropoiesis-stimulating agents such that they are no longer indicated for patients receiving myelosuppressive chemotherapy administered with curative intent. In the palliative setting, it is important for physicians to discuss with patients the potential benefits and risks of hematopoietic support with these agents.

Agents That Induce Fetal Hemoglobin (HbF)

Sickle cell disease is marked by acute pain crises, increased susceptibility to infection, and profound hemolytic anemia. Sickle hemoglobin (HbS)-containing erythrocytes are the root cause of these clinical manifestations of disease, which begins in childhood when HbS is first produced. Newborns and infants with sickle cell disease are asymptomatic because fetal globin gene expression persists for many months after birth, keeping fetal hemoglobin (HbF) levels high. (In patients with sickle cell disease, typical HbF levels are 15% of total hemoglobin as late as age 2 and 1–5% of total hemoglobin in adults.) Consistent with this observation, adults in whom HbF expression persists at high levels have less frequent pain crises and milder anemia than those with low HbF expression. These observations have made increasing HbF levels a tantalizing therapeutic goal.

In principle, there are two approaches for increasing HbF: stimulating HbF expression in adults and preventing the switch from fetal (HbF) to adult (HbS) hemoglobin expression in children. Two drugs in current clinical practice, **5-azacytidine** and **hydroxyurea**, use the first approach; the **butyrates**, a class of drugs that are still in clinical trials, may utilize both approaches. Early studies suggest that 5-azacytidine and hydroxyurea could be synergistic with butyrates and with erythropoietin, although erythropoietin should be used with caution in patients with sickle cell disease because it stimulates erythropoiesis in HbS- as well as HbF-containing cells.

5-Azacytidine and Decitabine

5-Azacytidine and its congener 5-aza-2′-deoxycytidine (**decitabine**) are DNA demethylating agents that can increase HbF production to greater than 20% of total globin expression in patients with sickle cell disease or β thalassemia. (Theoretical studies suggest that an HbF level of 30–40% would render a patient asymptomatic.) 5-Azacytidine and decitabine are thought to act by reversing methylation of the γ globin gene, but this mechanism remains unproven. Concern over the unknown mechanism of action and fear of long-term cancer risk (both agents also interfere with normal DNA synthesis; see Chapter 39, Pharmacology of Cancer: Genome Synthesis, Stability, and Maintenance) have hindered the acceptance of these drugs as a prophylactic therapy in sickle cell disease.

Hydroxyurea

The 1990s saw the first use of **hydroxyurea** to treat sickle cell disease. A cytostatic agent that blocks cell division by inhibiting ribonucleotide reductase, hydroxyurea had previously been used to treat clonal hematological disorders such as chronic myelogenous leukemia and polycythemia vera (see Chapter 39). From this experience, hydroxyurea was known to be relatively safe for long-term administration, even in children; suppression of white blood cell and platelet production was known to be its main adverse effect. The induction of HbF by hydroxyurea is slower than that by 5-azacytidine; nevertheless, hydroxyurea has proved to be effective in about 60% of patients with sickle cell disease. In these patients, hydroxyurea increases HbF levels to 20% or more, decreases the frequency of painful crises by 50% (from 4.5 to 2.5 per year, on average), and decreases the number of transfusions required by patients who have three or more crises per year. However, hydroxyurea does not prevent end-organ damage or stroke. In 1998, hydroxyurea was approved by the FDA for use in the treatment of sickle cell disease.

Despite its long history of use, hydroxyurea's mechanism of action in sickle cell disease remains uncertain. The current hypothesis is that hydroxyurea blocks the division of HbS-expressing erythroid precursors and that this somehow triggers reversion to a fetal pattern of hemoglobin expression in an attempt to maintain erythrocyte production. It has been shown that the mechanism by which hydroxyurea increases HbF expression is independent of ribonucleotide reductase inhibition.

Butyrates

Butyrates (e.g., arginine butyrate, phenylbutyrate) are short-chain fatty acids that inhibit histone deacetylases, the enzymes that modify DNA to make it inaccessible to transcription factors. Butyrates have increased HbF levels from 2% to more than 20% in early clinical trials, although these agents are apparently not effective in patients whose baseline HbF level is less than 1%. Butyrates prevent the switch from HbF to HbS in experimental animals, and children born to diabetic mothers (whose blood contains elevated levels of butyrates) have higher than normal levels of HbF. Butyrates are thought to act by allowing certain transcription factors to maintain or resume activity. Although this mechanism could explain the increased HbF production in response to butyrates, it does not explain the selectivity of butyrates for HbF over HbS production in patients with sickle cell disease.

Agents That Stimulate Leukocyte Production

A low neutrophil count, or **neutropenia**, is most often the result of interference with progenitor cell proliferation and differentiation into mature white blood cells (**myelosuppression**). Neutropenia frequently accompanies leukemia and other malignancies that invade the bone marrow, and it is a common adverse effect of cancer chemotherapy. Less common causes of neutropenia include bone marrow transplantation, congenital neutropenia, and HIV- or zidovudine-associated neutropenia. Three agents have been approved for use in the treatment of cancer- and chemotherapy-induced neutropenia: recombinant human G-CSF (**filgrastim**); its pegylated, long-acting form, PEG-G-CSF (**PEG-filgrastim**); and recombinant human GM-CSF (**sargramostim**).

Recombinant Human G-CSFs (Filgrastim and PEG-Filgrastim) and GM-CSF (Sargramostim)

Filgrastim and sargramostim are almost identical to the natural growth factors G-CSF and GM-CSF, respectively, and they act by the same mechanisms as the endogenous proteins. Although GM-CSF is a multilineage growth factor, the major clinical effect of GM-CSF or G-CSF administration is a dose-independent increase in the absolute neutrophil count. (GM-CSF also causes a mild and dose-dependent increase in eosinophils.) As noted above, G-CSF and GM-CSF enhance the microbicidal activity of neutrophils in addition to stimulating their production. For Mrs. M (see introductory case), PEG-filgrastim hastened the recovery of her neutrophils after chemotherapy and enhanced the ability of her neutrophils to combat infection. G-CSF and GM-CSF also mobilize hematopoietic stem cells from the bone marrow into the peripheral circulation; for this reason, they are often used before harvesting peripheral blood stem cells for transplantation. The immunostimulatory effects of GM-CSF have fostered research into its ability to increase antitumor immune activity.

A filgrastim analogue has been conjugated to polyethylene glycol (PEG). This analogue, PEG-filgrastim, is metabolized more slowly than the native molecule. PEG-filgrastim can therefore be administered as a single injection that is functionally equivalent to multiple daily doses of filgrastim.

The main adverse effect of recombinant human G-CSF is bone pain, which resolves upon discontinuation of the drug. The theoretical risk that G-CSF could induce acute myelogenous leukemia (AML) or myelodysplastic syndrome (MDS) remains controversial. In general, observational studies do not support an increased risk, but a study of breast cancer patients treated with chemotherapy did demonstrate a fivefold increased incidence of AML/MDS in patients who received G-CSF. Of note, however, these patients also received a higher dose of cyclophosphamide than patients who did not develop AML/MDS. GM-CSF is associated with fever, arthralgia, edema, and pleural and pericardial effusion. G-CSF and GM-CSF are proteins and must be administered parenterally, typically by daily injection over the course of several weeks.

Agents That Stimulate Platelet Production

A low platelet count, or **thrombocytopenia**, is an important adverse effect of many cancer chemotherapeutic agents, occasionally limiting the doses that can be delivered with acceptable safety and tolerability. The complications of thrombocytopenia include increased bleeding risk and platelet transfusion requirement; in turn, platelet transfusion is associated with an increased risk of infection, febrile reaction, and, rarely, graft-versus-host disease.

Research into the pharmacologic management of chemotherapy-induced thrombocytopenia initially focused on the thrombopoietin (TPO) analogues **recombinant human thrombopoietin (rhTPO)** and **pegylated recombinant human megakaryocyte growth and development factor (PEG-rHuMGDF)** (see below). To date, however, only **recombinant human IL-11 (rhIL-11 or oprelvekin)** has been approved by the FDA for this indication. These agents all have the potential to increase megakaryocytopoiesis (platelet production) in a dose-dependent manner; although these drugs stimulate some multipotent as well as committed precursor cells, they do not significantly increase the hematocrit or white blood cell count. Importantly, these agents must all be administered prophylactically because there is a 1–2 week delay from drug administration to a clinically significant increase in platelet count.

Thrombopoietin Receptor Agonists

Cloning of the thrombopoietin gene in 1994 led to the development of two thrombopoietin analogues. The first, rhTPO, was a full-length, glycosylated analogue; the second, PEG-rHuMGDF, consisted of the N-terminal 163 amino acids of thrombopoietin conjugated to polyethylene glycol (PEG). Like natural thrombopoietin, both rhTPO and PEG-rHuMGDF bind to Mpl (the endogenous receptor for thrombopoietin, named for its role in murine myeloproliferative leukemia), and activation of Mpl is the basis for the effect of these drugs. Both rhTPO and PEG-rHuMGDF were tested as prophylactic agents to minimize chemotherapy-induced thrombocytopenia, and both caused a twofold to tenfold increase in platelet count.

One potential caution was that stimulation of platelet production could lead to thrombosis if the platelets that are produced are also activated. A small trial of PEG-rHuMGDF suggested that this drug was safe to use in treating the thrombocytopenia associated with AML, even though AML cells may also express the TPO receptor. However, the heavily bioengineered variants of natural TPO (e.g., PEG-rHuMGDF) were dropped from clinical development because of an excess risk of developing anti-TPO autoantibodies, which could suppress natural platelet production. The testing of full-length rhTPO was subsequently dropped as well, even though there were no reports of neutralizing antibodies in patients who received this lightly bioengineered agent.

Two newer TPO receptor agonists are approved by the FDA for treatment of thrombocytopenia due to refractory immune thrombocytopenic purpura (ITP), an autoimmune disease caused by autoantibodies directed against the patient's own platelets. These drugs are **eltrombopag**, a small-molecule TPO receptor agonist, and **romiplostim**, a recombinant IgG1 Fc-peptide fusion protein that also binds and activates the TPO receptor. By activating the TPO receptor, both molecules induce a transient increase in the platelet count. However, worsening thrombocytopenia may develop after cessation of treatment with these agents, and bone marrow toxicity (manifesting as bone marrow fibrosis and other conditions) has also been reported.

Interleukin-11 (rhIL-11 [Oprelvekin])

Recombinant human IL-11 (rhIL-11), also called **oprelvekin**, is the only drug currently approved for the prevention of severe thrombocytopenia in patients receiving myelosuppressive chemotherapy. Oprelvekin is produced in *Escherichia coli* and differs from natural IL-11 only in its lack of the N-terminal proline residue. rhIL-11 causes a dose-dependent increase in the platelet count and in the number of megakaryocytes in the bone marrow. The practical goal of treatment with oprelvekin is to maintain the platelet count above $20,000/\mu L$ (normal range, $150,000–450,000/\mu L$) in order to minimize the risk of life-threatening bleeding. However, the use of rhIL-11 is associated with significant adverse effects, especially fatigue and fluid retention. Atrial fibrillation has also been observed, and rhIL-11 should be used with caution in any patient with underlying heart disease. The undesirable actions of rhIL-11 likely result from pleiotropic effects of this factor on receptors distributed outside the hematopoietic system. It is unclear whether the therapeutic benefit of this agent outweighs the risk of systemic adverse effects.

Immunomodulatory Agents with Antineoplastic Applications

Interferons

Clinical investigation has led to the use of interferons as therapeutic agents against a number of different malignancies, with moderate success. However, the multiple and overlapping effects of these proteins have made it difficult to determine the drugs' mechanism of action in any given clinical situation. Induction of antitumor-directed immunity, terminal differentiation of cycling tumor cells, and direct cytotoxic effects have all been hypothesized to play important roles in the treatment of different malignancies. Interferons are also used to treat certain viral infections and are discussed in greater detail in Chapter 38.

Levamisole

Levamisole was known as an antihelminthic agent for decades before its anticancer effects were discovered. In combination with the antimetabolite 5-fluorouracil (see Chapter 39), this drug is now approved for use in the treatment of colon cancer. Although its mechanism of action remains uncertain, levamisole is thought to cause macrophages and T cells to secrete cytokines (such as IL-1) and other factors that suppress tumor growth.

Interleukin-2

Interleukin-2 (IL-2) is approved by the FDA for the treatment of melanoma. At therapeutic doses, however, this cytokine has relatively low efficacy and relatively high toxicity. See Chapter 46, Pharmacology of Immunosuppression, for more information about IL-2.

Tretinoin

Tretinoin, or all-trans retinoic acid (ATRA), is a ligand of the retinoic acid receptor (RAR). ATRA is used in the treatment of acute promyelocytic leukemia. This disease is characterized by a translocation t(15;17) in which part of the *RARα* gene is fused to the *PML* gene, creating a fusion protein that induces a block to differentiation and thereby allows development of the leukemia. Treatment with ATRA stimulates differentiation of these cells into more normal granulocytes. In some patients, the induction of differentiation can lead to life-threatening overproduction of white blood cells. ATRA can also induce a rapidly progressive syndrome of fever, acute respiratory distress with pulmonary infiltrates, edema and weight gain, and multisystem organ failure. Therapy with high doses of glucocorticoids is often an effective treatment for this ATRA syndrome.

▌ CONCLUSION AND FUTURE DIRECTIONS

The production of cells of the hematopoietic system—red blood cells (erythrocytes), white blood cells (neutrophils, monocytes, lymphocytes, and other cell types), and platelets—is controlled by a variety of proteins called *growth factors* and *cytokines*. Cancer chemotherapy, malignant infiltration of the bone marrow, and other conditions can cause deficiencies in these cell populations (anemia, neutropenia, and/or thrombocytopenia). The agents currently used to treat these deficiencies are mainly recombinant analogues of the natural growth factors or agonists of the growth factor receptors. Thus, the erythropoietin analogues rhEPO, PEG-epoetin beta, and darbepoetin treat anemia; the G-CSF and GM-CSF analogues filgrastim, PEG-filgrastim, and sargramostim treat neutropenia; and rhIL-11 and the thrombopoietin receptor agonists eltrombopag and romiplostim treat thrombocytopenia. Several agents affecting the hematopoietic system are also used to treat sickle cell disease, a common autosomal recessive disease caused by a point mutation in the β globin gene. These agents (hydroxyurea, 5-azacytidine, and decitabine) increase expression of fetal hemoglobin (HbF) and thereby restore normal erythrocyte structure and function. Several other drugs, including recombinant forms of the immunostimulatory interferon proteins, levamisole, and retinoic acid, are used to treat certain cancers, although their precise mechanisms of action remain unknown.

Other agents that activate hematopoiesis continue to be identified. Animal studies suggest that pharmacologic inhibitors of the repressor BCL11A could potentially induce HbF and thereby ameliorate the hematologic and pathologic manifestations of sickle cell disease. Preclinical evidence suggests that daily injections of a parathyroid hormone analogue (PTH 1-34) promote blood cell development, perhaps by activating stimulatory receptors on osteoblasts that neighbor hematopoietic stem cells. These observations have led to clinical trials of PTH in enhancing stem cell production for transplantation and in protecting hematopoietic stem cells from the cytotoxic effects of chemotherapy. Studies designed to tease apart the complex overlapping functionalities of hematopoiesis-regulating proteins are likely to provide a source of more selective pharmacologic interventions in the future.

Suggested Reading

Bennett CL, Djulbegovic B, Norris LB, Armitage JO. Colony-stimulating factors for febrile neutropenia during cancer therapy. *N Engl J Med* 2013;368:1131–1139. (*Reviews the clinical uses of G-CSF and GM-CSF in cancer therapy.*)

Hankins J, Aygun B. Pharmacotherapy in sickle cell disease—state of the art and future prospects. *Br J Haematol* 2009;145:296–308. (*Reviews use of hydroxyurea and decitabine.*)

Kaushansky K. Lineage-specific hematopoietic growth factors. *N Engl J Med* 2006;354:2034–2045. (*Reviews hematopoietic growth factors.*)

Kuter DJ. The biology of thrombopoietin and thrombopoietin receptor agonists. *Int J Hematol* 2013;98:10–23. (*Reviews treatment of thrombocytopenia, including use of romiplostim and eltrombopag.*)

Pfeffer MA, Burdmann EA, Chen CY, et al. A trial of darbepoetin alfa in type 2 diabetes and chronic kidney disease. *N Engl J Med* 2009;361:2019–2032. (*Clinical trials of erythropoiesis-stimulating agents in patients with anemia and chronic kidney disease.*)

Singh AK, Szczech L, Tang KL, et al. Correction of anemia with epoetin alfa in chronic kidney disease. *N Engl J Med* 2006;355:2085–2098. (*Investigates quality of life in patients with chronic kidney disease treated with epoetin alfa to target hemoglobin levels of 13.5 g/dL vs. 11.3 g/dL.*)

Smith TJ, Khatcheressian J, Lyman GH, et al. Update of recommendations for the use of white blood cell growth factors: an evidence-based clinical practice guideline. *J Clin Oncol* 2006;24:3187–3205. (*American Society of Clinical Oncology guidelines for the use of myeloid growth factors.*)

Xu J, Peng C, Sankaran VG, et al. Correction of sickle cell disease in adult mice by interference with fetal hemoglobin switching. *Science* 2011;334:993–996. (*Evidence that inactivation of BCL11A could represent a viable therapeutic strategy for sickle cell disease.*)

DRUG SUMMARY TABLE: CHAPTER 45 Pharmacology of Hematopoiesis and Immunomodulation

DRUG	CLINICAL APPLICATIONS	*SERIOUS* AND COMMON ADVERSE EFFECTS	CONTRAINDICATIONS	THERAPEUTIC CONSIDERATIONS
AGENTS THAT STIMULATE ERYTHROCYTE PRODUCTION Mechanism—Activate the erythropoietin receptor and stimulate erythropoiesis				
Erythropoietin (epoetin alfa) **Methoxy polyethylene glycol (PEG)-epoetin beta** **Darbepoetin**	Cancer-associated anemia Chemotherapy-induced anemia Anemia of chronic kidney disease Blood product transfusion during surgical procedure	*Cardiac arrhythmia, heart failure, thrombotic disorder, immune hypersensitivity reaction, hypertensive crisis, tumor progression* Edema, rash, gastrointestinal upset, headache, arthralgia, cough, fever	Hypersensitivity to drug Uncontrolled hypertension and hypertensive encephalopathy Infants, neonates, or pregnant or nursing mothers	Darbepoetin has more sialic acid groups than epoetin alfa, giving it a longer half-life. PEG-epoetin beta has a polyethylene glycol coat, giving it a considerably longer half-life than epoetin alfa. Administration of epoetin or darbepoetin in nonanemic or mildly anemic patients can lead to polycythemia, blood hyperviscosity, and stroke or myocardial infarction. Consider use of erythropoiesis-stimulating agents (ESAs) when hemoglobin level of patients with chronic kidney disease is <10 g/dL. *Not* indicated for patients receiving myelosuppressive chemotherapy intended for cure. May be abused by athletes.
AGENTS THAT INDUCE FETAL HEMOGLOBIN Mechanism—5-Azacytidine and decitabine may reverse methylation of the γ globin gene, leading to increased HbF expression; hydroxyurea may block the division of HbS-expressing erythroid precursors, leading to increased HbF expression				
5-Azacytidine	See Chapter 39: Pharmacology of Cancer: Genome Synthesis, Stability, and Maintenance			
Decitabine	Myelodysplastic syndrome	*Atrial fibrillation, heart failure, myocardial infarction, Sweet's syndrome, anemia, febrile neutropenia, thrombocytopenia, bacteremia, intracranial hemorrhage, pleural effusion, pulmonary edema, infection* Peripheral edema, heart murmur, rash, hyperglycemia, electrolyte disturbances, gastrointestinal upset, leukopenia, arthralgia, asthenia, dizziness, headache, insomnia, shivering, cough, fatigue, fever	Hypersensitivity to decitabine	Decitabine and 5-azacytidine interfere with normal DNA synthesis and may pose a long-term cancer risk.
Hydroxyurea	Sickle cell anemia Refractory chronic myeloid leukemia Head and neck cancer Malignant melanoma Ovarian carcinoma	*Myelosuppression, skin ulcer, skin cancer, secondary leukemia with long-term use*	Hypersensitivity to hydroxyurea Severe bone marrow depression	Mechanism of therapeutic effect in cancer treatment appears to involve inhibition of ribonucleotide reductase. Mechanism of therapeutic effect in sickle cell anemia is uncertain.

continues

DRUG SUMMARY TABLE: CHAPTER 45 Pharmacology of Hematopoiesis and Immunomodulation *continued*

DRUG	CLINICAL APPLICATIONS	SERIOUS AND COMMON ADVERSE EFFECTS	CONTRAINDICATIONS	THERAPEUTIC CONSIDERATIONS
AGENTS THAT STIMULATE LEUKOCYTE PRODUCTION Mechanism—Multilineage (GM-CSF) or lineage-specific (G-CSF) growth factors that stimulate myelopoiesis. The major effect of GM-CSF and G-CSF is to raise neutrophil counts; GM-CSF also increases eosinophil counts.				
Filgrastim (rhG-CSF) **PEG-filgrastim**	Shared indication: Neutropenia Filgrastim only: Peripheral blood stem cell harvest	*Precipitation of sickle crisis, acute respiratory distress syndrome, splenic rupture (shared adverse effects); vasculitis of the skin, hemorrhage, myelodysplastic syndrome (filgrastim only)* Bone pain	Hypersensitivity to *E. coli*-derived proteins or to drug	PEG-filgrastim is a pegylated formulation with a longer half-life. G-CSF and GM-CSF enhance the microbicidal activity of neutrophils in addition to stimulating their production.
Sargramostim (rhGM-CSF)	Neutropenia Peripheral blood stem cell harvest Myeloid reconstitution after bone marrow transplant	*Capillary leak syndrome, cardiac arrhythmia, pericardial effusion, cerebral hemorrhage, renal failure* Chest pain, rash, hypercholesterolemia, hypomagnesemia, weight loss, gastrointestinal upset, increased bilirubin, arthralgia, bone pain, myalgia, asthenia, increased blood urea nitrogen, pharyngitis, fever, rigor	Hypersensitivity to GM-CSF or yeast-derived products Concomitant chemotherapy or radiation therapy (or within 24 hours before or after) Excess (>10%) leukemic myeloid blasts in the blood or bone marrow	GM-CSF causes a mild and dose-dependent increase in eosinophils.
AGENTS THAT STIMULATE PLATELET PRODUCTION Mechanism—See specific drug				
Eltrombopag	Idiopathic thrombocytopenic purpura unresponsive to corticosteroids, immunoglobulins, or splenectomy Thrombocytopenia due to chronic hepatitis C	*Hepatotoxicity, bleeding, thrombosis, acute renal failure* Nausea, diarrhea, anemia, fever, myalgia, fatigue, headache	None	Eltrombopag is a small-molecule TPO receptor agonist. Oral administration.
Romiplostim	Idiopathic thrombocytopenic purpura unresponsive to corticosteroids, immunoglobulins, or splenectomy	*Acute myeloid leukemia, bleeding, thrombosis, myelofibrosis* Arthralgia, myalgia, headache, dizziness, insomnia, paresthesia, upper respiratory infection, fatigue	None	Romiplostim is a recombinant IgG1 Fc-peptide fusion protein that binds and activates the TPO receptor. Subcutaneous injection once weekly.
Oprelvekin (rhIL-11)	Prevention of severe chemotherapy-induced thrombocytopenia	*Fluid retention, cardiac arrhythmia, cardiomegaly, hypokalemia, febrile neutropenia, anaphylaxis* Rash, oral candidiasis, nausea, vomiting, dizziness, fatigue, headache, conjunctival hyperemia, blurred vision, dyspnea	Hypersensitivity to oprelvekin	Differs from natural IL-11 in that it lacks the N-terminal proline residue. rhIL-11 causes a dose-dependent increase in the platelet count and in the number of megakaryocytes in the bone marrow.

IMMUNOMODULATORY AGENTS WITH ANTINEOPLASTIC APPLICATIONS
Mechanism—See specific drug

Interferons	See Drug Summary Table: Chapter 38 Pharmacology of Viral Infections		
Levamisole	Colon cancer (in combination with 5-fluorouracil)	*Leukopenia, neutropenia, thrombocytopenia, seizures, exfoliative dermatitis* Gastrointestinal disturbance, arthralgia, dizziness	Hypersensitivity to levamisole	Thought to cause macrophages and T cells to secrete cytokines (such as IL-1) and other factors that suppress tumor growth.
IL-2	See Drug Summary Table: Chapter 46 Pharmacology of Immunosuppression		
Tretinoin	Acute promyelocytic leukemia Acne vulgaris Fine wrinkles, hyperpigmentation, or skin roughness of the face (topical)	*Cardiac arrest, cardiomegaly, myocarditis, pericarditis, ATRA syndrome (fever, acute respiratory distress with pulmonary infiltrates, edema and weight gain, and multisystem organ failure), hemorrhage, disseminated intravascular coagulation, leukocytosis, stroke, acute promyelocytic leukemia syndrome, infection* Chest discomfort, flushing, severe skin and mucosal dryness, skin pigmentation, gastrointestinal upset, increased liver function tests, bone pain, dizziness, headache, paresthesia, visual disturbance, otalgia, anxiety, shivering	Hypersensitivity to tretinoin or parabens	Tretinoin is an all-trans retinoic acid (ATRA) that allows differentiation of promyelocytic cells into more normal granulocytes. Used widely to treat moderate to severe acne vulgaris.

46

Pharmacology of Immunosuppression

Elizabeth A. Brezinski, Lloyd B. Klickstein, and April W. Armstrong

INTRODUCTION

Patients with autoimmune disease and patients who have received transplanted tissues or organs typically require therapy with immunosuppressive drugs. Immunosuppressive agents have been in use for more than 50 years, beginning with corticosteroids, antimetabolites, and alkylating agents. These early agents assisted in the treatment of previously incurable conditions, but their lack of specificity led to many serious adverse effects. Over the past 20 years, the field of immunosuppression has shifted to specific inhibitors of immunity that affect distinct immune pathways. This shift is important both because of the greater efficacy and reduced toxicity of these agents and because, as the mechanisms of these agents are discovered, insights are gained into the operation of the immune system.

PATHOPHYSIOLOGY

Transplantation

The first transplant performed successfully in humans was a kidney transplant between identical twins. No immunosuppression was used, and the individuals did well. Currently, most organ transplantation occurs between unrelated individuals, termed an *allograft*. Donor and recipient tissues express different major histocompatibility complex (MHC) class I molecules, one class of alloantigens, and recipient immune cells therefore recognize the transplanted tissues as foreign. This is termed **alloimmunity**, and it occurs when the recipient's immune system attacks a transplanted organ. In the case of a bone marrow or stem cell transplant, **graft-versus-host disease (GVHD)** can result when donor lymphocytes mount an assault on recipient tissues.

Solid Organ Rejection

Transplant rejection of solid organs can be divided into three major phases according to the time to onset. These phases, **hyperacute**, **acute**, and **chronic rejection**, are caused by different mechanisms and are therefore treated differently. The following three sections examine each of these processes, and Table 46-1 summarizes their differences.

Hyperacute Rejection

Hyperacute rejection is mediated by preformed recipient antibodies against donor antigen. Because these antibodies are present at the time of organ implantation, hyperacute rejection occurs almost immediately after reperfusion of the transplanted organ. In fact, the surgeon can observe the changes in the organ minutes after restoration of blood flow. The normal, healthy, pink appearance of the transplanted organ rapidly

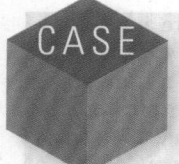
CASE

Mr. W is 59 years old when he undergoes right kidney transplantation in the spring of 2000 for chronic kidney failure resulting from long-standing uncontrolled hypertension. His induction immunosuppressant regimen consists of antithymocyte globulin. The antithymocyte globulin is co-administered with a glucocorticoid, an antihistamine, and an antipyretic. On postoperative day 1, he is transitioned to a maintenance immunosuppressant regimen of tacrolimus, mycophenolate mofetil, and prednisone. Progress during the first 2 months post-transplant is excellent, but then Mr. W develops headaches and laboratory testing shows an increase in his creatinine. The glucocorticoid dose is increased and his creatinine improves.

Three months after surgery, Mr. W is admitted to the hospital with fever, decreased urine output, and graft tenderness. Laboratory testing again shows increased serum creatinine and the tacrolimus serum level is within therapeutic limits. Infectious workup is negative and renal ultrasound shows no evidence of obstruction. A renal allograft biopsy demonstrates tubulitis and intimal arteritis, evidence of acute cellular rejection. He is treated with high-dose pulsed glucocorticoid therapy, which produces adverse effects of a metallic taste and abdominal discomfort. Mr. W's renal function improves and he is discharged. Over the next few weeks, his steroid dose is slowly tapered down to his maintenance dose.

In December 2010, Mr. W arrives at clinic for his regular annual examination. He is in good health on a maintenance immunosuppressant regimen of tacrolimus, mycophenolate mofetil, and prednisone, and his monthly creatinine values have remained normal. There has been no evidence of rejection since 2000. Renal ultrasound shows remarkably normal graft structure, perhaps as a result of the aggressive hypertension management by his physicians. However, his glucose levels are consistently elevated on routine laboratory testing, an indication that he may have developed new-onset diabetes after transplantation. Because of his new-onset diabetes, Mr. W's tacrolimus and prednisone doses are decreased and he is started on oral therapy to manage his diabetes. Over the next 2 years, his glucose and hemoglobin A1c levels remain at goal and he is able to enjoy time with his family.

Questions

1. How does each of the drugs prescribed for Mr. W reduce the likelihood of rejection?

2. Why is antithymocyte globulin administered with glucocorticoids, an antihistamine, and an antipyretic?

3. Why does Mr. W's pulsed steroid dose need to be slowly tapered down to his maintenance dose level?

4. What is the likely cause of Mr. W's new-onset diabetes? Why were his tacrolimus and prednisone doses decreased?

---

becomes cyanotic, mottled, and flaccid. This rapid change is the result of complement activation by antibody binding to endothelial cells of the transplanted organ, resulting in thrombosis and ischemia. Most commonly, hyperacute rejection is mediated by recipient antibodies that react with blood group antigens in donor organs (e.g., type AB donor in a type O recipient). Matching of blood types between donor and recipient prevents hyperacute rejection; therefore, drug therapy for hyperacute rejection is typically not necessary. Hyperacute rejection also occurs in xenotransplantation (i.e., organ transplantation between species, such as a pig heart transplanted into a human recipient), due to the presence of preformed human antibodies that react against antigenic proteins and carbohydrates expressed by the donor species.

Acute Rejection

Acute rejection has cellular and humoral components. **Acute cellular rejection** is mediated by cytotoxic T cells and causes interstitial as well as vascular damage. This cellular response is most commonly seen in the initial months after transplantation. Immunosuppression of T cells is highly effective at preventing or limiting activation of the recipient immune system by the transplanted organ, thereby preventing acute cellular rejection. In **acute humoral rejection**, recipient B cells become sensitized to donor antigens in the transplanted organ and produce antibodies against these alloantigens after a period of 7–10 days. The antibody response is typically directed against endothelial cells and is thus also known as **acute vascular rejection**. Like acute cellular rejection, acute humoral

---

TABLE 46-1 Modes of Immune Rejection

	HYPERACUTE REJECTION	ACUTE REJECTION	CHRONIC REJECTION
Mechanism	Preformed recipient antibodies react with donor antigen and activate complement	*Cellular*—Donor antigen activates recipient T cells *Humoral*—Donor antigen stimulates recipient antibody response	Unknown, but thought to be caused by chronic inflammation resulting from activated T-cell responses to donor antigen
Time course	Minutes to hours	Weeks to months	Months to years
How suppressed	Matching of donor and recipient blood types	Immunosuppression	Currently cannot be suppressed

rejection can usually be prevented by immunosuppression of the recipient after transplantation. Even with immunosuppression, however, episodes of acute rejection can occur months or even years after transplantation. Transplant recipients experiencing acute rejection are usually asymptomatic, and symptoms of fever or malaise are usually nonspecific.

Chronic Rejection

Chronic rejection is believed to be both cellular and humoral in nature and does not occur until months or years after transplantation. Because hyperacute and acute rejection are generally well controlled by donor/recipient matching and immunosuppressive therapy, chronic rejection is now the most common life-threatening pathology associated with organ transplantation.

Chronic rejection is thought to result from chronic inflammation caused by the response of activated recipient T cells to donor antigen. Activated T cells release cytokines that recruit macrophages into the graft. The macrophages induce chronic inflammation that leads to intimal proliferation of the vasculature and scarring of the graft tissue. The chronic changes eventually lead to irreversible organ failure. Other contributing nonimmune factors can include ischemia-reperfusion injury and infection.

No effective treatment regimens are currently available to eliminate chronic rejection. It is believed, however, that several experimental therapies have a reasonable chance of reducing chronic rejection. Especially promising is the possibility of developing tolerance through elimination of costimulation (see below).

Graft-Versus-Host Disease (GVHD)

Leukemia, primary immunodeficiency, and other conditions can be treated with bone marrow or peripheral stem cell transplantation. In this procedure, hematopoietic and immune function is restored after the patient's bone marrow has been eradicated by aggressive chemotherapy and/or radiation therapy. GVHD is a major complication of allogeneic bone marrow or stem cell transplantation. GVHD is an alloimmune inflammatory reaction that occurs when transplanted immune cells attack the cells of the recipient. The severity of GVHD ranges from mild to life-threatening and typically involves the skin (rash), gastrointestinal tract (diarrhea), lungs (pneumonitis), and liver (veno-occlusive disease). GVHD can often be ameliorated by removing T cells from the donor bone marrow before transplantation. Mild to moderate GVHD can also be beneficial when donor immune cells attack recipient tumor cells that have survived the aggressive chemotherapy and radiation therapy. (In the case of leukemia, this is called the **graft-versus-leukemia effect**, or **GVL**.) Therefore, although removing donor T cells from the "graft" reduces the risk of GVHD, this may not be the best approach for marrow transplants used in antineoplastic therapy.

Autoimmunity

Autoimmune diseases occur when the host immune system attacks its own tissues, mistaking self-antigen for foreign. The typical result is chronic inflammation in the tissue(s) expressing the antigen.

Autoimmune diseases are most commonly due to a breakdown of self-tolerance, both central and peripheral. **Central tolerance** refers to the specific clonal deletion of autoreactive T and B cells during their development from precursor cells in the thymus (T cells) and bone marrow (B cells). Central tolerance ensures that the majority of immature autoreactive T and B cells do not develop into self-reactive clones. The thymus and bone marrow do not express every antigen in the body, however; a number of proteins are expressed only in specific tissues. For this reason, **peripheral tolerance** is also important. Peripheral tolerance results from deletion of autoreactive T cells by Fas-Fas ligand-mediated apoptosis, activation of T suppressor cells, or induction of T-cell anergy due to antigen presentation in the absence of costimulation.

Although breakdown in tolerance lies at the center of virtually all autoimmune diseases, the inciting stimulus leading to loss of tolerance is often unknown. Genetic factors may play a role, in that the presence of certain MHC subtypes may predispose T cells to the loss of self-tolerance. For example, human leukocyte antigen (HLA)-B27 is causally related to many forms of autoimmune spondylitis. Several other autoimmune diseases are linked to specific HLA loci, supporting an association, if not a causal role, for genetic predisposition to autoimmunity. **Molecular mimicry**, in which epitopes from infectious agents are similar to self-antigens, can also lead to a breakdown of tolerance and may be the mechanism underlying poststreptococcal glomerulonephritis. Several other processes, including failure of T-cell apoptosis, polyclonal lymphocyte activation, and exposure of cryptic self-antigens, have also been hypothesized to lead to autoimmunity. The details of these mechanisms are beyond the scope of this book; however, the result of each is a *loss of tolerance*.

Once self-tolerance has been compromised, the specific expression of autoimmunity can take one of three general forms (Table 46-2). In some diseases, production of *autoantibodies* against a specific antigen causes antibody-dependent opsonization of cells in the target organ, with subsequent cytotoxicity. One example is Goodpasture's syndrome, which results from autoantibodies against collagen type IV in the renal glomerular basement membrane. In some autoimmune vasculitis syndromes, circulating antibody–antigen complexes deposit in blood vessels, causing inflammation and injury to the vessels. Two examples of *immune complex disease* are mixed essential cryoglobulinemia and systemic lupus erythematosus. Finally, *T-cell-mediated diseases* are caused by cytotoxic T cells that react with a specific self-antigen, resulting in destruction of the tissue(s) expressing that antigen. One example is type 1 diabetes mellitus, in which the cytotoxic T cells react against self-antigens in pancreatic β-cells.

The pharmacologic therapy for autoimmune diseases does not yet match the exquisite specificity of the offending biological process. Most currently available pharmacologic agents cause generalized immunosuppression and do not target the specific pathophysiology. Better understanding of the molecular pathways leading to autoimmune diseases should reveal new pharmacologic targets that can be used to suppress the specific autoimmune response before disease arises.

▌ PHARMACOLOGIC CLASSES AND AGENTS

Pharmacologic suppression of the immune system utilizes eight mechanistic approaches (Fig. 46-1):

1. Inhibition of gene expression to modulate inflammatory responses
2. Depletion of expanding lymphocyte populations with cytotoxic agents

TABLE 46-2 Representative Examples of Autoimmune Diseases, Categorized by Type of Tissue Damage

Antibody to Self-Antigen

SYNDROME	AUTOANTIGEN	CONSEQUENCE
Acute rheumatic fever	Streptococcal cell wall antigens that cross-react with cardiac muscle	Arthritis, myocarditis
Autoimmune hemolytic anemia	Rh blood group antigens	Destruction of erythrocytes
Goodpasture's syndrome	Renal glomerular basement membrane collagen type IV	Glomerulonephritis, pulmonary hemorrhage
Immune thrombocytopenic purpura	Platelet GPIIb-IIIa	Excessive bleeding
Pemphigus vulgaris	Epidermal cadherin	Blistering of skin

Immune-Complex Disease

SYNDROME	AUTOANTIGEN	CONSEQUENCE
Mixed essential cryoglobulinemia	Rheumatoid factor IgG complexes	Systemic vasculitis
Systemic lupus erythematosus	DNA, histones, ribosomes, snRNP, scRNP	Glomerulonephritis, vasculitis, arthritis

T-Cell-Mediated Disease

SYNDROME	AUTOANTIGEN	CONSEQUENCE
Experimental autoimmune encephalitis, multiple sclerosis	Myelin basic protein, proteolipid protein, myelin oligodendrocyte glycoprotein	Brain invasion by CD4 T cells, several CNS deficits
Rheumatoid arthritis	Unknown—possible synovial joint antigens	Joint inflammation and destruction
Type 1 diabetes mellitus	Pancreatic β-cell antigens	β-Cell destruction, insulin-dependent diabetes mellitus

Rh, Rhesus factor; DNA, deoxyribonucleic acid; IgG, immunoglobulin G; CNS, central nervous system; snRNP, small nuclear ribonucleoprotein; scRNP, small cytoplasmic ribonucleoprotein.

3. Inhibition of lymphocyte signaling to block activation of lymphocytes and expansion of lymphocyte populations
4. Neutralization of cytokines and cytokine receptors essential for mediating the immune response
5. Depletion of specific immune cells, usually via cell-specific antibodies
6. Blockade of costimulation to induce anergy
7. Blockade of cell adhesion to prevent migration and homing of inflammatory cells
8. Inhibition of innate immunity, including complement activation

Inhibitors of Gene Expression

Glucocorticoids

Glucocorticoids have broad anti-inflammatory effects. The intimate relationship between cortisol and the immune system is discussed in Chapter 29, Pharmacology of the Adrenal Cortex. Briefly, glucocorticoids are steroid hormones that exert their physiologic actions by binding to the cytosolic glucocorticoid receptor. The glucocorticoid–glucocorticoid receptor complex translocates to the nucleus and binds to glucocorticoid response elements (GREs) in the promoter region of specific genes, either up-regulating or down-regulating gene expression.

Glucocorticoids have important metabolic effects on essentially all cells of the body and, in pharmacologic doses, suppress the activation and function of innate and adaptive immune cells. Glucocorticoids down-regulate the expression of many inflammatory mediators, including key cytokines such as tumor necrosis factor (TNF)-α, interleukin-1 (IL-1), and IL-4. The role of glucocorticoids in suppressing eicosanoid biosynthesis and signaling is discussed in Chapter 43, Pharmacology of Eicosanoids. The overall effect of glucocorticoid administration is profoundly anti-inflammatory and immunosuppressive, explaining the use of glucocorticoids for the treatment of numerous inflammatory diseases such as rheumatoid arthritis and transplant rejection.

Long-term glucocorticoid administration has important adverse effects. Diabetes, reduced resistance to infection, osteoporosis, cataracts, increased appetite leading to weight gain, hypertension and its sequelae, and the masking of inflammation must all be closely monitored in patients receiving glucocorticoids. Abrupt cessation of glucocorticoid therapy can result in acute adrenal insufficiency because the hypothalamus and pituitary gland require weeks to months to reestablish adequate ACTH production. During this time, the underlying disease can worsen because of disinhibition of the immune system. To prevent the latter complications, glucocorticoid dosage should be tapered slowly as therapy is terminated. This is why Mr. W's dose of glucocorticoids was

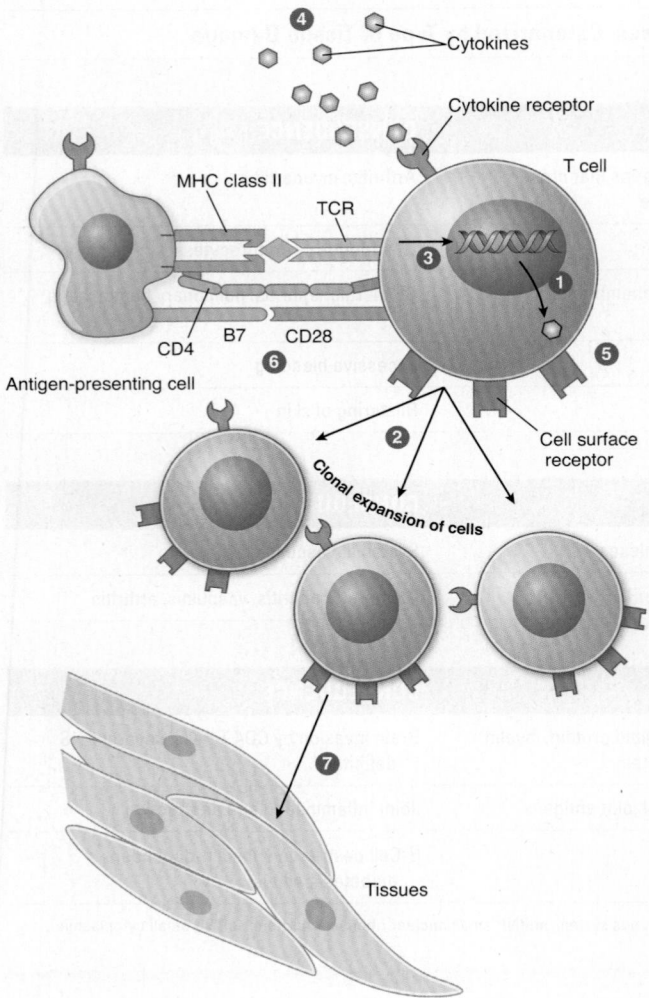

FIGURE 46-1. Overview of mechanisms of pharmacologic immunosuppression. The molecular mechanisms by which immune cells are activated and function provide eight major points for pharmacologic intervention by immunosuppressive agents. Blockade of T-cell activation can be accomplished by **(1)** inhibition of gene expression, **(2)** selective attack on clonally expanding lymphocyte populations, **(3)** inhibition of intracellular signaling, **(4)** neutralization of cytokines and cytokine receptors required for T-cell stimulation, **(5)** selective depletion of T cells (or other immune cells), **(6)** inhibition of costimulation by antigen-presenting cells, and **(7)** inhibition of lymphocyte–target cell interactions. Suppression of innate immune cells and complement activation may also block the initiation of immune responses (*not shown*).

tapered slowly after his pulsed steroid therapy for treatment of acute cellular rejection.

Cytotoxic Agents

Cytotoxic agents are used both for immunosuppression and for antineoplastic chemotherapy. The therapeutic goal in both cases is the elimination of pathogenic cells. Two classes of cytotoxic agents, **antimetabolites** and **alkylating agents**, are commonly used as immunosuppressants. Antimetabolites are structural analogues of natural metabolites that inhibit essential pathways involving these metabolites. Alkylating agents interfere with DNA replication and gene expression by alkylation of DNA.

Antimetabolites

Antimetabolites have been a mainstay of immunosuppressive treatment for many years. Their powerful suppressive effect on immune cells is accompanied by many adverse effects related to their lack of selectivity. The older antimetabolites, such as azathioprine and methotrexate, affect all rapidly dividing cells and can have toxic effects on the gastrointestinal mucosa and bone marrow. Newer antimetabolites, such as **mycophenolate mofetil** and **leflunomide**, cause fewer adverse effects. Mycophenolate mofetil may also be relatively selective for immune cells, further reducing its toxicity. Antimetabolites typically affect both cell-mediated and humoral immunity, rendering patients more susceptible to infection than would occur if only one of these immune systems were affected.

Antimetabolites are widely used in the treatment of cancer, and their mechanisms of action are described in detail in Chapter 39, Pharmacology of Cancer: Genome Synthesis, Stability, and Maintenance. Here, we focus on the antimetabolites used for immunosuppression and briefly discuss the anti-inflammatory aspects of their mechanisms of action.

Azathioprine

Azathioprine (AZA) was the first drug to be used for suppression of the immune system after organ transplantation, and it remains a mainstay for this indication. AZA is a prodrug of the purine analogue 6-mercaptopurine (6-MP), which is slowly released as AZA reacts nonenzymatically with sulfhydryl compounds such as glutathione (Fig. 46-2). *The slow release of 6-MP from AZA favors immunosuppression.* Although AZA prolongs organ graft survival, this drug is less efficacious than mycophenolate mofetil in improving the long-term survival of kidney allografts. AZA and 6-MP are also used as immunosuppressants in the treatment of inflammatory bowel disease, acute lymphoblastic leukemia, and autoimmune skin disorders.

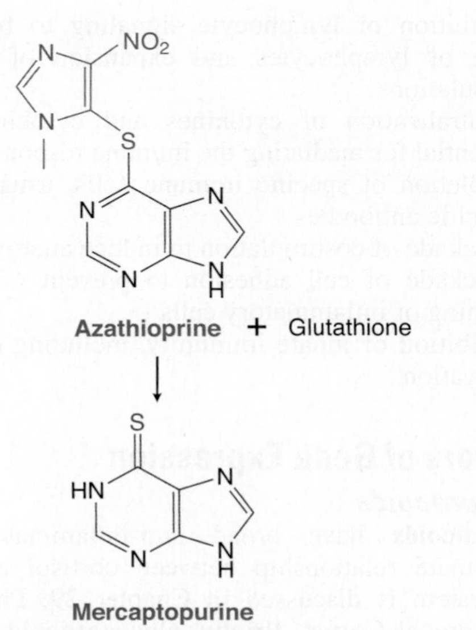

Azathioprine + Glutathione

Mercaptopurine

FIGURE 46-2. Formation of mercaptopurine from azathioprine. Azathioprine is a prodrug form of the antimetabolite 6-mercaptopurine. Mercaptopurine is formed by the cleavage of azathioprine in a nonenzymatic reaction with glutathione. Although mercaptopurine can also be used directly as a cytotoxic agent, azathioprine has higher oral bioavailability and a longer duration of action and is more immunosuppressive than mercaptopurine.

Methotrexate

Methotrexate is a folate analogue used since the 1950s to treat malignancies. Since that time, methotrexate has also become an extremely versatile drug in treating a wide variety of immune-mediated diseases, including rheumatoid arthritis and psoriasis. In addition, methotrexate is used for the prevention of GVHD.

The precise mechanism by which methotrexate exerts its anti-inflammatory effect is uncertain. Although methotrexate inhibits dihydrofolate reductase, the combination of methotrexate and low-dose folate is as effective as methotrexate alone in the treatment of rheumatoid arthritis. (High-dose folinic acid does interfere with the efficacy of methotrexate, however.) Methotrexate may also act as an anti-inflammatory agent by increasing adenosine levels. Adenosine is a potent endogenous anti-inflammatory mediator that inhibits neutrophil adhesion, phagocytosis, and superoxide generation. Methotrexate also causes apoptosis of activated CD4 and CD8 T cells but not of resting T cells. Other immunosuppressive agents, including 5-fluorouracil, 6-mercaptopurine, and mycophenolic acid, also promote apoptosis of activated T cells. Methotrexate may be such a versatile drug because of its combined antineutrophil, anti-T-cell, and antihumoral effects.

Mycophenolic Acid and Mycophenolate Mofetil

Mycophenolic acid (MPA) is an inhibitor of inosine monophosphate dehydrogenase (IMPDH), the rate-limiting enzyme in the formation of guanosine (see Fig. 39-3). Because MPA has low oral bioavailability, it is usually administered as a sodium salt or in its prodrug form, **mycophenolate mofetil (MMF)**, both of which have greater oral bioavailability (Fig. 46-3). MMF is increasingly used in the treatment of immune-mediated disease because of its high selectivity and profound effect on lymphocytes.

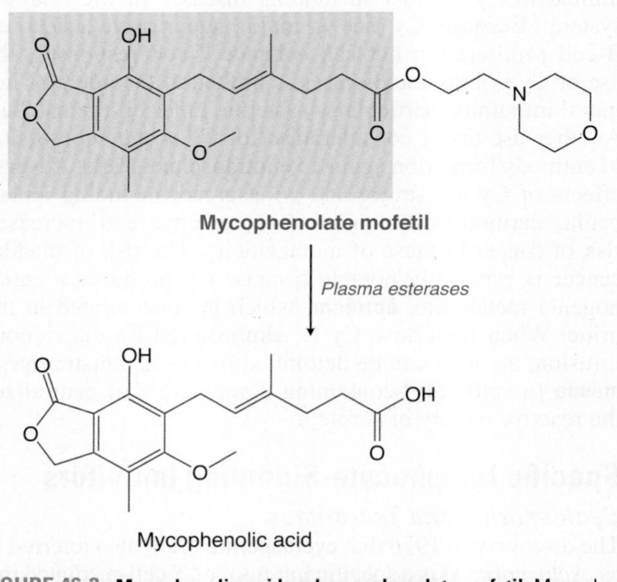

Mycophenolate mofetil

Plasma esterases

Mycophenolic acid

FIGURE 46-3. Mycophenolic acid and mycophenolate mofetil. Mycophenolate mofetil (MMF) has higher oral bioavailability than mycophenolic acid (MPA). Orally administered MMF is absorbed into the circulation, where plasma esterases rapidly cleave the ester bond to yield MPA. Both agents inhibit inosine monophosphate dehydrogenase type II (IMPDH II), an enzyme crucial for de novo synthesis of guanosine. Because of its higher oral bioavailability, MMF (or the sodium salt of MPA) is typically used.

MPA and MMF both act primarily on lymphocytes. Two main factors contribute to this selectivity. First, as discussed in Chapter 39, lymphocytes are dependent on the de novo pathway of purine synthesis, whereas most other tissues rely heavily on the salvage pathway. Because IMPDH is required for de novo synthesis of guanosine nucleotides but not for the salvage pathway, MPA selectively affects cells such as lymphocytes that rely on de novo purine synthesis. Second, IMPDH is expressed in two isoforms: type I and type II. MPA preferentially inhibits type II IMPDH, the isoform expressed mainly in lymphocytes. Together, these factors confer on MPA and MMF selectivity against T and B cells, with relatively low toxicity to other cells.

Inhibition of IMPDH by MPA reduces intracellular guanosine levels and increases intracellular adenosine levels, with many downstream effects on lymphocyte activation and activity. MPA has a cytostatic effect on lymphocytes and it can also induce apoptosis of activated T cells, leading to the elimination of reactive clones of proliferating cells. Because guanosine is required for some glycosylation reactions, the reduction in guanosine nucleotides leads to decreased expression of adhesion molecules that are required for recruitment of several immune cell types to sites of inflammation. Furthermore, because guanosine is a precursor of tetrahydrobiopterin (BH4), which regulates inducible nitric oxide synthase (iNOS), the reduction in guanosine levels leads to decreased NO production by neutrophils. Endothelial NOS (eNOS), which controls vascular tone and is regulated by Ca^{2+} and calmodulin, is not affected by changes in guanosine levels, again demonstrating the considerable selectivity of MPA.

As noted above, clinical studies comparing MMF and AZA have shown MMF to be more efficacious in preventing acute rejection of kidney transplants. Animal models show that chronic rejection is also reduced more effectively in recipients treated with MMF than in those treated with AZA or cyclosporine. The efficacy of MMF in treating chronic rejection may be related to its inhibition of both the lymphocyte and the smooth muscle cell proliferation characteristic of chronic rejection.

MMF is also efficacious in the treatment of autoimmune disease. In rheumatoid arthritis, levels of rheumatoid factor, immunoglobulin, and T cells are all reduced by treatment with MMF. MMF is frequently used in the initial therapy of lupus nephritis. There have also been isolated reports of successful treatment of myasthenia gravis, psoriasis, autoimmune hemolytic anemia, and inflammatory bowel disease with MMF.

The most common adverse effect of MMF is gastrointestinal discomfort, which is dose-dependent and can include nausea, diarrhea, soft stools, anorexia, and vomiting.

Leflunomide

Activated lymphocytes both proliferate and synthesize large quantities of cytokines and other effector molecules, and these processes require increased DNA and RNA synthesis. Therefore, agents that reduce intracellular nucleotide pools have suppressive effects on these activated cells. **Leflunomide** is an inhibitor of pyrimidine synthesis, specifically blocking the synthesis of uridylate (UMP) by inhibiting dihydroorotate dehydrogenase (DHOD). DHOD is a key enzyme in the synthesis of UMP (Fig. 46-4), which is essential for the synthesis of all pyrimidines. (See Chapter 39 for a review of

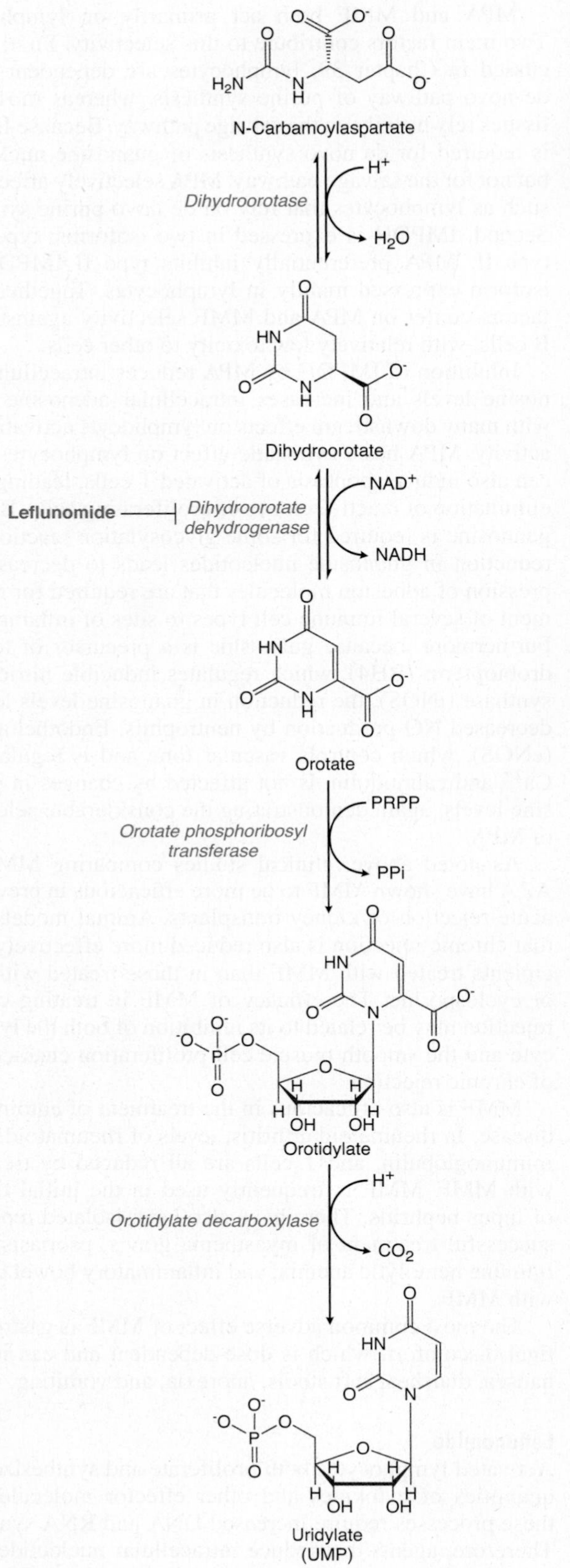

N-Carbamoylaspartate

Dihydroorotase

Dihydroorotate

Leflunomide ——| *Dihydroorotate dehydrogenase*

Orotate

Orotate phosphoribosyl transferase

Orotidylate

Orotidylate decarboxylase

Uridylate
(UMP)

FIGURE 46-4. Inhibition of pyrimidine synthesis by leflunomide. De novo pyrimidine synthesis depends on the oxidation of dihydroorotate to orotate, a reaction that is catalyzed by dihydroorotate dehydrogenase. Leflunomide inhibits dihydroorotate dehydrogenase and thereby inhibits pyrimidine synthesis. Because lymphocytes are dependent on de novo pyrimidine synthesis for cell proliferation and clonal expansion after immune cell activation, depletion of the pyrimidine pool inhibits lymphocyte expansion. Experimentally, leflunomide appears to inhibit preferentially the proliferation of B cells; the mechanism of this preferential action is unknown.

pyrimidine synthesis.) Experimentally, leflunomide has been shown to be most effective in reducing B-cell populations, and a significant effect on T cells has also been observed.

Leflunomide is currently approved for use in rheumatoid arthritis. The drug has also shown significant efficacy in the treatment of other immune diseases, including systemic lupus erythematosus and myasthenia gravis. Leflunomide has antiviral activity against cytomegalovirus (CMV) and has been used to treat this infection in cases of drug-resistant CMV and in transplant patients. Leflunomide prolongs transplant graft survival and limits GVHD in animal models.

The most significant adverse effects of leflunomide are diarrhea and reversible alopecia. Leflunomide undergoes significant enterohepatic circulation, resulting in a prolonged pharmacologic effect. If leflunomide must be removed quickly from a patient's system, cholestyramine may be administered. By binding to bile acids, cholestyramine interrupts the enterohepatic circulation and causes a rapid "washout" of leflunomide.

Alkylating Agents
Cyclophosphamide
Cyclophosphamide (Cy) is a highly toxic drug that alkylates DNA. The mechanism of action and uses of Cy are discussed extensively in Chapter 39; therefore, the discussion here is limited to Cy's utility in treating diseases of the immune system. Because Cy has a major suppressive effect on B-cell proliferation but can enhance T-cell responses, the use of Cy in immune diseases is limited to disorders of humoral immunity, particularly systemic lupus erythematosus. Another use under consideration for Cy is the suppression of antibody formation against xenotransplant grafts. Adverse effects of Cy are severe and widespread, including leukopenia, cardiotoxicity, pulmonary toxicity, and increased risk of cancer because of mutagenicity. The risk of bladder cancer is especially notable because Cy produces a carcinogenic metabolite, **acrolein**, which is concentrated in the urine. When high-dose Cy is administered by intravenous infusion, acrolein can be detoxified by co-administration of **mesna** (a sulfhydryl-containing compound that neutralizes the reactive moiety of acrolein).

Specific Lymphocyte-Signaling Inhibitors
Cyclosporine and Tacrolimus
The discovery in 1976 that **cyclosporine (CsA**; also referred to as *cyclosporin A*) is a specific inhibitor of T-cell-mediated immunity enabled widespread whole-organ transplantation. In fact, CsA made heart transplantation a legitimate alternative in the treatment of end-stage heart failure. CsA is a cyclic decapeptide isolated from a soil fungus, *Tolypocladium inflatum.*

CsA inhibits the production of IL-2 by activated T cells. IL-2 is an important cytokine that acts in an autocrine and

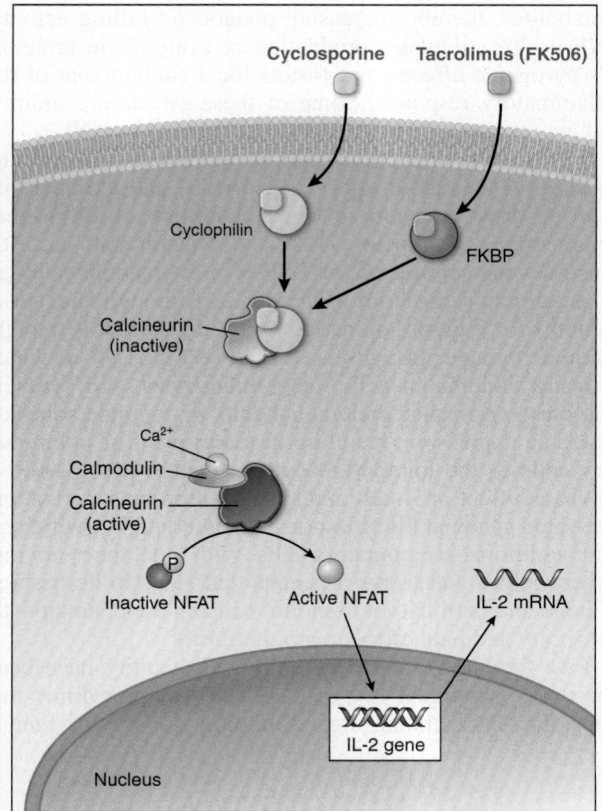

FIGURE 46-5. Mechanisms of action of cyclosporine and tacrolimus. The actions of cyclosporine and tacrolimus (also known as *FK506*) are mediated by blockade of intracellular T-cell signaling. In normal T-cell signaling **(bottom)**, stimulation of T cells increases the level of intracellular calcium, and Ca^{2+}/calmodulin activates the calcineurin-mediated dephosphorylation of the cytoplasmic transcription factor NFAT. Activated NFAT translocates to the nucleus, where it induces IL-2 gene transcription. Cyclosporine and tacrolimus cross the plasma membrane and bind to the cytoplasmic immunophilins cyclophilin and FK-binding protein (FKBP), respectively **(top)**. Both the cyclosporine–cyclophilin and tacrolimus–FKBP complexes bind to calcineurin, preventing the activation of calcineurin phosphatase activity by Ca^{2+}/calmodulin.

paracrine manner to cause activation and proliferation of T cells (Fig. 46-5). Activated T cells increase their production of IL-2 via a pathway that begins with dephosphorylation of a cytoplasmic transcription factor, **NFAT (nuclear factor of activated T cells)**. NFAT is dephosphorylated by the cytoplasmic phosphatase **calcineurin**. Upon dephosphorylation, NFAT translocates to the nucleus and enhances transcription of the IL-2 gene. CsA acts by binding to **cyclophilin**, and the CsA–cyclophilin complex binds to calcineurin and inhibits its phosphatase activity. By inhibiting calcineurin-mediated NFAT dephosphorylation, CsA prevents translocation of NFAT to the nucleus and thereby suppresses IL-2 production.

CsA is approved for use in organ transplantation, psoriasis, and rheumatoid arthritis. CsA is also used occasionally in the treatment of rare autoimmune diseases that are not responsive to other immunosuppressants. An ophthalmic preparation of CsA is approved for the treatment of chronic dry eyes.

The usefulness of CsA is limited by severe adverse effects, including nephrotoxicity, hypertension, infection, neurotoxicity, and hepatotoxicity. The mechanism of CsA toxicity is complex but may include stimulation of transforming growth factor-β (TGF-β) production. TGF-β causes cells to increase their biosynthesis of extracellular matrix components, resulting in interstitial fibrosis.

Tacrolimus (also known as *FK506*) is a more potent immunosuppressant than CsA; although its structure differs from that of CsA, it acts by a similar mechanism (Fig. 46-5). Tacrolimus is a macrocyclic triene isolated from the soil bacterium *Streptomyces tsukubaensis*. Tacrolimus acts by binding to **FK-binding proteins** (**FKBP**), and the tacrolimus–FKBP complex inhibits calcineurin. Tacrolimus inhibits IL-3, IL-4, IFN-γ, and TNF-α production in vitro, and it appears to inhibit cell-mediated immunity without suppressing B-cell or natural killer (NK) cell function. Tacrolimus is generally 50–100 times more potent than CsA, but, like CsA, it is nephrotoxic. Tacrolimus can also cause new-onset diabetes mellitus in post-transplant patients. In the introductory case, tacrolimus was a probable contributor to Mr. W's new-onset diabetes. This was the rationale for lowering both the tacrolimus and prednisone doses in Mr. W's immunosuppressive regimen after he developed diabetes mellitus.

Tacrolimus is approved as an immunosuppressant for transplantation. A topical formulation is used for the treatment of atopic dermatitis and other eczematous diseases.

mTOR Inhibitors

Sirolimus, also known as *rapamycin*, is a macrocyclic triene isolated from the soil bacterium *Streptomyces hygroscopicus*. Although they are structurally similar and are both used to prevent and treat organ rejection, tacrolimus and sirolimus have different mechanisms of action. Both bind to FKBP, but the sirolimus–FKBP complex does not inhibit calcineurin; instead, it blocks the IL-2 receptor signaling required for T-cell proliferation (Fig. 46-6). Sirolimus–FKBP binds to and inhibits molecular target of rapamycin (mTOR), a serine-threonine kinase that phosphorylates p70 S6 kinase and PHAS-1 (among other substrates). p70 S6 kinase and PHAS-1 regulate translation, the former by phosphorylating proteins (including the ribosomal S6 protein) involved in protein synthesis and the latter by inhibiting the activity of a factor (eIF4E) required for translation. By inhibiting mTOR, sirolimus–FKBP inhibits protein synthesis and arrests cell division in the G1 phase (Fig. 46-6).

Major adverse effects of sirolimus include hypertension, interstitial lung disease, and leukopenia. Notably, however, the nephrotoxicity associated with CsA and tacrolimus is not observed with sirolimus.

Everolimus and **zotarolimus** are mTOR inhibitors that are structurally related to sirolimus. Everolimus is approved for prevention of kidney transplant rejection and treatment of renal cell carcinoma, hormone-receptor positive, HER2-negative breast cancer, progressive neuroendocrine tumors of pancreatic origin, and renal angiomyolipoma and tuberous sclerosis complex, while zotarolimus is used only in drug-eluting stents. Recent studies have shown that sirolimus, everolimus, and zotarolimus inhibit mTOR complex 1 but are relatively weak inhibitors of mTOR complex 2; newer drugs are being developed to inhibit both complexes.

Sirolimus-, everolimus-, and zotarolimus-eluting stents have been approved for use in the treatment of coronary artery disease. In this unique drug delivery system, the mTOR inhibitor elutes from stents during the first few weeks after stent placement, locally inhibiting proliferation of coronary artery smooth muscle cells and thereby reducing the rate of in-stent restenosis that results from neointimal proliferation of vascular smooth muscle cells.

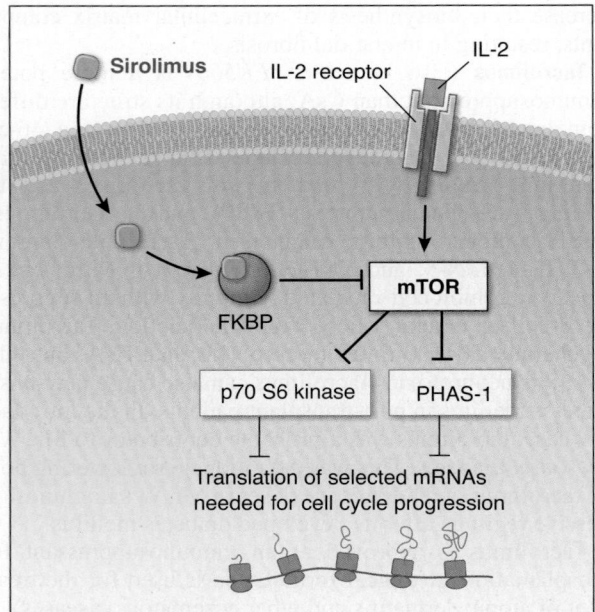

FIGURE 46-6. Mechanism of action of sirolimus. IL-2 receptor signal transduction involves a complex set of protein–protein interactions that lead to increased translation of selected mRNAs encoding proteins required for T-cell proliferation. Specifically, IL-2 receptor activation initiates an intracellular signaling cascade that leads to phosphorylation of the molecular target of rapamycin (mTOR). mTOR is a kinase that phosphorylates and thereby regulates the activity of PHAS-1 and p70 S6 kinase. PHAS-1 inhibits the activity of a factor (eIF4E) required for translation, and p70 S6 kinase phosphorylates proteins involved in protein synthesis (*not shown*). The net effect of mTOR activation is to increase protein synthesis, thereby promoting the transition from G1 to S phase of the cell cycle. Sirolimus (also known as *rapamycin*) crosses the plasma membrane and binds to intracellular FK-binding protein (FKBP). The sirolimus–FKBP complex inhibits mTOR, thereby inhibiting translation and causing T cells to arrest in G1. Everolimus and zotarolimus are sirolimus analogues that act by the same mechanism.

Cytokine and Cytokine Receptor Inhibition

Cytokines are critical signaling mediators in immune function. Cytokines are also pleiotropic; that is, they exert different effects depending on the target cell and overall cytokine milieu. For this reason, pharmacologic uses of cytokines or cytokine inhibitors may have unpredictable effects. Anticytokine therapy has been in clinical use for immunologically mediated diseases for more than a decade. The first anticytokine agent approved for use was **etanercept**, an anti-TNF drug developed for rheumatoid arthritis. During the initial clinical studies, some patients with severe, drug-refractory rheumatoid arthritis literally got up from their wheelchairs and walked after receiving etanercept. This dramatic efficacy ushered in a new era of biological therapies for autoimmune disease, and the number of new drugs that inhibit proinflammatory cytokines continues to grow rapidly. An alternative approach to block the action of inflammatory cytokines is to target the cytokine receptor.

TNF-α Inhibitors

Tumor necrosis factor (TNF)-α is a cytokine central to many aspects of the inflammatory response. Macrophages, mast cells, and activated T_H cells (especially T_H1 cells) secrete TNF-α. TNF-α stimulates macrophages to produce cytotoxic

metabolites, thereby increasing phagocytic killing activity. TNF-α also stimulates production of acute-phase proteins, has pyrogenic effects, and fosters local containment of the inflammatory response. Some of these effects are indirect and are mediated by other cytokines induced by TNF-α.

TNF-α has been implicated in numerous autoimmune diseases. Rheumatoid arthritis, psoriasis, and Crohn's disease are three disorders in which inhibition of TNF-α has demonstrated therapeutic efficacy. Rheumatoid arthritis illustrates the central role of TNF-α in the pathophysiology of autoimmune diseases (Fig. 46-7). Although the initial stimulus for joint inflammation is still debated, it is thought that macrophages in a diseased joint secrete TNF-α, which activates endothelial cells, other monocytes, and synovial fibroblasts. Activated endothelial cells up-regulate adhesion molecule expression, resulting in recruitment of inflammatory cells to the joint. Monocyte activation has a positive feedback effect on T-cell and synovial fibroblast activation. Activated synovial fibroblasts secrete interleukins, which recruit additional inflammatory cells. With time, the synovium hypertrophies and forms a pannus that leads to destruction of bone and cartilage in the joint, causing the characteristic deformity and pain of rheumatoid arthritis.

Five therapies interfering with TNF activity have been approved. **Etanercept** is a soluble TNF receptor dimer that links the extracellular, ligand-binding domain of human

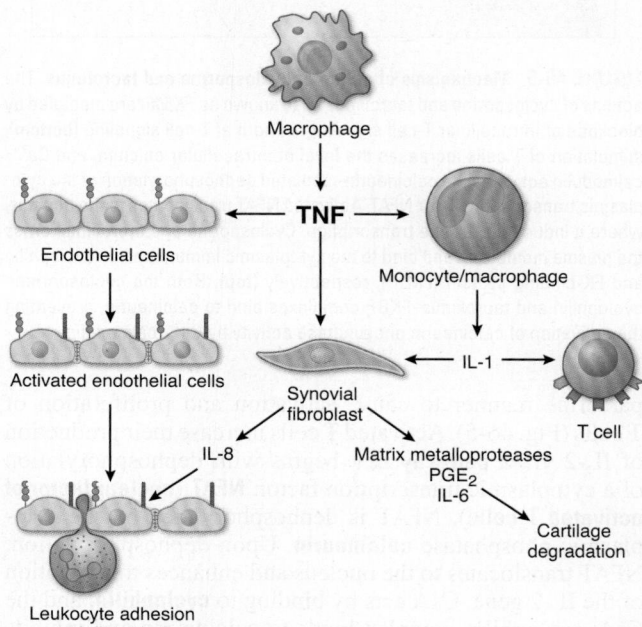

FIGURE 46-7. Proposed roles for tumor necrosis factor in rheumatoid arthritis. Tumor necrosis factor (TNF) is secreted by activated macrophages in an affected joint, where this cytokine has multiple proinflammatory effects. First, TNF activates endothelial cells to up-regulate their expression of cell surface adhesion molecules (*shown as projections on endothelial cells*) and undergo other phenotypic changes that promote leukocyte adhesion and diapedesis. Second, TNF has a positive feedback effect on nearby monocytes and macrophages, promoting their secretion of cytokines such as IL-1. In turn, IL-1 activates T cells (among other functions), and the combination of IL-1 and TNF stimulates synovial fibroblasts to increase their expression of matrix metalloproteases, prostaglandins (especially PGE₂), and cytokines (such as IL-6) that degrade the joint cartilage. Synovial fibroblasts also secrete IL-8, which promotes neutrophil diapedesis.

TNF receptor type II to the Fc domain of human immunoglobulin G1 (IgG1); **infliximab** is a partially humanized mouse monoclonal antibody directed against human TNF-α; and **adalimumab** is a fully human IgG1 monoclonal antibody directed against TNF-α (Fig. 46-8). **Certolizumab pegol** is a pegylated anti-TNF-α monoclonal antibody fragment that lacks the Fc portion of the antibody; as a result, unlike infliximab and adalimumab, certolizumab does not cause antibody-dependent cell-mediated cytotoxicity or fix complement in vitro. **Golimumab** is a fully human IgG1 monoclonal antibody directed against TNF-α that has a longer half-life than the other anti-TNF agents.

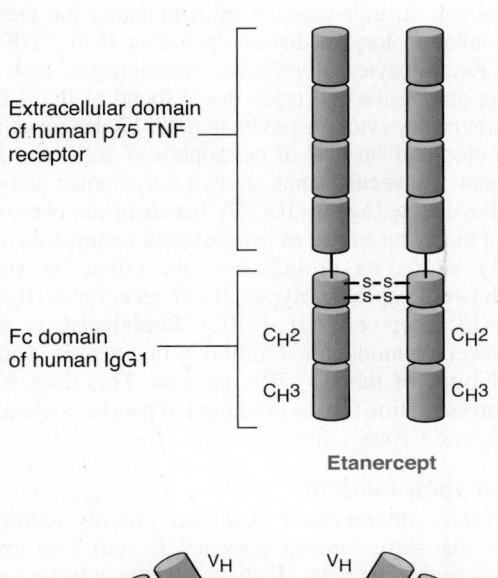

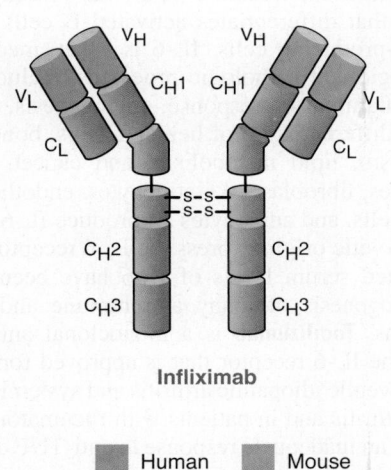

FIGURE 46-8. Anti-tumor necrosis factor agents. Shown is the molecular domain organization of etanercept and infliximab. Etanercept consists of the extracellular domain of the human tumor necrosis factor (TNF) receptor fused to the Fc domain of human IgG1. This "decoy" receptor binds TNF-α and TNF-β in the circulation, preventing the access of these cytokines to target tissues. Infliximab is a partially humanized monoclonal antibody directed against TNF-α. The variable heavy chain (V_H) and variable light chain (V_L) regions are derived from mouse antihuman sequences, while the remainder of the antibody (*the constant regions, denoted by C_H and C_L*) is composed of human antibody sequences. This modification of the original mouse anti-TNF monoclonal antibody reduces the likelihood of developing neutralizing antibodies against infliximab. Additional TNF inhibitors include adalimumab, a fully human monoclonal antibody; certolizumab pegol, a pegylated monoclonal antibody fragment; and golimumab, a fully human monoclonal antibody (*not shown*).

The monoclonal antibody-based TNF-α inhibitors illustrate the desirability of treatment with "humanized" or "fully human" antibodies as opposed to mouse or other nonhuman antibodies. Because mouse antibodies are foreign, treatment with them can induce the production of antibodies against the mouse-specific regions of the therapeutic antibody. The presence of these antibodies can reduce drug efficacy by sequestering the therapeutic antibody before it can exert its desired effect. To address this problem, one approach is to **humanize** therapeutic antibodies. In this approach, the portions of the antibody not involved in binding to the antigen are changed to the corresponding human sequences. Antibodies can be *partially* or *fully humanized*, depending on the extent of these changes. Humanization limits the likelihood of production of human antibodies against the therapeutic antibody, increasing the clinical effectiveness of the antibody and allowing its long-term use (see Chapter 54, Protein Therapeutics). A more recent approach to the preparation of therapeutic antibodies is to prepare the antibody in an experimental animal bearing a human immune system or to use an in vitro human antibody system. This strategy generates **fully human antibodies** that do not require further manipulation to render them nonimmunogenic.

Although all five of the anti-TNF agents target TNF-α, etanercept is somewhat less selective than the others because it binds to both TNF-α and TNF-β. Infliximab, adalimumab, certolizumab, and golimumab are selective for TNF-α and do not bind TNF-β. The Fc portions of infliximab, adalimumab, and golimumab may also have specific activity with respect to complement fixation and binding to Fc receptors on effector cells. The immune effector actions of these agents may be relevant to their mechanisms of action because TNF-α is expressed on the surface of cells, especially macrophages, and the cell surface form is cleaved to yield the soluble cytokine. Anti-TNF agents with immune effector functions may have biological effects different from those of agents that do not bind Fc receptors or fix complement.

The indications for TNF inhibitors have recently expanded to include conditions spanning the fields of dermatology, rheumatology, and gastroenterology. Etanercept is approved for use in rheumatoid arthritis, juvenile idiopathic arthritis, plaque psoriasis, psoriatic arthritis, and ankylosing spondylitis. Infliximab is approved for use in rheumatoid arthritis, Crohn's disease, ulcerative colitis, plaque psoriasis, psoriatic arthritis, and ankylosing spondylitis. Adalimumab is approved for use in rheumatoid arthritis, juvenile idiopathic arthritis, Crohn's disease, ulcerative colitis, plaque psoriasis, psoriatic arthritis, ankylosing spondylitis, and hidradenitis suppurtiva. Certolizumab is approved for the treatment of rheumatoid arthritis, Crohn's disease, psoriatic arthritis, and ankylosing spondylitis. Golimumab is approved for use in adults with rheumatoid arthritis (in combination with methotrexate), ulcerative colitis, psoriatic arthritis, and ankylosing spondylitis.

Although high levels of TNF-α are likely mediators of underlying pathophysiologic processes, treatment with an anti-TNF agent often improves disease symptoms without reversing the underlying pathophysiology. Therefore, upon drug discontinuation, maintenance of clinical response is uncertain. Etanercept, infliximab, adalimumab, certolizumab, and golimumab are proteins and must be administered parenterally. Orally active inhibitors of TNF-α and inhibitors of TNF-α converting enzyme (TACE) are under investigation.

Several important adverse effects must be considered when administering TNF inhibitors. All patients should undergo screening for tuberculosis before initiating therapy because of increased risk of reactivating latent tuberculosis. Any patient who develops an infection while taking a TNF inhibitor should undergo evaluation and aggressive antibiotic treatment. Additionally, patients diagnosed with a severe infection are recommended to temporarily interrupt treatment with TNF inhibitors. Epidemiologic surveillance has suggested that there may be an increased risk of demyelinating disease with anti-TNF therapy, although it has not yet been determined whether the relationship is causal.

IL-12/IL-23p40 Cytokine Inhibitors

New biological therapies for the treatment of T-cell-mediated diseases include antibodies to IL-12 and IL-23. IL-12 and IL-23 are cytokines involved in natural killer cell activation and CD4$^+$ T-cell differentiation and activation. IL-12, a heterodimer composed of p40 and p35 subunits, directs the differentiation of naïve T cells into T$_H$1 cells, which secrete IL-2, IFN-γ, and TNF-α. IL-23 is also a heterodimer that has the same p40 subunit covalently linked to a p19 subunit. IL-23 directs the differentiation of naïve T cells into T$_H$17 cells, which secrete IL-17 and IL-22. **Ustekinumab** is a high-affinity human IgG1 monoclonal antibody that binds to the p40 subunit shared by IL-12 and IL-23. Ustekinumab is approved for use in psoriasis and psoriatic arthritis and is in clinical trials for the treatment of Crohn's disease, sarcoidosis, and multiple sclerosis. Adverse effects include an *increased risk of infection*.

IL-1 Cytokine and IL-1 Receptor Inhibitors

Interleukin-1 (IL-1) is an ancient cytokine, expressed in both vertebrates and invertebrates, that serves as a bridge between innate and adaptive immunity. Two forms of IL-1, IL-1α and IL-1β, are encoded on different genes. In humans, IL-1β has primarily an immune role, while IL-1α may be involved in maintenance of epithelial cell function. Human genetic data and studies with IL-1β antagonists point to a nonredundant role for IL-1β as an inflammatory mediator. Hereafter, therefore, we use the term *IL-1* to refer to IL-1β.

Most IL-1 is generated by activated mononuclear cells. IL-1 stimulates IL-6 production, enhances adhesion molecule expression, and stimulates cell proliferation. Modulation of IL-1 activity in vivo is accomplished in part by an endogenous IL-1 receptor antagonist (IL-1ra).

Anakinra, a recombinant form of IL-1ra, is approved for use in rheumatoid arthritis. Anakinra has modest effects on pain and swelling but significantly reduces bony erosions, possibly because it decreases osteoclast production and blocks IL-1-induced metalloproteinase release from synovial cells. Several rare syndromes are mediated in part by increased levels of IL-1. Collectively, these syndromes are termed *cryopyrin-associated periodic syndromes (CAPS)*. Anakinra is approved for use in the CAPS syndrome neonatal-onset multisystem inflammatory disease, and the CAPS syndromes Muckle-Wells syndrome and Hibernian fever have also been treated effectively with anakinra. Anakinra may *cause neutropenia* and *increase susceptibility to infection*. The rapid clearance of this small recombinant peptide and its competitive binding mechanism may explain the need for daily injections of the drug to achieve efficacy.

Rilonacept is a recombinant, soluble IL-1 receptor Fc fusion protein that is approved for use in CAPS. Rilonacept binds both IL-1α and IL-1β and also endogenous IL-1ra. Possibly because of its binding to the endogenous receptor antagonist, once-weekly injections of rilonacept are sufficient for efficacy in the treatment of CAPS.

Canakinumab is a human IgG1 monoclonal antibody directed against IL-1β that is approved for use in CAPS and systemic juvenile idiopathic arthritis. Perhaps because of its specificity for IL-1β, canakinumab may be administered just once monthly and still exhibit full efficacy. No studies have been conducted to compare the efficacy of the three anti-IL-1β therapies.

IL-17 Cytokine and IL-17 Receptor Inhibitors

Interleukin-17 (IL-17, also known as *IL-17A*) is a cytokine that is mainly produced by IL-23-induced T$_H$17 cells. IL-17 plays a central role in inflammation by stimulating the production of key inflammatory mediators, including IL-6, TNF-α, and IL-1β. Keratinocytes, fibroblasts, macrophages, and neutrophils are among the cell types that respond to IL-17-induced proinflammatory cytokine production. IL-17 also stimulates the proliferation and survival of neutrophils, T cells, and B cells. **Ixekizumab** and **secukinumab** are two fully human monoclonal antibodies directed against IL-17A that are in late-phase clinical trials for the management of psoriasis and rheumatoid arthritis.

IL-17 exerts its proinflammatory effect by signaling through two receptor subtypes, IL-17 receptor A (IL-17RA) and IL-17 receptor C (IL-17RC). **Brodalumab** is an anti-IL-17 receptor monoclonal antibody that acts as a competitive inhibitor of the IL-17RA subunit. This drug is under active investigation for the treatment of psoriasis, rheumatoid arthritis, and Crohn's disease.

IL-6 Receptor Inhibitor

The cytokine **interleukin-6 (IL-6)** was initially identified as a factor that differentiates activated B cells into immunoglobulin-producing cells. IL-6 is a key mediator in many physiologic and pathologic processes, including the acute-phase inflammatory response, angiogenesis, neutrophil migration, differentiation of helper T cells, bone and cartilage metabolism, lipid metabolism, and cancer. Lymphocytes, monocytes, fibroblasts, keratinocytes, endothelial cells, mesangial cells, and adipocytes all produce IL-6, while cells of hematopoietic origin express the IL-6 receptor.

Elevated serum levels of IL-6 have been implicated in the pathogenesis of many autoimmune and inflammatory conditions. **Tocilizumab** is a monoclonal antibody directed against the IL-6 receptor that is approved for use in polyarticular juvenile idiopathic arthritis and systemic juvenile idiopathic arthritis and in patients with rheumatoid arthritis who have had an inadequate response to anti-TNF drugs. The drug is administered every 4 weeks as an intravenous infusion.

Depletion of Specific Immune Cells

Appropriately targeted antibodies deplete the immune system of reactive cells and thereby provide effective therapy for autoimmune diseases and transplant rejection. When the adaptive immune system reacts to an antigen, the resulting immunologic response includes the clonal expansion of cells specifically reactive against that antigen. Treatment with exogenous antibodies directed against cell surface molecules that are expressed selectively on reactive immune cells can preferentially deplete the immune system of these reactive cells. Antibodies that target cell surface receptors expressed selectively on malignant cells of immune origin are discussed in Chapter 40, Pharmacology of Cancer: Signal Transduction.

Polyclonal Antibodies
Antithymocyte Globulin

Antithymocyte globulin (ATG) is a preparation of antibodies induced by injecting rabbits or horses with human thymocytes. The rabbit or horse antibodies are polyclonal and target many antigens on human T cells. Because ATG targets essentially all T cells and leads to profound lymphocyte depletion, ATG treatment results in broad immunosuppression that can predispose to infection. ATG is approved for use in prevention or treatment of renal transplant rejection, and the equine-derived material is also approved for treatment of aplastic anemia. ATG is administered intravenously once daily for up to 28 days.

ATG therapy is often complicated by fever and headache as prominent manifestations of the **cytokine release syndrome**. This syndrome, common to many antibody drugs that target lymphocytes, results from activation of T cells and release of T-cell cytokines before the antibody-coated T cells can be cleared by macrophages. The cytokine release syndrome typically occurs after the first few doses of ATG therapy, and the syndrome dissipates as T cells are eliminated. However, administration of successive ATG doses can also be complicated by the development of antibodies against rabbit- or horse-specific epitopes on the administered immunoglobulins. ATG is generally co-administered with glucocorticoids, an antihistamine, and an antipyretic to mitigate infusion reactions. Note that Mr. W received medications in these three classes when starting induction ATG therapy after kidney transplant.

Monoclonal Antibodies
OKT3

OKT3 (muromonab-CD3, anti-CD3) is a mouse monoclonal antibody directed against human CD3, one of the cell surface signaling molecules important for activation of the T-cell receptor. CD3 is specifically expressed on T cells (both CD4 and CD8 cells). Treatment with OKT3 depletes the available pool of T cells via antibody-mediated activation of complement and clearance of immune cells. Because OKT3 targets all T cells, OKT3 treatment can result in profound immunosuppression. Also, because OKT3 binds to CD3, and CD3 is important for T-cell activation, OKT3 therapy can broadly activate T cells, resulting in the cytokine release syndrome. Another limitation is that OKT3 is a mouse antihuman antibody (see above). OKT3 was approved for use in acute renal transplant rejection but was subsequently (in 2010) withdrawn voluntarily from the market by the manufacturer.

Anti-CD20 mAb

Rituximab is a chimeric, partially humanized anti-CD20 monoclonal antibody. CD20 is expressed on the surface of all mature B cells, and administration of rituximab causes profound depletion of circulating B cells. Originally approved for the treatment of CD20$^+$ non-Hodgkin's lymphoma (see Chapter 40), rituximab has also been approved for use in rheumatoid arthritis refractory to TNF inhibitors, granulomatosis with polyangiitis, and microscopic polyangiitis. Several additional anti-CD20 antibodies are in clinical development; **ofatumumab** and **obinutuzumab** are fully human anti-CD20 monoclonal antibodies that recognize an epitope distinct from that bound by rituximab. Ofatumumab and obinutuzumab are approved for use in chronic lymphocytic leukemia.

Anti-CD25 mAb

Basiliximab is a monoclonal antibody directed against CD25, the high-affinity IL-2 receptor. IL-2 mediates early steps in T-cell activation. Because CD25 is expressed only on activated T cells, anti-CD25 antibody therapy selectively targets T cells that have been activated by an MHC-antigen stimulus.

Basiliximab is administered prophylactically in renal transplantation to inhibit acute organ rejection. It is also used as a component of general immunosuppressive regimens after organ transplantation. Basiliximab is typically administered in a two-dose regimen, with the first administration 2 hours before transplantation surgery and the second dose 4 days after transplantation. This type of dosing regimen, in which drug is administered for a limited period immediately after transplantation, is referred to as **induction therapy**. Daclizumab is another antibody with the same mechanism of action that was voluntarily withdrawn from the market by the manufacturer in 2009.

Anti-CD52 mAb

Campath-1 (CD52) is an antigen expressed on most mature lymphocytes and on some lymphocyte precursors. An antibody against this antigen was originally tested in rheumatoid arthritis and found to cause prolonged and sustained depletion of all T cells, often lasting for years. The reason for the sustained lymphocyte depletion is unknown. Anti-CD52 mAb therapy did lead to some improvement in the symptoms of arthritis; however, the sustained depletion of lymphocytes and concern about infections precluded further study of this antibody in autoimmune conditions. Under the generic name **alemtuzumab**, anti-CD52 monoclonal antibody had been approved as an adjunctive therapy in the treatment of B-cell chronic lymphocytic leukemia—a condition in which sustained suppression of the leukemic cells is desirable. However, alemtuzumab has been voluntarily withdrawn from the market in the United States and Europe.

LFA-3

LFA-3 (also called **CD58**) is the counter-receptor for CD2, an antigen expressed at high levels on the surface of memory effector T cells. Interaction of CD2 on T cells with LFA-3 on antigen-presenting cells promotes increased T-cell proliferation and enhanced T-cell-dependent cytotoxicity. Because the memory effector T-cell population is increased in patients with psoriasis, a pharmacologic agent that disrupts the CD2–LFA-3 interaction was tested for use in psoriasis.

Alefacept is an LFA-3/Fc fusion protein that interrupts CD2–LFA-3 signaling by binding to T-cell CD2 and thereby inhibits T-cell activation. Additionally, the Fc portion of alefacept may activate NK cells to deplete the immune system of memory effector T cells. Clinically, alefacept significantly decreases the severity of chronic plaque psoriasis. Because CD2 is expressed on other adaptive immune cells, however, administration of alefacept also causes a dose-dependent reduction in CD4 and CD8 T-cell populations. Patients taking alefacept may have an increased risk of serious infection and an increased risk of malignancy, primarily skin cancer. Alefacept was voluntarily withdrawn from the market by the manufacturer in 2011.

B-Lymphocyte Stimulator

Belimumab is a human monoclonal antibody directed against the B-lymphocyte stimulator (BLyS) cytokine. BLyS binding to normal B cells activates signaling cascades that stimulate cell survival and cell differentiation into antibody- and autoantibody-producing cells. Belimumab blocks the normal function of BLyS, resulting in B-cell apoptosis. As mentioned previously, autoantibodies against self-antigens are one mechanism of tissue injury and inflammation in systemic lupus erythematosus. Reducing the number of circulating B cells leads to a subsequent decrease in autoantibody production and reduced disease activity.

Antibody–Drug Conjugates

Brentuximab vedotin is a chimeric human monoclonal antibody–drug conjugate directed against CD30. CD30 is a membrane glycoprotein in the TNF receptor family that signals through multiple mechanisms, including the NFκB pathway, to promote cell proliferation and survival. CD30 is expressed on activated CD4 and CD8 T cells and on B cells. It is also highly expressed on Reed-Sternberg cells in Hodgkin's lymphoma and on anaplastic large cell lymphoma cells. The specific role of CD30 in the pathogenesis of lymphoma is under investigation. In brentuximab vedotin, the anti-CD30 antibody is linked to the antimitotic drug monomethyl auristatin E (MMAE) through a valine-citrulline dipeptide. This linker dipeptide is enzymatically cleaved after endocytosis at the target site to release MMAE into the cytoplasm. MMAE prevents microtubule polymerization, causing cell cycle arrest in the G2 to M phase and subsequent apoptosis in CD30-expressing cells.

Brentuximab vedotin is approved for the treatment of relapsing Hodgkin's lymphoma after failure of multi-agent chemotherapy or failure of autologous stem cell transplant. It is also approved for systemic anaplastic large cell lymphoma after failure of at least one multi-agent chemotherapy regimen. Additional anti-CD30 monoclonal antibodies, bispecific antibodies, and antibody–drug conjugates are under active investigation for the treatment of Hodgkin's lymphoma.

Inhibition of Costimulation

Costimulation refers to the paradigm that cells of the immune system typically require two signals for activation (see Chapter 42, Principles of Inflammation and the Immune System). If a first signal is provided in the absence of a second signal, the target immune cell may become anergic rather than activated. Because induction of anergy could lead to long-term acceptance of an organ graft or limit the extent of an autoimmune disease, inhibition of costimulation represents a viable strategy for immunosuppression. Several therapeutic agents inhibit costimulation by blocking the second signal required for cell activation, and more such agents are under development.

Abatacept

Abatacept consists of CTLA-4 fused to an IgG1 constant region. Abatacept complexes with costimulatory B7 molecules on the surface of antigen-presenting cells. When the antigen-presenting cell interacts with a T cell, MHC:antigen–TCR interaction ("signal 1") occurs, but the complex of B7 with abatacept prevents delivery of a costimulatory signal ("signal 2"), and the T cell develops anergy or undergoes apoptosis. By this mechanism, abatacept therapy appears to be effective in down-regulating specific T-cell populations.

Abatacept is approved for the treatment of juvenile idiopathic arthritis and rheumatoid arthritis that is refractory to methotrexate or TNF inhibitors. Clinically, abatacept significantly improves symptoms of rheumatoid arthritis in patients who fail to respond to methotrexate or TNF inhibitors.

The major adverse effects of abatacept are *exacerbations of preexisting chronic obstructive lung disease* and *increased susceptibility to infection*. Abatacept should not be administered concurrently with TNF inhibitors because the combination carries an unacceptably high risk of infection.

Belatacept

Belatacept is a close structural congener of abatacept that has increased affinity for B7-1 and B7-2. In a large clinical trial, belatacept was as effective as cyclosporine at inhibiting acute rejection in renal transplant recipients. Belatacept is approved as an immunosuppressant for renal transplantation in patients who are seropositive for Epstein-Barr virus (EBV).

Blockade of Cell Adhesion

The recruitment and accumulation of inflammatory cells at sites of inflammation is an essential element of most autoimmune diseases; the only exceptions to this rule are autoimmune diseases that are purely humoral, such as myasthenia gravis. Drugs that inhibit cell migration to sites of inflammation may also inhibit antigen presentation and cytotoxicity, thus providing multiple potential mechanisms of therapeutic action.

Natalizumab

Alpha-4 integrins are critical to immune-cell adhesion and homing. The $\alpha_4\beta_1$ integrin mediates immune-cell interactions with cells expressing vascular cell adhesion molecule 1 (VCAM-1), while the $\alpha_4\beta_7$ integrin mediates immune-cell binding to cells expressing mucosal addressin cell adhesion molecule 1 (MAdCAM-1). **Natalizumab** is a monoclonal antibody directed against α_4 integrin that inhibits immune-cell interactions with cells expressing VCAM-1 or MAdCAM-1.

Natalizumab was approved for the treatment of relapsing multiple sclerosis. During postmarketing surveillance of the drug, however, several patients treated with natalizumab developed progressive multifocal leukoencephalopathy (PML), a rare demyelinating disorder caused by infection with JC virus. This finding resulted in voluntary withdrawal of the drug. After further FDA investigation, it was decided to resume testing of natalizumab and to add a warning to the product label regarding the possible association. Natalizumab was subsequently reapproved for use in the treatment of multiple sclerosis and Crohn's disease.

Inhibition of Complement Activation

The complement system mediates multiple innate immune responses (see Chapter 42). Recognition of foreign proteins or carbohydrates leads to sequential activation of complement proteins and eventual assembly of the **membrane attack complex**, a multiprotein structure that can cause cell lysis. Patients with paroxysmal nocturnal hemoglobinuria (PNH) have acquired defects in complement regulatory proteins, leading to inappropriate activation of complement and complement-mediated lysis of erythrocytes. **Eculizumab** is a humanized monoclonal antibody directed against C5, a complement protein that mediates late steps in complement activation and triggers assembly of the membrane attack complex. Eculizumab is approved for treatment of PNH; it significantly decreases hemoglobinuria and the need for erythrocyte transfusions in patients with this disorder. Eculizumab is also approved for treatment of atypical hemolytic uremic syndrome. Genetic evidence indicates that complement activation may play an etiologic role in age-dependent macular degeneration, suggesting that inhibitors of the complement cascade could be useful local therapies for this disease.

Inhibition of Immune Checkpoints

As discussed above in the "Inhibition of Costimulation" section, the immune system uses costimulatory signals to activate antigen-specific immune responses (see also Chapter 42). The immune system also uses **immune checkpoint** signals to inhibit such responses. Inhibitory checkpoint molecules include cytotoxic T lymphocyte antigen 4 (CTLA-4), programmed cell death protein 1 (PD-1), and several others. In general, ligation of these molecules on T cells inhibits the immune response; the signaling pathways that mediate these inhibitory responses are subjects of active investigation. Some tumors have been found to up-regulate PD-1 ligands and thereby inhibit T-cell immune surveillance of tumors. Studies have shown that inhibition of CTLA-4 and/or PD-1 augments T-cell activation, proliferation, and cytokine production, and can be used to enhance the anti-tumor immune response.

CTLA-4 Blockade

Ipilimumab is a first-generation immune checkpoint inhibitor. This recombinant, humanized IgG1 monoclonal antibody binds to CTLA-4 and blocks the interaction of CTLA-4 with its ligands B7-1 and B7-2 (see Chapter 42). In clinical studies, ipilimumab showed an overall survival benefit in patients with unresectable or metastatic melanoma who had been previously treated with one or more anticancer therapies. Ipilimumab was approved for use in 2011 in advanced melanoma that is unresectable or metastatic. Patients taking ipilimumab should be monitored for possible immune-related hepatotoxicity and endocrinopathies.

PD-1 Blockade

Nivolumab and **pembrolizumab** are recombinant, humanized IgG4 monoclonal antibodies that bind to PD-1 and block the interaction of PD-1 with its ligands PD-L1 and PD-L2. By inhibiting the inhibition of T-cell proliferation and cytokine production that results from binding of PD-1 to PD-L1 and PD-L2, blockade of PD-1 by nivolumab and pembrolizumab releases PD-1 pathway-mediated inhibition of the immune response, including the anti-tumor immune response. In appropriate mouse tumor models, blocking PD-1 activity results in decreased tumor growth. Nivolumab and pembrolizumab are indicated for the treatment of unresectable or metastatic melanoma with disease progression following treatment with ipilimumab and, if the tumor is positive for a B-RAF V600 mutation, a B-RAF inhibitor. These therapies are also approved for metastatic non-small cell lung cancers that express PD-L1 and show disease progression on or after platinum-containing chemotherapy. For non-small cell lung cancer with sensitizing EGFR mutations or ALK rearrangements, disease progression on therapies targeted for these genomic tumor aberrations should be demonstrated prior to treatment with nivolumab or pembrolizumab.

■ CONCLUSION AND FUTURE DIRECTIONS

Several approaches are available for the pharmacologic suppression of adaptive immunity, ranging from the relatively low-selectivity approaches represented by glucocorticoids and cytotoxic agents to the more selective approaches represented by cell-signaling inhibitors and antibody therapies. *Glucocorticoids* induce profound suppression of the inflammatory response and immune system but cause many adverse effects, most of which are due to drug effects on cells outside the immune system. Glucocorticoid receptor modulators are being sought that retain the anti-inflammatory effects of glucocorticoids but have less severe adverse effects on metabolism and bone mineral homeostasis. *Cytotoxic agents* target DNA replication; although immune cells are highly susceptible to these drugs, so, too, are other normal cells such as those in the gastrointestinal epithelium. The cytotoxic agent mycophenolate mofetil is highly selective, both because lymphocytes depend on de novo purine synthesis and because mycophenolic acid preferentially targets the inosine monophosphate dehydrogenase isoenzyme expressed in lymphocytes. *Lymphocyte-signaling inhibitors*—such as cyclosporine, tacrolimus, sirolimus, and everolimus, which target intracellular signal transduction pathways necessary for T-cell activation—are also reasonably selective. Many new inhibitors of intracellular signaling in lymphocytes are under investigation; inhibition of the Janus kinase family appears particularly promising. *Cytokine inhibitors* interrupt soluble signals mediating immune-cell activation. TNF inhibitors—such as etanercept, infliximab, and adalimumab—represent an expanding class of drugs. Promising new targets include cytokine pathways associated with T_H17 cells, which are targeted by the IL-17A inhibitors ixekizumab and secukinumab and the IL-17 receptor antagonist brodalumab, among others. The concept of preventing immune-cell activation has been extended to the *blockade of costimulation* represented by abatacept and belatacept. *Specific depletion of B cells* is a well-established therapy for lymphomas and rheumatoid arthritis: belimumab, a first-in-its-class antibody against a crucial B-cell survival factor, is used in the treatment of systemic lupus erythematosus. *Specific depletion of T cells* may be beneficial in organ transplantation: antithymocyte globulin is directed against T-cell-specific epitopes. Several antibody therapeutics and small molecules are available that *block immune-cell adhesion* and homing, and more such agents are under development. *Immune checkpoint inhibitors* are an exciting new class of anticancer therapies.

Disclosure

Lloyd B. Klickstein is an employee and stockholder of Novartis, Inc., which manufactures or distributes drugs discussed in this chapter, including cyclosporine, mycophenolate sodium, everolimus, canakinumab, and basiliximab. April W. Armstrong serves as investigator and/or consultant to AbbVie, Amgen, Celgene, Janssen, Lilly, Merck, Novartis, and Pfizer.

Suggested Reading

Benedetti G, Miossec P. Interleukin 17 contributes to the chronicity of inflammatory diseases such as rheumatoid arthritis. *Eur J Immunol* 2014;44: 339–347. (*Discusses role that IL-17 may have in inflammatory diseases.*)

Intlekofer AM, Thompson CB. At the bench: preclinical rationale for CTLA-4 and PD-1 blockade as cancer immunotherapy. *J Leukoc Biol* 2013;94:25–39. (*Discusses the molecular mechanisms by which CTLA-4 and PD-1 function to turn off established immune responses.*)

Mahoney KM, Rennert PD, Freeman GJ. Combination cancer immunotherapy and new immunomodulatory targets. *Nat Rev Drug Discov* 2015;14:561–584. (*Discusses CTLA-4, PD-1, and other potential drug targets that mediate inhibition of the anti-tumor immune response.*)

Murphy K, Travers P, Walport M. *Janeway's immunobiology: the immune system in health and disease.* 8th ed. New York: Garland Publishing; 2012. (*Discussion of autoimmunity and transplantation immunity.*)

DRUG SUMMARY TABLE: CHAPTER 46 Pharmacology of Immunosuppression

DRUG	CLINICAL APPLICATIONS	SERIOUS AND COMMON ADVERSE EFFECTS	CONTRAINDICATIONS	THERAPEUTIC CONSIDERATIONS
INHIBITORS OF GENE EXPRESSION Mechanism—Inhibit COX-2 expression; induce lipocortins and activate endogenous anti-inflammatory pathways				
Prednisone Prednisolone Methylprednisolone Dexamethasone	See Drug Summary Table: Chapter 29 Pharmacology of the Adrenal Cortex			
CYTOTOXIC AGENTS Mechanism—See specific drug				
Mycophenolic acid Mycophenolate mofetil Mycophenolate sodium	Solid organ transplantation	*Gastrointestinal hemorrhage, leukopenia, myelosuppression, neutropenia, increased risk of infection or lymphoma, leukoencephalopathy, pleural effusion, pulmonary fibrosis* Hypertension, edema, hypercholesterolemia, electrolyte imbalance, gastrointestinal disturbance, headache, anxiety, asthenia, paresthesia	Hypersensitivity to mycophenolic acid, mycophenolate mofetil, or mycophenolate sodium Hypersensitivity to polysorbate 80 (IV formulation)	Inhibitor of inosine monophosphate dehydrogenase (IMPDH), the rate-limiting enzyme in the formation of guanosine. Avoid concurrent administration of oral iron because it markedly reduces the bioavailability of mycophenolate mofetil.
Leflunomide	Rheumatoid arthritis	*Stevens-Johnson syndrome, toxic epidermal necrolysis, pancytopenia, hepatotoxicity, interstitial lung disease* Alopecia, diarrhea, rash, mouth ulcer, dizziness, headache, infection	Hypersensitivity to leflunomide Pregnancy	Inhibits dihydroorotate dehydrogenase (DHOD), leading to inhibition of pyrimidine synthesis. Leflunomide undergoes significant enterohepatic circulation, resulting in a prolonged pharmacologic effect. Leflunomide has antiviral activity against cytomegalovirus (CMV) and can be used to treat resistant CMV and CMV in transplant patients.
Azathioprine Methotrexate Cyclophosphamide	See Drug Summary Tables: Chapter 33 Principles of Antimicrobial and Antineoplastic Pharmacology (methotrexate) and Chapter 39 Pharmacology of Cancer: Genome Synthesis, Stability, and Maintenance (azathioprine and cyclophosphamide)			
SPECIFIC LYMPHOCYTE-SIGNALING INHIBITORS Mechanism—See specific drug				
Cyclosporine	Solid organ transplantation Keratoconjunctivitis sicca (topical cyclosporine)	*Hyperkalemia, hypomagnesemia, nephrotoxicity, neurotoxicity, hepatotoxicity* Hypertension, gingival hyperplasia, hirsutism, headache, tremor, eye irritation, infection	Hypersensitivity to cyclosporine Abnormal renal function Uncontrolled hypertension Malignancies (rheumatoid arthritis and psoriasis patients) Concomitant PUVA or UVB therapy, methotrexate, immunosuppressive agents, coal tar, radiation therapy (psoriasis patients) Active ocular infection (topical cyclosporine)	Cyclosporine binds to cyclophilin, and the resulting complex inhibits the phosphatase activity of calcineurin, a cell-signaling protein that mediates T-cell activation. Cyclosporine inhibits the production of IL-2 by activated T cells. Danazol and other androgens can increase serum cyclosporine level. Rifampin and St. John's wort decrease serum cyclosporine level.

Drug	Clinical Applications	Serious and Common Adverse Effects	Contraindications	Therapeutic Considerations
Tacrolimus	Organ transplantation Atopic dermatitis (topical tacrolimus)	*Prolonged QT interval, atrial fibrillation, heart failure, diabetes mellitus, hyperkalemia, hypomagnesemia, gastrointestinal perforation, hepatotoxicity, neurotoxicity, nephrotoxicity, acute respiratory distress syndrome, increased risk of lymphoma or infection* Edema, alopecia, rash, gastrointestinal upset, anemia, leukocytosis, thrombocytopenia, headache, insomnia, paresthesia, tremor	Hypersensitivity to tacrolimus Hypersensitivity to hydrogenated castor oil (IV formulation)	Tacrolimus binds to FK-binding protein (FKBP), and the tacrolimus–FKBP complex inhibits calcineurin. Topical tacrolimus is used widely to treat atopic dermatitis and other eczematous dermatitis. Rifampin and St. John's wort markedly decrease serum tacrolimus level.
Sirolimus **Everolimus** **Zotarolimus**	Shared indication: Coronary artery disease (cardiac stents) Sirolimus and everolimus only: Prophylaxis for renal transplant rejection Everolimus only: Renal cell carcinoma Breast cancer Neuroendocrine tumors of pancreatic origin Renal angiomyolipoma or subependymal giant cell astrocytoma associated with tuberous sclerosis complex	*Thrombosis, pancytopenia, lymphocele, neurotoxicity, nephrotic syndrome, increased risk of infection or lymphoma, interstitial lung disease, angioedema* Edema, hypertension, rash, hyperlipidemia, gastrointestinal upset, arthralgia, headache, fever (shared adverse effects); electrolyte imbalance, amenorrhea, menorrhagia, stomatitis (everolimus only)	Hypersensitivity to sirolimus, everolimus, or zotarolimus	Sirolimus binds to FKBP, and the resulting sirolimus–FKBP complex inhibits mTOR, a regulator of protein translation; everolimus and zotarolimus act by similar mechanisms. Avoid co-administration of sirolimus or everolimus with drugs that induce or inhibit CYP3A4. Avoid co-administration of everolimus with cyclosporine.

TUMOR NECROSIS FACTOR INHIBITORS
Mechanism—Etanercept is a soluble TNF receptor dimer; infliximab, adalimumab, certolizumab, and golimumab are anti-TNF antibodies

Drug	Clinical Applications	Serious and Common Adverse Effects	Contraindications	Therapeutic Considerations
Etanercept	Rheumatoid arthritis Juvenile idiopathic arthritis Plaque psoriasis Psoriatic arthritis Ankylosing spondylitis	*Heart failure, myelosuppression, necrotizing fasciitis, Stevens-Johnson syndrome, toxic epidermal necrolysis, hepatotoxicity, optic neuritis, reactivation of tuberculosis, increased risk of infection or malignancy, demyelinating disease of central nervous system* Injection site reaction, upper respiratory infection, rhinitis	Sepsis	All patients should undergo screening for tuberculosis before initiating therapy with a TNF inhibitor because of a greatly increased risk of reactivating latent tuberculosis. Any patient developing an infection while taking a TNF inhibitor should undergo evaluation and aggressive antibiotic treatment. Etanercept is a soluble TNF receptor dimer that binds to both TNF-α and TNF-β, whereas infliximab, adalimumab, certolizumab, and golimumab are monoclonal antibodies that bind to TNF-α specifically.

continues

DRUG SUMMARY TABLE: CHAPTER 46 Pharmacology of Immunosuppression continued

DRUG	CLINICAL APPLICATIONS	SERIOUS AND COMMON ADVERSE EFFECTS	CONTRAINDICATIONS	THERAPEUTIC CONSIDERATIONS
TUMOR NECROSIS FACTOR INHIBITORS (continued) **Mechanism**—Etanercept is a soluble TNF receptor dimer; infliximab, adalimumab, certolizumab, and golimumab are anti-TNF antibodies				
Infliximab **Adalimumab** **Certolizumab** **Golimumab**	Shared indications: Rheumatoid arthritis Ankylosing spondylitis Psoriatic arthritis Infliximab, adalimumab, and certolizumab only: Crohn's disease Infliximab, adalimumab, and golimumab only: Ulcerative colitis Infliximab and adalimumab only: Plaque psoriasis Adalimumab only: Juvenile idiopathic arthritis	Similar to etanercept Additionally, gastrointestinal upset (infliximab only)	Hypersensitivity to infliximab Moderate to severe heart failure (infliximab doses >5 mg/kg)	Infliximab is a partially humanized mouse antibody against human TNF-α. Adalimumab and golimumab are fully human IgG1 antibodies against TNF-α; golimumab has a longer half-life than adalimumab. Certolizumab is a pegylated anti-TNF-α antibody fragment.
IL-12/IL-23p40 INHIBITORS **Mechanism**—Ustekinumab is a human IgG1 monoclonal antibody that binds to the p40 protein subunit shared by IL-12 and IL-23. IL-12 and IL-23 are cytokines involved in natural killer cell activation and CD4⁺ T-cell differentiation and activation.				
Ustekinumab	Plaque psoriasis Psoriatic arthritis	*Increased risk of infection or malignancy, leukoencephalopathy, angioedema* Nasopharyngitis, upper respiratory tract infection, headache, fatigue	Hypersensitivity to ustekinumab	After an initial loading dose, ustekinumab is administered subcutaneously every 3 months.
INTERLEUKIN-1 INHIBITORS **Mechanism**—Anakinra is a recombinant IL-1 receptor antagonist; rilonacept is a recombinant soluble IL-1 receptor Fc fusion protein; canakinumab is a human IgG1 monoclonal antibody to IL-1β				
Anakinra	Rheumatoid arthritis Cryopyrin-associated periodic syndromes, including neonatal-onset multisystem inflammatory disease	*Cardiorespiratory arrest, neutropenia, increased risk of infection or malignancy* Injection site reaction	Hypersensitivity to anakinra or *E. coli*-derived proteins	Reduces bony erosions, possibly by decreasing metalloproteinase release from synovial cells. Avoid administration of live vaccines.
Rilonacept **Canakinumab**	Shared indication: Cryopyrin-associated periodic syndromes, including familial cold autoinflammatory syndrome and Muckle-Wells syndrome Canakinumab only: Systemic juvenile idiopathic arthritis	*Gastrointestinal hemorrhage, neutropenia, meningitis (rilonacept only); macrophage activation syndrome, reactivation tuberculosis (canakinumab only)* Injection site reaction, upper respiratory infection (shared adverse effects); gastrointestinal upset, musculoskeletal pain, headache, vertigo (canakinumab only)	Hypersensitivity to rilonacept or canakinumab	Avoid administration in patients with active, recurring, or chronic infections. Avoid administration of live vaccines.

CYTOKINE RECEPTOR ANTAGONIST
Mechanism—Recombinant humanized monoclonal antibody to the IL-6 receptor

Drug	Indications	Adverse effects	Contraindications	Notes
Tocilizumab	Rheumatoid arthritis Polyarticular juvenile idiopathic arthritis Systemic juvenile idiopathic arthritis	*Serious infections, gastrointestinal perforation, thrombocytopenia, neutropenia, anaphylaxis* Hypertension, injection site reaction, gastrointestinal upset, abnormal liver function tests, dizziness, headache, nasopharyngitis	Hypersensitivity to tocilizumab	Avoid administration of live vaccines. All patients should undergo screening for tuberculosis before initiating therapy because of an increased risk of reactivating latent tuberculosis.

DEPLETION OF SPECIFIC IMMUNE CELLS
Mechanism—See specific drug

Drug	Indications	Adverse effects	Contraindications	Notes
Antithymocyte globulin	Renal transplantation Aplastic anemia	*Cytokine release syndrome (fever, shaking chills, myalgia, headache), hypertension, anemia, leukopenia, thrombocytopenia, increased risk of infection*	Acute infection History of allergy or anaphylaxis to rabbit or horse proteins	Polyclonal rabbit or horse antibodies against human T-cell epitopes. ATG treatment can result in broad immunosuppression that can lead to infection.
OKT3	Not applicable	Not applicable	Not applicable	Mouse monoclonal antibody against human CD3, a signaling molecule important for T-cell receptor–mediated cell activation. Voluntarily withdrawn by manufacturer in 2010.
Rituximab Ofatumumab Obinutuzumab	Shared indication: Chronic lymphocytic leukemia Rituximab only: B-cell non-Hodgkin's lymphoma Rheumatoid arthritis Granulomatosis with polyangiitis and microscopic polyangiitis	*Anemia, significant immunosuppression, leukoencephalopathy, tumor lysis syndrome (shared adverse effects); bowel obstruction, hepatitis, infusion reaction (rituximab and ofatumumab only); cardiac arrhythmia, heart failure, Stevens–Johnson syndrome, toxic epidermal necrolysis, keratitis, nephrotoxicity, pulmonary fibrosis, angioedema (rituximab only)* Rash, fever, fatigue (shared adverse effects); gastrointestinal upset (rituximab and ofatumumab only); hypotension, night sweats, arthralgia, myalgia, shivering (rituximab only)	None	Rituximab is a partially humanized anti-CD20 antibody; ofatumumab and obinutuzumab are fully human anti-CD20 antibodies. Avoid administration of live vaccines.
Basiliximab	Renal transplantation	Same as antithymocyte globulin	Hypersensitivity to basiliximab	Basiliximab is a chimeric mouse/human IgG1 monoclonal antibody to CD25, the high-affinity IL-2 receptor.
Alemtuzumab	Not applicable	Not applicable	Not applicable	Antibody to campath-1 (CD52), an antigen expressed on most mature lymphocytes and some lymphocyte precursors. Voluntarily withdrawn by manufacturer in the United States and Europe.
Alefacept	Not applicable	Not applicable	Not applicable	LFA-3/Fc fusion protein that interrupts CD2/LFA-3 signaling by binding to T-cell CD2, leading to inhibition of T-cell activation. Voluntarily withdrawn by manufacturer in 2011.

continues

DRUG SUMMARY TABLE: CHAPTER 46 Pharmacology of Immunosuppression *continued*

DRUG	CLINICAL APPLICATIONS	SERIOUS AND COMMON ADVERSE EFFECTS	CONTRAINDICATIONS	THERAPEUTIC CONSIDERATIONS
DEPLETION OF SPECIFIC IMMUNE CELLS *(continued)* Mechanism—See specific drug				
Belimumab	Systemic lupus erythematosus	*Susceptibility to infection or malignancy, infusion reaction, leukoencephalopathy, depression* Gastrointestinal upset, nasopharyngitis, fever	Previous anaphylaxis to belimumab	Fully human monoclonal antibody that inhibits B lymphocyte stimulator (BLyS), a factor that is required for the survival of B cells.
Brentuximab vedotin	Hodgkin's lymphoma Anaplastic large cell lymphoma	*Supraventricular arrhythmias, Stevens-Johnson syndrome, anemia, thrombocytopenia, neutropenia, neuropathy, leukoencephalopathy, pyelonephritis, pneumothorax, pulmonary embolism, pneumonitis, tumor lysis syndrome* Rash, gastrointestinal upset, upper respiratory infection, cough, fever, fatigue	Concomitant use of bleomycin due to pulmonary toxicity	Chimeric human monoclonal antibody–drug conjugate against CD30. CD30 is expressed on CD4 and CD8 T cells, B cells, and lymphoma cells. The drug monomethyl auristatin E (MMAE) is covalently attached to the antibody via a linker. MMAE functions as a microtubule-disrupting agent that induces cell cycle arrest and subsequent apoptosis. MMAE is a CYP3A4/5 inhibitor.
INHIBITION OF COSTIMULATION Mechanism—Abatacept and belatacept are CTLA-4 analogues fused to an IgG1 constant region. By forming a complex with cell surface B7 molecules, the drugs prevent delivery of a costimulatory signal and the T cell develops anergy or undergoes apoptosis.				
Abatacept	Rheumatoid arthritis Juvenile idiopathic arthritis	*Cellulitis, sepsis, pyelonephritis, pneumonia, acute exacerbation of chronic obstructive lung disease, susceptibility to malignancy* Nausea, headache, urinary tract infection, nasopharyngitis, upper respiratory infection	None	Abatacept should not be administered concurrently with TNF inhibitors due to increased risk of serious infection. Avoid administration of live vaccines. All patients should undergo screening for tuberculosis before initiating therapy.
Belatacept	Renal transplantation in patients who are EBV seropositive	*Post-transplant lymphoproliferative disorder, leukoencephalopathy, Guillain-Barre syndrome, anemia, leukopenia, serious infections* Hypertension, edema, electrolyte imbalance, gastrointestinal upset, cough, headache, fever	Patients who are EBV seronegative or with unknown EBV serostatus	Belatacept is a close structural congener of abatacept that has increased affinity for B7-1 and B7-2. May only be used in patients who are EBV seropositive. Avoid administration of live vaccines.
BLOCKADE OF CELL ADHESION Mechanism—Natalizumab is a monoclonal antibody against alpha-4 integrin that inhibits immune cell interaction with cells expressing VCAM-1 and MAdCAM-1				
Natalizumab	Multiple sclerosis, relapsing forms Crohn's disease	*Progressive multifocal leukoencephalopathy, bowel obstruction, hepatotoxicity, herpes encephalitis and meningitis, depression, suicidal ideation, pneumonia* Rash, gastrointestinal upset, arthralgia, headache, urinary tract infection, respiratory tract infection, fatigue	Hypersensitivity to natalizumab History of progressive multifocal leukoencephalopathy (PML) or existing PML	Infusion-related reactions may occur.

INHIBITOR OF COMPLEMENT ACTIVATION
Mechanism—Humanized monoclonal antibody against C5, a complement protein that mediates late steps in complement activation and assembly of the membrane attack complex

Eculizumab	Paroxysmal nocturnal hemoglobinuria Atypical hemolytic uremic syndrome	*Infections, leukopenia, anemia* Hypertension, gastrointestinal upset, headache, insomnia, nasopharyngitis, fever	Hypersensitivity to eculizumab *Neisseria meningitidis* infection No vaccination against *N. meningitidis*	All patients who discontinue eculizumab need to be monitored for signs and symptoms of intravascular hemolysis, including evaluation of serum lactate dehydrogenase levels.

INHIBITION OF IMMUNE CHECKPOINTS
Mechanism—Ipilimumab is a humanized monoclonal antibody against CTLA-4 and nivolumab and pembrolizumab are humanized monoclonal antibodies against PD-1. By inhibiting the interaction of CTLA-4 and PD-1 with their ligands B7-1/B7-2 and PD-L1/PD-L2, respectively, the drugs release checkpoint pathway-mediated inhibition of the anti-tumor immune response.

Ipilimumab	Unresectable or metastatic melanoma	*Pericarditis, endocrine disorder, enterocolitis, eosinophilia, anemia, hepatotoxicity, myositis, encephalitis, neuropathy, renal failure, iritis, uveitis, pneumonitis* Rash, diarrhea, fatigue	None	Administered intravenously every 3 weeks for a total of four doses.
Nivolumab Pembrolizumab	Unresectable or metastatic melanoma with disease progression following treatment with ipilimumab and, if indicated, a BRAF inhibitor Metastatic non-small cell lung cancers expressing PD-L1 and showing disease progression on or after platinum-containing chemotherapy	*Immune-mediated pneumonitis, colitis, hepatitis, endocrinopathies, nephritis, rash, encephalitis* Rash, fatigue, cough, musculoskeletal pain, decreased appetite, constipation	None	For non-small cell lung cancers with EGFR mutations or ALK rearrangements, disease progression on therapies targeted for these genomic aberrations should be demonstrated prior to treatment

47

Integrative Inflammation Pharmacology: Peptic Ulcer Disease

Dalia S. Nagel and Helen M. Shields

▮ INTRODUCTION

A peptic ulcer is a break in the mucosa of the stomach (gastric ulcer) or duodenum (duodenal ulcer). Four-and-a-half million people in the United States suffer from active peptic ulcer disease, and 500,000 new cases of peptic ulcer disease are diagnosed each year. The lifetime prevalence of peptic ulcer disease is approximately 10%, and the estimated annual cost for treatment exceeds $1 billion.

There are several pathophysiologic mechanisms for peptic ulcer disease, and clinical management often requires multiple pharmacologic strategies. This chapter describes the physiology of gastric acid secretion and the pathophysiology underlying the formation of peptic ulcers. The pharmacologic agents used in the treatment of peptic ulcer disease are then discussed in relation to the pathophysiology that is interrupted by these drugs.

▮ PHYSIOLOGY OF GASTRIC ACID SECRETION

Neurohormonal Control of Gastric Acid Secretion

Hydrochloric acid is secreted into the stomach by **parietal cells**, which are located in oxyntic glands in the fundus and body of the stomach. The parietal cell actively transports H^+ across its apical canalicular membranes via H^+/K^+ ATPases (proton pumps) that exchange intracellular H^+ for extracellular K^+. Three neurohormonal secretagogues regulate this process: **histamine**, **gastrin**, and **acetylcholine (ACh)**. Each of these secretagogues binds to and activates specific receptors on the basolateral membrane of the parietal cell, thereby initiating the biochemical changes necessary for active transport of H^+ out of the cell.

Histamine, released by **enterochromaffin-like (ECL) cells** located in and adjacent to the oxyntic glands and by **mast cells** in the lamina propria, binds to histamine **H$_2$ receptors** on the parietal cell. H$_2$ receptor activation stimulates adenylyl cyclase and increases intracellular cyclic adenosine monophosphate (cAMP). In turn, cAMP activates cAMP-dependent protein kinase (protein kinase A [PKA]). PKA phosphorylates and activates proteins responsible for trafficking of cytoplasmic tubulovesicles containing H^+/K^+ ATPase to the apical membrane of the cell. The H^+/K^+ ATPase does not pump H^+ into the tubulovesicles because the permeability of the vesicular membrane to K^+ is low. After fusion of the tubulovesicles with the apical membrane, the availability of extracellular K^+ allows the H^+/K^+ ATPase to pump H^+ from the parietal cell into the gastric lumen. Concurrent with the trafficking of cytoplasmic tubulovesicles to the apical membrane, cellular

---

CASE 1

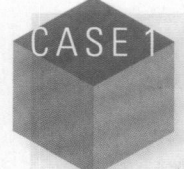

Tom is a 24-year-old graduate student. He is in good health, although he smokes approximately two packs of cigarettes and drinks five cups of coffee a day. He is currently under stress because of the impending deadline for his computer science thesis.

For the past 2 weeks, Tom has noted a burning pain in his upper abdomen that occurs 1–2 hours after eating. In addition, the pain frequently awakens him at approximately 3:00 AM. His pain is usually relieved by eating and by taking over-the-counter antacids.

When the pain increases in intensity, Tom decides to visit his internist, Dr. Smith, at University Health Services. Dr. Smith notes that the abdominal examination is normal except for epigastric tenderness. Dr. Smith discusses diagnostic options with Tom, including an upper gastrointestinal x-ray series and an endoscopic examination. Tom chooses to undergo the endoscopic examination. During the examination, an ulcer is identified in the proximal portion of the duodenum on the posterior wall. The ulcer is 0.5 cm in diameter. A mucosal biopsy of the gastric antrum is performed for detection of *Helicobacter pylori*.

Tom is diagnosed with a duodenal ulcer. Dr. Smith prescribes omeprazole, a proton pump inhibitor. The next day, when the pathology report indicates the presence of an *H. pylori* infection, Dr. Smith prescribes bismuth, clarithromycin, and amoxicillin in addition to the proton pump inhibitor. Dr. Smith also advises Tom to stop smoking and drinking coffee.

Questions

1. What risk factors did Tom have for the development of peptic ulcer disease? What is the role of *H. pylori* in this disease?
2. Why was Tom given clarithromycin rather than metronidazole for treatment of his *H. pylori* infection?
3. Why was Tom also treated with a proton pump inhibitor?

CASE 2

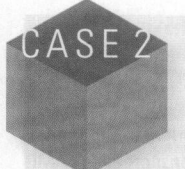

Marianne is a 54-year-old administrator in a printing shop who types 4–5 hours a day. She develops carpal tunnel syndrome and begins to take several aspirin daily for the pain. One month later, Marianne develops a burning pain in her upper abdomen. After vomiting "coffee grounds" material and noticing that her bowel movements are black, she decides to visit the emergency room of her local hospital. The on-call gastroenterologist performs an endoscopy and confirms that Marianne has a gastric ulcer that has recently bled. The gastroenterologist explains to Marianne that she has a peptic ulcer. Marianne's breath test is negative for *H. pylori*, and she is told that aspirin is the most likely cause. Marianne is treated with antacids and ranitidine (an H_2 receptor antagonist) and is told to stop taking nonsteroidal anti-inflammatory drugs (NSAIDs), including aspirin. The gastroenterologist reviews with Marianne the list of pain-relieving medications that are considered to be NSAIDs.

Two weeks pass. Marianne informs her gastroenterologist that the pain in her wrist has become unbearable and that she must continue taking aspirin to be able to type at work and keep her job. The gastroenterologist tells Marianne that she can take aspirin as long as she switches her antiulcer medication from an H_2 antagonist to a proton pump inhibitor.

Questions

4. Why was an H_2 antagonist prescribed for Marianne's ulcer, and why was her medication switched to a proton pump inhibitor when she insisted on using aspirin?

---

activation mobilizes an apical membrane K^+ channel to provide the extracellular K^+ for this process (Fig. 47-1).

Gastrin is secreted into the bloodstream by **G cells** in the gastric antrum, and **acetylcholine** is released from postganglionic nerves with cell bodies located in the submucosa (Meissner's plexus). Both of these secretagogues bind to their respective G protein-coupled receptors on the parietal cell and thereby activate phospholipase C and increase intracellular calcium levels (Ca^{2+}) (Fig. 47-1). Beyond the involvement of phospholipase C and intracellular Ca^{2+}, the signaling pathways by which parietal cell stimulation by gastrin and ACh leads to H^+/K^+ ATPase activation remain to be fully elucidated; protein kinase C is likely to be involved. In addition to its relatively minor role in stimulating the parietal cell directly, gastrin has a major role in stimulating the release of histamine by ECL cells (see below).

While histamine, gastrin, and ACh increase acid secretion by parietal cells, **somatostatin-secreting D cells** and **prostaglandins** limit the extent of gastric acid secretion. Somatostatin decreases acid secretion via three mechanisms: (1) inhibition of gastrin release from G cells by a paracrine mechanism, (2) inhibition of histamine release from ECL cells and mast cells, and (3) direct inhibition of parietal cell acid secretion. Prostaglandin E_2 (PGE_2) enhances mucosal resistance to tissue injury by (1) reducing basal and stimulated gastric acid secretion and (2) enhancing epithelial cell bicarbonate secretion, mucus production, cell turnover, and local blood flow.

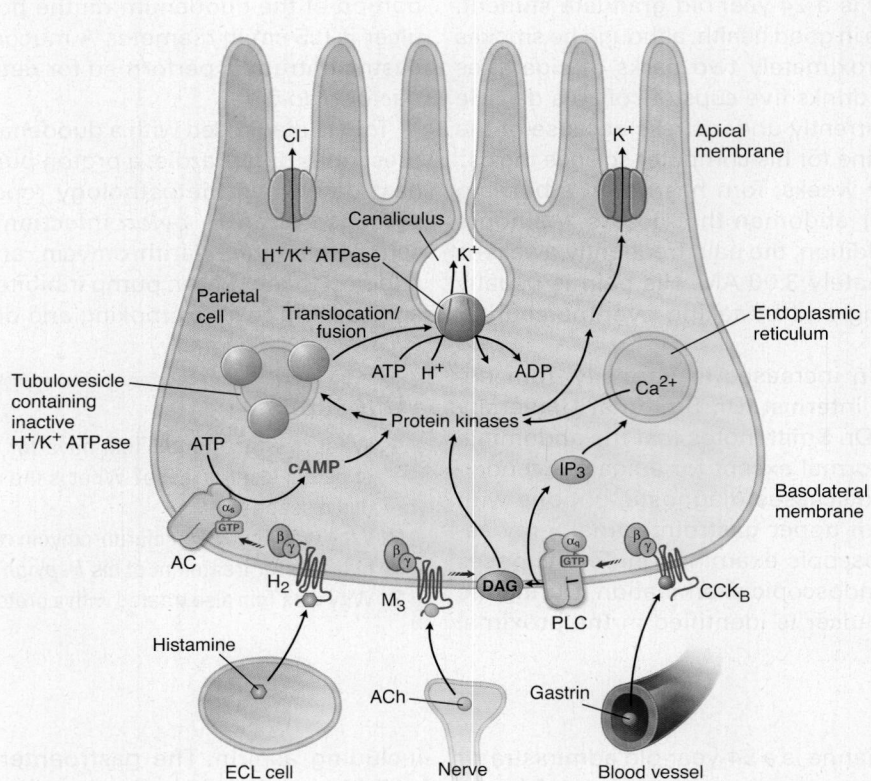

FIGURE 47-1. Control of parietal cell acid secretion. Stimulation of parietal cell acid secretion is modulated by paracrine (histamine), neuroendocrine (acetylcholine [ACh]), and endocrine (gastrin) pathways, which activate their respective receptors (H_2, M_3, and CCK_B). H_2 receptor activation increases cAMP, which activates protein kinase A. M_3 and CCK_B receptor activation stimulates release of Ca^{2+} by the G_q-mediated IP_3/DAG pathway; these signals may also stimulate protein kinase C activity. Protein kinase activation results in translocation of cytoplasmic tubulovesicles containing inactive H^+/K^+ ATPase to the apical membrane. Fusion of tubulovesicles with the apical membrane activates H^+/K^+ ATPase, which pumps H^+ ions into the stomach lumen. An apical membrane Cl^- channel couples Cl^- efflux to H^+ efflux, and an apical membrane K^+ channel recycles K^+ out of the cell. The net result of this process is the rapid extrusion of HCl into the stomach lumen. In addition to its direct effect on CCK_B receptors on parietal cells, gastrin also stimulates CCK_B receptors on ECL cells to promote histamine release (*not shown*).

Phases of Gastric Acid Secretion

Gastric secretions increase considerably during a meal. There are three phases of gastric acid secretion.

The **cephalic phase** includes responses to sight, taste, smell, and thought of food. "Sham feedings," experiments in which food is chewed but not swallowed, trigger an increase in acid secretion mediated by vagal stimulation and increased gastrin secretion.

Mechanical distension of the stomach and ingestion of amino acids and peptides stimulate the **gastric phase**. Distension activates stretch receptors in the wall of the stomach that are linked to short intramural nerves and vagal fibers. Luminal nutrients, such as amino acids, are strong stimulants for gastrin release. Gastrin travels via the blood to the oxyntic mucosa and stimulates ECL cells to release histamine. An important negative feedback on acid secretion in this phase is acid (pH <3)-mediated inhibition of gastrin release from antral G cells. Acid secretion is also inhibited by release of somatostatin from antral D cells.

The **intestinal phase** involves stimulation of gastric acid secretion by digested protein in the intestine. Gastrin plays a major role in mediating this phase as well.

Protective Factors

Factors that protect the gastric mucosa include gastric mucus, prostaglandins (discussed above and in Chapter 43, Pharmacology of Eicosanoids), gastric and duodenal bicarbonate, restitution (repair), and blood flow. The epithelial cells of the stomach secrete **mucus**, which acts as a lubricant that protects the mucosal cells from abrasions. Composed of hydrophilic glycoproteins that are viscous and have gel-forming properties, the mucus layer enables formation of an uninterrupted layer of water at the luminal surface of the epithelium. Together, the mucus and water layers attenuate potential damage due to the acidic environment of the gastric lumen. **Prostaglandins** stimulate mucus secretion, whereas NSAIDs and anticholinergic medications inhibit mucus production. In addition, *H. pylori* disrupts the mucus layer (see below).

Bicarbonate protects the gastric epithelium by neutralizing gastric acid. Bicarbonate is secreted by epithelial cells at the luminal surface of the gastric mucosa, in gastric pits, and at the luminal surface of the duodenal mucosa. Bicarbonate secretion in the duodenum serves to neutralize acid entering the intestine from the stomach.

Restitution refers to the ability of the gastric mucosa to undergo repair. Damage is repaired through migration of undamaged epithelial cells along the basement membrane to fill defects created by the sloughing of injured cells.

The final protective factor is **blood flow**. Blood flow to the gastric mucosa removes acid that has diffused across a damaged mucus layer.

PATHOPHYSIOLOGY OF PEPTIC ULCER DISEASE

A peptic ulcer is a break in the lining of the stomach or duodenum. The break can involve the mucosa, muscularis mucosa, submucosa, and in some cases, the deeper layers of the muscle wall. This compromise of mucosal integrity can cause pain, bleeding, obstruction, perforation, and even death. Peptic ulcers are caused by an imbalance between protective factors and damaging factors in the gastrointestinal mucosa. This section describes the main pathophysiologic mechanisms involved in ulcer formation, the two most common of which are *H. pylori* infection and NSAID use.

Helicobacter pylori

H. pylori, a Gram-negative, spiral-shaped bacterium, is the most common cause of non-NSAID-associated peptic ulcer disease. *H. pylori* has been found in the gastric antrum of a significant number of patients with duodenal ulcers and gastric ulcers, including Tom in the introductory case. Eradication of *H. pylori* leads to lower recurrence and relapse rates in patients with ulcers. The latter finding, together with the fact that many ulcer patients are infected with *H. pylori*, constitute the major evidence for *H. pylori*'s causal role in peptic ulcer disease.

H. pylori lives in the acidic environment of the stomach. The initial infection is transmitted by the oral route. Upon ingestion, the microaerophilic bacterium uses its four to six flagellae to move in corkscrew fashion through the gastric mucus layer. *H. pylori* attaches to adhesion molecules on the surface of gastric epithelial cells. In the duodenum, *H. pylori* attaches only to areas containing gastric epithelial cells that have arisen as a result of excess acid damage to the duodenal mucosa (gastric metaplasia). *H. pylori* is able to live in such a hostile environment partly because of its production of the enzyme **urease**, which converts urea to ammonia. The ammonia buffers the H^+ and forms ammonium hydroxide, creating an alkaline cloud around the bacterium and protecting it from the acidic environment of the stomach.

H. pylori's virulence factors cause damage to the host. Urease is one of these damaging factors because it is an antigen that causes a strong immune response. In addition, ammonium hydroxide produced by urease causes gastric epithelial cell injury. Other virulence factors include lipopolysaccharides (endotoxins), which are components of the bacteria's outer membrane, as well as a lipase and a protease that are secreted by the bacteria and degrade the gastric mucosa. Cytotoxicity caused by *H. pylori* has also been linked to two major proteins: cytotoxin-associated gene A (Cag A) and vacuolating cytotoxin (VacA). The *cag* pathogenicity island is linked to expression of Cag A. This pathogenicity island, which is present in the majority of *H. pylori* isolates, contains approximately 32 genes that encode a bacterial type IV secretion system. The secretion system inserts into gastric epithelial cells of the host and transports Cag A (and other virulence factors) into the epithelial cells. Once inside the host cell, Cag A undergoes tyrosine phosphorylation by host kinases. Both unphosphorylated and phosphorylated Cag A influence host signaling pathways and host cellular functions, including acid secretion, cytokine release, cellular proliferation and apoptosis, cell polarity, and cell motility. Compared to strains of *H. pylori* that do not express Cag A, *H. pylori* strains expressing Cag A have been linked to a higher incidence of duodenal ulcers, gastric ulcers, and gastric cancer.

The persistence of *H. pylori* can be traced, in part, to the inappropriate immune response that it elicits. Instead of the normal T_H2 mucosal immunity response, which controls luminal infections by means of secretory (IgA) antibody, the *H. pylori* organism elicits a T_H1 response. Cytokines associated with the T_H1 response induce inflammation and epithelial cell damage.

Several additional mechanisms characterize *H. pylori*-induced peptic ulcer disease (Fig. 47-2). Acid secretion is

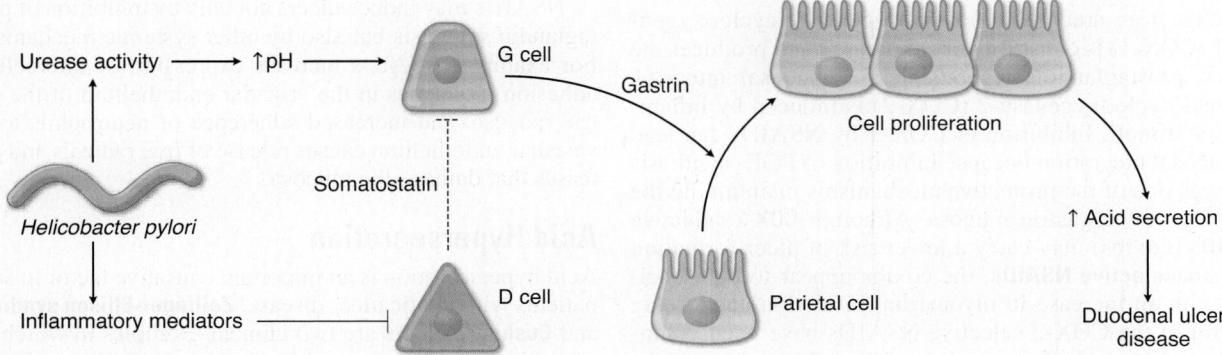

FIGURE 47-2. The role of *H. pylori* in duodenal peptic ulcer disease. Two of the mechanisms by which *H. pylori* infection predisposes to peptic ulcer disease are illustrated. First, the inflammatory mediators elicited by *H. pylori* inhibit somatostatin secretion by D cells in the antrum of the stomach. Decreased D cell somatostatin secretion causes disinhibition of gastrin release from G cells. Second, the ammonium hydroxide produced by *H. pylori*-derived urease increases gastric pH, which in turn stimulates gastrin secretion. Activation of gastrin release by both of these mechanisms leads to parietal cell proliferation, which increases the functional capacity of the gastric mucosa to secrete H^+ ions and thereby predisposes to the development of duodenal ulcer disease.

increased in patients with *H. pylori*-associated duodenal ulcers. This is thought to result from increased levels of circulating gastrin, causing parietal cell proliferation and increased acid production. Gastrin secretion is elevated by two mechanisms: (1) the ammonia generated by *H. pylori* produces an alkaline environment near the G cells and thereby stimulates gastrin release and (2) the number of antral D cells is lower than normal in *H. pylori*-infected patients, resulting in decreased somatostatin production and increased gastrin release. *H. pylori* also decreases duodenal bicarbonate secretion and thereby weakens the protective mechanisms of the duodenal mucosa.

The presence of *H. pylori* infection can be detected using the ^{13}C-urea breath test, which is based on the organism's production of urease. In this test, urease converts ingested ^{13}C-urea to ^{13}CO$_2$ if *H. pylori* is present in the stomach, and the ^{13}CO$_2$ is detected in the breath. The ^{13}C-urea breath test is currently the best diagnostic test for *H. pylori*; other methods of detection include a stool antigen test, histologic examination of a gastric mucosal biopsy (as was performed in Tom's case), and serologic testing for *H. pylori* antibodies. Serologic testing is of limited utility because the blood test for antibodies remains positive indefinitely. Thus, a positive serologic test does not differentiate an active infection from exposure to the organism in the distant past.

NSAIDs

More than 100,000 patients are hospitalized each year for NSAID-associated gastrointestinal complications, and gastrointestinal bleeding has a 5–10% mortality rate in these patients. The gastrointestinal tract is the most common target for the adverse effects of NSAID use.

NSAID-associated gastrointestinal damage is attributable to both *topical injury* and *systemic effects* of the NSAID (Fig. 47-3). Most NSAIDs are weak organic acids. In the acidic environment of the stomach, these drugs are neutral compounds that can cross the plasma membrane and enter gastric epithelial cells. In the neutral intracellular environment, the drugs are re-ionized and trapped. The resulting intracellular damage is responsible for the local gastrointestinal injury associated with NSAID use.

NSAIDs also cause systemic injury to the gastrointestinal lining, largely because of decreased mucosal prostaglandin synthesis. As described in detail in Chapter 43, two cyclooxygenase enzymes catalyze the formation of prostaglandins from arachidonic acid. In general, cyclooxygenase-1 (COX-1) is constitutively expressed and produces the gastric prostaglandins responsible for mucosal integrity, whereas cyclooxygenase-2 (COX-2) is induced by inflammatory stimuli. Inhibition of COX-1 by NSAIDs can lead to mucosal ulceration because inhibition of PGE$_2$ synthesis removes one of the protective mechanisms maintaining the integrity of the gastric mucosa. Although **COX-2 selective NSAIDs** (coxibs) may carry a lower risk of ulcer formation than **nonselective NSAIDs**, the coxibs appear to be associated with an increase in myocardial infarction and stroke. Several of the COX-2 selective NSAIDs have been voluntarily withdrawn (rofecoxib and valdecoxib), and use of the third has been voluntarily limited (celecoxib). The adverse cardiovascular effects of the COX-2 selective inhibitors may result from their suppression of prostacyclin production by vascular endothelial cells (catalyzed by COX-1 and COX-2), allowing thromboxane produced by platelets

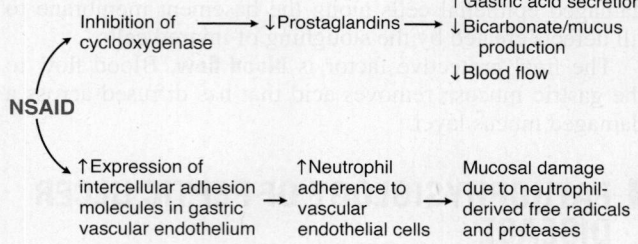

A Systemic effects

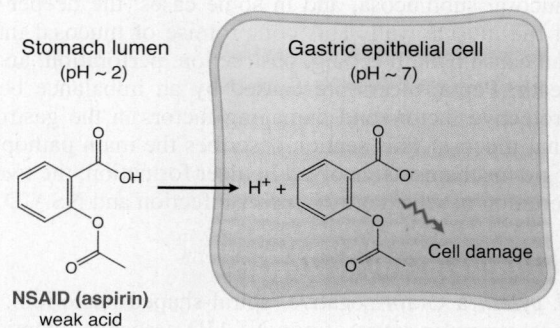

B Topical injury

FIGURE 47-3. Role of NSAIDs in peptic ulcer disease. NSAID-associated peptic ulcer disease is a result of both systemic effects and topical injury. **A.** Systemic effects: NSAIDs inhibit cyclooxygenase and thereby decrease the production of prostaglandins. Because prostaglandins activate G$_i$, and thereby decrease the generation of cAMP in gastric parietal cells, decreased prostaglandin production causes increased gastric acid secretion. Decreased prostaglandins also decrease bicarbonate production, mucus production, and blood flow in the stomach. An additional systemic effect involves the increased expression of intercellular adhesion molecules (ICAMs) in the vascular endothelium of the stomach, which increases neutrophil adherence to the vascular endothelial cells. Neutrophils release free radicals and proteases that cause mucosal damage. **B.** Topical effects: NSAIDs induce local injury via ion trapping. From the lumen of the stomach, the drug enters the gastric epithelial cell in its protonated (uncharged) form. In the neutral environment of the cytoplasm, the NSAID is ionized and trapped inside the cell, causing cell damage.

(catalyzed by COX-1) to exert an unopposed prothrombotic effect (see Chapter 43).

NSAIDs may induce ulcers not only by inhibition of prostaglandin synthesis but also by other systemic mechanisms. For example, NSAIDs increase expression of intercellular adhesion molecules in the vascular endothelium of the gastric mucosa, and increased adherence of neutrophils to the vascular endothelium causes release of free radicals and proteases that damage the mucosa.

Acid Hypersecretion

Acid hypersecretion is an important causative factor in some patients with peptic ulcer disease. **Zollinger-Ellison syndrome** and **Cushing's ulcers** are two clinical examples in which hyperacidity leads to peptic ulcer disease. In Zollinger-Ellison syndrome, a gastrin-secreting tumor of the non-beta cells of the endocrine pancreas leads to increased acid secretion. In Cushing's ulcers, seen in patients with severe head injuries, heightened vagal (cholinergic) tone causes gastric hyperacidity (see Fig. 47-1).

Other Factors

Gastric chief cells secrete pepsin, a digestive enzyme, as the inactive precursor pepsinogen. Studies have suggested a role for pepsin in ulcer formation. Cigarette smoking is associated with peptic ulcer disease; the mechanism is thought to involve impairment of mucosal blood flow and healing and inhibition of pancreatic bicarbonate production. Caffeine ingestion (increased acid secretion), alcoholic cirrhosis, glucocorticoid use, and genetic influences are also associated with peptic ulcer disease. Finally, chronic psychological stress may occasionally be an important cause of peptic ulcer disease. In Case 1, Tom smoked cigarettes, drank a lot of coffee, and was under stress to finish his computer science thesis. These factors may have contributed to his development of an ulcer.

▌ PHARMACOLOGIC CLASSES AND AGENTS

Several pathophysiologic mechanisms can lead to peptic ulcer disease, and clinical management requires consideration of multiple pharmacologic options. The available agents can be divided into drugs that (1) decrease acid secretion, (2) neutralize acid, (3) promote mucosal defense, and (4) modify risk factors (Fig. 47-4).

Agents That Decrease Acid Secretion

H₂ Receptor Antagonists

The discovery of **H₂ receptor antagonists** by Black and colleagues in the 1970s significantly changed the treatment of peptic ulcer disease. These investigators identified a second histamine receptor (H₁ was the first; see Chapter 44, Histamine Pharmacology) and elucidated its role in gastric acid secretion. H₂ receptor antagonists (also called **H₂ blockers**) reversibly and competitively inhibit the binding of histamine to H₂ receptors, resulting in suppression of gastric acid secretion. H₂ receptor antagonists also indirectly decrease gastrin- and acetylcholine-induced gastric acid secretion.

Four H₂ receptor antagonists are available: **cimetidine**, **ranitidine**, **famotidine**, and **nizatidine** (Fig. 47-5). H₂ receptor antagonists are absorbed rapidly from the small intestine. Peak plasma concentrations are achieved within 1–3 hours. Elimination of H₂ receptor antagonists involves both renal excretion and hepatic metabolism. It is therefore important to decrease the dose of these drugs in patients with liver or kidney failure. An exception is nizatidine, which is eliminated primarily by the kidney.

All four drugs are well tolerated in general. Occasional minor adverse effects include diarrhea, headache, muscle pain, constipation, and fatigue. H₂ receptor antagonists may

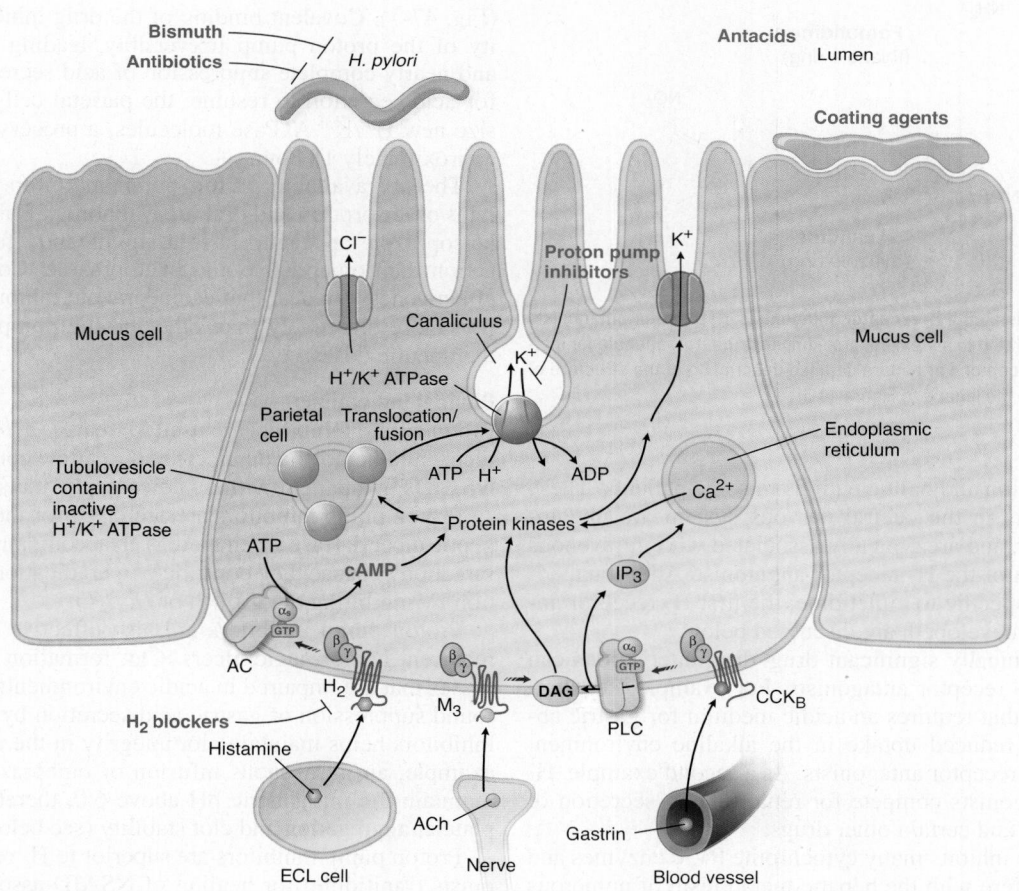

FIGURE 47-4. Sites of action of drugs used to treat peptic ulcer disease. H₂ receptor antagonists (H₂ blockers) inhibit activation of the histamine H₂ receptor by endogenous histamine. Proton pump inhibitors decrease the activity of the H⁺/K⁺ ATPase on the canalicular membrane of the parietal cell. Antacids neutralize acid in the stomach lumen. Coating agents provide a protective layer on the epithelial surface of the gastric mucosa. Bismuth and antibiotics act to eradicate *H. pylori* from the mucus layer coating the gastric mucosa. *H. pylori* infection is an important contributing factor in the pathogenesis of peptic ulcer disease.

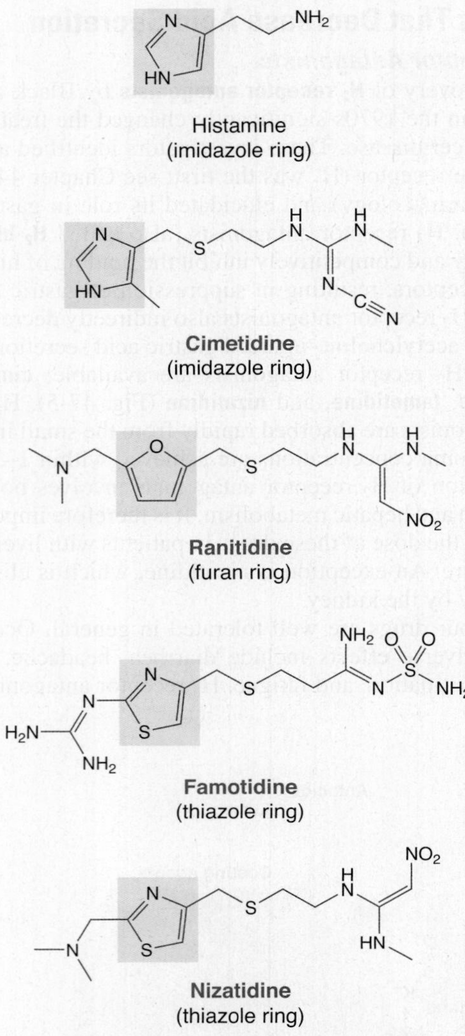

Histamine
(imidazole ring)

Cimetidine
(imidazole ring)

Ranitidine
(furan ring)

Famotidine
(thiazole ring)

Nizatidine
(thiazole ring)

FIGURE 47-5. Histamine H₂ receptor antagonists. H₂ receptor antagonists share moieties related to histamine, providing a structural rationale for inhibition of the H₂ receptor. For a more detailed description of the structure of these agents, see the legend to Figure 44-5.

induce confusion and hallucinations in some patients. These adverse effects in the central nervous system are uncommon, however, and are typically associated with intravenous administration of the H₂ receptor antagonist. Additional adverse effects specific to cimetidine, the first H₂ receptor antagonist to be developed, are discussed below.

Several clinically significant drug–drug interactions can occur with H₂ receptor antagonists. For example, ketoconazole, a drug that requires an acidic medium for gastric absorption, has reduced uptake in the alkaline environment created by H₂ receptor antagonists. As a second example, H₂ receptor antagonists compete for renal tubular secretion of procainamide and certain other drugs.

Cimetidine inhibits many cytochrome P450 enzymes and thus can interfere with the hepatic metabolism of numerous drugs. For example, cimetidine can decrease the metabolism of lidocaine, phenytoin, quinidine, theophylline, and warfarin, facilitating the accumulation of these drugs to toxic levels. Cimetidine appears to inhibit P450 enzymes to a greater extent than the other H₂ receptor antagonists, and

an H₂ receptor antagonist other than cimetidine may be preferred when the patient is prescribed multiple medications.

Cimetidine crosses the placenta and is secreted into breast milk and is therefore not recommended for use during pregnancy or when nursing. Cimetidine can have antiandrogenic effects because of its action as an antagonist at the androgen receptor, resulting in gynecomastia (enlarged breasts) and impotence in men and, rarely, galactorrhea (discharge of milk) in women.

Proton Pump Inhibitors

Proton pump inhibitors block the parietal cell H^+/K^+ ATPase (proton pump). Compared to H₂ receptor antagonists, proton pump inhibitors are superior at suppressing acid secretion and promoting peptic ulcer healing. **Omeprazole** is the prototype proton pump inhibitor. Several other proton pump inhibitors have also been developed, including **esomeprazole** (the [S]-enantiomer of omeprazole), **rabeprazole**, **lansoprazole**, **dexlansoprazole** (the [R]-enantiomer of lansoprazole), and **pantoprazole** (Fig. 47-6).

All of the proton pump inhibitors are prodrugs that require activation in the acidic environment of the parietal cell canaliculus. Oral formulations of these drugs are enteric-coated to prevent premature activation. The prodrug is converted to its active **sulfenamide** form in the acidic canalicular environment, and the sulfenamide reacts with a cysteine residue on the H^+/K^+ ATPase to form a covalent disulfide bond (Fig. 47-7). Covalent binding of the drug inhibits the activity of the proton pump irreversibly, leading to prolonged and nearly complete suppression of acid secretion. In order for acid secretion to resume, the parietal cell must synthesize new H^+/K^+ ATPase molecules, a process that requires approximately 18 hours.

The six available proton pump inhibitors have similar rates of absorption and oral bioavailability. Rabeprazole and lansoprazole appear to have a significantly faster onset of action than omeprazole and pantoprazole. Comparisons of effectiveness suggest that esomeprazole inhibits acid secretion more effectively than other proton pump inhibitors at therapeutic doses.

Clinical Indications

Proton pump inhibitors are used to treat *H. pylori*-associated ulcers and hemorrhagic ulcers and to allow continued use of NSAIDs in a patient with a known peptic ulcer.

Proton pump inhibitors are preferred for the treatment of peptic ulcer disease when there is an accompanying *H. pylori* infection because they contribute to eradication of the infection by inhibiting the growth of *H. pylori*.

Proton pump inhibitors are also effective in preventing recurrent hemorrhagic ulcers. Clot formation involves processes that are impaired in acidic environments, and the profound suppression of gastric acid secretion by proton pump inhibitors helps maintain clot integrity in the ulcer bed. For example, an intravenous infusion of omeprazole is able to maintain the intragastric pH above 6.0, thereby supporting platelet aggregation and clot stability (see below).

Proton pump inhibitors are superior to H₂ receptor antagonists (ranitidine) for healing of NSAID-associated gastric and duodenal ulcers when the patient continues NSAID use, most likely because proton pump inhibitors are better able to sustain a constant increase in gastric pH.

Several considerations may favor the use of H₂ receptor antagonists over proton pump inhibitors. H₂ receptor antagonists

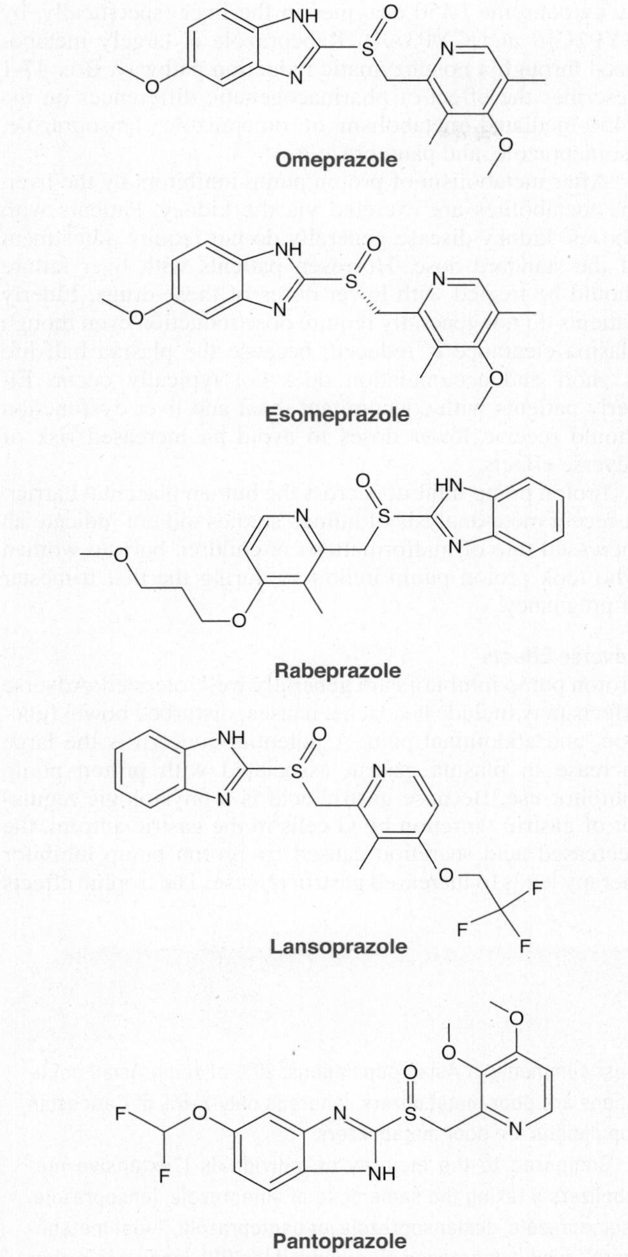

Omeprazole

Esomeprazole

Rabeprazole

Lansoprazole

Pantoprazole

FIGURE 47-6. Proton pump inhibitors. The proton pump inhibitors are a family of structurally related prodrugs that are all activated by the mechanism shown in Figure 47-7. Note that esomeprazole is the (S)-enantiomer of omeprazole, which is formulated as a racemic mixture of (R)- and (S)-enantiomers. Dexlansoprazole (*not shown*) is the (R)-enantiomer of lansoprazole.

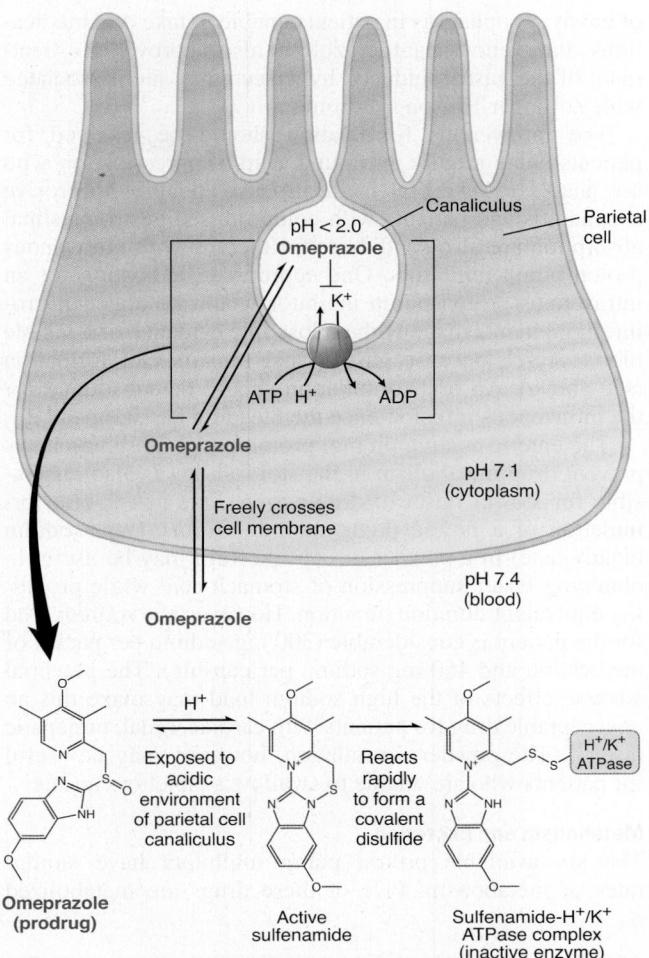

FIGURE 47-7. Mechanism of action of omeprazole, a proton pump inhibitor. Omeprazole freely enters the cytoplasm of the parietal cell (pH 7.1) in uncharged form. In the acidic environment of the parietal cell canalicular system (pH <2.0), omeprazole is converted to its active sulfenamide form. The sulfenamide reacts with a cysteine residue on the H^+/K^+ ATPase to form a covalent disulfide bond. Covalent modification of the H^+/K^+ ATPase inhibits the activity of the proton pump and thereby prevents acid secretion.

In Case 1, Tom was given a proton pump inhibitor because he was found to have an associated *H. pylori* infection. In Case 2, the gastroenterologist recommended a proton pump inhibitor to allow for the concomitant use of an NSAID.

Formulations

Four of the six proton pump inhibitors (omeprazole, esomeprazole, lansoprazole, and pantoprazole) are available in intravenous dosage forms. Intravenous formulations of proton pump inhibitors are useful clinically because this delivery route bypasses the harsh acidic environment of the stomach and upper duodenum. Intravenous delivery allows more of the drug to reach its site of action in the parietal cell canaliculus without degradation. For example, esomeprazole has a twofold higher peak concentration and a 66–83% greater area under the plasma concentration curve (AUC) when the dose is delivered intravenously instead of orally. The US Food and Drug Administration (FDA) has approved intravenous formulations of lansoprazole (7-day limit), esomeprazole (10-day limit), and pantoprazole (10-day limit) for treatment

have been in use longer than proton pump inhibitors, and their adverse effects are better studied. This may be an especially important consideration for pregnant women because H_2 receptor antagonists (with the exception of cimetidine) have proven to be safe in pregnancy, whereas the safety of proton pump inhibitors in pregnancy is less certain. In addition, H_2 receptor antagonists are generally less expensive than proton pump inhibitors. The possibility that proton pump inhibitors may cause gastric carcinoid tumors is sometimes raised as a concern for long-term proton pump inhibitor therapy, although this association has not been observed in humans.

of erosive esophagitis in patients unable to take oral medications. Intravenous pantoprazole is also approved for treatment of the gastrin-induced hypersecretory state associated with Zollinger-Ellison syndrome.

The intravenous formulation should be reserved for patients who require profound acid suppression or who are unable to take oral medications. Patients with erosive esophagitis and patients with compromised gastrointestinal absorption are also candidates for therapy with intravenous proton pump inhibitors. One appropriate indication for an intravenous proton pump inhibitor would be upper gastrointestinal hemorrhage with endoscopic evidence of a visible blood vessel, because gastric acid impairs clot formation (see above). An oral formulation should be substituted for the intravenous infusion once the bleeding has stopped.

The enteric coating on oral proton pump inhibitors helps prevent drug metabolism in the stomach but is also responsible for slower onset of drug action. One newer oral formulation of a proton pump inhibitor (omeprazole/sodium bicarbonate) in a powder or capsule form may be useful in obtaining faster suppression of stomach acid while providing equivalent duration of action. However, the sodium load for the patient is considerable (300 mg sodium per packet of medication and 460 mg sodium per capsule). The potential adverse effects of the high sodium load may make this an unacceptable drug for patients with cardiac, renal, or hepatic disease. The powder formulation, however, may be useful for patients who are unable to swallow a tablet or capsule.

Metabolism and Excretion
The six available proton pump inhibitors have similar rates of metabolism. Five of these drugs are metabolized

by cytochrome P450 enzymes in the liver (specifically, by CYP2C19 and CYP3A4). Rabeprazole is largely metabolized through a nonenzymatic reduction pathway. Box 47-1 describes the effect of pharmacogenetic differences on the P450-mediated metabolism of omeprazole, lansoprazole, esomeprazole, and pantoprazole.

After metabolism of proton pump inhibitors by the liver, the metabolites are excreted via the kidney. Patients with chronic kidney disease generally do not require adjustment of the standard dose. However, patients with liver failure should be treated with lower doses of these drugs. Elderly patients do not generally require dose reduction even though plasma clearance is reduced, because the plasma half-life is short and accumulation does not typically occur. Elderly patients with concomitant renal and liver dysfunction should receive lower doses to avoid an increased risk of adverse effects.

Proton pump inhibitors cross the human placental barrier. A recent meta-analysis of human studies did not indicate an increased rate of malformations in children born to women who took proton pump inhibitors during the first trimester of pregnancy.

Adverse Effects
Proton pump inhibitors are generally well tolerated. Adverse effects may include headache, nausea, disturbed bowel function, and abdominal pain. A potential concern is the large increase in plasma gastrin associated with proton pump inhibitor use. Because gastric acid is a physiologic regulator of gastrin secretion by G cells in the gastric antrum, the decreased acid secretion caused by proton pump inhibitor therapy leads to increased gastrin release. The trophic effects

BOX 47-1 Metabolism of Proton Pump Inhibitors

An individual's response to treatment with a proton pump inhibitor (PPI) may vary from a marked decrease in acid secretion to little change in acid secretion. The pharmacogenetics of drug metabolism is the major factor responsible for this variation. Omeprazole, lansoprazole, esomeprazole, dexlansoprazole, and pantoprazole are extensively metabolized in the liver to less active or inactive metabolites; of these five PPIs, omeprazole is the most extensively metabolized and pantoprazole is the least extensively metabolized. Metabolism of the PPIs involves two cytochrome P450 isoenzymes: CYP2C19 and CYP3A4 (also called *P450 2C19* and *P450 3A4*, respectively). CYP2C19 is responsible for the major metabolism of PPIs, while CYP3A4 functions as an ancillary metabolic pathway when the main pathway through CYP2C19 is saturated. Studies have shown that individuals have different rates of metabolism and clearance of these drugs because of genetic polymorphisms in their CYP2C19 isoenzymes.

Two polymorphisms of CYP2C19 (CYP2C19m1 and CYP2C19m2) are associated with decreased enzyme activity. Carriers of two copies of the polymorphisms are "poor metabolizers" of PPIs. Carriers of one copy of the polymorphisms are "intermediate to extensive metabolizers"; their rate of CYP2C19-mediated drug metabolism is reduced but not to the extent of individuals with two copies of the polymorphisms. These polymorphisms exist

most commonly in Asian populations: 20% of some Asian populations are poor metabolizers, whereas only 2–6% of Caucasian populations are poor metabolizers.

Compared to the majority of individuals ("extensive metabolizers") taking the same dose of omeprazole, lansoprazole, esomeprazole, dexlansoprazole, or pantoprazole, "poor metabolizers" exhibit decreased clearance of the PPI, leading to higher plasma concentrations of the drug and greater degrees of acid suppression. Fortunately, the standard recommended doses of PPIs take these differences into account, and most patients reach a sufficient degree of acid suppression regardless of the variability in metabolism of these drugs. Pharmacogenetic differences in PPI metabolism can lead to potentially significant drug–drug interactions, however. To date, only omeprazole has been found to interact with other drugs metabolized by CYP2C19. Although clinically significant interactions do not generally occur, awareness should be high if patients are taking omeprazole concomitantly with warfarin, phenytoin, diazepam, or carbamazepine. In the future, screening for the presence of CYP2C19 polymorphisms could allow physicians to determine which PPI is most appropriate for each patient and what dosage should most effectively favor acid suppression while avoiding drug–drug interactions. ■

of gastrin can induce hyperplasia of ECL cells and parietal cells in the gastric mucosa. Although rats treated for long periods with omeprazole developed gastric carcinoid tumors, these tumors have not been observed in humans. Patients with Zollinger-Ellison syndrome usually develop ECL and parietal cell hyperplasia, and some develop carcinoid tumors, but no increase in carcinoid tumors has been found in Zollinger-Ellison patients taking proton pump inhibitors. Hypergastrinemia can also result in rebound hypersecretion of acid upon discontinuation of the proton pump inhibitor.

Several recent studies suggest that proton pump inhibitors may decrease the clinical efficacy of the antiplatelet agent clopidogrel. One rationale for this potential drug–drug interaction could be that proton pump inhibitors and clopidogrel share a common metabolic pathway mediated by the cytochrome P450 isoenzyme CYP2C19 in the liver: most proton pump inhibitors are metabolized by CYP2C19 (see above), and clopidogrel is converted from a prodrug to the active drug form by the same enzyme. The clinical importance of this interaction remains uncertain, however, as observational studies have revealed conflicting results, and at least one large clinical trial has found no significant difference in adverse clinical outcomes (cardiovascular death, myocardial infarction, or stroke) between individuals treated with clopidogrel alone and individuals treated concomitantly with clopidogrel and a proton pump inhibitor.

Some studies suggest an increased risk of hip fracture in patients who take proton pump inhibitors for an extended period of time. Research on this topic has yielded conflicting evidence to date: some studies suggest that proton pump inhibitor therapy may decrease gastric absorption of insoluble calcium by raising gastric pH, but other studies suggest that omeprazole may decrease bone resorption by inhibiting osteoclastic vacuolar H^+/K^+ ATPase.

Use of proton pump inhibitors during hospital admission has been shown to increase the risk for hospital-acquired pneumonia, *Clostridium difficile* infection, and enteric infections with *Salmonella* and *Escherichia coli*. This increased risk may be related to compromise of a normal defense mechanism (i.e., gastric acid) by the proton pump inhibitor, allowing ingested organisms to escape acid-mediated destruction.

Theoretically, anticholinergic agents could be used to antagonize M_3 muscarinic ACh receptors on parietal cells and thereby decrease gastric acid secretion. However, anticholinergic agents are not used in the treatment of peptic ulcer disease because they are not as effective as H_2 receptor antagonists or proton pump inhibitors and they have many adverse anticholinergic effects.

Agents That Neutralize Acid

Antacids are used on an as-needed basis for symptomatic relief of dyspepsia. These agents neutralize hydrochloric acid by reacting with the acid to form water and salts. The most widely used antacids are mixtures of **aluminum hydroxide** and **magnesium hydroxide**. The hydroxide ion reacts with hydrogen ions in the stomach to form water, while the magnesium and aluminum react with bicarbonate in pancreatic secretions and with phosphates in the diet to form salts. Common adverse effects associated with these antacids include diarrhea (magnesium) and constipation (aluminum). When antacids containing aluminum and magnesium are taken together, constipation and diarrhea may be avoided. Antacids containing aluminum can bind phosphate; the resulting hypophosphatemia can cause weakness, malaise, and anorexia. In patients with chronic kidney disease, aluminum-containing antacids have been reported to cause neurotoxicity. Patients with chronic kidney disease should avoid magnesium-containing antacids because they can lead to hypermagnesemia.

Sodium bicarbonate reacts rapidly with HCl to form water, carbon dioxide, and salt. Antacids containing sodium bicarbonate have high amounts of sodium; in patients with hypertension or fluid overload, sodium-containing antacids can result in significant sodium retention.

Calcium carbonate is less soluble than sodium bicarbonate; it reacts with gastric acid to produce calcium chloride and carbon dioxide. Calcium carbonate is useful not only as an antacid but also as a calcium supplement for prevention of osteoporosis. The high calcium content of this antacid formulation may cause constipation.

Agents That Promote Mucosal Defense

Agents that promote mucosal defense are used in the symptomatic relief of peptic ulcer disease. These drugs include coating agents and prostaglandins.

Coating Agents

Sucralfate, a complex salt of sucrose sulfate and aluminum hydroxide, is a coating agent used to alleviate the symptoms of peptic ulcer disease. Sucralfate has little ability to alter gastric pH. Instead, in the acidic environment of the stomach, this complex forms a viscous gel that binds to positively charged proteins and thereby adheres to gastric epithelial cells (including areas of ulceration). The gel protects the luminal surface of the stomach from degradation by acid and pepsin. Because sucralfate is poorly soluble, there is little systemic absorption and no systemic toxicity. Constipation is one of the few adverse effects. In addition, sucralfate may bind to drugs such as quinolone antibiotics, phenytoin, and warfarin and thereby limit their absorption.

Colloidal bismuth is a second coating agent used in peptic ulcer disease. Bismuth salts combine with mucus glycoproteins to form a barrier that protects an ulcer from further damage by acid and pepsin. Bismuth agents may stimulate mucosal bicarbonate and prostaglandin E_2 secretion and thereby also protect the mucosa from acid and pepsin degradation. Colloidal bismuth has been found to impede the growth of *H. pylori* and is frequently used as part of a multidrug regimen for the eradication of *H. pylori*-associated peptic ulcers (see below).

Prostaglandins

Prostaglandins can be used in the treatment of peptic ulcer disease (see Chapter 43), specifically in the treatment of NSAID-induced ulcers. NSAIDs are ulcerogenic because they inhibit prostaglandin synthesis and thereby interrupt the "gastroprotective" functions of PGE_2, which include reduced gastric acid secretion and enhanced bicarbonate secretion, mucus production, and blood flow.

Misoprostol is a prostaglandin analogue used to prevent NSAID-induced peptic ulcers. Its most frequent adverse effects are abdominal discomfort and diarrhea. In clinical practice, these adverse effects often interfere with patient adherence. Misoprostol is contraindicated in women who are (or may be) pregnant because of the possibility of generating uterine contractions that could result in abortion (see Chapter 30, Pharmacology of Reproduction).

Agents That Modify Risk Factors

Diet, Tobacco, and Alcohol

As in Case 1, diet therapy typically involves recommendations to avoid caffeine-containing products because of their ability to increase acid secretion. Avoidance of alcohol and cigarette smoking is also advised. Excessive alcohol intake is directly toxic to the mucosa and is associated with erosive gastritis and an increased incidence of peptic ulcers. Cigarette smoking is thought to decrease the production of duodenal bicarbonate and diminish mucosal blood flow, leading to a delay in ulcer healing.

Treatment of H. pylori Infection

Elimination of *H. pylori* can lead to cure of *H. pylori*-associated peptic ulcers. Treatment for *H. pylori* infection uses broad-spectrum antibiotics, such as **amoxicillin** or **tetracycline** combined with **metronidazole** or **clarithromycin**, together with bismuth citrate and a proton pump inhibitor or ranitidine. Common regimens involve **triple therapy** with amoxicillin, clarithromycin, and a proton pump inhibitor, or **quadruple therapy** with tetracycline, metronidazole, a proton pump inhibitor, and bismuth.

H. pylori may develop resistance to antibiotic therapy. Metronidazole resistance has been reported in the United States in patients with *H. pylori* infections. Resistance to clarithromycin is less common. Three point mutations in the clarithromycin-binding site on *H. pylori* 23S rRNA (A2143G, A2142G, and A2142C) appear to be responsible for clarithromycin resistance, and the A2143G mutation has been associated with a very low bacterial eradication rate. Levofloxacin has recently been suggested as a useful alternative drug (together with amoxicillin) in second-line therapeutic regimens in patients with resistance to clarithromycin. In Case 1, Tom was given clarithromycin rather than metronidazole because the former drug is less commonly associated with drug resistance.

The adverse effects of therapy for *H. pylori* infection include hypersensitivity reactions to penicillin analogues, nausea, headache, and antibiotic-induced diarrhea caused by superinfection with *C. difficile*. These effects, together with the complicated dosing schedules associated with triple therapy and quadruple therapy, can lead to nonadherence. Resistance to *H. pylori* is a growing concern, and antibiotic regimens will need to evolve in order to meet the challenge.

▌CONCLUSION AND FUTURE DIRECTIONS

Peptic ulcer disease is responsible for significant morbidity and mortality in the United States. Because more than one pathophysiologic mechanism is often involved in the disease, multiple pharmacologic agents may be required for its prophylaxis and treatment (Fig. 47-4). Pharmacologic agents active against peptic ulcer disease decrease acid secretion, promote mucosal defense, and modify risk factors. Use of intravenous proton pump inhibitors and screening for cytochrome P450 polymorphisms may allow enhancement and customization of pharmacologic therapy for patients at risk. Improved treatment of *H. pylori* infection has the potential to decrease the overall incidence of peptic ulcer disease. COX-2 inhibitors have fallen short of expectations because of adverse cardiovascular effects. It remains to be seen whether new NSAIDs can be developed that do not promote peptic ulcer formation and have an acceptable cardiovascular effect profile.

Future directions will focus on unraveling and understanding the potential adverse effects that have recently been attributed to proton pump inhibitors. Given the prominence of this class of drugs in current medical practice, the interactions with thienopyridine antiplatelet agents (clopidogrel and prasugrel), the effects on bone formation and resorption, the risk of hospital acquired infections, and the risk of enteric infections will need to be carefully explored.

Suggested Reading

Barletta JF, Sclar DA. Proton pump inhibitors increase the risk for hospital-acquired *Clostridium difficile* infection in critically ill patients. *Crit Care* 2014;18:714–717. (*Case-control study showing that proton pump inhibitors are independent risk factors for the development of* Clostridium difficile *infection in ICU patients.*)

Cardoso RN, Benjo AM, DiNicolantonio JJ, et al. Incidence of cardiovascular events and gastrointestinal bleeding in patients receiving clopidogrel with and without proton pump inhibitors: an update meta-analysis. *Open Heart* 2015;2:e000248. (*Updated review of potential interaction of proton pump inhibitors and clopidogrel.*)

Chan FKL, Lau JYW. Treatment of peptic ulcer disease. In: Feldman M, Friedman LS, Brandt LJ, eds. *Sleisenger and Fordtran's gastrointestinal and liver disease.* 9th ed. Philadelphia: WB Saunders; 2010:869–886. (*Clinical overview of the management of peptic ulcer disease.*)

De Francesco V, Margiotta M, Zullo A, et al. Clarithromycin-resistant genotypes and eradication of *Helicobacter pylori. Ann Intern Med* 2006;144: 94–100. (*Discusses clarithromycin-resistant genotypes in H. pylori.*)

Forte JG, Zhu L. Apical recycling of the gastric parietal cell H,K-ATPase. *Annu Rev Physiol* 2010;72:273–296. (*Detailed review of the membrane recycling pathway responsible for translocation of cytoplasmic tubulovesicles and their fusion with the apical membrane of gastric parietal cells.*)

Herzig SJ, Howell MD, Ngo LH, Marcantonio ER. Acid-suppressive medication use and the risk for hospital-acquired pneumonia. *JAMA* 2009;301:2120–2128. (*Epidemiologic data suggesting an association between proton pump inhibitors and development of pneumonia.*)

Johnson DA, Oldfield EC. Reported side effects and complications of long-term proton pump inhibitor use: dissecting the evidence. *Clin Gastroenterol Hepatol* 2013;11:458–464. (*Recent evidence regarding possible adverse effects of proton pump inhibitors.*)

Kopic S, Murek M, Geibel JP. Revisiting the parietal cell. *Am J Physiol Cell Physiol* 2010;298:C1–C10. (*Detailed review of parietal cell physiology and ion transport, focusing on ion transporters in the apical and basolateral membranes.*)

McColl K. Effect of proton pump inhibitors on vitamins and iron. *Am J Gastroenterol* 2009;104:S5–S9. (*Physiology of proton pump inhibitors and absorption of nutrients.*)

Odenbreit S, Puls J, Sedlmaier B, Gerland E, Fischer W, Haas R. Translocation of *Helicobacter pylori* Cag A into gastric epithelial cells by type IV secretion. *Science* 2000;25:1487–1500. (*Study describing the mechanisms responsible for cagA virulence.*)

Targownik LE, Leslie WD, Davison KS, et al. The relationship between proton pump inhibitor use and longitudinal change in bone mineral density: a population-based study from the Canadian Multicentre Osteoporosis Study (CaMos). *Am J Gastroenterol* 2012;107:1361–1369. (*Clinical data on the possible association between proton pump inhibitors and osteoporosis.*)

DRUG SUMMARY TABLE: CHAPTER 47 Integrative Inflammation Pharmacology: Peptic Ulcer Disease

DRUG	CLINICAL APPLICATIONS	SERIOUS AND COMMON ADVERSE EFFECTS	CONTRAINDICATIONS	THERAPEUTIC CONSIDERATIONS
H₂ RECEPTOR ANTAGONISTS Mechanism—Decrease acid secretion by inhibiting histamine binding to H₂ receptors on parietal cells				
Cimetidine	Peptic ulcer disease Gastroesophageal reflux disease (GERD) Erosive esophagitis Gastric acid hypersecretion Systemic mast call disease Zollinger-Ellison syndrome	*Gastric cancer, necrotizing enterocolitis in fetus or newborn, pancreatitis, psychotic disorder* Gynecomastia	Hypersensitivity to cimetidine	Cimetidine inhibits the cytochrome P450-mediated metabolism of certain drugs, including theophylline, warfarin, phenytoin, lidocaine, and quinidine, delaying the clearance and increasing the plasma levels of these and other drugs.
Ranitidine Famotidine Nizatidine	Shared indications: Peptic ulcer disease Gastroesophageal reflux disease (GERD) Erosive esophagitis Gastric acid hypersecretion Ranitidine only: *Helicobacter pylori* gastrointestinal tract infection Zollinger-Ellison syndrome	*Stevens-Johnson syndrome, toxic epidermal necrolysis, necrotizing enterocolitis in fetus or newborn (shared adverse effects); agranulocytosis, aplastic anemia, pancytopenia, thrombocytopenia, hepatitis, liver failure (ranitidine only); nosocomial pneumonia (famotidine and nizatidine only); thrombocytopenia (nizatidine only)* Headache, abdominal pain, constipation, diarrhea	Hypersensitivity to ranitidine, famotidine, or nizatidine	Ranitidine can be given IV to treat hypersecretory conditions or to treat patients who are not able to tolerate the oral formulation. Bioavailability of nizatidine is higher than that of other H₂ receptor antagonists.
PROTON PUMP INHIBITORS Mechanism—Decrease acid secretion by irreversibly inhibiting H⁺/K⁺ ATPase on parietal cells				
Omeprazole Esomeprazole Rabeprazole Lansoprazole Dexlansoprazole Pantoprazole	Shared indications: Peptic ulcer disease Gastroesophageal reflux disease (GERD) Erosive esophagitis Gastric acid hypersecretion Omeprazole only: Stress ulcer Lansoprazole and pantoprazole only: Zollinger-Ellison syndrome	*Stevens-Johnson syndrome, toxic epidermal necrolysis, pancreatitis, hepatotoxicity, interstitial nephritis, liver failure, agranulocytosis, hemolytic anemia, possible interference with antiplatelet effects of clopidogrel, possible increased risk of hip, wrist, and spine fracture, rhabdomyolysis, hospital-acquired pneumonia and enteric infections including Clostridium difficile, Salmonella, and Escherichia coli (shared adverse effects); atrophic gastritis (pantoprazole only)* Headache, diarrhea, gastrointestinal discomfort, flatulence	Hypersensitivity to omeprazole, esomeprazole, rabeprazole, lansoprazole, dexlansoprazole, or pantoprazole	Proton pump inhibitors are metabolized in the liver by CYP2C19 and CYP3A4. Pantoprazole can be given IV as an alternative therapy in patients who are not able to tolerate oral pantoprazole. Drug interaction with ketoconazole or itraconazole due to the acid environment required for absorption of these azole drugs.
ANTACIDS Mechanism—Neutralize gastric acid				
Aluminum hydroxide	Symptomatic relief of dyspepsia associated with peptic ulcer disease, gastritis, gastroesophageal reflux disease (GERD), or hiatal hernia	*Phosphate depletion (severe weakness, malaise, anorexia)* Constipation, osteomalacia in patients with renal failure	Hypersensitivity to aluminum hydroxide	All antacids can potentially increase or decrease the rate or extent of absorption of concurrently administered oral drugs by changing transit time or by binding the drug.

continues

DRUG SUMMARY TABLE: CHAPTER 47 Integrative Inflammation Pharmacology: Peptic Ulcer Disease *continued*

DRUG	CLINICAL APPLICATIONS	SERIOUS AND COMMON ADVERSE EFFECTS	CONTRAINDICATIONS	THERAPEUTIC CONSIDERATIONS
ANTACIDS *(continued)* **Mechanism—Neutralize gastric acid**				
Magnesium hydroxide	Symptomatic relief of dyspepsia associated with peptic ulcer disease, gastritis, gastroesophageal reflux disease (GERD), or hiatal hernia	Diarrhea, hypermagnesemia (in patients with renal failure)	Hypersensitivity to magnesium hydroxide	Same as aluminum hydroxide.
Sodium bicarbonate	Diarrhea Indigestion Chronic metabolic acidosis Drug toxicity	*Cellulitis, skin ulcer, tissue necrosis, metabolic alkalosis*	Respiratory alkalosis Hypochloremia	Same as aluminum hydroxide. In addition, significant sodium retention in patients with hypertension or fluid overload.
Calcium carbonate	Calcium deficiency	*Myocardial infarction, urolithiasis, prostate cancer, milk alkali syndrome* Constipation, flatulence, swollen abdomen, hypercalcemia	Severe renal insufficiency	Same as aluminum hydroxide. In addition, hypercalcemia can occur in patients with impaired renal function.
COATING AGENTS **Mechanism—Coat gastric mucosa with a protective layer**				
Sucralfate	Peptic ulcer disease	*Hyperglycemia, bezoar, aluminum accumulation and toxicity (especially in patients with renal impairment)* Constipation	Hypersensitivity to sucralfate	Decreased effectiveness of quinolones (e.g., ciprofloxacin) because of chelation and decreased absorption.
Colloidal bismuth	Peptic ulcer disease Gastric ulcer disease Gastroesophageal reflux disease (GERD) Diarrhea with associated abdominal cramps *H. pylori* infection	Darkening of the tongue and/or stool, nausea, vomiting	Known allergy to aspirin or other nonaspirin salicylates	Frequently used as a component of a multidrug regimen for eradication of *H. pylori* because bismuth impedes growth of the organism. Reduces absorption of tetracyclines, likely through chelation or by reducing solubility as a result of increasing gastric pH. Acute bismuth intoxication is manifested by gastrointestinal disturbance, stomatitis, discoloration of mucous membranes, and potential for kidney and liver damage.
PROSTAGLANDINS **Mechanism—Reduce basal and stimulated gastric acid secretion; enhance bicarbonate secretion, mucus production, and blood flow**				
Misoprostol	See Drug Summary Table: Chapter 43 Pharmacology of Eicosanoids			

48

Integrative Inflammation Pharmacology: Asthma

Joshua M. Galanter and Stephen Lazarus

■ INTRODUCTION

Asthma is a chronic disease characterized by inflammation of the airways and exaggerated airway smooth muscle constriction. The symptoms of asthma include dyspnea and wheezing as well as mucus production and cough, particularly at night. Asthma is both an obstructive lung disease and an inflammatory disease; the obstructive component is characterized by bronchoconstriction, whereas the inflammatory component is marked by airway edema, goblet cell hyperplasia, mucus secretion, and infiltration and cytokine release by immune and inflammatory cells. Although the airway obstruction is generally reversible during acute asthma attacks, over time, the disease may cause airway remodeling and permanent deterioration in pulmonary function.

Medications used to treat asthma act in one of two ways: by relaxing bronchial smooth muscle or by preventing and reducing inflammation. This chapter approaches asthma as both a bronchoconstrictive and an inflammatory disease. After discussing the physiologic control of bronchial tone and the function of immune pathways in the airways, the chapter turns to the pathophysiology of asthma. Current therapies are then discussed, including the pharmacology of both bronchodilators and airway anti-inflammatory agents.

■ PHYSIOLOGY OF AIRWAY SMOOTH MUSCLE TONE AND IMMUNE FUNCTION

Asthma involves dysfunction in the pathways that regulate both smooth muscle tone and immune function in the airways. It is therefore important to review the normal physiology of these systems before discussing the pathophysiology of asthma.

Physiology of Airway Smooth Muscle Contraction

As discussed in Chapter 9, Principles of Nervous System Physiology and Pharmacology, involuntary responses of smooth muscle are regulated by the autonomic nervous system. In the airways, **sympathetic** (adrenergic) tone causes bronchodilation and **parasympathetic** (cholinergic) tone causes bronchoconstriction. Bronchial smooth muscle tone is also regulated by **nonadrenergic, noncholinergic (NANC)** fibers that innervate the respiratory tree.

Sympathetic innervation of the lung is concentrated primarily on pulmonary blood vessels and the submucosal glands. There is little direct sympathetic innervation of the bronchial smooth muscle. However, airway smooth muscle

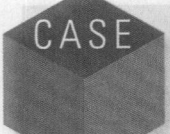

CASE

WY is a 51-year-old man with a long-standing history of asthma and allergies, first diagnosed at the age of 6. His asthma had been managed successfully for many years on a regimen of twice-daily inhaled fluticasone (an inhaled corticosteroid) and albuterol (a β-adrenergic agonist) as needed whenever he developed shortness of breath or wheezing. Over the past year, Mr. Y has noticed worsening symptoms and more frequent asthma attacks. He has had shortness of breath, wheezing, and chest tightness when running to catch the bus. He has also developed a significant amount of coughing, especially at night, and has found himself using albuterol several times a day.

One hazy, hot summer day, Mr. Y develops substantial coughing, wheezing, and shortness of breath at rest. He takes two puffs of his albuterol inhaler but finds that it provides only minimal relief. He calls his doctor but has trouble even speaking in full sentences. His doctor advises him to go to the emergency department (ED) immediately.

On presentation to the ED, Mr. Y is immediately given albuterol via nebulizer and a large dose of intravenous methylprednisolone (a corticosteroid). Although he is now more comfortable, he continues to "feel tight" and he has quiet breath sounds on exam. Fortunately, with continued administrations of nebulized albuterol and a treatment with inhaled ipratropium (an anticholinergic agent), Mr. Y begins to feel better over the next few hours. He is hospitalized for 2 days and sent home on a tapering dose of prednisone, an oral corticosteroid.

At a follow-up appointment with his pulmonologist, Mr. Y is concerned that his asthma has significantly worsened. Even though the acute event has passed, he continues to have frequent asthma symptoms, and his examination and pulmonary function tests suggest that his pulmonary function is significantly reduced. His pulmonologist discusses medication adherence and the proper way to use inhalers, including use of a spacer with the fluticasone inhaler and the need for Mr. Y to rinse his mouth after its use. Mr. Y's pulmonologist also increases the intensity of his drug regimen by adding salmeterol, a long-acting β-agonist, as well as montelukast, a cysteinyl leukotriene receptor antagonist.

Three months later, Mr. Y reports that his baseline symptoms have improved but that he has had an interval asthma exacerbation requiring treatment with prednisone. Because his asthma is still not under adequate control and his laboratory tests show an elevated IgE level, Mr. Y's physician recommends that he start omalizumab, an anti-IgE monoclonal antibody. Mr. Y now receives twice-monthly injections of omalizumab and he has had only one mild asthma exacerbation in the 6 months he has been on this therapy.

Questions

1. Why did Mr. Y develop asthma?
2. Why was Mr. Y initially managed with both an inhaled corticosteroid (fluticasone), taken twice daily, and a β-adrenergic agonist (albuterol), taken only as needed?
3. Why was it preferable to keep Mr. Y on a maintenance regimen of an inhaled corticosteroid (fluticasone) instead of a systemic corticosteroid? Why was it necessary to administer systemic corticosteroids (methylprednisolone intravenously and prednisone orally) to treat his asthma exacerbations?
4. How does omalizumab, an anti-IgE monoclonal antibody, prevent exacerbations of asthma?

cells express **β₂-adrenergic receptors** (and, to a lesser extent, β₁-adrenergic receptors) that are responsive to circulating catecholamines. β₂-Adrenergic receptors are activated by **epinephrine**, which is secreted by the adrenal medulla and causes bronchodilation. Exogenous epinephrine was one of the first pharmacotherapies for asthma and was available until recently in some over-the-counter formulations. Newer, β₂-selective adrenergic agonists, such as the **albuterol** used by Mr. Y, are now considered the first-line bronchodilators for treatment of acute asthmatic symptoms.

The vagus nerve provides parasympathetic innervation to the lungs. Airway smooth muscle cells express **muscarinic receptors**, especially the excitatory M₃ subtype of muscarinic receptor. Parasympathetic postganglionic neurons release acetylcholine, which stimulates these muscarinic receptors and induces bronchoconstriction. Parasympathetic neurons are dominant in maintaining airway smooth muscle tone, and **anticholinergic agents** can cause bronchorelaxation. These agents are used primarily in the treatment of chronic obstructive pulmonary disease (see Box 48-1) but can also be used in acute asthma exacerbations (as was the case with Mr. Y) or when β-adrenergic agonists are contraindicated.

Airway NANC fibers are primarily under parasympathetic control. These fibers can be either stimulatory (causing bronchoconstriction) or inhibitory (causing bronchodilation). NANC fibers do not release either norepinephrine or acetylcholine but instead release neuropeptides. Bronchoconstricting peptides released by NANC fibers include **neurokinin A**, **calcitonin gene-related peptide**, **substance P**, **bradykinin**, **tachykinin**, and **neuropeptide Y**; the bronchodilating peptide **vasoactive intestinal polypeptide (VIP)** is also released by NANC fibers, as is the bronchodilating gasotransmitter **nitric oxide (NO)**. Although no pharmacologic agents have yet been developed to take advantage of the NANC system, nitric oxide is a marker of the intensity of airway inflammation, and NO measurements have been used to assess the severity of asthma and titrate therapy accordingly.

BOX 48-1 Pharmacology of Chronic Obstructive Pulmonary Disease

Chronic obstructive pulmonary disease (COPD) describes a spectrum of disorders that result in obstructive lung disease. Unlike asthma, COPD is generally not reversible. COPD is caused by an abnormal inflammatory response to an inhaled environmental insult. In 90% of cases, this insult to the lungs is tobacco smoke. Clinically, COPD is divided into two frequently overlapping diseases: **emphysema** and **chronic bronchitis**. Pulmonary emphysema refers to alveolar enlargement caused by destruction of alveolar walls and loss of pulmonary elastic recoil, whereas chronic bronchitis is a clinical diagnosis made on the basis of a chronic cough for 3 or more months during 2 consecutive years that cannot be attributed to another cause.

As noted above, COPD is caused by an abnormal response to inhalation of tobacco smoke or other toxic agents. In contrast to asthma, where CD4$^+$ T lymphocytes, B lymphocytes, mast cells, and eosinophils are the primary inflammatory cells, the inflammatory response to tobacco smoke is primarily neutrophilic and monocytic. Tobacco smoke stimulates resident alveolar macrophages to produce chemokines that attract neutrophils. These neutrophils and resident macrophages release proteinases, particularly **matrix metalloproteinases**. The proteinases degrade elastin, which provides elastic recoil to the alveoli, as well as other proteins that compose the matrix supporting the lung parenchyma. Cell death follows, due to impaired attachment of alveolar cells to the degraded matrix and to the toxic actions of inflammatory cells and the environmental insult. The result is that alveoli degrade and coalesce, forming the characteristic enlargement of air spaces typical of emphysema. There is also enhanced mucus production and fibrosis, although the mechanisms underlying these pathologic phenomena have not been well characterized.

Although it is tempting to think that inflammation in COPD could be held in check by inhaled corticosteroids, steroids are unfortunately of limited benefit in this disease. The lack of steroid efficacy likely results from the fact that the inflammatory cells responsible for COPD are macrophages and neutrophils, which are less responsive than lymphocytes and eosinophils to the actions of corticosteroids. Moreover, the activity of histone deacetylase is impaired in COPD, so the inhibition of proinflammatory transcription factors is limited. A number of studies have examined the effects of inhaled corticosteroids on lung function in COPD, but none have found a statistically significant benefit. However, inhaled corticosteroids have been found to reduce the frequency and severity of acute exacerbations of COPD. Therefore, while corticosteroids are not routinely recommended for the treatment of COPD, they may be indicated in patients who develop frequent, severe exacerbations.

Because cysteinyl leukotrienes, mast cells, and IgE have no role in the pathophysiology of COPD, specific treatments for asthma that target these pathways are not useful in COPD. Interestingly, although **leukotriene B$_4$ (LTB$_4$)** is a potent chemotactic factor for neutrophils, clinical studies of LTB$_4$ antagonism have not shown a benefit to date.

Bronchodilators produce only a modest improvement in airflow in patients with COPD. However, even a small improvement in airflow can significantly improve symptoms in patients with COPD, especially in those whose lungs have become hyperinflated. Asthma is punctuated by acute attacks, while most patients with COPD have chronic breathlessness that is worsened with exertion. Therefore, short-acting "reliever" medications are less beneficial than long-acting drugs in COPD. Both β-adrenergic agonists and inhaled anticholinergic agents cause bronchodilation in COPD. However, many patients with COPD have concomitant coronary artery disease, so anticholinergic agents may be preferred in this subset of patients. There is evidence that the bronchodilatory effects of β-agonists and anticholinergic agents (and theophylline) are additive; therefore, patients with severe COPD may benefit from combination therapies such as formoterol and tiotropium. ■

Immune Function in the Airway

As described in Chapter 42, Principles of Inflammation and the Immune System, **T lymphocytes** play a key role in controlling the immune response. T lymphocytes are classified as CD8$^+$ **T$_C$ (cytotoxic) cells**, which are mediators of cellular adaptive immunity, and CD4$^+$ **T$_H$ (helper) cells**, which regulate adaptive immune responses. T$_H$ cells are subclassified as **T$_H$1** and **T$_H$2** cells based on the cytokines they produce. T$_H$1 cells, which produce predominantly **interferon-γ**, **IL-2**, and **TNF-α**, favor a cellular immune response involving T lymphocytes. T$_H$2 cells, on the other hand, produce **IL-4**, **IL-5**, **IL-6**, **IL-9**, **IL-10**, and **IL-13** and favor a humoral immune response involving antibody production by B cells. Because cytokines produced by activated T$_H$1 and T$_H$2 cells are mutually inhibitory, any given immune stimulus elicits predominantly one or the other response (Fig. 48-1).

All individuals continually inhale environmental aeroallergens such as pollens, cat dander, dust mites, and a host of other antigens. These allergens are phagocytosed by antigen-presenting cells lining the airways. The antigens are recognized as foreign by T$_H$ cells and generate a low-level T$_H$1 response mediated primarily by interferon-γ, as well as a low-level IgG antibody response. However, in asthma, an exaggerated T$_H$2 response often predominates, generating airway inflammation and bronchial hyperresponsiveness (Fig. 48-1).

PATHOPHYSIOLOGY OF ASTHMA

Asthma is a complex disease characterized by airway inflammation, airway smooth muscle hyperresponsiveness, and symptomatic bronchoconstriction. Because the most prominent clinical feature of asthma is bronchoconstriction, a simplistic approach to understanding the disease focuses on airway smooth muscle contraction. At its most fundamental level, however, asthma is an inflammatory

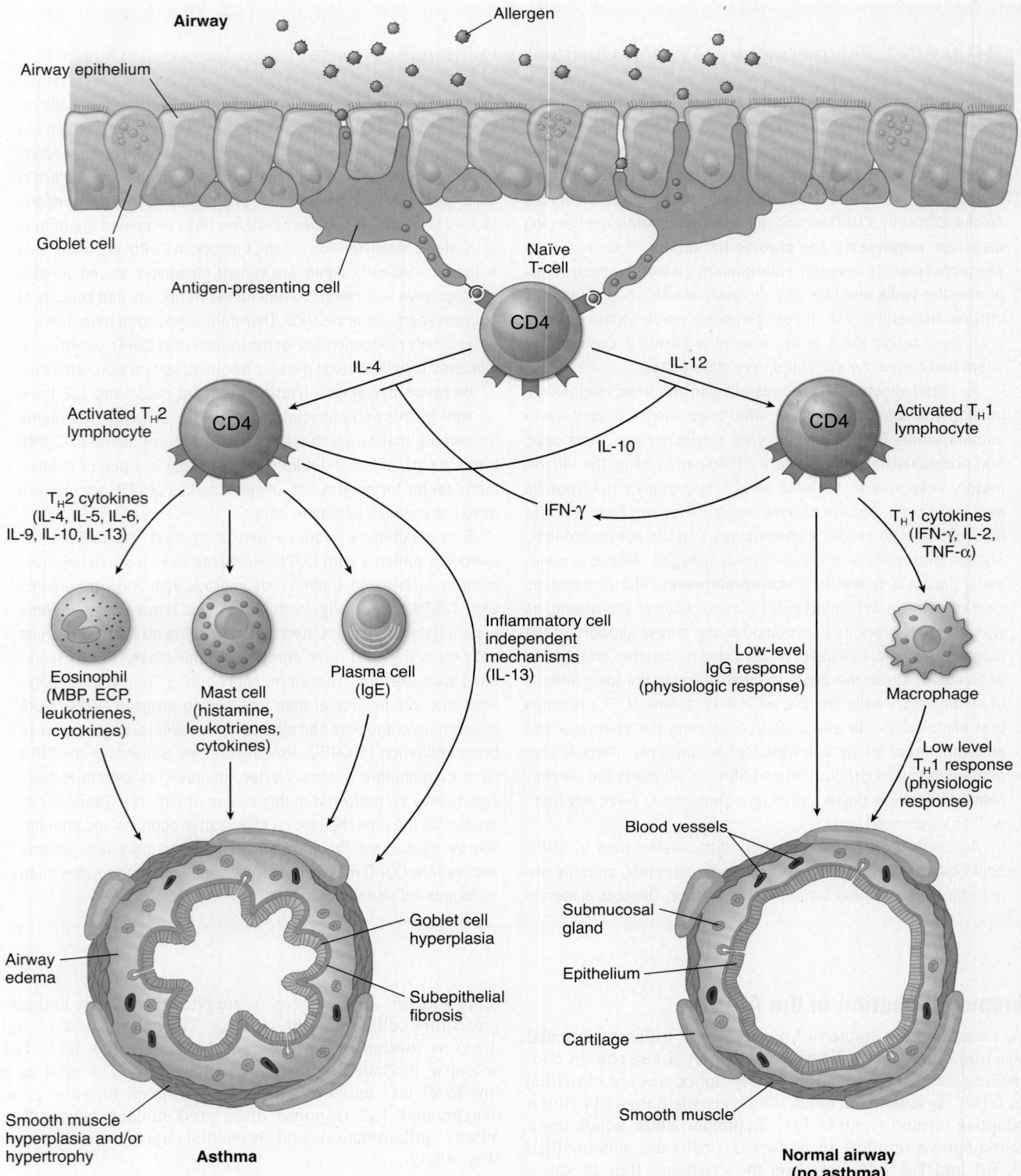

FIGURE 48-1. Origins of the asthmatic immune response. In nonatopic individuals, antigens derived from allergens are presented by antigen-presenting dendritic cells to engender a low-level, physiologic T_H1 response. This response does not cause airway inflammation or bronchoconstriction (**right side**). Interferon-γ, produced by activated T_H1 lymphocytes, inhibits a T_H2 response. In individuals susceptible to asthma, allergen-derived antigens that are presented to immature $CD4^+$ T cells cause these cells to differentiate into activated T_H2 lymphocytes. The T_H2 lymphocytes release cytokines that recruit other inflammatory cells, including eosinophils, mast cells, and IgE-producing B cells. Together, these cells produce an inflammatory response in the airway. Activated T_H2 cells also induce an asthmatic response directly, in part through release of IL-13. The net result—airway hyperresponsiveness, mucus production by goblet cells, airway edema, subepithelial fibrosis, and bronchoconstriction—constitutes the asthmatic response (**left side**).

disease of the airways, and treatment of the underlying inflammation is crucial to maintain normal airway function. Therefore, as detailed below, the treatment of asthma employs both bronchodilators and anti-inflammatory agents.

Asthma as a Bronchoconstrictive Disease

The propensity for the airways of asthmatic patients to constrict in response to a wide variety of stimuli, including allergens, environmental irritants, exercise, cold air, and infections, is termed **hyperresponsiveness**. Two features of airway hyperresponsiveness separate the response to stimuli in asthmatic patients from the nonasthmatic response: **hypersensitivity** and **hyperreactivity**. Hypersensitivity describes a normal response at abnormally low levels of stimuli (i.e., the airways of asthmatic patients constrict to stimuli that do not elicit a response in healthy individuals). Hyperreactivity describes an exaggerated response at normal levels of stimuli (i.e., the airways of asthmatic patients respond too vigorously). In Figure 48-2, hypersensitivity describes a shift of the stimulus–response curve to the left, while hyperreactivity describes an upward shift. The overall response to stimuli in asthmatic patients represents the combination of hypersensitivity and hyperreactivity.

The causes of airway hyperresponsiveness in asthma have not been completely elucidated. The hyperreactive response may be explained by alterations in airway smooth muscle mass due to the increase in size (hypertrophy) and number (hyperplasia) of myocytes that occurs in response to inflammation (Fig. 48-1). The hypersensitivity response is due to alterations in smooth muscle excitation–contraction coupling. Possible mechanisms of altered coupling in asthma include greater responsiveness of intracellular calcium release channels, increased calcium sensitization, and changes in the expression of ion channels, receptors, and second messengers.

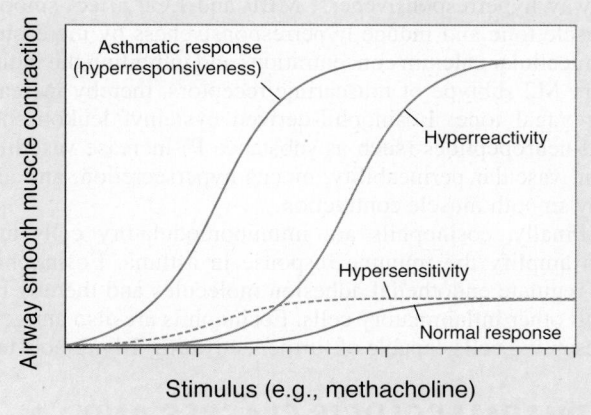

FIGURE 48-2. Airway hyperresponsiveness in asthma. Nonasthmatics have a low-level response to a stimulus that produces mild smooth muscle contraction at high exposures (normal response). An asthmatic patient has airways that manifest exaggerated smooth muscle contraction (bronchoconstriction) at low doses of stimulus (hyperresponsiveness). The two components of hyperresponsiveness are hypersensitivity (a normal response at abnormally low doses of stimulus) and hyperreactivity (an exaggerated response at normal doses of stimulus).

Asthma as an Inflammatory Disease

Although the primary symptoms (wheezing and shortness of breath) of most asthmatic patients are due to bronchoconstriction, the underlying cause of asthma is an allergic inflammation of the airways. The inflammatory process is visible histologically as airway edema, goblet cell hyperplasia, subepithelial fibrosis, mucus hypersecretion, and infiltration by a variety of inflammatory cells, including T_H2 lymphocytes, antigen-presenting cells, plasma cells, mast cells, neutrophils, and eosinophils (Fig. 48-1). Airway inflammation can lead to a chronic cough in asthmatic individuals, even in those who do not develop symptomatic bronchoconstriction (this diagnosis is known as **cough variant asthma**). Many inflammatory mediators and cytokines govern the interplay among the various immune cells. Anti-inflammatory medications, particularly corticosteroids, are mainstays in the pharmacologic treatment of asthma. As the complex pathophysiology of asthma has been further elucidated, more targeted therapies that block specific inflammatory pathways are being developed.

T_H2 Cells and the Origin of Asthma

Although the exact causes of asthma are not fully understood, one theory suggests that asthma, like other allergic diseases, is the result of an immune imbalance favoring T_H2 lymphocytes over T_H1 lymphocytes. T_H2 lymphocytes contribute to asthma through three mechanisms. First, in patients with a hereditary predisposition to **atopy** (from the Greek, meaning "out of place"), an allergen can trigger a **type I hypersensitivity** response. In normal (nonatopic) individuals, an allergen is phagocytosed by antigen-presenting cells, stimulating a low-level T_H1 response and the production of appropriate amounts of IgG antibodies directed against the allergen. In atopic individuals, however, the same allergen induces a strong T_H2 response mediated through the release of IL-4, which induces B cells to produce exaggerated amounts of IgE antibodies directed against the allergen (Fig. 48-1). The IgE antibodies bind to high-affinity IgE receptors on mast cells, and subsequent cross-linking of the IgE receptors upon reexposure to the allergen causes mast cell degranulation and triggers an allergic reaction (Fig. 48-2, and see below). Second, T_H2 cells can directly induce a **type IV hypersensitivity** reaction through the production of IL-13 (and, to a lesser degree, IL-4). In the airway, IL-13 causes goblet cell hyperplasia, increased mucus production, and smooth muscle hyperplasia and/or hypertrophy. IL-13 also stimulates B cells to produce IgE (Fig. 48-1). Third, T_H2 lymphocytes recruit **eosinophils** by producing IL-5 as well as GM-CSF and IL-4. These cytokines (especially IL-5) induce eosinophil proliferation and release from the bone marrow and promote eosinophil survival in the circulation and tissues. As in many patients with asthma, Mr. Y had a high level of circulating eosinophils and elevated levels of serum IgE.

What causes the imbalance between T_H1 and T_H2 lymphocytes in patients with asthma? Although the exact reasons remain to be fully elucidated, they likely involve environmental effects on genetically susceptible individuals. Epidemiologic studies have found that exposures to tuberculosis and viruses such as measles and hepatitis A are protective against the development of asthma. Having older siblings and/or encountering other children through attendance at a day care facility (both of which are associated with increased exposure to infectious agents) are also associated with a decreased incidence of asthma. Living in a rural environment (where there is substantial contact with bacterial endotoxins) is also protective. One leading theory suggests that a "Western lifestyle," including decreased exposure early in life to microbes that engender T_H1-lymphocyte responses, contributes to the development of asthma and other allergic diseases in susceptible individuals. Although this "hygiene hypothesis" is probably too simplistic to explain the origins of a complex disease such as asthma, it forms a useful model for thinking about the disease and is a possible explanation for the dramatic rise in the incidence of asthma in the Western hemisphere. It is impossible to know exactly what caused Mr. Y's asthma; however, the fact that he had allergic rhinitis and elevated levels of IgE suggests that he had an atopic predisposition triggered by environmental allergens.

Plasma Cells, IgE, Mast Cells, and Leukotrienes

As noted above, an IgE-mediated type I hypersensitivity response is one mechanism by which allergens cause the pathologic and clinical manifestations of asthma (Fig. 48-3). The allergic response is initiated when a dendritic cell phagocytoses an inhaled allergen. The dendritic cell presents the processed allergen to T_H2 cells and activates them. The activated T_H2 cells bind to and activate B lymphocytes via CD40 on the B-cell surface. Activated T_H2 cells also generate IL-4 and IL-13, which induce B-cell transformation into IgE-producing plasma cells.

IgE circulates briefly in the bloodstream before binding to **high-affinity IgE receptors (FcεRI)** on mast cells. Upon reexposure, the allergen binds to and cross-links the IgE–FcεRI complexes, thereby activating the mast cell. The activated mast cell degranulates, releasing its preformed inflammatory mediators. These molecules include **histamine**, proteolytic enzymes, and certain cytokines (such as **platelet-activating factor**). The activated mast cell also releases **arachidonic acid** from its plasma membrane and produces **leukotrienes** and **prostaglandin D$_2$** (Fig. 48-4).

Acutely, mast cell degranulation produces bronchoconstriction and airway inflammation. Histamine released by the mast cells promotes capillary leakage, leading to airway edema. Mast cells also release **leukotriene C$_4$ (LTC$_4$)**, which is subsequently converted into **LTD$_4$** and **LTE$_4$** (see Chapter 43, Pharmacology of Eicosanoids). These three leukotrienes, called **cysteinyl leukotrienes**, are central to the pathophysiology of asthma because they induce marked bronchoconstriction. *Leukotriene D$_4$ is 1,000 times more potent than histamine in producing bronchoconstriction.* Leukotrienes also cause mucus hypersecretion, capillary leakage, and vasogenic edema and recruit additional inflammatory cells. The effect of the leukotrienes, though slower in onset, is more powerful and sustained than that of the preformed mediators. Because of their delayed yet potent inflammatory effect, leukotrienes were once called **slow-reacting substance of anaphylaxis (SRS-A)** before their actual structures were identified.

Mast cells recruit other inflammatory cells via the release of cytokines. This produces a delayed reaction that develops 4 to 6 hours after exposure to allergen (Fig. 48-3). Mast cells also release **tryptase**, a protease that activates receptors on epithelial and endothelial cells, inducing the expression of adhesion molecules that attract eosinophils

and basophils. Tryptase is also a smooth muscle mitogen, causing hyperplasia of airway smooth muscle cells and contributing to airway hyperresponsiveness. The production of IL-1, IL-2, IL-3, IL-4, IL-5, GM-CSF, interferon-γ, and TNF-α by mast cells contributes to chronic inflammation and the chronic asthmatic reaction. Finally, mast cells release proteases and proteoglycans that act on supporting airway structures to produce chronic changes in the airway (also called **airway remodeling**). Unlike the reversible component of bronchoconstriction that characterizes the acute asthmatic reaction, airway remodeling induced by chronic inflammation may cause irreversible impairment in pulmonary function.

Eosinophils

The major physiologic role of eosinophils is to defend against parasitic infections. Eosinophils originate in the bone marrow and are stimulated by IL-4, IL-5, and GM-CSF produced by T_H2 lymphocytes and mast cells. Eosinophils migrate from the bloodstream to the airway by binding to specific adhesion molecules, particularly VCAM-1, and by traveling along chemokine gradients to sites of inflammation. Once recruited to the airway, eosinophils have a complex, multifunctional role in asthma. Activated eosinophils secrete cytotoxic granules that cause local tissue damage and induce airway remodeling, lipid mediators and neuromodulators that affect airway tone, and cytokines and chemokines that recruit other inflammatory cells.

The toxic granules of eosinophils contain a number of cationic proteins—including **major basic protein (MBP)**, **eosinophilic cationic protein (ECP)**, **eosinophil peroxidase**, and **eosinophil-derived neurotoxin**—that are directly damaging to the bronchial epithelium. For example, ECP can breach the integrity of target cell membranes by forming ion-selective, voltage-insensitive pores, and eosinophil peroxidase catalyzes the production of highly reactive oxygen species that oxidize target cell proteins and induce apoptosis. Eosinophils also produce **matrix metalloproteinases** that contribute to airway remodeling.

Eosinophils contribute both directly and indirectly to airway hyperresponsiveness. MBP and ECP affect smooth muscle tone and induce hyperresponsiveness by increasing intracellular calcium concentrations and inhibiting the inhibitory M2 subtype of muscarinic receptors, thereby increasing vagal tone. Eosinophil-derived cysteinyl leukotrienes and neuropeptides (such as substance P) increase vasodilation, vascular permeability, mucus hypersecretion, and airway smooth muscle contraction.

Finally, eosinophils are immunomodulatory cells that can amplify the immune response in asthma. Eosinophils up-regulate endothelial adhesion molecules and thereby recruit other inflammatory cells. Eosinophils are also antigen-presenting cells capable of further activating T lymphocytes.

▌ PHARMACOLOGIC CLASSES AND AGENTS

The pharmacologic agents used to treat asthma are divided into two broad categories: **relievers** and **controllers** (also called **preventers**). This distinction emphasizes the clinical uses of these agents and helps patients understand and adhere to the prescribed regimen. This classification scheme also relates to the mechanisms of action of drugs

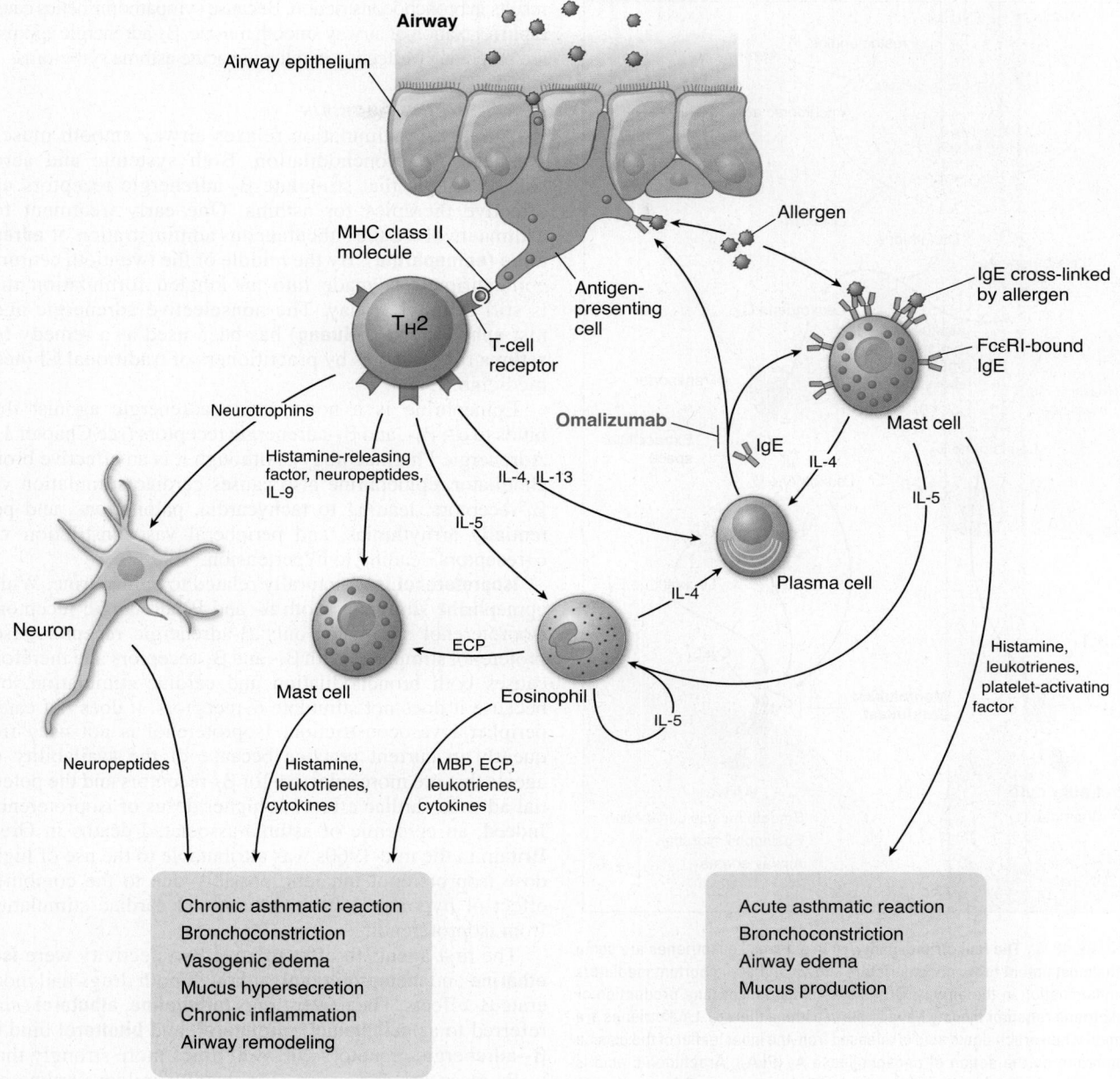

FIGURE 48-3. The allergic response in asthma. Asthma produces acute and chronic inflammatory responses in the airways. Antigen-presenting cells phagocytose and process allergens, presenting the antigens to CD4+ T cells. These cells differentiate into cytokine-producing T_H2 lymphocytes. The activated T_H2 cells release IL-4, IL-13, and IL-5, which recruit B cells and eosinophils. The B cells differentiate into IgE-producing plasma cells. The IgE binds to FcεRI receptors on mast cells and antigen-presenting cells. Upon reexposure to the allergen, the IgE-bound FcεRI is cross-linked, inducing the mast cell to degranulate and release preformed and newly generated inflammatory mediators including histamine, cysteinyl leukotrienes, platelet-activating factor, and other cytokines. These cytokines cause acute airway inflammation and produce acute asthmatic symptoms (an asthma "attack" or exacerbation). Chronically, activated T_H2 cells and mast cells produce circulating IL-5 that recruits eosinophils, and T_H2 cells release products that stimulate local mast cells and neurons. Together, the inflammatory mediators and catabolic enzymes produced by eosinophils, mast cells, and neurons cause chronic airway inflammation and lead to airway remodeling.

Omalizumab is a humanized monoclonal antibody directed against the FcεRI-binding domain of IgE. By preventing IgE from binding to the IgE receptor (FcεRI) on mast cells, omalizumab inhibits mast cell degranulation upon reexposure to allergen and thereby modulates the acute asthmatic reaction. Omalizumab also down-regulates FcεRI on antigen-presenting cells, thereby diminishing antigen processing and presentation to CD4+ lymphocytes. Because fewer immature T cells are induced by allergen to differentiate into T_H2 lymphocytes, the chronic asthmatic reaction is also blunted.

for asthma. *In general, bronchodilators, which alleviate smooth muscle bronchoconstriction, are used as relievers, and anti-inflammatory medications, which decrease airway inflammation, are used as controllers.* There is also evidence that some medications—**methylxanthines**, for example—have both bronchodilatory and anti-inflammatory effects. At the start of the introductory case, Mr. Y used fluticasone (an inhaled corticosteroid) as a controller, with albuterol (a short-acting β2-agonist) as a reliever.

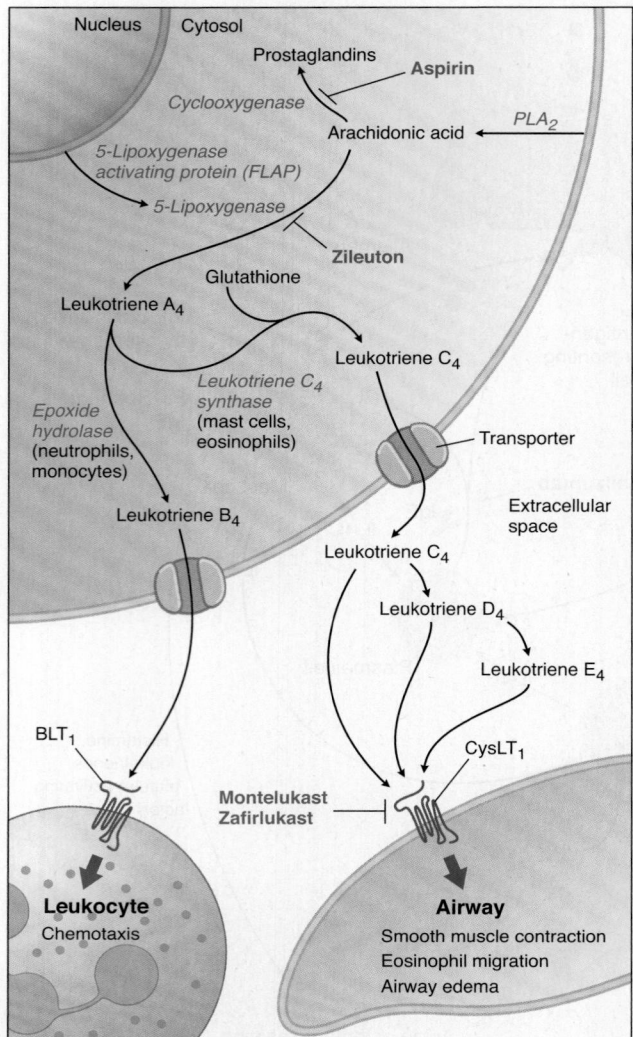

FIGURE 48-4. The leukotriene pathway in asthma. Leukotrienes are some of the most potent bronchoconstrictors known and are important mediators of inflammation in the airway. Drugs that inhibit leukotriene production or leukotriene receptor binding have a role in asthma therapy. Leukotrienes are formed when arachidonic acid is released from the inner leaflet of the plasma membrane by the action of phospholipase A_2 (PLA_2). Arachidonic acid is converted to leukotriene A_4 by the action of 5-lipoxygenase. 5-Lipoxygenase is activated by the membrane-bound enzyme 5-lipoxygenase activating protein (FLAP). Leukotriene A_4 is converted to leukotriene C_4 by the action of leukotriene C_4 synthase in mast cells and eosinophils, and leukotriene C_4 is transported out of the cell. Leukotriene C_4 is converted to leukotriene D_4 and then to leukotriene E_4; all three of these cysteinyl leukotrienes bind to $CysLT1$ receptors expressed on airway smooth muscle cells, leading to bronchoconstriction and airway edema. Leukotriene A_4 is converted to leukotriene B_4 by epoxide hydrolase in neutrophils and monocytes. Leukotriene B_4 is transported out of the cell and binds to $BLT1$ receptors expressed on leukocytes, leading to leukocyte chemotaxis and recruitment. The leukotriene pathway can be inhibited by the 5-lipoxygenase inhibitor zileuton or by the $CysLT1$ receptor antagonists montelukast and zafirlukast.

Bronchodilators

Bronchodilators affect airway smooth muscle tone by acting on autonomic nervous system receptors and signaling pathways. Sympathetic activation (mediated primarily by β_2-adrenergic receptors) results in bronchodilation, while parasympathetic stimulation (mediated by muscarinic acetylcholine receptors)

results in bronchoconstriction. Because sympathomimetics cause rapid relaxation of airway smooth muscle, β_2-adrenergic agonists are particularly effective in relieving acute asthma symptoms.

β-Adrenergic Agonists

β_2-Adrenergic stimulation relaxes airway smooth muscle and leads to bronchodilation. Both systemic and aerosolized agents that stimulate β_2-adrenergic receptors are effective therapies for asthma. One early treatment for asthma involved the subcutaneous administration of **adrenaline (epinephrine)**. By the middle of the twentieth century, epinephrine was made into an inhaled formulation that is still available today. The nonselective adrenergic agonist **ephedrine (Ma-Huang)** has been used as a remedy for asthma for centuries by practitioners of traditional Chinese medicine.

Epinephrine is a nonselective adrenergic agonist that binds to α-, β_1-, and β_2-adrenergic receptors (see Chapter 11, Adrenergic Pharmacology). Although it is an effective bronchodilator, epinephrine also causes cardiac stimulation via β_1-receptors, leading to tachycardia, palpitations, and potentially arrhythmias, and peripheral vasoconstriction via α-receptors, leading to hypertension.

Isoproterenol is structurally related to epinephrine. While epinephrine stimulates both α- and β-adrenergic receptors, isoproterenol stimulates only β-adrenergic receptors. Isoproterenol stimulates both β_1- and β_2-receptors and therefore causes both bronchodilation and cardiac stimulation, but because it does not stimulate α-receptors, it does not cause peripheral vasoconstriction. Isoproterenol is not used frequently in current practice because of the availability of agents that are more selective for β_2-receptors and the potential adverse cardiac effects at higher doses of isoproterenol. Indeed, an epidemic of asthma-associated deaths in Great Britain in the mid-1960s was attributable to the use of high-dose isoproterenol inhalers, possibly due to the combined effect of hypoxemia from asthma and cardiac stimulation from isoproterenol.

The first agents to offer relative β_2 selectivity were **isoetharine** and **metaproterenol**, although both drugs had moderate β_1 effects. The newer drugs **terbutaline**, **albuterol** (also referred to as **salbutamol**), **pirbuterol**, and **bitolterol** bind to β_2-adrenergic receptors 200–400 times more strongly than to β_1-receptors and cause significantly milder cardiac effects than the less selective adrenergic agonists. Albuterol was the first of the strongly β_2-selective agents to be available in inhaled form, further reducing systemic effects. Modern inhaled β_2-selective agonists were the first drugs to allow regular treatment of asthma with an acceptable adverse effect profile. Nonetheless, at high doses, especially if taken orally, even these drugs can cause cardiac stimulation and tachycardia. In addition, since β_2-adrenergic receptors are expressed in peripheral skeletal muscle, activation of these receptors by β_2-selective agents can result in a tremor.

Albuterol is a racemic mixture of two stereoisomers: R-albuterol (or **levalbuterol**) and S-albuterol. Levalbuterol, which is available as a pure enantiomer, has tighter binding to β_2-receptors and is more β_2-selective. In contrast, the S isomer induces airway hyperresponsiveness in animal models, although in clinical practice, this effect has not been significant. Although racemic albuterol and levalbuterol produce similar response and adverse effect profiles for most

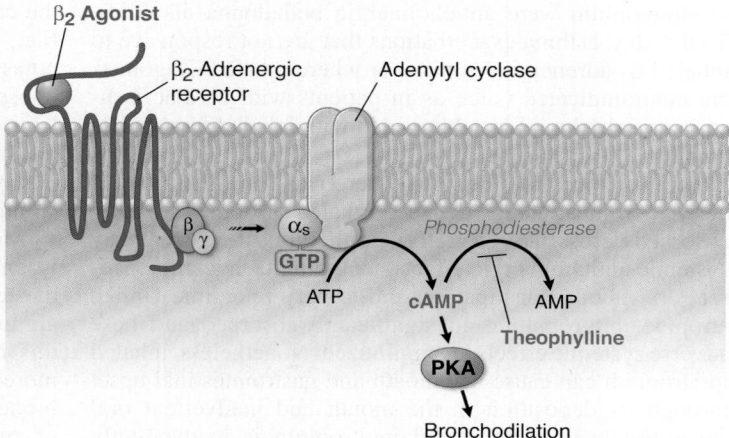

FIGURE 48-5. Mechanism of β₂-agonists and theophylline in asthma. In airway smooth muscle cells, activation of protein kinase A by cAMP leads to phosphorylation of a number of intracellular proteins and thus to smooth muscle relaxation and bronchodilation. Any therapy that increases the level of intracellular cAMP is expected to lead to bronchodilation. In practice, this is accomplished in one of two ways: by increasing the production of cAMP or by inhibiting the breakdown of cAMP. cAMP production is stimulated by β₂-agonist-mediated activation of β₂-adrenergic receptors, which are G protein-coupled receptors. cAMP breakdown is inhibited by theophylline-mediated inhibition of phosphodiesterase.

patients, a subset of patients may be more sensitive to the β₁ effects of *S*-albuterol and may experience decreased tachycardia and palpitations when taking levalbuterol.

β-Adrenergic receptors are coupled to the stimulatory G protein G$_s$ (see Chapter 11). The α subunit of G$_s$ activates adenylyl cyclase, which catalyzes the production of cyclic adenosine monophosphate (cAMP). In the lung, cAMP causes a decrease in the intracellular calcium concentration and, via activation of protein kinase A, inactivates myosin light chain kinase and activates myosin light chain phosphorylase (Fig. 48-5). In addition, the β₂-agonists open large-conductance calcium-activated potassium channels (K$_{Ca}$) and thereby hyperpolarize airway smooth muscle cells. The combination of decreased intracellular calcium, increased membrane potassium conductance, and decreased myosin light chain phosphorylation leads to smooth muscle relaxation and bronchodilation.

There is significant variability in clinical response among patients using β₂-agonists. Some of this variability may be mediated through variants in the gene for the β₂-adrenergic receptor. Researchers studying the effect of **single nucleotide polymorphisms (SNPs)** in the gene have found a common genetic variant that is associated with increased susceptibility to nocturnal asthma. Subjects homozygous for this genetic variant who receive regularly scheduled albuterol doses develop a decline in their peak expiratory flow rate (a measure of bronchoconstriction), while subjects without the polymorphism develop increased peak flow rates with scheduled albuterol use. Although the pharmacogenetics of the β₂-adrenergic receptor are complicated and have yielded inconsistent associations, it is likely that some of the variability in drug response results from genetic influences.

Most β₂-adrenergic agonists have a rapid onset of action (15 to 30 minutes), a peak effect at 30 to 60 minutes, and a duration of action of approximately 4 to 6 hours. This time course of drug action makes the β₂-agonists good candidates for use as asthma relievers (or rescue inhalers) during acute attacks. However, this profile also makes the β₂-agonists poor candidates for control of nocturnal asthma and for prevention of attacks, although they can be used prophylactically before exposure to a known trigger such as exercise. Several newer agents, **formoterol** (and its enantiomerically pure form **arformoterol**, approved only

for treatment of COPD), **salmeterol**, **vilanterol**, **indacaterol**, and **olodaterol** (the latter three approved only for treatment of COPD), are known as **long-acting beta-agonists (LABAs)**. The LABAs were engineered with lipophilic side chains that resist degradation. As such, these agents have a 12- to 24-hour duration of action, making them good candidates for prevention of bronchoconstriction. Although formoterol and salmeterol are reasonable asthma controllers, these agents do not treat the underlying inflammation. In fact, regular use of formoterol or salmeterol may be associated with an increase in asthma deaths. The exact mechanism for this observation is unknown, although it may occur because long-acting β-agonists can improve the chronic symptoms of asthma without affecting the underlying risk of a severe asthma exacerbation. Because patients may feel better on long-acting β-agonists, they may receive lower doses of inhaled corticosteroids or no inhaled corticosteroids at all. Since inhaled corticosteroids reduce the risk of asthma exacerbation (see below), the reduction or withdrawal of inhaled corticosteroids may place patients at increased risk of asthma hospitalization and fatal asthma attack. For this reason, a US Food and Drug Administration (FDA) advisory committee has recommended that formoterol and salmeterol should be used only in combination with an inhaled corticosteroid.

Because salmeterol has a slower onset of action than albuterol, it should not be used for acute asthma flares. Formoterol does have a rapid onset of action and can be used as a rescue inhaler, although it is not yet approved for this indication in the United States. One strategy has been to combine formoterol with an inhaled corticosteroid (budesonide) for use as needed in patients with mild asthma. Every time the patient uses this combination, the formoterol is available to provide acute relief of symptoms, and the patient also receives a dose of the inhaled corticosteroid to help quell the underlying inflammation.

Anticholinergics

Anticholinergic agents were the first medications used to treat asthma in Western medicine. As early as 1896, Stedman's *Twentieth Century Practice of Modern Medical Science* suggested that asthma attacks could be treated by smoking "asthma cigarettes" containing **stramonium** extracted from the plant *Datura stramonium*. The active ingredients in stramonium were anticholinergic belladonna alkaloids. To this day, asthma exacerbations that are not responsive to inhaled β_2-adrenergic agonists, or where inhaled β-agonists are contraindicated (such as in patients with cardiac ischemia or arrhythmia), can be treated with inhaled **ipratropium bromide**.

Ipratropium bromide is a quaternary ammonium salt derived from **atropine**. Because inhaled atropine is highly absorbed across the respiratory epithelium, it causes many systemic anticholinergic effects, including tachycardia, nausea, dry mouth, constipation, and urinary retention. Unlike atropine, ipratropium is not significantly absorbed, and these adverse systemic effects are minimized. Nonetheless, inhaled ipratropium can cause dry mouth and gastrointestinal upset through its deposition in the mouth and inadvertent oral absorption, and if nebulized ipratropium is inadvertently delivered to the eye, it can produce mydriasis (pupillary dilation) and increase intraocular pressure, resulting in angle-closure glaucoma.

Tiotropium (as well as the newer agents **umeclidinium** and **aclidinium**) is a long-acting anticholinergic agent that is used in the treatment of **chronic obstructive pulmonary disease** (**COPD**; Box 48-1). Like ipratropium, these long-acting anticholinergic agents are quaternary ammonium salts that produce few systemic effects because they are not systemically absorbed upon inhalation. Moreover, aclidinium is hydrolyzed rapidly in plasma, further reducing systematic exposure.

Antimuscarinic agents are competitive antagonists at muscarinic acetylcholine receptors. Of the four muscarinic receptor subtypes expressed in the lung (M_1, M_2, M_3, and M_4), the excitatory M_3 receptor is the most important in mediating smooth muscle contraction and mucus gland secretion in the airway. Ipratropium and the long-acting anticholinergic agents antagonize the effect of endogenous acetylcholine at M_3 receptors, leading to bronchorelaxation and decreased mucus secretion. Tiotropium, umeclidinium, and aclidinium have a long duration of action, which enables once-daily dosing, largely because of their slow dissociation from M_3 receptors.

Ipratropium and the long-acting antimuscarinic agents are used mainly to treat COPD, where the major reversible bronchoconstrictive component is mediated by cholinergic neural tone. In chronic asthma, cholinergic stimulation has only a secondary role in causing bronchoconstriction, although increased vagal stimulation at night may be an important contributor to nighttime symptoms. No anticholinergic agent is approved by the FDA for asthma, but studies have suggested therapeutic uses for ipratropium in the treatment of acute asthma exacerbations and as rescue therapy in the subset of patients who cannot tolerate β-adrenergic agonists or for whom therapy with sympathomimetics is contraindicated due to ischemic heart disease or tachyarrhythmia.

Methylxanthines and Phosphodiesterase Inhibitors

Two methylxanthines, **theophylline** and **aminophylline**, are occasionally used in asthma treatment. The mechanism of action of these drugs is complex, but their primary bronchodilatory effect appears to be due to nonspecific inhibition of phosphodiesterase isoenzymes. Inhibition of phosphodiesterase types III and IV prevents cAMP degradation in airway smooth muscle cells, leading to smooth muscle relaxation by

the cellular and molecular mechanisms detailed previously (i.e., decreased intracellular calcium, increased membrane potassium conductance, and decreased myosin light chain phosphorylation). As shown in Figure 48-5, the bronchodilatory effect of methylxanthines results from perturbation of the same pathway that is initiated by β_2-agonists, although methylxanthines act downstream of β_2-adrenergic receptor stimulation.

Methylxanthines also inhibit phosphodiesterase (PDE) isoenzymes in inflammatory cells. Inhibition of phosphodiesterase type IV in T lymphocytes and eosinophils has an immunomodulatory and anti-inflammatory effect. By this mechanism, theophylline can control chronic asthma more effectively than would be expected on the basis of its bronchodilatory effect alone. Some of the adverse effects of methylxanthines, including cardiac arrhythmias, nausea, and vomiting, are also mediated by phosphodiesterase inhibition, although the responsible isoenzymes remain to be elucidated.

Theophylline is a structural relative of **caffeine**, differing only by a single methyl group, and both caffeine and theophylline are adenosine receptor antagonists. Adenosine receptors are expressed on airway smooth muscle cells and mast cells, and antagonism of these receptors could play a role in preventing both bronchoconstriction and inflammation. In fact, caffeine (as coffee) has been used to treat asthma. However, experiments with specific adenosine receptor antagonists that do not inhibit phosphodiesterase have shown little bronchodilation, suggesting that phosphodiesterase inhibition is the primary mechanism of action of methylxanthines in asthma. Nonetheless, adenosine receptor antagonism is responsible for many secondary effects of theophylline, including increased ventilation during hypoxia, improved endurance of diaphragmatic muscles, and decreased adenosine-stimulated mediator release from mast cells. In addition, some adverse effects of theophylline, such as tachycardia, psychomotor agitation, gastric acid secretion, and diuresis, are mediated through adenosine receptor antagonism.

Because methylxanthines are nonselective and have multiple mechanisms of action, they cause multiple adverse effects and have a relatively narrow therapeutic index. Moreover, there is significant variation in the metabolism of theophylline by the P450 isoenzyme CYP3A, and theophylline use is susceptible to drug–drug interactions with CYP3A inhibitors such as cimetidine and the azole antifungals. At supratherapeutic levels, theophylline produces nausea, diarrhea, vomiting, headache, irritability, and insomnia. At even higher doses, seizures, toxic encephalopathy, hyperthermia, brain damage, hyperglycemia, hypokalemia, hypotension, cardiac arrhythmias, and death can occur. For this reason, the role of theophylline in the treatment of chronic asthma has diminished. Theophylline is still used occasionally with routine monitoring of plasma drug levels when β-adrenergic agonists and corticosteroids are ineffective or contraindicated.

A phosphodiesterase type IV inhibitor, **roflumilast**, has recently been approved for use in severe COPD (see Box 48-1), where it is associated with a small improvement in pulmonary function and a reduced likelihood of symptom exacerbation. Unfortunately, as with theophylline, off-target inhibition of PDE IV in the brain results in nausea, vomiting, and weight loss. Research is now focused on the development of PDE IV inhibitors with better inhaled formulations and fewer adverse effects.

Magnesium

Magnesium ions inhibit calcium transport into smooth muscle cells and can interfere with intracellular phosphorylation reactions that induce smooth muscle contraction. For this reason, **magnesium sulfate** is commonly used as a tocolytic to inhibit uterine contraction and delay preterm labor. Magnesium has similar effects on airway smooth muscle and has been used experimentally in acute asthma exacerbations. Although the results of clinical studies have been variable, two meta-analyses have suggested a benefit to using magnesium sulfate in patients with severe asthma exacerbations presenting to the emergency department. Magnesium was not used in the introductory case, but it would have been a reasonable therapeutic option at the time of Mr. Y's visit to the emergency department.

Anti-Inflammatory Agents

As detailed above, allergic inflammation of the airways forms the pathophysiologic basis for asthma. To control persistent asthma and prevent exacerbations of acute asthma, treatment of all but the mildest forms of the disease should generally include anti-inflammatory agents. Corticosteroids have long been mainstays of asthma treatment, although the profound adverse effects of systemically administered corticosteroids remained problematic until the development of inhaled formulations. Three additional classes of drugs with anti-inflammatory mechanisms of action are also used for the treatment of asthma: cromolyns, leukotriene pathway modifiers, and a humanized monoclonal anti-IgE antibody.

Corticosteroids

Inhaled corticosteroids are the chief preventive treatment for the vast majority of patients with asthma. Because inhaled corticosteroids produce higher local drug concentrations in the airway than an equivalent dose of systemically administered corticosteroids, a lower overall dose can be administered, reducing the likelihood of significant systemic effects.

Corticosteroids bind to the intracellular glucocorticoid receptor. The steroid–receptor complex translocates to the nucleus, where it binds to glucocorticoid response elements (GREs) in DNA, altering the transcription of dozens of genes. In general, corticosteroids increase the transcription of genes coding for the β_2-adrenergic receptor and a number of anti-inflammatory proteins such as IL-10, IL-12, and IL-1 receptor antagonist (IL-1Ra). Corticosteroids decrease the transcription of genes coding for many proinflammatory (and other) proteins; examples include IL-2, IL-3, IL-4, IL-5, IL-6, IL-11, IL-13, IL-15, TNF-α, GM-CSF, SCF, endothelial adhesion molecules, chemokines, inducible nitric oxide synthase (iNOS), cyclooxygenase (COX), phospholipase A_2, endothelin-1, and NK$_1$-2 receptor. As described above, IL-4 is important in inducing B-cell production of IgE, while IL-5 is an important recruiter of eosinophils (Fig. 48-3). *Therefore, inhibition of IL-4 and IL-5 markedly reduces the inflammatory response in asthma.* Moreover, corticosteroids induce apoptosis in a number of inflammatory cells, particularly eosinophils and T$_H$2 lymphocytes.

Corticosteroids do not directly affect mast cells, probably because most mast cell mediators are preformed; however, mast cells are indirectly inhibited over time as the overall inflammatory response is muted.

Corticosteroids reduce the number of inflammatory cells in the airways and decrease the damage to airway epithelium. Vascular permeability is also reduced, leading to resolution of airway edema. In addition, although steroids do not directly affect the contractile function of airway smooth muscle, over time, the reduced inflammation leads to a reduction in airway hyperresponsiveness. The net result is that corticosteroids reverse many of the features of asthma. Unfortunately, steroids merely suppress the inflammatory cascade and do not cure asthma, so they must be taken chronically. In addition, steroids cannot reverse airway remodeling caused by long-standing, poorly controlled asthma. Nonetheless, because the effects of these agents are so far-reaching, inhaled corticosteroids constitute the most important drug class for most patients with asthma.

Most systemic effects can be mitigated, if not eliminated, by delivering corticosteroids directly to the airway (i.e., by inhalation). Although all corticosteroids are active in asthma when given systemically, substitution at the 17α position increases topical absorption and allows such drugs to be active when given by inhalation (see Fig. 29-7). The currently available inhaled steroids include **beclomethasone**, **triamcinolone**, **fluticasone**, **budesonide**, **flunisolide**, **mometasone**, and **ciclesonide**. Even though only 10–20% of the administered dose is delivered to the airways by inhalation (the rest is deposited in the oropharynx and swallowed, unless the mouth is rinsed after using the inhaler), a much higher airway concentration of drug is produced than would occur with a similar dose administered systemically. Compared to systemic dosing, inhaled delivery allows a 100-fold decrease in the dose required to achieve a similar anti-inflammatory effect. In addition, the newer steroids (all but beclomethasone and triamcinolone) are subject to first-pass metabolism in the liver, such that much of the inadvertently swallowed dose does not reach the systemic circulation. Ciclesonide, the most recently approved inhaled corticosteroid, is an ester prodrug that is converted to its active compound, desisobutyrylciclesonide, by carboxyesterases and cholinesterases expressed in the upper and lower airway epithelium, thereby further limiting local oropharyngeal and systemic adverse effects.

The combination of lower dose and first-pass metabolism in the liver limits the incidence of adverse effects of inhaled corticosteroids. At sufficiently high doses, however, enough drug is absorbed through the gastrointestinal tract and pulmonary epithelium to cause systemic effects with prolonged use, including osteopenia or osteoporosis in adults and delayed growth in children. In addition, inhaled steroids can cause local adverse effects, such as oropharyngeal candidiasis from deposition into the oropharynx and hoarseness due to deposition into the larynx. These effects can be prevented by using a large-volume spacer to capture large droplets of steroid that would be deposited in the oropharynx and by rinsing the mouth after use.

Sometimes, however, inhaled corticosteroids are inadequate and systemic corticosteroids such as prednisone must be used as either a short "burst" for acute exacerbations or as long-term therapy when asthma cannot be controlled with other medication. For example, systemic steroids were necessary to control Mr. Y's symptoms during and after his asthma exacerbation. Systemic corticosteroids have a more widespread anti-inflammatory effect than inhaled corticosteroids. However, they also have a much more substantial adverse effect profile, as discussed in Chapter 29, Pharmacology of the Adrenal Cortex. For this reason, the use of systemic corticosteroids is typically limited to asthmatic patients with severe acute or chronic disease that cannot be otherwise controlled.

Cromolyns

Roger Altounyan was a physician with a predictable asthmatic response to guinea pig dander. In the 1960s, Dr. Altounyan tested a series of synthetic compounds based on a traditional Egyptian folk remedy for their ability to decrease his response to guinea pig dander extracts. These tests resulted in his discovery of a novel class of compounds, of which two—**cromolyn** (also known as **disodium cromoglycate**) and **nedocromil**—have since entered clinical practice.

Studies showed that cromolyn inhibits the immediate allergic response to an antigen challenge but does not relieve an allergic response once it has been initiated. Further studies found that cromolyn decreases the activity of mast cells, preventing release of their inflammatory mediators upon antigen challenge. For this reason, cromolyn is commonly viewed as a "mast cell stabilizing agent." This view is somewhat simplistic, however, as cromolyn also inhibits the release of mediators from eosinophils, neutrophils, monocytes, macrophages, and lymphocytes. The underlying molecular mechanism of action has not been fully elucidated but may involve inhibition of chloride transport, which in turn affects calcium gating and prevents mediator release from intracellular granules.

Because it prevents the acute allergic response in susceptible patients, cromolyn has found a role as a prophylactic therapy in patients with allergic asthma associated with specific triggers. It has also been useful in patients with exercise-induced asthma, as it can be taken immediately prior to exercise. Clinical experience has shown that cromolyn is more effective in children and young adults than in older patients.

Cromolyn has a better safety profile than any other asthma medication, largely due to its low systemic absorption. Cromolyn is administered by inhalation; less than 10% of the drug that reaches the lower airway is systemically absorbed, and less than 1% of the drug that reaches the gastrointestinal tract is absorbed. Unfortunately, cromolyn's clinical utility is limited because it is less effective than inhaled corticosteroids, particularly in cases of moderate and severe asthma, and it must be taken four times daily.

Leukotriene Pathway-Modifying Agents

The central role of leukotrienes in the pathogenesis of asthma suggests that inhibiting steps in the leukotriene pathway could serve as a treatment for the disease. 5-Lipoxygenase catalyzes the conversion of arachidonic acid to leukotriene A_4. Inhibition of 5-lipoxygenase by **zileuton** reduces the biosynthesis of LTA_4 and its active derivatives, the cysteinyl leukotrienes (Fig. 48-4). Downstream, **montelukast** and **zafirlukast** inhibit binding of LTC_4, LTD_4, and LTE_4 to the cysteinyl leukotriene receptor ($CysLT_1$) (Fig. 48-4). Finally, inhibition of the protein that activates 5-lipoxygenase (**5-lipoxygenase activating protein**, or **FLAP**) is being actively explored, although no currently approved agents work by this mechanism.

The leukotriene pathway inhibitors have two major clinical effects. In patients with moderate or severe asthma who have pulmonary function impairment at baseline, zileuton, montelukast, and zafirlukast produce an immediate, albeit small, improvement in lung function. This effect is likely due to antagonism of the abnormally constricted bronchial tone that results from cysteinyl leukotriene stimulation of $CysLT_1$ receptors at baseline. With chronic administration, the leukotriene-modifying agents reduce the frequency of exacerbations and improve control of asthma—as evidenced by fewer symptoms and less frequent use of inhaled β-agonists—even in patients who have mild asthma and only episodic symptoms. Nonetheless, compared to the effect of inhaled corticosteroids, the effect of leukotriene pathway modifiers on lung function and symptom control is limited. Because the leukotriene pathway is just one of several processes responsible for the inflammatory response in asthma, it is not surprising that leukotriene pathway modifiers are less effective than inhaled corticosteroids, which affect multiple inflammatory pathways and therefore have broader anti-inflammatory effects.

Leukotriene-modifying agents are particularly useful for treating the effects of **aspirin-exacerbated respiratory disease** (or aspirin-sensitive asthma). This condition is thought to result from the stimulation of the leukotriene pathway that results when synthesis of prostaglandin E_2 (PGE_2), which down-regulates the 5-lipoxygenase pathway, is reduced. Aspirin and other NSAIDs inhibit the cyclooxygenase pathway and decrease the synthesis of prostaglandins, including PGE_2. Patients with aspirin-sensitive asthma have an exaggerated leukotriene response to aspirin, and inhibition of the leukotriene pathway by leukotriene-modifying agents is an effective treatment.

Unlike many drugs used in the treatment of asthma, the leukotriene-modifying agents are all available as oral tablets rather than inhaled formulations. Although inhaled formulations generally decrease adverse effects by delivering the drug to the target organ directly, there are several advantages of the orally administered leukotrienes. First, many patients, particularly children, find it easier to take a tablet than use an inhaler, so adherence is frequently better. Second, because inhalers are often used improperly, there is a higher likelihood that the intended dose of a tablet is delivered. Finally, because orally delivered drugs are absorbed systemically, the drugs can be used to treat other coexisting allergic diseases, such as allergic rhinitis, that are also responsive to leukotriene pathway inhibition.

All three leukotriene-modifying agents are well tolerated and have few extrapulmonary effects, particularly compared to oral corticosteroids. Zileuton has a 4% incidence of hepatotoxicity, so periodic liver function testing is required. The leukotriene receptor antagonists are considered generally safe but have been associated with Churg-Strauss syndrome on rare occasions. Churg-Strauss syndrome is a serious granulomatous vasculitis affecting the small arteries and veins of the lungs, heart, kidneys, pancreas, spleen, and skin. Because Churg-Strauss syndrome is independently associated with asthma and eosinophilia, it is not clear whether the reported reactions represent a distinct effect of the drug or an unmasking of the preexisting syndrome due to the reduction in corticosteroid use allowed by the addition of a leukotriene receptor antagonist to the therapeutic regimen.

Anti-IgE Antibodies

The prominence of IgE-mediated allergic responses in asthma suggests that inactivation or removal of IgE antibodies from the circulation would mitigate the acute response to an inhaled allergen. **Omalizumab** is a humanized mouse monoclonal antibody that binds to the high-affinity IgE-receptor (FcεRI) binding domain on human IgE. Omalizumab both decreases the quantity of circulating IgE and blocks the remaining IgE from binding to mast cell FcεRI (Fig. 48-3). Because omalizumab does not cross-link FcεRI-bound IgE, the drug does not typically induce anaphylaxis. Furthermore, omalizumab affects both the early- and late-phase asthmatic responses to challenge by an inhaled allergen, since mast cells, basophils, and dendritic cells down-regulate the FcεRI receptor in response to the lower levels of circulating IgE. Receptor down-regulation reduces stimulation of T_H2 lymphocytes and decreases the late-phase asthmatic response beyond the decrease that could be expected from removal of the circulating IgE alone. These mechanisms decrease the frequency of asthma exacerbations in patients treated with omalizumab.

Because it is an antibody, omalizumab must be administered subcutaneously every 2–4 weeks. Although its high cost and the inconvenience of parenteral administration have limited the use of omalizumab to severe cases of asthma, the drug also reduces the dose of corticosteroids needed for disease control and decreases the frequency of exacerbations in moderate asthma (as in the case of Mr. Y). Despite the fact that omalizumab is a humanized antibody in which 95% of the original mouse amino acid sequence has been replaced by the corresponding human sequence, the drug is recognized as an antigen and triggers an immune response on rare occasions, so patients must be monitored closely for several hours after administration.

Drug Delivery

Many adverse effects of drugs used to treat asthma, especially the corticosteroids and β-agonists, can be minimized by delivery of the drug directly to the airway. There are three principal delivery systems for inhaled drugs: **metered-dose inhalers**, **dry powder inhalers**, and **nebulizers**. In a metered-dose inhaler, a compressed gas propels a fixed dose of drug out of the device upon activation of the canister. In the past, a chlorofluorocarbon (CFC) such as Freon® was used as the propellant. However, because of the environmental effects of CFCs on the ozone layer, these gases have been replaced by hydrofluoroalkane (HFA) propellants. Although the canisters are easy to use, they do require coordination between inhalation and actuation of the device and frequently require a 10-second breath hold, making them potentially challenging to use for young children and the elderly. This is not the case for dry powder inhalers, where the act of inspiration creates turbulent flow within the device that aerosolizes and scatters a dry powder. Some patients find dry powder inhalers easier to use than metered-dose inhalers, but others find the powder irritating or find that they cannot generate a sufficient inspiratory force to activate the device. Nebulizers

pass a compressed gas such as compressed air or oxygen through a liquid formulation of the medication to convert it into a mist that is then inhaled. Although nebulizers are not as portable as the other delivery devices, they can be used in a hospital or home setting for treatment of acute asthmatic exacerbations and are easier to use for the delivery of inhaled medication. For example, infants who cannot use metered-dose inhalers can be treated via nebulizer. Nebulizers are also useful in cases of acute exacerbation, where breathlessness can limit the patient's ability to perform a long breath hold.

Clinical Management of Asthma

Treatment of asthma should be based on the severity of disease. Current guidelines from the National Institutes of Health state that patients should use the smallest dose of medication needed for adequate control of symptoms. As a practical matter, this means adjusting the dose of medication to achieve adequate control and then reducing it to the lowest effective dose. A stepwise care approach has been advocated to facilitate the ambulatory treatment of asthma. This approach separates asthma into two domains: (1) impairment, a measure of ongoing asthma symptoms, and (2) risk, a measure of the frequency and severity of exacerbations. Patients are classified into one of four clinical categories based on their impairment and risk (Table 48-1). For example, patients with *mild intermittent* asthma have the following characteristics: no chronic impairment in lung function, symptoms occurring no more than twice a week and nocturnal awakenings due to asthma no more than twice a month, infrequent use of their rescue medication, and zero or one asthma exacerbations requiring systemic corticosteroids a year. Such patients can often be satisfactorily managed with inhaled β-agonists as needed for relief of symptoms or before exposure to known asthma triggers, and they require little or no ongoing controller medication. Patients with more frequent or severe symptoms, or with impairment in lung function, should be treated with regular preventive therapy, such as inhaled corticosteroids at escalating doses depending on severity of symptoms. Other medications, such as long-acting β-agonists or leukotriene-modifying agents, may be added to improve control. Combination agents that include an inhaled corticosteroid and a long-acting inhaled β-agonist (such as the fluticasone/salmeterol formulation ultimately given to Mr. Y) can improve adherence by reducing the number of inhalers needed.

As in Mr. Y's case, asthma management also involves avoiding environmental exposures known to provoke airway inflammation. For example, eliminating environmental tobacco smoke reduces symptoms and the frequency of asthma attacks in children whose parents or caregivers are cigarette smokers, and allergen reduction is an important component of patient education to maintain control of asthma symptoms.

▌CONCLUSION AND FUTURE DIRECTIONS

The increasing incidence of asthma entails a significant burden of disability, economic cost, and death. Nonetheless, biomedical research has uncovered key features of

TABLE 48-1 Clinical Management of Asthma

SEVERITY OF ASTHMA	CLINICAL CHARACTERISTICS	SHORT-TERM RELIEF	LONG-TERM CONTROL
Mild intermittent (Step 1)	Symptoms ≤2 times/week Nocturnal awakenings ≤2 times/month Exacerbations brief Lung function normal between exacerbations Limited peak flow variability	Short-acting β-agonist as needed for symptoms or prior to expected exposures	No medications necessary
Mild persistent (Step 2)	Symptoms >2 times/week Nocturnal awakenings >2 times/month Exacerbations brief and may affect activity Lung function normal when asymptomatic Peak flow decreased 20–30% when symptomatic	Short-acting β-agonist as needed for symptoms	Preferred: inhaled low-dose corticosteroid Alternative: leukotriene pathway modifier, mast cell stabilizer, or theophylline
Moderate persistent (Step 3)	Daily symptoms Nocturnal awakenings >1 time/week Frequent exacerbations lasting days, affecting activity Lung function 60–80% of predicted Peak flow variability >30%	Short-acting β-agonist as needed for symptoms	Preferred: low- to medium-dose inhaled steroid and long-acting inhaled β-agonist Alternatives: Medium-dose inhaled steroid alone; or low- to medium-dose inhaled steroid plus sustained-release theophylline; or low- to medium-dose inhaled steroid plus leukotriene pathway modifier
Severe persistent (Step 4)	Continual symptoms Limited activity Frequent nocturnal awakenings Frequent, severe exacerbations Lung function <60% of predicted Peak flow variability >30%	Short-acting β-agonist as needed for symptoms	Preferred: high-dose inhaled corticosteroid and long-acting inhaled β-agonist Oral corticosteroids if needed Addition of more controllers has not been studied adequately

asthma pathophysiology that can be exploited for pharmacologic management of the disease. At its core, asthma is a disease caused by an aberrant inflammatory response in the airways that leads to airway hyperresponsiveness and bronchoconstriction. There is no cure for asthma, but a therapeutic approach that treats both aspects of asthma, by using anti-inflammatory medications and bronchodilators, along with the avoidance of known triggers, can be successful in achieving long-term clinical control and enabling successful management of the disease in most patients.

As our understanding of the pathophysiology of asthma has improved, new targets for therapeutic intervention have become available. In general, research has focused on three areas: improving existing therapies by altering the ratio of benefit to adverse effect, devising new targeted therapies, and attempting to prevent or reverse permanent airway remodeling in long-standing asthma. One example of the first approach is the development of novel inhaled corticosteroids with reduced systemic effects, such as selective glucocorticoid receptor modulators that retain anti-inflammatory activity while minimizing adverse effects.

Recent research on new targeted therapies has involved further characterization of asthma on a molecular and phenotypic basis. Using both gene expression data and clinical characteristics, researchers have found a substantial amount of heterogeneity in the disease, with subsets of populations having different immunologic features. For example, while many asthmatic patients display a T_H2 response as described above in "Pathophysiology of Asthma," others show a much less active T_H2 response. This has opened the possibility of using biomarkers to identify the aberrant pathways in individual patients and targeting therapy for each patient that is most likely to be beneficial.

Inhibitors of inflammatory cytokines are under development as potential therapeutics to prevent airway remodeling in asthma. One example is the anti-IL-5 monoclonal antibody mepolizumab, which reduces the number of circulating and airway eosinophils in patients with asthma and appears to reduce the frequency of asthma exacerbations in a rare subgroup of patients with prednisone-dependent asthma and sputum eosinophilia. However, mepolizumab has shown no efficacy in the general population of patients with asthma, suggesting that reducing eosinophils alone may not significantly affect the disease in the majority of patients. A second example is pitrakinra, a variant of IL-4 that blocks binding of IL-4 and IL-13 to the IL-4 receptor alpha. This drug has shown promise in early-stage clinical studies. Lebrikizumab, an anti-IL-13 antibody, has also shown promise in early-stage clinical trials, particularly in patients with elevated levels of the biomarker periostin, which appears to signal an aberrant T_H2 pathway (Fig. 48-6). Finally, TNF-α (see Chapter 46, Pharmacology of Immunosuppression) is a cytokine that is up-regulated in asthma and that recruits neutrophils and eosinophils to the airways. The TNF pathway inhibitors etanercept (a recombinant fusion protein that inhibits TNF-α) and infliximab (an anti-TNF-α

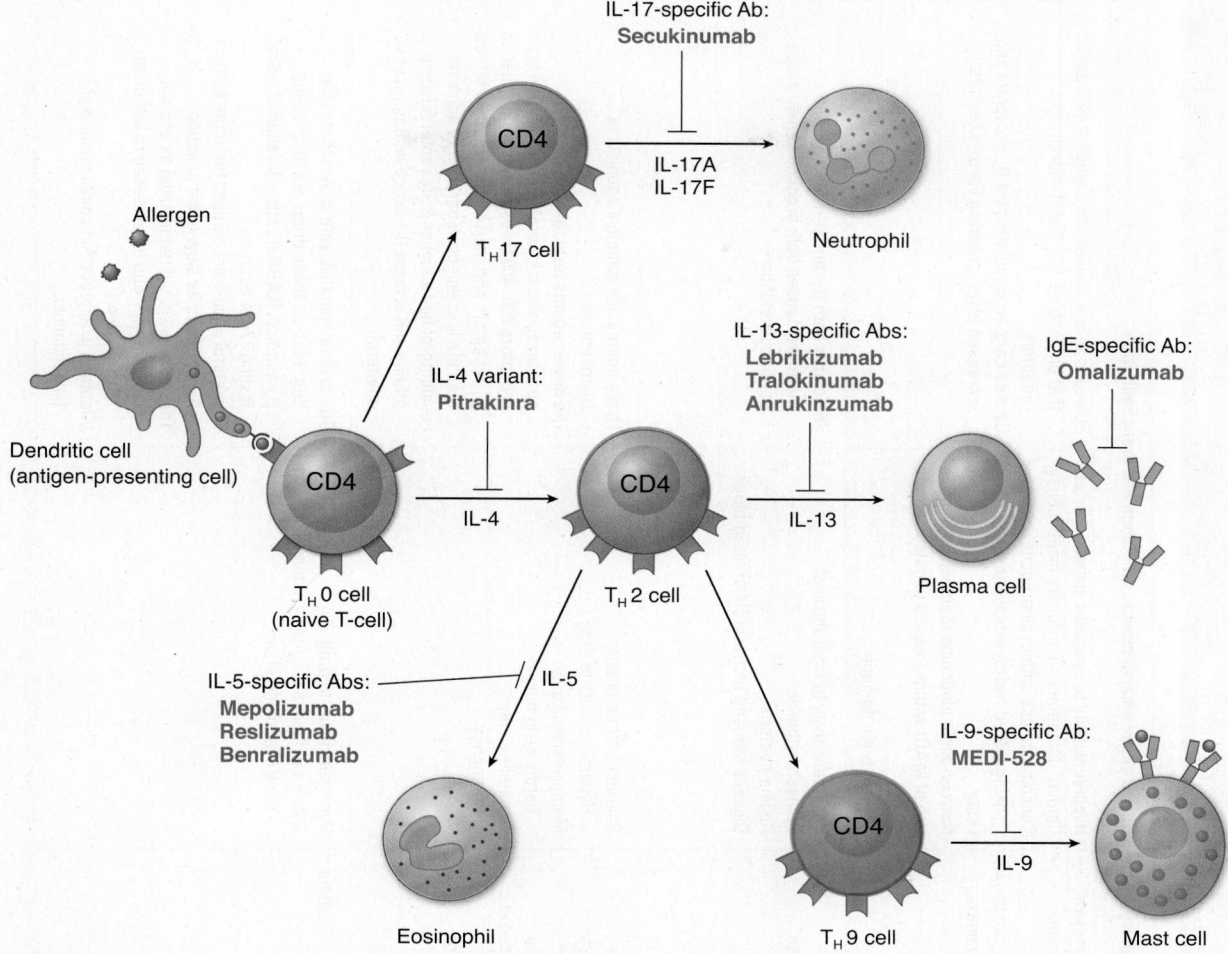

FIGURE 48-6. Targeted therapy for asthma cytokines. Much current research in asthma focuses on developing drugs that inhibit cytokines mediating the pathogenesis of asthma. These include variants of IL-4 such as pitrakinra; anti-IL-13 antibodies such as lebrikizumab, tralokinumab, and anrukinzumab; and anti-IL-5 antibodies such as mepolizumab, reslizumab, and benralizumab. Omalizumab, an approved monoclonal antibody, targets IgE before it can cross-link Fcε receptors on mast cells.

monoclonal antibody) have shown promising results in early clinical studies.

Suggested Reading

Barnes PJ. The cytokine network in asthma and chronic obstructive pulmonary disease. *J Clin Invest* 2008;118:3546–3556. (*Reviews the role of cytokines in the chronic asthmatic reaction and suggests targets for new drug development.*)

Fanta CH. Asthma. *N Engl J Med* 2009;360:1002–1014. (*Discusses the clinical management of asthma, focusing on commonly prescribed therapeutics.*)

Guidelines for the diagnosis and management of asthma (EPR-3). http://www.nhlbi.nih.gov/health-pro/guidelines/current/asthma-guidelines. (*This is the most recent set of practice guidelines for the diagnosis and treatment of asthma from the expert panel convened by the National Heart, Lung, and Blood Institute of the National Institutes of Health.*)

Locksley RM. Asthma and allergic inflammation. *Cell* 2010;140:777–783. (*Reviews the dysregulated interactions between airway epithelia and innate immune cells that initiate and maintain asthma.*)

Pelaia G, Vatrella A, Maselli R. The potential of biologics for the treatment of asthma. *Nat Rev Drug Discov* 2012;11:958–972. (*Describes approaches to individualized therapy for asthma and efforts to develop drugs targeting specific inflammatory pathways.*)

Rhen T, Cidlowski JA. Antiinflammatory action of glucocorticoids—new mechanisms for old drugs. *N Engl J Med* 2005;353:1711–1723. (*Discusses the molecular mechanisms by which glucocorticoids act and efforts to develop novel glucocorticoids with improved adverse effect profiles.*)

Vestbo J, Hurd SS, Agustí AG, et al. Global strategy for the diagnosis, management, and prevention of chronic obstructive pulmonary disease: GOLD executive summary. *Am J Respir Crit Care Med* 2013;187:347–365. (*Describes approaches for the diagnosis and treatment of chronic obstructive pulmonary disease.*)

DRUG SUMMARY TABLE: CHAPTER 48 Integrative Inflammation Pharmacology: Asthma

β-ADRENERGIC AGONISTS
Mechanism—Agonists at β-adrenergic receptors on airway smooth muscle; act through a stimulatory G protein (G$_s$) to cause smooth muscle relaxation and bronchodilation

DRUG	CLINICAL APPLICATIONS	SERIOUS AND COMMON ADVERSE EFFECTS	CONTRAINDICATIONS	THERAPEUTIC CONSIDERATIONS
Epinephrine	Asthma Anaphylaxis Blood coagulation disorders Cardiac arrest Open-angle glaucoma Congestion of mucosa Excessive uterine contraction Local anesthesia Syncope	*Cardiac arrhythmias, angina, hypertensive crisis, cerebral hemorrhage, pulmonary edema* Tachycardia, palpitations, sweating, nausea, vomiting, headache, asthenia, dizziness, tremor, nervousness, dyspnea	Hypersensitivity to sympathomimetic amines Cardiac dilatation and coronary insufficiency Concomitant use with cyclopropane or halogenated hydrocarbon anesthetics Labor Narrow-angle glaucoma (ophthalmic form) Use of MAOI within 2 weeks (inhalation form) Shock Organic brain damage	Epinephrine is a nonselective adrenergic agonist that binds to α$_1$-, β$_1$-, and β$_2$-adrenergic receptors. Causes cardiac stimulation via β$_1$-receptors and increased blood pressure via α-receptors.
Isoproterenol	Asthma Cardiac arrest Decreased vascular flow Heart block Heart failure Shock Stokes-Adams syndrome	*Coronary atherosclerosis* Tachyarrhythmia, syncope, confusion, headache, tremor, restlessness	Hypersensitivity to isoproterenol Tachyarrhythmias Angina pectoris Digitalis-induced tachycardia or heart block	Stimulates both β$_1$- and β$_2$-receptors and therefore causes both bronchodilation and cardiac stimulation.
Isoetharine Metaproterenol Terbutaline Albuterol (Salbutamol) Levalbuterol Pirbuterol Bitolterol	Asthma COPD	*Cardiac arrhythmia (shared adverse effect); paradoxical bronchospasm (metaproterenol, terbutaline, and pirbuterol only); pulmonary edema (terbutaline and albuterol only); diabetic ketoacidosis (albuterol only)* Palpitations, flushing, nausea, tremor, nervousness	Shared contraindication: Hypersensitivity to drug Metaproterenol only: Cardia arrhythmias Terbutaline only: Pregnancy	These agents are selective agonists at β$_2$-receptors. The newer agents terbutaline, albuterol, pirbuterol, and bitolterol bind to β$_2$-adrenergic receptors 200–400 times more strongly than to β$_1$-receptors and cause lesser cardiac effects than the less selective adrenergic agonists. Levalbuterol has a higher β$_2$-receptor binding affinity and is more β$_2$-selective than racemic albuterol.
Formoterol Salmeterol Arformoterol Vilanterol Indacaterol Olodaterol	Shared indication: COPD Formoterol and salmeterol only: Asthma	*Cardiac arrhythmias, exacerbation of asthma* Musculoskeletal pain, headache (salmeterol only)	Hypersensitivity to drug Asthma without a long-term asthma controller medication	Due to their lipophilic side chains that resist degradation, these drugs are long-acting β$_2$-agonists (LABAs) with a duration of action lasting 12–24 hours. Salmeterol should not be used for acute asthma flares due to its slow onset of action. These drugs should not be used as asthma monotherapy due to increased risk of death from asthma. Vilanterol is approved in combination with umeclidinium.

ANTICHOLINERGICS

Mechanism—Antagonists at muscarinic receptors on airway smooth muscle and glands, leading to decreased bronchoconstriction and mucus secretion

Drug	Clinical Applications	Serious and Common Adverse Effects	Contraindications	Therapeutic Considerations
Ipratropium **Tiotropium** **Umeclidinium** **Aclidinium**	Shared indication: COPD Ipratropium only: Nasal discharge	*Hypersensitivity reaction, stroke (ipratropium, tiotropium, and umeclidinium only); myocardial infarction (ipratropium and aclidinium only); bronchospasm (ipratropium and umeclidinium only); bowel obstruction (tiotropium only); angle-closure glaucoma (umeclidinium only)* Dry mouth, upper respiratory infection (shared adverse effects); abnormal taste, dry nasal mucosa (ipratropium only); urinary retention (umeclidinium only)	Shared contraindication: Hypersensitivity to drug Ipratropium only: Hypersensitivity to atropine Umeclidinium only: Hypersensitivity to soya lecithin or related food products (inhalation aerosol)	Tiotropium, umeclidinium, and aclidinium have a long duration of action because of slow dissociation kinetics from M_1 and M_3 receptors. Umeclidinium is only available in combination with vilanterol.

METHYLXANTHINES AND PHOSPHODIESTERASE IV RECEPTOR INHIBITORS

Mechanism—Theophylline and aminophylline: nonselective phosphodiesterase (PDE) inhibitors that prevent the degradation of cAMP; also act as adenosine receptor antagonists; the combined effect is smooth muscle relaxation and bronchodilation. Roflumilast: selective inhibitor of PDE IV

Drug	Clinical Applications	Serious and Common Adverse Effects	Contraindications	Therapeutic Considerations
Theophylline **Aminophylline**	Asthma COPD	*Atrial fibrillation, tachyarrhythmia, intracranial hemorrhage, seizure (shared adverse reactions); Stevens-Johnson syndrome (theophylline only); necrotizing enterocolitis in fetus or newborn, immune hypersensitivity reaction (aminophylline only)* Gastrointestinal upset, headache, insomnia, tremor, restlessness, irritability	Hypersensitivity to theophylline or aminophylline	Nonspecific inhibitors of phosphodiesterases that inhibit phosphodiesterase in both airway smooth muscle cells and inflammatory cells. Inhibition of phosphodiesterase types III and IV in smooth muscle cells results in bronchodilation, and inhibition of phosphodiesterase type IV in T cells and eosinophils causes immunomodulatory and anti-inflammatory effects. Plasma levels must be monitored to prevent toxic levels of these agents. Avoid co-administration with fluvoxamine, enoxacin, mexiletine, propranolol, or troleandomycin due to increased risk of theophylline toxicity. Avoid co-administration with zafirlukast because theophylline can decrease plasma concentration of zafirlukast.
Roflumilast	COPD	*Suicidal ideation* Weight loss, gastrointestinal upset, influenza, backache, dizziness, headache, insomnia	Hepatic impairment, Child-Pugh Class B or C	Selective inhibitor of PDE IV, approved for use in severe COPD. Results in small improvement in lung function and decreased risk of exacerbation.

MAGNESIUM

Mechanism—Inhibits calcium transport into smooth muscle cells, thereby inducing smooth muscle relaxation

Drug	Clinical Applications	Serious and Common Adverse Effects	Contraindications	Therapeutic Considerations
Magnesium sulfate	Atrial paroxysmal tachycardia Barium poisoning Cerebral edema Eclampsia Hypomagnesemia Seizure	*Heart block, hypotension, prolonged bleeding time, hyporeflexia, CNS depression, respiratory tract paralysis*	Heart block or myocardial damage	Tocolytic agent commonly used to cause uterine relaxation and to delay preterm labor. May benefit patients with acute asthma exacerbation.

DRUG SUMMARY TABLE: CHAPTER 48 Integrative Inflammation Pharmacology: Asthma *continued*

DRUG	CLINICAL APPLICATIONS	SERIOUS AND COMMON ADVERSE EFFECTS	CONTRAINDICATIONS	THERAPEUTIC CONSIDERATIONS
INHALED CORTICOSTEROIDS Mechanism—Inhibit COX-2 action and prostaglandin biosynthesis by inducing lipocortins; activate endogenous anti-inflammatory pathways; and other mechanisms				
Beclomethasone **Triamcinolone** **Fluticasone** **Budesonide** **Flunisolide** **Mometasone** **Ciclesonide**	See Drug Summary Table: Chapter 29 Pharmacology of the Adrenal Cortex			
CROMOLYNS Mechanism—Inhibit chloride transport, which in turn affects calcium gating to prevent granule release, possibly decreasing mast cell response to inflammatory stimuli				
Cromolyn **Nedocromil**	Shared indications: Asthma Conjunctivitis Cromolyn only: Allergic rhinitis Keratitis Keratoconjunctivitis Mast cell disorder	*Anaphylaxis, bronchospasm (cromolyn only)* Abnormal taste, burning sensation in eye, cough, throat irritation (shared adverse effects); gastrointestinal upset, dizziness, headache (nedocromil only)	Hypersensitivity to cromolyn or nedocromil	Used primarily as prophylactic therapy in patients with allergic asthma associated with specific triggers. Useful in patients with exercise-induced asthma; can be taken immediately prior to exercise. More effective in children and young adults than in older patients. Excellent safety profile but less efficacious than other asthma medications.
LEUKOTRIENE PATHWAY-MODIFYING AGENTS Mechanism—Zileuton inhibits 5-lipoxygenase, thereby decreasing synthesis of leukotrienes; montelukast and zafirlukast are cysteinyl leukotriene receptor antagonists				
Zileuton **Montelukast** **Zafirlukast**	See Drug Summary Table: Chapter 43 Pharmacology of Eicosanoids			
ANTI-IMMUNOGLOBULIN E ANTIBODIES Mechanism—Humanized mouse monoclonal antibody against the high-affinity IgE-receptor (FcεRI) binding domain on human IgE. Prevents IgE from binding to FcεRI on mast cells and antigen-presenting cells; also, decreases the quantity of circulating IgE. The combined effect is a decrease in the allergic response in asthma.				
Omalizumab	Asthma Idiopathic urticaria	*Eosinophilic disorder, thrombocytopenia, anaphylaxis* Injection site reaction, nausea, arthralgia, headache, cough, upper respiratory tract infection	Hypersensitivity to omalizumab	Affects both the early- and late-phase asthmatic responses to challenge by an inhaled allergen. Administered subcutaneously every 2–4 weeks. High cost limits its use to severe cases of asthma.

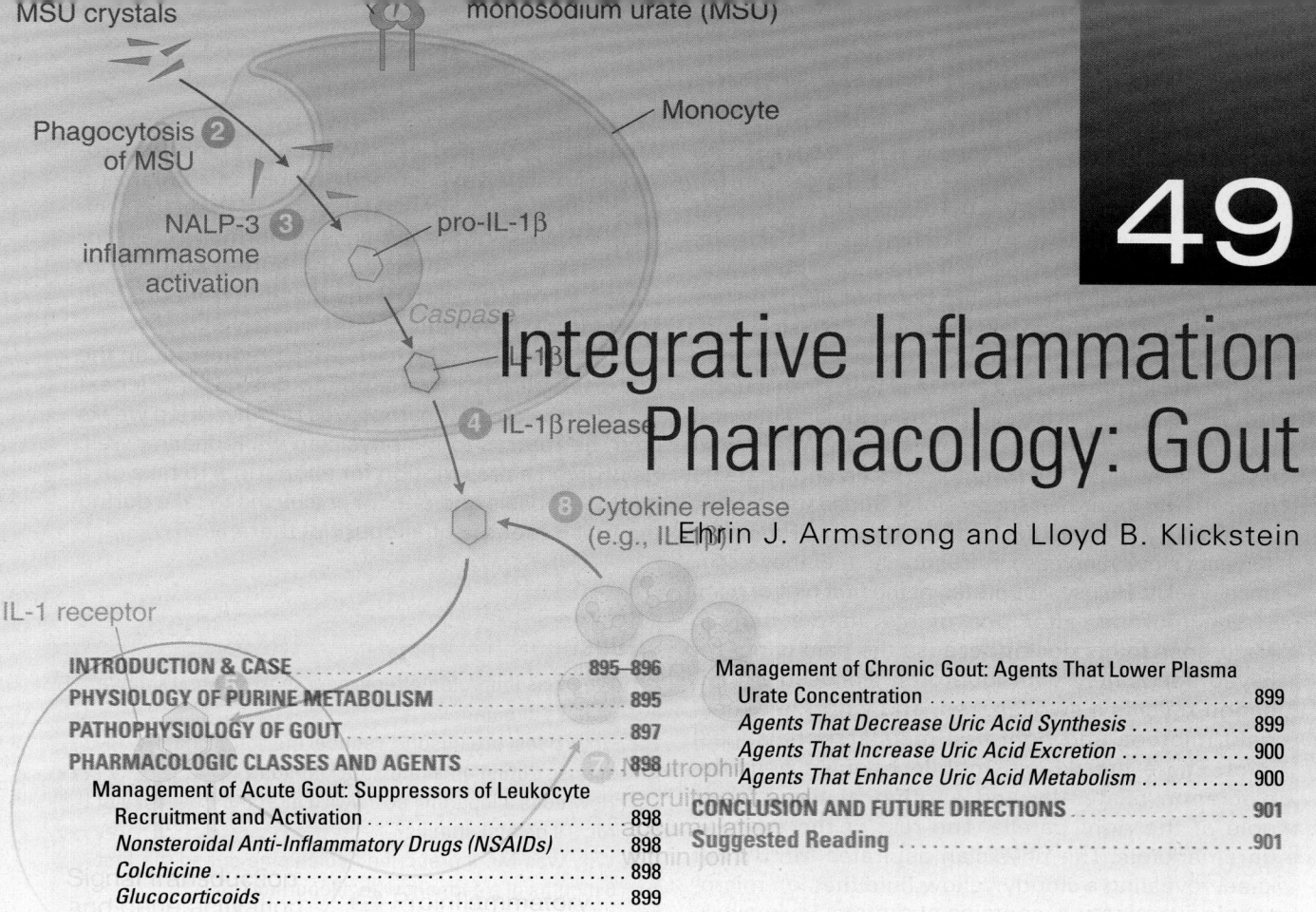

49

Integrative Inflammation Pharmacology: Gout

Ehrin J. Armstrong and Lloyd B. Klickstein

▌ INTRODUCTION

Gout is a uniquely human disease. Most mammals possess uricase, an enzyme that metabolizes purine breakdown products into a freely water-soluble substance, allantoin. Humans, in contrast, excrete most purines as sparingly soluble uric acid. High plasma levels of uric acid can lead to deposition of uric acid crystals in joints, most frequently the first metatarsophalangeal joint (great toe). Acute attacks of gout cause intense pain but typically occur infrequently.

A number of rational therapies exist for the treatment of gout. These therapies are broadly divided into two groups: those that treat acute gout attacks and those that prevent recurrent attacks. Drugs that suppress the immune response to crystal deposition or limit the extent of inflammation may be used for both indications, although they are more commonly used to treat acute attacks. Agents that reduce uric acid synthesis or increase the renal excretion of uric acid prevent monosodium urate crystal formation and are useful for prevention of recurrent attacks. These pharmacologic interventions provide effective therapy for most cases of gout.

▌ PHYSIOLOGY OF PURINE METABOLISM

Gout is caused by imbalances in purine metabolism. To understand the cause and treatment of gout, it is necessary to recall the principles of nucleotide biochemistry. Although pyrimidines such as cytosine, thymidine, and uracil are straightforward for the body to metabolize and excrete, it is a challenge to metabolize purines (most notably the

nucleotides guanine and adenine). The intermediates of purine metabolism are toxic to some cells, necessitating tight regulation of purine synthesis and degradation. Furthermore, the final breakdown product of purine metabolism is uric acid, which is barely soluble in blood or urine. Increased plasma levels of uric acid are the strongest risk factor for gout, although, for poorly understood reasons, not everyone with high plasma uric acid levels develops gout.

Purines are synthesized via two general pathways: **de novo synthesis** and the **salvage pathway** (Fig. 49-1). The first step in the de novo pathway is the reaction of phosphoribosyl pyrophosphate (**PRPP**, a ribose sugar with two pyrophosphates attached) with glutamine. PRPP provides the ribose sugar as one precursor for the nascent nucleotide. Hydrolysis of the pyrophosphate in a later step makes the de novo pathway irreversible. Glutamine is the precursor for inosine monophosphate (IMP), a precursor that is common to adenine and guanine biosynthesis. The reaction of PRPP with glutamine is catalyzed by the enzyme amidophosphoribosyltransferase (**amidoPRT**). AmidoPRT is activated allosterically by high levels of PRPP; PRPP is thus both a substrate and an activator of amidoPRT. In general, *the cellular level of PRPP is the most important determinant of de novo purine synthesis.* High PRPP levels result in enhanced de novo purine synthesis, whereas low PRPP levels decrease the rate of synthesis.

The salvage pathway is the second important route to purine synthesis. The first step in the salvage pathway is catalyzed by the key regulatory enzyme hypoxanthine-guanine phosphoribosyltransferase (**HGPRT**). HGPRT transfers PRPP to either hypoxanthine or guanine, resulting in the formation

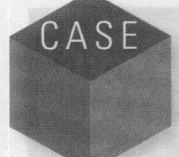

CASE

Mr. J, a 53-year-old man, awakens one morning with excruciating pain in his great toe. Even the weight of the bed sheet is enough to make him want to scream; he is unable to put on a sock or shoe. Worried that something terrible has occurred, Mr. J rushes to his doctor. Based on the history and physical findings, the physician diagnoses an acute attack of gout. The physician prescribes a course of high-dose ibuprofen, which improves his symptoms in the first day and relieves the pain after 3 days. Mr. J is then well until 5 years later, when the symptoms recur, and he treats himself with ibuprofen successfully. Subsequently, Mr. J learns to anticipate the attacks, which over the next 10 years slowly increase in frequency until they occur once weekly. He uses ibuprofen at the first hint of pain.

The morning after one of his attacks begins, Mr. J goes to his doctor because the pain is not relieved adequately with ibuprofen. Focused examination reveals a swollen, red, and warm left knee, right midfoot, and right first metatarsophalangeal joint. There are 0.5-cm mobile nodules near the olecranon bilaterally and another at the inferior pole of the right patella. The rest of the exam is unremarkable. The physician aspirates Mr. J's left knee, revealing a cloudy yellow fluid that, on microscopic examination, contains numerous leukocytes.

Abundant blue and yellow needle-shaped microscopic crystals are seen with the use of a polarizing filter with a red compensator, some of them intracellular. An x-ray of the left knee is normal except for the presence of an effusion; a film of the right foot shows a bony erosion of the distal first metatarsal. The culture of the joint fluid is negative.

Mr. J is treated with high-dose prednisone on the first day, followed by a tapering dose over the next 10 days. His condition improves rapidly. Three weeks later, he returns to his physician while feeling well. He is given a prescription for allopurinol to take on a long-term basis and one for colchicine to take during the first 6 months of allopurinol therapy.

Questions

1. Why was ibuprofen effective for most of Mr. J's acute attacks of pain?
2. How does prednisone reduce the inflammatory response during an acute attack of gout?
3. How does allopurinol act? Will it alter the frequency of Mr. J's painful attacks?
4. Why was Mr. J prescribed colchicine during the first 6 months of treatment with allopurinol?

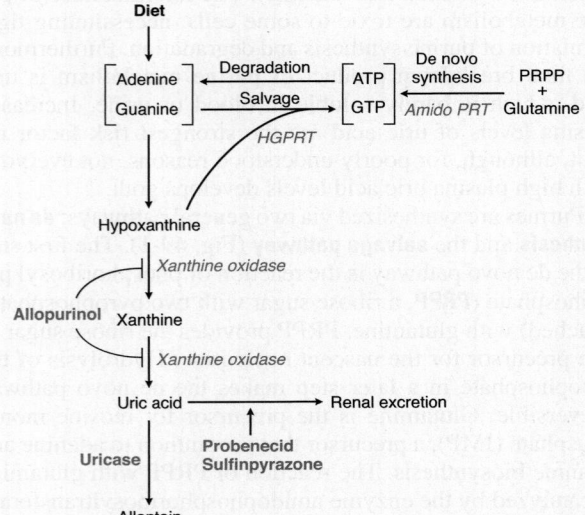

FIGURE 49-1. Purine metabolism. Purines are synthesized via de novo synthesis or via the salvage pathway. The de novo pathway utilizes the amino acid glutamine and phosphoribosyl pyrophosphate (PRPP) in a reaction catalyzed by amidophosphoribosyltransferase (amidoPRT). In the salvage pathway, hypoxanthine-guanine phosphoribosyltransferase (HGPRT) phosphorylates and ribosylates dietary adenine and guanine, forming the purine nucleotides (ATP and GTP) used for DNA and RNA synthesis. Degradation converts purines and purine nucleotides to hypoxanthine, and xanthine oxidase converts hypoxanthine to xanthine and ultimately to uric acid, which is excreted by the kidneys or gastrointestinal tract (*not shown*). Pharmacologic interventions that reduce plasma urate levels include reducing urate synthesis (allopurinol and its metabolite oxypurinol), increasing urate excretion (probenecid and sulfinpyrazone), or converting urate to the more soluble allantoin (uricase).

of IMP or guanosine monophosphate (GMP), respectively. Nucleotide interconversions can then yield adenosine triphosphate (ATP) and guanosine 5′-triphosphate (GTP).

Increased activity of the salvage pathway has two important consequences. First, increased scavenging activity depletes cells of PRPP, thus decreasing the rate of de novo purine synthesis. Second, the salvage pathway leads to the generation of more ATP and GTP. Increased levels of these nucleotides inhibit amidoPRT in a feedback manner, also resulting in decreased de novo purine synthesis.

Although purines can be synthesized by these two interrelated pathways, *degradation occurs via a convergent mechanism* (Fig. 49-1). Adenosine monophosphate (AMP) is deaminated, dephosphorylated, and deribosylated, forming hypoxanthine. GMP is also deaminated, dephosphorylated, and deribosylated, forming hypoxanthine. Hypoxanthine, which is moderately soluble, is oxidized to xanthine. Thus, xanthine is the common product of purine metabolism. A further oxidation step converts xanthine to uric acid. The enzyme **xanthine oxidase** catalyzes both the oxidation of hypoxanthine to xanthine and the oxidation of xanthine to uric acid.

Crosstalk between the de novo and salvage pathways is important for overall regulation of purine metabolism. The de novo pathway is the most important generator of purine breakdown products. *High de novo pathway activity increases purine turnover, resulting in higher plasma uric acid concentrations.* In contrast, increased salvage pathway activity leads to decreased de novo synthesis and reduced plasma uric acid levels.

The importance of crosstalk in purine metabolism is demonstrated by several inherited enzyme disorders. Certain genetic polymorphisms that increase PRPP synthase activity lead to increased intracellular levels of PRPP; because PRPP activates amidoPRT, high levels of PRPP cause increased de novo purine synthesis, leading to increased turnover and degradation of purines and increased plasma levels of uric acid. Similarly, genetic deficiencies of HGPRT (the critical enzyme in the salvage pathway) lead to decreased salvage pathway activity and increased de novo purine synthesis and degradation, resulting in increased uric acid levels. The inherited absence of HGPRT results in **Lesch-Nyhan syndrome**, a devastating disorder characterized by self-mutilation, mental retardation, and hyperuricemia. Partial defects in HGPRT (e.g., polymorphisms in the HGPRT gene that lead to decreased HGPRT synthesis or activity) are thought to explain some cases of hereditary gout.

Uric acid is eliminated by the kidney (65%) and gastrointestinal tract (35%). Uric acid is filtered and secreted by the kidney by the same mechanisms that process other organic anions. Approximately 90% of filtered uric acid is reabsorbed. The major mediator of uric acid reabsorption is urate transporter 1 (URAT1), a member of the organic anion transporter family (SLC22A12) that is expressed in the kidney proximal tubule (see Chapter 5, Drug Transporters). Recent genetic association studies have suggested that polymorphisms in URAT1 may predispose to the development of gout. Renal excretion is important for the maintenance of normal plasma uric acid levels, and kidney failure often leads to high plasma urate levels.

PATHOPHYSIOLOGY OF GOUT

The likelihood of developing gout correlates strongly with increased plasma uric acid levels. Uric acid is a weak acid ($pK_a = 5.6$); at physiologic pH, 99% of plasma uric acid is in the ionized, urate form. The normal urate concentration in human plasma is 4–6 mg/dL, reflecting a balance of urate synthesis, breakdown, and excretion. Urate is sparingly soluble: the plasma becomes saturated if urate levels exceed 6.8 mg/dL. A plasma level over 7.0 mg/dL for men or 6.0 mg/dL for women is classified clinically as hyperuricemia. The gender difference may be attributable to differences in urate excretion between women and men.

Any variable that decreases the solubility of urate can promote urate crystal deposition. Gout occurs most commonly in peripheral joints. Urate is less soluble at lower temperatures, which may explain the peripheral distribution of urate crystal deposition. Also, joint synovial fluid is more acidic than blood, favoring crystal formation. Nevertheless, a complete explanation for the pattern of joint involvement in gout remains elusive.

The pathogenesis of gout is thought to reflect deposition of urate crystals in the periarticular fibrous tissue of synovial joints after years of hyperuricemia. However, it is also possible to develop gout without hyperuricemia (e.g., due to an immune response to urate or to preferential deposition of urate in synovial fluid).

The natural history of gout has four stages (Table 49-1). First, asymptomatic hyperuricemia develops because of either increased purine breakdown or decreased urate excretion. Most cases of hyperuricemia never develop into gout, and there is no indication for treatment of hyperuricemia in the absence of gout. It is, however, important to determine the cause of marked hyperuricemia: such causes can include

TABLE 49-1 Natural History of Gout

STAGE	FEATURES	PHARMACOLOGIC INTERVENTION
1. Asymptomatic hyperuricemia	Plasma urate >6.0 mg/dL in women, >7.0 mg/dL in men	None
2. Acute gout	Acute arthritis Typically first metatarsophalangeal joint Excruciating pain	NSAIDs Colchicine Glucocorticoids
3. Intercritical phase	Asymptomatic hyperuricemia 10% may never have another acute attack	None
4. Chronic gout	Hyperuricemia Development of tophi Recurrent attacks of acute gout	Allopurinol Probenecid Sulfinpyrazone

The degree of hyperuricemia correlates with the likelihood of developing gout; however, developing gout without hyperuricemia is possible. No pharmacologic intervention is indicated for asymptomatic hyperuricemia, but the cause should be investigated.

lymphoma (increased purine turnover) and kidney failure (decreased urate excretion).

For patients with symptomatic gout, the second phase involves an acute attack of arthritis or, less frequently, renal colic due to a monosodium urate stone. The arthritis is typically manifested as a rapid onset of acute pain in a single joint, as occurred in Mr. J. More than 50% of patients with gout have their first attack in the first metatarsophalangeal joint (pain at this site is referred to as **podagra**), and most patients with recurrent, symptomatic gout have podagra at some point. Without treatment, an acute attack of gout may last for days to weeks but generally resolves spontaneously. It is not understood what causes the periodic onset of gout attacks, or why these attacks resolve spontaneously.

The end of an attack leads to the third, intercritical phase, characterized by hyperuricemia without acute symptomatic gout. Some individuals will experience only one acute attack of gout and remain in the intercritical phase for long periods or even for the remainder of their lives. Five years after his initial attack, Mr. J developed chronic, recurrent attacks of gout, the fourth phase. Typically, these attacks become polyarticular and more severe. Chronically high levels of plasma uric acid can also lead to deposition of urate crystals around synovial joints or at sites of tissue damage, called **tophi**. Mr. J's mobile olecranon and patellar nodules are tophi. Juxta-articular tophi may eventually destroy the synovial lining and cartilage.

Recent research has begun to elucidate the cellular and molecular mechanisms responsible for the inflammatory events that are initiated by deposition of urate crystals (Fig. 49-2). Interestingly, these mechanisms may represent a pathologic manifestation of a normal physiologic pathway in which uric acid released from injured and dying cells functions as a "danger signal" that initiates an inflammatory response, leading to tissue repair and host defenses.

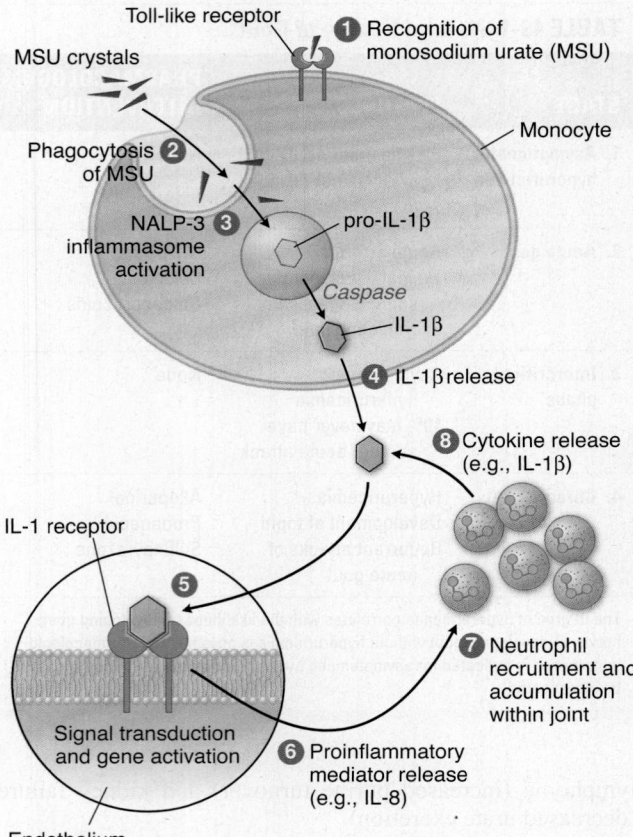

FIGURE 49-2. Mechanisms of the inflammatory response to urate crystals. In an acute attack of gout, monosodium urate (MSU) binds to toll-like receptors (TLRs) on monocytes (**1**). TLR activation initiates phagocytosis of MSU crystals (**2**), with subsequent assembly of intracellular inflammatory response enzymes referred to as the *NALP-3 inflammasome* (**3**). Assembly of the NALP-3 inflammasome activates caspase-1, an enzyme that cleaves inactive pro-IL-1β to the active cytokine IL-1β (**4**). IL-1β is released into the extracellular space, where it binds to receptors expressed on endothelial cells. Subsequent endothelial cell activation (**5**) leads to release of chemotactic factors such as IL-8 (**6**) that recruit neutrophils (**7**). Proinflammatory mediators released by activated endothelial cells and neutrophils complete a positive feedback loop of further IL-1β release, endothelial activation, and neutrophil recruitment (**8**).

In this model, pathologic urate crystals activate monocytes and synoviocytes by binding to toll-like receptors (TLRs), which are transmembrane signaling proteins that initiate an innate immune response. In monocytes, urate crystal binding and phagocytosis initiate assembly of an intracellular protein complex referred to as the *NALP-3 inflammasome*. Assembly of the inflammasome activates caspase-1, a proteolytic enzyme that cleaves inactive pro-IL-1β to active IL-1β. IL-1β is a potent cytokine that initiates a cascade of immune responses, including endothelial cell activation and increased neutrophil transmigration to the site of inflammation. Importantly, IL-1β up-regulates its own transcription and may provide positive feedback to amplify the initial innate immune response. Clinical trials of IL-1β antagonists and IL-1 receptor antagonists for the treatment of acute gout have shown some clinical benefit, but none of these drugs are approved by the US Food and Drug Administration (FDA) for use in the treatment of gout.

PHARMACOLOGIC CLASSES AND AGENTS

There are two main strategies for the treatment of gout: (1) management of acute attacks of gouty arthritis and (2) long-term management of chronic gout. Although some of the same drugs are used in treating acute and chronic gout, the aims of therapy differ in the two cases. The goal of acute gouty arthritis management is to control pain using drugs that limit joint inflammation. In contrast, therapy of the chronic disease aims to modify purine metabolism to achieve normal concentrations of plasma urate. Thus, pharmacologic agents for the treatment of chronic gout either decrease the production of urate or increase the renal clearance of urate.

Management of Acute Gout: Suppressors of Leukocyte Recruitment and Activation

Nonsteroidal Anti-Inflammatory Drugs (NSAIDs)
Metabolites of arachidonic acid play an important role in the inflammatory response to urate crystals in the joint. NSAIDs inhibit cyclooxygenase (COX) and thereby inhibit prostaglandin and thromboxane synthesis (see Chapter 43, Pharmacology of Eicosanoids). These drugs were effective for most of Mr. J's acute attacks of gout; his pain responded well to ibuprofen. Clinically, **indomethacin** is one of the NSAIDs used most often to treat acute attacks of gout. The choice of an NSAID or colchicine (see discussion below) for treatment of acute gout is generally based on the adverse effect profile, since the agents have similar efficacy. The serious adverse effects of NSAIDs include bleeding, salt and water retention, and renal insufficiency. COX-2 selective inhibitors are potentially useful for the management of acute gout attacks because they may be associated with a lower risk of gastrointestinal bleeding, although concerns about adverse cardiovascular effects limit their long-term use.

Colchicine
Colchicine binds to tubulin, inhibiting its polymerization and preventing the formation of microtubules. Colchicine inhibits cell division because microtubules are critical for the alignment and separation of chromosomes during mitosis (see Chapter 39, Pharmacology of Cancer: Genome Synthesis, Stability, and Maintenance). Microtubules are also essential in intracellular trafficking. In an acutely inflamed joint, colchicine limits the inflammatory response by inhibiting neutrophil activation. The mechanisms of neutrophil inhibition by colchicine include (1) decreased trafficking of phagocytosed particles to lysosomes; (2) decreased release of chemotactic factor; (3) decreased motility and adhesion of neutrophils; and (4) decreased tyrosine phosphorylation of neutrophil proteins, with a resulting decrease in leukotriene B$_4$ synthesis. Colchicine can also be administered in low doses as a prophylactic therapy for chronic gout to inhibit the occurrence of acute attacks. Drugs that alter urate homeostasis are often co-administered initially with colchicine to avoid precipitating an acute attack of gouty arthritis (see discussion below).

Colchicine causes several important adverse effects. Colchicine inhibits the turnover of epithelial cells in the gastrointestinal (GI) tract, and diarrhea is a common complication of moderate or high doses of the drug. Colchicine is myelosuppressive, particularly in high doses or in combination

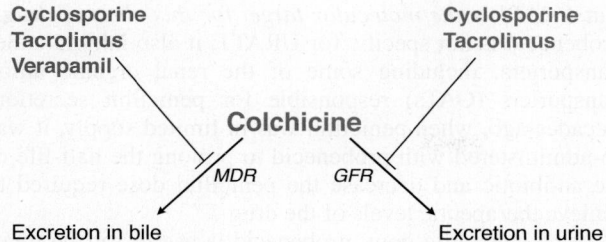

FIGURE 49-3. **Important drug interactions involving colchicine.** Cyclosporine and tacrolimus (immunosuppressant drugs frequently prescribed after organ transplantation) and verapamil (a Ca^{2+} channel blocker used to treat hypertension and some cardiac arrhythmias) each inhibit the activity of the multidrug-resistance (MDR) protein responsible for the hepatic excretion of colchicine. Cyclosporine and tacrolimus are also nephrotoxic, acting to reduce the glomerular filtration rate (GFR); this adverse effect can compromise the renal excretion of colchicine. Therefore, co-administration of colchicine with cyclosporine, tacrolimus, verapamil, or other inhibitors of hepatic MDR proteins can lead to systemic colchicine toxicity at the usual therapeutic doses; this systemic toxicity is not accompanied by the usual dose-limiting toxicity of diarrhea, because the drug is not redelivered to the GI tract via enterohepatic recirculation.

with other myelosuppressive agents such as ganciclovir or azathioprine. Colchicine undergoes extensive enterohepatic recirculation, and drug secretion into the bile is mediated by the liver multidrug-resistance (MDR) protein. Repeated delivery of colchicine from the liver to the GI tract (i.e., enterohepatic recirculation) likely explains why diarrhea is a common adverse effect of the drug. Drugs that inhibit the liver MDR protein, such as cyclosporine and verapamil, can significantly increase the fraction of a colchicine dose that is delivered to (and remains in) the systemic circulation (Fig. 49-3). By this mechanism, such drugs can cause systemic colchicine toxicity that may not be accompanied by diarrhea because the GI exposure to colchicine is decreased. Accordingly, the dose of colchicine should be lowered when the drug is administered concurrently with any drug known to inhibit MDR activity.

Glucocorticoids

Glucocorticoids have powerful anti-inflammatory and immunosuppressive effects (see Chapter 29, Pharmacology of the Adrenal Cortex). Glucocorticoids inhibit numerous steps in the inflammatory response during an acute attack of gout. Because they have widespread adverse effects when administered systemically, glucocorticoids are primarily reserved for use in the treatment of acute polyarticular gout, such as the most recent attack described for Mr. J, or when there are contraindications to other effective therapies, such as renal insufficiency. When an acute attack of gout occurs in a single joint and is unresponsive to NSAIDs or colchicine, depot preparations of prednisolone or another glucocorticoid can be injected directly into the joint to yield high local drug levels at the site of inflammation.

Management of Chronic Gout: Agents That Lower Plasma Urate Concentration

Agents That Decrease Uric Acid Synthesis

Allopurinol is an example of a drug designed to inhibit a well-understood biochemical pathway. Allopurinol is a structural analogue of xanthine. By inhibiting xanthine oxidase,

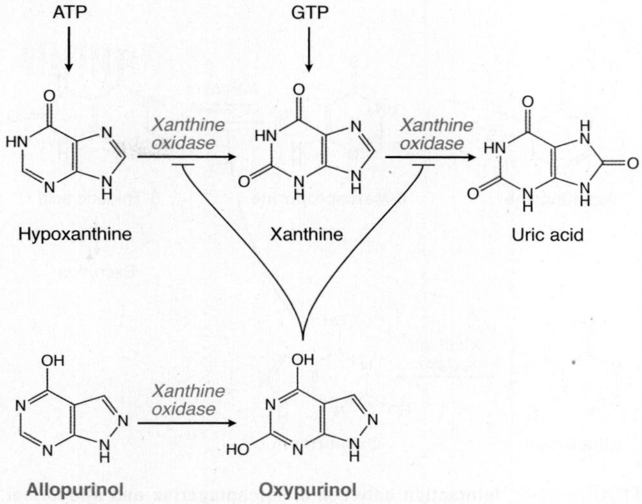

FIGURE 49-4. **Mechanism of allopurinol action.** Allopurinol is a structural analogue of hypoxanthine. Oxidation of allopurinol yields oxypurinol, a noncompetitive inhibitor of xanthine oxidase. (Although allopurinol is a competitive inhibitor of xanthine oxidase, oxypurinol is the more important inhibitor because of its much longer elimination half-life.) Inhibition of xanthine oxidase decreases the production of uric acid by inhibiting two steps in its synthesis. The increased plasma levels of xanthine and hypoxanthine are tolerated because these metabolites are more soluble than uric acid.

allopurinol decreases the concentration of uric acid in the blood (Fig. 49-4). Because of its close structural similarity to xanthine, allopurinol also acts as a substrate for xanthine oxidase. The oxidized form of allopurinol, known as **oxypurinol**, inhibits xanthine oxidase by preventing molybdenum in the active site of the enzyme from interconverting between the +4 and +6 oxidation states, essentially "freezing" the enzyme. Recall that xanthine oxidase is important for two sequential steps in purine degradation—oxidation of hypoxanthine to xanthine and oxidation of xanthine to uric acid. Therefore, inhibiting xanthine oxidase results in increased plasma levels of hypoxanthine and xanthine (see Fig. 49-1). Unlike uric acid, hypoxanthine and xanthine are moderately soluble in blood and can be filtered by the kidney without crystal deposition.

Allopurinol is used in the treatment of chronic gout, especially in cases caused by increased purine degradation. It should not be administered during an acute attack of gout because disruption of urate homeostasis can potentially worsen or precipitate acute attacks of gouty arthritis. Therefore, *an NSAID or colchicine is often co-administered during the first 4–6 months of allopurinol therapy to reduce the chance of precipitating an acute attack of gout.* This was the concern that prompted Mr. J's doctor to co-administer colchicine during his first 6 months of allopurinol therapy.

Because allopurinol inhibits purine degradation, caution should be used when a patient is taking other purine analogues. For example, azathioprine and its active form 6-mercaptopurine (see Chapter 39) are anticancer and immunosuppressive drugs that contain a purine backbone, and 6-mercaptopurine is metabolized by xanthine oxidase (Fig. 49-5). Inhibition of xanthine oxidase by allopurinol can result in toxic levels of co-administered mercaptopurine or azathioprine because of decreased degradation of the

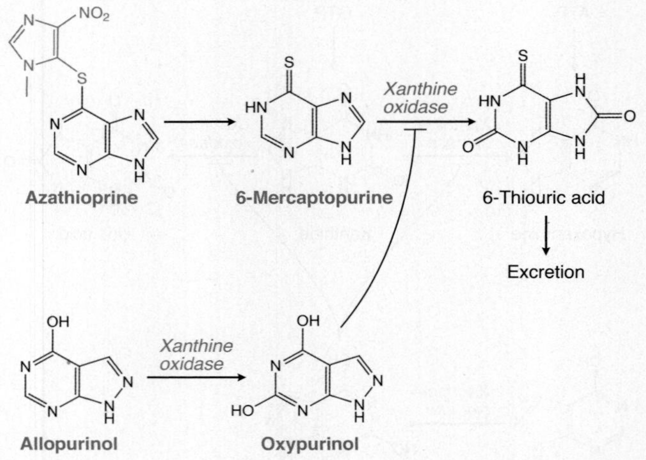

FIGURE 49-5. Interaction between 6-mercaptopurine and allopurinol. 6-Mercaptopurine and azathioprine (a prodrug) are metabolized and eliminated from the body via the same pathways as other purines. Allopurinol and its metabolite, oxypurinol, inhibit xanthine oxidase, thereby inhibiting the breakdown of 6-mercaptopurine. Decreased degradation causes plasma levels of 6-mercaptopurine to rise. When co-administering 6-mercaptopurine and allopurinol (e.g., in cancer chemotherapy), the dose of 6-mercaptopurine should be substantially reduced.

latter drugs. Therefore, the dose of mercaptopurine or azathioprine should be reduced by approximately 75% when allopurinol is co-administered. In some cases, switching from azathioprine to a nonpurine immunosuppressive drug, such as mycophenolic acid (see Chapter 46, Pharmacology of Immunosuppression), is another option.

Although allopurinol is generally well tolerated, several important adverse effects should be considered when prescribing this agent. A small percentage of patients taking allopurinol may develop a hypersensitivity reaction characterized by a rash that, in rare instances, can progress to Stevens-Johnson syndrome. For this reason, all patients who develop a cutaneous reaction to allopurinol should discontinue the drug. Rarely, allopurinol may also cause leukopenia, eosinophilia, and/or hepatic necrosis.

Febuxostat is a nonpurine small-molecule inhibitor of xanthine oxidase approved for the treatment of chronic gout. In a large clinical trial, febuxostat was as effective as allopurinol in preventing recurrent flares of gout. Unlike allopurinol, febuxostat undergoes extensive hepatic metabolism, and it may not require dose adjustment in renal insufficiency. Because of its nonpurine structure, febuxostat might not be associated with development of cutaneous reactions. As with allopurinol, initiation of febuxostat therapy should be accompanied by a suppressive medication such as colchicine in order to reduce the risk of gout flares in the first several months after initiation of urate-lowering therapy.

Agents That Increase Uric Acid Excretion

Because the kidney reabsorbs a substantial amount of filtered uric acid, pharmacologic agents that block tubular reabsorption increase uric acid excretion. Such drugs are called **uricosuric agents**.

Probenecid was one of the first drugs used to increase urate excretion. Individuals lacking the URAT1 anion transporter protein have very low serum uric acid levels and do not respond to uricosuric agents, including probenecid, indicating

that *URAT1 is the molecular target for this class of drugs.* Probenecid is not specific for URAT1; it also inhibits other transporters, including some of the renal organic anion transporters (OATs) responsible for penicillin secretion. Decades ago, when penicillin was in limited supply, it was co-administered with probenecid to prolong the half-life of the antibiotic and decrease the penicillin dose required to achieve therapeutic levels of the drug.

In patients with gout, probenecid is useful for the treatment of chronic hyperuricemia. Probenecid shifts the balance between renal excretion and endogenous production of urate, thereby lowering plasma urate levels. Uric acid levels lower than 6.0–6.5 mg/dL support dissolution of urate crystals, thereby reversing the process of crystal deposition in synovial joints. However, increasing renal urate excretion can predispose to formation of urate stones in the kidney or ureter. The likelihood of this complication can be diminished by recommending that patients increase their fluid intake and make their urine less acidic, commonly by co-administration of oral calcium citrate or sodium bicarbonate: uric acid has a pK_a of 5.6, and it remains predominantly in the more soluble neutral form if the urine pH is above 6.0. Because probenecid inhibits the secretion of many organic anions, the dose of other drugs excreted by this pathway should be reduced when probenecid is co-administered. Low-dose aspirin may antagonize probenecid action; the mechanism of this antagonism is unknown.

Sulfinpyrazone is a uricosuric agent that acts by the same mechanism as probenecid. It is more potent than probenecid, and it is effective in mild to moderate renal insufficiency. In addition to acting as a uricosuric, sulfinpyrazone has antiplatelet effects; it should therefore be used with caution in patients taking other antiplatelet agents or anticoagulants.

Benzbromarone is a uricosuric agent with a mechanism of action similar to that of probenecid and sulfinpyrazone. Benzbromarone may have greater uricosuric efficacy than probenecid and sulfinpyrazone, particularly in patients with impaired renal function. However, the frequent incidence of hepatotoxicity has limited widespread use of the drug, and it is currently not available in the United States.

Losartan is an angiotensin II receptor antagonist (see Chapter 22, Pharmacology of Vascular Tone) that has a modest uricosuric effect. Losartan may be a logical therapeutic choice in patients with both hypertension and gout, although no controlled studies have been performed to prove that losartan reduces the incidence of acute gout attacks.

Agents That Enhance Uric Acid Metabolism

Most mammals other than humans express the enzyme uricase. This enzyme oxidizes uric acid to allantoin, a compound that is easily excreted by the kidney (Fig. 49-1). In cancer chemotherapy, the rapid lysis of tumor cells can liberate free nucleotides and greatly increase plasma urate levels. By this mechanism, **tumor lysis syndrome** can lead to massive renal injury. Exogenous **uricase** can be co-administered with cancer chemotherapy to reduce plasma urate levels rapidly and thereby to prevent renal damage. Allopurinol can also be used to prevent this component of tumor lysis syndrome.

Currently, uricase is available in Europe as a protein purified from the fungus *Aspergillus flavus*. A recombinant version of the *Aspergillus* uricase, **rasburicase**, is available in the United States. A small percentage of patients have allergic reactions to the foreign protein and antidrug antibodies are common. **Pegloticase**, a pegylated formulation of recombinant porcine uricase, is approved for the treatment of gout refractory to conventional therapy.

CONCLUSION AND FUTURE DIRECTIONS

Gout can be thought of as a disorder of purine metabolism and excretion. An imbalance between urate synthesis and excretion leads to hyperuricemia; in some individuals, hyperuricemia progresses to gout. Acute therapeutic interventions are aimed at symptomatic treatment of gout attacks; these treatments interrupt inflammatory pathways by inhibiting neutrophil and monocyte activation. Treatments for chronic gout lower plasma urate levels by reestablishing the balance between urate synthesis and excretion. Allopurinol and febuxostat inhibit urate synthesis; probenecid increases renal urate excretion. Recombinant uricase rapidly decreases plasma urate levels by converting uric acid to allantoin, thereby preventing the adverse renal consequences of tumor lysis syndrome. New therapies are under development for the treatment of both acute and chronic gout. For example, IL-1 antagonists such as anakinra, canakinumab, and rilonacept are being studied for the treatment of acute gout flares unresponsive to standard therapies or for patients in whom standard therapies are contraindicated. Lesinurad is an investigational agent that inhibits URAT1 and OAT4, thereby limiting urate resorption.

Disclosure

Lloyd B. Klickstein is an employee and stockholder of Novartis, Inc., which manufactures or distributes drugs discussed in this chapter, including canakinumab.

Suggested Reading

Crittenden DB, Pillinger MH. New therapies for gout. *Annu Rev Med* 2013;64:325–337. (*Provides clinical and mechanistic details on febuxostat, URAT-1 inhibitors, and uricases.*)

Khanna PP, Gladue HS, Singh MK, et al. Treatment of acute gout: a systematic review. *Semin Arthritis Rheum* 2014;44:31–38. (*Clinical review suggesting similar efficacy of NSAIDs, corticosteroids, and colchicine in the treatment of acute gout.*)

Kingsbury SR, Conaghan PG, McDermott MF. The role of the NLRP3 inflammasome in gout. *J Inflamm Res* 2011;4:39–49. (*Detailed review of uric acid-induced inflammation and inflammasome biology.*)

Neogi T. Clinical practice. Gout. *N Engl J Med* 2011;364:443–452. (*Clinical practice review of gout.*)

Punzi L, Scanu A, Ramonda R, Oliviero F. Gout as an autoinflammatory disease: new mechanisms for more appropriate treatment targets. *Autoimmun Rev* 2012;12:66–71. (*Reviews advances in gout pathophysiology, including the role of IL-1 and development of IL-1 antagonists.*)

DRUG SUMMARY TABLE: CHAPTER 49 Integrative Inflammation Pharmacology: Gout

DRUG	CLINICAL APPLICATIONS	SERIOUS AND COMMON ADVERSE EFFECTS	CONTRAINDICATIONS	THERAPEUTIC CONSIDERATIONS
SUPPRESSORS OF LEUKOCYTE RECRUITMENT AND ACTIVATION Mechanism—Interrupt inflammatory pathways that cause inflammation in a gouty joint; see specific drug				
Colchicine	Acute gout Prevention of recurrent gout attacks Familial Mediterranean fever	*Myelosuppression* Diarrhea, nausea, vomiting	Hepatic or renal impairment Concomitant use of P-glycoprotein inhibitors or potent CYP3A4 inhibitors	Colchicine inhibits microtubule formation by binding to tubulin heterodimers; inhibition of microtubule assembly interrupts cellular motility and other processes necessary for neutrophil-mediated inflammatory response. Concomitant administration of cyclosporine, tacrolimus, or verapamil may increase plasma levels of colchicine.
Ibuprofen Indomethacin	See Drug Summary Table: Chapter 43 Pharmacology of Eicosanoids			
Prednisone Methylprednisolone	See Drug Summary Table: Chapter 29 Pharmacology of the Adrenal Cortex			Methylprednisolone may be injected into an inflamed joint for treatment of acute gout.
INHIBITORS OF URIC ACID SYNTHESIS Mechanism—Inhibit xanthine oxidase, the enzyme that converts hypoxanthine to xanthine and xanthine to uric acid; decreased uric acid levels lead to reduced urate crystal formation				
Allopurinol Oxypurinol	Prevention of recurrent gout attacks Cancer-related hyperuricemia Calcium and uric acid renal calculus	*Agranulocytosis, aplastic anemia, renal failure, hepatic necrosis, Stevens-Johnson syndrome, toxic epidermal necrolysis* Pruritus, rash, gastrointestinal disturbance	Hypersensitivity to drug Concomitant use with didanosine	Allopurinol is an inhibitor and substrate for xanthine oxidase; the product of allopurinol oxidation (oxypurinol) also inhibits xanthine oxidase. Oxypurinol is available on a compassionate use basis. Both drugs increase levels of azathioprine and 6-mercaptopurine. Amoxicillin, ampicillin, and thiazide diuretics may increase risk of severe rash.
Febuxostat	Prevention of recurrent gout attacks	*Myocardial infarction, Stevens-Johnson syndrome, thromboembolic disorder, hepatotoxicity, rhabdomyolysis, nephrotoxicity, angioedema* Abnormal liver enzymes, rash, nausea, arthralgia	Concomitant use with azathioprine or mercaptopurine	Nonpurine small-molecule inhibitor of xanthine oxidase. Initiation of febuxostat therapy should be accompanied by a suppressive medication such as colchicine to reduce the risk of gout flares in the first several months.

AGENTS THAT INCREASE URIC ACID EXCRETION
Mechanism—See specific drug

Drug	Clinical Applications	Serious and Common Adverse Effects	Contraindications	Therapeutic Considerations
Sulfinpyrazone **Probenecid**	Prevention of recurrent gout attacks	*Leukopenia, thrombocytopenia, bronchoconstriction in patients with asthma (shared adverse effects); aplastic anemia, hepatic necrosis, anaphylaxis, Stevens-Johnson syndrome, nephrotic syndrome (probenecid only)* Gastrointestinal disturbance	Shared contraindications: Hypersensitivity to drug Acute gout attack Blood dyscrasias Children under 2 years of age Co-administration of salicylates Uric acid kidney stones Sulfinpyrazone only: Radiation therapy for malignancy Cancer chemotherapy with agents causing rapid cytolysis	Sulfinpyrazone and probenecid inhibit the basolateral URAT1 anion exchanger in the kidney proximal tubule, leading to increased excretion of uric acid. Sulfinpyrazone and probenecid increase serum levels of penicillin and other organic anions; may also increase levels of nitrofurantoin. Probenecid increases the serum level of methotrexate.
Losartan	Hypertension (FDA-labeled indication) Prevention of recurrent gout attacks (non-FDA-labeled indication)	*Angioedema, rhabdomyolysis, hepatotoxicity, acute renal failure* Chest pain, hypotension, hyperkalemia, hypoglycemia, diarrhea, anemia, asthenia, dizziness, cough, fatigue	Hypersensitivity to drug Concomitant use with aliskiren in patients with diabetes	Losartan is an angiotensin II receptor antagonist with a modest uricosuric effect.

AGENTS THAT ENHANCE URIC ACID METABOLISM
Mechanism—Enzymes that convert sparingly soluble urate to the more soluble allantoin

Drug	Clinical Applications	Serious and Common Adverse Effects	Contraindications	Therapeutic Considerations
Rasburicase **Pegloticase**	Rasburicase only: Tumor lysis syndrome Pegloticase only: Treatment of gout unresponsive to standard therapies	*Hemolysis, methemoglobinemia, neutropenia, respiratory distress, sepsis (rasburicase only); anaphylaxis (pegloticase only)* Gastrointestinal disturbance (shared adverse effects); rash, headache, fever (rasburicase only); chest pain, nasopharyngitis (pegloticase only)	Hypersensitivity to drug Glucose-6-phosphate dehydrogenase (G6PD) deficiency	Rasburicase is a recombinant form of *Aspergillus* uricase that converts sparingly soluble urate to the more soluble allantoin. Pegloticase is a pegylated formulation with a longer half-life.

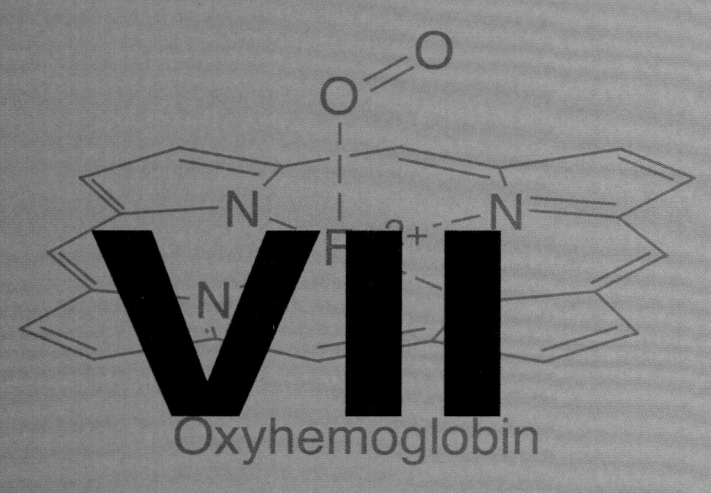

Oxyhemoglobin

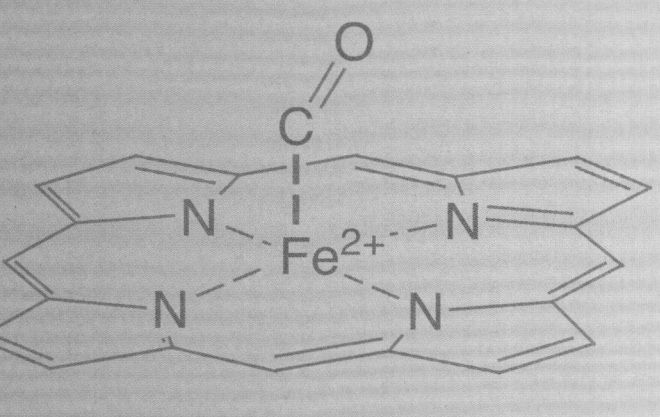

Carboxyhemoglobin

VII

Environmental Toxicology

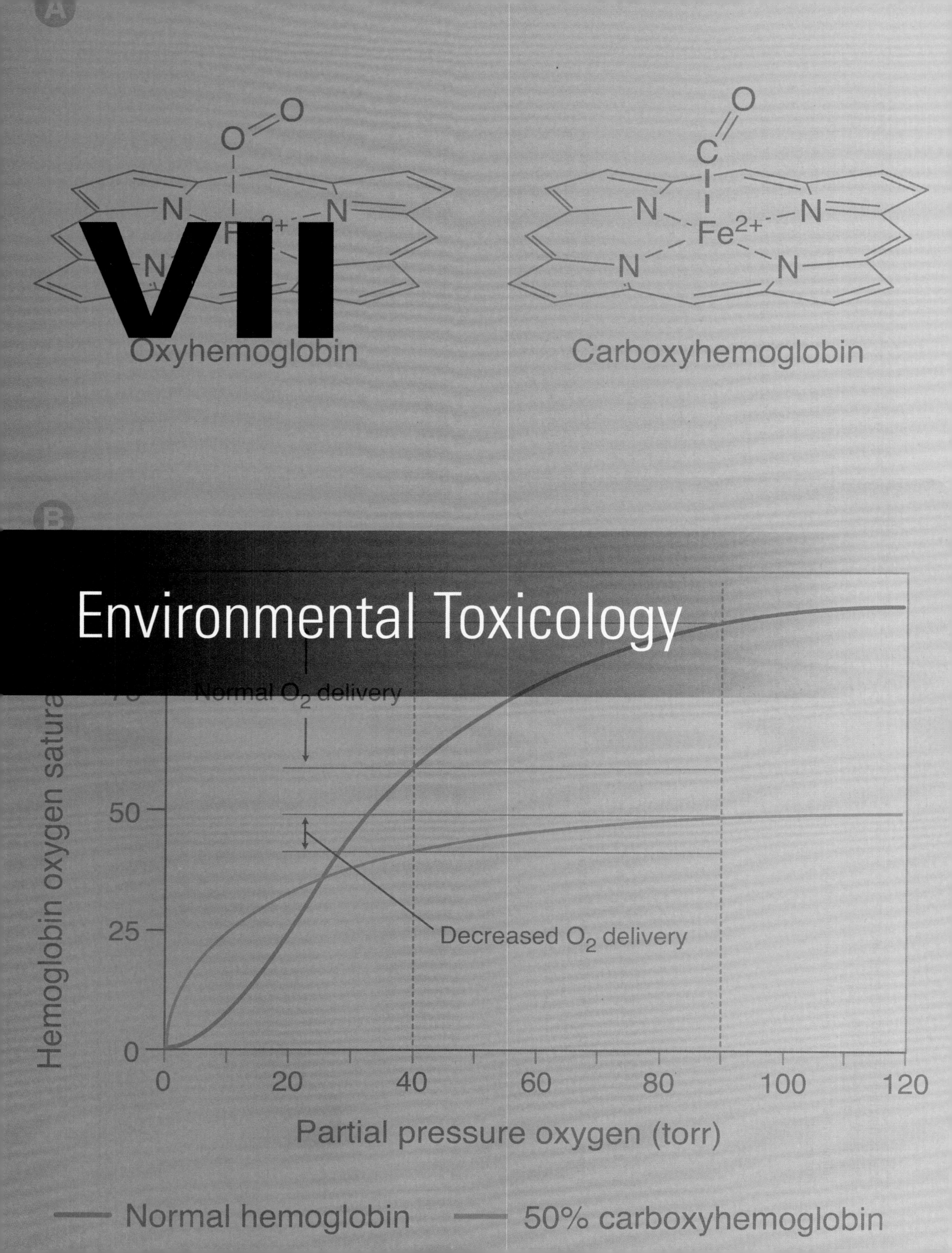

Hemoglobin oxygen saturation

Normal O$_2$ delivery

Decreased O$_2$ delivery

75

50

25

0

0   20   40   60   80   100   120

Partial pressure oxygen (torr)

Normal hemoglobin   50% carboxyhemoglobin

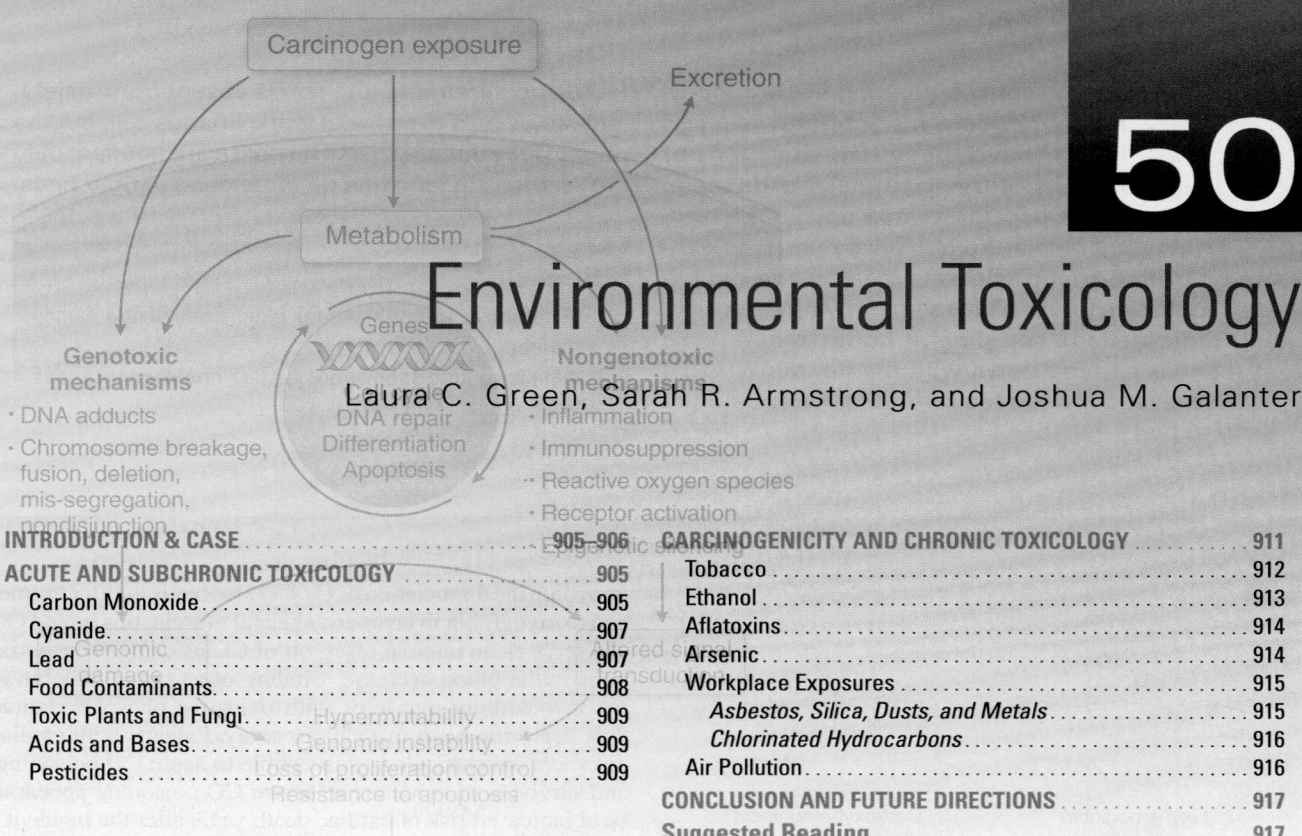

50

Environmental Toxicology

Laura C. Green, Sarah R. Armstrong, and Joshua M. Galanter

INTRODUCTION

Environmental toxicology is the study of deleterious effects of physical, chemical, or microbiological agents present in air, water, food, or other media. In this context, airborne exposures include those received by cigarette smokers and people working in various industries, as well as those received by all of us from pollutants. Many of the principles and mechanisms pertinent to drug toxicity, discussed in Chapter 6, Drug Toxicity, apply also to nondrug toxicants. In particular, the tenet of dose–response explains why low-level exposures to ubiquitous chemicals are typically harmless, while increasing levels of exposure confer increased risks of harm.

In the United States and elsewhere, actions by regulatory agencies such as the US Food and Drug Administration (FDA), the Occupational Safety and Health Administration, and the Environmental Protection Agency have resulted in foods, workplaces, and environments that are significantly safer than they were in the mid-twentieth century and earlier. Nonetheless, accidental poisonings, food poisoning, cigarette smoking, excessive consumption of alcoholic beverages, and the legacy of occupational overexposures to asbestos, silica, and other occupational carcinogens continue to be responsible for considerable burdens of disease. Similarly, although gross overexposures of children and others to the toxic metal lead are becoming less common in much of the world (due primarily to the removal of tetraethyl lead from gasoline and the reduced use of lead-based pigments), environmental sources of lead remain, and children deficient in iron and calcium in particular are at risk of lead-induced neurobehavioral disease. Worldwide, the prevalence of, and protections against, toxic agents vary widely, both across and within countries, such that the health of children, workers, and others may be considerably compromised. This is especially the case in groups suffering from malnutrition, chronic infections, and other insults that, per se and in concert with toxic exposures, harm health.

ACUTE AND SUBCHRONIC TOXICOLOGY

Numerous substances can cause serious acute illness and death. This section describes some common causes of acute and subchronic poisoning, the mechanisms by which they act, and, as appropriate, treatments.

Carbon Monoxide

The combustion of any organic material produces **carbon monoxide (CO)** gas and other products of incomplete combustion. Insufficiently vented home-heating furnaces, wood stoves, and other combustion sources can result in accumulation of CO in indoor air to toxic concentrations. The propane generator in the introductory case was not sufficiently ventilated, causing carbon monoxide to reach lethal concentrations. In the United States, some 15,000 emergency department visits and 500 deaths annually are caused by overexposures to CO. These deaths are exclusive of fire-related deaths, many of which are also caused in part by elevated concentrations of CO.

CO causes tissue hypoxia by binding more than 200-fold more tightly to the heme iron in hemoglobin than does O_2, thereby reducing the transport of oxygen in the blood (Fig. 50-1). In addition, **carboxyhemoglobin (COHb)** shifts the dissociation curve for oxyhemoglobin (OHb) to the left,

CASE

The W family is running out of money. Mr. W has lost his job, and Ms. W's hours have been cut back. After months of trying to make ends meet, Mr. W decides to stop paying the electricity bill. He borrows a propane generator from a friend and sets it up in the garage attached to the house. That evening, Mr. W, his wife, and their teenage son dine at home. Ms. W feels as if she is coming down with the flu, Mr. W has a headache, and the son feels irritable. All three retire early to bed.

The next morning, the son is absent from school, and Ms. W fails to arrive at work. Friends call, but the phone goes unanswered. The police are notified; they arrive, break in, and find all three dead in their beds.

Questions

1. What toxic agent(s) could have caused the family members' deaths?
2. Which routine laboratory test(s) could confirm the likely cause of death?

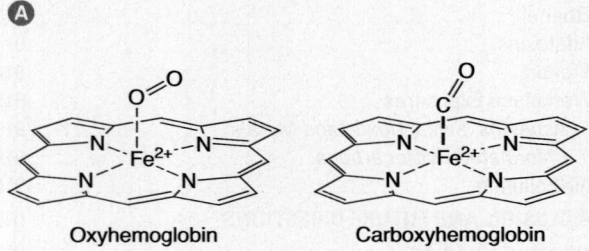

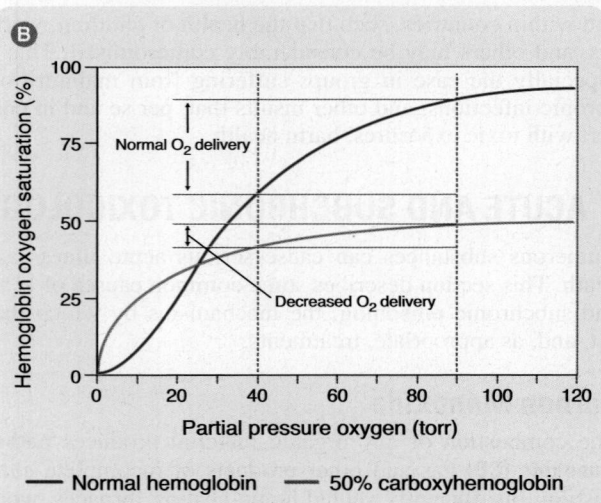

FIGURE 50-1. **Mechanism of carbon monoxide poisoning. A.** The ligand-binding site of hemoglobin is a ferrous heme that can reversibly bind oxygen. Carbon monoxide prevents oxygen binding by forming a bond to ferrous heme that is significantly stronger than the heme–oxygen bond (*shorter bold line*). **B.** Carbon monoxide interferes strongly with oxygen transport because it both prevents oxygen binding and increases the affinity of heme for oxygen. Under normal conditions (*blue line*), hemoglobin is 85% saturated with oxygen in the alveoli (where the partial pressure of oxygen is approximately 90 torr). At tissue partial pressures (40 torr), normal hemoglobin is 60% saturated with O_2. Thus, under normal conditions, 25% of the heme sites deliver their oxygen to the tissues. When 50% of oxygen binding sites are occupied by carbon monoxide (*red line*), hemoglobin oxygen saturation can be no more than 50% at a partial pressure of 90 torr. At tissue partial pressures (40 torr), the hemoglobin oxygen saturation is still greater than 35%, indicating that less than 15% of the heme sites can deliver their oxygen to the tissues.

impeding the dissociation of O_2. CO also binds to cytochromes and to myoglobin in heart and skeletal muscle; this bound CO can serve as an internal reservoir of CO as COHb concentrations in the blood decrease. Binding of CO to myoglobin in the myocardium interferes with oxidative phosphorylation, thus depriving heart muscle of energy. Patients with cardiac disorders are particularly susceptible to acute CO poisoning, and survivors of moderate to severe CO poisoning appear to be at increased risk of cardiac death years after the incident.

Because the initial symptoms of CO poisoning are non-specific, including headache, dizziness, and irritability, an accurate diagnosis is sometimes elusive. The W family did not react to the presence of carbon monoxide because it is odorless and nonirritating and because the symptoms they experienced shortly before sleep would not have been a cause of alarm. Had their house been equipped with a carbon monoxide detector, their deaths would almost certainly have been prevented. Measurement of COHb is straightforward, and concentrations higher than about 3% in nonsmokers and 5–10% in smokers indicate an unusual exposure. (Note that pO_2, the partial pressure of oxygen, is likely to be normal in a CO-poisoned patient.) Signs and symptoms of acute poisoning track approximately with COHb concentrations, with severe headache, vomiting, and visual disturbances at 30–40% COHb and collapse and convulsions at 50–60% COHb. Death is likely at 70% COHb and possible at lower concentrations.

Survivors of severe CO poisoning are at risk of brain damage; areas of the brain with high oxygen demand are most likely to be impaired, although the mechanisms and outcomes of CO poisoning differ from those of simple hypoxia. CO-induced neuropathy is due to marked cerebral vasodilation, mitochondrial dysfunction, cell death from apoptosis, and, upon reoxygenation, reperfusion injury.

The half-life of COHb is approximately 5 hours in room air and decreases to about 90 minutes in a 100% O_2 environment at normal pressure. Hyperbaric oxygen therapy (3 atmospheres, 100% O_2) can reduce the half-life to about 20 minutes and appears to protect against long-term brain damage by improving energy metabolism, minimizing lipid peroxidation, and decreasing neutrophil adherence. A rule of thumb is that victims with COHb concentrations above 25% (or above 15% in pregnant women) should receive hyperbaric oxygen therapy. However, COHb concentrations alone are only approximate indicators of risk, and use of hyperbaric oxygen therapy is preferred when available.

Cyanide

The cyanide ion ($C\equiv N^-$) is a highly toxic and frequently lethal poison. It may be inhaled, ingested, or absorbed through the skin from sources as diverse as hydrogen cyanide gas, cyanide salts, apricot pits, peach pits, cherry pits, cassava, fire smoke, and vapors from industrial metal plating operations. Cyanide is also a metabolite of nitriles and nitroprusside. Cyanide binds to the ferric iron in the heme a_3/Cu_B center of cytochrome c oxidase, thereby blocking aerobic respiration and preventing cellular use of oxygen. This causes a shift to anaerobic metabolism and a resulting metabolic acidosis. As with CO poisoning, cyanide poisoning damages tissues with high oxygen demand, such as the brain and heart.

Signs and symptoms of cyanide poisoning depend on dose and route of exposure and are somewhat nonspecific: headache, confusion, altered mental status, hypertension (early) or hypotension (late), nausea, and other symptoms are all possible. Pallor or cyanosis is not present (assuming that there is no co-exposure to carbon monoxide). Unless cyanide exposure is reported or witnessed, or is likely to have occurred given the patient's occupation or recent activities, diagnosis may be difficult. Sometimes, an odor of bitter almonds may be noted. Because cyanide is cleared rapidly from the blood, and because of technical challenges, measurements of cyanide in the blood may be both time-consuming and misleading. Moreover, some endogenous production of cyanide occurs in healthy individuals, and smokers' blood contains elevated cyanide concentrations. There is some debate about the blood concentrations of cyanide deemed toxic or potentially lethal, but 1 mg/L (39 μmol/L) is typically regarded as a potentially toxic level.

Treatment for acute cyanide poisoning may include decontamination, supportive therapy, and administration of an antidote. Decontamination may entail simply the removal of contaminated clothes, and care should be taken to avoid inadvertent exposure of responders to the cyanide-containing material. Supportive therapy, including supplemental oxygen, should aim to avoid organ failure and may be needed to address toxicities such as coma, lactic acidosis, hypotension, and respiratory failure.

The traditional antidotal treatment for acute cyanide poisoning in the United States is a cyanide antidote "kit" (CAK) that contains **amyl nitrite**, **sodium nitrite**, and **sodium thiosulfate**. The nitrites act by oxidizing hemoglobin to methemoglobin to provide a substrate that can compete with heme a_3 in cytochrome c oxidase for cyanide molecules. Amyl nitrite is usually given by inhalation and acts (and is cleared from the bloodstream) rapidly, while sodium nitrite is administered intravenously and has a longer duration of action. The methemoglobin-bound cyanide is oxidized to the relatively nontoxic thiocyanate by the enzyme **rhodanese** (also known as *transsulfurase*) and excreted in urine. Sodium thiosulfate provides a ready source of sulfur for the detoxication reaction and enhances cyanide metabolism.

Importantly, use of the CAK may pose significant risk to the patient, since a substantial fraction of hemoglobin must be converted to methemoglobin to compete effectively for the cyanide ion. Smoke inhalation victims (who have high levels of exposure to carbon monoxide) are sometimes presumed to have been poisoned by cyanide gas. Such patients may already be suffering from hypoxia before CAK treatment is begun. Exacerbation of hypoxia by forcing conversion of hemoglobin to methemoglobin may be detrimental to such patients. CAK should also be avoided in pregnant women and infants, who may carry fetal hemoglobin and have immature methemoglobin reductase activity. Furthermore, the CAK may cause severe hypotension and lead to cardiovascular collapse.

Concerns regarding possible terrorist use of cyanide led to the approval in 2006 by the FDA of an alternative antidote, hydroxocobalamin (Cyanokit®). This member of the vitamin B_{12} family is an endogenous compound that was already in use at lower doses for treatment of vitamin B_{12} deficiency. The mechanism of action of this drug differs from that of the compounds in the CAK: the cobalt moiety in hydroxocobalamin has high affinity for cyanide and competes directly with the ferric iron in cytochrome c oxidase for cyanide, forming nontoxic cyanocobalamin that is excreted in the urine. Hydroxocobalamin is generally well tolerated, but anaphylactic reactions are possible. The compound also causes urine to have a bright red color for about a week and may discolor the skin at the site of injection. Interference with spectrophotometric tests and assays for oxyhemoglobin, carboxyhemoglobin, and methemoglobin may also occur.

Lead

Lead is ubiquitous in the environment because of its persistence, its formerly widespread and unnecessary use as a gasoline additive, and its use in pigments, paints, plumbing, solder, and other products. Lead is toxic to the central nervous system, making exposure a particular concern for fetuses and children up to the age of about 7 years. Young children are also at risk because they are more likely than adults to ingest lead-contaminated paint dust and other nonfood materials. Despite a fivefold decrease in the exposure to lead in the United States and elsewhere since the mid-twentieth century, children today may still be at risk of developing lead-induced neurocognitive deficits. This is especially true for children who live near active, poorly controlled lead mines or smelters or in countries where leaded fuels are, or recently were, used. (Leaded gasoline was not banned in China until 2000, for example.) Lead-glazed clay cookware and solder remain common in some areas, and some of this lead contaminates food and water. Exposures to lead that present no overt symptoms may nonetheless be toxic, and testing young children's blood lead levels is essential. Although the half-life of lead in soft tissues is relatively short, its half-life in bone is more than 20 years; a substantial exposure in early childhood can result in elevated bone lead levels for decades.

Lead disrupts the blood–brain barrier, allowing both lead and other potential neurotoxins to reach the CNS. There, lead can block voltage-dependent calcium channels, interfere with neurotransmitter function, and, most importantly, interfere with cell–cell interactions in the brain; the latter effect causes permanent changes in neuronal circuitry. Overt lead encephalopathy, which is rare in the United States today, results in lethargy, vomiting, irritability, and dizziness and can progress to altered mental status, coma, and death. Low- and moderate-level exposures to young children are believed to result in IQ deficits of two to four points for every 10 μg/dL increase in blood lead concentration. Whether some blood lead levels are so low as to present essentially no risk of neurobehavioral deficit is a matter of debate and ongoing research.

Lead interferes with the synthesis of hemoglobin at multiple steps and thereby causes microcytic, hypochromic anemia. Specifically, lead inhibits **delta-aminolevulinic acid dehydratase (ALA-D)**, which catalyzes the synthesis of porphobilinogen, a heme precursor. Lead also inhibits the incorporation of iron into the porphyrin ring.

In the kidney, lead causes both reversible and irreversible toxicity. Lead can interfere reversibly with energy production in proximal tubular cells by interfering with mitochondrial function, resulting in decreased energy-dependent reabsorption of ions, glucose, and amino acids. Chronic exposure to lead results in interstitial nephritis, with the eventual development of fibrosis and chronic kidney disease.

When indicated clinically, body burdens of metals such as lead, mercury, or cadmium can be reduced using electron donors such as an amine, hydroxide, carboxylate, or mercaptan to form **metal–ligand complexes**. A **chelator**, which in Greek means "claw," is a multidentate structure with multiple binding sites (Fig. 50-2). Binding of the metal at multiple sites shifts the equilibrium constant in favor of metal ligation. High-affinity metal–ligand binding is critical because the chelator must compete with tissue macromolecules for binding. In addition, the chelator should be nontoxic and water-soluble, and the complex should be readily cleared. Finally, an ideal chelator should have a low binding affinity for endogenous ions such as calcium. To prevent the depletion of tissue calcium, many chelators are administered as calcium complexes. The target metal is then exchanged for calcium, and the body's calcium stores are not depleted.

The most important heavy metal chelators are **edetate disodium** (the calcium, disodium complex of EDTA), which can be used to bind lead; **dimercaprol** (also known as **British anti-Lewisite** or **BAL**), which binds gold, arsenic, lead, and mercury to its two thiol groups; and **succimer** (2,3-dimercaptosuccinic acid), which has supplanted dimercaprol for the removal of lead, cadmium, mercury, and arsenic. **Deferoxamine** is used for the removal of toxic levels of iron, such as would occur in accidental overdoses of iron-containing supplements or in patients with transfusion-dependent anemias. **Deferasirox** is an orally bioavailable iron chelator that may supplant deferoxamine for many conditions associated with chronic iron overload. Removal of copper, typically in patients with Wilson's disease, is accomplished with **penicillamine** or, for patients who do not tolerate penicillamine, **trientine**.

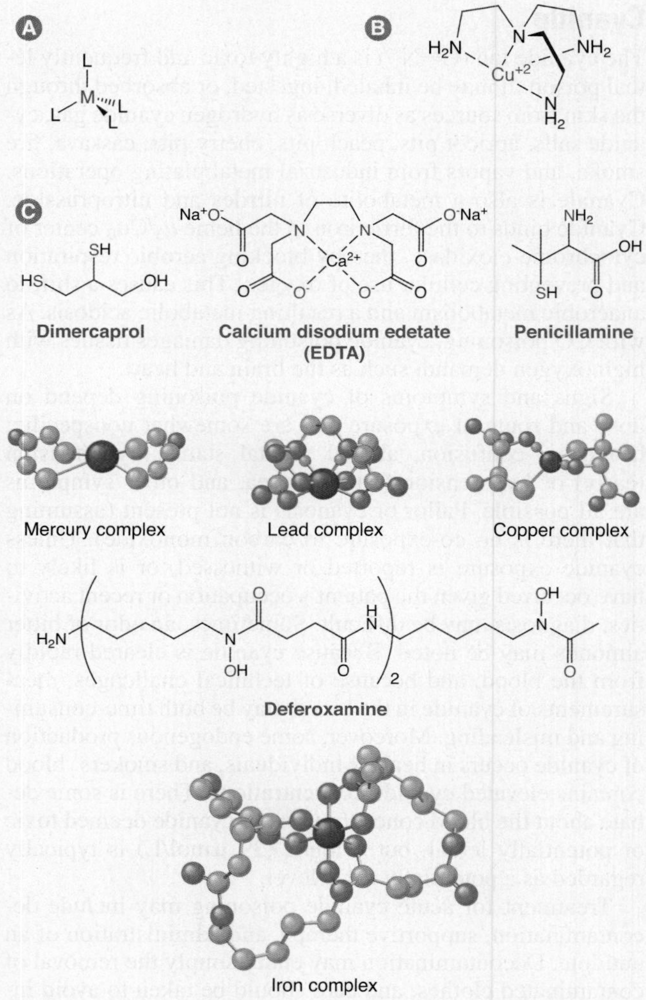

Food Contaminants

An estimated one in four Americans experience significant **food-borne illnesses** each year. The mechanisms of food poisoning involve either infection, which typically manifests one to several days after exposure, or intoxication from a preformed microbial or algal toxin, with symptoms occurring within a few hours of exposure. Infectious food poisoning is typically caused by species of *Salmonella*, *Listeria*, *Cryptosporidium*, or *Campylobacter*. Less common but quite virulent are poisonings by enteropathogenic *Escherichia coli*, which can cause sometimes-fatal hemorrhagic colitis and hemolytic uremic syndrome (HUS), likely through the uptake of pathologic bacterial proteins by host cells.

Food intoxication is often caused by toxins elaborated by *Staphylococcus aureus* or *Bacillus cereus* or by marine algal toxins ingested via seafood. *S. aureus* produces a variety of toxins; the staphylococcal enterotoxins (SE) induce emesis

FIGURE 50-2. Heavy metal chelators. A. A ligand (L) is a compound containing a Lewis base (such as amine, thiol, hydroxyl, or carboxylate groups) that can form a complex with a metal (M). **B.** A chelator is a multidentate ligand, that is, a ligand that can bind to a metal through multiple atoms, as in this example of a tetra-amino ligand bound to copper (Cu^{2+}) via its four amine groups. **C.** The structures of dimercaprol, calcium EDTA, penicillamine, and deferoxamine are shown; the atoms that form bonds with the metal are identified in *blue*. Three-dimensional structures of the mercury complex of dimercaprol, the lead complex of EDTA, the copper complex of penicillamine, and the iron complex of deferoxamine are also shown. Here, the heavy metal is highlighted in *red*. For simplicity, hydrogen atoms are not shown.

by stimulating receptors in the abdominal viscera. High-protein foods, such as meats, cold cuts, and egg and dairy products, are contaminated with *S. aureus* upon improper food handling after cooking, followed by poor refrigeration.

B. cereus, a common contaminant of cooked rice, produces several toxins that cause vomiting and diarrhea. Of particular concern is the production of **cereulide**, a small, cyclic peptide that stimulates intestinal 5-HT₃ receptors, resulting in emesis. The peptide is heat-stable to 259°F for up to 90 minutes, so reheating of contaminated cooked rice will typically not prevent intoxication.

Most algal toxins are neurotoxic and heat-stable, so, again, cooking leaves the toxins intact. Algal **saxitoxins** are a group of approximately 20 heterocyclic guanidine derivatives that bind with high affinity to the voltage-gated sodium channel, thus inhibiting neuronal activity and causing tingling and numbness, loss of motor control, drowsiness, incoherence, and, with sufficient doses (greater than about 1 mg), respiratory paralysis.

Many food-borne illnesses appear to be caused by pathogens that are not yet characterized. Moreover, novel pathogens can emerge because of changing ecologies or technologies or can arise via transfer of mobile virulence factors such as bacteriophages.

Toxic Plants and Fungi

Acute illness can also be caused by mistaken ingestion of nonfood items, such as poisonous mushrooms collected by amateur mycologists or any number of poisonous plants. The highly toxic "death cap" mushroom, for instance, *Amanita phalloides*, produces numerous cyclopeptide toxins that are not destroyed by cooking or drying, have no distinctive taste, and are taken up by hepatocytes. The **amatoxins** bind tightly to RNA polymerase II, substantially slowing RNA and protein synthesis and leading to hepatocyte necrosis. The somewhat less toxic **phallotoxins** and **virotoxins** interfere with F- and G-actins in the cytoskeleton. Consumption of *Amanita* species or their relatives can thus cause severe liver dysfunction, hepatic and renal failure, and death. Initial symptoms of poisoning, such as abdominal pain, nausea, severe vomiting and diarrhea, fever, and tachycardia, may occur 6–24 hours after consumption of the mushrooms. Hepatic and renal function may deteriorate even while the initial symptoms abate, leading to jaundice, hepatic encephalopathy, and fulminant liver failure; death may occur 4–9 days after consumption. There is no specific antidote.

An anticholinergic syndrome may be caused by deliberate or accidental ingestion of **jimson weed**, a plant belonging to the *Datura* family. All parts of the plant are toxic, but the seeds and leaves, in particular, contain atropine, scopolamine, and hyoscyamine. These compounds are rapidly absorbed and produce anticholinergic symptoms such as mydriasis, dry, flushed skin, agitation, tachycardia, hyperthermia, and hallucinations. The mnemonic for anticholinergic effects, "blind as a bat, dry as a bone, red as a beet, mad as a hatter, and hot as a hare," is applicable to jimson weed poisoning.

Some plants in the families *Umbelliferae* (such as parsley, parsnip, dill, celery, and giant hogweed), *Rutaceae* (such as limes and lemons), and *Moraceae* (such as figs) contain **psoralen isomers (furocoumarins)** in leaves, stems, or sap that can be absorbed into the skin after contact. Subsequent exposure to ultraviolet (UV) A radiation of wavelength >320 nm (generally via sunlight) can excite the furocoumarins, resulting in epidermal tissue damage. Within 2 days, burning, redness, and blistering are observed in areas of contact with the plant and light; after healing, hyperpigmentation may persist for months. The response is greater with increasing plant contact, humidity, and duration and intensity of radiation exposure. This nonallergic **phytophototoxic** mechanism is the basis of psoralen + UV-A (PUVA) therapy for eczema and other dermatologic disorders.

Acids and Bases

Strong acids, alkalis (caustic agents), oxidants, and reducing agents damage tissue by altering the structure of proteins, lipids, carbohydrates, and nucleic acids so severely that cellular integrity is lost. These substances, such as **potassium hydroxide** in drain cleaners and **sulfuric acid** in car batteries, produce **chemical burns** by hydrolyzing, oxidizing, or reducing biological macromolecules or by denaturing proteins. High concentrations of **detergents** can also cause nonspecific tissue damage by disrupting and dissolving the plasma membrane of cells.

Although some of these agents may target particular macromolecules, direct tissue-damaging agents tend to be relatively nonspecific. Thus, the systems most commonly affected are those most exposed to the environment. Skin and eyes are frequently affected by splashes or spills. The respiratory system is affected when toxic gases or vapors are inhaled, and the digestive system is affected by accidental or deliberate ingestion of toxic substances.

Many agents can cause damage to deep tissues after breaking through the barrier formed by the skin. Other agents are able to pass through the skin while causing relatively little local damage but destroy deeper tissues such as muscle or bone. For example, **hydrofluoric acid** (**HF**; found in, among other products, grout cleaner) causes milder skin burns than an equivalent amount of **hydrochloric acid** (**HCl**). However, once HF reaches deeper tissue, it destroys the calcified matrix of bone. In addition to the direct effects of the acid, the release of calcium stored in bone can cause life-threatening cardiac arrhythmias. For this reason, HF can be more dangerous than an equivalent amount of HCl.

Three characteristics determine the extent of tissue damage: the compound's identity, its concentration/strength, and its **buffering capacity**, or its ability to resist change in pH or redox potential. As mentioned above, HF is more injurious than an equivalent amount of HCl. In general, a stronger acid or base (measured by pH) or oxidant or reductant (measured by redox potential) will cause more damage than an equivalent compound at a more physiologic pH or redox potential. A solution of 10^{-2} M sodium hydroxide in water has a pH of 12 but has low capacity to cause tissue damage because it has a small buffering capacity and is rapidly neutralized by body tissue. In contrast, a buffered solution of pH 12, such as that found in wet ready-set concrete [made with buffered $Ca(OH)_2$], can cause more serious alkali burns because tissues cannot readily neutralize the material's extreme pH.

Pesticides

Pesticides include insecticides, herbicides, rodenticides, and other compounds designed to kill unwanted organisms in the environment. By their nature, pesticides—of which there are hundreds (vastly more natural than synthetic)—are biologically active; however, the degree of their specificity toward target organisms varies, and many of these compounds cause toxicity in humans and other nontarget organisms. Some of the more common acute poisonings involve organophosphate and pyrethroid insecticides and rodenticides.

Organophosphate insecticides, derived from phosphoric or thiophosphoric acid, include **parathion**, **malathion**, **diazinon**, **fenthion**, **chlorpyrifos**, and many other chemicals. These widely used compounds are acetylcholinesterase (AChE) inhibitors due to their ability to phosphorylate AChE at its esteratic active site (Fig. 50-3). Inhibition of AChE, and consequent accumulation of acetylcholine at cholinergic junctions in nerve tissue and effector organs, produces acute muscarinic, nicotinic, and central nervous system (CNS) effects such as bronchoconstriction, increased bronchial

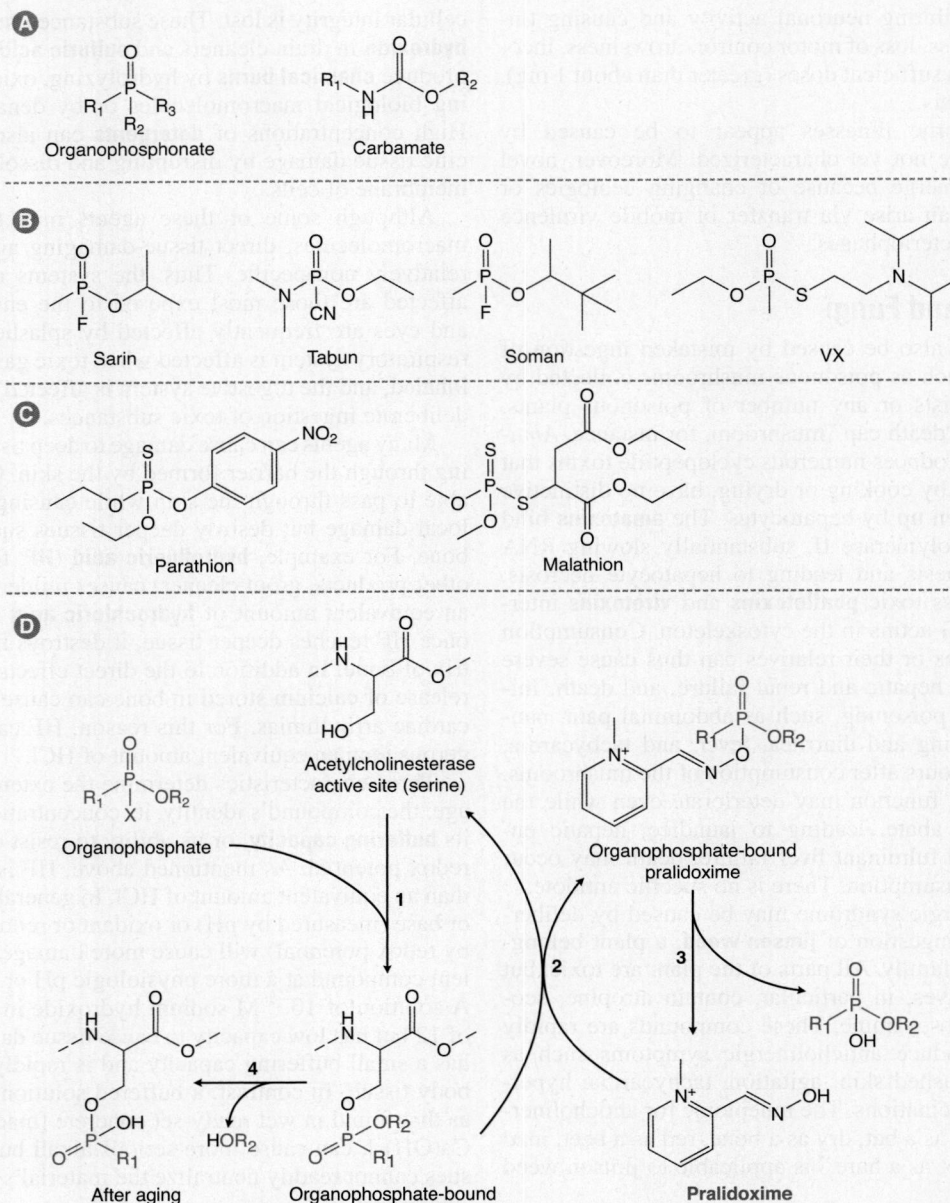

FIGURE 50-3. Structures and mechanisms of acetylcholinesterase inhibitors. A. Structures of typical acetylcholinesterase inhibitors, an organophosphonate on the left and a carbamate on the right. **B.** Structures of the principal nerve gases sarin, tabun, soman, and VX, which are potent inhibitors of human acetylcholinesterase. **C.** Structures of the organophosphate insecticides parathion and malathion. The thiophosphate bonds between sulfur and phosphorus are oxidized more efficiently by arthropod oxygenases than by mammalian oxygenases, so the compounds are less toxic to humans than the structurally related nerve gases. **D.** Organophosphates attack the serine active site in acetylcholinesterase, forming a stable phosphorus–oxygen bond *(1)*. Pralidoxime abstracts the organophosphate from serine, restoring active acetylcholinesterase *(2)*. Organophosphate-bound pralidoxime is unstable and spontaneously regenerates pralidoxime *(3)*. Organophosphate-bound acetylcholinesterase can lose an alkoxy group, in a process called *aging*. The end product of aging is more stable and cannot be detoxified by pralidoxime (*not shown*).

secretions, salivation, lacrimation, sweating, nausea, vomiting, diarrhea, and miosis (muscarinic signs), as well as twitching, fasciculations, muscle weakness, cyanosis, and elevated blood pressure (nicotinic signs). CNS effects can include anxiety, restlessness, confusion, and headache. Symptoms usually occur within minutes or hours of exposure and resolve within a few days in nonlethal poisonings.

Toxic exposures may occur by inhalation, ingestion, or dermal contact, depending on the product formulation and

manner of use or misuse. Toxic secondary exposures have occasionally occurred in people coming into close contact with the victim of direct exposure; for example, emergency responders and emergency department staff have suffered organophosphate toxicity after contacting—or simply being near—contaminated clothing, skin, secretions, or gastric contents.

Because the common organophosphate insecticides are metabolized and excreted relatively rapidly, the toxins do not accumulate in the body. However, the toxic effect may increase after repeated exposure because recovery of cholinesterase activity, either by dissociation of the phosphorylated AChE or de novo synthesis of the enzyme, is slow in the absence of treatment. Because the organophosphate insecticides are preferentially toxified by arthropod cholinesterases and/or preferentially detoxified by mammalian carboxyesterases, these compounds are more toxic to arthropods than to humans, an example of **selective toxicity**—although toxicity to humans exists as well.

Acute treatment for organophosphate poisoning involves restoration of the active site of the enzyme. While the administration of anticholinergic agents such as atropine can block the effect of excess acetylcholine at muscarinic receptors, it cannot restore the enzymatic function of AChE. As noted in Chapter 10, Cholinergic Pharmacology, **pralidoxime** can facilitate the hydrolysis of the serine–phosphate bond between the organophosphate and AChE, but this antidote must be administered before "aging" renders organophosphate inhibition essentially irreversible (Fig. 50-3).

Pyrethroid insecticides, such as **permethrin**, **deltamethrin**, **cypermethrin**, and **cyfluthrin**, are semisynthetic chemicals that are structurally related to the naturally occurring pyrethrins found in chrysanthemum flowers. The pyrethroids (and pyrethrins) have very high affinity for voltage-gated sodium channels, and, while they do not alter activation of sodium currents by membrane depolarization, they significantly delay termination of the action potential. Pyrethroids are common agricultural pesticides and are also found in some household products, including anti-lice shampoos.

Two classes of pyrethroids have been defined based on activity determined largely in laboratory experiments. Type I pyrethroids do not contain a cyano group, produce shorter duration sodium tail currents and repetitive discharges, and cause a **tremor (T) syndrome** in mammals that can include fine tremor, increased response to stimuli, and hyperthermia. Type II pyrethroids usually contain a cyano group, produce a longer duration sodium tail current and stimulus-dependent nerve depolarization and block, and cause a **choreoathetosis-with-salivation syndrome (CS)** that may include sinuous writhing (choreoathetosis) and salivation, coarse tremor, clonic seizures, and hypothermia. A few pyrethroids elicit intermediate syndromes. As in laboratory animals, T and CS signs are seen in people with large acute exposures to pyrethroids, as may occur during agricultural use of these insecticides. Pyrethroids are often formulated with a **synergist**, such as piperonyl butoxide, that inhibits insect cytochrome P450 enzymes (and thus pyrethroid metabolism) and increases pyrethroid toxicity.

Pyrethroid toxicity is relatively low in humans, but a small number of case reports of death in asthmatics exposed to pyrethroid-containing dog shampoos suggests a potential for exacerbation of asthma. Occupational exposure to pyrethroids often involves both inhalation and dermal exposure, since the insecticides are typically sprayed and workers may be caught in the drift. Absorption is rapid across the lung but very slow across the skin. Common symptoms include paresthesias (most frequently facial skin), dizziness, headache, blurred vision, nasal and laryngeal irritation, and shortness of breath. It is not clear to what extent other chemicals in the insecticidal formulation, such as petroleum hydrocarbons, contribute to these symptoms.

CARCINOGENICITY AND CHRONIC TOXICOLOGY

Environmental exposures are major causes of cancer. Consistent with the important role of environmental factors in carcinogenesis, the children of immigrants tend to develop cancers typical of their new, rather than ancestral, environs. Dietary factors differ according to locales and cultures, so that exposures to both procarcinogens and anticarcinogens in food are often different in adult immigrants relative to their offspring. Some of these environmental factors are, or work in concert with, carcinogenic viruses and other microorganisms, the prevalence and types of which vary remarkably from region to region. Thus, the prevalence of many types of cancer varies substantially among (and often within) countries.

Carcinogenic exposures (Table 50-1) include tobacco, alcoholic beverages, diet, chronic infections, radiation (ionizing and nonionizing), and occupational exposures to specific fibers, dusts, and chemicals. Carcinogenesis due to the toxic by-products of oxygen and other endogenous or unavoidable

TABLE 50-1 Some Environmental Exposures Known to Cause Cancer

EXPOSURE	TYPES OF CANCER
Acquired immunodeficiency syndrome (AIDS) due to human immunodeficiency virus (HIV)	Kaposi's sarcoma, non-Hodgkin's lymphoma, Hodgkin's disease, invasive cervical cancer
Aflatoxins (in diet)	Liver cancer
Alcoholic beverages	Oral, pharyngeal, laryngeal, esophageal, liver, colorectal, and female breast cancer
Arsenic (in water and in workplace air)	Lung, skin, and bladder cancer
Asbestos	Lung cancer, mesothelioma
Helicobacter pylori	Stomach cancer
Hepatitis B and C viruses	Liver cancer
Human T-lymphotropic virus type I	T-cell leukemia, T-cell lymphoma
Ionizing radiation	Leukemia, skin cancer, cancer of internal organs
Tobacco, smokeless	Oral cancer
Tobacco smoke	Cancer of lung, oro-, naso-, and hypopharynx, nasal cavity and paranasal sinuses, larynx, oral cavity, esophagus (adenocarcinoma and squamous cell carcinoma), stomach, colorectum, liver, pancreas, uterine cervix, ovary (mucinous), bladder, kidney (body and pelvis), and ureter; acute myelogenous leukemia
Ultraviolet radiation	Skin cancer

causes (such as spontaneous errors in DNA replication and repair) also accounts for a presumably sizable share of cancers that arise in humans and all other animals. All aerobic organisms, including bacteria, have developed defenses against oxidative and other damage to DNA, and these defenses work to counter at least low-level exposures to endogenous and many exogenous mutagens and carcinogens.

As outlined in Figure 50-4, carcinogens vary widely in their modes of action. Many organic chemical carcinogens are not genotoxic per se, but only via one or more electrophilic metabolites that form addition products—**adducts**—with one or more bases of DNA. These adducts can cause mutations, some of which lead ultimately to tumors. Interestingly, some such electrophiles have very short half-lives and so are mutagenic only in the organ, such as the liver or kidney, in which they are formed; others are stable enough to migrate to other tissues and organs, increasing risks of cancers at these distal sites. Carcinogenic metals can be directly toxic, or toxic via metabolism such as methylation, and can

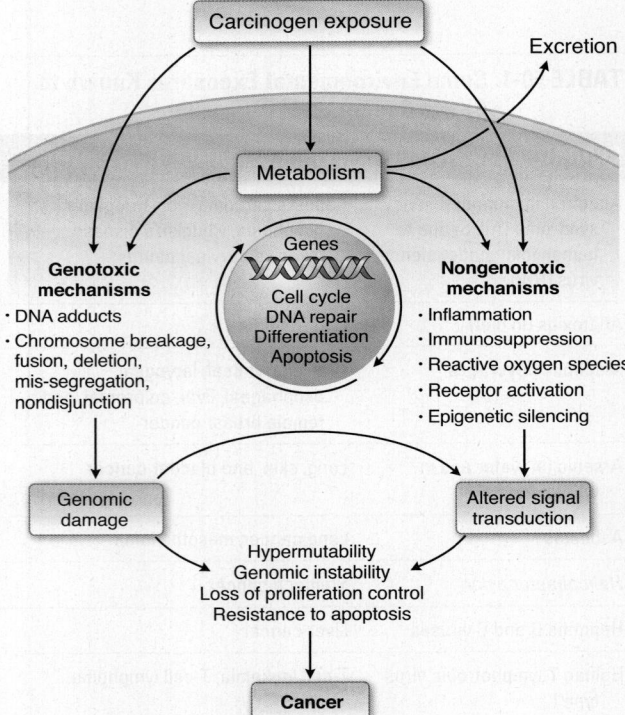

FIGURE 50-4. Overview of genotoxic and nongenotoxic effects of carcinogens. When chemical carcinogens are internalized by cells, they are often metabolized, and the resulting metabolic products are either excreted or retained. Retained carcinogens or their metabolic products can directly or indirectly affect the regulation and expression of genes involved in cell-cycle control, DNA repair, cell differentiation, and apoptosis. Some carcinogens act by genotoxic mechanisms, such as forming DNA adducts or inducing chromosome breakage, fusion, deletion, mis-segregation, and nondisjunction. Others act by nongenotoxic mechanisms such as induction of inflammation, immunosuppression, formation of reactive oxygen species (ROS), activation of receptors such as aryl hydrocarbon receptor (AhR) or estrogen receptor (ER), and epigenetic silencing. Together, these genotoxic and nongenotoxic mechanisms can alter signal transduction pathways, thus leading to hypermutability, genomic instability, loss of proliferation control, and resistance to apoptosis—some of the characteristic features of cancer cells.

alter chromosomal structure via hypermethylation of DNA and deacetylation of histones. Carcinogenic viruses and the carcinogenic bacterium, *Helicobacter pylori*, may act via many mechanisms, including induction of inflammation, itself a risk factor for cancer. Worldwide, chronic infections contribute to an estimated 15% of all cancers.

Carcinogenesis occurs via progressive stages broadly characterized as tumor initiation, promotion, and progression (Fig. 50-5). The sequence involves multiple rounds of stochastic mutations and selection, notably in proto-oncogenes and tumor suppressor genes. Infrequent mutations in other genes and cancer pathways are also involved, and determining which mutations are "cancer drivers" and which are mere passengers is a subject of active research.

The evolution from a normal cell to a clinically apparent tumor typically occurs over decades, so that cancer risk increases with age for the majority of cancers. Cigarette smokers, for example, develop lung cancer on average 30 years after first exposures. This explains why people who successfully quit smoking (a notoriously difficult task) reduce but do not eliminate their increased cancer risks relative to lifelong nonsmokers. Cancer deaths in dogs, cats, and laboratory rodents also occur largely in old age—and occur despite the animals' lack of deliberate exposures to exogenous chemical carcinogens. Exceptions to long latencies include cancers of childhood and acute myelogenous leukemias that develop secondary to treatment of another cancer with alkylating agents: such leukemias may arise in as short a time as 2–5 years after therapy.

Tobacco

It is difficult to overstate the toxicity of **tobacco**. Worldwide, tobacco kills 5 million people annually. **Cigarette smoke** is the most significant cause of cancer known: 30% of cancer deaths in developed countries are caused by cigarettes, and the burden of deaths due to cigarettes in developing nations is expected to rise in proportion to increasing prevalence of cigarette use. Smoking also causes nonmalignant pulmonary disease (such as COPD) and increases smokers' risks of cardiovascular disease and death, such that about half of all people addicted to tobacco die of tobacco-related diseases.

The carcinogenicity of cigarette smoke is due to the combined actions of at least 60 carcinogens and countless free radicals. Among the former are two "tobacco-specific" (that is, derived from nicotine) nitrosamines: 4-(methylnitrosamino)-1-(3-pyridyl)-1-butanone (NNK) and N'-nitrosonornicotine (NNN). Other carcinogenic components of cigarette smoke include polycyclic aromatic hydrocarbons (PAHs), aromatic amines, benzene, aldehydes and other volatile organic compounds, and various metals. Benzo[a]pyrene (Fig. 50-6) is among the carcinogenic PAHs in tobacco smoke and is also believed to account, in part, for the carcinogenicity of soots and coal tars. The important carcinogens and other toxins in tobacco smoke appear to be both in the solid "tar" phase of the smoke and in the gases and vapors. Thus, "low tar" cigarettes are apparently no less potent as carcinogens or causes of cardiovascular disease than are "regular" cigarettes.

Smokeless tobacco, which is variously "dipped," used as snuff, or chewed (alone, or with betel quid or other substances), contains significant concentrations of carcinogenic nitrosamines (and nicotine) and causes oral cancer as well as gum disease. The fraction of oral cancer that is attributable

A Tumor initiation

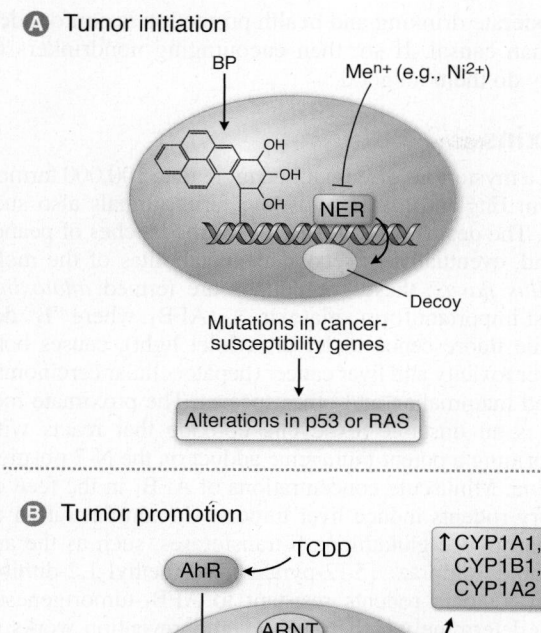

Mutations in cancer-susceptibility genes

↓

Alterations in p53 or RAS

B Tumor promotion

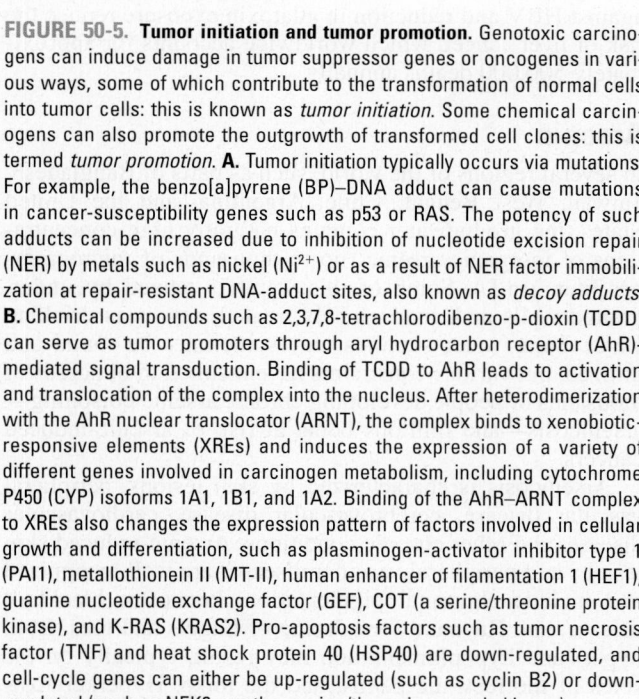

Extracellular signalling	Proliferation	Apoptosis	Cell cycle
↑PAI1	↑GEF	↓TNF	↑Cyclin B2
↑MT-II	↑COT	↓HSP40	↓NEK2
↑HEF1	↑KRAS2		

FIGURE 50-5. Tumor initiation and tumor promotion. Genotoxic carcinogens can induce damage in tumor suppressor genes or oncogenes in various ways, some of which contribute to the transformation of normal cells into tumor cells: this is known as *tumor initiation*. Some chemical carcinogens can also promote the outgrowth of transformed cell clones: this is termed *tumor promotion*. **A.** Tumor initiation typically occurs via mutations. For example, the benzo[a]pyrene (BP)–DNA adduct can cause mutations in cancer-susceptibility genes such as p53 or RAS. The potency of such adducts can be increased due to inhibition of nucleotide excision repair (NER) by metals such as nickel (Ni^{2+}) or as a result of NER factor immobilization at repair-resistant DNA-adduct sites, also known as *decoy adducts*. **B.** Chemical compounds such as 2,3,7,8-tetrachlorodibenzo-p-dioxin (TCDD) can serve as tumor promoters through aryl hydrocarbon receptor (AhR)-mediated signal transduction. Binding of TCDD to AhR leads to activation and translocation of the complex into the nucleus. After heterodimerization with the AhR nuclear translocator (ARNT), the complex binds to xenobiotic-responsive elements (XREs) and induces the expression of a variety of different genes involved in carcinogen metabolism, including cytochrome P450 (CYP) isoforms 1A1, 1B1, and 1A2. Binding of the AhR–ARNT complex to XREs also changes the expression pattern of factors involved in cellular growth and differentiation, such as plasminogen-activator inhibitor type 1 (PAI1), metallothionein II (MT-II), human enhancer of filamentation 1 (HEF1), guanine nucleotide exchange factor (GEF), COT (a serine/threonine protein kinase), and K-RAS (KRAS2). Pro-apoptosis factors such as tumor necrosis factor (TNF) and heat shock protein 40 (HSP40) are down-regulated, and cell-cycle genes can either be up-regulated (such as cyclin B2) or down-regulated (such as NEK2, another serine/threonine protein kinase).

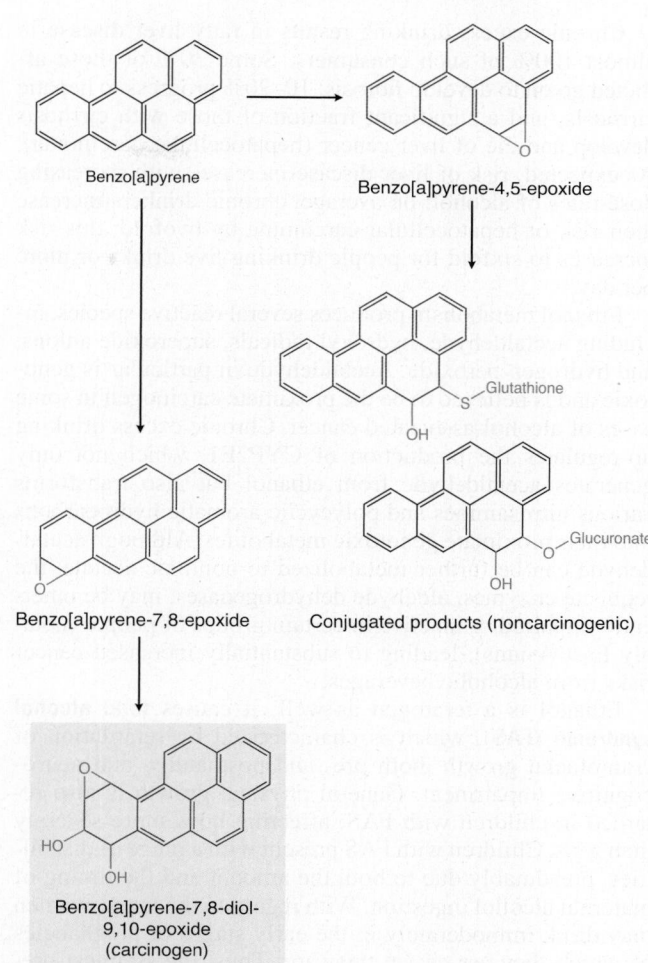

FIGURE 50-6. Metabolism of benzo[a]pyrene. Benzo[a]pyrene is metabolized into several products (*not all shown*). Epoxidation at carbons 4 and 5, followed by conjugation with glutathione or glucuronate, leads to nontoxic derivatives that are readily excreted. In contrast, oxidation at the "bay region" generates the proximate carcinogen benzo[a]pyrene-7,8-diol-9,10-epoxide, which goes on to form a repair-resistant adduct with guanine. Subsequent DNA replication, in the presence of this "bulky" polycyclic aromatic adduct, leads to G to T base pair transversions, including in the cancer genes p53 and RAS.

to smokeless tobacco in any given population depends on the prevalence of the habit, the potency of the local tobacco products (such as tobacco in betel quid and tobacco-areca nut mixtures), and competing causes of oral cancer. Thus, in the United States, smokeless tobacco accounts for 7% of oral cancer cases, while in India, more than 50% of oral cancers, in both men and women, are attributable to smokeless tobacco.

Ethanol

Excessive consumption of **ethyl alcohol** is a common and complex problem. Binge drinking occurs in a sizable minority of adolescents and young adults, at least in some cultures. In adults with coronary artery disease, binge drinking can cause myocardial ischemia and angina. Acutely, alcohol is a sedative and causes psychomotor retardation. A sizable fraction of morbidity and mortality from alcohol intoxication results from injuries suffered (and inflicted) while impaired.

Chronic excess drinking results in fatty liver disease in almost 100% of such consumers. Some 30% of those afflicted go on to develop fibrosis; 10–20% progress to hepatic cirrhosis; and a significant fraction of those with cirrhosis develop and die of liver cancer (hepatocellular carcinoma). As expected, risk of liver disease increases with increasing dose-rates of alcohol: on average, chronic drinkers increase their risk of hepatocellular carcinoma by twofold; this risk increases to sixfold for people drinking five drinks or more per day.

Ethanol metabolism produces several reactive species, including acetaldehyde, hydroxyl radicals, superoxide anions, and hydrogen peroxide. Acetaldehyde in particular is genotoxic and is believed to be the proximate carcinogen in some cases of alcohol-associated cancer. Chronic excess drinking up-regulates the production of CYP2E1, which not only generates acetaldehyde from ethanol but also transforms various nitrosamines and polycyclic aromatic hydrocarbons into their proximate genotoxic metabolites. Although acetaldehyde can be further metabolized to nontoxic acetate, the requisite enzymes, aldehyde dehydrogenases, may be inherently impaired or inactive in certain groups of people (notably East Asians), leading to substantially increased cancer risks from alcoholic beverages.

Ethanol is a teratogen as well; it causes **fetal alcohol syndrome** (**FAS**), which is characterized by retardation of craniofacial growth, both pre- and postnatally, and neurocognitive impairment. General physical growth is also retarded in children with FAS, affecting boys more severely than girls. Children with FAS present with a range of disabilities, presumably due to both the amount and the timing of maternal alcohol ingestion. With regard to the latter, women may drink immoderately in the early stages of pregnancies of which they are as yet unaware. Thus, the simplest prevention strategy (elimination of exposure) may not always be practical. FAS can be generated in laboratory rats and mice, and mechanistic studies using animal models have led to several working hypotheses. The facial abnormalities of FAS are believed to be due to apoptosis of neural crest cells during gastrulation or neurulation. Embryonic exposure to alcohol can result in reduced production of retinoic acid, and retinoic acid is essential for normal morphogenesis. Other postulated mechanisms involve ethanol-induced free-radical formation, altered gene expression, disruption of lipid bilayers in cell membranes, and interference with the activity of growth factors.

Excess drinking also increases the risks of pancreatitis, hemorrhagic stroke, and heart failure. The pathophysiology of alcoholic cardiomyopathy is complex and appears to involve cell death and pathologic changes in myocyte function.

Light to moderate ingestion of alcohol, on the other hand, appears to protect against cardiovascular disease. Red wine is believed by some to be particularly protective, perhaps because it contains not only ethanol but also resveratrol and other polyphenols; various cardioprotective mechanisms have been hypothesized, including improvements in endothelial function and effects on hemostasis. However, to the extent that evidence of the benefits of moderate drinking derives from observational rather than experimental studies, one must be mindful of the possibility that moderate drinkers are, by genetics or other habits or factors, less susceptible to cardiovascular disease in general, so that the association

with moderate drinking and health protection is confounded rather than causal. If so, then encouraging nondrinkers to start may do them no good.

Aflatoxins

In 1960, a mysterious disease killed more than 100,000 farmed turkeys in England; other birds and farm animals also succumbed. The deaths were linked to specific batches of peanut meal, and, eventually, to secondary metabolites of the mold *Aspergillus flavus*: these compounds are termed *aflatoxins*. The most important form, aflatoxin B_1 (AFB_1, where "B" denotes blue fluorescence under ultraviolet light), causes both acute liver toxicity and liver cancer (hepatocellular carcinoma) in myriad mammalian and other species. The proximate metabolite is an unstable, exocyclic epoxide that reacts with DNA, forming a potent mutagenic adduct on the N-7 position of guanine. Minuscule concentrations of AFB_1 in the feed of laboratory rodents induce liver tumors. Co-administration of drugs that induce glutathione S-transferases, such as the antihelminthic oltipraz [5-(2-pyrazinyl)-4-methyl-1,2-dithiol-3-thione], renders rodents resistant to AFB_1-tumorigenesis. Trials to determine whether such chemoprevention works in humans are ongoing.

As suggested above, various aflatoxin metabolites are nontoxic, including the glutathione conjugate and a hydrolysis product that binds to lysine residues on proteins such as serum albumin. Aflatoxin adducts and other biomarkers in blood and urine reflect a person's exposures to dietary aflatoxins over the prior 2–3 months and, in tropical regions where aflatoxin contamination is endemic and rural diets contain few foods, over many years. Epidemiological studies using these markers in populations in Africa and China have demonstrated that aflatoxin causes hepatocellular carcinoma, both directly and acting synergistically with liver damage due to hepatitis B virus (HBV). Both vaccination against HBV and reduction in aflatoxin exposure reduce the risk of liver cancer, which worldwide accounts for approximately 500,000 deaths annually.

Arsenic

In several regions of the world, such as parts of Bangladesh, Taiwan, West Bengal, Chile, Argentina, and the United States, the groundwater contains naturally high concentrations of inorganic arsenic (up to thousands of micrograms per liter, μg/L). Some of this water is tapped by underground wells and, inadequately treated, serves as drinking water. Safer water supplies may sometimes be found and utilized, but various constraints have resulted in hundreds of thousands of people developing chronic arsenic poisoning—arsenicosis—and millions being at risk of arsenic-induced cancers.

Arsenicosis is characterized by skin lesions, peripheral vascular disease, cerebrovascular disease, cardiovascular disease, and other chronic conditions. Arsenic-induced skin lesions and peripheral vascular diseases are well recognized and include abnormal pigmentation, keratoses, blackfoot disease, and Raynaud's syndrome of fingers and toes. Both hyper- and hypopigmentation may result, typically on the soles of the feet, the palms, and the torso. Hyperkeratosis also occurs on the soles and palms. Epidemiologic study suggests that these skin lesions may develop at lower arsenic concentrations (tens of μg/L) than do other arsenic-induced toxicities. Blackfoot disease used to be endemic in southwestern Taiwan, where arsenic was present at high concentration in artesian wells, and reached its highest incidence in the late 1950s before the introduction of tap water from safer sources. The disease has a typical progression: the first signs are preclinical peripheral vascular disease, followed by progressive discoloration of the skin from the toes toward the ankles. Feelings of numbness or coldness develop in the legs, followed by intermittent claudication, and eventually gangrene, ulceration, and surgical or spontaneous amputation. It is not clear why blackfoot disease is not seen in other regions with high, chronic oral exposures to arsenic.

Epidemiologic studies have indicated associations between exposure to high concentrations of arsenic (hundreds of μg/L) and various cardiovascular diseases such as hypertension and ischemic heart disease and between urinary levels of arsenic and levels of circulating markers of inflammation and endothelial damage, such as soluble intercellular adhesion molecule-1 (sICAM-1) and soluble vascular adhesion molecule-1 (sVCAM-1), both of which correlate with cardiovascular disease risk. In addition, studies of ApoE-knockout mice (which are vulnerable to development of atherosclerosis) exposed to inorganic arsenic support an association between this environmental contaminant and cardiovascular disease. Mechanisms remain to be elucidated, however, as does the degree of cardiovascular risk posed by drinking water containing lesser concentrations of arsenic.

Inorganic arsenic is a recognized human carcinogen that is causally associated with cancers of the skin, bladder, and lung. Associations with other cancers (e.g., liver, prostate) are less certain. The links to cancer were established in communities with extensive exposure to arsenic in drinking water, particularly in Taiwan and Chile, with clear dose–response patterns. Skin cancers may, but do not always, arise at sites of nonmalignant keratotic lesions and tend to be nonmelanomas. Interestingly, no adequate animal models have been identified for arsenic-induced cancers. However, experimental models have been used (and human cohorts have been observed) to shed light on the potential carcinogenic mechanisms: arsenic has indirect genotoxicity, effects on cell-cycle control, and the ability to cause oxidative damage, and it interferes with DNA repair or methylation. Other factors, such as nutritional status, genetic polymorphisms, and co-exposure to other toxins, may also influence the risk of arsenic-induced cancer.

Workplace Exposures

Various occupational exposures increase workers' risks of developing cancer and other diseases. As a general matter, exposure levels in industry are much higher than those in the general environment. To the extent that important and harmful occupational exposures have been characterized and minimized, the toll of occupational carcinogenesis has decreased. Needless to say, enforcement or even presence of occupational exposure limits is not guaranteed, and groups of workers in certain industries or nations continue to be at excess risk of developing one or more forms of cancer.

An eighteenth-century English surgeon, Percivall Pott, was among the first to recognize occupational carcinogenesis, deducing that "lodgment of soot in the rugae of the scrotum" caused scrotal cancer in young men employed as chimney sweeps (who typically worked naked, to avoid soiling their clothes). In the nineteenth and twentieth centuries,

industrial workers overexposed (1) to benzene were found to develop bone marrow disease, including aplastic anemia and acute myelogenous leukemia; (2) to 2-naphthylamine in dyemaking were at high risk for bladder cancer; (3) to various metals were susceptible to lung cancer; and (4) to asbestos developed lung cancer and mesothelioma. Other occupational carcinogens (including specific chemicals, industries, and industrial processes) were also identified.

Asbestos, Silica, Dusts, and Metals

Numerous cases of occupational lung injury are (or were) caused by inhalation of fibers or dusts—such as asbestos, crystalline silica, talc, and coal dust—and various metals. **Asbestos** is carcinogenic to the lung and mesothelium after long-term exposure to respirable fibers of specific dimensions. The formerly widespread use of asbestos-containing products in shipbuilding, construction, textiles, and other industries caused perhaps 200,000 cancer deaths in industrialized countries; because of latency, such deaths continue to occur. Current occupational exposures to asbestos are problematic in parts of India and elsewhere in Asia. Asbestos and cigarette smoking act synergistically, such that the risk of lung cancer (although, interestingly, not of mesothelioma, which is not caused by smoking) due to co-exposure is much larger than the risk from either factor alone. The toxic and carcinogenic potency of asbestos fibers and fiber types varies with their dimensions, surface chemistry, and biopersistence. The mechanisms by which asbestos fibers damage the lung or pleura involve production of reactive oxygen and nitrogen species by macrophages attempting to destroy the fibers. Asbestos also causes severe nonmalignant respiratory disease, **asbestosis**, characterized by fibrotic lesions in the lung parenchyma that impair gas exchange.

Black lung, or **coal worker's pneumoconiosis (CWP)**, is another nonmalignant (but potentially fatal) fibrotic lung disease induced by excessive exposure to coal dust. The simple form of CWP may not markedly impair respiration and may affect only small areas of the lung, whereas progressive CWP can develop and worsen even in the absence of continued exposure, leading to severe emphysema. Interestingly, coal dust does not appear to increase the risk of lung cancer. Although worker exposures to coal dust have been limited by US regulations in recent decades and underground mining is less common than in the past, thousands of coal miners in other countries, especially China, are at risk for CWP and related illnesses.

Occupational exposures to **metals** such as arsenic, cadmium, chromium (VI), and nickel increase workers' risks of cancers of the lung and, in some cases, nasal cavity and paranasal sinuses. A large number of mechanisms have been identified, both genetic and epigenetic.

Overexposures to certain metals can also cause nonmalignant disease. Chronic exposure to cadmium, for example, causes kidney disease. Abnormal renal function, characterized by proteinuria and decreased glomerular filtration rate (GFR), was first reported in cadmium workers in 1950 and has been confirmed in numerous investigations. The proteinuria consists of low-molecular-weight proteins such as β_2-microglobulin, retinol binding protein, lysozyme, and immunoglobulin light chains; these proteins are normally filtered in the glomerulus and reabsorbed in the proximal tubule. Cadmium-exposed workers also have a higher rate of kidney stone formation, perhaps due to disruption of calcium metabolism as a consequence of renal damage. Renal tubular dysfunction appears only after a threshold concentration of cadmium is reached in the renal cortex. The threshold varies among individuals but has been estimated to be approximately 200 μg/g wet weight. Several studies of the prevalence of proteinuria in worker populations suggest that inhalation exposure in excess of about 0.03 mg/m^3 for 30 years is associated with increased risk of tubular dysfunction. Unfortunately, removal from exposure does not necessarily halt disease in workers with cadmium-induced kidney damage; progressive decreases in GFR may occur and end-stage renal disease may develop. Progression of disease may depend on both the body burden of cadmium and the severity of proteinuria at last exposure. Unless renal damage is significant, urinary cadmium concentration reflects the body burden of the metal.

Although renal damage is clearly due to accumulation of cadmium in the kidney, the molecular mechanism responsible for this damage is unclear. Metallothionein may be involved; this cadmium-binding protein, which is synthesized in the liver and kidney, appears both to facilitate transport of cadmium to the kidney and to promote retention of cadmium in the kidney.

Chlorinated Hydrocarbons

Low-molecular-weight chlorinated hydrocarbons are widely used in industrial and other settings. Vinyl chloride, for example, is a gas used to make the plastic polyvinylchloride (PVC). Vinyl chloride gas is neither irritating nor acutely toxic (except at extremely high, narcotizing concentrations), and PVC workers were initially exposed to quite high concentrations. In the 1970s, exposures to vinyl chloride were found to cause angiosarcoma, a rare form of liver cancer, in both laboratory rats and workers; strict workplace exposure limits have since been imposed in most settings. Carcinogenesis is due to the epoxide metabolite of vinyl chloride. Some 98% of the DNA adducts formed from vinyl chloride epoxide are benign, but the other 2% are highly mutagenic etheno adducts with guanine and cytosine. Interestingly, these adducts are the same as those formed from everyday oxidative stress and lipid peroxidation. The ethenoguanine and ethenocytosine adducts are normally eliminated by base excision repair (see Chapter 39, Pharmacology of Cancer: Genome Synthesis, Stability, and Maintenance), but at sufficiently high rates of DNA damage, repair fails to be 100% effective. Thus, high-level exposures to vinyl chloride and similar genotoxins are demonstrably carcinogenic, while low-level exposures may not be. For example, laboratory rats exposed to low doses of vinyl chloride develop precancerous changes (altered hepatic foci) at rates indistinguishable from those seen in unexposed laboratory controls.

Trichloroethylene (TCE) and tetrachloroethylene (perchloroethylene) are solvents used for degreasing and dry cleaning. Essentially all humans are exposed to trace concentrations of TCE and perchloroethylene in ambient air. Exposures to high concentrations of TCE cause kidney tumors, but moderate- and low-level exposures apparently do not. This is because at low doses, trichloroethylene is converted to nontoxic metabolites that are readily eliminated, whereas at high doses, the detoxification pathway is saturated and a second metabolic pathway becomes operative. The latter pathway forms a nephrotoxic metabolite, S-(1,2-dichlorovinyl)-L-cysteine (DCVC), and the subsequent kidney damage appears to be a necessary precursor to TCE-induced kidney tumors. Nontoxic exposures to trichloroethylene up-regulate genes associated with stress, DCVC metabolism, cell proliferation and repair, and apoptosis, affording protection against renal tubular damage. Perchloroethylene does not appear to cause tumors in people, probably because virtually all of it is eliminated without metabolic activation.

Air Pollution

Toxicity due to ambient air pollution depends on both the types and concentrations of pollutants. As with other environmental exposures, air pollution takes much of its toll in regions lacking adequate environmental protection or resources. Combustion of fuels is an important source of air pollution; in most cities and suburbs, exhaust from gasoline- and diesel-powered vehicles is the largest source of pollutants. New and recently manufactured motor vehicles burn much more cleanly than vehicles made prior to the 1970s, but the number of vehicles in use continues to grow, and tailpipe emissions are, of course, close to ground level, limiting dilution into cleaner air.

Combustion of low-quality fuels indoors is not uncommon in some settings. For example, wood, soft coal, charcoal, or dried cow dung are burned for cooking and heating in poorly ventilated homes in some regions of Africa, Asia, and elsewhere. Measurements indicate indoor pollutant levels that exceed outdoor concentrations by two orders of magnitude. As a result of these residential exposures, women and children in particular are at risk of developing chronic bronchitis, dyspnea, and, eventually, interstitial lung disease. Moreover, the carcinogenic potency of soft coal smoke is 1,000 times greater than that of cigarette smoke (in a mouse skin-tumor assay). Women in China who use soft coal indoors have extraordinarily high body burdens of benzo[a]pyrene-adducted guanine, and their rates of death due to lung cancer are eight times higher than the national average for women.

Combustion generates thousands of chemicals, some of which depend on the material burned and others of which are inherent to combustion. These include carbon monoxide, organic irritants such as formaldehyde and acrolein, nitrogen oxides, sulfur dioxide, ammonia, hydrogen cyanide, and hydrogen fluoride, among other potentially toxic substances. Semi-volatile and nonvolatile chemicals also form in abundance and adsorb to the particle phase of smoke. Metals present in the combusted material are, of course, not destroyed by combustion and so may add to the acute and chronic toxicity of inhaled smoke.

Polluted air may become unusually acidic under certain meteorological and chemical conditions, and inhalation of acidic aerosols can induce bronchoconstriction and reduce the efficacy of mucociliary clearance. The action of ultraviolet radiation (sunlight) on reactive hydrocarbons and nitrogen oxides results in the formation of smog, containing significant concentrations of oxidizing chemicals such as ozone, peroxides, and peroxyacetyl nitrate. Acute and subchronic exposures to toxic levels of such oxidants can cause respiratory tract inflammation and irritation, sloughing of epithelium, and loss of cilia. Chronic overexposures can result in pulmonary fibrosis or chronic obstructive pulmonary disease, perhaps via altered metabolism of collagen and elastin.

The pulmonary effects of air pollutants depend in part on their water solubility. Sulfur dioxide, for example, dissolves readily in the mucous membranes of the upper airways and so does not typically reach the lung. Dissolution of the gas is not instantaneous, however, so that exercising or otherwise hyperventilating permits some of the inhaled sulfur dioxide to reach the lower respiratory tract, where, at sufficient concentrations, it can induce bronchoconstriction. Asthmatics are particularly sensitive to this effect.

■ CONCLUSION AND FUTURE DIRECTIONS

Much of the treatment for toxic exposures focuses on the acutely poisoned patient. Much of the morbidity associated with environmental factors, however, is caused by chronic exposures and may be clinically apparent only years or decades after the initial insult. In fact, there is generally no specific treatment for injury caused by chronic toxic exposures, and treatment modalities for cancers are independent of the underlying causes.

In theory, cancers and other chronic diseases caused by habits such as tobacco smoking and excessive drinking are entirely preventable, and although progress has been made in this regard, more remains to be done, although complete eradication of these threats seems unrealistic. Occupational exposures are well controlled in most of the developed world but remain problematic in industrializing nations. Epidemiologic evidence indicates that some specific foods—such as Chinese-style salted fish (containing high concentrations of the carcinogen dimethylnitrosamine) and foods contaminated with aflatoxins—increase people's risk of cancer, and that consumption of fruits and vegetables in general decreases risks of cancer, but the specific dietary components or characteristics that modify risk remain areas of active research. Obesity (and perhaps sedentary lifestyle) is an increasingly important risk factor for cancer, presumably in combination with environmental exposures or other factors.

Environmental exposures typically involve complex mixtures of only partially characterized chemicals. Traditional toxicological testing of individual chemicals or simple mixtures may yield results of incomplete or uncertain relevance. Additional information may be generated via microarray technologies and other tools of genomics, proteomics, and metabolomics applied to toxicological inquiry. Our microbiomes—that is, the microorganisms within us that, in toto, outnumber our own cells ten to one—presumably affect our responses to environmental exposures in many ways yet to be elucidated. More broadly, basic, mechanistic, and applied research is expected to continue to unravel the interconnections between and among genetic, environmental, and random factors involved in disease causation, with the hope that safer environments will lead to healthier lives.

Suggested Reading

Busl KM, Greer DM. Hypoxic-ischemic brain injury: pathophysiology, neuropathology and mechanisms. *NeuroRehabilitation* 2010;26:5–13. (*Reviews the pathophysiologic and molecular basis of hypoxic and cytotoxic brain injury.*)

Clower JH, Hampson NB, Iqbal S, Yip FY. Recipients of hyperbaric oxygen treatment for carbon monoxide poisoning and exposure circumstances. *Am J Emerg Med* 2012;30:846–851. (*Reviews data regarding 864 carbon monoxide-poisoned patients and makes recommendations for prevention and treatment.*)

Gordon SB, Bruce NG, Grigg J, et al. Respiratory risks from household air pollution in low and middle income countries. *Lancet Respir Med* 2014;2:823–860. (*Reviews evidence for association between household air pollution and infections, cancers, and chronic diseases of the respiratory system.*)

Hall AH, Saiers J, Baud F. Which cyanide antidote? *Crit Rev Toxicol* 2009;39:541–552. (*Reviews mechanisms, clinical efficacy, safety and tolerability, and supporting toxicology for antidotes to cyanide poisoning in use in the United States and elsewhere.*)

Hecht SS. Progress and challenges in selected areas of tobacco carcinogenesis. *Chem Res Toxicol* 2008;21:160–171. (*Review by a major researcher in the field.*)

International Agency for Cancer Research (IARC). Continuing series of monographs. http://monographs.iarc.fr/. (*As part of ongoing efforts since 1971, IARC convenes panels of experts charged with evaluating published evidence relevant to the determination of the established, probable, or possible carcinogenic effects of various chemical, biological, and physical agents and exposures. To date, some 116 substances and exposures have been characterized by IARC as carcinogenic to humans.*)

Klaassen CD, ed. *Casarett & Doull's toxicology: the basic science of poisons.* 8th ed. New York: McGraw-Hill; 2013. (*A comprehensive textbook of toxicology, this resource provides a solid foundation for the understanding of toxicology. It includes sections on general principles, toxicokinetics, nonspecific toxicity, organ-specific toxicity, toxic agents, environmental toxicology, and applications of toxicology, including a chapter on clinical toxicology.*)

Lang CH, Frost RA, Summer AD, Vary TC. Molecular mechanisms responsible for alcohol-induced myopathy in skeletal muscle and heart. *Int J Biochem Cell Biol* 2005;37:2180–2195. (*Reviews cellular and molecular mechanisms by which alcohol impairs skeletal and cardiac muscle function, with special emphasis on alterations in signaling pathways that regulate protein synthesis.*)

Luch A. Nature and nurture—lessons from chemical carcinogenesis. *Nat Rev Cancer* 2005;5:113–125. (*Reviews mechanisms of chemical carcinogenesis.*)

Pogribny IP, Rusyn I. Environmental toxicants, epigenetics, and cancer. *Adv Exp Med Biol* 2013;754:215–232. (*Reviews epigenetic changes caused by environmental carcinogens.*)

Schuhmacher-Wolz U, Dieter HH, Klein D, Schneider K. Oral exposure to inorganic arsenic: evaluation of its carcinogenic and non-carcinogenic effects. *Crit Rev Toxicol* 2009;39:271–298. (*Emphasizes findings with respect to risk of disease following relatively low exposures to arsenic.*)

Seitz HK, Stickel F. Risk factors and mechanisms of hepatocarcinogenesis with special emphasis on alcohol and oxidative stress. *Biol Chem* 2006;387:349–360. (*Review by major researchers in the field.*)

States JC, Srivastava S, Chen Y, Barchowsky A. Arsenic and cardiovascular disease. *Toxicol Sci* 2009;107:312–323. (*Reviews epidemiologic and experimental data.*)

Tauxe RV. Emerging foodborne pathogens. *Int J Food Microbiol* 2002;78:31–41. (*Overview of common sources of food poisoning.*)

Toxnet. http://toxnet.nlm.nih.gov/. (*This government resource, sponsored by the National Library of Medicine, contains a vast database of both toxic substances and articles in the field of toxicology.*)

Tzipori S, Sheoran A, Akiyoshi D, Donohue-Rolfe A, Trachtman H. Antibody therapy in the management of shiga toxin-induced hemolytic uremic syndrome. *Clin Microbiol Rev* 2004;17:926–941. (*Reviews the structure and mechanism of action of shiga toxins produced by E. coli O157:H7 and other enteropathic bacteria, the manifestations and treatment of hemolytic uremic syndrome, and the potential utility of antibody therapy.*)

Wogan GN, Hecht SS, Felton JS, Conney AH, Loeb LA. Environmental and chemical carcinogenesis. *Semin Cancer Biol* 2004;14:473–486. (*Review by major researchers in the field.*)

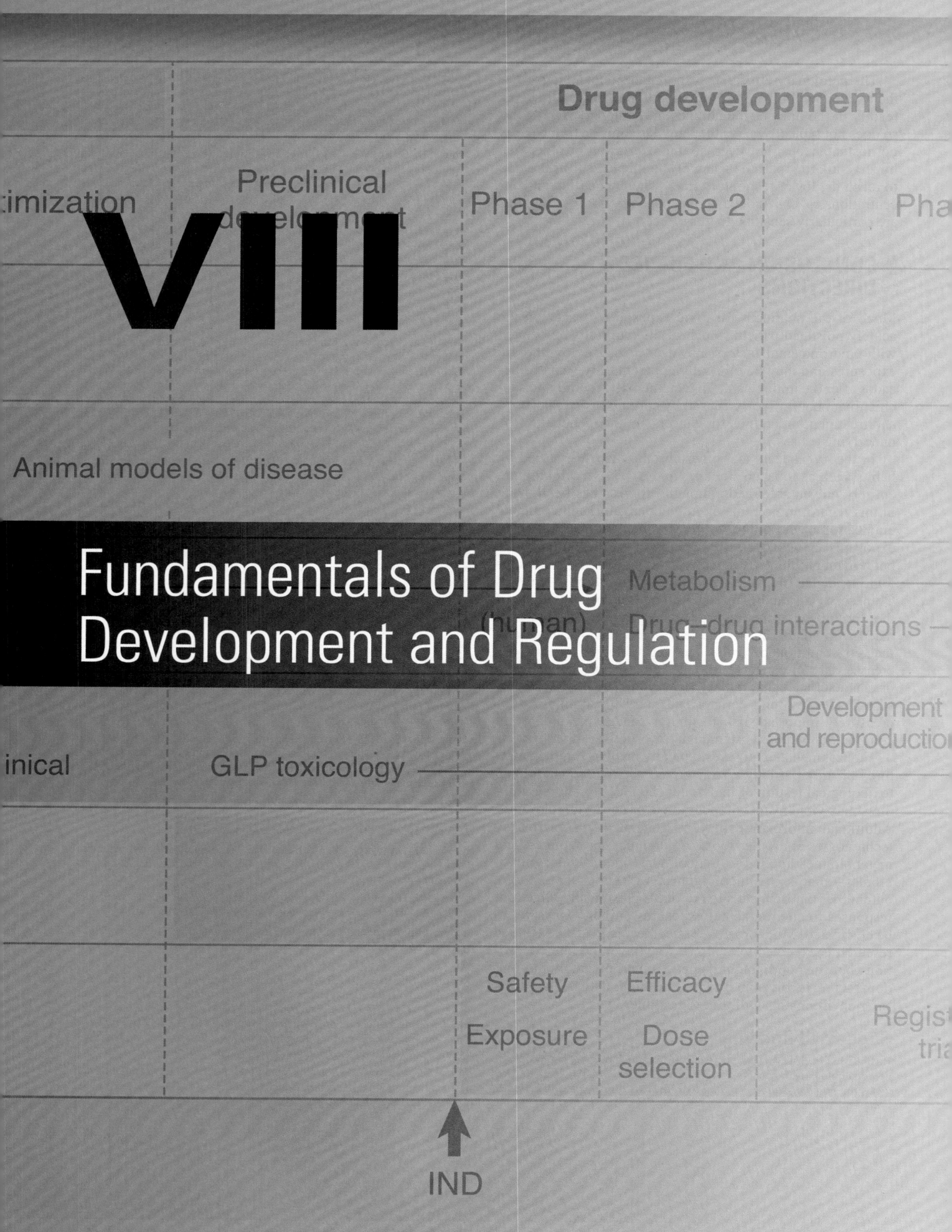

51

Drug Discovery and Preclinical Development

John L. Vahle, David L. Hutto, and Maarten Postema

INTRODUCTION

Over the past decade, the US Food and Drug Administration (FDA) has approved approximately 260 new therapeutics, including 220 new molecular entities (small molecules) and 42 biotherapeutics (generally, recombinant protein products). Many such therapies have enabled treatments for diseases that were previously untreatable. Others have yielded expanded treatment options because they are more efficacious and/or less toxic than previously available treatments. In the fight against infectious diseases, for example, pharmaceutical and biotechnology companies, university laboratories, and others have continued to develop new agents to treat diseases that have become resistant to existing treatments. With the availability of new technologies such as next-generation sequencing and novel protein engineering strategies, it is anticipated that important new classes of therapeutics will continue to be discovered and developed in the coming decades.

The development of a new drug is difficult and costly. Very few molecules that reach the development stage are ultimately approved as drugs: of 10,000 chemical compounds considered promising from the results of initial screening assays, fewer than 10 make it to clinical trials and only 2 are eventually approved. Furthermore, the costs associated with discovering and developing a new drug are estimated to be slightly over $1.2 billion, with some esti-

mates suggesting costs of up to $5 billion. Although the development of new drugs is a risky venture, successful drugs can be quite profitable for those willing to take such risks. The biggest commercial successes, such as **Abilify®**, have annual sales of more than $6 billion each.

Increased attention has recently been focused on the inability of the biomedical research community to produce innovative new therapies. The challenges involved in drug discovery and development were highlighted (along with potential solutions) in the 2004 report of the FDA Critical Path Initiatives (see "Suggested Reading"). This report noted that both the National Institutes of Health (NIH) budget and pharmaceutical company research and development spending approximately doubled over a 10-year period beginning in 1993. The added investment did not increase the rate of development of new medicines, however, as evidenced by a decline in major drug and biological product submissions to the FDA. While several potential solutions have been offered to address this issue, it is important to note that a joint report by the FDA and the Association of American Medical Colleges highlighted the critical role of physician-scientists in improving the effectiveness of drug discovery and development.

This chapter describes the phases of drug discovery and development and the scientific disciplines that are involved in these phases. **Drug discovery** spans the period from the identification of a potential therapeutic target to the selection

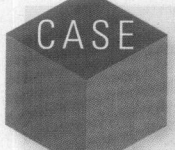

CASE

Drug discovery programs often start with a well-characterized biochemical or molecular target that is known to mediate a disease of interest. Drug discovery then involves the pursuit of a chemical compound (small molecule) or engineered macromolecule (generally, a protein) designed to modulate the pathway of interest. The following case provides an example of an alternative approach, in which an extensive genomics and bioinformatics program led to the identification of a novel protein (osteoprotegerin) and the discovery of a new pathway important in bone metabolism. These basic science discoveries then led to the development and commercialization of a novel protein therapeutic that is currently used to treat osteoporosis and bone destruction associated with cancer metastasis.

In the early 1990s, researchers at Amgen engaged in an extensive genomics program designed to identify novel genes and proteins in the anticipation that new biologic pathways and potential therapeutic targets would be identified. Full-length sequences were generated for specific genes of interest and were overexpressed in the livers of mice. These transgenic mice were then used in a phenotypic screen to identify biochemical, hematologic, radiographic, and histologic differences from wild-type control mice. Priority was given to genes encoding secreted proteins and genes encoding new members of families of proteins already known to have important roles in disease pathways. Through this process, investigators identified osteoprotegerin (OPG), a new protein with sequence homology to members of the tumor necrosis factor receptor (TNFR) family. Mice overexpressing OPG had a striking bone phenotype, with marked increases in bone that filled the medullary cavity. This increase in bone density was attributed to a marked reduction in osteoclast number. In 1995, Amgen patent filings identified OPG as an important regulator of bone metabolism. Starting from this discovery of OPG, investigators from Amgen and other laboratories elucidated a novel and critical pathway in osteoclast biology, including the discovery of receptor activator of NF-κB (RANK) and its ligand (RANKL).

Initial strategies to convert this biologic understanding into a useful therapeutic focused on OPG, including a fusion protein of OPG combined with a human immunoglobulin G1 (IgG1) Fc region. In animal models, this fusion protein was 200 times more active than full-length OPG, and, following safety testing in animals, it entered clinical trials in 1998. The initial Phase 1 study demonstrated dose-related reductions in bone turnover markers and provided proof of concept that modulation of the RANKL pathway could have beneficial effects on the human skeleton. Further optimization efforts led to the development of a similar molecule, derived from a mammalian cell line, with increased target affinity and a longer half-life. This molecule (AMGN-0007) entered clinical development; however, its development was halted based on the induction of an immune response to OPG in a clinical trial subject. Because of concerns regarding the potential for an OPG construct to induce an immune response and neutralize endogenous OPG, efforts to develop an OPG-based drug were discontinued.

Amgen had not limited its research program to an OPG-based therapeutic but had also capitalized on the significant progress that had been made in the area of monoclonal antibody generation technology to initiate development of a fully human monoclonal antibody targeting RANKL. These efforts led to the identification of AMG 162 (later known as *denosumab*). Because denosumab was not active in rodent species, studies in nonhuman primates were essential to demonstrate that denosumab had beneficial effects on the skeleton. Studies in nonhuman primates were also used to characterize the toxicity profile of denosumab, after which the drug entered clinical trials for the indication of osteoporosis in 2001. In the Phase 1 clinical program, denosumab demonstrated long-lasting reductions in bone turnover markers. Phase 2 studies demonstrated both increases in bone mineral density and reductions in bone turnover markers and were used to define the dose level to study in the Phase 3 program. The Phase 3 studies demonstrated robust reduction of fracture risk and, in 2010, led to the approval of denosumab as an agent to treat osteoporosis (Prolia®) in the United States.

It was hypothesized that RANKL is an important mediator of osteoclastic activity not only in osteoporosis but also in metastatic bone disease. Various rodent models of skeletal metastasis were found to have increases in stromal RANKL, and RANKL expression had been observed in some tumor types. Nonclinical studies conducted by Amgen and others established that RANKL inhibition can decrease osteoclast number and activity, limit the development of lytic bone lesions, and reduce skeletal tumor burden. Based on these positive findings from preclinical studies, a clinical development program was initiated and ultimately led, also in 2010, to the approval of denosumab (Xgeva®) for the prevention of skeletal-related events in patients with solid tumors.

of molecules for testing in humans. **Drug development** is generally defined as the period from the preclinical studies that support initial clinical trials through approval of the drug by regulatory authorities. The process of drug discovery and development is complex, requiring contributions from many otherwise disparate scientific disciplines (Fig. 51-1).

THE DRUG DISCOVERY PROCESS

The term **drug discovery** refers to the process by which pharmaceutical, biotechnology, academic, and government laboratories identify or screen compounds to find potentially active therapeutic agents. The discussion below is focused on the discovery of low-molecular-weight, chemically synthesized compounds. Many of the described concepts and principles are similar for the discovery of biotherapeutics (monoclonal antibodies and related molecules, oligonucleotide-based molecules, and others) but, generally, many fewer such molecules are interrogated during the screening process. Screening consists of testing many compounds in assays relevant to the disease in question: a compound that passes such a screen is called a **hit**. If the compound or its structural derivatives continue to show promise after further biological and chemical characterization, it becomes a **lead**. Drug discovery

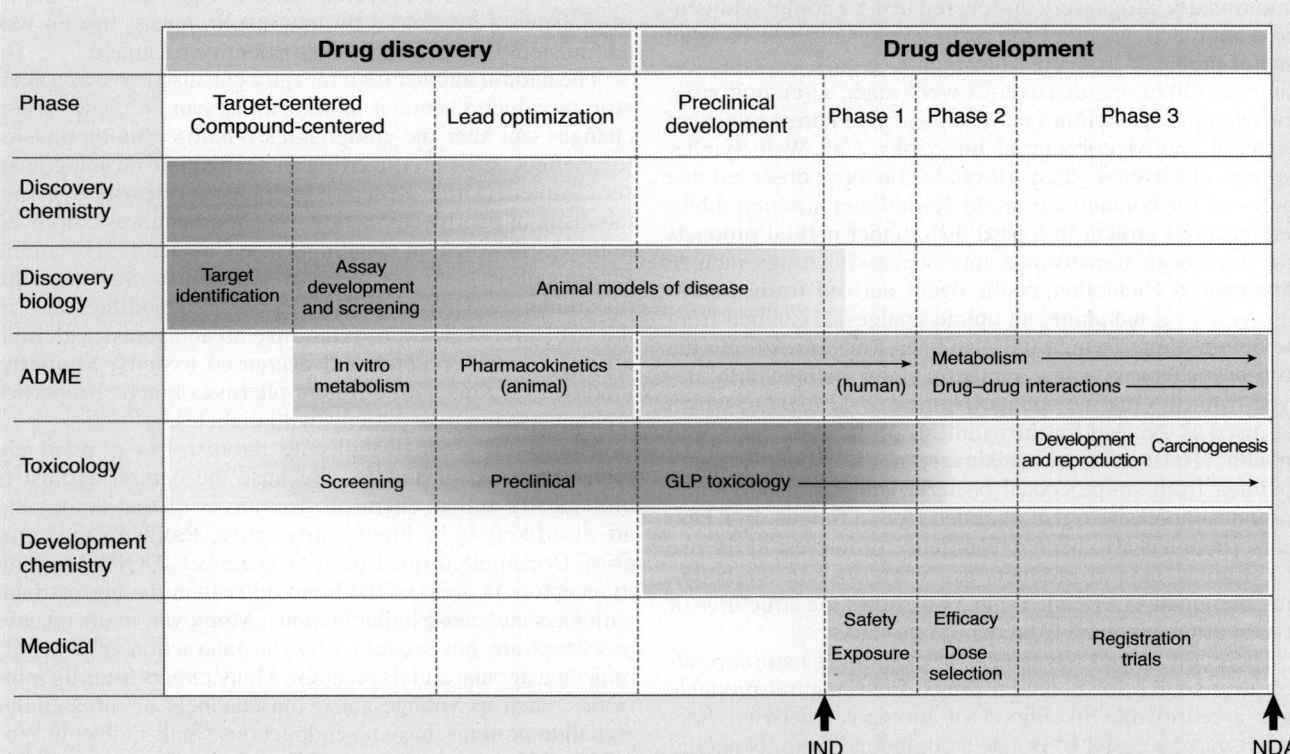

FIGURE 51-1. Sequence and phases of drug discovery and development. The important points to note are the general sequence of activities and the considerable overlap of functions with time. The process is highly interactive among multiple disciplines in an attempt to obtain the drug molecule with the greatest efficacy, least serious adverse effects, and greatest safety. The clinical trials and regulatory approval phases are described in Chapter 52. The entire process from hit to drug approval can take 8–12 years and cost more than $1 billion. IND, investigational new drug application; NDA, new drug application; ADME, absorption, distribution, metabolism, excretion; GLP, good laboratory practices.

should ideally be cost-effective, producing hits that have a high likelihood of conversion to leads and eventually to successful drugs (Fig. 51-1).

Two basic strategies are used to identify hits. In a **compound-centered** approach, a compound is identified by one of several methods (described below), and its biological profile is explored. If the compound displays desirable pharmacologic activity, it is refined and developed further. In a **target-centered** approach, which is now the more common mode, the putative drug target is identified first. The potential target could be a receptor thought to be involved in a disease process, a critical enzyme, or another biologically important molecule in the disease pathway. Once the target is identified, researchers search for compounds that interact with the target as agonists, antagonists, or modulators. The search may be systematic, using information about the structure of the target as a starting point (**structural biology-based approach** or simply **structure-based approach**), or it may take a **shotgun approach**, in which all the compounds in a large library of substances, synthesized via **combinatorial chemistry**, are tested in a high-speed automated assay. After any of these approaches identifies a hit, the hit is then often modified with the aid of specific knowledge about its target. For example, such knowledge can be used to design a high-throughput screen that will test the biologic activity of compounds generated by chemical modifications of the original hit.

Compound-Centered Drug Design

Natural and Synthetic Compounds

Traditionally, drugs were discovered using a compound-centered approach. Many of the earliest drugs discovered were **natural products** isolated from plants, molds, or other organisms. Often, the discoveries were made serendipitously. For example, **penicillin** (see Chapter 35, Pharmacology of Bacterial and Mycobacterial Infections: Cell Wall Synthesis) was discovered when Alexander Fleming observed that spores of the contaminant mold *Penicillium notatum* inhibited bacterial growth in a petri dish. Other natural products that have been transformed into successful drugs include **paclitaxel**, a chemotherapeutic agent derived from the Pacific yew tree; **morphine**, an opioid analgesic obtained from the opium poppy, which has also been transformed into the drug **oxycodone** in a few synthetic steps; **halichondrin**, derived from the marine sponge *Halichondria okadai*, which was used as the lead for the synthesis of the anticancer drug **eribulin** (Halaven®); **streptokinase**, a thrombolytic agent obtained from streptococcal bacteria; and **cyclosporine**, an immunosuppressive agent obtained from a fungus. In recent years, there has also been a resurgence of interest in the use of cytotoxic natural products as "warheads" in antibody–drug conjugates (ADCs). Table 51-1 shows the structures of several drugs obtained from natural products.

There are several advantages to examining natural products as a source for potential drugs. First, natural products have a reasonable likelihood of biological activity. Second, it may be easier to isolate a compound from its natural source than to synthesize a compound de novo, especially if the structure of the compound is complex or requires difficult synthetic manipulations. **Paclitaxel**, for example, has a complex structure that contains four fused rings, one of which contains eight carbons. A chemical synthesis of the

compound took over 50 steps to complete and had a total yield of less than 1%. Third, it may be feasible to use the natural compound as a starting point for synthetic fine-tuning (i.e., to form a **semisynthetic** product). Natural products also have disadvantages: it often takes significant effort to isolate a natural product, without a guarantee of success, and, even if it is found to be pharmacologically active, a natural product can be expensive to isolate and modify. Also, since the in vivo mechanism of action is often unknown for many natural products, establishing screening systems and identifying clinically feasible safety monitoring tools for these highly potent compounds present significant challenges in the current environment of targeted pharmaceutical therapies.

Synthetic compounds are now frequently used to search for new drugs. Researchers can construct a library consisting of thousands of compounds with differing structural characteristics, tailored for a particular type of investigation. A library could, for example, consist of numerous compounds that have a phenylalanine–proline bond or that are likely agonists or antagonists of a particular class of receptors.

Analogues of Natural Ligands

An alternative compound-centered approach uses the natural ligand (often an agonist) of a receptor as the starting point for drug development. For example, because lack of **dopamine** in the nigrostriatal pathways is associated with Parkinson's disease (see Chapter 14, Pharmacology of Dopaminergic Neurotransmission), one of the first effective treatments involved administering the drug **levodopa (L-DOPA)**, a metabolic precursor of dopamine. **Insulin** was developed in much the same way; once it was discovered that the signs and symptoms of diabetes were caused by low insulin levels, insulin was administered exogenously as an effective treatment.

The natural agonist for a receptor can also serve as a skeleton on which chemical modifications can be made. These changes can alter the compound's binding affinity, physiologic effect (such as converting an agonist into an antagonist; see Chapter 1, Drug–Receptor Interactions), distribution, metabolism, or pharmacokinetics. This approach was employed in the development of **cimetidine** (see Chapter 44, Histamine Pharmacology), an H_2 receptor antagonist. Starting with histamine, researchers made successive modifications in the structural skeleton to synthesize an antagonist with high affinity for the receptor and decreased toxicity. Similarly, modified insulins with different pharmacokinetic properties are now used to treat patients with diabetes.

Modifying a small-molecule agonist has a relatively high likelihood of success. Because the natural agonist is biologically active, chemical derivatives of that compound are also likely to be biologically active. Problems may also arise. Dopamine formed from exogenous L-DOPA can bind to receptors in areas of the brain other than the nigrostriatal pathways and cause hallucinations. Moreover, many disease processes are not mediated by the interaction of a small-molecule agonist and its receptor. Many targets for drug molecules, such as voltage-gated ion channels or intracellular signaling proteins, have no endogenous small-molecule agonists and hence are not amenable to the analogue approach.

Target-Centered Drug Design

In a target-centered approach to drug discovery and design, researchers use a biochemical or molecular target known to

TABLE 51-1 Examples of Natural Products Used as Drugs, Their Clinical Uses, and Sources

Natural Product	Drug	Clinical Use, Source, and Chapter Reference
Artemisinin	Artesunate	Antimalarial *Artemisia annua* (sweet wormwood) Chapter 37
Digoxin		Antiarrhythmic, cardiac inotrope *Digitalis lanata* (white foxglove), *Digitalis purpurea* (purple foxglove), numerous other plants Chapters 24, 25
Maytansine	Trastuzumab emtansine	Anticancer antibody–drug conjugate (ADC) *Maytenus* species (staff vine family) Chapter 40
Morphine	Oxycodone	Analgesic *Papaver somniferum* (poppy plant) Chapter 18
Paclitaxel		Anticancer microtubule inhibitor *Taxus brevifolia* (Pacific yew tree) Chapter 39

Portions of structures in *blue and bold* indicate semisynthetic additions to the natural product.

be essential in the disease of interest (a "validated" target) to search for hits. This approach has several advantages. First, if the target has been associated with a disease process, a hit that successfully interacts with the target has a relatively high likelihood of useful pharmacologic activity. Second, because the target is known, it may be easier to devise assays capable of isolating the effect of potential hits on the target. This is especially true for disease processes too complex to observe in cell or tissue preparations. For example, although a potential drug's effect on the process of atherosclerosis may be difficult to measure rapidly, it is relatively easy to measure whether the drug inhibits an enzyme known to be involved in the pathogenesis of atherosclerosis, such as HMG-CoA reductase (see Chapter 20, Pharmacology of Cholesterol and Lipoprotein Metabolism). As knowledge of the pathophysiology of disease processes has increased, target-centered approaches to drug discovery have become increasingly successful, and most new drugs have been discovered using target-centered methods. HIV protease inhibitors, such as **ritonavir**, are notable examples of a small-molecule drug class discovered using a target-centered approach (see Chapter 38, Pharmacology of Viral Infections). In a complementary target-centered approach, dissection of the underlying biological pathway has allowed the development of macromolecules, including antibodies, as novel pharmaceuticals to interrupt the pathway (Box 51-1).

High-Throughput Screening
The simplest target-centered approach involves rapidly screening many molecules using an assay based on the drug target. **High-throughput screening** uses a target-based assay and robotic automation to test many thousands of compounds in a few days.

Two aspects are critical in this approach. First, a large **library** of compounds must be available for screening.

Second, a robust **assay** that leads to rapid identification of true hits must be developed. The assay may be as simple as detecting the binding of drug candidates to a receptor (see Chapter 2, Pharmacodynamics), or it may be more sophisticated, involving complicated biochemical or cell-based biological readouts. The library is then "run through" the assay, and any hits giving a positive signal are examined more closely. An assay performed in a 96- or 384-well plate allows researchers to screen many compounds simultaneously. In addition, once a library of compounds has been assembled, the same library can be run through many different assays. The quality of the results is dependent on the quality of the assay and the compounds in the library, so a poorly designed assay or a limited library may result in false hits or may miss viable candidates. In practice, because high-throughput screening places a premium on rapid assays, false positives and false negatives are not uncommon and require follow up "validation" of potential hits. In addition, hits in a primary assay will often be "counter-screened" in second-tier assays designed to rule out binding of a hit to other related or unrelated targets. Even when a true hit is found, it will most likely need to be structurally refined to increase its binding affinity or to change its pharmacologic or pharmacokinetic properties (specificity, solubility, stability, kinetics, etc.); this process is called **hit-to-lead development**.

Combinatorial Chemistry
One important refinement in the process of high-throughput screening has been the introduction of **combinatorial chemistry**. In a strategy analogous to that used by nature to construct a wide variety of proteins from a relatively small number (approximately 20) of amino acids, combinatorial chemistry uses a relatively small number of precursor molecules to generate a large number of chemical compounds. Researchers are not limited to natural substances; instead, they

BOX 51-1 Macromolecular Biologics and Therapeutics

Increasingly, pharmaceutical and biotechnology companies are turning toward large molecules such as **peptides**, **peptidomimetics**, **proteins**, **antisense oligonucleotides**, and **monoclonal antibodies**. The pharmacologic properties and clinical utility of these therapies are described in Chapter 54, Protein Therapeutics.

The approach to the discovery and development of these molecules can differ significantly from that for small molecules. Consider, for example, the development of agents for the treatment of diseases related to an insufficiency or lack of an endogenous compound, such as **insulin** for diabetes, **erythropoietin** for anemia, or a coagulation factor (**factor VIII** or **factor IX**) for an inherited coagulopathy. In these situations, referred to as *replacement therapy*, it is not necessary to perform extensive screening of a large number of molecules to determine whether the endogenous molecule needs to be modified. Therefore, these agents may rapidly move into development and human testing.

Natural or modified macromolecules are increasingly used not only to replace but also to modulate physiologic processes, and engineered macromolecules such as antibodies are being used in the treatment of disease (Table 51-2). In the case of antibodies,

the drug discovery and development process may involve modifications that increase the affinity or specificity of the antibody for the desired molecular target or that "humanize" the antibody in order to minimize its immunogenic potential. Because these types of molecules must typically be administered parenterally, the need to screen for acceptable pharmacokinetic properties is lessened. Furthermore, the required discovery biology and animal toxicity testing may not be as extensive because toxicities for biotherapeutics are generally related to "hyperpharmacology" and there is often less risk of "off-target" toxicity (see Chapter 6, Drug Toxicity). Manufacturing a biologic product is much more expensive and more technically challenging than manufacturing a chemically synthesized molecule. Major challenges in development of a biologic product are to develop a system capable of producing the desired macromolecule in a bacterium, yeast, or mammalian cell and then to isolate the compound in pure form from the large mixture of metabolic products that often result from the synthesis. Faithfully reproducing the complex procedures involved in macromolecule synthesis and purification makes the preparation of generic biologic drugs a substantial challenge. ■

TABLE 51-2 Examples of Macromolecular Therapies

NAME	INDICATION	MOLECULAR CATEGORY	ORIGIN
Antivenin	Snake bite	Antibody	Equine or cell culture
Erythropoietin	Anemia	Growth factor	Bacteria (recombinant human)
Heparin	Anticoagulant	Glycosaminoglycan	Porcine or bovine
Human growth hormone	Growth retardation	Hormone	Bacteria (recombinant human)
Insulin	Diabetes	Hormone	Bacteria (recombinant human)
Parathyroid hormone	Osteoporosis	Hormone	Bacteria (recombinant human)
Streptokinase	Thrombolysis	Protein	*Streptococcus*
Trastuzumab	Cancer	Antibody	Chinese hamster ovary cell culture (humanized monoclonal antibody)

generally use a group of precursors with common functional groups and divergent side chains. For example, a researcher starting with three sets of 30 precursor building blocks can create 27,000 (30 × 30 × 30) different compounds in two synthetic steps (Fig. 51-2). One could theoretically create each compound individually in its own reaction well, but in practice, it is often easier to synthesize the molecules on a solid support phase such as a polystyrene bead. In a **parallel**

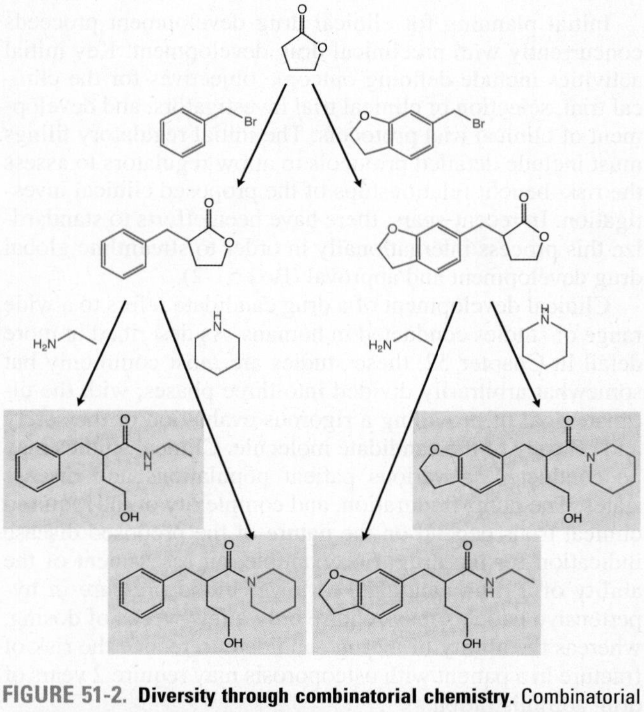

FIGURE 51-2. Diversity through combinatorial chemistry. Combinatorial chemistry uses simple building blocks to produce a complex library of compounds. In this example, the functionalized skeleton (*black*) has multiple sites of attachment. Two building blocks (*blue*) combine with the functionalized skeleton to produce a wide variety of products. In this example, two different side groups for each of the two building blocks results in four (2^2) possible products (*highlighted in blue boxes*). Combinatorial chemistry libraries use several building blocks, each with up to 20 or more different side groups, and can produce thousands of complex molecules using the same basic chemistry.

synthesis, the beads are split so that thousands are reacted at once and then successively recombined and split to undergo successive reactions. This strategy drastically reduces the number of reactions in the synthesis (30 at a time instead of 27,000 at a time, in the previous example). However, the challenge then becomes sorting the beads in order to know which compound has been synthesized on each bead. Researchers have solved this problem by **tagging** each bead with a unique chemical code, such as a ribonucleotide sequence, during each reaction. To identify a bead that bears a successful hit compound, the tag is cleaved, amplified by standard methods, and sequenced. The code then reveals which reactions the bead has been subjected to, and consequently the identity of the successful compound. Large chemical libraries can be synthesized in this manner and then screened in high-throughput assays for activity, sometimes with the compounds still attached to the beads.

The use of combinatorial chemistry and high-throughput screening is termed a **shotgun approach**, because researchers test a wide range of compounds blindly against a single target. This approach can also be modified to search for a particular result by using **biased libraries** for different types of targets. For example, researchers have synthesized large libraries of compounds that are more likely to interact with G protein-coupled receptors, proteolytic enzymes, kinases, or ion channels, based on the structural characteristics of each type of target.

Structure-Based Drug Design

Another target-centered approach is termed **structure-based drug design** or **rational drug design**. In this approach, a drug candidate is discovered using the three-dimensional structure of the target obtained through **nuclear magnetic resonance** (**NMR**) or **x-ray crystallography**. In theory, researchers could identify the active site within the structure of the target, use modeling algorithms to study the shape of the active site, and design a candidate drug molecule to fit into the active site. More commonly, though, the target is co-crystallized with a substrate analogue or receptor ligand (agonist or antagonist) in order to identify the structure of the active site. The structure of the analogue is then modified to increase the molecule's affinity, as was done in the case of the antiviral **ritonavir**. Alternatively, researchers can refine the structure of a new compound that binds to the target in a screening assay. By iteratively improving the fit of the prototypic molecule in the active site of the target, the binding affinity is increased.

There are several advantages to a structure-based drug design approach. The refined hit (also called *lead*) compounds are often extremely potent, with binding affinities in the nanomolar range. Moreover, only a limited number of candidates need to be tested because there is a high likelihood that one or more of the designed compounds will bind the target. In addition, iterative modification of the compound is relatively straightforward because it is known which parts of the molecule are critical for binding to the active site of the target. Thus, in comparison to a structure-blind approach, fewer analogues are prepared in a structure-based approach, but each analogue has a higher likelihood of activity. One disadvantage to this approach is that the modified compounds are often more difficult to synthesize because the molecular design demands specific functionalities in specific locations of the molecule. Another disadvantage is that obtaining a crystal structure of the target can be difficult, especially for membrane-bound proteins. Often, other methods of drug design yield hits long before the target can be crystallized. However, even if the initial hit compound results from another method, that hit can often be refined into a lead using a structure-based design approach.

As structure-based drug design gains feasibility, more drugs will be produced using structural information about the target even if the initial hits are discovered through other methods. Rational drug design has been critical for the development of HIV protease inhibitors such as ritonavir; structure-based methods have also been used to develop a second class of antiviral drugs, the neuraminidase inhibitors (see Chapter 38), as well as many tyrosine kinase inhibitors (TKIs) that are used widely in anticancer drug therapies (see Chapter 40, Pharmacology of Cancer: Signal Transduction).

Lead Optimization

The early drug discovery process typically identifies a promising group of lead molecules that appear to interact with the target in a desirable way. For these promising molecules, however, many of the critical physical, chemical, biological, pharmacologic, pharmacokinetic and safety properties that are important attributes of an effective drug have not been identified at the time of lead identification. **Lead optimization** is the stage of drug discovery where these properties are characterized and refined, with the ultimate goal of selecting a single molecule to enter into clinical testing and formal drug development.

In practice, most lead compounds have one or more characteristics (e.g., low solubility, low oral bioavailability, complex metabolism, off-target promiscuity) that make them poor candidates for clinical use. Using the data generated in lead optimization, it is often possible to modify the structure of the molecule to overcome these deficiencies. A variety of factors may cause a molecule to be terminated at the lead optimization stage. These include:

- Failure to demonstrate efficacy in a rigorous animal model of human disease
- Failure to attain adequate systemic exposures after oral administration (low bioavailability)

- Extensive or complex metabolism within the body, resulting in the generation of potentially dangerous reactive metabolites
- Extremely low solubility that prevents the preparation of a suitable formulation for dosing
- Negative effects in preliminary safety evaluation studies
- In vitro evidence that the molecule may damage DNA (genotoxicity)
- Extremely difficult chemical synthesis that cannot be scaled up in a cost-effective manner

■ PHASES OF DRUG DEVELOPMENT

The outcome of the lead optimization process is the selection of a molecule suitable for testing in humans. At this point, the molecule moves from drug discovery to drug development. Early drug development consists of preclinical activities designed to support clinical trials and clinical drug development. The initial preclinical phase of drug development includes the following activities:

- Manufacture, formulation, and packaging of a sufficient amount of high-quality drug material for both definitive animal safety testing and clinical trial use
- Animal toxicology and pharmacokinetic studies to define safe-use conditions of initial drug administration in humans
- Preparation of regulatory documents and submissions to regulatory authorities; these activities are described in more detail in Chapter 52, Clinical Drug Evaluation and Regulatory Approval.

Initial planning for clinical drug development proceeds concurrently with preclinical drug development. Key initial activities include defining outcome objectives for the clinical trial, selection of clinical trial investigators, and development of clinical trial protocols. The initial regulatory filings must include detailed protocols to allow regulators to assess the risk–benefit relationships of the proposed clinical investigation. In recent years, there have been efforts to standardize this process internationally in order to streamline global drug development and approval (Box 51-2).

Clinical development of a drug candidate refers to a wide range of studies conducted in humans. As described in more detail in Chapter 52, these studies are most commonly but somewhat arbitrarily divided into three phases, with the ultimate goal of providing a rigorous evaluation of the safety and efficacy of the candidate molecule. Clinical studies may be conducted in various patient populations and disease states. The number, duration, and complexity of the required clinical trials depend on the nature of the proposed disease indication for the drug. For example, an assessment of the ability of a drug candidate to lower blood pressure in hypertensive patients may require only a few weeks of dosing, whereas the ability of a drug candidate to reduce the risk of fracture in a patient with osteoporosis may require 2 years of drug administration.

Although evaluating the effects of the candidate molecule in humans is the primary focus of the drug development phase, extensive activities must also be completed by various scientific disciplines to support both these clinical trials and the ultimate regulatory approval of the drug. These activities are described in the following section, and they must be carefully coordinated in order for drug development to proceed as effectively as possible.

BOX 51-2 International Conference on Harmonization

The International Conference on Harmonization (ICH) brings together regulatory authorities and pharmaceutical industry experts from Japan, Europe, and the United States. The mission of the conference is to reach consensus on the scientific and technical aspects of drug development. The stated objective of the project is to create:

... a more economical use of human, animal and material resources, and the elimination of unnecessary delay in the global development and availability of new medicines whilst maintaining safeguards on quality, safety and efficacy, and regulatory obligations to protect public health.

The project is divided into four topic areas, including:

1. Quality – related to assuring the chemical qualities of the product
2. Safety – relating to safety testing in animals
3. Efficacy – relating to clinical studies in human subjects
4. Multidisciplinary – relating to topics involving multiple aspects of drug development

Each of the topic areas is articulated through a set of guidance documents. Before the existence of the ICH, it was not uncommon for different political jurisdictions (United States, Europe, Japan) to have different and conflicting regulatory requirements regarding preclinical and clinical drug development. Thus, a drug development "package" satisfying the requirements of one jurisdiction might not satisfy the requirements of another. As a result, a pharmaceutical company could spend years designing and completing a package to satisfy the requirements for one jurisdiction, only to find that another jurisdiction required additional, new, or reconfigured drug development activities.

The ICH is meant to unify and clarify drug development regulatory requirements across regulatory jurisdictions.

The preclinical safety guidelines of the ICH cover a range of topics, including:

1. Carcinogenicity – addressing the potential for the pharmaceutical to cause tumors
2. Genotoxicity – addressing the potential for damage of genetic material
3. Toxicokinetics and pharmacokinetics – addressing the need to characterize the ADME properties in animal species
4. Toxicity testing – addressing both acute and chronic toxicity in animals
5. Reproductive toxicity – addressing the potential of the molecule to impair fertility or cause developmental defects
6. Biotechnology products – addressing factors specific to preclinical studies for biotherapeutics
7. Pharmacology – addressing studies performed to characterize the acute effects on organ systems
8. Immunotoxicology – addressing studies performed to understand the impact on the structure and function of the immune system
9. Anticancer products – addressing special considerations for the preclinical safety assessment of anticancer drugs
10. Phototoxicity – addressing evaluation methods for determining whether a drug may cause toxicity after absorbing ultraviolet or visible light

In addition, a key multidisciplinary guidance describes when the above studies should be conducted in relationship to the clinical trials and product registration. This document also provides guidance on specialized topics such as understanding toxicity in juvenile animals. ■

KEY DISCIPLINES IN DRUG DISCOVERY AND DEVELOPMENT

Having discussed the overall process of drug discovery and development, we now turn to the fundamental tools—from basic chemistry and biology to manufacturing and formulation—that are crucial in the discovery and development of new therapeutic agents.

Discovery Chemistry

Chemists and biologists work hand in hand in the early phases of drug discovery. In compound-centered drug design, medicinal chemists begin the discovery process by preparing the molecules to be tested in biologic and pharmacologic assays. In target-centered design, the process begins with the identification of potential drug targets against which chemists then design and prepare the molecules for testing. Thus, in both approaches, there is close interaction and collaboration between chemists and biologists.

Initially, the amount of a drug candidate needed to run a simple screening assay is small—typically, less than 1 mg.

This is important because synthesizing or isolating even small amounts of a compound can be expensive, at least until the synthesis can be refined. Once a lead is identified, gram quantities are needed to carry out biological, toxicological, and chemical characterization studies. Kilogram quantities are required when a drug enters clinical trials, and if a drug is approved, plants need to manufacture material on a scale sufficient to meet expected clinical use. Quality and documentation of the specifications of the manufacturing process must be maintained throughout the scale-up (see Chapter 52).

Chemical characterization refers to the chemical properties of the drug candidate, including physical characteristics such as melting point, crystal form, and solubility, as well as purity and stability. The physical and chemical characteristics of a drug candidate are critical for determining how the drug could best be administered and stored (Table 51-3). The compound's chemical structure is commonly elucidated using a range of techniques, including mass spectrometry, which gives the compound's molecular weight; elemental analysis, which determines its atomic composition; NMR, which elucidates the types and connectivity patterns of atoms within

TABLE 51-3 Information Obtained in Chemical Characterization Studies

TYPE OF ASSAY	EXPERIMENTAL TECHNIQUE	CLINICAL IMPLICATIONS
Characterization, structure	Elemental analysis, mass spectrometry, NMR spectroscopy, IR spectroscopy, x-ray crystallography	Atomic composition, molecular weight, isomeric purity, compound structure
Impurities	HPLC, GC, mass spectrometry	Possible adverse reactions from impurities, toxicology
Partition coefficient	Octanol/water partition	Pharmacokinetics, including absorption, distribution, metabolism, and excretion; tissue distribution
Solubility	Solubility in various solvents	Pharmacokinetics, including absorption, distribution, metabolism, and excretion; formulations
Stability	Stability measurements under different conditions (heat, cold, humidity, light)	Shelf life, degradation products

NMR, nuclear magnetic resonance; IR, infrared; HPLC, high-performance liquid chromatography; GC, gas chromatography.

the molecule; and x-ray crystallography, which determines its three-dimensional structure. It is also important to distinguish among various isomers of the same compound, because biologic activity is often stereoisomer-selective. For example, propranolol (see Chapter 11, Adrenergic Pharmacology) is a mixture of (−) and (+) stereoisomers, but only the (−) isomer acts as a β-adrenergic receptor antagonist.

Chemists also characterize physical properties of the molecule that are used in developing the formulation, such as the pKa of an acidic or basic drug (see below). In addition, the drug's solubility is measured in a variety of solvents, especially water, to provide information on the molecule's likely oral bioavailability and possible hepatic metabolism. The partition coefficient describes the distribution of a molecule between an aqueous solvent, analogous to blood, and a hydrophobic solvent, analogous to the plasma membrane. Finally, the compound's stability over time and its impurity profiles must be determined.

Discovery Biology: Biochemical Assays, Cellular Assays, and Animal Models

The goal of discovery biology is to determine whether a molecule is likely to be effective in a particular disease state. Effectiveness may be assessed at the biochemical, cell, tissue, organ, and organism levels. If undesirable biologic properties are found, it may be possible to modify the structure of the molecule so as to improve its pharmacologic profile. In general, biochemical and cell-based assays are used early in the drug discovery process, while more complex organ and whole-animal studies are used in the lead optimization phase to characterize the pharmacologic properties of the molecule.

Biochemical assays evaluate the mechanism of action of the drug candidate at a molecular level. **Receptor binding assays** measure both the binding affinity and selectivity of the molecule for the target receptor. **Enzyme activity assays** measure the ability of the drug to inhibit the activity of a target enzyme. Selectivity for the desired target is critically important in the design and testing of lead molecules. Development of these assays is often a costly and rate-limiting step in the drug discovery process, since assay development requires identification and synthesis of key reagents and extensive optimization and validation of the assay.

In **cellular** or **biologic assays**, researchers aim to determine whether the lead molecule(s) acts appropriately in an environment that more closely approximates its in vivo use. For example, if the drug is designed to act in the cytoplasm, then it is essential to determine whether the drug can cross the plasma membrane. Early identification of potential safety problems may be assessed by incubating the lead molecule with a variety of receptors, ion channels, tissues, or cells, including induced pluripotent stem cells (iPS) or human embryonic stem cells (hES), either of which may be differentiated by culture techniques to cardiomyocytes or neuron-like cells to assess potential safety issues in those organ systems. Drug-induced changes in complex patterns of gene expression can be assessed using gene-array chips capable of measuring mRNA levels for thousands of genes simultaneously.

Finally, at the highest level of complexity, the effects of the drug candidate on whole organisms are established. Ideally, **animal models** are used that mirror the critical aspects of human pathophysiology for the target disease. For example, cancer chemotherapeutic agents can be tested in nude (T-cell-deficient) mice that have had human tumor cells implanted subcutaneously. Similarly, drugs for the treatment of postmenopausal osteoporosis can be tested in rats that have been ovariectomized to mimic the postmenopausal state. Table 51-4 describes some of the many animal models used by pharmaceutical researchers.

Absorption, Distribution, Metabolism, and Excretion (ADME)

Studies characterizing the fate of a molecule after its administration are critical to understand the potential effectiveness as well as the safety of that molecule. Such studies collectively describe the ADME (absorption, distribution, metabolism, and excretion) profile of the molecule. These studies are initially conducted using *in silico* and in vitro methods as well as animal studies, and more definitive information is obtained during clinical drug development. The basic principles investigated in the course of these studies are described in Chapters 3 (Pharmacokinetics) and 4 (Drug Metabolism).

The systemic exposure of a drug candidate in animals is typically determined in pharmacokinetic studies, in which the concentration of drug in the systemic circulation is

TABLE 51-4 Examples of Efficacy Models Used in Drug Discovery

DISEASE	ANIMAL MODEL	DRUG EXAMPLE
Cancer	Tumor xenografts in nude mice	Cisplatin
Diabetes	Genetically predisposed rodents (Zucker Diabetic Fatty Rat)	Insulin Metformin Thiazolidinediones
Hypercholesterolemia	Genetically hypercholesterolemic rats/mice Diet-induced hypercholesterolemia	Statins
Obesity	db/db and ob/ob rats	Orlistat Rimonabant Sibutramine
Postmenopausal osteoporosis	Ovariectomized rats	Bisphosphonates SERMs (raloxifene) Teriparatide
Rheumatoid arthritis	Collagen-induced arthritis	Anti-TNF antibodies

SERM, selective estrogen receptor modulator; TNF, tumor necrosis factor.

measured at various time points after administration. Important parameters include the maximal level of systemic exposure (C_{max}), the time after drug administration at which the maximal systemic exposure occurs (T_{max}), the overall systemic exposure during a treatment interval (area under the time-concentration curve [AUC]), and the length of time over which the drug remains in the circulation (half-life or $T_{1/2}$). These parameters are measured for different administered dose levels and are also evaluated for acute (single-dose) and chronic (repeat-dose) administrations. The tissues to which the drug distributes and the routes of excretion of the drug are typically measured by administering radiolabeled drug and then measuring the radioactivity levels in the different organs and body fluids.

As described in Chapter 4, metabolism or biotransformation refers to the processes by which biochemical reactions alter drugs within the body. As drug discovery and development proceeds, there is a continual accrual of data to understand these processes for a candidate drug. Initial studies are often conducted in vitro, using animal and human liver microsomes (cellular fractions containing smooth endoplasmic reticulum) or hepatocytes as the source of the drug-metabolizing enzymes. Measured parameters include the metabolic stability of the drug and its ability to inhibit or induce important drug-metabolizing enzymes and cellular drug transporters. The latter studies help to assess the potential of the molecule to cause metabolic drug–drug interactions. Later in drug development, studies are conducted to characterize the metabolic fate of the candidate drug in both animals and humans. In addition, formal drug–drug interaction clinical studies are performed to determine whether the candidate drug is likely to affect the metabolism of other drugs that are already in clinical use for the indicated disease state.

Toxicology

Animal toxicity studies are conducted to determine the conditions (doses, dosing regimen, route of administration) under which it is safe to initiate clinical trials with the drug candidate and ultimately to market the drug in the intended patient population. Studies of increasing duration and complexity are completed as the molecule proceeds through clinical drug development. The animal toxicity testing program is customized based on the desired therapeutic goal. For example, a drug designed to be used acutely in a critical care setting would require only short-term animal studies, whereas an agent intended for chronic use would require studies encompassing nearly the lifetime of the animal. Because these animal toxicity studies are critical for an accurate assessment of the potential risks to clinical trial subjects from administration of the drug candidate, they are governed by a complex set of regulations. To ensure the quality of the study data, pivotal toxicology studies that directly support a clinical trial must be conducted under regulations called the *Good Laboratory Practices (GLP)*.

Many drug discovery organizations will perform an initial, limited assessment of the molecule's toxicity during lead optimization. At this stage, the toxicity assays may involve in vitro assays designed to assess cytotoxicity or screen for off-target receptor binding, *in silico* and in vitro studies designed to assess the potential of the molecule to alter DNA (genotoxicity testing), in vitro and in vivo studies of the potential of the molecule to affect the cardiovascular system (cardiovascular pharmacology testing), and studies of the toxicity of the molecule in short-term animal studies. These studies may provide insights into the nature and mechanisms of potential toxic effects of the molecule. Unacceptable target-organ toxicity (functional and/or histopathologic) may be a frequent source of molecule termination at this phase of drug development.

As a molecule proceeds into the testing required for clinical trial authorizations, a more comprehensive set of toxicity studies is conducted. Some of the most important safety data derive from **repeat-dose toxicity studies**. In general, these studies are conducted in both a rodent (e.g., rat or mouse) and a nonrodent (e.g., dog or monkey) species. For small-molecule drugs, the species are chosen most often based on the similarity of the number and identity of metabolites produced during *ex vivo* exposure of the drug to human and animal liver microsomes and/or hepatocytes. Toxicity species for biotherapeutics are chosen based on demonstration of the pharmacologic responsiveness of the species to the drug. Animals in these studies are administered various dose levels of the molecule for periods of time that depend on the duration of the proposed clinical trial (e.g., 2 weeks to 1 year). Repeat-dose toxicity studies evaluate body weight, clinical signs, and clinical laboratory parameters (hematology, clinical chemistry, and urinalysis). Histologic evaluation of all organ systems is also performed. Safety pharmacology studies are employed to assess potential adverse drug effects on the central nervous, cardiovascular, and respiratory systems. Genotoxicity is thoroughly assessed by evaluating drug effects on mutational status (nucleotide sequence changes) and clastogenicity (chromosomal damage). Animal studies are also performed to characterize effects on fertility, reproduction, and development and to study the ability of the drug to induce tumors in animal models. If unique human metabolites are identified that are not produced by the selected toxicity species, the potential toxicity of those metabolites must be assessed in a separate toxicology study.

In sum, the results of these comprehensive animal studies identify the potential toxicities that could occur upon administration of the drug to humans and assess the systemic exposures and durations of treatment that could potentially be related to those adverse effects. An additional desired outcome is to identify clinically translatable biomarkers that would enable monitoring of patients for early detection of the toxicities that have been identified in the animal studies.

Development Chemistry: Chemical Synthesis, Scale-Up, and Manufacturing

An effective chemical synthesis must satisfy several requirements. Ideally, it should require few synthetic steps. Each additional step in a synthesis increases the possibility of impurities, decreases the yield (the amount of material obtained at the end of the synthesis), and increases the cost. If multiple isomers of a compound are possible products of the synthesis, then a synthesis that produces only the target isomer is preferable. Finally, the synthesis should be amenable to scale-up.

Two techniques, **retrosynthetic analysis** and **convergent synthesis**, aid in the establishment of an effective synthetic scheme. In a retrosynthetic analysis, key steps are developed by examining important structural elements in the final product and figuring out how specific reactions could lead to the product (Fig. 51-3A). This procedure is performed iteratively so that a complex final molecule is reduced to

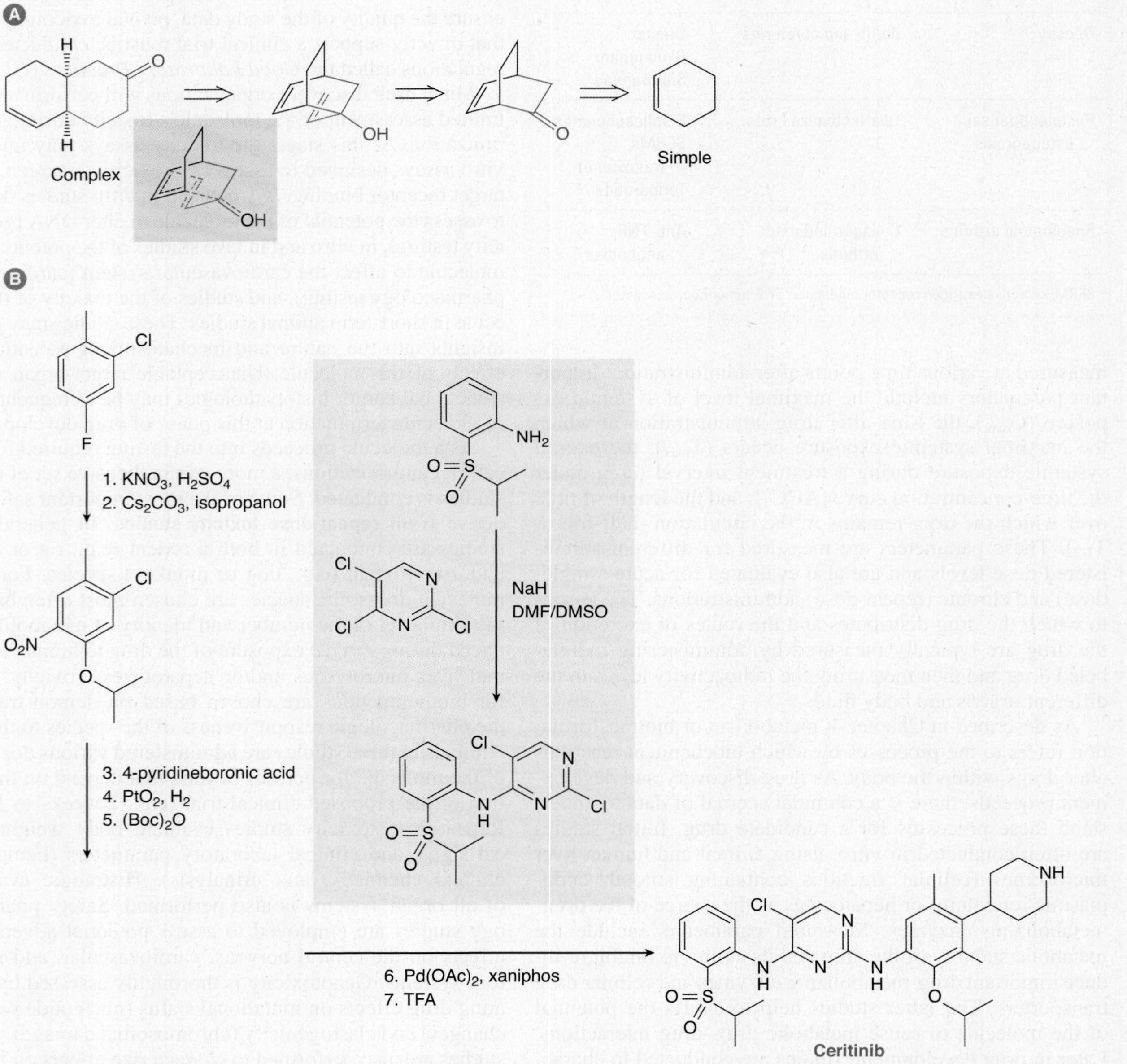

FIGURE 51-3. Retrosynthetic analysis and convergent synthesis of a complex molecule. A. A retrosynthetic analysis of a complex molecule, such as the illustrated bicyclic compound, allows the identification of simple starting materials such as cyclohexene. Analysis of the structural element (*blue*) demonstrates the creative process required to envision how a complex structure could be deconstructed into its component parts. The structure in the *blue box* illustrates the thinking required when deconstructing a molecule. These simple starting materials can then be combined in a series of steps to create the complex molecule. **B.** Retrosynthetic analysis and subsequent convergent synthesis were used to synthesize the ALK pathway inhibitor ceritinib (see Chapter 40).

simpler intermediates, as was done in the convergent synthesis of the ALK pathway inhibitor ceritinib (Fig. 51-3B). **Flow chemistry** is a new technology that has greatly simplified process chemistry practices. Each flow reactor contains reagents and catalysts to effect a single chemical reaction. As the starting material flows through the first reactor, it is transformed to the desired end product and is then ready to flow into the next reactor, poised for the next chemical transformation. This technology can be applied to a linear synthesis or a convergent synthesis; in a convergent synthesis, two or more individual parts of a molecule are synthesized separately, and the parts are assembled only near the end of the synthesis (Fig. 51-4; see also Fig. 51-3B). Convergent synthesis increases the overall yield of the synthesis by reducing the number of linear steps required and allows the synthesis of each key component of the final product to be optimized individually. Retrosynthetic analysis and convergent synthesis are complementary and are often employed together in planning the chemical synthesis of a compound. Flow chemistry can also be developed in a discovery-chemistry setting and then transferred to the process-chemistry setting.

For early drug development, the goal of development chemistry is to generate enough product to meet the demands of chemical and biological characterization, particularly for animal toxicology and formulation studies. As the scale of the need increases, the synthesis strategy must evolve. For example, a chemical synthesis often starts out using available raw materials, which may include expensive specialty chemicals. However, as the scale of the synthesis increases, these reagents must be replaced with cheaper (and/or safer) alternatives. Furthermore, in an early synthetic scheme, each intermediate is typically isolated, purified, and characterized to ensure that each sequential step of the synthesis is effective. However, as chemists gain more experience with the synthesis, multiple steps may be combined without isolating intermediates or purifying the products of each reaction, in a so-called **one-pot synthesis**.

Once the synthesis strategy of a drug candidate has been fully developed, process chemists must then adapt the synthesis for large-scale commercial manufacturing. This process must be initiated before a drug is approved, because the approval process requires that several batches of the drug be successfully manufactured, formulated (see below), and rigorously tested for quality and stability. A pharmaceutical company must also be prepared to meet market demands immediately after approval, which means that a manufacturing process must be established before the commercial launch of the drug.

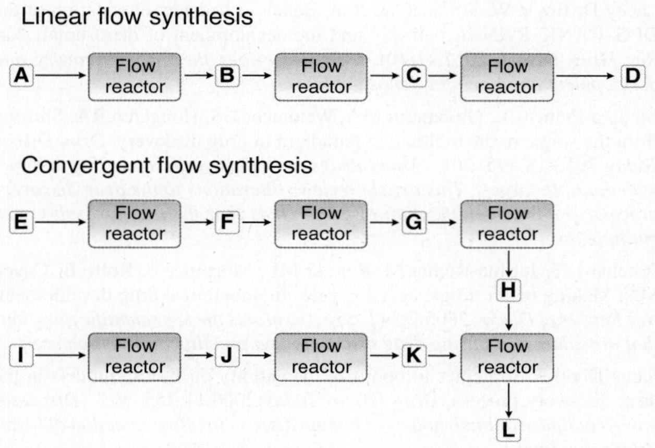

The process chemist must also ensure that the synthesis is safe and meets environmental regulations for emissions and disposal of waste. This may preclude the use of certain solvents that are commonly used by synthetic chemists in small-scale syntheses.

Formulation

Drugs must be manufactured in a form that can be administered to animals and humans in a measured dose. The type of formulation depends on the intended route of administration (Table 51-5). **Enteral formulations**, which include oral, sublingual, and rectal dosage forms, are designed to be absorbed across portions of the digestive tract. **Parenteral formulations** include intravenous, intramuscular, and subcutaneous injections; transdermal patches; and inhaled agents. The preferred route of administration is determined by many variables, including the drug's stability and its pharmacokinetic properties of absorption, distribution, metabolism (including first-pass metabolism), and excretion. Oral dosage forms are favored for drugs that are relatively stable in the digestive tract, are not rapidly metabolized in the liver, have high oral bioavailability, and do not require an immediate action. Parenteral dosage forms are preferred for drugs that must be fast-acting and are more reliably absorbed by nonenteral than by enteral routes. Macromolecules, which generally have little or no oral bioavailability, are typically administered via injection (see Chapter 54, Protein Therapeutics).

Most drugs are administered orally in either tablet or capsule form. In addition to the measured dose of the drug, most tablets contain **binders**, which keep the components together, and **stabilizers**, which enhance the drug's shelf life. For acid-sensitive drugs, it is often possible to coat the tablet with an **enteric coating** that is acid-resistant but dissolves in the intestine. Formulation chemists can also manipulate the rate at which the tablet or capsule dissolves or releases its contents, thus enabling "sustained-release" formulations in which the drug is released slowly over the course of hours (see Chapter 55, Drug Delivery Modalities). Drugs formulated into **liposomes** are also being increasingly used as mechanisms for controlling drug release in vivo. **Doxil®** is a liposome-encapsulated form of doxorubicin used to treat Kaposi's sarcoma.

A drug's absorption profile and first-pass metabolism are typically not issues for drugs delivered intravenously. However, the drug must be dissolved in a vehicle, usually water. Moreover, the solution must be made isotonic with plasma by adding osmotically active compounds such as saline, dextrose, or mannitol, so that the solution does not cause hemolysis. The solution must also be sterile for intravenous injection. Finally, a drug is often less stable in solution than as a solid, so formulation chemists must test its stability in solution. If the drug is unstable, it may be prepared as a **lyophilized powder** that can be dissolved in water or buffer immediately before administration.

Linear flow synthesis

Convergent flow synthesis

FIGURE 51-4. Flow chemistry. Each flow reactor contains reagents and catalysts to effect a single chemical reaction. Flow chemistry can be applied to linear synthesis or convergent synthesis of the desired compound. In a linear synthesis, each component is added sequentially. In a convergent synthesis, each component is assembled separately and then combined in the last step. The convergent synthesis approach generally results in higher yields. The *arrows* indicate sequential synthetic reactions.

TABLE 51-5 Advantages and Disadvantages of Common Formulations

FORMULATION	ADVANTAGES	DISADVANTAGES	EXAMPLES
Enteral			
Oral	Ease of administration	Slow absorption First-pass metabolism Reduced bioavailability	Acetaminophen Oxycodone Pravastatin
Sublingual	Rapid action No first-pass metabolism	Few drugs are absorbed by this route	Nitroglycerin
Rectal	Rapid action No first-pass metabolism	Uncomfortable	Morphine
Parenteral			
Intravenous	Rapid action High bioavailability Can control dose easily	Risk of infection Uncomfortable Must be administered by trained personnel	Lidocaine Morphine Tissue plasminogen activator
Intramuscular	Sustained release possible	Uncomfortable Adverse reaction possible	Meperidine Growth hormone
Subcutaneous	Slow action	Poor adherence	Insulin
Transdermal	Sustained release No first-pass metabolism	Poor absorption Slow action	Estrogen Nicotine (patch)
Inhalation	Large surface area for absorption Convenience (no injection)	Inconvenience (device)	Albuterol Glucocorticoids (asthma)

CONCLUSION AND FUTURE DIRECTIONS

The discovery and development of new drugs is a complex, interdisciplinary process that often requires 10 or more years and up to or exceeding a billion dollars. Researchers start by searching for a biologically active compound. This may involve a compound-centered approach or a target-centered approach. New pharmacologic targets are currently being identified by gene sequencing, by analysis of genetic factors that predispose to disease, by gene knockout experiments in laboratory animals, and by other techniques. In addition, information about genetic polymorphisms may enable the products of specific, mutant genes to be the targets of new drugs (see Chapter 7, Pharmacogenomics). Methods to assess potential safety are also rapidly evolving and significant emphasis is being placed on developing in vitro methods that model complex physiologic systems (e.g., organ-on-a-chip) more accurately than current cell-based assays. *In silico* systems, already used to provide information regarding the potential of a chemical to cause genotoxicity, continue to evolve and be implemented to make predictions regarding a variety of toxicologic outcomes.

Acknowledgment

We thank the late Armen H. Tashjian, Jr. for his invaluable contributions to this chapter in the First, Second, and Third Editions of *Principles of Pharmacology: The Pathophysiologic Basis of Drug Therapy*.

Suggested Reading

Cook D, Brown D, Alexander R, et al. Lessons learned from the fate of AstraZeneca's drug pipeline: a five dimensional framework. *Nat Rev Drug Discov* 2014;13:419–431. (*One major pharmaceutical company's insightful analysis of their research and development productivity, including a discussion of key technical determinants of project success.*)

Drews J. Drug discovery: a historical perspective. *Science* 2000;287: 1960–1964. (*Historical description of the major methods of drug discovery.*)

International Conference on Harmonization: guidance on nonclinical safety studies for the conduct of human clinical trials and marketing authorization for pharmaceuticals 2009. http://www.ich.org/fileadmin/Public _Web_Site/ICH_Products/Guidelines/Multidisciplinary/M3_R2/Step4 /M3_R2__Guideline.pdf. (*Describes the types of animal studies required by regulatory authorities to support clinical testing and registration of pharmaceuticals.*)

Lacey D, Boyle W, Simonet W, et al. Bench to bedside: elucidation of the OPG–RANK–RANKL pathway and the development of denosumab. *Nat Rev Drug Discov* 2012;11:401–419. (*Describes the drug discovery and development approach for denosumab.*)

Medina-Franco JL, Giulianotti MA, Welmaker GS, Houghten RA. Shifting from the single to the multitarget paradigm in drug discovery. *Drug Discov Today* 2013;18:495–501. (*Many drugs are effective because they interact with multiple targets. This article reviews alterations to the drug discovery process to allow identification of compounds that interact favorably with multiple targets.*)

Pritchard JF, Jurima-Romet M, Reimer ML, Mortimer E, Rolfe B, Cayen MN. Making better drugs: decision gates in nonclinical drug development. *Nat Rev Drug Discov* 2003;2:542–553. (*Explores the key scientific questions that are addressed during drug discovery and preclinical development.*)

Sams-Dodd F. Strategies to optimize the validity of disease models in the drug discovery process. *Drug Discov Today* 2006;11:355–363. (*Discusses how to optimize animal models of human disease to allow selection of better drug candidates.*)

U.S. Food and Drug Administration, U.S. Department of Health and Human Services. Innovation or stagnation: challenge and opportunity on the critical path to new medical products. March 2004. http://www.fda.gov/oc /initiatives/criticalpath/whitepaper.pdf. (*Discusses current challenges and opportunities in the development of new drugs, biologic products, and medical devices.*)

Drug discovery
(3–6 years)

Drug development
(5–9 years)

Post-approval
regulation

hemistry and biology

Compound identification
and optimization

Biological
characterization

Toxicology

Toxicology
studies

Clinical

IND
filed

Manufacturing

Develop manufacturing
Develop QA/QC program, GMP practices

52

Clinical Drug Evaluation and Regulatory Approval

Mark A. Goldberg and Alexander E. Kuta

■ INTRODUCTION

Controlled clinical trials provide the scientific and legal basis by which regulatory authorities around the world evaluate new prescription drugs and approve them for sale. In the United States, the regulatory review of drugs and devices is the responsibility of the **US Food and Drug Administration (FDA)**. Over the past 50 years, improved methods for large-scale clinical studies have precipitated a shift toward evidence-based medicine. The increased emphasis on clinical trials to appropriately assess the safety and efficacy of new drugs has resulted in a dramatic rise in the costs associated with drug development. According to the Pharmaceutical Manufacturers of America (PhRMA), the overall drug development process from discovery to approval of a new drug takes an average of 10–15 years and an estimated cost of $1 to $2 billion; the clinical development phase of this work is typically in the range of 6 to 7 years. Moreover, only about 1 in 10 drugs that enters the clinic for testing ultimately receives regulatory approval and is marketed. Given the tremendous cost and duration of clinical drug development, it is imperative that every effort is made to plan carefully and

execute effectively. Drug development programs must be well designed not only to appropriately demonstrate safety and clinical efficacy but also, through the use of appropriate biomarkers, pharmacodynamic markers, and safety monitoring, to allow for the early discontinuation of development of drugs that are destined to fail.

This is an exciting and challenging time to be involved in drug development. Major advances in the biological sciences have yielded a much greater understanding of the molecular basis of many diseases and provide the opportunity to have an unprecedented impact on the alleviation of human suffering. However, translating these scientific advances into new and more effective therapies for human diseases has proven to be daunting. In the 10 years between 1994 and 2003, there was an average of 33.6 new drugs approved per year by the FDA; in the following 10 years up to 2013, there has been an average of slightly more than 26 approvals per year, suggesting a relative stagnation in the rate of new drugs being approved and made available to patients. To close this apparent gap between the acceleration of innovative basic-science discoveries and the stagnating rate of approvals of innovative new therapies will require diligent clinical drug development programs that

933

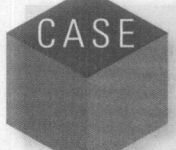

CASE

For most of the latter half of the twentieth century, advances in the pharmacologic treatment of malignancies relied primarily on the use of cytotoxic agents that target various aspects of cellular viability and proliferation, with only a narrow window between the doses necessary for the killing of tumor cells and those that kill normal cells (i.e., the therapeutic window). In the 1970s and 1980s, studies by scientists such as Michael Bishop and Harold Varmus led to the identification of retroviral oncogenes, which are mutated forms of normal cellular genes that control cell viability, differentiation, and proliferation. Many of these oncogenes were shown to encode mutated protein kinases involved in the pathogenesis of human malignancies. Chronic myelogenous leukemia (CML) is one such malignancy that is fairly well understood at the molecular level. CML has been demonstrated to depend on a chromosomal translocation, the so-called Philadelphia chromosome, characterized by a reciprocal translocation between the long arms of chromosomes 9 and 22, which leads to the rearrangement and dysregulation of a particular tyrosine kinase called *c-abl*.

These findings set the stage for an extraordinarily successful collaboration between Brian Druker, an academic oncologist at Oregon Health Sciences University, and Nick Lydon, a pharmaceutical researcher at Novartis. Druker had a research focus on tyrosine kinase biology with an emphasis on finding an effective treatment for CML by targeting the c-abl tyrosine kinase, and Lydon had a research focus on identifying specific inhibitors of protein tyrosine kinases. Druker and Lydon identified a small molecule, codenamed STI-571 (**imatinib**), that effectively inhibited c-abl as well as at least two other tyrosine kinases, c-kit and platelet-derived growth factor receptor B. Studies in cell culture demonstrated selective toxicity of STI-571 in cells containing dysregulated c-abl, and preclinical studies in the appropriate animal models confirmed this activity. Preclinical toxicology studies in rats, dogs, and monkeys described the hematological, renal, and hepatobiliary toxicity of imatinib. A phase 1 study in 83 CML patients showed that oral dosing in the range from 25 to 1,000 mg/day did not cause dose-limiting toxicity. Additionally, the study demonstrated that imatinib had excellent oral bioavailability and a pharmacokinetic profile such that once-daily oral dosing could

achieve sustained plasma levels at concentrations that had been sufficient to inhibit c-abl in preclinical models. Three open-label, single-arm phase 2 studies in 1,027 CML patients at various stages of disease progression all showed marked imatinib activity, as assessed by high cytogenetic response rates and hematological response rates, with less toxicity than that typically observed with the available standard of care (interferon-alpha).

Based on the marked activity of imatinib in patients with advanced disease and in patients who had failed first-line therapy with interferon-alpha, imatinib received accelerated approval by the FDA in May 2001, after only 3 months of review. This represented one of the fastest reviews ever performed by the FDA and also marked the approval of the first selectively targeted cancer therapy (i.e., therapy directed at a target that is specifically dysregulated in CML cells compared to normal cells). Accelerated approval was granted rather than full approval since cytogenetic responses and hematological responses are surrogate clinical endpoints thought to predict clinical benefit with a reasonable likelihood but are not an ultimate clinical endpoint such as survival. Under accelerated approval, the sponsor (in this case, Novartis) was required to conduct post-approval studies to verify and confirm the clinical benefit of imatinib. Novartis then conducted and submitted for approval a randomized phase 3 study comparing imatinib to combination therapy with interferon-alpha and cytarabine in patients with newly diagnosed CML, with a primary endpoint of overall survival. Novartis also committed to perform phase 1 and phase 2 studies of imatinib in children. Based on long-term follow-up of patients from the earlier phase 2 trials as well as new data from the phase 3 trial and the pediatric trials, imatinib ultimately received full approval for all stages of CML in both adults and children.

Questions

1. What ethical standards govern the relationship between physicians and patients in clinical research?
2. What are the critical elements to be considered in developing a clinical trial protocol?
3. What data do the FDA review when considering approval of a new drug?

include rigorous, well-controlled trials, integrated clinical development plans, the use of novel statistical methods, adaptive clinical trial designs, and the inclusion of novel pharmacodynamic and other biomarkers at the various stages of drug development. Coordinated teams of experts will be needed to integrate these clinical development programs with the related processes of drug discovery, preclinical development, regulatory approval, and ultimately patient treatment. In addition,

major health authorities such as the FDA have implemented programs to work more effectively with industry in drug development while preserving their remit to protect the public health.

Drug discovery and development remains a lengthy, high-risk, and complex process. It has been estimated that of every 5,000 to 10,000 chemically synthesized molecules that are screened as potential drugs, only one becomes an approved drug. The previous chapter (Chapter 51, Drug Discovery and Preclinical Development) outlines the preclinical phase of drug development from target identification to candidate selection. This chapter describes the process by which new candidate drug molecules are evaluated in clinical trials and approved for marketing and sale in the United States.

HISTORY OF US FOOD AND DRUG LAW

Drug development, testing, and approval is a lengthy process, the major milestones of which are shown in Figure 52-1. Achievement of each of these milestones requires the cooperation of researchers, clinicians, patients, pharmaceutical or biotechnology companies, and government regulators. The development of a new drug or biotherapeutic is a highly regulated process that has evolved considerably during the last century. Several public health crises have led to the development of current laws and regulations, including:

1. The public outcry over the unsanitary and unsafe conditions of the meatpacking industry: this resulted in the **Pure Food and Drugs Act** in 1906, which prohibited interstate commerce in adulterated and misbranded food and drugs.
2. The death of more than 100 people after consuming "Strep-Elixir," an untested product containing a sulfonamide and a chemical analogue of antifreeze: this resulted in the passage of the **Food, Drug, and Cosmetic Act** in 1938, which, among other things, required approval of all new drugs by the FDA prior to marketing. Sponsors submitted an application for approval and, unless the FDA determined that the drug was unsafe within 180 days, the drug could be marketed.
3. The discovery that thalidomide, used to treat morning sickness, caused birth defects in large numbers of babies born in Europe: this resulted in passage of the **Kefauver-Harris Amendments** in 1962, which required proof of efficacy in addition to safety prior to drug approval and mandated reporting of adverse events. Additionally, the Amendments stated that patients must provide informed consent to participate in clinical trials, gave the FDA authority to regulate prescription drug advertising, and introduced good manufacturing practice standards.
4. In response to widely publicized safety issues with COX-2 inhibitors and several other drugs, Congress passed the **FDA Amendments Act (FDAAA)** of 2007. One aspect of the FDAAA provides enhanced authority to the FDA to manage the safety of approved drugs. In particular, the FDA has focused on the implementation of Risk Evaluation and Mitigation Strategies (REMS) for selected new drugs as well as drugs that are already approved. The objective of REMS is to put in place measures to ensure that a drug or biologic product is dispensed and utilized in such a manner as to ensure that its benefits outweigh its risks.
5. The **FDA Safety and Innovation Act (FDASIA) of 2012** expanded FDA authority in several ways. It reauthorized prescription drug and medical device user fees and implemented generic drug and biosimilar biologic products user fees. These fees are mandated by law and are used, in part, to support the FDA's review of marketing applications. FDASIA also introduced a new mechanism to expedite development and review of promising new drugs for serious and life-threatening diseases. These drugs are given Breakthrough Therapy designation. This mechanism builds on past FDA programs to assist sponsors in drug development. Additionally, FDASIA expands the FDA's ability to obtain patient input into the drug development and review process and, recognizing the increasing globalization of drug supply and sourcing (for both finished product and active ingredients), it expands FDA authority to ensure the safety and availability of this supply.

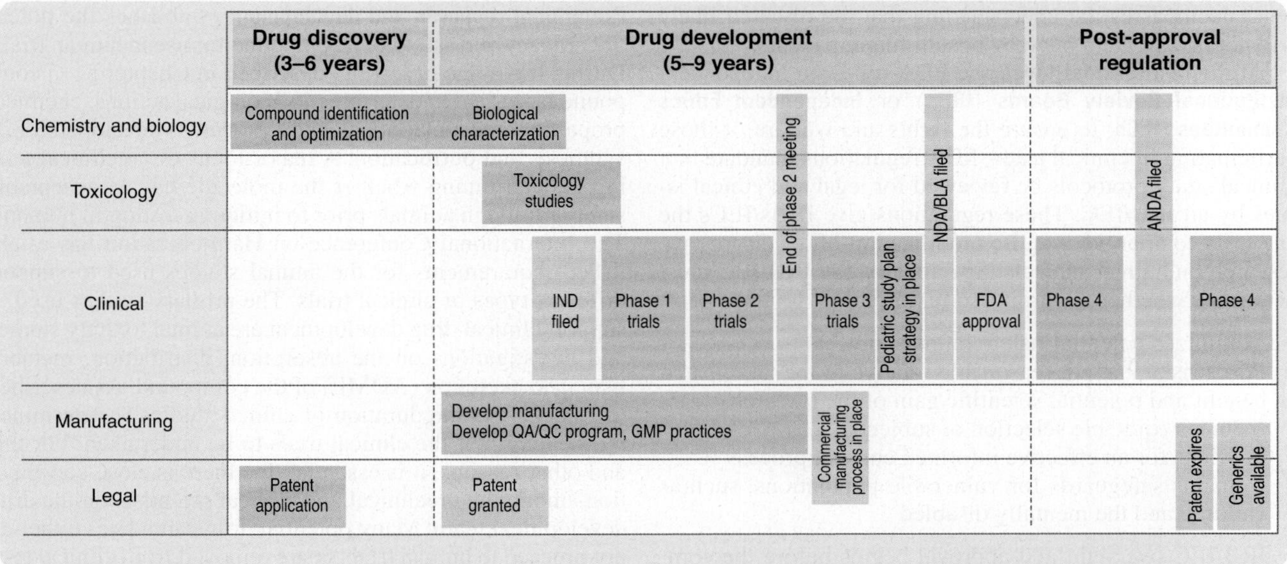

Drug discovery (3–6 years)
Drug development (5–9 years)
Post-approval regulation
Chemistry and biology
Toxicology
Clinical
Manufacturing
Legal
Compound identification and optimization
Biological characterization
Toxicology studies
IND filed
Phase 1 trials
Phase 2 trials
End of phase 2 meeting
Phase 3 trials
Pediatric study plan strategy in place
NDA/BLA filed
FDA approval
Phase 4
ANDA filed
Phase 4
Develop manufacturing
Develop QA/QC program, GMP practices
Commercial manufacturing process in place
Patent application
Patent granted
Patent expires
Generics available

FIGURE 52-1. Life cycle of drug approval. The life cycle of approval for a new drug is complex, ranging from 8 to 15 years for completion. Drug discovery, discussed in Chapter 51, produces a new drug molecule. The first patents are usually filed at this stage and are granted several years later. The drug development process requires that biological characterization and toxicology studies in animals are conducted before an IND can be filed. In turn, an IND is required for the start of clinical trials. At the conclusion of successful clinical development, a drug company files a NDA/BLA, which is reviewed by the FDA. Once a drug is approved, it must be monitored for safety for the remainder of its lifespan (postmarketing surveillance). The first of the drug's patents expires 20 years after its application. ANDA, Abbreviated New Drug Application; FDA, US Food and Drug Administration; GMP, Good Manufacturing Practice; IND, Investigational New Drug application; NDA/BLA, New Drug Application/Biologics License Application; QA/QC, quality assurance and quality control.

In the United States, the FDA Center for Drug Evaluation and Research (CDER) and the FDA Center for Biologics Evaluation and Research (CBER) are responsible for regulating the development and approval of new medicines.

ETHICS IN CLINICAL DRUG INVESTIGATION

The development of new therapeutics to treat human diseases requires research to be conducted on human subjects, either normal volunteers (typically in phase 1 trials) or in patients with the disease for which the new treatment is being investigated. Any time research is conducted in humans, it is essential that every effort is made to protect their safety. Regulatory agencies around the world have codified standards of ethical behavior for all parties involved in clinical research, including clinicians, pharmaceutical companies, and medical institutions. The ethical relationship is governed by the notion that clinical trial research represents a partnership between investigator (physician) and subject (volunteer or patient). Four major ethical principles, established by the **International Conference on Harmonization** and the **Declaration of Helsinki**, support this partnership. These principles are as follows:

- The trial must minimize the risks for participants.
- Provisions must be made for the overall care of the patient.
- The investigator is responsible for terminating the trial when the risks become incompatible with the goals of the trial.
- Adverse events must be reported immediately to an ethics or safety committee.

Investigators must obtain subjects' **informed consent**. Informed consent is not just a signed document but rather a process in which patients (1) are made aware of the potential risks and benefits of the trial and (2) must make an informed decision to participate voluntarily in a clinical study. For patients with poor prognoses and for normal volunteers, informed consent encompasses the understanding that the research likely will not benefit them but may benefit future patients.

At the institutional level, the FDA relies on independent **Institutional Review Boards** (**IRBs**) or **Independent Ethics Committees** (**IECs**) to ensure the rights and welfare of those participating in clinical trials. FDA regulations mandate that clinical study protocols be reviewed for legal and ethical issues by an IRB/IEC. These regulations give IRBs/IECs the authority to approve, require modification of, or disapprove research on human subjects. Specifically, the IRB/IEC must determine whether the proposed research:

- Minimizes potential risk to human subjects
- Poses risks that are reasonable relative to the anticipated benefit and potential scientific gain of the research
- Includes equitable selection of subjects
- Provides for an effective informed consent process
- Contains safeguards for vulnerable populations, such as children and the mentally disabled

IRB/IEC oversight and approval begins before the commencement of human trials and continues for the duration of clinical trials. The membership of an IRB/IEC consists of five or more experts and laypersons from various backgrounds. Federal regulations stipulate that IRB membership must include at least one member whose primary expertise is in a scientific area, one member whose primary expertise is in a nonscientific area, and one member who is not affiliated with the institution overseeing the clinical research protocol. In addition, the other members' qualifications must be such that the IRB is able to evaluate research protocols in terms of institutional requirements, applicable law, standards of professional practice, and community attitudes. Thus, many IRBs include clergy, social workers, and attorneys as well as physicians, scientists, and other health care professionals.

Clinical trials must be appropriately designed and rigorously executed in order to optimize the ratio of benefit to risk and to satisfactorily answer the scientific questions under study. Scientific clinical trial design must include appropriate control or comparator arm(s), randomization and blinding, and sample size, among other elements (see below). Some institutions have a scientific review committee that must approve all protocols involving human subjects to ensure that the protocol is appropriately designed to answer the questions being asked. To further assure that the findings of clinical trials are accurate and credible and that the rights of clinical trial subjects are protected, regulatory agencies require that clinical trials leading to the approval of new drugs be conducted according to **good clinical practices (GCP)**. Guidelines for GCP have been developed by the International Conference on Harmonization to provide a standard for the design, conduct, recording of findings, monitoring of data, analysis, auditing, and reporting of results of clinical trials.

DRUG EVALUATION AND CLINICAL DEVELOPMENT

The investigation of a new drug candidate comprises several phases, beginning with preclinical evaluation and typically proceeding through phase 3 clinical studies. At the conclusion of this process, the FDA may consider the molecule for approval as a new drug.

Authorizations to Initiate Clinical Trials

Preclinical research and development establishes the potential efficacy and safety of a compound for use in human trials. During this stage of testing, described in Chapter 51, a compound is studied to determine its biological actions, chemical properties, and metabolism, and a process is developed for its synthesis and purification. A major focus of preclinical testing is determining whether the molecule has an acceptable safety profile in animals prior to initiating testing in humans. The International Conference on Harmonization has established requirements for the animal studies used to support different types of clinical trials. The primary studies used to support clinical drug development are animal toxicity studies and investigations on the absorption, distribution, metabolism, and excretion (ADME) of the compound. As described in Chapter 51, the duration of animal studies is determined by the length of the clinical trials to be undertaken. For this and other reasons, it is essential that there is close coordination among the preclinical and clinical scientists on the drug development team. Many potential drug candidates either do not proceed to human trials or are removed from clinical testing due to adverse safety findings in animal studies. The preclinical research phase is also an important time to explore potentially important pharmacodynamic markers and other biomarkers that could help facilitate clinical development.

The mechanism for seeking approval to initiate clinical trials in the United States is the submission of an **Investigational**

New Drug application (**IND**) to the FDA. The IND contains data from the preclinical studies, data from prior clinical investigations (if available), the proposed protocol for human trials, and other background information. The IND also contains a document referred to as the **Investigator's Brochure** (**IB**). The IB is provided to regulators, clinical investigators, and IRBs/IECs; it represents a summary of all available information on the investigational drug and may be several hundred pages in length. The IND must also contain information on characterization, manufacture, and quality of the drug. INDs can be submitted by commercial sponsors with the ultimate goal of obtaining approval for marketing and sale of a new drug product or by individual investigators and academic centers. The latter are typically referred to as **Investigator Sponsored INDs**. The IND is a "living document" and, at a minimum, is updated annually.

The FDA must review the IND within 30 days and decide whether human trials may begin. Figure 52-2 is a flowchart representing the process used by the FDA to review an IND.

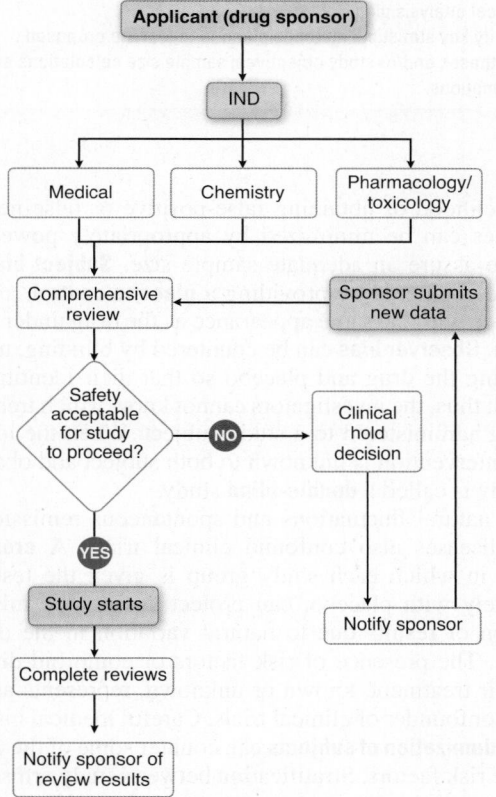

FIGURE 52-2. Process of Investigational New Drug (IND) review. When an IND is filed by a sponsor, the FDA has 30 days to review the application. The flow diagram shows the process of internal review. Various disciplines within the FDA review the sponsor's data package. These reviews culminate in a decision by the FDA as to whether the proposed clinical protocol is acceptable to proceed. If the safety is not deemed acceptable, the sponsor is notified that the IND is on clinical hold and trials may not proceed. The sponsor may submit additional data to support the safety of the proposed trial and a subsequent round of safety review is initiated. If the safety is deemed acceptable, the study may proceed after the 30-day review period. The FDA then completes its reviews and may provide the sponsor with additional comments on issues that may need to be addressed in later stages of drug development. *Colored boxes* correspond to actions by the drug sponsor; *white boxes* correspond to actions by the FDA.

The areas of review include a **chemistry review**, a **pharmacology/toxicology review**, and a **medical review**. If the IND review does not identify any safety concerns, the IND is considered open or active after the 30-day wait period. If the review reveals the potential for unreasonable risk to participants, the FDA contacts the sponsor, and a **clinical hold** is issued, preventing initiation of human studies. The sponsor must address any issues in question before the clinical hold is lifted. A clinical hold may be issued at any time during clinical drug development; this can be based on issues such as new findings from animal studies, clinical data indicating an unacceptable risk profile, or a finding that a sponsor did not accurately disclose the risk of the study to investigators or subjects.

Clinical Development

Given the time, cost, and risks associated with clinical drug development, it is imperative to plan carefully and execute meticulously. The goals of clinical drug development include:

■ Assessment of the dose–response profile
■ Assessment of the toxicity profile for a given dosing regimen
■ Assessment of pharmacokinetic/pharmacodynamic relationships
■ Establishment of the safety and efficacy profile in well-controlled studies in well-defined patient populations

These goals are accomplished through the conduct of clinical trials. Each clinical trial must be designed to answer specific questions. In turn, each trial should be part of an integrated development plan leading to the ultimate demonstration of safety and efficacy in well-controlled trials.

Target Product Profile

The target product profile (TPP) articulates the goal of the clinical development program. The key elements of the target product profile include the primary indication, target patient population, route of administration, pharmaceutical formulation, dosing schedule, efficacy assessments, expected primary endpoint in pivotal trial(s), expected safety profile, and key product characteristics, including those that may allow differentiation compared to products already available. As the development plan unfolds, data from clinical trials and product development inform the TPP and, as a result, aspects of the TPP are likely to evolve. However, it is important to understand what the minimally acceptable target product profile is and to have the discipline to terminate development as quickly and responsibly as possible if it becomes clear that the minimally acceptable TPP will not be attainable.

Development of a Clinical Trial

By definition, clinical trials involve studies of human subjects. The subjects may be normal volunteers or patients with specific diseases; the trials may be interventional (i.e., patients receive therapies and/or undergo tests or procedures) or observational (e.g., a study of the natural history of a disease). No matter what the situation, the clinical investigator has an ethical responsibility to the subjects to ensure that all elements of a trial are optimally designed to maximize what will be learned. The key elements for consideration when developing any clinical trial are detailed in Table 52-1.

TABLE 52-1 Elements of a Clinical Trial Design

1. Title of study
2. Study hypothesis(es) including methods to test hypothesis(es)
3. Study objectives
4. Study design
   - Indicate any proposed substudies and their design aspects.
   - Indicate whether interim analyses are planned and their objectives (e.g., early dose selection, futility, stopping for success).
5. Study rationale
   - Include how study fits into overall product development plan.
6. Study population
   - Specify all inclusion and exclusion criteria.
   - Geographical considerations.
   - Special regional regulatory considerations.
   - Does trial design fit with usual medical practice in the region?
7. Sample size
   - Calculated sample size, number of sites required, and number of subjects per site.
   - Parameters used to determine sample size estimate, including the detectable difference and a power statement.
8. Enrollment period
   - Total projected time for enrollment period, including detailed timing for various periods (e.g., screening).
   - Are there any requirements for site enrollment rate?
9. Study duration
   - Specify both the study duration and the duration of treatment.
10. Randomization (if any)
    - Specify randomization scheme or ratio.
11. Rationale for dose selection
12. Study medications (or product)
    - Specify all (test and comparator) medications to be used and how they will be obtained.
13. Study medication administration
    - Specify how and when medication will be administered (if titration or other dose modification is permitted or to be used also, explain).
14. Pharmacokinetic/pharmacodynamic measures
    - Specify pharmacokinetic/pharmacodynamic measures, including any special procedures involved.
15. Efficacy measures
    - Specify details of all primary and secondary efficacy measures, including any special procedures.
    - If measure is a detailed scale or questionnaire, provide it in an appendix.
16. Safety measures
    - Specify all safety measures, including specific clinical laboratory tests.
    - Identify any other procedures or measurements to be done.
17. Statistical analysis plan
    - Specify key statistical methods planned to test the proposed hypotheses and/or study objectives; sample size calculations and assumptions.

Trial protocols must be structured to provide reliable answers to specific questions. Each test and procedure in the study should have a clearly defined purpose that fits into the integrated development plan. Among the most important issues to consider are:

- Determination of the appropriate balance for the inclusion and exclusion criteria. It is often desirable to have a relatively homogeneous patient population to allow for better planning and interpretation of study results. However, this needs to be balanced by the understanding that patients and diseases are frequently heterogeneous. By restricting study participation too severely, one runs the risk of developing a trial that will be difficult to enroll and the results of which may be applicable only to a narrow subset of patients with a particular disease, when, in fact, a broader population could potentially benefit. Furthermore, product labeling typically reflects only those patients with characteristics matching those in the clinical trials in which safety and efficacy were demonstrated.

It is not uncommon for regulatory authorities to raise the following issues during discussion and review of trials designed to support marketing approval:

- Which prospectively defined outcome variables are feasible to measure and are scientifically valid
- Whether a control group is feasible and what comparator drugs, if any, need to be used in control-group subjects
- The ease with which subjects and investigators may be blinded (see the following discussion)
- The numbers of participating trial sites and subjects

When developing a clinical trial protocol, one must assess chance, bias, and other confounding factors that might affect the trial and incorporate measures to address these issues.

The likelihood of obtaining false-positive or false-negative outcomes can be minimized by appropriately powering a study to assure an adequate sample size. **Subject bias** can often be countered by providing a **placebo control**, an inert substance with the same appearance as the drug under investigation. **Observer bias** can be countered by blinding, usually by coding the drug and placebo so that their identities are masked; thus, the investigators cannot know which treatment is being administered to a study subject. When the identity of the intervention is unknown to both subject and observer, the study is called a **double-blind** study.

The natural fluctuations and spontaneous remissions of many diseases also confound clinical trials. A **crossover design**, in which each study group is given the test drug alternately with placebo, can protect against the misinterpretation of results due to natural variation in the disease process. The presence of risk factors or comorbid diseases and their treatment, known or unknown, represents another major confounder of clinical trials. Careful medical histories and **randomization of subjects** can counter some of the effects of these risk factors. Stratification between study arms based on known clinically important covariates, and/or prospectively defining in the statistical analysis plan how corrections will be made for imbalances in clinically important covariates, can also help to minimize the impact of potentially confounding variables. In addition to the strategies mentioned above—use of placebo controls, blinded studies, crossover design, and randomization—a large **sample size** can help to minimize the effect of these factors. Phase 3 trials, the key studies that typically form the primary basis for regulatory approval, are often referred to as **pivotal trials** and are usually *randomized, well-controlled studies*.

Finally, it is essential to ensure that the required schedule of tests is feasible in the practice settings in which the trial will be conducted. This may be accomplished by extensive

TABLE 52-2 Clinical Drug Testing in Humans

PHASE	NUMBER OF SUBJECTS	LENGTH OF PHASE	PURPOSE
Phase 1	20–100	Several months	Safety, pharmacokinetics, and pharmacodynamics
Phase 2	Up to several hundred	Several months to 2 years	Effectiveness, safety, dose ranging
Phase 3	Several hundred to several thousand	1–4 years	Safety, dosage, effectiveness

discussions with physicians, nurses, and study coordinators who are being considered to conduct the trial. Central laboratories may be employed, especially for conduct of novel tests or evaluation of disease-associated biomarkers. Additionally, central laboratories are commonly used when conducting multicenter phase 2 and phase 3 trials to better ensure standardization of data among study sites.

Once the IND is active and an IRB or IEC approves the study protocol, clinical studies proceed in three phases. Table 52-2 summarizes the typical number of subjects, length of time required, and purpose of each phase of clinical trials, although these can vary considerably based on multiple factors.

Phase 1 Studies

Phase 1 studies are primarily intended to establish the safety and tolerability of a drug, including determination of the maximum-tolerated dose (MTD) and dose-limiting toxicity (DLT). Single-dose trials in phase 1A often precede repeat-dose trials in phase 1B. To protect patient safety, phase 1 trials are typically dose escalation trials. Subjects are divided into dosing groups, or cohorts. The initial cohort is administered a dose of the study drug that is anticipated to have little to no effect; subsequent subject cohorts receive increasing doses of study drug until either a DLT is reached or a relevant pharmacodynamic endpoint is achieved. Alternatively, and less commonly, intrapatient dose escalation may be employed. However, this can make interpretation of toxicity difficult if the study medication has delayed adverse effects. Part of phase 1 investigation also involves study of the drug's pharmacokinetic properties, including absorption, distribution, metabolism, and excretion (ADME). Although phase 1 trials focus on safety, tolerability, and pharmacokinetics, **pharmacodynamic assessments** are increasingly being used to provide data early in drug development on the potential effectiveness of the molecule.

Phase 1 studies frequently involve between 20 and 100 subjects. These may often be healthy normal volunteers. However, if high levels of toxicity are expected, such as with many cancer drugs, patients with the target condition may be used instead of healthy volunteers. Phase 1 studies usually involve **nonblinded trials**, in which subject and investigator are both aware of what is being administered. Phase 1 studies must yield sufficient information about a drug's pharmacokinetics to inform the design of scientifically valid phase 2 studies. For example, knowing the drug's volume of distribution and clearance enables study designers to determine an appropriate maintenance dose and dosing frequency for phase 2 and 3 trials (see Chapter 3, Pharmacokinetics).

Phase 2 Studies

Phase 2 studies may involve up to several hundred subjects with the medical condition of interest. Phase 2 clinical trials have multiple objectives, including the acquisition of preliminary data regarding the effectiveness of the drug for treatment of a particular condition. Like phase 1 trials, phase 2 trials continue to monitor safety. Because phase 2 studies enroll more patients, they are capable of detecting less common adverse events. Phase 2 studies also evaluate **dose–response** and dosing regimens, which are critically important in establishing the optimum dose or doses and frequency of administration of the drug.

A typical phase 2 design may involve either **single-blind** or **double-blind** trials in which the drug of interest is evaluated against placebo and/or an existing therapy. The trial usually compares several dosing regimens to obtain optimum dose range and toxicity information. The results of phase 2 studies are critically important in evaluating whether or not to proceed to phase 3 and, if so, establishing a phase 3 study design. Specifically, phase 2 studies should be designed to obtain a reasonable estimate of the size of the treatment effect of the experimental therapy; these data will then inform the appropriate sample size for phase 3 studies. Phase 2 results can also be used to pinpoint additional data that must be collected in phase 3 trials, such as monitoring of liver function tests if phase 2 data suggest possible hepatotoxicity.

During the drug development process, IND sponsors have multiple opportunities to consult with regulatory agencies through formal meetings. After the completion of phase 2 studies and before the initiation of phase 3 (pivotal) studies, the sponsor will typically request a meeting with the FDA to discuss the results obtained to date and to present the phase 3 program design. Given the time and expense of phase 3 clinical trials, it is critical that there is agreement between the FDA and the sponsor on the appropriate trial design(s) before the trial is initiated. Currently, the FDA provides the option of allowing the sponsor to use the Special Protocol Assessment (SPA) process to reach formal agreement on the design of the study that will be used to support approval provided that the study is successful.

Phase 3 Studies

Phase 3 studies involve several hundred to several thousand patients and are conducted at multiple sites and in settings similar to those in which the drug will ultimately be used. Phase 3 studies utilize specific **clinical endpoints** as the primary endpoints of the trial to establish efficacy of a drug. Examples of accepted clinical endpoints include survival, reduction or prevention of disease relapse, improvement in patient functional status, or improvement in how patients feel (e.g., pain, health-related quality-of-life assessments). **Surrogate endpoints** that have been validated in prior clinical trials (e.g., reduction in serum LDL cholesterol as a surrogate for clinically meaningful improvement in cardiac outcomes) may be acceptable endpoints in phase 3 pivotal trials. Examples of surrogate endpoints include markers for decreased disease burden, such as a reduction in the plasma levels of biochemical markers (e.g., glucose), an increase in cardiac output, or a reduction in size of a tumor.

In situations of life-threatening diseases for which no acceptable therapy is available, surrogate endpoints that are reasonably likely to predict clinical benefit (but that are not yet validated) may be used as endpoints in pivotal trials. In such instances, the FDA may use the **Accelerated Approval** mechanism to approve drugs that demonstrate a favorable impact on surrogate endpoints. Accelerated approval allows the drug to be developed more quickly and to be made available to patients in a timelier manner. It is important to note that "accelerated" refers to the development process, not the FDA review timeline; however, drugs being considered for accelerated approval may also be given **priority review** status (6 months, compared to the 10-month standard review). This approach has been used to approve drugs for the treatment of acquired immunodeficiency syndrome (AIDS) and several types of cancer, among other indications. Under accelerated approval, the sponsor is required to conduct post-approval phase 4 studies to verify and confirm the clinical benefit of the drug. In the introductory case, imatinib was granted accelerated approval based on the surrogate clinical endpoints of hematological and cytogenetic response rates and was then granted full approval after the successful completion of post-approval studies demonstrating increased survival compared to the current standard of care.

Clinical Pharmacology

Many pharmaceutical and biotechnology companies have developed groups dedicated to studying the clinical pharmacology of their products in development. These groups may be called by names such as Experimental Medicine, Molecular Medicine, or Clinical Pharmacology. The groups typically investigate aspects of the drug's clinical pharmacology, including fasting and fed single-dose and repeat-dose pharmacokinetics; drug–drug interactions, with a special emphasis on the role of cytochrome P450 isoforms on drug metabolism; and the impact of renal or hepatic impairment on drug metabolism. They perform thorough QT studies to assess the impact of the drug on cardiac electrophysiological function (see Chapter 6, Drug Toxicity). The groups make careful assessments of immunogenicity, particularly if the drug is a protein therapeutic, and of the drug's clinical pharmacology in pediatric patients and in specific ethnic groups such as Asian populations. Clinical pharmacology groups also work closely with preclinical scientists to develop appropriate biomarkers to better assess the impact of the drug at the earliest stages of clinical development. Biomarker assessments may take a variety of forms, including exploration of the population of patients most likely to benefit or most likely to be susceptible to toxicity as well as pharmacodynamic markers of drug activity. The groups may attempt to correlate gene polymorphisms or expression profiles with responsiveness. These and other clinical pharmacology studies are performed throughout the clinical development program and are incorporated into phase 1, 2, and 3 studies.

Pediatric Studies

Both the European Union regulatory authority, called the European Medicines Agency (EMA), and the US FDA have placed increased emphasis on performing studies of drug safety, pharmacokinetics, and efficacy in pediatric populations whenever possible and appropriate. The EMA requires approval of a pediatric investigation plan, or PIP, by its pediatric committee prior to submission of a marketing application for a new drug or biologic. Similarly, under FDASIA, the FDA now has the authority and responsibility

to promulgate regulations relating to pediatric study plans (PSPs) in order to identify the required pediatric studies early in drug development and to begin planning for these studies, often prior to the filing of the NDA/BLA.

Challenges in the Development of Drugs to Treat Rare Diseases

Historically, pharmaceutical companies had typically been disinterested in developing products for diseases with small patient populations, since the cost of developing drugs for small markets was similar to that for developing drugs for larger patient populations but the resulting revenues were smaller. In an attempt to encourage development of drugs for rare diseases, Congress passed the **Orphan Drug Act** in 1983. The legislation offers financial incentives to companies that develop drugs for **orphan diseases**, which are defined as diseases that affect fewer than 200,000 individuals in the United States. In addition, an orphan drug enjoys exclusive approval for the orphan indication for 7 years following approval. This legislation has proven to be very successful in stimulating the development of new drugs for rare diseases. Since 1983, the FDA has approved more than 460 drugs to treat orphan diseases. Examples include **imiglucerase** for Gaucher disease type 1, **epoetin alfa** for anemia associated with end-stage renal disease, **imatinib** for chronic myelogenous leukemia, and **mipomersen** and **lomitapide** for homozygous familial hypercholesterolemia.

Even with orphan drug legislation, the development of drugs for very rare diseases presents several special challenges. FDA regulations require the same degree of rigor in the development of such drugs as that for non-orphan indications, including the appropriate demonstration of safety and statistically significant efficacy in well-controlled clinical trials. Designing trials for patient populations that might be as small as 5,000 patients worldwide can prove challenging. The testing required in many of these trials may be highly specialized and may best be conducted at only a small number of centers of excellence in the world. Hence, patients, and in some instances their care providers, may need to be transported to remote clinical trial sites and housed far from their homes and support systems for extended periods of time. Additionally, even with a very effective drug, if the disease in question has a long natural history, enrolling a sufficient number of patients for a long enough period of time to demonstrate a statistically significant difference from the placebo control may present major feasibility challenges. Furthermore, if a rare disease is heterogeneous in its clinical course, then the expected treatment effect of the new drug may be confounded by a less-than-solid understanding of the disease's natural history. This, in turn, makes it difficult to determine the sample size necessary to ensure that the trial is designed with sufficient power to observe a statistically significant difference between study arms. In some instances, sponsors have conducted natural history studies in parallel with traditional early-phase interventional studies in order to better understand the natural history of the disease and thereby inform the design of the subsequent pivotal trials.

The challenges of drug development for rare diseases may gain increasing attention in the coming years as advances in the basic sciences continue to allow diseases to be better understood and defined at the molecular level. The result of this improved understanding will likely be that a group of heterogeneous diseases, which until now has been considered as one disease entity encompassing many patients, will be categorized into smaller, orphan-sized subgroups based on specific molecular markers or mutations.

Adaptive Trial Designs

As discussed earlier, it usually takes many years and many millions of dollars to successfully develop a new therapeutic. In order to be as efficient as possible, much attention has recently been given to the development of adaptive clinical trial designs. This methodology allows for modification of such variables as trial duration, cohort assignment, or number of patients enrolled based on examination and analysis of the accumulated data at one or more prospectively defined points in the trial. Adaptive designs may not only be more efficient but may also increase the chances of demonstrating an effect of the investigational agent (if one exists). In all cases, it is important that such designs are developed in close collaboration with regulatory authorities to ensure that they will be deemed acceptable.

Successful Drug Development: Design and Execution

Successful drug development requires not only a thoughtful, well-conceived, strategic development plan but also rigorous, responsible execution. This, in turn, requires a strong organization, competent leadership, adequate resources, and a highly functioning, multidisciplinary global team. It cannot be emphasized enough that successful drug development requires intensive and extensive collaboration among many people in a wide array of disciplines. Table 52-3 lists many of the most important clinical study activities that require extensive planning. Careful planning is critical since errors that either result in the need for protocol amendments or endanger the integrity of the results will cost significant time and money, jeopardize the results obtained, and, most importantly, have the potential to place patients at inappropriate risk. Clinical study operations include study site start-up and initiation, interim site monitoring, interim site management, and site closeout at the conclusion of the study. Each of these activities requires the successful completion of many smaller activities, as illustrated in Table 52-3.

TABLE 52-3 Elements to Be Considered in Clinical Trial Operations: Planning and Execution

Study Management

- Case report form design and printing (unless electronic data capture is employed)
- Projected (or required) enrollment rates
- Health economics issues
- Use of independent Data Monitoring Committees (DMCs), special monitoring, or adjudication committees (include proposed charter and/or proposed procedure)
- Are special laboratories needed?
- Will the study use a contract research organization (CRO) for all or key parts of study conduct?
- Are there any special sample handling or supply shipping concerns?
- Investigator meeting planning

- Database development
- Data management
- Medical writing
- Clinical monitoring
- Medical monitoring
- Paper/electronic submission
- Publication analysis and writing
- Pharmacovigilance plans, including risk evaluation and mitigation strategies (REMS)
- Randomization system
- Central clinical laboratories/diagnostics
- Clinical trial material labeling and handling

Site Start-up

- Obtain confidentiality agreements.
- Obtain clinical trial agreements.
- Distribute study documents.
- Perform qualification visits.
- Assist with ethics committee or Institutional Review Board (IRB) approvals.

- Collect study documents.
- Ship study drug and case report forms.
- Hold investigator meeting.
- Initiate sites (visit).

Interim Site Monitoring

- Review enrollment.
- Review signed informed consents.
- Review regulatory binder (required documents).
- Perform drug accountability.
- Verify data from source documentation (CRF vs. medical record).

- Review serious adverse event reporting.
- Assess protocol and GCP/ICH compliance.
- Assess adequacy of personnel and facilities.
- Communicate findings to study personnel.
- Typically, monitor sites every 4–6 weeks.

Interim Site Management

- Track patient enrollment.
- Ongoing site support.
- Track and supply study drug.
- Review monitoring reports/data error frequency.

- Review protocol deviations/violations.
- Assess need for protocol amendments.
- Support QA audits.

Site Closeout

- Perform final drug accountability.
- Ship study drug for destruction.
- Verify data from source documentation, if needed.
- Ensure documentation on site complete.

- Obtain copies of site files.
- Inform site regarding communicating FDA audits to sponsor.
- Review record retention and publication policy.

CRF, case report form; GCP, good clinical practices; ICH, International Conference on Harmonization; QA, quality assurance; FDA, US Food and Drug Administration.

Mechanisms to Expedite Development of Therapeutics for Serious Conditions

Four principal mechanisms are supported by the FDA to expedite drug development for serious unmet needs. These include (1) Fast Track designation, (2) Breakthrough Therapy designation, (3) Accelerated Approval, and (4) Priority Review. Each program targets drugs intended to treat serious conditions; the qualifying criteria and advantages of the programs are differentiated as follows:

- **Fast Track** designation requires nonclinical or clinical data that demonstrate the potential to address a serious unmet medical need. Advantages include opportunities for frequent FDA interactions, rolling review (allows the sponsor to submit portions of the application for approval on a rolling basis as the documents become available rather than submitting all of the many thousands of pages at one time), and eligibility for priority review.
- **Breakthrough Therapy** designation requires preliminary clinical data that indicate the drug may demonstrate substantial improvement over existing therapies in a clinically significant endpoint(s). Advantages include early and intensive guidance, involvement of FDA senior staff, rolling review, and eligibility for priority review.
- **Accelerated Approval**, as described in "Phase 3 Studies" above, requires that the product provides a meaningful advantage over available therapy and demonstrates an effect in a surrogate endpoint.
- **Priority Review** criteria stipulate that the product, if approved, would provide a significant improvement in safety or effectiveness. The advantage of priority review is that it provides for a 6-month review period from the time of filing of the application with the FDA to a decision rather than the standard 10-month review period.

It is important to note that a development program can fit more than one of these expedited development mechanisms. In addition, even with such expedited development opportunities, adequate data must be provided to fulfill the FDA's statutory requirements for a product to demonstrate safety and efficacy.

▍DRUG APPROVAL PROCESS

FDA Review

Approval of new drugs in the United States is based on the New Drug Application (NDA) in the case of a small-molecule therapeutics or the Biologics License Application (BLA) in the case of a biotherapeutic. The NDA/BLA must contain all relevant data collected by a sponsor during research and development of the proposed new drug. As such, data gathered for the IND are integrated into the NDA/BLA. The FDA mandates that every NDA/BLA must contain the following sections: index, summary, chemistry, manufacturing and quality control, samples, methods validation, package and labeling, nonclinical pharmacology and toxicology, human pharmacokinetics, metabolism and bioavailability, microbiology, clinical data, safety update report (typically submitted 120 days after NDA/BLA submission), statistical information, case report tabulations, case report forms, patent information, patent certification, and other information. The typical NDA/BLA submission is comprehensive and may consist of thousands of pages in multiple volumes. To facilitate the submission of these data to regulatory agencies in multiple countries, the data are presented in a format referred to as the **Common Technical Document (CTD)**. With the passage of FDASIA in 2012, all CTDs will ultimately be required to be submitted in electronic format.

Upon receipt of an NDA/BLA, the FDA has 60 days to assess an application's acceptability to be filed for review. The review is organized into several categories, which may include the following: **medical review**, **biopharmaceutical review**, **pharmacology review**, **statistical review**, **chemistry review**, and **microbiology review**. Within each of these groups, FDA experts review the data package submitted to the agency and provide an assessment of the safety and efficacy of the proposed new drug. Figure 52-3 is a flowchart representing the process used by the FDA to evaluate an NDA/BLA.

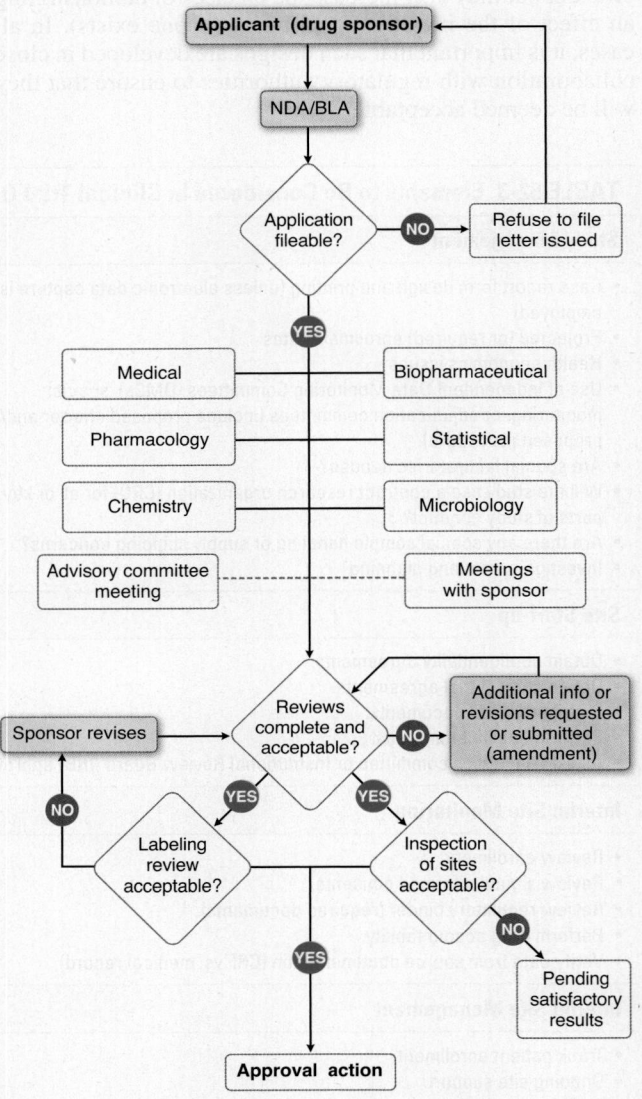

FIGURE 52-3. Process of New Drug Application/Biologics License Application (NDA/BLA) review. When a new drug application is filed, the drug sponsor provides data regarding the drug's medical, pharmacologic, chemical, biopharmaceutical, statistical, and microbiological characteristics; these data are reviewed by separate committees at the FDA. If the review is complete and acceptable, then the drug application is reviewed for acceptable labeling (official instructions for use). The manufacturing sites and sites where significant clinical trials were performed also undergo inspections and audits. *Colored boxes* correspond to actions by the drug sponsor; *white boxes* correspond to actions by the FDA.

In addition to reviews internal to the agency, the FDA may also call on an **external advisory committee** for input on an NDA/BLA. These committees provide medical and scientific input and allow for consultation with outside experts in a particular field. Although the FDA usually incorporates advisory committee recommendations into its decisions, these external opinions are not binding. The FDA may also engage external experts as needed during the review process for specific technical issues.

During the review process, the FDA maintains ongoing communication with the sponsor regarding scientific or other issues that arise during review. Regular correspondence (including face-to-face meetings if necessary) occurs between the sponsor and the agency, particularly if additional data are needed. The FDA frequently asks the sponsor questions in writing, and the sponsor may submit additional data or a new analysis of previously available data to assist in addressing these questions. Substantial amounts of new information are considered an amendment to the NDA/BLA and can prolong the time to approval.

FDA Approval

The FDA may take one of two possible actions following the review of an NDA/BLA—approval of the application or issuance of a Complete Response Letter (CRL) to the sponsor of the application. A Complete Response Letter is issued when the FDA determines that an application has deficiencies to such a degree that approval should not be granted; in response, a sponsor must notify the FDA of its intent to resubmit the application, withdraw it, or request a hearing. In the CRL, the FDA must list all of the specific deficiencies in the application that need to be satisfactorily addressed in order for the application to be reconsidered for approval. Often, the FDA will meet with the sponsor to discuss the steps that must be taken to secure approval. In some cases, these revisions may require significant new studies to be undertaken. The sponsor then must decide whether to generate new data or abandon a particular development program. If a sponsor fails to act on a CRL within 1 year of its issue, the FDA considers this lack of response to represent a request by the sponsor to withdraw the NDA/BLA.

Approval in Other Countries

Before drugs may be sold in countries outside the United States, they must first be evaluated and approved by the appropriate regulatory authorities in those regions. In some countries, this may include a comprehensive review of all data, similar to the NDA/BLA review. In other countries, a more limited review may occur if the drug has already been approved in one of the major foreign markets (United States, European Union, Japan). During these reviews, a regulatory authority may require additional types of data or analyses that were not required for US approval. In addition, different regulatory agencies may have different approaches to the type and amount of data required in product labeling. In the European Union, many drugs are first evaluated by the **European Medicines Agency** (**EMA**) and then approved by the **European Commission** if approval is recommended by the EMA. In Canada, **Health Canada** administers the regulations embodied in the **Canadian Food and Drugs Act**. In Japan, approval of new drugs is granted by the **Ministry of Health and Welfare**. Importantly, Japanese regulatory authorities require studies to be performed in ethnic Japanese patients in order to demonstrate that the pharmacokinetic and safety profiles observed in a Japanese population are similar to those observed in a Western population. Demonstration of efficacy in Japanese patients may also be required.

Expanded Access of an Investigational Drug or an Approved Drug with Restricted Distribution

The FDA has established several mechanisms for the "compassionate use" of investigational drugs for patients with serious or immediately life-threatening conditions for which there are no alternative therapies. Examples of compassionate use may include when a patient fails to meet established inclusion criteria for an ongoing trial of an investigational drug; when a patient seeks access to an investigational drug after a pivotal study is completed to support a marketing application; or when access is sought for an approved drug whose distribution is controlled due to safety reasons. In all cases, three criteria must be met: (1) patients to be treated must have a serious or life-threatening condition with no therapeutic alternatives; (2) the potential benefit must outweigh the potential risk of the drug; and (3) providing the drug will in no way interfere with ongoing clinical development of the drug.

Drug Labeling

Each region's regulatory body has an established format and organization for drug labeling. A **drug label** must include the drug's proprietary and chemical name, formula and ingredients, clinical pharmacology, indications and usage, contraindications, warnings, precautions, adverse reactions, drug abuse/dependence potential, overdosage, dosage, rate and route of administration, and how the drug is supplied. In the United States, this information is also known as the drug's **package insert**. When a new drug approaches approval, the FDA reviews and negotiates the final package insert with the sponsor to ensure that the labeling is justified by the data submitted in the NDA/BLA. To provide more accessible and informative drug information, in 2006, the FDA instituted the Physician Labeling Rule, which provides key information important to prescribers in a standardized format.

Regulatory agencies may use additional methods to ensure that important attributes of the drug are clearly communicated. For example, in the United States, package inserts for drugs that have certain safety risks include a **"black box" warning**, in which key safety information is prominently displayed. In addition, the FDA may require sponsors to create **Medication Guides** for mandatory distribution to patients; these guides communicate critical safety information in language that is readily understandable.

Drug Naming

Another facet of drug approval involves the determination of a drug's name. A drug is known by two principal names, the **generic name** and the **brand name** (or **trade name**). A drug's generic name is based on its chemical name and is unprotected by a trademark. The generic name is also known as the *International Nonproprietary Name* or *INN*. In contrast, a drug's brand name refers to the exclusive name of a substance or drug product owned by a company under trademark law.

For example, the generic name of the drug discussed in the introductory case is imatinib mesylate, while the brand name is Gleevec®.

Additional Indications

Once a drug is approved, physicians and certain other healthcare professionals are permitted to prescribe the drug according to the various labeled doses or dosage regimens. Providers may modify dosing and also prescribe the drug for indications other than that for which it was originally approved; this is known as **"off-label" use**.

Physicians are also permitted to conduct investigational studies with the drug, provided that they follow the rules of informed consent and obtain IRB approval for the studies. However, in many instances, the investigator may be required to file an IND, particularly if the investigation involves a route of administration, dose, patient population, or other factor that has not been well studied and may significantly increase the risk associated with the use of the drug product.

Pharmaceutical companies may not market the drug for any indications other than those for which it has been approved by the FDA. Current regulations prohibit pharmaceutical companies from proactively providing any marketing materials, including scientific articles, on the off-label use of a drug, unless such materials are requested by a physician. In order to market a drug for a new indication, a pharmaceutical company must conduct an additional program of development to prove that the drug is safe and efficacious for the new indication. These data are then submitted to regulatory authorities as a **supplemental NDA/BLA (sNDA/sBLA)** and subjected to additional review prior to the granting of approval for the new indication. Product labeling may then be modified accordingly.

REGULATORY ASPECTS OF DRUG PRODUCTION AND QUALITY CONTROL

In addition to demonstrating a drug's safety and efficacy, manufacturers must also comply with FDA regulations for manufacturing as a requirement for drug approval and subsequent distribution. The **Good Manufacturing Practice** (**GMP**) guidelines govern quality management and control for all aspects of drug manufacturing, and the FDA has the authority to inspect manufacturing facilities in order to determine compliance. FDA regulations require sponsors to establish manufacturing process controls, product quality attributes, and quality control procedures in order to ensure a product's purity, potency, and identity.

A company must obtain prior FDA approval before implementing any manufacturing change that is determined by the FDA to have substantial potential to affect the safety or efficacy of a drug through alterations in its identity, strength, quality, purity, or potency. Other changes may be implemented either with or without submission of a supplemental NDA/BLA. GMP criteria apply whether a sponsor manufactures its own products or uses contract manufacturers.

GENERIC DRUGS

The FDA also oversees approval of **generic drugs**, which the agency defines as drugs that are comparable to innovator drugs in dosage form, safety, strength, route of administration, quality, performance characteristics, and intended use. Under the **Drug Price Competition and Patent Term Restoration Act of 1984**, also known as the **Hatch-Waxman Act**, a company may submit an **Abbreviated New Drug Application (ANDA)** before the patent governing the brand name drug expires. However, the company must wait for the original drug's patent to expire before it can market a generic version. The first company to file an ANDA has the exclusive right to market the generic drug for 180 days.

ANDAs for generic drugs are not required to provide data establishing safety and efficacy, because this has been established in the NDA for the innovator drug. To establish **bioequivalence**, which is required in the ANDA, sponsors may submit a formulation comparison, comparative dissolution testing (where there is a known correlation between in vitro and in vivo effects), in vivo bioequivalence testing (comparing the rate and extent of absorption of the generic with that of the reference product), and, for nonclassically absorbed products, a head-to-head evaluation of comparative effectiveness based on clinical endpoints. In addition, an ANDA sponsor must provide evidence that its manufacturing processes and facilities, as well as any outside testing or packaging facilities, are in compliance with federal GMP regulations.

"Generic" versions of biologic drugs, primarily proteins, present much greater challenges than generic versions of small-molecule drugs. Whereas small molecules can readily be shown to be comparable to the innovator drug as described above, this is not so easy with recombinant proteins, which usually have many post-translational modifications. Seemingly minor changes in post-translational modifications may result in marked differences from the innovator drug in safety and efficacy. Changes in cell lines used to manufacture such proteins and changes in any step of the production process may alter post-translational modifications.

As a result, the precise regulatory path for the development of "biosimilars" was less than clear. The **Biologics Price Competition and Innovation Act** of 2009 (**BPCIA**), the analogue of the Hatch-Waxman act for biological products, authorized the approval pathway for **biosimilar** products. The **Biosimilar User Fee Act**, as authorized by FDASIA in 2012, provides the FDA with the resources and staff to review and approve biosimilar products. The FDA has issued several documents providing guidance on the development of biosimilars, including a Scientific Considerations document, a Quality Considerations document, and a Questions and Answers (Q&A) document on Implementation of the BPCIA. In 2013, guidance was issued outlining formal procedures for holding meetings with the FDA on biosimilar development. During 2014 and 2015, the FDA issued additional guidances on clinical pharmacology data, scientific considerations, and quality considerations to support biosimilarity to a reference product, as well as a revision to the Q&A document.

NONPRESCRIPTION DRUGS AND SUPPLEMENTS

The 1951 **Durham-Humphrey Amendment** to the Food, Drug, and Cosmetic Act defined prescription drugs as drugs that are unsafe for use except under professional supervision. In determining which drugs do not require a prescription, the FDA examines a drug's toxicity and the facility with which a condition may be self-diagnosed. Because **over-the-counter (OTC)** drugs are sold in lower doses than their prescription counterparts and are used primarily to treat symptoms of disease, the FDA requires their labels to contain the following:

- Intended uses of the product, as well as the product's effects
- Adequate directions for use
- Warnings against unsafe use
- Adverse effects

Although OTC products present a potential danger of misuse or misdiagnosis in the absence of physician oversight, the increased availability of these products has provided many US citizens with access to effective and relatively inexpensive treatments.

The **Dietary Supplement Health and Education Act** of 1994 defines a **dietary supplement** as any product intended for ingestion as a supplement to the diet, including vitamins, minerals, herbs, botanicals, other plant-derived substances, amino acids, concentrates, metabolites, and constituents and extracts of these substances. The FDA oversees the safety, manufacturing, and health claims made by dietary supplements. The FDA does not, however, evaluate the efficacy of supplements as it does for drugs. The FDA may restrict or halt the sale of unsafe supplements, but it must demonstrate that such supplements are unsafe before taking action. This occurred in February 2004, when the FDA announced a rule banning dietary supplements containing ephedrine alkaloids (**ephedra**) after reviewing the substantial number of adverse events (including deaths) associated with these products.

■ CONCLUSION AND FUTURE DIRECTIONS

Specific laws and regulations have been established to provide for the development of new drugs, while at the same time ensuring privacy and safety for the individuals participating in clinical trials. Regulatory approval of new drugs follows a disciplined process of preclinical and clinical studies in parallel with product characterization and manufacturing process development. Each phase of development provides critical information that informs subsequent phases of investigation. Industry, academia, and health authorities strive to balance safety and clinical benefit with speed of drug availability for patients in need. However, no amount of analytical, animal, and clinical trial data can provide a completely accurate prediction of the safety profile of a drug after it is introduced to the marketplace. Thus, the FDA and drug manufacturers continue to monitor the adverse effects, manufacturing processes, and overall safety of a drug for its lifetime (see Chapter 53, Systematic Detection of Adverse Drug Events).

Acknowledgment

We thank the late Armen H. Tashjian, Jr. for his valuable contribution to this chapter in the Second Edition of *Principles of Pharmacology: The Pathophysiologic Basis of Drug Therapy.*

Suggested Reading

Adams CP, Brantner VV. Estimating the cost of new drug development: is it really 802 million dollars? *Health Aff* 2006;25:420–428. (*Finds that developing a new drug costs between $500 million and $2 billion, depending on the indication.*)

Center for Drug Evaluation and Research, U.S. Food and Drug Administration, U.S. Department of Health and Human Services. The CDER handbook. Revised 03/16/98. http://www.fda.gov/downloads/AboutFDA/CentersOffices/CDER/UCM198415.pdf. (*Describes the processes by which the FDA evaluates and regulates drugs, including new drug evaluation and postmarketing monitoring of drug safety and effectiveness.*)

Cohen MH, Williams G, Johnson JR, et al. Approval summary for imatinib mesylate capsules in the treatment of chronic myelogenous leukemia. *Clin Cancer Res* 2002;8:935–942. (*Summarizes the approval of imatinib mesylate, the drug discussed in the introductory case.*)

DiMasi JA, Grabowski HG. The cost of biopharmaceutical R&D: is biotech different? *Manage Decis Econ* 2007;28:469–479. (*First paper to estimate costs of biopharmaceutical development compared to costs of traditional pharmaceutical development.*)

Dixon JR. The International Conference on Harmonization Good Clinical Practice guideline. *Qual Assur* 1999;6:65–74. (*Guidelines for standard design of drug development.*)

Food and Drug Administration Strategic Priorities 2014–2018. http://www.fda.gov/downloads/AboutFDA/ReportsManualsForms/Reports/UCM403191.pdf. (*A draft document for public comment that provides an overarching view of how the FDA is addressing and plans to address the public health challenges facing the United States in the next 5 years.*)

Kesselheim AS, Darrow JJ. Drug development and FDA approval, 1938–2013. *N Engl J Med* 2014;360:e39. (*Interactive presentation of the major legislative and regulatory events related to the approval of new drugs by the FDA, including drug approvals.*)

Long G, Works J. *Innovation in the biopharmaceutical pipeline: a multidimensional view.* Boston, MA: Analysis Group; 2013. www.analysisgroup.com/uploadedFiles/Publishing/Articles/2012_Innovation_in_the_Biopharmaceutical_Pipeline.pdf. (*Descriptive information about the development of innovative medicines in multiple therapeutic areas.*)

Pharmaceutical Research and Manufacturers of America. 2014 biopharmaceutical research industry profile. Washington, DC: Pharmaceutical Research and Manufacturers of America; 2014. http://www.phrma.org/sites/default/files/pdf/2014_PhRMA_PROFILE.pdf. (*Overview of the current status of the pharmaceutical industry with respect to innovations in research and development and impact on patients and society, published by the Pharmaceutical Research and Manufacturers of America [PhRMA].*)

Swann JP. FDA's origin and functions. http://www.fda.gov/AboutFDA/WhatWeDo/History/Origin/ucm124403.htm. (*An excellent overview of the evolution of the FDA from its beginnings in 1848.*)

U.S. Food and Drug Administration, U.S. Department of Health and Human Services. Innovation or stagnation: challenge and opportunity on the critical path to new medical products. March 2004. http://www.fda.gov/ScienceResearch/SpecialTopics/CriticalPathInitiative/CriticalPathOpportunitiesReports/ucm077262.htm. (*An FDA report that addresses the slowdown in innovative drug development.*)

53

Systematic Detection of Adverse Drug Events

Jerry Avorn

	Adverse outcome	No adverse outcome
Drug exposure	**A** Exposure + Outcome +	**B** Exposure + Outcome −
No drug exposure	**C** Exposure − Outcome +	**D** Exposure − Outcome −

INTRODUCTION

Because medications act by interfering with one or more aspects of molecular and cellular function, it is difficult to do so without also causing an undesirable effect either by that perturbation or by another (perhaps unexpected) drug action. Because all drugs have risks, the goal of pharmacotherapy cannot be to prescribe a risk-free regimen. Instead, it is to ensure that the risks of drug therapy are as low as possible and are acceptable in the context of a medication's clinical benefit.

Some adverse effects of a drug are apparent during its early development and often result from the same on-target mechanism responsible for its therapeutic effect (e.g., cytotoxic cancer chemotherapy). Even in such situations, however, it is necessary to know how those expected adverse effects will be manifested when the drug is in routine use—in terms of both their frequency and their severity. After a drug has been approved for clinical use, the goal becomes detecting and quantifying the risks as quickly and rigorously as possible.

Serious or even life-threatening adverse effects have led to the withdrawal of widely used drugs. This has heightened the sensitivity of clinicians and patients to the growing field of pharmacoepidemiology—the measurement of drug effects in large, "real-world" populations of patients. Advances in informatics and analytic techniques in this field hold promise for enhancing our understanding of drug risks so that they can be better understood and managed, with the goal of putting a drug's benefits into context and guiding clinical decision making and regulatory action.

CHALLENGES IN THE ASCERTAINMENT OF DRUG SAFETY

The randomized controlled trial (RCT) is the gold standard for determining the efficacy of a drug and is the main criterion used by regulatory agencies, such as the US Food and Drug Administration (FDA), in deciding whether to approve a new medication for use. But this valuable tool also has limits, and it is important to understand those limits when assessing the benefits and risks of a given agent.

Study Size and Generalizability

Compared to the number of patients who eventually use a drug, the number of subjects in clinical trials supporting the approval of that drug is relatively modest. Approval decisions are generally made on the basis of trials that include 2,000–4,000 participants, or fewer for rare conditions. If a particular adverse event occurs just once in every 1,000 patients, it may not occur at all during clinical trials,

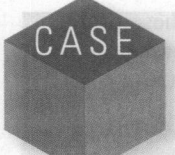

CASE

Mr. Keeley is a 67-year-old man with severe degenerative joint disease of both hips. He brings to his doctor several magazine ads and newspaper clippings that describe the nonsteroidal anti-inflammatory drug rofecoxib. These ads claim that rofecoxib provides excellent relief of arthritic pain with a lower risk of gastrointestinal toxicity. Rofecoxib selectively inhibits cyclooxygenase-2, which mediates pain and inflammation, rather than cyclooxygenase-1, which maintains gastrointestinal mucosal integrity and whose inhibition can cause gastrointestinal bleeding. This drug is widely hailed as a "super-aspirin" with minimal gastrointestinal toxicity and is heavily promoted. Mr. Keeley's physician decides to prescribe rofecoxib, and the patient reports that it works better than the acetaminophen he had previously been using.

The patient continues to experience good relief of his arthritic pain. In the ensuing months, he develops mild hypertension that is easily managed with a thiazide medication but is otherwise well. Nine months after Mr. Keeley begins taking rofecoxib, his wife calls to report that her husband has been hospitalized with a myocardial infarction. He survives several episodes of arrhythmia and cardiogenic shock and is discharged to home. His physician is not surprised at this report, since the patient was an active smoker, had elevated serum cholesterol, and has a recent diagnosis of hypertension.

Two years after Mr. Keeley's myocardial infarction, rofecoxib is withdrawn from the market when a randomized controlled trial reveals that rofecoxib nearly doubles the risk of myocardial infarction and stroke.

Questions

1. How do regulatory agencies such as the US Food and Drug Administration assess the safety of medications before they are approved?
2. How do physicians, patients, and the FDA learn about the adverse effects of drugs once they are in widespread use?
3. How can observational studies be used to determine the adverse effects of drugs that are in widespread use?
4. What issues must be considered in interpreting and acting on the results of such analyses?

or if it does occur, it may be difficult or impossible to determine whether its rate of occurrence is meaningfully higher among study subjects compared to controls. One in 1,000 may seem like a rare event, but if 10 million people take a drug each year, that rate would result in 10,000 occurrences of the adverse event annually. For a life-threatening adverse effect such as fulminant hepatotoxicity, this could have important clinical and public health consequences.

Subjects in clinical trials of new drugs are nearly always volunteers—people who have come forward to participate in medical research and have given their informed consent to take part in the study. There is ample evidence that such people tend to be different from typical patients who will receive the drug when it is in routine use; study subjects tend to be younger, healthier, better educated, and of higher socioeconomic status. This problem is often exacerbated by strict exclusion criteria in preapproval study protocols. Some of these exclusions prohibit participation of patients over a given age cutoff (such as 65 or 70), even if the drug is expected to be used disproportionately by the elderly. Other entry criteria may exclude patients who have important comorbidities in addition to the disease being studied (thereby also excluding those who are taking multiple other medications). While this may be the "cleanest" way to test the efficacy of a new agent, there is growing concern that the data thus generated have limited generalizability to the populations who ultimately use these medications. Other kinds of patients may be excluded for unassailable ethical reasons, such as not allowing pregnant women or children into most preapproval drug trials. However, when such patients then take these drugs in routine care, there is little information to guide their use.

By definition, clinical trials are conducted by physicians and support staff who have experience in clinical research and who work in settings accustomed to such activities. Their actions are guided by study protocols that often require close monitoring for adverse effects as well as efficacy. Such protocols also ensure that patients are taking the prescribed product as directed. This, too, is far different from routine care in typical settings, in which both patient adherence and the intensity of surveillance for early detection of adverse events are generally lower.

Surrogate Outcomes and Comparators

It would be difficult to postpone the approval of every new antihypertensive drug until it had been shown to reduce stroke rates, or not to allow a new statin lipid-lowering drug on the market until it had been shown to prevent myocardial infarctions. Such a requirement could delay the availability of potentially useful new therapies, as well as further increase their cost. As a consequence, new products may be approved on the basis of their effect on "surrogate outcomes," such as blood pressure for antihypertensives, hemoglobin A1c level for drugs used to manage diabetes, serum LDL cholesterol level for statins, intraocular pressure for drugs used to treat glaucoma, or biomarkers of tumor growth for oncology therapies. *While such a metric can be useful in making drug approval quicker and more efficient, its utility depends on the association between the surrogate marker and the clinical outcome of concern.* These may correlate well, but not always. For example, the antiarrhythmics **encainide** and **flecainide** reduced the surrogate outcome of ventricular ectopy after myocardial infarction, but a larger study (the CAST trial) demonstrated that they actually increased mortality in such patients, despite their success in "treating" the surrogate marker. Similarly, **rosiglitazone** (Avandia®) was approved based on its capacity to reduce hemoglobin A1c levels in preapproval trials. However, once the drug was in widespread use, meta-analysis of those trials found that it increased the risk of myocardial infarction.

When feasible, placebos are the comparison treatment preferred by manufacturers and the FDA for premarket trials used to determine approval. Such comparisons provide the clearest contrasts and the most straightforward statistical analysis, and there is no possibility of confusion resulting from therapeutic or adverse events caused by an active agent used in the control group. Placebo controls also facilitate the approval of new products whose efficacy is similar to that of existing drugs; performing "equivalency" or "non-inferiority" studies against active therapies requires larger numbers of patients and is more demanding statistically. If it is ethically or pragmatically impossible to conduct placebo-controlled trials (e.g., with a new AIDS drug or an antibiotic for a serious bacterial infection), then an active comparator is used.

However, while the "better than placebo" comparison may be sufficient for a manufacturer to meet the FDA's legal requirements for drug approval, the data it yields often fall short of what the clinician, patient, or payor needs to know about a new drug's safety or comparative effectiveness. A new drug may work better than placebo, but is it better than an existing treatment the physician may choose instead? Or is it even as good? The new drug may produce a serious adverse effect (e.g., rhabdomyolysis with a statin), but is the rate of occurrence of the effect higher or lower than that seen with older therapies? And even if it poses a higher risk of a given adverse effect, does the new drug also provide greater efficacy (in this case, prevention of ischemic cardiac events)? If so, the trade-off might possibly be acceptable; if not, it would not be. But if no such comparative data exist, the question cannot even be considered.

Duration and Post-Approval Studies

The duration of efficacy trials for certain new drugs can be as short as 8–16 weeks, if the comparator is placebo and surrogate endpoints are used to meet a legal definition of efficacy. However, such short-term trials may yield little useful information about benefits and risks that occur beyond this time frame. The FDA requires a minimum of 6 months of safety testing for a new drug that is designed for chronic use (where chronic is defined as any period longer than 6 months), although even this duration of safety testing may be too short for a chronically administered medication that may be taken for many years.

In approving a new drug for widespread use, the FDA may ask the manufacturer to conduct additional postmarketing studies (**phase IV studies**) to address questions that were not resolved by the evidence submitted prior to approval. Sometimes, useful new data about a drug's benefits and risks are obtained in this way. But until 2007, the agency had little authority to oblige a drug's sponsor to complete these studies, since its main regulatory power, once a drug had been approved, had been confined to the "nuclear option" of threatening to take it off the market—an action that was often not possible in the absence of additional data. Each year, the agency reports how well such "postmarketing commitments" are being met by manufacturers. A report by the Government Accountability Office noted that up to half of the "mandated" postmarketing safety studies requested by the agency had not been initiated, even years after the drugs

had entered widespread use. Concern about these problems was intensified by public concern over several prominent drug safety problems, particularly **rofecoxib** (Vioxx®). The drug had been used widely for 5 years before it was withdrawn from the market following a study demonstrating that it nearly doubled the risk of myocardial infarction or stroke. A 2006 report by the Institute of Medicine recommended sweeping changes in the way the FDA addresses drug safety (see below).

PHARMACOEPIDEMIOLOGY

Pharmacoepidemiology is the study of drug outcomes as documented in observations of clinical data from large populations of typical patients receiving routine care. To understand this approach, it is necessary to think about drug effects in ways that are different from those of conventional pharmacology (Table 53-1). This perspective considers the *population* as the experimental system being studied. Medications can be considered to be variables introduced into this system much as they might be studied in an individual patient, in tissue culture, or in an isolated single-cell preparation. The differences are that, in populations, true randomization does not occur, the intervening decision making and behavior of doctors and patients can alter the drug's effect, outcomes are measured in terms of probabilities (or rates) of events, and the magnitude of drug experience in the analysis is much larger than that of conventional pharmacology, ranging to millions of patients and millions of person-years of exposure.

The importance of pharmacoepidemiology is highlighted by a number of prominent drug withdrawals in recent years. Each of these withdrawals was preceded by severe or fatal adverse effects that had been unrecognized or underappreciated at the time of approval (Table 53-2). Using the tools of pharmacoepidemiology, it is possible to identify adverse effects that may be overlooked in randomized trials because those adverse effects are uncommon, represent an increase in risk from an already high baseline (e.g., an increase in risk of myocardial infarction or stroke in older patients), occur primarily in patient groups underrepresented in clinical trials (e.g., the elderly, children, or pregnant women), require many months or years to develop, occur primarily with co-administration of specific other drugs, and/or occur primarily in patients with a specific comorbidity or genotype.

TABLE 53-1 Conventional Pharmacology Compared to Pharmacoepidemiology

CONVENTIONAL PHARMACOLOGY	PHARMACOEPIDEMIOLOGY
Modest number of patients studied	Large populations of patients studied
Direct dose–response relationships	Define *probabilities* of benefit and risk
Focus on biology	Focus on behavior of prescribers and patients as well as biology
Outcomes over short time frame	Longer time frame of study
Rare events difficult to study	Able to identify rare events

TABLE 53-2 Important Withdrawals of Widely Used Drugs

TRADE NAME (GENERIC NAME)	REASON FOR WITHDRAWAL
Duract (bromfenac)	Hepatotoxicity
Posicor (mibefradil)	Hypotension, bradycardia
Fen-phen (fenfluramine/ phentermine)	Pulmonary hypertension, cardiac valvulopathy
Rezulin (troglitazone)	Hepatotoxicity
Baycol (cerivastatin)	Rhabdomyolysis
PPA (phenylpropanolamine)	Intracerebral hemorrhage
Vioxx (rofecoxib)	Myocardial infarction, stroke
Bextra (valdecoxib)	Stevens-Johnson syndrome, myocardial infarction

Sources of Pharmacoepidemiologic Data

Once a drug is in routine use, information about its adverse effects can come from a variety of sources. These include (1) spontaneous reports submitted to the FDA or manufacturer by physicians, other health professionals, or patients; (2) analysis of data sets assembled by large health care systems, government programs, or private insurers in the course of paying for prescriptions and clinical services; (3) ongoing registries of patients given a specific medication or with a given disease; and (4) individual ad hoc studies designed to answer a specific question. Each approach has its strengths and weaknesses, which must be considered in assessing the quality of the evidence derived from a particular source.

Spontaneous Reports

By default, spontaneous reports have been one of the most heavily relied-upon sources of information used by the FDA to track the adverse effects of marketed drugs. Such reports are submitted by practitioners or patients to drug makers or to the FDA, describing an adverse event in a single patient that may have been drug related. A strength of spontaneous reports is that they are often the first signal of an effect that was not previously suspected (e.g., cardiac valvulopathy in patients taking fenfluramine-type diet aids).

While such reports can be useful to generate new hypotheses, they have important limitations. First, the majority (90–99%) of drug-induced illness is never reported; this is true even for previously unknown, serious adverse effects. The rate of reporting is influenced heavily by the newness of a drug, by reports in the medical literature and lay media, and by other factors. Because such reports originate in undefined populations of users, it is difficult to learn much from their frequency—an important issue in trying to compare the rates of a particular known adverse effect between one drug and other members of the same class. Limited availability of clinical data about the reported case can also hamper efforts to assess confounders that may have distorted the drug–outcome relationship (see discussion below).

Automated Databases

Automated health care utilization databases have become increasingly important for defining associations among medications and adverse effects. Nearly all prescriptions filled by patients are recorded in computerized databases, often for billing purposes, making such databases some of the best "wired" components of the health care system. For many patients, individual clinical encounters (e.g., physician visits, hospitalizations, procedures, and diagnostic tests) are recorded for the same reason, usually with one or more associated diagnoses, in separate billing databases. Even when these services are delivered in an uncoordinated manner (as for most Medicare and Medicaid patients), the data trail produced makes it possible to measure the frequency of use of a given drug in a defined population of patients, as well as the frequency of specific outcomes (desired or undesired) in users of such drugs.

If a population is relatively well defined and stable (as may be the case in many public insurance programs and some nongovernmental health care systems), it is possible to evaluate exposures and outcomes systematically. The increasing availability of adequate clinical information in such data sets (e.g., diagnosis and number and length of hospitalizations for specific reasons) makes it possible to conduct rigorous studies of specific drug–outcome relationships, as described below. In the past, an important concern with the use of such utilization-based databases has been the limited and often unvalidated nature of the diagnostic information, particularly in the outpatient setting. Care is required in evaluating this diagnostic information. Whereas a filled prescription for a 30-day supply of simvastatin 30 mg is specified unambiguously in a pharmacy data file, the presence (or absence) of a code for depression or drug allergy or heart failure may represent a much wider spectrum of clinical reality. Some diagnoses can be made with certainty from computer-based claims data, such as a hip fracture repaired surgically or a hospitalization for myocardial infarction. Others may require validation of a computer-based diagnosis by reviewing the primary medical record. Fortunately, the quantity and quality of such information are growing, with more opportunities each year to link data from the text of medical notes, laboratory test results, and other elements of the patient record.

Patient Registries

For some drugs, the manufacturer is asked by the FDA to keep track of all patients (or a sample of all patients) who use the drug. This request may be made both to define and to prevent specific dangerous adverse effects (e.g., the agranulocytosis that can result from use of the antipsychotic medication **clozapine**).

Ad Hoc Studies

Some important questions in pharmacoepidemiology cannot be addressed by these methods but must instead be answered by collecting data de novo on particular groups of patients with a given disease or patients taking a particular class of medications. One example is the definition of sudden uncontrollable somnolence (sometimes called *sleep attacks*) in patients taking dopamine agonists for Parkinson's disease (PD). Such events were not systematically documented in most large clinical trials of these drugs and were not likely to be recorded as a new diagnosis in an office visit.

Determining whether some drugs are more likely to cause this problem than others required interviewing a large sample of PD patients using different classes of medications to define the details of the risk and point to means of reducing it (e.g., dose reduction).

Study Strategies

Once a source of pharmacoepidemiologic data has been identified, statistical methods are used to evaluate those data and reach conclusions about the associations between a drug and possible adverse effects. The two most common types of analyses used to evaluate these observational data are cohort studies and case-control studies. Each is designed to evaluate the likelihood that a particular adverse outcome is caused by use of a given drug.

Cohort and Case-Control Studies

In cohort studies, one identifies a group of patients exposed to a given drug (e.g., patients with arthritis treated with a particular NSAID) and a second group of patients who are as similar as possible to the exposed group but did not take the drug of interest (e.g., patients with arthritis of comparable severity who were treated with a different NSAID). Both groups are then followed over time to determine how many in each group develop an adverse effect of interest (e.g., myocardial infarction; Fig. 53-1). While this can be done on a real-time basis, more commonly, exposure (or nonexposure) that occurred in the past is defined from an existing database, so that subsequent events can be analyzed retrospectively. Cohort studies make it possible to measure actual incidence rates (i.e., the likelihood of a given outcome following use of a particular drug) and to track multiple outcomes. They also make it possible to restrict analyses to new users of a given medication, since "veteran" (prevalent) users are more likely to include those who have not experienced an adverse effect (or even died) as a result of the drug exposure. Such new-user designs also parallel the structure of a clinical trial more closely.

By contrast, in case-control studies, one first specifies the case-defining outcome event (e.g., myocardial infarction) and identifies a group of patients who have experienced that event; these are the cases. The controls are patients in the same population who are as similar as possible to the cases but have not had the outcome of interest (e.g., patients of similar age and gender, and with similar cardiac risk factors, who have not had a myocardial infarction). One then looks back in time prior to the occurrence of the event of interest (or its nonoccurrence, for controls) to review all the medications that were taken by cases and by controls to determine whether use of a given drug was higher than expected among cases than among controls (Fig. 53-1). The case-control design is more efficient than the cohort design if the outcome of interest is rare and one has to interview all study participants, because it is possible to focus on a selected group of patients known to have had the outcome of interest.

Evaluation of Risk

At the most basic level, cohort and case-control studies yield data that can be seen as comprising a *2 × 2* table defining the presence or absence of exposure to the drug of interest as well as the presence or absence of the adverse outcome. The data can be arranged in four cells, as shown in Figure 53-2: patients who took the drug of interest and had the outcome *(A)*, patients who took the drug but did not have

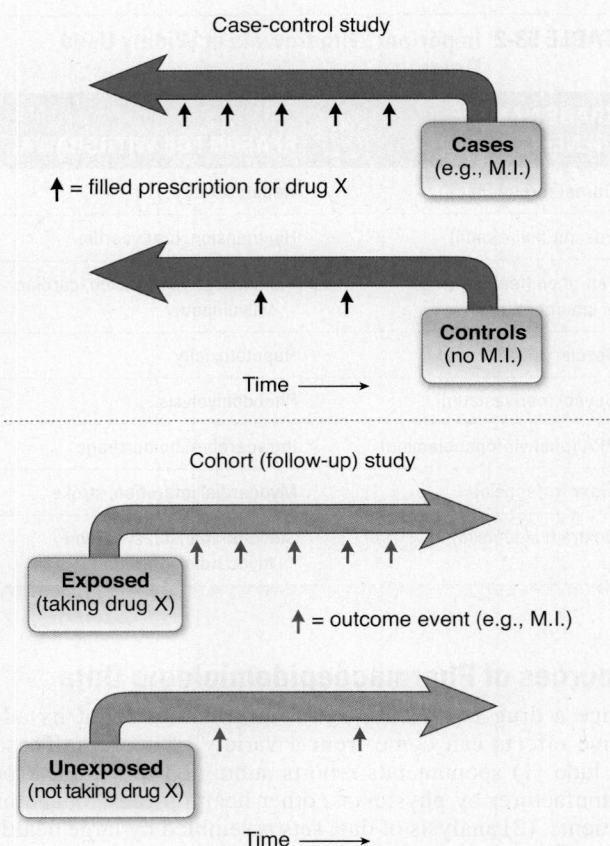

FIGURE 53-1. Schematic design of case-control and cohort studies. Top. In a case-control study, cases are identified as patients in a population who have experienced the outcome event of interest (e.g., myocardial infarction [*M.I.*]); controls are patients in the same population who are as similar as possible to the cases but have not had that outcome. All medications taken by cases and controls are then reviewed retrospectively to determine whether use of a given medication was higher among cases than among controls. **Bottom.** In a cohort study, two groups of patients are identified: those who are taking a given drug and another group who are as similar as possible to the exposed group but are not taking the drug of interest. All patients are followed over time to determine how many in each group develop a specified outcome event of interest (e.g., myocardial infarction).

the outcome *(B)*, patients who did not take the drug but had the outcome anyway *(C)*, and patients who did not take the drug and did not have the outcome *(D)*.

Cells *A* and *D* are concordant for the drug–outcome relationship, and cells *B* and *C* are discordant for this association. In simple terms, the product *A × D* divided by the product *B × C* reflects the strength of such an association. For cohort studies, this is referred to as the **relative risk**; for case-control studies (provided that the case outcome is not common), this is known as the **odds ratio**. A relative risk (or odds ratio) of 2 means that patients using the drug are twice as likely to have the outcome as patients not using the drug; a relative risk or odds ratio of 0.5 means that users of the drug are half as likely as nonusers to experience the outcome (i.e., the drug has a protective effect for that outcome).

Issues in Study Design and Interpretation

Although pharmacoepidemiology provides the capacity to assess drug outcomes in large populations of typical patients,

FIGURE 53-2. Basic analysis of data from case-control and cohort studies. The *2 × 2* table is defined by the presence or absence of exposure to the drug of interest as well as the presence or absence of the outcome of concern. Cells *A* to *D* include, respectively, patients who took the drug and had the outcome *(A)*, patients who took the drug but did not have the outcome *(B)*, patients who did not take the drug but had the outcome anyway *(C)*, and patients who did not take the drug and did not have the outcome *(D)*. In simple terms, the product *A × D* divided by the product *B × C* reflects the strength of the drug–outcome association. For case-control studies (provided that the case outcome is not common), this ratio is termed the *odds ratio*; for cohort studies, this ratio is termed the *relative risk*.

it should be noted that the use of one drug rather than another in routine care is determined by individual decisions—not at random, as would occur in a controlled clinical trial. This decision bias introduces the potential problem that patients given Drug A could differ systematically from those given Drug B—and that those differences, rather than differences in the drugs, could lead to a higher incidence of a particular outcome. Epidemiologists and statisticians have developed several strategies to correct for this problem of **confounding**, which is inherent in observational studies. The goal is to address the possibility that the drug does not cause the outcome of interest but appears associated with it because both are associated with a third confounding factor. For example, lung cancer is more common among coffee drinkers; this is not because coffee causes lung cancer, but because coffee drinkers are more likely to be smokers. To address confounding, researchers attempt to learn as much as possible about the characteristics of patients who use each drug regimen under study. Were the patients who were prescribed one drug older than patients given a comparator drug? Or sicker? Or more likely to be taking (or not taking) other medications that could influence the likelihood of a given outcome? For example, in a study comparing rates of myocardial infarction in patients taking **rofecoxib** (Vioxx®) with those taking **celecoxib** (Celebrex®), **ibuprofen** (Motrin®), or no NSAID, one would want to know as much as possible about the patients' history of cardiovascular disease as well as their cardiac risk factors. If these characteristics were evenly balanced across the users of the various drugs, there would not likely be a problem. However, if not (for example, if users of rofecoxib were more likely to be smokers than users of celecoxib, or less likely to take prophylactic doses of aspirin), this would have to be adjusted for in the analysis. Such adjustment can be accomplished by statistical techniques that include multiple regression, propensity scores, or instrumental variable methods.

Confounding by Indication

In a randomized trial, subjects are assigned arbitrarily to one treatment versus another. If the study is large enough and the randomization works adequately, differences in outcomes between subjects in the various study arms are likely to be the result of the different treatments they received because they were (by definition) similar in all other respects. By contrast, in an observational study, the researcher is obliged to study outcomes in patients for whom a physician has already chosen to prescribe one drug versus another versus no drug. It is therefore necessary to move beyond the simple *2 × 2* formulation described above, adjusting the observed relationships so as to control for differences that may have existed before the patients took the drugs under study.

For example, patients who take antihypertensive medications are likely to have more cardiovascular disease than a group of age- and sex-matched people in the same community who do not take antihypertensive medications. Of course, this is not because blood pressure medicines cause heart disease; on the contrary, antihypertensive medications reduce the risk of cardiovascular disease (including heart failure, myocardial infarction, and stroke) in such patients. But while these medications reduce the risk of heart disease, they do not reduce it to zero. Furthermore, many patients with hypertension start therapy later in life, or do not adhere adequately to their prescribed regimens. As a result, antihypertensive medication users overall have a *higher* rate of heart disease than demographically identical individuals who do not take blood pressure medication. This problem is known as *confounding by indication*.

Selection Bias

A second problem is produced by the fact that in routine care, patients' drug use is determined by their physicians and not by a research protocol. For example, when **fluoxetine** (Prozac®) first introduced the selective serotonin reuptake inhibitor (SSRI) class of antidepressants in the late 1980s, reports emerged that depressed patients given the new drug were more likely to commit suicide than patients taking older antidepressants such as the tricyclic antidepressants (**amitriptyline**, **nortriptyline**, **desipramine**). Indeed, concern persists (based on placebo-controlled randomized trials) that SSRIs may precipitate suicidal thoughts or attempts in some patients, especially adolescents and children. However, the early reports of increased risk suggest that **selection bias** could provide an alternative explanation for suicide in fluoxetine users. Patients doing well on older antidepressants would have been less likely to be switched to the newer drug when it was first marketed; use of a novel medication would have occurred disproportionately more in depressed patients who were not doing well—including, perhaps, those who were continuing to consider suicide. Moreover, the lethal dose (LD_{50}; see Chapter 2, Pharmacodynamics) for the older drugs is low because of their cardiovascular toxicity, whereas it is much more difficult to ingest enough SSRI for a fatal overdose. Thus, a physician would prefer a potentially suicidal patient to have a supply of fluoxetine at home rather than a supply of tricyclic antidepressant. Whatever the underlying risk of suicide caused by either drug, these factors alone would combine to create a profile of higher suicide rates among new fluoxetine users compared to tricyclic antidepressant users in an observational assessment.

The Healthy User Effect

Several epidemiologic studies of drug use and outcomes have defined relationships that have not been borne out in randomized controlled trials. These include reduced rates of cardiac disease, incontinence, and depression in women taking postmenopausal estrogen and reduced rates of cancer and Alzheimer's disease in patients taking statins. Such studies are often flawed by what has been called the "healthy user" effect. Patients who are regular users of any preventive medication appear to be different from those who do not exhibit this behavior: they are more likely to visit their doctor seeking preventive therapy, or are at least open to receiving it, and their physicians are sufficiently prevention oriented to write such a prescription. Such patients are probably also more likely to engage in other health-promoting behaviors, such as tobacco avoidance, weight control, exercise, and adherence to their other prescribed drug regimens. These characteristics likely exist to an even greater extent among patients who adhere faithfully to the prescribed regimen for a prolonged period of time.

Several large randomized trials have proven a similar point: patients randomized to placebo who adhere well to their dummy pill "regimen" have better outcomes (including mortality) than patients who do not adhere well to their placebo "regimen." Because the content of the placebo could not have produced this effect, these findings provide clear evidence that patients who consistently behave in a health-promoting manner are more likely to have better clinical outcomes, apart from any therapeutic effect of a specific drug in their regimen. To address this issue in observational studies, some research groups use only "active controls" as comparator groups—for example, comparing patients adherent to statin regimens with patients adherent to regimens of other preventive drugs rather than simply comparing such patients with patients who are not regular statin users.

Interpreting Statistical Significance

In evaluating the results of both observational studies and randomized trials, it is conventional to use a p value of 0.05 as a threshold or benchmark for statistical significance. This criterion is often mistakenly interpreted to mean that a finding is "real" if the p value for the difference between groups is less than that value and "not real" if it is greater than that value. However, more sophisticated readers of the literature understand that such a cut point is largely arbitrary (compared to, for example, a p value of 0.03 or 0.07), and that attention must also be paid to the magnitude of the difference. For example, a $p < 0.05$ difference between a new drug and placebo may be clinically meaningless if there is only a 2% difference in effect size.

The situation is even more critical in assessing the statistical significance of data about adverse events, whether from a randomized trial or from an observational analysis. It is useful to recall that the p value is determined by both sample size and the magnitude of an observed difference. Most clinical trials are powered to be large enough to detect a difference between a study drug and its comparator in producing a clinical outcome that is relatively common (e.g., reduction in blood pressure or LDL cholesterol level). As a result, however, such studies are not likely to have adequate power to find a statistically significant difference between groups for outcomes that are much more rare (e.g., hepatotoxicity). Adherence to a "$p < 0.05$" standard for uncommon adverse effects can lead to dismissal of important risks that a study may not have been powered to detect.

The solution is not to embrace all differences in adverse effect rates regardless of their statistical properties. Instead, it is to consider such rate differences thoughtfully and to seek additional evidence to clarify worrisome relationships even if they are not "significant" in p-value terms. For example, when the FDA was evaluating the risk of suicidal thoughts and actions in adolescents and children taking SSRI antidepressants in placebo-controlled trials, the rates of these relatively rare outcomes were generally higher in the treated patients than in those randomized to placebo. Each individual study did not find a $p < 0.05$ level of significance for these differences. However, when the data from all such trials were aggregated (in some cases, years after the studies were completed), it became clear that the risk across all studies was clear and consistent (and also met the conventional $p < 0.05$ level).

The opposite problem arises when considering the statistical significance of data from large population-based epidemiologic studies. Here, sample size (power) is not a limitation, especially when studies employ data on several hundred thousand patients through use of an automated claims database. A 4% or 5% difference in rates of a given effect (either therapeutic or adverse) may achieve a p value < 0.001, simply because of the huge size of the population studied. But here, even if the finding appears to have statistical significance, a difference of such small magnitude may have little or no clinical importance.

ADVERSE DRUG EFFECTS AND THE HEALTH CARE SYSTEM

The series of safety-related withdrawals of commonly used drugs in the 1990s and early 2000s led to renewed interest in developing ways to prevent such problems, or at least to limit the number of patients exposed to risk by identifying adverse effects earlier. As a result, the concept of *risk management* has become an important theme in drug development and regulation.

Balancing Benefits and Risks

As noted above, new products are often not compared with existing alternatives when they are evaluated for approval, and such studies are not commonly performed after approval either. For drugs with known risks, it is therefore difficult to know whether an adverse effect occurs more commonly with a new drug than with another drug in the same class (e.g., gastrointestinal hemorrhage with nonselective NSAIDs, or rhabdomyolysis with statins). A higher rate of a given adverse event might be acceptable for a particular drug if it were accompanied by substantially higher efficacy. In this case, however, the absence of head-to-head clinical trials makes it difficult to make such an evaluation. Thus, in most instances, the individual clinician is left to make therapeutic decisions without the data needed to make such choices rigorously. A recent development designed to remedy this problem is the movement toward **comparative effectiveness** research—a program of publicly funded studies that systematically evaluate therapies against one another. This program was initiated in 2009 with a $1.1 billion federal investment and is expected to be an important ongoing component of the research agendas of several federal agencies.

The clinical use of medications is heavily influenced by the $30 billion spent annually by the pharmaceutical industry to market its products. This expenditure is heavily "front-end loaded," with vast sums spent soon after a drug is launched in order to maximize sales for as many years as possible while the company's patent is still in effect. Ironically, this means that the heaviest promotion of a drug occurs during the period in which there is least experience with its use and effects in the population as a whole. At the time of approval, there may not be much (or even any) information in the peer-reviewed literature about a drug's efficacy and safety, so promotional sources of information are often the primary means by which physicians learn about new products. Industry critics have argued that these materials often emphasize therapeutic benefits more persuasively than they communicate risk. As an alternative, several innovative programs have emerged that provide prescribers with noncommercial, publicly funded "marketing" of evidence-based data about drug benefits, risks, and costs, known as *academic detailing* (e.g., see www.NaRCAD.org and www.alosafoundation.org).

Role of the FDA

Just as the thalidomide tragedy of the early 1960s helped spark a wave of regulatory reforms that gave the FDA new authority to demand proof of efficacy before a drug was approved, the 2004 withdrawal of rofecoxib (Vioxx®) also led to calls for regulatory reform, particularly in the way adverse events are detected and followed up. One area of vigorous debate was the FDA's lack of clear authority to require postmarketing studies of drug risks. While the agency holds considerable sway over manufacturers during the initial drug approval process, it has had little power to compel further study of a drug once it is on the market. Governmental reviews have demonstrated that, even when postmarketing safety studies are mandated at the time of approval, they are often not completed or even initiated (see above). This helps explain the tardiness with which important adverse effects have been detected and acted on. Rationalizing the national response to this problem has become a key goal for public policy. In 2007, the **FDA Amendments Act** gave the agency the authority and responsibility to perform its own systematic surveillance of adverse events of marketed drugs, to alter a drug's official labeling to warn of safety risks (such authority was previously in the hands of the manufacturer), and to compel drug companies to conduct follow-up studies of potential safety concerns. That legislation also mandated and funded the creation of a nationwide "Sentinel System" to use large existing automated data sets from a variety of health care delivery systems to conduct ongoing postmarketing drug safety surveillance. Within a few years, the system was expanded to include data describing the medication use and clinical encounters of more than 100 million (anonymized) patients, making it a valuable tool for the systematic detection of adverse drug effects far earlier than had previously been possible.

Legal and Ethical Issues

The drug safety controversies of recent years (see Table 53-2) have caused many in the medical profession, the government, and the public to ask how responsibility should be apportioned for discovering and acting on important adverse effect data. There is a growing consensus that, in addition to greater vigilance on the part of the FDA, a drug's manufacturer should also be expected to serve as "steward of its molecule," responsible for proactive research into possible harms beyond the minimum required by law. Juries and courts have agreed with this notion; legal settlements exceeded $1 billion for **cerivastatin** (Baycol®) and $21 billion for **dexfenfluramine** (Redux®), even in the absence of criminal convictions.

■ CONCLUSION AND FUTURE DIRECTIONS

Increasing availability and detail of electronic data defining drug use and clinical events in very large populations, coupled with advances in epidemiology and developments in the fields of informatics and data processing, have made it possible to perform sophisticated surveillance of the outcomes of routine medication use with rigor and efficiency. These data are being made even more useful by advanced methodological tools, such as propensity scores and instrumental variables, to improve control for confounding in observational studies. Pharmacoepidemiologic analyses based on these developments can form the foundation for decisions—made both at the bedside and at policy levels—based on science rather than on hunches, fear, or hype. These databases and epidemiologic tools also hold potential for defining comparative drug effectiveness by using the same tools to measure desired clinical outcomes across agents. Thus, observational studies make possible the head-to-head comparison of medications that is not required by the approval process but that is central to the informational needs of prescribers, patients, and payors.

From a biological perspective, the systematic detection of adverse effects will further benefit from the development of research tools to predict the toxicities of new compounds more accurately and to flag them for intensive surveillance once a drug is marketed. In addition, pharmacogenomics (see Chapter 7, Pharmacogenomics) is addressing many of these questions from the perspective of inherited differences in drug metabolism (pharmacokinetics) and drug responses (pharmacodynamics).

Suggested Reading

Avorn J. *Powerful medicines: the benefits, risks, and costs of prescription drugs.* New York: Knopf; 2005. (*An examination of the interrelationships among pharmacology, clinical practice, epidemiology, industry, and drug policy.*)

Avorn J. The promise of pharmacoepidemiology in helping clinicians assess drug risk. *Circulation* 2013;128:745–748. (*An assessment of how observational methods can be used to define medication safety problems, using anticoagulants as an example.*)

Eichler HG, Oye K, Baird LG, et al. Adaptive licensing: taking the next step in the evolution of drug approval. *Clin Pharmacol Ther* 2012;91:426–437. (*A proposal to integrate epidemiologic assessment into the evaluation of drug effectiveness and toxicity.*)

Gagne JJ, Wang SV, Rassen JA, Schneeweiss S. A modular, prospective, semi-automated drug safety monitoring system for use in a distributed data environment. *Pharmacoepidemiol Drug Saf* 2014;23:619–627. (*A new method for automating analysis of large clinical data sets to detect adverse effects more rapidly.*)

Psaty BM, Breckenridge AM. Mini-Sentinel and regulatory science—big data rendered fit and functional. *N Engl J Med* 2014;370:2165–2167. (*An overview of current programs to harness routine clinical data to monitor drug safety.*)

Schneeweiss S, Rassen JA, Glynn RJ, Avorn J, Mogun H, Brookhart MA. High-dimensional propensity score adjustment in studies of treatment effects using health care claims data. *Epidemiology* 2009;20:512–522. (*Description of an innovative approach to use large-scale electronic databases to study the outcomes of marketed drugs.*)

Strom BL, Kimmel SE, Hennessey S, eds. *Textbook of pharmacoepidemiology.* West Sussex, United Kingdom: Wiley-Blackwell; 2013. (*A comprehensive textbook of pharmacoepidemiology.*)

IX

Surface erosion

Bulk erosion

Frontiers in Pharmacology

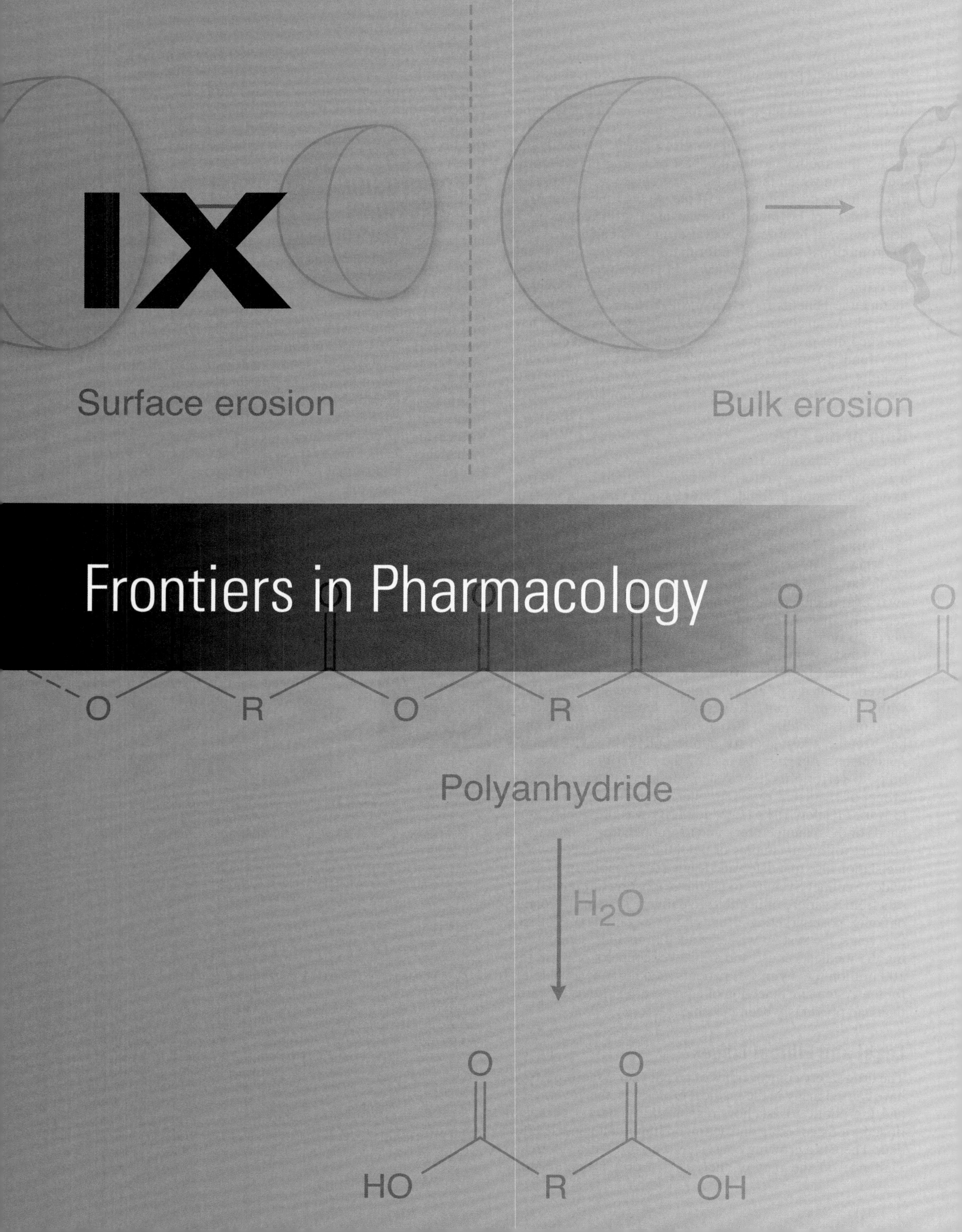

Polyanhydride

H_2O

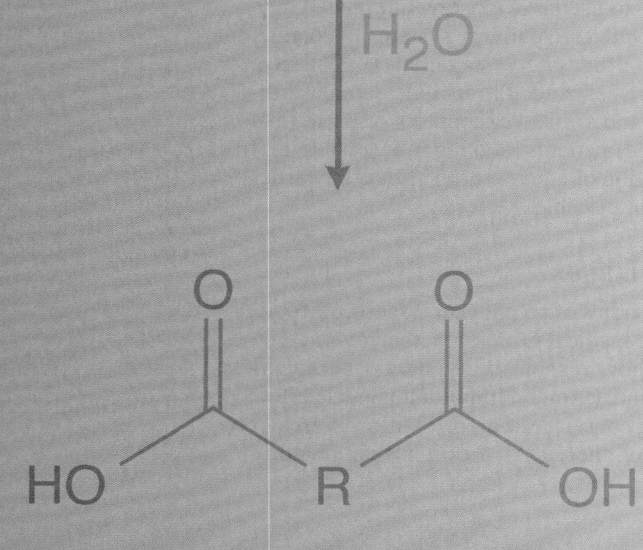

PROTEIN	TRADE NAME	FUNCTION	EXAMPLES OF CLINICAL
Endocrine Disorders (Hormone Deficiencies)			
Insulin	Humulin Novolin	Regulates blood glucose, shifts potassium into cells	Diabetes mellitus, diabetic ketoacidosis, hyperkalemia
Insulin human inhalation	Exubera (withdrawn from market in 2008) Afrezza (FDA approved in 2014)	Insulin formulated for inhalation with faster onset of action	
Insulin aspart Insulin glulisine Insulin lispro	Novolog (aspart) Apidra (glulisine) Humalog (lispro)	Insulin analogues with faster onset of action and shorter duration of action	Diabetes mellitus
Isophane insulin	NPH	Insulin protamine crystalline formulation with somewhat slower onset of action and longer duration of action	Diabetes mellitus
Insulin detemir Insulin glargine	Levemir (detemir) Basaglar (glargine) Lantus (glargine)	Insulin analogues with slower onset of action and longer duration of action	Diabetes mellitus
Insulin zinc extended	Lente Ultralente	Insulin zinc hexameric complex with slower onset of action and longer duration of action	Diabetes mellitus
Pramlintide	Symlin	Mechanism unknown	... combinat...

54

Protein Therapeutics

Quentin J. Baca, Benjamin Leader, and David E. Golan

◼ INTRODUCTION

Proteins have the most dynamic and diverse roles of any macromolecules in the body, catalyzing biochemical reactions, constituting receptors and channels in membranes, providing intracellular and extracellular scaffolding support, and transporting molecules within a cell or from one organ to another. According to current estimates, there are approximately 19,000–20,000 protein-coding genes in the human genome, and with alternative splicing of genes and post-translational modification of proteins (e.g., by cleavage, phosphorylation, acylation and glycosylation), the number of functionally distinct proteins is likely to be greater than 100,000. Viewed from the perspective of disease mechanisms, these estimates pose an immense challenge to modern medicine, as disease may result when any one of these proteins contains mutations or other abnormalities or is present in an abnormally high or low concentration. Viewed from the perspective of therapeutics, however, these estimates represent a tremendous opportunity in terms of harnessing protein therapeutics to alleviate disease. At present, more than 206 different proteins or peptides are approved for clinical use by the US Food and Drug Administration (FDA), and many more are in development.

Protein therapeutics have several advantages over small-molecule drugs. First, proteins often serve a highly specific and complex set of functions that cannot be mimicked by simple chemical compounds. Second, because the action of proteins is highly specific, there is often less potential for protein therapeutics to interfere with normal biological processes and cause adverse effects. Third, because the body naturally produces many of the proteins that are used as therapeutics, these agents are often well tolerated and are less likely to elicit immune responses. Fourth, for diseases in which a gene is mutated or deleted, protein therapeutics can provide effective replacement treatment without the need for gene therapy, which is not currently available for most genetic disorders. Fifth, the clinical development and FDA approval time of protein therapeutics may be faster than that of small-molecule drugs. A study published in 2003 showed that the average clinical development and approval time was more than 1 year faster for 33 protein therapeutics approved between 1980 and 2002 than for 294 small-molecule drugs approved during the same time period. Sixth, because proteins are unique in form and function, companies are able to obtain far-reaching patent protection for protein therapeutics. Seventh, many protein therapeutics address unmet needs for rare diseases and are eligible for orphan drug designation, which can provide priority review by the FDA and extended patent protection terms. Last, the total sales of protein therapeutics are continuing to trend upward. In the year 2000, no protein therapeutics were represented in the top 20 drugs sold in the United States. In 2013, protein therapeutics comprised four of the top ten pharmaceuticals by sales in the United States and seven of the top ten pharmaceuticals by sales worldwide. The last four advantages make proteins attractive from a financial perspective compared with small-molecule drugs.

A relatively small number of protein therapeutics are purified from their native sources, such as **pancreatic enzymes** from hog and pig pancreas and **α-1-proteinase inhibitor** from pooled human plasma. Instead, most therapeutic proteins are now produced by recombinant DNA technology and purified from a wide range of organisms. Production systems for recombinant proteins include bacteria, yeast, insect cells, mammalian cells, and transgenic animals and plants. The system of choice can be dictated by the cost of production or the modifications of the protein (e.g., glycosylation, phosphorylation, or proteolytic cleavage) that are required for biological activity. For example, bacteria do not perform glycosylation reactions, and each of the other biological systems listed above produces a different type or pattern of glycosylation. Protein glycosylation patterns can have a dramatic effect on the activity, half-life, and immunogenicity

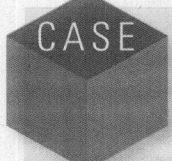

CASE

MR is a 55-year-old traveling salesman who presents to the emergency department of a small rural hospital with left-sided chest pain and light-headedness. The pain started suddenly 1 hour ago when he was carrying a large box. At first, MR felt as if he was going to pass out, but the pain and light-headedness improved at rest and eventually resolved after 20 minutes. MR denies any other symptoms, and he has no history of medical problems. He takes no medications, he is not a smoker, and his father died unexpectedly in a car accident at age 53. On physical exam, MR is afebrile with heart rate 100 beats/min, blood pressure 150/90 mm Hg, and respiratory rate 16 breaths/min. His pulse oximeter displays 96% with oxygen flowing at 2 liters per minute by nasal cannula. He appears to be comfortable, and the remainder of his physical exam is notable only for an S4 heart sound. His ECG demonstrates sinus tachycardia with no ST segment elevation. His chest x-ray is normal. His STAT chemistry panel shows normal sodium, potassium, chloride, bicarbonate, blood urea nitrogen (BUN), and creatinine levels. Cardiac biomarkers and coagulation studies are pending. MR is given aspirin, metoprolol, and sublingual nitroglycerin upon his arrival in the emergency department.

While waiting in the emergency department, MR's troponin T level returns at 1.34 ng/mL (normal, 0–0.1 ng/mL), he again develops chest pain, and a repeat EKG shows 2-mm ST segment depression in

leads V1–V3. At this time, he is also given heparin, abciximab, and clopidogrel, and his chest pain resolves. He is admitted to the hospital and his clinical course is stable overnight.

The next day, however, MR develops crushing substernal chest pain and diaphoresis, and his ECG shows 4-mm ST segment elevation in leads V2–V4. Because cardiac catheterization is not available at the regional cardiac center for at least 4 hours, MR is given tenecteplase in the coronary care unit, and his aspirin, metoprolol, nitroglycerin, heparin, and clopidogrel are continued. He stabilizes on this regimen.

After an otherwise uneventful 5-day hospitalization, MR is transferred to the regional cardiac center for catheterization, with a diagnosis of unstable angina that evolved into an ST elevation myocardial infarction. Outpatient plans include cardiac rehabilitation and treatment with aspirin, metoprolol, enalapril, spironolactone, and sublingual nitroglycerin as needed.

Questions

1. By what mechanism does tenecteplase act?
2. How does the action of tenecteplase differ from that of heparin?
3. By what mechanism does abciximab act?
4. How could abciximab augment the function of clopidogrel and aspirin in this case?

---

of the recombinant protein in the body. For example, the half-life of native **erythropoietin**, a growth factor important in erythrocyte production, can be lengthened by increasing the glycosylation of the protein. **Darbepoetin-α** is an erythropoietin analogue that is engineered to contain two additional amino acids that are substrates for N-linked glycosylation reactions. When expressed in Chinese hamster ovary cells, the analogue is synthesized with five rather than three N-linked carbohydrate chains; this modification causes the half-life of darbepoetin to be three times longer than that of erythropoietin.

Perhaps the best example of trends in the production and use of protein therapeutics is provided by the history of insulin in the treatment of **type 1** and **type 2 diabetes mellitus**. Untreated, type 1 diabetes is a disease that leads to severe wasting and death due to lack of the protein hormone insulin, which signals cells to perform numerous functions related to glucose homeostasis and intermediary metabolism. In 1922, insulin was first purified from bovine and porcine pancreas and used as a life-saving daily injection for patients with type 1 diabetes. At least three problems hindered the widespread use of this protein therapy: first, the availability of animal pancreases for purification of insulin; second, the cost of insulin purification from animal pancreas; and third, the immunological reaction of some patients to animal insulin. These problems were addressed by isolating the human

insulin gene and engineering *Escherichia coli* to express human insulin by using recombinant DNA technology. By growing vast quantities of these bacteria, large-scale production of human insulin was achieved. The resulting insulin was abundant, inexpensive, of low immunogenicity, and free from other animal pancreatic substances. **Recombinant insulin**, approved by the FDA in 1982, was the first commercially available recombinant protein therapeutic and has been the major therapy for type 1 diabetes (and a major therapy for type 2 diabetes) ever since.

Recombinantly produced proteins can have several further benefits compared with nonrecombinant proteins. First, transcription and translation of an exact human gene can lead to a higher specific activity of the protein and a decreased chance of immunological rejection. Second, recombinant proteins are often produced more efficiently and inexpensively and in potentially limitless quantity. One striking example is found in the protein-based therapy for Gaucher's disease, a chronic congenital disorder of lipid metabolism caused by a deficiency of the enzyme **β-glucocerebrosidase** (also known as *glucosylceramidase*) that is characterized by an enlarged liver and spleen, increased skin pigmentation, and painful bone lesions. At first, β-glucocerebrosidase purified from human placenta was used to treat this disease, but this requires purification of protein from 50,000 placentas per patient per year, which clearly places a practical limit on the amount of purified protein available. A recombinant form of β-glucocerebrosidase was subsequently developed and introduced, which is not only available in sufficient quantities to treat many more patients with the disease but also eliminates the risk of transmissible (e.g., viral or prion) diseases associated with purifying the protein from human placentas. This also illustrates a third benefit of recombinant proteins over nonrecombinant proteins—the reduction of exposure to animal or human diseases.

A fourth advantage is that recombinant technology allows the modification of a protein or the selection of a particular gene variant to improve function or specificity. Again, recombinant β-glucocerebrosidase provides an interesting example. When this protein is made recombinantly, a change of amino acid arginine-495 to histidine allows the addition of mannose residues to the protein. The mannose is recognized by endocytic carbohydrate receptors on macrophages and many other cell types, allowing the enzyme to enter these cells more efficiently and to cleave the intracellular lipid that has accumulated in pathological amounts, which results in an improved therapeutic outcome. Last, recombinant technology allows the engineering and production of proteins that provide a novel function or activity, as discussed below.

The more than 30 years since the approval of recombinant insulin by the FDA have seen a remarkable expansion in the number of therapeutic applications of proteins. More than 206 unique proteins (over 160 of which are produced recombinantly) are currently approved for clinical use by the FDA, and many more are in development.

USES OF PROTEINS IN MEDICINE

An appreciation of the many therapeutic uses of proteins may be facilitated by categorizing such therapies according to their mechanism of action. In this chapter, we summarize currently approved protein therapeutics using a classification system that is based on their pharmacologic action (Box 54-1). Examples of protein therapeutics in each category and clinical conditions in which they are used are discussed in the text, and a listing of FDA-approved protein therapies and their functions and clinical uses is presented in Tables 54-1 through 54-5. Examples of protein-based vaccines and diagnostics, which also highlight

---

BOX 54-1 Functional Classification of Protein Therapeutics

Protein therapeutics in the tables are organized by function and therapeutic application. The numbers of therapeutics per group reflect the relative difficulty associated with drug development across the various classes of protein therapeutics. Every effort has been made to include in these tables all US Food and Drug Administration (FDA)-approved Group I and Group II protein-based therapies. Groups III and IV present selected examples that highlight the use of proteins in vaccines and diagnostic agents.

Group I: Enzymes and Regulatory Proteins

- Ia: Replacing a protein that is deficient or abnormal (Table 54-1)
- Ib: Augmenting an existing pathway (Table 54-2)
- Ic: Providing a novel function or activity (Table 54-3)

Endocrine and metabolic disorders with defined molecular etiologies dominate Group Ia. As more diseases are linked to deficiencies of specific proteins, this class will continue to grow. Group Ib is dominated by therapies that augment hematological and endocrine pathways and immune responses. The many interferon and growth factor therapies in Group Ib effectively treat disease even when their precise pharmacologic mechanism of action is unknown. Group Ic demonstrates the rational use of naturally occurring proteins to modify the pathophysiology of human diseases. The future growth of this class depends on understanding protein function in human physiology as well as protein function in other organisms.

Group II: Targeted Proteins

- IIa: Interfering with a molecule or organism (Table 54-4)
- IIb: Delivering other compounds or proteins (Table 54-5)

Group IIa therapeutics use their special targeting activity to interfere with molecules or organisms by binding specifically to them and blocking their function, targeting them for destruction, or stimulating a signaling pathway. This group has grown as monoclonal antibody technology has matured and will expand further as signaling pathways and etiologies of disease are more clearly identified. Group IIb therapeutics deliver other compounds or proteins to a specific site. This class has great potential to grow, as demonstrated by the breadth of the specifically targeted Group IIa therapies.

Group III: Protein Vaccines

- IIIa: Protecting against a deleterious foreign agent (Table 54-6)
- IIIb: Treating an autoimmune disease (Table 54-6)
- IIIc: Treating cancer (Table 54-6)

Although this is currently a small class of therapies, there is great potential for the production of recombinant vaccines that provide broad protection against infectious agents. Similarly, individualized vaccines against cancers are likely to be in great demand. Selected examples of the more than 80 FDA-approved vaccines in Table 54-6 highlight the use of recombinant protein technology in vaccine production. Many of the FDA-approved vaccines protect against multiple infectious agents and include synthetic, recombinant, and purified protein components. A complete list of FDA-approved vaccines may be found at http://www.fda.gov/BiologicsBloodVaccines/Vaccines/ApprovedProducts.

Group IV: Protein Diagnostics

Protein diagnostics, of which selected examples are shown in Table 54-7, are a class that powerfully affects clinical decision making. These diagnostics use technology and therapeutics developed in other classes to answer clinical questions. This table presents primarily in vivo protein diagnostics, but in vitro protein diagnostics are also critical to medical decision making and are too numerous to address comprehensively here. ■

the growing importance of proteins in medicine, are provided in Tables 54-6 and 54-7.

Group I: Enzymes and Regulatory Proteins

Protein therapeutics in this group function by a classic paradigm in which a specific endogenous protein is deficient, and the deficit is then remedied by treatment with exogenous protein. Protein therapeutics classified in Group Ia are used to replace a particular activity in cases of protein deficiency or abnormal protein production. These proteins are used in a range of conditions, from providing lactase in patients lacking this gastrointestinal enzyme to replacing vital blood-clotting factors such as **factor VIII** and **factor IX** in hemophiliacs. A classic example, as mentioned above, is the use of **insulin** for the treatment of diabetes. Another important example is in the treatment of **cystic fibrosis**, a common and often lethal genetic disorder. In this disease, defects in the chloride channel encoded by the *CFTR* gene lead to abnormally thick secretions, which can (among other effects) block pancreatic enzymes from travelling down the pancreatic duct into the duodenum. This prevents food from being properly digested and results in malnutrition. Patients with cystic fibrosis are often treated with a combination of pancreatic enzymes isolated from pigs—including lipases, amylases, and proteases—that allow the digestion of lipids, sugars, and proteins. Patients who have had their pancreas removed or who suffer from chronic pancreatitis can also benefit from this therapy. Other striking examples include various diseases caused by metabolic enzyme deficiencies, such as Gaucher's disease as mentioned above, mucopolysaccharidosis, **Fabry disease**, and others. Additional protein therapies that replace a particular activity are listed in Table 54-1.

It may sometimes be desirable to enhance the magnitude or timing of a particular normal protein activity, and protein therapeutics classified in Group Ib are administered to achieve this. Such protein therapeutics have been successful in treating hematopoietic defects; the most prominent example is recombinant **erythropoietin**, a protein hormone secreted by the kidney that stimulates erythrocyte production in the bone marrow. In patients with chemotherapy-induced anemia, recombinant erythropoietin is used to increase erythrocyte production and thereby ameliorate the anemia. In patients with chronic kidney disease, whose levels of endogenous erythropoietin are below normal, recombinant protein is administered to correct this deficiency. Another example is provided by the use of **granulocyte** or **granulocyte-macrophage colony-stimulating factor** (**G-CSF** or **GM-CSF**, respectively) to treat patients with chemotherapy-induced neutropenia. G-CSF and GM-CSF stimulate the bone marrow to increase the number of neutrophils produced, which allows these patients to better combat microbial infections. Similarly, patients with chronic immune thrombocytopenia can be treated with **romiplostim**, a thrombopoietin receptor agonist that increases platelet production and thereby prevents bleeding complications.

In vitro fertilization (IVF) is another area in which Group Ib proteins are applied. Increased levels of **follicle-stimulating hormone** (**FSH**) are normally produced by the anterior pituitary gland just before ovulation. These high levels of FSH can be enhanced by treatment with recombinant FSH, leading to maturation of an increased number of follicles and to an increased number of oocytes available for IVF. Similarly, recombinant **human chorionic gonadotropin** (**HCG**) is used in assisted reproductive technology to promote follicle rupture, a process that must occur before the oocytes can be transported into the fallopian tubes for fertilization.

Group Ib proteins can also have life-saving effects on thrombosis and hemostasis. **Alteplase** (recombinant tissue plasminogen activator [tPA]) is used to treat life-threatening blood clots in conditions such as coronary artery occlusion, acute ischemic stroke, and pulmonary embolism. Endogenous tPA is secreted by the endothelial cells that line blood vessels. The secreted tPA normally cleaves plasminogen to plasmin, which then degrades fibrin and thereby lyses fibrin-based clots. Although endogenous tPA may be present at normal or even increased levels near the site of a blood clot, administration of relatively large amounts of exogenous tPA may be required to disrupt these clots. **Reteplase**, a genetically modified form of recombinant tPA, is used to treat acute myocardial infarction, and **tenecteplase**, another genetically engineered derivative of tPA, has greater specificity than tPA for binding to plasminogen and therefore causes more efficacious lysis of fibrin in blood clots. In the introductory case, MR received tenecteplase when his unstable angina evolved into an ST elevation myocardial infarction. Supraphysiologic levels of coagulation **factor VIIa** may catalyze thrombosis and thereby stop life-threatening bleeding in patients with **hemophilia A** or **B**. Studies have suggested that recombinant **activated protein C** can improve immunoregulation and prevent excessive clotting reactions in patients with severe, life-threatening sepsis and organ dysfunction. Many other Group Ib protein therapeutics are also used for immunoregulation—chronic **hepatitis B** and **C**, **Kaposi's sarcoma**, melanoma, and some types of leukemia and lymphoma have been treated with various forms of **interferon**, as noted in Table 54-2. Other disease states treated with Group Ib proteins are summarized in Table 54-2.

Occasionally, the activity of a particular protein is desirable even though the body does not normally express that activity. Protein therapeutics classified in Group Ic include foreign proteins with novel functions and endogenous proteins that act at a novel time or place in the body. **Papain**, for example, is a protease purified from the *Carica papaya* fruit. This protein is used therapeutically to degrade proteinaceous debris in wounds. **Collagenase**, obtained from fermentation by *Clostridium histolyticum*, can be used to digest collagen in the necrotic base of wounds. The protease-mediated debridement or removal of necrotic tissue is useful in the treatment of burns, pressure ulcers, postoperative wounds, carbuncles, and other types of wounds. Collagenase can also be used to digest subcutaneous collagen that contributes to the debilitating hand deformity known as *Dupuytren's contracture*. Recombinant human **deoxyribonuclease I** (**DNAse1**) has an interesting novel use. Normally found inside human cells, this recombinant enzyme can be used to degrade the DNA left over from dying neutrophils in the respiratory tract of patients with cystic fibrosis. Such DNA could otherwise form mucus plugs that obstruct the respiratory tract and lead to pulmonary fibrosis, bronchiectasis, and recurrent pneumonias. Thus, recombinant protein technology has allowed the therapeutic application of a normally intracellular enzyme in a novel extracellular environment.

There are many other successful examples of this approach to protein therapy. For instance, certain forms of acute lymphoblastic leukemia are unable to synthesize asparagine and therefore require the availability of this amino acid to survive.

TABLE 54-1 Protein Therapeutics Replacing a Protein That Is Deficient or Abnormal (Group Ia)

PROTEIN	TRADE NAME	FUNCTION	EXAMPLES OF CLINICAL USE
Endocrine Disorders (Hormone Deficiencies)			
‡Insulin	Humulin Novolin	Regulates blood glucose, shifts potassium into cells	Diabetes mellitus, diabetic ketoacidosis, hyperkalemia
‡Insulin human inhalation	Exubera (withdrawn from market in 2008) Afrezza (FDA approved in 2014)	Insulin formulated for inhalation with faster onset of action	Diabetes mellitus
‡Insulin aspart ‡Insulin glulisine ‡Insulin lispro	Novolog (aspart) Apidra (glulisine) Humalog (lispro)	Insulin analogues with faster onset of action and shorter duration of action	Diabetes mellitus
‡Isophane insulin	NPH	Insulin protamine crystalline formulation with somewhat slower onset of action and longer duration of action	Diabetes mellitus
‡Insulin detemir ‡Insulin glargine	Levemir (detemir) Basaglar (glargine) Lantus (glargine)	Insulin analogues with slower onset of action and longer duration of action	Diabetes mellitus
‡Insulin zinc extended	Lente Ultralente	Insulin zinc hexameric complex with slower onset of action and longer duration of action	Diabetes mellitus
Pramlintide	Symlin	Mechanism unknown; recombinant synthetic peptide analogue of human amylin (a naturally occurring neuroendocrine hormone regulating postprandial glucose control)	Diabetes mellitus, in combination with insulin
Metreleptin	Myalept	Synthetic analogue of the hormone leptin, which regulates satiety and metabolic rate	Leptin deficiency, in addition to diet, in patients with congenital generalized lipodystrophy or acquired generalized lipodystrophy
‡Growth hormone (GH), somatotropin, somatropin, somatrem	Genotropin Humatrope Norditropin NorlVitropin Nutropin Omnitrope Protropin Saizen Serostim Valtropin Zorbtive	Anabolic and anticatabolic effector	Growth failure due to GH deficiency or chronic renal insufficiency, Prader-Willi syndrome, Turner syndrome
‡Mecasermin	Increlex	Recombinant insulin-like growth factor 1 (IGF-1) induces mitogenesis, chondrocyte growth, and organ growth, which combine to restore appropriate statural growth	Growth failure in children with GH gene deletion or severe primary IGF-1 deficiency
‡Mecasermin rinfabate	IPlex	Similar to mecasermin; IGF-1 bound to IGF binding protein 3 (IGFBP-3) is thought to keep the hormone inactive until it reaches its target tissues, thereby decreasing hypoglycemia-like adverse effects	Growth failure in children with GH gene deletion or severe primary IGF-1 deficiency
Hemostasis and Thrombosis			
Factor VIII	Bioclate Helixate Kogenate Novoeight Recombinate ReFacto XYNTHA	Coagulation factor	Hemophilia A

continues

TABLE 54-1 Protein Therapeutics Replacing a Protein That Is Deficient or Abnormal (Group Ia) *continued*

PROTEIN	TRADE NAME	FUNCTION	EXAMPLES OF CLINICAL USE
Factor VIII-Fc fusion protein	Eloctate	Coagulation factor conjugated to human Fc protein to prolong circulation time and decrease dosing frequency	Hemophilia A
Factor IX	Benefix Rixubis	Coagulation factor	Hemophilia B
Factor IX-Fc fusion protein	Alprolix	Coagulation factor conjugated to human Fc protein to prolong circulation time and decrease dosing frequency	Hemophilia B
*Factor XIII	Corifact	Coagulation factor purified from human plasma	Congenital factor XIII deficiency
Factor XIII A-subunit	Tretten	Coagulation factor	Routine prophylaxis of bleeding in patients with congenital factor XIII A-subunit deficiency
*Von Willebrand factor/ coagulation factor VIII complex	Wilate	Coagulation factor complex purified from human plasma	Treatment of bleeding in patients with severe von Willebrand disease
*Fibrinogen	RiaSTAP	Coagulation factor purified from human plasma	Control of acute bleeding in patients with congenital fibrinogen deficiency
*Prothrombin complex concentrate	Kcentra	Mixture of vitamin K-dependent coagulation factors purified from pooled human plasma; includes factors II, VII, IX, and X as well as antithrombotic protein C and protein S	Urgent reversal of acquired coagulation factor deficiency induced by vitamin K antagonist (VKA; e.g., warfarin)
Antithrombin III *Antithrombin III	ATryn (recombinant human antithrombin III [AT-III]) Thrombate III (human AT-III purified from pooled plasma)	In a reaction catalyzed by endogenous or exogenous heparin, AT-III inactivates thrombin by forming a covalent bond between the catalytic serine residue of thrombin and an arginine-reactive site on AT-III; AT-III replacement therapy prevents inappropriate blood clot formation	Treatment of thromboembolism and prevention of perioperative and postpartum thromboembolic events in patients with hereditary antithrombin III deficiency
*Protein C concentrate	Ceprotin	After activation by the thrombin–thrombomodulin complex, protein C inhibits coagulation factors Va and VIIIa	Treatment and prevention of venous thrombosis and purpura fulminans in patients with severe hereditary protein C deficiency
*C1 esterase inhibitor	Berinert Cinryze	Serine protease inhibitor purified from human plasma; restores serum levels of C1 esterase inhibitor and prevents inappropriate activation of complement and coagulation pathways that can lead to bradykinin generation and increased vascular permeability	Prophylaxis against angioedema attacks in patients with hereditary angioedema (HAE)
C1 esterase inhibitor	Ruconest	Recombinant human analogue of C1 esterase inhibitor; prevents inappropriate activation of complement and coagulation pathways that can lead to bradykinin generation and increased vascular permeability	Treatment of acute attacks of hereditary angioedema (HAE)
Metabolic Enzyme Deficiencies			
β-Glucocerebrosidase *β-Glucocerebrosidase	Cerezyme Ceredase (purified from pooled human placenta)	Hydrolyzes glucocerebroside to glucose and ceramide	Gaucher's disease
Taliglucerase alfa (biosimilar to glucocerebrosidase)	Elelyso	Recombinant glucocerebrosidase produced from a plant-based expression system	Gaucher's disease

TABLE 54-1 **Protein Therapeutics Replacing a Protein That Is Deficient or Abnormal (Group Ia)** *continued*

PROTEIN	TRADE NAME	FUNCTION	EXAMPLES OF CLINICAL USE
Velaglucerase alfa (biosimilar to glucocerebrosidase)	Vpriv	Recombinant glucocerebrosidase	Gaucher's disease
Alglucosidase alfa	Lumizyme Myozyme	Degrades glycogen by catalyzing the hydrolysis of α-1,4 and α-1,6 glycosidic linkages of lysosomal glycogen	Pompe disease (glycogen storage disease type II)
Laronidase	Aldurazyme	α-L-iduronidase is an enzyme that digests endogenous glycosaminoglycans (GAGs) within lysosomes and thereby prevents an accumulation of GAGs that can cause cellular, tissue, and organ dysfunction	Hurler and Hurler–Scheie forms of mucopolysaccharidosis I (MPS I)
Idursulfase	Elaprase	Iduronate-2-sulfatase cleaves the terminal 2-O-sulfate moieties from the GAGs dermatan sulfate and heparan sulfate, thereby allowing their digestion and preventing GAG accumulation	Mucopolysaccharidosis II (Hunter syndrome)
Elosulfase alfa	Vimizim	N-acetylgalactosamine-6-sulfatase cleaves a sulfate from the GAG keratan sulfate, thereby allowing its digestion and preventing its accumulation in lysosomes	Mucopolysaccharidosis IV
Galsulfase	Naglazyme	N-acetylgalactosamine-4-sulfatase cleaves the terminal sulfate from the GAG dermatan sulfate, thereby allowing its digestion and preventing GAG accumulation	Mucopolysaccharidosis VI
Human α-galactosidase A, Agalsidase β	Fabrazyme	Enzyme that hydrolyzes globotriaosylceramide (GL-3) and other glycosphingolipids, reducing deposition of these lipids in capillary endothelium of the kidney and certain other cell types	Fabry disease; prevents accumulation of lipids that could lead to renal and cardiovascular complications
Pulmonary and Gastrointestinal Tract Disorders			
*α-1-Proteinase inhibitor	Aralast Glassia Prolastin	Inhibits elastase-mediated destruction of pulmonary tissue; purified from pooled human plasma	Congenital α-1-antitrypsin deficiency
*Lactase	Lactaid	Digests lactose; purified from fungus *Aspergillus oryzae*	Gas, bloating, cramps, diarrhea due to inability to digest lactose
*Pancreatic enzymes (lipase, amylase, protease)	Arco-Lase Cotazym Creon Donnazyme Pancrease Pertzye Ultresa Viokase Zenpep Zymase	Digests food (protein, fat, and carbohydrate); purified from hogs and pigs	Cystic fibrosis, chronic pancreatitis, pancreatic insufficiency, post-Billroth II gastric bypass surgery, pancreatic duct obstruction, steatorrhea, poor digestion, gas, bloating
Immunodeficiencies			
*Adenosine deaminase	Adagen (pegademase bovine, PEG-ADA)	Metabolizes adenosine, prevents accumulation of adenosine; purified from cows	Severe combined immunodeficiency disease (SCID) due to adenosine deaminase (ADA) deficiency
*Pooled immunoglobulins	Bivigam Octagam Privigen Vivaglobin	Intravenous immunoglobulin preparation	Primary immunodeficiencies and chronic immune thrombocytopenic purpura (ITP)

continues

TABLE 54-1 Protein Therapeutics Replacing a Protein That Is Deficient or Abnormal (Group Ia) *continued*

PROTEIN	TRADE NAME	FUNCTION	EXAMPLES OF CLINICAL USE
Other			
*Human albumin	Albumarc Albumin (Human) Albuminar AlbuRx Albutein Buminate Flexbumin Plasbumin	Increases circulating plasma osmolarity, thereby restoring and maintaining circulating blood volume	Decreased production of albumin (hypoproteinemia), increased loss of albumin (nephrotic syndrome), hypovolemia, hyperbilirubinemia

Protein-based therapies derive their specificity and function from their structure. Molecules ranging from large and complex enzymes to short peptide sequences have specific biological activity due to their amino acid-based secondary and tertiary structure. For example, somatostatin is active as either a 14- or 28-amino-acid chain, and its even shorter synthetic analogues share a characteristic hairpin loop structure that defines their specificity and biological activity. Some very short peptide therapeutics are better thought of as small-molecule drugs, since they lack secondary and tertiary structures that define their biological activity. For this reason, therapeutics such as glatiramer acetate (a four-amino-acid peptide consisting of acetate with L-Glu, L-Ala, L-Tyr, L-Lys) are not addressed in this chapter. Protein therapeutics are recombinant unless otherwise stated. * Nonrecombinant. ‡ Also classed in Group Ib.

TABLE 54-2 Protein Therapeutics Augmenting an Existing Pathway (Group Ib)

PROTEIN	TRADE NAME	FUNCTION	EXAMPLES OF CLINICAL USE
Hematopoiesis			
Erythropoietin, epoetin alfa	Epogen Procrit	Stimulates erythropoiesis	Anemia due to chronic kidney disease or chemotherapy, preoperative preparation
Darbepoetin alfa	Aranesp	Modified erythropoietin with longer half-life; stimulates red blood cell production in the bone marrow	Treatment of anemia in patients with chronic kidney disease (+/− dialysis)
Methoxy polyethylene glycol-epoetin beta	Mircera	Erythropoietin conjugated to methoxy polyethylene glycol (PEG) butanoic acid; stimulates erythropoiesis	Anemia associated with chronic kidney disease
Peginesatide acetate	Omontys	Synthetic peptide analogue of erythropoietin, conjugated to polyethylene glycol (PEG)	Product recalled in 2013 and US FDA New Drug Application (NDA) voluntarily withdrawn by manufacturer in 2014
Granulocyte colony-stimulating factor (G-CSF), filgrastim	Neupogen	Stimulates neutrophil proliferation, differentiation, and migration	Neutropenia in AIDS or after chemotherapy or bone marrow transplantation, severe chronic neutropenia
Tbo-Filgrastim	Granix	Stimulates neutrophil proliferation, differentiation, and migration (minor structural differences from filgrastim)	Shorten the duration of neutropenia after chemotherapy
Peg-G-CSF, pegfilgrastim	Neulasta	Stimulates neutrophil proliferation, differentiation, and migration	Neutropenia in AIDS or after chemotherapy or bone marrow transplantation, severe chronic neutropenia
Granulocyte-macrophage colony-stimulating factor (GM-CSF), sargramostim	Leukine	Stimulates proliferation and differentiation of neutrophils, eosinophils, and monocytes	Leukopenia, myeloid reconstitution after bone marrow transplantation, HIV/AIDS
Interleukin-11 (IL-11), oprelvekin	Neumega	Stimulates megakaryocytopoiesis and thrombopoiesis	Prevention of severe thrombocytopenia, especially after myelosuppressive chemotherapy

TABLE 54-2 Protein Therapeutics Augmenting an Existing Pathway (Group Ib) *continued*

PROTEIN	TRADE NAME	FUNCTION	EXAMPLES OF CLINICAL USE
Romiplostim	Nplate	Fc-peptide fusion protein (peptibody) that acts as a thrombopoietin receptor agonist; stimulates platelet production	Treatment of thrombocytopenia in patients with chronic immune (idiopathic) thrombocytopenic purpura (ITP)
Fertility			
Human follicle-stimulating hormone (FSH)	Gonal-F / Follistim	Stimulates ovulation	Assisted reproductive technology for infertility
Human chorionic gonadotropin (HCG)	Ovidrel	Stimulates ovarian follicle rupture and ovulation	Assisted reproductive technology for infertility
Lutropin alfa	Luveris	Recombinant human luteinizing hormone (LH) increases estradiol secretion, thereby supporting follicle-stimulating hormone (FSH)-induced follicular development	Infertility with LH deficiency
Immunoregulation			
*ACTH (repository corticotropin)	H.P. Acthar	Mechanism unknown; immunoregulator	Infantile spasms (West syndrome), multiple sclerosis relapse, dermatomyositis, systemic lupus erythematosus (SLE)
Type I alpha-interferon, interferon alfacon-1, consensus interferon	Infergen	Mechanism unknown; immunoregulator	Chronic hepatitis C
Interferon alpha-2a (IFNα-2a)	Roferon-A	Mechanism unknown; immunoregulator	Hairy cell leukemia, chronic myelogenous leukemia, Kaposi's sarcoma, chronic hepatitis C
Peginterferon alfa-2a	Pegasys	Mechanism unknown; immunoregulator	Adults with chronic hepatitis C who have compensated liver disease and who have not been previously treated with interferon alpha; used alone or in combination with ribavirin (Copegus)
Interferon alfa-2b (IFNα-2b)	Intron A	Mechanism unknown; immunoregulator	Hepatitis B, melanoma, Kaposi's sarcoma, follicular lymphoma, hairy cell leukemia, condylomata acuminata, hepatitis C
Peginterferon alfa-2b	Peg-Intron	Recombinant interferon alpha-2b conjugated to polyethylene glycol (PEG) in order to increase half-life	Adults with chronic hepatitis C who have compensated liver disease and have not been treated previously with interferon alpha
*Interferon alfa-n3 (IFNα-n3)	Alferon N	Mechanism unknown; nonrecombinant human interferon alfa-n3 purified from pooled human leukocytes	Condylomata acuminata (genital warts caused by human papillomavirus)
Interferon beta-1a (rIFN-β)	Avonex Rebif	Mechanism unknown; antiviral and immunoregulator	Multiple sclerosis
Interferon beta-1b (rIFN-β)	Betaseron Extavia	Mechanism unknown; antiviral and immunoregulator	Multiple sclerosis
Peginterferon beta-1a	Plegridy	Recombinant interferon beta-1a conjugated to polyethylene glycol (PEG) in order to increase half-life	Multiple sclerosis
Interferon gamma-1b (IFN-γ)	Actimmune	Increases inflammatory and antimicrobial response	Chronic granulomatous disease (CGD), severe osteopetrosis

continues

TABLE 54-2 Protein Therapeutics Augmenting an Existing Pathway (Group Ib) *continued*

PROTEIN	TRADE NAME	FUNCTION	EXAMPLES OF CLINICAL USE
Interleukin-2 (IL-2), epidermal thymocyte activating factor (ETAF), aldesleukin	Proleukin	Stimulates T and B cells, natural killer cells, and lymphokine-activated killer (LAK) cells	Metastatic renal cell cancer, melanoma
Hemostasis and Thrombosis			
Tissue plasminogen activator (tPA), alteplase	Activase	Promotes fibrinolysis by binding fibrin and converting plasminogen to plasmin	Pulmonary embolism, myocardial infarction, acute ischemic stroke, occlusion of central venous access devices
Reteplase (deletion mutein of plasminogen activator [tPA])	Retavase	Contains the nonglycosylated kringle 2 and protease domains of human tPA; functions similarly to tPA	Management of acute myocardial infarction, improvement of ventricular function
‡Tenecteplase	TNKase	Tissue plasminogen activator with greater specificity for plasminogen conversion; has amino acid substitutions of Thr103 to Asp, Asp117 to Gln, and Ala for amino acids 296–299	Acute myocardial infarction
*Urokinase	Abbokinase	Nonrecombinant plasminogen activator derived from human neonatal kidney cells	Pulmonary embolism
Factor VIIa	NovoSeven	Prothrombotic (activated factor VII; initiates the coagulation cascade)	Hemorrhage in patients with hemophilia A or B and inhibitors to factor VIII or factor IX
Activated protein C, drotrecogin alfa	Xigris	Antithrombotic (inhibits coagulation factors Va and VIIIa), anti-inflammatory	Severe sepsis with a high risk of death Voluntarily withdrawn from the market in 2011 due to lack of efficacy
Thrombin (human recombinant) *Thrombin (pooled from human plasma)	Recothrom Evithrom	Cleaves fibrinogen to fibrin and activates the coagulation cascade	Hemostasis aid in surgical situations; applied topically to accelerate coagulation
*Fibrin sealant (fibrinogen and thrombin mixture)	Artiss Evarrest TachoSil	Two-component fibrin sealant purified from pooled human plasma; when combined, the fibrinogen and thrombin mimic the final stage of blood coagulation	Adheres autologous skin grafts to surgically prepared wound beds resulting from burns; used to control bleeding during surgery
Endocrine Disorders			
Calcitonin-salmon	Fortical (recombinant) Miacalcin (synthetic)	Mechanism unknown; inhibits osteoclast function	Postmenopausal osteoporosis
Human parathyroid hormone residues 1–34, teriparatide	Forteo	Markedly enhances bone formation; administered as a once-daily injection	Severe osteoporosis
§‡Exenatide	Byetta	Incretin mimetic with actions similar to glucagon-like peptide-1 (GLP-1); increases glucose-dependent insulin secretion, suppresses glucagon secretion, slows gastric emptying, decreases appetite (first identified in saliva of the Gila monster *Heloderma suspectum*)	Type 2 diabetes resistant to treatment with metformin and a sulfonylurea
§‡Liraglutide	Victoza	Recombinant, acylated, and modified human glucagon-like peptide-1 (GLP-1) agonist with amino acid sequence homology to GLP-1 residues 7–37; increases insulin secretion	Type 2 diabetes

TABLE 54-2 **Protein Therapeutics Augmenting an Existing Pathway (Group Ib)** *continued*

PROTEIN	TRADE NAME	FUNCTION	EXAMPLES OF CLINICAL USE
§‡Albiglutide	Tanzeum	GLP-1 agonist conjugated to human albumin to increase half-life and allow once-weekly dosing	Type 2 diabetes
Growth Regulation			
§Octreotide	Sandostatin	Potent somatostatin analogue; inhibits growth hormone, glucagon, and insulin	Acromegaly, symptomatic relief of vasoactive intestinal peptide (VIP)-secreting adenomas and metastatic carcinoid tumors
§Lanreotide	Somatuline depot	Cyclical somatostatin analogue formulated for sustained release	Long-term treatment of acromegaly
Recombinant human bone morphogenic protein 2 (rhBMP-2), dibotermin alfa	Infuse	Mechanism unknown	Spinal fusion surgery, bone injury repair
Recombinant human bone morphogenic protein 7 (rhBMP-7)	Osteogenic protein-1	Mechanism unknown	Tibial fracture nonunion, lumbar spinal fusion
†§Gonadotropin-releasing hormone (GnRH): Goserelin Histrelin Leuprolide Nafarelin Tesamorelin	Egrifta Eligard Lupaneta Lupron Supprelin LA Synarel Vantas Viadur Zoladex	Synthetic analogue of human GnRH; acts as a potent inhibitor of gonadotropin secretion when administered continuously by causing reversible down-regulation of GnRH receptors in the pituitary and desensitizing pituitary gonadotropes	Precocious puberty, endometriosis, breast cancer, prostate cancer, lipodystrophy associated with treatment for HIV infection
Keratinocyte growth factor (KGF), palifermin	Kepivance	Recombinant analogue of KGF; stimulates keratinocyte growth in skin, mouth, stomach, and colon	Severe oral mucositis in patients undergoing chemotherapy
Platelet-derived growth factor (PDGF), becaplermin	Regranex	Promotes wound healing by enhancing granulation tissue formation and fibroblast proliferation and differentiation	Debridement adjunct for diabetic ulcers
Other			
*Trypsin	Granulex	Proteolysis	Decubitus ulcer, varicose ulcer, debridement of eschar, dehiscent wound, sunburn
Nesiritide	Natrecor	Recombinant B-type natriuretic peptide	Acute decompensated heart failure
Linaclotide	Linzess	Peptide agonist of guanylate cyclase 2C; increases chloride and bicarbonate secretion into intestinal lumen and decreases constipation	Irritable bowel syndrome
Ocriplasmin	Jetrea	Truncated version of human serine protease plasmin; proteolytic activity against fibronectin and laminin allows release of adherent macula and vitreous	Symptomatic vitreomacular adhesion of the eye
Teduglutide	Gattex kit	Peptide analogue of glucagon-like peptide-2 (GLP-2) with one amino acid substitution to increase half-life; promotes intestinal mucosal growth	Short bowel syndrome

Proteins are recombinant unless otherwise stated. * Nonrecombinant. § Synthetic. ‡ Also classed in Group Ic. † Also classed in Group IIa.

L-Asparaginase, purified from *E. coli*, can be used to lower serum levels of asparagine in such patients and thereby inhibit cancer cell growth. A key component of many chemotherapy regimens is the folate analogue **methotrexate**, which inhibits dihydrofolate reductase. Lethal concentrations of methotrexate can develop in patients with renal failure or patients who are inadvertently overdosed with the drug. This potentially fatal complication can be corrected with **glucarpidase**, a recombinant bacterial carboxypeptidase G2 that degrades methotrexate into inactive metabolites. Studies of the medical leech, *Hirudo medicinalis*, revealed that its salivary gland produces hirudin, a potent thrombin inhibitor. The gene for this protein was then identified, cloned, and used recombinantly to provide a new protein therapy, **lepirudin**, which prevents clot formation in patients with heparin-induced thrombocytopenia. Other organisms can also be used to produce proteins that are capable of breaking up clots that have already formed; for example, **streptokinase** is a plasminogen-activating protein produced by group C β-hemolytic streptococci. Many more therapeutic proteins that provide a novel function or activity are presented in Table 54-3.

Group II: Targeted Proteins

The exquisite binding specificity of monoclonal antibodies and immunoadhesins can be exploited in numerous ways using recombinant DNA technology. Many protein therapeutics in Group IIa use the antigen recognition sites of immunoglobulin (Ig) molecules or the receptor-binding domains of native protein ligands to guide the immune system to destroy specifically targeted molecules or cells. Other monoclonal antibodies and immunoadhesins neutralize molecules by simple physical blocking of a functionally important region of the molecule. Immunoadhesins combine the receptor-binding domains of protein ligands with the Fc region of an Ig. The Fc region can target a soluble molecule for destruction because cells of the immune system can recognize the Fc region, endocytose the attached molecule, and break down the molecule chemically and enzymatically. When an immunoadhesin is bound to specifically recognized molecules on the surface of a cell, the Fc region can target the cell for destruction by the immune system. Cell killing can be mediated by macrophages, by other immune cells, or by complement fixation.

Several Group IIa protein therapeutics have been approved for the treatment of inflammatory diseases, such as the immunoadhesin **etanercept**, which is a fusion between two human proteins: tumor necrosis factor (TNF) receptor and the Fc region of the human antibody protein IgG1. The TNF receptor portion of the molecule binds excess TNF in the plasma, while the Fc portion of the molecule targets the bound complex for destruction. By combining these two functions, etanercept neutralizes the deleterious effects of TNF (a cytokine that stimulates increased activity of the immune system) and thereby provides an effective therapy for inflammatory arthritis and **psoriasis**. Another Group IIa protein that targets TNF is **adalimumab**. This recombinantly produced monoclonal antibody binds to TNF-α and is used to neutralize the action of TNF-α in a variety of inflammatory conditions including **rheumatoid arthritis**, **psoriasis**, and **inflammatory bowel disease**. Adalimumab was the *top selling therapeutic worldwide* in 2013, with more than $11 billion in sales—a distinction that, until recently, had always been held by a small-molecule drug.

Some Group IIa proteins are used to treat infectious diseases. Patients at high risk for severe respiratory syncytial virus (RSV) infection, one of the leading causes of hospital admissions for pediatric respiratory illness, are given a recombinant monoclonal antibody, **palivizumab**, which binds to the RSV F protein and thereby directs the immune-mediated clearance of the virus from the body. **Enfuvirtide** is an example of a Group IIa protein therapeutic that is not a monoclonal antibody or an immunoadhesin. By binding to gp120/gp41—the HIV envelope protein responsible for fusion of the virus with host cells—this 36-amino-acid peptide prevents the conformational change in gp41 that is required for viral fusion and thereby inhibits viral entry into the cell.

Group IIa antibodies are of growing importance in oncology. For example, **rituximab** is a human/mouse chimeric monoclonal antibody that binds to CD20, a transmembrane protein expressed on >90% of B-cell non-Hodgkin's lymphomas, and targets the cells for destruction by the body's immune system. Although rituximab is most often used in combination with anthracycline-based chemotherapy, it is one of the few monoclonal antibody anticancer therapies that is approved as a monotherapy. **Cetuximab** is a monoclonal antibody used to treat colorectal cancer and head and neck cancer; this monoclonal antibody binds epidermal growth factor receptor (EGFR) and impairs cancer cell growth and proliferation. Other recently developed Group IIa protein therapeutics are listed in Table 54-4, and many more protein therapeutics utilizing the exquisite specificity of monoclonal antibodies are in development, especially for cancer and inflammatory diseases.

Many important processes are modulated by cell surface receptors that are activated upon binding of their cognate ligands. By binding to such receptors, targeted protein therapeutics may activate cell signaling pathways and profoundly affect cell function. Outcomes may range from cell death (through the induction of apoptosis), to down-regulation of cell division, to increased cell proliferation. Although it has been difficult to prove that a particular target-binding protein mediates an in vivo effect through the modulation of a particular signaling pathway, in vitro evidence suggests that this type of modulation is involved in the mechanism of action of certain therapeutic proteins. For example, treatment of certain breast cancers, in which the malignant cells express the HER2/neu (also known as ERBB2) cell surface receptor, is enhanced by the addition of **trastuzumab** (an anti-HER2/neu monoclonal antibody) to the therapeutic regimen. Although trastuzumab contains an Fc region that facilitates antibody-dependent cellular cytotoxicity mediated by natural killer cells, it seems unlikely that this is trastuzumab's only mechanism of action. Other monoclonal antibodies, with similar Fc regions and abilities to target breast cancer cells, have failed to show efficacy in vivo. Trastuzumab, however, has been shown in vitro to induce intracellular signaling events that control the growth of breast cancer cells. It is therefore likely that a combination of mechanisms accounts for the therapeutic activity of trastuzumab, including inhibition of the phosphatidylinositol 3-kinase (PI3K) pathway, inhibition of angiogenesis, and inhibition of HER2 receptor cleavage. The complex action of trastuzumab highlights the fact that, while modulation of cell physiology through simple receptor binding may play a role in the activity of some targeted therapies, the relative contribution of receptor binding to the overall efficacy of the therapeutic may be difficult to dissect.

TABLE 54-3 Protein Therapeutics Providing a Novel Function or Activity (Group Ic)

PROTEIN	TRADE NAME	FUNCTION	EXAMPLES OF CLINICAL USE
Enzymatic Degradation of Macromolecules			
*Botulinum toxin type A	Botox Dysport Xeomin	Cleaves SNAP-25 at neuromuscular junction to disrupt SNARE complex and prevent acetylcholine release, causing flaccid paralysis	Many types of dystonia, particularly cervical; cosmetic uses
*Botulinum toxin type B	Myobloc	Cleaves synaptobrevin at neuromuscular junction to disrupt SNARE complex and prevent acetylcholine release, causing flaccid paralysis	Many types of dystonia, particularly cervical; cosmetic uses
*Collagenase	Collagenase Santyl	Collagenase obtained from fermentation by *Clostridium histolyticum*; digests collagen in necrotic base of wounds	Debridement of chronic dermal ulcers and severely burned areas
*Collagenase	Xiaflex	Mixture of two collagenases (AUX-I and AUX-II) obtained from fermentation by *Clostridium histolyticum*; digests subcutaneous collagen	Treatment for Dupuytren's contracture
Human deoxyribonuclease I, dornase alfa	Pulmozyme	Degrades DNA in purulent pulmonary secretions	Cystic fibrosis; decreases respiratory tract infections in selected patients with forced vital capacity (FVC) greater than 40% of predicted
*Hyaluronidase Hyaluronidase	Amphadase (bovine) Hydase (bovine) Vitrase (ovine) Hylenex (recombinant human)	Catalyses the hydrolysis of hyaluronic acid to increase tissue permeability and allow faster drug absorption	Used as an adjuvant to increase the absorption and dispersion of injected drugs, particularly anesthetics in ophthalmic surgery and certain imaging agents
*Papain	Accuzyme Panafil	Protease from the *Carica papaya* fruit	Debridement of necrotic tissue or liquefaction of slough in acute and chronic lesions, such as pressure ulcers, varicose and diabetic ulcers, burns, postoperative wounds, pilonidal cyst wounds, carbuncles, and other wounds
Enzymatic Degradation of Small-Molecule Metabolites			
*L-asparaginase	ELSPAR	Provides exogenous asparaginase activity, removing available asparagine from serum; purified from *E. coli*	Acute lymphoblastic leukemia (ALL), which requires exogenous asparagine for proliferation
*Asparaginase *Erwinia chrysanthemi*	Erwinaze	Provides exogenous asparaginase activity, removing available asparagine from serum; purified from *E. chrysanthemi*	Acute lymphoblastic leukemia (ALL), which requires exogenous asparagine for proliferation
*Peg-asparaginase	Oncaspar	Provides exogenous asparaginase activity, removing available asparagine from serum; purified from *E. coli* and conjugated to polyethylene glycol (PEG) to decrease immunogenicity and increase half-life	Acute lymphoblastic leukemia (ALL), which requires exogenous asparagine for proliferation
Glucarpidase	Voraxaze	Recombinant carboxypeptidase G2 degrades methotrexate into inactive metabolites	Treatment of supratherapeutic levels of methotrexate
Rasburicase	Elitek	Catalyzes enzymatic oxidation of uric acid into an inactive, soluble metabolite (allantoin); originally isolated from *Aspergillus flavus*	Pediatric patients with leukemia, lymphoma, and solid tumors who are undergoing anticancer therapy that may cause tumor lysis syndrome

continues

TABLE 54-3 Protein Therapeutics Providing a Novel Function or Activity (Group Ic) *continued*

PROTEIN	TRADE NAME	FUNCTION	EXAMPLES OF CLINICAL USE
Pegloticase	Krystexxa	Recombinant uricase conjugated to polyethylene glycol (PEG) to increase half-life; metabolizes uric acid to allantoin	Chronic gout that is refractory to conventional therapy
Hemostasis and Thrombosis			
Lepirudin Desirudin	Refludan Iprivask	Recombinant hirudin, a thrombin inhibitor from salivary gland of medicinal leech *Hirudo medicinalis*	Heparin-induced thrombocytopenia (HIT), prophylaxis against deep vein thrombosis in patients undergoing elective hip replacement surgery
§Bivalirudin	Angiomax	Synthetic hirudin analogue; specifically binds both the catalytic site and the anion-binding exosite of circulating and clot-bound thrombin	Reduce blood clotting risk in coronary angioplasty and heparin-induced thrombocytopenia (HIT)
*Streptokinase	Streptase	Converts plasminogen to plasmin; produced by group C β-hemolytic streptococci	Acute evolving ST elevation myocardial infarction, pulmonary embolism, deep vein thrombosis, arterial thrombosis or embolism, occlusion of arteriovenous cannula
*Anistreplase, anisoylated plasminogen streptokinase activator complex (APSAC)	Eminase	Converts plasminogen to plasmin; p-anisoyl group protects the catalytic center of the plasminogen–streptokinase complex and prevents premature deactivation, thereby providing longer duration of action than streptokinase	Thrombolysis in patients with unstable angina
Protamine	Protamine sulfate	Inactivates heparin by forming a stable 1:1 protamine:heparin complex	Heparin overdose

Proteins are recombinant unless otherwise stated. * Nonrecombinant. § Synthetic.

TABLE 54-4 Protein Therapeutics Interfering with a Molecule or Organism (Group IIa)

PROTEIN	TRADE NAME	FUNCTION	EXAMPLES OF CLINICAL USE
Cancer			
Bevacizumab	Avastin	Humanized monoclonal antibody (mAb) that binds all isoforms of vascular endothelial growth factor A (VEGF-A)	Colorectal cancer
Ziv-aflibercept (same functional entity as aflibercept; see below)	Zaltrap	Recombinant fusion protein with the extracellular domains of human VEGF receptors 1 and 2 fused to the Fc portion of human IgG1; inhibits neovascularization	Metastatic colorectal cancer
Ramucirumab	Cyramza	Fully human mAb (IgG1) targeting vascular endothelial growth factor receptor 2 (VEGFR2)	Advanced gastric cancer
Cetuximab	Erbitux	MAb targeting epidermal growth factor receptor (EGFR)	Colorectal cancer, head and neck cancer
Panitumumab	Vectibix	MAb that competitively inhibits ligand interactions with epidermal growth factor receptor (EGFR)	Metastatic colorectal cancer
Degarelix (GnRH receptor antagonist)	Firmagon	Synthetic linear decapeptide containing seven unnatural amino acids; GnRH receptor competitive antagonist that prevents GnRH binding to pituitary receptors and thereby decreases downstream testosterone production	Advanced prostate cancer

TABLE 54-4 Protein Therapeutics Interfering with a Molecule or Organism (Group IIa) *continued*

PROTEIN	TRADE NAME	FUNCTION	EXAMPLES OF CLINICAL USE
Alemtuzumab	Campath	Humanized mAb directed against CD52 antigen on T and B cells	Voluntarily withdrawn by manufacturer in United States and Europe
Rituximab	Rituxan	Chimeric (human/mouse) mAb that binds CD20, a transmembrane protein found on more than 90% of B-cell non-Hodgkin's lymphomas; synergistic effect with some small-molecule chemotherapeutic agents has been demonstrated in lymphoma cell lines	CD20-positive B-cell non-Hodgkin's lymphoma, diffuse large B-cell CD20-positive non-Hodgkin's lymphoma, rheumatoid arthritis, Wegener's granulomatosis, microscopic polyangiitis
Obinutuzumab	Gazyva	Humanized mAb targeting CD20 on B cells; mediates cell death via multiple mechanisms, including engagement of immune effector cells, activation of intracellular apoptosis pathways, and activation of the complement cascade	Chronic lymphocytic leukemia
Ofatumumab	Arzerra	Human mAb targeting CD20; inhibits early-stage B lymphocyte activation	Chronic lymphocytic leukemia
Trastuzumab	Herceptin	MAb that binds HER2/neu cell surface receptor and controls cancer cell growth	HER2-positive breast cancer; HER2-positive metastatic gastric adenocarcinoma
Pertuzumab	Perjeta	MAb that inhibits HER dimerization and thereby prevents receptor activation	HER2-positive breast cancer (used in combination with trastuzumab)
Ipilimumab	Yervoy	MAb targeting and blocking CTLA-4, thereby inhibiting CTLA-4 interactions with CD80 and CD86 and augmenting T-cell activation and proliferation	Metastatic melanoma
Denosumab	Xgeva (same functional entity as Prolia; see below)	MAb that inhibits RANKL; inhibits osteoclast maturation and decreases bone turnover	Prevention of skeletal fracture in patients with solid tumors metastatic to bone, treatment of giant cell tumor of bone
Immunoregulation			
Adalimumab	Humira	Binds to TNF-α and blocks its interaction with p55 and p75 cell surface TNF receptors, resulting in decreased levels of inflammation markers including CRP, ESR, and IL-6	Rheumatoid arthritis, psoriasis, Crohn's disease
Certolizumab	Cimzia	Recombinant humanized Fab antibody fragment conjugated to polyethylene glycol (PEG); binds to and neutralizes TNF-α	Crohn's disease
Etanercept	Enbrel	Dimeric fusion protein composed of recombinant soluble tumor necrosis factor receptor (TNFr) linked to Fc portion of human IgG1	Moderate to severe active rheumatoid arthritis (RA) after failing other therapies, moderate to severe active polyarticular juvenile RA
Golimumab	Simponi	Human IgG/κ mAb that binds and neutralizes TNF-α	Rheumatoid arthritis, psoriatic arthritis, ankylosing spondylitis
Infliximab	Remicade	MAb that binds and neutralizes TNF-α, preventing induction of proinflammatory cytokines	Rheumatoid arthritis, Crohn's disease
Abatacept	Orencia	Selective costimulation modulator composed of the extracellular domain of human CTLA-4 linked to the Fc portion of human IgG1; inhibits T-cell activation by binding to CD80 and CD86, thereby blocking interaction with CD28 and inhibiting autoimmune T-cell activation	Rheumatoid arthritis (especially when refractory to TNF-α inhibition)

continues

TABLE 54-4 **Protein Therapeutics Interfering with a Molecule or Organism (Group IIa)** *continued*

PROTEIN	TRADE NAME	FUNCTION	EXAMPLES OF CLINICAL USE
Tocilizumab	Actemra	Recombinant humanized antihuman interleukin-6 (IL-6) receptor mAb	Moderate to severe active rheumatoid arthritis in adults who have failed one or more anti-TNF therapy
Anakinra	Antril Kineret Synergen	Recombinant interleukin-1 receptor antagonist	Moderate to severe active rheumatoid arthritis in adults who have failed one or more disease-modifying antirheumatic drug
Canakinumab	Ilaris	Recombinant human IgG1/κ mAb that binds and sequesters IL-1β	Cryopyrin-associated periodic syndromes (CAPS), including familial cold autoinflammatory syndrome (FCAS) and Muckle-Wells syndrome (MWS)
Rilonacept	Arcalyst	Interleukin-1β decoy receptor; dimeric fusion protein consisting of the ligand-binding domains of the extracellular portions of the human interleukin-1 receptor component (IL-1RI) and IL-1 receptor accessory protein (IL-1RAcP) linked to the Fc portion of human IgG1	Cryopyrin-associated periodic syndromes (CAPS), including familial cold autoinflammatory syndrome (FCAS) and Muckle-Wells syndrome (MWS)
Siltuximab	Sylvant	Recombinant chimeric mAb targeting IL-6	Castleman's disease (a lymphoproliferative disorder)
Alefacept	Amevive	MAb that binds CD2 on the surface of lymphocytes and inhibits interaction with leukocyte function-associated antigen 3 (LFA-3)	Voluntarily withdrawn by manufacturer in 2011
Efalizumab	Raptiva	Humanized mAb directed against CD11a	Adults with chronic moderate to severe plaque psoriasis who are candidates for systemic therapy
Ustekinumab	Stelara	Human IgG/κ mAb that disrupts IL-12 and IL-23 signaling by binding to their common p40 subunit	Plaque psoriasis
Natalizumab	Tysabri	Mechanism unknown: binds to the α4 subunit of α4β1 and α4β7 integrins, blocking their interactions with vascular cell adhesion molecule-1 (VCAM-1) and mucosal addressin cell adhesion molecule-1 (MadCAM-1), respectively	Relapsing multiple sclerosis
Vedolizumab	Entyvio	Mechanism unknown: binds to α4β7 integrin on T cells, blocking its interaction with MadCAM-1 and thus preventing adhesion of T cells to the ileal endothelium	Ulcerative colitis, Crohn's disease
Belimumab	Benlysta	Human mAb that inhibits B-cell activating factor	Systemic lupus erythematosus
Eculizumab	Soliris	Humanized mAb that binds complement protein C5 and inhibits its cleavage to C5a and C5b, preventing the formation of the terminal complement complex C5b-9	Paroxysmal nocturnal hemoglobinuria (PNH)
Transplantation			
*Antithymocyte globulin (rabbit)	Thymoglobulin	Selective depletion of T cells; exact mechanism unknown	Acute kidney transplant rejection, aplastic anemia
Basiliximab	Simulect	Chimeric (human/mouse) IgG1 mAb that blocks cellular immune response in graft rejection by binding the alpha chain of CD25 (IL-2 receptor) and thereby inhibiting the IL-2-mediated activation of lymphocytes	Prophylaxis against allograft rejection in renal transplant patients receiving an immunosuppressive regimen including cyclosporine and corticosteroids

TABLE 54-4 Protein Therapeutics Interfering with a Molecule or Organism (Group IIa) *continued*

PROTEIN	TRADE NAME	FUNCTION	EXAMPLES OF CLINICAL USE
Belatacept	Nulojix	Fusion protein composed of the extracellular domain of human CTLA-4 linked to the Fc portion of human IgG1; inhibits T-cell activation (differs from abatacept by two amino acids)	Prophylaxis of organ rejection in kidney transplantation
Daclizumab	Zenapax	Humanized IgG1 mAb that blocks cellular immune response in graft rejection by binding the alpha chain of CD25 (IL-2 receptor) and thereby inhibiting the IL-2-mediated activation of lymphocytes	Prophylaxis against acute allograft rejection in patients receiving renal transplants
Muromonab-CD3	Orthoclone OKT3	MAb that binds CD3 and blocks T-cell function	Voluntarily withdrawn by manufacturer in 2010
*Hepatitis B immune globulin	HepaGam B	Prepared from purified gamma globulins from human plasma; binds surface components on hepatitis B virus and provides passive immunization; complete mechanism not understood	Prevention of hepatitis B recurrence after liver transplant in hepatitis B-infected patients; postexposure prophylaxis against hepatitis B infection
Pulmonary Disorders			
Omalizumab	Xolair	IgG mAb that inhibits IgE binding to the high-affinity IgE receptor on mast cells and basophils, decreasing activation of these cells and release of inflammatory mediators	Adults and adolescents with moderate to severe persistent asthma who have a positive skin test or in vitro reactivity to a perennial aeroallergen and whose symptoms are inadequately controlled with inhaled corticosteroids
Palivizumab	Synagis	Humanized IgG1 mAb that binds the A antigenic site of the F protein of respiratory syncytial virus	Prevention of respiratory syncytial virus infection in high-risk pediatric patients
Infectious Diseases†			
Enfuvirtide	Fuzeon	36-Amino-acid peptide that inhibits HIV entry into host cells by binding to the HIV envelope protein gp120/gp41	Adults and children with advanced HIV infection
Raxibacumab	Raxibacumab	MAb that targets the protective antigen of anthrax toxin to prevent intracellular entry of the anthrax lethal factor and edema factor	Prophylaxis and treatment of inhaled anthrax
Hemostasis and Thrombosis			
Abciximab	ReoPro	Fab fragment of chimeric (human/mouse) mAb 7E3 that inhibits platelet aggregation by binding to the glycoprotein IIb/IIIa integrin receptor	Adjunct to aspirin and heparin for prevention of cardiac ischemia in patients undergoing percutaneous coronary intervention or patients about to undergo percutaneous coronary intervention with unstable angina not responding to medical therapy
Ecallantide	Kalbitor	Polypeptide inhibitor of plasma and tissue kallikreins, enzymes that catalyze the generation of bradykinin as part of the final common pathway of edema formation in hereditary angioedema (HAE)	Hereditary angioedema (HAE)
Icatibant	Firazyr	Peptidomimetic antagonist of bradykinin B2 receptor; blocks the final common pathway of edema formation in HAE	Hereditary angioedema (HAE)

continues

TABLE 54-4 Protein Therapeutics Interfering with a Molecule or Organism (Group IIa) *continued*

PROTEIN	TRADE NAME	FUNCTION	EXAMPLES OF CLINICAL USE
Endocrine Disorders			
‡Gonadotropin-releasing hormone (GnRH) receptor antagonists: Cetrorelix Ganirelix	Antagon Cetrotide Orgalutran	Suppresses premature LH surges in the early to mid-follicular phase of the menstrual cycle	Assisted reproductive technology (controlled ovarian hyperstimulation) for infertility
Pegvisomant	Somavert	Recombinant human growth hormone conjugated to PEG; blocks the growth hormone receptor	Acromegaly
Denosumab	Prolia (same functional entity as Xgeva; see above)	MAb that inhibits RANKL; inhibits osteoclast maturation and decreases bone turnover	Osteoporosis
Other§			
*Crotalidae polyvalent immune Fab (ovine)	Crofab	Mixture of Fab fragments of IgG that bind and neutralize venom toxins of 10 clinically important North American Crotalidae snakes	Crotalidae envenomation (Western diamondback, Eastern diamondback, Mojave rattlesnakes, and water moccasins)
*Digoxin immune serum, Fab (ovine)	Digifab	Monovalent fragment antigen-binding (Fab) immunoglobulin fragment obtained from sheep immunized with a digoxin derivative	Digoxin toxicity
Aflibercept (same functional entity as ziv-aflibercept; see above)	Eylea	Recombinant fusion protein with the extracellular domains of human VEGF receptors 1 and 2 fused to the Fc portion of human IgG1; inhibits neovascularization	Wet macular degeneration
Ranibizumab	Lucentis	Binds isoforms of vascular endothelial growth factor A (VEGF-A)	Neovascular age-related macular degeneration

Proteins are recombinant unless otherwise stated. * Nonrecombinant. ‡ Also classed in Group Ib. † Purified immune globulins can also be used to mitigate the acute effects of exposure to an infectious agent. Human immune globulins targeting botulism, cytomegalovirus, hepatitis B, rabies, tetanus, vaccinia, and varicella have been approved by the FDA. § Three additional antivenins have been approved by the FDA: antivenin immune globulin (equine)—*Latrodectus mactans* (black widow spider), antivenin immune globulin (equine)—*Micrurus fulvius* (North American coral snake), and antivenin immune F(ab')₂ (equine)—*Centruroides sculpturatus* (Arizona bark scorpion). CHOP, cyclophosphamide, hydroxydaunorubicin (doxorubicin), Oncovin® (vincristine), prednisone/prednisolone; CTLA4, cytotoxic T-lymphocyte-associated antigen 4; CVP, cyclophosphamide, vincristine, prednisone; EGFR, epidermal growth factor receptor; LFA-3, leukocyte function-associated antigen 3; mAb, monoclonal antibody; MadCAM1, mucosal addressin cell adhesion molecule 1; TNF, tumor necrosis factor; VCAM1, vascular cell adhesion molecule-1; VEGF-A, vascular endothelial growth factor A.

One of the great challenges in drug therapy is the selective delivery of small-molecule drugs and proteins to the intended therapeutic target. The body normally uses proteins to achieve specialized transport and delivery of many different molecules. An active area of current research is focused on understanding the principles of protein-based, targeted delivery of molecules, so that these principles can be applied to modern pharmacotherapy. This strategy is exploited by protein therapeutics in Group IIb (Table 54-5), such as **gemtuzumab ozogamicin**, which links the binding region of a monoclonal antibody directed against CD33 with calicheamicin, a small-molecule chemotherapeutic agent. By using this therapy, the toxic compound is selectively delivered to CD33-expressing acute myelogenous leukemia cells, resulting in the selective killing of these cells. Similarly, refractory CD20-expressing non-Hodgkin's lymphoma cells can be destroyed selectively by **ibritumomab tiuxetan**, a monoclonal antibody directed against CD20 and linked to a radioactive yttrium isotope (Y-90). Another example is provided by **denileukin diftitox**, which uses a monoclonal antibody

directed against the CD25 component of the IL-2 receptor to deliver cytocidal diphtheria toxin to T-cell lymphoma cells that express this receptor.

A unique challenge in targeted, protein-based delivery of small, toxic molecules is the choice of the chemical linker that bridges the protein and the small molecule. Many approaches to linker chemistry have used functional groups that are designed to break apart in the intracellular environment, which is mildly more acidic than the extracellular environment. However, in some cases, preclinical testing has demonstrated nonspecific release of the cytotoxic conjugates prior to cellular uptake, causing increased systemic toxicity in animal models. Recently approved therapeutics, such as **trastuzumab emtansine**, demonstrate the use of more mature linker chemistry that may serve as a platform technology to facilitate the development of additional targeted therapies. Trastuzumab emtansine uses a heterodimeric crosslinker, abbreviated SMCC (succinimidyl trans-4-(maleimidylmethyl)cyclohexane-1-carboxylate), to link the cytotoxic maytansine molecule to the targeting antibody (see Table 51-1). This crosslinker

TABLE 54-5 Protein Therapeutics Delivering Other Compounds or Proteins (Group IIb)

PROTEIN	TRADE NAME	FUNCTION	EXAMPLES OF CLINICAL USE
Brentuximab vedotin	Adcetris	Chimeric monoclonal antibody (mAb) targeting CD30 (brentuximab) conjugated to the small-molecule antimitotic agent monomethyl auristatin E	Hodgkin's lymphoma and systemic anaplastic large cell lymphoma
Denileukin diftitox	Ontak	Directs the cytocidal action of diphtheria toxin to cells expressing the IL-2 receptor	Persistent or recurrent cutaneous T-cell lymphoma expressing the CD25 component of the IL-2 receptor
Gemtuzumab ozogamicin	Mylotarg	Humanized anti-CD33 IgG4 kappa mAb conjugated to calicheamicin, a small-molecule chemotherapeutic agent	Relapsed CD33-expressing acute myelogenous leukemia. Voluntarily withdrawn from the US market in 2010 due to high rate of fatal toxicity seen in post-approval study
‡Ibritumomab tiuxetan	Zevalin	MAb portion recognizes CD20-expressing B cells and induces apoptosis, while the chelation site allows either imaging (In-111) or cellular damage by beta emission (Y-90)	Relapsed or refractory low-grade, follicular, or transformed B-cell non-Hodgkin's lymphoma (NHL), including rituximab-refractory follicular NHL
‡Tositumomab / I-131 tositumomab	Bexxar / Bexxar I-131	MAb that binds CD20 surface antigen and stimulates apoptosis / MAb coupled to radioactive iodine-131; binds CD20 surface antigen and delivers cytotoxic radiation (used after tositumomab without I-131)	CD20-expressing follicular non-Hodgkin's lymphoma, with and without transformation, in patients whose disease is refractory to rituximab and has relapsed following chemotherapy; tositumomab and then I-131 tositumomab are used sequentially in the Bexxar treatment regimen
‡Trastuzumab emtansine	Kadcyla	Trastuzumab conjugated to the cytotoxic agent maytansine both inhibits HER2 signaling and delivers maytansine to cancer cells that overexpress the HER2 receptor	HER2 positive metastatic breast cancer

All proteins are recombinant. ‡ Also classed in Group IIa. MAb, monoclonal antibody.

binds to the cytotoxic molecule via a covalent thioester bond, which is chemically stable and is unlikely to be degraded in the circulation before reaching the target cells. The antibody–drug conjugate is endocytosed selectively by the target cell, and within the cell, the antibody is sufficiently degraded that the maytansine moiety is exposed and allowed to exert its cytotoxic effect.

In addition to these current examples, interesting developments are in progress that illustrate where the field might be heading. One active area of research involves the delivery of proteins and other macromolecules to the CNS, which is challenging owing to the highly selective blood–brain barrier (BBB). Animal experiments have demonstrated, however, that fusion proteins combining a therapeutic protein with a protein that naturally has specific penetration through the BBB can allow successful delivery of the therapeutic protein to the CNS. For example, a fragment of the tetanus toxin protein that naturally crosses the BBB has been shown in animal experiments to deliver the enzyme superoxide dismutase (SOD) to the CNS. Alternatively, antibodies that target endogenous protein receptors in the BBB, such as the insulin receptor or the transferrin receptor, can bypass the BBB using existing transport mechanisms. These carrier antibodies can be conjugated to other proteins or small molecules to allow them to bypass the BBB. Finally, experiments in mice suggest that targeted inhibitors of the Mfsd2a protein could potentially be used to locally disrupt

the BBB by allowing transcytosis of protein-containing vesicles across CNS endothelial cells. These types of therapeutics could potentially be used to treat neurological disorders such as **amyotrophic lateral sclerosis**, in which CNS levels of SOD are reported to be low. Exciting prospects also exist for the treatment of other disorders of the CNS in which levels of a particular protein are abnormal.

Group III: Protein Vaccines

As recombinant DNA technology was being developed, great strides were also being made in understanding the molecular mechanisms that allow the immune system to protect the body against infectious diseases and cancer. Armed with this new understanding, proteins in Group III have been successfully applied as prophylactic or therapeutic vaccines. Table 54-6 provides selected examples.

For humans to develop effective immunity against foreign organisms or cancer cells, immune cells such as helper T cells must be activated. Immune cell activation is mediated by antigen-presenting cells, which display on their surface specific oligopeptides that are derived from proteins found in foreign organisms or cancer cells. Vaccination against certain organisms such as polio or measles has most often been achieved by injecting heat-killed or attenuated forms of these pathogens. Unfortunately, these methods have involved a certain amount of unavoidable risk of infection or

TABLE 54-6 Protein Vaccines (Group III)

PROTEIN	TRADE NAME	FUNCTION	EXAMPLES OF CLINICAL USE
Protecting Against a Deleterious Foreign Agent (Group IIIa)			
HBsAg	Engerix Recombivax HB	Noninfectious protein on surface of hepatitis B virus	Hepatitis B vaccination
HPV vaccine	Gardasil	Quadrivalent HPV recombinant vaccine (strains 6, 11, 16, 18); contains major capsid proteins from four HPV strains	Prevention of HPV infection
OspA	LYMErix	Noninfectious lipoprotein on outer surface of *Borrelia burgdorferi*	Lyme disease vaccination
Treating an Autoimmune Disease (Group IIIb)			
Anti-Rh IgG	Rhophylac	Neutralizes Rh antigens that could otherwise elicit anti-Rh antibodies in an Rh-negative individual	Routine antepartum and postpartum prevention of Rh(D) immunization in Rh(D)-negative women; Rh prophylaxis in case of obstetric complications or invasive procedures during pregnancy; suppression of Rh immunization in Rh(D)-negative individuals transfused with Rh(D)-positive red blood cells
Treating Cancer (Group IIIc)			
Sipuleucel-T	Provenge	Antigen-presenting cells are extracted from the patient and then incubated *ex vivo* with prostatic acid phosphatase (an antigen expressed on prostate cancer cells) and GM-CSF to stimulate the cells. The activated cells are then infused into the patient, and they activate an in vivo immune response against the prostate cancer cells.	Metastatic hormone-refractory prostate cancer

Selected vaccines highlight the use of recombinant protein technology in vaccine production. Vaccines for the following agents or diseases are currently approved by the FDA: anthrax, acellular pertussis, BCG (for childhood TB protection), diphtheria, hepatitis A and B, human papillomavirus types 6, 11, 16, and 18, influenza types A, B, and H5N1, Japanese encephalitis, Lyme disease, measles, meningococcus, mumps, plague, pneumococcus, polio, rabies, rotavirus, rubella, smallpox, tetanus, typhoid, varicella-zoster, and yellow fever (see http://www.fda.gov/cber/vaccine/licvacc.htm).

adverse reaction. By specifically injecting the appropriate immunogenic (but nonpathogenic) protein components of a microorganism, vaccines can hopefully be created that provide immunity in an individual without exposing that individual to the risks of infection or toxic reaction.

Proteins in Group IIIa are used to generate protection against infectious diseases or toxins. One successful example is the **hepatitis B vaccine**. This vaccine was created by producing recombinant hepatitis B surface antigen (HBsAg), a noninfectious protein of the hepatitis B virus. When immunocompetent humans are challenged and rechallenged with this protein, significant immunity results in the large majority of individuals. Similarly, the noninfectious lipoprotein (OspA) on the outer surface of *Borrelia burgdorferi* has been engineered into a vaccine for **Lyme disease**. A recently approved vaccine against human papillomavirus (HPV) combines the major capsid proteins from four HPV strains that commonly cause genital warts (strains 6 and 11) and **cervical cancer** (strains 16 and 18).

In addition to generating protection against foreign invaders, recombinant proteins can induce protection against an overactive immune system that attacks its own body or "self." One theory is that administration of large amounts of this self-protein causes the body's immune system to develop tolerance to that protein by eliminating or deactivating cells that react against the self-protein. Proteins in Group IIIb are used

to treat patients with disorders that arise from this type of autoimmune phenomenon. Immunological acceptance of a fetus during pregnancy represents a special situation with respect to vaccine use. Occasionally, a pregnant woman can reject a fetus after she has been immunized against certain antigens carried by a fetus from a previous pregnancy. Administration of an **anti-Rhesus D antigen Ig** prevents the sensitization of an Rh-negative mother at the time of delivery of an Rh-positive neonate. Because the woman fails to develop antibodies directed against the fetal Rh antigens, immune reactions and pregnancy loss do not occur in subsequent pregnancies, even if the new fetus carries the Rh antigens.

Proteins in Group IIIc include therapeutic anticancer vaccines. The first protein therapeutic in this class, **sipuleucel-T**, was approved in 2010, and promising clinical trials are underway using a variety of approaches to develop additional patient-specific cancer vaccines. Sipuleucel-T is designed to train the immune system to detect and attack **metastatic prostate cancer** cells. This is accomplished by first isolating dendritic cells (antigen-presenting cells) from a patient's peripheral blood and then incubating the cells with a fusion protein composed of prostatic acid phosphatase (PAP; an antigen that is present on most prostate cancer cells), conjugated to GM-CSF (which promotes maturation of the dendritic cells). The activated dendritic cells, which now recognize the PAP antigen, are then transfused back into the patient, where they help direct the immune system to destroy the prostate cancer cells. In another example in development, a vaccine for **B-cell non-Hodgkin's lymphoma** uses transgenic tobacco plants (*Nicotiana benthamiana*). Each patient with this type of lymphoma has a malignant proliferation of an antibody-producing B cell that displays a unique antibody on its surface. By subcloning the idiotype region of this tumor-specific antibody and expressing the region recombinantly in tobacco plants, a tumor-specific antigen is produced that can be used to vaccinate a patient. This process requires 6–8 weeks from biopsy of the lymphoma to a ready-to-use, patient-specific vaccine. As the genomes of infectious organisms and the pathophysiology of autoimmune diseases and cancer are more fully elucidated, more recombinant proteins will undoubtedly be developed for use as vaccines.

Group IV: Protein Diagnostics

Proteins in Group IV are not used to treat disease, but purified and recombinant proteins used for medical diagnostics (both in vivo and in vitro) are mentioned here because they are invaluable in the decision-making process that guides the treatment and management of many diseases. Table 54-7 provides selected examples.

A classic example of an in vivo diagnostic is the **purified protein derivative (PPD) test**, which determines whether an individual has been exposed to antigens from *Mycobacterium tuberculosis*. In this example, a noninfectious protein component of the organism is injected under the skin of an immunocompetent individual. An active immune reaction is interpreted as evidence that the patient has been previously infected by *M. tuberculosis* or exposed to the antigens of this organism.

Several stimulatory protein hormones are used to diagnose endocrine disorders. **Growth hormone releasing hormone (GHRH)** stimulates somatotroph cells of the anterior pituitary gland to secrete growth hormone. Used as a diagnostic, GHRH can help to determine whether pituitary growth hormone secretion is defective in patients with clinical signs of growth hormone deficiency. Similarly, the recombinant human protein **secretin** is used to stimulate pancreatic secretions and gastrin release and thereby aid in the diagnosis of pancreatic exocrine dysfunction or gastrinoma. In patients with a history of thyroid cancer, recombinant **thyroid-stimulating hormone (TSH)** is an important component of the surveillance methods used to detect residual thyroid cancer cells. Before the advent of recombinant TSH, patients with a history of thyroid cancer were required to stop taking replacement thyroid hormone in order to develop a hypothyroid state to which the anterior pituitary would respond by releasing endogenous TSH. TSH-stimulated cancer cells could then be detected by radioactive iodine uptake. Unfortunately, this method required patients to experience the adverse consequences of hypothyroidism. Use of recombinant TSH instead of endogenous TSH not only allowed patients to remain on replacement thyroid hormone but also resulted in the improved detection of residual thyroid cancer cells.

Imaging agents are a broad group of protein diagnostics that can be used to help identify the presence or localization of a pathologic condition. For example, **apcitide** is a technetium-labeled synthetic peptide that binds glycoprotein IIb/IIIa receptors on activated platelets and is used to image acute venous thrombosis. **Capromab pendetide** is an indium-111-labeled anti-PSA (prostate-specific antigen) antibody that can be used to detect **prostate cancer**. Protein-based imaging agents are often used to detect otherwise hidden disease so it can be treated early, when treatment is most likely to succeed. Imaging agents are currently used to detect cancer, image myocardial injury, or identify sites of occult infection; these agents are presented in more detail in Table 54-7.

There are numerous in vitro protein diagnostics, and two are presented here as examples of a much larger class. Natural and recombinant HIV antigens are essential components of common screening (enzyme immunoassay) and confirmatory (Western blot) tests for HIV infection. In these tests, the antigens serve as "bait" for specific antibodies to HIV *gag*, *pol*, and *env* gene products that have been elicited in the course of infection. Hepatitis C infection is diagnosed by using recombinant hepatitis C antigens to detect antibodies directed against this virus in the serum of potentially infected patients.

CHALLENGES FOR PROTEIN THERAPEUTICS

There are by now many examples in which proteins have been used successfully in therapy. Nonetheless, potential protein therapies that have failed far outnumber the successes, in part owing to several important challenges that are faced in the development and use of protein therapeutics.

First, protein solubility, route of administration, distribution, and stability are all factors that can hinder the successful application of a protein therapy. Proteins are large molecules with both hydrophilic and hydrophobic properties that can make entry into cells and other compartments of the body difficult, and the half-life of a therapeutic protein can be drastically affected by proteases, protein-modifying chemicals, or other clearance mechanisms. One example of how such challenges are being addressed is through the production of PEGylated versions of therapeutic proteins. For example, **PEG-interferon** is a modified form of interferon in which the polymer polyethylene glycol (PEG) is added to prolong the absorption, decrease the renal clearance, retard the enzymatic degradation, increase the elimination half-life, and reduce the immunogenicity of interferon.

A second challenge is that the body may mount an immune response against the therapeutic protein. In some cases, this immune response can neutralize the protein and can even cause a harmful reaction in the patient. For example, immune responses can be generated against Group Ia therapeutic proteins used to replace a factor that has been missing since birth, as illustrated by the development of **anti-factor VIII antibodies** (inhibitors) in patients with severe hemophilia A who are treated with recombinant human factor VIII. More commonly, however, immune responses are generated against proteins of nonhuman origin. Until recently, the widespread clinical application of monoclonal antibodies had been limited by the rapid induction of immune responses against this class of therapeutic proteins. The need for antibody therapeutics that evade immune surveillance and response has been a driving force in the maturation of antibody production technology. Recombinant technology and other advances have allowed the development of various antibody products that are less likely to provoke an immune response than unmodified murine antibodies. In *humanized*

TABLE 54-7 Protein Diagnostics (Group IV)

PROTEIN	TRADE NAME	FUNCTION	EXAMPLES OF CLINICAL USE
In Vivo Infectious Disease Diagnostics			
DPPD	Recombinant purified protein derivative (DPPD)	Noninfectious protein from *Mycobacterium tuberculosis*	Diagnosis of tuberculosis exposure
Hormones			
§Cosyntropin (ACTH 1-24)	Cortrosyn	Fragment of ACTH that stimulates cortisol release by the adrenal cortex	Diagnosis of primary versus secondary adrenal insufficiency
*Glucagon	GlucaGen	Pancreatic hormone that increases blood glucose by stimulating the liver to convert glycogen to glucose	Diagnostic aid to slow gastrointestinal motility in radiographic studies; reversal of hypoglycemia
‡Growth hormone-releasing hormone (GHRH)	Geref	Recombinant fragment of GHRH that stimulates growth hormone (GH) release by somatotroph cells of the pituitary gland	Diagnosis of defective growth hormone secretion
§Secretin	ChiRhoStim (synthetic human peptide) SecreFlo (synthetic porcine peptide)	Stimulation of pancreatic secretions and gastrin	Aids in the diagnosis of pancreatic exocrine dysfunction or gastrinoma; facilitates identification of the ampulla of Vater and accessory papilla during endoscopic retrograde cholangiopancreatography
Thyroid-stimulating hormone (TSH), thyrotropin	Thyrogen	Stimulates thyroid epithelial cells or well-differentiated thyroid cancer tissue to take up iodine and produce and secrete thyroglobulin, triiodothyronine, and thyroxine	Adjunctive diagnostic for serum thyroglobulin testing in the follow-up of patients with well-differentiated thyroid cancer
Imaging Agents, Cancer			
Capromab pendetide	ProstaScint	Imaging agent; indium-111-labeled anti-PSA antibody; recognizes intracellular PSA	Prostate cancer detection
§Indium-111-octreotide	OctreoScan	Imaging agent; indium-111-labeled octreotide	Neuroendocrine tumor and lymphoma detection
Satumomab pendetide	OncoScint	Imaging agent; indium-111-labeled mAb specific for tumor-associated glycoprotein (TAG-72)	Colon and ovarian cancer detection
Arcitumomab	CEA-scan	Imaging agent; technetium-labeled anti-CEA antibody	Colon and breast cancer detection
Nofetumomab	Verluma	Imaging agent; technetium-labeled antibody specific for small cell lung cancer	Small cell lung cancer detection and staging
Imaging Agents, Other			
§Apcitide	Acutect	Imaging agent; technetium-labeled synthetic peptide; binds GPIIb/IIIa receptors on activated platelets	Imaging of acute venous thrombosis
Imciromab pentetate	Myoscint	Imaging agent; indium-111-labeled antibody specific for human cardiac myosin	Detects presence and location of myocardial injury in patients with suspected myocardial infarction
Technetium fanolesomab	NeutroSpec	Imaging agent; technetium-labeled anti-CD15 antibody; binds neutrophils that infiltrate sites of infection	Diagnostic agent (used in patients with equivocal signs and symptoms of appendicitis)
Examples of In Vitro Diagnostics			
HIV antigens	Enzyme immunoassay (EIA) Western blot OraQuick Uni-Gold	Detects human antibodies to HIV	Diagnosis of HIV infection
Hepatitis C antigens	Recombinant immunoblot assay (RIBA)	Detects human antibodies to hepatitis C virus	Diagnosis of hepatitis C exposure

Protein diagnostics are recombinant unless otherwise stated. * Also classed in Group Ib. ‡ Also classed in Group Ia. § Synthetic. ACTH, adrenocorticotropic hormone; CEA, carcinoembryonic antigen; mAb, monoclonal antibody; PSA, prostate-specific antigen.

antibodies, portions of the antibody that are not critical for antigen-binding specificity are replaced with human Ig sequences that confer stability and biological activity on the protein but do not provoke an anti-antibody response. *Fully human antibodies* can be produced using transgenic animals or phage display technologies.

The field of cancer therapeutics illustrates the pace of advances in monoclonal antibody development. In the 1980s, most of the monoclonal cancer therapeutics were murine, although there were a few examples of chimeric antibodies and isolated instances of humanized and human antibodies in clinical development. During the 1990s, humanized and fully human antibodies became the most common types of antibodies introduced into clinical trials. Since 2000, there has been a further increase in the proportion of antibodies that are fully human, and the proportion of murine and chimeric antibodies introduced into clinical trials has decreased. Fully human antibodies are especially well represented in recent FDA-approved protein therapeutics.

More heavily engineered protein therapies that are based on human antibodies have also been developed over the past 10–20 years. One example is the "minibody" **romiplostim**, which is approved for the treatment of immune thrombocytopenic purpura. This construct consists of an Fc region of a human antibody with two copies of a peptide sequence linked to each of its IgG1 heavy chains. The peptide sequence was selected to stimulate the thrombopoietin receptor, yet the sequence has no similarity to its endogenous analogue thrombopoietin. The Fc portion extends the half-life of romiplostim in the circulation, and the lack of sequence homology to thrombopoietin will ideally prevent the development of cross-reactive anti-thrombopoietin antibodies—a serious adverse effect that had been seen with a PEGylated version of thrombopoietin.

A third issue is that for a protein to be physiologically active, post-translational modifications such as glycosylation, phosphorylation, and proteolytic cleavage are often required. These requirements may dictate the use of specific cell types that are capable of expressing and modifying the protein appropriately. In addition, recombinant proteins must be synthesized in a genetically engineered cell type for large-scale production. The host system must produce not only biologically active protein but also a sufficient quantity of this protein to meet clinical demand. Also, the system must allow purification and storage of the protein in a therapeutically active form for extended periods of time. The protein's stability, folding, and tendency to aggregate may be different in large-scale production and storage systems than in smaller scale systems used to produce the protein for animal testing and clinical trials. Some have proposed engineering host systems that co-express a chaperone or foldase with the therapeutic protein of interest, but these approaches have had limited success.

Potential solutions could include the development of systems in which entire cascades of genes involved in protein folding are induced together with the therapeutic protein; the impetus for this work is the observation that plasma cells, which are natural protein production "facilities," use such gene cascades to produce large quantities of monoclonal antibody. Compared to bacteria and yeast, which are generally considered easy to culture, certain mammalian cell types can be more difficult and more costly to culture. Other methods of production, such as genetically engineered

animals and plants, could provide a production advantage. Transgenic cows, goats, and sheep have been engineered to secrete protein in their milk, and transgenic chickens that lay eggs filled with recombinant protein are anticipated in the future. Transgenic plants can inexpensively produce vast quantities of protein without waste or bioreactors, and potatoes can be engineered to express recombinant proteins and thereby make edible vaccines. The first available protein therapeutic produced in plants is **taliglucerase alfa**, a glucocerebrosidase used to treat Gaucher's disease; this drug was approved by the FDA in 2012. Finally, by using fluid-shaking bioreactors, microliter-sized culture systems might be able to predict the success of large-scale culture systems and thereby provide substantial cost savings by focusing investment on systems that are more likely to succeed.

A fourth important challenge is the costs involved in developing protein therapies. Although switching to recombinant methodology from laborious purification of placentally derived protein has allowed the production of sufficient β-glucocerebrosidase to treat Gaucher's disease in many patients, the cost of the recombinant protein can be more than $100,000 per patient per year.

The example of Gaucher's disease also illustrates aspects of a fifth issue associated with protein therapeutics: ethics (although these ethical issues are not exclusive to protein therapeutics). For example, the possibility of efficacious but expensive protein therapeutics for small but severely ill patient populations, such as patients with Gaucher's disease, can present a dilemma with respect to allocation of financial resources of health care systems. In addition, the definition of illness or disease could be challenged by protein therapeutics that can "improve upon" conditions previously viewed as variants of normal. For example, the definition of short stature may begin to change with the possibility of using growth hormone to increase the height of a child.

Finally, the regulatory landscape that governs protein therapies will likely continue to have a significant impact on the development of new therapies and their cost. As the field of protein therapeutics matures and certain therapies lose patent protection, the role of follow-on or generic protein therapies in medicine will be decided. Only in 2010 was a regulatory pathway established in the United States that addresses the development of generic versions of protein therapeutics (so-called **biosimilars**), and it remains unclear how effective this pathway will be at reducing the cost and effort required to bring a biosimilar to market. Due to the complexity of protein manufacture and the costs and risks associated with protein therapeutic development and testing, relatively small changes in the regulatory landscape may have strong impacts on the investment in and development of protein therapeutics.

CONCLUSION AND FUTURE DIRECTIONS

Medicine is entering a new era in which approaches to managing disease are at the level of the genetic and protein information that underlies all biology, and protein therapeutics are playing an increasingly important role. Already, recombinant human proteins make up the majority of FDA-approved biotechnology medicines, which include monoclonal antibodies, natural interferons, vaccines, hormones, modified natural enzymes, and various cell therapies. The future potential for such therapies is huge, given the thousands of proteins produced by the human body and the many thousands of proteins produced by other organisms.

Furthermore, recombinant proteins not only provide alternative (or the only) treatments for particular diseases but can also be used in combination with small-molecule drugs to provide additive or synergistic benefit. Treatment of EGFR-positive colon cancer is illustrative of this point: combination therapy with the small-molecule drug **irinotecan**, which prevents DNA repair by inhibiting DNA topoisomerase, and the recombinant monoclonal antibody **cetuximab**, which binds to and inhibits the extracellular domain of EGFR, results in increased survival in patients with colorectal cancer. The therapeutic synergy between irinotecan and cetuximab may be due to the fact that both drugs inhibit the same EGFR signaling pathway, with one drug (cetuximab) inhibiting the initiation of the pathway and the other drug (irinotecan) inhibiting a target downstream in the pathway.

A small-molecule drug recently approved for use in the treatment of cystic fibrosis may point the way to a new conceptual approach to protein therapeutics. **Ivacaftor** is a potentiator of the cystic fibrosis transmembrane conductance regulator (CFTR) protein. This drug is indicated for the treatment of cystic fibrosis in patients who have a G551D mutation in the *CFTR* gene. Ivacaftor facilitates increased chloride transport through the CFTR chloride channel by increasing the open channel probability of the G551D-CFTR protein. Thus, instead of replacing the abnormal (nonconducting) G551D-CFTR protein with its normal (conducting) counterpart, *the drug restores normal function to the abnormal protein*. This paradigm may be increasingly employed in the coming years to treat diseases associated with the expression of abnormal proteins.

A second new concept in protein therapeutics is exemplified by **mipomersen**, the first antisense oligonucleotide to be approved by the FDA. This agent targets the messenger RNA for apolipoprotein B100 (apoB); by binding to apoB mRNA, mipomersen inhibits translation of apoB and thereby decreases production of apoB and secretion of very-low-density lipoprotein (VLDL) particles. Mipomersen is used to treat patients with homozygous familial hypercholesterolemia (see Chapter 20, Pharmacology of Cholesterol and Lipoprotein Metabolism). Additional antisense oligonucleotide therapeutics are in development.

The early success of recombinant insulin production in the 1970s created an atmosphere of enthusiasm and hope, which was unfortunately followed by an era of disappointment when the vaccine attempts, nonhumanized monoclonal antibodies, and cancer trials in the 1980s were largely unsuccessful. Despite these setbacks, significant progress has been made recently. Some of the major successes with protein therapeutics are described in this chapter, and new production methods are changing the scale, cost, and even route of administration of recombinant protein therapeutics. With the large number of protein therapeutics both in current clinical use and in clinical trials for a range of disorders, one can confidently predict that protein therapeutics will have an expanding role in medicine for years to come.

Acknowledgment

We thank the late Armen H. Tashjian, Jr. for many helpful discussions in developing this chapter for the First, Second, and Third Editions of *Principles of Pharmacology: The Pathophysiologic Basis of Drug Therapy*. Portions of this chapter have been published as a review article (Leader B, Baca QJ, Golan DE. Protein therapeutics: a summary and pharmacological classification. *Nat Rev Drug Discov* 2008;7:21–39) and are adapted with permission.

Suggested Reading

Ben-Zvi A, Lacoste B, Kur E, et al. Mfsd2a is critical for the formation and function of the blood–brain barrier. *Nature* 2014;509:507–511. (*Identifies Mfsd2a as a key regulator of blood–brain barrier function.*)

Keen H, Glynne A, Pickup JC, et al. Human insulin produced by recombinant DNA technology: safety and hypoglycaemic potency in healthy men. *Lancet* 1980;2:398–401. (*A milestone in the use of a recombinantly produced protein therapeutic.*)

Mascelli MA, Zhou H, Sweet R, et al. Molecular, biologic, and pharmacokinetic properties of monoclonal antibodies: impact of these parameters on early clinical development. *J Clin Pharmacol* 2007;47:553–565. (*Discusses trends in antibody formulation and how specific properties of candidate drugs guide early drug development.*)

Nelson AL, Dhimolea E, Reichert JM. Development trends for human monoclonal antibody therapeutics. *Nat Rev Drug Discov* 2010;9:767–774. (*Describes the development of human monoclonal antibodies and their increasing role as protein therapeutics.*)

Walsh CT. *Posttranslational modification of proteins: expanding nature's inventory*. Greenwood Village, CO: Roberts & Company; 2005. (*Reviews mechanisms and biological roles of covalent modifications of proteins.*)

Woodcock J, Griffin J, Behrman R, et al. The FDA's assessment of follow-on protein products: a historical perspective. *Nat Rev Drug Discov* 2007;6:437–442. (*Discusses challenges of developing protein therapeutics, including difficulties in demonstrating bioequivalence in follow-on protein therapeutics.*)

55

Drug Delivery Modalities

Joshua D. Moss and Robert Langer

▌ INTRODUCTION

Drugs are typically administered in either pill or injection form, with limited control over release rate and localization. More advanced drug delivery systems have recently been developed, however. The goal of these new technologies is to alter four pharmacokinetic properties: (1) absorption of the drug, including the period of time over which it is released into the systemic circulation or at its final site of action; (2) distribution of the drug, whether it be to the entire body or to a specific tissue or organ system; (3) metabolism of the drug, either to be avoided entirely or used to convert a prodrug to an active form; and (4) elimination of the drug.

This chapter describes several existing and emerging delivery modalities and discusses how these modalities influence one or more of these four properties. The field of drug delivery is large and encompasses many disciplines, and this discussion will highlight approaches that illustrate these properties rather than provide an exhaustive description of all ongoing practice and research. The highlighted modalities include the novel use of existing delivery routes, polymer-based delivery systems, and liposome-based delivery systems.

▌ NOVEL USE OF EXISTING DELIVERY ROUTES

Oral Delivery

Oral administration of small molecules is currently the most common method of drug delivery. The main advantages of oral delivery are ease of use and relatively low cost, both of which can improve patient adherence. However, incomplete absorption, metabolism of the drug during absorption, and metabolism of the drug during the first pass through the liver can decrease bioavailability of the drug. The variability of these factors, as well as limitations in dosing frequency, also affect the ability to maintain a therapeutic drug concentration in the blood. In addition, only relatively small molecules can be used in conventional pills: the intestine generally cannot absorb large molecules intact. Intact peptide and protein drugs, such as insulin, are poorly absorbed orally because of proteolysis in the digestive tract. Recent advances and ongoing research in oral drug delivery are beginning to address these issues.

Sustained or **extended-release formulations** can prolong plasma drug concentrations with less frequent doses. In early approaches to sustained release, pill or capsule solubility was modified with one or more inert substances known as **excipients**. By formulating the drug in an emulsion or suspension that is relatively difficult to digest, the period of time over which the drug dissolves and is absorbed can be extended. Similar results have been achieved by coating the drug with substances such as cellulose derivatives or wax. This approach is used in a wide variety of both prescription and over-the-counter medications. Another successful and more recent approach to sustained release oral formulations involves an osmotic pump capsule (see below).

Techniques are also being developed for delivery of larger molecules, such as proteins and DNA, in oral formulations. Several designs make use of drug-carrying vehicles, including liposomes and microspheres. **Liposomes**, small vesicles with lipid bilayer membranes, are lipophilic and can be taken up by intestinal Peyer's patches when targeted to M cells (specialized epithelial cells) with appropriate ligands. Certain types of liposomes have been moderately successful in experimental oral vaccine delivery; their use in intravenous delivery systems is discussed below. Polyanhydride **microspheres**, which adhere strongly

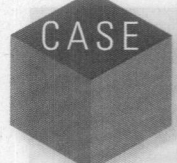

CASE

March 1988: Mr. F is 13 years old. His parents begin to notice that he is tired much of the time, despite getting plenty of sleep. He can no longer participate on his school's track team because he becomes exhausted in the middle of races—the same races he had often won less than a year earlier. Also, Mr. F complains of being thirsty constantly and, as a result, consumes large quantities of water. Mr. F goes to his family physician, who measures his blood glucose level at 650 mg/dL (approximately six times normal levels) and makes an initial diagnosis of type 1 diabetes mellitus. The diagnosis is confirmed in the hospital, where Mr. F's physicians stabilize his blood glucose and develop an insulin therapy regimen. He is taught how to draw a drop of blood from his fingertip to measure his blood glucose and how to give himself subcutaneous injections of insulin. Each day, Mr. F injects recombinant human insulin before breakfast and before dinner.

January 1997: Throughout high school and most of college, Mr. F rarely monitors his glucose levels and purposely keeps them higher than recommended. He wants to be as "normal" as possible, which for him means never allowing his glucose level to fall so low as to require food in the middle of a class or at other unusual times. As Mr. F becomes older, he begins to appreciate that avoiding the long-term consequences of poorly controlled diabetes—atherosclerosis, retinopathy, nephropathy, and peripheral neuropathy, among others—is worth the inconvenience of better control. He switches to a regimen involving four injections a day and begins checking his blood glucose four to five times a day. Eventually, he switches from multiple subcutaneous injections (MSI) to continuous subcutaneous insulin infusion (CSII) with an insulin pump.

The pump delivers a constant basal level of insulin that can be supplemented with bolus releases before meals, thereby more closely approximating the body's physiologic control of blood glucose levels.

September 2024: Back in 1997, Mr. F used his insulin pump for only about 3 months, deciding that the small machine he needed to keep constantly attached to his body was not compatible with his active lifestyle or self-image. He resumed MSI therapy for several more years, until he began participating in human trials for a new, implantable insulin delivery system. Now, a 2-year supply of insulin is incorporated into a polymer matrix that can be implanted in the subcutaneous fat of the abdomen. A device in Mr. F's wristwatch constantly measures his glucose levels transdermally, and it transmits instructions to a magnetic oscillator implanted near the polymer delivery system. The dosing advantages of the insulin pump are thus achieved without Mr. F feeling limited or tied to a machine in any way. He simply has the polymer system replaced every 2 years and makes minor daily adjustments to the programmed delivery parameters in his wristwatch device. Mr. F is looking forward to receiving a transplant of pancreatic beta cells, developed from his own stem cells, that will cure his diabetes.

Questions

1. Why is oral administration of insulin not practical?
2. Which other routes of insulin administration have been tried?
3. Which technologies may make it possible to monitor blood glucose levels transdermally?
4. How can polymers be used to optimize and simplify administration of some drugs?

to the intestinal mucosal surface, have been shown to penetrate intestinal epithelium. After the microspheres are absorbed, presumably because they can stay in contact with the intestinal epithelium for long periods of time, the complex molecules carried within them can be released into the blood.

Another potential approach to delivering proteins orally involves targeting the drug to the colon, which has lower levels of protease activity than the upper gastrointestinal tract. For example, microsphere delivery vehicles can be synthesized from polymers that have enzymatically degradable azoaromatic cross-links. The colon has a relatively high concentration of azoreductases, facilitating degradation of the microspheres and protein release within the colon. Substances that transiently increase the permeability of colonic epithelium, possibly co-incorporated in the microspheres, may improve the absorption of proteins delivered to the colon. Another approach involves carrier molecules that may

be able to shuttle large molecules across the epithelial lining of the intestine.

Pulmonary Delivery

Patients suffering from asthma and other respiratory diseases have long been able to treat their condition by inhaling aerosols of drugs directly into their lungs: β_2-adrenergic agonists, such as albuterol, and glucocorticoid analogues are widely used examples of such locally delivered drugs. In early metered-dose inhaler designs, many of which are still used, the drug is delivered in liquid form using a high velocity chlorofluorocarbon (CFC) propellant. With this technique, very little drug is reproducibly delivered to the lung—often less than 10%. Particles often accumulate in the mouth and throat, and many are immediately exhaled. Components of the immune system and macrophages in the lung can also clear some of the drug before it can act. In addition, many patients use their inhalers incorrectly; common mistakes include not shaking the inhaler well enough, pressing the inhaler too early or too late during inhalation, or using an empty inhaler. Incorrect use further reduces delivery efficiency.

Inhaler design continues to improve. Recent advances include more consistent dosing, greater ease of use via electronic breath actuation, and non-CFC propellants. The aerosol formulations have also been improved by adjusting several properties of the particles themselves. For example, optimized particle chemistry and surface morphology can minimize undesirable particle–particle aggregation. Similarly, particle solubility can be modified to influence the rate of therapeutic release once delivered. Dry powder aerosol clouds that reach deep into the lungs can be generated by blowing compressed air into a drug powder, breaking the powder into tiny (1–5 μm) particles inside the inhaler. Devices that take advantage of these improvements have reduced both dosing frequency and cost for local applications of pulmonary drug delivery in patients with asthma and cystic fibrosis.

The lung also offers several potential advantages for noninvasive, systemic delivery of molecules. The large alveolar surface area, thin tissue lining, and limited numbers of proteolytic enzymes make the lung an ideal tissue for proteins and peptides to enter the bloodstream. One dry powder aerosol device has been approved for the pulmonary delivery of insulin but is not currently manufactured or marketed due to poor acceptance among patients and physicians. Insulin remains an attractive candidate for inhalation therapy, however, as do other biotherapeutics that are currently administered subcutaneously—such as growth hormone, glucagon, and α_1-antitrypsin.

One approach to achieving increased delivery efficiency is the design of large, highly porous aerosol particles with very low densities. Such particles tend to aggregate less than smaller, denser particles, resulting in more efficient aerosolization. In addition, these particles have an "aerodynamic diameter," a parameter based on both density and actual particle dimensions, similar to conventional aerosol particles; thus, they can reach the deep parts of the lung through an airstream, despite their relatively large (5–20 μm) size. Once deposited, the particles can escape clearance by alveolar macrophages, because phagocytosis of particles by macrophages diminishes with increasing particle size beyond 2–3 μm. Thus, drugs can be delivered more efficiently over longer periods of time. In one study, insulin was encapsulated in biodegradable polymer microspheres. Some of the microspheres were small and nonporous, and some were large and porous (low density), but both types had similar aerodynamic diameters. When the microspheres were delivered into the lungs, the relative bioavailability of the large, porous insulin particle was about seven times greater, and the total time of insulin release into the systemic circulation was about 24 times longer, than that of the conventional particle.

Transdermal Delivery

The stratum corneum, composed of lipids and keratinocytes, is the outermost skin layer and the major barrier to transdermal transport. Small, lipophilic drugs have been successfully delivered through the skin into the systemic circulation by passive diffusion at low flux rates, thereby avoiding first-pass metabolism by the liver. Currently, passive transdermal patches are available for hormone replacement and for pharmacologic treatment of motion sickness, angina, nicotine withdrawal, hypertension, pain, and other conditions.

In addition to providing higher bioavailability while remaining noninvasive, transdermal delivery systems are often associated with fewer adverse effects than conventional oral dosage forms. For example, potential liver damage during first-pass metabolism is avoided when a drug is delivered by the transdermal route. Thus, more sophisticated transdermal systems are under development in an attempt to provide these advantages for drug molecules that are otherwise unable to penetrate the skin. **Iontophoresis** is one approach to enhancing the transport of charged, low-molecular-mass molecules through the skin. Iontophoresis involves the application of low-voltage electric pulses for long time periods; this technology is already used clinically for local applications, such as therapy for hyperhidrosis (excessive perspiration), and is under development for systemic delivery of small-molecule analgesic drugs. The use of high-voltage pulses for a short time period—on the order of milliseconds—is also being explored. In human cadaver skin, which is commonly used as a model for skin transport, such high-voltage pulses have been shown to induce temporary pores. This phenomenon, known as **electroporation**, will potentially allow systemic delivery of large, charged molecules, such as heparin and oligonucleotides. **Microneedles** are also being studied.

Ultrasound enhancement of drug delivery through the skin, termed **sonophoresis**, is also being explored for molecules such as insulin, interferon, and erythropoietin. Application of ultrasound to the skin results in cavitation, the formation of tiny air-filled spaces in lipid bilayers of the stratum corneum. The net result of cavitation is disordering of the lipid bilayers, enhancing diffusivity of the drug through the skin by up to 1,000 times. Sonophoresis does not damage the skin, which typically regains its normal structure within 2 hours, and no undesirable effects have been observed in early clinical trials.

Sonophoresis can also be used to remove diagnostic samples from the extracellular space under the stratum corneum. Experiments have been devised in which a reservoir was placed between an ultrasound transducer and a rat's skin, and interstitial fluid was extracted. Theophylline, glucose, cholesterol, urea, and calcium could be measured in the sample; the glucose measurements were sufficiently accurate to be used as a surrogate for blood glucose monitoring in diabetics. With a portable ultrasound transducer, this technique could be incorporated in a futuristic device such as the one Mr. F used in 2024.

◼ POLYMER-BASED DELIVERY SYSTEMS

General Mechanisms

Polymer-based drug delivery systems gradually release drugs into their surroundings. Polymer delivery mechanisms are widely used in diverse applications such as birth control, chemotherapy, and antiarrhythmic therapy. These systems offer advantages in both controlled release and targeting of drugs and are thus the focus of much research. Drug delivery from a polymer-based system can be achieved via three general mechanisms: (1) diffusion, (2) chemical reaction, and (3) solvent activation (Fig. 55-1).

Diffusion

Diffusion from either a reservoir or a matrix is the most common release mechanism. In a reservoir system, the drug is contained within a polymer membrane through which it diffuses over time (Fig. 55-1A). Norplant®, a long-term contraceptive system (no longer marketed in the United States), acts by this principle. **Levonorgestrel**, a synthetic

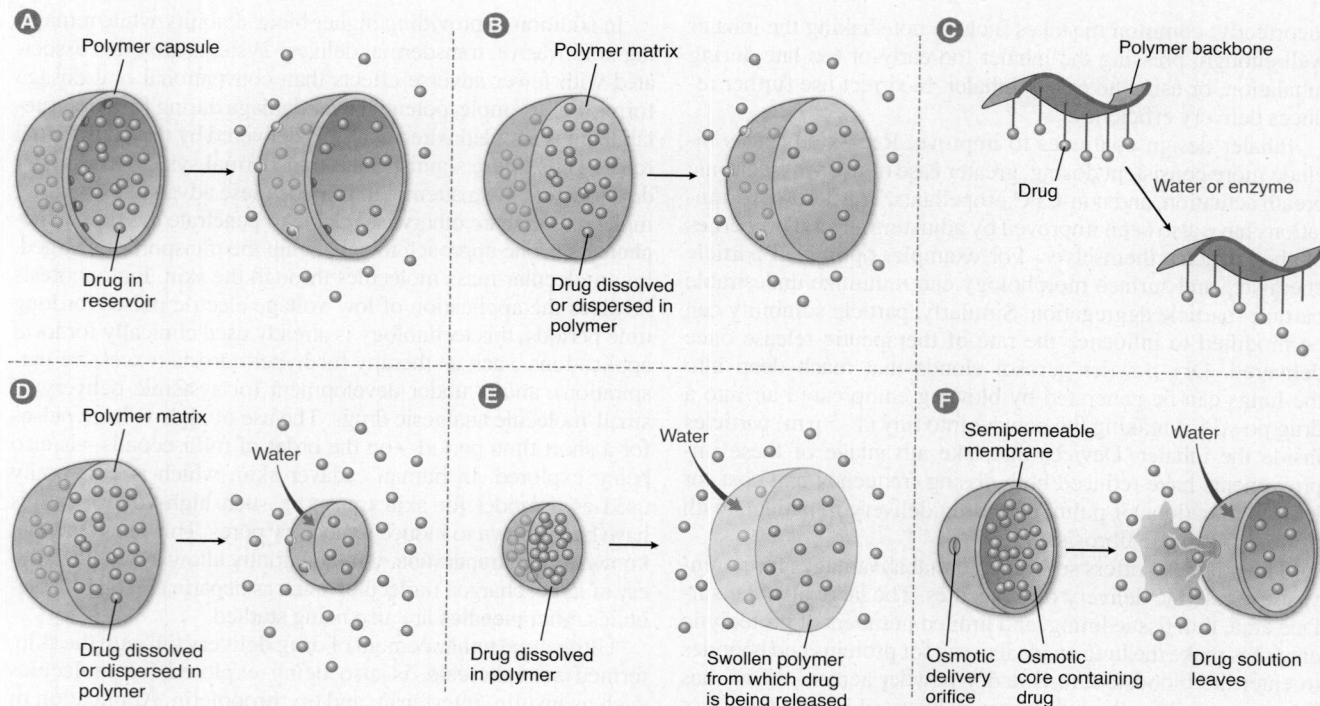

FIGURE 55-1. Polymer release mechanisms. In all panels except *C*, the simplified diagrams represent polymeric systems in cross section. The most common release mechanism is diffusion, whereby the drug migrates from its initial location in the polymer system to the polymer's outer surface and then to the body. **A, B.** Diffusion can occur from a reservoir, in which a drug core is surrounded by a polymer film, or from a matrix, where the drug is uniformly distributed through the polymeric system. **C, D.** Drugs can also be released by chemical mechanisms such as cleavage of the drug from a polymer backbone or hydrolytic degradation of the polymer. **E.** Exposure to a solvent can also activate drug release. For example, the drug can be retained in place by polymer chains; upon exposure to environmental fluid, the outer polymer regions begin to swell, allowing the drug to diffuse outward. **F.** An osmotic system in the form of a tablet with a laser-drilled hole in the polymer surface can provide constant drug release rates. Water diffuses through the semipermeable membrane into the tablet along its osmotic gradient, swelling the osmotic core inside the tablet and forcing drug solution out through the hole. Combinations of these approaches are also possible. Release rates can be controlled by the nature of the polymeric material and the design of the system.

progestin, is stored in small silicone tubes implanted in the arm. The drug diffuses slowly through the polymer capsule over the course of 5 years, providing effective long-term contraception. (For a further discussion of progestin action on the menstrual cycle, see Chapter 30, Pharmacology of Reproduction.) However, such reservoir systems are limited by the size of the drug molecules being delivered. Molecules larger than approximately 300 daltons (Da) are unable to diffuse through the polymer shell.

In one common matrix system design, the drug is contained in a series of interconnecting pores within the polymer rather than in one large reservoir (Fig. 55-1B). This system is less limited by the size of the drug molecules because each pore can accommodate molecules with molecular weights of several million daltons. The rate of diffusion between the pores—and thus through the matrix and out of the system—is controlled architecturally; tight constrictions and tortuous connections between pores prevent rapid release of the stored drug. One such system is used clinically to administer **gonadotropin-releasing hormone (GnRH) analogues.** GnRH analogues are peptide hormones that, when administered continuously, inhibit anterior pituitary gland production of gonadotropins (LH and FSH) and are useful in the treatment of sex-hormone-dependent diseases such as prostate cancer. A major previous limitation of this therapeutic approach was the short in vivo half-life of GnRH analogues following intramuscular injection. When the drug is incorporated into

polymer microcapsules and the capsules are injected intramuscularly, the half-life of GnRH is extended significantly, so that therapeutic concentrations are maintained over a period of 1–4 months. Drug delivery by the microcapsule system utilizes two mechanisms: first, the drug diffuses out of the microcapsules; and second, the polymer matrix itself degrades slowly. The second mechanism of polymer-based drug delivery involves a chemical reaction between the polymer and water (see below).

Chemical Reaction

In **chemical reaction-based systems**, part of the system is designed to degrade over time. Degradation can involve either a chemical or enzymatic reaction. In some designs, covalent bonds that connect the drug to a polymer are cleaved in the body by endogenous enzymes (Fig. 55-1C). Such polymer–drug complexes are typically administered intravenously, and the use of water-soluble polymers such as polyethylene glycol (PEG) increases the biological half-life of the drug considerably. For example, PEG-Intron®, a pegylated form of **interferon-α2b**, has been approved by the US Food and Drug Administration (FDA) for weekly administration; this treatment for hepatitis C infection previously required injections three times as often. In the case of the intramuscular GnRH microcapsules discussed above, the polymer itself is degraded in a reaction with water (Fig. 55-1D).

Most insoluble polymers considered for these applications exhibit bulk erosion (i.e., the entire matrix dissolves at the same rate), which results in larger pores and a more sponge-like and unstable structure. This pattern of degradation makes constant release rates difficult to achieve and creates the potential risk of undesirable "dose dumping." Novel polymers have been designed to overcome this problem by optimizing degradation for controlled drug delivery (i.e., through surface erosion). For example, a polymer with desirable erosion properties can be engineered by using hydrophobic monomers connected by anhydride bonds. The hydrophobic monomers exclude water from the interior of the polymer matrix, eliminating bulk erosion. In contrast, the anhydride bonds are highly water reactive, allowing surface erosion in the aqueous environment of the body. This design allows the polymer to degrade from the outside only (Fig. 55-2). The rate of degradation can be controlled by using a combination of monomers, one more hydrophobic than the other. The length of time over which the polymer persists is specified by the ratio of monomers used, and a drug that is uniformly distributed within such a polymer matrix will be released constantly over time. Based on these principles, Gliadel® has become the first local controlled-release system for an anticancer drug to receive FDA approval. After surgeons remove glioblastoma multiforme, an aggressive form of brain cancer, they place up to eight small polymer–drug wafers at the tumor site. As the polymer surface erodes over 1 month, the drug **carmustine** (an alkylating agent; see Chapter 39, Pharmacology of Cancer: Genome Synthesis, Stability, and Maintenance) is slowly released.

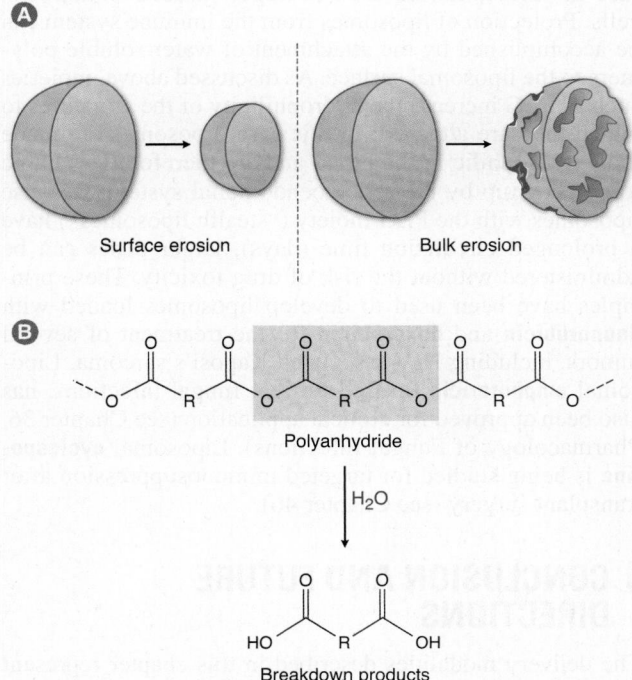

FIGURE 55-2. Surface erosion using polyanhydride polymers. A. Surface erosion of degradable polymer delivery devices allows for more accurately controlled release rates and is therefore preferable to bulk erosion. **B.** Polyanhydrides are used to promote surface erosion. They have hydrophobic monomers that exclude water from the interior of the polymer matrix and prevent bulk erosion. However, the monomers are linked by water-soluble anhydride bonds, allowing breakdown at exposed surfaces.

The concentration of carmustine at the tumor site is maintained at a level sufficiently high to kill many of the remaining tumor cells, while adverse effects of systemic delivery are avoided. This treatment significantly prolongs the lives of patients with this cancer.

Solvent Activation

The third mechanism for polymer-based drug delivery is **solvent activation**, in which the solvent does not react with the polymer chemically but rather initiates drug release via swelling (Fig. 55-1E) or **osmosis** (Fig. 55-1F) of the system. One widely used example of such a system is an extended-release oral formulation of **nifedipine**, a calcium channel blocker (see Chapter 22, Pharmacology of Vascular Tone). The drug is mixed with an osmotically active agent, such as a salt, and coated with a membrane that is permeable to water but not the drug. A laser is then used to drill a small hole in the capsule membrane. After ingestion, the constant osmotic influx of water through the membrane forces the drug out of the pill through the hole, thereby controlling release. This delivery technique, when compared to conventional (immediate release) oral formulations, provides patients greater relief from ischemic events with fewer adverse effects. Concerta®, an extended-release formulation of **methylphenidate**, uses a similar system to treat children with attention-deficit hyperactivity disorder (ADHD).

Intelligent Delivery

There are situations in which pulsatile delivery is desirable to mimic the body's natural pattern of synthesizing and releasing compounds (e.g., hormones). In the case of Mr. F, the insulin pump he wore provided a constant, basal rate of insulin to maintain his blood glucose levels between meals. When Mr. F ate, he could set the pump to provide an additional bolus of insulin and thereby prevent a sudden, excessive rise in blood glucose concentration. Several innovative approaches have been taken to incorporate such versatility in polymer-based drug delivery systems, which have traditionally been designed to deliver drugs at constant or decreasing release rates.

In one early design, magnetic beads were incorporated in the polymer matrix together with a 2-year supply of insulin. The system was then implanted subcutaneously in rats, where the insulin was slowly released by diffusion out of the matrix, as discussed above. When an oscillating magnetic field was applied externally, movement of the magnetic beads within the matrix caused alternating expansion and contraction of the drug-carrying pores. The insulin could thus be effectively squeezed out of the matrix, resulting in higher dose delivery for as long as the oscillating magnetic field was applied. This system significantly lowered blood glucose levels in the treated rats compared to control rats and may eventually become a viable method of insulin delivery. In Mr. F's hypothetical future, the implanted magnetic oscillator allowed him to administer a rapid bolus of insulin simply by selecting the appropriate program on his wristwatch controller, which sent the instructions to the implanted device via a radiofrequency signal.

Other methods of increasing the rate of drug diffusion from a polymer matrix include the application of either ultrasound or electric current. Ultrasound delivered at an appropriate frequency can have an effect similar to that of the magnetic bead system. Ultrasound causes cavitation (the formation of tiny air pockets) in the polymer, disrupting the porous architecture to facilitate faster drug release. Applying an electric current to certain polymers can induce electrolysis of water at the polymer surface, lowering local pH and disrupting hydrogen bonding within the complex. The polymer subsequently degrades at a faster than normal rate, allowing transient release of larger drug doses. Pulsatile delivery can also be achieved in response to local environmental stimuli. For example, hydrogels (materials composed of polymers and water) can be designed to sense changes in temperature, pH, and even specific molecules by virtue of their structure.

A silicon microchip delivery system that offers even more control over release rates has also been designed. The microchip contains up to 1,000 tiny drug reservoirs, each covered with a thin gold film. Applying a small external voltage to an individual implanted reservoir dissolves the gold film electrochemically, releasing the drug stored in that reservoir. Because the reservoirs can be loaded and opened individually, almost limitless possibilities exist for both dosing of single drugs and combining multiple drugs.

Targeting

Accurate targeting allows for larger, more effective doses to reach the tissues of interest without risking the toxic effects of systemic delivery. The first variable that can be controlled is the anatomic placement of the polymer-based drug delivery system; the carmustine wafer delivery system discussed earlier makes use of this basic consideration. Other notable examples include Estring®, a vaginal ring that delivers **estradiol** for vaginal dryness; Vitrasert®, an eye implant that delivers **ganciclovir** for the treatment of cytomegalovirus retinitis in AIDS patients (see Chapter 38, Pharmacology of Viral Infections); and drug-eluting stents that deliver **sirolimus**, **everolimus**, **zotarolimus**, or **paclitaxel** for the prevention of in-stent restenosis in coronary angioplasty (see Chapter 46, Pharmacology of Immunosuppression). Many tissues are accessed practically only via the bloodstream, however, making targeted delivery more difficult. Both passive and active targeting techniques have been developed to direct polymer-based systems to specific tissues following intravenous administration.

Passive targeting exploits vascular differences between the target tissue and other tissues to deliver drugs selectively. For example, high-molecular-mass polymer–drug complexes accumulate in some tumor tissues to a greater extent than in normal tissues because the tumor has more permeable capillary beds. Therefore, rather than using lower doses of low-molecular-mass anticancer drugs, which rapidly diffuse through all cell membranes and distribute throughout the body, larger and more effective doses of high-molecular-mass polymer–drug conjugates can be used to target tumors. In addition, the polymer–drug conjugates can be constructed in such a way as to allow enzymatic cleavage of the drug after the complex has left the bloodstream and been taken up by tumor cells (Fig. 55-1C). In one example of such a system, the anticancer drug **doxorubicin** (see Chapter 39) is conjugated to a water-soluble, nonimmunogenic polymer through a peptidyl linker. The polymer–drug complex accumulates in mouse melanoma tumors at concentrations up to 70 times higher than in normal tissue because of the relatively leaky microvasculature in the tumor. Once inside the tumor cells, the peptidyl linker is cleaved by lysosomal proteases, releasing the cytotoxic drug. The polymer portions of the complex either degrade or are excreted by the kidneys.

In **active targeting**, the polymer–drug conjugate is linked to a molecule that is recognized specifically by cell surface receptors in the tissue of interest. For example, a human IgM antibody directed against a tumor-associated antigen can be used to target a polymer–doxorubicin complex to malignant tissues. Linked to the polymer with an acid-labile bond, the doxorubicin is selectively released in the acidic environment of the tumor. In another system, galactose is used to target a polymer–drug complex to the liver via the hepatocyte cell surface asialoglycoprotein receptor.

LIPOSOME-BASED DELIVERY SYSTEMS

Drugs attached to a single polymer chain are stable structures that can remain in the circulation for long periods of time; the drug–polymer complexes discussed above in the context of tissue targeting are examples of such systems. However, these polymer chains can accommodate only small amounts of drug, thus limiting the dose per unit volume administered. The potentially high drug-carrying capacity of **liposomes**, small vesicles with lipid bilayer membranes, makes them an attractive option for a circulating drug delivery system.

Important considerations in the design of liposome-based delivery systems include tissue targeting and protection from the immune system. Highly specific antibodies, analogous to those used for active targeting of polymer–drug complexes, can be used to improve tissue targeting. For example, antibodies against the *HER2* proto-oncogene, implicated in the progression of breast cancer and other cancers, are being explored for tumor targeting. Similarly, antibodies against E-selectin, an endothelial-specific surface molecule, can be used to target vascular endothelial cells. Protection of liposomes from the immune system can be accomplished by the attachment of water-soluble polymers to the liposomal surface. As discussed above, moieties such as PEG increase the hydrophilicity of the structures to which they are attached; in this case, liposomes are made more hydrophilic in the blood and are therefore less liable to be taken up by the reticuloendothelial system. Because liposomes with the PEG moiety ("stealth liposomes") have a prolonged circulation time (days), larger doses can be administered without the risk of drug toxicity. These principles have been used to develop liposomes loaded with **daunorubicin** and **doxorubicin** for the treatment of several tumors, including HIV-associated Kaposi's sarcoma. Liposomal **amphotericin B**, used to treat fungal infections, has also been approved for clinical application (see Chapter 36, Pharmacology of Fungal Infections). Liposomal **cyclosporine** is being studied for targeted immunosuppression after transplant surgery (see Chapter 46).

CONCLUSION AND FUTURE DIRECTIONS

The delivery modalities described in this chapter represent selected novel approaches to optimizing absorption, distribution, metabolism, and excretion of drugs. There are several advantages of improved drug delivery:

- Drug levels can be continuously maintained in a therapeutically desirable range. Sustained-release oral formulations, large particles that can be inhaled, and many polymer-based designs have this desirable property.

- Harmful adverse effects can be reduced by preventing transient high peak blood levels of drug. Designs that alter absorption kinetics, targeted delivery systems (e.g., antibody-conjugated polymer–drug complexes), and systems that avoid first-pass liver metabolism (e.g., transdermal delivery of drugs that are otherwise taken orally) achieve this goal.
- The total amount of drug required can be reduced, as with advanced inhaler designs. Both a decrease in the number of required dosages and a less invasive administration route contribute to improved patient adherence. Mr. F's case illustrates the influence of lifestyle factors on patient adherence.
- Pharmaceuticals with short half-lives, such as peptides and proteins, can be successfully delivered using controlled-release polymer-based delivery systems.

Advanced drug delivery technologies also introduce new concerns that must be considered in their design. For example, each material put in the body, as well as its degradation products, must be evaluated for toxic effects; this factor is especially important for synthetic materials such as polymers. Other potential dangers must be avoided, such as unwanted rapid release of the drug from a system intended for sustained release. Discomfort caused by the delivery system or its insertion is another potential disadvantage: Mr. F's insulin pump, while providing better control of his diabetes, was uncomfortable to him. Finally, advanced technology is often accompanied by increased cost, which can be a problem for patients, their insurance companies, and hospitals.

Despite these obstacles, advanced drug delivery technologies play an increasingly valuable role in making the pharmacologic management of disease safer, more effective, and more agreeable to patients.

Suggested Reading

Edwards DA, Ben-Jebria A, Langer R. Recent advances in pulmonary drug delivery using large, porous inhaled particles. *J Appl Physiol* 1998;85:379–385. (*Review of aerodynamic diameter principles and the potential advantages and applications of large, porous inhaled particles.*)

Farra R, Sheppard N, McCabe L, et al. First in-human testing of a wirelessly controlled drug delivery microchip. *Sci Transl Med* 2012;4:122ra21. (*First report of an implantable microchip-based device used to deliver parathyroid hormone.*)

Hrkach J, Von Hoff D, Mukkaram Ali M, et al. Preclinical development and clinical translation of a PSMA-targeted docetaxel nanoparticle with a differentiated pharmacological profile. *Sci Transl Med* 2012;4:128ra39. (*Development of a polymeric nanoparticle for delivery of docetaxel.*)

Langer R. Drug delivery and targeting. *Nature* 1998;392:5–10. (*Review of drug delivery techniques, with emphasis on polymer and liposome-based systems as well as novel use of delivery routes.*)

Langer R. Where a pill won't reach. *Sci Am* 2003;288:50–57. (*Broad overview of concepts in drug delivery.*)

Langer R, Weissleder R. Nanotechnology. *JAMA* 2015;313:135–136. (*Reviews use of nanotechnology for therapeutics, diagnostics, and imaging.*)

Leong KW, Brott BC, Langer R. Bioerodible polyanhydrides as drug-carrier matrices. I: characterization, degradation, and release characteristics. *J Biomed Mater Res* 1985;19:941–955. (*Good starting point for learning more about polymer matrix design.*)

Prausnitz M, Langer R. Transdermal drug delivery. *Nat Biotechnol* 2008;26:1261–1268. (*Reviews advances in transdermal drug delivery.*)

Santini JT Jr, Cima MJ, Langer R. A controlled-release microchip. *Nature* 1999;397:335–338. (*More detailed information about intelligent drug delivery using silicon microchips with arrays of drug reservoirs.*)

Credit List

Figure 1-1: Adapted from an illustration (http://www.genome.gov/Glossary/resources /protein.pdf) on the National Human Genome Research Institute website: http://www.nhgri.nih.gov.

Figure 1-2: Data used to render the image in panel A were deposited in the RCSB Protein Data Bank (http://www.rcsb.org/pdb, PDB ID: 1FPU) by Schindler T, Bornmann W, Pellicena P, et al. Structural mechanism for STI-571 inhibition of Abelson tyrosine kinase. *Science* 2000;289:1938–1942, Figure 1. Panels B and C were adapted with permission from Schindler et al. (ibid., Figures 1 and 2).

Figure 2-7A: Adapted with permission from Stephenson RP. A modification of receptor theory. *Brit J Pharmacol* 1956;11:379–393, Figure 10.

Figure 2-7B: Data used to generate the dose–response curves for morphine and buprenorphine were published in Cowan A, Lewis JW, Macfarlane IR. Agonist and antagonist properties of buprenorphine, a new antinociceptive agent. *Brit J Pharmacol* 1977;60:537–545.

Figure 3-1: Adapted with permission from Hardman JG, Limbird LE, eds. *Goodman & Gilman's the pharmacological basis of therapeutics*. 10th ed. New York: McGraw-Hill; 2001:3, Figure 1-1.

Figure 3-7: Adapted with permission from Katzung BG, ed. *Basic & clinical pharmacology*. 7th ed. New York: Lange Medical Books/McGraw-Hill; 1998:38, Figure 3-2.

Figure 4-2A: Adapted with permission from Katzung BG, ed. *Basic & clinical pharmacology* (7th ed.). New York: Lange Medical Books/McGraw-Hill; 1998:52, Figure 4-3.

Figure 5-1: Adapted with permission from Giacomini KM, Huang SM. Transporters in drug development and clinical pharmacology. *Clin Pharmacol Ther* 2013;94:3–9, Figure 1.

Figure 5-2: Adapted with permission from Mariana Ruiz Villarreal (LadyofHats). Image created February 4, 2007, "Simple diffusion in cell membrane." In Public Domain. Archived at https://en.wikipedia.org/wiki/Passive_transport

Figure 5-3: Adapted with permission from Mariana Ruiz Villarreal (LadyofHats). Image created February 4, 2007, "Facilitated diffusion in cell membrane." In Public Domain. Archived at https://en.wikipedia.org/wiki/Facilitated_diffusion

Figure 5-4A: Adapted with permission from Mariana Ruiz Villarreal (LadyofHats). Image created February 23, 2007, "Sodium potassium pump." In Public Domain. Archived at https://en.wikipedia.org /wiki/Active_transport

Figure 5-4B: Adapted with permission from Hundal HS, Taylor PM. Amino acid transporters: gate keepers of nutrient exchange and regulators of nutrient signaling. *Am J Physiol Endocrinol Metab* 2009;296:E603–E613, Figure 2, and Sweet DH, Bush KT, Nigam SK. The organic anion transporter family: from physiology to ontogeny and the clinic. *Am J Physiol Renal Physiol* 2001;281:F197–F205, Figure 1.

Figure 6-3A: Adapted with permission from Grattagliano I, Bonfrate L, Diogo CV, et al. Biochemical mechanisms in drug-induced liver injury: certainties and doubts. *World J Gastroenterol* 2009;15:4865–4876, Figure 1.

Figure 6-3B: Adapted with permission from Grattagliano I, Bonfrate L, Diogo CV, et al. Biochemical mechanisms in drug-induced liver injury: certainties and doubts. *World J Gastroenterol* 2009;15:4865–4876, Figure 2.

Figure 7-1A: Adapted with permission from Bertilsson L, Lou YQ, Du YL, et al. Pronounced differences between native Chinese and Swedish populations in the polymorphic hydroxylations of debrisoquin and S-mephenytoin. *Clin Pharmacol Ther* 1992;51:388–397 [Erratum, *Clin Pharmacol Ther* 1994;55:648].

Figure 7-1B: Photo of the AmpliChip CYP450 array was provided by Roche Diagnostics.

Figure 7-2A: Adapted with permission from Jin Y, Desta Z, Stearns V, et al. CYP2D6 genotype, antidepressant use, and tamoxifen metabolism during adjuvant breast cancer treatment. *J Natl Cancer Inst* 2005;97:30–39.

Figure 7-2B: Adapted with permission from Goetz MP, Knox SK, Suman VJ, et al. The impact of cytochrome P450 2D6 metabolism in women receiving adjuvant tamoxifen. *Breast Cancer Res Treat* 2007;101:113–121.

Figure 7-3: Adapted with permission from Weinshilboum RM, Sladek SL. Mercaptopurine pharmacogenetics: monogenic inheritance of erythrocyte thiopurine methyltransferase activity. *Am J Human Genet* 1980;32:651–662, and Weinshilboum R, Wang L. Pharmacogenomics: Bench to bedside. *Nature Rev Drug Discovery* 2004;3:739–748.

Figure 7-5: Adapted with permission from Ingelman-Sundberg M, Zhong X-B, Hankinson O, et al. Potential role of epigenetic mechanisms in the regulation of drug metabolism and transport. *Drug Metab Dispos* 2013;41:1725–1731, Figure 1.

Figure 8-9: Adapted with permission from Rizo J, Rosenmund C. Synaptic vesicle fusion. *Nat Struct Mol Biol* 2008;15:665–674.

Figure 9-14: Adapted with permission from Goldstein GW, Laterra J. Appendix B: Ventricular organization of cerebrospinal fluid: blood–brain barrier, brain edema, and hydrocephalus. In: Kandel ER, Schwartz JH, Jessell TM, eds. *Principles of neural science*. 4th ed. New York: McGraw-Hill; 2000:1291, Figure B-4.

Figure 10-2: Adapted with permission from Changeux JP. Chemical signaling in the brain. *Sci Am* 1993;269:58–62.

Figure 10-4: Adapted with permission from Kandel ER, Schwartz JH, Jessell TM, eds. *Principles of neural science*. 4th ed. New York: McGraw-Hill; 2000:188, Figure 11-1.

Table 10-5: Adapted with permission from Hardman JG, Limbird LE, eds. *Goodman & Gilman's the pharmacological basis of therapeutics*. 10th ed. New York: McGraw-Hill; 2001:159, Table 7-1.

Table 11-1: Adapted with permission from Hardman JG, Limbird LE, eds. *Goodman & Gilman's the pharmacological basis of therapeutics*. 10th ed. New York: McGraw-Hill; 2001:137, Table 6-3.

Table 12-1: Adapted with permission from Carpenter RL, Mackey DC. Local anesthetics. In: Barash PG, Cullen BF, Stoelting RK, eds. *Clinical anesthesia*. 2nd ed. Philadelphia: Lippincott; 1992:509–541.

Figure 13-2B: Adapted with permission from Cooper JR, Bloom FE, Roth RN. *Biochemical basis of neuropharmacology*. 7th ed. New York: Oxford University Press; 1996: Figures 6-1 and 6-11.

Figure 13-4: Adapted with permission from Neelands TR, Greenfield J, Zhang J, et al. GABA$_A$ receptor pharmacology and subtype mRNA expression in human neuronal NT2-N cells. *J Neurosci* 1998;18:4993–5007, Figure 1a.

Figure 14-4: Adapted with permission from Hardman JG, Limbird LE, eds. *Goodman & Gilman's the pharmacological basis of therapeutics*. 10th ed. New York: McGraw-Hill; 2001:554, Figure 22-5.

Figure 14-5: Adapted with permission from Seeman P. Dopamine receptor sequences. Therapeutic levels of neuroleptics occupy D2 receptor, clozapine occupies D4. *Neuropsychopharmacology* 1992;7:261–284, Figure 2.

Figure 14-9: Adapted with permission from Seeman P. Dopamine receptors and the dopamine hypothesis of schizophrenia. *Synapse* 1987;1:133–152.

Figure 16-3: Adapted with permission from Lothman EW. Pathophysiology of seizures and epilepsy in the mature and immature brain: cells, synapses and circuits. In: Dodson WE, Pellock JM, eds. *Pediatric epilepsy: diagnosis and therapy.* New York: Demos; 1993:1–15.

Figure 16-4: Adapted with permission from Lothman EW. The neurobiology of epileptiform discharges. *Am J EEG Technol* 1993;33:93–112.

Figure 16-5A: Adapted with permission from Kandel ER, Schwartz JH, Jessell TM, eds. *Principles of neural science.* 4th ed. New York: McGraw-Hill; 2000:899, Figure 45-9.

Figure 17-2: Adapted from Miller KW. General anesthetics. In: Wolff ME, ed. *Burger's medicinal chemistry and drug discovery, Volume 3: therapeutic agents.* 5th ed. Hoboken, NJ: John Wiley & Sons; 1996: Figure 36-2. This material used by permission of John Wiley & Sons, Inc.

Figure 17-6: Adapted with permission from Eger EI. *Anesthetic uptake and action.* Baltimore: Williams & Wilkins; 1974: Figure 4-7.

Figure 17-7: Adapted from Eger EI. Uptake and distribution. In: Miller RD, ed. *Anesthesia.* 5th ed. Philadelphia: Churchill Livingstone; 2000: Figure 4-2. With permission from Elsevier.

Figure 17-9: Adapted with permission from Eger EI. *Anesthetic uptake and action.* Baltimore: Williams & Wilkins; 1974: Figures 7-1 and 7-8.

Figure 17-10: Adapted from Eger EI. Uptake and distribution. In: Miller RD, ed. *Anesthesia.* 5th ed. Philadelphia: Churchill Livingstone; 2000: Figure 4-10. With permission from Elsevier.

Figure 17-12: Adapted with permission from Eger EI. *Anesthetic uptake and action.* Baltimore: Williams & Wilkins; 1974: Figure 14-8.

Figure 17-13: Adapted with permission from Trevor AJ, Miller RD. General anesthetics. In: Katzung BG, ed. *Basic & clinical pharmacology.* 7th ed. New York: Lange Medical Books/McGraw-Hill; 1998:421, Figure 25-6.

Figure 19-6: Adapted from Jones RT. The pharmacology of cocaine smoking in humans. In: Chiang CN, Hawks RL, eds. *NIDA research monograph 99 (research findings on smoking of abused substances).* Washington, DC: U.S. Department of Health and Human Services; 1990:30–41.

Figure 20-1: Adapted from Larsen PR, Kronenberg HM, Melmed S, et al., eds. *Williams textbook of endocrinology.* 10th ed. Philadelphia: WB Saunders; 2003: Figure 34-5. With permission from Elsevier.

Figure 20-2: Adapted with permission from Scapa EF, Kanno K, Cohen DE. Lipoprotein metabolism. In: Benhamou JP, Rizzetto M, Reichen J, et al, eds. *The textbook of hepatology: from basic science to clinical practice.* 3rd ed. Oxford, United Kingdom: Blackwell; 2007: Figure 2.

Figure 20-6B: Adapted with permission from Mahley RW, Ji ZS. Remnant lipoprotein metabolism: Key pathways involving cell-surface heparan sulfate proteoglycans and apolipoprotein E. *J Lipid Res* 1999;40:1–16.

Figure 20-8: Adapted with permission from Quinn MT, Parthsarathy S, Fong LG, Steinberg D.

Oxidatively modified low density lipoproteins: a potential role in recruitment and retention of monocyte/macrophages during atherogenesis. *Proc Natl Acad Sci USA* 1987;84:2995–2998, Figure 1.

Figure 20-9B: Adapted with permission from Scapa EF, Kanno K, Cohen DE. Lipoprotein metabolism. In: Benhamou JP, Rizzetto M, Reichen J, et al, eds. *The textbook of hepatology: from basic science to clinical practice.* 3rd ed. Oxford, United Kingdom: Blackwell; 2007: Figure 6B.

Figure 20-11: Adapted from Vaughan CJ, Gotto AM Jr, Basson CT. The evolving role of statins in the management of atherosclerosis. *J Am Coll Cardiol* 2000;35:1–10. With permission from Elsevier.

Table 20-1: Adapted from Jonas A. Lipoprotein structure. In: Vance DE, Vance JE, eds. *Biochemistry of lipids, lipoproteins and membranes* 4th ed. Amsterdam: Elsevier; 2002:483–504. With permission from Elsevier.

Figure 21-10: Adapted from Skorecki KL, Brenner BM. Body fluid homeostasis in congestive heart failure and cirrhosis with ascites. *Am J Med* 1982;72:323–338, Figure 1. With permission from Elsevier.

Figure 21-11: Adapted with permission from Seldin DW, Giebisch G, eds. *The kidney: physiology and pathophysiology.* 3rd ed. Philadelphia: Lippincott Williams & Wilkins; 2000:1494, Figure 54-8.

Figure 21-12: Adapted with permission from Katzung BG, ed. *Basic & clinical pharmacology.* 8th ed. New York: Lange Medical Books/McGraw-Hill; 2001:173, Figure 11-6.

Figure 22-1: Adapted with permission from Greineder K, Strichartz GR, Lilly LS. Basic cardiac structure and function. In: Lilly LS, ed. *Pathophysiology of heart disease.* 2nd ed. Baltimore: Williams & Wilkins; 1998:9, Figure 1.7, and adapted from Berne RM, Levy MN. Control of cardiac output: coupling of heart and blood vessels. In: *Cardiovascular physiology.* St. Louis: Mosby Year Book; 1997: Figure 9.2. With permission from Elsevier.

Figure 22-10: Adapted with permission from Benowitz NL. Antihypertensive agents. In: Katzung BG, ed. *Basic & clinical pharmacology.* 7th ed. New York: Lange Medical Books/McGraw-Hill; 1998:168, and Kalkanis S, Sloane D, Strichartz GR, Lilly LS. Cardiovascular drugs. In: Lilly LS, ed. *Pathophysiology of heart disease.* 2nd ed. Baltimore: Williams & Wilkins; 1998:360, Figure 17.7.

Figure 23-1A–D: Adapted from Cotran RS, Kumar V, Collins T, eds. *Robbins pathologic basis of disease.* 6th ed. Philadelphia: WB Saunders; 1999: Figure 5-5. With permission from Elsevier.

Figure 23-1E: Courtesy of James G. White.

Figure 23-2: Adapted from Cotran RS, Kumar V, Collins T, eds. *Robbins pathologic basis of disease.* 6th ed. Philadelphia: WB Saunders; 1999: Figure 5-7. With permission from Elsevier.

Figure 23-3: Adapted from Cotran RS, Kumar V, Collins T, eds. *Robbins pathologic basis of disease.* 6th ed. Philadelphia: WB Saunders; 1999: Figure 5-7. With permission from Elsevier.

Figure 23-11: Adapted from Cotran RS, Kumar V, Collins T, eds. *Robbins pathologic basis of disease.* 6th ed. Philadelphia: WB Saunders; 1999: Figure 5-12. With permission from Elsevier.

Figure 23-15: Adapted from Lefkovits J, Topol EJ. Direct thrombin inhibitors in cardiovascular medicine. *Circulation* 1994;90:1522–1536, Figure 1.

Figure 24-1: Adapted from Ackerman M, Clapham DE. Normal cardiac electrophysiology. In: Chien KR, Breslow JL, Leiden JM, et al, eds. *Molecular basis of cardiovascular disease: a companion to Braunwald's heart disease.* Philadelphia: WB Saunders; 1999:282, Figure 12-1. With permission from Elsevier.

Figure 24-2: Adapted from Ackerman M, Clapham DE. Normal cardiac electrophysiology. In: Chien KR, Breslow JL, Leiden JM, et al, eds. *Molecular basis of cardiovascular disease: a companion to Braunwald's heart disease.* Philadelphia: WB Saunders; 1999:284, Figure 12-2. With permission from Elsevier.

Figure 24-3: Adapted from Ackerman M, Clapham DE. Normal cardiac electrophysiology. In: Chien KR, Breslow JL, Leiden JM, et al, eds. *Molecular basis of cardiovascular disease: a companion to Braunwald's heart disease.* Philadelphia: WB Saunders; 1999:282,284, Figures 12-1 and 12-2. With permission from Elsevier.

Figure 24-5: Adapted with permission from Lilly LS, ed. *Pathophysiology of heart disease.* 2nd ed. Baltimore: Williams & Wilkins; 1998:241, Figure 11.7.

Figure 24-6: Adapted with permission from Lilly LS, ed. *Pathophysiology of heart disease.* 2nd ed. Baltimore: Williams & Wilkins; 1998:241, Figure 11.8.

Figure 24-7: Adapted with permission from Lilly LS, ed. *Pathophysiology of heart disease.* 2nd ed. Baltimore: Williams & Wilkins; 1998:243, Figure 11.9.

Figure 24-9A: Adapted with permission from Lilly LS, ed. *Pathophysiology of heart disease.* 2nd ed. Baltimore: Williams & Wilkins; 1998:371, Figure 17.11B.

Figure 24-10: Adapted with permission from Lilly LS, ed. *Pathophysiology of heart disease.* 2nd ed. Baltimore: Williams & Wilkins; 1998:371, Figure 17.11A.

Figure 24-11: Adapted with permission from Lilly LS, ed. *Pathophysiology of heart disease.* 2nd ed. Baltimore: Williams & Wilkins; 1998:376, Figure 17.12.

Figure 24-12: Adapted with permission from Lilly LS, ed. *Pathophysiology of heart disease.* 2nd ed. Baltimore: Williams & Wilkins; 1998:377, Figure 17.13.

Figure 24-13: Adapted with permission from Lilly LS, ed. *Pathophysiology of heart disease.* 2nd ed. Baltimore: Williams & Wilkins; 1998:380, Figure 17.14.

Figure 25-1: Adapted with permission from Katz AM. Congestive heart failure: role of altered myocardial cellular control. *N Engl J Med* 1975;293:1184–1191, and Lilly LS, ed. *Pathophysiology of heart disease.* 2nd ed. Baltimore: Williams & Wilkins; 1998:11, Figure 1.9.

Figure 25-2: Adapted with permission from Katz AM. *Physiology of the heart.* 2nd ed. New York: Raven Press; 1992:187, Figure 8.4.

Figure 26-2: Adapted with permission from Deshmukh R, Smith A, Lilly LS. Hypertension. In: Lilly LS, ed. *Pathophysiology of heart disease.* 2nd ed. Baltimore: Williams & Wilkins; 1998:270, Figure 13.3.

Figure 26-3: Adapted with permission from Deshmukh R, Smith A, Lilly LS. Hypertension. In: Lilly LS, ed. *Pathophysiology of heart disease.* 2nd ed. Baltimore: Williams & Wilkins; 1998:286, Figure 13.10.

Figure 26-6: Adapted with permission from Lilly LS, ed. *Pathophysiology of heart disease.* 2nd ed. Baltimore: Williams & Wilkins; 1998:141, Figure 6.5.

Figure 26-7: Adapted from Gould KL, Lipscomb K. Effects of coronary stenoses on coronary flow reserve and resistance. *Am J Cardiol* 1974;34:48–55, Figure 2. With permission from Elsevier.

Figure 26-8: Adapted with permission from Libby P. Current concepts of the pathogenesis of acute coronary syndromes. *Circulation* 2001;104:365–372.

Figure 26-10: Adapted with permission from Libby P. Current concepts of the pathogenesis of acute coronary syndromes. *Circulation* 2001;104:365–372.

Figure 26-11: Adapted with permission from Frankel SK, Fifer MA. Heart failure. In: Lilly LS, ed. *Pathophysiology of heart disease.* 2nd ed. Baltimore: Williams & Wilkins; 1998:199, Figure 9.5.

Figure 26-12: Adapted with permission from Harvey RA, Champe PC, eds. *Lippincott's illustrated reviews: pharmacology.* Philadelphia: Lippincott Williams & Wilkins; 1992:157, Figure 16-6.

Table 26-3: Adapted from Kaplan NM. Systemic hypertension: therapy. In: Zipes DP, Libby P, Bonow RO, Braunwald E, eds. *Braunwald's heart disease.* 7th ed. Philadelphia: Elsevier Saunders; 2005: Table 38-4. With permission from Elsevier.

Figure 29-2: Adapted from Cotran RS, Kumar V, Collins T, eds. *Robbins pathologic basis of disease.* 6th ed. Philadelphia: WB Saunders; 1999: Figure 26-27. With permission from Elsevier.

Figure 29-8: Adapted from Cotran RS, Kumar V, Collins T, eds. *Robbins pathologic basis of disease.* 6th ed. Philadelphia: WB Saunders; 1999: Figure 26-27. With permission from Elsevier.

Figure 30-5: Adapted with permission from Thorneycroft IH, Mishell DR Jr, Stone SC, et al. The relation of serum 17-hydroxyprogesterone and estradiol-17β levels during the human menstrual cycle. *Am J Obstet Gynecol* 1971;111:947–951.

Figure 30-8: Structures were deposited in the Protein Data Bank (http://www.rcsb.org/pdb/; structures 1ERE and 1ERR) by Brzozowski AM, Pike ACW, Dauter Z, et al. Molecular basis of agonism and antagonism in the oestrogen receptor. *Nature* 1997;389:753–758, and are reproduced with permission.

Figure 31-4: Adapted with permission from Braunwald E, Fauci AS, et al, eds. *Harrison's principles of internal medicine.* 15th ed. New York: McGraw-Hill; 2001: Figure 33-34.

Figure 33-5: Adapted from Haskell CM, ed. *Cancer treatment.* 3rd ed. Philadelphia: WB Saunders; 1990:5, Figure 1.2. With permission from Elsevier.

Figure 34-2C: Data used to render the image were deposited in the RCSB Protein Data Bank (http://www.rcsb.org/pdb; PDB ID: 1AFZ) by Zegar IS, Stone MP. Solution structure of an oligodeoxynucleotide containing the human N-Ras codon 12 sequence refined from 1H NMR using molecular dynamics restrained by nuclear overhauser effects. *Chem Res Toxicol* 1996;9:114–125.

Figure 34-3: Adapted with permission from Dekker NH, Rybenkov VV, et al. The mechanism of type IA topoisomerases. *Proc Natl Acad Sci USA* 2002;99:12126–12131, Figure 1.

Figure 34-4: Adapted with permission from Berger JM, Gamblin SJ, Harrison SC, Wang JC. Structure and mechanism of DNA topoisomerase II. *Nature* 1996;379:225–232, Figure 5.

Figure 34-7: Adapted with permission from PharmAid. Copyright 2003, Jeffrey T. Joseph and David E. Golan.

Figure 34-13A: Adapted with permission from Schlunzen F, Zarivach R, Harms J, et al. Structural basis for the interaction of antibiotics with the peptidyl transferase centre in eubacteria. *Nature* 2001;413:814–821, Figure 5.

Figure 34-13B: Adapted with permission from Schlunzen F, Zarivach R, Harms J, et al. Structural basis for the interaction of antibiotics with the peptidyl transferase centre in eubacteria. *Nature* 2001;413:814–821, Figure 4.

Figure 37-1: Adapted with permission from Miller LH, Baruch DI, Marsh K, Doumbo OK. The pathogenic basis of malaria. *Nature* 2002;415:674–679, Figure 2.

Figure 37-4: Adapted from http://www.cdc.gov /ncidod/emergplan/box23.htm.

Figure 37-6: Adapted with permission from Huston CD, Haque R, Petri WA. Molecular-based diagnosis of Entamoeba histolytica infection. *Expert Rev Mol Med* 1999:1–11, Figure 1.

Figure 38-3: Adapted from an illustration kindly provided by Professor Stephen Harrison, Department of Biological Chemistry and Molecular Pharmacology, Harvard Medical School.

Figure 38-4: Adapted from Hay AJ. The action of adamantanamines against influenza A viruses: inhibition of the M2 ion channel protein. *Sem Virol* 1992;3:21–30, Figure 3. With permission from Elsevier.

Figure 38-5A: Adapted with permission from Knipe DM, Howley PM, eds. *Fields virology.* 6th ed. Philadelphia: Lippincott Williams & Wilkins; 2013: Figure 27-2.

Figure 38-9A: Adapted with permission from Knipe DM, Howley PM, eds. *Fields virology.* 5th ed. Philadelphia: Lippincott Williams & Wilkins; 2007: Figure 57-18.

Figure 38-9C: Adapted from an illustration kindly provided by Professor Peter Cherepanov, Department of Medicine, Imperial College, London, United Kingdom.

Figure 38-11C: Data used to render the image were deposited in the RCSB Protein Data Bank (http://www.rcsb.org/pdb; PDB ID: 1HXW) by Kempf DJ, Marsh KC, Denissen JF, et al. ABT-538 is a potent inhibitor of human immunodeficiency virus protease and has high oral bioavailability in humans. *Proc Natl Acad Sci USA* 1995;92:2484–2488.

Figure 38-12A: Data used to render the image were deposited in the RCSB Protein Data Bank (http://www.rcsb.org/pdb; PDB ID: 2BAT) by Varghese JN, McKimm-Breschkin JL, Caldwell JB, et al. The structure of the complex between influenza virus neuraminidase and sialic acid, the viral receptor. *Proteins* 1992;14:327–332.

Figure 38-12C: Adapted with permission from Lave WG, Bischofberger N, Webster RG. Disarming flu viruses. *Sci Amer* 1999;280:78–87.

Figure 39-8: Adapted with permission from Shiloh Y. ATM and related protein kinases: safeguarding genome integrity. *Nat Rev Cancer* 2003;3:155–168, Box 2.

Figure 39-9: Adapted with permission from de Lange T. Shelterin: the protein complex that shapes and safeguards human telomerases. *Genes Dev* 2005;19:2100–2110, Figure 2.

Figure 39-11: Adapted with permission from Lodish H, Berk A, Zipursky SL, et al, eds. *Molecular cell biology.* 4th ed. New York: W.H. Freeman and Company/Worth Publishers; 2000:797, Figure 19-2.

Figure 39-12: Adapted with permission from Lodish H, Berk A, Zipursky SL, et al, eds. *Molecular cell biology.* 4th ed. New York: W.H. Freeman and Company/Worth Publishers; 2000:806, Figure 19-15.

Figure 39-21A: Data used to render the image were deposited in the RCSB Protein Data Bank (http://www.rcsb.org/pdb; PDB ID: 1AO1) by Caceres-Cortes J, Sugiyama H, Ikudome K, et al. Interactions of cobalt(III) pepleomycin (green form) with DNA based on NMR structural studies. *Biochemistry* 1997;36:9995–10005.

Figure 39-21B: Data used to render the image were deposited in the RCSB Protein Data Bank (http://www.rcsb.org/pdb; PDB ID: 1AIO) by Takahara PM, Rosenzweig AC, Frederick CA, Lippard SJ. Crystal structure of double-stranded DNA containing the major adduct of the anticancer drug cisplatin. *Nature* 1995;377:649–652.

Figure 39-21C: Data used to render the image were deposited in the RCSB Protein Data Bank (http://www.rcsb.org/pdb; PDB ID: 1D10) by Frederick CA, Williams LD, Ughetto G, et al. Structural comparison of anticancer drug/DNA complexes adriamycin and daunomycin. *Biochemistry* 1990;29:2538–2549.

Figure 39-22: Adapted with permission from Downing KH. Structural basis for the interaction of tubulin with proteins and drugs that affect microtubule dynamics. *Annu Rev Cell Dev Biol* 2000;16:89–111, Figure 9.

Figure 40-4A: Adapted with permission from Mani A, Gelmann EP. The ubiquitin-proteasome pathway and its role in cancer. *J Clin Oncol* 2005;23:4776–4789, Figure 1.

Figure 42-1: Adapted with permission from Janeway CA, Travers P, Walport M, eds. *Immunobiology: the immune system in health and disease.* 4th ed. New York: Garland Publishing, Inc; 1999:4, Figure 1.3.

Figure 42-4: Adapted from Abbas AK, Lichtman AH, Pober JS. *Cellular and molecular immunology.* 4th ed. Philadelphia: WB Saunders; 2000:169, Figure 8-3. With permission from Elsevier.

Figure 42-5: Adapted from Abbas AK, Lichtman AH, Pober JS. *Cellular and molecular immunology.* 4th ed. Philadelphia: WB Saunders; 2000:173, Figure 8-5. With permission from Elsevier.

Figure 42-6: Adapted with permission from Janeway CA, Travers P, Walport M, eds. *Immunobiology: the immune system in health and disease.* 4th ed. New York: Garland Publishing, Inc; 1999:378, Figure 10.11.

Table 42-2: Adapted from Cotran RS, Kumar V, Collins T, eds. *Robbins pathologic basis of disease.* 6th ed. Philadelphia: WB Saunders Company; 1999: Table 3-7. With permission from Elsevier.

Figure 43-2: Adapted with permission from Serhan CS. Eicosanoids. In: Kooperman WJ, ed. *Arthritis and allied conditions: a textbook of rheumatology.* 14th ed. Philadelphia: Lippincott Williams & Wilkins; 1999:516, Figure 24.2.

Figure 43-4: Adapted with permission from Serhan CS. Eicosanoids. In: Kooperman WJ, ed. *Arthritis and allied conditions: a textbook of rheumatology.* 14th ed. Philadelphia: Lippincott Williams & Wilkins; 1999:524, Figure 24.6.

Figure 44-2: Adapted with permission from Janeway CA, Travers P, Walport M, eds. *Immunobiology: the immune system in health and disease.* 4th ed. New York: Garland Publishing, Inc; 1999:474, Figure 12.12.

Figure 44-3: Adapted with permission from Leurs R, Church MK, Taglialatela M. H1 antihistamines: inverse agonism, anti-inflammatory actions and cardiac effects. *Clin Exp All* 2002;32:489–498, Figure 1.

Figure 45-1: Adapted from Cotran RS, Kumar V, Collins T, eds. *Robbins pathologic basis of disease.* 6th ed. Philadelphia: WB Saunders Company; 1999: Figure 14-1. With permission from Elsevier.

Figure 46-7: Adapted with permission from Fox DA. Cytokine blockade as a new strategy to treat rheumatoid arthritis: inhibition of tumor necrosis factor. *Arch Intern Med* 2000;160:437–444, Figure 1.

Figure 46-8: Adapted with permission from Fox DA. Cytokine blockade as a new strategy to treat rheumatoid arthritis: inhibition of tumor necrosis factor. *Arch Intern Med* 2000;160:437–444, Figure 2.

Figure 48-1: Adapted from Mason RJ, Broaddus VC, Murray JF, Nadel J, eds. *Murray and Nadel's textbook of respiratory medicine.* 4th ed. Philadelphia: WB Saunders Company; 2005. With permission from Elsevier.

Figure 48-3: Adapted from Mason RJ, Broaddus VC, Murray JF, Nadel J, eds. *Murray and Nadel's textbook of respiratory medicine.* 4th ed. Philadelphia: WB Saunders Company; 2005. With permission from Elsevier.

Figure 48-4: Adapted with permission from Drazen JM. Treatment of asthma with drugs modifying the leukotriene pathway. *N Engl J Med* 1999;340: 197–206, Figure 1.

Figure 48-6: Adapted with permission from Pelaia G, Vatrella A, Maselli R. The potential of biologics for the treatment of asthma. *Nat Rev Drug Discov* 2012;11:958–972, Figure 2.

Figure 49-2: Adapted with permission from So A, Busso N. A magic bullet for gout? *Ann Rheum Dis* 2009;68:1517–1519, Figure 2.

Figure 50-4: Adapted with permission from Luch A. Nature and nurture—lessons from chemical carcinogenesis. *Nat Rev Cancer* 2005;5:113–125, Figure 3.

Figure 50-5: Adapted with permission from Luch A. Nature and nurture—lessons from chemical carcinogenesis. *Nat Rev Cancer* 2005;5:113–125, Figure 4.

Figure 51-3A: Adapted with permission from Schreiber SL. Target-oriented and diversity-oriented organic synthesis in drug discovery. *Science* 2000;287:1964–1969.

Figure 51-3B: Adapted with permission from Marsilje TH, Pei W, Chen B, et al. Synthesis, structure-activity relationships, and in vivo efficacy of the novel potent and selective anaplastic lymphoma kinase (ALK) inhibitor 5-chloro-N2-(2-isopropoxy-5-methyl-4-(piperidin 4-yl) phenyl)-N4-(2-(isopropylsulfonyl)phenyl) pyrimidine-2,4-diamine (LDK378) currently in phase 1 and phase 2 clinical trials. *J Med Chem* 2013;56:5675–5690.

Figure 52-2: Adapted from the CDER handbook by the U.S. Food and Drug Administration, available at http://www.fda.gov/.

Figure 52-3: Adapted from the CDER handbook by the U.S. Food and Drug Administration, available at http://www.fda.gov/.

Table 52-2: Adapted from http://www.fda.gov /fdac/special/newdrug/testtabl.html.

Index